a **LANGE** medical book

CURRENT

Surgical Diagnosis & Treatment

a **LANGE** medical book

CURRENT
Surgical Diagnosis
& Treatment

Tenth Edition

Lawrence W. Way, MD
Professor of Surgery
University of California School of Medicine
San Francisco
Chief of Surgical Service,
Veterans Affairs Medical Center,
San Francisco

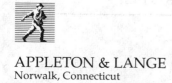

APPLETON & LANGE
Norwalk, Connecticut

94 95 96 97 98 / 10 9 8 7 6 5 4 3 2

Prentice Hall International (UK) Limited, *London*
Prentice Hall of Australia Pty. Limited, *Sydney*
Prentice Hall Canada, Inc., *Toronto*
Prentice Hall Hispanoamericana, S.A., *Mexico*
Prentice Hall of India Private Limited, *New Delhi*
Prentice Hall of Japan, Inc., *Tokyo*
Simon & Schuster Asia Pte. Ltd., *Singapore*
Editora Prentice Hall do Brasil Ltda., *Rio de Janeiro*
Prentice Hall, *Englewood Cliffs, New Jersey*

ISSN: 0894–2277

Acquisitions Editor: Martin J. Wonsiewicz
Production Editor: Christine Langan
Designer: Penny Kindzierski

ISBN 0-8385-1439-1

90000

9 780838 514399

PRINTED IN THE UNITED STATES OF AMERICA

Table of Contents

---

*Deceased.

The Authors

John E. Adams, MD
Guggenheim Professor Emeritus of Neurological Surgery, University of California, San Francisco.

N. Scott Adzick, MD
Associate Professor of Surgery, Division of Pediatric Surgery, University of California, San Francisco.

Jeffrey M. Arbeit, MD
Assistant Professor of Surgery, University of California, San Francisco.

Allen I. Arieff, MD
Professor of Medicine, University of California, San Francisco; Chief, Geriatrics Research, Veterans Affairs Medical Center, San Francisco.

Nancy L. Ascher, MD, PhD
Professor of Surgery, Chief, Transplant Service, University of California, San Francisco.

Nicholas M. Barbaro, MD
Associate Professor in Residence, Department of Neurological Surgery, University of California, San Francisco.

Samuel W. Beenken, MD
Assistant Professor of Surgery, University of Alabama at Birmingham; Head, Section of Head and Neck Surgery, Veterans Affairs Medical Center, Birmingham.

Edward G. Biglieri, MD
Professor of Medicine, University of California, San Francisco; Director of the Clinical Study Center and Chief of the Endocrine Service, San Francisco General Hospital, San Francisco.

John H. Boey, MD
Former Reader in Surgery, University of Hong Kong, Hong Kong.

David S. Bradford, MD
Chair and Professor, Department of Orthopedic Surgery, University of California, San Francisco.

Orlo H. Clark, MD
Professor and Vice Chairman, Department of Surgery, University of California, San Francisco; and Chief of Surgery, Mount Zion Medical Center, San Francisco.

Howard A. Cohen, MD
Assistant Clinical Professor, Department of Orthopedic Surgery, University of California, San Francisco

Lorraine Day, MD
Rancho Mirage, California

Alfred A. deLorimier, MD
Professor of Surgery, Division of Pediatric Surgery, University of California, San Francisco.

Robert H. Demling, MD
Professor of Surgery, Harvard Medical School, Boston; and Director of the Longwood Area Trauma/Burn Center, Boston.

Karen Deveney, MD
Professor of Surgery and Director, Surgical Education, Oregon Health Sciences University, Portland.

James F. Donovan, MD
Associate Professor of Urology, University of Iowa School of Medicine, Iowa City, Iowa.

Quan-Yang Duh, MD
Assistant Professor of Surgery, University of California, San Francisco.

J. Englebert Dunphy, MD*
Formerly Professor of Surgery Emeritus, University of California, San Francisco.

Michael F.B. Edwards, MD
Professor of Neurosurgery and Pediatrics; Director, Division of Pediatric Neurosurgery, University of California, San Francisco.

*Deceased.

David J. Effeney, MB, BS, FRACS
Professor of Surgery, University of Queensland, Brisbane, Australia.

Nicholas J. Feduska, MD
Director, Kidney Transplant Program, Pacific Transplant Institute, California Pacific Medical Center, San Francisco.

Karen K. Fu, MD
Professor of Radiation Oncology, University of California, San Francisco.

Armando E. Giuliano, MD
Professor of Surgery, University of California, Los Angeles, Chief of Surgical Oncology and Director, Breast Center, John Wayne Cancer Institute, Saint John's Hospital and Health Center, Santa Monica, California.

Jerry Goldstone, MD
Professor and Vice Chairman, Department of Surgery; Chief, Division of Vascular Surgery, University of California, San Francisco; and Staff Surgeon, Department of Veterans Affairs Medical Center, San Francisco.

William H. Goodson III, MD
Associate Professor of Surgery in Residence, University of California, San Francisco.

William P. Graham III, MD
Attending Plastic Surgeon, Carlisle Hospital, Carlisle Pennsylvania.

Michael R. Harrison, MD
Professor of Surgery and Pediatrics; Chief, Division of Pediatric Sugery; and Director, The Fetal Treatment Center, University of California, San Francisco.

Hani A. Hennein, MD
Chief Resident in Cardiothoracic Surgery, University of California, San Francisco.

Michael S. Hickey, MD
Associate Clinical Professor of Surgery, University of California, San Francisco; Surgical Director, San Francisco General Hospital Nutrition Support Center, San Francisco.

Robert F. Hickey, MD
Professor of Anesthesia, University of California, San Francisco.

Edward C. Hill, MD
Professor Emeritus of Obstetrics & Gynecology, University of California, San Francisco.

Julian T. Hoff, MD
Professor of Surgery and Head of Neurosurgery, University of Michigan, Ann Arbor.

David C. Hohn, MD
Professor of Surgery, U.T.M.D. Anderson Cancer Center, Houston, Texas.

James W. Holcroft, MD
Professor of Surgery, University of California Davis Medical Center, Sacramento, California.

Serena S. Hu, MD
Assistant Professor, Department of Orthopedics, University of California, San Francisco.

Michael H. Humphreys, MD
Professor of Medicine, University of California, San Francisco; and Chief, Division of Nephrology, San Francisco General Hospital, San Francisco.

Thomas K. Hunt, MD
Professor of Surgery, Vice Chair for Research Affairs, Department of Surgery, University of California, San Francisco.

Ernest Jawetz, MD, PhD
Professor Emeritus of Microbiology and Medicine, University of California, San Francisco.

James O. Johnston, MD
Clinical Professor of Orthopedic Surgery, University of California, San Francisco.

Fraser M. Keith, MD
Assistant Professor of Surgery, Division of Cardiothoracic Surgery, University of California, San Francisco.

Eugene S. Kilgore, Jr., MD
Clinical Professor of Surgery, University of California, San Francisco.

Marcus A. Krupp, MD
Clinical Professor of Medicine Emeritus, Stanford University School of Medicine, Stanford, California; and Director (Emeritus) of Research Institute, Palo Alto Medical Foundation for Health Care, Research and Education, Palo Alto, California.

William C. Krupski, MD
Professor of Surgery; and Chief, Vascular Surgery Section, University of Colorado Health Sciences Center, Denver.

Frank R. Lewis, Jr., MD
Chairman, Department of Surgery, Henry Ford Hospital, Detroit.

Edmund T. Lonergan, MD
Clinical Professor of Medicine, San Francisco General Hospital, San Francisco.

James R. Macho, MD
Assistant Professor of Surgery, University of California, San Francisco; Director of Surgical Critical Care, Mount Zion Hospital, San Francisco.

Robert E. Markison, MD
Assistant Clinical Professor of Surgery, University of California, San Francisco.

Barry M. Massie, MD
Professor of Medicine, University of California, San Francisco; Associate Staff Member, Cardiovascular Research Institute; Chief, Hypertension Unit; and Director, Coronaries Care Unit, San Francisco Veterans Affairs Medical Center, San Francisco.

Juliet S. Melzer, MD
Associate Professor of Surgery, Transplant Service, University of California, San Francisco.

Ronald D. Miller, MD
Professor and Chairman, Department of Anesthesia, University of California, San Francisco.

Reid V. Mueller, MD
Chief Resident, Department of Surgery, University of California, San Francisco.

Sean J. Mulvihill, MD
Associate Professor of Surgery and Chief, Division of General Surgery, University of California, San Francisco.

Jack Nagan, JD
Office of Veterans Affairs Regional Counsel, Veterans Affairs Medical Center, San Francisco.

Russ P. Nockels, MD
Assistant Professor of Neurosurgery, University of California, San Francisco.

Christopher J. O'Brien, MD
Attending Surgeon, Department of Head and Neck Surgery, Royal Prince Alfred Hospital, Sydney, Australia.

Robert S. Pashman, MD
Clinical Instructor, Department of Orthopedics, University of California, San Francisco; and Attending Surgeon, West Coast Spine Institute, Los Angeles.

Carlos A. Pellegrini, MD
Professor and Chairman, Department of Surgery, University of Washington, Seattle.

Theodore L. Phillips, MD
Professor and Chairman, Department of Radiation Oncology, University of California, San Francisco.

Lawrence H. Pitts, MD
Professor and Vice Chairman, Department of Neurological Surgery, University of California, San Francisco; and Chief, Neurosurgery Service, San Francisco General Hospital, San Francisco.

J. Scott Rankin, MD
Professor and Chief, Division of Cardiothoracic Surgery, University of California, San Francisco.

Howard A. Reber, MD
Professor and Vice Chairman, Department of Surgery, University of California Los Angeles School of Medicine; and Chief, Surgical Service, Sepulveda Veterans Affairs Medical Center, Los Angeles.

John Andrew Ridge, MD, PhD
Chief, Head and Neck Surgery Section, Department of Surgical Oncology, Fox Chase Cancer Center, Philadelphia.

John Paul Roberts, MD
Associate Professor of Surgery, University of California, San Francisco.

Harold Rosegay, MD
Clinical Professor, Neurological Surgery, University of California, San Francisco.

Mark L. Rosenblum, MD
Chairman of Neurosurgery, Henry Ford Hospital, Detroit, Michigan.

Donald A. Ross, MD
Assistant Professor of Surgery, Section of Neurological Surgery, University of Michigan, Ann Arbor.

Lee D. Rowe, MD
Associate Clinical Professor of Otolaryngology, Thomas Jefferson School of Medicine, Philadelphia.

Thomas R. Russell, MD
Chairman, Department of Surgery, California Pacific Medical Center, San Francisco; and Clinical Professor of Surgery, University of California, San Francisco.

Theodore R. Schrock, MD
Professor of Surgery, University of California, San Francisco.

Marvin D. Siperstein, MD, PhD
Professor of Medicine, Univeristy of California, San Francisco; and Chief, Metabolism Section, Veterans Affairs Medical Center, San Francisco.

Harry B. Skinner, MD, PhD
Professor of Orthopedic Surgery, University of California, San Francisco; and Professor of Mechanical Engineering, University of California, Berkeley.

Samuel D. Spivack, MD
Clinical Professor of Medicine and Radiology; and Research Associate, Cancer Research Institute, University of California, San Francisco.

Khalid F. Tabbara, MD, FCOphth
Professor and Chairman, Department of Ophthalmology, College of Medicine, King Saud University, Riyadh, Saudi Arabia.

Pearl T.C.Y. Toy, MD
Professor, Department of Laboratory Medicine; and Chief, Blood Bank and Donor Center, University of California, San Francisco.

Kevin Turley, MD
Chief, Pediatric Cardiovascular Surgery, California Pacific Medical Center, San Francisco.

J. Blake Tyrrell, MD
Clinical Professor of Medicine, Director of Endocrine Clinic; and Associate Director of the Metabolic Research Unit, University of California, San Francisco.

Marshall M. Urist, MD
Professor and Director, Division of General Surgery; Chief, Section of Surgical Oncology, University of Alabama School of Medicine, Birmingham.

Henry C. Vasconez, MD
Associate Professor, Division of Plastic Surgery, University of Kentucky, Lexington.

Luis O. Vasconez, MD
Professor of Surgery and Chief of the Division of Plastic and Reconstructive Surgery, University of Alabama School of Medicine, Birmingham.

Edward D. Verrier, MD
Professor and Chief, Division of Cardiothoracic Surgery, University of Washington, Seattle.

Robert S. Warren, MD
Assistant Professor, Department of Surgery, University of California, San Francisco.

Lawrence W. Way, MD
Professor of Surgery, University of California, San Francisco; and Chief of Surgical Service, Veterans Affairs Medical Center, San Francisco.

Philip E. Weinstein, MD
Professor of Neurosurgery and Vice Chairman, Department of Neurosurgery, University of California, San Francisco; and Chief, Neurosurgical Service, Veterans Affairs Medical Center, San Francisco.

Richard D. Williams, MD
Professor and Head, Department of Urology, University of Iowa Hospitals and Clinics, Iowa City.

Charles B. Wilson, MD
Professor and Chairman, Department of Neurological Surgery, University of California, San Francisco.

David H. Wisner, MD
Associate Professor of Surgery, Chief of Trauma Surgery, University of California, Davis Medical Center.

Preface

Current Surgical Dianosis & Treatment is intended to serve as a ready source of information about diseases managed by surgeons. Like other books in this Lange series, it emphasizes quick recall of major diagnostic features and brief descriptions of disease processes, followed by procedures for definitive diagnosis and treatment. Epidemiology, pathophysiology, and pathology are discussed to the extent that they contribute to the book's ultimate purpose—patient care.

Not quite a third of the book is given over to general medical and surgical topics important in the management of all patients.

References to the current journal literature are provided for the reader who wishes to explore specific matters in greater detail than would be appropriate in a concise text of this sort.

OUTSTANDING FEATURES

- Revised and updated biennially. With each revision, particular subjects are completely, substantially, partially, or minimally rewritten as called for by the progress in each field.
- With each new edition, the journal literature is scanned for useful references to support the text.
- Illustrations have been judiciously chosen to clarify anatomic and surgical concepts.
- Over 1000 diseases and disorders are covered.
- Thorough coverage of the role of the many new minimally invasive surgical procedures in treatment.

INTENDED AUDIENCE

Students will find this book to be an authoritative introduction to surgery as it is taught and practiced at major teaching institutions.

House officers will find many occasions to refer to the concise discussions of the diseases they must deal with every day as well as less common ones calling for quick study on the spot.

Medical practitioners who must occasionally deal with surgical problems or counsel patients needing surgical referrals will have many uses for this book, as will practicing surgeons as a guide to the most current management strategies.

ORGANIZATION

This book is organized chiefly by organ system. Lists of subjects taken up in the longer chapters are presented in the table of contents, but for some users the more convenient portal of entry to the text will be the index.

Early chapters provide general information about the relationship between surgeons and their patients (Chapter 1), preparation for surgery (Chapter 2), postoperative care (Chapter 3), and surgical complications (Chapter 4). Chapter 5 deals with the problems of medically ill patients who require surgery. Chapter 6 summarizes the main features of the surgeon's legal obligations and tort law. Then follow chapters on wound healing (Chapter 7), inflammation, infection, and antibiotics (Chapter 8), fluid and electrolyte management (Chapter 9), surgical metabolism and nutrition (Chapter 10), anesthesia (Chapter 11), and shock and acute pulmonary failure (Chapter 12). Chapter 13 discusses management of trauma and Chapter 14, management of burns. The main series of body system topics begins with Chapter 15 (head and neck tumors) and ends with Chapter 45 (hand surgery). Pediatric surgery (Chapter 46), oncology and cancer chemotherapy (Chapter 47), and organ transplantation (Chapter 48) round out the main text. An appendix contains reference material on chemical analysis of body fluids, therapeutic serum levels of drugs, and schedules of controlled drugs.

NEW TO THIS EDITION

Along with the customary revision of all sections as called for by changing concepts in each field covered in this book, the following can be mentioned specifically:

- Thorough coverage on the role of laparoscopy in surgical therapy.
- Chapter 19, Heart, has been completely rewritten.
- Chapter 10, Surgical Metabolism & Nutrition, has been completely rewritten.
- Esophagus & Diaphragm (Chapter 20) has been extensively revised.
- Pancreas (Chapter 27) has been extensively revised.
- Stomach & Duodenum (Chapter 23) has been extensively rewritten.
- Portal Hypertension (Chapter 25) has been extensively revised.
- Biliary Tract (Chapter 26) has been extensively revised.

ACKNOWLEDGEMENTS

The editor and the contributors continue to acknowledge their gratitude to J. Englebert Dunphy, MD for his inspiration and lifetime of service to the practice and teaching of surgery. We further wish to acknowledge the important contributions that James Ransom, who has served as copy editor for over 20 years, has made to the quality of this text. We are grateful also to our colleagues and readers who have offered comments and criticisms for our guidance in preparing future editions. We hope that anyone with an idea, suggestion, or criticism regarding this book will write to us at Appleton & Lange, 25 Van Zant Street, P.O. Box 5630, Norwalk, CT 06856-5630.

Lawrence W. Way, MD

San Francisco, California
September, 1993

Approach to the Surgical Patient

J. Englebert Dunphy, & Lawrence W. Way, MD

The management of surgical disorders requires not only the application of technical skills and training in the basic sciences to the problems of diagnosis and treatment but also a genuine sympathy and indeed love for the patient. The surgeon must be a doctor in the old-fashioned sense, an applied scientist, an engineer, an artist, and a minister to his or her fellow human beings. Because life or death often depends upon the validity of surgical decisions, the surgeon's judgment must be matched by courage in action and by a high degree of technical proficiency.

THE HISTORY

At their first contact, the surgeon must gain the patient's confidence and convey the assurance that help is available and will be provided. The surgeon must demonstrate concern for the patient as a person who needs help and not just as a "case" to be processed through the surgical ward. This is not always easy to do, and there are no rules of conduct except to be gentle and considerate. Most patients are eager to like and trust their doctors and respond gratefully to a sympathetic and understanding person. Some surgeons are able to establish a confident relationship with the first few words of greeting; others can only do so by means of a stylized and carefully acquired bedside manner. It does not matter how it is done, so long as an atmosphere of sympathy, personal interest, and understanding is created. Even under emergency circumstances, this subtle message of sympathetic concern must get across.

Eventually, all histories must be formally structured, but much can be learned by letting the patient ramble a little. Discrepancies and omissions in the history are often due as much to overstructuring and leading questions as to the unreliability of the patient. The enthusiastic novice asks leading questions; the cooperative patient gives the answer that seems to be wanted; and the interview concludes on a note of mutual satisfaction with the wrong answer thus developed.

BUILDING THE HISTORY

History taking is detective work. Preconceived ideas, snap judgments, and hasty conclusions have no place in this process. The diagnosis must be established by inductive reasoning. The interviewer must first determine the facts and then search for essential clues, realizing that the patient may conceal the most important symptom—eg, the passage of blood by rectum—in the hope (born of fear) that if it is not specifically inquired about or if nothing is found to account for it in the physical examination, it cannot be very serious.

Common symptoms of surgical conditions that require special emphasis in the history taking are discussed in the following paragraphs.

Pain

A careful analysis of the nature of pain is one of the most important features of a surgical history. The examiner must first ascertain how the pain began. Was it explosive in onset, rapid, or gradual? What is the precise character of the pain? Is it so severe that it cannot be relieved by medication? Is it constant or intermittent? Are there classic associations, such as the rhythmic pattern of small bowel obstruction or the onset of pain preceding the limp of intermittent claudication?

One of the most important aspects of pain is the patient's reaction to it. The overreactor's description of pain is often obviously inappropriate, and so is a description of "excruciating" pain offered in a casual or jovial manner. A patient who shrieks and thrashes about is either grossly overreacting or suffering from renal or biliary colic. Very severe pain—due to infection, inflammation, or vascular disease—usually forces the patient to restrict all movement as much as possible.

Moderate pain is made agonizing by fear and anxiety. Reassurance of a sort calculated to restore the patient's confidence in the care being given is often a more effective analgesic than an injection of morphine.

Vomiting

What did the patient vomit? How much? How often? What did the vomitus look like? Was vomiting

1

projectile? It is especially helpful for the examiner to see the vomitus.

Change in Bowel Habits

A change in bowel habits is a common complaint that is often of no significance. However, when a person who has always had regular evacuations notices a distinct change, particularly toward intermittent alternations of constipation and diarrhea, colon cancer must be suspected. Too much emphasis is placed upon the size and shape of the stool—eg, many patients who normally have well-formed stools may complain of irregular small stools when their routine is disturbed by travel or a change in diet.

Hematemesis or Hematochezia

Bleeding from any orifice demands the most critical analysis and can never be dismissed as due to some immediately obvious cause. The most common error is to assume that bleeding from the rectum is attributable to hemorrhoids. The character of the blood can be of great significance. Does it clot? Is it bright or dark red? Is it changed in any way, as in the coffee-ground vomitus of slow gastric bleeding or the dark, tarry stool of upper gastrointestinal bleeding? The full details and variations cannot be included here but will be emphasized under separate headings elsewhere.

Trauma

Trauma occurs so commonly that it is often difficult to establish a relationship between the chief complaint and an episode of trauma. Children in particular are subject to all kinds of minor trauma, and the family may attribute the onset of an illness to a specific recent injury. On the other hand, children may be subjected to severe trauma though their parents are unaware of it. The possibility of trauma having been inflicted by a parent must not be overlooked.

When there is a history of trauma, the details must be established as precisely as possible. What was the patient's position when the accident occurred? Was consciousness lost? Retrograde amnesia (inability to remember events just preceding the accident) always indicates some degree of cerebral damage. If a patient can remember every detail of an accident, has not lost consciousness, and has no evidence of external injury to the head, brain damage can be excluded.

In the case of gunshot wounds and stab wounds, knowing the nature of the weapon, its size and shape, the probable trajectory, and the position of the patient when hit may be very helpful in evaluating the nature of the resultant injury.

The possibility that an accident might have been caused by preexisting disease such as epilepsy, diabetes, coronary artery disease, or hypoglycemia must be explored.

■   ■   ■

When all of the facts and essential clues have been gathered, the examiner is in a position to complete the study of the present illness. By this time, it may be possible to rule out (by inductive reasoning) all but a few possible diagnoses. A novice diagnostician asked to evaluate the causes of shoulder pain in a given patient might include ruptured ectopic pregnancy in the list of possibilities. The experienced physician will automatically exclude that possibility on the basis of sex or age.

Family History

The family history is of great significance in a number of surgical conditions. Polyposis of the colon is a classic example, but diabetes, Peutz-Jeghers syndrome, chronic pancreatitis, multiglandular syndromes, other endocrine abnormalities, and cancer are often better understood and better evaluated in the light of a careful family history.

Past History

The details of the past history may illuminate obscure areas of the present illness. It has been said that people who are well are almost never sick, and people who are sick are almost never well. It is true that a patient with a long and complicated history of diseases and injuries is likely to be a much poorer risk than even a very old patient experiencing a major surgical illness for the first time.

In order to make certain that important details of the past history will not be overlooked, the system review must be formalized and thorough. By always reviewing the past history in the same way, the experienced examiner never omits significant details. Many skilled examiners find it easy to review the past history by inquiring about each system as they perform the physical examination on that part of the body.

In reviewing the past history, it is important to consider the nutritional background of the patient. There is an increasing awareness throughout the world that the underprivileged malnourished patient responds poorly to disease, injury, and operation. Indeed, there is some evidence that various lesions such as carcinoma may be more fulminating in malnourished patients. Malnourishment may not be obvious on physical examination and must be elicited by questioning.

Acute nutritional deficiencies, particularly fluid and electrolyte losses, can be understood only in the light of the total (including nutritional) history. For example, a low serum sodium may be due to the use of diuretics or a sodium-restricted diet rather than to acute loss. In this connection, the use of any medications must be carefully recorded and interpreted.

A detailed history of acute losses by vomiting and diarrhea—and the nature of the losses—is helpful in estimating the probable trends in serum electrolytes. Thus, the patient who has been vomiting persistently with no evidence of bile in the vomitus is likely to have acute pyloric stenosis associated with benign ulcer, and hypochloremic alkalosis must be anticipated. Chronic vomiting without bile—and particularly with evidence of changed and previously digested food—is suggestive of chronic obstruction, and the possibility of carcinoma should be considered.

It is essential for the surgeon to think in terms of nutritional balance. It is often possible to begin therapy before the results of laboratory tests have been obtained, because the specific nature and probable extent of fluid and electrolyte losses can often be estimated on the basis of the history and the physician's clinical experience. Laboratory data should be obtained as soon as possible, but a knowledge of the probable level of the obstruction and of the concentration of the electrolytes in the gastrointestinal fluids will provide sufficient grounds for the institution of appropriate immediate therapy.

The Patient's Emotional Background

Psychiatric consultation is seldom required in the management of surgical patients, but there are times when it is of great help. Emotionally and mentally disturbed patients require surgical operations as often as others, and full cooperation between psychiatrist and surgeon is essential. Furthermore, either before or after an operation, a patient may develop a major psychotic disturbance that is beyond the ability of the surgeon to appraise or manage. Prognosis, drug therapy, and overall management require the participation of a psychiatrist.

On the other hand, there are many situations in which the surgeon can and should deal with the emotional aspects of the patient's illness rather than resorting to psychiatric assistance. Most psychiatrists prefer not to be brought in to deal with minor anxiety states. As long as the surgeon accepts the responsibility for the care of the whole patient, such services are superfluous.

This is particularly true in the care of patients with malignant disease or those who must undergo mutilating operations such as amputation of an extremity, ileostomy, or colostomy. In these situations, the patient can be supported far more effectively by the surgeon and the surgical team than by a consulting psychiatrist.

Surgeons are becoming increasingly more aware of the importance of psychosocial factors in surgical convalescence. Recovery from a major operation is greatly enhanced if the patient is not worn down with worry about emotional, social, and economic problems that have nothing to do with the illness itself. Incorporation of these factors into the record contributes to better total care of the surgical patient.

THE PHYSICAL EXAMINATION

The complete examination of the surgical patient includes the physical examination, certain special procedures such as gastroscopy and esophagoscopy, laboratory tests, x-ray examination, and follow-up examination. In some cases, all of these may be necessary; in others, special examinations and laboratory tests can be kept to a minimum. It is just as poor practice to insist on unnecessary thoroughness as it is to overlook procedures that may contribute to the diagnosis. Painful, inconvenient, and costly procedures should not be ordered unless there is a reasonable chance that the information gained will be useful in making clinical decisions.

THE ELECTIVE PHYSICAL EXAMINATION

The elective physical examination should be done in an orderly and detailed fashion. One should acquire the habit of performing a complete examination in exactly the same sequence, so that no step is omitted. When the routine must be modified, as in an emergency, the examiner recalls without conscious effort what must be done to complete the examination later. The regular performance of complete examinations has the added advantage of familiarizing the beginner with what is normal so that what is abnormal can be more readily recognized.

All patients are sensitive and somewhat embarrassed at being examined. It is both courteous and clinically useful to put the patient at ease. The examining room and table should be comfortable, and drapes should be used if the patient is required to strip for the examination. Most patients will relax if they are allowed to talk a bit during the examination, which is another reason for taking the past history while the examination is being done.

A useful rule is to first observe the patient's general physique and habitus and then to carefully inspect the hands. Many systemic diseases show themselves in the hands (cirrhosis of the liver, hyperthyroidism, Raynaud's disease, pulmonary insufficiency, heart disease, and nutritional disorders).

Details of the examination cannot be included here. The beginner is urged to consult special texts.

Inspection, palpation, and auscultation are the time-honored essential steps in appraising both the normal and the abnormal. Comparison of the two sides of the body often suggests a specific abnormality. The slight droop of one eyelid characteristic of Horner's syndrome can only be recognized by careful comparison with the opposite side. Inspection of the female breasts, particularly as the patient raises and lowers her arms, will often reveal slight dimpling indicative of an infiltrating carcinoma barely detectable on palpation.

Successful palpation requires skill and gentleness. Spasm, tension, and anxiety caused by painful examination procedures may make an adequate examination almost impossible, particularly in children.

Another important feature of palpation is the laying on of hands that has been called part of the ministry of medicine. A disappointed and critical patient often will say of a doctor, "He hardly touched me." Careful, precise, and gentle palpation not only gives the physician the information being sought but also inspires confidence and trust.

When examining for areas of tenderness, it may be necessary to use only one finger in order to precisely localize the extent of the tenderness. This is of particular importance in examination of the acute abdomen.

Auscultation, once thought to be the exclusive province of the physician, is now more important in surgery than it is in medicine. Radiologic examinations, including cardiac catheterization, have relegated auscultation of the heart and lungs to the status of preliminary scanning procedures in medicine. In surgery, however, auscultation of the abdomen and peripheral vessels has become absolutely essential. The nature of ileus and the presence of a variety of vascular lesions are revealed by auscultation. Bizarre abdominal pain in a young woman can easily be ascribed to hysteria or anxiety on the basis of a negative physical examination and x-rays of the gastrointestinal tract. Auscultation of the epigastrium, however, may reveal a murmur due to obstruction of the celiac artery.

Examination of the Body Orifices

Complete examination of the ears, mouth, rectum, and pelvis is accepted as part of a complete examination. Palpation of the mouth and tongue is as essential as inspection. Inspection of the rectum with a sigmoidoscope is now regarded as part of a complete physical examination. Every surgeon should acquire familiarity with the use of the ophthalmoscope and sigmoidoscope and should use them regularly in doing complete physical examinations.

THE EMERGENCY PHYSICAL EXAMINATION

In an emergency, the routine of the physical examination must be altered to fit the circumstances. The history may be limited to a single sentence, or there may be no history if the patient is unconscious and there are no other informants. Although the details of an accident or injury may be very useful in the total appraisal of the patient, they must be left for later consideration. The primary considerations are the following: Is the patient breathing? Is the airway open? Is there a palpable pulse? Is the heart beating? Is massive bleeding occurring?

If the patient is not breathing, airway obstruction must be ruled out by thrusting the fingers into the mouth and pulling the tongue forward. If the patient is unconscious, the respiratory tract should be intubated and mouth-to-mouth respiration started. If there is no pulse or heartbeat, start cardiac resuscitation.

Serious external loss of blood from an extremity can be controlled by elevation and pressure. Tourniquets are rarely required.

Every victim of major blunt trauma should be suspected of having a vertebral injury capable of causing damage to the spinal cord unless rough handling is avoided.

Some injuries are so life-threatening that action must be taken before even a limited physical examination is done. Penetrating wounds of the heart, large open sucking wounds of the chest, massive crush injuries with flail chest, and massive external bleeding all require emergency treatment before any further examination can be done.

In most emergencies, however, after it has been established that the airway is open, the heart is beating, and there is no massive external hemorrhage—and after antishock measures have been instituted, if necessary—a rapid survey examination must be done. Failure to perform such an examination can lead to serious mistakes in the care of the patient. It takes no more than 2 or 3 minutes to carefully examine the head, thorax, abdomen, extremities, genitalia (particularly in females), and back. If cervical cord damage has been ruled out, it is essential to turn the injured patient and carefully inspect the back, buttocks, and perineum.

Tension pneumothorax and cardiac tamponade may easily be overlooked if there are multiple injuries.

Upon completion of the survey examination, control of pain, splinting of fractured limbs, suturing of lacerations, and other types of emergency treatment can be started.

LABORATORY & OTHER EXAMINATIONS

Laboratory Examination

Laboratory examinations in surgical patients have the following objectives: (1) screening for asymptomatic disease that may affect the surgical result (eg, unsuspected anemia or diabetes); (2) appraisal of diseases that may contraindicate elective surgery or require treatment before surgery (eg, diabetes, heart failure); (3) diagnosis of disorders that require surgery (eg, hyperparathyroidism, pheochromocytoma); and (4) evaluation of the nature and extent of metabolic or septic complications.

Patients undergoing major surgery, even though they seem to be in excellent health except for their surgical disease, should have a complete blood and urine examination. A history of renal, hepatic, or heart disease requires detailed studies. Latent, asymptomatic renal insufficiency may be missed, since many patients with chronic renal disease have varying degrees of nitrogen retention without proteinuria. A fixed urine specific gravity is easily overlooked, and preoperative determination of the blood urea nitrogen and creatinine is frequently required. Patients who have had hepatitis may have no jaundice but may have severe hepatic insufficiency that can be precipitated into acute failure by blood loss or shock.

Medical consultation is frequently required in the total preoperative appraisal of the surgical patient, and there is no more rewarding experience than the thorough evaluation of a patient with heart disease or gastrointestinal disease by a physician and a surgeon working together. It is essential, however, that the surgeon not become totally dependent upon a medical consultant for the preoperative evaluation and management of the patient. The total management must be the surgeon's responsibility and is not to be delegated. Moreover, the surgeon is the only one with the experience and background to interpret the meaning of laboratory tests in the light of other features of the case—particularly the history and physical findings.

Imaging Studies

Modern patient care calls for a variety of critical radiologic examinations. The closest cooperation between the radiologist and the surgeon is essential if serious mistakes are to be avoided. This means that the surgeon must not refer the patient to the radiologist, requesting a particular examination, without providing an adequate account of the history and physical findings. Particularly in emergency situations, review of the films and consultation are needed.

When the radiologic diagnosis is not definitive, the examinations must be repeated in the light of the history and physical examination. Despite the great accuracy of x-ray diagnosis, a negative gastrointestinal study still does not exclude either ulcer or a neoplasm; particularly in the right colon, small lesions are easily overlooked. At times, the history and physical findings are so clearly diagnostic that operation is justifiable despite negative imaging studies.

Special Examinations

Special examinations such as cystoscopy, gastroscopy, esophagoscopy, colonoscopy, angiography, and bronchoscopy are often required in the diagnostic appraisal of surgical disorders. The surgeon must be familiar with the indications and limitations of these procedures and be prepared to consult with colleagues in medicine and the surgical specialties as required.

2

Preoperative Care

Robert H. Demling, MD

The care of the patient with a major surgical problem commonly involves distinct phases of management that occur in the following sequence:

(1) **Preoperative care**
   Diagnostic workup
   Preoperative evaluation
   Preoperative preparation
(2) **Anesthesia and operation**
(3) **Postoperative care**
   Postanesthetic observation
   Intensive care
   Intermediate care
   Convalescent care

DEFINITIONS & OBJECTIVES

Preoperative Care

The **diagnostic workup** is concerned primarily with determining the cause and extent of the present illness. **Preoperative evaluation** consists of an overall assessment of the patient's general health in order to identify significant abnormalities that might increase operative risk or adversely influence recovery. **Preoperative preparation** includes procedures dictated by the findings on diagnostic workup and preoperative evaluation and by the nature of the expected operation.

Postoperative Care

The **postanesthetic observation** phase of management comprises the few hours immediately after operation during which the acute reaction to operation and the residual effects of anesthesia are subsiding. A recovery room with special staff and equipment is usually provided for this purpose. Patients who need continued cardiopulmonary support or continued invasive monitoring and critical care to avoid major morbidity and death should be transferred to the intensive care unit. For most postoperative patients, the duration of stay in the ICU is 1–2 days. However, a stay in excess of 2 weeks can result if organ failure develops, usually as a result of infection.

Uncomplicated operations for appendicitis and other problems of similar magnitude ordinarily require only a few days of hospitalization and an inter-mediate level of care on a regular nursing unit. Operations for hernias, anal conditions, and plastic procedures are now usually performed as an outpatient procedure.

Postoperative can be described as that normally available on the regular nursing units of the hospital. This type of care, and the **convalescent care** provided to the ambulatory patient outside the hospital, will not be reviewed here, because they pose no special problems not discussed in Chapters 3, 4, and 12.

The Continuum of Surgical Care

The continuum of surgical care has been represented above as progressing through a series of pre- and postoperative phases. In practice, these phases merge, overlap, and vary in relative importance from patient to patient. Complications, death, and the therapeutic end result in the surgical patient depend upon the competence with which each succeeding phase is managed. The rapid progression and severe episodic stress of major surgical illness leave small margin for errors of management. The care immediately preceding and following operation, which includes preoperative evaluation and preparation and postanesthetic observation and intensive care, is especially critical. The increased complexity of surgical critical care has resulted in a team approach to the ICU patient, with management directed by the primary surgeon and the surgical directors of the ICU, whose role it is to maintain optimum care.

PREOPERATIVE EVALUATION

General Health Assessment

The initial diagnostic workup of the surgical patient is concerned chiefly with determining the cause of the presenting complaints. Except in strictly minor surgical illness, this initial workup should be supplemented by a complete assessment of the patient's general health. Such an evaluation, which should be completed prior to all major operations, seeks to identify abnormalities that may influence operative risk or may have a bearing on the patient's future well-being. Preoperative evaluation thus involves a comprehensive examination and should include at least a complete history and physical examination, urinalysis, complete blood count, and posteroanterior and lateral chest x-rays. In patients over 40, it is advisable also to obtain an electrocardiogram, a stool test for occult blood, and a blood chemistry screening battery. The risk of reinfarction during even elective operative procedures done within 3 months after myocardial infarction exceeds 30%, while the infarction rate decreases to 4.5% after 6 months. Therefore, it is recommended that elective surgery be postponed and that urgent surgery be preceded by coronary artery bypass for correction of possible myocardial ischemia. Open wounds and infections usually require culture and determination of antibiotic sensitivity. Surface cultures of open wounds are usually of little help, particularly when closure of the wound with a skin graft is contemplated or primary closure will be allowed to occur. Quantitative cultures of punch biopsies from the wound are much more precise indicators. Greater than 10^5 organisms per gram of tissue correspond to a greater than 50% graft failure, whereas values below 10^5 organisms per gram correspond to a greater than 80% graft take. To minimize cost, much of this workup should be done before admission.

In addition to the foregoing studies, all significant specific complaints and physical findings should be adequately evaluated by appropriate special tests, examinations, and consultations. The adequacy of circulating blood volume needs to be evaluated and can be determined by the adequacy of peripheral perfusion, the fullness of neck veins in the supine and partially erect positions, and tests for orthostatic changes in blood pressure and pulse. Severe cardiovascular disease will make these parameters much more difficult to interpret. Patients (other than those with acute blood loss) who are prone to a hypovolemic state preoperatively are those with significant weight loss as a result of cancer, gastrointestinal disease, or drugs such as diuretics. The level of hemoglobin concentration cannot be used as a valid criterion of volume if the anemia is chronic. Under these circumstances, blood volume may be relatively normal. A hemoglobin of 10 g/dL is considered to be physiologically safe for tissue oxygen delivery. However, this may be inadequate in the patient with reduced cardiac output. Preoperative transfusions should be performed slowly and cautiously if anemia is chronic, in view of the potential for producing a hypervolemic state prior to operation. The adequacy of liver and kidney function should be tested if impairment is suspected, as both organs play a major role in the response to and clearance of various anesthetic agents both preoperatively and intraoperatively. Selection of the ideal agent depends on recognition of liver or renal impairment in the preoperative period. Bleeding tendencies, medications currently being taken, and allergies and reactions to antibiotics and other agents should be noted and prominently displayed on the chart. Psychiatric consultation should be considered in patients with a past history of significant mental disorder that may be exacerbated by operation and in patients whose complaints may have a psychoneurotic basis.

The physical examination should be thorough and must include neurologic examination and check of peripheral arterial pulses (carotid, radial, femoral, popliteal, posterior tibial, and dorsalis pedis). If a carotid bruit is found, other studies may be indicated to determine the need and timing of carotid surgery. A rectal examination should always be done, and a pelvic examination should be performed unless contraindicated by age, virginity, or other valid reason. A Papanicolaou smear of the cervix should be obtained in women over 30 years of age. Sigmoidoscopy is required for completeness of evaluation when there are rectal or colonic complaints.

In summary, the preoperative evaluation should be comprehensive in order to assess the patient's overall state of health, to determine the risk of the impending surgical treatment, and to guide the preoperative preparation.

Specific Factors Affecting Operative Risk

A. The Compromised or Altered Host: Patients may be considered compromised or altered hosts if significant impairment of systems and tissues does not allow a normal response to operative trauma or infection. Preoperative recognition of an abnormal nutritional or immune state is of obvious importance.

1. Nutritional assessment–It has long been documented that malnutrition leads to a significant increase in the operative death rate. Weight loss of more than 20% caused by illness such as cancer or intestinal disease not only results in a higher death rate but also a greater than 3-fold increase in the postoperative infection rate. Although there is still no uniformity of opinion about the best way to determine nutritional status, it is clear that dietary history is of major importance in the assessment, as is a working knowledge of the basic nutritional deficiencies associated with certain disease states, particularly vitamin deficiencies. Standard biochemical parameters that indicate impairment in the visceral protein mass include a serum albumin of less than 3 g/dL or a serum transferrin of less than 150 mg/dL.

Even when malnutrition is diagnosed, there is no uniformity of opinion about when short-term (7–10 days) preoperative hyperalimentation is indicated. It is known that nutrition can improve wound healing and immune function. Current indications for supportive measures before elective surgery include a history of weight loss in excess of 10% of body weight or an anticipated prolonged postoperative recovery period during which the patient will not be fed orally.

2. Assessment of immune competence–Increased knowledge and appreciation of immune defenses has led to a greater awareness of the increased postoperative rates of complication and death due to infection in patients with immune deficiency disorders. Many immune deficiency states are linked to malnutrition, as previously described. Total lymphocyte count and cell-mediated immunity measurement are the two most commonly performed tests. Anergy or impaired immunity is diagnosed if no response is noted to any of the skin tests, whereas a positive response (5 mm or more of induration at test site) to one or more skin tests indicates normal lymphocyte activity. Anergy is associated with an increased susceptibility to infectious complications. Other more specific tests include neutrophil chemotaxis and measurements of specific lymphocyte populations. Patients at high risk for immune deficiency in whom this information is helpful include elderly patients and those with malnutrition, severe trauma or burns, or cancer. Other than for a course of preoperative hyperalimentation, no stimulants of the immune system are consistently being used in the preoperative period, although research activity in this area is extensive. The AIDS patient is also severely immunocompromised and presents a risk to health care workers. Since preoperative AIDS testing is not required, even for high-risk patient groups, universal precautions are practiced, especially when dealing with blood and body secretions.

3. Other factors leading to increased infection—Certain drugs may reduce the patient's resistance to infection by interfering with host defense mechanisms. Corticosteroids, immunosuppressive agents, cytotoxic drugs, and prolonged antibiotic therapy are associated with an increased incidence of invasion by fungi and other organisms not commonly encountered in infections. A combination of irradiation and corticosteroid therapy is found experimentally to predispose to lethal fungal infections. It is possible that the synergistic combination of irradiation, corticosteroids, and serious underlying disease may set the stage for clinical fungal infection. A high rate of wound, pulmonary, and other infections is seen in renal failure, presumably as a result of decreased host resistance. Granulocytopenia and diseases that may produce immunologic deficiency—eg, lymphomas, leukemias, and hypogammaglobulinemia—are frequently associated with septic complications. The uncontrolled diabetic is also observed clinically to be more susceptible to infection (see Chapter 5).

B. Pulmonary Dysfunction: The patient with compromised pulmonary function preoperatively is susceptible to postoperative pulmonary complications, including hypoxia, atelectasis, and pneumonia. Preoperative evaluation of the degree of respiratory impairment is necessary in patients at high risk for postoperative complications. These include a history of heavy smoking and cough, obesity, advanced age, major intrathoracic or upper abdominal surgery, and known pulmonary disease. Pertinent factors in the history include the presence and character of cough and excessive sputum production, history of wheezing, and exercise tolerance. Pertinent physical findings include the presence of wheezing or prolonged expiration. A chest x-ray, ECG, blood gases, and some basic pulmonary function tests are indicated. Although an evaluation of arterial oxygen tension is very helpful, the major reason for obtaining preoperative blood gases is to determine whether CO_2 retention is present. This indicates severe pulmonary dysfunction, and the need for an elective operative procedure must be reevaluated. If surgery is necessary, oxygen must be used carefully in the postoperative period, as overuse will accentuate CO_2 retention and aggravate concomitant respiratory acidosis. The most helpful screening pulmonary function tests are forced vital capacity (FVC) and forced expiratory volume in 1 second (FEV_1). Values less than 50% of predicted outcome based on age and body size indicate significant airway disease with a high risk for complications.

Preoperative pulmonary preparation for a period as short as 48 hours has been shown to significantly decrease postoperative complications. Even a few days of abstinence from smoking will decrease sputum production. Oral or inhaled bronchodilators along with twice-daily chest physical therapy and postural drainage will help clear inspissated secretions from the airway. Before surgery, patients should be instructed in techniques of coughing, deep breathing, and use of one of the incentive spirometry devices that increase inspiratory effort. The use of intermittent positive pressure breathing (IPPB) treatments has been found to be no more effective than the much less expensive incentive spirometers when used properly.

C. Delayed Wound Healing: This problem can be anticipated in certain categories of patients whose tissue repair process may be compromised. Many factors have been alleged to influence wound healing. However, only a few are of possible clinical significance. These include protein depletion, ascorbic acid deficiency, marked dehydration or edema, and severe anemia. It has been shown experimentally that hypovolemia, vasoconstriction, increased blood viscosity, and increased intravascular aggregation and erythrostasis resulting from remote trauma will interfere with wound healing by reducing tissue oxygen tension. The most important component is maintenance of adequate blood volume and perfusion. Decreased perfusion results in a marked decrease in tissue oxygen tension, which in turn impairs collagen deposition. Often the decrease is not clinically evident, but it can be expected to occur in patients receiving chronic diuretic therapy or those with underlying myocardial dysfunction. Large doses of corticosteroids have been shown to depress wound healing in humans. It is therefore reasonable to assume that wounds in patients who have received appreciable doses of corticosteroids preoperatively should be closed with special care to prevent disruption and managed postoperatively as though healing will be delayed.

Operation may be required on a patient receiving cancer chemotherapy with cytotoxic drugs. These drugs usually interfere with cell proliferation and (theoretically at least) tend to decrease the tensile strength of the surgical wound. Although experimental evidence to support this assumption is equivocal, it is wise to manage wounds in patients receiving cytotoxic drugs as though healing will be slower than normal.

Decreased vascularity and other local changes occur after a few weeks or months in tissues that have been heavily irradiated. These are potential deterrents to wound healing, a point that should be kept in mind in planning surgical incisions in patients who have been irradiated. Radiation therapy at levels of 3000 cGy or more are injurious to skin and to connective and vascular tissues. Chronic changes include scarring, damage to fibroblasts and collagen, and degenerative changes with subsequent hyalinization in the walls of blood vessels. Angiogenesis, seen as the capillary budding in granulation tissue and collagen formation, is inhibited when these changes are well established, so that surgical wounds in heavily irradiated tissues will heal slowly or may break down in the presence of infection. When radiation is given prior to operation, it is generally agreed that there is an optimal delay period (2–12 weeks) after completion of the radiation therapy before operation is performed, in order to minimize wound complications. Technical problems in correctly timed operations for cancer are not usually increased by low-dosage (2000–4000 cGy) adjunctive radiotherapy. With radiation dosage in the therapeutic range (5000–6000 cGy), an increased incidence of wound complications can be expected, although this can be minimized by careful surgical technique and proper timing.

D. Drug Effects: Drug allergies, sensitivities, and incompatibilities and adverse drug effects that may be precipitated by operation must be foreseen and, if possible, prevented. A history of skin or other untoward reactions or sickness after injection, oral administration, or other use of any of the following substances should be noted so that they can be avoided:

Penicillin or other antibiotic
Morphine, codeine, meperidine, or other narcotic
Procaine or other anesthetic
Aspirin or other analgesic
Barbiturates
Sulfonamides
Tetanus antitoxin or other serums
Iodine, thimerosal (Merthiolate), or other germicide
Any other medication
Any foods such as eggs, milk, or chocolate
Adhesive tape

A personal or strong family history of asthma, hay fever, or other allergic disorder should alert the surgeon to possible hypersensitivity to drugs.

Drugs currently or recently taken by the patient may require continuation, dosage adjustment, or discontinuation. Medications such as digitalis, insulin, and corticosteroids must usually be maintained and their dosage carefully regulated during the operative and postoperative periods. Prolonged use of corticosteroids such as cortisone (even though discontinued 1 month or more preoperatively) may be associated with hypofunction of the adrenal cortex, which impairs the physiologic responses to the stress of anesthesia and operation. The standard dose of hydrocortisone (100 mg three times daily) is more than twice that required during surgical stress. Such a patient should receive a corticosteroid immediately before, during, and after operation. The standard dose of hydrocortisone (100 mg three times daily) is more than twice that required during surgical stress. Anticoagulant drugs are an example of a medication that is to be strictly monitored or eliminated preoperatively.

The anesthesiologist is concerned with the long-term preoperative use of central nervous system dep (eg, barbiturates, opiates, and alcohol) which may be associated with increased tolerance for anesthetic drugs; tranquilizers (eg, phenothiazine derivatives such as chlorpromazine); and antihypertensive agents (eg, rauwolfia derivatives such as reserpine), which may be associated with hypotension in response to anesthesia.

E. Risks of Thromboembolism: Increased risk factors for deep vein thrombophlebitis and pulmonary embolus include cancer, obesity, myocardial dysfunction, age over 45 years, and a prior history of thrombosis. Prophylaxis and treatment of venous thrombolic disease is discussed in Chapter 37.

F. The Pediatric Patient: See Chapter 46.

G. The Elderly Patient: (See also discussion in Chapter 5.) Operative risk should be judged on the basis of physiologic rather than chronologic age, and an elderly patient should not be denied a needed operation because of age alone. The hazard of the average major operation for the patient over age 60 years is increased only slightly provided there is no cardiovascular, renal, or other serious systemic disease. Assume that every patient over 60—even in the absence of symptoms and physical signs—has some generalized arteriosclerosis and potential limitation of myocardial and renal reserve. Accordingly, the preoperative evaluation should be comprehensive. Occult cancer is not infrequent in this age group; therefore, even minor gastrointestinal and other complaints should be thoroughly investigated by the physician.

Administer intravenous fluids with care so as not to overload the circulation. Monitoring of intake, output, body weight, serum electrolytes, and central venous pressure is important in evaluating cardiorenal response and tolerance in this age group.

Aged patients generally require smaller doses of strong narcotics and are frequently depressed by routine doses. Codeine is usually well tolerated. Sedative and hypnotic drugs often cause restlessness, mental confusion, and uncooperative behavior in the elderly and should be used cautiously. Preanesthetic medications should be limited to atropine or scopolamine in the debilitated elderly patient, and anesthetic agents should be administered in minimal amounts.

H. The Obese Patient: Obese patients have an increased frequency of concomitant disease and a high incidence of postoperative wound complications. A controlled preoperative weight loss program is often beneficial before elective procedures.

Consultations

The opinion of a qualified consultant should be obtained when it may be of benefit to the patient, when requested by the patient or family members, or when it may be of medicolegal importance. The physician should take the initiative in arranging consultation when the treatment proposed is controversial or exceptionally risky, when dangerous complications occur, or when the physician senses that the patient or family members are unduly apprehensive regarding the plan of management or the course of events. Consultation with cardiac or other medical or surgical specialists preoperatively is important if the patient has abnormal findings in their fields of competence. It is also beneficial for the specialist consultant to become acquainted with the patient and the condition preoperatively when the possibility exists that the consultant will be called upon for advice later in connection with a postoperative complication or development. Second-opinion programs for elective surgery have recently become more popular, with many programs being initiated by insurance companies. The purpose is to assist patients in making an informed decision when elective surgery has been recommended. The second opinion can be requested either by the patient or by the physician and is of particular assistance in difficult cases.

Anesthesia consultation is always requested prior to major surgery if an anesthesiologist is available. In poor-risk patients, this consultation should be requested several days in advance of operation if possible. The patient's prospects for a smooth and uncomplicated anesthetic experience are greatly improved by the anesthesiologist's preoperative evaluation and advice. Respiratory, cardiovascular, and other complications related to anesthesia are forestalled or minimized when the anesthesiologist has an opportunity to adapt the anesthesia to the patient's special circumstances.

Preoperative Note

When the diagnostic workup and preoperative evaluation have been completed, all details should be reviewed and a preoperative note written in the chart. This is usually done on the day before the operation. The note summarizes the pertinent findings and decisions, gives the indications for the operation proposed, and attests that a discussion of the complications and the risks of operation has occurred between surgeon and patient (ie, informed consent). This constitutes a final check on the adequacy of the analysis of the patient's problem, the need for treatment, and the patient's understanding of these facts.

PREOPERATIVE PREPARATION

Major operations create surgical wounds and cause severe stress, subjecting the patient to the hazard of infection and metabolic and other derangements. Appropriate preoperative preparation facilitates wound healing and systemic recovery by making certain that the patient's condition is optimal. Operation also results in psychic trauma to the patient and to family members and has significant medicolegal implications, all of which deserve special consideration preoperatively to avoid postoperative repercussions. In emergency conditions, time for preparation is limited but is usually sufficient to permit the principles of good surgical preparation to be followed. In elective operation, meticulous preoperative preparation is both possible and mandatory and includes the following steps.

Informing the Patient

Surgery is a frightening prospect for both patient and family. Their psychologic preparation and reassurance should begin at the initial contact with the surgeon. Appropriate explanation of the nature and purpose of preoperative studies and treatments establishes confidence. When all pertinent information has been gathered, it is the surgeon's responsibility to describe the planned surgical procedure and its risks and possible consequences in understandable terms to the patient and usually also to the next of kin. The potential need for blood transfusion must also be addressed. Preferably, the patient has already donated his or her own blood before scheduled surgery. This discussion must be documented in the chart. It is also very helpful to explain to the patient what will happen in the operating room before induction of anesthesia and in the recovery room. The patient should be told that an endotracheal tube may be in place and that speech may not be possible for that reason. Similarly, prompt postoperative interpretation of pertinent findings and prospects to patient and family contributes to rapport and to cooperation during the recovery period.

Operative Permit

The patient or the legal guardian of the patient must sign (in advance) a permit authorizing a major or minor operation or a procedure such as thoracentesis, lumbar puncture, or sigmoidoscopy. The nature, risk, and probable result of the operation or procedure must be made clear to the patient or a legally responsible relative or guardian so that the signed permit will constitute informed consent. A separate anesthesia consent is usually required. A signed consent is not ordinarily valid except for the specific operation or procedure for which it was obtained.

Therapeutic abortions and operations that adversely affect the sexual or childbearing functions should usually be undertaken with the concurrence in writing of the marital partner.

Emergency lifesaving operations or procedures may have to be done without a permit. In such cases, every effort should be made to obtain adequate consultation, and the director of the hospital should be informed in advance if possible.

Legal and institutional requirements regarding permits vary. It is essential that the physician know and follow local regulations.

Preoperative Orders

On the day before operation, orders are written that assure completion of the final steps in the preoperative preparation of the patient. These orders will usually include the following:

A. Skin Preparation: See below.

B. Diet: Omit solid foods for 12 hours and fluids for 8 hours preoperatively. Special orders are written for diabetics and for infants and children.

C. Enema: Enemas need not be given routinely. Patients with well-regulated bowel habits do not require a preoperative enema except in the case of operations on the colon, rectum, and anal regions or operations (chiefly abdominal) likely to be followed by paralytic ileus and delayed bowel function.

Constipated patients and those scheduled for the above types of operations should be given a flushing enema 8–12 hours preoperatively with 500–1500 mL of warm tap water or, preferably, physiologic saline, or with 120–150 mL of hypertonic sodium phosphate solution conveniently available in a commercial kit (Fleet Enema). Tap water enemas are contraindicated in congenital megacolon because of the danger of excessive water absorption. When thorough cleaning of the bowel is not essential, satisfactory evacuation on the evening before operation can usually be accomplished by use of a 10-mg bisacodyl (Dulcolax) rectal suppository. A hypertonic sodium phosphate enema or bisacodyl rectal suppository, or both, may also be effective in the rapid preparation of the colon and rectum for sigmoidoscopy.

D. Bedtime and Preanesthetic Medication: The physician anesthesiologist, if responsible for anesthesia, will usually examine the patient and write the premedication order. Otherwise, follow the guidelines set forth in Chapter 11.

E. Special Orders: In addition to the above more or less routine preoperative orders required for most major operative procedures, additional special orders related to the type and severity of the operation should be written. Examples are given below.

1. Blood transfusion–If blood transfusions may be needed during or after operation, have the patient typed and arrange for a sufficient number of units to be cross-matched and available prior to operation. Most hospitals now have a blood bank program whereby the patient can donate blood prior to admission or family members or friends can donate blood in the name of the patient to replace the units used. In some hospitals this program is mandatory owing to shortages of blood.

2. Nasogastric tube–A nasogastric tube on suction may be needed after operations on the gastrointestinal tract to prevent distention due to paralytic ileus. However, routine use is not necessary, especially for procedures such as cholecystectomy. If the patient has gastrointestinal obstruction with possible gastric residual, a nasogastric tube is passed preoperatively and the stomach aspirated or placed on continuous suction to reduce the possibility of regurgitation and aspiration during induction of anesthesia. When there is no indication for nasogastric intubation prior to operation and the patient is to be under general anesthesia, the anesthesiologist can pass the tube into the stomach after the patient is unconscious.

3. Bladder catheter–If it appears the patient will need hourly monitoring of urinary output during or after operation or if postoperative urinary retention is anticipated, a Foley catheter is inserted for constant bladder drainage. If bladder distention will interfere with exposure in the pelvis (eg, during abdominoperineal resection), a catheter should be placed preoperatively. Catheterization can be done on the nursing or preoperative holding unit just before the patient leaves for the operating room or after anesthetization.

4. Venous access and hemodynamic monitoring–Operations associated with marked blood loss call for preoperative placement of one or two 14- or 16-gauge intravenous plastic catheters for rapid administration of blood, fluids, or medication. Percutaneous insertion is usually possible; if not, a cutdown should be done to expose a vein, usually the antecubital. Central venous pressure monitoring may be required for assessment of the circulation during certain procedures such as complicated cardiovascular and pulmonary operations. A Swan-Ganz catheter is necessary for intraoperative monitoring when cardiopulmonary disease decreases the usefulness of central venous pressure as an indicator of left atrial pressure. If catheter placement is via the subclavian or internal jugular vein, it is often safer to place the lines before operation. This is done to avoid the risk of converting an unrecognized pneumothorax into a tension pneumothorax during anesthesia as a result of positive pressure breathing. Arterial catheterization or cannulation, usually of the radial artery, is done primarily for monitoring blood pressure and obtaining blood gas measurements during and after operation in selected patients in whom repeated accurate measurement of these parameters is essential. Continuous assessment of arterial hemoglobin oxygen saturation, using the noninvasive technique of pulse oximetry, is now used in virtually all patients undergoing general anesthesia.

5. Preoperative hydration–In large vascular procedures where adequate renal perfusion is essential or when a patient is thought to be relatively hypovolemic before a major operation—as frequently occurs in the cancer patient with weight loss or one with gastrointestinal disease—preoperative intravenous hydration with crystalloid beginning the night before surgery is indicated.

6. Continuing medications–Certain patients will be receiving continuing medications whose dosage or route of administration must be altered as the result of operation. Insulin and corticosteroids are examples of hormone preparations requiring special preoperative orders. Digitalis, other cardiac drugs, antibiotics, etc, may require a shift to the parenteral route of administration and altered dosage in the immediate preoperative period and during operation. Foresight in the adjustment of medication orders will minimize the possibility of underdosage or overdosage of potent and essential drugs.

7. Prophylactic antibiotics–See Chapter 8.

Asepsis & Antisepsis in the Prevention of Wound Infection

Protection of the surgical patient from infection is a primary consideration throughout the preoperative, operative, and postoperative phases of care. The factor of host resistance that influences the individual patient's susceptibility to infection has been discussed above. The incidence and severity of infection, particularly wound sepsis, are related also to the bacteriologic status of the hospital environment and to the care with which basic principles of asepsis, antisepsis, and surgical technique are implemented. The entire hospital environment must be protected from undue bacterial contamination in order to avoid colonization and cross-infection of surgical patients with virulent strains of bacteria that will invade surgical wounds in the operating room in spite of aseptic precautions taken during operation. Prevention of wound infection therefore involves both application of general concepts and techniques of antisepsis and asepsis in the hospital at large, and the use of specific procedures in preparation for operation.

A. Sterilization: The only completely reliable methods of sterilization in wide current use for surgical instruments and supplies are (1) steam under pressure (autoclaving), (2) dry heat, and (3) ethylene oxide gas.

1. Autoclaving–Saturated steam at a pressure of 750 mm Hg (14.5 psi above atmospheric pressure) at a temperature of 120 °C destroys all vegetative bacteria and most resistant dry spores in 13 minutes. Sterilization time is markedly shortened by the high-vacuum or high-pressure autoclaves now widely used.

2. Dry heat–Exposure to continuous dry heat at 170 °C for 1 hour will sterilize articles that would be spoiled by moist heat or are more conveniently kept dry. If grease or oil is present on instruments, safe sterilization calls for 4 hours' exposure at 160 °C.

3. Gas sterilization–Liquid and gaseous ethylene oxide as a sterilizing agent will destroy bacteria, viruses, molds, pathogenic fungi, and spores. It is also flammable and toxic, and it will cause severe burns if it comes in contact with the skin. Gas sterilization with ethylene oxide is an excellent method for sterilization of most heat-sensitive materials, including telescopic instruments, plastic and rubber goods, sharp and delicate instruments, and miscellaneous items such as electric cords and sealed ampules. It has largely replaced soaking in antiseptics as a means of sterilizing materials that cannot withstand autoclaving. Gas sterilization is normally carried out in a pressure vessel (gas autoclave) at slightly elevated pressure and temperature. It requires $1\frac{3}{4}$ hours for sterilization in a gas autoclave utilizing a mixture of 12% ethylene oxide and 88% dichlorodifluoromethane (Freon 12) at a temperature of 55 °C and a pressure of 410 mm Hg (8 psi above atmospheric pressure). Following sterilization, a variable period of time is required for dissipation of the gas from the materials sterilized. Solid metal or glass items such as knives, drills, and thermometers may be used immediately following sterilization. Lensed instruments and packs including cloth, paper, rubber, and other porous items must usually be kept on the shelf exposed to air for 24–48 hours before use. Certain types of materials or complex instruments, such as a cardiac pacemaker, may require 7 days of exposure to air before use.

B. Skin Antiseptics: The most important applications of skin antisepsis are the hand scrub of the operating team and the preparation of the operative field.

1. Hand scrub routine–Although the duration of the hand scrub is not universally defined, a 5-minute scrub before the first case—provided a brush is used—appears to be sufficient. Greatest attention should be paid to the fingertips and nails, since these areas harbor the greatest numbers of bacteria. A 2-minute scrub is adequate in between cases. Solutions containing chlorhexidine or one of the iodophors appear to be the most effective.

2. Preparation of the operative field–Initial preparation of the skin is usually done in the afternoon or evening before operation. The area should be washed with soap and water, making sure that it is grossly quite clean. A shower or tub bath is satisfactory. The type of soap used makes little difference. Soap is a weak antiseptic and is useful because of its nonirritating detergent action, especially when washing is combined with mechanical friction.

For elective operations involving areas with high levels of resident bacteria (eg, hands, feet) or likely to be irritated by strong antiseptics (eg, face, genitalia), preoperative degerming of the skin can be improved by repeated use of chlorhexidine gluconate (Hibiclens). Instruct the patient to wash the area several times daily with one of these preparations (and with nothing else) for 3–5 days before operation. It has been well established that shaving the surgical area the night before or within several hours of surgery increases the skin bacterial flora. Therefore, it is recommended that shaving be performed immediately before the operation, preferably in an adjacent preparation area. Shaving may be eliminated if only fine hairs are present, as their presence has not been found to increase the incidence of infection.

3. In the operating room–A 1-minute skin preparation using either 70% alcohol or 2% iodine in 90% alcohol—followed by a polyester adherent wound drape—has been shown to be as effective in controlling wound infections as the more traditional 5- to 10-minute wound scrub with povidone-iodine.

Iodine is one of the most efficient skin antiseptics available. It rarely causes skin reactions in this concentration. Avoid streaming of iodine outside of the operative field. Do not use iodine on the perineum, genitalia, or face; on irritated or delicate skin (eg, small children); or when the patient has a history of iodine sensitivity. For iodine-sensitive patients, one can use 80% isopropyl or 70% ethyl alcohol. Apply to the skin with a gauze swab for 3 minutes and allow to dry before draping. Alternatively, tinted tincture of benzalkonium (1:750) may be used.

For sensitive areas (perineum, around the eyes, etc), apply iodophor, chlorhexidine, or 1:1000 aqueous benzalkonium solution.

The adherent drape is an important component of infection control. Using drapes that simply lie over the skin is associated with a higher infection rate than using drapes that are firmly adherent.

Disease transmission to patients and health care workers—especially with the hepatitis virus and the AIDS virus—is a major problem in the operating room environment. Both can be transmitted to the patient and care providers by blood. Transmission to the surgeon or nurse via a needle or cut is of major concern because of the frequent occurrence of accidental punctures. Since the infected patient cannot readily be detected in the absence of a mandatory preoperative testing program, universal precautions are required, including the following:

a. All health care workers should routinely use appropriate barrier precautions—gloves, masks, goggles, etc—to prevent skin and mucous membrane exposure when contact with blood or body fluids is anticipated. The added safety of double gloving is still not clear.

b. Immediate hand and other skin surface washing is necessary if contamination occurs.

c. Special precautions must be taken to avoid accidental injuries, eg, needle punctures and cuts.

d. Workers who have any open wounds should avoid direct patient contact.

e. If a glove is torn, it should be removed and changed as promptly as patient safety permits and the needle or instrument removed from the sterile field.

C. Control of Hospital Environment: Hospital cross-infection with hemolytic, coagulase-positive *Staphylococcus aureus* and other organisms is always a potential problem. Strains endemic in hospitals are often resistant to many antimicrobial drugs as a consequence of the widespread use of these agents. Relaxation of aseptic precautions in the operating room and an unwarranted reliance on "prophylactic" antibiotics contribute to the development of resistant strains. The result may be a significant increase in the incidence of hospital-acquired wound infection, pneumonitis, and septicemia, the latter two complications especially affecting infants, the aged, and the debilitated.

Although the pyogenic cocci are major offenders, the enteric gram negative bacteria (particularly the coliform and *Proteus* groups and *Pseudomonas aeruginosa*) are increasingly prominent in hospital-acquired infections.

1. Hospital administration–

a. The surgical infection control program should be coordinated closely with that of other services through a hospital infection committee set up to promulgate and enforce regulations.

b. All significant infections must be reported immediately. A clean wound infection rate of more than 1% indicates a need for more effective control measures. The wound infection rate should be continuously monitored on the surgical services.

2. Cultures–Obtain culture and antibiotic sensitivity studies on all significant infections.

3. Isolation–Isolate every patient with a significant source of communicable bacteria; every case of suspected communicable infection until the diagnosis has been ruled out; and every patient in whom cross-infection will be serious.

4. Aseptic technique–

a. Operating room–The operating room should be considered an isolation zone that may be entered only by persons wearing clean operating attire (which may not be worn elsewhere).

b. Patient unit procedures–All open wounds should be aseptically dressed to protect them from cross-infection and to prevent heavy contamination of the environment. Eliminate dressing carts containing supplies and equipment for multiple bedside dressings.

c. Hand washing–Hand washing before and after each contact with a patient is a simple but important routine measure in control of infection.

5. Antibiotics–Prophylactic antibiotics are indicated for clean contaminated or contaminated cases.

Even for clean cases, prophylactic antibiotics appear to decrease the rate of infection. When possible, antibiotic therapy should be based on sensitivity studies. Antibiotics should be given in adequate doses and discontinued as soon as it is appropriate to do so.

6. Epidemiology–

a. Personnel with active staphylococcal infections should be excluded from patient contact until they have recovered. Personnel carrying staphylococci in their nasal passages or gastrointestinal tracts must observe personal hygiene but need not be removed from duty unless they prove to be a focus of infection. The advisability of treatment of the carrier is uncertain, since the carrier state is frequently transient or recurrent in spite of treatment.

b. Every significant infection acquired in the hospital should be investigated to determine its origin and spread, possible contacts and carriers, and whether improper techniques may have been responsible.

Postoperative Care

3

Sean J. Mulvihill, MD, & Carlos A. Pellegrini, MD

The recovery from major surgery can be divided into three phases: (1) an immediate, or postanesthetic phase; (2) an intermediate phase, encompassing the hospitalization period; and (3) a convalescent phase. During the first two phases, care is principally directed at maintenance of homeostasis, treatment of pain, and prevention and early detection of complications. The convalescent phase is a transition period from the time of hospital discharge to full recovery. The trend toward earlier postoperative discharge after major surgery has added new importance to this period.

THE IMMEDIATE POSTOPERATIVE PERIOD

The major causes of early complications and death following major surgery are acute pulmonary, cardiovascular and fluid derangements. The postanesthetic recovery room is staffed by specially trained personnel and provided with equipment for early detection and treatment of these problems. All patients undergoing major procedures should be initially monitored in this specialized unit. While en route from the operating room to the recovery room, the patient should be accompanied by a physician and other qualified attendants. In the recovery room, the anesthesiologist generally exercises primary responsibility for the patient's cardiopulmonary function. The surgeon is responsible for the operative site and all other aspects of the patient's care not directly related to the effects of anesthesia. The patient can be discharged from the recovery room when cardiovascular, pulmonary, and neurologic function has returned to baseline, which usually occurs 2–4 hours following operation. Patients who require continuing ventilatory or circulatory support or who have other conditions that require frequent monitoring are transferred to the intensive care unit. In this setting, nursing personnel specially trained in the management of respiratory and cardiovascular emergencies are available, and the staff:patient ratio is higher than on the wards. Monitoring equipment is available to ensure early detection of cardiorespiratory derangements.

Postoperative Orders

Detailed treatment orders should be written upon arrival in the recovery room. Unusual or particularly important orders should also be communicated to the nursing team orally. The nursing team must also be advised of the nature of the operation and the patient's condition. Postoperative orders should cover the following:

A. Monitoring:

1. Vital signs–Blood pressure, pulse, and respiration should be recorded every 15–30 minutes until stable and then hourly until discharge from the recovery room. The frequency of vital sign measurements thereafter depends upon the nature of the operation and the patient's course in the recovery room. When an arterial catheter is in place, blood pressure and pulse should be monitored continuously. Continuous electrocardiographic monitoring is indicated in most patients in the recovery room. Any major changes in vital signs should be communicated to the anesthesiologist and surgeon immediately.

2. Central venous pressure–Central venous pressure should be recorded periodically in the early postoperative period if the operation has entailed large blood losses or fluid shifts. A Swan-Ganz catheter for measurement of pulmonary artery wedge pressure is indicated under these conditions if the patient has borderline cardiac or respiratory function.

3. Fluid balance–A record is maintained by the anesthesiologist of all fluid administered and all blood loss and urine output during the operation. This record should be continued in the postoperative period and should also include fluid losses from drains and stomas. This information aids in assessing hydration and guides intravenous fluid replacement. In operations where fluid shifts are great or when renal function is marginal, a bladder catheter should be placed for frequent measurement of urine output. In the absence of a bladder catheter, the surgeon should be notified if the patient is unable to void within 6–8 hours after operation.

4. Other types of monitoring–Depending on the nature of the operation and the patient's preexisting conditions, other types of monitoring may be necessary. Examples include measurement of intracranial pressure and level of consciousness following cranial surgery and monitoring of distal pulses following vascular surgery or in patients with casts.

B. Respiratory Care: In the early postoperative

period, the patient may remain mechanically ventilated or treated with supplemental oxygen by mask or nasal prongs. These orders should be specified. In intubated patients, tracheal suctioning or other forms of respiratory therapy should be ordered as required. Patients who are not intubated should be encouraged to take deep breaths frequently to prevent atelectasis.

C. Position in Bed and Mobilization: The postoperative orders should describe any required special positioning of the patient. Unless contraindicated, the patient should be turned from side to side every 30 minutes until conscious and then hourly for the first 8–12 hours to minimize atelectasis. Early ambulation is encouraged to reduce venous stasis. Venous stasis may also be minimized by intermittent compression of the calf by a pneumatic device (see Chapter 37).

D. Diet: Patients undergoing thoracic or abdominal surgery and critically ill patients should have nothing by mouth until normal gastrointestinal function has returned (usually within 4 days). Other patients usually can tolerate liquids by mouth shortly after full return to consciousness.

E. Administration of Fluid and Electrolytes: Orders for postoperative intravenous fluids should be based on maintenance needs and the replacement of gastrointestinal losses from drains, fistulas, or stomas (see Chapter 9).

F. Drainage Tubes: The care required for drains should be included in the postoperative orders. Details such as type and pressure of suction, irrigation fluid and frequency, and skin exit site care should be specified. The surgeon should examine drains frequently, since the character or quantity of drain output may herald the development of postoperative complications such as bleeding or fistulas.

G. Medications: Orders should be written for antibiotics, analgesics, and sedatives. If appropriate, preoperative medications should be reinstituted. Careful attention should be paid to replacement of corticosteroids in patients at risk, since postoperative adrenal insufficiency may be life-threatening. Gastric stress ulcer prophylaxis with antacids or histamine H_2 receptor antagonists should be considered for patients in the intensive care unit. The incidence of stress ulcer formation is too low to justify the use of these agents routinely after all elective operations. Other medications such as antipyretics, laxatives, and stool softeners should not be ordered routinely but should be used selectively as indicated.

H. Laboratory Examinations and Imaging: The use of postoperative laboratory and radiographic examinations should be aimed at the detection of specific abnormalities in high-risk groups. Routine use of daily chest radiographs, blood counts, electrolytes, and renal or liver function panels is not indicated.

THE INTERMEDIATE POSTOPERATIVE PERIOD

The intermediate phase starts with complete recovery from anesthesia and lasts for the rest of the hospital stay. During this time, the patient recovers most basic functions and becomes self-sufficient and able to continue convalescence at home.

Care of the Wound

Within hours after a wound is closed, the wound space fills with an inflammatory exudate. Epidermal cells at the edges of the wound begin to divide and migrate across the wound surface. By 48 hours after closure, deeper structures are completely sealed off from the external environment. Sterile dressings applied in the operating room provide protection during this period. Dressings over closed wounds should be removed on the third or fourth postoperative day. If the wound is dry, dressings need not be reapplied; this simplifies periodic inspection. Dressings should be removed earlier if they are wet, because soaked dressings increase bacterial contamination of the wound. Dressings should also be removed if the patient has manifestations of infection (eg, fever, unusual wound pain). The wound should then be inspected and the adjacent area gently compressed. Any drainage from the wound should be examined by culture and Gram-stained smear. Removal of the dressing and handling of the wound during the first 24 hours should be done with aseptic technique. Medical personnel should wash their hands before and after caring for any surgical wound. When the wound is sealed, gloves need not be used during changing of dressings, but gloves should always be used with open wounds and fresh wounds.

Generally, skin sutures or skin staples may be removed by the fifth or sixth postoperative day and replaced by tapes. Sutures should be left in longer (eg, for 2 weeks) with incisions across creases (eg, groin, popliteal area), incisions closed under tension, in some incisions in the extremities (eg, the hand), and in debilitated patients. Sutures should be removed if suture tracts show signs of infection. If the incision is healing normally, the patient may be allowed to take a shower or bath by the seventh postoperative day.

Fibroblasts proliferate in the wound space quickly, and by the end of the first postoperative week, new collagen is abundant in the wound. On palpation of the wound, connective tissue can be felt as a prominence (the healing ridge) and is evidence that healing is normal. Tensile strength is minimal for the first 5 days. It increases rapidly between the fifth and 20th postoperative days and more slowly thereafter. Wounds continue to gain tensile strength slowly for about 2 years. In otherwise healthy patients, the wound should be subjected only to minor stress for 6–8 weeks. When wound healing is expected to be slower than normal (eg, in elderly or debilitated patients or those taking corticosteroids), activity should be delayed even further.

Adequate tissue perfusion is important for wound healing. In a patient with venous stasis, for example, tissue perfusion will increase, and a wound of the lower extremity will heal faster if the extremity is elevated and edema is eliminated. Oxygen tension has a profound effect on healing tissue. Indolent healing in an amputation stump may be substantially improved by arterial surgery that increases blood supply to the extremity.

When a wound has been contaminated with bacteria during surgery, it is often best to leave the skin and subcutaneous tissues open and to either perform delayed primary closure or allow secondary closure to occur. The wound is loosely packed with fine-mesh gauze in the operating room and is left undisturbed for 4–5 days; the packing is then removed. If at this time the wound contains only serous fluid or a small amount of exudate, the skin edges can be approximated with tapes. If drainage is considerable or infection is present, the wound should be allowed to close by secondary intention. In this case, the wound should be packed with moist-to-dry dressings, which are changed once or twice daily. The patient can usually learn how to care for the wound and should be discharged as soon as his or her general condition permits. Most patients do not require visiting nurses to assist with wound care at home.

Wound healing is faster if the state of nutrition is normal and there are no specific nutritional deficits. For example, vitamin C deficiency interferes with collagen synthesis and vitamin A deficiency decreases the rate of epithelialization. Deficiencies of copper, magnesium, and other trace metals decrease the rate of scar formation. Supplemental vitamins and minerals should be given postoperatively when deficiencies are suspected, but wound healing cannot be accelerated beyond the normal rate by nutritional supplements.

Wound problems should be anticipated in patients taking corticosteroids, which inhibit the inflammatory response, fibroblast proliferation, and protein synthesis in the wound. Maturation of the scar and gain of tensile strength occur more slowly. Extra precautions include using nonabsorbable suture materials for fascial closure, delaying removal of skin stitches, and avoiding stress in the wound for 3–6 months.

Deuel TF et al: Growth factors and wound healing: Platelet-derived growth factor as a model cytokine. Annu Rev Med 1991;42:567.

Jensen JA, Hunt TK: The wound healing curve as a practical teaching device. Surg Gynecol Obstet 1991;173:63.

Jonsson K, Hunt TK, Mathes SJ: Oxygen as an isolated variable influences resistance to infection. Ann Surg 1988;208:783.

Laufman H: Current use of skin and wound cleansers and antiseptics. Am J Surg 1989;157:359.

Longaker MT, Adzick NS: The biology of fetal wound healing: A review. Plast Reconstr Surg 1991;87:788.

Moesgaard F et al: Intraincisional antibiotic in addition to systemic antibiotic treatment fails to reduce wound infection rates in contaminated abdominal surgery: A controlled clinical trial. Dis Colon Rectum 1989;32:36.

Management of Drains

Drains are used to prevent accumulation of fluid following operation or to drain pus, blood, or other fluids. Thus, they are used either to prevent or to treat an unwanted accumulation of fluid. Drains are also used to evacuate air from the pleural cavity so that the lungs can reexpand. When used prophylactically, drains are usually placed in a sterile intra-abdominal location. Strict precautions must be taken to prevent bacteria from entering the abdomen through the drainage tract in these situations. The external portion of the drain must be handled with aseptic technique, and the drain must be removed as soon as it is no longer useful. When drains have been placed in an infected area, there is a smaller risk of retrograde infection of the peritoneal cavity, since the infected area is usually walled off. Drains should usually be brought out through a separate incision, because drains through the operative wound increase the risk of wound infection.

Soft latex drains are held in place by skin stitches and are prevented from slipping into the abdominal cavity by a safety pin placed through the external part of the drain or a suture between the drain and the skin. If the amount of drainage is expected to be more than about 50 mL every 8 hours, a bag should be placed over the drain site. The quantity and quality of drainage may be noted, and contamination is minimized. If drainage is scant, drains may be covered with a dressing, which should be changed often enough to prevent it from becoming soaked through or at least once every 24 hours. When drains are no longer needed, they may be withdrawn entirely at one time if there has been little or no drainage or may be progressively withdrawn over a period of a few days. Penrose drains should not be left in place longer than about 14 days, since at this point, the drain tract will begin to firm up and a soft pliable drain will act as a plug. If drains are needed beyond 2 weeks, soft drains should be replaced with rubber catheters, which can be irrigated periodically.

Closed drainage is possible with a firm catheter that passes through a small, snug hole in the skin. Closed drainage minimizes retrograde movement of bacteria from the external environment into the area being drained. Flow through the tube may be aided with suction, but unless a sump tube is used, the drain often becomes plugged if drainage is thicker than a thin serous fluid. Closed drainage is ideal when drainage is serous and in a location especially vulnerable to infection (eg, the subcutaneous space after mastectomy). Rigid tubes in the abdomen may erode into adjacent intestine after approximately 4 weeks and should therefore be positioned carefully during surgery.

Sump drains have an airflow system that keeps the lumen of the drain open when fluid is not passing through it, and they must be attached to a suction device. Sump drains are especially useful when the amount of drainage is large or when drainage is likely to plug other kinds of drains. Some sump drains have an extra lumen through which saline solution can be infused to aid in keeping the tube clear. There is evidence that continuous perfusion of sump drains with saline prevents early encapsulation and isolation of the drain, which preserves drainage of wider areas for longer periods. When an abscess cavity requires frequent irrigations, however, it is better to leave a firm catheter in place for periodic lavage. Several times each day, the large-bore catheter can be removed and a smaller catheter inserted in its place so that the cavity can be flushed with irrigating solution. Debris and secretions are thereby washed from the interior of the space being drained. After irrigation, the large-bore catheter is replaced. After infection has been controlled and the discharge is no longer purulent, the large-bore catheter is progressively replaced with smaller catheters, and the cavity eventually closes.

Cameron SE et al: Suction drainage of the axilla: A prospective randomized trial. Br J Surg 1988;75:1211.

Galandiuk S, Fazio VW: Postoperative irrigation-suction drainage after pelvic colonic surgery: A prospective randomized trial. Dis Colon Rectum 1991;34:223.

Monson JR et al: Cholecystectomy is safer without drainage: The results of a prospective, randomized clinical trial. Surgery 1991;109:740.

Smulders YM et al: How soon should drainage tubes be removed after cardiac operations? Ann Thorac Surg 1989;48:540.

Wihlborg O, Bergljung L, Martensson H: To drain or not to drain in thyroid surgery: A controlled clinical study. Arch Surg 1988;123:40.

Postoperative Pulmonary Care

The changes in pulmonary function observed following anesthesia and surgery are principally the result of decreased vital capacity, functional residual capacity (FRC), and pulmonary edema. Vital capacity decreases to about 40% of the preoperative level within 1–4 hours after major intra-abdominal surgery. It remains at this level for 12–14 hours, slowly increases to 60–70% of the preoperative value by 7 days, and returns to the baseline level during the ensuing week. FRC is affected to a lesser extent. Immediately after surgery, FRC is near the preoperative level, but by 24 hours postoperatively, it has decreased to about 70% of the preoperative level. It remains depressed for several days and then gradually returns to its preoperative value by the tenth day. These changes are accentuated in patients who are obese, who smoke heavily, or who have preexisting lung disease. Elderly patients are particularly vulnerable because they have decreased compliance, increased closing volume, increased residual volume, and increased dead space, all of which enhance the risk of postoperative atelectasis. In addition, reduced FEV_1 impairs the aged patient's ability to clear secretions and increases the chance of infection postoperatively.

The postoperative decrease in FRC is caused by a breathing pattern consisting of shallow tidal breaths without periodic maximal inflation. Normal human respiration includes inspiration to total lung capacity several times each hour. If these maximal inflations are eliminated, alveolar collapse begins to occur within a few hours and atelectasis with transpulmonary shunting is evident shortly thereafter. Pain is thought to be one of the main causes of shallow breathing postoperatively. Complete abolition of pain, however, does not completely restore pulmonary function. Neural reflexes, abdominal distention, obesity, and other factors that limit diaphragmatic excursion appear to be as important.

The principal means of minimizing atelectasis is deep inspiration. Periodic hyperinflation can be facilitated by using an incentive spirometer. This is particularly useful in patients with a higher risk of pulmonary complications (eg, elderly, debilitated, or markedly obese patients). Intermittent positive pressure breathing (IPPB) has lost popularity because it is expensive and no more effective than simpler measures. *Early mobilization, encouragement to take deep breaths (especially when standing), and good coaching by the nursing staff suffice for most patients.*

Postoperative pulmonary edema is caused by high hydrostatic pressures (due to left ventricular failure, fluid overload, decreased oncotic pressure, etc), increased capillary permeability, or both. Edema of the lung parenchyma narrows small bronchi and increases resistance in the pulmonary vasculature. In addition, pulmonary edema may increase the risk of pulmonary infection. Adequate management of fluids postoperatively and early treatment of cardiac failure are important preventive measures.

Systemic sepsis increases capillary permeability and leads to pulmonary edema. In the absence of deranged cardiac function or fluid overload, the development of pulmonary edema postoperatively should be regarded as evidence of sepsis.

RESPIRATORY FAILURE

Most patients tolerate the postoperative changes in pulmonary function described above and recover from them without difficulty. Patients who have marginal preoperative pulmonary function may be unable to maintain adequate ventilation in the immediate postoperative period and may develop respiratory failure. In these patients, the operative trauma and the effects of anesthesia lower respiratory reserve below levels that can provide adequate gas exchange. In contrast to acute respiratory distress syndrome (see Chapter 12), early postoperative respiratory failure (which develops within 48 hours after the operation) is usually only a mechanical problem, ie, there are minimal alterations of the lung parenchyma. However, this problem is life-threatening and requires immediate attention.

Early respiratory failure develops most commonly in association with major operations (especially on the chest or upper abdomen), severe trauma, and preexisting lung disease. In most of these patients, respiratory failure develops over a short period (minutes to 1–2 hours) without evidence of a precipitating cause. By contrast, late postoperative respiratory failure (which develops beyond 48 hours after the operation) is usually triggered by an intercurrent event such as pulmonary embolism, abdominal distention, or opioid overdose.

Respiratory failure is manifested by tachypnea above 25–30 breaths per minute with a low tidal volume of less than 4 mL/kg. Laboratory indications are acute elevation of P_{CO_2} above 45 mm Hg, depression of P_{O_2} below 60 mm Hg, or evidence of low cardiac output. Treatment consists of immediate endotracheal intubation and ventilatory support with a volume ventilator to assure adequate alveolar ventilation. As soon as the patient is intubated, it is important to determine whether there are any associated pulmonary problems such as atelectasis, pneumonia, or pneumothorax that require immediate treatment.

Prevention of respiratory failure requires careful postoperative pulmonary care. Atelectasis must be minimized using the techniques described above. Patients with preexisting pulmonary disease must be carefully hydrated to avoid hypovolemia. These patients must hyperventilate in order to compensate for the inefficiency of the lungs. This extra work causes greater evaporation of water and dehydration. Hypovolemia leads to dry secretions and thick sputum, which are difficult to clear from the airway. High F_{IO_2} in these patients removes the stabilizing gas N_2 from the alveoli, predisposing to alveolar collapse. In addition, it may impair the function of the respiratory center, which is driven by the relative hypoxemia, and thus further decrease ventilation. The use of epidural blocks or other methods of local analgesia in patients with COPD may prevent respiratory failure by relieving pain and permitting effective respiratory muscle function.

Chuter TAM et al: Effect of incentive spirometry on diaphragmatic function after surgery. Surgery 1989;105: 488.

Cooper MH, Primrose JN: The value of postoperative chest radiology after major abdominal surgery. Anesthesia 1989;44:306.

Hall JC et al: Incentive spirometry versus routine chest physiotherapy for prevention of pulmonary complications after abdominal surgery. Lancet 1991;337:953.

Hedenstierna G: Mechanisms of postoperative pulmonary dysfunction. Acta Chir Scand 1989;550(Suppl):152

Jackson CV: Preoperative pulmonary evaluation. Arch Int Med 1988;148;2120.

Lawrence VA, Page CP, Harris GD: Preoperative spirometry before abdominal operations: A critical appraisal of its predictive value. Arch Intern Med 1989;149:280.

Pett SB, Wernly JA: Respiratory function in surgical patients: Perioperative evaluation and management. Surg Annu 1988;20:311.

Ross WB et al: Intercostal blockade and pulmonary function after cholecystectomy. Surgery 1989;105:166.

Sabanathan S, Eng J, Mearns AJ: Alterations in respiratory mechanics following thoracotomy. J R Coll Surg Edinb 1990;35:144.

Warner MA et al: Role of preoperative cessation of smoking and other factors in postoperative pulmonary complications: A blinded prospective study of coronary artery bypass patients. Mayo Clin Proc 1989;64:609.

Postoperative Fluid & Electrolyte Management

Postoperative fluid replacement should be based on the following considerations: (1) maintenance requirements, (2) extra needs resulting from systemic factors (eg, fever, burns), (3) losses from drains, and (4) requirements resulting from tissue edema and ileus (third-space losses). Daily maintenance requirements for sensible and insensible loss in the adult are about 1500–2500 mL, depending on the patient's age, sex, weight, and body surface area. A rough estimate can be obtained by multiplying the patient's weight in kilograms times 30 (eg, 1800 mL/24 h in a 60-kg patient). Maintenance requirements are increased by fever, hyperventilation, and conditions that increase the catabolic rate.

For patients requiring intravenous therapy for a short period (most postoperative patients), it is not necessary to measure serum electrolytes at any time during the postoperative period, but measurement is indicated in complicated cases (patients with extra fluid losses, sepsis, preexisting electrolyte abnormalities, or other factors). Assessment of the status of fluid balance requires accurate records of fluid intake and output and is aided by weighing the patient daily.

Usually, 2000–2500 mL of 5% dextrose in normal saline or in lactated Ringer's solution is given daily. Potassium should usually not be added during the first 24 hours after surgery, because increased amounts of potassium enter the circulation during this time as a result of operative trauma and increased aldosterone activity.

In most patients, fluid lost through a nasogastric tube is less than 500 mL/d and can be replaced by increasing the infusion used for maintenance by a similar amount. About 20 meq of potassium should be added to every liter of fluid used to replace these losses. One must remember, however, that with the exception of urine, body fluids are isosmolar, and if large volumes of gastric or intestinal juice are replaced with normal saline solution, electrolyte imbalance will eventually result. Whenever external losses from any site amount to 1500 mL/d or more, electrolyte concentrations in the fluid should be measured periodically, and the amount of replacement fluids should be adjusted to equal the amount lost. Table 3–1 lists the compositions of the most frequently used solutions.

Losses that result from fluid sequestration at the operative site are usually adequately replaced during operation, but in patients with a large retroperitoneal dissection, severe pancreatitis, etc, third-space losses may be substantial and should be considered when postoperative fluids are given.

Fluid requirements must be evaluated frequently. Intravenous orders should be rewritten every 24 hours or more often if indicated by special circumstances. Following an extensive operation, fluid needs on the first day should be reevaluated every 4–6 hours. Other aspects of fluid and electrolyte therapy are discussed in Chapter 9. Postoperative nutrition is discussed in Chapter 10.

Postoperative Care of the Gastrointestinal Tract

Following laparotomy, gastrointestinal peristalsis temporarily decreases. Peristalsis returns in the small intestine within 24 hours, but gastric peristalsis returns more slowly. Function returns in the right colon by 48 hours and in the left colon by 72 hours. After operations on the stomach and upper intestine, propulsive activity of the upper gut remains disorganized for 3–4 days. In the immediate postoperative period, the stomach may be decompressed with a nasogastric tube. Nasogastric intubation was once used in almost all patients undergoing laparotomy, to avoid gastric distention and vomiting, but it is now recognized that routine nasogastric intubation is unnecessary and may cause postoperative atelectasis and pneumonia. For example, following cholecystectomy, pelvic operations, and colonic resections, nasogastric intubation is not needed in the average patient, and it is

probably of marginal benefit following operations on the small bowel. On the other hand, nasogastric intubation is probably useful after esophageal and gastric resections and should always be used in patients with marked ileus or a very low level of consciousness (to avoid aspiration) and in patients who manifest acute gastric distention or vomiting postoperatively.

The nasogastric tube should be connected to low intermittent suction and irrigated frequently to ensure patency. The tube should be left in place for 2–3 days or until there is evidence that normal peristalsis has returned (eg, return of appetite, audible peristalsis, or passage of flatus). The nasogastric tube enhances gastroesophageal reflux, and if it is clamped overnight for assessment of residual volume, there is a slight risk of aspiration.

Once the nasogastric tube has been withdrawn, fasting is usually continued for another 24 hours, and the patient is then started on a liquid diet. Opioids may interfere with gastric motility and should be stopped in patients who have evidence of gastroparesis beyond the first postoperative week.

Gastrostomy and jejunostomy tubes should be connected to low intermittent suction or dependent drainage for the first 24 hours after surgery. Absorption of nutrients and fluids by the small intestine is not affected by laparotomy, and enteral nutrition through a jejunostomy feeding tube may therefore be started on the second postoperative day even if motility is not entirely normal. Gastrostomy or jejunostomy tubes should not be removed before the third postoperative week, because firm adhesions should be allowed to develop between the viscera and the parietal peritoneum.

After most operations in areas other than the peritoneal cavity, the patient may be allowed to resume a regular diet as soon as the effects of anesthesia have completely worn off.

Livingston EH, Passaro EP Jr: Postoperative ileus. Dig Dis Sci 1990;35:121.

Pricolo VE et al: Decompression after gastric surgery. Gastrostomy vs nasogastric tube. Am Surg 1989;55:413.

Tollesson PO et al: Treatment of postoperative paralytic ileus with cisapride. Scand J Gastroenterol 1991;26:477.

Wolff BG et al: Elective colon and rectal surgery without

Table 3–1. Composition of frequently used intravenous solutions.

Solution	Glucose g/L	Na$^+$ meq/L	Cl$^-$ meq/L	HCO$_3^-$ meq/L	K$^+$ meq/L
Dextrose 5% in water	50	...	...	...	...
Dextrose 5% and sodium chloride 0.45%	50	77	77	...	...
Sodium chloride 0.9%	...	154	154	...	...
Sodium chloride 0.45%	...	77	77	...	...
Lactated Ringer's solution	...	130	109	28	4
Sodium chloride 3%	...	513	513	...	...

nasogastric decompression: A prospective, randomized trial. Ann Surg 1989;209:670.

Postoperative Pain

Severe pain is a common sequela of intrathoracic, intraabdominal, and major bone or joint procedures. About 60% of such patients perceive their pain to be severe, 25% moderate, and 15% mild. In contrast, following superficial operations on the head and neck, limbs, or abdominal wall, less than 15% of patients characterize their pain as severe. The factors responsible for these differences include duration of surgery, degree of operative trauma, type of incision, and magnitude of intraoperative retraction. Gentle handling of tissues, expedient operations, and good muscle relaxation help lessen the severity of postoperative pain.

While factors related to the nature of the operation influence postoperative pain, it is also true that the same operation produces different amounts of pain in different patients. This varies according to individual physical, emotional, and cultural characteristics. Much of the emotional aspect of pain can be traced to anxiety. Feelings such as helplessness, fear, and uncertainty contribute to anxiety and may heighten the patient's perception of pain.

It was once thought that anesthesia and analgesia in neonates and infants was too risky and that these young patients did not perceive pain. It is now known that reduction of pain with appropriate techniques actually decreases morbidity from major surgery in this age group.

The physiology of postoperative pain involves transmission of pain impulses via splanchnic (not vagal) afferent fibers to the central nervous system, where they initiate spinal, brain stem, and cortical reflexes. Spinal responses result from stimulation of neurons in the anterior horn, resulting in skeletal muscle spasm, vasospasm, and gastrointestinal ileus. Brain stem responses to pain include alterations in ventilation, blood pressure, and endocrine function. Cortical responses include voluntary movements and psychologic changes, such as fear and apprehension. These emotional responses facilitate nociceptive spinal transmission, lower the threshold for pain perception, and perpetuate the pain experience.

Postoperative pain serves little useful purpose and may cause alterations in pulmonary, circulatory, gastrointestinal, and skeletal muscle function that set the stage for postoperative complications. Pain following thoracic and upper abdominal operations, for example, causes voluntary and involuntary splinting of thoracic and abdominal muscles and the diaphragm. The patient may be reluctant to breath deeply, promoting atelectasis. The limitation in motion due to pain sets the stage for venous stasis, thrombosis, and embolism. The release of catecholamines and other stress hormones by postoperative pain causes vasospasm and hypertension, which may in turn lead to complications such as stroke, myocardial infarction, and bleeding. Prevention of postoperative pain is thus important for reasons other than the pain itself. Effective pain control may improve the outcome of major operations. Management of postoperative pain includes the following:

A. Physician-Patient Communication: Close attention to the patient's needs, frequent reassurance, and genuine concern help minimize postoperative pain. A few minutes spent with the patient every day in frank discussions of progress and any complications does more to relieve pain than many physicians realize.

B. Parenteral Opioids: Opioids administered intramuscularly are the mainstay of therapy for postoperative pain. Their analgesic effect is via two mechanisms: (1) a direct effect on opiate receptors and (2) stimulation of a descending brain stem system that contributes to pain inhibition. Although substantial relief of pain may be achieved with opioids, they do not modify reflex phenomena associated with pain, such as muscle spasm. Opioids administered intramuscularly, while convenient, result in wide variations in plasma concentrations. This, as well as the wide variations in dosage required for analgesia among patients, reduces efficacy. Physician and nurse attitudes reflect a persistent misunderstanding of the pharmacology and psychology of pain control. Frequently, the dose of opioid prescribed or administered is too small and too infrequent. When opioid usage is limited to temporary treatment of postoperative pain, drug addiction is extremely rare.

Morphine is the most widely used opioid for treatment of postoperative pain. Adequate pain relief with minimal side effects is achieved in about two-thirds of patients with severe pain following an intramuscular dose of 10 mg. The remaining one-third of patients require higher doses. The peak analgesic effect occurs in 1–2 hours after intramuscular injection. The recommended dosing interval is every 3–4 hours.

Morphine may also be administered intravenously, either intermittently or continuously. Except as discussed below in the section on patient-controlled analgesia, these last methods require close supervision and are impractical except in the recovery room or intensive care unit. Side effects of morphine include respiratory depression, nausea and vomiting, and clouded sensorium. In the setting of severe postoperative pain, however, respiratory depression is rare, because pain itself is a powerful respiratory stimulant.

Meperidine is a opioid with about one-eighth the potency of morphine. It provides a similar quality of pain control with similar side effects. The usual dosage of meperidine in the treatment of severe pain is 75–100 mg intramuscularly. The duration of pain relief is somewhat shorter than with morphine. The dosing interval should be no longer than every 3 hours. Like morphine, meperidine may be given intravenously, but the same requirements for monitoring apply.

Other opioids useful for postoperative analgesia include hydromorphone and methadone. Hydromorphone is usually administered in a dose of 1–2 mg intramuscularly every 2–3 hours. Methadone is given intramuscularly or orally in an average dose of 10 mg every 4–6 hours. The main advantage of methadone is its long half-life (6–10 hours) and its ability to prevent withdrawal symptoms in patients with morphine dependence.

Pentazocine is a potent analgesic with mixed opiate agonist and antagonist properties. This was once thought to reduce the likelihood of development of dependence. Compared with 10 mg of morphine, 30 mg of pentazocine produces an equivalent analgesic effect but with a somewhat shorter duration of action. Pentazocine produces more local reactions at the injection site and may cause dizziness or hallucinations.

C. Nonopioid Parenteral Analgesics: Ketorolac tromethamine is a nonsteroidal anti-inflammatory drug (NSAID) with potent analgesic and moderate anti-inflammatory activities. It is available in injectable form suitable for postoperative use. In controlled trials, ketorolac (30 mg) has demonstrated analgesic efficacy roughly equivalent to that of morphine (10 mg). A potential advantage over morphine is its lack of respiratory depression. Gastrointestinal ulceration, impaired coagulation, and reduced renal function—all potential complications of NSAID use—have not yet been reported with short-term perioperative use of ketorolac.

D. Other Agents: Hydroxyzine is an anxiolytic and ataractic occasionally useful as an adjunct to potent opioids for postoperative pain. Hydroxyzine potentiates the analgesic (and respiratory depressant) properties of morphine. It produces a calming effect and has antiemetic properties.

E. Oral Analgesics: Within several days following most abdominal surgical procedures, the severity of pain decreases to a point where oral analgesics suffice. Aspirin should be avoided as an analgesic postoperatively, since it interferes with platelet function, prolongs bleeding time, and interferes with the effects of anticoagulants. For most patients, a combination of acetaminophen with codeine (eg, Tylenol No. 3) or propoxyphene (Darvocet-N 50 or -N 100) suffices. Hydrocodone with acetaminophen (Vicodin) is a synthetic opioid with properties similar to those of codeine. For more severe pain, oxycodone is available in combination with aspirin (Percodan) or acetaminophen (Percocet, Tylox). Oxycodone is an opioid with slightly less potency than morphine. As with all opioids, tolerance develops with long-term use.

F. Patient-Controlled Analgesia: Prospective surveys of postoperative patients indicate that up to 40% have inadequate analgesia with conventional techniques such as intermittent subcutaneous opioid injections. This prompted the development of patient-controlled analgesia (PCA), which puts the frequency of analgesic administration under the patient's control but within safe limits. A device containing a timing unit, a pump, and the analgesic medication is connected to an intravenous line. By pressing a button, the patient delivers a predetermined dose of analgesic (usually morphine, 1–3 mg). The timing unit prevents overdosage by interposing an inactivation period (usually 6 minutes) between patient-initiated doses. The possibility of overdosage is also limited by the fact that the patient must be awake in order to search for and push the button that delivers the morphine. The dose and timing can be changed by medical personnel to accommodate the needs of the patient. This method appears to improve pain control and even reduces the total dose of opioid given in a 24-hour period. The addition of a background continuous infusion to the patient-directed administration of analgesic appears to offer no advantage over PCA alone.

G. Continuous Epidural Analgesia: Opioids are also effective when administered directly into the epidural space. Topical morphine does not depress proprioceptive pathways in the dorsal horn, but it does affect nociceptive pathways by interacting with opiate receptors. Therefore, epidural opioids produce intense, prolonged segmental analgesia with relatively less respiratory depression or sympathetic, motor, or other sensory disturbances. In comparison with parenteral administration, epidural administration requires similar dosage for control of pain, has a slightly delayed onset of action, provides substantially longer pain relief (eg, 10 mg of epidural morphine produces satisfactory analgesia in 90% of patients for 15–16 hours), and is associated with better preservation of pulmonary function. Epidural morphine is usually administered as a continuous infusion at a rate of 0.2–0.8 mg/h with or without the addition of 0.25% bupivacaine. Analgesia produced by this technique is superior to that of intravenous or intramuscular opioids. Patients managed in this way are more alert and have better gastrointestinal function. Side effects of continuous epidural administration of morphine include pruritus, nausea, and urinary retention. Respiratory depression may occur. Because the patient is unable to urinate, bladder catheterization is almost always required. Since a catheter must be left in the epidural space, this technique is practical only for the first 48–72 hours postoperatively.

H. Intercostal Block: Intercostal block may be used to decrease pain following thoracic and abdominal operations. Since the block does not include the visceral afferents, it does not relieve pain completely, but it does eliminate muscle spasm induced by cutaneous pain and helps to restore respiratory function. It does not carry the risk of hypotension—as does continuous epidural analgesia—and it produces analgesia for periods of 3–12 hours. The main disadvantage of intercostal blocks is the risk of pneumothorax and the need for repeated injections. These problems can be minimized by placing a catheter in the intercostal space or in the pleura through which a continuous infusion of bupivacaine 0.5% is delivered at a rate of 3–8 mL/h.

Ahn H et al: Effects of continuous postoperative epidural anesthesia on intestinal motility. Br J Surg 1988;75:1176.

Anand KJS, Hickey PR: Halothane-morphine compared with high-dose sufentanil for anesthesia and postoperative analgesia in neonatal cardiac surgery. N Engl J Med 1992;326:1.

Breslow MJ et al: Epidural morphine decreases postoperative hypertension by attenuating sympathetic nervous system hyperactivity. JAMA 1989;261:3577.

Burns JW et al: The influence of patient characteristics on the requirements for postoperative analgesia: A reassessment using patient-controlled analgesia. Anaesthesia 1989;44:2.

Campbell C: Epidural opioids: The preferred route of administration. (Editorial.) Anesth Analg 1989;68:710.

El-Naggar MA, Schaberg FJ Jr, Phillips MR: Intrapleural regional analgesia for pain management in cholecystectomy. Arch Surg 1989;124:568.

Ellis DJ, Miller WL, Reisner LS: A randomized double-blind comparison of epidural versus intravenous fentanyl infusion for analgesia after cesarean section. Anesthesiology 1990;72:981.

Marlowe S, Engstrom R, White PF: Epidural patient-controlled analgesia (PCA): An alternative to continuous epidural infusions. Pain 1989:37:97.

Parker RK, Holtmann B, White PF: Patient-controlled analgesia. Does a concurrent opioid infusion improve pain management after surgery? JAMA 1991;266:1947.

Perez-Woods R et al: Pain control after cesarean birth. Efficacy of patient-controlled analgesia vs traditional therapy (IM morphine). J Perinatol 1991;11:174.

Postoperative pain relief and non-opioid analgesics: Lancet 1991;337:524.

Power I et al: Comparison of i.m. ketorolac trometamol and morphine sulphate for pain relief after cholecystectomy. Br J Anaesth 1990;65:448.

Ross WB et al: Intercostal blockade and pulmonary function after cholecystectomy. Surgery 1989;105:166.

Smith G: Management of post-operative pain. Can J Anaesth 1989;36:S1.

REFERENCES

Gagner M: Value of preoperative physiologic assessment in outcome of patients undergoing major surgical procedures. Surg Clin North Am 1991;71:1141.

Gluck R, Munoz E, Wise L: Preoperative and postoperative medical evaluation of surgical patients. Am J Surg 1988;155:730.

Machiedo GW, Suval WD: Detection of sepsis in the postoperative patient. Surg Clin North Am 1988;68:215.

Tweedle D, Nightingale P: Anesthesia and gastrointestinal surgery. Acta Chir Scand 1989;550(Suppl);131.

Ulrich RS: View through a window may influence recovery from surgery. Science 1984;224:420.

Warner MA et al: Surgical procedures among those > 90 years of age. A population based study in Olmsted County, Minnesota, 1975–1985. Ann Surg 1988;207:380.

4

Postoperative Complications

Sean J. Mulvihill, MD, & Carlos A. Pellegrini, MD

Postoperative complications may result from the primary disease, the operation, or unrelated factors. Occasionally, one complication will result from another previous one (eg, myocardial infarction following massive postoperative bleeding). The usual clinical signs of disease are often blurred in the postoperative period. Early detection of postoperative complications requires repeated evaluation of the patient by the operating surgeon and other team members.

Prevention of complications starts in the preoperative period with evaluation of the patient's disease and risk factors. Efforts should be made to improve the health of the patient before surgery. For example, cessation of smoking for 6 weeks before surgery decreases the incidence of postoperative pulmonary complications from 50% to 10%. Correction of gross obesity decreases intra-abdominal pressure and the risk of wound and respiratory complications and improves ventilation postoperatively. The surgeon should explain the operation and the expected postoperative course to the patient at this time. The preoperative hospital stay should be as short as possible to minimize exposure to antibiotic-resistant microorganisms. Adequate training in respiratory exercises should be provided, as this substantially decreases the incidence of postoperative pulmonary complications. At operation, good technique practiced by a disciplined team is critical to the prevention of complications.

Early mobilization, proper respiratory care, and careful attention to fluid and electrolyte needs are important postoperatively. On the evening after surgery, the patient should be encouraged to sit up, cough, breathe deeply, and walk. The upright position permits expansion of basilar lung segments, and walking increases the circulation of the lower extremities and lessens the danger of venous thromboembolism. In severely ill patients, complications may be avoided by continuous monitoring of systemic blood pressure and cardiac performance. Other aspects of prevention of complications are discussed in Chapters 3 and 5.

WOUND COMPLICATIONS*

Hematoma

Wound hematoma, a collection of blood and clots in the wound, is one of the most common wound complications and is almost always caused by imperfect hemostasis. Patients receiving aspirin or minidose heparin have a slightly higher risk of developing this complication. The risk is much higher in patients who have been given anticoagulants and those with preexisting coagulopathies. Vigorous coughing or marked arterial hypertension immediately after surgery may contribute to the formation of a wound hematoma.

Hematomas produce elevation and discoloration of the wound edges, discomfort, and swelling. Blood sometimes leaks through skin sutures. Neck hematomas following operations on the thyroid, parathyroid, carotid artery, etc, are particularly dangerous, because they may expand rapidly and compress the trachea. Hematomas in this area must be evacuated early, before ventilation is compromised. Small hematomas may resorb, but they increase the incidence of wound infection. Treatment in most cases consists of evacuation of the clot under sterile conditions, ligation of bleeding vessels, and reclosure of the wound.

Seroma

A seroma is a fluid collection in the wound other than pus or blood. Seromas often follow operations that involve elevation of skin flaps and transection of numerous lymphatic channels (eg, mastectomy, operations in the groin). Seromas delay healing and increase the risk of wound infection. Those located under skin flaps can usually be evacuated by needle aspiration. Compression dressings should then be applied to seal lymphatic leaks and prevent reaccumulation. Small seromas that recur may be treated by evacuation and injection of tetracycline (1 g in 150 mL saline) as a sclerosant solution. Seromas of the groin, which are common after vascular operations,

---

*Postoperative wound infection and other aspects of wound sepsis are discussed in Chapter 8.

are best left alone, since the risks of introducing a needle (infection, disruption of vascular structures, etc) are greater than the risk associated with the seroma itself. If seromas persist—or if they start leaking through the wound after several days—the wound should be explored in the operating room and the lymphatics ligated.

Wound Dehiscence

Wound dehiscence is partial or total disruption of any or all layers of the operative wound. Rupture of all layers of the abdominal wall and extrusion of abdominal viscera is called evisceration. Wound dehiscence occurs in 1–3% of abdominal surgical procedures. Systemic and local factors contribute to the development of this complication.

A. Systemic Risk Factors: Dehiscence is rare in patients under age 30 but affects about 5% of patients over age 60 having laparotomy. It is more common in patients with diabetes mellitus, uremia, immunosuppression, jaundice, sepsis, hypoalbuminemia, and cancer; in obese patients; and in those receiving corticosteroids.

B. Local Risk Factors: The three most important local factors predisposing to wound dehiscence are inadequate closure, increased intra-abdominal pressure, and deficient wound healing. Dehiscences often result from a combination of these factors rather than from a single one. The kind of incision (transverse, longitudinal, etc) does not influence the incidence of dehiscence.

1. Adequacy of closure–This is the single most important factor. The fascial layers give strength to a closure, and when fascia disrupts, the wound separates. Accurate approximation of anatomic layers is essential for adequate wound closure. Most wounds dehisce because the sutures cut through the fascia. Prevention of this problem includes performing a neat incision, avoiding devitalization of the fascial edges by careful handling of the tissues during the operation, placing and tying sutures correctly, and selecting the proper suture material. Sutures must be placed 2–3 cm from the wound edge and about 1 cm apart. *Dehiscence is often the result of using too few stitches and placing them too close to the edge of the fascia.* Modern synthetic suture materials (polyglycolic acid, polypropylene, and others) are clearly superior to catgut for fascial closure. In infected wounds, polypropylene and polyglyconate sutures are more resistant to degradation than polyglycolic acid sutures and have lower rates of wound disruption. Wound complications are decreased by obliteration of dead space. Ostomies and drains should be brought out through separate stab incisions to reduce the rate of wound infection and disruption.

2. Intra-abdominal pressure–After any intra-abdominal operation, some degree of ileus is inevitable. High abdominal pressures may occur in patients with chronic obstructive pulmonary disease who use their abdominal muscles as accessory muscles of respiration. In addition, coughing produces sudden increases in intra-abdominal pressure. Other factors contributing to increased abdominal pressure are postoperative bowel obstruction, obesity, and cirrhosis with ascites formation. Extra precautions are necessary to avoid dehiscence in such patients.

3. Deficient wound healing–Infection is an associated factor in more than half of wounds that rupture. The presence of drains, seromas, and wound hematomas also delays healing. Normally, a "healing ridge" (a palpable thickening extending about 0.5 cm on each side of the incision) appears near the end of the first week after surgery. The presence of this ridge is clinical proof that healing is adequate, and it is invariably absent from wounds that rupture.

C. Diagnosis and Management: Although wound dehiscence may occur at any time following wound closure, it is most commonly observed between the fifth and eighth postoperative days, when the strength of the wound is at a minimum. Wound dehiscence may occasionally be the first manifestation of an intra-abdominal abscess. The first sign of dehiscence is discharge of serosanguineous fluid from the wound, or, in some cases, sudden evisceration. The patient often describes a popping sensation associated with severe coughing or retching. Thoracic wounds, with the exception of sternal wounds, are much less prone to dehiscence than are abdominal wounds. When a thoracotomy closure ruptures, it is heralded by leakage of pleural fluid or air and paradoxic motion of the chest wall. Sternal dehiscences, which are almost always associated with infection, produce an unstable chest and require early treatment. If infection is not overwhelming and there is minimal osteomyelitis of the adjacent sternum, the patient may be returned to the operating room for reclosure. Continuous mediastinal irrigation through small tubes left at the time of closure appears to reduce the failure rate. In cases of overwhelming infection, the wound is best treated by debridement and closure with a pectoralis major flap, which increases vascular supply to the area.

Patients with dehiscence of a laparotomy wound and evisceration should be returned to bed and the wound covered with moist towels. With the patient under general anesthesia, any exposed bowel or omentum should be rinsed with Ringer's lactate solution containing antibiotics and then returned to the abdomen. After mechanical cleansing and copious irrigation of the wound, the previous sutures should be removed and the wound reclosed using full-thickness retention sutures of No. 22 wire or heavy nylon. Evisceration carries a 10% mortality rate due to both contributing factors (eg, sepsis and cancer) and resulting infections.

Wound dehiscence without evisceration is best managed by prompt elective reclosure of the incision. If a partial disruption (ie, the skin is intact) is stable and the patient is a poor operative risk, treatment may be delayed and the resulting incisional hernia accepted. It is important in these patients that skin stitches not be removed before the end of the second postoperative week and that the abdomen be wrapped with a binder or corset to prevent further enlargement of the fascial defect or sudden disruption of the covering skin. When partial dehiscence is discovered during treatment of a wound infection, repair should be delayed if possible until the infection has been controlled, the wound has healed, and 6–7 months have elapsed. In these cases, antibiotics specific for the organisms isolated from the previous wound infection must be given at the time of hernia repair.

Recurrence of evisceration after reclosure of dehisced wounds is rare, though incisional hernias are later found in about 20% of such patients—usually those with wound infection in addition to dehiscence.

Miscellaneous Problems of the Operative Wound

Every new operative wound is painful, but those subject to continuous motion (eg, incisions that cross the costal margin) may be more painful than others. In general, the pain of an operative wound decreases substantially during the first 4–6 postoperative days. Chronic pain localized to one portion of an apparently healed wound may indicate the presence of a stitch abscess, a granuloma, or an occult incisional hernia. Abnormalities on examination of the wound usually allow for easy diagnosis; when this is difficult, ultrasound scanning may help detect a fascial defect or a collection of fluid associated with granulomas or abscesses. Rarely, a neuroma in the wound is responsible for focal pain and tenderness late in the postoperative course. Persistent localized pain is best treated by exploring the area, usually under local anesthesia, and removing a stitch, draining an abscess, or closing a hernia defect. Small sinus tracts usually result from stitch abscesses. The infected stitch can usually be removed with a clamp or crochet hook passed down the tract. If drainage continues, it is occasionally necessary to reopen the skin for better exposure and to remove a series of infected stitches.

Patients with ascites are at risk of fluid leak through the wound. Left untreated, **ascitic leaks** increase the incidence of wound infection and, through retrograde contamination, may result in peritonitis. Prevention in susceptible patients involves closing at least one layer of the wound with a continuous suture and taking measures to avoid the accumulation of ascites postoperatively. If an ascitic leak develops, the wound should be explored and the fascial defect closed. The rest of the wound, including the skin, should also be closed.

Broadwater JR et al: Mastectomy following preoperative chemotherapy: Strict operative criteria control operative morbidity. Ann Surg 1991;213:126.

Dawson I et al: Effect of shoulder immobilization on wound seroma and shoulder dysfunction following modified radical mastectomy: A randomized prospective clinical trial. Br J Surg 1989;76–311.

Hugh TB et al: Is closure of the peritoneal layer necessary in the repair of midline surgical abdominal wounds? World J Surg 1990; 14:231.

Johnson JA et al: Wound complications after infrainguinal bypass: Classification, predisposing factors, and management. Arch Surg 1988;123:859.

Larsen PN et al: Closure of the abdominal fascia after clean and clean-contaminated laparotomy. Acta Chir Scand 1989; 155:461.

Lewis RT, Wiegand FM: Natural history of vertical abdominal parietal closure: Prolene versus Dexon. Can J Surg 1989;32:196.

Lievy E et al: Septic necrosis of the midline wound in postoperative peritonitis. Successful management by debridement, myocutaneous advancement, and primary skin closure. Ann Surg 1988;207:470.

Vinton AL, Traverso LW, Jolly PC: Wound complications after modified radical mastectomy compared with tylectomy with axillary lymph node dissection. Am J Surg 1991;161:584.

RESPIRATORY COMPLICATIONS*
(See also Chapter 5.)

Respiratory complications are the largest single cause of morbidity after major surgical procedures and the second most common cause of postoperative death in patients older than 60 years. Patients undergoing chest and upper abdominal operations are particularly prone to pulmonary complications. The incidence is lower after pelvic surgery and even lower after extremity or head and neck procedures. Pulmonary complications are more common after emergency operations. Special hazards are posed by preexisting chronic obstructive pulmonary disease (chronic bronchitis, emphysema, asthma, pulmonary fibrosis). Elderly patients are at much higher risk because they have decreased compliance, increased closing and residual volumes, and increased dead space, all of which predispose to atelectasis.

Atelectasis

Atelectasis, the most common pulmonary complication, affects 25% of patients who have abdominal surgery. It is more common in patients who are elderly or overweight and in those who smoke or have symptoms of respiratory disease. It appears most frequently in the first 48 hours after operation and is responsible for over 90% of febrile episodes during that period. In most cases, the course is self-limited and recovery uneventful.

The pathogenesis of atelectasis involves obstruc-

---

*Pulmonary embolism is discussed in Chapter 37. Acute respiratory distress syndrome is discussed in Chapter 12.

tive and nonobstructive factors. Obstruction may be caused by secretions resulting from chronic obstructive pulmonary disease, intubation, or anesthetic agents. Occasional cases may be due to blood clots or malposition of the endotracheal tube. In most instances, however, the cause is not obstruction but closure of the bronchioles. Small bronchioles (≤ 1 mm) are prone to close when lung volume reaches a critical point (closing volume). Portions of the lung that are dependent or compressed are the first to experience bronchiole closure, since their regional volume is less than that of nondependent portions. Shallow breathing and failure to periodically hyperinflate the lung result in small alveolar size and decreased volume. The closing volume is higher in older patients and in smokers owing to the loss of elastic recoil of the lung. Other nonobstructive factors contributing to atelectasis include decreased functional residual capacity and loss of pulmonary surfactant.

The air in the atelectatic portion of the lung is absorbed, and since there is minimal change in perfusion, a ventilation/perfusion mismatch results. The immediate effect of atelectasis is decreased oxygenation of blood; its clinical significance depends on the respiratory and cardiac reserve of the patient. A later effect is the propensity of the atelectatic segment to become infected. In general, if a pulmonary segment remains atelectatic for over 72 hours, pneumonia is almost certain to occur.

Atelectasis is usually manifested by fever (pathogenesis unknown), tachypnea, and tachycardia. Physical examination may show elevation of the diaphragm, scattered rales, and decreased breath sounds, but it is often normal. Postoperative atelectasis can be largely prevented by early mobilization, frequent changes in position, encouragement to cough, and use of an incentive spirometer. Preoperative teaching of respiratory exercises and postoperative execution of these exercises prevents atelectasis in patients without preexisting lung disease. Intermittent positive pressure breathing is expensive and less effective than these simpler exercises.

Treatment consists of clearing the airway by chest percussion, coughing, or nasotracheal suction. Bronchodilators and mucolytic agents given by nebulizer may help in patients with severe chronic obstructive pulmonary disease. Atelectasis from obstruction of a major airway may require intrabronchial suction through an endoscope, a procedure that can usually be performed at the bedside with moderate sedation.

Pulmonary Aspiration

Aspiration of oropharyngeal and gastric contents is normally prevented by the gastroesophageal and pharyngoesophageal sphincters. Insertion of nasogastric and endotracheal tubes and depression of the central nervous system by drugs interferes with these defenses and predisposes to aspiration. Other factors, such as gastroesophageal reflux, food in the stomach, or position of the patient, may play a role. Trauma victims are particularly likely to aspirate regurgitated gastric contents when consciousness is depressed. Patients with intestinal obstruction and pregnant women—who have increased intra-abdominal pressure and decreased gastric motility—are also at high risk of aspiration. Two-thirds of cases of aspiration follow thoracic or abdominal surgery, and of these, one-half result in pneumonia. The death rate for grossly evident aspiration and the subsequent pneumonia is about 50%.

Minor amounts of aspiration are frequent during surgery and are apparently well tolerated. Methylene blue placed in the stomach of patients undergoing abdominal operations can be found in the trachea at the completion of the procedure in 15% of cases. Radionuclide techniques have shown aspiration of gastric contents in 45% of normal volunteers during sleep.

The magnitude of pulmonary injury produced by aspiration of fluid, usually from gastric contents, is determined by the volume aspirated, its pH, and the frequency of the event. If the aspirate has a pH of 2.5 or less, it causes immediate chemical pneumonitis, which results in local edema and inflammation, changes that increase the risk of secondary infection. Aspiration of solid matter produces airway obstruction. Obstruction of distal bronchi, although well tolerated initially, may lead to atelectasis and pulmonary abscess formation. The basal segments are affected most often. Tachypnea, rales, and hypoxia are usually present within hours; less frequently, cyanosis, wheezing, and apnea may appear. In patients with massive aspiration, hypovolemia caused by excessive fluid and colloid loss into the injured lung may lead to hypotension and shock.

Aspiration has been found in 80% of patients with tracheostomies and may account for the predisposition to pulmonary infection in this group. Patients who must remain intubated for long periods should have a low-pressure, high-volume type of cuff on their tube, as this type prevents aspiration and avoids pressure necrosis of the trachea.

Aspiration can be prevented by preoperative fasting, proper positioning of the patient, and careful intubation. A single dose of cimetidine before induction of anesthesia may be of value in situations where the risk of aspiration is high. Treatment of aspiration involves reestablishing patency of the airway and preventing further damage to the lung. Endotracheal suction should be performed immediately, as this procedure confirms the diagnosis and stimulates coughing, which helps to clear the airway. Bronchoscopy may be required to remove solid matter. Fluid resuscitation should be undertaken concomitantly. Hydrocortisone, 30 mg/kg/d intravenously, may be useful for the first 3 days. Antibiotics are used initially when the aspirate is heavily contaminated; they are used later to treat pneumonia.

Postoperative Pneumonia

Pneumonia is the most common pulmonary complication among patients who die after surgery. It is directly responsible for—or contributes to—death in more than half of these patients. Patients with peritoneal infection and those requiring prolonged ventilatory support are at highest risk for developing postoperative pneumonia. Atelectasis, aspiration, and copious secretions are important predisposing factors.

Host defenses against pneumonitis include the cough reflex, the mucociliary system, and activity of alveolar macrophages. After surgery, cough is usually weak and may not effectively clear the bronchial tree. The mucociliary transport mechanism is damaged by endotracheal intubation, and the functional ability of the alveolar macrophage is compromised by a number of factors that may be present during and after surgery (oxygen, pulmonary edema, aspiration, corticosteroid therapy, etc). In addition, squamous metaplasia and loss of ciliary coordination further hamper antibacterial defenses. More than half of the pulmonary infections that follow surgery are caused by gram-negative bacilli. They are frequently polymicrobial and usually acquired by aspiration of oropharyngeal secretions. Although colonization of the oropharynx with gram-negative bacteria occurs in only 20% of normal individuals, it is frequent after major surgery as a result of impaired oropharyngeal clearing mechanisms. Aggravating factors are azotemia, prolonged endotracheal intubation, and severe associated infection.

Occasionally, infecting bacteria reach the lung by inhalation—eg, from respirators. *Pseudomonas aeruginosa* and *Klebsiella* can survive in the moist reservoirs of these machines, and these pathogens have been the source of epidemic infections in intensive care units. Rarely, contamination of the lung may result from direct hematogenous spread from distant septic foci.

The clinical manifestations of postoperative pneumonia are fever, tachypnea, increased secretions, and physical changes suggestive of pulmonary consolidation. A chest x-ray usually shows localized parenchymal consolidation. Overall mortality rates for postoperative pneumonia vary from 20% to 40%. Rates are higher when pneumonia develops in patients who had emergency operations; are on respirators; or develop remote organ failure, positive blood cultures, or infection of the second lung.

Maintaining the airway clear of secretions is of paramount concern in the prevention of postoperative pneumonia. Respiratory exercises, deep breathing, and coughing help prevent atelectasis, which is a precursor of pneumonia. Although postoperative pain is thought to contribute to shallow breathing, neither intercostal blocks nor epidural narcotics prevent atelectasis and pneumonia when compared with traditional methods of postoperative pain control. The prophylactic use of antibiotics does not decrease the incidence of gram-negative colonization of the oropharynx or that of pneumonia. Treatment consists of measures to aid the clearing of secretions and administration of antibiotics. Sputum obtained directly from the trachea, usually by endotracheal suctioning, is required for specific identification of the infecting organism.

Postoperative Pleural Effusion & Pneumothorax

Formation of a very small pleural effusion is fairly common immediately after upper abdominal operations and is of no clinical significance. Patients with free peritoneal fluid at the time of surgery and those with postoperative atelectasis are more prone to develop effusions. In the absence of cardiac failure or a pulmonary lesion, appearance of a pleural effusion late in the postoperative course suggests the presence of subdiaphragmatic inflammation (subphrenic abscess, acute pancreatitis, etc). Effusions that do not compromise respiratory function should be left undisturbed. If there is a suspicion of infection, the effusion should be tapped. When an effusion produces respiratory compromise, it should be drained with a thoracostomy tube.

Postoperative pneumothorax may follow insertion of a subclavian catheter or positive pressure ventilation, but it sometimes appears after an operation during which the pleura has been injured (eg, nephrectomy or adrenalectomy). Pneumothorax should be treated with a thoracostomy tube.

Chuter TA et al: Effects of incentive spirometry on diaphragmatic function after surgery. Surgery 1989;105: 488.

Hall JC et al: Incentive spirometry versus routine chest physiotherapy for prevention of pulmonary complications after abdominal surgery. Lancet 1991;337:953.

Lawrence VA, Page CP, Harris GD: Preoperative spirometry before abdominal operations: A critical appraisal of its predictive value. Arch Int Med 1989;149:280.

LoCicero J: Bronchopulmonary aspiration. Surg Clin North Am 1989;69:71.

Mock CN et al: Surgical intensive care unit pneumonia. Surgery 1988;104:494.

Ross WB et al: Intercostal blockade and pulmonary function after cholecystectomy. Surgery 1989;105:166.

Roukema JA, Carol EJ, Prins JG: The prevention of pulmonary complications after upper abdominal surgery in patients with noncompromised pulmonary status. Arch Surg 1988;123:30.

Sabanathan S, Eng J, Mearns AJ: Alterations in respiratory mechanics following thoracotomy. J R Coll Surg Edinb 1990;35:144.

Warner MA et al: Role of preoperative cessation of smoking and other factors in postoperative pulmonary complications: A blinded prospective study of coronary artery bypass patients. Mayo Clin Proc 1989;64:609.

Windsor JA, Hill GL: Risk factors for postoperative pneumonia: The importance of protein depletion. Ann Surg 1988;208:209.

FAT EMBOLISM

Fat embolism is relatively common but only rarely causes symptoms. Fat particles can be found in the pulmonary vascular bed in 90% of patients who have had fractures of long bones or joint replacements. Fat embolism can also be caused by exogenous sources of fat, such as blood transfusions, intravenous fat emulsion, or bone marrow transplantation. **Fat embolism syndrome** consists of neurologic dysfunction, respiratory insufficiency, and petechiae of the axilla, chest, and proximal arms. It was originally described in trauma victims—especially those with long bone fractures—and was thought to be a result of bone marrow embolization. However, the principal clinical manifestations of fat embolism are seen in other conditions. The existence of fat embolism as an entity distinct from posttraumatic pulmonary insufficiency has been questioned.

Fat embolism syndrome characteristically begins 12–72 hours after injury but may be delayed for several days. The diagnosis is clinical. The finding of fat droplets in sputum and urine is common after trauma and is not specific. Decreased hematocrit, thrombocytopenia, and other changes in coagulation parameters are usually seen.

Once symptoms develop, supportive treatment should be provided until respiratory insufficiency and central nervous system manifestations subside. Respiratory insufficiency is treated with positive end-expiratory pressure ventilation and diuretics. The prognosis is related to the severity of the pulmonary insufficiency.

Chastre J et al: Bronchoalveolar lavage for rapid diagnosis of the fat embolism syndrome in trauma patients. Ann Intern Med 1990;113:583.

Laub DR Jr, Laub DR: Fat embolism syndrome after liposuction: A case report and review of the literature. Ann Plast Surg 1990;25:48.

Levy D: The fat embolism syndrome: A review. Clin Orthop 1990;261:281.

CARDIAC COMPLICATIONS
(See also Chapter 5.)

Cardiac complications following surgery may be life-threatening. Their incidence is reduced by appropriate preoperative preparation.

Dysrhythmias, unstable angina, heart failure, or severe hypertension should be corrected before surgery whenever possible. Valvular disease—especially aortic stenosis—limits the ability of the heart to respond to increased demand during operation or in the immediate postoperative period. When aortic stenosis is recognized preoperatively—and assuming that the patient is monitored adequately (Swan-Ganz, central venous pressure, etc)—the incidence of major perioperative complications is small. Thus, patients with preexisting heart disease should be evaluated by a cardiologist preoperatively. Determination of cardiac function, including indirect evaluation of the left ventricular ejection fraction, identifies patients at higher risk for cardiac complications. Continuous electrocardiographic monitoring during the first 3–4 postoperative days detects episodes of ischemia or dysrhythmia in about a third of these patients. Oral anticoagulant drugs should be stopped 3–5 days before surgery, and the prothrombin time should be allowed to return to normal. The patient should receive heparin until approximately 6 hours before the operation, when heparin should be stopped. If needed, heparin can be restarted 36–48 hours after surgery along with oral anticoagulation.

General anesthesia depresses the myocardium, and some anesthetic agents predispose to dysrhythmias by sensitizing the myocardium to catecholamines. Monitoring of cardiac activity and blood pressure during the operation detects dysrhythmias and hypotension early. In patients with a high cardiac risk, regional anesthesia may be safer than general anesthesia for procedures below the umbilicus.

The duration and urgency of the operation and uncontrolled bleeding with hypotension have been individually shown to correlate positively with the development of serious postoperative cardiac problems. In patients with pacemakers, the electrocautery current may be sensed by the intracardiac electrode, causing inappropriate pacemaker function.

Noncardiac complications may affect the development of cardiac complications by increasing cardiac demands in patients with a limited reserve. Postoperative sepsis and hypoxemia are foremost. Fluid overload can produce acute left ventricular failure. Patients with coronary artery disease, dysrhythmias, or low cardiac output should be monitored postoperatively in the intensive care unit.

Dysrhythmias

Most dysrhythmias appear during the operation or within the first 3 postoperative days. They are especially likely to occur after thoracic procedures.

A. Intraoperative Dysrhythmias: The overall incidence of intraoperative cardiac dysrhythmias is 20%. The incidence is higher in patients with preexisting dysrhythmias and in those with known heart disease (35%). About one-third of dysrhythmias occur during induction of anesthesia. These dysrhythmias are usually related to anesthetic agents (eg, halothane, cyclopropane), sympathomimetic drugs, digitalis toxicity, and hypercapnia.

B. Postoperative Dysrhythmias: These dysrhythmias are generally related to reversible factors such as hypokalemia, hypoxemia, alkalosis, digitalis toxicity, and stress during emergence from anesthesia. Occasionally, postoperative dysrhythmias may be the first sign of myocardial infarction. Most postoperative dysrhythmias are asymptomatic, but occasionally the patient complains of chest pain, palpitations, or dyspnea.

Supraventricular dysrhythmias usually have few serious consequences but may decrease cardiac output and coronary blood flow. Patients with atrial flutter or fibrillation with a rapid ventricular response who are in shock require cardioversion. If they are hemodynamically stable, they should be given digitalis. Propranolol and verapamil are also helpful, provided that myocardial function is not substantially reduced. Associated hypokalemia should be treated promptly.

Ventricular premature beats are often precipitated by hypercapnia, hypoxemia, pain, or fluid overload. They should be treated with oxygen, sedation, analgesia, and correction of fluid or electrolyte abnormalities. Ventricular dysrhythmias have a more profound effect on cardiac function than supraventricular dysrhythmias and may lead to fatal ventricular fibrillation. Immediate treatment is with lidocaine, 1 mg/kg intravenously as a bolus, repeated as necessary to a total dose of 250 mg, followed by a slow intravenous infusion at a rate of 1–2 mg/min. Higher doses of lidocaine may cause seizures.

Postoperative complete heart block is usually due to serious cardiac disease and calls for the immediate insertion of a pacemaker. First- or second-degree heart block is usually well tolerated.

Postoperative Myocardial Infarction

Approximately 0.4% of all patients undergoing an operation in the USA develop postoperative myocardial infarction. The incidence increases to 5–12% in patients undergoing operations for other manifestations of atherosclerosis (eg, carotid endarterectomy, aortoiliac graft). Other important risk factors include preoperative congestive heart failure, ischemia identified on dipyridamole-thallium scan or treadmill exercise test, and age over 70 years. In selected patients with angina, consideration should be given to performing a coronary artery bypass graft before proceeding with a major elective operation on another organ.

Postoperative myocardial infarction may be precipitated by factors such as hypotension or hypoxemia. Clinical manifestations include chest pain, hypotension, and cardiac dysrhythmias. Over half of postoperative myocardial infarctions, however, are asymptomatic. The absence of symptoms is thought to be due to the residual effects of anesthesia and to analgesics administered postoperatively.

Diagnosis is substantiated by electrocardiographic changes and elevated serum creatine kinase levels, especially the MB isoenzyme. The mortality rate of postoperative myocardial infarction is as high as 67% in high-risk groups. The prognosis is better if it is the first infarction and worse if there have been previous infarctions. Prevention of this complication includes postponing elective operations for 3 months or preferably 6 months after myocardial infarction, treating congestive heart failure preoperatively, and controlling hypertension perioperatively.

Patients with postoperative myocardial infarction should be monitored in the intensive care unit and provided with adequate oxygenation and precise fluid and electrolyte replacement. Anticoagulation, though not always feasible after major surgery, prevents the development of mural thrombosis and arterial embolism after myocardial infarction. Congestive heart failure should be treated with digitalis, diuretics, and vasodilators as needed.

Postoperative Cardiac Failure

Left ventricular failure and pulmonary edema appear in 4% of patients over age 40 undergoing general surgical procedures with general anesthesia. Fluid overload in patients with limited myocardial reserve is the most common cause. Postoperative myocardial infarction and dysrhythmias producing a high ventricular rate are other causes. Clinical manifestations are progressive dyspnea, hypoxemia with normal CO_2 tension, and diffuse congestion on chest x-ray.

Clinically inapparent ventricular failure is frequent, especially when other factors predisposing to pulmonary edema are present (massive trauma, multiple transfusions, sepsis, etc). The diagnosis may be suspected from a decreased Pa_{O_2}, abnormal chest x-ray, or elevated pulmonary artery wedge pressure. The treatment of left ventricular failure depends on the hemodynamic state of the patient. Those who are in shock require transfer to the intensive care unit, placement of a pulmonary artery line, monitoring of filling pressures, and immediate pre- and afterload reduction. Preload reduction is achieved by diuretics (and nitroglycerin if needed); afterload reduction, by administration of sodium nitroprusside. Dopamine is the best drug for inotropic support. Patients who are not in shock may, instead, be digitalized. Rapid digitalization (eg, divided intravenous doses of digoxin to a total of 1–1.5 mg over 24 hours, with careful monitoring of the serum potassium level), fluid restriction, and diuretics may be enough in these cases. Fluids should be restricted, and diuretics may be given. Respiratory insufficiency calls for ventilatory support with endotracheal intubation and a mechanical respirator. Although pulmonary function may improve with the use of positive end-expiratory pressure, hemodynamic derangements and decreased myocardial reserve preclude it in most cases.

Lette J et al: Postoperative myocardial infarction and cardiac death: Predictive value of dipyridamole-thallium imaging and five clinical scoring systems based on multifactorial analysis. Ann Surg 1990;211:84.

Mark DB et al: Prognostic value of a treadmill exercise score in outpatients with suspected coronary artery disease. N Engl J Med 1991;325:849.

Pedersen T, Eliasen K, Henriksen E: A prospective study of mortality associated with anaesthesia and surgery: Risk indicators of mortality in hospital. Acta Anaesthesiol Scand 1990;34:176.

Raby KE et al: Correlation between preoperative ischemia and major cardiac events after peripheral vascular surgery. N Engl J Med 1989;321:1296.

PERITONEAL COMPLICATIONS

Hemoperitoneum*

Bleeding is the most common cause of shock in the first 24 hours after abdominal surgery. Postoperative hemoperitoneum—a rapidly evolving, life-threatening complication—is usually the result of a technical problem with hemostasis, but coagulation disorders may play a role. For example, most of these patients have experienced substantial intraoperative blood loss, and several transfusions have already been given. As a consequence, changes usually observed after transfusion, such as thrombocytopenia, may be present. Other causes of coagulopathy such as mismatched transfusion, administration of heparin, etc, should also be ruled out. In these cases, bleeding tends to be more generalized, occurring in the wound, venipuncture sites, etc.

Hemoperitoneum usually becomes apparent within 24 hours after the operation. Its manifestations are those of hypovolemia: tachycardia, decreased blood pressure, decreased urine output, and peripheral vasoconstriction. If bleeding continues, abdominal girth may increase. Changes in the hematocrit are usually not obvious for 4–6 hours and are of limited diagnostic help in patients with rapid blood loss.

The manifestations may be so subtle that the diagnosis is overlooked. Only a high index of suspicion, frequent examination of patients at risk, and a systematic investigation of patients with postoperative hypotension will result in early recognition of the problem. Preexisting disease and drugs taken before surgery as well as those administered during the operation may cause hypotension. The differential diagnosis of immediate postoperative circulatory collapse also includes pulmonary embolism, cardiac dysrhythmias, pneumothorax, myocardial infarction, and severe allergic reactions. Infusions to expand the intravascular volume should be started as soon as other diseases have been ruled out. If hypotension or other signs of hypovolemia persist, one must reoperate promptly. At operation, bleeding should be stopped, clots evacuated, and the peritoneal cavity rinsed with saline solution.

Complications of Drains

Postoperative drainage of the peritoneal cavity is indicated to prevent fluid accumulation such as bile or pancreatic juice or to treat established abscesses. Drains may be left to evacuate small amounts of blood, but this process cannot be used to provide a reliable estimate of the rate of bleeding. The trend recently has been away from the use of drains in uncomplicated operations such as splenectomy and cholecystectomy. The use of drains in these settings increases the rate of postoperative intra-abdominal and wound infection. These problems can be minimized with the use of closed suction drains brought out of the abdomen through separate stab incisions. Latex Penrose drains, which were once popular, should be avoided because of the risk of introducing infection. Large rigid drains may erode into adjacent viscera or vessels and cause fistula formation or bleeding. This risk is lessened with the use of softer, Silastic drains which are removed as early as possible. Drains should not be left in contact with intestinal anastomoses, as they promote anastomotic leakage and fistula formation.

Flint LM: Early postoperative acute abdominal complications. Surg Clin North Am 1988;68:445.

Monson JR et al: Cholecystectomy is safer without drainage: The results of a prospective, randomized clinical trial. Surgery 1991;109:740.

Smulders YM et al: How soon should drainage tubes be removed after cardiac operations? Ann Thorac Surg 1989;48:540.

POSTOPERATIVE PAROTITIS

Postoperative parotitis—a rare but serious staphylococcal infection of the parotid gland—is limited almost entirely to elderly, debilitated, malnourished patients with poor oral hygiene. It appears in the second postoperative week and is associated with prolonged nasogastric intubation. The triggering factors are dehydration and poor oral hygiene, and the pathogenesis consists of a decrease in the secretory activity of the gland with inspissation of parotid secretions that become infected by staphylococci or gram-negative bacteria from the oral cavity. This results in inflammation, accumulation of cells that obstruct large and medium-sized ducts, and, eventually, formation of multiple small abscesses. These lobular abscesses, separated by fibrous bands, may dissect through the capsule and spread to the periglandular tissues to involve the auditory canal, the superficial skin, and the neck. If the disease is not treated at this stage, it may produce acute respiratory failure from tracheal obstruction.

Clinically, parotitis first appears as pain or tenderness at the angle of the jaw. With progression, high fever and leukocytosis develop, and there is swelling and redness in the parotid area. The parotid usually feels firm, and even after abscesses have formed, fluctuation is uncommon.

---

*Coagulation disorders are discussed in Chapter 5.

Prophylaxis includes adequate fluid intake, avoiding the use of anticholinergics, minimizing trauma during intubation, and, most importantly, good oral hygiene (frequent gargles, mouth irrigation, and other mouth cleansing and moistening measures). Stimulation of salivary flow with chewing gum, hard candy, etc, may also be useful. Routine observance of these simple preventive measures has virtually eliminated parotitis, which was once a common postoperative complication.

When signs of acute parotitis appear, fluid obtained from Stensen's duct by gentle compression of the gland should be cultured. Vancomycin should be started while the results of cultures are awaited. Warm moist packs and mouth irrigations may be helpful. In most instances, the disease responds promptly to these measures. If the disease progresses, the parotid must be surgically drained. The procedure consists of elevating a skin flap over the gland and making multiple small incisions parallel to the branches of the facial nerve. The wound is then packed open.

Matlow A et al: Parotitis due to anaerobic bacteria. Rev Infect Dis 1988;10:420.

COMPLICATIONS CAUSED BY POSTOPERATIVE ALTERATIONS OF GASTROINTESTINAL MOTILITY

The presence, strength, and direction of normal peristalsis is governed by the enteric nervous system. Anesthesia and surgical manipulation result in a decrease of the normal propulsive activity of the gut, or **postoperative ileus.** Several factors worsen ileus or prolong its course. These include medications—especially opioids—electrolyte abnormalities, inflammatory conditions such as pancreatitis or peritonitis, and pain.

Gastrointestinal peristalsis returns within 24 hours after most operations that do not involve the abdominal cavity. After laparotomy, gastric peristalsis returns in about 48 hours. Colonic activity returns after 48 hours, starting at the cecum and progressing caudally. The motility of the small intestine is affected to a lesser degree, except in patients who had small bowel resection or who were operated on to relieve bowel obstruction. Normal postoperative ileus leads to slight abdominal distention and absent bowel sounds. Return of peristalsis is often noted by the patient as mild cramps, passage of flatus, and return of appetite. Feedings should be withheld until there is evidence of return of normal gastrointestinal motility. Although there is no specific therapy for postoperative ileus, cisapride appears to shorten its duration, probably because of prokinetic effects on colonic motility (the principal component of postoperative ileus).

Gastric Dilatation

Gastric dilatation, a rare life-threatening complication, consists of massive distention of the stomach by gas and fluid. Predisposing factors include asthma, recent surgery, gastric outlet obstruction, and absence of the spleen. Infants and children in whom oxygen masks are used in the immediate postoperative period and adults subjected to forceful assisted respiration during resuscitation are also at risk. Occasionally, gastric dilatation develops in patients with anorexia nervosa or during serious illnesses without a specific intercurrent event.

As the air-filled stomach grows larger, it hangs down across the duodenum, producing a mechanical gastric outlet obstruction that contributes further to the problem. The increased intragastric pressure produces venous obstruction of the mucosa, causing mucosal engorgement and bleeding and, if allowed to continue, ischemic necrosis and perforation. The distended stomach pushes the diaphragm upward, which causes collapse of the lower lobe of the left lung, rotation of the heart, and obstruction of the inferior vena cava. The acutely dilated stomach is also prone to undergo volvulus.

The patient appears ill, with abdominal distention and hiccup. Hypochloremia, hypokalemia, and alkalosis may result from fluid and electrolyte losses. When recognized early, treatment consists of gastric decompression with a nasogastric tube. In the late stage, gastric necrosis may require gastrectomy.

Bowel Obstruction

Failure of postoperative return of bowel function may be the result of paralytic ileus or mechanical obstruction. Mechanical obstruction is most often caused by postoperative adhesions or an internal (mesenteric) hernia. Most of these patients experience a short period of apparently normal intestinal function before manifestations of obstruction supervene. About half of cases of early postoperative small bowel obstruction follow colorectal surgery, probably owing to the more extensive peritoneal stripping involved.

Diagnosis may be difficult, because the symptoms are difficult to differentiate from those of paralytic ileus. If plain films of the abdomen show air-fluid levels in loops of small bowel, mechanical obstruction is a more likely diagnosis than ileus. Enteroclysis or an ordinary small bowel series with barium sulfate may aid diagnosis.

Strangulation is uncommon, because the adhesive bands are broader and less rigid than in the average case of late small bowel obstruction. The death rate is high (about 15%), however, probably because of delay in diagnosis and the postoperative state. Treatment consists of nasogastric suction for several days and, if the obstruction does not resolve spontaneously, laparotomy.

Small bowel intussusception is an uncommon

cause of early postoperative obstruction in adults but accounts for 10% of cases in the pediatric age group. Ninety percent of postoperative intussusceptions occur during the first 2 postoperative weeks, and more than half are in the first week. Unlike idiopathic ileocolic intussusception, most postoperative intus-susceptions are ileoileal or jejunojejunal. They most often follow retroperitoneal and pelvic operations. The cause is unknown. The symptom complex is not typical, and x-ray studies are of limited help. The physician should be aware that intussusception is a possible explanation for vomiting, distention, and ab-dominal pain after laparotomy in children and that early reoperation will avoid the complications of per-foration and peritonitis. Surgery is the only treatment, and provided the bowel is viable, reduction of the in-tussusception is all that is needed.

Postoperative Fecal Impaction

Fecal impaction after operative procedures is the result of colonic ileus and impaired perception of rec-tal fullness. It is principally a disease of the elderly but may occur in younger patients who have predis-posing conditions such as megacolon or paraplegia. Postoperative ileus and the use of opioid analgesics and anticholinergic drugs are aggravating factors. Early manifestations are anorexia and obstipation or diarrhea. In advanced cases, marked distention may cause colonic perforation. The diagnosis of postoper-ative fecal impaction is made by rectal examination. The impaction should be manually removed, enemas given, and digital examination then repeated.

Barium remaining in the colon from an examina-tion done before surgery may harden and produce **barium impaction.** This usually occurs in the right colon, where most of the water is absorbed, and is a more difficult management problem than fecal im-paction. The clinical manifestations are those of bowel obstruction. Treatment includes enemas and purgation with polyethylene glycol-electrolyte solu-tion (eg, CoLyte, GoLYTELY). Diatrizoate sodium (Hypaque), a hyperosmolar solution that stimulates peristalsis and increases intraluminal fluid, may be effective by enema if other solutions fail. Surgery is rarely needed.

Dehn TC, Nolan DJ: Enteroclysis in the diagnosis of intes-tinal obstruction in the early postoperative period. Gas-trointest Radiol 1989;14:15.

Fabri PJ, Rosemurgy A: Reoperation for small intestinal ob-struction. Surg Clin North Am 1991;71:131.

Livingston EH, Passaro EP Jr: Postoperative ileus. Dig Dis Sci 1990;35:121.

Menzies D, Ellis H: Intestinal obstruction from adhesions: How big is the problem? Ann R Coll Surg Engl 1990;72:60.

Wattwil M et al: Epidural analgesia with bupivacaine re-duces postoperative paralytic ileus after hysterectomy. Anesth Analg 1989;68:353.

West KW et al: Postoperative intussusception: Experience with 36 cases in children. Surgery 1988;104:781.

POSTOPERATIVE PANCREATITIS

Postoperative pancreatitis accounts for 10% of all cases of acute pancreatitis. It occurs in 1–3% of pa-tients who have operations in the vicinity of the pan-creas, and with higher frequency after operations on the biliary tract. For example, pancreatitis occurs in about 1% of patients undergoing cholecystectomy and in 8% of patients undergoing common bile duct exploration. In the latter cases, it does not appear re-lated to the performance of intraoperative cholangio-grams or choledochoscopy. Postoperative pancreati-tis after biliary surgery is worse in patients who have had biliary pancreatitis preoperatively. Pancreatitis is occasionally observed following cardiopulmonary bypass, parathyroid surgery, and renal transplanta-tion. Postoperative pancreatitis is frequently of the necrotizing type. Infected pancreatic necrosis and other complications of pancreatitis develop with a frequency three to four times greater than in biliary and alcoholic pancreatitis. The reason postoperative pancreatitis is so severe is unknown, but the mortality rate is 30–40%.

The pathogenesis in most cases appears to be me-chanical trauma to the pancreas or its blood supply. Nevertheless, manipulation, biopsy, and partial re-section of the pancreas are usually well tolerated, so why some patients develop pancreatitis is unclear. Prevention of this complication includes careful han-dling of the pancreas and avoidance of forceful dila-tion of the choledochal sphincter or obstruction of the pancreatic duct. The 2% incidence of pancreatitis fol-lowing renal transplantation is probably related to special risk factors such as use of corticosteroids or azathioprine, secondary hyperparathyroidism, or viral infection. Acute changes in serum calcium are thought to be responsible for pancreatitis following parathyroid surgery. Hyperamylasemia develops in about half of patients undergoing heart surgery with extracorporeal bypass, but clinical evidence of pan-creatitis is present in only 5% of these patients.

The diagnosis of postoperative pancreatitis may be difficult in patients who have recently had an abdom-inal operation. Hyperamylasemia may or may not be present. One must be alert to renal and respiratory complications and the consequences of necrotizing or hemorrhagic pancreatitis. Because of the high fre-quency with which complications develop, frequent monitoring of the pancreas and retroperitoneum with CT scans is useful.

See Chapter 27 for diagnosis and treatment of acute pancreatitis.

Fernandez del Castillo C et al: Risk factors for pancreatic cellular injury after cardiopulmonary bypass. N Engl J Med 1991;325:382.

Watson CJ et al: Early abdominal complications following heart and heart-lung transplantation. Br J Surg 1991;78:699.

POSTOPERATIVE HEPATIC DYSFUNCTION

Hepatic dysfunction, ranging from mild jaundice to life-threatening hepatic failure, follows 1% of surgical procedures performed under general anesthesia. The incidence is greater following pancreatectomy, biliary bypass operations, and portacaval shunt. Postoperative hyperbilirubinemia may be categorized as prehepatic jaundice, hepatocellular insufficiency, and posthepatic obstruction (Table 4–1).

Prehepatic Jaundice

Prehepatic jaundice is caused by bilirubin overload, most often from hemolysis or reabsorption of hematomas. Fasting, malnutrition, hepatotoxic drugs, and anesthesia are among the factors that impair the ability of the liver to excrete increased loads of bilirubin in the postoperative period.

Increased hemolysis may result from transfusion of incompatible blood but more often reflects destruction of fragile transfused red blood cells. Other causes include extracorporeal circulation, congenital hemolytic disease (eg, sickle cell disease), and effects of drugs.

Hepatocellular Insufficiency

Hepatocellular insufficiency, the most common cause of postoperative jaundice, occurs as a consequence of hepatic cell necrosis, inflammation, or massive hepatic resection. Drugs, hypotension, hypoxia, and sepsis are among the injurious factors. Although posttransfusion hepatitis is usually observed much later, this complication may occur as early as the third postoperative week.

Table 4–1. Causes of postoperative jaundice.

I. Prehepatic jaundice (bilirubin overload)
  Hemolysis (drugs, transfusions, sickle cell crisis)
  Reabsorption of hematomas
II. Hepatocellular insufficiency
  Viral hepatitis
  Drug-induced (anesthesia, others)
  Ischemia (shock, hypoxemia, low-output states)
  Sepsis
  Liver resection (loss of parenchyma)
  Others (total parenteral nutrition, malnutrition)
III. Posthepatic obstruction (to bile flow)
  Retained stones
  Injury to ducts
  Tumor (unrecognized or untreated)
  Cholecystitis
  Pancreatitis

Benign postoperative intrahepatic cholestasis is a vague term used to denote jaundice following operations that often involve hypotension and multiple transfusions. Serum bilirubin ranges from 2 to 20 mg/dL and serum alkaline phosphatase is usually high, but the patient is afebrile and postoperative convalescence is otherwise smooth. The diagnosis is one of exclusion. Jaundice clears by the third postoperative week.

Hepatocellular damage is occasionally seen after intestinal bypass procedures for morbid obesity. Cholestatic jaundice may develop in patients receiving total parenteral nutrition.

Posthepatic Obstruction

Posthepatic obstruction can be caused by direct surgical injury to the bile ducts, retained common duct stones, tumor obstruction of the bile duct, or pancreatitis. Acute postoperative cholecystitis is associated with jaundice in one-third of cases, though mechanical obstruction of the common duct is usually not apparent.

One must determine if a patient with postoperative jaundice has a correctable cause that requires treatment. This is particularly true for sepsis (where decreased liver function may sometimes be an early sign), lesions that obstruct the bile duct, and postoperative cholecystitis. Liver function tests are not helpful in determining the cause and do not usually reflect the severity of disease. Liver biopsy, ultrasound and CT scans, and transhepatic or endoscopic retrograde cholangiograms are the tests most likely to sort out the diagnostic possibilities. Renal function must be monitored closely, since renal failure may develop in these patients. Treatment is otherwise expectant.

Ray DC, Drummond GB: Halothane hepatitis. Br J Anaesth 1991;67:84.

Read AE et al: Hepatitis C in patients undergoing liver transplantation. Ann Intern Med 1991;114:282.

POSTOPERATIVE CHOLECYSTITIS

Acute postoperative cholecystitis may follow any kind of operation but is more common after gastrointestinal procedures. Acute cholecystitis develops shortly after endoscopic sphincterotomy in 3–5% of patients. Chemical cholecystitis has been observed in patients undergoing hepatic arterial chemotherapy with mitomycin and floxuridine with such frequency that cholecystectomy should always be performed before infusion of these agents is begun. Fulminant cholecystitis with gallbladder infarction may follow percutaneous embolization of the hepatic artery for malignant tumors of the liver or for arteriovenous malformation involving this artery.

Postoperative cholecystitis differs in several respects from the common form of acute cholecystitis:

It is frequently acalculous (70–80%), more common in males (75%), progresses rapidly to gallbladder necrosis, and is not likely to respond to conservative therapy. The cause is clear in cases of chemical or ischemic cholecystitis but not in other forms. Factors thought to play a role include biliary stasis (with formation of sludge), biliary infection, and ischemia. Diagnosis and treatment are discussed in Chapter 26.

Inoue T, Mishima Y: Postoperative acute cholecystitis: A collective review of 494 cases in Japan. Jap J Surg 1988;18:35.

Ziv Y et al: Acute cholecystitis complicating unrelated disease: Etiological considerations. Am J Gastroenterol 1987;82:1165.

CLOSTRIDIUM DIFFICILE COLITIS

Postoperative diarrhea due to *Clostridium difficile* is a common nosocomial infection in surgical patients. The spectrum of illness ranges from asymptomatic colonization to—rarely—severe toxic colitis. Transmission from hospital personnel probably occurs. The main risk factor is perioperative antibiotic use. The diagnosis is established by identification of a specific cytopathic toxin in the stool or culture of the organism from stool samples or rectal swabs. In severely affected patients, colonoscopy reveals **pseudomembranes.** Prevention is accomplished by strict handwashing, enteric precautions, and minimizing antibiotic use. Treatment of established infection is with oral vancomycin or metronidazole.

Johnson S et al: Nosocomial *Clostridium difficile* colonisation and disease. Lancet 1990;336:97.

McFarland LV et al: Nosocomial acquisition of *Clostridium difficile* infection. N Engl J Med 1989;320:204.

Yee J et al: *Clostridium difficile* disease in a department of surgery. The significance of prophylactic antibiotics. Arch Surg 1991;126:241.

URINARY COMPLICATIONS*

Postoperative Urinary Retention

Inability to void postoperatively is common, especially after pelvic and perineal operations or operations under spinal anesthesia. Factors responsible for postoperative urinary retention are interference with the neural mechanisms responsible for normal emptying of the bladder and overdistention of the urinary bladder. When its normal capacity of approximately 500 mL is exceeded, bladder contraction is inhibited. Prophylactic bladder catheterization should be performed whenever an operation is likely to last 3 hours or longer or when large volumes of intravenous fluids

are anticipated. The catheter can be removed at the end of the operation if the patient is expected to be able to ambulate within a few hours. When bladder catheterization is not performed, the patient should be encouraged to void immediately before coming to the operating room and as soon as possible after the operation. During abdominoperineal resection, operative trauma to the sacral plexus alters bladder function enough so that an indwelling catheter should be left in place for 4–5 days. Patients with inguinal hernia who strain to void as a manifestation of prostatic hypertrophy should have the prostate treated before the hernia.

The treatment of acute urinary retention is catheterization of the bladder. In the absence of factors that suggest the need for prolonged decompression, such as the presence of 1000 mL of urine or more, the catheter may be removed.

Urinary Tract Infection

Infection of the lower urinary tract is the most frequently acquired nosocomial infection. Preexisting contamination of the urinary tract, urinary retention, and instrumentation are the principal contributing factors. Bacteriuria is present in about 5% of patients who undergo short-term (< 48 hours) bladder catheterization, though clinical signs of urinary tract infection occur in only 1%. Cystitis is manifested by dysuria and mild fever and pyelonephritis by high fever, flank tenderness, and, occasionally, ileus. Diagnosis is made by examination of the urine and confirmed by cultures. Prevention involves treating urinary tract contamination before surgery, prevention or prompt treatment of urinary retention, and careful instrumentation when needed. Treatment includes adequate hydration, proper drainage of the bladder, and specific antibiotics.

Anderson JB, Grant JB: Postoperative retention of urine: A prospective urodynamic study. Br Med J 1991;302:894.

Meares EM Jr: Current patterns in nosocomial urinary tract infections. Urology 1991;37(3 Suppl):9.

Petros JG et al: Factors influencing postoperative urinary retention in patients undergoing elective inguinal herniorrhaphy. Am J Surg 1991; 161:431.

CEREBRAL COMPLICATIONS

Postoperative Cerebrovascular Accidents

Postoperative cerebrovascular accidents are almost always the result of ischemic neural damage due to poor perfusion. They often occur in elderly patients with severe atherosclerosis who become hypotensive during or after surgery (from sepsis, bleeding, cardiac arrest, etc). Normal regulatory mechanisms of the cerebral vasculature can maintain blood flow over a wide range of blood pressures down to a mean pressure of about 55 mm Hg. Abrupt hypotension, how-

---

*Postoperative renal failure is described in Chapter 5.

ever, is less well tolerated than a more gradual pressure change. Irreversible brain damage occurs after about 4 minutes of total ischemia.

Strokes occur in 1–3% of patients after carotid endarterectomy and other reconstructive operations of the extracranial portion of the carotid system. Embolization from atherosclerotic plaques, ischemia during carotid clamping, and postoperative thrombosis at the site of the arteriotomy or of an intimal flap are usually responsible. Aspirin, which inhibits platelet aggregation, may prevent immediate postoperative thrombosis.

Open heart surgery using extracorporeal circulation or deep cooling is also occasionally followed by stroke. The pathogenesis of stroke is thought to be related to hypoxemia, emboli, or poor perfusion. The presence of a carotid bruit preoperatively increases the risk of postoperative stroke after coronary bypass by a factor of 4. Previous stroke or transient ischemic attacks and postoperative atrial fibrillation also increase the risk. For patients undergoing noncardiac, noncarotid surgery, the risk of stroke has been estimated at 0.2%. Predictors of risk in these patients are the presence of cerebrovascular, cardiac, or peripheral vascular disease and arterial hypertension.

Convulsions

Epilepsy, metabolic derangements, and medications may lead to convulsions in the postoperative period. For unknown reasons, patients with ulcerative colitis and Crohn's disease are peculiarly susceptible to convulsions with loss of consciousness after surgery. Convulsions should be treated as soon as possible to minimize their harmful effects.

Archie JP: The relationship of early hypertension following carotid endarterectomy to intraoperative cerebral ischemia. Ann Vasc Surg 1988;2:108.

Landercasper J et al: Perioperative stroke risk in 173 consecutive patients with a past history of stroke. Arch Surg 1990;125:986.

Michenfelder JD, Cucchiara RF, Sundt TM Jr: Influence of intraoperative antibiotic choice on the incidence of early post-craniotomy seizures. J Neurosurg 1990;72:703.

Reed GL III et al: Stroke following coronary-artery bypass surgery: A case control estimate of the risk from carotid bruits. N Engl J Med 1988;319:1246.

PSYCHIATRIC COMPLICATIONS

Anxiety and fear are normal in patients undergoing surgery. The degree to which these emotions are experienced depends upon diverse cultural and psychologic variables. Underlying depression or a history of chronic pain may serve to exaggerate the patient's response to surgery. The boundary between the normal manifestations of stress and **postoperative psychosis** is difficult to establish, since the latter is not really a distinct clinical entity.

Postoperative psychosis develops in about 0.5% of patients having abdominal operations. It is more common after thoracic surgery, in the elderly, and in those with chronic disease. About half of these patients suffer from mood disturbances (usually severe depression). Twenty percent have delirium. Drugs given in the postoperative period may play a role in the development of psychosis; meperidine, cimetidine, and corticosteroids are most commonly implicated. Patients who develop postoperative psychosis have higher plasma levels of β-endorphin and cortisol than those who do not. These patients also lose, temporarily, the normal circadian rhythms of β-endorphin and cortisol. Specific psychiatric syndromes may follow specific procedures, such as visual hallucinations and the "black patch syndrome" after ophthalmic surgery. Preexisting psychiatric disorders not apparent before the operation sometimes contribute to the motivation for surgery (eg, circumcision or cosmetic operations in schizophrenics).

Clinical manifestations are rare on the first postoperative day. During this period, patient appear emotionless and unconcerned about changes in the environment or in themselves. Most overt psychiatric derangements are observed after the third postoperative day. The symptoms are variable but often include confusion, fear, and disorientation as to time and place. Delirium presents as altered consciousness with cognitive impairment. These symptoms may not be readily apparent to the surgeon, as this problem is usually seen in sick patients whose other problems may mask the manifestations of psychosis. Early psychiatric consultation should be obtained when psychosis is suspected so that adequate and prompt assessment of consciousness and cognitive function can be done and treatment instituted. The earlier the psychosis is recognized, the easier it is to correct. Metabolic derangements or early sepsis (especially in burned patients) must be ruled out as the cause. Severe postoperative emotional disturbances may be avoided by appropriate preoperative counseling of the patient by the surgeon. This includes a thorough discussion of the operation and the expected outcome, acquainting the patient with the intensive care unit, etc. Postoperatively, the surgeon must attend to the patient's emotional needs, offering frequent reassurance, explaining the postoperative course, and discussing the prognosis and the outcome of the operation.

Special Psychiatric Problems

A. The ICU Syndrome: The continuous internal vigilance that results from pain and fear and the sleep deprivation from bright lights, monitoring equipment, and continuous noise causes a psychologic disorganization known as ICU psychosis. The patient whose level of consciousness is already decreased by illness and drugs is more susceptible than a normal individual, and the result is decreased ability to think, perceive, and remember. When the cognitive processes are thoroughly disorganized, delirium occurs. The manifestations include distorted visual, auditory, and tactile perception; confusion; restlessness; and inability to differentiate reality from fantasy. Prevention includes isolation from the environment, decreased noise levels, adequate sleep, and removal from the intensive care unit as soon as possible.

B. Postcardiotomy Delirium: Mental changes that occasionally follow open heart surgery include impairment of memory, attention, cognition, and perception and occasionally hysteria, depressive reaction, and anxiety crisis. The symptoms most often appear after the third postoperative day. The type of operation, the presence of organic brain disease, prolonged medical illness, and the length of time on extracorporeal circulation are related to the development of postcardiotomy psychosis. Mild sedation and measures to prevent the ICU syndrome may prevent this complication. In more severe cases, haloperidol (Haldol) in doses of 1–5 mg given orally, intramuscularly, or intravenously may be required. Haloperidol is preferred over phenothiazines in these patients because it is associated with a lower incidence of cardiovascular side effects.

C. Delirium Tremens: Delirium tremens occurs in alcoholics who stop drinking suddenly. Hyperventilation and metabolic alkalosis contribute to the development of the full-blown syndrome. Hypomagnesemia and hypokalemia secondary to alkalosis or nutritional deficits may precipitate seizures. Readaptation to ethanol-free metabolism requires about 2 weeks, and it is during this period that alcoholics are at greatest risk of developing delirium tremens.

The prodrome includes personality changes, anxiety, and tremor. The complete syndrome is characterized by agitation, hallucinations, restlessness, confusion, overactivity, and, occasionally, seizures and hyperthermia. The syndrome also causes a hyperdynamic cardiorespiratory and metabolic state. For example, cardiac index, oxygen delivery, and oxygen consumption double during delirium tremens and return to normal 24–48 hours after resolution. The wild behavior may precipitate dehiscence of a fresh laparotomy incision. Diaphoresis and dehydration are common, and exhaustion may herald death.

Withdrawal symptoms may be prevented by giving small amounts of alcohol, but benzodiazepines are the treatment of choice. Vitamin B_1 (thiamine) and magnesium sulfate should also be given.

The aims of treatment are to reduce agitation and anxiety as soon as possible and to prevent the development of other complications (eg, seizures, aspiration pneumonia). General measures should include frequent assessment of vital signs, restoration of nutrition, administration of vitamin B, correction of electrolyte imbalance or other metabolic derangements, and adequate hydration. Physical restraint, although necessary for seriously violent behavior,

should be as limited as possible. With proper care, most patients improve within 72 hours.

D. Sexual Dysfunction: Sexual problems commonly occur after certain kinds of operations, such as prostatectomy, heart surgery, and aortic reconstruction. The pathogenesis is unclear. In abdominoperineal resection, severance of the peripheral branches of the sacral plexus may cause impotence. It is important to discuss this possibility with the patient before any operation with a risk of impotence is performed. When sexual dysfunction is psychogenic, reassurance is usually all that is needed. If psychogenic impotence persists beyond 4–6 weeks, psychiatric consultation is indicated.

Craven JL: Cyclosporine-associated organic mental disorders in liver transplant recipients. Psychosomatics 1991;32:94.

Cryns AG, Gorey KM, Goldstein MZ: Effects of surgery on the mental status of older persons: A meta-analytic review. J Geriatr Psychiatry Neurol 1990;3:184.

Romach MK, Sellers EM: Management of the alcohol withdrawal syndrome. Annu Rev Med 1991;42:323.

Smith LW, Dimsdale JE: Postcardiotomy delirium: Conclusions after 25 years? Am J Psychiatry 1989;146:452.

COMPLICATIONS OF INTRAVENOUS THERAPY & HEMODYNAMIC MONITORING

Air Embolism

Air embolism may occur during or after insertion of a venous catheter or as a result of accidental introduction of air into the line. Embolized air lodges in the right atrium, preventing adequate filling of the right heart. This is manifested by hypotension, jugular venous distention, and tachycardia. This complication can be avoided by placing the patient in the Trendelenburg position when a central venous line is inserted. Emergency treatment consists of aspiration of the air with a syringe. If this is unsuccessful, the patient should be positioned right side up and head down, which will help dislodge the air from the right atrium and return circulatory dynamics to normal.

Phlebitis

A needle or a catheter inserted into a vein and left in place will in time cause inflammation at the entry site. When this process involves the vein, it is called phlebitis. Factors determining the degree of inflammation are the nature of the cannula, the solution infused, bacterial infection, and venous thrombosis. Phlebitis is one of the most common causes of fever after the third postoperative day. The symptomatic triad of induration, edema, and tenderness is characteristic. Visible signs may be minimal. Prevention of phlebitis is best accomplished by observance of aseptic techniques during insertion of venous catheters, frequent change of tubing (ie, every 48–72 hours), and rotation of insertion sites (ie, every 4 days). Silastic catheters, which are the least reactive, should be used when the line must be left in for a long time. Hypertonic solutions should be infused only into veins with substantial flow, such as the subclavian, jugular, or vena cava. Venous catheters should be removed at the first sign of redness, induration, or edema. Because phlebitis is most frequent with cannulation of veins in the lower extremities, this route should be used only when upper extremity veins are unavailable. Removal of the catheter is adequate treatment.

Suppurative phlebitis may result from the presence of an infected thrombus around the indwelling catheter. Staphylococci are the most common causative organisms. Local signs of inflammation are present, and pus may be expressed from the venipuncture site. High fever and positive blood cultures are common. Treatment consists of excising the affected vein, extending the incision proximally to the first open collateral, and leaving the wound open.

Cardiopulmonary Complications

Perforation of the right atrium with cardiac tamponade has been associated with the use of central venous lines. This complication can be avoided by checking the position of the tip of the line, which should be in the superior vena cava, not the right atrium. Complications associated with the use of the flow-directed balloon-tipped (Swan-Ganz) catheter include cardiac perforation (usually of the right atrium), intracardiac knotting of the catheter, and cardiac dysrhythmias. Pulmonary hemorrhage may result from disruption of a branch of the pulmonary artery during balloon inflation and may be fatal in patients with pulmonary hypertension. Steps in prevention include careful placement, advancement under continuous pressure monitoring, and checking the position of the tip before inflating the balloon.

Ischemic Necrosis of the Finger

Continuous monitoring of arterial blood pressure during the operation and in the intensive care unit requires insertion of a radial or femoral arterial line. The hand receives its blood supply from the radial and ulnar arteries, and because of the anatomy of the palmar arches, patency of one of these vessels is usually enough to provide adequate blood flow through the hand. Occasionally, ischemic necrosis of the finger has followed use of an indwelling catheter in the radial artery. This serious complication can usually be avoided by evaluating the patency of the ulnar artery (Allen's test) before establishing the radial line and by changing arterial line sites every 3–4 days. After an arterial catheter is withdrawn, a pressure dressing should be applied to avoid formation of an arterial pseudoaneurysm.

Corona ML et al: Infections related to central venous catheters. Mayo Clin Proc 1990;65:979.

Hammond JS, Varas R, Ward CG: Suppurative thrombophlebitis: A new look at a continuing problem. South Med J 1988;81:969.

Purdue GF, Hunt JL: Placement and complications of monitoring catheters. Surg Clin North Am 1991;71:723.

Sladen A: Complications of invasive hemodynamic monitoring in the intensive care unit. Curr Probl Surg (Feb) 1988;25:69.

Swan HJ: The pulmonary artery catheter. Dis Mon (Aug) 1991;37:473.

POSTOPERATIVE FEVER

Fever occurs in about 40% of patients after major surgery. In most patients the temperature elevation resolves without specific treatment. However, postoperative fever may herald a serious infection, and it is therefore important to evaluate the patient clinically. Features often associated with an infectious origin of the fever include preoperative trauma, ASA class above 2, fever onset after the second postoperative day, an initial temperature elevation above 38.6 °C (101.5 °F), a postoperative white blood cell count greater than 10,000/μL, and a postoperative serum urea nitrogen of 15 mg/dL or greater. If three or more of the above are present, the likelihood of associated bacterial infection is nearly 100%.

Fever within 48 hours after surgery is usually caused by atelectasis. Reexpansion of the lung causes body temperature to return to normal. Because laboratory and radiologic investigations are usually unrevealing, an extensive evaluation of early postoperative fever is rarely appropriate if the patient's convalescence is otherwise smooth.

When fever appears after the second postoperative day, atelectasis is a less likely explanation. The differential diagnosis of fever at this time includes catheter-related phlebitis, pneumonia, and urinary tract infection. A directed history and physical examination complemented by focused laboratory and radiologic studies usually determine the cause.

Patients without infection are rarely febrile after the fifth postoperative day. Fever this late suggests wound infection or, less often, anastomotic breakdown and intra-abdominal abscesses. A diagnostic workup directed to the detection of intra-abdominal sepsis is indicated in patients who have high temperatures (> 39 °C [102.2 °F]) and wounds without evidence of infection 5 or more days postoperatively. CT scan of the abdomen and pelvis is the test of choice and should be performed early, before overt organ failure occurs.

Fever is rare after the first week in patients who had a normal convalescence. Allergy to drugs, transfusion-related fever, septic pelvic vein thrombosis, and intra-abdominal abscesses should be considered.

Freischlag J, Busuttil RW: The value of postoperative fever evaluation. Surgery 1983;94:358.

Mellors JWW et al: A simple index to estimate the likelihood of bacterial infection in patients developing fever after abdominal surgery. Am Surg 1988;54:558.

Theuer CP, Bongard FS, Klein SR: Are blood cultures effective in the evaluation of fever in perioperative patients? Am J Surg 1991;162:615.

REFERENCES

Entrup MH, Davis FG: Perioperative complications of anesthesia. Surg Clin N Amer 1991;71:1151.

Keats AS: Anesthesia mortality in perspective. Anesth Analg 1990;71:113.

Meguid MM et al: Complications of abdominal operations for malignant disease. Am J Surg 1988;156:341.

Velanovich V: The value of routine preoperative laboratory testing in predicting post-operative complications: A multivariate analysis. Surgery 1991;109:236.

Special Medical Problems in Surgical Patients

ENDOCRINE DISEASE & THE SURGICAL PATIENT

Marvin D. Siperstein, MD

DIABETES MELLITUS

Diabetic patients no doubt undergo more surgical procedures than do nondiabetics, and the management of the diabetic patient before, during, and after surgery is an important responsibility. Fortunately, because of the close control of fluids, electrolytes, glucose, and insulin that is now possible in the operating room, control of blood glucose levels during the perioperative period is usually relatively simple. Attempts must be made to avoid marked hyperglycemia during surgery; the greater danger, however, is from severe unrecognized hypoglycemia.

Preoperative Workup

Blood glucose concentrations tend to be elevated in diabetic patients during the preoperative period. Physical trauma, if present, combined with the emotional and physiologic stress of the illness may cause epinephrine and cortisol levels to rise, in each case resulting in increased blood glucose levels. If exogenous cortisol is being administered (eg, to a renal or pancreatic transplant recipient), marked insulin resistance and elevations of blood glucose levels regularly result. Infections may also increase blood glucose concentrations, occasionally to dangerous levels. Inactivity in bedridden patients can increase blood glucose levels by causing insulin resistance. Hypokalemia—frequently the result of diuretic therapy but also of epinephrine release induced by trauma—may prevent B cells from secreting adequate amounts of insulin and may thereby raise blood glucose levels in patients with non-insulin-dependent diabetes.

The preoperative workup of patients with diabetes mellitus should include a thorough physical examination, with special care taken to discover occult infections; an ECG to rule out myocardial infarction; and a chest x-ray to identify hidden pneumonia or pulmonary edema. A complete urinalysis should be done to rule out urinary tract infection and proteinuria, the earliest sign of diabetic renal disease. Serum potassium levels should be measured to check for hypokalemia or hyperkalemia, the latter usually resulting from hyporeninemic hypoaldosteronism, a relatively common syndrome in diabetics. Serum creatinine levels should be measured to assess renal function. The serum glucose concentration should ideally be between 100 and 200 mg/dL, but surgery is safe when it is as high as 350–400 mg/dL preoperatively.

Preoperative & Intraoperative Management of Diabetic Patients

A. Non-Insulin-Dependent (Type 2) Diabetes Mellitus: Approximately 85% of diabetics over age 50 years have only a moderately decreased ability to produce and secrete insulin, and when at home they can usually be controlled by diet or by sulfonylureas. If the serum glucose level is below 250 mg/dL on the morning of surgery, sulfonylureas should be withheld; long-acting sulfonylurea drugs—glipizide, glyburide, and chlorpropamide—should be discontinued on the day before surgery; and 5% glucose solution should be administered intravenously at a rate of about 100 mL/h. This means that over a 10-hour period, only 50 g of glucose would be given; by contrast, during an average day, a diabetic on a normal diet would consume 4–5 times as much carbohydrate (ie, 200–250 g). During any but the most extensive surgery, the pancreas should be able to produce enough insulin to handle this modest glucose load and at the same time prevent undue gluconeogenesis.

If the fasting glucose level is above 250–300 mg/dL or if the patient is taking small doses of insulin but does not actually require insulin to prevent ketoacidosis, an alternative approach would be to add 5 units of insulin directly to each liter of 5% glucose solution being given at 100 mL/h. If the operation is lengthy, blood glucose levels should be measured every 3–4 hours during surgery to ensure adequate glucose control. The goal is to maintain glucose levels between 100 and 200 mg/dL, but there is little harm in allowing them to go as high as 250 mg/dL.

B. Insulin-Dependent (Type 1) Diabetes Mellitus: These patients require insulin during surgery. It can be administered by any of the following methods: (1) subcutaneous administration of long-acting insulin; (2) constant infusion of a mixture of glucose and insulin; or (3) separate infusions of glucose and insulin. Intravenous boluses of regular insulin are rarely, if ever, indicated. The effect of single boluses of insulin given intravenously typically lasts only minutes, leading to the danger of acute hypoglycemia followed shortly by recurrent hyperglycemia. With each technique, blood glucose levels should be monitored at least every 2 hours during the procedure to avoid hypoglycemia below 60 mg/dL and hyperglycemia above 250 mg/dL. Blood glucose levels can be measured rapidly during surgery with the small portable electronic glucose analyzers now available.

1. Conventional procedure for insulin administration—The first and still most widely used method of controlling blood glucose levels during surgery is to administer subcutaneously, on the morning of the operation, one-third to one-half the patient's usual dose of long-acting insulin plus one-third to one-half the usual dose of short-acting insulin. This is followed by intravenous infusion of 5% or even 10% glucose at a rate of 100 mL/h preoperatively and intraoperatively. If the operation is prolonged, potassium chloride should be added at a rate of 20 meq/h.

There are a number of disadvantages to this procedure, which results in giving the full day's insulin requirement preoperatively. First, after subcutaneous administration, the absorption of NPH and regular insulin varies greatly in individual patients, especially when they are inactive. Second, although surgeons are aware that operations on diabetics should be scheduled early in the day, all too often the procedure must be delayed until afternoon. The relatively small amounts of glucose being administered are then inadequate to compensate for the 18–20 hours the patient has been without food, with the result that the insulin causes severe afternoon hypoglycemia. In the average diabetic, the peak action of regular insulin occurs about 6 hours after its administration—not 1–2 hours afterward, as stated in older textbooks. Therefore, if regular insulin is given subcutaneously at 7 AM, its peak action in an average patient will occur at about 1 PM. As a result, following subcutaneous administration of regular insulin in the early morning, the patient's glucose concentration may be inadequately controlled early in the morning; and if surgery is delayed, the peak action of regular insulin in the early afternoon and of NPH insulin in the later afternoon may result in severe hypoglycemia. If surgery must be delayed, it is imperative that blood glucose levels be carefully monitored for hypoglycemia and additional glucose given as necessary.

2. Intravenous infusion of insulin in glucose solution—There is an increasing tendency to treat type 1 diabetics undergoing surgery by giving an infusion of 5% or 10% glucose solution containing 5, 10, or even 15 units of insulin per liter, depending on the patient's initial blood glucose concentration. At an infusion rate of 100 mL/h, insulin is thereby administered at a rate of 0.5, 1, or 1.5 units/h, respectively. In patients receiving corticosteroids, as much as 20 units per liter of insulin may be required.

There are a number of advantages to this regimen. First, the problem of absorption of insulin is avoided, since it is given intravenously. As a result, instead of an average 6-hour lag for maximal response to regular insulin, the effect starts within 10–15 minutes and is relatively constant. Second, unlike the fixed insulin dose with subcutaneous administration, the insulin infusion can be changed at any time in response to changes in blood glucose levels. Third, the dangers of hypo- and hyperglycemia are minimized, because if the intravenous solution is stopped (if the needle is inadvertently removed or the tubing clamped), both the glucose and the insulin are discontinued simultaneously. Since only 10% of insulin adsorbs to glass or plastic, the resulting reduction in dosage is of little therapeutic importance. A similar continuous intravenous infusion of insulin has also become the most common way to treat diabetic ketoacidosis.

3. Use of insulin "piggy-backed" into the glucose infusion—Instead of mixing insulin in the same bottle as the glucose, an insulin solution is infused ("piggy-backed") into the tubing delivering the 5% or 10% glucose. Generally, 50 units of regular insulin are mixed with 500 mL of normal saline—a solution containing 1 unit of insulin per 10 mL of solution. The glucose solution is given at a rate of 100 mL/h, and the insulin infusion is adjusted (usually by IVAC pump) to deliver a total of 5 mL (0.5 units), 10 mL (1 unit), 30 mL (30 units) per hour, etc, depending on the results of blood glucose determinations obtained approximately hourly during the surgical procedure. Of the three techniques, this one is the most flexible, allows the closest control of blood glucose levels, and is therefore increasingly being recommended as the method of choice. It requires careful monitoring of the pump delivery rate, because too rapid infusion of insulin will cause hypoglycemia. A number of simple algorithms have been recommended for adjusting the rate of insulin infusion according to the previous plasma glucose levels. This approach is especially useful during prolonged operations. The simplest and most practical is to give no insulin if plasma glucose is less than 90 mg/dL. Above values of 90 mg/dL, the dosage of regular insulin in units per hour should equal 1% of the previous hour's plasma glucose (mg/dL)—eg, at a glucose level of 200 mg/dL, give 2 units/h at 300 mg/dL, give 3 units/h, etc.

Postoperative Care

With either of the intravenous infusion techniques,

it is best to continue the glucose-insulin infusion until the patient is eating. Hypoglycemia, the most common postoperative complication, most often follows the use of long-acting insulin given subcutaneously before surgery. Although hypoglycemia may also occur if the intravenous insulin infusion is excessive in relation to that of the glucose, an infusion of 1.5 units or less of insulin per hour, when given with 5% glucose, rarely results in hypoglycemia. Blood glucose levels should be measured every 2–4 hours and the patient monitored for signs and symptoms of hypoglycemia (eg, anxiety, tremulousness, profuse sweating without fever). When hypoglycemia is detected, the amount of glucose infused should be promptly increased and the insulin decreased. It is rarely advisable to stop the insulin infusion completely for mild hypoglycemia, since a smoother transition to euglycemia results if the insulin is continued but at a lower dose.

The use of a "sliding scale" based on urine glucose values to judge insulin requirements is no longer justified for postoperative diabetic management. Problems of urine retention, failure to obtain a double-voided specimen, and variations in the renal threshold for glucose excretion confuse the interpretation of urine glucose values; this makes it extremely dangerous to base insulin requirements on these measurements. Therefore, adjustments in the rate of glucose or insulin administration must be based on *blood* glucose levels. Many instruments are available for bedside monitoring of glucose that are easy to use, accurate, and provide quick measurements (ie, it takes 2–3 minutes to obtain a result). A finger-stick provides the single drop of blood required.

Hyperosmolar Coma

Hyperosmolar coma, the result of severe dehydration, may occur in undiagnosed diabetics who have been given large amounts of glucose during surgery. The resulting osmotic diuresis leads to disproportionate water loss, dehydration, and hyperosmolarity. Hyperosmolar coma is rarely seen until the serum glucose level exceeds 800 mg/dL and the osmolarity exceeds 340 meq/L. Hyperosmolar coma may be best avoided by monitoring fluid input and output, measuring blood glucose levels, and instituting treatment promptly if the value exceeds 400 mg/dL.

A marked increase in glucose and insulin requirements postoperatively suggests the presence of occult infection (eg, wound infection, cellulitis at the intravenous site, urinary tract infection, or unrecognized aspiration pneumonia).

Gavin LA: Management of the diabetic patient during surgery. West J Med 1989;151:525.

Rosenstock J et al: Practical guidelines for diabetes management. Clin Diabetes 1987;5:49.

Schade DS: Surgery and diabetes. Med Clin North Am 1988;72:1531.

Watts NB et al: Postoperative management of diabetes mellitus: Steady-state glucose control with bedside algorithm for insulin adjustment. Diabetes Care 1987;10:722.

THYROID DISEASE

Both hyper- and hypothyroidism represent serious problems for patients undergoing surgery. It may be difficult to establish an adequate airway in patients with large goiters. The hyperthyroid patient undergoing surgery is apt to develop hypertension, severe cardiac dysrhythmias, congestive heart failure, and hyperthermia.

Life-threatening thyrotoxicosis (thyroid storm) may be precipitated by any operation but especially by thyroidectomy, which accentuates thyroxine release. It is therefore preferable to bring hyperthyroid patients into a euthyroid state before surgery. This takes 1–6 weeks and is best accomplished by treatment with propylthiouracil, 800–1000 mg/d for about 1 week, followed by a maintenance dose of 200–400 mg/d. If emergency surgery is required, adequate sedation and potassium iodide plus a β-adrenergic blocking agent such as propranolol should be given in addition to propylthiouracil.

Hypothyroid patients are subject to acute hypotension, shock, and hypothermia during surgery; if the patient is allowed to breathe spontaneously, severe CO_2 retention may result from hypoventilation. **Myxedema coma** should be suspected in patients who fail to awaken promptly from anesthesia and who manifest CO_2 retention, even to the point of CO_2 narcosis, accompanied by hypothermia. Increased tissue friability, poor wound healing, and even wound dehiscence may also occur. It is highly advisable to treat myxedematous patients with levothyroxine before elective surgery. In an emergency (eg, severe myxedema requiring immediate surgery), treatment should consist of levothyroxine sodium, 500 μg (0.5 mg) intravenously, by nasogastric tube, or orally. If there is no emergency, the euthyroid state may be gradually restored with levothyroxine, 25 μg/d, with the dose increased over several weeks to a maintenance dose of 150–200 μg/d. It is also always advisable to obtain a baseline cortisol level before treatment of myxedema to rule out coexistent Addison's disease (Schmidt's syndrome), since levothyroxine therapy can precipitate addisonian crisis in this setting.

Finlayson DC, Kaplan JA: Myxoedema and open heart surgery: Anaesthesia and intensive care unit experience. Can Anaesth Soc J 1982;29:543.

Ladenson PW et al: Complications of surgery in hypothyroid patients. Am J Med 1984;77:261.

Moley JF et al: Hypothyroidism abolishes the hyperdynamic phase and increases susceptibility to sepsis. J Surg Res 1984;36:265.

Murkin JM: Anesthesia and hypothyroidism: A review of thyroxine physiology, pharmacology, and anesthetic implications. Anesth Analg 1982;61:371.

ADRENAL INSUFFICIENCY

Patients with adrenal insufficiency undergoing the stress of operation are at risk of addisonian crisis, manifested by salt wastage, decreased blood volume, hypotension, shock, and death. For at least 2–3 days preoperatively, they should receive fluid and sodium chloride replacement intravenously (usually 1–3 L of normal saline per day) and cortisol therapy (20 mg each morning and 10 mg each afternoon). On the day of surgery, 100 mg of cortisol is administered intramuscularly or intravenously just before the operation, followed by 50–100 mg every 6 hours during surgery, a regimen that mimics the normal endogenous cortisol response to stress (up to 300 mg/d). Saline is continued postoperatively at a rate of at least 2–3 L/d, with careful monitoring of blood pressure, serum electrolyte concentrations, and urine output. In the absence of complications, the cortisol dosage can be decreased by half each day, until the usual maintenance dose of about 30 mg/d is reached.

Patients receiving chronic corticosteroid therapy may present with severe hypokalemia and at times serious hypertension, both of which should be corrected before surgery. Stress doses of cortisol (approximately 300 mg/d) must be administered during surgery, according to the protocol described for addisonian patients. If the patient is diabetic, large doses of insulin (eg, 3 units/h) may be required to control blood glucose levels during surgery. Postoperatively, slow wound healing and a predisposition to infection should be anticipated. Infections in these patients may occur without fever.

PITUITARY INSUFFICIENCY

Patients with **panhypopituitarism** must be treated for thyroid and adrenocorticosteroid insufficiency with the doses of levothyroxine and cortisol set forth in the preceding sections.

HEART DISEASE & THE SURGICAL PATIENT

Barry M. Massie, MD

Anesthesia and surgery present a finite risk to any patient, but this risk is increased in the patient with preexisting heart disease, whether clinically apparent or undiagnosed. Indeed, complications related to heart disease are the major cause of nonsurgical perioperative deaths.

Cardiac disease may be exacerbated by many of the physiologic changes accompanying surgery, including fluctuations in heart rate, blood pressure, blood volume, oxygenation, pH, and coagulability. These may lead to myocardial ischemia due to increased myocardial O_2 demand or reduced coronary blood flow, impaired myocardial contractility, and altered cardiac performance due to changes in preload or afterload. Increased circulating catecholamines or sympathetic nervous system activity may precipitate arrhythmias as well as increase heart rate and blood pressure. Anesthesia and medications such as vagolytics and muscle relaxants have direct effects on myocardial contractility, automaticity, and conduction.

While it is often felt that the operative period itself is the most stressful, intraoperative cardiac complications are in fact relatively uncommon as a result of careful monitoring and improved understanding of the risk of the accompanying hemodynamic alterations. The greatest risk occurs in the first 72 hours after operation, when fluid volume shifts, fluctuations in heart rate and blood pressure, and medication changes are greatest and the ability to control them is less. The best approach to minimizing cardiac complications is to maintain one's awareness of the presence and severity of preexisting heart disease and of the risk of asymptomatic and unrecognized disease.

Given this information, the medical consultant, anesthesiologist, and surgeon can weigh the following key questions: (1) Is the operation urgent, essential but with elective timing, or optional? (2) Does the patient have heart disease, manifest or silent? (3) What additional risk does heart disease impose? (4) Can this risk be reduced by additional treatment or by delaying surgery? The answers to these questions will determine the appropriate management strategy. Urgent surgery must proceed, so the problem for the consultant and anesthesiologist is to minimize risk. Elective surgery may need to be delayed or canceled, depending on the risk:benefit ratio.

Cardiac Conditions Masquerading as Surgical Illnesses

It is important to recognize that cardiovascular diseases may occasionally produce symptoms that mimic surgical conditions, and this possibility must be considered before operation. Such presentations include the following:

(1) Myocardial infarction or angina pectoris presenting with epigastric pain, suggesting peptic ulcer, gallbladder disease, or other surgical abdominal disease.

(2) Right heart failure presenting as right upper

quadrant pain due to hepatic congestion, suggesting gallbladder disease.

(3) Nonspecific gastrointestinal symptoms such as anorexia, nausea, early satiety, and weight loss due to severe heart failure, suggesting cancer or other abdominal surgical disease.

(4) Ascites due to heart failure or pericardial disease.

(5) Dysphagia due to left atrial enlargement or diseases of the aorta.

(6) Back and abdominal pain due to aortic dissection.

(7) Abdominal pain due to splenic, renal, or mesenteric emboli from infective endocarditis, emboli of cardiac origin, or atrial myxoma.

(8) Upper abdominal pain and even jaundice due to pulmonary infarction.

Most of these conditions will be readily recognized if they are considered. More typical associated symptoms are usually present. The ECG should reveal evolving or recent infarction, and the physical examination and chest x-ray should demonstrate heart failure or signs of pericardial disease. Echocardiography will confirm the presence of left or right ventricular failure, valvular disease, and pericardial disease and may reveal a source of emboli.

Preoperative Evaluation of the Surgical Patient for Cardiovascular Disease

All patients should be evaluated for possible cardiovascular disease preoperatively. The extent of this evaluation will depend on the statistical likelihood of previously unrecognized disease if the patient is asymptomatic and the nature of the heart condition if the diagnosis is known. A careful history is the primary screening procedure. Key areas of inquiry include the presence of dyspnea, exercise tolerance (and what limits it), chest discomfort and other ischemic equivalents (epigastric, throat, shoulder, or arm discomfort), edema, syncope or presyncope, or a history of heart murmur, hypertension, or failing an employment or insurance physical examination. Patients with a family history of premature coronary disease or with associated peripheral vascular disease should be assumed to be at high risk for ischemic heart disease, as should patients with a long history of diabetes. Patients with hyperlipidemia or hypertension are also at increased risk.

The physical examination will occasionally demonstrate a previously unrecognized heart murmur, mitral valve prolapse, irregular heart rhythm, or hypertension. In patients with heart disease, it will reveal the severity and degree of compensation of heart failure and provide a guide to the severity of valvular disease.

Most patients should have a preoperative ECG, though the yield is low in young patients with negative histories and examinations. Important findings include abnormal rhythms and conduction, left ventricular hypertrophy, myocardial infarction, and "nonspecific" ST segment and T wave abnormalities. A routine preoperative chest x-ray has a low yield in healthy subjects but may be useful in patients with symptoms or an abnormal physical examination. Additional noninvasive tests such as echocardiography, exercise testing, stress (exercise or dipyridamole) thallium scintigraphy, radionuclide ejection fraction measurements, and ambulatory monitoring may be indicated to diagnose and define the severity of cardiac abnormalities. In some patients, cardiac catheterization and coronary arteriography are indicated to determine the severity of heart disease and the need for additional medical or other intervention before surgery.

The evaluation and management of specific cardiac diseases and abnormalities are discussed below.

Relative Contraindications to Surgery

There are no absolute contraindications to surgery, but a number of cardiac conditions substantially increase the risks and become relative contraindications. These include recent myocardial infarction, an unstable or progressive pattern of angina pectoris, decompensated heart failure, severe aortic or mitral stenosis, and severe hypertension. Most heart diseases do not themselves prohibitively increase the surgical risk, but when they are progressive, unstable, or decompensated, the level of risk rises abruptly.

Several approaches have been proposed for quantifying operative risk. The most widely used of these is the Goldman Index, which provides a point score for findings associated with additional risk:

Finding	Points
S_3 gallop or elevated venous pressure	11
Myocardial infarction in previous 6 months	10
>5 VPCs/min on any ECG	7
Nonsinus rhythm or APCs on last ECG	7
Age >70 years	5
Emergency operation	4
Intrathoracic, intraperitoneal, or aortic surgery	3
Significant aortic stenosis	3
Poor general medical condition	3

The risk of cardiac death and life-threatening cardiac complications rises progressively with the total point score—from less than 1% when the score is 0–5 points, to 7% for 6–12 points, 13% (2% mortality rate) with 13–25 points, to 78% (including a 56% mortality rate) in patients with scores over 26 points.

Detsky has modified this multifactorial index to take into account the nature of the operation. However, it should be recognized that these indices serve two functions: to identify factors of risk and to provide probabilities for populations. In assessing the individual patient, the physician must make a judgment based upon the specific cardiac disease, its severity, and its stability.

Specific Cardiac Conditions

A. Coronary Artery Disease: Coronary artery disease is the most common cardiac disease and the major cause of morbidity and mortality in patients undergoing surgery. Several categories of patients must be considered: those with prior myocardial infarction, those with angina pectoris, and those with possible asymptomatic coronary disease. Virtually all patients who have had a myocardial infarction have coronary artery disease and are at risk for further ischemia or reinfarction. This risk is highest in patients in whom the infarction is most recent, declining from approximately 20–30% (or higher in earlier studies) in the first 3 months, to 10–15% after 4–6 months and 5% thereafter. With advances in medical therapy, better diagnostic testing, and improved perioperative management, these numbers are falling, but it is still preferable to delay elective surgery for 3–6 months after myocardial infarction. In the absence of heart failure, the propensity for ischemia and reinfarction are higher following nontransmural infarctions, in which the volume of residual ischemic myocardium is greater. If the infarction is recent, such patients should undergo stress testing with exercise or dipyridamole thallium scintigraphy to identify individuals with large areas of ischemia before major surgery; these patients should undergo coronary angiography and revascularization if indicated. It may be helpful to assess left ventricular function noninvasively in patients with anterior transmural infarctions, since they may have significantly decreased ejection fractions in the absence of symptomatic heart failure.

Angina pectoris also reflects underlying coronary artery disease and is just as important an indicator of risk as is prior infarction. When the pattern is progressive or unstable or the threshold is very low, operation should be postponed at least until the angina can be stabilized by medical therapy. If major noncardiac surgery is planned, coronary arteriography is usually indicated to detect critical lesions.

Patients with *stable* mild to moderate angina pectoris, old myocardial infarction, or multiple risk factors but no overt coronary artery disease represent a group with intermediate perioperative risk. When major surgery (especially vascular procedures) is planned or if additional risk factors such as age ≥ 70 years, diabetes mellitus, or heart failure are present, further evaluation may be warranted—but only if the detection of significant ischemia would alter the management of the patient (eg, result in cancellation of surgery or a different approach to perioperative care). Since exercise testing is often not feasible, pharmacologic stress with dipyridamole or adenosine in association with perfusion scintigraphy are usually employed. Individuals with demonstrable ischemia, especially when it involves multiple or large areas, are at increased risk; coronary arteriography or additional medical therapy may be indicated. However, data are not available to support prophylactic revascularization in stable patients, and the combined morbidity of revascularization plus that of the required surgery must be balanced against the risk of the surgery alone. Furthermore, recent data indicate that as these tests are more widely employed, they have not been as accurate in defining high- and low-risk groups as in early reports (Table 5–1).

Patients with coronary artery disease or a high probability of coronary artery disease need to be managed carefully. Preoperative medications—including beta-blockers in particular but also nitrates and calcium channel blockers—should be continued throughout the perioperative period. Aspirin should be continued unless concerns about hemostasis are overriding; addition of aspirin postoperatively may be useful, since many infarcts may be caused by a postoperative hypercoagulable state. Excessive tachycardia, hypertension, and hypotension should be avoided. Complications are most common in the second to fifth postoperative days, so vigilance must be maintained.

B. Congestive Heart Failure: Severe or decompensated congestive heart failure is probably the greatest risk factor for perioperative cardiac death. Surgery should be postponed until congestive heart failure is stable, pulmonary edema is absent, and excessive fluid is eliminated. A stable regimen of diuretics, angiotensin-converting enzyme inhibitors, and digoxin when indicated should be instituted. Underlying reversible causes (such as valvular lesions, ischemia, or uncontrolled hypertension) should be identified and treated. For major surgery, hemodynamic monitoring intraoperatively and postoperatively is essential. Decompensation is most common during and after the second postoperative day, when extravascular fluid begins to be mobilized. Weights, fluid balance, and oxygenation must be followed closely and diuretic therapy reinstituted early unless hypotension is present.

C. Valvular Heart Valvular heart disease in the absence of congestive heart failure is usually well tolerated during surgery. The exceptions are critical aortic stenosis and mitral stenosis. The former can be associated with hypotension and heart failure, while the latter often causes pulmonary edema when the heart rate increases, atrial fibrillation occurs, or excessive fluid volume is administered. Nonetheless, patients with moderate obstructions (eg, aortic valve area > 0.8 cm^2; mitral area > 1.2 cm^2) usually do well, and those with even more severe stenoses can be managed successfully with careful monitoring if the need for surgery is urgent. Mitral valve prolapse is an indication for antibiotic prophylaxis in nonsterile procedures but does not increase the risk of surgery.

Table 5–1. Significance of a reversible dipyridamole $^{201}T1$ defect.

Author	Reference	N	Sensitivity (%)	Specificity (%)	PPV (%)	NPV (%)	RR
Boucher	N Engl J Med 1985;312:389	48	100	80	50	100	16.0
Cutler	J Vasc Surg 1987;5:91	101	100	69	23	100	14.3
Leppo	J Am Coll Cardiol 1987;9:269	89	93	62	33	98	15.7
Eagle	JAMA 1987;257:2185	200	83	66	30	96	7.2
Mangano	Circulation 1991;84:493	60	46	66	27	82	1.5
Marwick[1]	Clin Cardiol 1990;13:14	86	30	75	14	89	1.2
Fleisher	Anesthesiology 1990;73(3A):A75	19	0	46	0	38	0
Bertrand[2]	Anesthesiology 1990;73(3A):A85	71	43	77	55	63	1.3

[1]Fixed or reversible defect considered positive.
[2]Compared with coronary arteriography.

PPV = Predictive value of a positive test for subsequent outcome event.
NPV = Predictive value of a negative test for absence of an outcome event.
RR = Relative risk for an outcome event of patients with a positive test compared with those with a negative test.

D. Dysrhythmias and Conduction Abnormalities: Supraventricular arrhythmias can usually be managed with agents such as verapamil and esmolol as well as with digoxin. Frequent ventricular ectopy does indicate increased risk, but this usually reflects associated myocardial disease, which should be sought and evaluated. It is not necessary to suppress asymptomatic nonsustained ventricular arrhythmias preoperatively. Increased ectopy and ventricular tachycardia occurring during or after surgery can be managed with intravenous lidocaine or procainamide.

Left bundle branch block or bifascicular block also indicate higher risk, since they often indicate myocardial disease. However, progression to advanced atrioventricular block during surgery is rare. Prolonged PR intervals, Mobitz I (Wenckebach) atrioventricular block, or sinus bradycardia (heart rate less than 45–50/min) often reflect excessive medication effect from digoxin, β-adrenergic blocking agents, and calcium channel blocking agents. These should be adjusted if possible. Higher degrees of atrioventricular blockade should usually be managed with temporary or permanent pacing.

E. Congenital Heart Disease: Space does not permit discussion of the impact of various congenital lesions on perioperative risk. In general, if these lesions are associated with heart failure, severe pulmonary hypertension (systolic pulmonary pressure above 80 mm Hg), or hypoxemia, the risk of surgery is high.

F. Hypertension: Patients with uncomplicated and controlled hypertension usually tolerate surgery well. The presence of left ventricular hypertrophy with repolarization changes indicates mildly increased risk, perhaps because of a higher incidence of associated coronary artery disease. Indeed, untreated and suboptimally treated hypertension do not appear to significantly increase risk when the pressure is below 160/105 mm Hg, since it is relatively easy to reduce it with anesthesia and parenteral agents. When the pressure exceeds 180/110 mm Hg, the incidence of severe perioperative hypertension increases along with the need for prolonged parenteral treatment and observation as well as the risk of complications.

Antihypertensive medications should be continued to avoid withdrawal syndromes, especially when the patient is receiving central sympatholytics or beta-blockers. This can usually be accomplished with oral medication, but transdermal clonidine, sublingual nifedipine, and intravenous calcium channel blockers (verapamil and diltiazem) and parenteral beta-blockers and converting enzyme inhibitors are available.

Special Issues Related to Monitoring & Anesthesia

A. Medications: As noted above, it is feasible and desirable to continue most medications in the perioperative period. This is especially true with medications for coronary artery disease, congestive heart failure, and hypertension. If additional medications are needed, parenteral therapy is optimal.

B. Hemodynamic Monitoring: Hemodynamic monitoring of high risk patients during major surgical procedures has become routine. This is essential in patients with congestive heart failure, impaired left ventricular function (ejection fraction below 40%), critical valve disease, and recent myocardial infarction when the surgery is major. It probably is not necessary in patients at risk for ischemia with preserved left ventricular function, except in the case of major vascular procedures. Perhaps the most valuable period for hemodynamic monitoring in high-risk patients is the immediate postoperative period, when appropriate parameters for fluid administration and blood pressure can be difficult to define.

C. Transesophageal Echocardiography: This technique is being increasingly used in the operating room. It permits excellent visualization of the left ventricle and can provide continuous monitoring of cavity size, contractile function, and segmental wall motion. In experienced hands, transesophageal echocardiography allows early detection of heart failure and myocardial ischemia, but its additional value beyond hemodynamic monitoring in noncardiac surgery has not been proved.

D. Choice of Anesthetics: There is no conclusive evidence that the choice of anesthetics affects outcome in patients with heart disease, and the selection of the route of anesthesia and the choice of agent are best left to the anesthesiologist. Epidural anesthesia may be preferable when a low spinal level is adequate for the procedure, but hypotension is a problem with higher levels. Narcotics have little myocardial depressant action and may be preferable to the volatile gases in patients with diminished contractility.

E. Antibiotic Prophylaxis: Patients with valvular heart disease and prosthetic heart valves require antibiotic prophylaxis for potentially bacteremic events, including genitourinary, gastrointestinal, oropharyngeal, and gallbladder surgery. The usual regimen is ampicillin, 2 g intravenously, plus gentamicin, 1.5 mg/kg intravenously 30 minutes before operation. This may be repeated after 8 hours. Vancomycin, 1 g intravenously over 60 minutes, may be substituted in patients allergic to penicillin.

F. Anticoagulation: Patients with prosthetic valves and other heart conditions may be receiving chronic anticoagulation. In the former case, interruption of anticoagulation should be as brief as possible. Such patients should have their warfarin withdrawn 5 days prior to surgery and be maintained on intravenous heparin from the time their prothrombin time falls below 1½ times control until 6 hours before operation. Heparin can usually be resumed 12 hours postoperatively. Anticoagulation for other indications can usually be withdrawn safely for the perioperative period.

Abraham S et al: Coronary risk of noncardiac surgery. Prog Cardiovasc Dis 1991;34:205.

Detsky AS et al: Predicting cardiac complications in patients undergoing non-cardiac surgery. J Gen Intern Med 1986;1:211.

Eagle KA et al: Combining clinical and thallium data optimizes preoperative assessment of cardiac risk before major vascular surgery. Ann Intern Med 1989;110:859.

Freeman WK, Gibbons RJ, Shub C: Preoperative assessment of cardiac patients undergoing noncardiac surgical procedures. Mayo Clin Proc 1989;64:1105.

Goldman L: Multifactorial index of cardiac risk in noncardiac surgery: Ten-year status report. (Review article.) J Cardiothorac Anesth 1987;1:237.

Mangano DT et al: Association of perioperative myocardial ischemia with cardiac morbidity and mortality in men undergoing non-cardiac surgery. N Engl J Med 1990;323:1781.

Mangano DT et al: Dipyridamole thallium-201 scintigraphy as a preoperative screening test: A reexamination of its predictive potential. Circulation 1991; 84:493.

Salem DN, Chuttani K, Isner JM: Assessment and management of cardiac disease in the surgical patient. Curr Probl Cardiol 1989;14:171.

Wong T, Detsky A: Perioperative cardiac risk assessment for patients having peripheral vascular surgery. Ann Intern Med 1992;116:745.

RESPIRATORY DISEASE & THE SURGICAL PATIENT

Robert F. Hickey, MD

Risk Factors

The most common perioperative complications involve the pulmonary system. The relatively high incidence of pulmonary complications is associated with anesthesia and surgery, and the two primary determinants are the operative site and the presence of lung disease. The correlation between the site of surgical incision and the incidence of pulmonary complications—from high to low—is thoracotomy, upper abdomen, lower abdomen, and periphery. Pulmonary complications are least common in patients with normal lung function who are undergoing peripheral surgery. Any treatment that lessens preexisting pulmonary disease also lessens the incidence of perioperative pulmonary complications.

Factors that contribute to perioperative pulmonary complications include pulmonary aspiration, retention of tracheobronchial secretions, respiratory depression from drugs, decreased lung volume with development of atelectasis, and immobility. Upper abdominal surgery has also been shown to produce diaphragmatic dysfunction, which predisposes to pulmonary complications.

Secondary determinants of perioperative pulmonary complications include age, obesity, cooperativeness of the patient in postoperative care, and a history of smoking. These factors foster the development of lung disease, decrease the ability of the patient to cooperate in maneuvers that prevent or treat pulmonary complications, and compromise laryngeal integrity.

Specific Diseases & Problems

A. Acute Upper Respiratory Tract Infections: Both anesthesia and surgery provide an opportunity for the spread of infection because respiratory defense mechanisms are compromised and instrumentation of the airway may be required. Therefore, the presence of a cold, pharyngitis, or tonsillitis is a relative contraindication to elective surgery, since viral infections decrease defense mechanisms against bacterial infections. If surgery is absolutely necessary, an appropriate antibiotic should be administered prophylactically and manipulation of the infected area avoided to the extent possible.

B. Acute Lower Respiratory Tract Infections (Tracheitis, Bronchitis, Pneumonia): These infections are absolute contraindications to elective surgery. If emergency surgery is necessary, therapy for pulmonary disease includes humidification of inhaled gases, removal of lung secretions, and continued administration of bronchodilators and antibiotics.

C. Chronic Obstructive Pulmonary Disease (COPD) (Bronchitis, Emphysema, Bronchiectasis): In patients with chronic obstructive pulmonary disease, the frequency and severity of postoperative pulmonary complications are related to the extent of compromised lung function. Preoperative preparation should consist of applying the following measures for 2–7 days before surgery: cessation of smoking, administration of antibiotics for purulent sputum, administration of bronchodilators, and physical therapy. For operations on parts of the body other than the thorax, lung disease has not been shown to influence the frequency of pulmonary complications unless it is very severe (eg, severe enough to result in elevated $PaCO_2$ levels).

D. Bronchial Asthma: Patients with bronchial asthma who are undergoing surgery are at increased risk of pulmonary complications. Preoperative management includes adjustment of bronchodilator medication, cessation of smoking, and treatment of infection. Intraoperative bronchoconstriction from mechanical stimulation of the airway must be prevented by giving appropriate anesthetics in adequate concentrations. Adverse interactions between anesthetic agents and bronchodilators must be avoided. Many patients with bronchial asthma are receiving corticosteroids and require corticosteroid therapy in the perioperative period.

E. Restrictive Lung Disease (Caused by Pulmonary Fibrosis and Obesity): Restrictive lung disease reduces lung volume and decreases arterial oxygen tension; the decrease in arterial oxygen tension is particularly noticeable with exercise. Preoperative preparation is similar to that for other lung diseases: treatment of infection, removal of sputum, and discontinuance of smoking. When mechanically controlled ventilation is required for patients with pulmonary fibrosis, it may be necessary to use smaller tidal volumes and more rapid respiratory rates than normal.

The effects of obesity on the development of perioperative pulmonary complications are most evident in the massively obese patient. Obesity is defined as body weight more than 1.2 times normal; in massive obesity, body weight is more than twice the calculated ideal weight. In obese patients, pulmonary compromise is mostly due to reduced lung volumes, which leads to hypoxemia, airway obstruction from soft tissue encroachment, and possibly an increase in gastric contents and acidity. If problems are recognized and treated preoperatively, complications can be minimized. The massively obese patient should be mobilized as soon as possible after surgery.

Patients with pulmonary fibrosis as a consequence of bleomycin therapy are particularly susceptible to oxygen toxicity, so inspired oxygen concentrations should be carefully controlled.

Preoperative Evaluation of Pulmonary Function

The purpose of preoperative pulmonary evaluation is to assess the risk of perioperative lung complications. The information obtained not only guides perioperative pulmonary care but also selects patients for specific preoperative treatment intended to decrease the risk of pulmonary complications and the length of the hospital stay.

Pulmonary evaluation should be performed by the referring physician or surgeon (or both) at the time surgery is first proposed. The site of surgery is a major consideration in the decision to perform pulmonary function tests and institute treatment. Other indications for pulmonary function testing are found in the history and physical examination and include manifestations of lung disease, such as exertional dyspnea, exercise tolerance, cough, production of sputum, history of smoking, previous pulmonary complications, asthma, age, and body weight. Patients with mild pulmonary compromise who will be undergoing surgery other than on the abdomen or thorax probably do not require pulmonary function testing. When testing is indicated, spirometry with measurement of forced expiratory airflow is usually all that is required. If airflow on forced expiration is reduced significantly, the response to bronchodilators should be measured and arterial blood gases determined. More complex tests such as measurement of diffusion capacity, radioisotopic ventilation-perfusion scans, and pulmonary artery catheterization are largely confined to patients with pulmonary hypertension or life-threatening lung disease or for those who require thoracic surgery.

Many studies have been performed to determine which pulmonary function tests are the most sensitive and reliable indicators of surgical and anesthetic risk. As yet there is no way to define absolute criteria for operability. Tests can provide guidelines but are not entirely reliable predictors for the following reasons:

(1) Although the incidence is low, patients with normal pulmonary function may develop perioperative pulmonary complications.

(2) Criteria developed for one surgical procedure (eg, thoracotomy) may not be accurate for another procedure.

(3) Pulmonary function tests cannot take into account intangibles such as patient cooperativeness. The available tests cannot measure the amount of

sputum produced or predict the likelihood of pulmonary aspiration.

In general, spirometry with measurement of the degree of impairment of airflow provides the best and least expensive screening test. Patients undergoing thoracic surgery without lung resection are at increased risk if the FEV_1 or maximum breath capacity is less than 50% of normal. For peripheral surgery, these values are lower (about 30% of predicted normal values). If the arterial CO_2 tension is greater than 45 mm Hg and the patient is not receiving drugs that depress ventilation, abdominal or thoracic operations impose a risk of life-threatening pulmonary complications. Surgery on such individuals should proceed only after thorough and careful consultation. In peripheral surgery as well, elevated $Paco_2$ levels indicate a greater likelihood of pulmonary complications and the possible need for postoperative mechanical ventilation and special monitoring.

Azaro KS et al: Preoperative evaluation and general preparation for chest-wall operations. Surg Clin North Am 1989;69:899.

Bechard D, Wetstein L: Assessment of exercise oxygen consumption as preoperative criterion for lung resection. Ann Thorac Surg 1987;44:344.

Gomez MN, Tinker JH: Smoking, anesthesia, and coronary bypass operation: A witches' cauldron? Mayo Clin Proc 1989;64:708.

Jackson CV: Preoperative pulmonary evaluation. Arch Int Med 1988;148:2120.

Jayr C et al: Postoperative pulmonary complications: General anesthesia with postoperative parenteral morphine compared with epidural analgesia. Surgery 1988;104:57.

Lawrence VA, Page CP, Harris GD: Preoperative spirometry before abdominal operations: A critical appraisal of its predictive value. Arch Intern Med 1989;149:280.

LoCicero J: Bronchopulmonary aspiration. Surg Clin North Am 1989;69:71.

Roukema JA, Carol EJ, Prins JG: The prevention of pulmonary complications after upper abdominal surgery in patients with noncompromised pulmonary status. Arch Surg 1988;123:30.

Vodinh J et al: Risk factors of postoperative pulmonary complications after vascular surgery. Surgery 1989;105:360.

Wahi R et al: Determinants of perioperative morbidity and mortality after pneumonectomy. Ann Thorac Surg 1989;48:33.

Warner MA et al: Role of preoperative cessation of smoking and other factors in postoperative pulmonary complications: A blinded prospective study of coronary artery bypass patients. Mayo Clin Proc 1989;64:609.

Wolfe WG: Preoperative assessment of pulmonary function. Ann Thorac Surg 1987;44:562.

RENAL DISEASE & THE SURGICAL PATIENT

Allen I. Arieff, MD

More patients with renal disease are undergoing surgery now than in the past, largely because of new techniques for the management of patients with acute or chronic renal failure. Because of these advances, elective surgery is not usually deferred when renal disease is present. In most cases, a simple workup will suffice to screen patients for the presence of unsuspected renal disease. A complete urinalysis and measurement of serum creatinine, albumin, and blood urea nitrogen, when combined with the history and physical examination, will disclose impaired renal function. Suggestive findings include hematuria, proteinuria, hypoalbuminemia, and elevated blood urea nitrogen or serum creatinine.

If potential complications are anticipated, renal disease per se is rarely a contraindication to surgery. In patients with chronic renal failure, who do not require maintenance dialysis (GFR > 15 mL/min; serum creatinine < 6 mg/dL), preoperative hydration and blood transfusion to raise the hematocrit above 32% are usually all that is required. During surgery, strict attention to fluid balance is essential, since dehydration can precipitate acute renal failure.

In patients maintained by intermittent dialysis (GFR < 5 mL/min), transfusion to a hematocrit above 32% is usually necessary preoperatively. These patients are more susceptible to infection, and because they are anephric, fluid and electrolyte management is more difficult. Patients on dialysis tend to be hypercatabolic and malnourished, and this tendency will be accentuated by surgery. Excessive accumulation of toxic metabolites can be minimized by performing dialysis the day before surgery and as soon postoperatively as allowed by considerations of hemostasis.

Certain renal diseases present unique hazards. Patients with renal insufficiency due to diabetes mellitus are more susceptible to infection and cardiovascular complications such as stroke and acute myocardial infarction and demonstrate poorer wound healing. Diagnostic procedures that would be safe in most patients can be disastrous in the diabetic. Acute renal failure may occur as a complication of intravenous contrast media given for radiographic studies. Major risk factors include age over 65 years, nephrotic syndrome, dehydration, diabetes mellitus, and serum creatinine level above 2 mg/dL. In patients with two or more of these risk factors, the amount of contrast medium should be kept at an absolute minimum by using digital subtraction angiography instead of arteriography and ultrasound instead of intravenous urography whenever possible. The abrupt onset of acute renal failure following intra-arterial invasive procedures (eg, cardiac catheterization, aortography) may be due to atheromatous emboli. Differentiation between this condition and dye-induced renal failure may be difficult, but renal failure caused by atheroemboli is more likely to be irreversible. Patients with macroglobulinemia, multiple myeloma, and amyloid renal disease are prone to develop acute renal failure after intravenous contrast procedures. Patients with obstructive jaundice have a higher than expected incidence of postoperative renal failure.

Drugs & the Kidney

Many drugs are toxic to the kidney. Therapeutic agents whose dosage should be modified in patients with renal disease include antibiotics, antituberculosis agents, anti-inflammatory agents, hypoglycemic agents, analgesics and anesthetics, hypnotics, and antineoplastic drugs. The worst offenders are antibiotics such as gentamicin, methicillin, tetracyclines, and amphotericin B; gold salts; analgesics such as indomethacin and phenacetin; hypoglycemic drugs; and anesthetic drugs, including methoxyflurane. In some normal subjects and in patients with chronic renal failure, administration of nonsteroidal anti-inflammatory agents, which inhibit prostaglandin synthesis, may lead to acute renal failure. All of the aforementioned drugs are potentially even more toxic when used in combination. For example, salicylates are usually not nephrotoxic when used alone, but the combination of a salicylate and ibuprofen, or similar agents, may lead to acute renal failure.

Digitalis preparations deserve special mention, because they are used so frequently in elderly patients who may require surgery. Although these drugs are largely protein-bound, excretion (with the exception of digitoxin) is mainly (85%) through the kidneys, and dosage must be modified in patients with renal insufficiency. A number of techniques for dosage modification based on the patient's creatinine clearance and body weight have been devised. With normal renal function, about 20% of body digoxin stores are lost daily, whereas with a 50% reduction in renal function, only 10% will be lost each day. Thus, maintenance digoxin dosage should be decreased proportionate to the decline in GFR. While renal function (GFR) is usually estimated from serum creatinine, in patients with renal disease, serum creatinine measurements may lead to overestimation of GFR by as much as 3-fold. In such patients, measurement of GFR by more precise methods may be necessary. Digitoxin, unlike digoxin, is not significantly excreted by the kidneys.

Postoperative Renal Insufficiency

Postoperative renal insufficiency is usually diagnosed on the basis of a rising serum creatinine level. The differential diagnosis includes atheromatous renal disease, dye-induced renal failure, and acute glomerulonephritis (which is often secondary to systemic infection or undetected abscesses). Although atheromatous renal disease often presents as fulminant renal failure after an intra-arterial catheter study, it more often presents as chronic slowly progressive renal insufficiency. AIDS can also affect the kidney and lead to renal insufficiency. The most common cause of postoperative renal insufficiency, however, is acute renal failure.

Acute Oliguria & Acute Renal Failure

Acute oliguria (urine output < 20 mL/h) can be of intrinsic (renal) or extrinsic origin. The more common extrinsic causes include reduced effective blood volume (prerenal), which may be due to external fluid loss (eg, hemorrhage, dehydration, diarrhea) or to internal, third-space accumulation of fluid (eg, bowel obstruction, pancreatitis, extensive soft tissue trauma). Postrenal extrinsic causes of oliguria include prostatic hypertrophy, retroperitoneal tumor, and unilateral stone or tumor in a solitary kidney. Oliguria due to intrinsic renal damage is called acute renal failure. Acute renal failure with a normal 24-hour urine volume is called nonoliguric acute renal failure. Renal failure complicating abdominal sepsis is often secondary to acute glomerulonephritis and may resolve with treatment of the abdominal infection. Acute pancreatitis is also frequently a cause of acute renal failure, but the mechanism is unclear.

There are several simple tests that should enable the physician to distinguish between extrinsic and intrinsic causes of oliguria. If the cause is intrinsic (ie, acute renal failure), the urine sediment usually contains renal tubular cells and renal tubular cell casts, and the urine sodium concentration usually exceeds 40 meq/L. Urine sodium is below 20 meq/L in patients with prerenal azotemia. In most patients with prerenal azotemia, the urine/plasma creatinine ratio exceeds 40:1 and the urine/plasma osmolar ratio exceeds 1.1:1. Enough intravenous fluids should be given to raise the central venous pressure to 15–20 cm water. If the response is inadequate, an attempt should be made to bring about diuresis by giving intravenous furosemide, 100–200 mg; mannitol, 12.5 g; or dopamine, 5 μg/kg/min. Although diuresis does not correct acute tubular necrosis, it may convert oliguric to nonoliguric renal failure, which has a better prognosis. An increase of urine volume to over 40 mL/h within 2 hours is strong evidence that oliguria has an extrinsic cause. Postrenal causes of oliguria (obstruction) may be sought by catheterizing the bladder, performing ultrasonography or CT scan to look for caliceal dilatation, or performing retrograde urography.

Over the past decade there has been a reappraisal of the use of dialysis therapy for patients with acute renal failure. Whereas such patients had previously been dialyzed only as a means of managing symptoms (hyperkalemia, pericardial effusion, obtundation), the trend now is toward early dialysis regardless of symptoms or the results of blood chemical analyses. In addition, dialysis is usually performed every 2–3 days, regardless of the results of blood chemical tests. Such prophylactic dialysis has been found to decrease the death rate and rate of complications (eg, gastrointestinal bleeding, sepsis). Dialysis has not been shown to prolong life in patients with renal failure and AIDS.

The first step in preparing an arteriovenous shunt or fistula for vascular access if hemodialysis is to be done, or insertion of a peritoneal cannula if peritoneal dialysis is selected. Whether peritoneal dialysis or hemodialysis is the best means of treating acute renal failure is not resolved, with certain advantages claimed for each procedure. Relative contraindications to peritoneal dialysis include an abdominal vascular prosthetic graft (eg, aortic graft) and systemic hypotension (because of reduced peritoneal blood flow), whereas a pronounced bleeding tendency constitutes a relative contraindication to hemodialysis. Although dialysis has markedly altered the treatment of patients with acute renal failure, the physician should not forget the other fundamentals of treatment, including prevention and treatment of infection, maintenance of fluid and electrolyte balance, and adequate nutrition. Hyperalimentation using essential amino acids may reverse the negative nitrogen balance often associated with acute renal failure and improve survival. (See Chapter 10.)

Postoperative Electrolyte Disorders

Hyponatremia, alkalosis, and hypokalemia are well-known postsurgical water and electrolyte problems. Two syndromes that have only recently come to be recognized as specific entities that may result in death or permanent brain damage are symptomatic postoperative hyponatremia with respiratory arrest and postoperative hypernatremia. In the former, healthy individuals undergoing elective surgery abruptly stop breathing. The cause is usually excessive administration of 5% dextrose in water associated with an idiosyncratic response to high postoperative levels of vasopressin (ADH), leading to retention of most of the fluid being administered. Serum sodium in these patients has been in the range of 90–120 mmol/L, and all cases have ended in death or permanent brain damage.

Postoperative hypernatremia, associated with a serum sodium of 150–185 mmol/L, is related to a number of postoperative events, including diarrhea, nasogastric or T-tube drainage, or excessive administration of isotonic sodium chloride or hypertonic sodium bicarbonate. The common denominator is loss of isotonic or hypotonic fluid without adequate replacement of free water. Among postoperative patients with serum sodium levels above 148 mmol/L, the overall mortality rate is about 50%.

Arieff AI: Hyponatremia, convulsions, respiratory arrest, and permanent brain damage after elective surgery in healthy women. N Engl J Med 1986;314:1529.

Cigarroa RG et al: Dosing of contrast material to prevent contrast nephropathy in patients with renal disease. Am J Med 1989;86:649.

Miller DC, Myers BD: Pathophysiology and prevention of acute renal failure associated with thoracoabdominal or abdominal aortic surgery. J Vasc Surg 1987;5:518.

Myers BD, Moran SM: Hemodynamically mediated acute renal failure. N Engl J Med 1986;31:97.

Papadakis MA, Arieff AI: Unpredictability of clinical evaluation of renal function in cirrhosis. Am J Med 1987;82:945.

Parfrey PS et al: Contrast material-induced renal failure in patients with diabetes mellitus, renal insufficiency, or both: A prospective controlled study. N Engl J Med 1989;320:143.

Porter GA: Contrast-associated nephropathy. Am J Cardiol 1989;64:22E.

Russell JD, Churchill DN: Calcium antagonists and acute renal failure. Am J Med 1989;87:306.

Svensson LG et al: Appraisal of adjuncts to prevent acute renal failure after surgery on the thoracic or thoracoabdominal aorta. J Vasc Surg 1989;10:230.

HEMATOLOGIC DISEASE & THE SURGICAL PATIENT

Pearl T.C.Y. Toy, MD

PREOPERATIVE HEMOSTATIC EVALUATION

(1) All patients should be asked if they have ever experienced prolonged bleeding after dental extractions, tonsillectomy, or any other kind of surgery or after minor cuts; if they have ever had large bruises in the absence of an injury; or if massive swelling of the lips or tongue has ever occurred after they have bitten themselves. They should also be asked if there are any bleeders in the family.

(2) Patients with positive bleeding histories require a platelet count, prothrombin time (PT), partial thromboplastin time (PTT), and hematology consultation. The bleeding time does not predict surgical bleeding.

(3) The cause of an abnormal platelet count, PT, or PTT must be determined before surgery in order to determine appropriate therapy.

Borzotta AP: Value of preoperative history as an indicator of hemostatic disorders. Ann Surg 1984;200:648.

Bowie EJ, Owen CA: Clinical and laboratory diagnosis of hemorrhagic disorders. In: *Disorders of Hemostasis.* Ratnoff OD, Forbes CD (editors). Saunders, 1991.

Lind SE: The bleeding time does not predict surgical bleeding. Blood 1991;77:2547.

SURGERY IN PATIENTS WITH ANEMIA

In general, moderate anemia (hematocrit > 30%) does not increase the hazards associated with surgery. If time permits, deficiencies of iron, folic acid, and vitamin B_{12} should be repaired before surgery. In the case of megaloblastic anemias (pernicious anemia and folic acid deficiency), surgery should be deferred if possible until specific therapy (vitamin B_{12} or folic acid) has repaired the generalized tissue defect, because in these two conditions all the cells of the body are affected by the vitamin deficiency, and transfusions alone do not render surgery safe. It probably takes 1–2 weeks to reach adequate tissue levels.

In patients with sickle cell disease, sickling may be precipitated by anoxia and acidosis. Although this occurs infrequently during surgery with careful anesthesia administration, partial exchange with normal packed red cells decreases the concentration of sickle hemoglobin and may be considered before general anesthesia in patients with sickle cell disease.

The decision to transfuse a specific patient should take into consideration the duration of anemia, the intravascular volume, the extent of the operation, the probability of massive blood loss, and the presence of coexisting conditions such as impaired pulmonary function, inadequate cardiac output, myocardial ischemia, or cerebrovascular or peripheral circulatory disease. These factors are representative of the universe of considerations that comprise clinical judgment.

No single measure can replace good clinical judgment as the basis for decisions regarding perioperative transfusion. However, current experience suggests that otherwise healthy patients with hemoglobin values of 10 g/dL or greater rarely require perioperative transfusion, whereas those with acute anemia with resulting hemoglobin values of less than 7 g/dL frequently will require red blood cell transfusions. The decision to transfuse red blood cells will depend on clinical assessment aided by laboratory data such as arterial oxygenation, mixed venous oxygen tension, cardiac output, the oxygen extraction ratio, and blood volume, when indicated.

NIH Consensus Conference: Perioperative red blood cell transfusion. JAMA 1988;260:2700.

Practice strategies for elective red blood cell transfusion. American College of Physicians. Ann Intern Med 1992;116:403.

HEMATOLOGIC DISORDERS THAT MAY SIMULATE ACUTE ABDOMINAL SURGICAL CONDITIONS

Sickle Cell Anemia

Painful abdominal crises in sickle cell anemia may suggest appendicitis, cholecystitis, a ruptured viscus, or other acute abdominal conditions. In a patient with this kind of pain, helpful diagnostic points are the following: (1) In sickle cell anemia, although the abdomen may be rigid and tender, peristalsis is usually normal. (2) The leukocytosis in sickle cell anemia has a relatively normal differential count—eg, with a white count of 20,000/μL, only 65% granulocytes. (3) Leukocyte counts above 20,000/μL are seen in many patients with sickle cell anemia who are not acutely ill. An elevated leukocyte alkaline phosphatase level suggests infection rather than painful crisis.

Henoch-Schönlein or Nonthrombocytopenic Purpura

These conditions are usually associated with obvious skin lesions or perhaps hematuria but may on occasion present with acute abdominal pain. The symptoms are apparently due to bleeding into the bowel wall. Intussusception may occur and may require operation. No reliably effective treatment is available to prevent or treat abnormal bleeding, although prednisone may be tried.

Lead Poisoning

Lead poisoning may cause acute abdominal pain. A history of possible exposure to lead may be of great importance. Laboratory clues are moderate anemia with striking stippling and a marked elevation of urinary coproporphyrin. The diagnosis is established by finding elevated lead levels in blood and urine.

Abdominal Wall Hemorrhage

Hemorrhage into the abdominal wall may simulate acute appendicitis in patients with thrombocytopenia, hemophilia, or other severe coagulation disorders.

SURGERY IN PATIENTS WITH HEMATOLOGIC MALIGNANT DISORDERS

It is occasionally necessary to operate on patients who have leukemia, lymphoma, myeloma, or related disorders. Such patients can always undergo surgery without increased risk if they are in hematologic remission, and surgery may be relatively safe in partial remission. In acute leukemia, the risk of surgery is low if the white count is not excessive, the hemoglobin is over 10 g/dL, and the platelet count is near 100,000/μL. Other coagulation factors are not usually disturbed in acute leukemia.

In patients with chronic myelocytic leukemia with platelet counts in excess of 1 million/μL or white counts above 100,000/μL, bleeding may be a problem. In patients with chronic lymphatic leukemia and a normal platelet count, even white counts in excess of 100,000/μL are no contraindication to surgery.

Very high platelet counts may be encountered in polycythemia vera and essential thrombocythemias. If surgery is urgently necessary, platelet pheresis to a platelet count below 1 million/µL may be considered before surgery. If surgery can be deferred for a week, therapy with hydroxyurea, 30 mg/kg/d orally, may be used.

Patients with polycythemia vera have a greatly increased incidence of bleeding and thromboses. In patients with very high packed cell volumes (over 60%), prothrombin time and partial thromboplastin time will appear falsely prolonged unless allowance is made for the relatively small plasma volume by reducing the amount of citrate in the test tube. Similarly, fibrinogen may be too low for the volume of whole blood. When blood counts have become normal (after phlebotomy, radiotherapy, or chemotherapy), surgery is safer, but the incidence of complications is still increased.

Patients with multiple myeloma or macroglobulinemia may bleed excessively in surgery, because their elevated abnormal globulin may interfere with the coagulation process. Plasmapheresis before surgery should be considered.

Patients with all of the above have no increased difficulty with wound healing or postoperative infections as long as their total granulocyte count is at least 1500/µL. The common anticancer chemotherapeutic agents—mercaptopurine, busulfan, melphalan, methotrexate, and cyclophosphamide—do not interfere with wound healing.

SURGERY IN PATIENTS RECEIVING ANTICOAGULANTS

Heparin

Since the average dose of heparin (5000 units intravenously) maintains the whole blood clotting time at twice the control value for only 3–4 hours, a short wait will let the coagulation time return to normal. If a large dose has been administered, it may be necessary to neutralize its effect in a patient who suddenly becomes a candidate for emergency surgery.

Immediately after an intravenous dose of heparin, the amount of protamine sulfate required (in milligrams) is equal to 1/100 the last dose of heparin (in units). The biologic half-life of heparin is less than 1 hour. The dose of protamine is reduced if some time has elapsed since the last dose of heparin: in 30 minutes, only about half the amount of protamine is required; in 4–6 hours, there is seldom need for neutralization. Protamine should always be given by slow intravenous injection. Rapid injection may cause thrombocytopenia. If given in excessive amounts, protamine may act as a weak anticoagulant.

During open heart surgery and extracorporeal circulation, large doses of heparin are required to prevent coagulation in the pump oxygenator and the patient's circulatory system; at the end of the procedure, the heparin must be neutralized. The dose of protamine should be based on the amount of heparin

used. Heparin neutralization is not required in some vascular operations if the protamine dosage is calculated and timed so as to lose its effect at the end of the operation.

Coumarin Anticoagulants

Surgery in patients given coumarin derivatives for anticoagulation is relatively safe when the prothrombin time is 25% or greater, or less than 1½ times prolonged. In patients with lower values, prophylactic measures are in order if surgery is necessary. Vitamin K_1, 5 mg orally or parenterally, will return the prothrombin time to safe levels (40% or better) in approximately 4 hours and to normal levels in 24–48 hours. However, its administration may render the patient refractory to all coumarin therapy for a week or more. For immediate, transient (a few hours') restoration of normal prothrombin values, one may infuse 500–1000 mL of plasma. Factors II, VII, IX, and X—the factors lowered by coumarin therapy—are quite stable in banked plasma. Blood products that can be transfused for warfarin reversal include fresh frozen plasma and liquid plasma.

SURGERY IN PATIENTS WITH DISORDERS OF HEMOSTASIS

Platelet Disorders

A. Thrombocytopenia: In general, even major surgery can be performed safely in patients with platelet counts as low as 50,000/µL, especially if they have shown no clinical signs of bleeding (eg, purpura, ecchymoses) before the operation. Occasionally, the spleen must be removed in patients with immune thrombocytopenia or hypersplenism, despite the presence of very low platelet counts. Preoperative platelet transfusions are futile until the splenic pedicle has been clamped. The indications for splenectomy in various hematologic diseases are discussed in Chapter 28.

B. Qualitative Platelet Defects: Aspirin and nonsteroidal anti-inflammatory agents may cause slight prolongation of bleeding time, but this is of no clinical significance in normal persons.

Renal failure is frequently associated with severe platelet dysfunction; patients with bleeding require dialysis to improve platelet function. Desmopressin, 0.3 units/kg, may reverse the defect. Administration of conjugated estrogens, 0.6 mg/kg intravenously daily for 5 days, is also useful.

Surgery in patients with congenital disorders of platelet function requires preoperative platelet transfusions.

Thrombocytopenia with or without abnormal platelet function may develop in patients who have undergone cardiac bypass surgery. Desmopressin, 0.3 units/kg intravenously postbypass, increases von Willebrand factor levels and reduces blood loss in patients undergoing complex cardiac operations. Prophylactic platelet concentrates are not indicated, but if diffuse microvascular oozing occurs at raw wounds, mucosa, and puncture sites, platelet concentrates may be given.

Patients with uremia are often anemic and have platelet dysfunction, with or without mild thrombocytopenia. Consultation is recommended with hematologists or transfusion medicine experts knowledgeable about the use of erythropoietin, estrogens, and platelet transfusion. For major elective surgery with large anticipated blood loss, anemia can be corrected with the preoperative administration of recombinant erythropoietin. In addition, platelet dysfunction should be treated preoperatively with dialysis. Conjugated estrogens, 0.6 mg/kg intravenously daily for 5 days, also improve platelet dysfunction for about 14 days; the mechanism of action is unclear. Mild thrombocytopenia can also occur in patients with uremia, and the platelet count should probably be maintained at 70,000–100,000/μL with platelet transfusions if necessary; the higher level of platelet count may compensate for the partially dysfunctional platelets. Intraoperatively, desmopressin acetate, 0.3 μg/kg administered intravenously, may release factor VIIIR (von Willebrand factor) from the blood vessel wall. The effect occurs within 30 minutes and lasts several hours. One or two doses can be repeated every 12–24 hours. Postoperatively, dialysis is the treatment of choice for uremic platelet dysfunction, when estrogens and desmopressin have been used before and during the procedure.

Bolan CD, Alving BM: Pharmacologic agents in the management of bleeding disorders. Transfusion 1990; 30:541.

Wooley AC: Platelet dysfunction in uremia. The Kidney 1987;19:15.

Coagulation Factors

Patients with hemophilia may have surgery if enough antihemophilic factor (AHF) concentrate is given to bring the preoperative factor VIII level to 75%; most commercial concentrates contain 200–250 AHF units per package. To calculate the amount of AHF required to bring blood levels to 75%, multiply the desired percentage by the normal plasma volume (40 mL/kg). For example, for a 75-kg man, 75% AHF = 75 × 40 = 3000 units, or 12 bottles of 250 AHF units each; the dose is repeated at 12 hours, and half the amount is then given again every 12 hours for 7–10 days.

Nilsson IM et al: The use of blood components in the treatment of congenital coagulation disorders. World J Surg 1987;11:14.

SPECIAL PROBLEMS IN PATIENTS WITH LIVER DISEASE

Bleeding from the gastrointestinal tract in patients with cirrhosis of the liver is not usually due to abnormal coagulation but to esophageal varices, gastritis, or hemorrhoids. Plasma levels of all coagulation factors may be reduced, but rarely to clinically important levels (below 20%). Factor VIII is not lowered by liver disease.

Platelets may be severely reduced, below 30,000/μL, in acute alcoholism and may be responsible for bleeding problems, but they rise spontaneously to normal levels in a few days when alcohol is withdrawn. Moderate thrombocytopenia (50,000–100,000/μL) that does not remit spontaneously may be a sign of hypersplenism secondary to cirrhosis. Platelet dysfunction may occur.

A rare hemorrhagic complication of liver disease is acute generalized oozing. There are three causes: (1) Disseminated intravascular coagulation (DIC), characterized by prolonged PT and thrombin time, greatly prolonged PTT, low plasma fibrinogen, a low platelet count, a poor clot, the presence of fibrin degradation products (FDP), and fibrin monomer. (2) primary fibrinolysis, in which the necrotic liver fails to clear plasminogen activators. In general, platelets and factors V and VIII are less strikingly reduced than in DIC. Elevated levels of FDP are not diagnostic; their clearance may be impaired by severe liver disease without bleeding. (3) acute hemodilution, in which blood loss is replaced by packed red blood cells and saline. Because these patients already have decreased levels of coagulation factor, further hemodilution can result in significant further reduction in coagulation factors.

Clotting factor deficiency resulting from liver damage does not respond to vitamin K even when it is given parenterally in large doses. If fresh frozen plasma (FFP) is used, two to four units are necessary. The peak effect on coagulation times is within 2 hours posttransfusion. PT and PTT should be measured before and within 2 hours post-FFP transfusion. Desmopressin acetate (DDAVP), 0.3 μg/kg, shortens the bleeding time in cirrhotics.

Ratnoff OD: Hemostatic defects in liver and biliary tract disease and disorders of vitamin K metabolism. In: Disorders of Hemostasis. Ratnoff OD,. Forbes CA (editors). Saunders, 1991.

DISSEMINATED INTRAVASCULAR COAGULATION
(Defibrination Syndrome, DIC)

The coagulation mechanism in disseminated intravascular coagulation differs from normal clotting in three principal ways: (1) It is diffuse instead of localized; (2) it damages the site of clotting instead of protecting it; and (3) it consumes enough of some clotting factors that plasma concentrations fall and diffuse bleeding may occur.

Disseminated intravascular coagulation is seen following acute hemolytic transfusion reactions, some types of surgery (particularly involving the lung, brain, or prostate), and certain obstetric catastrophes. It sometimes occurs in patients with malignant tumors (especially of the prostate) and in patients with septicemia. Many patients with severe liver disease have some degree of disseminated intravascular coagulation.

The most common clinical manifestation is diffuse bleeding from many sites at surgery and from needle punctures. Uncontrollable postpartum hemorrhage may be a manifestation. In the laboratory, a combination of reduced platelets on the blood smear and a prolonged prothrombin time is very suggestive. The PTT is greatly prolonged and fibrinogen levels severely decreased, usually well below 75 mg/dL. The thrombin time is prolonged, and fibrin monomer and fibrin degradation fragments are present.

In the differential diagnosis, a prolonged prothrombin time and PTT may be due to vitamin K deficiency, so a trial of vitamin K may be indicated. On rare occasions, circulating anticoagulants and accidental excessive heparin administration may simulate disseminated intravascular coagulation.

When the fibrinogen deficiency is severe, cryoprecipitate must be given. A unit of cryoprecipitate contains about 250 mg of fibrinogen; one unit per 10 kg is usually necessary to correct the defect. Occasionally, platelet transfusions are also necessary. On rare occasions, it may be necessary to use heparin to stop the pathologic clotting. A reduced dose of heparin is used (a loading dose of 5000 units, followed by 7.5 units/kg, by continuous intravenous drip). Hematology consultation should be obtained.

TRANSFUSION OF BLOOD, BLOOD COMPONENTS, & PLASMA SUBSTITUTES

Transfusion of blood, blood components, and plasma substitutes for surgical patients may be required for one or more of the following reasons: (1) to restore and maintain normal blood volume, (2) to correct severe anemia, or (3) to correct bleeding and coagulation disorders. Certain other blood abnormalities such as granulocytopenia or hypoalbuminemia cannot be satisfactorily corrected by blood transfusion.

Decisions about the need for transfusion and selection of the proper type and amount of transfusion material must be based upon careful evaluation of the individual patient. Urgency of need and the availability of diagnostic and therapeutic resources are obvi-

ously the determining factors. Attention must be given to the total clinical picture.

Rossi EC, Simon TL, Moss GS (editors): *Principles of Transfusion Medicine.* Williams & Wilkins, 1991.
Rudowski WJ: Blood transfusions yesterday, today, and tomorrow. World J Surg 1987;11:86.

Prehospital Donation for Autologous Transfusion

Autologous transfusion is the safest transfusion. Patients who should predeposit are those whose arm veins can accommodate a 16-gauge needle, whose hematocrit is above 34%, and who will require transfusion for an elective procedure. The number of units to be predeposited is the number of cross-matched units recommended for the procedure by the maximum surgical blood order schedule. Healthy patients can donate a unit a week starting 5 weeks before surgery if given ferrous sulfate, 325 mg orally three times daily between meals. The longer the donation period, the greater the amount of red blood cell regeneration before surgery.

National Blood Resource Education Program Expert Panel: The use of autologous blood. JAMA 1990;263:414.
Toy PTCY et al: Predeposited autologous blood for elective surgical patients: A National Multicenter Study. N Engl J Med 1987;316:517.

Intraoperative Autotransfusion

Intraoperative autotransfusion may be a valuable adjunct in the management of vascular surgery and major trauma. Several commercially available devices can be used to implement this procedure. Intracavitary blood is incoagulable; it has virtually no fibrinogen; systemic anticoagulation is unnecessary; and emboli should be entirely preventable when the available devices are used properly. Because of the equipment needed, autotransfusions are not really less expensive than bank blood. Washed cell-saver red blood cells contain virtually no platelets or coagulation factors, and the platelet count, PT, and PTT should be monitored.

Autotransfusion then and now. (Editorial.) Lancet 1991; 338:418.
Pittman RD, Inahara T: Eliminating homologous blood transfusions during abdominal aortic aneurysm repair. Am J Surg 1990;159:522.

WHOLE BLOOD

When banked blood is transfused, cells damaged from storage (10% after 2 weeks' storage) are removed within 24 hours, and the remainder survive normally. Whole blood can be stored for up to 35 days and is the product of choice for massive transfusions. The increased content of lactic acid, inorganic phosphate, ammonia, and potassium in stored blood is usually clinically insignificant. Except for patients with severe hepatic or renal impairment, the use of acceptable aged blood imposes no significant metabolic burden on the recipient.

Most coagulation factors are stable in stored blood, but platelets and factors V and VIII deteriorate. Bank blood that has been stored in the refrigerator for more than 2 days is essentially devoid of viable platelets. Massive replacement with this blood (eg, giving 15–20 units in rapid succession) often results in mild thrombocytopenia. Loss of other clotting factors is usually less important. For factor V, only 5–10% of normal levels is adequate for hemostasis; reductions to this level rarely result from multiple transfusions if whole blood is used.

Serologic Considerations (Blood Typing)

A. Emergency Transfusions: In an emergency, type-specific packed red cells or whole blood is the product of choice. The patient's ABO and Rh types can be determined in 5 minutes, and type-specific blood can be issued in 10 minutes. Although O-negative packed red cells can be transfused to any patient, only 6% of the population are O-negative, and this rare universal donor blood should therefore be reserved for critically bleeding patients from whom a blood sample cannot be obtained.

B. Elective Transfusions: When red cell transfusion can be postponed for an hour, maximal compatibility of donor red cells is ensured by performing an antibody screen and cross-match. In the antibody screen, the patient's serum is tested for red cell antibodies other than those in the ABO system. The antibody screen takes about 45 minutes. If the antibody screen is negative, donor red cells are cross-matched with patient serum in 5 minutes, and cross-matched compatible blood can be issued in 10 minutes. In elective surgical patients in whom a type and screen has been performed within the last 48 hours, if the antibody screen is negative, cross-matched blood can be available in 10 minutes.

Amount of Blood for Transfusion

A. Adults: One unit of packed red cells will raise the hemoglobin by 1 g/dL and the hematocrit by 3% in the average adult (70 kg).

B. Children: The amount of whole blood to be given is as follows: Children over 25 kg, 50 mL/kg; children under 25 kg, 20 mL/kg; and premature infants, 10 mL/kg.

Rate of Transfusion

Blood is normally given at a rate of 500 mL in 1½–2 hours. In patients with heart disease, one should allow 2–3 hours for the transfusion. For rapid transfusions in emergencies, it is best to use a 15-gauge plastic cannula and allow the blood to run freely. The use of added pressure to increase flow is dangerous unless it can be applied by gentle compression of collapsible plastic blood containers. Central venous pressure monitoring is a safeguard against overtransfusion; it is a measure of the heart's ability to handle venous return.

Massive Transfusions

Bleeding from one site is usually due to a structural defect and should be corrected by sutures and cautery. Bleeding from multiple sites suggests a hemostatic disorder, which is usually manifested by diffuse microvascular oozing from raw wounds, mucosa, and puncture sites. Development of abnormal bleeding correlates strongly with the duration of hypotension. Primary treatment of coagulopathy due to hypoperfusion is by restoring blood volume.

Platelet concentrates are indicated in patients with diffuse microvascular bleeding and thrombocytopenia. Prophylactic administration of platelet concentrates in the absence of abnormal bleeding is not recommended. Platelet counts rarely fall below 50,000/μL on the basis of hemodilution alone unless 15–20 units have been given.

If diffuse microvascular bleeding occurs and hypofibrinogenemia is present, cryoprecipitate can be given. If hypofibrinogenemia is not present and the PT or PTT is more than 1½ times normal, FFP can be administered. If whole blood is administered in massive transfusion, prophylactic use of FFP is not necessary.

Leslie SD, Toy PTCY: Laboratory hemostatic abnormalities in massively transfused patients given red blood cells and crystalloid. Am J Clin Path 1991;96:770.

Reed LR et al: Prophylactic platelet administration during massive transfusion: A prospective, randomized, double-blind clinical study. Ann Surg 1986;203:40.

Intraoperative Autotransfusion

Intraoperative autotransfusion may be a valuable adjunct in the management of major trauma, intra-abdominal vascular surgery, liver transplantation, and orthopedic surgery. Several commercially available devices can be used to implement this procedure. Intracavitary blood is incoagulable; it has virtually no fibrinogen; systemic anticoagulation is unnecessary; and emboli should be entirely preventable when the available devices are used properly. Because of the equipment needed, autotransfusions are not always less expensive than bank blood.

Williamson KR, Taswell HF: Intraoperative blood salvage: A review. Transfusion 1991;31:662.

Complications of Blood Transfusion

Acute hemolysis due to transfusion of the wrong unit of blood to the wrong patient is the most common cause of immediate deaths due to transfusion. Hepatitis is the most common cause of late deaths.

(1) Hemolytic reactions are a serious complication of blood transfusion. The most severe immediate reactions are due to ABO incompatibility, but serious hemolytic delayed (a week after transfusion) reactions may also be due to antibodies resulting from isoimmunization following previous transfusion or pregnancy. Symptoms may include apprehension, headache, fever, chills, pain at the injection site or in the back, chest, and abdomen, and shock; but in the anesthetized patient, spontaneous bleeding from different areas and changes in vital signs may be the only clinical evidence of transfusion reactions. Posttransfusion blood counts fail to show the anticipated rise in hemoglobin. Free hemoglobin can be detected in the plasma within a few minutes. Hemoglobinuria and oliguria may occur. Exact identification of the offending antibody should be made, and this is usually possible when the Coombs test is positive.

Some studies suggest that osmotic diuretics such as mannitol can prevent renal failure following a hemolytic transfusion reaction. After an apparent reaction and in oliguric patients, a test dose of 12.5 g of mannitol (supplied as 25% solution in 50-mL ampules) is administered intravenously over a period of 3–5 minutes; this dose may be repeated if no signs of circulatory overload develop. A satisfactory urinary output following the use of mannitol is 60 mL/h or more. Mannitol can be safely administered as a continuous intravenous infusion; each liter of 5–10% mannitol should be alternated with 1 L of normal saline to which 40 meq of KCl have been added to prevent serious salt depletion. If oliguria develops despite these efforts, treat as for acute renal failure.

(2) Fever is the most common immediate transfusion reaction and is due chiefly to recipient reaction against white cells in the donor blood. Treatment is with antipyretics. If fever occurs after transfusion of three different units despite pretreatment with antipyretics, leukocyte-poor blood products should be used.

(3) Allergic reactions occur in about 1% of transfusions. They are usually mild and associated with itching, urticaria, and bronchospasm, but they may be severe or even fatal. (The reaction results from an antigen-antibody reaction between a protein in the donor plasma and a corresponding antibody in the patient. Some of these reactions are caused by an antibody to IgA.) If reactions are mild, the transfusion may be cautiously continued. Antihistamines, epinephrine, and corticosteroids may be required.

(4) Too rapid transfusions of large quantities of blood may result in circulatory complications (eg, cardiac or respiratory failure). This is particularly true of elderly or debilitated patients. Careful monitoring should help prevent this complication.

(5) Viral hepatitis C acquired from the donor is the commonest lethal complication of blood transfusion. The risk of contracting hepatitis is unknown but is es-

timated to be 1:3300 per unit. Among patients who develop hepatitis and who survive their primary illness, it is estimated that half develop chronic liver disease. About 10% of those with chronic liver disease develop cirrhosis.

(6) Concern has been expressed about the possibility of contracting AIDS from transfused blood. The risk of HIV infection after 1985, when testing began in the USA, is estimated to be 1:225,000 to 1:60,000.

Contribution of HIV infection to the risk of death from transfusion, expressed in days of life expectancy lost, has become extremely small over the last several years. It is estimated that the risk of HIV infection contributes only 0.1 day of life lost with transfusion of two units of blood in a 50-year-old patient.

(7) Bacterial contamination of blood may occur through improper collection, storage, and administration. Reactions—noted early in the course of transfusions—are serious and may be fatal. Treat as for septic shock. Patients develop fever, chills, and hypotension after the contaminated transfusion.

Carson JL et al: The risks of blood transfusion: The relative influence of acquired immunodeficiency syndrome and non-A, non-B hepatitis. Am J Med 1992;92:45.

Dodd R: The risk of transfusion-transmitted infection. N Engl J Med 1992;327:419.

Seyfried H, Walewska I: Immune hemolytic transfusion reactions. World J Surg 1987;11:25.

PACKED RED BLOOD CELLS

Packed red cells have a storage (shelf) life of 42 days. They are the treatment of choice for anemia without hypovolemia. Most blood transfusions can be given as packed red cells, even in patients with moderate degrees of blood loss, if adequate crystalloid is given concomitantly. A hematocrit of 30% or a hemoglobin concentration of 10 g/dL is considered acceptable in surgical patients. However, lower levels may be acceptable, because renal transplant patients with hematocrit levels in the low 20s undergo surgery safely.

In assessing the need for perioperative red blood cell transfusion, the patient's age, cardiopulmonary status, the hemoglobin concentration, and the amount of anticipated further perioperative blood loss should be considered. In selected patients with little or no further bleeding, a hemoglobin level of 8 g/dL may be adequate.

Anemia does not adversely affect wound healing, provided that peripheral perfusion is maintained by adequate volume replacement. Human and animal studies show that collagen deposition did not correlate with postoperative hematocrit but correlated with oxygen tension in wounds.

Audet AM, Goodnough L: Practice strategies for elective red blood cell transfusion. (Clinical guidelines.) Ann Intern Med 1992;116:403.

Jonsson K et al: Tissue oxygenation, anemia, and perfusion in relation to wound healing in surgical patients. Ann Surg 1991;214:605.

Welch WG, Meehan K, Goodnough L: Prudent strategies for elective red blood cell transfusion. Ann Intern Med 1992;116:393.

Perioperative red cell transfusion. (NIH Consensus Conference.) JAMA 1988;260:2700.

PLATELET TRANSFUSION

The goal of platelet transfusion is to achieve a hemostatic level of platelets in the circulation. Generally, a platelet count of 50,000/µL is adequate for surgical hemostasis. The platelet count should be maintained higher—above 100,000/µL—during the perioperative period of patients undergoing surgery in a critical area (eg, brain, eye, upper airway). Platelet transfusions should be given, when necessary, 4 hours or less before the surgical procedure, and a 10-minute to 1-hour posttransfusion platelet count should be done to document efficacy of the platelet transfusion. The usual adult dose is six units, which should raise the patient's platelet count by approximately 40,000/µL. Absence of a rise in platelet count after platelet transfusion is a serious finding and may be due to alloantibody, autoantibody, posttransfusion purpura, DIC, or other causes of platelet consumption. To determine the reason for refractoriness to platelet transfusion, hematology consultation is recommended.

Platelet transfusion therapy. (NIH Consensus Conference.) JAMA 1987;257:1777.

COAGULATION FACTOR CONCENTRATES

Heated factor VIII concentrates and recombinant factor VIII are the products of choice for patients with severe hemophilia A. Wet heat treatment of factor VIII concentrates inactivates HIV and the hepatitis viruses. However, factor IX concentrates are dry-heated and still transmit hepatitis, may cause thrombosis, and are contraindicated in patients with DIC.

Cryoprecipitate, a concentrate prepared by freeze-thawing the plasma from a single donor, contains 80–120 units of factor VIII, 250 mg of fibrinogen, and an unknown amount of von Willebrand's factor per bag (15–25 mL). It is effective in the treatment of classic hemophilia and von Willebrand's disease and the rare case of fibrinogen deficiency in need of therapy. One unit of the cryoprecipitate for each 6 kg body weight raises the AHF level to 50%—enough for most surgical procedures. For difficult cases, it may have to be

followed by half that amount every 12 hours given as long as necessary. An adequate dose for hypofibrinogenemia is 5 g, or 20 bags.

Fibrin glue is a blood product that has high concentrations of fibrinogen which when mixed with thrombin forms a fibrin clot at the site of bleeding. Fibrin glue is usually made by freeze-thawing of plasma and can be made from the patient's own (autologous) blood donated at least 3 days before surgery. Fibrin glue is a useful operative sealant in a variety of procedures, including cardiovascular surgery (mediastinal spray application, sealing of vascular anastomoses and prostheses), thoracic surgery (treatment of bronchopleural fistula), trauma management (repair of liver or splenic injury), transplantation procedures (transplant of partial hepatectomy specimen), plastic repair (skin grafts), central nervous system repair (repair of dural or peripheral nerve injury, pituitary tumor removal), and orthopedic operations (repair of osteochondral fracture or of the Achilles tendon). Fibrin glue has achieved hemostasis in a few patients with coagulation disorders. In patients with coagulopathy due to multiple coagulation deficiency, fibrin glue was effective in controlling liver hemorrhage and bleeding from splenorrhaphy. Unless fibrin glue is made from the patient's own blood, it carries the same risks of viral transmission as are associated with administration of other blood products.

Gibble JW, Ness PM: Fibrin glue: The perfect operative sealant? Transfusion 1990;8:741.

Lusher JM et al: Recombinant factor VIII for the treatment of previously untreated patients with hemophilia A. N Engl J Med 1993;328:453.

Pierce GF et al: The use of purified clotting factor concentrates in hemophilia. JAMA 1989;261:3434.

PLASMA

The proper use of plasma is confined to the management of certain coagulation problems. Indications for use of fresh-frozen plasma include the following:

(1) For patients in whom the effects of warfarin must be reversed rapidly. Immediate hemostasis can be achieved in patients receiving anticoagulant therapy who are actively bleeding or who require emergency surgery.

(2) As an adjunct to massive blood transfusions when only packed red cells are available. Bleeding in patients whose entire blood volume has been replaced over a few hours can be due to thrombocytopenia or depletion of coagulation factors, and when a factor deficiency occurs, as demonstrated by a greater than 1½ times prolonged prothrombin time or PTT, fresh-frozen plasma can be used for correction.

(3) In surgical patients with liver disease who still have abnormal prothrombin times after administra-

tion of vitamin K, fresh-frozen plasma may be given, although it often fails to correct the abnormality.

(4) In patients requiring replacement of specific factors such as antithrombin III, factor XI, or factor XIII, and in the management of thrombotic thrombocytopenic purpura.

There is no justification for the use of fresh-frozen plasma as a volume expander or as a nutritional source, because safer and cheaper alternatives exist. For volume expansion, crystalloid solutions are preferable to fresh-frozen plasma.

Fresh frozen plasma. (NIH Consensus Conference.) JAMA 1985;253:551.

BLOOD SUBSTITUTES

Artificial Colloids

Artificial colloids (dextran, gelatin, hetastarch [hydroxyethyl starch]) are inexpensive, effective plasma expanders without infectious risks. They have been used extensively in Europe. Their infrequent use in the USA has been due to the anaphylactoid/anaphylactic reactions of all these colloids, the antithrombotic effect of the dextrans, and the unknown long-term effects of hetastarch, which remains in the reticuloendothelial system. Recently, hetastarch was found to be a cheaper and safe alternative to albumin in abdominal aortic aneurysm surgery.

Gold MS et al: Comparison of hetastarch to albumin for perioperative bleeding in patients undergoing abdominal aortic aneurysm surgery: A prospective, randomized study. Ann Surg 1990;211:482.

Electrolyte Solutions

Experimental and clinical studies have shown that substantial blood losses can be effectively replaced with balanced salt solutions. With careful monitoring of central venous pressure, vital signs, urinary output, and serum electrolyte determinations, specific fluid and electrolyte abnormalities may be corrected and normal blood volume maintained. The volume of normal salt replacement solutions used must be 2–3 times the volume lost.

Future Blood Substitutes

Red cell substitutes are not yet available, but research is being performed on hemoglobin solutions, encapsulated hemoglobins, and perfluorocarbons. It is unlikely that synthetic products will replace the use of donor red cells or platelets in the foreseeable future.

Looker D et al: Human recombinant haemoglobin designed for use as a blood substitute. Nature 1992;356:258.
Urbaniak SJ: Artificial blood. Br Med J 1991;303:1348.

PREGNANCY & THE SURGICAL PATIENT

Edward C. Hill, MD

The incidence of surgical illness is the same in pregnant women as in nonpregnant women of the same age group, ranging from 1:500 to 1:50 gestations. Pregnancy may alter or mask the signs and symptoms of the disease, so that recognition is more difficult. Furthermore, the fetus must be considered in planning a surgical procedure, and pregnancy may modify the timing of a semielective operation or the surgical approach of an emergency abdominal procedure. Purely elective surgery should be deferred until the postpartum period. Any major operation represents a risk not only to the mother but to the fetus as well. Although there is no firm evidence that congenital anomalies are induced in the developing fetus by anesthesia, semielective procedures should be deferred until the second trimester of pregnancy, exercising the greatest precautions to prevent hypoxia and hypotension.

Despite these measures, prematurity and intrauterine growth retardation rates are increased in fetuses whose mothers have had nonobstetric surgery during pregnancy. The illness requiring the operation may be a factor as well.

Diagnostic radiologic examinations of the lower abdomen and pelvis should be avoided during pregnancy, if possible, especially during the first 6 weeks of gestation, when the fetus is particularly susceptible to irradiation. There is statistical evidence that mothers of leukemic children had a higher incidence of abdominal radiologic studies during pregnancy. Radioactive isotopes pose a particular hazard to the fetus when they are used in the pregnant patient. Radioactive iodine or pertechnetate for thyroid scanning and bone scanning with radioactive strontium or calcium are contraindicated because these agents cross the placenta and are taken up by the fetal tissues. Sonography and MRI have proved to be useful diagnostic alternatives in many circumstances. The use of MRI should be limited to circumstances in which sonography is inadequate. These two techniques are considered safe for use during pregnancy.

The following surgical problems that may occur in pregnant women are discussed briefly in the following paragraphs: acute appendicitis, cholecystitis and cholelithiasis, intestinal obstruction, hernias, breast cancer, and ovarian tumors.

Doll DC, Ringenberg QS, Yarbro JW: Management of cancer during pregnancy. Arch Intern Med 1988;148:2058.
Hunt MJ et al: Perinatal aspects of abdominal surgery for non-obstetric disease. Am J Perinatol 1989;6:412.

James FM 3rd: Anesthesia for nonobstetric surgery during pregnancy. Clin Obstet Gynecol 1987;30:621.

Kammerer WS: Nonobstetric surgery in pregnancy. Med Clin North Am 1987;71:551.

Mazze RI. Källén B: Reproductive outcome after anesthesia and operation during pregnancy: A registry study of 5,405 cases. Am J Obstet Gynecol 1989;161:1178.

Appendicitis

Acute appendicitis occurs about once in every 2000 pregnancies. The signs and symptoms are the same as those that occur in nonpregnant women, but they may be considerably modified. Because of the nausea and vomiting and lower abdominal discomfort that are seen frequently in the first and second trimesters of normal pregnancy, as well as the moderate leukocytosis and elevated sedimentation rate, errors in diagnosis are more frequently made. The differential diagnosis includes ectopic pregnancy, ruptured corpus luteum cyst, adnexal torsion, round ligament syndrome, degenerating myoma, cholecystitis, and pyelonephritis. Moreover, the enlarging uterus often carries the appendix higher in the abdomen, so that McBurney's point can no longer be used as a point of reference, and maximal tenderness is proportionately higher. For the same reason, the presence of the gravid uterus may effectively block off the omentum and loops of small intestine and thus hinder the walling-off process, particularly in the third trimester. Therefore, rupture of the appendix is more often associated with widespread dissemination of infection, generalized peritonitis, and a high death rate. If an abscess does form following perforation, the gravid uterus forms the medial wall of the abscess. The intense inflammatory process often initiates uterine contractions, with premature labor and the loss of the fetus. With evacuation, there is a sudden reduction in the size of the uterus; the abscess then ruptures into the free peritoneal cavity.

Because of the flaccidity of the anterior abdominal wall in the last trimester, there may be relatively little rigidity associated with inflammation of the appendix, and rebound tenderness may be hard to define, so that one cannot rely upon these physical findings. Adler's sign may be helpful. The pain is located while the patient is in the supine position. If the pain shifts to the left when she turns on her left side, the cause may be uterine or adnexal. If the pain remains in the same location, appendicitis should be suspected. A positive Bryan sign, indicative of acute appendicitis, is exacerbation of pain when the uterus is shifted to the right side. Ultrasonographic imaging of the appendix may be useful in confirming the diagnosis.

The treatment of acute appendicitis during pregnancy is immediate operation. Because of the extreme seriousness of perforation when it occurs, it is better to remove a normal appendix when the diagnosis is in doubt than to wait for typical signs or symptoms and risk the consequences. Perforation of the appendix is seen most commonly in the third trimester and is often associated with a delay in performing laparotomy. If generalized peritonitis exists, it is probably best to deliver the baby by cesarean section as the incidence of premature labor is high and fetal death in utero due to bacterial toxemia is not uncommon.

Regional anesthesia is preferred, and the transverse or oblique muscle-splitting incision should be placed somewhat higher than in the nonpregnant individual. In fact, late in the third trimester the appendix may be in the right upper quadrant of the abdomen, and a right paramedian incision is more appropriate. Although premature labor is not common following an uncomplicated appendectomy, when the operation is performed after 23 weeks of gestation the risk of delivery within a week of operation is increased. There is no further increase in this risk if the pregnancy continues beyond 1 week.

Appendicitis in pregnancy. (Editorial.) Lancet 1986;1:195.

Blaakaer J et al: Abruptio placentae as complication to acute appendicitis. Int J Gynaecol Obstet 1989;29:179.

Brennan DF, Harwood-Nuss AL: Postpartum abdominal pain. Ann Emerg Med 1989;18:83.

Dornhoffer JL, Calkins JW: Appendicitis complicating pregnancy. Kans Med 1988;89:139.

Masse RI, Källé B: Appendectomy during pregnancy: A Swedish Registry study of 778 cases. Obstet Gynecol 1991;77:835.

Richards C, Daya S: Diagnosis of acute appendicitis in pregnancy. Can J Surg 1989;32:358.

Schwerk WB et al: Ultrasonography in the diagnosis of acute appendicitis: A prospective study. Gastroenterology 1989;97:630.

Cholecystitis & Cholelithiasis

Acute cholecystitis in pregnancy occurs less often than acute appendicitis, the prevalence being about one in 3500–6500 pregnancies. It is associated with gallstones in 50% of cases.

The symptoms are the same as in the nonpregnant patient, with an abrupt onset of colicky right upper quadrant abdominal pain radiating to the right scapula, low-grade fever, and nausea and vomiting. Cholecystitis may be difficult to distinguish from acute appendicitis, with the high position of the appendix associated with the third trimester of pregnancy. Ultrasound may be helpful in making the diagnosis.

Unlike appendicitis, however, acute cholecystitis in the first trimester of pregnancy is best managed conservatively, with hospitalization, parenteral fluids, nasogastric suction, antispasmodics, analgesics, and broad-spectrum antibiotics. In three out of four patients thus treated, there will be a definite improvement within 2 days, and a definitive surgical procedure can be deferred until the second trimester or the postpartum period. Surgery should be done whenever there is doubt regarding the differentiation from acute appendicitis or if there is no response to conservative therapy as manifested by an enlarging mass (empyema), jaundice (common duct obstruction), evidence of rupture, or associated pancreatitis. Gallstone-induced pancreatitis increases both fetal and maternal death rates. Cholecystectomy is the procedure of choice, but cholecystostomy may be performed if technical difficulties warrant it, the excision of the gallbladder being delayed until the puerperium.

DeVore GR: Acute abdominal pain in the pregnant patient due to pancreatitis, acute appendicitis, cholecystitis or peptic ulcer disease. Clin Perinatol 1980;7:349.

Dixon NP, Faddis DM, Silberman H: Aggressive management of cholecystitis during pregnancy. Am J Surg 1987;154:292.

Landers D et al: Acute cholecystitis in pregnancy. Obstet Gynecol 1987;69:131.

Intestinal Obstruction

Intestinal obstruction occurs infrequently during pregnancy, but it should be considered in the differential diagnosis of any pregnant patient with an abdominal scar who develops abdominal pain and vomiting. Adhesive bands are the most common cause of intestinal obstruction, and displacement of the intestine is most likely to occur when uterine growth carries the pregnancy into the abdomen around the fourth or fifth month of gestation; near term, when lightening occurs; or postpartum, with sudden reduction in the size of the uterus. The most frequent causes of postoperative adhesions are appendectomies and gynecologic operations. Other causes of intestinal obstruction during pregnancy are volvulus, intussusception, and large bowel cancer.

The symptoms and signs of intestinal obstruction are the same as those that occur in the nonpregnant woman, although the clinical picture may be obscured by the nausea and vomiting of early pregnancy, round ligament pain, and the abdominal distention already produced by the pregnancy. X-ray examination of the abdomen may be diagnostic and must be obtained.

When operation is indicated, it should be performed without delay, and the pregnancy should be a secondary consideration. Near term, a cesarean section may be required to obtain necessary exposure.

Hernias

Hiatal hernia is common during pregnancy; perhaps 15–20% of pregnant women develop this condition as a result of pressure against the stomach by the enlarging uterus. The principal symptom is reflux esophagitis with severe heartburn, aggravated by recumbency or ingestion of a large meal and relieved by an upright position or antacids. Very rarely, hematemesis may result from ulceration of the esophageal mucosa.

Elevation of the upper half of the body while reclining; frequent small meals; and antacids given liberally are usually effective treatment. Most hiatal hernias disappear following the pregnancy. Surgical correction is required only for those that persist and remain symptomatic.

Umbilical, inguinal, and ventral hernias usually are unaffected by pregnancy. Repair can be carried out electively after delivery. Surgery during pregnancy is indicated only in the rare event of an incarcerated or strangulated hernia.

Kurzel RB, Naunheim KS, Schwartz RA: Repair of symptomatic diaphragmatic hernia during pregnancy. Obstet Gynecol 1988;71:869.

Cancer of the Breast

Cancer of the breast occurs infrequently during pregnancy, complicating one in 3000 pregnancies. The breast changes that occur during gestation make detection of early breast carcinoma much more difficult. As there is considerable delay in diagnosis, most cases are advanced by the time the diagnosis is made. Fine-needle aspiration will serve to distinguish cysts and galactoceles from solid tumors and may be diagnostic of cancer. Mammography is not very helpful during pregnancy, because of the increased radiographic density of the breast. Biopsy and appropriate surgical treatment should be undertaken as soon as the cancer is suspected. If the cancer is confined to the breast, the prognosis is good; if the axillary nodes are involved, the outlook is poor. Breast cancer has no direct effect on the fetus, though metastases to the placenta have been reported.

The overall cure rate for breast cancer developing during pregnancy or lactation is significantly lower than that of nonpregnant women of comparable age, primarily because of delay in diagnosis, resulting in more advanced disease. Cure rates of 90% have been achieved in pregnant patients with stage I disease.

Therapeutic abortion is not indicated in the patient with localized disease of a favorable microscopic type. Interruption of an early pregnancy as part of estrogen ablation may be of some palliative benefit to the woman with advanced disease, but if the pregnancy has progressed beyond the 20th week, the life of the fetus should take precedence.

Pregnancies subsequent to treatment of breast carcinoma are best deferred for 3–5 years, after the period of greatest risk of recurrence is past.

Donegan WL: Cancer and pregnancy. CA 1983;33:194.

Finley JL, Silverman JF, Lannin DR: Fine-needle aspiration cytology of breast masses in pregnant and lactating women. Diagn Cytopathol 1989;5:255.

Greene FL: Gestational breast cancer: A ten-year experience. South Med J 1988;81:1509.

Gallenberg MM, Loprinzi CL: Breast cancer and pregnancy. Semin Oncol 1989;16:369.

Parente JT et al: Breast cancer associated with pregnancy. Obstet Gynecol 1988;71(Part 1):861.

Tretli S et al: Survival of breast cancer patients diagnosed during pregnancy or lactation. Br J Cancer 1988;58:382.

Ovarian Tumors

A cystic corpus luteum is the most frequent cause of ovarian enlargement during pregnancy. This structure rarely exceeds 6 cm in diameter and gradually diminishes in size as the pregnancy progresses. It is usually asymptomatic, and only careful observation is required to distinguish it from a proliferative type of cystic enlargement.

True ovarian neoplasms are encountered in 1:1000 pregnancies, the majority being detected during the first trimester. Some are not found until the immediate postpartum period, when the uterine size no longer masks their presence and the abdominal wall is flaccid. Most ovarian neoplasms are cystic; solid tumors are quite rare. Frequently, they are silent, producing few symptoms unless there is hemorrhage into the tumor, rupture of the cyst, or torsion of the pedicle—complications that are definitely increased during pregnancy (see Chapter 42).

The cystic neoplasms most often seen during pregnancy are benign cystic teratomas (about 40% are of this variety), serous and mucinous cystadenomas, and endometrial cysts. Dysgerminoma is the most frequently encountered solid tumor. Malignant ovarian neoplasms rarely complicate pregnancy, occurring in one in 9000–25,000 pregnancies. Serous and mucinous cystadenocarcinomas and endometrioid carcinomas are the most common histologic types.

Because of the danger of inducing an abortion during the first trimester, surgical removal of a suspected true neoplasm should be deferred until the fourth month of gestation except in the event of an acute abdominal emergency caused by torsion, rupture, or hemorrhage. When a neoplasm is discovered during the immediate postpartum period, removal should be done as soon as possible to avoid the complications of infection, hemorrhage, rupture, and torsion.

Jolles CJ: Gynecologic cancer associated with pregnancy. Semin Oncol 1989;16:417.

Schwartz RP et al: Endodermal sinus tumor in pregnancy: Report of a case and review of the literature. Gynecol Oncol 1983;15:434.

MANAGEMENT OF THE OLDER SURGICAL PATIENT

Edmund T. Lonergan, MD

Advances in perioperative management have made surgery available for a growing number of persons 65 years of age and older, and recent figures show more than 600,000 operations in the USA on geriatric patients each year. Despite a 50% improvement in surgical mortality for this population since the 1960s, older patients constitute about 70% of postoperative deaths and complications. Diminished physiologic reserves associated with aging may contribute to complications, but most of the increased risk is due to chronic illness.

Older patients should undergo the same preoperative and postoperative evaluations as younger adults, but a number of other factors also should receive attention, including (1) age-related changes in organ function, (2) functional status, and (3) special problems of the aged.

AGE-RELATED CHANGES IN ORGAN FUNCTION

The most important of these are summarized in Table 5–2. As a rule, organ function decreases with aging, though it usually remains adequate to meet the stress of surgery, and age, as such, is rarely a contraindication to surgical procedures.

A. Pulmonary Function: Decreased pulmonary function due to aging should pose no risk to surgical candidates who are otherwise free of pulmonary disease. However, diminished pulmonary reserve may exaggerate conditions that would be better tolerated by younger patients, with attendant risk of postoperative hypoxia, atelectasis, and pneumonia. Pain, oversedation, infection, and intrathoracic or upper abdominal surgical procedures may increase this risk. The following guidelines are helpful in managing the pulmonary problems of older surgical patients.

1. Pulmonary function tests should be considered before surgery in older patients, and a complete pulmonary function evaluation should be performed in any older patient whose history (chronic cough, dyspnea on exertion, chronic exposure to tobacco) suggests pulmonary disease. COPD and preoperative respiratory infection, however minor, increase the risk of postoperative pulmonary failure. At highest risk are patients with an arterial PCO_2 of more than 50 mm Hg 50, or FEV_1/FVC (1 second timed vital capacity/forced vital capacity) ratio of less than 0.5.

2. Postoperative confusion in a geriatric patient should stimulate a search for hypoxia or hypercapnia and correction of the cause (eg, infection, atelectasis, oversedation, pulmonary embolus, bronchial plugging).

3. To improve bronchial toilet, cigarette smoking should be stopped 6 weeks or more before elective surgery. Lesser periods not only have no value but paradoxically, may even increase susceptibility to complications. Treatment of bronchial constriction and infection with bronchodilators and antibiotics will improve pulmonary function in patients with COPD, and inhalation of humidified gases and chest physiotherapy (including blow-bottles) will reduce

Table 5–2. Age-related changes in selected organ systems.

Organ System	Change With Age	Potential Clinical Consequences
Pulmonary	Decreased compliance of thorax. Increase in dead space, residual volume, closing volume (>age 45). FEV_1 decreases by 10 mL/yr >age 30.	Increased alveolar-arterial PO_2 gradient; increased vulnerability to hypoxia. Decreased clearance of secretions.
Cardiovascular	Decreased sinus node P cells; decreased cells in AV node, bundle of His, Purkinje network. Decreased response to catecholamines; blunted baroreceptor activity (especially >age 75). Increased rigidity of arterial tree; decreased LV compliance.	Increased risk of arrhythmias. Increased vulnerability to volume loss, postural hypotension. Diminished response to volume overload.
Renal	≥30% decrease in GFR (note exceptions). Decreased ability to concentrate or dilute urine. Decreased formation of NH_4^+. Decreased renin response to volume loss.	Increased risk of renal failure. Decreased excretion of some drugs. Increased vulnerability to dehydration and to overhydration. Decreased defense against acidosis. Increased vulnerability to volume depletion.
Central nervous system	Decreased cerebral blood flow autoregulation >age 65. Decreased acetylcholine stores (especially Alzheimer's disease).	Increased vulnerability to cerebral ischemia with hypotension. Increased risk of confusion with anticholinergic drugs.

the risk of pulmonary insufficiency. Patients receiving supplemental oxygen (Ventimask; nasal prongs) for hypoxia may require endotracheal intubation if CO_2 retention occurs.

B. Cardiovascular Function: (Table 5–2.) In healthy older persons, cardiac output rises in response to exercise well into the ninth decade. Since the maximal heart rate is diminished in the aged (220 – Age) and increased cardiac output depends upon stroke volume, cardiac performance is vulnerable to volume depletion (hemorrhage, dehydration, excessive diuresis).

Diminished sinus node activity and loss of cardiac conducting tissue increase the likelihood of arrhythmias. Decreased responsiveness to catecholamines, heightened vascular resistance, and reduced left ventricular compliance may limit the ability of the aging cardiovascular system to cope with stress. Blunted baroreceptor reflexes increase the risk of postural hypotension, especially during ambulation shortly after surgery.

Older patients have less tolerance of depletion or expansion of intravascular volume, so they must be monitored closely for hypotension or pulmonary edema.

A history of myocardial infarction or angina is a major risk factor. Postoperative myocardial infarction has a mortality rate of 50% and occurs in 30% of operated patients following a fresh infarct—down to 6% after 6 months. The prevalence of arteriosclerotic heart disease (often asymptomatic) in men aged 60 or older is about 20%, rising to 40% after age 80.

Arrhythmias, heart failure, myocardial ischemia (often asymptomatic) and infarction, and thromboembolism are the most serious cardiovascular problems in older patients.

1. In addition to the classic findings, cardiac problems in the aged may be manifested as acute confusion, weakness and hypotension, severe fatigue, dyspnea, neurologic changes, arrhythmias, and pulmonary edema. Any of these states should be investigated (eg, by CK, serial ECGs, isotope studies) as possible signs of myocardial ischemia. The hours immediately after surgery are especially dangerous for patients with ischemic heart disease, and during this time the patient should be monitored with great care for pain, hypoxia, hypotension, and other conditions that may increase cardiac work.

2. The risk of postoperative cardiac failure is increased in the presence of an S_3 gallop or distended external jugular veins, a heart rate of less than 100/min after 2 minutes of bicycle exercise in the supine position, or the presence of ischemic changes (which may occur in the absence of symptoms) on the ECG in the immediate postoperative period.

3. Patients at increased risk for postural hypotension often have elevated systolic blood pressures and may be identified by a drop of 20 mm Hg or more in systolic pressure after 2–3 minutes in the upright position following a 5-minute period in the supine position. If postural hypotension is detected, ambulation should be allowed with caution. Volume status and hypotensive drugs must be attended to in the immediate postoperative period.

4. Control of hypertension, arrhythmias, angina, and cardiac failure will reduce perioperative mortality and morbidity in older patients. Unless contraindicated, cardiac medications should be continued until the morning of surgery. Monitoring of cardiovascular status following surgery (eg, blood gases, Swan-Ganz line, ECGs) is often necessary and should be instituted earlier for suspected cardiac embarrassment in patients age 65 and above.

5. Good management of pain decreases catecholamine release and arrhythmias, but it is equally important to guard against oversedation and hypoxia.

6. Early ambulation of older patients protects them against deconditioning, and together with low-dose heparin prophylaxis (5000 units every 8–12 hours) reduces the frequency of thromboembolism.

C. Renal Function: (Table 5–2.) Most persons experience a decline in glomerular filtration rate (GFR) of at least 30% by the eighth decade, although one-third of older persons who are free of renal and cardiovascular disease have a well-preserved GFR, as reflected by serial creatinine clearances. A reduction in GFR and renal blood flow may predispose geriatric patients to postoperative renal failure and toxicity from drugs cleared by the kidney. Impaired thirst perception, decreased urine concentration, and reduced renin response to volume contraction weaken the older patient's defense against hypotension when challenged by hemorrhage, nasogastric drainage, third-space sequestration of fluid, or dehydration.

Decreased dilutional capacity may lead to overhydration and hyponatremia after vigorous fluid administration, with serious cardiovascular (pulmonary edema) or central nervous system (cerebral edema) complications. Reduced NH_4^+ secretion impairs the aged patient's ability to correct acidosis.

A history of renal disease is present in a minority of patients who develop postoperative renal failure; detection of subclinical renal insufficiency in older surgical candidates is an important priority to protect them against this potentially catastrophic event (mortality rate about 60%).

1. Because muscle mass and creatinine production are much less in many older patients, serum creatinine levels may be normal despite a 60% or more decline in GFR. Nomograms and formulas that estimate creatinine clearance without the need for urine collections have proved unreliable. Therefore, if incipient renal failure is suspected, a 12- to 24-hour creatinine clearance determination should be obtained before nonemergent surgery.

2. A 50% or more reduction in GFR (< 50–60 mL/min) reflects in increased risk of postoperative renal failure. Operations lasting more than 3 hours or involving clamping of the aorta above the renal arteries are extra risk factors.

3. Avoiding volume depletion or overhydration, limiting the use of nephrotoxic drugs or drugs cleared by the kidney, monitoring acid-base status and urine output, and maintaining urine volume at 1 mL/min all help minimize renal complications postoperatively.

D. Central Nervous System Function: The aged brain (Table 5–2) has a diminished ability to maintain cerebral blood flow during hypotension and a decreased acetylcholine content in many areas of the cerebrum and associated structures.

1. Because autoregulatory control of cerebral blood flow is impaired in older patients, signs of cerebral ischemia may appear when mean arterial pressure (MAP = 0.33 × [systolic blood pressure – diastolic blood pressure] + diastolic blood pressure) falls below 80 mm Hg. Geriatric surgical patients whose systolic blood pressure is 105 mm Hg or less should be closely monitored for cognitive impairment or confusion, and corrective action should be taken as appropriate (eg, decrease vasodilator therapy, improve volume status).

2. The risk of bladder obstruction in older men with enlarged prostates who receive anticholinergic drugs (eg, diphenhydramine, some antidepressants, opioids) is well known, but these drugs may also lead to acute confusion in the elderly (especially those with Alzheimer's disease) as a consequence of age-related depletion of acetylcholine in the cerebrum and elsewhere in the central nervous system. Postoperatively, older patients receiving anticholinergics should be examined for acute confusion, and these drugs should be used only when absolutely required.

FUNCTIONAL STATUS OF OLDER PATIENTS

About 23% of older persons are unable to perform one or more activities of daily living (ADLs) (Table 5–3). This is true for only 7% of those under age 74, but the percentage rises to 50% or more after age 85.

Pre- and postoperative evaluation of persons age 65 and older should include attention to ADLs; rehabilitation therapy and appropriate support (eg, home care, visiting nurse) should be provided when patients are deficient in one or more activities of self-care. For example, an older patient who is unable to move from bed to chair after successful surgery may have to be rehospitalized or admitted to a nursing home if the disability is not corrected or no provision is made to assist the family or the patient's aged spouse with the necessary care.

SPECIAL PROBLEMS OF OLDER PATIENTS
(Table 5–4)

Altered Drug Disposition

Changes in body composition, renal function, hepatic function, and nutritional status may lead to in-

Table 5–3. Activities of daily living.

Bathing
Feeding oneself
Dressing
Grooming
Being continent of stool and urine
Transferring from bed to chair
Going to the toilet

Table 5–4. Special problems of older patients.

Decreased drug metabolism and elimination
Delirium
Falls
Pressure sores
Infection

creased risks when older surgical patients receive drugs.

A. Changes in Body Composition: Increased fat and decreased muscle mass in old age result in diminished total body water and a contracted volume of distribution for water-soluble drugs such as nitrates, aminoglycosides, and some antihypertensive agents. To avoid overdosing with water-soluble drugs, therapy should begin at the low end of the dosage scale, with regular monitoring of drug levels in older subjects.

B. Diminished Renal Function: Diminished renal function is common in old age, and unless this is borne in mind patients may receive excessive doses of nephrotoxic agents (eg, nonsteroidal anti-inflammatory agents, aminoglycosides) or drugs cleared by the kidney (eg, digoxin, some calcium channel blockers) that accumulate and cause side effects.

C. Decreased Liver Function: Hepatic mass and function decline by about 30% by the eighth decade. This poses little danger unless it is exacerbated by decreased blood flow (hypotension, volume contraction) or by drugs that inhibit hepatic enzymes (eg, cimetidine) or that reduce liver blood flow (eg, cimetidine, propranolol). In such cases, there is a risk of toxicity from drugs (eg, nitrates, propranolol, morphine) cleared by rapid hepatic inactivation.

D. Malnutrition: Malnutrition is present in 20% of hospitalized older patients, and decreased serum albumin levels associated with malnutrition (or with acute phase reactions to infection) may lead to an increase in the free serum levels of drugs that are highly protein-bound (eg, quinidine, warfarin, rifampin, propranolol), with attendant risks of toxicity. Patients with hypoalbuminemia who receive such drugs should be monitored closely for toxic side effects.

Delirium

Postoperative confusion and delirium are common in the aged and occur more often among patients with diminished cognition. Delirium carries a poor prognosis in older patients. Although it is often self-limited, all patients with delirium should be examined for reversible causes (oversedation, hypoxia, infection, pain, decreased cardiac output, anticholinergic drugs). Low-dose haloperidol (0.5 mg every 8–12 hours) may be useful for severe agitation, but on occasion it will increase confusion in cognitively impaired patients.

Falls

One-third of the geriatric population experience a fall at least once each year, with a resulting one million fractures. Weakness, hypotension, deconditioning, and pain on movement may increase the risk of falling among older postoperative patients. Surgical candidates should be questioned closely for a history of falls (a predictor of subsequent falls); the blood pressure should be taken while standing in all subjects aged 75 or older (to detect positional hypotension); and patients should be examined for postural defects, awkwardness on arising from a chair, and ataxic gait.

Pressure Sores
(See also Chapter 44.)

Immobilization, urinary and fecal incontinence, and malnutrition expose aged patients to the development of pressure sores. Patients with predisposing factors should have daily inspection of pressure points for evidence of early skin ischemia (blanching erythema), stage I pressure sores (nonblanching erythema; shallow ulcers), or more extensive dermal defects. Patients at high risk should be protected by being kept dry, by frequent turning to relieve skin pressure, and by the use of air or foam mattresses. Treatment of skin ulcers involves wet-to-dry dressings to remove dead tissue, protective coverings, and surgical debridement and skin grafting for advanced lesions.

Infection

Patients of advanced age who are infected in the perioperative period may have atypical or nonspecific manifestations, including failure to develop elevated core temperatures. Often, the presenting picture is one of slowness to recover function after surgery, cognitive impairment, or persistent weakness. If infection is suspected, the triad of fever, leukocytosis, and elevated band count strongly support the diagnosis of bacterial invasion, and the absence of these indicators is good evidence against infection.

Gerson MC et al: Prediction of cardiac and pulmonary complications related to elective abdominal and noncardiac thoracic surgery in geriatric patients. Am J Med 1990; 88:101.

Gustafson Y et al: A geriatric-anesthesiologic program to reduce acute confusional states in elderly patients treated for femoral neck fracture. J Am Geriatric Soc 1991;39: 655.

Koruda MJ, Sheldon GF: Surgery in the aged. Adv Surg 1991;24:293.

Lipowski ZJ: Delirium in the elderly patient. N Engl J Med 1989;320:578.

Lonergan ET (editor): *Extending Life, Enhancing Life. A National Research Agenda on Aging.* National Academy Press, 1991.

Lonergan ET, Schmucker D: Drug therapy in older patients.

In: Katzung BG (editor). *Drug Therapy*. Appleton & Lange, 1991.

Macpherson DS, Snow R, Lofgren RP: Preoperative screening: value of previous tests. Ann Intern Med 1990; 113:969.

Mangano DT et al: Association of perioperative myocardial ischemia with cardiac morbidity and mortality in men undergoing noncardiac surgery. N Engl J Med 1990;323: 1781.

Manning FC: Preoperative management of the elderly patient. Am Fam Phys 1989;39:123.

Merrill WH et al: Cardiac surgery in patients age 80 years or older. Ann Surg 1990;211:772.

Ramanathan KB et al: Interactive effects of age and other risk factors on long-term survival after coronary artery surgery. Am J Cardiol 1990;15:1493.

Rorbackmadsen M et al: General surgery in patients 80 years and older. Br J Surg 1992;79:1216.

Suter-Gut D et al: Post-discharge care planning and rehabilitation of the elderly surgical patient. Clin Geriatr Med 1990;6:669.

Tinetti M et al: Risk factors for falls among elderly persons living in the community. N Engl J Med 1988;319:1701.

Wasserman M et al: Utility of fever, white blood cells, and differential count in predicting bacterial infections in the elderly. J Am Geriatr Soc 1989;37:537.

Legal Medicine for the Surgeon

6

Jack Nagan, JD

Surgery entails risks. The surgeon recognizes that a good outcome is never certain, even in the most skilled hands, but this is not always appreciated by patients. Bad results, whether real or perceived, generate malpractice litigation against 40% of all physicians in the USA at some point during their careers. Many others serve as expert witnesses or peer reviewers. Consequently, most physicians eventually become involved in legal proceedings developed to determine medical liability. To reduce the chances of being sued, to increase the chances of successfully defending a lawsuit, and to maximize the effectiveness of one's efforts, all physicians should understand the legal principles of medical practice. This chapter is intended to sharpen awareness of those principles, to be supplemented by advice from legal counsel as the need arises.

OVERVIEW: CIVIL & CRIMINAL LAW

There are two kinds of law: civil and criminal. Medical malpractice belongs in the former category. When lay people discuss medical negligence, however, the two areas are often confused. For example, one is not *guilty* of negligence but *liable for* negligence; guilt is a criminal finding, and negligence is a civil wrong. Other essential distinctions between civil and criminal law should also be kept in mind. For example, the party who brings the complaint is always the *plaintiff*, but the civil complainant is a person or entity seeking redress for a personal injury whereas in criminal law the people bring the action against the defendant. That is why criminal cases bear titles such as *People versus Smith* and civil cases *Jones versus Smith*. The victim in a criminal case is said to be the state–ie, even though a particular individual may have been murdered or raped, the crime is, in theory, one against society.

The purpose of the criminal suit is punishment and deterrence of crime; the object of civil litigation is generally to remedy a wrong so as to place the plaintiff in the same position he or she would have occupied if the wrong had not occurred. The idea is to make the plaintiff whole. Thus, civil redress is usually seen in terms of compensation, although there are certain narrowly restricted situations in which

punishment is allowed in the form of exemplary damages (discussed below).

The scale used to judge the plaintiff's allegations differs in criminal and civil law. In both criminal and civil law, of course, the plaintiff bears the burden of proving each element of the case. Every cause of action, whether it be a complaint for murder, robbery, negligence, or breach of contract, is composed of certain required elements which, taken as a whole, are known as the prima facie case for that cause of action. Both the civil and the criminal plaintiff bear the burden of establishing their prima facie case, but the standard by which the plaintiff's case is judged is different in civil and criminal proceedings. In a criminal case, the defendant is assumed to be innocent until and unless the state can prove each element of its prima facie case beyond a reasonable doubt. In a civil action, the defendant remains blameless and free of liability until and unless the plaintiff can establish each element of the prima facie case by a preponderance of the evidence. Obviously, there is a significant difference between the two standards, although an exact definition of reasonable doubt remains elusive. It is quite clear that "beyond a reasonable doubt" is meant to be very close to certainty, as opposed to a "preponderance of the evidence," which requires only that a fact be established as more likely to be true than not to be true.

The sanctions imposed for criminal guilt and civil liability are also different. Criminal guilt may be punished by death, imprisonment, or fine, whereas civil liability in most cases is imposed in the form of a judgment for money damages.

It is possible that the same act may involve both a criminal and a civil wrong, as, for instance, in the case of rape. That act may be prosecuted in a criminal court as rape and may also be the subject of a civil action for the intentional tort of battery. Where an act results in the possibility of both criminal and civil actions, the two cases must be tried separately and, given the difference in the required levels of proof, might well result in a judgment for damages but a verdict of not guilty on the criminal charge.

LITIGATION

The legal process in the USA is characterized by the adversary system. The adversary system does not guarantee justice, just as the physician practicing medicine does not guarantee a cure. Both the legal and medical systems employ sets of procedures that have been tested and found by experience to be sound. All of these procedures are constantly under review and are continually being refined in an attempt to improve the result. In the adversary system, the assumption is that a contest between two equally knowledgeable and equally well prepared adversaries, judged by an impartial third party, affords a thorough airing of each issue of fact and law, which in most cases leads to a finding or reconstruction of what actually happened. It is this process that is the immediate goal of the legal system, with "justice" generally appearing as the ultimate product. It is well to remember that in law the result depends on what is *proved* rather than what *is*.

The roles of the participants in a civil trial are easily explained. Each client's attorney presents evidence of facts most favorable to that side, minimizing by deletion or explanation any unfavorable evidence and rebutting damaging evidence produced by opposing counsel. Testimonial evidence is presented by witnesses to fact (called percipient witnesses), who relate their first-hand experience of relevant subjects within lay comprehension. As to matters outside lay understanding, testimony is limited to expert witnesses (eg, physicians), who alone can offer opinions as evidence. Where there is a judge and a jury, the judge sits as the trier of law only; it is not the judge's task to decide which evidence presented, whether testimonial or physical, is true and which is not true. That decision is reserved for the jury, which sits as the trier of fact. After all of the evidence has been presented, the jury decides which are the facts based on the evidence. It disbelieves some evidence, believes other evidence, and weighs every piece of evidence according to each juror's knowledge, experience, and understanding.

The judge, as trier of law, controls the conduct of the trial and, most importantly, determines the admissibility of evidence sought to be presented to the jury by counsel for each side. If, at the completion of the plaintiff's presentation of the case, the judge finds that the plaintiff has not met the burden of proof in establishing a prima facie case, a nonsuit against the plaintiff may be directed, which terminates the action in favor of the defendant. The judge may also find that, although the plaintiff's presentation has met the burden of proof, the defendant's presentation substantially rebutted the plaintiff's evidence, and the judge may thus direct a verdict in favor of the defendant. The defendant may fail so completely to rebut the plaintiff's case that a directed verdict is entered by the judge in favor of the plaintiff. The judge also

has the option of allowing the jury to reach its own verdict, but even then, if the judge believes that there is no rational basis for the jury's decision, a judgment may be directed "notwithstanding the verdict" in favor of either party.

When the plaintiff and defendant have concluded their presentations and the judge has decided to let the case go to the jury, it is the judge's duty to instruct the jury on matters of law relevant to the case. These instructions are generally framed to indicate that certain findings of fact by the jury require certain conclusions of law. The judge even has the power to reduce the amount of the jury's money verdict (remittitur) or to increase it (additur). Although there must be agreement by the plaintiff to remittitur and agreement by the defendant to additur, the judge can "jaw-bone" the agreement of either party by indicating that unless agreement is reached, a motion for a new trial will be granted and the judgment of the jury set aside. There are, of course, numerous other decisions of law that must be made by the judge, such as matters of jurisdiction, venue, and appropriateness of parties to the action, which can greatly affect the initiation, location, and outcome of the litigation.

In cases where there is no jury, the judge acts as finder of fact as well as trier of law.

The physician's defense counsel in a medical negligence action may prefer to present the case to a judge sitting as trier of fact as well as of law. A trial to the judge alone is conducted with a great deal more flexibility than a trial before a judge and jury, because the judge is not concerned so much about evidence that may be prejudicial. That is, a jury of lay people may be somewhat dumbfounded by emotionally charged or complex evidence. The evidence may be so technical, as in many medical malpractice cases, that it is hopelessly beyond lay understanding (perhaps even with the assistance of expert witnesses). The judge is probably better informed than the average juror and may be familiar with medical terminology from other cases. The judge is much less likely to be influenced by emotional testimony or evidence that might be prejudicial to one of the parties. As a result, questions of admissibility before a judge alone are more likely to be resolved in favor of admission, whereas a judge might hesitate to admit the same evidence in a jury trial because of the possibility of an effect on the jury out of proportion to the real weight of the evidence.

The matter of appeal is sometimes misunderstood by those unfamiliar with the legal process. When a case is appealed, the facts are no longer in dispute. The trier of fact has already heard all of the evidence and made its decision, and the facts are as found. Unless it can be said that there was no rational basis for the finding of fact, which is an exceedingly difficult standard to meet, the findings as to facts will stand on appeal. The issues being contested by an appeal are questions of law decided by the trial judge. Any of the trial judge's decisions referred to above may become the basis for an appeal to a higher court. It then becomes a question of the opinion of an appellate judge, or panel of appellate judges, against that of the trial judge. Trial judges do not like to be overruled on appeal, so they try to make their decisions and instructions on law conform to acceptable, frequently used standards.

Although criminal law in the USA is almost exclusively governed by the state penal codes, civil law is still largely based on the common law system, which began with decisions of English courts and acts of Parliament and was adopted by the American states at the time of the Revolution. This inherited body of common law has since been augmented by decisions of appellate courts at both the state and federal levels. The key to understanding the common law system is the doctrine of stare decisis, which is the rule of legal precedent requiring lower courts to adopt decisions of higher courts. When the issue is "on all fours" with an earlier appellate court decision in the same jurisdiction, the earlier decision will control the present case.

CONTRACT BASIS OF THE PHYSICIAN-PATIENT RELATIONSHIP

Civil law obligations are of three types: contract, quasi-contract, and tort. A basic understanding of these areas is useful to physicians because the doctor-patient relationship is a complex one that may involve all of them. The essence of a contractual relationship is voluntary agreement between the parties, expressed orally or in writing, or implied by conduct. A quasi-contractual relationship is the result of a voluntary commitment of only one of the parties and the imposition of an agreement on the other party to avoid unjust enrichment. The ordinary purchase of goods or services is the simplest example of a contractual relationship, where one party agrees to furnish the goods or services and the other party agrees to pay for them. An example of a quasi-contractual situation is providing essential medical care for a patient who is incapable of contractual assent, such as an unconscious person, a minor, or an incompetent. The law will impose a quasi-contractual obligation on the patient or his or her legal representative (eg, parent or guardian) to pay for the medical care (*Greenspan v Slate,* 97 A2d 390 [NJ 1957]).

If the doctor and patient enter into a written contract for treatment, or if a verbal exchange takes place in which the patient promises to pay and the physician promises to treat, or if there is conduct in place of a promise (patient comes to doctor's office, doctor treats), the doctor-patient relationship is contractual. Subsequent failure of the patient to pay would amount to a breach of contract. Once having undertaken the obligation to treat the patient, a physician

who fails to do so commits a particular type of breach known as abandonment. This is true no matter how the physician-patient relationship was created. The fact of that relationship imposes the obligation.

The relationship that is formed is one of fiduciary trust, based on the unavoidable reliance of the lay person on the professional. This means that, unlike the usual "arm's length" sales transaction, there is a special obligation on the part of the physician: a duty of affirmative disclosure. Physicians deal with patients at all times in the context of this special trust. The relationship continues in the ordinary course of events until the treatment is completed. However, there may be situations where the patient wishes to terminate earlier. The patient can terminate at any time without notice or may decide at any time for any reason not to see that doctor any more, and that is the end of it.

There is, however, the possibility that a patient who demonstrates an intent to terminate unilaterally might later claim abandonment by the physician when, for example, an incision is slow in healing or the doctor's bill is higher than expected. To guard against this situation, the physician should confirm the patient's intent to terminate by written notification to the patient with a return receipt to document the change in relationship for the office file

The physician can also terminate the relationship unilaterally, but special conditions apply. Notice must first be given to the patient and information on past treatment provided to the new physician. In one case, a patient was brought to an emergency room with a gunshot wound in the neck. The patient was examined, admitted, and sent to the ward by the surgeon, who then went home. The surgeon was called shortly thereafter and told that the patient was having difficulty breathing and needed a tracheostomy. The admitting physician failed to return, and by the time another surgeon got the patient to the operating room it was too late. The patient died 4 hours after admission. Even though only a few hours had passed and there had been no formed intent on the part of the admitting doctor to permanently discontinue treatment, the court nevertheless ruled that the doctor had abandoned the patient (*Johnson v Vaughn,* 370 SW2d 591 [Ky 1963]). So the definition of abandonment is highly flexible. For instance, if a fracture has been set by an orthopedic surgeon, treatment might include checking the patient every few months until healing and rehabilitation are complete. Even though there is no contact between doctor and patient for months, the relationship remains intact. Thus, for a doctor to be protected in terminating the physician-patient relationship, notice must first be given to the patient. How much notice is required varies with the case. In general, the courts have held that 30 days is sufficient.

Of course, there are difficult situations, like the doctor who is working in a small community where there is literally no other doctor available, in which case termination may be impossible. The period of reasonable notice is based in large part on the availability of adequate medical coverage; it is the responsibility of the terminating physician not only to give the patient enough notice to find another physician but also to furnish information to the successor fast enough so that there is no delay in treatment. What constitutes unreasonable delay may also vary with the details of the illness. In the average case, a routine mailing of the records to the new physician and being available for telephone consultation would be sufficient.

It is important to understand the legal distinction between referral and consultation. A referral usually transfers responsibility for care of the patient to a new physician. The referring doctor (legally) drops out of the picture (after documenting that the new physician has accepted responsibility for care). A consultation does not shift responsibility from one physician to another. Instead, it adds another doctor to the treating team until the consultation is complete. Thereafter, there is no continuing relationship between consultant and patient—only the original physician-patient relationship remains.

Occasionally, a physician who does not intend to terminate care waits too long to start the necessary treatment, with resultant injury to the patient. In this case, the legal issue concerns a possible breach of the standard of care. There are situations where abandonment may result in both contractual liability and tort liability, and damages may be recovered for either.

Once the doctor-patient relationship is formed, the obligation of the physician is defined as the possession and application of care, skill, and knowledge common to other physicians of good standing. However, a physician may increase the level of this obligation by expressly promising or "warranting" a particular result or a cure, in which event the failure to achieve the promised result will render the physician liable in contract for breach of warranty. The prima facie case for breach of contract is simple, since it only requires proof of the contract and that the physician made a particular promise and then substantially failed to perform. Thus, there is a considerable legal difference between the obstetrician who promises to perform a tubal ligation and one who promises to sterilize the patient. However successful the surgeon's experience with a given procedure, the discussion of treatment objectives with the patient should be limited to the results expected and hoped for, the statistical probabilities, and the sincere promise to spare no effort to achieve a satisfactory outcome.

Money judgments for breach of contract in most states are limited to the value of the patient's "loss of the bargain" (which assumes that the promised treatment was obtained elsewhere at a greater cost) or "out of pocket" cost to the patient for securing the treatment elsewhere. A minority of jurisdictions do, however, allow recovery of money damages for pain and suffering where it was foreseeable at the time of the breach that failure of the doctor to perform, or delay in performance, would result in such pain and suffering for the patient. Actions for breach of contract against physicians are rare. They may be brought by patients who wish to "punish" a physician for a bad result although they know the physician was not negligent, or may be the only recourse in instances where a negligence action is barred by the shorter statute of limitations for tort.

INTENTIONAL TORTS

The third—and by far the most important—area of civil law for the physician is tort law. There are two kinds of tort: intentional and negligent. Although some categories of torts involve invasions of property rights, our concern here will be solely with invasions of personal rights, ie, those of the patient.

The category of intentional torts includes assault, battery, false imprisonment, defamation, invasion of privacy, infliction of emotional distress, and intentional misrepresentation. The prima facie case for the intentional torts is established by proving that the defendant's conduct was deliberate. If the conduct results in actual injury to the plaintiff, it is compensable in money damages. If conduct is established but injury is not, the damages will be limited to a nominal sum. But if the act (or omission) was particularly outrageous, punitive damages may be awarded in addition to compensatory or nominal damages. It should be emphasized that the only intent required for the commission of an intentional tort is the intent to commit the act, not an intent to bring about the ultimate injury. Another way of saying this is that the intention to bring about the ultimate injury is presumed from the commission of the act.

The act required to establish an **assault** is that which places another in immediate apprehension of harm. Traditionally, words alone without supporting gestures do not establish a cause of action for assault. A **battery** is simply an unauthorized touching of another. Of course, the authorization or consent for contact may not always be expressed. For instance, the fact that a patient has visited a physician for treatment implies consent to reasonable physical contact necessary for the examination. However, when the physician's treatment entails more than such customary contact, as in surgery, invasive diagnostic procedures, and drug treatment involving the risk of special harm, the consent of the patient to the specific procedures must first be obtained. In the absence of such consent, treatment by the physician would be battery, as would also be the case where consent was obtained to operate on a specific site and the consent was exceeded by operating on a different site, either instead of or in addition to the area of original consent. In situations where the issue is not whether any consent was obtained from the patient but rather whether the physician disclosed *enough* information for a reasonable patient to make an intelligent choice, the trend of the courts is to view the lack of so-called informed consent as a form of negligence in the disclosure of information by the physician. The matter of informed consent has been the subject of so much attention that it will be discussed below under its own heading.

The intentional tort of **false imprisonment** consists of an invasion of the personal interest in freedom from restraint of movement. Thus, a physician who orders a patient placed in restraints or drugged to the point of immobility by mistake or without a good medical reason may be liable for damages for false imprisonment. The physician most often involved in false imprisonment actions is the psychiatrist who orders involuntary commitment.

The intentional tort of **defamation** consists of injury to reputation by means of slanderous (oral) or libelous (written) statements to another person that diminish the respect in which the plaintiff is held by others and lessen his or her standing in the community. The extent of the injury caused by verbal defamation must be proved by the plaintiff except in the case of slander involving an accusation of criminal conduct, loathsome disease (eg, syphilis, leprosy), acts incompatible with one's business, trade, or profession, or unchastity of a woman. These are the four categories of slander per se from which general damages are presumed to result without need of proof.

Special (actual) damages need not be proved in the case of libel inherent on the face of a publication, but where reference to extrinsic information is needed to create the libelous meaning (known as libel per quod), general damages will be presumed only in the same four areas as above. Otherwise, special injury must be proved to establish the prima facie case of libel. The defendant may avoid liability for defamation by establishing a privilege of immunity that covers the statement or by establishing that the statement was true. It should be noted that one who repeats or "republishes" defamatory statements faces the same liability as the original purveyor.

Invasion of privacy is a new and still developing area of tort law dating in broad acceptance from the 1930s. The types of invasion recognized in this category are public use for profit of personal information about another or some type of intrusion on one's physical solitude. The most common defenses to an action for invasion of privacy are the privileges that exist for publication of information of public interest or concerning public figures. Specific state statutes define exceptions to the restrictions of defamation and invasion of privacy law. Such laws, known as **reporting statutes,** commonly include specific communicable diseases, gunshot and stab wounds, seizure disorders, and child abuse. (*Examples:*

California Penal Codes 11160, 11161; California Health and Safety Codes 410, 3125.) Giving out details of medical treatment concerning patients (eg, celebrities), even if the information is truly newsworthy, can exceed the privilege. Without a signed release from the patient or a court order, caution is the rule: "If in doubt, don't give it out." The same caution extends to identifying a patient if a description of the case is published. Also, no outsiders are allowed in the operating room without the patient's advance consent. (Standard consent forms usually allow observers to view surgery for educational purposes.)

Infliction of mental distress as a cause of action independent of contemporaneous physical injury has only recently achieved judicial recognition. The conduct or language must be outrageous and extreme and the emotional upset apparent (most successful suits have involved resulting physical illness). The law requires an individual to be somewhat tough-skinned, and annoyance or insult alone is not actionable. Nevertheless, the special closeness and reliance that characterized the fiduciary relationship between doctor and patient add weight to possible liability for ill considered conduct by physicians, who have a duty to protect and comfort their patients.

Intentional torts are not covered by professional insurance and are not included in the protection afforded by governmental immunity statutes. Where liability for an intentional tort is established, the judgment comes out of the doctor's own pocket.

NEGLIGENT TORTS

Although few physicians will ever have to face a suit for intentional tort, fewer still will complete a career without some involvement in a medical negligence action, whether as defendant, percipient witness, expert witness, or forensic consultant. A basic understanding of negligence law lessens the physician's chances of becoming a defendant and increases the prospects for making an effective, rational response if a legal proceeding does become necessary.

The prima facie case for negligence consists of four elements: duty, breach, causation, and damages. Each of these elements must be proved by the plaintiff by a preponderance of the evidence, and failure to do so will be fatal to the plaintiff's cause of action. In the case of a medical negligence action, the duty owed is coextensive with the doctor-patient relationship. It consists of the obligation on the doctor's part to acquire and maintain the same level of skill, care, and knowledge possessed by other members of the profession in good standing and to exercise that skill, care, and knowledge in the treatment of patients. There is no duty to accept a patient for treatment, and the physician may refuse to accept any person as a patient for any reason or for no reason at all.

There is one situation in which a physician may

undertake treatment of an individual without creating a doctor-patient relationship and thus without incurring the obligation to treat, ie, by rendering emergency treatment outside the normal scope of practice. Public policy in favor of physicians stopping to aid accident victims is so strong that the states have enacted special statutes, known generally as Good Samaritan Acts, which provide immunity from liability arising out of ordinary negligence in treatment of such victims and often even for injury due to gross negligence. In addition, some states have enacted special statutes that provide for immunity of medical specialists who are called in emergencies as consultants to "bail out" another physician whose patient has deteriorated despite (or as a result of) earlier treatment. The following statutes enacted in California are typical examples: Section 2395 of the Business and Professions Code, entitled "Emergency Care at Scene of Accident," contains the following wording: "No licensee, who in good faith renders emergency care at the scene of an emergency, shall be liable for any civil damages as result of any acts or omissions by such person in rendering the emergency care." Note that "scene of an emergency" encompasses not only location but also normal scope of employment. Therefore, if a doctor treats a patient while performing normal duties in the emergency room or as part of the responding "crash cart" team in a hospital, the Good Samaritan statute would not apply (*Colby v Schwartz,* 144 *California Reporter* 624 [1978]; *McKenna v Cedars of Lebanon Hospital,* 155 *California Reporter* 631 [1979]).

Section 2396 of the Business and Professions Code, entitled "Emergency Care for Complication Arising From Prior Care by Another," reads as follows: "No licensee, who in good faith upon the request of another person so licensed, renders emergency medical care to a person for medical complication arising from prior care by another person so licensed, shall be liable for any civil damages as a result of any acts or omissions by such licensed person in rendering such emergency medical care." Scene of an emergency is defined as above.

One problem under the general heading of the physician's duty is the *unintentional* formation of a physician-patient relationship. This situation usually arises where a doctor is consulted very briefly and usually very casually by an individual seeking a quick (and free) "curbstone opinion." Where such an opinion is rendered by a physician in surroundings that quite clearly indicate that no professional relationship was intended, such as a social gathering, the courts have not found the existence of a doctor-patient relationship. The findings may be otherwise, however, where the doctor is consulted in the hospital and—for example—instead of telling the questioner to come to the office for a regular appointment or referring to another doctor for medical advice, or even saying nothing at all, gives an opinion on which the

"patient" relies. Even late-at-night advice by telephone to call another doctor in the morning may be held to constitute treatment, since it assumes that the patient can afford to wait until morning before seeking care. The best course to follow when confronted with such a request, unless the doctor does intend to treat the patient, is to offer no advice at all other than an immediate referral to another source of medical treatment (eg, a hospital emergency room).

The physician's duty to the patient is performed within the "standard of care," and it is the failure of a physician to meet the standard of care in a given case that constitutes the "breach" element of the prima facie case for negligence. In the great majority of medical negligence cases, determining what the specific standard of care should be is beyond the comprehension of the lay persons on the jury. In these cases, the law requires that the standard be established by expert medical testimony. This method of setting the standard requires a physician to take the witness stand and testify about the treatment required in the particular case. Although technically any physician may testify as an expert on any medical specialty, in practice, the medical expert will be of the particular specialty appropriate to the facts of the case.

At one time the standard of care was established by comparison with good medical practice in the same community in which the defendant was practicing. This so-called **locality rule** has undergone extensive change, until today most jurisdictions have broadened the standard to include treatment by physicians in good standing **under similar circumstances**–one of those circumstances being similarity of locale in terms of proximity to major medical centers and accessibility of medical information generally. Some states have gone so far as to abolish the locality rule entirely, holding that dissemination of medical advances, especially in the newer specialties, is so effective today that there is, in effect, a national standard of care for those fields of medicine. The well-established trend is away from the narrow confines of the locality rule and toward a national standard (and perhaps, eventually, an international standard of care, beginning with English-speaking countries). Obviously, it is the efficacy of the treatment that is important in setting the standard of care and not the country or city where the treatment occurred. The courts have increasingly recognized that geographic isolation should not offer protection for the use of modes of treatment that have been discredited and discarded by physicians in general.

Even in situations where one mode of therapy is preferred by the majority of specialists in the field, the law does not require that this particular form of treatment be adopted as the standard of care by which all physicians in that field shall be judged. It is sufficient that the treatment actually rendered be approved by a respected school of medical thought in order for it to come within the standard of care.

The requirement of expert medical testimony to establish the standard of care has one well-established exception, ie, where the alleged negligence is within the lay understanding of the jury. In such cases, which include the "foreign object" cases, the judge must decide as a matter of law whether a medical expert will be required to establish the prima facie case in any particular respect. The judge may let the jury decide whether leaving a sponge, needle, clamp, or other object inside the patient is negligent (ie, a breach of the standard of care) but may require medical expert testimony on the element of causation.

The standard of care based on the modes of treatment employed by members of the medical specialty group in good standing is a **minimum standard.** There are two situations in which that minimum standard can be raised to require a higher level of treatment by a medical defendant. The first is that a physician who has made representations to the patient of greater skill or experience than is the case will be bound by them. In other words, a generalist who claims to possess the skill and experience of a specialist (or, if a specialist, that of a subspecialist) will be bound as a matter of law by the higher standard of care. The second situation arises in rare cases when the court itself determines that the standard of treatment in current use is simply not high enough to protect society. The likelihood of such a finding by a court is increased in cases where the added burden on the physician in meeting the higher standard proposed is very slight and the benefit to patients is very great. Where the existing standard of care is not adequate to protect the patient, the court may impose a stricter standard. This type of reasoning was demonstrated in the informed consent case of *Cobbs v Grant,* 502 P2d 1, 8 (Cal 1972).

It is plain from the decisions on standard of care that the law requires every physician to know his or her own limitations. The physician who attempts too much in a nonemergency case is risking liability for failure to consult or refer.

The element of causation has been the source of considerable confusion in the law. The plaintiff's case must include two types of causation: causation in fact and proximate cause. The test used most often in determining the presence of factual causation is simply that the defendant's conduct must be a substantial factor in bringing about the injury complained of. A minority of jurisdictions approach factual causation somewhat differently and require that the defendant's conduct be an indispensable antecedent to the plaintiff's injury, but in most cases the result is the same whichever test is used. Under either of these tests, the substance of the factual causation element is the same: proof of a sequence of events that connects breach of duty to conform to the standard of care with injury to the plaintiff.

The importance of the factual causation element is demonstrated by cases in which the treatment rendered is palliative and does not affect the course of the underlying disease process. In such cases where the patient dies as a result of the disease, a breach of the standard of care by the physician in administering the palliative treatment does not as a matter of law lead to liability for the death because the treatment was not a cause in fact of the patient's death.

For the purposes of this discussion, it is best to think of the second type of causation, known as either proximate cause or legal cause, as a set of limitations on causation in fact. Having established causation in fact, the court may nevertheless fail to find liability if the injury is too far removed from the physician's conduct or where some abnormal force intervenes to break the chain of events connecting the conduct with the result. The effect of the proximate cause requirement is that, in addition to proving the chain of events connecting the conduct and the result, the plaintiff must also establish a close and direct relationship between the conduct and the result.

RES IPSA LOQUITUR

The three elements of duty, breach, and causation are commonly referred to collectively as the liability aspect of a negligence case. With two basic exceptions, the plaintiff must establish the defendant's liability by a preponderance of the evidence in order to recover. The first of these exceptions is the doctrine of **res ipsa loquitur** ("the thing speaks for itself"). Considering the reams of print and judicial contention that have been generated by this doctrine, its origin was rather prosaic. The term was first applied by Baron Pollack in the 1863 case of *Byrne v Boadle* (2 H & C 772, 159 *English Reports* 299 [1863]), tried on appeal before the English Court of Exchequer. In the words of Pollack: "There are certain cases of which it may be said res ipsa loquitur, and this seems one of them." In some cases the courts have held that the mere fact of the accident having occurred is evidence of negligence: ". . .The present case upon the evidence comes to this, a man is passing in front of the premises of a dealer in flour, and there falls down upon him a barrel of flour. I think it apparent that the barrel was in the custody of the defendant who occupied the premises, and who is responsible for the acts of his servants who had the control of it; and in my opinion the fact of its falling is prima facie evidence of negligence."

The doctrine evolved steadily from that case down to the landmark decision of the California Supreme Court in *Ybarra v Spangard* (154 P2d 687 [Cal 1944]), a case which applied the doctrine of res ipsa loquitur to medical negligence. The holding of the court in *Ybarra* was that "where a plaintiff receives unusual injuries while unconscious and in the course of medical treatment, all those defendants who had any control over his body or the instrumentalities which might have caused the injuries may properly be called upon to meet the inference of negligence by giving an explanation of their conduct."

The doctrine itself serves as a substitute for the elements of breach and causation, although the plaintiff must still establish the existence of the duty element and must show damages. In order to gain the benefit of this substitution, the plaintiff must establish, first, that the accident is of a kind that ordinarily does not occur in the absence of someone's negligence; second, that it must be caused by an instrumentality within the exclusive control of the defendant; and third, that it must not have been due to any voluntary action on the plaintiff's part. If the court finds as a matter of law that these requirements have been met by the plaintiff, the court will instruct the jury that it may infer breach and causation by the defendant unless the inference is successfully rebutted by defendant's proof. As an inference of negligence, the doctrine of res ipsa loquitur operates as a substitute for evidence that would be especially difficult for the plaintiff to produce. The threshold issue—whether the injury is of a type that ordinarily does not occur in the absence of negligence—may itself call for expert testimony. If such testimony establishes that the injury occurs as an inherent risk in a documented percentage of cases not involving negligence, the doctrine will not be applied.

VICARIOUS LIABILITY

The other method of bypassing the prima facie case for negligence against a particular defendant is by imputed negligence. This method relies on the rule of law known as **respondeat superior,** which holds the principal responsible for the acts of his or her agents. This doctrine is manifested in the operating room in the form of the so-called captain of the ship doctrine. As the captain of the ship, the surgeon is held responsible for negligent injury to the patient while the surgeon is directing the operation. It is the exercise of control over others by the surgeon that is the key to the application of the doctrine. For this reason, the actions of the anesthesiologist are generally not imputed to the surgeon. Of course, to the extent that the surgeon issues specific orders to the anesthesiologist, a secondary liability is assumed if the anesthesiologist is negligent in carrying out the orders. In addition, in a medical partnership, the negligence of one partner is imputed to the other partners, and all partners become equally liable for damages that ensue. These instances of vicarious liability are exceptions to the general rule requiring that the elements of the prima facie case be established against the particular defendant only in the sense that once

they are established as to one defendant, they may fix liability on another defendant as well, based on the legal relationship of the parties.

DAMAGES

Of course, even when the plaintiff has established the elements of duty, breach, and causation by a preponderance of the evidence as to each, there is still the requirement of proving the last element of the prima facie case: damages. Considering that the average cost today of bringing a medical malpractice case through trial is over $25,000, it is plainly impractical for a plaintiff's attorney to bring a case to trial unless the alleged injury to the plaintiff has been substantial and offers a potential money judgment well in excess of expenses incurred.

The two categories of compensatory damages in personal injury cases are general damages, which include such intangible elements as pain and suffering; and special damages, which include documented economic loss from costs of medical care and diminished income. Because there are no mathematical formulas or other objective criteria for placing a dollar value on pain and suffering, this type of damage award is a frequent target for tort reform. In fact, since 1975, more than half of the states have enacted statutory limits or "caps" on medical malpractice damage awards for pain and suffering. In a wrongful death action, the general damages do not include pain and suffering but do include the family's loss of "comfort and society"; and the special damages include loss of economic support along with funeral expenses. In both personal injury and wrongful death actions, proof of gross negligence or especially outrageous conduct may result in exemplary (punitive) damages, which are fixed in relation to the wealth of the defendant.

DEFENSES

Common defenses to medical negligence actions are the statutes of limitations and contributory or comparative negligence. The purpose of **statutes of limitations** is to avoid litigation over stale claims by requiring a plaintiff to initiate suit within a fixed number of years after the negligent act or omission. Although the number of years varies from state to state, the effect of the running of the statutory period is the same everywhere—the plaintiff is forever barred from instituting suit based on that particular act or omission. The period begins to run on the date of the occurrence of the alleged negligence unless the negligence results in an injury that the plaintiff would typically be unaware of, such as the foreign body type of case. To cover this situation, most states and all federal jurisdictions apply the "discovery rule," under which the statutory period does not begin to run until the plaintiff knows, or in the exercise of reasonable diligence should have known, that the injury suffered was the result of treatment. Also, in many states the statutory period is tolled (suspended) by a legal disability on the part of the plaintiff such as minority or incompetency, by misrepresentation of the facts surrounding the treatment by the defendant physician, or by the "continuing care rule," which tolls the statute until the physician-patient relationship is terminated. The importance of a detailed medical record to the maintenance of a statute of limitations defense cannot be overemphasized.

The defense of **contributory negligence** operates in a minority of jurisdictions as a complete bar to the maintenance of the plaintiff's action when it is established that the injury was in any way the result of the plaintiff's negligence. Thus, even if it were found that the surgeon was 75% responsible for the injury and the plaintiff only 25% responsible, a verdict for the defendant must result. A bare majority of states now employ the **comparative negligence** approach, which apportions the total amount of damages according to the relative negligence of the plaintiff and the defendant. Thus, in comparative negligence jurisdictions, if it is found that the plaintiff has been injured to the extent of $100,000 in damages but was 25% negligent, the defendant would be accessed $75,000 in damages.

INFORMED CONSENT

Much attention has been paid to the topic of informed consent in recent years, but, for all the reams of analysis, the new case law on consent does not actually affect the basic process of securing consent for medical treatment. The big question has always been, "How much should the patient be told?"

The new cases on consent, founded on *Canterbury v Spence* (464 F2d 772 [DC Cir 1972]) and *Cobbs v Grant* (supra), do not change the priority of the question; neither do they answer it. Common sense is still the best guideline. The exchange between physician and patient in securing consent need be no different for any given treatment now than it was 15 years ago. The requirements are a description of the procedure, its chances of success, the risks, and the alternatives. The physician has always compared risks and benefits in deciding what mode of treatment to recommend. Explaining them to the patient in plain language is all that was ever required and is as sound in law today as it has always been good medical practice.

Traditionally, courts in the USA have used the "customary practice" standard to determine whether enough information was presented to the patient to support a rational decision. The new line of cases, which now constitutes a growing minority trend, holds that reliance on the custom of doctors in good standing is an illusory standard. These courts have substituted a standard of materiality to the patient. Under this minority approach, the test becomes whether a reasonable person would have refused the treatment if the risk of the complication that occurred had been clearly explained.

The effect of this materiality test is that the more important the procedure is to the patient's health, the less credible the claim that the procedure would have been refused. Conversely, the less important the procedure, the more credible will be a later complaint that it would have been refused had the risks been fully identified.

Put in its simplest form, a fully detailed informed consent is less crucial where the procedure may save life or limb and more important where the treatment objective is cosmetic. The principle finds its ultimate expression in the long-established rule that consent is implied in a medical emergency. There is one caveat to the rule of implied consent: the physician cannot assume that consent is implied if a competent adult refuses treatment.

The above discussion of the consent process is rooted in two basic premises. The first is that the physician determines which forms of treatment are appropriate for the patient's condition. The second is that once these therapeutic options have been explained to the patient, the patient will decide which of the options (including the option of no treatment at all) will be elected. The legal right of a competent adult to accept or decline proposed medical treatment has its foundation in the common-law and constitutionally guaranteed right of personal privacy. The patient's right to refuse treatment is not affected by the gravity of the consequences of refusal. Even if pain, disability, or death will be a probable consequence of a refusal of consent, a competent adult has the legal right to make that decision.

The first court decisions on cessation of life support generally involved patients in a persistent vegetative state being maintained on respirators. These cases, beginning with *Matter of Quinlan,* 355 A2d 647 (1976), sided with the patient's (or legal representative's) right to refuse such treatment. Later cases have involved patients who were seriously ill but not curable (or whose prognoses could not be improved) and refused less intrusive life support such as nasogastric tube feeding or intravenous hydration, further refining the patient's right to refuse treatment. From these cases has evolved what is now known as the **doctrine of proportionality,** which states that artificial life support should be initiated and maintained so long as it constitutes "proportionate treatment," ie, treatment which, in the patient's view, has at least a reasonable chance of providing benefits to the patient that outweigh the burdens attendant upon treatment. Thus, even if a proposed course of treatment might be extremely painful or intrusive, it would still be proportionate treatment if the prognosis was for complete cure or significant improvement in the patient's condition. On the other hand, a treatment course that is only minimally painful or intrusive may nonetheless be considered disproportionate to the potential benefits if the prognosis is virtually hopeless for any significant improvement in condition. *Barber v Superior Court,* 147 Cal App 3d 1006, 1019 (1983).

The words of the patient himself in one of these cases impressed the court and are instructive here: "While I have no wish to die, I find intolerable the living conditions forced upon me by my deteriorating lungs, heart and blood vessel systems, and I find intolerable my being continuously connected to this ventilator, which sustains my every breath and my life for the past six and one-half . . . weeks. Therefore, I wish this court to order that the sustaining of my respiration by this mechanical device violates my constitutional right, is contrary to my every wish, and constitutes a battery upon my person. I fully understand that my request to have the ventilator removed and discontinued, which I have frequently made to my wife and my doctors, will very likely cause respiratory failure and ultimately lead to my death. I am willing to accept that risk rather than to continue the burden of this artificial existence which I find unendurable, degrading and dehumanizing." *Bartling v Superior Court,* 163 Cal App 3d 186, 191 (1984).

In October 1990, the United States Supreme Court decided its first "right-to-die" case, *Cruzan v Director, Missouri Department of Health,* 110 S.Ct. 2841 (1990), confirming the right of a competent adult to accept or refuse medical care but leaving to the states the power to set the standard of proof for evidence that a patient has made such a decision. The best way to prove that treatment has been refused is by means of a written, signed, and witnessed instruction by the patient, executed while competent. Instructions such as this are termed **advance directives** and include durable powers of attorney for health care, living wills, and natural death directives, depending on state law. There is now a new federal law, the Patient Self-Determination Act, effective December 1, 1991 (42 U.S. Code 1395cc et seq), that requires Medicare or Medicaid providers to give their adult patients information on advance directives at the time of initial care or admission under applicable state law. The law does not change the rights of the patient. It does make the health care provider responsible for informing the patient of those rights.

In cases involving patients whose condition is irreversibly and imminently terminal, there may be no treatment the physician can offer. Where there is a consensus among the treatment team, next-of-kin, and the known wishes of the patient, a "do-not-resuscitate" or "no code" order may be appropriate. If such an order is given by the attending physician, it should be a written order in the patient's chart. The order should be supported with a progress note that includes diagnosis and prognosis, wishes (if known) of the patient and family, consensus of the treatment team, and confirmation of the patient's competence.

If a person in need of medical treatment is incapable of giving informed consent, substituted consent must be obtained from the next of kin. In most states, the order of intestate succession controls the identity of next of kin. The order is generally spouse, adult child, parent, sibling. For a person who has been adjudicated incompetent, consent of the court-appointed guardian must be obtained. If a minor is in need of care, consent of one parent is required. The courts have recognized, however, that refusal by parents to consent to emergency care for a child is subject to judicial review.

The signed consent form is merely evidence that the consent process occurred. It should always be backed up by the physician's own brief entry in the progress notes, with date and time. If the need to alter an entry arises, there is only one safe method: Line out the error (without obliterating it), initial and date the deletion, and enter the correct information.

MEDICAL INSURANCE

Discussions of the present status of availability of medical malpractice insurance are usually phrased in terms of crisis. For the physician approaching private practice, sufficient understanding of the basics of professional insurance is imperative so that at least the right questions can be asked.

The insurance crisis was generated by the loss of profitability of medical liability insurance. This resulted from reduction of surpluses owing to investment losses by the insurance companies, large increases in the cost to the primary insurer of reinsurance (beginning in 1970), and the combination of unpredictability of occurrence claims and the small physician base from which to generate the premium pool. Of the many proposals to remedy the problem, several have found nationwide application. First, there has been a direct shift in the type of policy written from "occurrence" to "claims made."

Briefly, an occurrence policy provides coverage for events that become the basis for claims in the year that the event occurs, while the claims made policy provides coverage only for the year in which a claim is presented to the insurer, regardless of when the underlying event took place. The practical effect of the change from occurrence to claims made policies is that the physician is only secure so long as coverage continues to be purchased every year without lapse. For claims made policies, therefore, it is imperative that the insurance contract include provision for purchase by the doctor of the "tail" of coverage. In other words, there must be liability coverage for the years following the doctor's retirement or change in practice from patient care to nonpatient care. Care should also be taken that "presentation" of a claim under a claims made policy be defined, since some contracts allow presentation only by a third party (plaintiff or attorney) and not by the physician. Attention must also be given to exclusions from coverage, which may place certain high-risk operations outside the scope of the policy.

The purposes of medical liability insurance are protection against costs of defending a suit (commonly as high as $25,000) and payment of adverse judgments. Any physician considering "going bare" (practicing without liability coverage) must weigh the potential impact of these costs. As difficult to achieve as it is, attaining "judgment-proof" status (eg, irrevocable transfer of assets to another person prior to threat of suit) only protects against payment of a judgment. The only way to avoid litigation costs as well would be to submit to default judgment. The hazards of going bare thus make the cost of insurance more palatable.

Following the medical liability insurance "crisis" of the mid 1970s, the number of malpractice claims filed actually leveled off between the years 1976 to 1978. Unfortunately, claims-filed activity rose again in 1979 and has continued to rise steadily. We are faced now with a new crisis in medical insurance. Largely because of the growth of doctor-owned insurance companies, there is no availability problem. There is, however, a serious affordability problem, which is getting worse. With increasing claims activity and the uncertainty of long "tail" coverage, the cost of liability insurance may actually prevent newly licensed physicians from practicing in high-risk surgical specialties. One possible solution that has worked well in some areas is state-sponsored reinsurance pools for coverage of awards over a certain amount (eg, $250,000). Another solution may be found in state-run physician-supported patient compensation funds set up to cover amounts over a statutory limit on what can be awarded.

HOSPITAL STAFF PRIVILEGES

The nature of the physician-hospital relationship has changed drastically since the turn of the century as the hospital's status has graduated from that of essentially a quarantine facility for the isolation of the ill to the modern health care center. With this development, the importance of access to the hospital facility (ie, staff privileges) by the individual physician has become a professional and economic necessity. Until the Illinois Supreme Court decision in *Darling v Charleston Community Memorial Hospital,* 211 NE2d 253 (1965), *cert denied* 383 US 946 (1966), it was generally accepted by the courts that the private physician with staff privileges was an independent contractor with the hospital and that the hospital would not be vicariously liable for contractors' mal-

practice under the doctrine of respondeat superior. This left no cause of action at all against the hospital. *Darling* and its progeny now represent the majority position in the USA, creating a cause of action for direct hospital liability for failure to adequately supervise the quality of care in the hospital, including evaluation of the abilities of the physicians granted staff privileges. Since the *Darling* decision, the Joint Committee on Accreditation of Health Organizations has increased pressure on hospitals to tailor staff privileges to the ability of the individual physician in order the raise the quality of care. There has also been increased emphasis by medical malpractice insurance carriers on the limitation of privileges in the hope of reducing exposure from high-risk specialties. These factors will undoubtedly result in closer scrutiny by hospitals of applications for new privileges and for renewal of privileges. Those applications that are granted will be more narrowly drawn than in the past to match the applicants' education, training, and experience. We can also expect to see a proliferation of "closed shop" specialty units in hospitals, such as hemodialysis and cardiac intensive care units.

The physician whose application for staff privileges has been denied or restricted is entitled to a fair hearing before a reasonably impartial tribunal of the hospital with adequate notice of the reasons for denial or restriction; a right to examine documentary evidence in the case; and a right to cross-examine adverse witnesses. Such a hearing provides the minimum procedural due process without which the denial or restriction of privileges would constitute an improper infringement of the physician's liberty or property interests under the 14th Amendment of the US Constitution. The standard the hospital must meet when restricting or denying staff privileges is that there must be a rational basis for the action which is reasonably related to the hospital's operation. Hospital action that is unreasonable, arbitrary, or capricious is likely to be reversed on judicial review.

FEES FOR MEDICAL WITNESSES

The single most common source of dispute between physicians and attorneys is the medical witness fee. This is due to the lack of understanding by doctors of the rights and duties of such witnesses and the willingness of the trial bar to take advantage of that ignorance. A treating physician is a percipient witness in any suit in which the patient's condition is at issue, and in that role the physician has the same duty to testify as if, for example, an automobile accident were witnessed by the physician. If subpoenaed, the physician must testify. That is the obligation of every citizen, and the standard witness fee (presently $40 per day and 25 cents per mile in federal courts) is all the physician is entitled to.

On the other hand, if a physician is hired by either

side as a medical expert to analyze and render an opinion on treatment rendered to the patient by others, reasonable compensation is justified. A physician who is approached by an attorney seeking the services of a medical expert to testify or a medical consultant to evaluate the case and report to the attorney should reach agreement with the attorney *in advance and in writing* on hourly charges for medicolegal services. The hourly fee paid by the federal government for medical expert and consultant services in 1989 is up to $200 per hour for consultation and $800 per trial day for testimony. Remember that the AMA Code of Medical Ethics does not allow a physician to charge a fee contingent on the outcome of the trial.

Today, most local medical societies have panels of physicians available to the trial bar for the impartial review of medicolegal cases. If these panels find substandard care, they will furnish medical experts to testify in the case. The establishment of such panels should be supported by all physicians because the panels benefit patients deserving compensation, the public image of the medical profession, and the private conscience of the expert medical witness.

CORONER'S INVESTIGATION

The coroner is a county government officer acting under statutory authority to investigate certain classes of deaths. These classes generally include violent deaths such as homicide, suicide, and accidents. Also included are deaths for which no physician can certify the cause, either because no physician was in attendance, the physician was in attendance for less than 24 hours before death, or the physician is *unable* to state the cause of death. (*Note:* This means truly unable, not merely unwilling.) Often the coroner is charged with investigation of deaths in operating rooms, deaths where a patient has not fully recovered from an anesthetic, and deaths in which the patient is comatose throughout the period of the physician's attendance. When a death falls within one of these statutory classes, it must be reported promptly to the coroner. The coroner makes a brief inquiry, perhaps by telephone, and decides whether to take jurisdiction over the case. Thus, simply reporting the case to the coroner does not make it a "coroner's case." The coroner may decide not to take the case and may instruct the reporting physician to sign the death certificate. When a physician is instructed by the coroner to sign the certificate, the contact, the instruction, and the identity of the coroner's official must be immediately entered in the physician's or hospital's patient chart.

MALPRACTICE

The most comprehensive study yet published on medical malpractice in the USA is the Report of the Secretary's Commission on Medical Malpractice (DHEW Publication No. [OS] 73-88, 1973). The commission found that the primary factor generating medical malpractice claims was injurious or adverse results of treatment. Factors such as poor physician-patient rapport, patient frustration with the handling of specific complaints concerning treatment and complications, unrealistic expectations about what can be achieved with treatment, and increased patient suit-consciousness are of only secondary importance. A rational prescription for curing the medical malpractice problem would be to reduce patient injury by instituting aggressive risk management programs (especially in the hospital setting), improving personal communication between health care providers and their patients, and adoption of arbitration provisions at the outset of the physician-patient relationship.

When the physician recognizes that the patient has been injured as a result of iatrogenic error, the best course is to tell the patient right away and in plain language exactly what happened. The explanation should stick to the facts and avoid opinions and conclusions of law (such as admissions of negligence). It is essential to document in writing that this discussion has occurred, because the statute of limitations in most jurisdictions is much shorter when the patient has knowledge of the treatment error than when the patient is left to discover that a mistake has been made.

REFERENCES

American College of Legal Medicine: *Legal Medicine: Legal Dynamics of Medical Encounters.* Mosby, 1988.

Blackman NS, Bailey CP: *Liability in Medical Practice: A Reference for Physicians.* Harwood, 1990.

Citation: *A Medicolegal Digest for Physicians.* American Medical Association. [Biweekly publication.]

Dix A: *Law for the Medical Profession.* Butterworth, 1988.

Ficarra BJ: *Medicolegal Examination, Evaluation, and Report.* CRC Press, 1987.

Gee DJ, Mason JK: *The Courts and the Doctor.* Oxford Univ Press, 1990.

Halley M: *Medical Malpractice Solutions.* Thomas, 1989.

Halley MM et al (editors): *Medical Malpractice Solutions: Systems and Proposals for Injury Compensation.* Thomas, 1989.

Harsha WN: *Medical Malpractice: Handling Orthopedic Cases.* McGraw-Hill, 1990

Health Law Handbook. Clark Boardman, 1989.

Hirsch DJ, Goldstein C: *Current Issues in Law and Medicine.* Defense Research Institute, 1987.

Journal of Legal Medicine. Pharmaceutical Communications, Inc. [Quarterly publication.]

Mann A: *Medical Negligence Litigation: Medical Assessment Of Claims.* Redfern, NSW/Legal Books, International Business Communications, 1989.

Morris LA: *Communicating Therapeutic Risks.* Springer-Verlag, 1990.

Nora PF (editor); *Professional Liability/Risk Management: A Manual for Surgeons.* American College of Surgeons, 1991

Robertson JD, Keavy WT: *Plastic Surgery Malpractice and Damages.* Wiley Law Publications, 1990.

Rosenblum JB, Curry CL: *Medical Malpractice: Handling Cardiology and Cardiovascular Surgery Cases.* McGraw-Hill, 1991.

Scott WL (editor): *Medicolegal Glossary.* Medical Economics, 1989.

Shiffman MA: *Medical Malpractice: Handling General Surgery Cases.* McGraw-Hill, 1990.

Sloan FA et al: *Insuring Medical Malpractice.* Oxford Univ Press, 1991.

Southby RMF, Hirsh HL: *Health Care Law and Ethics.* George Washington Univ Press, 1989.

Tomes JP: *Healthcare Records: A Practical Legal Guide.* Kendall/Hunt, 1990

Van Oosten F: *The Doctrine of Informed Consent in Medical Law.* Peter Lang, 1991.

Vevaina JR, Bone RC, Kassoff E: *Legal Aspects of Medicine.* Springer-Verlag, 1989.

Weiler PC: *Medical Malpractice on Trial.* Harvard Univ Press, 1991

7 Wound Healing

Thomas K. Hunt, MD, Reid V. Mueller, MD, & William H. Goodson III

Only a century ago, complicated and incomplete healing after injury was the rule rather than the exception. Surgeons had little choice but to accept draining wounds and invasive infections. The evolution of wound care and antisepsis in the 18th and 19th centuries changed surgery as dramatically as the discovery of anesthesia. Even so, poor healing, infection, and excessive scarring continue to be leading causes of disability and death.

Knowledge of the basic mechanisms of healing has grown rapidly. A detailed knowledge of these mechanisms allows surgeons to influence healing and anticipate and prevent problems of infection and incomplete or excessive repair.

FORMS OF HEALING

Surgeons customarily divide types of wound healing into first and second "intention." **First intention (primary) healing** occurs when tissue is cleanly incised and reapproximated and repair occurs without complication. **Second intention (secondary) healing** occurs in open wounds through formation of granulation tissue* and eventual coverage of the defect by spontaneous migration of epithelial cells. Most infected wounds and burns heal in this manner. Primary healing is simpler and requires less time and material than secondary healing. It sometimes happens that primary healing is possible but there is insufficient reserve to support secondary healing. For example, an ischemic limb may heal primarily, but if the wound opens and becomes secondarily infected, it may not heal. These two forms may be combined in **delayed primary closure,** when a wound is allowed to heal open for about 5 days and is then closed as if primarily. Such wounds are less likely to become infected than if closed immediately.

THE NATURE OF REPAIR
(Figure 7–1)

Injury profoundly disrupts the chemical environment and architecture of tissues. The postinjury environment, characterized by impaired perfusion coinciding with inflammation, invokes a number of fundamental biochemical, physiologic, and cellular coping mechanisms. The subsequent struggle to restore normality (ie, healing) involves a sequence that includes coagulation, inflammation, angiogenesis, epithelialization, fibroplasia, matrix deposition, and contraction. The cells that perform this transformation are platelets, leukocytes (especially macrophages), fibroblasts, vascular endothelial cells, and epithelial cells. The signals that direct these cells—growth factors and cytokines (Table 7–1)—traverse the local extracellular fluid. Growth factors are a class of peptides that signal cells to proceed through their replicative cycle. In as yet mysterious ways, these substances guide growth, development, and reparative processes from conception to death. Growth factors particularly pertinent to wound healing include insulin, insulin-like growth factors (IGFs), transforming growth factors (TGFs), fibroblast growth factors (FGFs), leukocyte-derived growth factors (LDGFs), platelet-derived growth factors (PDGFs), and others. The term "growth factor," however, is a misnomer. In vivo, these molecules may also behave as chemoattractants, inhibitors of differentiation, and stimulants of specific protein synthesis. In higher doses, they may be cytolytic.

Cytokines—messenger molecules originating in and usually targeted at leukocytes—also contribute to this process. They include interleukins, of which at least 12 have been defined (IL-1, IL-2, etc), and tumor necrosis factor (TNF). Many have been found in wounds, and IL-1, IL-2, and IL-6 appear to contribute to repair. The overlap with growth factors is considerable.

The following describes the complex and often redundant process in which wound cells, a unique injury environment, and specific signal molecules secrete a new vascularized connective tissue matrix and appropriate epithelium that eventually returns the extracellular environment to normal.

---

*Granulation tissue is the red, granular, moist tissue that appears during healing of open wounds. Microscopically, it contains new collagen, new blood vessels, fibroblasts, and inflammatory cells, especially macrophages.

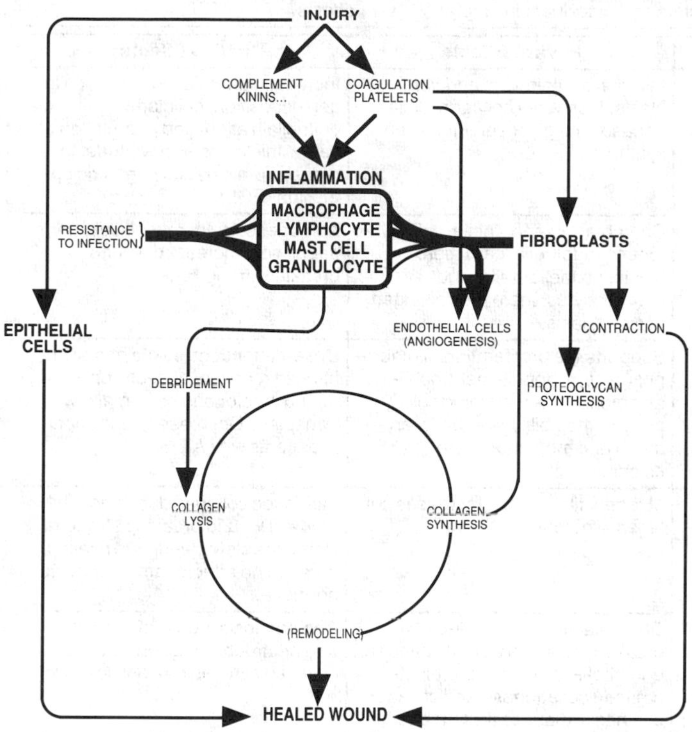

Figure 7–1. Schematic diagram of the sequence of events in wound healing. (Modified and reproduced, with permission, from Hunt TK, van Winkle W Jr: *Fundamentals of Wound Management.* Vol 1. Chirurgecom Press, 1976.)

THE INITIAL RESPONSE: COAGULATION & INFLAMMATION

Clotting of blood contributes the first reparative signals. Fibrinopeptides and thrombin attract macrophages into injured tissue, and activated platelets release PDGF, IGF-1, and TGFβ, all of which prepare local cells to multiply. Later, fibrin itself activates macrophages to release more reparative signals.

Inflammation begins as damaged endothelial cells release cytokines, which induce integrin and integrin receptor expression in passing leukocytes. The leukocytes adhere to local endothelial cells and enter the injured extravascular space, attracted by tissue complement factors, fibrinopeptides, growth factors, and cytokines. Initially, inflammatory components such as histamine, serotonin, and kinins cause vessels to constrict as an aid to hemostasis and then to dilate a short time later. Under their influence, vessels become porous and release cells and blood plasma into the injured area.

The newly arrived inflammatory cells increase metabolic demand. Since the local microvasculature has been damaged, a local energy sink results, and Po_2 falls while CO_2 and lactate accumulate. Lactate in particular plays a critical role. These conditions persist throughout repair, and—together with other stimulants such as fibrin, foreign bodies, etc—they direct leukocytes, particularly macrophages, to release a variety of cytokines, chemoattractants, and growth factors.

These events trigger reparative processes and ensure their continuation, because macrophages, which secrete growth-promoting products, assume the control of repair as the flood of coagulation-mediated growth substances begins to ebb. Furthermore, macrophages, stimulated by fibrin and hypoxia, release large quantities of lactate even in the presence of oxygen, thereby maintaining the environment of injury. The environment causes them to release growth promoters and more lactate, which in turn stimulates angiogenesis and collagen deposition.

By the third or fourth day after injury, the reparative cells become loosely arranged in a characteristic spatial relationship as shown in Figure 7–2, a diagram of a wound made in a rabbit's ear and enclosed in a thin, optically clear chamber and allowed to heal for a week. Unless the wound becomes infected, its granulocyte population, which dominated on the first day, has diminished. Macrophages now cover the cut surface. Immature fibroblasts, the product of growth signals, lie just beneath, mixed with buds of new vessels. More mature fibroblasts are scattered behind. The spatial relations of cells with respect to oxygen and lactate concentrations define zones of reparative activities.

These spatial relationships show how macrophages condition a highly lactated, hypoxic, acidotic growth

Table 7–1. Growth factors and cytokines: in vitro and in vivo effects.

Peptide	Site of Synthesis	Target Cells	In Vitro Effects	In Vivo Effects
EGF, TGFα	Brain keratinocytes, macrophages, submaxillary gland	Chondrocytes, endothelial cells, epithelial cells, fibroblasts, smooth muscle	Mitogen for epithelial and fibroblasts. Increases collagen, collagenase, and glycosaminoglycan synthesis.	Increased granulation tissue, collagen deposition, cellularity, epithelialization, and granulation of partial thickness skin wounds. Increased proliferation of gastric epithelium (EGF).
FGF	Endothelial cells, fibroblasts, macrophages	Chondrocytes, endothelial cells, epithelial cells, fibroblasts	Chemotactic: endothelial cells. Mitogen: endothelial cells, fibroblasts, epithelial cells, and chondrocytes. Increases collagenase synthesis.	Angiogenesis. Increased collagen deposition. Increased wound breaking strength.
GM-CSF	Endothelial cells, fibroblasts, T lymphocytes (cytokine)	Granulocyte, erythrocyte, monocyte, megakaryocyte progenitor cells (CFU-GEMM, CFU-MEG, CFU-Eo, CFU-GM)	Supports the proliferation of macrophage-, eosinophil-, neutrophil-, and monocyte-containing colonies. Some ability to support erythroid and megakaryocyte colonies.	Dose-dependent leukocytosis. Enhanced recovery of neutrophils during autologous bone marrow transplant. Decreased neutropenia in patients with AIDS.
IGF-1	Fibroblasts, hepatocytes, macrophages, platelets	Bone chondrocytes, endothelial cells, fibroblasts, macrophages	Mitogen: fibroblasts. Increases collagen synthesis.	Increased collagen deposition. Increased wound breaking strength. Reverses steroid-induced healing defect. The effector arm of growth hormone.
IL-1	Endothelial cells, lymphocytes, keratinocytes, macrophages (cytokine)	Endothelium, fibroblasts, neutrophils	Chemotactic: neutrophils; increases respiratory burst. Mitogen: endothelial cells and fibroblasts; increased collagenase and collagen synthesis; induces IL-8 production.	Angiogenesis. Local inflammation and neutrophil influx. Enhanced collagen synthesis in low doses.
IL-8	Endothelial cells, fibroblasts, lymphocytes, monocytes (cytokine)	Basophils, neutrophils, T lymphocytes	Chemotactic: neutrophils; increases respiratory burst.	Neutrophil accumulation.
NGF	Schwann cells, tissues innervated by sympathetic and sensory neurons	Peripheral sympathetic and sensory neurons	Stimulates neurite extension. Promotes neuron survival. Promotes differential phenotype.	Sympathetic and sensory nerve growth toward the NGF source.
PDGF	Endothelial cells, fibroblasts, macrophages, platelets, smooth muscle, skeletal muscle	Endothelial cells, fibroblasts, macrophages, neutrophils, smooth muscle cells	Chemotactic: neutrophils, monocytes, fibroblasts, smooth muscle, and endothelial cells (BB homodimer). Mitogen: endothelial cells; increases collagenase and glycosaminoglycan synthesis.	Angiogenesis. Increased fibroblast influx. Increased collagen deposition. Increased wound breaking strength. Activation of neutrophil and monocyte respiratory burst.
TNFα	Lymphocytes, macrophages, transformed cell lines (cytokine)	Endothelial cells, monocytes, neutrophils	Chemotactic: endothelial cells; increases respiratory burst, phagocytosis. Mitogen: fibroblasts; cytolytic to some cells.	Angiogenesis. Systemic administration produces many symptoms of sepsis.
TGFβ	Almost all cells. Platelets and bone are the major source.	Almost all cells	Chemotactic: monocytes, neutrophils, and fibroblasts; inhibits endothelial cell chemotaxis; inhibits endothelial cell and keratinocyte proliferation; increases collagen and thymocyte mutagenic protein; decreases collagenase.	Angiogenesis. Increased collagen deposition. Increased wound breaking strength. Reverses steroid-induced healing defect. Reverses doxorubicin-induced healing defect.

Key:

EGF	= Epidermal growth factor		IL	= Interleukin
FGF	= Fibroblast growth factor		NGF	= Nerve growth factor
GM-CSF	= Granulocyte macrophage colony-stimulating factor		PDGF	= Platelet-derived growth factor
			TGF	= Transforming growth factor
IGF	= Insulin-like growth factor		TNF	= Tumor necrosis factor

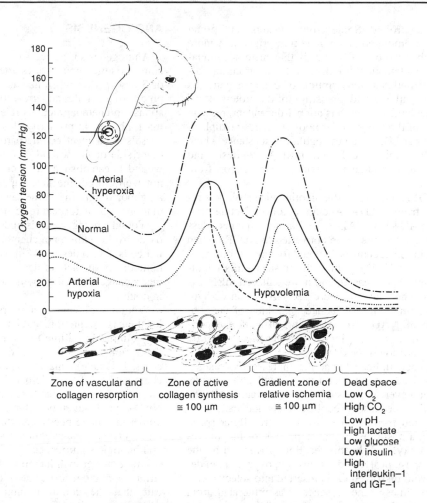

Figure 7–2. Schematic plot of oxygen tension as measured in a healing wound in a rabbit ear chamber. The gradient zone advances into the dead space, and behind it the neovasculature resorbs as the reparative tissue advances. The oxygen tension plot illustrates the effects of hyperoxia, hypoxia, and hypovolemia. Since oxygen is required for repair, little progress can be expected during hypovolemia.

environment to construct a growth center. Farther back toward the uninjured tissue, young fibroblasts are still highly lactated but are much better oxygenated and therefore more suited to matrix deposition.

FIBROPLASIA & MATRIX DEPOSITION

Fibroplasia

During the course of healing, fibroplasia (replication of fibroblasts) is stimulated by multiple mechanisms, starting with PDGF, IGF-1, and TGFβ released by platelets and continuing with cytokines released by macrophages. Fibroblasts appear to release IGF-1. Epidermal growth factor and IGF-1 are also delivered by blood.

Dividing fibroblasts are seen mainly near the wound edge, where they are exposed to the growth environment and to an oxygen tension of approximately 40 mm Hg in normally healing wounds. In cell culture, this Po_2 is optimal for fibroblast replication.

Fibroblasts originate locally by replication. However, if there is such a thing as a fibrocyte, it is not recognized. Smooth muscle cells are likely progenitors because fibroblasts seem to stream from the adventitia and media of vessels. Lipocytes, pericytes, and others are also candidates. Perhaps all contribute.

Matrix Deposition

The newly replicated fibroblasts secrete the collagen and proteoglycans of the connective tissue matrix that weld wound edges together. Both assume high-molecular-weight polymeric forms and become the physical basis of wound strength. Collagen synthesis is not a constitutive property of fibroblasts but is highly controlled. Some growth factors (TGFβ and IGF-1) promote collagen gene transcription. A more basic observation, however, is that mere accumulation of lactate in the extracellular environment directly stimulates transcription of collagen genes as well as synthesis and deposition of the protein itself. This mechanism, which is not pH-dependent, rests on the size of the intracellular pool of adenosine diphosphoribose (ADPR), a key regulatory substance which normally inhibits collagen mRNA synthesis and other vital steps that facilitate collagen export from fibroblasts.

ADPR results when the nicotinamide moiety is removed from NAD+. Accumulation of lactate converts NAD+ to NADH. As a consequence, less NAD+ is available to be converted to ADPR. When ADPR in the nucleus is depleted for any reason—as it is when the NAD+ pool is diminished—this inhibitory control is released, and more collagen mRNA is formed. The cause of decreased NAD+ can be hypoxia, accumulation of lactate, inhibition of the conversion of NAD+ to ADPR, or, in culture experiments, the artifactual increase of the NAD+ pool by simple addition of NAD+.

Evidence indicates that the increase in collagen mRNA leads to an increased procollagen peptide. This, however, is not sufficient to increase collagen deposition because procollagen peptide cannot be transported from the cell to the extracellular space until, in a posttranslational step, some of its prolines are hydroxylated. In this reaction, performed by the dioxygenase prolyl hydroxylase, an oxygen atom derived from dissolved O_2 is inserted into selected collagen prolines in the presence of ascorbic acid, iron, and α-ketoglutarate. The activity of this enzyme is normally suppressed by cytoplasmic ADPR. Thus, accumulation of lactate—or any other process that decreases the NAD+ pool—leads to production of collagen mRNAs, increased collagen peptide synthesis, and (provided enough ascorbate and oxygen is present) increased posttranslational modification and secretion of collagen monomers into the extracellular space.

Another dioxygenase, lysyl hydroxylase, hydroxylates a number of the procollagen lysines and sets the stage for later lysyl to lysyl cross-binding between collagen molecules and fibers, thereby endowing them with considerable strength. It too requires adequate amounts of ascorbate and oxygen. These oxygenase reactions proceed only as fast as the local concentration of oxygen (Po_2) will allow. The rates are half-maximal at about 20 mm Hg and maximal at about 200 mm Hg. They can be forced to supernormal rates by tissue hyperoxia.

ANGIOGENESIS

Angiogenesis is a necessary feature of repair. It becomes visible about 4 days after injury but begins 2 or 3 days earlier when new capillaries sprout out of preexisting venules and grow toward the injury in response to chemoattractants released by platelets and macrophages. In primarily closed wounds, sprouting vessels soon meet counterparts migrating from the other side of the wound, and blood flow across the wound is established. In unclosed wounds or those not well closed, the new capillaries fuse only with neighbors migrating in the same direction, and granulation tissue is formed instead (Figure 7–3).

Wound angiogenesis is inducible in unwounded tissue by the addition of chemoattractants to endothelial cells. Examples found in wounds include the BB homodimer of platelet-derived growth factor and a macrophage-derived growth factor whose identity is in doubt.

Wound angiogenesis appears to be a response to local energy depletion, and its mechanism is remarkably similar in outline to the regulation of collagen deposition. In reducing conditions (hypoxia or increased lactate), macrophages secrete a peptide chemoattractant to endothelial cells that causes angiogenesis in a corneal assay. Maintenance of the NAD+ pool severely inhibits the process. Thus, unmet metabolic needs lead through a growth factor mechanism to an anatomic response probably of general biologic significance.

Numerous growth factors and cytokines are said to stimulate angiogenesis, but animal experiments indicate that the dominant angiogenic stimulants in wounds are derived first from platelets in response to coagulation and then from macrophages in response to hypoxia or high lactate, fibrin, etc.

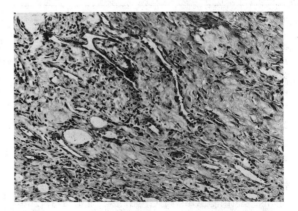

Figure 7–3. Photomicrograph of granulation tissue grown into a dead space surrounded by wire mesh. All the tissue is newly made. Note the rich vascular network, especially at the edge of the tissue in the upper left corner, where several open capillaries are leaking red cells into the wound.

EPITHELIALIZATION

Epithelial cells respond to many of the same stimuli as do fibroblasts and endothelial cells. A variety of growth factors regulate replication. TGFβ, for instance, tends to keep epithelial cells from differentiating and thus may potentiate and perpetuate mitogenesis, though it is not itself a mitogen for these cells. TGFα is an epithelial cell mitogen.

In healing, mitoses appear in epithelium a few cells away from the wound edge. The new cells migrate over the cells at the edge and into the unhealed area, perhaps attracted by a growth factor or cytokine, and anchor on the first unepithelized place, forming a new wound edge. The Po_2 on the underside of the cell at the anchor point is likely to be low. Low Po_2 stimulates squamous epithelial cells to produce TGFβ, presumably hindering terminal differentiation and favoring mitosis. This process repeats itself until the wound is closed.

Squamous epithelialization and differentiation proceed maximally when the local Po_2 approaches about 700 mm Hg and when surface wounds are kept moist.

Contrary to classic thought, even short periods of drying can impair the process. The exudate from acute, uninfected, superficial wounds also contains growth factors and lactate and therefore recapitulates the growth environment found internally.

COLLAGEN FIBER MATURATION, LYSIS, & CONTRACTION

Replacement of an extracellular matrix is a complex process. First, fibroblasts replace the provisional fibrin extracellular matrix with collagen monomers. Extracellular enzymes, some of which are Po_2-dependent, quickly polymerize these monomers but in a pattern that is much more random than normal, thus leaving young wounds weak and brittle. This brittleness is overcome when the hastily placed matrix is replaced with a more mature one consisting of larger, better organized, stronger, and more durable fibers (Figure 7–4).

Turnover and reorganization of new matrix is an important feature of healing, and fibroblasts and leukocytes secrete collagenases that ensure the lytic component. Turnover occurs rapidly at first and then more slowly. Even in simple wounds, increased turnover can be detected chemically for as long as 18 months. Healing is successful when a net excess of matrix is deposited despite concomitant lysis. Lysis, being destructive, is less dependent upon energy and nutrition. If synthesis is impaired, lysis weakens wounds. In some tissues (eg, colon), lysis unnecessarily weakens tissue structure, and inhibition of lysis with orally administrable agents leads to quicker gain of tensile strength. This is one of many features of healing that has not yet been clinically exploited.

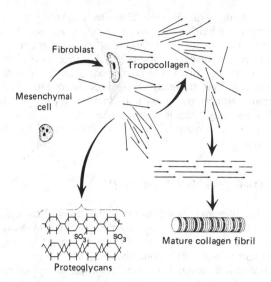

Figure 7–4. Schematic representation of collagen synthesis, deposition, and polymerization. The molecules polymerize with a "three-fourths stagger" overlap, which accounts for the cross banding visible on electron microscopy.

During rapid turnover, wounds gain strength and durability but also are vulnerable to contraction and stretching. Fibroblasts provide the motive force for contraction. Receptors in fibroblast membranes attach to collagen molecules and pull them together when the cell membranes shorten as the fibroblasts migrate. The fibers are then fixed in the packed positions, probably by a variety of cross-linking mechanisms. Both open and closed wounds tend to contract if not subjected to a superior distorting force. The phenomenon is best seen in surface wounds, which in areas of loose skin may close 90% or more by contraction alone. The result of a large open wound on the back of the neck, for instance, may be a very small area of reepithelialization. On the back, the buttock, or the neck, this is often a beneficial process, whereas in the face and about joints, the results may be disabling or disfiguring. This undesirable result is usually termed a contracture or a stricture. Skin grafts, especially thick ones, impede but do not totally stop the process. Dynamic splints, passive or active stretching, or insertion of flaps containing dermis and subdermis may be needed to counteract contraction. The force can be quite strong, though even severely contracted joints can usually be straightened with countertraction. Contraction occurs as long as collagen deposition is active, and chronic, slowly healing wounds (eg, as in ischemic tissues) are particularly likely to contract. Prevention of a stricture in a ureteric repair, for example, depends on ensuring that the opposing tissue edges are well perfused so that healing can proceed quickly to completion.

Healing wounds may also stretch during active turnover when tension overcomes contraction. This may account for the laxity of scars in ligaments of injured but unsplinted joints and the tendency for hernia formation in abdominal wounds of obese patients. If wounds are traumatized when passively stretched, contraction or weakness may continue for long periods and may become troublesome.

Even with remodeling, the net result of healing is still a scar.

COMPLETION OF HEALING

Healing and growth of malignancies are strikingly similar processes. As opposed to their role in oncogenesis, however, growth factors in wound healing generally obey basic controls, and healing stops at an appropriate point. Normally, the final stimuli to release of growth factors and cytokines seem to be local hypoxia and lactic acidosis. When these stimuli disappear as the new microcirculation matures, healing should stop.

Keloids, local overgrowths of connective tissue, and hypertrophic scars, which occur particularly in pigmented skin, probably represent a loss of normal control over the healing process, but few facts are known. Hypertrophic scars are generally self-limited and may regress after a year or so. The last areas of a burn to heal are the ones most often hypertrophic, but traction and reinjury due to tension also play a role. Therefore, prolonged inflammatory reactions are probably the common cause.

ROLE OF TISSUE HYPOXIA

Healing is not a unique process. The injury environment recruits normal cellular mechanisms, which become redundant and self-reinforcing. Partly because of its redundancy, healing is almost foolproof. The few vulnerable spots are related to perfusion and oxygenation, nutrition, and aberrations of inflammation.

Impaired perfusion and oxygenation are the most frequent causes of healing failure. Oxygen is required for successful inflammation, angiogenesis, epithelialization, and matrix deposition. The critical oxygenases involved have Km values for oxygen of about 20 mm Hg and maxima of about 200 mm Hg, which means that their reaction rates are governed by Pao_2 and blood perfusion throughout the entire physiologic range. The Po_2 of wound fluid in human wounds is about 30–40 mm Hg, implying that these enzymes normally function just beyond half capacity. Furthermore, wound Po_2 is depressed by blood volume deficiency, catecholamine infusion, or cold. On the other hand, under ideal conditions, wound fluid Po_2 can be raised above 100 mm Hg by improved perfusion and breathing of oxygen. Collagen deposition in human wounds is proportionate to wound Po_2. Human healing is profoundly influenced by local blood supply, vasoconstriction, and all other factors that govern perfusion and blood oxygenation.

Cardiopulmonary diseases affect wound healing, but vasoconstriction due to sympathetic nervous system activity is the principal source of clinical problems. Prevention or resolution of problems can be achieved by turning off sympathetic activity by correcting blood volume deficits, alleviating pain, and avoiding hypothermia. Wounds in highly vascularized tissues (eg, head, anus) heal fast and are quite resistant to infection.

IMPAIRED HEALING IN DISORDERS OF INFLAMMATION

The growth signals and lytic enzymes released by inflammatory cells are necessary for repair. Excessive and inadequate inflammatory responses can pose problems. Failure to heal is common in patients taking anti-inflammatory corticosteroids, immune suppressants, or cancer chemotherapeutic agents and whose inflammatory responses are blunted. Open wounds suffer more than primarily healing ones. The administration of these agents after inflammation is established is less detrimental. Healing impaired by inadequate inflammation, especially that due to corticosteroids, can be accelerated by vitamin A systemically or locally. In experiments, some of the growth factors also have had an effect. Both growth factors and vitamin A increase the number of inflammatory cells in the wound.

Inflammation may also be excessive. A mild excess may produce a hypertrophic scar. A major excess (eg, in response to endotoxin) can excite inflammatory cells to produce cytolytic amounts of cytokines and large amounts of proteinases. In gram-negative wound infections or septic shock, granulation tissue may not develop or it may be lysed. Prolonged inflammation due to infection or foreign bodies is a common cause of excess scarring.

Massive injuries give rise to large inflammatory reactions, and cytokines from large but otherwise uncomplicated wounds can produce systemic symptoms. Extensive wounds can produce large amounts of lactate that must be reconverted to glucose in the liver—a process that contributes to the hypermetabolism of trauma.

Debridement of damaged tissue and early immobilization of fractures minimize the above effects. Stimulation of the reticuloendothelial system, major amounts of injured tissue, and failure to debride can produce the systemic inflammatory response syndrome (SIRS) even in the absence of infection.

EFFECT OF MALNUTRITION

Malnutrition impairs healing, since healing depends on cell replication, specific organ function (liver, heart, lungs), and matrix synthesis. Weight loss and protein depletion have been shown experimentally to be risk factors. Still, healing may be normal in patients who have lost weight over a long period. Deficient healing is seen mainly in patients with acute malnutrition (ie, in the weeks just before or after an injury or operation). Even a few days of starvation measurably impairs healing, and an equally short period of repletion can reverse the deficit. Wound complications increase in severe malnutrition. A period of preoperative total parenteral nutrition is generally recommended for patients who have recently lost 10% or more of their body weight. This subject is covered in detail in Chapter 10.

HEALING OF SPECIALIZED TISSUES

Nerves

The brain heals largely through connective tissue scar formation in which glial and perivascular cells seem to differentiate into fibroblasts. When a peripheral nerve is severed, the distal nerve degenerates, leaving the axon sheaths to heal together by inosculation. The axon then regenerates from the nerve cell through the rejoined sheaths, advancing as much as 1 mm/d. Unfortunately, because individual neural sheaths have no means of seeking out their original distal ends, the axon sheaths reconnect randomly, and motor nerve axons may regenerate in vain into a sensory distal sheath and end organ. The functional result of neural regeneration, therefore, is more satisfactory in the purer peripheral nerves and in nerves rejoined by microscopic surgical techniques. Recent advances in growth factor technology and the ischemic, hypoxic nature of wounds suggests that means may be devised to improve nerve regeneration. This is currently one of the forefronts of surgical research.

Intestine

The rate of repair varies from one part of the intestine to the other in proportion to vascularity. Anastomoses of the colon and esophagus are precarious and likely to leak, whereas leakage of stomach or small intestine anastomoses is rare. Intestinal anastomoses usually regain strength rapidly. By 1 week they resist bursting more strongly than the more normal surrounding tissue. However, the surrounding intestine participates in the reaction to injury, loses a large portion of its collagen by lysis, and consequently loses strength. For this reason, leakage is about as likely to occur a few millimeters from the anastomosis as it is in the anastomosis itself, especially at the site of excessively tight sutures or staples. Drugs such as fluo-

rouracil limit lysis and in experimental conditions appear to prevent the early loss of strength.

Any event that delays collagen synthesis or exaggerates collagen lysis is likely to increase the risk of perforation and leakage (Figure 7–5). The danger of leakage is greatest from the fourth to seventh days, when tensile strength normally would rise rapidly but is prevented from doing so by increased lysis or compromised collagen deposition. Local infection, which often occurs near esophageal and colonic anastomoses, promotes lysis and delays synthesis, thus increasing the likelihood of perforation.

Though the surgeon aims for primary healing in anastomoses, much of the healing actually occurs by second intention in both sutured and stapled anastomoses. Fine surgical technique is more likely to promote primary repair.

Adhesions are assumed to be an almost inevitable consequence of abdominal surgery. While they are common, they are not inevitable. The most powerful stimuli are ischemic tissues (which attract a new blood supply that takes the form of vascularized adhesions), abscesses, and foreign bodies. All attract nests of macrophages which are activated to generate a fibrotic process.

Simple peritoneal defects are insufficient to cause adhesions, but when trauma, large defects, infection, ischemia, or foreign bodies are added, the process becomes more intense. Trauma and inflammation excite plasma leaks and deposition of fibrin. If allowed to remain, the fibrin increases the volume of ischemic tissue. Peritoneum normally produces plasminogen activator, which quickly leads to fibrin lysis. Exogenous plasminogen activator has decreased the occurrence of adhesions in experimental circumstances.

Attempts to prevent adhesions by suturing peritoneal defects usually worsen the problem by causing local ischemia and suture granulomas. Starch powder used in most surgical gloves as a lubricant was a great improvement over talc, but severe peritoneal (as well as pericardial, pleural, and meningeal) inflammatory

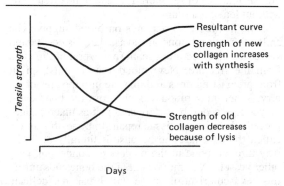

Figure 7–5. Tensile strength is the resultant between the strength of old collagen as affected by lysis and new collagen as affected by synthesis and lysis.

reactions due to starch and leading to adhesions have been well documented.

Bone

Bone healing is controlled by many of the same mechanisms that control soft tissue healing. It too occurs in three morphologic stages: an inflammatory stage, a reparative stage, and a remodeling stage. The duration of each stage varies depending on the location and nature of the fracture.

Injury (fracture) leads to hematoma formation from the damaged blood vessels of the periosteum, endosteum, and surrounding tissues. Within hours, an inflammatory infiltrate of neutrophils and macrophages is recruited into the hematoma as in soft tissue injuries. Monocytes and granulocytes debride and digest necrotic tissue and debris, including bone, on the fracture surface. This process continues for days to weeks depending on the amount of necrotic tissue.

During the reparative stage, the hematoma is gradually replaced by specialized granulation tissue with the power to form bone. This tissue, known as callus, develops from both sides of the fracture and is composed of fibroblasts, endothelial cells, and bone-forming cells (chondroblasts, osteoblasts). The extent to which callus forms from the medulla, the periosteum, or cortical bone depends upon the site of fracture, the degree of immobilization, and the type of bone injured. Within days after injury, mesenchymal tissue, which subsequently differentiates into chondroblasts and osteoblasts, proliferates. As macrophages phagocytose the hematoma and injured tissue, fibroblasts deposit a collagenous matrix, and chondroblasts deposit mucopolysaccharides in a process called enchondral bone formation. This step, prominent in some bones, is then converted to bone as osteoblasts condense hydroxyapatite crystals on specific points on the collagen fibers, and endothelial cells form a vasculature characteristic of bone with an end result analogous to reinforced concrete. Eventually the fibrovascular callus is completely replaced by new bone. Unlike healing of soft tissue, bone healing has features of regeneration, and bone often heals without leaving a scar.

Bone healing also depends on blood supply. The ends of fractured bone are avascular. Osteocyte and vessel lacunae become vacant for several millimeters from the fracture. New blood vessels must sprout from preexisting ones and migrate into the area of injury. When new blood vessels cross the bone ends, they are preceded by osteoclasts just as macrophages precede them in soft tissue repair. In bone, this unit is called the cutting cone because it literally bores its way through bone in the process of connecting with other vessels. Any movement of the bone ends during this revascularization stage will break the delicate new vessels and delay healing. Osteomyelitis originates most often in ischemic bone fragments. Hyperoxygenation hastens fracture healing and aids in the cure of osteomyelitis. Acute or chronic hypoxia slows bone repair.

Once the fracture has been bridged by new bone, it remodels in response to the mechanical stresses upon it, with restoration to normal or near-normal strength. During this process, as in soft tissue, bone and its vascular network are simultaneously removed and replaced. Increased bone turnover may be detected as long as 6–9 years after injury. Although remodeling is efficient, it cannot correct deformities of angulation or rotation in misaligned fractures. Careful fracture reduction is still necessary.

Fibroblasts, chondroblasts, and osteoblasts in healing fractures are derived from surrounding primitive mesenchyme. The origin of the mesenchyme is less clear. It seems to arise from muscle, fascia, periosteum, endothelium, marrow, even from circulating cells, as well as directly from fibrous tissue. The differentiation of these mesenchymal cells into bone-forming cells appears to be governed by specific growth factors such as bone morphogenetic protein (BMP), TGFβ, IGF-1, GM-CSF, and PDGF, all of which stimulate proliferation and induce the differentiation of osteoblasts in cell culture. BMP (which belongs to the TGFβ supergene family) appears to be the most specific for bone and is found in large quantity in bone matrix. BMP induces ectopic bone formation in the absence of preexisting bone and induces cartilage formation in vivo.

Bone repair may occur through primary or secondary intention. Primary repair can occur only when the fracture is stable and aligned and its surfaces closely apposed. This situation is rarely present in normal bone healing but is the goal of ridged plate fixation. When these conditions are met, capillaries can grow across the fracture and rapidly reestablish a vascular supply. Little or no callus forms. Secondary repair with abundant callus is more common.

Bone repair can be manipulated. Electrical stimulation, growth factors, and distraction osteogenesis are three promising new tools for this purpose. Electrical currents applied directly (through implanted electrodes) or induced by external alternating electromagnetic fields accelerate repair by inducing new bone formation in much the same way as small piezoelectric currents produced by mechanical deformation of intact bone controls remodeling along lines of stress. The technique of electrical stimulation has been used successfully to treat nonunion of bone (where new bone formation between bone ends fails, often requiring long periods of bed rest). BMP-impregnated implants have accelerated bone healing in animals and have been used with encouraging results to treat large bony defects and nonunions.

The **Ilizarov technique** of distraction osteogenesis can lengthen bones, transport bone across a defect, or correct defects of angulation. The Ilizarov device is an external fixator attached to the bones through metal pins or wires. A surgical break is created and then slowly pulled apart (1 mm/d) or reangulated. The vascular supply and subsequent new bone formation migrate along with the moving segment of bone.

SUTURES

The ideal suture material would be flexible, strong, easily tied, and securely knotted. It would excite little tissue reaction and would not serve as a nidus for infection.

Stainless steel wire is inert and maintains strength for a long time. It is difficult to tie and may have to be removed late postoperatively because of pain. It does not harbor bacteria, and it can be left in granulating wounds, when necessary, and will be covered by granulation tissue without causing abscesses.

Silk is an animal protein but is relatively inert in human tissue. It is commonly used because of its favorable handling characteristics. It loses strength over long periods and is unsuitable for suturing arteries to plastic grafts or for insertion of prosthetic cardiac valves. Silk sutures are multifilament and provide a potential haven for bacteria. Occasionally, silk sutures form a focus for small abscesses that migrate and "spit" through the skin, forming small sinuses that will not heal until the suture is removed.

Catgut (made from the submucosa of bovine intestine) will eventually resorb, but the resorption time is highly variable. It excites considerable inflammatory reaction and tends to potentiate infections. Catgut also loses strength rapidly and unpredictably in the intestine and in infected wounds as a consequence of acid and enzyme hydrolysis. There is little use for catgut suture in modern surgery.

Synthetic nonabsorbable sutures are generally inert and retain strength longer than wire. However, their handling characteristics are not as good as those of silk, and they must usually be knotted at least four times, resulting in large amounts of retained foreign body. Multifilament plastic sutures are just as apt to become infected and migrate to the surface as silk sutures. Monofilament plastic, like wire, will not harbor bacteria. Nylon monofilament is extremely nonreactive, but it is difficult to tie. Monofilament polypropylene is intermediate in all of these properties. Plastic sutures are required for cardiovascular work because they are not absorbed. Vascular anastomoses to prosthetic vascular grafts rely indefinitely on the strength of sutures; therefore, use of absorbable sutures may lead to aneurysm formation. Even monofilament sutures will "spit." However, this disadvantage is generally confined to sizes of 00 and larger.

Synthetic absorbable sutures are strong, have predictable rates of loss of tensile strength, incite a minimal inflammatory reaction, and may have special usefulness in gastrointestinal, urologic, and gynecologic surgery. Compared with catgut, polyglycolic acid and polyglactin retain tensile strength

longer in gastrointestinal anastomoses. Polydioxanone sulfate sutures are monofilament and lose about half their strength in 50 days, thus solving the problem of premature breakage in fascial closures.

Tapes are the skin closure of choice for clean or contaminated wounds. They minimize the probability of infection by not introducing a foreign body in the form of a skin suture that connects the skin surface to the wound dead space. They cannot be used on actively bleeding wounds or wounds with complex surfaces, such as those in the perineum.

Staples, whether for internal use or skin closure, are mainly steel-tantalum alloys, which incite a minimal tissue reaction. The technique of staple placement is different from sutures, but the same basic rules pertain. There are no real differences in the healing that follows suture or stapled closures. Stapling devices tend to minimize errors in technique, but at the same time they do not offer a feel for tissue and have limited ability to accommodate to exceptional circumstances.

Staples are preferable to sutures for skin closure, since they do not penetrate the skin and do not provide a conduit for contaminating organisms. Staples are not preferable to skin tapes.

IMPLANTABLE MATERIALS

Although prosthetic materials are constantly being improved, none are ideal in regard to tissue compatibility, permanent fixation, and resistance to infection. Two principles are paramount: biocompatibility and a fabric that is incorporated into tissue. Biocompatibility is the foremost consideration. Both specific and nonspecific immune mechanisms are involved in the inflammatory reaction to foreign materials. Highly incompatible materials, such as wood splinters, are rejected immediately with an acute inflammatory process that includes massive local release of proteolytic enzymes. Consequently, the foreign body is never incorporated and lies loosely in a fibrous pocket. Mechanical irritation may induce a similar reaction, which accounts for the occasional spontaneous rejection of large (usually larger than 00), stiff suture materials from soft tissue sites. In less severe incompatibility, rejection is not so vigorous and proteolysis not so prominent. Mononuclear cells—the major component of inflammatory tissue—direct a response that creates a fibrous capsule which may be acceptable in a joint replacement but which may distort a breast reconstruction severely.

Most implants must become anchored to adjacent normal tissues by allowing ingrowth of fibrous tissue or bone. This requires biocompatibility and interstices large enough to incite ingrowth just as in a wound and to allow pedicles of vascularized tissue to enter and join similar units.

In bone this imparts stability. In vascular grafts, the

invading tissue supports neointima formation, which retards mural thrombosis and distal embolization. Soft tissue will grow into pores larger than about 50 μm in diameter and even faster into much larger ones. Of the vascular prostheses, woven Dacron is best for tissue incorporation. In bone, sintered, porous metallic surfaces are best. Large-screen polypropylene mesh can be used to support the abdominal wall or chest even in the presence of infection and is usually well incorporated into the granulation tissue that penetrates the mesh.

Unfortunately, when the mechanical properties of the implant do not match those of the host tissue, shear forces may overcome delicate biologic unions, with loosening of anchoring sites, especially with orthopedic prostheses.

The implantation space remains vulnerable to infection for years and is a particular problem in implants that cross the body surface. Mesh cuffs that incite incorporation have successfully forestalled infection for months, but infections that arise from bacteria entering the body along "permanently" implanted foreign bodies which traverse the skin surface remain an unsolved problem.

Plastic implants are often chosen for texture and flexibility. Silastic materials are highly compatible, but fixation and material fatigue are problems. Cosmetic implants—particularly silicone breast implants—have a low but troublesome incidence of deforming fibrotic capsule formation. In addition to idiosyncratic healing responses, there is also the problem of toxic responses to trace components such as plasticizers and hardeners. Potential complications include cancers if materials such as asbestos are present even in small amounts.

DECUBITUS & OTHER CHRONIC ULCERS

Decubitus Ulcers

Decubitus ulcers are disastrous complications of immobilization. They result from prolonged pressure that robs tissue of its blood supply. Irritative or contaminated injections and prolonged contact with moisture, urine, and feces also play a prominent role. Most patients who develop decubitus ulcers are also poorly nourished. Pressure ulcers are common in drug addicts who take overdoses and lie immobile for many hours. The ulcers vary in depth and often extend from skin to a bony pressure point such as the greater trochanter or the sacrum.

Most decubitus ulcers are preventable. Hospital-acquired ulcers are nearly always the result of inadequate nursing care.

Treatment is difficult and usually prolonged. The first important step is to incise and drain any infected spaces or necrotic tissue. Dead tissue is then debrided until the exposed surfaces are viable and granulating. Many will then heal spontaneously. However, deep ulcers may require surgical closure, sometimes with removal of underlying bone. The defect may require closure by judicious movement of thick, well-vascularized tissue into the affected area. Musculocutaneous flaps are the treatment of choice when chronic infection and significant tissue loss are combined.

Chronic Wounds

Chronically unhealed wounds, especially on the lower extremity, are common in the setting of vascular, immunologic, and neurologic disease. Venous ulcers, largely of the medial lower leg, reflect poor perfusion and perivascular leakage of plasma into tissue. This is the result of venous hypertension produced by incompetent venous valves. Most venous ulcers will heal if the venous congestion and edema are relieved by bed rest, compression stockings, or surgical procedures that eliminate incompetent feeding vessels.

Arterial or ischemic ulcers, which tend to occur on the lateral ankle or foot, are best treated by revascularization. Hyperbaric oxygen, which provides a temporary source of oxygen and enhances angiogenesis, is an effective though expensive alternative when revascularization is not possible. Useful information can be obtained by transcutaneous oximetry. Tissues with a low Po_2 will not heal spontaneously. However, if oxygen tension can be raised into a relatively normal range by oxygen administration, the lesion will probably respond to oxygen therapy. Sensory loss, especially of the feet, leads to ulceration and bony deformities due to fractures, the so-called Charcot deformity. Ulcers in patients with diabetes mellitus may have two causes. Patients with neuropathic ulcers usually have good circulation, and their lesions will heal if protected from weight trauma by bed rest, special shoes, or splints. Recurrences are common, however. Diabetics with ischemic disease, whether they have neuropathy or not, are at risk for gangrene, and they frequently require amputation if revascularization is not possible. Insulin dressings have been advocated.

In pyoderma gangrenosum, granulomatous inflammation with or without arteritis kills skin and subcutaneous skin, possibly by a mechanism involving excess cytokine release. These ulcers are associated with inflammatory bowel disease and certain types of arthritis and chondritis. Corticosteroids or other anti-inflammatory drugs are helpful. Anti-inflammatory corticosteroids can also contribute to poor healing by inhibiting cytokine release. Topical or systemic vitamin A restores the inflammatory mechanism and may induce healing of the lesions. Distinguishing between these possibilities in patients with inflammatory bowel disease may be difficult.

Infection may contribute to the lack of healing of chronic ulcers or may be a complication. Antibiotics should be part of initial therapy in most cases. They are not effective as continuous therapy in chronic wounds, however.

The first principle in managing chronic wounds is to diagnose and treat any underlying circulatory disease. The second principle is never to allow open wounds to dry (ie, use moist dressings). Moist dressings may also relieve pain. A third principle is to control any infection with systemic antibiotics. Topical barriers to infection are useful but not always necessary. A fourth principle is to recognize that chronically scarred tissue is usually poorly perfused. Debridement of unhealthy tissue, often followed by skin grafting, may be required for healing.

Compared with healing wounds, fluid collected from chronic wounds is often deficient in growth factors or cytokines. This area of investigation has great promise. A number of growth factors have been shown to accelerate healing of acute wounds in animals. They include FGFs, TGFβ, IGF-1, PDGF, and EGF, and the list is growing. However, in the setting of chronic human wounds, with the perfusion problems noted above, "proof" of efficacy has been difficult to develop, and no clear-cut advantage to any formulation has yet been convincingly demonstrated.

SURGICAL TECHNIQUE

The most important means of achieving optimal healing after operation is good surgical technique. Many cases of healing failure are due to technical errors. Tissue should be protected from drying and internal or external contamination. The surgeon should use fine instruments; should perform clean, sharp dissection; and should make minimal, skillful use of electrocautery, ligatures, and sutures. All these precautions contribute to the most important goal of surgical technique—gentle handling of tissue. Even the best ligature or suture is a foreign body that may strangulate tissue if tied tightly. The skillful operator who uses sutures minimally and gently will be rewarded with the best results. Good hemostasis is a laudable objective, but excessive sponging, electrocautery, and tying of small vessels are traumatic and invite infection.

Wound Closure

As with many other surgical techniques, the exact method of wound closure may be less important than how well it is performed. The tearing strength of sutures from fascia is no greater than 3–4 kg. There is little reason for use of sutures of greater strength than this. Excessively tight closure strangulates tissue and leads to hernia formation and infection.

If surgeons could foresee the future, dehiscence (undesired spontaneous separation of wound edges) would not occur, since techniques to prevent it are well known. The surgeon can choose the techniques to meet the needs and risks of the individual wound (Figures 7–6 and 7–7). The most common technical

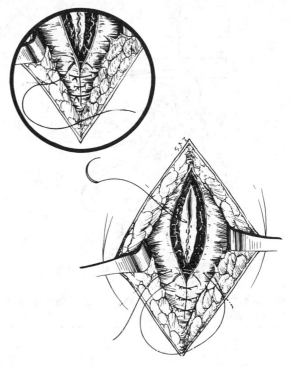

Figure 7–6. Closure of peritoneum with continuous sutures. Fascia closure with figure-of-eight sutures (top) and simple interrupted sutures (bottom) is illustrated. "Running" closures are also useful, and the suture "bites" should be similar to those illustrated, 1 and 1.5 cm apart and 1–1.5 cm apart.

causes of dehiscence are infection and excessively tight sutures.

The ideal closure for small wounds in healthy patients is with fine interrupted sutures placed loosely and conveniently close to the wound edge. In abdominal wounds, the peritoneum need not be sutured, but posterior and anterior fasciae are sutured with nonabsorbable or slowly absorbable sutures.

Unfortunately, surgeons often must operate on patients who have impaired wound healing. In these cases, closures must be stronger to avoid dehiscence. A more secure closure begins with a running or mattress absorbable suture in the posterior sheath, joint capsule, or submucosa. The closure is continued with simple buried retention sutures through the fascia in which the farthest point of penetration is at least 1 cm from the wound edge. When the tension is placed this far back, the fascial fibers that become weakened by postinjury collagen lysis are not expected to provide critical support. The lytic effect extends for about 5 mm to each side of the wound edge. The skin is preferably closed with adhesive strips unless bleeding from the wound or an uneven surface makes adherence of the strips precarious, in which case staples are the next choice. With this fascial closure, the skin can

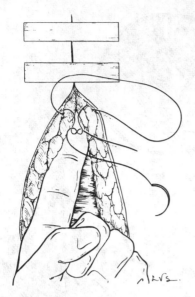

Figure 7–7. Skin closure with interrupted subdermal sutures and Steri-Strips.

Table 7–2. Controllable factors affecting healing.

I. Factors that decrease collagen synthesis
    Starvation (protein depletion)
    Steroids
    Infection[1]
    Associated injuries
    Hypoxia and hypovolemia
    Radiation injury
    Uremia
    Diabetes
    Drugs: dactinomycin, fluorouracil, methotrexate, etc
    Advanced age
II. Operative factors
    Tissue injury
    Poor blood supply
    Poor apposition of surrounding tissues (pelvic anastomosis, unreduced fracture, unclosed dead space)
III. Factors that increase collagen lysis
    Starvation
    Severe trauma
    Inflammation
    Infection
    Steroids

[1]Some infections may in time cause excess collagen deposition.

easily be left open for delayed primary or secondary closure. Subcutaneous tissues rarely need to be sutured closed.

In all closures, sutures should be placed as far apart as possible consistent with approximation of tissue. Sutures placed too tightly and too close together obstruct blood supply to the wound. In most cases of dehiscence, suture material cuts through tissue and is not broken or untied.

It is useful to assess wound risk in advance, so that the proper choice of closure can be made easily (Table 7–2).

Delayed primary closure is a technique by which the wound is held open for 4–5 days and then closed with skin tapes. The environs of the wound are inspected daily to be sure that invasive infection is absent, but if there is no need to disturb the dressing, it is left in place until the fourth or fifth day, when, under sterile conditions, the wound is closed, usually with skin tapes. During the delay period, angiogenesis and healing start, and bacteria are cleared from the wound. The success of this method depends on the ability of the surgeon to detect minor signs of infection. Merely leaving the wound open for 4 days does not guarantee that it will not become infected, and some wounds (eg, fibrin-covered or inflamed wounds) should not be closed by a delayed primary closure.

POSTOPERATIVE CARE

The appearance of delayed wound infection—weeks to years after operation—emphasizes that all wounds are contaminated and that the line between apparent infection and apparent normal repair is a fine one. A minor setback such as a period of cardiac failure or of malnutrition will often allow infection to become established. Most frequently, however, poor tissue perfusion and oxygenation of the wound during the postoperative period are the causes of weakened host resistance. Maintenance of perfusion is the essence of postoperative care; however, there are few ways of measuring perfusion of subcutaneous tissue and fascia. Urine output, central venous pressure, wedge pressures, etc, are all poor indices. Better indicators are the speed of capillary return (normal: < 1.5 seconds on the forehead or 5 seconds on the knee), thirst, and postural changes in vital signs. New means of measuring perfusion (eg, subcutaneous or transcutaneous oximetry and postcapillary Po_2 determinations) are now being developed to assure good perfusion, and they are relevant to wound management. Proper fluid balance and nutritional status should be maintained to ensure the kind of perfusion that will support repair and resist infection. Hypothermia is a potent source of vasoconstriction and should be corrected.

Postoperative care of the wound also involves cleanliness, protection from trauma, and maximal support of the patient. Even closed wounds can be infected by surface contamination of bacteria, particularly within the first 2–3 days. Bacteria gain entrance most easily through suture tracts. If a wound is likely to be traumatized or contaminated, it should be protected during this time. Such protection may require special dressings such as occlusive sprays or repeated cleansings as well as dressings.

Some mechanical stress enhances healing. Even fracture callus formation is greater if slight motion is allowed. Patients should move and stress their wounds a little. Early ambulation and return to normal activity are, in general, good for repair.

The ideal care of the wound begins in the preoper-ative period and ends only months later. The patient must be prepared so that optimal conditions exist when the wound is made. Surgical technique must be clean, gentle, skillful, and ingenious. Postoperatively, wound care includes maintenance of nutrition, blood volume, and oxygenation. Although wound healing is in many ways a local phenomenon, ideal care of the wound is essentially ideal care of the patient.

REFERENCES

Aaronson SA et al: Growth factor-regulated pathways in epithelial cell proliferation. Am Rev Respir Dis 1990;142(6 Part 2):S7.

Amento EP, Beck LS: TGF-beta and wound healing. Ciba Found Symp 1991;167:115.

Anderson TL, Gorstein F, Osteen KG: Stromal-epithelial cell communication, growth factors, and tissue regulation. Lab Invest 1990;62:519.

Border JR, Bone LB: Multiple trauma: Major extremity wounds; their immediate management and its consequences. Adv Surg 1988;21:263.

Brand R, Rubin C: *Fracture Healing: The Scientific Basis of Orthopaedics.* Appleton & Lange, 1987.

Buckley A, Davidson J, Kamerath C: Epidermal growth factor increases granulation tissue formation dose dependently. J Surg Res 1987;43:322.

Burgess AW: Epidermal growth factor and transforming growth factor alpha. Br Med Bull 1989;45:401.

Clark S, Kamen R: The human hematopoietic colony-stimulating factors. Science 1987;236:1229.

Ehrlich HP, Rajaratnam JB: Cell locomotion forces versus cell contraction forces for collagen lattice contraction: An in vitro model of wound contraction. Tissue Cell 1990;22:407.

Ellis H, Bucknall T, Cox P: Abdominal incisions and their closure. Curr Probl Surg 1985;22:1.

Ford H et al: Characterization of wound cytokines in the sponge matrix model. Arch Surg 1989;124:1422.

Gallin J, Goldstein I, Snyderman R (editors): *Inflammation: Basic Principles and Clinical Correlates.* Raven Press, 1988.

Ghezzi P et al: Hypoxia increases production of interleukin-1 and tumor necrosis factor by human mononuclear cells. Cytokine 1991;3:189.

Hammarlund C, Svedman C, Svedman P: Hyperbaric oxygen treatment of healthy volunteers with u.v.-irradiated blister wounds. Burns 1991;17:296.

Herndon DN et al: Effects of recombinant human growth hormone on donor-site healing in severely burned children. Ann Surg 1990;212:424.

Hussain MZ, Ghani QP, Hunt TK: Inhibition of prolyl hydroxylase by poly(ADP-ribose) and phosphoribosyl-AMP: Possible role of ADP-ribosylation in intracellular prolyl hydroxylase regulation. J Biol Chem 1989;264:7850.

Ignotz R, Endo T, Massague J: Regulation of fibronectin and type I collagen mRNA levels by transforming growth factor-b. J Biol Chem 1987;262:6443.

Jensen J et al: Wound healing in anemia. West J Med 1986;144:465.

Jensen JA et al: Effect of lactate, pyruvate, and pH on secretion of angiogenesis and mitogenesis factors by macrophages. Lab Invest 1986;54:574.

Jonsson K, Jiborn H, Zederfeldt B: Collagen metabolism in small intestinal anastomosis. Am J Surg 1987;154:288.

Klagsbrun M: The fibroblast growth factor family: Structural and biological properties. Prog Growth Factor Res 1989;1:207.

Levi-Montalcini R: The nerve growth factor 35 years later. Science 1987;237:1154.

Mohan S, Baylink D: Bone growth factors. Clin Orthop 1991;263:30.

Mueller R et al: The role of IGF-I and IGFBP-3 in wound healing. In: *Modern Concepts of Insulin-Like Growth Factors.* Spencer EM (editor). Elsevier, 1991.

Paty P, Banda M, Hunt T: Fibrin activation of macrophages: One mechanism of angiogenesis in wound healing: Highlights of Second International Forum. In: *Fibrinolysis and Angiogenesis.* Steward A et al (editors). Excerpta Medica, 1987.

Pepicello J, Novorek H: Five year experience with tape closure of abdominal wounds. Surg Gynecol Obstet 1989;169:310.

Poole G: Mechanical factors in abdominal wound closure: The prevention of fascial dehiscence. Surgery 1986;97:631.

Quaglino DJ et al: Transforming growth factor-beta stimulates wound healing and modulates extracellular matrix gene expression in pig skin: I. Excisional wound model. Lab Invest 1990;63:307.

Rappolee DA et al: Wound macrophages express TGF-alpha and other growth factors in vivo: Analysis by mRNA phenotyping. Science 1988;241:708.

Thiebaud D et al: Insulinlike growth factor 1 regulates mRNA levels of osteonectin and pro-alpha 1(I)collagen in clonal preosteoblastic calvarial cells. J Bone Miner Res 1990;5:761.

Tompkins RG, Burke JF: Progress in burn treatment and the use of artificial skin. World J Surg 1990;14:819.

8

Inflammation, Infection, & Antibiotics

Thomas K. Hunt, MD, & Reid V. Mueller, MD

SURGICAL INFECTIONS

A surgical infection is an infection that (1) is unlikely to respond to nonsurgical treatment (it usually must be excised or drained) and occupies an unvascularized space in tissue or (2) occurs in an operated site. Common examples of the first group are appendicitis, empyema, gas gangrene, and most abscesses.

Surgeons are regrettably familiar with the vicious circle of operation or injury, infection, malnutrition, immunosuppression, organ failure, reoperation, further malnutrition, and further infection. One of the fine arts of surgery is to know when to intervene with excision, drainage, physiologic support, antibiotic therapy, and nutritional therapy. For infections arising in a space or in dead tissue, by far the most important aspect of treatment is to establish surgical drainage.

Pathogenesis

Three elements are common to surgical infections: (1) an infectious agent, (2) a susceptible host, and (3) a closed, unperfused space.

A. The Infectious Agent: Although a few pathogens cause most surgical infections, many organisms are capable of doing so. Among the aerobic organisms, streptococci may invade even minor breaks in the skin and spread through connective tissue planes and lymphatics. *Staphylococcus aureus* is the most common pathogen in wound infections and around foreign bodies. *Klebsiella* often invades the inner ear and enteric tissues as well as the lung. Enteric organisms, especially *Escherichia coli* and enterococci, are often found together with anaerobes. Among the anaerobes, *Bacteroides* species and peptostreptococci are often present in surgical infections, and *Clostridium* species are major pathogens in ischemic tissue.

Pseudomonas and *Serratia* are usually nonpathogenic surface contaminants but may be opportunistic and even lethal invaders in immunosuppressed patients. Some fungi (*Histoplasma* and *Coccidioides*) and yeasts *(Candida),* along with *Nocardia* and *Actinomyces,* cause abscesses and sinus tracts, and even

animal parasites (amebas and *Echinococcus*) may cause abscesses, especially in the liver. Destructive granulomas, such as tuberculosis, once required excision, but antibiotic therapy has now superseded operation for this purpose in most cases. Nevertheless, tuberculosis and brucellosis of the intestinal tract still must be treated surgically on occasion. Other rare diseases such as cat-scratch fever, psittacosis, and tularemia may cause suppurative lymphadenitis and require drainage or excision.

Identification of the pathogen by smear and culture remains a cardinal step in therapy. The surgeon must inform the microbiologist of peculiar circumstances associated with any given specimen, so that appropriate smears and cultures can be done; serious errors may otherwise result.

B. The Susceptible Host: Surgical infections such as appendicitis and furuncles occur in patients whose only defect in immunity is a closed space in tissue. However, patients with suppressed immune systems are being seen with increasing frequency, and their problems have become a major surgical challenge. **Immunosuppression** seems a simple concept but in fact usually represents a combination of defects of the multifaceted immune mechanism.

1. Specific immunity–The immune process that depends upon prior exposure to an antigen involves detection and processing of antigen by macrophages, mobilization of T and B lymphocytes, synthesis of specific antibody, and other functions. Its relative importance is illustrated in acquired immunodeficiency syndrome (AIDS), transplant immunosuppression, and agammaglobulinemia, each of which is associated with only a slight increase in the frequency and severity of some surgical infections. Specific abnormalities of cell-mediated and humoral immunity have been reported in almost every imaginable form of surgical infection. For instance, major burns incite suppressor cell activity and the appearance of immunosuppressor substances in blood. Burn victims are highly susceptible to infection. Unfortunately, the clinical significance of this and other isolated defects of specific immunity is obscure, and their clinical importance in the complex immune system is difficult to determine. In general, isolated defects contribute little to the severity of ordinary surgical infections. Major defects contribute substantially, but only to long-term morbidity and to deaths due to more widespread infections such as pneumonia, meningitis, and viral diseases, for which specific immune mechanisms constitute the principal mode of defense.

2. Nonspecific immunity–Despite the emphasis in the literature on specific immune mechanisms, nonspecific immunity, which depends on phagocytic leukocytes seeking out, ingesting, and killing microorganisms, is the principal means by which the host defends against abscess-forming and necrotizing infections. This includes wound infections.

The importance of nonspecific immunity is illustrated by granulocytopenia, which frequently leads to acute bacterial infection and septicemia and often results in death. Similarly, defective phagocyte chemotaxis is accompanied by infection after trauma and burns and operations on malnourished patients. Phagocytic defects such as Job's syndrome, for example, are rare but devastating. Without antibiotic support, children with defective intraphagocytic killing due to chronic granulomatous disease die in infancy or childhood, often from multiple abscesses.

a. Chemoattraction and phagocytosis–Granulocytes move from the bloodstream toward sites in tissues at which organisms contact and activate chemoattractive complement molecules. They adhere to the organisms by means of specific antibodies or nonspecific opsonins such as complement 3b or fibronectin and internalize them by engulfment in a phagocytic vacuole. These steps require little or no oxygen, but chemotaxis is vulnerable to a number of disorders, particularly anti-inflammatory steroid hormones and malnutrition, which reduce the number of granulocytes that arrive at a contaminated site in a given time.

b. Killing mechanisms–Once the phagosome is formed, other cytoplasmic granules (lysosomes) fuse with it and release into it preformed and increasingly acidic proteolytic solutions that kill most bacteria and fungi.

A second process, termed "oxidative killing," is particularly important to the killing of organisms such as staphylococci which are commonly responsible for surgical infections. This mechanism consumes and requires molecular oxygen, which it converts to superoxide anion. In this process, a membrane-bound NADPH oxidase is activated, and a burst of respiration (oxygen consumption) follows. Part of the consumed oxygen is converted to a series of oxygen radicals (including superoxide, hydroxyl radical, and hypochlorite), which are released into phagosomes and assist in bacterial killing. This process is progressively inhibited when extracellular oxygen tension falls below about 30 mm Hg. When oxygen tension is 0 mm Hg, the antibacterial capacity of normal granulocytes for S $aureus$ and E $coli$, for instance, falls by half—to the same capacity observed in granulocytes

taken from victims of chronic granulomatous disease, which results from the genetic absence of membrane-bound oxidase and which without aggressive antibiotic therapy is lethal in early childhood.

Whether a given inoculum will establish an infection and become invasive depends to a great extent on how well tissue perfusion—and therefore oxygenation—can meet the increased metabolic demands of the granulocytes. Inflammatory signals from complement factors and histamine, for instance, dilate vessels and help direct blood flow to infected areas, but if blood volume or regional vascular supply is so poor that tissue perfusion cannot increase, invasive infection soon follows. Tissue oxygen supplies can often be raised by increasing blood volume and arterial Po_2 and are lowered by hypovolemia and pulmonary insufficiency. Tests in animals show that correcting arterial hypoxia aborts bacterial infections as effectively as does use of specific antibiotics and that antibiotics are far more effective when phagocytes have an adequate oxygen supply.

Patients with pulmonary disease, severe trauma, congestive heart failure, hypovolemia, or excessive levels of vasopressin, angiotensin, or catecholamines have hypoxic peripheral tissues and are unusually susceptible to infection. They are truly immunosuppressed. Support of the circulation is just as important to immune defense as is nutrition or antibiotic therapy.

3. Anergy–Anergy is defined as the lack of inflammatory response to skin test antigens. It characterizes a population of immunosuppressed patients who tend to develop infections and die from them. The skin tests used to diagnose anergy are those often used to test recall antigens and delayed hypersensitivity—but in fact they test much of the spectrum of antibacterial immunologic events, including antigen detection and processing by macrophages, release of lymphokines, antibody synthesis, and the inflammatory response, including leukocyte chemotaxis. One event they do not detect is, conspicuously, the final crucial step of actually killing bacteria. Anergy has many causes, including defective T and B lymphocytes, the presence of excess anti-inflammatory corticosteroids, defective antigen processing, and increased numbers of suppressor T cells. Infection itself suppresses skin test responses, which often become active again after incision and drainage of an infective focus. However, among surgical patients, malnutrition and disorders of leukotaxis are among the most powerful and common causes of anergy, and skin testing has become a useful research tool because it assays elements of both nonspecific and specific immunity.

4. Immunity in diabetes mellitus–Diabetes mellitus impairs immunity. Well-controlled diabetics resist infection normally except in tissues made ischemic by arterial disease, while uncontrolled diabetics do not. The mechanism is unknown, except that leukocytes from poorly controlled diabetics adhere, migrate, and kill bacteria poorly. They improve their performance when control is regained. Leukocytes also function poorly without insulin, and insulin is consumed in wounds and other poorly perfused spaces, resulting in low ambient insulin levels.

C. The Closed Space: Most surgical infections start in a susceptible, usually poorly vascularized place in tissue such as a wound or a natural space. The common denominators are poor perfusion, local hypoxia, hypercapnia, and acidosis. Some natural spaces with narrow outlets, such as those of the appendix, gallbladder, and intestines, are especially prone to becoming obstructed and then infected.

The peritoneal and pleural cavities are not normally spaces, and their surfaces slide over one another, thereby dispersing contaminating bacteria. However, foreign bodies, dead tissue, and injuries interfere with this mechanism and predispose to infection. Fibrin inhibits the clearing of bacteria. It polymerizes around bacteria, trapping them; this encourages abscess formation but at the same time prevents dangerous spread of infection.

Foreign bodies may have spaces in which bacteria can reside. Infarcted tissue is markedly susceptible to infection. Thrombosed veins, for example, rarely become infected unless intravenous catheters enter them and act as entry points for bacteria.

Spread of Surgical Infections

Surgical infections usually originate as a single focus and become dangerous by spreading and releasing toxins. Spreading occurs by several mechanisms.

A. Necrotizing Infections: Necrotizing infections tend to spread along anatomically defined paths. Clostridial myonecrosis, for instance, spreads by progressive necrosis of muscle. Necrotizing fasciitis spreads along poorly perfused fascial and subcutaneous planes, its toxins causing thrombosis even of large vessels ahead of the necrotic area, thus creating more ischemic and vulnerable tissue.

B. Abscesses: If not promptly drained, abscesses enlarge, killing more tissue in the process. Natural boundaries can be breached; eg, intestinal cutaneous fistulas may form, or blood vessel walls may be penetrated. Leukocytes contribute to necrosis by releasing lysosomal enzymes during phagocytosis.

C. Phlegmons and Superficial Infections: Phlegmons contain little pus but much edema. They spread along fat planes and by contiguous necrosis, combining features of both of the above kinds of spread. Superficial infections may spread along skin not only by contiguous necrosis but also by metastasis.

D. Spread of Infection via the Lymphatic System: Streptococcal and sometimes staphylococcal infections may spread along lymphatic pathways. Lymphangitis produces red streaks in the skin and travels proximally along major lymph vessels. However, it may also occur in hidden places such as the retroperitoneum in puerperal sepsis.

E. Spread of Infection via the Bloodstream: Empyema and endocarditis caused by intravenously injected contaminated drugs are now common. Brain abscesses resulting from infections elsewhere in the body (especially the face) occur in infants and diabetics. Liver abscesses may complicate appendicitis and inflammatory bowel disease, sometimes as a result of suppurative phlebitis of the portal vein (pylephlebitis).

Complications

A. Fistulas and Sinus Tracts: Fistulas and sinus tracts often result when abdominal abscesses contiguous to bowel open to the skin. Actinomycosis, in particular, leads to chronic sinus tracts in the neck, chest, and lower abdomen after operations for infected lung cysts, diverticulitis, or appendicitis. When tissue necrosis compounds the development of sinus tracts and erodes major blood vessels, severe bleeding may occur. This is most troublesome in irradiated tissue of nonhealing neck wounds and in infected groin wounds after vascular surgery.

Some intestinal fistulas originate in poorly fashioned or necrotic suture lines, and some result from contiguous abscesses that eventually penetrate both bowel and skin, often helped along by the surgeon who must drain the abscess.

B. Suppressed Wound Healing: Suppressed wound healing is a consequence of infection. The mechanism is probably stimulation by bacteria of interleukin-1, which in turn stimulates proteolysis, especially collagenase production.

C. Immunosuppression and Superinfection: Immunosuppression and superinfection are common consequences of surgical infection. There is no clear explanation of why infection sometimes suppresses immunity, nor is there ever likely to be a simple one, but consumptive immunopathy and toxicity have been invoked to explain it. Superinfection occurs when immunosuppression provides an opportunity for invasion by opportunistic, often antibiotic-resistant organisms.

Some Definitions

The term "bacteremia" denotes the presence of bacteria in blood. The significance of septicemia is variable, and it is often harmless. It frequently follows dental work, and in that context is hazardous only for patients with damaged heart valves and impaired immune systems. It occurs predictably during instrumentation of the infected urinary tract and should be prevented in those circumstances by prior administration of appropriate antibiotics. Gram-positive bacteremia is usually less significant than gram-negative bacteremia and has less unfavorable prognostic implications. In burns, for example, an episode of gram-positive bacteremia entails little risk of death, while an episode of gram-negative bacteremia entails a considerable risk.

"Septicemia" usually means bacteremia plus leukocytosis, but operationally this has little meaning since leukopenia may also accompany infection.

"Sepsis" has come to denote significant infection in which bacteria, bacterial toxins, or inflammatory mediators escape the control of the immune system, enter the bloodstream, and incite a systemic response. Chills, fever (due to the stimulating effect of interleukin-1 [IL-1] on prostanoid synthesis in the hypothalamus), and sometimes pulmonary failure or shock reflect the release of bacterial toxins and "inflammatory mediators" (mainly cytokines).

Cytokines & The Systemic Inflammatory Response

Severe infection with leukocytosis and fever may be accompanied by failure of one or more organs, including, in decreasing order of frequency, the lungs, kidneys, liver, gastrointestinal tract, immune system, heart, and nervous system. The organ failure is secondary to damage by inflammatory mediators or cytokines from injured or infected tissue and cells of the reticuloendothelial system. Macrophages of the reticuloendothelial system release cytokines under the influence of endotoxin or the effects of shock, tissue hypoxia, or extensive trauma. Cytokines are joined by products of the classic inflammatory pathway—such as complement, histamine, and bradykinin—and the sympathetic nervous system to produce hemodynamic, inflammatory, and metabolic derangements.

These events are highly exaggerated coping mechanisms, which under less severe circumstances are useful to destroy infecting organisms and elicit reparative mechanisms in wounded tissue. Organ failure, however, is the result of excessive amounts of cytokines interfering with microcirculatory perfusion and cellular metabolism.

Cytokines are a group of loosely related substances, largely peptides, whose normal function is communication between cells of the inflammatory and reticuloendothelial systems. They include the interleukins (IL-1–13), tumor necrosis factor (TNF-α), granulocyte-macrophage colony-stimulating factor (GM-CSF), and the interferons. TNF-α and GM-CSF have somewhat deceptive names because they were discovered in the context of oncologic and hematologic research. Like many of the interleukins, they act as growth factors in low concentrations and are cytolytic in high concentrations. The interleukins are a chemically similar but functionally dissimilar group of peptides. Interleukin-1 (Table 8–1) has a number of effects, including stimulation of the liver to synthesize and release acute-phase proteins and stimulation of the hypothalamus to release prostanoids, which cause fever. Interleukin-2 is mainly a

growth factor for clonal expansion of stimulated lymphocytes. Interleukin-6 stimulates the production of granulocytes from bone marrow (Table 8–1). IL-1, IL-8, and TNF-α may be part of the mechanism by which lymphocytes kill tumor cells and bacteria.

The Systemic Inflammatory Response Syndrome & Multiple Organ Failure

The systemic inflammatory response syndrome results from release of gram-negative endotoxins from urologic or gastrointestinal infections. Endotoxins, taken up by reticuloendothelial cells throughout the body, stimulate a secondary release of cytokines, which up-regulate integrins on leukocyte cell membranes and the receptors for integrins on endothelial cells. The end result is that leukocytes and platelets adhere to endothelial cells. This has two major consequences. First, local microvascular perfusion is impaired. The consequent hypoxic damage causes reticuloendothelial cells to release more cytokines, adding to the inflammatory cascade and depressing organ function. The second effect is local release of lethal concentrations of growth factors, cytokines, and high-energy oxygen radicals, which may injure the endothelial cells, causing fluids to leak from blood to tissue. As fluid losses increase, hypovolemia, release of catecholamines, and release of nitric oxide from endothelial cells may exaggerate the basic problem. Poor perfusion of vital organs coexists with vasodilation in other vascular beds and low peripheral resistance. The patient appears flushed, and high cardiac output shock results. Organ failure shortly appears, most often with fluid extravasation into the lungs and pulmonary failure.

While infection and endotoxemia are the most common causes of this syndrome, hemorrhagic shock can also induce the response if it lasts long enough and does enough damage. Hypoxic endothelial damage leads to margination and activation of leukocytes and platelets, which themselves are quite tolerant of hypoxia. Leukocytes migrate into tissue, led there by complement activated by distressed cells. The combination of damaged cells, hypoxia, and lactic acidosis causes these leukocytes to release more cytokines, including IL-1, TNF-α, TGF-β, and perhaps others, which on occasion reach the bloodstream. The effects are as listed above with organ failure. The risks of organ failure in this case are proportionate to the duration and severity of shock and the age and basic health of the patient.

Massive tissue injury, such as pancreatitis or burns, excites a similar cascade of tissue damage, which may produce shock and a similar cascade of events.

The target organs of cytokines (ie, the susceptible tissues) include the lung, cardiovascular system, liver, kidney, nervous system, gastrointestinal tract, and the reticuloendothelial and immune systems themselves.

The gastrointestinal tract is a pivotal organ that,

Table 8–1. Cytokines.

Peptide	Site of Synthesis	Regulation	Target Cells	Effects
G-CSF	Fibroblasts, monocytes	Induced by IL-1, LPS, IFNα.	Committed neutrophil progenitors (CFU-G, Gran)	Supports the proliferation of neutrophil-forming colonies. Stimulates respiratory burst.
GM-CSF (IL-3 has almost identical effects)	Endothelial cells, fibroblasts, macrophages, T lymphocytes, bone marrow	Induced by IL-1, TNF.	Granulocyte-erythrocyte-monocyte-megakaryocyte progenitor cells (CFU-GEMM, CFU-MEG, CFU-Eo, CFU-GM)	Supports the proliferation of macrophage-, eosinophil-, neutrophil-, and monocyte-containing colonies. $t_{1/2} = 2$ minutes, ruling out possibility of long-range bone marrow stimulation.
IFNα, -β, -γ	Epithelial cells, fibroblasts, lymphocytes, macrophages, neutrophils	Induced by viruses (foreign nucleic acids), microbes, microbial foreign antigens, cancer cells.	Lymphocytes, macrophages, infected cells, cancer cells	Inhibits viral multiplication. Activates defective phagocytes, direct inhibition of cancer cell multiplication, activation of killer leukocytes, inhibition of collagen synthesis.
IL-1	Endothelial cells, keratinocytes, lymphocytes, macrophages	Induced by TNFα, IL-1, IL-2, C5a. Suppressed by IL-4, TGFβ.	Monocytes, macrophages, T cells, B cells, NK cells, LAK cells	Stimulates T cells, B cells, NK cells, LAK cells. Induces tumoricidal activity and production to other cytokines, endogenous pyrogen (via PGE$_2$ release). Induces steroidogenesis, acute-phase proteins, hypotension; chemotactic neutrophils. Stimulates respiratory burst.
IL-1ra	Monocytes	Induced by GM-CSF, LPS, IgG.	Blocks type I IL-1 receptors on T cells, fibroblasts, chondrocytes, endothelial cells.	Blocks type I IL-1 receptors on T cells, fibroblasts, chondrocytes, endothelial cells. Ameliorates animal models of arthritis, septic shock, and inflammatory bowel disease.
IL-2	Lymphocytes	Induced by IL-1, IL-6.	T cells, NK cells, B cells, activated monocytes	Stimulates growth of T cells, NK cells, and B cells.
IL-4	T cells, NK cells, mast cells	Induced by cell activation, IL-1.	All hematopoietic cells and many others express receptors	Stimulates B cell and T cell growth. Induces HLA class II molecules.
IL-6	Endothelial cells, fibroblasts, lymphocytes, some tumors	Induced by IL-1, TNFα.	T cells, B cells, plasma cells, keratinocytes, hepatocytes, stem cells	B cell differentiation. Induction of acute-phase proteins, growth of keratinocytes. Stimulates growth of T cells and hematopoietic stem cells.
IL-8	Endothelial cells, fibroblasts, lymphocytes, monocytes	Induced by TNF, IL-1, LPS, cell adherence (monocytes).	Basophils, neutrophils, T cells	Induces expression of endothelial cell LECAM-1 receptors, β$_2$ integrins, and neutrophil transmigration. Stimulates respiratory burst.
M-CSF	Endothelial cells, fibroblasts, monocytes	Induced by IL-1, LPS, IFN-α.	Committed monocyte progenitors (CFU-M, Mono)	Supports the proliferation of monocyte-forming colonies. Activates macrophages.
MCP-1, MCAF	Monocytes. Some tumors secrete a similar peptide.	Induced by IL-1, LPS, PHA.	Unstimulated monocytes	Only known chemoattractant specific for monocytes.
TNF-α (LT has almost identical effects)	Macrophages, NK cells, T cells, transformed cell lines, B cells (LT)	Suppressed by PGE$_2$, TGF-β, IL-4. Induced by LPS.	Endothelial cells, monocytes, neutrophils	Stimulates T cell growth. Direct cytotoxin to some tumor cells. Profound proinflammatory effect via induction of IL-1 and PGE$_2$. Systemic administration produces many symptoms of sepsis. Stimulates respiratory burst and phagocytosis.

Key:

CFU	= Colony-forming unit		MCAF	= Monocyte chemotactic and activating factor
G-CSF	= Granulocyte colony-stimulating factor		M-CSF	= Macrophage colony-stimulating factor
GM-CSF	= Granulocyte-macrophage colony-stimulating factor		MCPO-1	= Monocyte chemotactic peptide-1
IFN	= Interferon		NK	= Natural killer
IL	= Interleukin		PHA	= Phytohemagglutinin
IL1ra	= Interleukin-1 receptor antagonist		TGF-β	= Transforming growth factor beta
LPS	= lipopolysaccharide		TNF-α	= Tumor necrosis factor alpha
LT	= Lymphotoxin			

when involved, amplifies the cascade of cytokines. The gastrointestinal mucosa normally contains and excludes from contact with other tissues an enormous number of bacteria. Some pathogens—*Salmonella* and *Listeria,* for example—easily penetrate this barrier and cause serious illness. However, most bacteria translocate across this barrier into blood or lymph only rarely. Translocation is increased after shock or when the gastrointestinal tract is under attack by cytokines and gram-negative organisms. Consequently, endotoxins are released into the visceral circulation more rapidly and find their way to the liver, spleen, etc. Translocation appears to occur through the gut epithelial cells more so than between them.

The large numbers of reticuloendothelial cells in the liver and spleen release yet more cytokines in response to endotoxins and in that way further amplify the inflammatory response. These cells, excited by cytokines and phagocytosis, send signals to hepatocytes and spleen cells. Hepatocytes shut off albumin synthesis and increase production of acute-phase proteins, which normally are part of the immune system response. Nitric oxide appears to be a tertiary mediator of the signaling process. The gastrointestinal tract, therefore, becomes a potent amplifier of inflammatory mediators and has been termed by some the "motor" of multiple organ failure.

One pernicious effect of some cytokines (IL-1, IL-2, TNF-α) is excessive production of nitric oxide by vascular endothelium. Nitric oxide is a powerful smooth muscle relaxant that is involved in regulating vascular tone. Excessive production leads to reduced peripheral resistance and probably accounts for the low peripheral resistance seen in endotoxic shock. The effects of nitric oxide can be overcome by catecholamines, but the balance of vascular tone is clinically elusive and probably irrelevant to much of the malperfusion that occurs in this syndrome. Nitric oxide also triggers metabolic changes, especially in liver cells.

The final pathways of organ dysfunction are not yet fully understood. Metabolic alterations induced by TNF-α must be one. Unregulated oxygen radical production is another. Leukocytes are stimulated to increase oxygen consumption manyfold by ingestion of bacteria and by some cytokines. This probably accounts for a significant portion of the increased total body oxygen consumption seen in sepsis. Normally, this oxygen would be used to kill bacteria in phagosomes and in highly controlled chemical reactions. Under extreme stimulation of the reticuloendothelial system, radicals escape compartmentalization, overcome normal scavenging mechanisms, and damage nearby cells as well as the cell of generation.

The immune system itself is also a target organ. Whether by exhaustion or other secondary effects of cytokine assault, the immune system fails. T and B cells are depressed. T suppressor cells are stimulated, and vulnerability to infection increases.

One somewhat curious property of the reticuloendothelial system is that it can be primed or potentiated. An infection occurring soon after a major burn is more likely to produce pulmonary failure than the same infection alone. Each new insult is likely to produce a greater effect than the last. The priming effect lasts a few weeks in declining degrees after stimulation stops.

The basic principles of treatment are paramount: prompt treatment of shock, debridement or drainage of inflamed or infected tissue, immobilization of fractures, and early specific antibiotic therapy. Despite the application of these fundamentals, many patients experience multiple organ failure. The goal of specific therapy is to interrupt steps in the cascade. Polymyxin B has been given to absorb or inactivate endotoxin, antibodies to endotoxin or to TNF-α or IL-1, or antibodies to their receptors on somatic cells. Efforts to prevent the generation of or to scavenge oxygen radicals or inhibit prostanoid synthesis have been effective in experimental studies but not clinically.

When only one organ is affected—usually the lung or kidney—the prognosis is fairly good, and about 70% of patients recover. If two organs are involved, the recovery rate falls to about 50%, and if three or more organs are affected or the central nervous system, the heart, the liver, or the immune system, the prognosis is grim. The prognosis is also related to the age and health status of the victim.

Diagnosis

The aim of management is to detect and treat sepsis before it evolves into more advanced stages.

A. Physical Examination: Physical examination is the easiest way to diagnose a surgical infection. When infection is suspected but cannot be found initially, repeated examination will often reveal subtle warmth, erythema, induration, tenderness, or splinting due to a developing abscess. Failure to repeat the physical examination is the most common reason for delayed diagnosis and therapy.

B. Laboratory Findings:

1. General findings–Laboratory data are only of limited value. Leukocytosis may give way to leukopenia. Acidosis is helpful in diagnosis, and signs of disseminated intravascular coagulation are useful as well. Otherwise unexplained respiratory, hepatic, renal, and gastric (ie, stress ulcers) failure is strong evidence for sepsis.

2. Blood cultures–Blood cultures often provide the best evidence of sepsis. In rapidly advancing cases, two separate blood cultures should be taken within 15 minutes. In less urgent situations, three blood cultures should be taken over a 24-hour period, and six should be taken if the patient has a cardiac or joint prosthesis or vascular shunt or if antibiotics are being given. It is often wise to discontinue antibiotics for 12–24 hours while blood for cultures is being drawn. For each culture, 10 mL of blood is taken, half to be used for aerobic cultures and half for anaerobic cultures. False-negative results occur in about 20% of cases. False-positive results are difficult to define, since skin commensals (even some diphtheroids and *S albus*), regarded as contaminants in the past, have proved occasionally to be true pathogens. Arterial blood cultures may be necessary to detect fungal endocarditis.

C. Imaging Studies: Radiologic examination is frequently helpful, particularly for the diagnosis of pulmonary infections. An elevated and immobile diaphragm is a clue to the presence of subphrenic abscess. Obliteration of the psoas shadow frequently indicates an appendiceal abscess. Whenever infection is close to bone, radiologic examination is indicated to detect early signs of osteomyelitis, which might require aggressive surgical therapy. CT scanning—particularly of the liver or brain—is useful for detecting abscesses in these organs. CT scanning and ultrasonography are particularly useful in localizing occult infection. Numerous radionuclide scans have been tested all with fair results. The best radionuclides for labeling leukocytes are gallium Ga 67 and indium In 111.

D. Source of Infection: An early diagnosis of septicemia is usually based on a combination of suspicion and inconclusive evidence, since the results of blood cultures are often unavailable during this stage. An important initial step is to identify the source. Surgical or traumatic wounds, surgical infections in the abdomen or thorax, and clostridial infections are all common, but so are urinary tract infections, pneumonia, and even sinus infections. Once identified, any septic focus amenable to surgical therapy should be excised or drained.

Treatment

A. Incision and Drainage: Abscesses must be opened and bacteria, necrotic tissue, and toxins drained to the outside. The pressure and the number of bacteria in the infected space are lowered; this decreases the spread of toxins and bacteria.

An abscess with systemic manifestations is a surgical emergency. Fluctuation is a reliable but late sign of a subcutaneous abscess. Abscesses in the parotid or perianal area may never become fluctuant, and if the surgeon waits for this sign, serious sepsis may result. Drainage creates an open wound, but the tissue will heal by second intention with remarkably little scarring. Deep abscesses difficult to drain surgically may be drained by a catheter placed percutaneously under guidance by CT scanning or ultrasonography.

It may appear that a patient with septicemia cannot withstand operation. In fact, operation to drain an abscess may be the most important of all therapeutic measures. One can hardly imagine delaying removal of infarcted bowel because the patient is in shock. There is no substitute for obliteration of the focus of infection when it is surgically accessible.

B. Excision: Some surgical infections may be excised (eg, an infected appendix or gallbladder). In these cases, drainage may not be necessary, and the patient is cured on the operating table. Clostridial myositis may require amputation of the infected limb. The success of such operations is greatly facilitated by intensive specific antimicrobial therapy.

C. Circulatory Enhancement: Just as infections due to vascular ischemia are cured by restoring arterial patency, chronic infections in poorly vascularized areas, as in osteoradionecrosis, may be cured by transplanting a functioning vascular bed (eg, a musculocutaneous flap or omental transposition) into the affected area.

D. Antibiotics: Antibiotics are not necessary for simple surgical infections that respond to incision and drainage alone—furuncles and uncomplicated wound infections. Infections likely to spread or persist require antibiotic therapy, best chosen on the basis of sensitivity tests.

In "toxic" infections, including septic shock, antibiotics must be started promptly and empirically and the regimen modified later from the results of blood cultures. The choice of drugs must take into account the organisms most often cultured from similar infections in previous patients, the results of gram-stained smears, and specific characteristics of the patient. When the responsible organism is not known, the initial regimen should consist of a penicillinase-resistant penicillin (eg, nafcillin or oxacillin) and gentamicin, tobramycin, or netilmicin. If the presence of enterococci is suspected, ampicillin or penicillin G should be added. Another good regimen for initial treatment is a combination of a cephalosporin with gentamicin, tobramycin, or netilmicin. Vancomycin should be considered if the infecting organism is thought to be a methicillin- or nafcillin-resistant *Staphylococcus* species. Carbenicillin, ticarcillin, azlocillin, mezlocillin, or piperacillin (often combined with an aminoglycoside) is indicated for infections due to *Pseudomonas*. To treat disease due to fecal anaerobes, metronidazole, clindamycin, and cefoxitin are effective. Anaerobic coverage is essential in patients with abscesses associated with disease of the gastrointestinal tract.

Because of their nephrotoxicity, aminoglycosides must be used cautiously in the presence of existing or imminent renal failure. If sepsis is hospital-acquired, the regimen may be tailored to attack the organisms responsible for infections seen previously in that institution. Cancer patients are more likely than others to have anaerobic infections. Initially, the killing of many gram-negative bacteria (which releases endotoxin) may exacerbate the problem. Therefore, supportive measures are particularly important and include fluid administration (often massive) and control of fever to diminish metabolic requirements. The management of circulatory and respiratory dysfunction is discussed in Chapter 12.

E. Nutritional Support: In malnourished, septic, or severely traumatized patients, the ability to ward off or recover from infection is often enhanced by aggressive nutritional therapy. Specific measurable effects include improved immunocompetency and blunting or reversal of catabolism. Protection or restoration of visceral and skeletal muscle allows the patient to cough better and be more mobile and helps avoid sepsis-induced failure of the liver, kidneys, lungs, heart, and stomach.

Prognosis

The mortality rate ranges from 10% in septic patients with manifestations limited to fever, chills, and toxicity, to almost 100% in those who manifest shock and multiple organ failure. Factors that have independent influences on outcome include the causative microorganism, blood pressure, body temperature (inverse relationship), primary site of infection, age, predisposing factors, and place of acquisition of infection (hospital or home). In patients who respond to therapy, the risk of a septic relapse is about 20% if the temperature is normal; 3% if the temperature and leukocyte count are normal; and virtually nil if the temperature and leukocyte count are normal and the proportion of granulocytes is less than 73%. Of patients with low-grade fever and an elevated leukocyte count after antibiotics have been discontinued, 60% will have a relapse. Nevertheless, continuation of antibiotics in questionable cases is often contraindicated because it only delays recognition of infection and may enhance its morbidity.

Bohnen JMA et al: APACHE II score and abdominal sepsis. A prospective study. Arch Surg 1988;123:225.

Bone RC: A critical evaluation of new agents for the treatment of sepsis. JAMA 1991;266:1686.

Border JR: Hypothesis: Sepsis, multiple systems organ failure, and the macrophage. Arch Surg 1988;123:285.

Burchard KW et al: *Enterobacter* bacteremia in surgical patients. Surgery 1986;100:857.

Carrico CJ et al: Multiple organ failure syndrome. Arch Surg 1986;121:196.

Cerra FB et al: Selective gut decontamination reduces nosocomial infections and length of stay but not mortality or organ failure in surgical intensive care unit patients. Arch Surg 1992;127:163. (See also discussion on p 167.)

Curran RD et al: Multiple cytokines are required to induce hepatocyte nitric oxide production and inhibit total protein synthesis. Ann Surg 1990;212:462. (See also discussion on p 470.)

Damas P et al: Cytokine serum level during severe sepsis in human IL-6 as a marker of severity. Ann Surg 1992;215:356.

Deitch EA, Winterton J, Berg R: Effect of starvation, malnutrition, and trauma on the gastrointestinal tract flora and bacterial translocation. Arch Surg 1987;122:1019.

Duignan JP et al: The association of impaired neutrophil chemotaxis with postoperative surgical sepsis. Br J Surg 1986;73:238.

Gerzof SG, Oates ME: Imaging techniques for infections in the surgical patient. Surg Clin North Am 1988;68:147.

Gould IM, Wise R: *Pseudomonas aeruginosa:* Clinical manifestations and management. Lancet 1985;2:1224.

Hau T et al: Antibiotics fail to prevent abscess formation secondary to bacteria trapped in fibrin clots. Arch Surg 1986;121:163.

Hibbs JJ et al: Evidence for cytokine-inducible nitric oxide synthesis from L-arginine in patients receiving interleukin-2 therapy. J Clin Invest 1992;89:867.

Knaus WWA et al: Prognosis in acute organ system failure. Ann Surg 1985;202:685.

Lamas S et al: Nitric oxide synthesis in endothelial cells: Evidence for a pathway inducible by TNF-alpha. Am J Physiol 1991;261(4 Part 1):C634.

Lundsgaard-Hansen P et al: Purified fibronectin administration to patients with severe abdominal infections. Ann Surg 1985;202:745.

Marshall JC et al: The microbiology of multiple organ failure: The proximal gastrointestinal tract as an occult reservoir of pathogens. Arch Surg 1988;123:309.

Michie HR, Guillou PJ, Wilmore DW: Tumour necrosis factor and bacterial sepsis. Br J Surg 1989;76:670.

Neu HC: Infections due to gram negative bacteria: An overview. Rev Infect Dis 1985;7(Suppl 4):S778.

Polk HC Jr: Non-specific host defence stimulation in the reduction of surgical infection in man. Br J Surg 1987;74:969.

Pruitt BA: Host opportunist interactions in surgical infection. Arch Surg 1986;121:13.

Rackow EC, Astiz ME: Pathophysiology and treatment of septic shock. JAMA 1991;266:548.

Sleigh JD, Peutherer JF: Changing patterns of bacterial and viral infections in surgery. Br Med Bull 1988;44:403.

Sullivan JS et al: Correlation of plasma cytokine elevations with mortality rate in children with sepsis. J Pediatr 1992;120(4 Part 1):510.

Tennenberg SD, Solomkin JS: Neutrophil activation in sepsis: The relationship between fmet-leu-phe receptor mobilization and oxidative activity. Arch Surg 1988;213:171.

Tracy KG et al: Anti-cachectin/TNF monoclonal antibodies prevent septic shock during lethal bacteraemia. Nature 1987;330:662.

Watters JM et al: Both inflammatory and endocrine mediators stimulate host responses to sepsis. Arch Surg 1986;121:179.

Waydhas C et al: Inflammatory mediators, infection, sepsis, and multiple organ failure after severe trauma. Arch Surg 1992;127:460.

NOSOCOMIAL INFECTIONS & INFECTION CONTROL

Patients may acquire infection in hospital through contact with the surgical team or a nonsterile operating room, or infection may develop from bacteria harbored by the patient before operation.

The Surgical Team as a Source of Infection

Most nosocomial infections are transmitted through human contact. In order to minimize transmission in hospital, rules made for surgical behavior, dress, and hygiene should be obeyed.

Any break in operative technique noted by any member of the operating team should be corrected immediately. Members of the team should not operate if they have cutaneous infections or upper respiratory or viral infections that may cause sneezing or coughing.

Scrub suits should be worn only in the operating room and not in other areas of the hospital. If they must be worn outside the operating room, they should be changed before reentering. Physicians and nurses should always wash their hands between patients. Careful hand washing should follow all contact with infected patients. For preoperative preparation, hands should be scrubbed for 5–10 minutes with any approved agent if the surgeon has not scrubbed within the past week. Shorter scrubs are allowable between operations. Traffic and talking in the operating room should be minimized.

Unwashed hands are by far the most frequent sources of nosocomial infections such as pneumonia, intravenous catheter sepsis, burn wound infections, and even pseudomembranous enterocolitis. Hand washing should be a matter of reflex conditioning. In today's atmosphere, failure to wash one's hands between patient contacts in a hospital is essentially an unethical act.

The Operating Room as a Source of Infection

Though many parts of the operating environment are sterile, the operative field is not—it is merely as sterile as it can be made. Attempts to achieve a level of sterility beyond normal standards have not led to further reductions in wound infection. This reflects the fact that bacteria are also present in the patient, and immune variables are also important determinants of infection not affected by more aggressive attempts to achieve sterility.

Many special and expensive techniques have been advised to minimize bacteria in the operating room. Ultraviolet light, laminar flow ventilation, and elaborate architectural and ventilation schemes have been advocated. Each scheme has its proponents, but in general, none of them have proved more effective than common sense and surgical discipline.

The only completely reliable methods for sterilization of surgical instruments and supplies are steam under pressure (autoclaving), dry heat, and ethylene oxide gas. Saturated steam at 2 atm pressure and a temperature of 120 °C destroys all vegetative bacteria and most resistant dry spores in 13 minutes, but exposure of surgical instrument packs should usually be extended to 30 minutes to allow heat and moisture to penetrate the center of the package. Shorter times are allowable for unwrapped instruments with the vacuum-cycle or high-pressure autoclaves now widely used. Continuous dry heat at 170 °C for 1 hour sterilizes articles that cannot tolerate moist heat. If grease or oil is present on instruments, safe dry-heat sterilization requires 4 hours at 160 °C.

Gaseous ethylene oxide destroys bacteria, viruses, fungi, and various spores. It is used for heat-sensitive materials, including telescopic instruments, plastic and rubber goods, sharp and delicate instruments, electrical cords, and sealed ampules. It damages certain plastics and pharmaceuticals. The technique requires a special pressurized-gas autoclave, with 12% ethylene oxide and 88% Freon 12 at 55 °C, 8 psi pressure above atmospheric pressure. Most items must be aerated in sterile packages on the shelf for 24–48 hours before use in order to rid them of the dissolved gas. Implanted plastics should be stored for 7 days before use. Ethylene oxide is toxic and represents a safety hazard unless it is used according to strict regulations.

Miscellaneous sterilization procedures include soaking in antiseptics, such as 2% glutaraldehyde, to remove viruses from instruments with lenses. Total sterilization by this method requires 10 hours. Chemical antiseptics are often used to clean operating room surfaces and instruments that need not be totally sterile. Other disinfectant solutions include synthetic phenolics, polybrominated salicylanilides, iodophors, alcohols, other glutaraldehyde preparations, and 6% stabilized hydrogen peroxide. These agents maintain high potency in the presence of organic matter and usually leave excellent residual antibacterial activity on surfaces. They are also used to clean anesthetic equipment that cannot be sterilized. Prepackaged instruments and supplies can be sterilized with gamma radiation by manufacturers. Synthetic fabrics have now proved to be superior barriers to bacteria and less costly than the traditional cotton. They can be used in gowns and drapes.

The Patient as a Source of Infection

Patients themselves are often the most important source of infection.

When possible, preexisting infections should be treated before surgery. Secretions from patients with respiratory tract infections should be cultured and appropriate treatment given. The urinary tract should be cultured and specific antibiotics administered before instruments are introduced; this precaution has eliminated septic shock as a complication of urologic surgery. The colon should be prepared as discussed in Chapter 31.

Commensal bacteria on the patient's skin are a common cause of infection. Preoperative showers or baths with antiseptic soap diminish infections in clean wounds by 50%. Shaving of the operative field hours prior to incision is associated with a 50% increase in wound infections and should not be done. If the patient has a heavy growth of hair, an area just large enough to accommodate the wound and its closure should be clipped rather than shaved immediately before operation. Razor shaving more than a few minutes before operation clearly raises the wound infection rate.

The skin to be included in the operating field should be cleansed with antiseptic. Nonirritating agents such as benzalkonium salts should be used in or around the nose or eyes. Perineal skin is best cleansed with chlorhexidine or povidone-iodine. For other skin areas, 0.5% aqueous iodine should be used, care being taken not to allow drips (which burn if the water evaporates, thus concentrating the iodine) and to remove excess iodine. If used carefully, this is as effective as any other agent and less expensive.

Isolation Procedures: Universal Precautions

Traditionally, patients with infection were individually isolated. More recently—partly in response to the AIDS epidemic—a more general kind of isolation, called "universal precautions," has been substituted. In this system, *any* procedure involving close contact with *any* patient—and especially those involving contact with blood, urine, feces, or saliva—is performed by hospital personnel wearing gloves and other protective devices. The need for handwashing is not diminished by this system.

Antibiotic Prophylaxis for Surgical Infection

The principles of antibiotic prophylaxis are simple: (1) Choose antibiotics for the expected type of contamination. (2) Use antibiotics only if the risk of infection justifies their use. (3) Give antibiotics in appropriate doses and at appropriate times. (4) Stop dosing before the risk of side effects outweighs benefits.

Antibiotics for preventive use must not be highly toxic and should not be "first-line" antibiotics for treatment of established infection. Because resistance to antibiotics may develop quickly, agents that have been used frequently for prophylaxis are likely to lose their effectiveness for later treatment. Prophylactic agents should be chosen for cost-effectiveness and safety as well as for efficacy.

Prophylactic antibiotics should be selected to combat the organisms most likely to be encountered in the anticipated operative procedure. In urologic surgery, agents must be chosen on the basis of preoperative urine cultures; for colon surgery, agents should be effective against anaerobes and gram-negative aerobes; and in gynecologic surgery, agents should effective against anaerobic bacteria. For clean operations in which prostheses or other foreign bodies will be placed, antibiotics should be chosen to combat the bacteria most troublesome in the individual hospital (in most cases, staphylococci).

Antibiotic prophylaxis cannot eliminate bacteria. Use of multiple antibiotics increases the risk of drug reactions, diminishes effectiveness in the long run by promoting the emergence of resistant strains, and increases costs. Antibiotics should be given only when a significant rate of infection is encountered without them or when the consequences of infection would be disastrous, as with placement of vascular, cardiac, or joint prostheses. Operations commonly followed by inconsequential infection, such as anal or oral procedures, generally should not be preceded by prophylactic antibiotics unless the patient has rheumatic heart disease or a prosthetic heart valve.

The surgeon may be tempted to give every patient antibiotics in order to have an infection-free record, but there are several reasons why this strategy is not appropriate: (1) Clean wounds may become infected with organisms for which prophylactic antibiotics are ineffective. (2) Resistant organisms will eventually develop, creating a higher risk of infection within the hospital. (3) The expense and risks associated with antibiotics (eg, kidney failure, hearing loss, anaphylaxis, skin rashes, fungal infections, enterocolitis) overshadow the minimal beneficial effects of using antibiotics in clean cases. The number of antibiotic-resistant strains has been correlated with the number of kilograms of antibiotics used in any given hospital.

Antibiotics should be given intravenously or intramuscularly just long enough before operation to achieve a therapeutic level in the blood, ie, so the fibrin clots that trap bacteria will contain a therapeutic concentration of antibiotic. Antibiotics given more than 2 hours before operation are wasted unless there is old infection in the operative area. In this case, antibiotics should be chosen to treat the old infection.

In the usual case, prophylactic antibiotics should be stopped a few hours after operation. If contamination will be possible for an extended period, as when intravascular lines remain in patients with cardiac prostheses, prophylaxis may be continued. However, the longer the period of contamination, the less effective will be the antibiotics.

Control of Infection Within the Hospital

The Joint Commission on Accreditation of Hospitals in the USA requires each hospital to have an infection control committee. This committee is expected to establish infection control procedures, with rules for isolation of infected patients and for protection of hospital personnel exposed to infection. In addition, the committee establishes procedures for disposal of materials contaminated by bacteria, as well as guidelines for limiting the spread of infection. Usually, infection control personnel record and analyze patterns of infection. Isolates of bacteria cultured from patients are routinely analyzed for potential significance to the hospital environment. Attempts are made to determine the source of "epidemics." Considering the cost of infection in both lives and money, infection control appears to be a sound investment.

Antimicrobial prophylaxis in surgery. Med Lett Drugs Ther 1992;34:5.

Condon RE et al: Does infection control control infection? Arch Surg 1988;123:250.

Guidelines for prevention of transmission of human immunodeficiency virus and hepatitis B virus to health-care and public-safety workers. MMWR 1989;38:S–6.

Pollock AV: Surgical prophylaxis: The emerging picture. Lancet 1988;1:225.

Protection against viral hepatitis. Recommendations of the Immunization Practices Advisory Committee (ACIP). MMWR 1990;39(RR-2):1.

Van Scoy RE, Wilkowske CJ: Prophylactic use of antimicrobial agents in adult patients. Mayo Clin Proc 1987;62: 1137.

SPECIFIC TYPES OF SURGICAL INFECTIONS

POSTOPERATIVE & IATROGENIC INFECTIONS

Patients undergoing major surgery are almost by definition immunosuppressed. Rates of infection in surgical patients are as high as 50% in intensive care and burn units.

1. POSTOPERATIVE WOUND INFECTION

Postoperative wound infection results from bacterial contamination during or after a surgical procedure. The space is the wound. Infection usually is confined to the subcutaneous tissues. Despite every effort to maintain asepsis, most surgical wounds are contaminated to some extent. However, infection rarely develops if contamination is minimal, if the wound has been made without undue injury, if the subcutaneous tissue is well perfused and well oxygenated, and if there is no dead space.

Operative wounds can be divided into four categories: (1) clean (no gross contamination from exogenous or endogenous sources); (2) lightly contaminated (clean-contaminated); (3) heavily contaminated; and (4) infected (in which obvious infection has been encountered during operation). The infection rate is about 1.5% in clean cases. Clean-contaminated wounds (eg, with gastric or biliary surgery) are infected about 2–5% of the time. Heavily contaminated wounds, as in operations on the unprepared colon or emergency operations for intestinal bleeding or perforation, may have an infection risk of 5–30%. Wise use of isolation techniques, preoperative antibiotics, and delayed primary closure will keep rates of wound infection within acceptable limits. Since even a minor postoperative wound infection prolongs hospitalization and increases economic loss, all reasonable efforts must be made to keep the infection rate low.

The risk of wound infection is not entirely determined by the degree of contamination, however. Many physiologic and immunologic factors limit the patient's resistance. Risk can be more precisely assessed by giving one point for each of the following ("SENIC score"): (1) abdominal operation, (2) operation lasting more than 2 hours, (3) contaminated operation, and (4) more than three diagnoses exclusive of wound infection. A total score of 0 indicates a risk of 1%, 1 indicates 3%, 2 indicates 8%, 3 indicates 17%, and 4 indicates 28%.

The susceptibility of the host is usually but not always local. Susceptibility is also proportionate to the oxygen tension in the operative wound, and wound oxygen tension is inversely and significantly proportionate to the above scores. Wound tissue Po_2 in turn is proportionate to arterial Po_2 and the perfusion rate. The perfusion rate is generally determined by the cardiac output and by the tone of the sympathetic nervous system. Sympathetic tone, ie, the degree of peripheral vasoconstriction, is determined by the patient's surface temperature, the degree of pain, the blood volume, and the degree of fear. Therefore, susceptibility to infection can be reduced by such simple methods as rapid infusion of additional fluids, warming, better pain control, and oxygen administration (but only after perfusion has been ensured). The rate of peripheral perfusion is extremely important and can be estimated clinically by noting the rate of capillary return over the forehead (< 1.5 seconds) and patellae (< 5 seconds), postural changes in pulse and blood pressure (there should be none), eye globe turgor, and thirst. Contrary to popular opinion, urinary output correlates poorly with the incidence of wound infection. When the infection risk is high, wound tissue Po_2 can be measured, monitored, and supported. Appropriate technology is available.

Clinical Findings

Wound infections usually appear between the fifth and tenth days after surgery, but they may appear as early as the first postoperative day or even years later. The first sign is usually fever, and postoperative fever requires inspection of the wound. The patient may complain of wound pain. The wound rarely appears severely inflamed, but edema may be obvious because the skin sutures appear tight.

Palpation of the wound may disclose an abscess. A good method is to pour surgical soap on the wound and, using it as a lubricant, palpate gently with the gloved hand. Firm or fluctuant areas, crepitus, or tenderness can be detected with minimal pain and contamination. The rare infection deep to the fascia may be difficult to recognize. In doubtful cases, one can carefully open the wound in the suspicious area. If no pus is present, the wound can be closed immediately with skin tapes. Cultures even of clean wounds that are successfully reclosed are often positive.

Differential Diagnosis

Differential diagnosis includes all other causes of postoperative fever, wound dehiscence, and wound herniation (see Chapter 4).

Prevention

There are three main aspects to prevention of infection: (1) careful, gentle, clean surgery; (2) reduction of contamination; and (3) support of the patient's defenses, including use of antibiotics. The surgeon who traumatizes tissue, leaves foreign bodies or hematomas in wounds, uses too many ligatures, and exposes the wound to drying or pressure from retractors is exposing patients to needless risks of infection.

The purpose of sutures is to approximate tissues and hold them securely, and the right number to use is as few as will accomplish this aim. Since sutures strangulate tissue, they should be tied as loosely as the requirements of approximation permit. Subcutaneous sutures should be used rarely. Using skin tapes instead of skin sutures or staples lowers infection rates, especially in contaminated wounds.

Severely contaminated wounds in which subcutaneous infection is likely to develop are best left open initially and managed by delayed primary closure. This means that the deep layers are closed while skin and subcutaneous tissues are left open, dressed with sterile gauze, inspected on the fourth or fifth day, and then closed (preferably with skin tapes) if no sign of infection is seen. A clean granulating open wound is preferable to a wound infection. Scarring from secondary healing is usually minimal.

The value of prophylactic antibiotics is discussed on p 116. Prophylactic antibiotics are indicated whenever wound contamination during the operation can be predicted to be high (eg, operations on the colon). Excessively liberal use of antibiotics is not reasonable. The incidence of postoperative infections in clean operations is not diminished by administration of antimicrobials, and the prophylactic use of these drugs must be reserved for selected cases at high risk for infection.

Treatment

The basic treatment of established wound infection is to open the wound and allow it to drain. Antibiotics are not necessary unless the infection is invasive. Culture should be performed to help locate the source and prevent further infection in other patients; to gain a preview of bacterial flora in case other infections develop deep to the wound or in case the existing infection becomes invasive; and to select preoperative antibiotics in case the wound must be entered again.

Prognosis

Most wound infections make illness more severe. Wound infection correlates positively with death rates but is not often the cause of death. It may tip the scales against successful operation.

Bergamini TM, Polk HC Jr: The importance of tissue antibiotic activity in the prevention of operative wound infection. J Antimicrob Chemother 1989;23:303.

Cruse PJE, Foord R: The epidemiology of wound infection: A 10-year prospective study of 62,939 wounds. Surg Clin North Am 1980;60:27.

Culver DH et al: Surgical wound infection rates by wound class, operative procedure, and patient risk index. National Nosocomial Infections Surveillance System. Am J Med 1991;91:152S.

Daschner F: Cost-effectiveness in hospital infection control: Lessons for the 1990s. J Hosp Infect 1989;13:325.

Farber BF, Kaiser DL, Wenzel RP: Relation between surgical volume and incidence of postoperative wound infection. N Engl J Med 1981;305:200.

Gorse GH, Messner RL, Stephens ND: Association of malnutrition with nosocomial infection. Infect Control Hosp Epidemiol 1989;10:194.

Haley RW et al: Identifying patients at high risk of surgical wound infection: A simple multivariate index of patient susceptibility and wound contamination. Am J Epidemiol 1985;121:206.

Larsen RA et al: Improved perioperative antibiotic use and reduced surgical wound infections through use of computer decision analysis. Infect Control Hosp Epidemiol 1989;10:316.

Penin BG, Ehrenkranz JN: Priorities for surveillance and cost-effective control of postoperative infection. Arch Surg 1988;123:1305.

Windsor JA, Hill GL: Protein depletion and surgical risk. Aust NZ J Surg 1988;58:711.

2. OTHER POSTOPERATIVE INFECTIONS

Subphrenic abscess is discussed in Chapter 22. Urinary tract infection is discussed in Chapters 4 and 41. Infections due to foreign bodies are discussed in chapters on specific parts of the body.

FURUNCLE, CARBUNCLE, & HIDRADENITIS

Furuncles and carbuncles are cutaneous abscesses that begin in skin glands and hair follicles. Furuncles are the most common surgical infections, but carbuncles are rare.

Furuncles can be multiple and recurrent (furunculosis). Furunculosis usually occurs in young adults and is associated with hormonal changes resulting in impaired skin function. The commonest organisms are staphylococci and anaerobic diphtheroids.

Hidradenitis suppurativa is a serious skin infection

of the axillae or groin consisting of multiple abscesses of the apocrine sweat glands. The condition often becomes chronic and disabling.

Furuncles usually start in infected hair follicles, although some are caused by retained foreign bodies and other injuries. Hair follicles normally contain bacteria. If the pilosebaceous apparatus becomes occluded by skin disease or bacterial inflammation, the stage is set for development of a furuncle. Because the base of the hair follicle may lie in subcutaneous tissue, the infection can spread as a cellulitis, or it can form a subcutaneous abscess. If a furuncle results from confluent infection of hair follicles, a central core of skin may become necrotic and will slough when the abscess is drained. Furuncles may take a phlegmonous form, ie, extend into the subcutaneous tissue, forming a long, flat abscess.

Clinical Findings

Furuncles itch and cause pain. The skin first becomes red and then turns white and necrotic over the top of the abscess. There is usually some surrounding erythema and induration. Regional nodes may become enlarged. Systemic symptoms are rare.

Carbuncles usually start as furuncles, but the infection dissects through the dermis and subcutaneous tissue in a myriad of connecting tunnels. Many of these small extensions open to the surface, giving the appearance of large furuncles with many pustular openings. As carbuncles enlarge, the blood supply to the skin is destroyed and the central tissue becomes necrotic. Carbuncles on the back of the neck are seen almost exclusively in diabetic patients. The patient is usually febrile and mildly toxic. This is a serious problem that demands immediate surgical attention. Diabetes must be suspected and treated when a carbuncle is found.

Differential Diagnosis

On occasion, the surgeon may be confronted with a localized area of erythema and induration without obvious suppuration. Many such lesions will go on to central suppuration and become obvious furuncles. On the other hand, when these lesions are located near joints or over the tibia or when they are widely distributed, one must consider such differential diagnoses as rheumatoid nodules, gout, bursitis, synovitis, erythema nodosum, fungal infections, some benign or malignant skin tumors, and inflamed (but not usually infected) sebaceous or epithelial inclusion cysts.

Hidradenitis is differentiated from furunculosis by skin biopsy, which shows typical involvement of the apocrine sweat glands. One suspects hidradenitis when abscesses are concentrated in the apocrine gland areas, ie, the axillae, groin, and perineum. Carbuncles are rarely confused with any other condition.

Complications

Any of these infections may cause suppurative phlebitis when located near major veins. This is particularly important when the infection is located near the nose or eyes. Central venous thrombosis in the brain is a serious complication, and abscesses on the face usually must be treated with antibiotics as well as prompt incision and drainage.

Hidradenitis may disable the patient but rarely has systemic manifestations. Carbuncles on the back of the neck may lead to epidural abscess and meningitis.

Treatment

The classic therapy for furuncle is drainage, not antibiotics. Invasive carbuncles, however, must be treated by excision and antibiotics. Between these two extremes, the use of antibiotics depends on the location of the abscess and the extent of infection.

Patients with recurrent furunculosis may be diabetic or immune-deficient. Frequent washing with soaps containing hexachlorophene or other disinfectants is advisable. It may also be necessary to advise extensive laundering of all personal clothing and disinfection of the patient's living quarters in order to reduce the reservoirs of bacteria. Furunculosis associated with severe acne may benefit from tetracycline, 250 mg orally once or twice daily.

When an abscess fails to resolve after a superficial incision, the surgeon must look for a small opening to a deeper and larger subcutaneous abscess, ie, a **collar-button abscess.**

Hidradenitis is usually treated by drainage of the individual abscess followed by careful hygiene. The patient must avoid astringent antiperspirants and deodorants. Painting with mild disinfectants is sometimes helpful. Fungal infections should be searched for if healing after drainage does not occur promptly. If none of these measures are successful, the apocrine sweat-bearing skin must be excised and the deficit filled with a skin graft.

Carbuncles are often more extensive than the external appearance indicates. Incision alone is almost always inadequate, and excision with electrocautery is required. Excision is continued until the many sinus tracts are removed—usually far beyond the cutaneous evidence of suppuration. It is sometimes necessary to produce a large open wound. This may appear to be drastic treatment, but it achieves rapid cure and prevents further spread. The large wound usually contracts to a small scar and does not usually require skin grafting, because carbuncles tend to occur in loose skin on the back of the neck and on the buttocks, where contraction is the predominant form of repair.

CELLULITIS

Cellulitis is a common invasive nonsuppurative infection of connective tissue. The term is loosely used and often misapplied. The microscopic picture is one of severe inflammation of the dermal and subcutaneous tissues. Although PMNs predominate, there is no gross suppuration except perhaps at the portal of entry.

Clinical Findings

Cellulitis usually appears on an extremity as a brawny red or reddish-brown area of edematous skin. It advances rapidly from its starting point, and the advancing edge may be vague or sharply defined (eg, in erysipelas). A surgical wound, puncture, skin ulcer, or patch of dermatitis is usually identifiable as a portal of entry. The disease often occurs in susceptible patients, eg, alcoholics with postphlebitic leg ulcers. Most cases are caused by streptococci, but other bacteria have been involved. A moderate or high fever is almost always present.

Lymphangitis arising from cellulitis produces red, warm, tender streaks 3 or 4 mm wide leading from the infection along lymphatic vessels to the regional lymph nodes. There is no suppuration. Bacteria are difficult to obtain for culture, but blood culture is sometimes positive.

Differential Diagnosis

Since the visible features of cellulitis are all due to inflammation, the words inflammation and cellulitis have sometimes been used imprecisely as synonyms. Some forms of inflammation are associated with suppuration requiring incision and drainage, whereas cellulitis as such is not.

Thrombophlebitis is often difficult to differentiate from cellulitis, but phlebitic swelling is usually greater, and tenderness may localize over a vein. Homans' sign does not always make the differentiation—nor does lymphadenopathy. Fever is usually greater with cellulitis, and pulmonary embolization does not occur in cellulitis.

Contact allergy, such as poison oak, may mimic cellulitis in its early phase, but dense nonhemorrhagic vesiculation soon discloses the allergic cause.

Chemical inflammation due to drug injection may also mimic streptococcal cellulitis.

The appearance of hemorrhagic bullae and skin necrosis suggests necrotizing fasciitis.

Treatment

Hot packs actually elevate subcutaneous temperature, and if regional blood supply is normal, they can raise local oxygen tension.

Therapy should entail rest, elevation, massive hot wet packs, and penicillin, 2.4 million units per day intramuscularly (600,000 units every 6 hours). If a clear response has not occurred in 12–24 hours, one should suspect an abscess or consider the possibility that the causative agent is a staphylococcus or other resistant organism. The patient must be examined one or more times daily to detect a hidden abscess masquerading within or under cellulitis.

PYOMYOSITIS

Pyomyositis is an acute pyogenic infection of muscles—usually gluteal, quadriceps, or calf—occurring mostly in hot climates and after intense muscular activity. It accounts for about 3% of all surgical admissions in Africa and is being reported more frequently in nontropical countries.

The most common form, usually due to *Staphylococcus aureus,* begins insidiously with localized pain progressing to fever, induration, and abscess formation. An acute variety, caused usually by streptococci, may progress in hours or days and resembles infection with non-gas-forming clostridial organisms.

Neither the pathogenesis nor the source of the bacteria is entirely clear. The usual portal for entry of bacteria is a local injury, but spread via the bloodstream into a fatigued or injured muscle has also been postulated. Since normal muscle is very difficult to infect, some preceding predisposing event or condition is suspected.

The diagnosis is facilitated by sonography or CT scan.

Antibiotics effective against staphylococci and streptococci are given empirically until culture and sensitivity test results are reported. Prompt treatment may prevent abscess formation, but surgical drainage is usually required in the acute form. Delays in surgery have led to loss of limb or even to death due to sepsis.

Chiedozi LC: Pyomyositis: Review of 205 cases in 112 patients. Am J Surg 1979;137:255.
Widrow CA et al: Pyomyositis in patients with the human immunodeficiency virus: An unusual form of disseminated bacterial infection. Am J Med 1991;91:129.

CLOSTRIDIAL INFECTIONS

1. CLOSTRIDIAL INFECTIONS OTHER THAN TETANUS

Gas gangrene is closely associated with grossly contaminated war injuries. However, it is also an important problem in civilian surgical practice. The rising rate of civilian trauma and the appreciable incidence of clostridial infection after elective surgery—especially after biliary and colon operations—make the prevention and treatment of gas gangrene a matter of major concern. The break in immunity is unperfused, hypoxic tissue.

A broad spectrum of disease is caused by clostridia, ranging from negligible surface contamination through invasive cellulitis of connective tissue to invasive anaerobic infection of muscle with massive tissue necrosis and profound toxemia.

Six species cause infection in humans. Several species may be found in the same lesion. *Clostridium perfringens (Clostridium welchii)* is recovered in about 80%, *Clostridium novyi (Clostridium oedematiens)* in 40%, and *Clostridium septicum* in 20%.

Pathophysiology & Bacteriology

Clostridia are saprophytes. Vegetative and spore forms are widespread in soil, sand, clothing, and feces. They are, generally, fastidious anaerobes requiring a low redox potential to grow and to initiate conversion of the spores to vegetative, toxin-producing pathogens.

Tissue redox potentials are diminished by impaired blood supply, muscle injury, pressure from casts, severe local edema, foreign bodies, or oxygen-consuming organisms. Clostridial infections frequently occur in the presence of other bacteria, especially gram-negative bacilli. Cancer patients are particularly susceptible.

Clostridia proliferate and produce toxins that diffuse into the surrounding tissue. The toxins destroy local microcirculation. This allows further invasion, which can advance at an astonishing rate. The alpha toxin, a necrotizing lecithinase, is thought to be particularly important in this sequence, but other toxins, including collagenase, hyaluronidase, leukocidin, protease, lipase, and hemolysin, also contribute. When the disease has advanced sufficiently, toxins enter the systemic circulation, causing the systemic features of pallor, anxiety, restlessness, delirium, severe tachycardia, jaundice, and, ultimately, shock and death. The progress of the local lesion can be judged by the general state of the patient as well as by the local signs.

Clinical Findings

Clostridial infections are classified, in ascending order of lethal potential, as simple contamination, gas abscess, clostridial cellulitis, localized clostridial myositis, diffuse clostridial myositis, and edematous gangrene. The term gas gangrene is reserved to denote clostridial myositis with gas production.

A. Simple Contamination: Many open wounds are superficially infected or contaminated with clostridia without developing significant infections. There is often a brown seropurulent exudate. The condition is not invasive, because the surrounding tissue is basically healthy and the clostridia are confined to necrotic surface tissue. Debridement of dead surface tissue is usually the only treatment necessary. Simple clostridial contamination can change to inva-

sive gangrene if a severe hemodynamic abnormality or further injury decreases the oxidation-reduction potential of the surrounding tissue and allows invasion.

B. Gas Abscess (Welch's Abscess): Gas abscess is a localized infection not usually thought of as invasive. Muscle is not involved. The incubation period is usually a week or more. There is usually little pain; the edema is moderate; and the patient does not appear toxic, though fever and tachycardia may be present. The wound, however, has the characteristic brown seropurulent exudate and the characteristic autopsy room odor, and gas may be present. Except for the involved area, the tissue appears well perfused. Treatment usually consists of incision and drainage and administration of penicillin.

C. Crepitant Clostridial Cellulitis: This type ("anaerobic cellulitis") is an invasive infection of subcutaneous tissue that has been made susceptible by injury or ischemia. It usually follows appendectomy. Invasion is superficial to the deep fascia and may spread very fast, often producing discoloration of the skin and edema as well as crepitus. The systemic symptoms and signs are much less pronounced than the surface appearance and extent of gas production might indicate, and this picture distinguishes cellulitis from myositis. The differentiation is important, since adequate therapy for cellulitis is far less aggressive than that for myositis.

D. Localized Clostridial Myositis: Localized clostridial myositis is rare. The injury and infection involve muscle, but the infection is not invasive. The wound has the characteristic odor, edema, crepitation, and appearance, but the changes are localized and the region appears well perfused, with intact pulses. The systemic reaction may include fever and tachycardia but not severe prostration, delirium, and other signs of toxemia.

E. Diffuse Clostridial Myositis (Gas Gangrene): Diffuse clostridial myositis usually begins less than 3 days after the injury, with rapid increase of pain in the wound, edema, and a brown seropurulent exudate, often containing bubbles. There is marked tachycardia, but fever is variable. Crepitus may or may not be present. Profound toxemia often appears early and progresses to delirium and hemolytic jaundice. The surface edema, necrosis, and discoloration are usually less extensive than the underlying muscle necrosis. The disease characteristically progresses rapidly with loss of blood supply to the infected muscle. The swelling and edema may produce ischemia under tight dressings or plaster casts. Delayed or inadequate debridement of injured tissue after devascularizing injury is the most common setting. Since gas gangrene often develops under plaster casts, a sudden deterioration within 3–4 days after injury, an autopsy room odor, and a brown exudate are indications that removal or windowing of the cast is necessary.

F. Edematous Gangrene: Edematous gangrene is a variant caused by *C novyi (C oedematiens)*. No gas is produced, but edema of muscle is prominent. This is a particularly aggressive and often fatal infection requiring rapid and aggressive therapy.

Differential Diagnosis

Diffuse clostridial myositis (gas gangrene) is confused with other gas-producing infections, which are usually due to mixtures of gram-negative bacilli and gram-positive cocci. These mixed infections are not usually as virulent as gas gangrene and respond well to incision and drainage. Crepitant cellulitis should not be confused with clostridial gangrene, since it, too, is well treated by lesser means (see below). Gas in the tissues is not a good differentiating point, since some species (eg, *C novyi*) do not produce gas, nonclostridial organisms (eg, *Escherichia coli*) often produce gas, and air can enter tissues through a penetrating wound or from the chest.

The diagnosis must be made early and rests upon the clinical appearance of the wound and the presence of large gram-positive rods on stained smears of exudate or tissue. *C perfringens* in tissue may not exhibit spores, but other clostridia often do.

Prevention

Almost all clostridial infections are preventable. The keystone of prevention is early debridement of dead tissue and support of the circulation.

Suspicion should be directed at any wound incurred out of doors and contaminated with a foreign body, soil, or feces and any wound in which tissue (particularly muscle) has been extensively injured. This type of wound should be carefully examined, with the patient under sufficient anesthesia to permit full inspection and debridement. The minimum criteria for tissue viability are that the tissue bleeds freely when it is cut and that muscle contracts when gently pinched.

Early antibiotic treatment after injury is valuable. Penicillin is most often used, though many antibiotics have prevented gas gangrene in laboratory animals. However, *no antibiotic can prevent gas gangrene without adequate surgical debridement.*

Treatment

The major emphasis in treatment is inevitably surgical. Antibiotics are often essential but are ineffective without surgical control of the disease.

A. Surgical Treatment: The wound must be opened, and dead and severely damaged tissue must be excised. Tight fascial compartments must be decompressed. Immediate amputation is necessary when there is diffuse myositis with complete loss of blood supply or when adequate debridement would leave a useless limb.

Surgical treatment for clostridial cellulitis must often be aggressive, *but amputation is not necessary.*

Extensive debridement may be performed, with excision of necrotic skin or subcutaneous tissue, or both. Wide-open drainage is essential. One must be careful to determine whether muscle is involved, because myositis and cellulitis may coexist. Daily debridement under anesthetic may be required, since these lesions are extensive. If skin is viable, surprising amounts can be saved after debridement of subcutaneous tissue.

When clostridial infections follow penetrating injuries of the colon and rectum, diverting proximal colostomy with wide drainage of the flanks, buttocks, or perineum is required. On occasion, clostridial infections involve tissues that cannot be extensively debrided, such as spinal cord, brain, or retroperitoneal tissues, and greater reliance must be placed on antibiotics and hyperbaric oxygenation.

B. Hyperbaric Oxygenation: Hyperbaric oxygenation is beneficial in treating clostridial infections, but it cannot replace surgical therapy, since no amount of increased arterial PO_2 can force oxygen into dead tissue. Hyperbaric oxygen inhibits bacterial invasion but does not eliminate the focus of infection. It probably prevents production of alpha toxin by bacteria in environments where PO_2 can be raised enough. Treatment for 1 or 2 hours at 3 atm repeated every 6–12 hours is recommended, and only three to five exposures are usually necessary. If large hyperbaric chambers are available, operation and hyperbaric oxygenation can be accomplished simultaneously. Early use of hyperbaric oxygen, sometimes prior to debridement, can reduce tissue losses.

Because even hyperbarically administered oxygen will fail to reach the tissues in hypovolemic patients, vigorous support of blood volume is necessary. Many patients with gas gangrene and extensive injuries require multiple blood transfusions. Fresh blood should be given early, and serum phosphate levels should be kept within the normal range.

C. Antibiotics: Penicillin, 20–40 million units/d, is given intravenously. In patients allergic to penicillin, clindamycin or metronidazole is administered. Combinations of beta-lactam inhibitor antibiotics such as ampicillin together with sulbactam or ticarcillin plus clavulanate are other alternatives. In mixed infections, one has the choice between the traditional multiple antibiotics and imipenem.

Prognosis

Clostridial cellulitis and myositis are potentially lethal diseases. With adequate treatment, deaths should occur only when treatment is delayed or when patients are already severely ill with other diseases or have advanced invasion of vital structures. The death rate is currently about 20%.

The prognosis for salvage of functioning limbs is not so favorable. When clostridial myonecrosis is added to injury, affected limbs often become useless and must be amputated to save life.

Ahrenholz DH: Necrotizing soft-tissue infections. Surg Clin North Am 1988;68:199.

Bretzke ML, Bubrick MP, Hitchcock CL: Diffuse spreading *Clostridium septicum* infection, malignant disease, and immune suppression. Surg Gynecol Obstet 1988;166: 197.

Close P et al: Clostridial gas gangrene: A review of 48 consecutive cases. Acta Clin Belg 1988;43:411.

Colles JG: Concepts of anaerobic infection in relation to prevention and management. Scand J Infect Dis 1985;46: 82.

Davison AJ, Rotsetein OD: The diagnosis and management of common soft-tissue infections. Can J Surg 1988;31: 333.

Finch R: Skin and soft-tissue infections. Lancet 1988;1:164.

Hirn M, Niinikoski J: Hyperbaric oxygen in the treatment of clostridial gas gangrene. Ann Chir Gynaecol 1988;77:37.

Kingston D, Seal DV: Current hypotheses on synergistic microbial gangrene. Br J Surg 1990;77:260.

Kirk CR, Dogran JC, Hart CA: Gas gangrene: Cautionary tale. Br Med J 1988;296:1236.

Riseman JA et al: Hyperbaric oxygen therapy for necrotizing fasciitis reduces mortality and the need for debridements. Surgery 1990;108:847.

Russotti GM, Sim GH: Missile wounds of the extremities: A current concepts review. Orthopedics 1985;8:1106.

2. TETANUS

Essentials of Diagnosis

- Limitation of movements of the jaw, with painful muscle spasm and spasm of the facial muscles.
- Laryngospasm and stiffness of the neck.
- Tonic spasms and generalized convulsions.
- Presence of penetrating wounds that have not been debrided.

General Considerations

Tetanus is a specific anaerobic infection that is mediated by the neurotoxin of *Clostridium tetani* and leads to nervous irritability and tetanic muscular contractions. The causative organism enters and flourishes in hypoxic wounds contaminated with soil or feces. The tetanus-prone wound is usually a puncture wound or one containing devitalized tissue or a foreign body.

Symptoms of tetanus may occur as soon as 1 day following exposure or as long as several months later; the average incubation period is 8 days. The longer the delay between injury and debridement and immune globulin, the sooner symptoms are likely to appear.

Neonatal tetanus due to infection of the umbilical cord is common in cultures that practice poultice application to the umbilicus.

Clinical Findings

A. Symptoms and Signs: The first symptoms are usually pain or tingling in the area of injury, lim-

itation of movements of the jaw (lockjaw), and spasms of the facial muscles (risus sardonicus). These are followed by stiffness of the neck, difficulty in swallowing, and laryngospasm. Hesitancy in micturition due to sphincter spasm is also seen. In more severe cases, spasms of the muscles of the back produce opisthotonos. Spasms become increasingly frequent and involve more and more muscle groups. As chest and diaphragm spasms occur, longer and longer periods of apnea follow. The temperature is normal or slightly elevated. Sweating may be profuse. Marked rise in pulse rate is a grave sign. The severity of cases varies widely; some are very mild and barely recognizable.

B. Laboratory Findings: Polymorphonuclear leukocytosis may be present.

Prevention

Every child should be actively immunized with tetanus toxoid, beginning with routine childhood immunization and continuing with booster injections (Td) every 7–10 years. As shown in Table 8–2, tetanus prophylaxis in injured patients depends on the history of immunization and the type of wound. A Td booster, tetanus immune globulin (TIG), or both may be indicated.

The dose of TIG is 250 units intramuscularly. Equine or other tetanus antitoxin should be used only if TIG is not available and only after testing for hypersensitivity to the product.

Individuals not previously immunized should receive the following doses:

(1) Clean, minor wounds (tetanus unlikely): Give 0.5 mL of adsorbed tetanus toxoid as initial immunizing dose. The patient is then given a written record and instructed to complete the immunization schedule. Basic immunization with precipitated toxoid requires three injections: one initially and two at intervals of 4–6 weeks.

(2) Wounds with tetanus risk: Give 0.5 mL intramuscularly of adsorbed tetanus toxoid as the initial immunizing dose plus 250 units intramuscularly of

Table 8–2. Guide to tetanus prophylaxis in wound management.[1]

History of Tetanus Immunization	Clean, Minor Wounds		All Other Wounds	
	Td[2]	TIG[3]	Td[2]	TIG[3]
Uncertain, or less than 2 doses	Yes	No	Yes	Yes
Three or more doses; last dose within 10 years	No	No	Yes[4]	No

[1]Reproduced and modified, with permission, from Ann Intern Med 1981;95:726.
[2]Td = tetanus toxoid and diphtheria toxoid, adult form. Use only this preparation (Td-adult) in children older than 6 years of age.
[3]TIG = tetanus immune globulin.
[4]Unless last Td dose was within the past year.

TIG—in a different syringe and at a different site—and consider the use of antibiotics. Plan to complete the toxoid series.

Caution: Tetanus antitoxin is gamma globulin. It should *never* be given intravenously.

Treatment

Intensive treatment should be started soon, since respiratory paralysis may advance rapidly. Treatment often becomes extremely complicated and requires the combined efforts of a surgeon, an anesthesiologist, and an internist or clinical pharmacologist.

Treatment of tetanus is usually arranged in a sequence of priorities:

(1) Neutralize toxin with TIG. The usual dose of tetanus immune globulin for established tetanus is 3000–6000 units intramuscularly, given preferably in the proximal portion of the wounded extremity or in the vicinity of the wound. Repeated doses may be necessary since the half-life of the antibody is about 3 weeks and established tetanus often lasts longer.

(2) Excise and debride the suspected wound, with the patient under anesthesia appropriate to a complete and unhurried excision. Ordinarily, surgery should be done after systemic serotherapy has been started. The wound must be left open and may be treated with hydrogen peroxide.

(3) The patient should be protected from sudden stimuli, unnecessary movement, and excitement. Barbiturates or other sedatives may be employed, but overdoses often cause cardiorespiratory failure. Diazepam may reduce the amount of barbiturate necessary to control spasms. Curarization is preferable to cardiosuppressant doses of barbiturates even though curarization necessitates the use of mechanical ventilation. Cardiac dysrhythmias, pyrexia, peripheral vasoconstriction, and increased catecholamine excretion have been notable features in certain cases. When these manifestations of intense sympathetic nervous system activity occur, they can and should be reversed with peripheral alpha- or beta-blocking agents (or both).

(4) The patient with respiratory problems may require tracheostomy, since mechanical ventilation, once it becomes necessary, must be continued for weeks. The patient should be intubated as soon as respiratory problems appear.

(5) Aqueous penicillin G, 10–40 million units a day, should be given by intermittent intravenous bolus injection. The penicillin is given to kill clostridial organisms and prevent the release of more neurotoxin. Penicillin has no effect on liberated toxin. Again, imipenem is an alternative.

(6) Doses of all drugs are lower for neonatal tetanus.

Prognosis

The death rate is 30–60% in established tetanus with respiratory insufficiency. The death rate is inversely proportionate to the length of the incubation period and directly proportionate to the severity of symptoms.

An attack of tetanus does not confer lasting immunity, and patients who have recovered from the disease require active immunization according to the usual recommended schedules.

Centers for Disease Control: Tetanus—United States, 1987 and 1988. JAMA 1990;263:1192, 1195.

The diagnosis of tetanus. (Editorial.) Lancet 1980;1:1066.

Edmondson RS, Flowers MW: Intensive care in tetanus: Management, complications, and mortality in 100 cases. Br Med J 1979;1:1401.

Flowers MW, Edmondson RS: Long-term recovery from tetanus: A study of 50 survivors. Br Med J 1980;280:303.

Lindsay D: Tetanus prophylaxis: Do our guidelines assure protection? J Trauma 1984;24:1063.

New recommended schedule for active immunization of normal infants and children. MMWR 1986;35:577.

Perez-Stable EJ: Immunizations for adults. West J Med 1986;144:616.

Postoperative tetanus. (Editorial.) Lancet 1984;2:964.

Trujillo MJ et al: Tetanus in the adult: Intensive care and management experience with 233 cases. Crit Care Med 1980;8:419.

3. PSEUDOMEMBRANOUS ENTEROCOLITIS

This is a severe ulcerating mucosal infection of bowel, especially colon, in which a pseudomembrane of necrotic mucosa is often formed. It is characterized by fever, abdominal distention, and usually copious diarrhea in postoperative patients who are being given antibiotics. Stool smear shows many leukocytes and may show many gram-positive bacilli. The stool shows a rising titer of *Clostridium difficile* toxin.

Treatment includes intravenous fluids, correction of electrolyte disorders, withdrawal of antibiotics, and sometimes repopulation of the gastrointestinal tract with lactobacilli. Severe cases may require therapy with oral metronidazole or vancomycin.

The disorder occurs when the gastrointestinal flora is disturbed, when gastrointestinal perfusion is low, and when the patient is inoculated with the causal agent, *C difficile*. Antibiotics and starvation disturb the gastrointestinal flora. The disease may occur in the absence of antibiotics or after almost any antibiotic has been given for a few days. Spread is nosocomial, and poor hand washing has been implicated in several outbreaks.

Shellito PC: Pseudomembranous colitis. N Engl J Med 1992;326:1059.

Treatment of *Clostridium difficile* diarrhea. Med Lett Drugs Ther 1989;31:94.

Yee J et al: *Clostridium difficile* disease in a department of surgery: The significance of prophylactic antibiotics. Arch Surg 1991;126:241.

NECROTIZING FASCIITIS

Necrotizing fasciitis, an invasive infection of fascia, is usually due to multiple pathogens. It is characterized by infectious thrombosis of vessels passing between the skin and deep circulation, producing skin necrosis superficially resembling ischemic vascular or clostridial gangrene.

Clinical Findings

Fasciitis usually begins in a localized area such as a puncture wound, leg ulcer, or surgical wound. The infection spreads along the relatively ischemic fascial planes, meanwhile causing the penetrating vessels to thrombose. The skin is thus devascularized. Externally, hemorrhagic bullae are usually the first sign of skin death. The fascial necrosis is usually wider than the skin appearance indicates. The bullae and skin necrosis are surrounded by edema and inflammation. Crepitus is occasionally present, and the skin may be anesthetic. The patient often seems alert and unconcerned but appears toxic and has fever and tachycardia.

Gram-stained smears and bacteriologic cultures are helpful for diagnosis and treatment. The infection usually involves a mixed microbial flora, often including microaerophilic streptococci, staphylococci, gram-negative bacteria, and anaerobes, especially peptococci, peptostreptococci, and *Bacteroides*. Clostridia may be present, and the disease may clinically resemble clostridial cellulitis. At surgery, the finding of edematous, dull-gray, and necrotic fascia and subcutaneous tissue confirms the diagnosis. Thrombi in penetrating vessels are often visible. Frozen-section biopsy showing dense inflammation, arteritis, or obliterative thrombosis of arteries and veins may hasten the diagnosis.

One may encounter related infections in which severe fascial or muscle gangrene may occur with relatively little evidence that such a severe process is occurring. Muscle necrosis may be encountered and should always be suspected. Necrotic tissue can usually be removed with limited excision.

Differential Diagnosis

Although it is essential to avoid underestimating the severity of the disease and confusing it with cellulitis, localized abscess, and phlebitis, it is also necessary not to confuse necrotizing fasciitis with clostridial myositis or vascular gangrene and thereby overestimate and overtreat it. Fasciitis advances rapidly; Meleney's ulcer (chronic progressive cutaneous gangrene) advances very slowly.

Treatment

Prevention of postoperative fasciitis requires blood volume support, adequate debridement, and preventive antibiotics. Treatment consists of surgical debridement, antibiotics, and support of the local and general circulation.

A. Surgical Treatment: Debridement—under general or spinal anesthesia—must be thorough, with removal of all avascular skin and fascia. This may require extensive denudation. Where necrotic fascia undermines viable skin, longitudinal skin incisions (not too close together) aid debridement of fascia without sacrificing excessive amounts of skin. It is essential to avoid confusing fasciitis with deep gangrene. It is a tragic error to amputate an extremity when removal of dead skin and fascia will suffice. A functional extremity can usually be salvaged in fasciitis; if not, amputation can be safely performed later.

It is often difficult to distinguish necrotic from edematous tissue. Careful daily inspections of the wound will demonstrate whether repeated debridements will be necessary. If possible, all obviously necrotic tissue should be removed the first time. When viability of the remaining tissue is assured and the infection has been controlled, homografting is sometimes useful until autografting can be performed.

B. Antibiotics: Penicillin, 20–40 million units/d intravenously, is begun as soon as material has been taken for smear and culture. Because gram-negative bacteria are so often seen in this disease, another appropriate antibiotic (eg, gentamicin, 5 mg/kg/d; amikacin, 15 mg/kg/d) should be added and changed if indicated by reports of antibiotic sensitivity.

C. Circulatory Support: Blood volume must be maintained by transfusions of blood or plasma. Debridement often leaves a large raw surface that may bleed extensively. Since tissue oxygenation is critical, early transfusion with fresh blood is a rational procedure. Diabetes mellitus, if present, must be treated appropriately.

Prognosis

Reliable data on prognosis are not available, since the proper diagnosis is so often missed. Death often results, especially in elderly patients.

Gozal D et al: Necrotizing fasciitis. Arch Surg 1986;121:233.

Pessa ME, Howard RJ: Necrotizing fasciitis. Surg Gynecol Obstet 1985;161:357.

Rogers JM et al: Usefulness of computerized tomography in evaluating necrotizing fasciitis. South Med J 1984; 77:782.

Stamenkovic I, Lew PD: Early recognition of potentially fatal necrotizing fasciitis: The use of frozen-section biopsy. N Engl J Med 1984;310:1689.

Sudarsky LA et al: Improved results from a standardized approach in treating patients with necrotizing fasciitis. Ann Surg 1987;206:661.

Wang KC, Shih CH: Necrotizing fasciitis of the extremities. J Trauma 1992;32:179.

OTHER ANAEROBIC INFECTIONS

A number of bacteria can cause the typical features of anaerobic infection. Microaerophilic streptococci, peptococci, gram-negative bacilli, and *Bacteroides fragilis* are frequently seen. Some of these are gas-producing, and others are not. In general, they are less aggressive than clostridia. These bacteria usually occur in combinations.

RABIES

Rabies is a viral encephalitis usually transmitted through the saliva of an infected animal, though aerosol spread has been reported. About 30% of victims have no memory or evidence of a bite. Humans are usually inoculated by the bite of a rabid bat, skunk, raccoon, fox, wolf, dog, cat, or other animal. Since the established disease is almost invariably fatal, early preventive measures are essential.

The incubation period varies in humans from 10 days to many years. Clinical symptoms begin with pain and numbness around the site of the wound, followed by fever, irritability, malaise, dysphagia, hydrophobia, and pharyngeal spasms. Paralysis and convulsions occur terminally. About 20% of cases are characterized by progressive paralysis and sensory disturbances without a hyperactive phase.

Rabies and tetanus have many features in common. The history is the most useful differentiating point. The paralytic form must be distinguished from poliomyelitis.

Prevention

The wound should be flushed immediately and cleaned repeatedly with soap and water. Tetanus prophylaxis should be given. For severe exposure, the area around the wound should be infiltrated with anti-rabies serum (half the total dose).

If the animal has escaped, try to determine if the bite was provoked. If so, treatment with vaccine and serum becomes less urgent. A bite by a bat mandates antiserum. Consultation with local health authorities about the prevalence of rabies may facilitate the decision whether to use serum or vaccine.

If the animal is a dog or cat and can be captured, do not kill it but confine it under veterinary observation for 10 days. If it becomes rabid, the animal should be killed and its brain examined for rabies antigen by immunofluorescence. If the animal dies of any cause or if it is killed before 10 days have passed, the head should be sent to the nearest public health or other competent laboratory for examination. Wild animals should be killed immediately, not quarantined 10

days, and tested for rabies. Consult local health authorities to determine if any animal rabies has been reported recently in the area.

The physician must reach a decision based on the recommendations of the USPHS Advisory Committee but should also be influenced by the circumstances of the bite, the extent and location of the wound, the presence of rabies in the region, the type of animal responsible for the bite, etc.* Treatment includes both passive antibody and vaccine. The optimal form of passive immunization is human rabies immune globulin (20 IU/kg). Up to 50% of the globulin should be used to infiltrate the wound; the rest is administered intramuscularly. If human gamma globulin is not available, equine rabies antiserum (40 IU/kg) can be used after appropriate tests for horse serum sensitivity. Active immunization is accomplished with the human diploid cell rabies vaccine, which is given as five injections intramuscularly on days 0, 3, 7, 14, and 28 after exposure. The vaccine effectively produces an antibody response. Few side effects have occurred. The vaccine can be obtained through state health departments.

Preexposure prophylaxis with three injections of diploid cell vaccine is recommended for persons at high risk of exposure (veterinarians, animal handlers, etc).

Treatment

This very severe illness with an almost universally fatal outcome requires skillful intensive care with attention to the airway, maintenance of oxygenation, and control of seizures.

Prognosis

Once the symptoms have appeared, death almost inevitably occurs after 2–3 days as a result of cardiac or respiratory failure or generalized paralysis.

Eng TR et al: Rabies surveillance, United States, 1988. MMWR CDC Surveill Summ 1989;38:1.

Koprowski H: Rabies oral immunization. Curr Top Microbiol Immunol 1989;146:137.

Lakhanpal U, Sharma RC: An epidemiological study of 177 cases of human rabies. Int J Epidemiol 1985;14:614.

Rabies prevention—United States, 1991. Recommendations of the Immunization Practices Advisory Committee (ACIP). MMWR 1991;3:1.

Remington PL et al: A recommended approach to the evaluation of human rabies exposure in an acute care hospital. JAMA 1985;254:67.

Spriggs DR: Rabies pathogenesis: Fast times at the neuromuscular junction. J Infect Dis 1985;152:1362.

Udwadia ZF et al: Human rabies: Clinical features, diagnosis, complications, and management. Crit Care Med 1989;17:834.

*Consultation is provided by the Rabies Investigation Unit, Centers for Disease Control, Atlanta.

TYPHOID FEVER

Typhoid fever often causes necrosis of lymphoid tissue of the intestine. This develops into ulcers, usually of the ileum, which occasionally perforate. The signs of typhoid perforation may be occult but often are obvious, with abdominal pain and signs of spreading peritonitis. The diagnosis is confirmed by the discovery of free air on x-ray of the abdomen. Significant hemorrhage sometimes results from the mucosal ulcer and may itself require emergency operation. Small perforations can be simply closed if bacteriologic control has been achieved. Larger lesions may require resection or exteriorization of the intestinal segment.

Although acute cholecystitis due to typhoid is rare, chronic typhoid infection of the gallbladder is a fairly common cause of the carrier state. When patients continue to excrete *Salmonella typhi* in the stool despite adequate treatment, cholecystectomy may be indicated.

The other common surgical complications of typhoid are osteomyelitis and chondritis.

Either chloramphenicol (2–3 g/d orally), ampicillin, or trimethoprim-sulfamethoxazole may be effective, but drug resistance is emerging. Trimethoprim-sulfamethoxazole is less toxic and more likely to be effective. Third-generation cephalosporins are also effective.

In Asia, recrudescence of typhoid fever is a fairly common complication of abdominal surgery.

Achampongg EQ: Tropical diseases of the small bowel. World J Surg 1985;9:887.

Gibney EJ: Typhoid perforation. Br J Surg 1989;76:887. (And see comments.)

Gutpa SP et al: Current clinical patterns of typhoid fever: A prospective study. J Trop Med Hyg 1985;88:377.

Meier DE, Imediegwu OO, Tarpley JL: Perforated typhoid enteritis: Operative experience with 108 cases. Am J Surg 1989;157:423.

ECHINOCOCCOSIS
(Hydatid Disease)

Echinococcosis is caused by a tapeworm, *Echinococcus granulosus,* which forms larval cysts in human tissue. Dogs and, in some areas, foxes are the definitive hosts that harbor adult worms in their intestines. Ova are passed in the feces and are ingested by intermediate hosts such as cattle, humans, rodents, and particularly sheep. Dogs become infected by eating uncooked sheep carcasses that contain hydatid cysts.

Most human infection occurs in childhood, following ingestion of materials contaminated with dog feces. The ova penetrate the intestine and pass via the portal vein to the liver and then to the lung or other tissues. In the tissue, the ovum develops into a cyst filled with clear fluid. Brood capsules containing scoleces bud into the cyst lumen. Such "endocysts" may cause secondary intraperitoneal cyst formation if spilled into the peritoneal cavity.

The disease may cause systemic allergic manifestations or local symptoms due to pressure by the cyst. The patient may complain of hives or, if the cyst ruptures, may go into anaphylactic shock. Eosinophilia is present in about 40% of infected patients. Sixty percent of patients have one cyst. About 50% are located in the liver, 30% in the lung, and 20% in other organs. Forty percent of patients with a lung cyst have a liver cyst, and 25% of those with a liver cyst have one in the lung. In 25% of patients, the parasite dies, the cyst wall calcifies, and therapy is not required.

Diagnosis may be substantiated by serologic tests. The Casoni skin test is 80–90% accurate. Hemagglutination inhibition and complement fixation tests are accurate and useful, since they become negative if treatment eradicates the parasite. The overall death rate is about 15%, but it is only 4% in surgically treated cases.

Hydatid Disease of the Liver

Hydatid disease of the liver usually presents with hepatomegaly and chronic right upper quadrant pain in a past resident of an endemic area. Many cases are first seen after the cyst has ruptured into the bile ducts, in which case biliary colic and jaundice are present. Liver scanning will outline the cyst or cysts, usually in the right lobe. In about 15% of cases, there are two cysts. Ultrasonography and CT scanning readily demonstrate the cyst in the liver. ERCP can be used preoperatively to determine if the cyst communicates with the biliary tree.

Surgical treatment of cysts is effective in most cases. Because of the dangers of anaphylaxis or implantation, care must be taken to avoid rupturing the cyst and spilling its contents into the peritoneal cavity. In some cases, the cyst fluid can be aspirated and replaced by a scolicidal agent such as hypertonic (10–20%) sodium chloride solution or 0.5% sodium hypochlorite solution. More often, this is impossible because debris repeatedly plugs the needle as attempts are made to apply suction. Formalin and phenol, which have been used in the past, should not be injected into the cyst, because they can severely damage the bile ducts if a communication exists.

The cyst can sometimes be shelled out intact by developing a cleavage plane between the endocyst and ectocyst layers. Otherwise the contents must be removed piecemeal. The residual cavity can be drained and filled with omentum. Hepatic lobectomy is required rarely for especially large or multiple cysts. If the patient has been jaundiced preoperatively or if ERCP has demonstrated hydatid debris in the bile duct, a common duct exploration should be performed.

Albendazole or praziquantel is recommended postoperatively to prevent recurrence and as primary therapy for patients with disseminated disease or recurrence of a surgically inaccessible cyst or for those who are too ill to undergo surgery. These drugs must be used cautiously and the patients followed carefully for bone marrow depression or other signs of toxicity.

Hydatid Disease of the Lungs

Hydatid cysts of the lung cause chest pain and dyspnea. They may secondarily communicate with bronchioles and become infected. Oral expulsion of the cyst fluid may follow rupture into a bronchus, after which an air-fluid level can be seen on chest x-ray.

Removal of pulmonary cysts presents fewer technical difficulties than removal of liver cysts. The lung is incised over the cyst, and while the anesthesiologist inflates the lung, the cyst can be slowly delivered intact. Large cysts may be managed by lobectomy, but pneumonectomy is rarely necessary. Secondary bacterial infection and abscess formation should be treated as for pulmonary abscess in general.

Belli L et al: Improved results with pericystectomy in normothermic ischemia for hepatic hydatidosis. Surg Gynecol Obstet 1986;163:127.

Demirci S et al: Comparison of the results of different surgical techniques in the management of hydatid cysts of the liver. World J Surg 1989;13:88.

Dogan R et al: Surgical treatment of hydatid cysts of the lung: Report on 1055 patients. Thorax 1989;44:192.

Drugs for parasitic infections. Med Lett Drugs Ther 1992;34:17.

Karavias D et al: Improved techniques in the surgical treatment of hepatic hydatidosis. Surg Gynecol Obstet 1992;174:176.

Lewall DB, McCorkell SJ: Rupture of echinococcal cysts: Diagnosis, classification, and clinical implications. AJR 1986;146:391.

Magistrelli P et al: Surgical treatment of hydatid disease of the liver: A 20-year experience. Arch Surg 1991;126:518. (See discussion on p 523.)

Miguet JP, Bresson-Hadni S: Alveolar echinococcosis of the liver. J Hepatol 1989;8:373.

Morel P, Robert J, Rohner A: Surgical treatment of hydatid disease of the liver: A survey of 69 patients. Surgery 1988;104:859.

Musio F, Linos D: Echinococcal diseases in an extended family and review of the literature. Arch Surg 1989;124:741.

Todorov T et al: Experience in the chemotherapy of severe, inoperable echinococcosis in man. Infection 1992;20:19.

AMEBIASIS

Amebiasis is caused by the protozoal parasite *Entamoeba histolytica*. Ten percent of the world's population is infected. The active vegetative forms—the trophozoites—often inhabit the colon, where they subsist on bacteria, usually without causing symptoms. The trophozoites may develop into more resistant cystic forms that are passed in stools. The infection is transmitted by oral-fecal contact. Invasion by trophozoites produces disease principally in the colon and liver. The skin, brain, vagina, and other organs are involved rarely.

Clinical Findings

A. Intestinal Amebiasis: When amebas invade the colon, they burrow through and undermine the colonic mucosa, producing ulcers. The resulting colitis may vary in severity from chronic and indolent to acute and fulminating.

1. Amebic dysentery–The usual case begins with intermittent cramps. After weeks to months, mild diarrhea with blood-stained mucus develops. Fever is usually less than 38.5 °C (101.3 °F), and the patient is rarely seriously ill. Tenderness is present to palpation in both lower quadrants, and the liver is often slightly enlarged.

2. Severe amebic colitis–This form of the disease may progress to colonic perforation and peritonitis. It may begin suddenly with severe diarrhea of blood and mucus. Abdominal pain, cramps, tenesmus, and dehydration are severe. The patient is toxic, with fever from 39 to 40 °C (102.2–104 °F) and leukocytosis in the range of 25,000/µL. The stools often contain sloughs of colonic mucosa.

Sigmoidoscopy demonstrates the typical small, white-capped amebic ulcers, but the examination must be performed gently to avoid perforation. Stool or mucosa obtained by sigmoidoscopy may reveal the trophozoites. Colonic dilatation may resemble acute megacolon of ulcerative colitis. This distinction is critical, because administration of corticosteroid drugs severely aggravates amebic colitis and colectomy is frequently lethal, whereas amebicides and tetracycline usually control the disease. Very rarely, operation may be necessary for perforation or obstruction.

3. Localized intestinal disease–Amebas may invade only a short segment—usually the cecum and sigmoid colon—and lead to stricture formation or a granulomatous mass called **ameboma.** The cecum, sigmoid, and transverse colon are involved in that order of frequency. The typical patient presents with pain in the right lower quadrant and an enlarged and tender cecum and ascending colon. A history of dysentery is usually obtained, and trophozoites may be demonstrated in stool specimens. Barium enema shows concentric narrowing of the affected bowel. Resection may be indicated for intestinal obstruction, but in most cases drug therapy is curative. After treatment, a follow-up barium enema should be obtained to make sure the mass has resolved and did not represent cancer.

Amebic rectal strictures may be confused with neoplasms or lymphogranuloma venereum.

B. Hepatic Amebiasis: Hepatic abscess, which results from seeding via the portal vein, develops in fewer than 10% of cases of amebic dysentery. The abscess is usually solitary and in 90% of cases involves the right lobe. The liver remote from the abscess is normal. The concept of amebic hepatitis, implying diffuse hepatic inflammation, is not supported by histologic evidence. The abscess contains sterile pus (anchovy paste) that varies from pink to chocolate-brown. Trophozoites may occasionally be found at the active periphery of the abscess. Amebic abscess and dysentery rarely occur simultaneously, and only about 20% of patients with an abscess have a history suggesting previous dysentery.

Fever usually ranges from 38 to 39 °C (100.4–102.2 °F), and the white count is elevated to 15,000–25,000/µL. The liver is enlarged, and there is tenderness in the right upper quadrant over the abscess. Motion makes the pain worse. Serum bilirubin is usually normal unless secondary pyogenic infection occurs. The serum alkaline phosphatase is often increased, and albumin is decreased. X-rays show an elevated right diaphragm and pleural fluid in the right hemithorax. Ultrasonography, CT scanning, and technetium-99m scanning will usually demonstrate the abscess. Gallium-67 and indium-111 scans are usually negative until bacterial superinfection occurs.

The distinction from pyogenic abscess may be difficult. The presence of infection elsewhere in the abdomen in a severely toxic patient suggests a bacterial abscess. A positive hemagglutination titer, sterile pus in the abscess, and trophozoites in the stool or the abscess suggest amebic abscess.

The abscess may burst into the peritoneal cavity, the pleural space, or the peritoneum.

Diagnosis

Trophozoites are present in the stool during active intestinal disease, but there are many pitfalls in demonstrating them. The stool specimen must be handled properly and either examined within 1 hour of passage or preserved with polyvinyl alcohol. Laxatives, antacids, antibiotics, bismuth, kaolin compounds, and barium x-ray studies may interfere with demonstration of the parasite for as long as 2 weeks.

The indirect hemagglutination titer, the best serologic test, is positive in 85% of patients with symptomatic intestinal amebiasis and in 98% of those with extraintestinal disease. After successful treatment of amebiasis, the titer may remain high indefinitely.

Treatment

Parenteral metronidazole is used in patients with ileus or vomiting from severe colitis. Some experts recommend needle aspiration of all abscesses that can be localized (about two-thirds of cases); others reserve aspiration for especially large abscesses

thought to be in imminent danger of rupturing. Aspiration of left lobe abscesses is more urgent, since they may penetrate the pericardium. Rarely, operation may be required, usually for multiple abscesses that become superinfected with bacteria.

Conter RL et al: Differentiation of pyogenic from amebic hepatic abscesses. Surg Gynecol Obstet 1986;162:114.
Drugs for parasitic infections. Med Lett Drugs Ther 1992;34:17.
Hai AA et al: Amoebic liver abscess: Review of 220 cases. Int Surg 1991;76:81.
Hossain A et al: Indirect haemagglutination (IHA) test in the serodiagnosis of amoebiasis. J Hyg Epidemiol Microbiol Immunol 1989;33:91.
Korelitz BI: When should we look for amebas in patients with inflammatory bowel disease? J Clin Gastroenterol 1989;11:373.
Krogstad DJ: Isoenzyme patterns and pathogenicity in amebic infection. N Engl J Med 1986;315:390.
Sarda AK et al: Intraperitoneal rupture of amoebic liver abscess. Br J Surg 1989;76:202.
Singh JP, Kashyap A: A comparative evaluation of percutaneous catheter drainage for resistant amebic liver abscesses. Am J Surg 1989;158:58.
Thompson JE et al: Amebic abscess of the liver: Surgical aspects. West J Med 1982;136:103.
Variyam EP et al: Nondysenteric intestinal amebiasis: Colonic morphology and search for *Entamoeba histolytica* adherence and invasion. Dig Dis Sci 1989;34:732.

ACTINOMYCOSIS & NOCARDIOSIS

These are chronic, slowly progressive infections that may involve many tissues, resulting in the formation of granulomas and abscesses that drain through sinuses and fistulas. The lesions resemble those produced by fungi, but the organisms are true bacteria.

Actinomycosis

Actinomycetes are gram-positive, non-acid-fast, filamentous organisms that usually show branching and may break up into short bacterial forms. They are strict anaerobes and part of the normal flora of the human oropharynx and tonsils.

Inflammatory nodular masses, abscesses, and draining sinuses occur most commonly on the head and neck. One-fifth of the cases have primary lesions in the chest and an equal proportion in the abdomen, most commonly involving the appendix and cecum. Multiple sinuses are commonly formed, and the discharging pus may contain "sulfur granules," yellow granules of tangled filaments. The inflammatory lesions are often hard and relatively painless and nontender. Systemic symptoms, including fever, are variably present. The discharging sinus tracts or fistulas usually become secondarily infected with other bacteria.

Abdominal actinomycosis may give rise to appendicitis, and early appendectomy may be curative. If the appendix perforates, multiple lesions and sinuses of the abdominal wall form. Thoracic actinomycosis may give rise to cough, pleural pain, fever, and weight loss, simulating mycobacterial or mycotic infection. Later in the course of the disease, the sinuses perforate the pleural cavity and the chest wall, often involving ribs or vertebrae.

All forms of actinomycosis are treated with penicillin (5–20 million units daily) for many weeks. In addition, surgical extirpation or drainage of lesions—or repair of defects—may be required for cure.

Nocardiosis

Nocardiae are gram-positive, branching, filamentous organisms that may be acid-fast. The filaments often fragment into bacillary forms. They are aerobes that are rarely found in the normal flora of the respiratory tract. Nocardiae are not susceptible to penicillin but are often inhibited by sulfonamides.

Nocardiosis may present with two forms. One is localized, chronic granuloma, with suppuration, abscess, and sinus tract formation resembling actinomycosis. A specialized disorder occurs in the extremities as **Madura foot** (mycetoma), with extensive bone destruction but little systemic illness.

A second form is a systemic infection, beginning as pneumonitis with suppuration and progressing via the bloodstream to involvement of other organs, eg, meninges or brain. Systemic nocardiosis produces fever, cough, and weight loss and resembles mycobacterial or mycotic infections. It is particularly apt to occur as a complication of immunodeficiency in lymphoma or drug-induced immunosuppression.

Nocardiosis is best treated with sulfonamides (eg, sulfamethoxazole, 6–8 g daily orally) for many weeks. The simultaneous administration of minocycline (200–400 mg daily orally) may be advantageous. Surgical drainage of abscesses, excision of fistulas, and repair of defects are essential features of management.

Heffner JE: Pleuropulmonary manifestations of actinomycosis and nocardiosis. Semin Respir Infect 1988;3:352.

Jensen BM, Kruse-Andersen S, Andersen K: Thoracic actinomycosis. Scand J Thorac Cardiovasc Surg 1989;23:181.

Lerner PI: The lumpy jaw: Cervicofacial actinomycosis. Infect Dis Clin North Am 1988;2:203.

McGinnis MR, Fader RC: Mycetoma: A contemporary concept. Infect Dis Clin North Am 1988;2:939.

INFECTIONS RESULTING FROM DRUG ABUSE

The recent increase of drug abuse has resulted in a number of atypical infections that demand unusual expertise from the surgeon.

Clinical Findings

Infections associated with drug abuse commonly result from intravascular or extravascular needle injection of drugs with irritating or even necrotizing foreign substances that may contain bacteria. In many cases, the local lesion is complicated by large areas of necrosis, bacteremia, and inflammation. Needles may penetrate the fascia, causing deep space infections in which fluctuation or other external signs of abscess may be absent. The most common causative organisms are staphylococci and streptococci, which account for almost all monomicrobial infections, but gram-negative enteric organisms are commonly seen in mixed infections. The patients are often malnourished, and complicating immune disorders are common (eg, acquired immunodeficiency syndrome [AIDS]). Gamma globulin levels are high. Helper/suppressor cell ratios tend to be inverted. Addicts are often dehydrated and may have been hypotensive for a period after the contaminating injection. Drugs are often mixed with foreign substances such as talcum powder, milk, lighter fluid, barbiturates, and even amphetamines. The drugs themselves are often vasoconstrictors (methamphetamine, cocaine) and therefore facilitate infection. The addict may give an inaccurate history and may use drugs even while under treatment.

A typical problem is a grossly swollen, tense, immobile forearm that is acutely tender but shows no localizing signs of infection. Fever and tachycardia are usually not severe. Many such acute, possibly sterile reactions will subside with rest, elevation, and hot packs. On the other hand, if sepsis is suspected on the basis of the systemic effects, surgical drainage is mandatory even though localization may be difficult. Sonograms and CT scans are extremely useful in finding hidden abscesses. Unfortunately, addicts have many reasons for fever, including other drug-related problems such as withdrawal, pneumonia, empyema, hepatitis, or endocarditis.

Complications

Infections complicating drug abuse are multiple. The most important are pneumonia (from aspiration), hepatitis, endocarditis, meningitis, tetanus, suppurative phlebitis, and empyema. AIDS greatly complicates both the diagnosis and the treatment, and evidence of it should be sought in virtually every drug-associated infection.

Treatment

Drainage of abscesses is essential, but they are often difficult to find. When the abscess is not found in the subcutaneous tissue, the deep fascia and muscle compartments must be opened. Neurologic findings may help; eg, median nerve paresis is an indication for extensive deep exploration if the injection was in the antecubital fossa. Infection may spread along a vein and necessitate its removal up to the next major tributary. Necrotic skin indicates extensive deeper damage requiring extensive excision. Fever that does not respond to drainage within 24 hours indicates additional sites of infection or inflammation. Sonography is helpful in delineating the extent of the disease.

Prolonged use of amphetamines may lead to arterial aneurysms, often in the visceral arteries. Concomitant bacteremia may result in mycotic endarteritis. Arteriograms followed by excision during specific antibiotic therapy may be required. Coexisting endocarditis (bacterial or candidal) must be considered. Drug-related cardiac valvulitis has been treated with emergency excision and replacement, but long-term survivors are few. Early diagnosis and aggressive therapy are extremely important.

Tetanus is also prevalent in addicts, and immunization is imperative.

Intra-arterial injection of barbiturates or methamphetamine may cause acute vascular obstruction that may at first mimic cellulitis or abscess. Heroin is often diluted with barbiturates, and inadvertent arterial injection of heroin may cause a serious reaction. Pentazocine injections produce a severe, local sterile inflammation that can destroy muscles, nerves, and tendons and for which there is no known cure or prevention.

Prognosis

The prognosis for long-term survival is poor in heroin or methamphetamine addicts who have destroyed their veins to the point where extravasation occurs or they are reduced to "skin popping" (subcutaneous injection). Many limbs have been crippled or lost as a result of this pattern of abuse. Complications and recurrences are usually due to continued drug abuse.

Bradley S: Drugs of abuse and infections. Adv Exp Med Biol 1991;288:119.
Cregler LL, Mark H: Medical complications of cocaine abuse. N Engl J Med 1986;315:1495.
Reyes F: Infections secondary to intravenous drug abuse. Hand Clin 1989;5:629.

SEXUALLY TRANSMITTED DISEASES

Sexually transmitted diseases are treated principally by medical means, but complications may require surgery.

Syphilis

Syphilis is rarely a surgical disease, but the cutaneous lesions of syphilis may masquerade as skin tumors or as stubborn infectious lesions. The primary ulcer (chancre) occurs most often on the genitalia, face, or anus and is self-limited. Secondary lesions usually begin as indurated nodules that break down to form punched-out, sometimes oval ulcers with sharp epidermal edges. They may occur anywhere but are particularly common on the legs.

Syphilis is known as "the great imitator." It produces gummas (tumorous granulomas specific to syphilis) that may involve the gastrointestinal tract, skin, bones, joints, or nose and throat. They may invade tissues such as the nasal septum, where perforations occur, and may cause masses in liver or in bone.

The diagnosis is made by darkfield or immunofluorescent examination of smears or exudates and by serologic tests.

Treatment is with penicillin G, 2.4 million units intramuscularly as a single injection; or erythromycin, 500 mg orally four times daily for 15 days.

Hook EW 3rd: Syphilis and HIV infection. J Infect Dis 1989;160:530.
Kunloch-de-Loes S, Radeff B, Saurat JH: AIDS meets syphilis: Changing patterns of the syphilitic infection and its treatment. Dermatologica 1988;177:261.

Yaws

Yaws (frambesia) is not sexually transmitted but is closely related to syphilis, since it is caused by *Treponema pertenue*. It causes ulcerating papules resembling those of syphilis. The disease is endemic, particularly among children, in hot tropical countries.

Diagnosis and treatment are as for syphilis.

Browne SG: Yaws. Int J Dermatol 1982;21:220.
Sehgal VN: Leg ulcers caused by yaws and endemic syphilis. Clin Dermatol 1990;8:166.
Yaws again. (Editorial.) Br Med J 1980;281:1090.

Gonorrhea

Although gonorrhea usually begins with urethritis, producing a creamy exudate, it may also cause a painful proctitis—now commonly seen both in women and in homosexual males. It may also cause epididymitis and prostatitis, may involve the joints or even the meninges, and may cause serious systemic symptoms. Surgery is rarely needed except for gonococcal strictures of the urinary tract or for excision of tubo-ovarian abscess.

The diagnosis is made by finding gram-negative intracellular diplococci on smear, which is positive in most men but only 60% of women with the disease. Culture for *Neisseria gonorrhoeae* is also usually necessary.

The recommended treatment is with ceftriaxone, 250 mg intramuscularly as a single dose. Spectinomycin, cefixime, ciprofloxacin, or procaine penicillin G may also be used. However, because treatment with ceftriaxone alone results in a high rate of residual chlamydial infection, a 7-day course of doxycycline should be given to cover the possibility of coincidental infection.

Britigan BE et al: Gonococcal infection: A model of molecular pathogenesis. N Engl J Med 1985;312:1683.

Handsfield HH: Recent developments in gonorrhea and pelvic inflammatory disease. J Med 1983;14:281.

Platt R et al: Risk of acquiring gonorrhea and prevalence of abnormal adnexal findings among women recently exposed to gonorrhea. JAMA 1983;250:3205.

Rice RJ, Thompson SE: Treatment of uncomplicated infections due to Neisseria gonorrhoeae. JAMA 1986;255:1739.

Speedy diagnosis of gonorrhea. (Editorial.) Lancet 1983;1:684.

Stamm WE et al: Effect of treatment regimens for Neisseria gonorrhoeae on simultaneous infection with Chlamydia trachomatis. N Engl J Med 1984;310:545.

Washington AE et al: The economic cost of pelvic inflammatory disease. JAMA 1986;255:1735.

Chlamydia trachomatis Infection

Chlamydial infection is the most common bacterial sexually transmitted disease, responsible for nongonococcal urethritis and epididymitis in men and cervicitis, urethritis, and pelvic inflammatory disease in women. Most infections in women are asymptomatic. Chlamydia is responsible for complications of pregnancy such as premature rupture of the fetal membranes, premature delivery, and postpartum endometritis.

Lymphogranuloma venereum is a systemic disease also caused by Chlamydia trachomatis. It usually presents with inguinal adenopathy progressing to suppuration. Ulcerative proctitis, a common presentation in women and homosexual males, may progress to anal or rectal stricture formation.

The laboratory diagnosis of chlamydial infections is best accomplished with cell culture or fluorescein-conjugated monoclonal antibody staining of mucosal exudates. Antibody titers may be the only feasible diagnostic procedure for chronic syndromes.

Treatment consists of doxycycline (100 mg twice daily) or erythromycin (500 mg four times daily) for 7 days. The drugs are given in the same dosages for lymphogranuloma venereum. Ciprofloxacin is also an alternative.

Bell TA et al: Centers for Disease Control guidelines for prevention and control of Chlamydia trachomatis infections. Ann Intern Med 1986;104:524.

Chlamydia in women: A case for more action? Lancet 1986;1:892.

Sanders LL et al: Treatment of sexually transmitted chlamydial infections. JAMA 1986;255:1750.

Chancroid

In its primary phase, chancroid can be differentiated from syphilis on the basis of its angular, very shallow genital ulceration, with purulent discharge and pain—as opposed to the usually painless chancre, with raised edges, of syphilis. Chancroid does not give a positive serologic test for syphilis, but patients with chancroid may have or have had syphilis. Darkfield examination is negative. Smear reveals a mixed flora including gram-negative rods in chains. The major organism is Haemophilus ducreyi. Ceftriaxone, 250 mg intramuscularly as a single injection, is the treatment of choice. Erythromycin, 500 mg orally four times daily for 7 days, is an alternative.

Schmid GP et al: Chancroid in the United States: Reestablishment of an old disease. JAMA 1987;258:3265.

Granuloma Inguinale

Granuloma inguinale is a relatively uncommon infection caused by Donovania (Calymmatobacterium) granulomatis. The lesion usually begins as a pustule in or around the genitalia. It soon ulcerates, produces a milky secretion, and slowly invades the adjacent skin. Although it is an infectious disease, it can behave almost in a malignant fashion when not treated. It rarely causes pain or tenderness and usually advances radially from the genitalia or from the anus.

Diagnosis is best made by finding "Donovan bodies" in biopsy material. Treatment is usually with tetracyclines. Streptomycin and ampicillin are second-choice drugs.

Faro S: Lymphogranuloma venereum, chancroid, and granuloma inguinale. Obstet Gynecol Clin North Am 1989;16:517.

Growdon WA et al: Granuloma inguinale in a white teenager: A diagnosis easily forgotten, poorly pursued. West J Med 1985;143:105.

Kuberski T: Granuloma inguinale (donovanosis). Sex Transm Dis 1980;7:29.

Condylomata Acuminata (Venereal Warts)

Venereal warts are usually seen around the genitalia and anus as painful cauliflower-like papillomas with a rough papillated surface. The etiologic agent is a papillomavirus. Rarely, these warts invade the urethra and bladder or rectum. When this occurs, extensive operative procedures may be needed to eradicate the warts and their obstructive effects.

The differential diagnosis includes syphilitic or lymphogranulomatous condylomas, hemorrhoids, and skin and anal cancer. Warts that fail to respond to podophyllum resin should be biopsied.

Most external venereal warts are best treated by painting with tincture of podophyllum resin. This is extremely effective, but it may be painful, and extensive cases should be treated in segments. Warts within the urethra, bladder, anal canal, or rectum usually require electrofulguration. Recurrences are common. Intralesional injections of alpha interferon are also effective and are synergistic with cryotherapy and podophyllum resin. This combination therapy may become useful in the treatment of refractory cases. Fluorouracil is an alternative topical application.

Douglas JJ et al: A randomized trial of combination therapy with intralesional interferon alpha 2b and podophyllin versus podophyllin alone for the therapy of anogenital warts. J Infect Dis 1990;162:52.
Drugs for sexually transmitted diseases. Med Lett Drugs Ther 1991;33:119.
Eron LJ et al: Interferon therapy for condylomata acuminata. N Engl J Med 1986;315:1059.
Handley JM et al: Subcutaneous interferon alpha 2a combined with cryotherapy vs cryotherapy alone in the treatment of primary anogenital warts: A randomised observer blind placebo controlled study. Genitourin Med 1991;67:297.

SNAKEBITE*

Only four venomous snakes are indigenous to the USA. Three of these—the rattlesnake, the cottonmouth, and the copperhead—are pit vipers. The fourth is the coral snake, a member of the family Elapidae (cobra-like), which produces a venom unrelated to that of the pit vipers. Pit vipers can be distinguished from nonvenomous snakes by a round mouth and a pit between the eyes and the nares on each side.

Snake venom contains proteolytic enzymes, peptides, and metalloproteins that, when injected through the hollow fangs of the snake, can cause local tissue destruction and necrosis of blood vessels and profound neurotoxic or hemotoxic systemic reactions. Secondary edema spreads rapidly and may contribute to ischemia of an extremity. Bites on the fingers or toes may cause destruction of digits, muscle compartments, and subcutaneous tissues. When intravascular injection occurs, bleeding secondary to low fibrinogen and platelet levels may ensue. Hemorrhage into tissue will exacerbate local pressure effects. Hemolysis may occur and produce acute tubular necrosis. Myonecrosis, shock, and pituitary failure are other possible manifestations.

A bite by a venomous snake results in envenomation in only 50–70% of cases. Envenomation may be mild (scratch followed by minimal swelling and not much pain); moderate (fang marks, local swelling, and definite pain); or severe (fang marks, severe and progressive swelling and pain).

Treatment

A. First Aid Measures: Apply a broad, firm constricting bandage over the bite, and wrap as much of the bitten limb as possible. Splint the limb and transport the patient to a medical facility.

Tourniquets, incision and suction, application of

ice, and cryotherapy as first aid measures to the bite wound are of no proved value. The most important objective of early management in the field is to get the patient to a hospital as quickly as possible.

B. Definitive Treatment: Antivenin is the mainstay of therapy. The earlier it can be administered, the more effective it will be, but because of potential side effects, antivenin should be given only when the bite is likely to be significant or after early signs of envenomation have appeared.

In the USA, two kinds of antivenin are available, one for North American pit vipers and another for Eastern coral snakes. Antivenin for other poisonous snakes not indigenous to the USA can usually be obtained from any large zoo.

All antivenins are horse sera, so immediate (anaphylaxis) and late (serum sickness) allergic reactions are not uncommon. Epinephrine and antihistamines should be on hand. The dose of antivenin required varies with the type of snake and the amount of envenomation. The range is from five vials to as much as 40–50 vials intravenously for severe or intravenous pit viper bites.

Surgical excision of the bite is no longer recommended, because it is unnecessary except in rare instances. Pressure should be measured in fascial compartments if swelling becomes significant, and fasciotomy should be performed in the uncommon case where pressure rises above 30–40 mm Hg.

Prognosis

The death rate following snakebite should be no more than 7% if adequate supportive care and specific antivenin are given.

Banner W Jr: Bits and stings in the pediatric patient. Curr Probl Pediatrics 1988;18:1.
Curry SC et al: The legitimacy of rattlesnake bites in central Arizona. Ann Emerg Med 1989;18:658.
Jamieson R, Pearn J: An epidemiological and clinical study of snake-bites in childhood. Med J Aust 1989;150:698.
Nelson BK: Snake envenomation: Incidence, clinical presentation and management. Med Toxicol Adverse Drug Exp 1989;4:17.
Wasserman GS: Wound care of spider and snake envenomations. Ann Emerg Med 1988;17:1331.
White RR, Weber RA: Poisonous snakebite in central Texas: Possible indicators for antivenin treatment. Ann Surg 1991;213:466. (See discussion on p 471.)

ARTHROPOD BITES*

Stings and bites of arthropods are most often merely a nuisance. Some arthropods, however, can

---

*Consultations on complex cases of snakebite or bites of other poisonous animals may be obtained through the Poison Control Center, University of Arizona Health Sciences, Tucson, Arizona.

*Consultations on complex cases of snakebite or bites of other poisonous animals may be obtained through the Poison Control Center, University of Arizona Health Sciences, Tucson, Arizona.

produce death by direct toxicity or by hypersensitivity reactions. Because of their prevalence and widespread distribution, bees and wasps kill more people than any other venomous animal, including snakes.

Bees & Wasps

When a bee stings, it becomes anchored by the two barbed lancets, so that withdrawal is impossible. In the struggle, a bee will usually avulse its stinging apparatus and die. After being stung by a bee, one should scrape the exuded poison sac with a sharp knife. Any attempt to pull the poison apparatus out will simply cause more venom to be squeezed into the tissue. The stinger, once embedded, remains present. If this has occurred in an eyelid, it may irritate the globe of the eye months after the sting.

The stinging lancets of the wasp are not barbed and can easily be withdrawn by the insect to allow it to reinsert or to escape. It is unusual, therefore, to find a stinger left in place after a wasp sting. The females of the variety called yellow jackets are very aggressive. These insects sometimes bite before stinging.

The venom of bees and wasps contains histamine, basic protein components of high molecular weight, free amino acids, hyaluronidase, and acetylcholine. Antigenic proteins are species-specific and may lead to cross-reactivity between insects. Symptoms of arthropod stings may vary from minimal erythema to a marked local reaction of severe systemic toxicity (especially from multiple stings). Infection may occur. A generalized allergic reaction has been described that resembles serum sickness.

Early application of ice packs to reduce swelling is indicated. Elevation of the extremity is also useful. Oral antihistamines may be of some use in reducing urticaria. Parenteral corticosteroids may reduce delayed inflammation. If infection occurs, treatment consists of local debridement and antibiotics. Moderately severe reactions will present as generalized syncope or urticarial reactions. If an anaphylactic reaction or severe reaction is present, aqueous epinephrine, 0.5–1 mL of 1:1000 solution, should be given intramuscularly. A repeat dose may be given in 5–10 minutes, followed by 5–20 mg of diphenhydramine slowly intravenously. Administration of corticosteroids and general supportive measures such as oxygen administration, plasma expanders, and pressor agents may be required in case of shock. Previously sensitized patients should carry identifying tags and a kit for emergency intramuscular injection of epinephrine.

It is possible to immunize persons against bee and wasp stings, but cost-benefit analyses indicate that this is rarely if ever indicated.

Spiders

All spiders have poison glands for killing insects, but only a few are potent enough to be harmful to humans. In humans, the bite of *Loxosceles* (eg, brown recluse spider) causes local necrosis, while the toxic effects of *Latrodectus* (eg, black widow spider) bites are principally systemic. *Latrodectus* bites, the most serious, result in a death rate of about 5%. Individual species of both *Latrodectus* and *Loxosceles* are distributed throughout the world. The following descriptions apply to the two common examples of potentially dangerous spiders found in the USA. Contrary to common belief, the bites of the tarantula spiders *Lycosa tarentula,* found in the Mediterranean region, and Theraphosidae, found principally in North America, are not dangerous.

A. Black Widow Spider *(Latrodectus mactans)*: The female black widow spider is characterized by a shiny black body with a red hourglass design on the underside of the abdomen. The male is smaller, less dark, and does not bite. The bite is usually followed by pain and muscular rigidity. Symptoms begin within 10 minutes to 1 hour. Within 24 hours, abdominal pain becomes severe and the abdomen often board-like. Convulsions, hypertension, and delirium may follow. Severe symptoms usually subside within 48 hours, but the untreated illness lasts for about a week. The death rate may be as high as 5%. Symptoms are usually self-limited. Debridement of the bite or use of a tourniquet is of no value, since the dissemination of black widow spider venom is instantaneous. Ice packs will reduce the pain. Intravenous injections of 10% calcium gluconate will relieve muscle pain and spasm. A specific antivenin (horse serum) packaged in sterile water is available. Horse serum sensitivity testing and, if necessary, desensitization must precede its use. The usual dose is 2.5 mL of reconstituted serum given intramuscularly.

B. Brown Recluse Spider (Violin Spider; *Loxosceles reclusa)*: The brown spider is dark tan and has three pairs of eyes on the anterior part of the cephalothorax and a violin-shaped marking on the dorsal carapace. Immediately after being bitten, there is little local pain. In minor envenomation, the local reaction consists of erythema and edema. At the site of a more serious bite, an erythematous hemorrhagic bulla develops within 24–48 hours, surrounded by a patch of ischemia. This usually evolves into an indolent ulcer that may take weeks to heal. Systemic symptoms may include fever, urticaria, nausea and vomiting, and, rarely, hemolysis or disseminated intravascular coagulation.

Treatment is largely supportive. If the local reaction is progressing rapidly or if an ulcer has appeared, the patient may be treated with dapsone, 50–100 mg/d. This drug may prevent ulceration or accelerate healing of an established ulcer. Death is rare, but tissue loss is common, and early excision is followed by poor repair.

Amital Y et al: Scorpion sting in children: A review of 51 cases. Clin Pediatr 1985;24:136.

Binder LS: Acute arthropod envenomation: Incidence, clinical features, and management. Med Toxicol 1989;4:163.

Golden DA, Schwartz HJ: Guidelines for venom immunotherapy. J Allergy Clin Immunol 1986;77:727.

Golden DBK et al: Epidemiology of insect venom sensitivity. JAMA 1989;262:240.

King LE Jr, Rees RS: Management of brown recluse spider bite. JAMA 1984;251:889.

Rees RS et al: Brown recluse spider bites: A comparison of early surgical excision versus dapsone and delayed surgical excision. Ann Surg 1985;202:659.

Rosson CL, Tolle SW: Management of marine stings and scrapes. West J Med 1989;150:97.

Stawiski MA: Insect bites and stings. Emerg Med Clin North Am 1985;3:785.

Timms PK, Gibbons RB: Latrodectism: Effects of the black widow spider bite. West J Med 1986;144:315.

Wilson DC, King LE Jr: Spiders and spider bites. Dermatol Clin 1990;8:277.

Young VL, Pin P: The brown recluse spider bite. Ann Plast Surg 1988;20:447.

ANTIMICROBIAL CHEMOTHERAPY

Ernest Jawetz, MD, PhD

PRINCIPLES OF SELECTION OF ANTIMICROBIAL DRUGS

Selection of an Antimicrobial Drug on Clinical Grounds

For optimal treatment of an infectious process, a suitable antimicrobial must be administered as early as possible. This involves a series of decisions: (1) The surgeon decides, on the basis of a clinical impression, that a microbial infection probably exists. (2) Analyzing the symptoms and signs, the surgeon makes a guess as to which microorganisms are most likely to cause the suspected infection; an etiologic diagnosis is attempted on clinical grounds. (3) The surgeon selects the drug most likely to be effective against the suspected organisms ("empiric therapy"); ie, a specific drug is aimed at a specific organism. (4) Before ordering the drug, the surgeon must secure specimens likely to provide a microbiologic diagnosis. (5) The surgeon observes the clinical response to the prescribed antimicrobial. Upon receipt of laboratory identification of a possible important microorganism, this new information is weighed against an original "best guess" of etiologic organism and drug. (6) The surgeon may choose to change the drug regimen then or upon receipt of further laboratory information on drug susceptibility of the isolated organism. However, laboratory data need not always overrule a decision based on clinical and empiric grounds, especially when the clinical response supports the initial etiologic diagnosis and drug selection.

Selection of an Antimicrobial Drug by Laboratory Tests

When an etiologic pathogen has been isolated from a meaningful specimen, it is often possible to select the drug of choice on the basis of current clinical experience. Such a listing of drug choices is given in Table 8–3. At other times, laboratory tests for antimicrobial drug susceptibility are necessary, particularly if the isolated organism is of a type that often exhibits drug resistance, eg, enteric gram-negative rods.

Antimicrobial drug susceptibility tests may be done on solid media as disk tests, in broth in tubes, or in wells of microdilution plates. The latter method yields results expressed as the MIC (minimal inhibitory concentration), and the technique can be modified to also permit determination of the MBC (minimal bactericidal concentration). The latter is of value in situations where host defenses cannot control infection (eg, endocarditis, osteomyelitis, meningitis) or when the patient is immunodeficient or immunosuppressed. When performed in a well-controlled setting, disk tests indicate whether a microbial culture is susceptible or resistant to drug concentrations achievable in vivo with conventional dosage regimens. This can provide valuable guidance in selecting therapy. At times, however, there is a marked discrepancy between the results of the test and the clinical response of the patient treated with the chosen drug. Some possible explanations for such discrepancies are listed below.

(1) The organism isolated from the specimen may not be the one responsible for the infectious process. The usual cause is failure to culture tissue instead of pus.

(2) There may have been failure to drain a collection of pus, debride necrotic tissue, or remove a foreign body. Antimicrobials can never take the place of surgical drainage and removal.

(3) Superinfection occurs fairly often in the course of prolonged chemotherapy. New microorganisms may have replaced the original infectious agent. This is particularly common with open wounds or sinus tracts.

(4) The drug may not reach the site of active infection in adequate concentration. The pharmacologic properties of antimicrobials determine their absorption and distribution. Certain drugs penetrate phagocytic cells poorly and thus may not reach intracellular organisms. Some drugs may diffuse poorly into the eye, central nervous system, or pleural space unless injected directly into the area.

(5) At times, two or more microorganisms participate in an infectious process but only one may have been isolated from the specimen. The antimicrobial being used may be effective only against the less virulent organism.

Table 8–3. Drugs of choice for suspected or proved microbial pathogens, 1992.
(± = alone or combined with)

Suspected or Proved Etiologic Agent	Drug(s) of First Choice	Alternative Drug(s)
Gram-negative cocci		
Moraxella catarrhalis	Amoxicillin-clavulanic acid or TMP-SMZ[1]	Newer cephalosporins,[2] erythromycin,[3] tetracycline[4]
Gonococcus	Ceftriaxone	Cefixime, ciprofloxacin, spectinomycin
Meningococcus	Penicillin[5]	Newer cephalosporins,[2] ampicillin, chloramphenicol
Gram-positive cocci		
Pneumococcus *(Streptococcus pneumoniae)*	Penicillin[5]	Erythromycin,[3] cephalosporin,[6] vancomycin
Streptococcus, hemolytic, groups A, B, C, G	Penicillin[5]	Erythromycin,[3] cephalosporin,[6] vancomycin
Streptococcus viridans	Penicillin[5] + aminoglycosides[7]	Cephalosporin,[6] vancomycin
Staphylococcus, methicillin-resistant	Vancomycin + gentamicin or rifampin (or both)	TMP-SMZ, ciprofloxacin
Staphylococcus, non-penicillinase-producing	Penicillin	Cephalosporin, vancomycin
Staphylococcus, penicillinase-producing	Penicillinase-resistant penicillin[8]	Vancomycin, cephalosporin[6]
Streptococcus faecalis (enterococcus)	Ampicillin + gentamicin	Vancomycin + gentamicin
Gram-negative rods		
Acinetobacter	Aminoglycoside[7] + imipenem	Minocycline, TMP-SMZ[1]
Bacteroides, oropharyngeal strains	Penicillin,[5] clindamycin	Metronidazole, cephalosporin[2,6]
Bacteroides, gastrointestinal strains	Metronidazole	Cefoxitin, chloramphenicol, clindamycin
Brucella	Tetracycline[4] + streptomycin	TMP-SMZ[1]
Campylobacter	Erythromycin[3]	Tetracycline,[4] ciprofloxacin
Enterobacter	TMP-SMZ,[1] aminoglycoside[7]	Imipenem, newer cephalosporins[2]
Escherichia coli (sepsis)	Aminoglycoside,[7] newer cephalosporins[2]	Ampicillin, TMP-SMZ[1]
Escherichia coli (first urinary infection)	Sulfonamide,[9] TMP-SMZ[1]	Ampicillin, cephalosporin[6]
Haemophilus (meningitis, respiratory infections)	Newer cephalosporins[2]	Ampicillin and chloramphenicol[1]
Klebsiella	Newer cephalosporins[2]	TMP-SMZ, 1 aminoglycoside[7]
Legionella sp (pneumonia)	Erythromycin[3] + rifampin	TMP-SMZ[1]
Pasteurella (Yersinia) (plague, tularemia)	Streptomycin, tetracycline[4]	Chloramphenicol
Proteus mirabilis	Ampicillin	Newer cephalosporins,[2] aminoglycoside[7]
Proteus vulgaris and other species	Newer cephalosporins[2]	Aminoglycoside[7]
Pseudomonas aeruginosa	Aminoglycoside[7] + antipseudomonal penicillin[10]	Ceftazidime or cefoperazone + aminoglycoside; imipenem + aminoglycoside; aztreonam
Pseudomonas pseudomallei (melioidosis)	Ceftazidime	Chloramphenicol, tetraacycline,[4] TMP-SMZ[1]
Pseudomonas mallei (glanders)	Streptomycin + tetracycline[4]	Chloramphenicol + streptomycin
Salmonella	Ceftriaxone	TMP-SMZ,[1] ciprofloxacin, ampicillin, chlorampenicol
Serratia, Providencia	Newer cephalosporins,[2] aminoglycoside[7]	TMP-SMZ[1]
Shigella	TMP-SMZ[1]	Ampicillin, tetracycline,[4] ciprofloxacin, chloramphenicol
Vibrio (cholera, sepsis)	Tetracycline[4]	TMP-SMZ[1]
Gram-positive rods		
Actinomyces	Penicillin[5]	Tetracycline[4]
Bacillus (eg, anthrax)	Penicillin[5]	Erythromycin[3]
Clostridium (eg, gas gangrene, tetanus)	Penicillin[5]	Metronidazole, chloramphenicol, clindamycin
Corynebacterium diphtheriae	Erythromycin[3]	Penicillin[5]
Corynebacterium jeikeium	Vancomycin	Ciprofloxacin
Listeria	Ampicillin + aminoglycoside[7]	TMP-SMZ[1]
Acid-fast rods		
Mycobacterium tuberculosis	INH + rifampin + pyrazinamide	Other antituberculous drugs
Mycobacterium leprae	Dapsone + rifampin, clofazimine	Ethionamide
Mycobacterium kansasii	INH + rifampin + ethambutol	Other antituberculous drugs
Mycobacterium avium-intracellulare	Ethambutol + rifampin + clofazimine + ciprofloxacin + amikacin	Other antituberculous drugs
Mycobacterium fortuitum-chelonei	Amikacin + doxycycline	Cefoxitin, erythromycin, sulfonamide
Nocardia	Sulfonamide,[9] TMP-SMZ[1]	Minocycline

(continued)

Table 8–3. Drugs of choice for suspected or proved microbial pathogens, 1992.
(± = alone or combined with) (continued)

Suspected or Proved Etiologic Agent	Drug(s) of First Choice	Alternative Drug(s)
Spirochetes		
Borrelia (Lyme disease, relapsing fever)	Tetracycline,[4] ceftriaxone	Penicillin,[5] erythromycin[3]
Leptospira	Penicillin[5]	Tetracycline[4]
Treponema (syphilis, yaws, etc)	Penicillin[5]	Erythromycin,[3] tetracycline[4]
Mycoplasmas	Erythromycin[3] or tetracycline[4]	
Chlamydiae		
C psittaci	Tetracycline[4]	Chloramphenicol
C trachomatis (urethritis or pelvic inflammatory disease)	Doxycycline or erythromycin[3]	Ofloxacin or azithromycin
C pneumoniae	Tetracycline[4]	Erythromycin[3]
Rickettsiae	Tetracycline[4]	Chloramphenicol

[1]TMP-SMZ is a mixture of 1 part trimethoprim and 5 parts sulfamethoxazole.

[2]Newer cephalosporins (1992) include cefotaxime, cefuroxime, ceftriaxone, ceftazidime, ceftizoxime, and others.

[3]Erythromycin estolate is best absorbed orally but carries the highest risk of hepatitis; erythromycin stearate and erythromycin ethylsuccinate are also available.

[4]All tetracyclines have similar activity against microorganisms. Dosage is determined by rates of absorption and excretion of various preparations.

[5]Pencillin G is preferred for parenteral injection; penicillin V for oral administration—to be used only in treating infections due to highly sensitive organisms.

[6]Older cephalosporins are cephalothin, cefazolin, cephapirin, and cefoxitin for parenteral injection; cephalexin and cephradine can be given orally.

[7]Aminoglycosides—gentamicin, tobramycin, amikacin, netilmicin—should be chosen on the basis of local patterns of susceptibility.

[8]Parenteral nafcillin or oxacillin; oral dicloxacillin, cloxacillin, or oxacillin.

[9]Oral sulfisoxazole and trisulfapyrimidines are highly soluble in urine; parenteral sodium sulfadiazine can be injected intravenously in treating severely ill patients.

[10]Antipseudomonal penicillins: ticarcillin, carbenicillin, mezlocillin, azlocillin, pipericillin.

[11]First choice for previously untreated urinary tract infection is a highly soluble sulfonamide (see Note 9). TMP-SMZ (see Note 1) is acceptable.

(6) In the course of drug administration, resistant microorganisms may have been selected from a mixed population, and these drug-resistant organisms continue to grow in the presence of the drug.

Assessment of Drug & Dosage

An adequate therapeutic response is an important but not always sufficient indication that the right drug is being given in the right dosage. Proof of drug activity in serum or urine against the original infecting organisms may provide important support for a selected drug regimen even if fever or other signs of infection are continuing. If drug therapy is adequate, the patient's serum will be markedly bactericidal in vitro against the organism isolated from that patient prior to therapy. Such a serum assay must be performed with special diluents and using a defined inoculum; drug levels are adequate when a serum dilution of 1:10 or more is able to kill 99.9% of the inoculum. In infections limited to the urinary tract, the patient's urine must exhibit marked activity against the organism originally isolated from it.

Determining Duration of Therapy

The duration of drug therapy is determined in part by clinical response and past experience and in part by laboratory indications of suppression or elimina-

tion of infection. Ultimate recovery must be verified by careful follow-up. In evaluating the patient's clinical response, the possibility of adverse reactions to drugs must be kept in mind. Such reactions may mimic continuing activity of the infectious process by causing fever, skin rashes, central nervous system disturbances, and changes in blood and urine. In the case of many drugs, it is desirable to assess liver and kidney function at intervals. Abnormal findings may force the surgeon to reduce the dose or even discontinue a given drug.

Oliguria & Renal Failure

Oliguria and renal failure have an important influence on antimicrobial drug dosage, since most of these drugs are excreted—to a greater or lesser extent—by the kidneys. Only minor adjustments in dosage or frequency of administration is necessary with relatively nontoxic drugs (eg, penicillins) or with drugs that are detoxified or excreted mainly by the liver (eg, erythromycins or chloramphenicol). On the other hand, aminoglycosides (eg, tobramycin), tetracyclines, and vancomycin must be drastically reduced in dosage or frequency of administration if toxicity is to be avoided in the presence of nitrogen retention. Some general guidelines for the administration of such drugs to patients with renal failure are given in Tables 8–4 and 8–5. The administration of particularly nephrotoxic antimicrobials such as aminoglycosides to patients in renal failure may have to be guided by direct, frequent assay of drug concentrations in serum.

In the newborn or premature infant, excretory mechanisms for some antimicrobials are poorly developed, and for this reason, special dosage schedules must be used in order to avoid accumulation of drugs.

Intravenous Antibiotics

When an antibiotic must be administered intravenously (eg, for life-threatening infection or for maintenance of very high blood levels), the following cautions should be observed:

(1) Give in neutral solution (pH 7.0–7.2) of isotonic sodium chloride (0.9%) or dextrose (5%) in water.

(2) Give alone without admixture of any other drug in order to avoid chemical and physical incompatibilities (which can occur frequently).

(3) Administer by intermittent (every 2–6 hours) addition to the intravenous infusion to avoid inactivation (by temperature, changing pH, etc) and prolonged vein irritation from high drug concentration, which favors thrombophlebitis.

(4) Change the infusion site every 48–72 hours to reduce the chance of superinfection.

ANTIMICROBIAL DRUGS USED IN COMBINATION

Indications

Possible reasons for employing two or more antimicrobials simultaneously instead of a single drug are as follows:

(1) Prompt treatment in desperately ill patients suspected of having a serious microbial infection. A good guess about the most probable two or three pathogens is made, and drugs are aimed at those organisms. Before such treatment is started, it is essential that adequate specimens be obtained for identifying the etiologic agent in the laboratory. Gram-negative sepsis is the most important disease in this category at present.

(2) To delay the emergence of microbial mutants resistant to one drug in chronic infections by the use of a second or third non-cross-reacting drug. The most prominent example is active tuberculosis of any organ with large microbial populations.

(3) Mixed infections, particularly those following massive trauma. Each drug is aimed at an important pathogenic microorganism likely to cause bacteremia.

(4) To achieve bactericidal synergism (see below). In a few infections, eg, enterococcal sepsis, a combination of drugs is more likely to eradicate the infection than either drug used alone. Unfortunately,

such synergism is unpredictable, and a given drug pair may be synergistic for only a single microbial strain.

Disadvantages

The following disadvantages of using antimicrobial drugs in combinations must always be considered:

(1) The surgeon may feel that since several drugs are already being given, nothing more can be done for the patient. This attitude leads to relaxation of the effort to establish a specific diagnosis. It may also give the surgeon a false sense of security.

(2) The more drugs administered, the greater the chance for drug reactions to occur or for the patient to become sensitized to drugs.

(3) Combined drug regimens may be unnecessarily expensive.

(4) Antimicrobial combinations often accomplish no more than an effective single drug.

(5) On rare occasions, one drug may antagonize a second drug given simultaneously. Antagonism resulting in increased rates of illness and death has been observed mainly in bacterial meningitis when a bacteriostatic drug (eg, tetracycline or chloramphenicol) was given with (or prior to) a bactericidal drug (eg, penicillin or ampicillin). However, antagonism can usually be overcome by giving a larger dose of one of the drugs in the pair and is therefore an infrequent problem in clinical therapy.

Synergism

Antimicrobial synergism occurs in the situations listed below. Synergistic drug combinations must be selected by specialized laboratory procedures.

(1) One drug inhibits a microbial enzyme that might destroy a second drug. For example, clavulanic acid inhibits bacterial β-lactamase and protects simultaneously given amoxicillin from destruction.

(2) Sequential block of a metabolic pathway. Sulfonamides inhibit utilization of extracellular p-aminobenzoic acid by susceptible bacteria. Trimethoprim inhibits the reduction of folates, the next metabolic step. Simultaneous use of sulfamethoxazole and trimethoprim can be strikingly more effective in some bacterial infections than use of either drug alone. Similarly, sulfamethoxazole plus pyrimethamine has greatly enhanced activity in *Pneumocystis* and *Toxoplasma* parasitic infections.

(3) One drug enhances greatly the uptake of a second drug. Cell-wall inhibitor (β-lactam) drugs enhance the penetration of various bacteria by aminoglycosides and thus greatly increase the overall bactericidal effect. Eradication of infections by enterococci (*Streptococcus faecalis*) requires simultaneous use of penicillin and an aminoglycoside. Similarly, the control of sepsis by *Pseudomonas* and other gram-negative rods may be enhanced by using ticarcillin plus an aminoglycoside.

Table 8–4. Use of antibiotics in patients with renal failure[1] and hepatic failure.

	Principal Mode of Excretion of Detoxifi-cation	Approximate Half-Life in Serum		Proposed Dosage Regimen in Renal Failure		Removal of Drug by Hemodialysis	Dose After Hemodi-alysis	Dosage in Hepatic Failure
		Normal	Renal Failure[2]	Initial Dose[3]	Maintenance Dose			
Acyclovir	Renal	2.5–3.5 hours	20 hours	2.5 mg/kg	2.5 mg/kg q24h	Yes	2.5 mg/kg	No change
Ampicillin	Tubular se-cretion	0.5–1 hour	8–12 hours	1 g	1 g q8–12h	Yes	1 g	No change
Azlo-, mezlo-, piperacillin	Renal 50–70%; biliary 20–30%	1 hour	3–6 hours	3 g	2 g q6–8h	Yes	1 g	1–2 g q8h
Aztreonam	Renal	1.7 hours	6 hours	1–2 g	0.5–1 g q6–8h	Yes	0.5–1 g	No change
Carbenicillin	Tubular se-cretion	1 hour	16 hours	4 g	2 g q12h	Yes	2 g	No change
Chloramphenicol	Mainly liver	3 hours	4 hours	0.5 g	0.5 g q6h	Yes	0.5 g	0.25–0.5 g q12h
Ciprofloxacin	Renal and liver	4 hours	8.5 hours	0.5 g	0.25–0.75 g q24h	No	None	No change
Clindamycin	Liver	2–4 hours	2–4 hours	0.6 g IV	0.6 g q8h	No	None	0.3–0.6 g q8h
Erythromycin	Mainly liver	1.5 hours	1.5 hours	0.5–1 g	0.5–1 g q6h	No	None	0.25–0.5 g q6h
Fluconazole	Renal	30 hours	98 hours	0.2 g	0.1 g q24h	Yes	Give q24h dose	No change
Ganciclovir	Renal	3 hours	11–28 hours	1.25 mg/kg	1.25 mg/kg q24h	Yes	Give q24h dose	No change
Imipenem	Glomerular filtration	1 hour	3 hours	0.5 g	0.25–0.5 g q12h	Yes	0.25–0.5 g	No change
Metronidazole	Liver	6–10 hours	6–10 hours	0.5 g IV	0.5 g q8h	Yes	0.25 g	0.25 g q12h
Nafcillin	Liver 80%; kidney 20%	0.75 hours	1.5 hours	1.5 g	1.5 g q5h	No	None	2–3 g q12h
Penicillin G	Tubular se-cretion	0.5 hours	7–10 hours	1–2 mil-lion units	1 million units q8h	Yes	500,000 units	No change
Ticarcillin	Tubular se-cretion	1.1 hour	15–20 hours	3 g	2 g q6–8h	Yes	1 g	No change
Trimethoprim-sulfamethoxa-zole	Some liver	TMP 10–12 hours; SMZ 8–10 hours	TMP 24–48 hours; SMZ 18–24 hours	320 mg TMP + 1600 mg SMZ	80 mg TMP + 400 mg SMZ every 12 hours	Yes	80 mg TMP + 400 mg SMZ	No change
Vancomycin	Glomerular filtration	6 hours	6–10 days	1 g	1 g q6–10d based on serum levels[4]	None	None	No change

[1]For cephalosporins, see text and Table 34–7; for aminoglycosides, see Table 34–8.
[2]Considered here to be marked by creatinine clearance of 10 mL/min or less.
[3]For a 70-kg adult with a serious systemic infection.
[4]When serum levels reach 5–10 μg/mL, another dose should be given.

Table 8–5. Pharmacology of the cephalosporins.

Drug	Peak Serum Level (μg/mL) After 1 g IV	Serum Half-Life (min)	Total Daily Dose (hours)	Dosage Interval (hours)	Moderate (Cl$_{cr}$ 10–50 mL/min)	Severe (Cl$_{cr}$ <10 mL/min)	Post-hemodialysis Dose
Cephalothin, cephapirin	40–60	40	50–200	4–6	1–2 g every 6–12 hours	1 g every 12 hours	1 g
Cefazolin	90–120	90	25–100	8	0.5–1 g every 12 hours	0.5 g daily	0.5 g
Cephalexin cephradine[1]	15–20	50–60	15–30	6	0.25–0.5 g every 8–12 hours	0.25–0.5 g daily	0.5 g
Cefadroxil[1]	15	75	15–30	12–24	1 g daily	0.5 g daily	0.5 g
Cefamandole	60–80	45	75–200	6–8	1 g every 12 hours	1–2 g daily	0.5 g
Cefuroxime	80–100	80	50	6–12	1 g every 12 hours	1–2 g daily	0.5 g
Cefuroxime axetil[1]	6–8	75	5–15	12	0.5 g every 24 hours	0.25 g daily	0.25 g
Cefonicid	200–250	240	15–30	24	0.5 g daily	1 g every 72 hours	0.25 g
Ceforanide	125	180	15–30	12	1 g daily	1 g every 48 hours	0.25 g
Cefaclor[1]	15–20	50	20–40 children, 10–15 adults	6–8	0.5 g every 8–12 hours	0.25–0.5 g every 12–24 hours	0.25–0.5 g
Cefixime[1]	3–5	180–240	8 (with maximum of 0.4 g/d total)	12–24	0.4 g daily	0.1 g daily	None
Cefotetan	60–80	150	50–100	8–12	1 g every 8–12 hours	0.5–1 g daily	0.5 g
Cefotaxime	40–60	60	50–75	6–8	1–2 g every 6–8 hours	1–2 g every 12 hours	1–2 g
Cefoxitin	60–80	60	50–100	6–8	1 g every 12 hours	1–2 g daily	0.5 g
Cefmetazole	70–100	60–80	50–100	6–8	1 g every 12–24 hours	1–2 g every 24–48 hours	1 g
Ceftizoxime	80–100	100	5–75	8–12	0.5–1 g every 8–12 hours	0.25–0.5 g every 12–24 hours	0.5 g
Ceftriaxone	150	480	30–50	12–24	1–2 g daily	1–2 g daily	None
Ceftazidime	100–120	120	50–75	8–12	1 g every 12 hours	0.5–1 g daily	0.5 g
Cefoperazone	150	120	30–200	8–12	1–2 g every 12 hours	1–2 g every 12 hours	None
Moxalactam	60–100	120	50–200	6–12	0.5–1 g every 12 hours	0.25–0.5 g every 12 hours	0.5 g

[1]Oral agents. Serum levels based on 0.5 g oral dose.

REFERENCES

Bergamini TM, Polk HC Jr: Pharmacodynamics of antibiotic penetration of tissue and surgical prophylaxis. Surg Gynecol Obstet 1989;168:283.

Donowitz GR, Mandell GL: Beta-lactam antibiotics. (Two parts.) N Engl J Med 1988;318:419, 490.

Drugs for parasitic infections. Med Lett Drugs Ther 1990;32:23.

Terrell CL, Hermans PE: Antifungal agents used for deep-seated mycotic infections. Mayo Clin Proc 1987;62:1116.

The choice of antimicrobial drugs. Med Lett Drugs Ther 1990;32:41.

Treatment of sexually transmitted diseases. Med Lett Drugs Ther 1990;32:5.

Van Scoy RE, Wilson WR: Antimicrobial agents in adult patients with renal insufficiency: Initial dosage and general recommendations. Mayo Clin Proc 1987;62:1142.

Wise R: Antimicrobial agents: A widening choice. Lancet 1987;2:1251.

Fluid & Electrolyte Management

Michael H. Humphreys, MD

The surgical patient is liable to develop numerous disorders of body fluid volume and composition, some of which may be iatrogenic. Understanding the physiologic mechanisms that regulate the composition and volume of the body fluids and the principles of fluid and electrolyte therapy is therefore essential for patient management.

BODY WATER & ITS DISTRIBUTION

Total body water comprises 45–60% of body weight; the percentage in any individual is influenced by age and the lean body mass, but in health it remains remarkably constant from day to day. Table 9–1 lists the average values of total body water as a percentage of body weight for men and women of different ages. Total body water is divided into intracellular (ICF) and extracellular (ECF) compartments. Intracellular water represents about two-thirds of total body water, or 40% of body weight. The remaining one-third of body water is extracellular. ECF is divided into two compartments: (1) plasma water, comprising approximately 25% of ECF, or 5% of body weight; and (2) interstitial fluid, comprising 75% of ECF, or 15% of body weight.

The solute composition of the intracellular and extracellular fluid compartments differs markedly (Figure 9–1). ECF contains principally sodium, chloride, and bicarbonate, with other ions in much lower concentrations. ICF contains mainly potassium, organic phosphate, sulfate, and various other ions in lower concentrations.

Even though plasma water and interstitial fluid have similar electrolyte compositions, plasma water contains more protein than interstitial fluid. This results in slight differences in electrolyte concentrations, as governed by the Gibbs-Donnan equilibrium. The plasma proteins, chiefly albumin, account for the high colloid osmotic pressure of plasma, which is an important determinant of the distribution of fluid between vascular and interstitial compartments, as defined by the Starling relationships.

The kidneys maintain constant volume and composition of body fluids by two distinct but related mechanisms: (1) filtration and reabsorption of sodium, which adjusts urinary sodium excretion to match changes in dietary intake; and (2) regulation of water excretion in response to changes in secretion of antidiuretic hormone. These two mechanisms allow the kidneys to keep the volume and osmolality of body fluid constant within a few percentage points despite wide variations in intake of salt and water. A corollary is that analysis of the composition and volume of the urine usually provides valuable clues in the diagnosis of disorders of body fluid volume and composition.

Although the movement of certain ions and proteins between the various body fluid compartments is restricted, water is freely diffusible. Consequently, the osmolality (total solute concentration) of all the body compartments is identical—normally, about 290 mosm/kg H_2O. The solutes dissolved in body fluids contribute to total osmolality in proportion to their molar concentration: In ECF, sodium and its salts account for most of the osmolality, whereas in ICF salts of potassium are chiefly responsible. Control of osmolality occurs through regulation of water intake (thirst) and water excretion (urine volume, insensible loss, and stool water), with the kidneys being the chief regulator. If water intake is low, the kidneys can reduce urine volume and raise urine solute concentration fourfold above plasma (ie, to 1200–1400 mosm/kg H_2O). If water intake is high, the kidneys can excrete a large volume of dilute (50 mosm/kg H_2O) urine.

Concentrations of electrolytes are usually expressed as equivalent weights: A 1-molar (M) solution contains 1 gram molecular weight of a compound dissolved in 1 liter (L) of fluid; 1 equivalent (eq) of an ion is equal to 1 mole (mol) multiplied by the valence of the ion. For example, in the case of the monovalent sodium ion, 1 eq is equal to 1 mol. In the case of calcium, which is divalent, 1 eq is equal to 0.5 mol. In the relatively dilute conditions of body fluids, the sum of the molar concentrations of ions is approximately equal to total fluid osmolality. However, because the chemical activities of these solutes differ, it is usually more accurate to estimate osmolality by multiplying the serum sodium concentration by 2.

The sensitive regulation of salt and water excretion by the kidney produces an intimate relationship between body fluid osmolality and volume. Edelman and his coworkers showed that the osmolality of

Table 9–1. Total body water (as percentage of body weight) in relation to age and sex.

Age	Male	Female
10–18	59	57
18–40	61	51
40–60	55	47
Over 60	52	46

plasma or any other body fluid can be closely approximated by the sum of exchangeable sodium (Na_e^+) and its anions (A^-) plus exchangeable potassium (K_e^+) and its anions divided by total body water (TBW):

$$\text{Osmolality} = \frac{(Na_e^+ + A^-) + (K_e^+ + A^-)}{\text{TBW}} \quad \ldots (1)$$

The plasma sodium concentration (P_{Na}) can be determined by the expression shown in equation 2:

$$P_{Na} = \frac{(Na_e^+) + (K_e^+)}{\text{TBW}} \quad \ldots (2)$$

Although it is neither practical nor necessary to measure exchangeable sodium, exchangeable potassium, or total body water routinely, equation 2 illustrates the major factors that affect the serum sodium concentration and helps one to understand the cause and therapy of many fluid and electrolyte disturbances.

In a steady state, the volume and composition of the urine depend upon the intake of water and dietary solutes. An average North American diet generates about 600 mosm of solute daily that must be excreted by the kidneys. Most people ingest more than 5 g of sodium chloride per day, equivalent to about 85 meq of Na^+ (1 g NaCl = 17 meq Na^+). Potassium excretion averages 40–60 meq/d. Water intake is more variable but usually amounts to about 2 L/d; an additional 400 mL of water per day is generated from cellular metabolism. Extrarenal (insensible) water loss amounts to 10 mL/kg body weight/24 h equally divided among losses from the lungs, from the skin, and in the stool. Losses from the lungs and skin may vary under physiologic conditions, but stool water rarely exceeds 200 mL/d in health. Thus, a typical 24-hour urine volume is 1500 mL and has the approximate solute concentrations shown in Table 9–2.

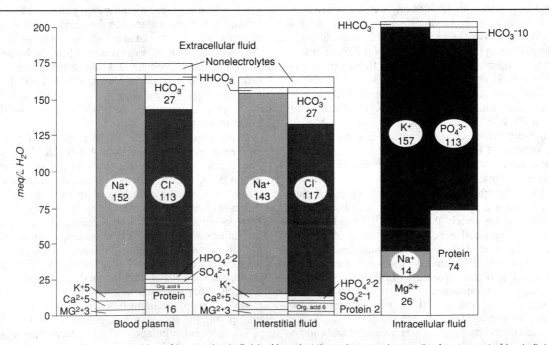

Figure 9–1. Electrolyte composition of human body fluids. Note that the values are in meq/L of water, not of body fluid. (Reproduced, with permission, from Leaf A, Newburgh LH: *Significance of the Body Fluids in Clinical Medicine,* 2nd ed. Thomas, 1955.)

Table 9–2. Typical daily solute balances in normal subjects.

	Concentration	Total Amount
Intake		
Water		
Ingested	...	2 L
Cell metabolism	...	0.4 L
Total solute	...	600 mosm
Sodium	...	100 meq
Potassium	...	60 meq
Urinary excretion		
Water		1.5 L
Total solute	400 mosm/kg H$_2$O	600 mosm
Sodium	60 meq/L	90 meq[1]
Potassium	36 meq/L	54 meq[1]

[1]Small amounts of sodium and potassium are lost extrarenally (stool, sweat).

VOLUME DISORDERS

RECOGNITION & TREATMENT OF VOLUME DEPLETION

Since volume depletion is common in surgical patients, a general approach to the diagnosis and treatment of volume depletion should be developed and applied to each patient systematically. The clinical manifestations of volume depletion are low blood pressure, narrow pulse pressure, tachycardia, poor skin turgor, and dry mucous membranes. The history may suggest the reason for volume depletion. Records of intake and output, changes in body weight, urine specific gravity, and analysis of the chemical composition of the urine should confirm the clinical impression and be useful when a treatment plan is being devised. Therapy must aim to correct the volume deficit and associated aberrations in electrolyte concentrations.

VOLUME DEPLETION

The simplest form of volume depletion is water deficit without accompanying solute deficit. However, in surgical patients, water and solute deficits more often occur together. Pure water deficits occur in patients who are unable to regulate intake. They may be debilitated or comatose or may have increased insensible water loss from fever. Patients given tube feedings without adequate water supplementation and those with diabetes insipidus may also develop this syndrome. Pure water deficit is reflected biochemically by hypernatremia; the magnitude of the deficit can be estimated from the P$_{Na}$ (equations 2, 3).

Associated findings are an increase in the plasma osmolality, concentrated urine, and a low urine sodium concentration (< 15 meq/L) despite hypernatremia. The clinical manifestations are chiefly caused by hypernatremia, which can depress the central nervous system, resulting in lethargy or coma. Muscle rigidity, tremors, spasticity, and seizures may occur. Since many patients suffering from water deficit have primary neurologic disease, it is often difficult to tell if the symptoms were caused by hypernatremia or by the underlying disease.

Treatment involves replacement of enough water to restore the plasma sodium (P$_{Na}$) concentration to normal. The excess sodium for which water must be provided can be estimated from the following expression:

$$\Delta Na = (140 - P_{Na}) \times TBW \qquad ...(3)$$

The Δ Na represents the total milliequivalents of sodium in excess of water. Divide Δ Na by 140 to obtain the amount of water required to return the serum sodium concentration to 140 meq/L. Because of the dehydration, an estimate of total body water (TBW) should be used that is somewhat lower than the normal values listed in Table 9–1. In addition to correction of the existing water deficit, ongoing obligatory water losses (due to diabetes insipidus, fever, etc) must be satisfied. Treat the patient with 5% dextrose in water unless hypotension has developed, in which case hypotonic saline should be used. Rarely, isotonic saline may be indicated to treat shock due to dehydration even though the patient is hypernatremic.

VOLUME & ELECTROLYTE DEPLETION

Combined water and electrolyte depletion may occur from gastrointestinal losses due to nasogastric suction, enteric fistulas, enterostomies, or diarrhea. Other causes are excessive diuretic therapy, adrenal insufficiency, profuse sweating, burns, and body fluid sequestration following trauma or surgery. Diagnosis of combined volume and electrolyte deficiency can be made from the history, physical signs, and records of intake and output. The clinical findings are similar to those of pure volume depletion. However, the urine Na$^+$ concentration is often less than 10 meq/L, a manifestation of renal sodium conservation resulting from the action of aldosterone on the renal tubule. The urine is usually hypertonic (sp gr > 1.020), with an osmolality greater than 450–500 mosm/kg. The decreased blood volume diminishes renal perfusion and often produces prerenal azotemia, reflected by elevated blood urea nitrogen (BUN) and serum creatinine. Prerenal azotemia is characterized by a disproportionate rise of BUN compared to creatinine; the normal BUN/creatinine ratio of 10:1 is exceeded and may go as high as 20–25:1. This relationship helps differentiate prerenal azotemia from acute tubular necrosis, in which the BUN/creatinine ratio remains close to normal as the serum levels of both substances rise.

Combined water-electrolyte deficits are corrected by restoring volume and the deficient electrolytes. The magnitude of the volume deficit can be estimated by serial measurements of body weight, since acute changes in body weight primarily reflect changes in body fluid. Central venous or pulmonary artery pressure may be low in blood volume deficits and may be useful for monitoring replacement therapy.

The composition of the replacement fluid should take into account the plasma sodium concentration: If the P_{Na} is normal, fluid and electrolyte losses are probably isotonic, and the replacement fluid should be isotonic saline or its equivalent. Hyponatremia may result from salt loss exceeding water loss (ie, the decrease in Na^+ will be greater than the decrease in TBW; equation 2) or from previous administration of hypotonic solutions. In this situation, the magnitude of the salt deficit can be calculated from equation 3.

Replacement therapy should be planned in two steps: (1) the sodium deficit should be calculated, and (2) the volume deficit should be estimated from clinical signs and changes in body weight. From these calculations, a hypothetical replacement solution can be devised in which the sodium deficit is administered as NaCl and the volume deficit as isotonic NaCl solution. Then administer isotonic NaCl solutions containing appropriate amounts of additional NaCl and monitor the patient's response (ie, urine volume and composition, serum electrolytes, and clinical signs). When replacement is adequate, renal function and serum Na^+ and Cl^- concentrations will return to normal.

VOLUME OVERLOAD

Hormonal and circulatory responses to surgery result in postoperative conservation of sodium and water by the kidneys that is independent of the status of the ECF volume. Antidiuretic hormone, released during anesthesia and surgical stress, promotes water conservation by the kidneys. Renal vasoconstriction and increased aldosterone activity reduce sodium excretion. Consequently, if fluid intake is excessive in the immediate postoperative period, circulatory overload may occur. The tendency for water retention may be exaggerated if heart failure, liver disease, renal disease, or hypoalbuminemia is present. Clinical manifestations of volume overload include edema of the sacrum and extremities, jugular venous distention, tachypnea (if pulmonary edema develops), increased body weight, and elevated pulmonary artery and central venous pressure. A gallop rhythm would indicate cardiac failure.

Volume overload may precipitate prerenal azotemia and oliguria. Examination of the urine usually shows low sodium and high potassium concentrations consistent with enhanced tubular reabsorption of Na^+ and water.

Management of volume overload depends upon its severity. For mild overload, sodium restriction will usually be adequate. If hyponatremia is present, water restriction will also be necessary. Diuretics must be used for severe volume overload. If cardiac failure is present, digitalis must be given.

Inappropriate secretion of antidiuretic hormone (which may occur with head injury, some cancers, and burns) will produce a syndrome characterized by hyponatremia, concentrated urine, elevated urine sodium concentration, and a normal or mildly expanded ECF volume. The serum Na^+ values may drop below 110 meq/L and produce confusion and lethargy. In most cases, restriction of water intake alone will be sufficient to correct the abnormality. Occasionally, a potent diuretic (eg, furosemide) should be given and intravenous isotonic saline infused at a rate equal to the urine output; this will rapidly correct the hyponatremia.

SPECIFIC ELECTROLYTE DISORDERS

SODIUM

Regulation of the sodium concentration in plasma or urine is intimately associated with regulation of total body water (equation 2) and clinically reflects the balance between total body solute and TBW.

Hypernatremia represents chiefly loss of water; this condition has been discussed above.

In addition to dilutional hyponatremia and isotonic dehydration, apparent hyponatremia may develop in patients with marked hyperlipidemia or hyperproteinemia, because fat and protein contribute to plasma bulk even though they are not dissolved in plasma water. The sodium concentration of plasma water in this situation is usually normal.

Hyponatremia in severe hyperglycemia results from the osmotic effects of the elevated glucose concentration, which draws water from the intracellular space to dilute ECF sodium. In hyperglycemia, the magnitude of this effect can be estimated by multiplying the blood glucose concentration in mg/dL by 0.016 and adding the result to the existing serum sodium concentration. The sum represents the predicted serum sodium concentration if the hyperglycemia were corrected.

Acute, severe hyponatremia occasionally develops

in patients undergoing elective surgery. In these patients, the hyponatremia results from excessive intravenous sodium-free fluid administration coupled with the postsurgical stimulation of antidiuretic hormone release and causes severe permanent brain damage. This outcome underscores the need to limit postoperative free water administration and monitor serum electrolytes.

In most cases, hyponatremia can be successfully treated by administering the calculated sodium needs in isotonic solutions. Infusion of hypertonic saline solutions is rarely indicated and could precipitate circulatory overload. Only when severe hyponatremia (usually with $P_{Na} < 110$ meq/L) produces mental obtundation and seizures should the patient be treated with hypertonic sodium solutions. Hyponatremia with volume overload usually indicates impaired renal ability to excrete sodium.

POTASSIUM

The potassium in extracellular fluids constitutes only 2% of total body potassium (Figure 9–1); the remaining 98% is within body cells.

The serum potassium concentration ($[K^+]$) is determined primarily by the pH of ECF and the size of the intracellular K^+ pool (Figure 9–2). With extracellular acidosis, a large proportion of the excess hydrogen is buffered intracellularly by an exchange of intracellular K^+ for extracellular H^+; this movement of K^+ may

produce dangerous hyperkalemia. Alkalosis has an opposite effect: as the pH rises, K^+ moves into cells.

In the absence of an acid-base disturbance, serum K^+ reflects the total body pool of potassium (Figure 9–2). With excessive external losses of potassium (eg, from the gastrointestinal tract) (Table 9–3), the serum $[K^+]$ falls: A loss of 10% of total body K^+ drops the serum $[K^+]$ from 4 to 3 meq/L at a normal pH.

Although pH and body composition influence potassium metabolism, measurement of potassium intake and urinary potassium excretion allows the clinician to control potassium balance. Renal excretion of potassium is regulated by mineralocorticoid (aldosterone) levels. Renal failure—particularly acute oliguric renal failure—results in potassium retention and hyperkalemia. Adrenal insufficiency may produce hyperkalemia through impaired renal excretion. Hypokalemia from excessive renal excretion may follow administration of diuretics, adrenal steroid excess, and certain renal tubular disorders associated with potassium wasting. Rarely, potassium deficiency can arise from deficient dietary potassium intake, as in alcoholic patients or in those receiving total parenteral nutrition with inadequate potassium replacement.

1. HYPERKALEMIA

Hyperkalemia is a treatable problem that may prove fatal if undiagnosed. Blood potassium levels must be closely monitored in susceptible patients such as those with severe trauma, burns, crush injuries, renal insufficiency, or marked catabolism from other causes. Hyperkalemia may also be due to Addison's disease. Clinical evidence of significant hyperkalemia is usually not present. Nausea and vomiting, colicky abdominal pain, and diarrhea may occur. The electrocardiographic changes are the most helpful indicators of the severity of the disorder: Early changes include peaking of the T waves, widening of the QRS complex, and depression of the ST segment. With further elevation of the blood potassium level, the QRS widens to such a degree that the tracing resembles a sine wave, a finding that portends imminent cardiac standstill.

A number of factors must be rapidly considered in assessing the hyperkalemic patient. First, one should determine whether the serum potassium level is a true metabolic abnormality or has been elevated by hemolysis, marked leukocytosis, or thrombocytosis. Platelet counts greater than 1 million/µL may elevate the serum potassium, since the ion is liberated from platelets as they are consumed during clotting. Second, the acid-base status should be assessed to ascertain its influence (Figure 9–2). Finally, the rapidity with which the elevated serum potassium should be corrected must be determined.

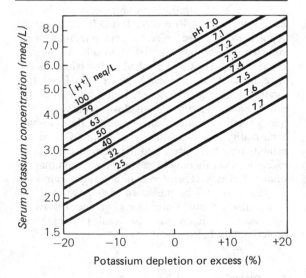

Figure 9–2. Relationship of serum potassium to total body potassium stores at different blood pH levels. (Reprinted, with permission, from: *University of Washington Teaching Syllabus for the Course on Fluid and Electrolyte Balance.* Edited by Belding Scribner, MD.)

Table 9–3. Volume and electrolyte content of gastrointestinal fluid losses.[1]

	Na+ (meq/L)	K+ (meq/L)	Cl- (meq/L)	HCO3- (meq/L)	Volume (mL)
Gastric juice, high in acid	20 (20–30)	10 (5–40)	120 (80–150)	0	1000–9000
Gastric juice, low in acid	80 (70–140)	15 (5–40)	90 (40–120)	5–25	1000–2500
Pancreatic juice	140 (115–180)	5 (3–8)	75 (55–95)	80 (60–110)	500–1000
Bile	148 (130–160)	5 (3–12)	100 (90–120)	35 (30–40)	300–1000
Small bowel drainage	110 (80–150)	5 (2–8)	105 (60–125)	30 (20–40)	1000–3000
Distal ileum and cecum drainage	80 (40–135)	8 (5–30)	45 (20–90)	30 (20–40)	1000–3000
Diarrheal stools	120 (20–160)	25 (10–40)	90 (30–120)	45 (30–50)	500–17,000

[1]Average values/24 h with range in parentheses.

There are three general approaches to the treatment of hyperkalemia. Initially, an intravenous infusion of 100 mL of 50% dextrose solution containing 20 units of regular insulin will lower extracellular K^+ by promoting its intracellular transport in association with glucose. Intravenous $NaHCO_3$ solutions will lower serum Na^+ as acidosis is corrected. Calcium antagonizes the tissue effects of potassium; an infusion of calcium gluconate will transiently reverse cardiac depression from hyperkalemia without changing the serum potassium concentration. A slower method of controlling hyperkalemia is to administer the cation exchange resin sodium polystyrene sulfonate (Kayexalate) orally or by enema at a rate of 40–80 g/d. This drug binds potassium in the intestine, in exchange for sodium. It is often given with sorbitol to induce osmotic diarrhea and enhance the rate of potassium removal. Finally, when hyperkalemia is a manifestation of renal failure, peritoneal dialysis or hemodialysis is often necessary.

2. HYPOKALEMIA

Hypokalemia may be associated with alkalosis through either of two mechanisms: (1) intracellular shift of potassium in exchange for hydrogen or (2) renal wasting of potassium. The clinical manifestations of hypokalemia relate to neuromuscular function: Decreased muscle contractility and muscle cell potential develop, and in extreme cases death may result from paralysis of the muscles of respiration.

When the clinician assesses hypokalemia, the initial goal is to identify the cause. If alkalosis is the cause of hypokalemia, the K^+ needs can be determined from the nomogram in Figure 9–2. If there is no acid-base imbalance, or if hypokalemia persists after alkalosis is corrected, renal losses are probably excessive. Urine potassium excretion of more than 30 meq/24 h associated with a serum $[K^+]$ under 3.5 meq/L indicates renal potassium wasting. The primary problem in this situation is usually diuretic therapy, alkalosis, or increased aldosterone activity. If renal potassium excretion is less than 30 meq/24 h, the kidneys are conserving potassium appropriately, and hypokalemia reflects a total body deficit.

Treatment consists of correcting the cause of hypokalemia and administering potassium. If the patient is able to eat, potassium should be given orally; otherwise, it should be given intravenously. Usually, potassium concentrations in intravenous solutions should not exceed 40 meq/L. In moderate to severe hypokalemia ($[K^+] < 3$ meq/L), potassium may be administered at a rate of 20–30 meq/h. With mild hypokalemia ($[K^+]$ 3–3.5 meq/L), potassium should be replaced slowly to avoid hyperkalemia. Potassium should usually be administered intravenously as the chloride salt; in metabolic alkalosis, potassium chloride is specific, since it helps to correct the acid-base abnormality as well as the hypokalemia. Occasional patients may have persistent hypokalemia refractory to replacement therapy because of coexistent magnesium deficiency. Therefore, serum magnesium concentration should be measured in hypokalemic patients, particularly since many of the causes of potassium deficiency will also result in magnesium depletion (see below).

CALCIUM

Calcium is an important mediator of neuromuscular function and cellular enzyme processes even though most of the body calcium is contained in the skeleton. The usual dietary intake of calcium is 1–3 g/d, most of which is excreted unabsorbed in the feces.

The normal serum calcium concentration (8.5–10.3 mg/dL, 4.2–5.2 meq/L) is maintained by humoral factors, mainly vitamin D, parathyroid hormone, and calcitonin. Acidemia increases and alkalemia decreases the serum ionized calcium concentration. Approximately half of the total serum calcium is bound to plasma proteins, chiefly albumin; a small amount is complexed to plasma anions, such as citrate; and the remainder (approximately 40%) of the total serum calcium is free, or ionized, calcium, which is the fraction responsible for the biologic effects. The ionized calcium usually remains constant when the total serum calcium concentration changes with different serum albumin concentrations. Unless the ionized calcium is measured, the serum calcium can only be reliably assessed if accompanied by measurement of the serum albumin concentration.

Severe disturbances of calcium concentration are uncommon in surgical patients, although transient asymptomatic hypocalcemia is common. After operations on the thyroid or parathyroids, the serum calcium concentration should be measured at regular intervals to detect hypocalcemia early if it appears.

1. HYPOCALCEMIA

Hypocalcemia occurs in hypoparathyroidism, hypomagnesemia, severe pancreatitis, chronic or acute renal failure, severe trauma, crush injuries, and necrotizing fasciitis. The clinical manifestations are neuromuscular: hyperactive deep tendon reflexes, a positive Chvostek sign, muscle and abdominal cramps, carpopedal spasm, and, rarely, convulsions. Hypocalcemia is reflected in the ECG by a prolonged QT interval.

The initial step is to check the whole blood pH; if alkalosis is present, it should be treated. Intravenous calcium, as calcium gluconate or calcium chloride, may be needed for the acute problem (eg, after parathyroidectomy). Chronic hypoparathyroidism requires vitamin D, oral calcium supplements, and often aluminum hydroxide gels to bind phosphate in the intestine.

2. HYPERCALCEMIA

Hypercalcemia most frequently is caused by hyperparathyroidism, cancer with bony metastases, ectopic production of parathyroid hormone, vitamin D intoxication, hyperthyroidism, sarcoidosis, milk-alkali syndrome, or prolonged immobilization (especially in young patients or those with Paget's disease). It is also a rare complication of thiazide diuretics.

The symptoms of hypercalcemia are fatigability, muscle weakness, depression, anorexia, nausea, and constipation. Long-standing hypercalcemia may impair renal concentrating mechanisms, resulting in polyuria and polydipsia and in metastatic deposition of calcium. Severe hypercalcemia can cause coma and death. *A serum concentration above 12 mg/dL should be regarded as a medical emergency!*

With severe hypercalcemia ($Ca^{2+} > 14.5$ mg/dL), intravenous isotonic saline should be given to expand ECF, increase urine flow, enhance calcium excretion, and reduce the serum level.

Furosemide and intravenous sodium sulfate are other methods of increasing renal calcium excretion. Mithramycin is particularly useful for hypercalcemia associated with metastatic cancer. Adrenal corticosteroids are useful for hypercalcemia associated with sarcoidosis, vitamin D intoxication, and Addison's disease. Calcitonin is indicated in patients with impaired renal and cardiovascular function. When renal failure is present, hemodialysis may be required.

MAGNESIUM

Magnesium is largely present in bone and cells, where it serves an important role in cellular energy metabolism. The normal plasma magnesium concentration is 1.5–2.5 meq/L. Magnesium is excreted primarily by the kidneys. The serum magnesium concentration reflects total body magnesium. Serum magnesium levels may be elevated in hypovolemic shock as magnesium is liberated from cells.

1. HYPOMAGNESEMIA

Hypomagnesemia occurs with poor dietary intake, intestinal malabsorption of ingested magnesium, or excessive losses from the gut (eg, severe diarrhea, enteric fistulas, use of purgatives, or nasogastric suction). It may also be caused by excessive urinary losses (eg, from diuretics), chronic alcohol abuse, hyperaldosteronism, and hypercalcemia. Hypomagnesemia occasionally develops in acute pancreatitis, in diabetic acidosis, in burned patients, or after prolonged total parenteral nutrition with insufficient magnesium supplementation. The clinical manifestations resemble those of hypocalcemia: hyperactive tendon reflexes, a positive Chvostek sign, and tremors that may progress to delirium and convulsions.

The diagnosis of hypomagnesemia depends on clinical suspicion with confirmation by measurement of the serum magnesium. Treatment consists of administering magnesium, usually as the sulfate or chloride. In moderate magnesium deficiency, oral replacement is adequate. In more severe deficits, parenteral magnesium must be administered intravenously (40–80 meq of $MgSO_4$ per liter of intravenous fluid).

When large doses are infused intravenously, there is a risk of producing hypermagnesemia, with tachycardia and hypotension. The ECG should be inspected for prolongation of the QT interval. Magnesium should be administered cautiously to oliguric patients or those with renal failure and only after magnesium deficiency has been unequivocally documented. Magnesium deficiency may also be accompanied by refractory hypokalemia.

2. HYPERMAGNESEMIA

Hypermagnesemia usually occurs in patients with renal disease; it is rare in surgical patients. In patients with renal insufficiency, serum magnesium levels should be monitored closely. Strict attention must be paid to excess magnesium intake, which can occur from a variety of commonly administered antacids and laxatives and which may produce severe and even fatal hypermagnesemia in renal insufficiency.

The initial signs and symptoms of hypermagnesemia are lethargy and weakness. Electrocardiographic changes resemble those in hyperkalemia (widened QRS complex, ST segment depression, and peaked T waves). When the serum level reaches 6 meq/L, deep tendon reflexes are lost; with levels above 10 meq/L, somnolence, coma, and death may ensue.

Treatment of hypermagnesemia consists of giving intravenous isotonic saline to increase the rate of renal magnesium excretion. This may be accompanied by slow intravenous infusion of calcium, since calcium antagonizes some of the neuromuscular actions of magnesium. Patients with hypermagnesemia and severe renal failure may need dialysis.

PHOSPHORUS

Phosphorus is primarily a constituent of bone, but it is also an important intracellular ion with a role in energy metabolism. The serum phosphorus level is only an approximate indicator of total body phosphorus and can be influenced by a number of factors, including the serum calcium concentration and the pH of blood. In urine, phosphorus is an important buffer that facilitates the excretion of acids formed by intermediary metabolism. Urine phosphate buffer is reflected by the excretion of titratable acid.

1. HYPOPHOSPHATEMIA

Clinically important hypophosphatemia may follow poor dietary intake (especially in alcoholics), hyperparathyroidism, and antacid administration (antacids bind phosphate in the intestine). Hypophosphatemia was at one time a frequent complication of total parenteral nutrition until phosphate sup-plementation became routine. Clinical manifestations appear when the serum phosphorus level falls to 1 mg/dL or less. Neuromuscular manifestations include lassitude, fatigue, weakness, convulsions, and death. Red blood cells hemolyze, oxygen delivery is impaired, and white cell phagocytosis is depressed. Chronic phosphate depletion has been implicated in the development of osteomalacia.

2. HYPERPHOSPHATEMIA

Hyperphosphatemia most often develops in severe renal disease, after trauma, or with marked tissue catabolism. It is rarely caused by excessive dietary intake. Hyperphosphatemia is usually asymptomatic. Because it raises the calcium-phosphorus product, the serum calcium concentration is depressed. A high calcium-phosphate product predisposes to metastatic calcification of soft tissues. Treatment of hyperphosphatemia is by diuresis to increase the rate of urinary phosphorus excretion. Administration of phosphate-binding antacids, such as aluminum hydroxide gels, will diminish the gastrointestinal absorption of phosphorus and lower the serum phosphorus concentration. In patients with renal disease, dialysis may be required.

ACID-BASE BALANCE

NORMAL PHYSIOLOGY

During the course of daily metabolism of protein and carbohydrate, approximately 70 meq (or 1 meq/kg of body weight) of hydrogen ion is generated and delivered into the body fluids. In addition, a large amount of carbon dioxide is formed that combines with water to form carbonic acid (H_2CO_3). If efficient mechanisms for buffering and eliminating these acids were not available, the pH of body fluids would fall rapidly. Although mammals have a highly developed system for handling daily acid production, disturbances of acid-base balance are common in disease.

Hydrogen ions generated from metabolism are buffered through two major systems. The first involves intracellular protein, eg, the hemoglobin in red blood cells. More important is the bicarbonate/carbonic acid system, which can be understood from the Henderson-Hasselbalch equation:

$$pH = pK + \log \frac{[HCO_3^-]}{0.03 \times P_{CO_2}} \qquad \cdots (4)$$

where pK for the $\dfrac{HCO_3^-}{H_2CO_3}$ system is 6.1.

Hydrogen ion concentration is related to pH in an inverse logarithmic manner. The following transformation of equation 4 is easier to use, because it eliminates the logarithms:

$$[H^+] = \frac{24 \times P_{CO_2}}{[HCO_e^-]} \qquad \ldots (5)$$

There is an approximately linear inverse relationship between pH and hydrogen ion concentration over the pH range of 7.9–7.50: For each 0.01 decrease in pH, the hydrogen ion concentration increases 1 nmol. Remembering that a normal blood pH of 7.40 is equal to a hydrogen ion concentration of 40 nmol/L, one can calculate the approximate hydrogen ion concentration for any pH between 7.10 and 7.50. For example, a pH of 7.30 is equal to a hydrogen ion concentration of 50 nmol/L. This estimation introduces an error of approximately 10% at the extremes of this pH range.

A consideration of the right-hand side of equation 5 demonstrates that hydrogen ion concentration is determined by the ratio of the P_{CO_2} to the plasma bicarbonate concentration. In body fluids, CO_2 is dissolved and combines with water to form carbonic acid, the acid part of the acid-base pair. If any two of these three variables are known, the third can be calculated using this expression.

Equation 5 also illustrates how the body excretes acid produced from metabolism. Blood P_{CO_2} is normally controlled within narrow limits by pulmonary ventilation. The plasma bicarbonate concentration is regulated in the renal tubules by three major processes: (1) Filtered bicarbonate is reabsorbed, mostly in the proximal tubule, to prevent excessive bicarbonate loss in the urine; (2) hydrogen ions are secreted as titratable acid to regenerate the bicarbonate that was buffered when these hydrogen ions were initially produced and to provide a vehicle for excretion of about one-third of the daily acid production; and (3) the kidneys also excrete hydrogen ion in the form of ammonium ion by a process that regenerates bicarbonate initially consumed in the production of these hydrogen ions. Volume depletion, increased P_{CO_2}, and hypokalemia all favor enhanced tubular reabsorption of HCO_3^-.

ACID-BASE ABNORMALITIES

The management of clinical acid-base disturbances is facilitated by the use of a nomogram (Figure 9–3) that relates the three variables in equation 5.

Primary respiratory disturbances cause changes in the blood CO_2 (the numerator in equation 5) and pro-

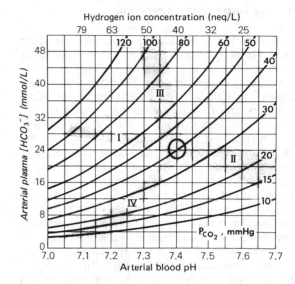

Figure 9–3. Acid-base nomogram for use in evaluation of clinical acid-base disorders. Hydrogen ion concentration (top) or blood pH (bottom) is plotted against plasma HCO_3^- concentration; curved lines are isopleths of CO_2 tension (P_{CO_2}, mm Hg). Knowing any two of these variables permits estimation of the third. The circle in the center represents the range of normal values; the shaded bands represent the 95% confidence limits of four common acid-base disturbances: I, acute respiratory acidosis; II, acute respiratory alkalosis; III, chronic respiratory acidosis; IV, sustained metabolic acidosis. Points lying outside these shaded areas are mixed disturbances and indicate two primary acid-base disorders. (Courtesy of Anthony Sebastian, MD, University of California Medical Center, San Francisco.)

duce corresponding effects on the blood hydrogen ion concentration. Metabolic disturbances primarily affect the plasma bicarbonate concentration (the denominator in equation 5). Whether the disturbance is primarily respiratory or metabolic, some degree of compensatory change occurs in the reciprocal factor in equation 5 to limit or nullify the magnitude of perturbation of acid-base balance. Thus, changes in blood P_{CO_2} from respiratory disturbances are compensated for by changes in the renal handling of bicarbonate. Conversely, changes in plasma bicarbonate concentration are blunted by appropriate respiratory changes.

Because acute changes allow insufficient time for compensatory mechanisms to respond, the resulting pH disturbances are often great and the abnormalities may be present in pure form. By contrast, chronic disturbances allow the full range of compensatory mechanisms to come into play, so that blood pH may remain near normal despite wide variations in the plasma bicarbonate or blood P_{CO_2}.

1. RESPIRATORY ACIDOSIS

Acute respiratory acidosis occurs when respiration suddenly becomes inadequate. CO_2 accumulates in the blood (the numerator in equation 5 increases), and hydrogen ion concentration increases. This occurs most often in acute airway obstruction, aspiration, respiratory arrest, certain pulmonary infections, and pulmonary edema with impaired gas exchange. There is acidemia and an elevated blood P_{CO_2} but little change in the plasma bicarbonate concentration. Over 80% of the carbonic acid resulting from the increased P_{CO_2} is buffered by intracellular mechanisms—about 50% by intracellular protein and another 30% by hemoglobin. Because relatively little is buffered by bicarbonate ion, the plasma bicarbonate concentration may be normal. An acute increase in the P_{CO_2} from 40 to 80 mm Hg will increase the plasma bicarbonate by only 3 meq/L. This is why the 95% confidence band for acute respiratory acidosis (I in Figure 9–3) is nearly horizontal; ie, increases in P_{CO_2} directly decrease pH with little change in plasma bicarbonate concentration. Treatment involves restoration of adequate ventilation. If necessary, tracheal intubation and assisted ventilation or controlled ventilation with morphine sedation should be employed.

Chronic respiratory acidosis arises from chronic respiratory failure in which impaired ventilation gives a sustained elevation of blood P_{CO_2}. Renal compensation raises plasma bicarbonate to the extent illustrated by the 95% confidence limits in Figure 9–3 (the area marked by III). Rather marked elevations of P_{CO_2} produce small changes in blood pH, because of the increase in plasma bicarbonate concentration. This is achieved primarily by increased renal excretion of ammonium ion, which enhances acid excretion and regenerates bicarbonate, which is returned to the blood. Chronic respiratory acidosis is generally well tolerated until severe pulmonary insufficiency leads to hypoxia. At this point, the long-term prognosis is very poor. Paradoxically, the patient with chronic respiratory acidosis appears better able to tolerate additional acute increases in blood P_{CO_2}.

Treatment of chronic respiratory acidosis depends largely on attention to pulmonary toilet and ventilatory status. Rapid correction of chronic respiratory acidosis, as may occur if the patient is placed on controlled ventilation, can be dangerous, since the P_{CO_2} is lowered rapidly and the compensated respiratory acidosis may be converted to a severe metabolic alkalosis.

2. RESPIRATORY ALKALOSIS

Acute hyperventilation lowers the P_{CO_2} without concomitant changes in the plasma bicarbonate concentration and thereby lowers the hydrogen ion concentration (II in Figure 9–3). The clinical manifestations are paresthesias in the extremities, carpopedal spasm, and a positive Chvostek sign. Acute hyperventilation with respiratory alkalosis may be an early sign of bacterial sepsis.

Chronic respiratory alkalosis occurs in pulmonary and liver disease. The renal response to chronic hypocapnia is to decrease the tubular reabsorption of filtered bicarbonate, increasing bicarbonate excretion, with a consequent lowering of plasma bicarbonate concentration. As the bicarbonate concentration falls, the chloride concentration rises. This is the same pattern seen in hyperchloremic acidosis, and the two can only be distinguished by blood gas and pH measurements. Generally, chronic respiratory alkalosis does not require treatment.

3. METABOLIC ACIDOSIS

Metabolic acidosis is caused by increased production of hydrogen ion from metabolic or other causes or from excessive bicarbonate losses. In either case, the plasma bicarbonate concentration is decreased, producing an increase in hydrogen ion concentration (see equation 5). With excessive bicarbonate loss (eg, severe diarrhea, diuretic treatment with acetazolamide or other carbonic anhydrase inhibitors, certain forms of renal tubular disease, and in patients with ureterosigmoidostomies), the decrease in plasma bicarbonate concentration is matched by an increase in the serum chloride, so that the anion gap (the sum of chloride and bicarbonate concentrations subtracted from the serum sodium concentration) remains at the normal level, below 15 meq/L. On the other hand, metabolic acidosis from increased acid production is associated with an anion gap exceeding 15 meq/L. Conditions in which this occurs are renal failure, diabetic ketoacidosis, lactic acidosis, methanol ingestion, salicylate intoxication, and ethylene glycol ingestion. The lungs compensate by hyperventilation, which returns the hydrogen ion concentration toward normal by lowering the blood P_{CO_2}. In long-standing metabolic acidosis, minute ventilation may increase sufficiently to drop the P_{CO_2} to as low as 10–15 mm Hg. The shaded area marked IV on the nomogram (Figure 9–3) represents the confidence limits for sustained metabolic acidosis.

Treatment of metabolic acidosis depends on identifying the underlying cause and correcting it. Often, this is sufficient. In some conditions, particularly when there is an increased anion gap, alkali administration is required. The amount of sodium bicarbonate required to restore the plasma bicarbonate concentration to normal can be estimated by subtracting the existing plasma bicarbonate concentration from the normal value of 24 meq/L and multiplying the resulting number by half the estimated total body water. This is a useful empiric formula. In practice, it is not usually wise to administer enough bicarbonate to return the plasma bicarbonate completely to normal. It is better to raise the plasma bicarbonate concentration by 5 meq/L initially and then reassess the clinical situation. The administration of sodium bicarbonate may cause fluid overload from the large quantity of sodium and may overcorrect the acidosis. The long-term management of patients with metabolic acidosis entails providing adequate alkali, either as supplemental sodium bicarbonate tablets or by dietary manipulation. In all cases, attempts should be made to minimize the magnitude of bicarbonate loss in patients with chronic metabolic acidosis.

4. METABOLIC ALKALOSIS

Metabolic alkalosis is probably the most common acid-base disturbance in surgical patients. In this condition, the blood hydrogen ion concentration is decreased as a result of accumulation of bicarbonate in plasma. The pathogenesis is complex but involves at least three separate factors: (1) loss of hydrogen ion, usually as a result of loss of gastric secretions rich in hydrochloric acid; (2) volume depletion, which is often severe; and (3) potassium depletion, which almost always is present.

HCl secretion by the gastric mucosa returns bicarbonate ion to the blood. Gastric acid, after mixing with ingested food, is subsequently reabsorbed in the small intestine, so that there is no net gain or loss of hydrogen ion in this process. If secreted hydrogen ion is lost through vomiting or drainage, the result is a net delivery of bicarbonate into the circulation. Normally, the kidneys are easily able to excrete the excess bicarbonate load. However, if volume depletion accompanies the loss of hydrogen ion, the kidneys work to preserve volume by increasing tubular reabsorption of sodium and whatever anions are also filtered. Consequently, because of the increased sodium reabsorption, the excess bicarbonate cannot be completely excreted. This perpetuates the metabolic alkalosis. At first, some of the filtered bicarbonate escapes reabsorption in the proximal tubule and reaches the distal tubule. Here it promotes potassium secretion and enhanced potassium loss in the urine. The urine pH will be either neutral or alkaline, because of the presence of bicarbonate. Later, as volume depletion becomes more severe, the reabsorption of filtered bicarbonate in the proximal tubule becomes virtually complete. Now, only small amounts of sodium, with little bicarbonate, reach the distal tubule. If potassium depletion is severe, sodium is reabsorbed in exchange for hydrogen ion. This results in the paradoxically acid urine sometimes observed in patients with advanced metabolic alkalosis.

Assessment should involve examination of the urine electrolytes and urine pH. In the early stages, bicarbonate excretion will obligate excretion of sodium as well as potassium, so the urine sodium concentration will be relatively high for a volume-depleted patient and the urine pH will be alkaline. In this circumstance, the urine chloride will reveal the extent of the volume depletion: A urine chloride of less than 10 meq/L is diagnostic of volume depletion and chloride deficiency. Later, when bicarbonate reabsorption becomes virtually complete, the urine pH will be acid, and urine sodium, potassium, and chloride concentrations will all be low. The ventilatory compensation in metabolic alkalosis is variable, but the maximal extent of compensation can only raise the blood P_{CO_2} to about 55 mm Hg. A P_{CO_2} greater than 60 mm Hg in metabolic alkalosis suggests a mixed disturbance also involving respiratory acidosis.

To treat metabolic alkalosis, fluid must be given, usually as saline solution. With adequate volume repletion, the stimulus to tubular sodium reabsorption is diminished, and the kidneys can then excrete the excess bicarbonate. Most of these patients are also substantially potassium-depleted and will require potassium supplementation. This should be administered as KCl, since chloride depletion is another hallmark of this condition and potassium given as citrate or lactate will not correct the potassium deficit.

5. MIXED ACID-BASE DISORDERS

In many situations, mixed disorders of acid-base balance develop. The most common example in surgical patients is metabolic acidosis superimposed on respiratory alkalosis. This problem can arise in patients with septic shock or hepatorenal syndrome. Since the two acid-base disorders tend to cancel each other, the disturbance in hydrogen ion concentration is usually small. The reverse situation, ie, respiratory acidosis combined with metabolic alkalosis, is less common. Combined metabolic and respiratory acidosis occurs in cardiorespiratory arrest and obviously constitutes a medical emergency. Circumstances involving both metabolic and respiratory alkalosis are rare. The clue to the presence of a mixed acid-base disorder can come from plotting the patient's acid-base data on the nomogram in Figure 9–3. If the set of data falls outside one of the confidence bands, then by definition the patient has a mixed disorder. On the other hand, if the acid-base data fall within one of the confidence bands, it suggests (but does not prove) that the acid-base disturbance is pure or uncomplicated.

PRINCIPLES OF FLUID & ELECTROLYTE THERAPY

The development of a rational plan of fluid and electrolyte therapy requires an understanding of the principles developed earlier in this chapter. First, maintenance fluid requirements must be determined. Second, existing deficits of volume or composition should be calculated. This involves the analysis of four aspects of the patient's fluid and electrolyte status based on weight changes, serum electrolyte concentrations, and blood pH and P_{CO_2}: (1) the magnitude of the volume deficit present, (2) the pathogenesis and treatment of abnormal sodium concentration, (3) assessment of any potassium requirement, and (4) management of any coexistent acid-base disturbance. Finally, therapy must also recognize the presence of ongoing obligatory fluid losses and include these losses in the daily plan of treatment.

Normal maintenance requirements can be determined using the guidelines in Table 9–2. Fever or elevated ambient temperature will increase insensible losses and thereby increase these requirements. The normal response to the stress of surgery is to conserve water and electrolytes, so maintenance requirements are decreased in the immediate postoperative period. In addition, increased catabolism will deliver more potassium to the circulation, so that this ion can be omitted from maintenance solutions for several days postoperatively.

Correction of preexisting deficits must be based on the four factors listed above. Volume deficit is best estimated on the basis of acute changes in weight or from clinical estimates; the clinician should remember that deficits less than 5% of body water will not be detectable and that loss of 15% of body water will be associated with severe circulatory compromise. The relationship of net sodium to net fluid deficit is given by the serum sodium concentration according to equation 3. If the serum sodium concentration is normal, fluid losses have been isotonic; if hyponatremia is present, more sodium than water has been lost. In either case, initial replacement should be with isotonic saline solutions. Any potassium excess or deficit must be assessed in the light of the blood pH according to Figure 9–2. If hypokalemia exists at normal pH, the magnitude of the total body potassium deficit can also be estimated using Figure 9–2. For example, a serum potassium concentration of 2.5 meq/L at pH 7.40 suggests a 20% depletion of total body potassium. A normal human has a potassium capacity of 45 meq/kg body weight; a moderately wasted patient, 35 meq/kg. For a normal 70-kg man, total potassium capacity is 45×70, or 3150 meq; the deficit is 20% of this, or 630 meq, and this amount must be considered in therapy calculations. Principles of acid-base therapy have already been outlined.

Two rules of thumb should be applied in prescribing parenteral therapy for fluid and electrolyte deficits. The first is that for most problems, half of the calculated deficits should be replaced in a 24-hour period, with subsequent reassessment of the clinical situation. The second is that a fluid or electrolyte abnormality should take as long to correct as it took to develop. By adherence to these guidelines, overly vigorous replacement will be avoided and, along with it, the production of a different (iatrogenic) electrolyte abnormality.

Ongoing losses must be considered also in the daily fluid therapy plan, with regard to both volume and composition. Characteristic measurements for fluids removed from different segments of the gastrointestinal tract are shown in Table 9–3.

ILLUSTRATIVE EXAMPLE

A 40-year-old man whose normal weight is 70 kg is admitted to the hospital after 5 days' protracted vomiting, during which time he has been able to ingest nothing but an occasional glass of water. Physical examination shows evidence of dehydration, and diagnostic studies confirm the admitting impression of a duodenal ulcer with pyloric obstruction. Weight on admission is 65 kg. Initial laboratory studies include the following:

Serum Na^+ 122 meq/L, K^+ 2 meq/L, Cl^- 80 meq/L, HCO_3^- 35 meq/L, urea nitrogen 42 mg/dL, creatinine 1.7 mg/dL.
Arterial blood pH 7.50, P_{CO_2} 44 mm Hg.
Urine Na^+ 27 meq/L, Cl^- 8 meq/L, K^+ 64 meq/L, pH 7.0.

Discussion

Volume depletion is suggested by weight loss of 5 kg, evidence of volume depletion, elevation of BUN and creatinine, and urine Cl^- less than 10 meq/L. The underlying abnormality is metabolic alkalosis and chloride depletion from loss of gastric juice. Hyponatremia results from loss of sodium (gastric juice and urine) with ingestion only of water. Urine pH is neutral because of bicarbonate excretion, obligating sodium excretion, and the high urine potassium is reflective of the potassium wasting occurring in metabolic alkalosis despite hypokalemia.

Parenteral fluid therapy for the first 24 hours should consider the following:

Maintenance requirements will be unchanged from normal in the absence of fever. Based on weight, the volume deficit is about 5 L. The sodium deficit, calculated from equation 3, is 585 meq; this amount is required to restore the serum sodium concentration to

140 meq/L. To this must be added the amount of sodium in 5 L of isotonic replacement fluid, or 700 meq, for a total sodium deficit of 1285 meq. The serum potassium, when corrected to normal pH, would be about 2.4 meq/L, consistent with a 20% deficit, or about 630 meq. The alkalosis in this setting will be responsive merely to volume replacement and requires no special therapy; sodium and potassium replacements, however, must be with chloride as the anion. If gastric losses via nasogastric suction continue in the hospital, they should be included in the plan (Table 9–3). These considerations result in the following:

	Volume (L)	Na⁺ (meq/L)	K⁺ (meq/L)
Maintenance	2	100	60
Correction of deficit	5	1285	630
Ongoing losses (estimated)	2	40	20

Using the rule of thumb that half of deficits should be replaced in 24 hours, the physician should issue initial orders for intravenous therapy of about 6.5 L of fluid, 780 meq of sodium, and 260 meq of potassium; this last figure is not sufficient to replace half of the potassium deficit but limits the potassium concentration in intravenous fluid to 40 meq/L, the highest concentration routinely advisable. This combination can be approximated with 4 L of 5% dextrose in isotonic sodium chloride and 2.5 L of 5% dextrose in 0.5 N saline, with potassium added to each bottle to achieve a concentration of 40 meq/L. These fluids should then be administered at a rate of 250 mL/h and the situation then reassessed after 24 hours.

REFERENCES

General

Brenner BM, Rector RC (editors): *The Kidney,* 4th ed. Saunders, 1991.

Cogan MG: *Fluid and Electrolytes: Physiology and Pathophysiology.* Appleton & Lange, 1991.

Fluid Volume

Anderson RJ: Hospital associated hyponatremia. Kidney Int 1986;29:1237.

Arieff AI: Hyponatremia, convulsions, respiratory arrest, and permanent brain damage after elective surgery in healthy women. N Engl J Med 1986;314:1529.

Ayus JC, Krothapalli RK, Arieff AI: Changing concepts in treatment of severe symptomatic hyponatremia. Am J Med 1985;78:8972.

Ayus JC, Krothapalli RK, Arieff AI: Treatment of symptomatic hyponatremia and its relation to brain damage. N Engl J Med 1987;317:1190.

Ayus JC, Wheeler JM, Arieff AI: Postoperative hyponatremic encephalopathy in menstruant women. Ann Intern Med 1992;117:891.

Daniels BS, Ferris TF: The use of diuretics in nonedematous disorders. Semin Nephrol 1988;8:342.

Daugirdas JT et al: Hyperosmolar coma: Cellular dehydration and the serum sodium concentration. Ann Intern Med 1989;100:8557.

Fraser CL, Arieff AI: Fatal central diabetes mellitus and insipidus resulting from untreated hyponatremia. Ann Intern Med 1990;112:113.

Hura CE, Kunau RT Jr, Stein JH: Use of diuretics in salt-retaining states. Semin Nephrol 1988;8:318.

Katz MA: Hyperglycemia-induced hyponatremia: Calculation of expected serum sodium depression. N Engl J Med 1973;289:843.

Narins RG, Riley LJ: Polyuria: Simple and mixed disorders. Am J Kidney Dis 1991;17:237.

Oh MS, Carroll HJ: Disorders of sodium metabolism: Hypernatremia and hyponatremia. Crit Care Med 1992;20:943.

Schrier RW: Body fluid volume regulation in health and disease: A unifying hypothesis. Ann Intern Med 1990;113:155.

Schrier RW: Pathogenesis of sodium and water retention in high-output and low-output cardiac failure, nephrotic syndrome, cirrhosis, and pregnancy. (Two parts.) N Engl J Med 1988;319:1065, 1127.

Siperstein MD: Diabetic ketoacidosis and hyperosmolar coma. Endocrinol Metab Clin North Am 1992;21:415.

Snyder NA, Feigal DW, Arieff AI: Hypernatremia in elderly patients: A heterogeneous, morbid, and iatrogenic entity. Ann Intern Med 1987;107:309.

Sterns RH: Severe symptomatic hyponatremia: Treatment and outcome. Ann Intern Med 1987;107:656.

Tien R et al: Hyponatremic encephalopathy: Is central pontine myelinolysis a component? Am J Med 1992;92:513.

Acid-Base & Potassium

Adrogue JH, Madias NE: Changes in plasma potassium concentration during acute acid-base disturbances. Am J Med 1981;71:456.

Bouchama A et al: Refractory hypercapnia complicating massive pulmonary embolism. Am Rev Resp Dis 1988;138:466.

Brown RS: Extrarenal potassium homeostasis. Kidney Int 1986;30:116.

Chan JC, Alon U: Tubular disorers of acid-base and phosphate metabolism. Nephron 1985;40:257.

Ethier JH et al: Evaluation of the renal response to hypokalemia and hyperkalemia. Am J Kidney Dis 1990;15:309.

Fine A: Application of principles of physiology and biochemistry to the bedside: Metabolic alkalosis and hypokalamia. Clin Invest Med 1990;13:47.

Hertford JA, McKenna JP, Chamovitz BN: Metabolic acidosis with an elevated anion gap. Am Fam Physician 1989;39:159.

Kruse JA, Carlson RW: Rapid correction of hypokalemia using concentrated intravenous potassium chloride infusions. Arch Intern Med 1990;150:613.

Kushner RF: Total parenteral nutrition-associated metabolic acidosis. J Parentr Entral Nutr 1986;10:306.

Okusawa S, Aikawa N, Abe O: Postoperative metabolic alkalosis following general surgery: Its incidence and possible etiology. Jpn J Surg 1989;19:312.

Potkin RT, Swenson ER: Resuscitation from severe acute hypercapnia: Determinants of tolerance and survival. Chest 1992;102:1742.

Rimmer JM, Horn JF, Gennari FJ: Hyperkalemia as a complication of drug toxicity. Arch Intern Med 1987;147:867.

Rocher LL, Tannen RL: The clinical spectrum of renal tubular acidosis. Annu Rev Med 1986;37:319.

Schoolwerth AC: Regulation of renal ammoniagenesis in metabolic acidosis. Kidney Int 1991;40:961.

Tannen RL: Disorders of potassium balance. In: *The Kidney,* 4th ed. Brenner BM, Rector RC (editors). Saunders, 1991.

Ventriglia WJ: Arterial blood gases. Emerg Med Clin North Am 1986;4:235.

Warnock DG: Uremic acidosis. Kidney Int 1988;34:278.

Whang R, Whang DD, Ryan MP: Refractory potassium repletion: A consequence of magnesium deficiency. Arch Intern Med 1992;152:40.

Wright FS: Renal potassium handling. Semin Nephrol 1987;7:174.

Calcium, Phosphorus, & Magnesium

Bilezikian JP: Management of acute hypercalcemia. N Engl J Med 1992;326:11963.

Bilezikian JP: Parathyroid hormone-related peptide in sickness and in health. N Engl J Med 1990;322: 1151.

Chernow B et al: Hypomagnesemia in patients in postoperative intensive care. Chest 1989;95:391.

Desai TK, Carlson RW, Geheb MA: Hypocalcemia and hypophosphatemia in acutely ill patients. Crit Care Clin 1987;3:927.

Fassler CA et al: Magnesium toxicity as a cause of hypotension and hypoventilation. Arch Intern Med 1985;145:1604.

Ferdinandus J, Pederson JA, Whang R: Hypermagnesemia as a cause of refractory hypotension, respiratory depression, and coma. Arch Intern Med 1981;141: 669.

Halvey J, Buluik S: Severe hypophosphatemia in hospitalized patients. Arch Intern Med 1988;148:153.

Knochel JP: Hypophosphatemia and phosphorus deficiency. In: Brenner BM, Rector FC: *The Kidney,* 4th ed. Saunders, 1991.

Lentz RD, Brown DM, Kjellstrand CM: Treatment of severe hypophosphatemia. Ann Intern Med 1978;89: 941.

Molloy DW: Magnesium and respiratory muscle power. Am Rev Respir Dis 1984;129:497.

Oster JR, Epstein M: Management of magnesium depletion. Am J Nephrol 1988;8:349.

Ralston SH et al: Cancer-associated hypercalcemia: Morbidity and mortality. Clinical experience in 126 treated patients. Ann Intern Med 1990;112: 4994.

Ritch PS: Treatment of cancer-related hypercalcemia. Semin Oncol 1990;2(Suppl 5):26.

Singer F: Role of the bisphosphonate etidronate in the therapy of cancer-related hypercalcemia. Semin Oncol 1990;17(Suppl 5):34.

Singer FR et al: Treatment of hypercalcemia of malignancy with intravenous etidronate: A controlled, multicenter study. Arch Intern Med 1991;151:471.

Whang R, Whang DD, Ryan MP: Refractory potassium repletion: A consequence of magnesium deficiency. Arch Intern Med 1992;152:40.

Whang R: Magnesium deficiency: Pathogenesis, prevalence, and clinical implications. Am J Med 1987;82 (Suppl 3A):24.

Yu GC, Lee DB: Clinical disorders of phosphorus metabolism. West J Med 1987;147:569.

Zaloga GP, Chernow B: Hypocalcemia in critical illness. JAMA 1986;256:1924.

Surgical Metabolism & Nutrition

10

Michael S. Hickey, MD, Jeffrey M. Arbeit, MD, & Lawrence W. Way, MD

Malnutrition is common in surgical patients and predisposes to a variety of postoperative complications, especially in patients who have lost more than 10 lb or 10% of their usual body weight. Since malnutrition can be diagnosed and treated, an understanding of normal and abnormal nutrition is important for surgeons.

NUTRITIONAL ASSESSMENT
(Tables 10–1, 10–2, 10–3)

A proper nutritional assessment includes (1) a history and physical examination, (2) determination of protein (visceral and somatic) and fat reserves, (3) a 24-hour nitrogen balance determination, (4) assessment of gastrointestinal function, and (5) calculation of the daily caloric and protein requirements.

History & Physical Examination

The cornerstone of nutritional assessment is the history and physical examination. The dietary history provides a good estimate of the patient's caloric, protein, vitamin, and trace metal intake. In most cases, the possibility of malnutrition is suggested by the underlying disease or by a history of recent weight loss. Liver and kidney diseases are often associated with deficiencies of protein, vitamins, and trace metals. Patients with renal failure who require hemodialysis also lose amino acids, vitamins, trace metals, and carnitine in the dialysate. Patients with inflammatory bowel disease—especially those with ileal involvement—often suffer from deficiencies of protein (due to a combination of poor intake, chronic diarrhea, and treatment with corticosteroids), fat, vitamins, calcium, magnesium, and trace elements. About 30% of patients with cancer have protein, calorie, and vitamin deficiencies due either to the underlying disease or to antimetabolite chemotherapy (eg, methotrexate). Patients infected with the human immunodeficiency virus (HIV) are frequently malnourished and have protein, trace metal (selenium and zinc), mineral, and vitamin deficiencies.

The physical examination provides information regarding the extent of malnutrition. The amount of subcutaneous tissue on the extremities and buttocks

and in the buccal fat pads reflects caloric intake. Protein status is evaluated from the bulk and strength of the extremity muscles and visible evidence of temporal muscle wasting. Vitamin malnutrition may be manifested by changes in the texture of the skin, the presence of follicular plugging or a skin rash, corneal vascularization, cracks at the corners of the mouth (cheilosis), hyperemia of the oral mucosa (glossitis), cardiac enlargement and murmurs, altered sensation in the hands and feet, absence of vibration and position sense (dorsal and lateral column deficits), and abnormal quality and texture of the hair. Trace metal deficiencies produce abnormalities similar to those associated with vitamin deficiency plus changes in mental status.

Protein (Visceral & Somatic) & Fat Reserve

The visceral protein reserve is estimated from the serum total protein, albumin, and transferrin levels; total lymphocyte count; and antigen skin testing. The serum albumin level provides a rough estimate of the patient's nutritional status. Because albumin has such a long half-life (18 days), other serum proteins such as transferrin, prealbumin, retinol-binding protein, and ceruloplasmin, which have half-lives of a few hours, are more sensitive indices of acute changes in nutritional status. Unfortunately, their serum levels are also influenced by other factors, so they have limited utility.

Somatic (skeletal) protein reserve—most protein resides in skeletal muscle—is estimated by measuring the midarm circumference. This measurement is corrected to account for subcutaneous tissue (TSF), which gives the midarm muscle circumference (MAMC). The result is compared with normal values for the patient's age and sex to determine the extent of protein depletion or reserve.

Fat reserve is estimated from the thickness of the triceps skin fold (TSF) (Tables 10–1 and 10–2.)

24-Hour Nitrogen Balance Determination

Protein synthesis or breakdown can be determined by measuring the nitrogen balance (nitrogen intake minus nitrogen excretion) (Figure 10–1). Nitrogen intake is the sum of nitrogen delivered from enteral and parenteral feedings. Nitrogen output is the sum of

Table 10–1. Nutritional assessment.

HISTORY

Present illness = $\dfrac{\text{Actual weight} \times 100}{\text{Ideal weight}}$

Percentage usual body weight = $\dfrac{\text{Actual weight} \times 100}{\text{Usual weight}}$

Past illness predisposing to malnutrition

PHYSICAL EXAMINATION
  Skin: Quality, texture, rash, follicles, hyperkeratosis, nail deformities
  Hair: Quality, texture, recent loss
  Eyes: Keratoconjunctivitis, night blindness
  Mouth: Cheilosis, glossitis, mucosal atrophy, dentition
  Heart: Chamber enlargement, murmurs
  Abdomen: Hepatomegaly, abdominal mass, ostomy, fistulas
  Rectum: Stool color, perineal fistula
  Neurologic: Peripheral neuropathy, dorsolateral column dificit
  Extremities: Muscle size and strength, pedal edema

LABORATORY TESTS
  CBC: Hemoglobin, hematocrit, red cell indices, white count and differential, total lymphocyte count,[1] platelet count
  Electrolytes: Sodium, potassium, chloride, calcium, phosphate, magnesium
  Liver function tests: AST (SGOT), ALT (SGPT), alkaline phosphatase, bilirubin, albumin,[2] prealbumin,[3] retinol-binding protein,[4] prothrombin
  Miscellaneous: BUN, creatinine, triglycerides, cholesterol, free fatty acids, ketones, uric acid, calcium, copper, zinc, magnesium, transferrin[5]

[1]Total lymphocyte count (normal = 1500–4000 cells/μL)
  Mild malnutrition: 1200–2000 cells/μL
  Moderate malnutrition: 800–1200 cells/μL
  Severe malnutrition: < 800 cells/μL
[2]Albumin (normal = > 3.5 g/dL)
  Mild malnutrition: 2.8–3.2 g/dL
  Moderate malnutrition: 2.1–2.7 g/dL
  Severe malnutrition: < 2.1 g/dL
[3]Prealbumin (normal = 17–42 mg/dL): Values < 17 mg/dL represent malnutrition
[4]Retinol-binding protein (normal = 4.1–6.1 mg/dL): Values < 4.1 mg/dL represent malnutrition
[5]Transferrin (normal = > 250 mg/dL)
  Mild malnutrition: 200–250 mg/dL
  Moderate malnutrition: 100–200 mg/dL
  Severe malnutrition: < 100 mg/dL

nitrogen excreted in urine, fistula drainage, diarrhea, etc. The usual approach is to measure the urea nitrogen concentration of an aliquot of a 24-hour urine collection and then calculate nitrogen content from the urine volume. A correction factor is added to account for nitrogen losses in the stool and from skin exfoliation. The difference in nitrogen intake minus output estimates the 24-hour nitrogen balance. The result is not very precise, however, because it represents a small difference between two large numbers. Accuracy can be improved if the calculations are extended to cover a period of several weeks. When losses of nitrogen are large (eg, diarrhea, hematochezia, protein-losing enteropathy, fistula, or burn exudate), measurements of nitrogen balance lose accuracy because of the difficulty in collecting all of the secretions. Despite these shortcomings, a 24-hour urine collection for nitrogen balance determination is the best practical means of measuring net protein synthesis and breakdown.

A nitrogen balance determination should be routine for patients receiving nutritional therapy and should be performed weekly in critically ill patients.

In general, patients in positive nitrogen balance do not require nutritional therapy, whereas those in negative nitrogen balance do.

The urinary excretion of 3-methylhistidine is a more precise measurement of protein status. The amino acid histidine is irreversibly methylated in muscle. During tissue breakdown histidine (ie, within 3-methylhistidine) is not reincorporated into protein, so the urinary excretion of 3-methylhistidine correlates well with muscle protein breakdown. Unfortunately, measuring 3-methylhistidine is too expensive to use as a clinical test (Figure 10–3).

Gastrointestinal Function

Well-nourished critically ill patients with normal gut function can usually tolerate an oral or nasointestinal enteral diet. These patients rarely require special amino acid or polypeptide enteral or parenteral formulas. In contrast, patients who are malnourished or have gut dysfunction rarely tolerate oral or enteral formula diets and need these special diets.

Table 10–2. Clinical staging of malnutrition.

Clinical and Laboratory Parameters	Extent of Malnutrition		
	Mild	Moderate[1]	Severe[1]
Albumin (g/dL)[2]	2.8–3.2	2.1–2.7	< 2.1
Transferrin (mg/dL)[2]	200–250	100–200	< 100
Total lymphocyte count (cells/μL)[2]	1200–2000	800–1200	< 800
Creatinine/height index (%)[3]	60–80	30–60	< 40
Ideal body weight (%)	80–90	70–80	< 70
Usual body weight (%)	85–95	75–85	< 75
Weight loss/unit time	< 5%/month < 7.5%/3 months < 10%/6 months	< 2%/week > 5%/month > 7.5%/3 months > 10%/6 months	> 2%/week
Skin tests (No. reactive ÷ No. placed)	4/4 (normal)	1–2/4 (weak)	0/0 (anergic)
Normal anthropometric measurements	**Male**	**Female**	
Triceps skin fold(mm)[4]	12.5	16.5	
Midarm circumference (cm)	29.3	28.5	

[1]Nutritional therapy indicated.
[2]Visceral protein reserve.
[3]Somatic protein reserve (see Table 10–3).
[4]Fat reserve.

Determining Energy Requirements

Adult daily caloric requirements are estimated as follows:

Goal	kcal/kg/d
Weight loss	20–25
Weight maintenance	30–35
Weight gain	35–40

The adult daily caloric requirement is calculated by using the total energy expenditure (TEE) equation, which is a modified version of the Harris-Benedict equation (Table 10–4). It includes three variables: height (cm), weight (kg), and age (yr); and makes allowances for specific activity, injury factors, and gender.

Indirect calorimetry is the most accurate method for determining an adult's daily caloric requirements. It calculates the production of O_2 ($\dot{V}O_2$) and CO_2 ($\dot{V}CO_2$) from the timed volumetric collection of expired O_2, CO_2, and urinary nitrogen. The resting energy expenditure (REE) in kilocalories (kcal) per minute is derived from the **Weir formula:**

$$\text{kcal/min} = 3.9(\dot{V}O_2) + 1.1(\dot{V}CO_2) - 2.2(\text{urine N})$$

$$\text{Nonprotein RQ} = \frac{\dot{V}CO_2 - 4.8(\text{urine N})}{\dot{V}O_2 - 5.9(\text{urine N})}$$

where $\dot{V}O_2$ and $\dot{V}CO_2$ are oxygen consumption and CO_2 production in mL/min and urine nitrogen is in g/min.

The nonprotein respiratory quotient (RQ) is the percentage of carbohydrate and fat used for energy production. When the RQ is 1, pure carbohydrate is being oxidized. When the RQ is 0.7, only fat is being oxidized. The nonprotein RQ is used to gauge the patient's metabolic response to nutritional therapy. Theoretically, the administration of large amounts of glucose to patients with sepsis and chronic obstructive pulmonary disease (COPD) could result in CO_2 retention due to the increased $\dot{V}CO_2$ (Table 10–3).

NUTRIENT REQUIREMENTS

Calories

The body requires an energy source to remain in a steady state. About 50% of the basal metabolic rate (BMR) reflects the work of ion pumping; 30% represents protein turnover; and the remainder represents recycling of amino acids, glucose, lactate, and pyruvate. Total energy expenditure is the sum of energy consumed in basal metabolic processes, physical activity, the specific dynamic action of protein, and extra requirements resulting from injury, sepsis, or burns. Energy consumed in physical activity constitutes 10–50% of the total in normal subjects but drops to 10–20% for hospitalized patients. The increment above basal needs resulting from injury or trauma is about 10% for elective operations, 10–30% for trauma, 50–80% for sepsis, and 100–200% for burns (depending on the extent of the wound).

Calories can come from glucose or fat. The metabolism of 1 g glucose yields 3.4 kcal. The metabolism

Table 10–3. Special tests for nutritional assessment.

1. **Anthropometrics:**
   Triceps skin fold (TSF)
   Midhumeral circumference (MHC)

   $$\text{Arm muscle circumference} = \frac{\text{MHC} - (\pi)(\text{TSF})}{10}$$

   $$\text{Creatinine-height index} = \frac{\text{24-hour urine creatinine excretion}}{\text{Ideal creatinine excretion for height}}$$

2. **Energy:**
   Total energy expenditure (Table 10–4)
   Weir formula (REE): kcal/min = 3.9 $(\text{V}_{O_2})^1$ + 1.1 (V_{CO_2})—2.2 (urine N)[1]

   $$\text{Nonprotein RQ: } \frac{\dot{\text{V}}_{CO_2}\ \dot{\text{V}}_{CO_2} - 4.8\ (\text{urine N})}{\text{V}_{O_2} - 5.9\ (\text{urine N})}$$

3. **Protein:**
   Nitrogen balance = Nitrogen intake – Nitrogen output (refer to text for equation)
   3-Methylhistidine urinary excretion
   Isotopic determination of protein turnover (^{15}N glycine, ^{15}N lysine, and ^{4}C leucine infusion)

4. **Body Composition:**
   Total body water (TBW): ^{3}H or ^{2}H H_2O isotope dilution
   Extracellular water (ECW): ^{22}Na isotope dilution

   $$\text{Lean body mass (LBW): } \frac{\text{TBW}}{0.73}$$

   Body cell mass (BCM): $(K_e)(0.083)$ or (TBN)(6.25)(4)
   Total body potassium: ^{42}K isotope dilution; ^{40}K whole body counting; K_e (exchangeable potassium)
   Total body nitrogen (TBN): Neutron activation

5. **Immunologic testing:**
   Skin tests   Immunoglobulin levels
   Lymphocyte blastogenesis   Complement levels
   Mixed lymphocyte response   Lymphokine production

6. **Miscellaneous laboratory tests:**
   Prealbumin[2]
   Retinol-binding protein[3]
   Transferrin[4]

[1]$\dot{\text{V}}_{O_2}$ and $\dot{\text{V}}_{CO_2}$ are oxygen consumption and CO_2 production in mL/min; urine nitrogen is in g/min.
[2]Prealbumin (normal = 17–42 mg/dL): Values < 4.1 mg/dL represent malnutrition.
[3]Retinol-binding protein (normal = 4.1–6.1 mg/dL): Values <4.1 mg/dL represent malnutrition.
[4]Transferrin (normal = >250 mg/dL):
   Mild malnutrition: 200–250 mg/dL
   Moderate malnutrition: 100–200 mg/dL
   Severe malnutrition: <100 mg/dL

of 1 g fat yields 9.2 kcal. Glucose, the primary source of calories, stimulates insulin secretion, which in turn influences protein synthesis. Fat can be used to provide as much as 60% of daily caloric requirements, but more than that could impair polymorphonuclear, macrophage, and reticuloendothelial cell function.

Protein

Protein balance reflects the sum of protein synthesis and breakdown. By changing the levels of metabolic substrates, hormones, or cytokines, the body adjusts protein stores in response to changes in the basal state, level of activity, operations, trauma, sepsis, or

$$\text{Nitrogen balance} = \text{Nitrogen}^{(\text{intake})} - \text{Nitrogen}^{(\text{output})}$$

$$\text{Nitrogen}^{(\text{intake})} = \frac{\text{g Protein}}{6.25\ \text{g Protein/g Nitrogen}}$$

$$\text{Nitrogen}^{(\text{output})} = \text{UUN}^1 \times \frac{1000\ \text{mL}}{\text{L}} \times 24\text{-hour Urine volume (L)} \times \frac{\text{g Nitrogen}}{1000\ \text{mg Nitrogen}} + 3$$

$$^1\text{UUN} = \frac{\text{mg Nitrogen}}{100\ \text{mL Urine}}$$

Figure 10–1. Twenty-four-hour nitrogen balance determination.

Table 10–4. Total energy expenditure equation for adults.

Estimated:
 Calories (total kcal) (male or female)
  25–30/kg (weight loss)
  30–35/kg (weight maintenance)
  35–40/kg (weight gain)
 Protein (g) (male or female)
  0.8–2.0/kg

Calculated:
 Calories (total kcal) for weight maintenance
  Male $= [66.5 + (13.7 \times \text{wt kg}) + (5 \times \text{ht cm}) - (6.7 \times \text{age yr})] \times AF^1 \times IF^2$
  Female $= [665.1 + (9.6 \times \text{wt kg}) + (1.8 \times \text{ht cm}) - (4.7 \times \text{age yr})] \times AF^1 \times IF^2$
  Note: Add 500 kcal to the above equations for weight gain.
 Protein (g)

$$\text{Male or female} = \text{Total kcal} \times \frac{\text{g nitrogen}}{150 \text{ kcal}} \times \frac{6.25 \text{ g protein}}{\text{g nitrogen}}$$

[1]Activity factor		[2]Injury factor	
Confined to bed	1.2	Surgery	1.1–1.2
Ambulatory	1.3	Infection	1.2–1.6
Fever factor (>37 °C)	1.3	Trauma	1.1–1.8
		Sepsis	1.4–1.8

burns. Because protein turnover is in constant flux, the published requirements for protein, amino acids, and nitrogen are only approximations.

The quality of a protein is related to its amino acid composition. The 20 amino acids are divided into essential amino acids (EAA) and nonessential amino acids (NEAA), depending on whether they can be synthesized de novo in the body. They are further divided into aromatic (AAA), branched chain (BCAA), and sulfur-containing amino acids. Amino acids contain highly reactive thiol, imidazole, aromatic, and dicarboxylic acid groups, which catalyze chemical reactions and help determine the tertiary structures of protein molecules via polar, hydrophobic, nonionic, disulfide, and hydrogen bonds. Certain amino acids have unique metabolic functions. For example, alanine and glutamine participate in a cycle with glucose that preserves carbon during starvation; leucine stimulates protein synthesis and inhibits catabolism; and BCAAs are the fuels preferred by cardiac and skeletal muscle during starvation.

Glutamine

Glutamine is a nonessential, neutral amino acid that can be synthesized by virtually all tissues. Several unique properties suggest that glutamine plays an important role in the metabolically stressed patient.

Following injury, operation, sepsis, and other catabolic events, intracellular glutamine stores may decrease by greater than 50% and plasma levels by 25%. The decline exceeds that of any other amino acid and persists during recovery after the concentrations of other amino acid have returned to normal.

Glutamine is avidly consumed by replicating cells, such as fibroblasts, lymphocytes, tumor cells, and intestinal epithelial cells. Catabolic states, such as trauma, sepsis, major burns, and uncontrolled diabetes mellitus, are characterized by accelerated skeletal muscle proteolysis and translocation of amino acids from the periphery to the visceral organs. Glutamine accounts for a major portion of the amino acids released by muscle in these states.

Gastrointestinal uptake of glutamine occurs in the epithelial cells of the small bowel villi. Glutamine is the major energy substrate for the gut. Glutamine also appears to be important in maintaining normal intestinal structure and function.

Arginine

Arginine, a semiessential amino acid, enhances T lymphocyte activation in response to concanavalin A and phytohemagglutinin, and it increases the mean CD4 phenotype of patients with impaired cellular immunity. Thus, arginine is a vital nutrient for the immune system.

Nucleotides

Nucleotides are precursors of DNA and RNA and participate in a number of metabolic reactions fundamental to cellular activity.

Nucleotides increase delayed hypersensitivity responses, resistance to infection, and interleukin-2 production. These immunologic effects are directly related to a requirement for nucleotides for T cell maturation and expression of phenotype markers.

Vitamins

Vitamins are involved in metabolism, wound healing, and immune function. They are essential parts of the diet because they cannot be synthesized de novo. The normal requirements for vitamins (Table 10–5) may increase in disease. For example, increased amounts of vitamins are excreted in the urine of patients with trauma, burns, and sepsis.

Table 10–5. Daily electrolyte, trace element, vitamin, and mineral requirements for adults.

	Enteral	Parenteral
Electrolytes		
Sodium	90–150 meq	90–150 meq
Potassium	60–90 meq	60–90 meq
Trace elements		
Chromium[1,2]	5–200 µg	10–15 µg
Copper[1,2]	2–3 mg	0.15–0.5 mg
Manganese[1,2]	2.5–5.0 mg	0.15–0.8 mg
Zinc[1]	15 mg	2.5–4.0 mg
Iron	10 mg	2.5 mg
Iodine	150 µg	. . .
Fluoride[2]	1.5–4.0 mg	. . .
Selenium[2]	0.05–0.20 mg	20–40 µg
Molybdenum[2]	0.15–0.50 mg	20–120 µg
Tin[3]	. . .	. . .
Vanadium[3]	. . .	. . .
Nickel[3]	. . .	. . .
Arsenic[3]	. . .	. . .
Silicon[3]	. . .	. . .
Vitamins		
Ascorbic acid (C)[4]	60 mg	100 mg
Retinol (A)[4]	1000 µg	3300 IU
Vitamin D[4]	5.0 µg	200 IU
Thiamine (B_1)[4]	1.4 mg	3.0 mg
Riboflavin (B_2)[4]	1.7 mg	3.6 mg
Pyridoxine (B_6)[4]	2.2 mg	4.0 mg
Niacin[4]	19 mg	40 mg
Pantothenic acid[4]	4–7 mg	15 mg
Vitamin E[4]	10.0 mg	10 IU
Biotin[2,4]	100–200 µg	60 µg
Folic acid[2]	400 µg	400 µg
Cyanobalamin (B_{12})[4]	2.0 µg	5.9 µg
Vitamin K[5]	70–149 µg	10 mg
Minerals		
Calcium	800 mg	0.20–0.30 meq/kg
Phosphorus	800 mg	300–400 mg/kg
Magnesium	350 mg	0.34–0.45 meq/kg
Sulfur	2–3 g	. . .

[1]Multitrace 5 mL provides the normal daily requirement.
[2]Estimated safe and adequate dose.
[3]No data available regarding human requirements.
[4]M.V.I.-12 10 mL parenterally provides the normal daily requirement.
[5]Weekly requirement.

A. Fat-Soluble Vitamins: Vitamins A, D, E, and K are absorbed in the proximal small bowel in association with bile salt micelles and fatty acids. After absorption, they are delivered to the tissues in chylomicrons and stored in large quantities in the liver (vitamins A and K) or subcutaneous tissue and skin (vitamins D and E). Fat-soluble vitamins participate in immune function and wound healing.

B. Water-Soluble Vitamins: Vitamins B_1, B_2, B_6, vitamin B_{12}, C, niacin, folate, biotin, and pantothenic acid are absorbed in the duodenum and proximal small bowel, transported in portal vein blood, and utilized in the liver and peripherally. Only vitamin B_{12} is stored to any extent. Water-soluble vitamins serve as cofactors that facilitate reactions involved in the generation and transfer of energy and in amino acid and nucleic acid metabolism. Because of their limited storage, water-soluble vitamin deficiencies are common.

Trace Elements

The daily requirements for the trace elements (Table 10–5) vary geographically owing to differences in soil composition. Trace elements have important functions in metabolism, immunology, and wound healing. Subclinical trace element deficiencies occur in many common diseases.

Iron, which is essential for hemoglobin synthesis, serves as the core of the heme prosthetic group in hemoglobin and the respiratory chain cytochromes. Impaired cerebral, muscular, and immunologic function can occur in patients with iron deficiency before anemia becomes evident.

Zinc is a cofactor for a number of metalloenzymes involved in carbohydrate, fat, amino acid, and nucleic acid metabolism. Deficiency may develop in patients with large fecal losses (eg, AIDS) or after prolonged total parenteral nutrition (TPN) in the absence of zinc supplements. Clinically, zinc deficiency is characterized by a diffuse maculopapular rash (similar to that of acrodermatitis enteropathica), poor wound healing, cutaneous anergy, hair loss, and taste and smell disturbances.

Copper is a component of a number of metalloenzymes, including cytochrome oxidase (the terminal enzyme of the electron transport chain), dopamine hydroxylase (a key enzyme in catecholamine metabolism), and lysyl oxidase (which is involved in collagen cross-linkage). Copper deficiency is manifested by anemia (unresponsive to iron) or pancytopenia.

Chromium forms a complex with a small peptide containing nicotinic acid to produce glucose tolerance factor (GTF). GTF facilitates the binding of insulin to membrane receptors. Chromium may improve glucose tolerance in patients with adult-onset diabetes mellitus. Chromium deficiency presents as sudden glucose intolerance during prolonged unsupplemented TPN without evidence of sepsis, in which case chromium therapy returns glucose tolerance to normal.

Selenium is part of the enzyme glutathione peroxidase. A decrease in the activity of this enzyme leads to peroxidation of membrane lipids, resulting in elevated concentrations of pentane in expired air. Selenium deficiency, which can occur in patients receiving TPN for a prolonged period, is manifested by proximal neuromuscular weakness or cardiac failure with electrocardiographic changes.

Manganese is the cofactor for the metalloenzymes pyruvate carboxylase and manganese-superoxide dismutase, being involved in the initial step in gluconeogenesis and in cellular antioxidant capability. Manganese deficiency is associated with weight loss, altered hair pigmentation, nausea, and low plasma levels of phospholipids and triglycerides.

Molybdenum is involved in uric acid, purine, and amino acid metabolism as a cofactor for the metalloenzymes xanthine oxidase and aldehyde oxidase. Deficiency results in elevated plasma methionine levels and depressed uric acid concentrations, producing a syndrome consisting of nausea, vomiting, tachycardia, and central nervous system disturbances.

Iodine is a key component of thyroid hormone. Deficiency is rare in the USA because of the widespread use of iodized salt. Chronically malnourished patients can become iodine-deficient, and since thyroxine participates in the neuroendocrine response to trauma and sepsis, iodine should be included in TPN solutions.

Essential Fatty Acids

The essential polyunsaturated fatty acids (PUFAs) are grouped into two families: ω-6 and ω-3 fatty acids. Linoleic acid is an example of the ω-6 PUFAs; α-linolenic acid of the ω-3 PUFAs. Vegetable oils, such as corn, safflower, sunflower, and soybean oils are good sources of linoleic acid (ω-6 PUFA). Linseed, canola, walnut, and soybean oils are good sources of α-linolenic acid (ω-3 PUFA). Cold water fish are a rich source of ω-3 fatty acids, specifically eicosapentaenoic acid (EPA) and docosahexaenoic acid (DHA). Linoleic acid (ω-6 PUFA) is desaturated by δ-6 desaturase and elongated to form arachidonic acid. Arachidonic acid is a precursor to the synthesis of eicosanoids, specifically the series-2 prostaglandins and series-4 leukotrienes. Eicosanoids are potent biochemical mediators of cell-to-cell communication and are involved in inflammation, infection, tissue injury, and immune system modulation.

Delta-6 desaturase also regulates the conversion of α-linolenic acid (ω-3 PUFA) to EPA, a precursor of less potent eicosanoids, the series-3 prostaglandins, and series-5 leukotrienes. These mediators compete with or inhibit the effects of the eicosanoids produced by the ω-6 PUFA.

Efficient functioning of the immune system depends upon a balance of eicosanoid production between the ω-6 and ω-3 PUFA. Eicosanoids modulate numerous events involving cell-mediated and humoral immunity and can be synthesized in varying amounts by all immune cells, especially macrophages and monocytes. Diets high in ω-6 fatty acids suppress immune function by inhibiting mitogenesis due to increased prostaglandin E_2 synthesis, which inhibits T cell proliferation. The administration of additional ω-3 PUFAs negates this effect.

NUTRITIONAL PATHOPHYSIOLOGY

Physiologic processes, immunocompetence, wound healing, and recovery from critical illness depend upon adequate nutrient intake. A working knowledge of nutritional pathophysiology is essential in planning nutritional regimens.

Starvation

After an overnight fast, liver glycogen is rapidly depleted because of a fall in insulin and a rise in glucagon levels in plasma (Figure 10–2). Concomitantly, there is an increase in hepatic gluconeogenesis from amino acids derived from the breakdown of muscle protein. Hepatic glucose production must satisfy the energy demands of the hematopoietic system and the central nervous system, particularly the brain, which is dependent on glucose oxidation during acute starvation. The release of amino acids from muscle is regulated by insulin, which stimulates amino acid uptake, polyribosome formation, and protein synthesis. The periodic rise and fall of insulin associated with ingestion of nutrients stimulates muscle protein synthesis and breakdown. During starvation, chronically low insulin levels result in a net loss of amino acids from muscle (ie, protein synthesis drops while protein catabolism remains unchanged). Hepatic gluconeogenesis requires energy, which is supplied by the oxidation of FFA. The fall in insulin along with a rise in plasma glucagon levels results in an increase in the concentration of cAMP in adipose tissue, which stimulates a hormone-sensitive lipase to hydrolyze triglycerides and release FFA. Gluconeogenesis and FFA mobilization require the presence of ambient cortisol and thyroid hormone (a permissive effect).

During starvation, the body attempts to conserve substrate by recycling metabolic intermediates. The hematopoietic system utilizes glucose anaerobically and increases lactate production. Lactate is recycled back to glucose in the liver via the glucogenic (not gluconeogenic) Cori cycle (Figure 10–3). The glycerol released during peripheral triglyceride hydrolysis is converted into glucose via gluconeogenesis. Alanine and glutamine are the preferred substrates for hepatic gluconeogenesis from amino acids, and they contribute 75% of the amino acid carbon for glucose production. Alanine and glutamine also constitute about 75% of the amino acids released from skeletal muscle during starvation.

Branched-chain amino acids are unique because they are secreted rather than taken up by the liver during starvation; they are oxidized by skeletal and cardiac muscle to supply a portion of the energy requirements of these tissues; and they stimulate protein synthesis and inhibit catabolism. The amino groups, which are derived from oxidation of BCAAs or transamination of other amino acids, are donated to pyruvate or α-ketoglutarate to form alanine and glutamine. Glutamine is taken up by the small bowel, transaminated to form additional alanine, and released into the portal circulation. These amino acids plus glucose participate in the glucose-alanine/glutamine-BCAA cycle, which shuttles amino groups and

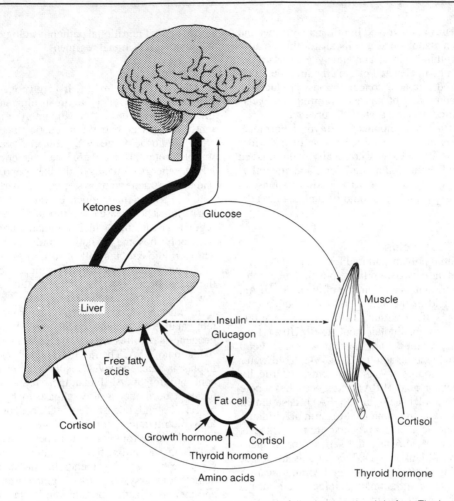

Figure 10–2. The plasma substrate concentrations and hormone levels following an overnight fast. The brain is dependent on glucose, which is supplied by gluconeogenesis from amino acids. These amino acids are derived from the breakdown of skeletal muscle protein.

carbon from muscle to liver for conversion into glucose.

Gluconeogenesis from amino acids results in a urinary nitrogen excretion of 8–12 g/d, predominantly as urea, which is equivalent to a loss of 340 g/d of lean tissue. At this rate, 35% of the lean body mass would be lost in 1 month, a uniformly fatal amount. Starvation can be survived for 2–3 months, however, as long as water is available. The explanation is that during prolonged starvation, the body adapts by decreasing energy expenditure and shifting the substrate preference of the brain (Figure 10–4). The BMR decreases by slowing the heart rate and reducing stroke work, while voluntary activity declines owing to weakness and fatigue. The nonprotein RQ, which in early starvation is 0.85 (reflecting mixed carbohydrate and fat oxidation), falls to 0.70–0.73. Blood ketone levels rise sharply, accompanied by increased cerebral ketone oxidation. Brain glucose utilization drops from 140 g/d to 60–80 g/d, decreasing the demand for gluconeogenesis. Ketones also inhibit hepatic gluconeogenesis, and urinary nitrogen excretion falls to 2–3 g/d. The main component of urine nitrogen is now ammonia (rather than urea), derived from renal transamination and gluconeogenesis from glutamine, and it buffers the acid urine that results from ketonuria.

Acute or chronic starvation is characterized by hormone and fuel alterations orchestrated by changing blood substrate levels and can be thought of as "substrate-driven" processes. In summary, the adaptive changes in uncomplicated starvation are a decrease in energy expenditure, a change in type of fuel consumed (which maximizes the caloric potential), and preservation of protein.

Elective Operation or Trauma

The effects of elective operations and trauma (Fig-

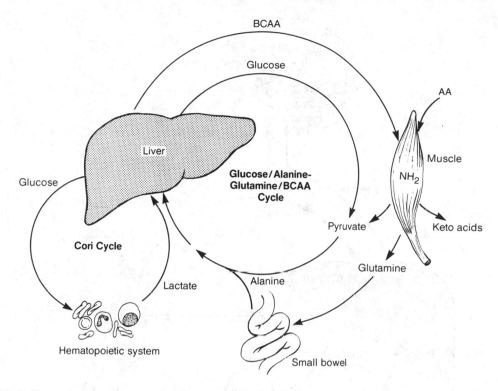

Figure 10–3. The cycles that preserve metabolic intermediates during fasting. Lactate is recycled to glucose via the Cori cycle, while pyruvate is transaminated to alanine in skeletal muscle and converted to glucose by hepatic gluconeogenesis.

ure 10–5) differ from those of simple starvation due to activation of neural and endocrine systems, which accelerates the loss of lean tissue and inhibits adaptation. Following injury, neural impulses carried via spinothalamic pathways activate the brain stem, thalamic centers, and cortical centers, which in turn stimulate the hypothalamus. The control center for the sympathetic nervous system and the trophic nuclei of the pituitary is in the hypothalamus. Consequently, hypothalamic stimulation triggers a combined neural and endocrine discharge. Norepinephrine is released from sympathetic nerve endings, epinephrine from the adrenal medulla, aldosterone from the adrenal cortex, ADH from the posterior pituitary, insulin and glucagon from the pancreas, and ACTH, TSH, and growth hormone from the anterior pituitary. This causes secondary elevations of cortisol, thyroid hormone, and somatomedins. This heightened neuroendocrine secretion produces (1) peripheral lipolysis, by the synergistic activation of hormone-sensitive lipase by glucagon, epinephrine, cortisol, and thyroid hormone; (2) accelerated catabolism, consisting of a rise in proteolysis, stimulated by cortisol; and (3) decreased peripheral glucose uptake due to insulin antagonism by growth hormone and epinephrine. These peripheral effects result in a marked rise in plasma concentrations of FFA, glyc-

erol, glucose, lactate, and amino acids. The liver responds by an increase in substrate uptake and glucose production, owing to glucagon-stimulated glycogenolysis and to enhanced gluconeogenesis induced by cortisol and glucagon.

This accelerated glucose production, along with inhibited peripheral uptake, produces the **glucose intolerance of trauma.** The kidney avidly retains water and sodium because of the effects of ADH and aldosterone. Urinary nitrogen excretion increases to 15–20 g/d in severe trauma, equivalent to a lean tissue loss of 750 g/d. Without exogenous nutrients, the median survival under these circumstances is about 15 days.

The difference in the metabolic response to accidental trauma and to elective operation is related to the intensity of the neuroendocrine stimulus. The REE rises only 10% in postoperative patients, compared with 25–30% after severe accidental trauma. The liberal use of analgesia and immobilization of injured extremities decreases the intensity of neuroendocrine stimuli, helping to spare the loss of lean body tissue.

The neuroendocrine response to trauma results in an exaggerated mobilization of metabolic substrates and a loss of the adaptive decrease in REE and nitrogen excretion seen in starvation. In contrast to the

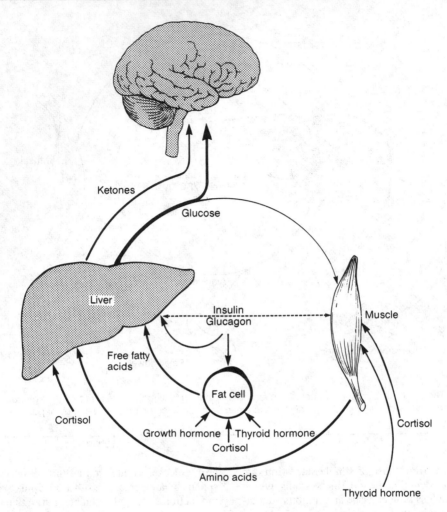

Figure 10–4. The metabolic adaptation to chronic starvation whereby the brain shifts its substrate preference to ketones produced by the liver. Hepatic gluconeogenesis falls and protein breakdown is diminished, which conserves lean tissue.

substrate dependency of uncomplicated starvation, operation and trauma are "neuroendocrine-driven" processes.

Sepsis

The metabolic changes during sepsis are somewhat different (Figure 10–6). The REE rises 50–80% above control values, and urinary nitrogen excretion reaches 20–30 g/d, equivalent to a median survival of 10 days without nutritional input. The plasma glucose, amino acid, and FFA levels increase more than in trauma, while there is an enormous increase in muscle protein catabolism along with a profound depression of protein synthesis. Hepatic protein synthesis is stimulated, with both enhanced secretion of export and accumulation of structural protein. The nonprotein RQ falls to 0.69–0.71, indicative of intense FFA oxidation. This enhanced FFA oxidation is

unresponsive to exogenous nutrients. During nutritional therapy, septic patients fail to demonstrate a rise in RQ to 1 or greater, indicating FFA synthesis from glucose. This unresponsiveness of the RQ can result in large increases in V_{CO_2} and can even precipitate respiratory failure when these patients are supported with a glucose-based TPN system. Septic patients also have an abnormal plasma amino acid pattern (ie, increased levels of AAA and decreased levels of BCAA) similar to that of patients with liver failure. Terminal sepsis results in a further increase in plasma amino acids and a fall in glucose concentration, as hepatic amino acid clearance declines and gluconeogenesis stops.

Burns

Thermal injury has a tremendous impact on metabolism because of prolonged, intense neuroendocrine

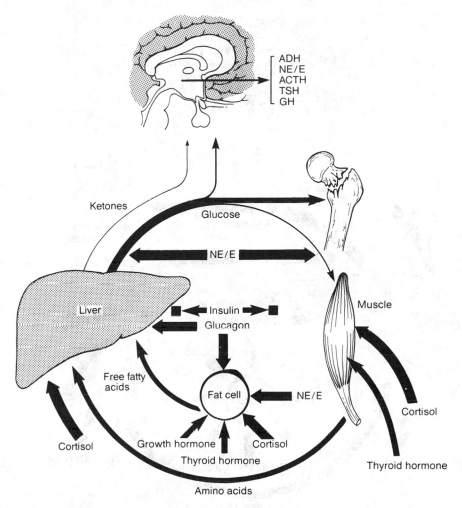

Figure 10–5. The metabolic response to trauma is a result of neuroendocrine stimulation, which accelerates protein breakdown, stimulates gluconeogenesis, and produces glucose intolerance.

stimulation. Extensive burns raise the REE 100–200% above baseline and urinary nitrogen excretion to 30–40 g/d, equivalent to a loss of 1500 g/d of lean tissue and a median survival of 7–10 days without nutritional support. The increase in metabolic demands following thermal injury is proportionate to the extent of ungrafted body surface. The principal mediator of burn hypermetabolism is elevated levels of catecholamines, which return to baseline only when skin coverage is complete. Decreasing the intensity of neuroendocrine stimulation by providing analgesia and thermoneutral environments lowers the accelerated metabolic rate in many of these patients and helps to decrease catabolic protein loss until the burned surface can be grafted.

Burned patients are also prone to infection, and cytokines activated by sepsis augment catabolism. The keratinized layer of skin contains large amounts of interleukin-1, which are released during thermal

injury, and cytokine activity may be an important stimulus of burn catabolism.

Because infection so often complicates TPN therapy in burn patients, enteral nutrition is preferred whenever tolerated. Aggressive enteral feeding should be started within the first 6–12 hours postburn to reduce the hypermetabolic response and improve postburn survival. Gastric ileus is not a problem if the tip of the nasointestinal feeding tube is passed into the duodenum.

Burn patients have increased caloric requirements (Table 10–6). In addition to maintenance needs (females, 22 kcal/kg/d; males, 25 kcal/kg/d), they require an additional 40 kcal per percent of total body surface area burned. During the hypermetabolic phase of burn injury (0–14 days), the ability to metabolize fat is restricted, so a diet that derives calories primarily from carbohydrate is preferable. Following the hypermetabolic phase, the metabolism of fat be-

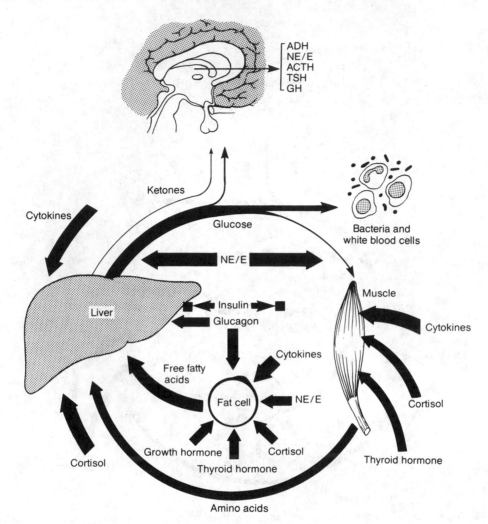

Figure 10–6. During sepsis, cytokines (IL-1, IL-2, TNF) released by lymphocytes and macrophages contribute to catabolism of muscle protein and adipose tissue and amplify the neuroendocrine response to antecedent trauma.

comes normal. The burn patient should also be given supplemental arginine, nucleotides, and ω-3 polyunsaturated fat to maintain and stimulate immunocompetence.

Cancer

Patients with cancer may have abnormal energy, protein, or carbohydrate metabolism. REE increases by 20–30% in certain malignant tumors, yet in the absence of other disease, neuroendocrine activity is normal. The increase in REE can even occur in patients with extreme cachexia, in whom a similar degree of uncomplicated starvation would produce a profound decrease in REE. Whether or not the increase in REE is proportionate to the extent of disease and volume of tumor is unsettled.

Patients with cancer avidly retain nitrogen despite losses in most lean tissue. Animal carcass analysis has shown that the retained nitrogen resides in the tumor, which behaves as a nitrogen trap. Synthesis, catabolism, and turnover of body protein are all increased, but the change in catabolism is greatest.

The changes in carbohydrate metabolism consist of impaired glucose tolerance, elevated glucose turnover rates, enhanced Cori cycle activity, and gluconeogenesis from alanine. Patients with extensive tumors are susceptible to lactic acidosis when given large glucose loads during TPN, owing to the high rate of anaerobic glucose metabolism in the neoplastic tissue.

Treatment of malnutrition with TPN does not increase tolerance to chemotherapy, response to therapy, or long-term survival, and in the absence of antineoplastic therapy, TPN therapy may even stimulate tumor growth. TPN administered postoperatively may decrease the incidence of complications in mal-

Table 10–6. Daily caloric and protein requirements for burn patients.

Estimated:
Calories (total kcal) (male or female)
    Maintenance + 40 kcal per % TBSA[1] burned
Protein (g) (male or female)
    1.5–2.5/kg

Calculated:
Calories (total kcal) for weight maintenance
    Male   = (25 kcal × preburn wt kg × BMR[2]age factor) + (40 kcal × % TBSA[1] burn)
    Female = (22 kcal × preburn wt kg × BMR[2]age factor) + (40 kcal × % TBSA[1] burn)
    Note: Add 500 kcal to the above equations for weight gain.
Protein (g)
    Male or female = (1 g protein × preburn wt kg) + (3 × % TBSA[1] burn)

[1]TBSA = Total body surface area.
[2]BMR = Basal metabolic rate:
    20–40 yr = 1.00
    40–50 yr = 0.95
    50–75 yr = 0.90
    >75 yr = 0.80

nourished patients with cancer, but the data are inconclusive.

Renal Failure

Whether intensive nutritional support improves the outcome of acute renal failure is difficult to determine because the metabolism of renal failure is so complex.

Patients with acute renal failure can have a normal or increased metabolic rate. Renal failure precipitated by x-ray contrast agents, antibiotics, aortic or cardiac surgery, or moderate periods of hypotension is associated with a normal or slightly elevated REE and a moderately negative nitrogen balance (4–8 g/d). When renal failure follows severe trauma, rhabdomyolysis, or sepsis, the REE may be markedly increased and the nitrogen balance sharply negative (15–25 g/d). When dialysis is frequent, losses into the dialysate of amino acids, vitamins, glucose, trace metals, and lipotrophic factors can be substantial.

The method of measuring nitrogen balance in renal failure is presented in Table 10–7. Nitrogen output is calculated from the urea nitrogen appearance (UNA) and the application of a correction factor for nitrogen loss in stool, skin, and feces. The UNA is the differ-

Table 10–7. Calculation of nitrogen balance in renal failure.

Nitrogen balance (g/d) = Nitrogen intake – Nitrogen output

Nitrogen output (g/d) = (0.97) (UNA) + 1.93

UNA (g/d) = Urine urea nitrogen + Dialysate urea nitrogen[1] +
    Change in body urea nitrogen

Change in body urea nitrogen = $(BUN_f - BUN_i) (BW_i)^2 (0.6)^3$
    + $(BW_f - BW_i) (BUN_f)^4$

[1]UNA (urea nitrogen appearance) is determined between dialysis runs, so this term can be dropped in final calculations.
[2]BW = body weight.
[3]0.6 = the volume of distribution of urea.
[4]f = final; i = initial.

ence in BUN levels between dialysis intervals multiplied by a factor for the volume of distribution of urea in total body water plus the change in weight (assuming weight change is due entirely to water).

Patients in renal failure (serum creatinine > 2 mg/dL) with a normal metabolic rate (UNA 4–8 g/d) who cannot undergo dialysis should receive a concentrated (maximum calories and protein per milliliter of diet) enteral or parenteral diet containing just the essential amino acids (EAA), dextrose, and limited amounts of sodium, potassium, magnesium, and phosphate.

In contrast, patients with a normal metabolic rate who can undergo dialysis should receive a concentrated enteral or parenteral diet that contains a combination of EAA and nonessential amino acids (NEAA), dextrose, and limited amounts of sodium, potassium, phosphate, and magnesium.

Hepatic Failure

Most patients with hepatic failure present with acute decompensation superimposed on chronic hepatic insufficiency. Liver disease or poor diet has usually contributed to depletion of protein, vitamins, and trace elements. Total body protein is often diminished because of poor dietary habits (eg, in alcoholics) or iatrogenic protein restriction intended to control encephalopathy. Water-soluble vitamins, including folate, ascorbic acid, niacin, thiamine, and riboflavin, are especially likely to be deficient. Fat-soluble vitamin deficiency may be a result of malabsorption due to bile acid insufficiency (vitamins A, D, K, and E), deficient storage (vitamin A), inefficient utilization (vitamin K), or failure of conversion to active metabolites (vitamin D). Hepatic iron stores may be depleted either from poor intake or as a result of gastrointestinal blood loss. Total body zinc is decreased owing to the above factors plus increased urinary excretion.

The contribution of amino acid abnormalities to hepatic encephalopathy is discussed in Chapter 24.

The use of BCAA-enriched amino acid formulations for TPN in patients with liver disease is controversial, because the results of controlled trials are inconclusive. Patients without clinical signs of encephalopathy should receive a concentrated enteral or parenteral diet that has a reduced carbohydrate content, a combination of EEA and NEAA, and limited amounts of sodium and potassium. In contrast, patients with clinical signs of encephalopathy should receive a concentrated enteral or parenteral diet that has a reduced carbohydrate content, only branched-chain amino acids, and limited amounts of sodium and potassium.

Hepatorenal Failure

Hepatorenal failure patients who cannot undergo dialysis and have clinical signs of encephalopathy should receive a concentrated enteral or parenteral diet that has a reduced carbohydrate content, only BCAA, and limited amounts of sodium, potassium, magnesium, and phosphate.

Cardiac Disease

Myocardial dysfunction may complicate malnutrition, especially in the late stages, and fatal cardiac failure can develop in extreme cachexia.

Cardiac muscle uses FFA and BCAA as preferred metabolic fuels instead of glucose. During starvation, the heart rate slows, cardiac size decreases, and the stroke volume and cardiac output fall. As starvation progresses, cardiac failure ensues, along with chamber enlargement and anasarca.

The profound nutritional depletion that may accompany chronic heart failure, particularly in valvular disease, is the result of anorexia from chronic disease and passive congestion of the liver; malabsorption due to venous engorgement of the small bowel mucosa; and enhanced peripheral proteolysis due to chronic neuroendocrine secretion.

Attempts at aggressive nutritional repletion in patients with cardiac cachexia, before or after operation, have produced inconclusive results. Concentrated dextrose (eg, 35% rather than 25%) and 7.5% amino acid preparations should be used to avoid fluid overload. Nitrogen balance should be measured to ensure adequate nitrogen intake. Lipid emulsions should be administered cautiously because they can produce myocardial ischemia and negative inotropy.

Gastrointestinal Disease

Gastrointestinal disease (eg, inflammatory bowel disease, fistula, pancreatitis) often presents nutritional problems due to intestinal obstruction, malabsorption, or anorexia. In each situation, the patient would benefit from nutritional therapy.

Chronic involvement of the ileum in inflammatory bowel disease leads to malabsorption of fat-soluble and water-soluble vitamins, calcium and magnesium, anions (phosphate), and the trace elements iron, zinc, chromium, and selenium. Protein-losing enteropathy, accentuated by transmural destruction of lymphatics, can add to protein depletion. The REE is increased by 25–30%, which prevents the adaptive hypometabolism of chronic starvation and causes a negative caloric balance. Treatment with sulfasalazine can produce folate deficiency, and glucocorticoid administration may accelerate breakdown of lean tissue and enhance glucose intolerance owing to stimulation of gluconeogenesis. Patients with inflammatory bowel disease who require elective surgery should be evaluated, and those with a recent loss of 10% of body weight should be given nutritional therapy preoperatively.

Parenteral nutrition therapy for 4–6 weeks combined with bowel rest, metronidazole, and sulfasalazine is the treatment of choice for patients with acute exacerbations of inflammatory bowel disease without bowel obstruction or perforation. Patients who fail to respond to medical therapy or develop intestinal obstruction or perforation require operation and postoperative parenteral diet therapy.

Patients with gastrointestinal fistulas can develop electrolyte, protein, fat, vitamin, and trace metal deficiencies; dehydration; and acid-balance imbalance. They require fluid replacement and aggressive nutritional therapy.

Antidiarrheal agents usually fail to reduce fluid losses from enterocutaneous fistulas, but octreotide acetate, a synthetic octapeptide analogue of somatostatin, is more effective. Octreotide suppresses the secretion of serotonin, vasoactive intestinal polypeptide, gastrin, insulin, glucagon, growth hormone, secretin, and pancreatic polypeptides and exerts widespread effects on gastrointestinal function. It prolongs intestinal transit, regulates intestinal water and electrolyte transport, and decreases splanchnic blood flow. In a dose of 50–300 μg every 6 hours (intravenously or subcutaneously) it is quite useful in the management of high-output fistulas.

Patients with fistulas also require nutritional therapy, which differs depending on the level of bowel involved. Patients with a proximal enterocutaneous fistula (ie, from the stomach to the mid ileum) should receive TPN with no oral intake. Patients with a low enterocutaneous fistula (ie, distal ileum or colon) should receive TPN initially, but after infection is brought under control, they can often be switched to an enteral formula or even a low-residue diet. The management of enterocutaneous fistulas is discussed further in Chapter 30.

Pancreatic Disease

Patients with acute pancreatitis who present with fewer than three Ranson criteria (see Chapter 27) should be treated with fluid replacement, nasogastric suction, and bowel rest for at least a week before considering parenteral nutrition. Most of these patients can resume an oral diet and do not benefit from TPN. Patients with more than three Ranson criteria should receive TPN. Enteral diets, including elemental and polypeptide formulas, are not recommended because they stimulate the pancreas and may aggravate the disease.

AIDS

Patients with AIDS develop protein-calorie malnutrition and lose weight. Many factors contribute to deficiencies of electrolytes (sodium and potassium), trace metals (copper, zinc, and selenium), and vitamins (A, C, E, pyridoxine, and folate). Dehydration occurs as a consequence of refractory diarrhea.

Enteropathy may impair fluid and nutrient absorption and produce a voluminous life-threatening diarrhea. Standard antidiarrheal agents do not control the diarrhea in AIDS patients, but octreotide often helps.

Malnourished AIDS patients require 35–40 kcal and 2.0–2.5 g protein/kg/d. In addition to the required electrolytes, vitamins, and minerals, they should receive glutamine, arginine, nucleotides, ω-3 polyunsaturated fats, branched-chain amino acids, and trace metal supplements. Those with normal gut function should be given a high-protein, high-calorie, low-fat, lactose-free oral diet. Patients with compromised gut function require an enteral (amino acid, polypeptide or immuno-enriched) diet or TPN.

ENTERAL NUTRITIONAL THERAPY

The appropriate enteral dietary regimen depends upon the patient's diagnosis, nutritional status, nutrient and fluid requirements, and alimentary tract function. In general, enteral (tube feeding) is preferable to parenteral therapy because of its lower cost and greater simplicity of administrations, because it preserves bowel immunologic function, and because it is associated with fewer technical and septic complications.

Enteral Diets

Enteral feedings may be used as a supplement or the sole source of nutrients. There are two kinds of commercial preparations—standard and special—based upon protein content or clinical application.

Standard enteral diets (Table 10–8) contain intact protein and require normal gut function for digestion and absorption. They are recommended for patients experiencing minimal metabolic stress who have normal gut function.

Special enteral diets (Table 10–8) contain protein in the form of low-molecular-weight free amino acids or polypeptides. Amino acid (elemental) and polypeptide diets are efficiently absorbed in the presence of compromised gut function. Consequently, they may be used in patients with moderate or severe metabolic stress and abnormal gut function. Also included in the special enteral ducts are those formulated for specific clinical situations (eg, pulmonary, renal, or hepatic failure or immune dysfunction).

The available preparations (Table 10–8) vary in (1) caloric and protein content; (2) protein, carbohydrate, and fat composition; (3) nonprotein carbohydrate calorie-to-gram nitrogen ratio; (4) osmolality; (5) content of minor trace metals (selenium, chromium, and molybdenum); (6) glutamine or glutamic acid (glutamate) content; and (7) branched-chain amino acid content.

Enteral Diet Administration

Enteral diets are administered via a nasointestinal feeding tube whose tip has been positioned radiographically in the proximal duodenum. Nasointestinal feeding is used for short-term (< 6 weeks) nutritional therapy and is administered continuously through a tube with a volumetric pump. Bolus and gravity feedings are not recommended because of the risk of gastric distention and aspiration. A nasogastric feeding tube (ie, a tube whose distal tip is in the stomach) should be avoided because of the risk of gastric distention and aspiration. Percutaneous gastrostomy and jejunostomy feeding tubes are recommended for long-term (> 6 weeks) nutritional therapy.

Before infusing an enteral diet, one should confirm radiographically that the tip of the feeding tube is in the duodenum.

The infusion schedule depends on the formula's osmolality. Isosmolar diets are initially infused full-strength via pump at a rate of 40 mL/h. The rate is then advanced according to the schedule in Table 10–9. Hyperosmolar diets are initially infused one-quarter strength at a rate of 40 mL/h. The infusion rate is then advanced according to the schedule in Table 10–9. The final infusion rate depends on the patient's estimated caloric and protein requirements, age, and cardiovascular status.

Enteral nutritional therapy orders should indicate the desired formula and monitoring guidelines. The protocol in the box on the next page is an example.

PARENTERAL NUTRITIONAL THERAPY

When the gastrointestinal tract cannot be used, nutrients must be given parenterally. Since parenteral nutrition is more expensive is associated with more technical, metabolic, and septic complications, and requires more expertise than enteral nutrition, it should only be used when the gut cannot be used. Parental formulas deliver 75–150 nonprotein carbohydrate calories per gram of nitrogen infused, a ratio that maximizes carbohydrate and protein assimilation and minimizes metabolic complications (aminoacid-

---

PROTOCOL FOR NASOGASTRIC FEEDING

1. Insert a nasointestinal feeding tube.
2. Obtain a stat portable KUB postinsertion to confirm the position of the nasointestinal feeding tube in the small bowel. Notify the physician when a plain film of the abdomen (KUB) is completed.
3. Begin _____ (enteral diet) at _____ (strength) at a rate of _____ mL/h continuously per volumetric pump via the nasointestinal feeding tube when notified by the physician that the feeding tube is positioned in the small bowel.
4. Elevate the head of the bed 30 degrees or more while administering the enteral diet.
5. Only liquid medications or powdered solids suspended in liquid by a pharmacist should be administered via the feeding tube.
6. Flush the feeding tube every 4 hours with 20 mL of sterile water.
7. Check on the amount of residual fluid by aspirating the feeding tube every 4 hours. If the residual is > 150 mL, discontinue the infusion for 2 hours. After 2 hours, recheck again for residual. If the residual is < 150 mL, restart the enteral diet infusion. If the residual remains > 150 mL, do not restart the infusion until the physician is notified.
8. Inform the physician about persistent residuals >150 mL, increasing abdominal distention, nausea, vomiting, diarrhea, or an oral temperature > 38 °C (100.4 °F).
9. Record intake and output (I/O) with strict accuracy. Total the I/O every 24 hours.
10. Record the patient's weight weekly on the vital signs sheet.
11. Check the urine for sugar and acetone daily and record the results on the vital signs sheet. If the urine sugar is 4+, obtain a stat serum glucose determination. If the serum glucose is > 160 mg/dL, contact the physician for treatment orders.
12. Begin (per the nasointestinal feeding tube):
    a. Neutra-Phos (phosphate supplement): 1 or 2 capsules (250 mg/capsule) dissolved in 75–150 mL of the enteral diet 4 times daily.
    b. Zinc sulfate (zinc supplement): 200 mg added to the enteral diet twice daily.
    c. Titralac (calcium supplement): 2 tsp added to the enteral diet twice daily.
13. Routine enteral diet laboratory samples are to be drawn weekly on the day and at the times specified below:

    Thursday AM: CBC, SMAC-20, copper, zinc, magnesium, transferrin, and triglyceride.

---

uria, hyperglycemia, and hepatic glycogenesis). There are two methods: peripheral parenteral nutrition (PPN) and total parenteral nutrition (TPN). In addition to route of administration, the two differ in 1) the dextrose and amino acid (protein) content of the parenteral solution, 2) primary caloric source (glucose vs. fat), 3) frequency of fat administration, 4) infusion schedule and 5) potential complications (Table 10–10).

1. PERIPHERAL PARENTERAL NUTRITION (PPN)

Indications

PPN therapy is indicated for patients with compromised gut function who require short-term (< 10 days) nutrition because they are unable to ingest adequate nutrients. It is contraindicated for patients who can be nourished via the gut.

PPN Solution Formulation

One liter of standard PPN solution contains $D_{20}W$, 500 mL; 10% amino acids, 500 mL; plus electrolytes, vitamins, minerals, and trace metals. $D_{20}W$ contains 20 g glucose per 100 mL (100 g per 500 mL). Since the metabolism of 1 g glucose yields 3.4 kcal, the metabolism of 500 mL of $D_{20}W$ yields 340 kcal. Therefore, 1 L of standard PPN solution ($D_{20}W$ 500 mL + 10% amino acids 500 mL) provides 340 kcal.

A 10% amino acid solution contains 10 g protein per 100 mL or 50 g protein per 500 mL. Since 1 g of nitrogen is equivalent to 6.25 g of protein, 50 g of protein is equivalent to 8 g of nitrogen. Therefore, 1 L of standard PPN solution ($D_{20}W$ 500 mL + 10% amino acids 500 mL) provides approximately 8 g of nitrogen.

The ratio of nonprotein carbohydrate calories to grams of nitrogen in 1 L of standard PPN solution is approximately 43:1 (340 kcal per 8 g nitrogen = 43 kcal/g nitrogen).

Since 1 L of standard PPN solution contains adequate nitrogen but inadequate calories, the daily PPN regimen should also include 500 mL of 20% fat emulsion (2 kcal/mL). Table 10–11 lists the various PPN additives and gives the basic formulation of a standard liter of PPN solution. By giving PPN solution at 125 mL/h and supplementing it with 500 mL of 20% fat emulsion daily, PPN provides about 2200 kcal and 150 g protein (24 g nitrogen) daily.

Fat is an excellent source of calories, but, as mentioned earlier, it should not be used to provide more

Table 10–8. Standard and special enteral diets.

Name	kcal/mL	NPC:N$_2$ Ratio[1]	mosm/kg H$_2$O	g protein/mL	g fat/mL	Na$^+$ (meq/mL)	K$^+$ (meq/mL)
Intact protein, lactose-free							
Nutren 1.0	1.00	131:1	300	.040	.038	.022	.032
Nutren 1.0 with fiber	1.00	131:1	303	.040	.038	.022	.032
Replete	1.00	75:1	350	.063	.033	.022	.040
Ensure	1.06	153:1	450	.037	.037	.037	.040
Ensure HN	1.06	125:1	470	.044	.035	.040	.040
Isocal	1.06	167:1	300	.034	.044	.023	.034
Osmolite	1.06	153:1	300	.037	.038	.028	.026
Osmolite HN	1.06	125:1	310	.044	.037	.040	.040
Intact protein, lactose-free, high density							
Nutren 1.5	1.50	131:1	410	.060	.068	.033	.048
Nutren 2.0	2.00	131:1	710	.080	.106	.044	.064
Isocal HCN	2.00	145:1	690	.075	.091	.035	.036
Isotein HN	1.20	86:1	300	.068	.034	.027	.027
TwoCal HN	2.00	126:1	740	.083	.091	.046	.059
Blenderized meat-based							
Compleat Modified Formula	1.07	131:1	300	.043	.037	.029	.036
Compleat Regular Formula	1.07	131:1	405	.043	.043	.056	.036
Vitaneed	1.00	154:1	310	.035	.040	.022	.032
Free amino acid							
Vivonex T.E.N.	1.00	149:1	630	.038	.003	.020	.020
Stresstein	1.20	97:1	910	.070	.028	.028	.028
Polypeptide							
Peptamen	1.00	131:1	270	.040	.039	.022	.032
Vital HN	1.00	125:1	460	.041	.011	.020	.034
Pepti 2000	1.00	156:1	490	.040	.010	.029	.029
Specific organ failure							
Pulmonary							
Nutrivent	1.50	115:1	450	.068	.095	.033	.057
Pulmocare	1.50	125:1	490	.062	.092	.057	.049
Renal							
Travasorb Renal	1.35	363:1	590	.023	.018	. . .	. . .
Amin-Aid	1.00	830:1	1095	.019	.046	<.015	<.006
Hepatic							
Travasorb Hepatic	1.10	218:1	600	.029	.015	.010	.023
Hepatic-Aid	1.10	148:1	560	.044	.036	<.015	<.006
Immuno-enriched							
Impact	1.00	71:1	375	.056	.028	.046	.032

[1]NPC:N$_2$ ratio = ratio of nonprotein calories to nitrogen.

than 60% of the patient's estimated daily caloric requirement.

Administration

PPN is infused via an 18-gauge intravenous cannula in a peripheral vein. A 16-gauge single-lumen central venous catheter (SLCVC) positioned in the superior vena cava via the subclavian or internal jugular vein may also be used. A peripheral PPN catheter site is dressed like any other peripheral intravenous site. A central PPN catheter site is dressed like a TPN catheter site (discussed below). Standard PPN therapy orders (Figure 10–7) should include the administration schedule for the PPN solution and fat supplement as well as explicit catheter care orders and monitoring guidelines.

Special PPN Solutions

A. Concentrated: Since the final dextrose concentration of a PPN solution cannot exceed 12.5%, it is impossible to formulate a concentrated PPN solution for patients on restricted fluid intake (eg, cardiac disease, renal failure). Consequently, PPN is contraindicated in the treatment of fluid-restricted patients.

B. Nonoliguric Renal Failure: Patients in nonoliguric renal failure (serum creatinine > 2 mg/dL) who can tolerate the PPN regimen of 3500 mL daily and who cannot be dialyzed should receive a special renal failure PPN solution and daily fat supplements. One liter of this solution should contain a combination of $D_{20}W$ 500 mL and renal failure amino acids (essential amino acids only) 500 mL plus limited amounts of sodium, potassium, magnesium, and phosphate.

Table 10–9. Enteral diet infusion schedule.

Hours	Strength	Rate (mL/h via pump)
ISOSMOLAR (280–300 mosm/kg water)		
24	Full	40
24	Full	80
24	Full	100–125[1]
HYPEROSMOLAR (> 300 mosm/kg water)		
24	One-fourth	40
24	One-half	40
24	Full	40
24	Full	80
24	Full	100–125[1]

[1]The final infusion rate is dependent upon the patient's calculated total caloric and protein requirements, overall cardiovascular status, and toleration of the diet.

C. Hepatic Failure: Patients with hepatic encephalopathy who can tolerate the daily 3500 mL infusion should receive a special hepatic failure PPN solution that contains $D_{20}W$ 500 mL and hepatic failure amino acids (primarily branched-chain amino acids) 500 mL plus additives, with the exception that sodium content is limited to < 40 meq/L.

2. TOTAL PARENTERAL NUTRITION (TPN)

Indications

TPN is indicated for patients who cannot be nourished enterally and need more than 10 days of nutritional support.

Solution Formulation

One liter of standard TPN solution contains $D_{50}W$ 500 mL, 8.5% amino acids 500 mL, plus electrolytes, vitamins, minerals, and trace metals.

$D_{50}W$ contains 50 g of glucose per 100 mL or 250 g per 500 mL (and thus 850 kcal). An 8.5% amino acid solution contains 8.5 g of protein per 100 mL or 42.5 of protein (or 6.8 g of nitrogen) per 500 mL. Therefore, 1 L of standard TPN solution ($D_{50}W$ 500 mL + 8.5% amino acids 500 mL) provides approximately 1000 kcal and 6.8 g of nitrogen; and the ratio of nonprotein carbohydrate calories to grams of nitrogen is approximately 125:1.

Patients receiving TPN should also receive 3–5% of their daily caloric requirement as fat in order to prevent a fatty acid deficiency. This is accomplished by giving 500 mL of 20% fat emulsion (2 kcal/mL) intravenously over 6–8 hours at least three times per week. TPN therapy also includes additives as listed in Table 10–12.

1. PPN components:

ROUTINE ADDITIVES	Recommended Dosage Ranges per Liter PPN	BAG #___	BAG #___	BAG #___
D₂₀W	500 mL	500 mL	500 mL	500 mL
AA 10%	500 mL	500 mL	500 mL	500 mL
NaCl	0–140 meq	meq	meq	meq
NaPO₄	0–20 mmol	mmol	mmol	mmol
K⁺Cl	0–40 meq	meq	meq	meq
MgSO₄	0–12 meq	meq	meq	meq
Ca gluconate	4.5 or 9 meq	meq	meq	meq
MVI-12®	10 mL/d	10 mL		
Multitrace®	5 mL/d	5mL		
OPTIONAL ADDITIVES				
Na acetate	0–140 meq	meq	meq	meq
K⁺ acetate	0–40 meq	meq	meq	meq
Regular insulin	0–40 units	units	units	units
H₂ antagonist**				
NURSE'S SIGNATURE				

* TOTAL POTASSIUM CONTENT PER LITER OF PPN SHOULD NOT EXCEEED 40 meq.
** DIVIDE THE DAILY DOSAGE EQUALLY INTO EACH LITER OF PPN.

RATE: __100–125__ mL/h via pump.
Final dextrose concentration __10_ % Final AA concentration __10__ %

2. Pharmacy to add vitamin K 10 mg to 1 L of PPN solution every Mon. and Thurs.
3. Insert at least an 18-gauge peripheral IV and begin the PPN infusion at 100–125 mL/h per pump.
4. Infuse 500 mL 20% fat emulsion daily IVPB over 6–8 hours via at least an 18-gauge peripheral IV.
5. Strict I/O every shift. Total the I/O every 24 hours.
6. Record the daily weight in kilograms on the vital signs sheet.
7. Check the urine for sugar and acetone every shift and record on the vital signs sheet. If the urine sugar is 4+, request a STAT serum glucose measurement to be drawn by the physician. If the serum glucose is > 160 mg/dL, contact the physician for treatment orders.
8. Notify the physician if the oral temperature is >38°C (>100.4°F).
9. Routine PPN laboratory tests are to be drawn weekly on the days and times specified below:
   - Sun. AM: CBC, SMAC-20
   - Tues. AM: Electrolytes, BUN, creatinine, and glucose
   - Thurs. AM: CBC, SMAC-20, copper, zinc, magnesium, transferrin, and triglycerides
10. Begin a 24-hour urine collection for urinary urea nitrogen (UUN) at 6:00 AM every Mon. for nitrogen balance determination.
11. PPN catheter dressing and tubing changes per the hospital IV protocol.
12. Contact the physician for all problems related to PPN.
13. All changes in PPN therapy must be approved by the physician.

Figure 10–7. PPN therapy orders.

Administration

In patients over age 10, TPN solutions are routinely administered via a single-lumen central venous catheter (SLCVC) with a Luer-Lok connection. The distal port of a triple-lumen central venous catheter (TLCVC) may be used, but this results in a higher incidence of catheter infection.

The TPN catheter is inserted either into the superior vena cava via the internal jugular or subclavian vein or into the inferior vena cava via the femoral vein. Because of the discomfort and increased risk of infection associated with neck and groin insertions, they are not recommended. The TPN catheter site is dressed with a sterile gauze or transparent, occlusive, polyurethane dressing.

Table 10–10. Partial (PPN) versus total (TPN) therapy: Indications, contraindications, and characteristic features.

	Standard PPN Therapy	Standard TPN Therapy
Clinical indications	Short-term (< 10 days) supplemental or total nutritional therapy.	Long-term (> 10 days) supplemental or total nutritional therapy.
Clinical contraindications	(1) Patients who are able to consume their daily caloric, protein, and other required nutrients per oral or enteral feedings. (2) Patients who require long-term (> 10 days) total nutritional therapy because of gut dysfunction.	(1) Patients who are unable to consume their daily caloric, protein, and other required nutrients per oral or enteral feedings. (2) Patients who require short-term (< 10 days) total nutritional therapy because of gut dysfunction.
Primary source of calories	Fat metabolism.	Dextrose metabolism.
Dextrose content	$D_{20}W$	$D_{50}W$
Protein content	10% amino acids (essential and nonessential).	8.5% amino acids (essential and nonessential).
Fat therapy	Fat emulsion 20% 500 mL daily.[1]	Fat emulsion 20% 500 mL every Monday, Wednesday, and Friday.
Route of administration	Peripheral 18-gauge intravenous cannula or a central intravenous infusion catheter with the distal tip positioned in the superior or inferior vena cava.	Central intravenous infusion catheter with the distal tip positioned in the superior or inferior vena cava.
Infusion schedule (mL/h via pump)	Day 1: 100–125[3]	Day 1: 40
Therapeutic monitoring	CBC, blood chemistries, and 24-hour nitrogen balance determination.[4]	CBC, blood chemistries, and 24-hour nitrogen balance determination.[1]
Complications	Technical, infectious, and metabolic (Tables 10–13 and 10–15).[5]	Technical, infectious, and metabolic (Tables 10–13 and 10–15).[5]
Rebound hypoglycemia	No risk.[6]	Risk.[7]

[1]Fat emulsion therapy provides the major source of calories.

[2]Fat emulsion 20% 500 mL is administered intravenously via at least an 18-gauge peripheral intravenously or central venous catheter positioned in the superior vena cava per pump over 4–6 hours. Fat therapy should provide at least 4–6% of the daily caloric requirement to prevent the development of a fatty acid deficiency. The frequency and quantity of fat administered weekly may be increased depending on the patient's estimated daily caloric requirement.

[3]The final infusion rate is dependent upon the patient's calculated daily caloric and protein requirements, age, and overall cardiovascular status.

[4]Sunday AM: CBC and SMAC-20; Monday (6:00 AM): Begin 24-hour urine collection for urinary urea nitrogen (UUN) and nitrogen balance determination; Tuesday AM: electrolytes, BUN, creatinine, and glucose; and Thursday AM: CBC, SMAC-20, copper, zinc, magnesium, transferrin, triglyceride, prealbumin, and retinol-binding protein.

[5]Phlebitis is the most common complication.

[6]PPN therapy can be discontinued at any time without the risk of rebound hypoglycemia.

[7]The discontinuance of central TPN therapy may result in rebound hypoglycemia if the patient is either NPO or has inadequate enteral caloric intake. To avoid rebound hypoglycemia in these patients, the central TPN solution must be tapered or replaced with a $D_{10}W$ infusion at the previous infusion rate.

The solution is initially infused at a rate of 40 mL/h via a constant infusion pump. The rate should be 40 mL/h on the first day, 80 mL/h on the second day, and 100–125 mL/h on the third day. The final rate, achieved within 72 hours, depends on the patient's daily caloric and protein requirements, age, and cardiovascular status. Standard TPN therapy orders (Figure 10–8) should include the administration schedule for the TPN solution and fat supplement as well as explicit catheter care orders and monitoring guidelines.

Special TPN Solutions

A. Concentrated: The TPN solution must be more concentrated for patients who require fluid restriction (eg, those with pulmonary and cardiac failure). One liter of concentrated TPN solution usually contains a combination of $D_{60}W$ or $D_{70}W$ 500 mL and 10% or 15% amino acids 500 mL plus additives.

B. Renal Failure: Patients in renal failure (serum creatinine > 2 mg/dL) who cannot be dialyzed and who require fluid restriction should receive a special renal failure TPN solution. Each liter of solution contains a combination of $D_{60}W$ or $D_{70}W$ 500 mL and renal failure amino acids (essential amino acids only) 500 mL plus limited amounts of sodium, potassium, magnesium, and phosphate.

Patients in renal failure who can undergo dialysis should receive a TPN solution that contains $D_{60}W$ or $D_{70}W$ and 8.5% standard amino acids (a combination of essential and nonessential) 500 mL plus additives, with limited amounts of sodium, potassium, magnesium, and phosphate.

C. Hepatic Failure: Patients with hepatic en-

Table 10–11. PPN solution formulation.

Components in 1 L of PPN:	
Routine additives	
$D_{20}W$[1]	500 mL
10% amno acid[1]	500 mL
Sodium chloride[2]	0–140 meq
Sodium phosphate[3]	0–20 mmol
Potassium chloride[4]	0–40 meq
Magnesium sulfate[5]	0–12 meq
Calcium gluconate[5,6]	4.5 or 9.0 meq
M.V.I.-12[7]	10 mL
Multitrace[7]	5 mL
Optional additives	
Sodium acetate[2]	0–140 meq
Potassium acetate[4]	0–40 meq
H_2 antagonist[8]	Variable[8]
Regular insulin[9]	0–40 units

Administration schedule for standard PPN:

Day of Therapy	Rate (mL/h)
1	40
2	80
3	100–125[10]

Fat emulsion schedule:

Infuse a 20% fat emulsion 500 mL intravenously via pump over 6–8 hours at least daily via either an 18-gauge peripheral intravenous cannula or piggyback per the central infusion catheter.

[1]The solution is formulated to deliver 43 nonprotein carbohydrate calories per gram of nitrogen infused.
[2]Add sodium chloride if the serum $CO_2 > 25$ meq/L. Add sodium acetate if the serum $CO_2 \leq 25$ meq/L.
[3]The total phosphate dosage should not exceed 20 mmol/L or 60 mmol daily.
[4]Add KCl if the serum $CO_2 > 25$ meq/L. Add potassium acetate if the serum $CO_2 \leq 25$ meq/L. The potassium dosage should not exceed 40 meq/L.
[5]Added to each liter.
[6]Add calcium gluconate 9 meq to each liter if the serum calcium < 8.5 meq/L. Add 4.5 meq if the serum calcium ≥ 8.5 meq/L.
[7]Administered in only 1 L per day.
[8]Dosage depends upon the H_2 antagonist selected. Divide the daily dosage equally in all liters of PPN administered.
[9]Total dosage should not exceed 40 units/L.
[10]The final infusion rate is dependent upon the patient's calculated daily caloric and protein requirements and overall cardiovascular status.

Table 10–12. TPN solution formulation.

Components in 1 L of standard TPN:	
Routine additives	
$D_{50}W$[1]	500 mL
8.5% amino acid[1]	500 mL
Sodium chloride[2]	0–140 meq
Sodium phosphate[3]	0–20 mmol
Potassium chloride[4]	0–40 meq
Magnesium sulfate[5]	0–12 meq
Calcium gluconate[5,6]	4.5 or 9.0 meq
M.V.I.-12[7]	10 mL
Multitrace[7]	5 mL
Optional additives	
Sodium acetate[2]	
Potassium acetate[4]	0–140 meq
H_2 antagonist[8]	0–40 meq
Regular insulin[9]	Variable[8]
	0–40 units

Administration schedule for standard TPN:

Day of Therapy	Rate (mL/h)
1	40
2	80
3	100–125[10]

Fat emulsion schedule:

Infuse a 20% fat emulsion 500 mL intravenously via pump over 6–8 hours at least 3 times per week via either an 18-gauge peripheral intravenous cannula or piggyback per the central infusion catheter.

[1]The solution is formulated to deliver 125 nonprotein carbohydrate calories per gram of nitrogen infused.
[2]Add sodium chloride if the serum $CO_2 > 25$ meq/L. Add sodium acetate if the serum $CO_2 \leq 25$ meq/L.
[3]The total phosphate dosage should not exceed 20 mmol/L or 60 mmol daily.
[4]Add KCl if the serum $CO_2 > 25$ meq/L. Add potassium acetate if the serum $CO_2 \leq 25$ meq/L. The potassium dosage should not exceed 40 meq/L.
[5]Added to each liter.
[6]Add calcium gluconate 9 meq to each liter if the serum calcium < 8.5 meq/L. Add 4.5 meq if the serum calcium ≥ 8.5 meq/L.
[7]Administered in only 1 L per day.
[8]Dosage depends upon the H_2 antagonist selected. Divide the daily dosage equally in all liters of TPN administered.
[9]Total dosage should not exceed 40 units/L.
[10]The final infusion rate is dependent upon the patient's calculated daily caloric and protein requirements and overall cardiovascular status.

cephalopathy should receive a hepatic failure TPN solution that contains a combination of $D_{30}W$ or $D_{40}W$ 500 mL and a special hepatic failure amino acid solution (branched-chain amino acids) 500 mL plus additives, with the exception of limited amounts of sodium (< 40 meq/L).

COMPLICATIONS OF NUTRITIONAL THERAPY

1. ENTERAL THERAPY
(Tables 10–13 and 10–14)

Technical complications occur in about 5% of enterally fed patients and include plugging of the tube; esophageal, tracheal, bronchial, or duodenal perforation; and tracheobronchial intubation with tube feeding aspiration. The tip of the feeding tube must be positioned in the duodenum radiographically; any other method is unreliable and runs the risk of a gastric infusion and its potential complications.

Functional complications—including nausea, vom-

1. TPN components:

ROUTINE ADDITIVES	Recommended Dosage Ranges per Liter TPN	BAG #___	BAG #___	BAG #___
$D_{50}W$	500 mL	500 mL	500 mL	500 mL
AA 8.5%	500 mL	500 mL	500 mL	500 mL
NaCl	0–140 meq	meq	meq	meq
$NaPO_4$	0–20 mmol	mmol	mmol	mmol
K^+Cl	0–40 meq	meq	meq	meq
$MgSO_4$	0–12 meq	meq	meq	meq
Ca gluconate	4.5 or 9 meq	meq	meq	meq
MVI-12®	10 mL/d	10 mL		
Multitrace®	5 mL/d	5mL		
OPTIONAL ADDITIVES				
Na acetate	0–140 meq	meq	meq	meq
K^+ acetate	0–40 meq	meq	meq	meq
Regular insulin	0–40 units	units	units	units
H_2 antagonist**				
25% albumin***	25 g	g	g	g
NURSE'S SIGNATURE				

* TOTAL POTASSIUM CONTENT PER LITER OF TPN SHOULD NOT EXCEEED 40 meq.
** DIVIDE THE DAILY DOSAGE EQUALLY INTO EACH LITER OF TPN.
*** ONLY IF THE SERUM ALBUMIN < 2.5g/dL AND ENTERAL DIET THERAPY IS ANTICIPATED.

RATE: ___40___ mL/h via pump.
Final dextrose concentration __25_% Final AA concentration _4.25_%

2. Pharmacy to add vitamin K 10 mg to 1 L of TPN solution every Mon. and Thurs.
3. Fat emulsion 20% 500 mL every Mon., Wed., and Fri. IVPB per pump over 6–8 hours via at least an 18-gauge peripheral IV or via the subclavian catheter.
4. STAT upright and expirational portable chest x-ray to check the position of the subclavian catheter and to rule out a pneumothorax. Notify the physician when the chest x-ray is completed.
5. Heparin lock the TPN catheter with 2 mL of heparin (100 units/mL) until notified by the physician to start the first liter of TPN solution.
6. Strict I/O every shift. Total the I/O every 24 hours.
7. Record the daily weight in kilograms on the vital signs sheet.
8. Check the urine for sugar and acetone every shift and record on the vital signs sheet. If the urine sugar is 4+, request a STAT serum glucose measurement to be drawn by the physician. If the serum glucose is > 160 mg/dL, contact the physician for treatment orders.
9. Notify the physician if the oral temperature is >38°C (>100.4°F).
10. Routine TPN laboratory tests are to be drawn weekly on the days and times specified below:
    Sun. AM: CBC, SMAC-20
    Tues. AM: Electrolytes, BUN, creatinine, and glucose
    Thurs. AM: CBC, SMAC-20, copper, zinc, magnesium, transferrin, and triglycerides
11. Begin a 24-hour urine collection for urinary urea nitrogen (UUN) at 6:00 AM every Mon. and Thurs. for nitrogen balance determination.
12. TPN catheter dressing and tubing changes per the hospital TPN protocol.
13. Contact the physician for all problems related to TPN.
14. All changes in TPN therapy must be approved by the physician.

Figure 10–8. TPN therapy orders.

iting, abdominal distention, constipation, and diarrhea—occur in 25% of tube-fed patients and are the main reason for intolerance to enteral diets. Nausea, vomiting, and abdominal distention can be minimized by infusing into the duodenum rather than the stomach and giving the diet continuously rather than as a bolus.

Diarrhea is usually the result of polypharmacy (eg, multiple antibiotics), mechanical gut dysfunction (eg, partial small bowel obstruction), intestinal bacterial overgrowth (eg, *Clostridium difficile*), protein con-

tent or osmolality of the diet, intrinsic bowel disease (eg, inflammatory bowel disease), or systemic disease (eg, HIV infection, amyloidosis). Treatment consists of stopping any medications at fault, correcting gut dysfunction, giving appropriate antibiotics, modifying the protein content (intact protein vs. amino acid or polypeptide formula) or osmolality of the diet, adding pectin or fiber to the diet, or administering antidiarrheal agents.

Electrolyte abnormalities (principally hyper- and hyponatremia; hyper- and hypokalemia; hypophosphatemia; and hypomagnesemia) occur in about half of patients. Hyperglycemia severe enough to cause hyperosmolar nonketotic acidosis may occur.

2. PARENTERAL NUTRITION

PPN Therapy
(Tables 10–13 and 10–15)

Technical complications of PPN are few. The most common problem is maintenance of venous access. Because it causes phlebitis, the PPN infusion catheter must often be moved to another site. Since most patients have few usable peripheral veins, prolonged PPN (> 10 days) is rarely possible. The addition of fat, heparin, or corticosteroids to PPN solutions has not decreased the incidence of phlebitis.

Infectious complications such as catheter site skin infection and septic phlebitis develop in 5% of patients.

TPN Therapy (Table 13–15)

Technical, infectious, and metabolic complications each occur in 5% of patients, and the overall mortality rate directly attributable to TPN is 0.2%.

The most common technical complications are inability to cannulate the subclavian vein, malposition of the catheter, pneumothorax bleeding, and air embolism.

Air embolism—a rare but often lethal complication of subclavian vein catheterization—is characterized by sudden, severe respiratory distress (tachypnea), hypotension, and a cogwheel murmur. To prevent air embolism, the subclavian line should be inserted only with the patient tilted into a head-down position. It is also critical that the line not be disconnected when the patient is upright. This is easier to ensure if Luer-Lok connections are used.

Treatment of air embolism involves placing the patient with left side down, head down, and feet (Durant position) elevated and aspirating blood and air through the subclavian catheter (Figure 10–9).

Catheter site infection is characterized by mild fever (37.5–38 °C [99.5–100.4 °F]), pus around the catheter tract, and erythema and tenderness of the surrounding skin. Late changes include induration of the skin and systemic sepsis.

Primary line (catheter) infection is more difficult

Table 10–13. Nutritional therapy complications.

Enteral Nutrition	Total Parenteral Nutrition
Technical	**Technical**
Abscess of nasal septum	Air embolus
Acute sinusitis	Arterial laceration
Aspiration pneumonia	Brachial plexus injury
Bacterial contamination of formula	Arteriovenous fistula
Esophagitis-ulceration-stenosis	Brachial plexus injury
Gastrointestinal perforation	Cardiac perforation
Gastrostomy/jejunostomy dislodgment	Catheter embolism
Hemorrhage	Catheter malposition
Hoarseness	Pneumothorax
Inadvertent tracheobronchial intubation	Subclavian vein thrombosis
Intestinal obstruction	Thoracic duct laceration
Intracranial passage of tube	Venous laceration
Knotting of tube	
Laryngeal ulceration	
Nasal erosions	
Necrotizing enterocolitis	
Otitis media	
Pneumatosis intestinalis	
Rupture of varices	
Skin excoriation	
Tracheoesophageal fistula	
Functional	**Infectious**
Nausea	Catheter fever
Vomiting	Catheter tip
Abdominal distension	Catheter exit site
Constipation	Catheter tip with bacteremia
Diarrhea	
Metabolic	**Metabolic**
Dehydration	Azotemia
EFA deficiency	EFA deficiency
Hyperglycemia	Fluid overload
Hyperkalemia	Hyperchloremic metabolic acidosis
Hypernatremia	Hypercalcemia
Hyperosmolar nonketotic coma	Hyperkalemia
Hyperphosphatemia	Hypermagnesemia
Hypokalemia	Hypernatremia
Hypocupremia	Hyperosmolar nonketotic coma
Hypoglycemia	Hyperphosphatemia
Hypomagnesemia	Hypervitaminosis A
Hyponatremia	Hypervitaminosis D
Hypophosphatemia	Hypocalcemia
Hypozincemia	Hypokalemia
Liver function test elevation	Hypomagnesemia
Overhydration	Hyponatremia
Vitamin K deficiency	Hypophosphatemia
	Liver function test elevation
	Metabolic bone disease
	Trace element deficiency
	Ventilatory failure

to diagnose than is local catheter site infection. Because catheter infections are twice as common (10% versus 5%) with triple-lumen than with single-lumen catheters, the latter are much preferred. The principal findings are (1) unexplained hyperglycemia (serum glucose > 160 mg/dL), (2) a plateau pattern of fever (38–38.5 °C [100.4–101.3 °F]) for 12–24 hours, (3) leukocytosis (> 10,000/μL), and (4) positive blood cultures from a remote vein as well as from the suspect catheter. Skin changes are rare.

Patients with a suspected catheter infection who have negative blood cultures and no cardiovascular compromise should have the catheter exchanged over a guide-wire and the tip sent for bacterial and fungal cultures. If the fever resolves and subsequent cultures are negative (colony count < 15), no further therapy is necessary. If the patient remains febrile after the catheter exchange or continues to have positive blood or catheter cultures, a new central catheter should be inserted at another site. The most common metabolic complications (Tables 10–13 and 10–15) are hyperglycemia (serum glucose > 160 mg/dL), electrolyte and mineral abnormalities, and acidosis.

Patients with severe malnutrition and weight loss

Table 10–14. Management of complications of enteral nutrition.

Complication	Treatment
Diarrhea	(1) Check the actual serum albumin (ASA) level. If the level < 2.5 g/dL, calculate the albumin deficit (AD) by means of the **Andrassy formula:** $$AD = (2.5 - ASA) \times 0.3 \times 10 \times \text{wt kg}$$ Then administer 25% albumin 25 g intravenously every 6 hours until the calculated albumin deficit is replaced. Recheck the serum albumin. If the serum albumin level ≥ 2.5 g/dL, no further albumin therapy is necessary. If the level < 2.5 g/dL, recalculate the albumin deficit and administer additional albumin intravenously until the serum albumin ≥ 2.5 g/dL. *or* Hetastarch 250 mL/d for 1 or 2 days. (2) Administer antidiarrheal agents: Deodorized tincture of opium 15–20 drops orally or by nasointestinal tube every 4–6 hours as needed. *or* Diphenoxylate with atropine 1 or 2 tablets (2.5 mg/tab) orally every 4–6 hours or 5–10 mL (2.5 mg/5 mL) per nasointestinal tube every 4–6 hours as needed. *or* Loperamide 1 or 2 caps (2 mg/cap) orally every 4–6 hours or 10–20 mL (1 mg/5 mL) per nasointestinal tube every 4–6 hours as needed. *or* Ocreotide acetate 50–350 mg subcutaneously or intravenously every 6 hours as needed. (3) If the above measures fail, discontinue the current enteral diet and begin Peptamin or Compleat Modified Formula (full strength) enteral diet at 40 mL/h per pump. If tolerated (no diarrhea), increase the infusion rate per the Isosmolar Enteral Diet Infusion Schedule. (4) If the above measures fail, discontinue enteral nutritional therapy and begin parenteral nutritional therapy.
Residuals (> 150 mL)	(1) Examine the patient and rule out the possibility of either a mechanical intestinal obstruction or paralytic ileus. (2) Confirm the position of the feeding tube in the small bowel per KUB. (3) Check the serum potassium and calcium levels. (4) Consider a pharmacologic etiology.
Hyperglycemia (> 160 mg/dL)	Reduce the oral glucose intake and administer regular insulin subcutaneously per a sliding scale regimen. If this fails to maintain the serum glucose ≤ 160 mg/dL, discontinue the current full-strength enteral diet and begin either a less concentrated infusion of the current diet or begin a new full-strength diet that has a lower glucose content (consult the *Physician's Desk Reference*) at the previous infusion rate.
Hypoglycemia (< 65 mg/dL)	Administer one ampule of $D_{50}W$ intravenously and then recheck the serum glucose. If the serum glucose remains < 70 mg/dL, administer additional $D_{50}W$ until the serum glucose ≥ 70 mg/dL. If the patient continues to require intravenous glucose supplements, discontinue the current full-strength enteral diet and begin a new full-strength diet that has a greater glucose content (consult the *Physician's Desk Reference*) at the previous infusion rate.
Hypernatremia (> 145 meq/L)	Evaluate need for increasing or decreasing water intake. If needed, reduce or discontinue all oral and intravenous sodium intake. If this fails to maintain the serum sodium ≤ 145 meq/L, discontinue the current full-strength enteral diet and begin either a less concentrated infusion of the current diet or begin a new full-strength diet that has a lower sodium content (consult the *Physician's Desk Reference*) at the previous infusion rate.
Hyponatremia (< 135 meq/L)	Evaluate need for increasing or decreasing water intake. If needed, administer additional sodium intravenously until the serum sodium ≥ 135 meq/L. If intravenous sodium supplementation fails to correct the hyponatremia, discontinue the full-strength enteral diet and begin a new full-strength diet that has a greater sodium content (consult the *Physician's Desk Reference*) at the previous infusion rate.
Hyperkalemia (> 5 meq/L)	Discontinue all oral and intravenous potassium intake. If this fails to maintain the serum potassium ≤ 5 meq/L, discontinue the current full-strength enteral diet and begin a new full-strength diet that has a lower potassium content (consult the *Physician's Desk Reference*) at the previous infusion rate.
Hypokalemia (< 3.5 meq/L)	Administer additional potassium orally or intravenously until the serum potassium ≥ 3.5 meq/L. If the patient continues to require excessive oral or intravenous potassium supplements, discontinue the currrent full-strength enteral diet and begin a new full-strength diet that has a greater potassium content (consult the *Physician's Desk Reference*) at the previous infusion rate.

(continued)

Table 10–14. Management of complications of enteral nutrition. (continued)

Complication	Treatment
Hyperphosphate-mia (> 4.5 mg/dL)	Discontinue all oral and intravenous phosphate intake. If this fails to maintain the serum phosphate ≤ 4.5 mg/dL, discontinue the current full-strength enteral diet and begin a new full-strength diet that has a lower phosphate content (consult the *Physician's Desk Reference*) at the previous infusion rate.
Hypophosphatemia (< 2.5 mg/dL)	Administer additional phosphate either orally as Neutra-Phos 1 or 2 capsules (250 mg/cap) dissolved in 75–150 mL of tube feeding 2–4 times daily (consult the *Physician's Desk Reference* for additional enteral phosphate preparations) or iv4 times daily (consult the *Physician's Desk Reference* for additional enteral phosphate preparations) or intravenously as sodium or potassium phosphate to maintain the serum phosphate ≥ 2.5 mg/dL. (***Note:*** *The daily intravenous phosphate dosage should not exceed 60 mmol.*)
Hypermagnesemia (> 3 mg/dL)	Discontinue all intravenous and oral magnesium intake. If this fails to maintain the serum magnesium ≤ 3 mg/dL, discontinue the current full-strength enteral diet and begin either a less concentrated infusion of the current diet or begin a new full-strength diet that has a lower magnesium content (consult the *Physician's Desk Reference*) at the previous infusion rate.
Hypomagnesemia (< 1.6 mg/dL)	Administer additional magnesium either orally or intravenously to maintain the serum magnesium ≥ 1.6 mg/dL. Consult the *Physician's Desk Reference* for the various enteral and parenteral magnesium preparations.
Hypercalcemia (> 10.5 mg/dL)	Discontinue all oral and intravenous calcium supplements. If this fails to maintain the serum calcium ≤ 10.5 mg/dL. If this fails to maintain the serum sodium ≤ 145 meq/L, discontinue the current full-strength enteral diet and begin a new full-strength diet that has a lower calcium content (consult the *Physician's Desk Reference*) at the previous infusion rate.
Hypocalcemia (< 8.5 mg/dL)	Administer additional calcium either orally or as Titralac 2 tsp added to the tube feeding twice daily or intravenously as calcium gluconate 10–30 meq daily to maintain the serum calcium ≥ 8.5 mg/dL. Consult the *Physician's Desk Reference* for additional enteral and parenteral calcium preparations.
High serum zinc (> 150 µg/dL)	Discontinue all oral and intravenous zinc intake until the serum zinc ≤ 150 µg/dL.
Low serum zinc (< 50 µg/dL)	Administer additional zinc either orally as zinc sulfate 200 mg 3 or 4 times daily or intravenously as elemental zinc 2–5 mg daily to maintain a serum zinc ≥ 50 µg/dL. Consult the *Physician's Desk Reference* for additional enteral and parenteral zinc preparations.
High serum copper (> 140 µg/dL)	Discontinue all oral and intravenous copper intake until the serum copper ≤ 140 µg/dL.
Low serum copper (< 70 µg/dL)	Administer additional copper either orally (consult the *Physician's Desk Reference* for the various enteral copper preparations) or intravenously as elemental copper 2–5 mg daily to maintain a serum copper > 70 µg/dL.

(> 30% of their usual weight) may develop sudden cardiopulmonary failure during TPN, a complication known as the "refeeding syndrome." In starvation, energy is derived principally from fat metabolism. TPN results in a shift from fat to glucose as the predominant fuel, which increases the production of phosphorylated intermediates of glycolysis and inhibits fat metabolism, thereby trapping phosphate and resulting in hypophosphatemia. Hypophosphatemia decreases ventricular stroke work and mean arterial pressure and produces severe congestive cardiomyopathy as a consequence of deficient ATP production and subsequent cell and tissue damage.

Because of these risks, the rate of TPN for a severely malnourished patient (< 70% of usual weight) should be slowly increased over several days. Instead of trying to meet the patient's nutritional requirements within 72 hours, the infusion should be raised by increments of 5–10 mL daily and only if the patient's heart rate is less than 100 beats/min.

Severely malnourished patients should also receive intravenous fat supplements and sodium phosphate, the latter to prevent hypophosphatemic cardiomyopathy. The daily phosphate dosage should not exceed 60 mmol. When oral nutrient intake is low, discontinuation of TPN may cause rebound hypoglycemia unless the infusion is decreased gradually.

The recommended tapering schedule for a patient with no oral nutrient intake (NPO) who is receiving TPN at an infusion rate of 125 mL/h is as follows: Start an infusion of $D_{10}NS$ at 40 mL/h via pump into a peripheral vein. Then proceed as follows: (1) Decrease the TPN infusion rate to 80 mL/h and continue the $D_{10}NS$ at 40 mL/h for 2 hours; (2) then decrease the TPN infusion rate to 40 mL/h and increase the $D_{10}NS$ infusion rate to 80 mL/h for 2 hours; and, finally, (3) discontinue the TPN infusion and increase the $D_{10}NS$ infusion rate to 125 mL/h. Once the TPN infusion is discontinued, the central catheter can be used to infuse the $D_{10}NS$ (peripheral intravenous catheter is removed or preserved with a heparin lock).

The TPN infusion rate does not need to be tapered if the patient has adequate oral nutrient intake.

Table 10–15. Complications of TPN.

Complication	Treatment

Catheter sepsis
Incidence
  Single-lumen catheter: 3–5%
  Triple-lumen catheter: 10%
Diagnosis:
  • Unexplained hyperglycemia (> 160 mg/dL)
  • "Plateau" temperature elevation (> 38 °C) for several hours or days. (**Note:** *An isolated spike or "picket fence" temperature pattern is usually not indicative of an infected catheter.*)
  • Leukocytosis (> 10,000/μL)
  • Exclusion of other potential sources of infection,
 	
      or
 	
  • A positive blood culture (> 15 colony count) aspirated via the TPN catheter or obtained peripherally,
 	
      or
 	
  • Catheter site induration, erythema, or purulent drainage.
	Algorithms:
	Negative blood cultures and no cardiovascular signs of sepsis:
	(1) Aspirate a blood specimen via the TPN catheter and peripherally for bacterial and fungal culture and then sterilely exchange the preexisting TPN catheter for a new catheter over a guidewire; submit the previous catheter tip for bacterial and fungal culture and colony count; and continue the TPN infusion.
	
	        then
	
	(2) Monitor the patient's temperature closely. If the patient defervesces, no further therapy is necessary. If the fever continues or recurs, remove the catheter and insert a new one on the contralateral side and continue the TPN infusion.
	
	Positive blood culture or cardiovascular signs of sepsis:
	(1) Aspirate a blood specimen via the TPN catheter and peripherally for bacterial and fungal culture. Then remove the catheter immediately, and submit the catheter tip for bacterial and fungal culture and colony count.
	
	        then
	
	(2) Insert a new TPN infusion catheter on the contralateral side and continue the TPN infusion.
	
	        then
	
	(3) Initiate appropriate antibiotic therapy.

Hyperglycemia
(> 160 mg/dL)
	Algorithms:
	(1) Maintain the current TPN infusion rate and begin adding regular insulin to the TPN solution in 10-unit increments until the serum glucose is maintained at ≤ 160 mg/dL. (**Note:** *The maximum allowable insulin dosage per liter of TPN is 40 units.*) Until the hyperglycemia is controlled by adding insulin to the TPN solution, simultaneously administer intravenous regular insulin. (**Note:** *One unit of regular insulin results in an approximately 10 mg/dL increase in the serum glucose. The maximum intravenous dose of regular insulin should not exceed 15 units.*) If the serum glucose remains > 160 mg/dL despite the addition of a total of 40 units of regular insulin per liter of TPN and intravenous regular insulin therapy,
	
	        then
	
	(2) Maintain the current TPN infusion rate but begin gradually decreasing the final dextrose concentration of the TPN solution. (**Note:** *The lower limit for the final dextrose concentration is 15%.*) In addition, begin adding regular insulin to the TPN solution in 10-unit increments until the serum glucose is maintained at ≤ 160 mg/dL or the maximum allowable insulin dosage (40 units) is reached. Regular insulin should also be simultaneously administered intravenously as in (1) above until the hyperglycemia is controlled by adding insulin to the TPN solution. If the serum glucose remains > 160 mg/dL despite the addition of 40 units of regular insulin per liter of TPN solution, decreasing the final TPN dextrose concentration to 15%, and intravenous regular insulin therapy,
	
	        then
	
	(3) Restart the original TPN solution as in (1) above but begin decreasing the TPN infusion rate. Also begin insulin therapy as discussed in (2) above while simultaneously increasing the frequency of fat emulsion therapy from every Monday, Wednesday and Friday to daily to provide adequate caloric intake.

Hypoglycemia (< 65 mg/dL)	May occur with the sudden discontinuance of TPN infusion. If the TPN infusion administered to either an NPO patient or a patient consuming inadequate oral calories is suddenly discontinued, immediately begin an infusion of $D_{10}NS$ at the previous TPN infusion rate via either the TPN catheter or a peripheral IV to prevent rebound hypoglycemia.
Hypernatremia (> 145 meq/L)	Determine the cause. Hypernatremia secondary to dehydration is treated by administering additional "free water" and providing only the daily maintenance sodium requirements (90–150 meq/L) via the TPN infusion. Hypernatremia secondary to increased sodium intake is treated by reducing or deleting sodium from the TPN solution until the serum sodium ≤ 145 meq/L.

(continued)

Table 10–15. Complications of TPN. (continued)

Complication	Treatment
Hyponatremia (< 135 meq/L)	Determine the cause. Hyponatremia secondary to dilution is treated by fluid restriction and by providing only the daily maintenance sodium requirements (90–150 meq/L). Hyponatremia secondary to inadequate sodium intake is treated by increasing the sodium content of the TPN solution until the serum sodium ≥ 135 meq/L. (***Note:** The maximum sodium content per liter of TPN should not exceed 154 meq.*)
Hyperkalemia (> 5 meq/L)	Immediately discontinue the current TPN infusion containing potassium and begin an infusion of $D_{10}NS$ at the previous TPN infusion rate. Then reorder a new TPN solution without potassium and continue to delete potassium from the TPN solution until the serum potassium ≤ 5 meq/L.
Hypokalemia (< 3.5 meq/L)	A TPN solution should not be utilized for the primary treatment of hypokalemia. The potassium content per liter of TPN solution should not exceed 40 meq. If additional potassium is necessary, it should be administered via another route, eg, IV interrupts.
Hyperphosphatemia (> 4.5 mg/dL)	Immediately discontinue the present phosphate-containing TPN infusion and begin an infusion of $D_{10}NS$ at the previous infusion rate. Then reorder a new TPN solution without phosphate and continue to delete phosphate from the TPN solution until the serum phosphate ≤ 4.5 mg/dL.
Hypophosphatemia (< 2.5 mg/dL)	Increase the phosphate content of the TPN solution to a maximum of 20 mmol/L. (***Note:** The total daily phosphate dosage should not exceed 60 mmol.*)
Hypermagnesemia (> 3 mg/dL)	Immediately discontinue the present magnesium-containing TPN infusion and begin an infusion of $D_{10}NS$ at the previous infusion rate.
Hypomagnesemia (< 1.6 mg/dL)	Increase the magnesium content of the TPN solution to a maximum of 12 meq/L. (***Note:** The total daily dosage of magnesium should not exceed 36 meq.*)
Hypercalcemia (> 10.5 mg/dL)	Immediately discontinue the present calcium-containing TPN infusion and begin an infusion of $D_{10}NS$ at the previous TPN infusion rate. Then reorder a new TPN solution without calcium and continue to delete calcium from the TPN dilution until the serum calcium ≤ 10.5 mg/dL.
Hypocalcemia (< 8.5 mg/dL)	Increase the calcium content of the TPN solution to a maximum of 9 meq/L. (***Note:** The total daily calcium dosage should not exceed 27 meq.*)
High serum zinc (> 150 µg/L)	Discontinue the trace metal supplement (Multitrace 5 mL) in the TPN solution until the serum zinc ≤ 150 µg/L.
Low serum zinc (< 550 µg/dL)	Add elemental zinc 2–5 mg daily to 1 L of TPN solution only until the serum zinc ≥ 55 µg/dL. (***Note:** The elemental zinc is added in addition to the daily supplement.*)
High serum copper (> 140 µg/dL)	Discontinue the trace metal supplement in the TPN solution until the serum copper ≤ 140 µg/dL.
Low serum copper (< 70 µg/dL)	Add elemental copper 2–5 mg daily to 1 L of TPN solution only until the serum copper ≥ 70 µg/dL. (***Note:** The elemental copper is added in addition to the daily Multitrace 5 mL.*)
Hyperchloremic metabolic acidosis (CO_2 < 22 mmol/L and Cl^- > 110 meq/L)	Reduce the chloride intake by administering the Na^+ and K^+ in the acetate form as either sodium or potassium acetate (or both) until the acidosis resolves (serum CO_2 ≥ 22 mmol/L) and the serum chloride level returns to normal (< 110 meq/L).

DIETS

Optimal Diet

An optimal diet (Table 10–15) should have the following distribution of energy sources: carbohydrate 55–60%, fat 30%, protein 10–15%. Refined sugar should constitute no more than 15% of dietary energy and saturated fats no more than 10%, the latter balanced by 10% monounsaturated and 10% polyunsaturated fats. Cholesterol intake should be limited to about 300 mg/d (one egg yolk contains 250 mg of cholesterol). The amount of salt in the average American diet, 10–18 g, far exceeds the recommended 3 g. For Western societies to meet the criteria for an optimal diet, consumption of fat would have to decrease (from 40%) and carbohydrate (principally complex

carbohydrates such as potatoes and whole grain bread) would have to increase. As a source of protein, meat is presently overemphasized at the expense of grain, legumes, and nuts. Diets that chronically include substantial fish intake have been associated with a decrease in numbers of deaths from cardiovascular disease. The active ingredient is ω-3 fatty acids, principally eicosapentaenoic and docosahexaenoic acids.

Many adults, particularly those who drink no milk, consume inadequate amounts of calcium. In women this may result in calcium deficiency and skeletal calcium depletion, which in later years predispose to osteoporosis and possibly fractures (eg, of the hip or vertebrae).

The amount of fiber in Western diets averages 25

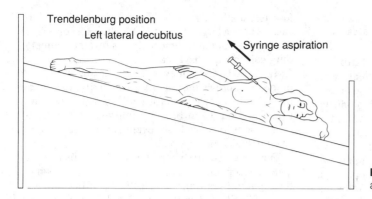

Figure 10–9. Durant position for treatment of air embolism.

g/d, but some persons ingest as little as 10 g/d. Fiber is a chemically complex group of indigestible carbohydrate polymers, which includes cellulose, hemicellulose, lignins, pectins, gums, and mucilages. It is thought that people who consume low-fiber diets are more prone to the development of chronic constipation, appendicitis, diverticular disease, diabetes mellitus, colonic neoplasms, and the irritable bowel syndrome. Thus, increased fiber intake would probably be beneficial, though the evidence for this is not conclusive. Fiber can be obtained in the form of bran in cereals and bread. It can also be obtained from fruit, potatoes, rice, and leafy vegetables.

Many therapeutic diets are archaic and based on currently unaccepted concepts of illness. For example, low-residue diets are no longer considered to be useful for diverticulitis. The "progressive diet," designed for postoperative feeding and consisting of a clear liquid (high in sodium), then a full liquid (high in sucrose), then a regular diet, is based on outmoded concepts. When peristalsis returns after operation, as evidenced by bowel sounds and ability to tolerate water, most patients are able to ingest a regular diet. The following paragraphs describe briefly the therapeutic diets most commonly prescribed in clinical practice.

Regular Diets

Regular diets have an unrestricted spectrum of foods and are most attractive to the patient. An average regular hospital diet for 1 day contains 230–275 g of carbohydrate, 70–75 g of fat, and 95–110 g of protein, with a total caloric content of 2000–2500 kcal. This composition reflects the nutritional needs of healthy persons of average height and weight and will not meet the increased demands imposed by malnutrition or disease.

Soft Diet

A soft diet is nutritionally the same as a regular diet, but high-fiber vegetables and meats or shellfish with a tough texture are omitted.

Bland Diet

In a bland diet, caffeine, spices, alcohol, and hot or cold foods have been eliminated from the regular diet. Contrary to former belief, a bland diet has no specific therapeutic usefulness in peptic ulcer disease or any other condition.

Low-Residue Diet

Low-residue diets are restricted in the amounts of fibrous vegetables, raw fruits, nuts, and milk. They emphasize lean meat, starchy vegetables, refined cereals, and simple carbohydrates. Low-residue diets are expensive because of the large amounts of meat. Constipation may require stool softeners, bulk-forming agents such as psyllium (Metamucil, etc), or cathartics.

Clear Liquid Diets:

Clear liquid diets contain easily digestible carbohydrates, small amounts of protein, and a caloric concentration of about 600 kcal per 2000 mL. A clear liquid diet is often prescribed for 1–2 days after an abdominal operation before the patient can resume a less restricted diet. There is no rationale for this practice, which deprives the patient of adequate nutrition for a few days longer than necessary. The diet is inadequate in all nutrients except for Vitamin C.

Full Liquid Diets

Full liquid diets include a wide spectrum of juices and other foods that remain liquid at body temperature. Caloric content is about 1700 kcal per 2500 mL, with 45 g of protein, 60 g of fat, and 240 g of carbohydrates. This diet may be useful for patients with an anatomic or neurologic esophageal abnormality.

Sodium-Restricted Diets

Sodium-restricted diets are often indicated for patients with cardiovascular or renal disease. Daily sodium intake in an unrestricted diet ranges from 4 to 6 g (174–261 meq Na^+). In general, a 2000-mg sodium diet is enough restriction for most patients; more severe restriction is indicated for refractory cases.

Lactose Intolerance & Lactose-Free Diets

A lactose-free diet is indicated for patients who have symptoms such as diarrhea, bloating, or flatulence after the ingestion of milk or milk products. Lactose intolerance is genetically determined and in adults is found in 5–10% of European Caucasians, 60% of Ashkenazic Jews, and 70% of blacks. A previously subclinical lactose intolerance commonly becomes unmasked by an unrelated disease or operation on the gastrointestinal tract. For example, following gastrectomy, symptomatic relief from nonspecific complaints may be obtained by interdicting lactose-containing foods. Similar advice is often useful in managing patients with Crohn's disease, ulcerative colitis, and AIDS. The frequency of lactose intolerance is high enough in the general population that it should be considered as a possible cause of flatulence and diarrhea in many clinical circumstances. The efficiency of lactose digestion and absorption can be measured by giving 100 g of lactose orally and measuring the blood lactose concentration at 30-minute intervals for 2 hours. Patients with lactose intolerance exhibit a rise in blood glucose of 20 mg/dL or less. However, unpredictable variations in gastric emptying interfere with the reliability of this test, so in most cases it is better to observe the results of eliminating lactose from the diet than to perform a lactose tolerance test. A lactose-free diet may be deficient in Ca^{2+}, vitamin D, and riboflavin.

OBESITY

Massively obese patients—those who weigh more than twice the calculated ideal weight—are handicapped physically, emotionally, socially, and economically. This degree of excessive weight has been termed **morbid obesity** to emphasize the life-threatening seriousness of the condition. Complications such as arthritis, hypertension, diabetes mellitus, hyperlipidemia, and Pickwickian syndrome may develop. The death rate is greater for morbidly obese people than for people of average weight.

Obesity is quantified according to the body mass index (BMI), which is calculated as follows:

$$BMI = \frac{Weight\ (kg)}{Height\ (m)^2}$$

The average BMI in our society is 25; 28 is considered the threshold for obesity.

The standard approach to therapy for obesity begins with reducing diets and medical counseling. Unfortunately, these measures are almost uniformly unsuccessful in patients with severe obesity. Weight loss is usually disappointing, and in the 5–10% of cases where a large amount of weight is lost on a rigid dieting program, it is almost always regained quickly. Surgical therapy is acceptable for patients whose BMI exceeds 40 if they strongly desire surgery in order to improve the quality of their lives. Surgery may also be appropriate for patients with a BMI between 30 and 40 in order to improve serious comorbid conditions, such as severe sleep apnea or obesity-related cardiomyopathy.

The first operation for obesity that gained widespread acceptance was jejunoileal bypass, in which the jejunum was transected 14 inches from the ligament of Treitz and anastomosed to the terminal ileum 4 inches from the ileocecal valve. Weight loss resulted from malabsorption due to the shortened bowel and from deceased food intake. However, late follow-up demonstrated an unacceptable rate of serious metabolic complications. Protein deficiency occurred in about 25% of patients, sometimes causing liver disease that occasionally progressed to hepatic cirrhosis. Renal stones were very common. Consequently, jejunoileal bypass is now rarely used. Patients suffering from late complications of a jejunoileal bypass should have the bypassed intestine put back into continuity. A concomitant gastric bypass is necessary if weight loss from the earlier procedure is to be maintained.

Gastric Bypass & Gastroplasty

The operations now in use for weight control are designed to decrease food intake. One way to accomplish this is to wire the patient's jaws shut so that intake is restricted to fluids. Experience has shown that when the wires are removed, however, the patient regains the weight.

Operations on the stomach can permanently curtail food intake and are more acceptable to the patient than is wiring of the jaws. The three types of gastric operations that have been used to treat obesity are (1) horizontal gastroplasty, (2) gastric bypass, and (3) vertical banded gastroplasty.

A. Horizontal Gastroplasty: Horizontal gastroplasty involves placing a row of staples across the proximal stomach to create a small (50 mL) proximal pouch and a small (1 cm) channel for the passage of food. The channel is made by removing a few staples from either the lesser or greater curvature end of the staple line or by constructing a small side-to-side anastomosis between the proximal and distal gastric pouches. Because of stomal dilatation or staple line separation, the late results of horizontal gastroplasty are not as good as those of the other two gastric procedures, so it cannot be recommended.

B. Gastric Bypass and Vertical Banded Gastroplasty: (Figure 10–10.) Gastric bypass is performed by placing four rows of staples across the proximal stomach to form a small (eg, 30–50 mL) pouch and then constructing a Roux-en-Y gastrojeju-

Vertical banded
gastroplasty

Roux-en-Y
gastric bypass

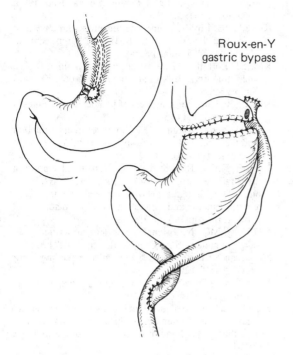

Figure 10–10. Operations for obesity.

brings the patient within 30% of the ideal weight. Thereafter, the weight tends to remain stable unless the stoma has dilated. In general, patients who lose at least 25% of their preoperative weight benefit from the procedure.

The failure rate of vertical banded gastroplasty (due to staple disruption, etc) appears to be higher than for gastric bypass. In one prospective randomized study, success (defined as loss of more than 50% of excess weight) was 17% for horizontal gastroplasty, 48% for vertical banded gastroplasty, and 67% for gastric bypass. Success also depends greatly upon continued cooperation of the patient in avoiding high-calorie liquid foods, such as milkshakes. In addition to the cosmetic benefits, patients who lose large amounts of weight following surgery have a decreased risk of obesity-related disease (eg, cardiac, pulmonary, metabolic).

Supplemental B vitamins, iron, and folate must be given postoperatively.

Benotti PN: Vertical banded gastroplasty in the treatment of severe obesity. Mayo Clin Proc 1991;66:862.
Cates JA et al: Reoperative surgery for the morbidly obese. Arch Surg 1990;125:1400.
Dean P, Joshi S, Kaminski DL: Long-term outcome of reversal of small intestinal bypass operations. Am J Surg 1990;159:118.
Garrow J: Importance of obesity. Br Med J 1991;303:704.
Gastrointestinal surgery for severe obesity: Consensus Development Conference Panel. Ann Intern Med 1991;115:956.
Gleysteen JJ, Barboriak JJ, Sasse EA: Sustained coronary-risk-factor reduction after gastric bypass for morbid obesity. Am J Clin Nutr 1990;51:774.
Goodrick GK, Foreyt JP: Why treatments for obesity don't last. J Am Diet Assoc 1991;91:1243.
Hall JC et al: Gastric surgery for morbid obesity. Ann Surg 1990;211:419.
Hirsch J, Leibel RL: A biological basis for human obesity. J Clin Endocrinol Metab 1991;73:1153.
MacLean LD, Rhode BM, Forse RA: Late results of vertical banded gastroplasty for morbid and super obesity. Surgery 1990;107:20.
Mason EE, Scott DH: Reoperation for failed gastric bypass procedures for obesity. Surg Clin North Am 1991;71:45.
Nightengale ML et al: Prospective evaluation of vertical banded gastroplasty as the primary operation for morbid obesity. Mayo Clin Proc 1991;66:773.
Yale CE, Weiler SJ: Weight control after vertical banded gastroplasty for morbid obesity. Am J Surg 1991;162:13.
Zimmerman ME et al: Alterations in body composition after gastroplasty for morbid obesity. Scand J Gastroenterol 1990;25:263.

nostomy to the pouch with a stoma 1 cm in diameter. The distal part of the stomach is left out of continuity with the path of food.

Vertical banded gastroplasty involves the creation of a small (eg, 30 mL) gastric pouch with a restricted outlet along the lesser curvature distal to the gastroesophageal junction. During surgery, a 32F dilator is passed orally and positioned along the lesser curvature. Two 10-cm rows of staples are placed adjacent to each other, parallel to and just at the left border of the dilator. Finally, a 5-cm ring of plastic (eg, Silastic; polypropylene) tubing or mesh is sutured around the lower end of this channel to prevent it from dilating.

Patients are restricted to liquids for a few weeks postoperatively and are then given a blenderized diet. Solid foods are allowed after 2 months. In most cases, the amount of weight lost in the first 1–2 years following gastric bypass or vertical banded gastroplasty

REFERENCES

Nutritional Therapy

Baue AE: Nutrition and metabolism in sepsis and multisystem organ failure. Surg Clin North Am 1991; 71:549.

Becker WK, Pruitt BA Jr: Parenteral nutrition in the thermally injured patient. Compr Ther 1991;17:47.

Benya R, Mobarhan S: Enteral alimentation: Administration and complications. J Am Coll Nutr 1991;10:209.

Bounos G: Elemental diets in the prophylaxis and therapy for intestinal lesions: An update. Surgery 1989; 105:571.

Bower RH: Nutritional and metabolic support of critically ill patients. JPEN J Parentr Enteral Nutr 1990;14(5 Suppl):S257.

Burzstein S, Elwyn DH, Kvetan V: Nutritional and metabolic support. Crit Care Clin 1991;7:451.

Chandra RK: Nutrition and immunity: Lessons from the past and new insights into the future. Am J Clin Nutr 1991;53:1087.

Christou N: Perioperative nutritional support: Immunologic defects. JPEN J Parentr Enteral Nutr 1990; 14(Suppl):186.

Compher C, Mullen JL, Barker CF: Nutritional support in renal failure. Surg Clin North Am 1991;71:597.

Conly JM et al: A prospective, randomized study comparing transparent and dry gauze dressings for central venous catheters. J Infect Dis 1989;159:310.

Cortes V, Nelson LD: Errors in estimating energy expenditure in critically ill surgical patients. Arch Surg 1989;124:287.

Daly JM et al: Dietary protein prevents bacterial translocation from the gut. JPEN J Parentr Enteral Nutr 1991;15:295.

Daly JM et al: Nutritional support of patients with cancer of the gastrointestinal tract. Surg Clin North Am 1991;71:523.

Douglas RG, Shaw JHF: Metabolic response to sepsis and trauma. Br J Surg 1989;76:115.

Dudrick PS, Souba WW: Amino acids in surgical nutrition: Principles and practice. Surg Clin North Am 1991;71:459.

Ellis LM, Copeland EM 3d, Souba WW: Perioperative nutritional support. Surg Clin North Am 1991;71:493.

Feliciano DV et al: Enteral versus parenteral nutrition in patients with severe penetrating abdominal trauma. Contemp Surg 1991;39:3036.

Fischer JE: Branched-chain-enriched amino acid solutions in patients with liver failure. JPEN J Parentr Enteral Nutr 1990;14(Suppl):226.

Good RA, Lorenz E: Influence of energy levels and trace metals on health and life span. JPEN J Parentr Enteral Nutr 1990;14(5 Suppl):S230.

Gorlin R: The biological actions and potential clinical significance of dietary omega-3 fatty acids. Arch Intern Med 1988;148:2043.

Hickey MS: Nutritional support of patients with AIDS. Surg Clin North Am 1991;71:645.

Hickey MS: Enteral and parenteral nutrition. In: *Drug Therapy,* 2nd ed. Katzung BG (editor). Appleton & Lange, 1991.

Hwang TL et al: Effects of intravenous fat emulsion on respiratory failure. Chest 1990;97:934.

Jeejeebhoy KN, Detsky AS, Baker JP: Assessment of nutritional status. JPEN J Parentr Enteral Nutr 1990; 14(5 Suppl):S193.

Kinsella JE: Lipids, membrane receptors and enzymes: Effects of dietary fatty acids. JPEN J Parentr Enteral Nutr 1990;14(5 Suppl):S200.

Kirk SJ, Barbul A: Role of arginine in trauma. sepsis. and immunity. JPEN J Parentr Enteral Nutr 1990;14(5 Suppl):S226.

Klasing K: Nutritional aspects of leukocytic cytokines. J Nutr 1988;118:1436.

Kotler DP et al: Magnitude of body-cell-mass depletion and the timing of death from wasting in AIDS. Am J Clin Nutr 1989;50:444.

Latifi R, Killam RW, Dudrick SJ: Nutritional support in liver failure. Surg Clin North Am 1991;71:567.

Lipman TO: Clinical trials of nutritional support in cancer: Parenteral and enteral therapy. Hematol Oncol Clin North Am 1991;5:91.

McCarthy MC: Nutritional support in the critically ill surgical patient. Surg Clin North Am 1991;71:83.

Mobarhan S, Trumbore LS: Enteral tube feeding. Nutr Rev 1991;49:129.

Mobarhan S, Trumbore LS: Nutritional problems of the elderly. Clin Geriatr Med 1991;7:191.

Ng EH, Lowry SF: Nutritional support and cancer cachexia. Evolving concepts of mechanisms and adjunctive therapies. Hematol Oncol Clin North Am 1991; 5:161.

Payne-James JJ, Silk DB: Hepatobiliary dysfunction associated with total parenteral nutrition. Dig Dis Sci 1991;9:106.

Phelps SJ et al: Toxicities of parenteral nutrition in the critically ill. Crit Care Clin 1991;7:725.

Pingleton SK, Harmon GS: Nutritional management in acute respiratory failure. JAMA 1987;257:3094.

Robinson EN, Fogel R: SMS 201-995, a somatostatin analogue, and diarrhea in the acquired immunodeficiency syndrome (AIDS). (Letter.) Ann Intern Med 1988;109:680.

Sax HC: Practicalities of lipids: ICU patient, autoimmune disease, and vascular disease. JPEN J Parentr Enteral Nutr 1990;14(5 Suppl):S223.

Schlag P, Decker-Baumann C: Strategies and needs for nutritional support in cancer surgery. Recent Results Cancer Res 1991;121:233.

Shikora SA, Blackburn GL: Nutritional consequences of major gastrointestinal surgery: Patient outcome and starvation. Surg Clin North Am 1991;71:509.

Shizgal HM: Parenteral and enteral nutrition. Annu Rev Med 1991;42:549.

Smith LC, Mullen JL: Nutritional assessment and indications for nutritional support. Surg Clin North Am 1991;71:449.

Taylor L, O'Neill JA Jr: Total parenteral nutrition in the pediatric patient. Surg Clin North Am 1991;71:477.

Van Way CW 3d: Nutritional support in the injured patient. Surg Clin North Am 1991;71:537.

The Veterans Affairs Total Parenteral Nutrition Cooperative Study Group: Perioperative total parenteral nutrition in surgical patients. N Engl J Med 1991; 325:527.

Wilmore DW: Catabolic illness. Strategies for enhancing recovery. N Engl J Med 1991;325:695.

Windsor JA, Hill GL: Weight loss with physiological impairment: A basic indicator of surgical risk. Ann Surg 1988;207:290.

Oral Nutrition in General

ADA Timely Statement on Nutrition and Your Health: Dietary guidelines for Americans. J Am Diet Assoc 1990;90:1720.

Bal DG, Foerster SB: Changing the American diet: Impact on cancer prevention. Cancer 1991;67:2671.

Bingham S: Dietary aspects of a health strategy for England. Br Med J 1991:303:353.

Hegsted DM: Recommended dietary intakes of elderly subjects. Am J Clin Nutr 1989;50(5 Suppl):1190. [See also discussion on p 1231.]

Hill JO et al: Nutrient balance in humans: Effects of diet composition. Am J Clin Nutr 1991;54:10.

Kritchevsky D: Diet and cancer. CA 1991;41:328.

Lactose intolerance. (Editorial.) Lancet 1991;338:663.

Nelson RC, Franzi LR: Nutrition and aging. Med Clin North Am 1989;73:1531.

Peterkin BB: Dietary guidelines for Americans, 1990 edition. J Am Diet Assoc 1990;90:1725.

Truswell S: Who should take vitamin supplements? Br Med J 1990;301:135.

Ulbricht TL, Southgate DA: Coronary heart disease: Seven dietary factors. Lancet 1991;338:985.

Weinhouse S et al: American Cancer Society guidelines on diet, nutrition, and cancer. CA 1991;41:334.

Whitehead RG: Vitamins, minerals, schoolchildren, and IQ. Br Med J 1991;302:548.

Willett W, Sacks FM: Chewing the fat: How much and what kind? N Engl J Med 1991;324:121.

Ziegler RG: Vegetables, fruits, and carotenoids and the risk of cancer. Am J Clin Nutr 1991;53(Suppl 1):251S.

11

Anesthesia

Ronald D. Miller, MD

Anesthesiology is concerned not only with the administration of anesthesia for surgery but also with many other areas of patient care, including critical care medicine, management of chronic pain, and respiratory therapy. In this chapter, the discussion will be limited to anesthesia during surgery and the overall perioperative period.

The development of anesthesia represents one of the most interesting aspects of United States medical history. In 1842, Crawford Long was the first physician to administer diethyl ether by inhalation to produce surgical anesthesia, but his work went largely unrecognized. In 1846, a dentist, William Morton, administered diethyl ether for the removal of a submandibular tumor by surgeon John Warren. This event took place at the Massachusetts General Hospital before an audience of surgeons, medical students, and a newspaper reporter and was therefore well publicized. Another dentist, Horace Wells, allowed nitrous oxide to be administered to him by Gardner Colton, a showman, while a fellow dentist performed a painless tooth extraction. Unfortunately, Wells failed to appreciate the marginal potency of nitrous oxide and was unable to reproduce surgical anesthesia during a demonstration at the Massachusetts General Hospital. Between 1844 and 1886, nitrous oxide continued to be used by showmen who staged public displays of the exhilarating effects of the gas. Diethyl ether was often used for similar purposes. Since then, many techniques for general anesthesia have been developed and improved upon.

In the late 19th century, within a year after Karl Koller, a Viennese surgeon, discovered the topical anesthetic properties of cocaine, William Halsted, of Johns Hopkins University, gave the drug by injection for the production of peripheral nerve block. In 1898, after a trial on himself that led to the first-described lumbar puncture headache, August Bier, in Germany, administered the first spinal anesthetic. In the years that followed, the development of local anesthetics with different durations of action led to the widespread use of regional anesthesia.

Kitz RJ, Vandam LD: A history and the scope of anesthetic practice. In: *Anesthesia,* 3rd ed. Miller RD (editor). Churchill Livingstone, 1990.

OVERALL ANESTHETIC RISK

Anecdotal reports of anesthetic mishaps are difficult to evaluate, partly because morbidity and mortality resulting from problems related to the anesthesia itself are difficult to distinguish from those due to the surgical procedure. Yet, in an age of increasing assessment and accountability, data bases are being analyzed to determine the benefit and hazards of surgery in general and anesthesia specifically. The results of several of these types of analysis indicate a death rate of 0.4–1 in 10,000 operative deaths entirely due to the anesthetic and about 2 in 10,000 due in major part to the anesthetic is a reasonable estimate of the overall anesthetic risk.

Many deaths or cases of severe morbidity related exclusively to the anesthetic occur because of the physician's failure to recognize a problem or deal with it effectively. For example, the mortality rate from anesthetic cardiac arrest was found to be 0.9 per 10,000 in one series of 163,240 anesthetic mishaps reviewed over 15 years. In another analysis of 250,543 anesthetics, there was an incidence of 4.6 per 10,000 of anesthetic-induced cardiac arrests with a mortality rate of 0.4 per 10,000. Ventilatory problems leading to hypoxia are the most common cause of anesthetic cardiac arrest in nearly all studies. Another approach is analysis of closed malpractice claims files. A review of 1004 law suits showed that unrecognized esophageal intubation and nerve damage related to positioning during surgery or needle trauma were the most common problems.

Despite these problems, with proper care, the overall anesthetic risk is extremely low, leading one writer to state that "perhaps the most insidious hazard of anesthesia is its relative safety." (See Cooper reference, below.)

Cooper JB et al: An analysis of major errors and equipment failures in anesthesia management. Anesthesiology 1984;60:34.

Cheney FW et al: Standard of care and anesthesia liability. JAMA 1989;261:1599.

Eichhorn JH: Prevention of intraoperative anesthesia accidents and severe injury through safety monitoring. Anesthesiology 1989;70:572.

Gaba DM, DeAnda A: The response of anesthesia trainees to simulated critical incidents. Anesth Analg 1989; 68:444.

Keenan RL, Boyan CP: Cardiac arrest due to anesthesia: A study of incidence and causes. JAMA 1985;253:2373.

Relman AS: Assessment and accountability: The third revolution in medical care. N Engl J Med 1988;319:1220.

Ross AF, Tinker JM: Anesthesia risk. In: *Anesthesia,* 3rd ed. Miller RD (editor). Churchill Livingstone, 1990.

PREOPERATIVE PROCEDURES ASSOCIATED WITH ANESTHESIA

Preoperative Evaluation for Anesthetic Risk

Anesthetic risk is difficult to ascertain precisely in most cases. Perioperative complications and deaths are frequently caused by a combination of factors, including concurrent disease, complexity of the operation, and adverse effects of anesthesia. A few complications are due entirely to anesthesia, such as aspiration pneumonitis and hypoxemia due to failure to maintain a patent airway. The patient's physical status can be classified according to the criteria given in Table 11–1. This classification system was not specifically designed to estimate anesthetic risk but does provide a "common language" of evaluation for use by different institutions.

A. History and Physical Examination: The history should include a review of the patient's previous experiences with anesthesia, and data should be elicited regarding any allergic reactions, delayed awakening, prolonged paralysis from neuromuscular blocking agents, and jaundice. The presence and severity of any concurrent diseases (eg, hepatitis), coagulopathies, endocrine abnormalities (eg, diabetes mellitus), or cardiorespiratory dysfunction should be noted.

The physical examination should focus on the cardiovascular system, lungs, and upper airway. It should include measurements of heart rate and of arterial blood pressure obtained in both the supine and standing positions and auscultation for cardiac murmurs, carotid artery bruits, or abnormal breathing. If abnormalities are found, additional tests (electrocardiography, pulmonary function tests, etc) may be indicated. The airway, head, and neck should be examined for factors that could make endotracheal intubation difficult, eg, fat or short neck, limited temporomandibular mobility. Peripheral venous sites, including the external jugular vein, should also be checked. If regional anesthesia is planned, the proposed site of injection should be examined for abnormalities and signs of infection, and a limited neurologic examination should also be performed.

B. Evaluation of Concurrent Drug Therapy: Concurrent drug therapy must be reviewed, since many drugs can interact with anesthetic agents (Table 11–2). For example, acute cocaine intoxication can increase anesthetic requirements; long-term use of an antihypertensive drug can reduce anesthetic requirements; and ethanol use can either increase (long-term use) or decrease (acute intoxication) the requirements. Smoking and alcohol are well-known factors influencing anesthetic requirement. Antiarrhythmics, local anesthetics, and especially antibiotics may enhance the neuromuscular blockade from neuromuscular blocking drugs. Tricyclic antidepressants exaggerate the sympathomimetic response of many vasopressors, but antihypertensive and antiarrhythmic drugs can decrease peripheral sympathetic activity and augment the depressant effect of anesthetics. In the past, it was recommended that antihypertensives be discontinued for 2 weeks before an operation, but this practice exposed the patient to the risk of untreated hypertension during this period. Current practice is to continue therapy until the evening before surgery and to anticipate the need for less anesthetic agent, including monoamine oxidase inhibitors. Barbiturates can enhance the metabolism of anesthetic drugs and thereby increase the possibility of a toxic reaction. Echothiophate may prolong the response to neuromuscular blocking drugs. Obviously, the safety of continuing drug therapy depends on awareness of potential drug interactions.

C. Laboratory Tests: In the past, hospital rules mandated that a large battery of screening laboratory

Table 11–1. Physical status classification of the American Society of Anesthesiologists.

Class	Physical Status
1	Patient has no organic, physiologic, biochemical, or psychiatric disturbance.
2	Patient has mild to moderate systemic disturbance that may or may not be related to the disorder requiring surgery (eg, essential hypertension, diabetes mellitus).
3	Patient has severe systemic disturbance that may or may not be related to the disorder requiring surgery (eg, heart disease that limits activity, poorly controlled essential hypertension).
4	Patient has severe systemic disturbance that is life-threatening with or without surgery (eg, congestive heart failure, persistent angina pectoris).
5	Patient is moribund and has little chance for survival, but surgery is to be performed as a last resort (resuscitative effort) (eg, uncontrolled hemorrhage, as from a ruptured abdominal aneurysm).
E	Patient requires emergency operation.

Table 11–2. Mechanisms by which drugs may influence the effects of anesthesia.

Anesthetic requirements may be increased or decreased.
Neuromuscular blockade from muscle relaxants may be enhanced.
Cardiovascular response to sympathomimetics and anesthetics may be exaggerated.
Peripheral sympathetic nervous system activity may be reduced, and cardiovascular depressant reactions to anesthetics may be augmented.
Metabolism may be enhanced or impaired.

tests be given prior to anesthesia; however, many of these tests have been found to be unnecessary, and the advisability of others has been questioned. For example, one common rule is that elective surgery should not be performed if the hemoglobin concentration is less than 10 g/dL. There is no evidence, however, that correction of normovolemic anemia decreases perioperative morbidity and mortality rates. More important is the need to determine why the patient is anemic. Administering blood preoperatively in an effort to increase the hemoglobin concentration above 10 g/dL is questionable medical therapy, since the risk of hepatitis from blood transfusion (3–10%) exceeds any risks imposed by anemia.

The history and physical examination are the most valuable guides for determining which laboratory tests are necessary (eg, a long history of smoking dictates a thorough examination of pulmonary status by means of pulmonary function tests). Men aged 40 years or younger with no history of problems with anesthesia and normal findings on physical examination usually require no laboratory tests; women of this age and health status usually require only hemoglobin measurements.

Questionnaires are a useful means of identifying patients likely to have complications who would therefore benefit from preoperative laboratory testing. This is especially important with increasing emphasis on same-day surgery. Blue Cross/Blue Shield estimates that several billion dollars a year are wasted in the USA on unnecessary preoperative tests and subsequent evaluation of trivial abnormal results. Excessive testing can even be hazardous, because borderline abnormalities may lead to additional—sometimes invasive—tests or therapy. An example is potassium treatment for borderline low potassium levels.

Cohen MM, Duncan PG, Tate RB: Does anesthesia contribute to operative mortality? JAMA 1988;260:2859.

El-Ganzowie A et al: Monoamine oxidase inhibitors: Should they be discontinued preoperatively? Anesth Analg 1985;64:592.

Gluck R, Muñoz E, Wise L: Preoperative and postoperative medical evaluation of surgical patients. Am J Surg 1988;155:730.

Kaplan EB et al: The usefulness of preoperative laboratory screening. JAMA 1985;253:3576.

McKee RF, Scott EM: The value of routine preoperative investigations. Ann R Coll Surg Engl 1987;69:160.

Rohrer MJ, Michelotti MC, Nahrwold DL: A prospective evaluation of the efficacy of perioperative coagulation testing. Ann Surg 1988;208:554.

Turnbull JM, Buck C: The value of preoperative screening investigations in otherwise healthy individuals. Arch Intern Med 1987;147:1101.

Wyatt WJ, Reed DN Jr, Apelgren KN: Pitfalls in the role of standardized pre-admission laboratory screening for ambulatory surgery. Am Surg 1989;55:343.

Informed Consent

Informed consent involves advising the patient of what to expect from administration of anesthesia and of possible adverse effects and risks. The general scenario of the perioperative period should be described, and the patient should be allowed to ask questions. Table 11–3 lists concerns that the anesthesiologist should routinely address. A signed consent form should be obtained, and the physician should make notes and file them in the patient's medical record (see Chapter 6).

"Informed consent" is a term that is becoming increasingly difficult to define for both surgery and anesthesia. While one might argue that a patient should be informed of every possible complication, in actuality this is not practical and may even be harmful by causing undue worry. In anesthesia, patient autonomy must be balanced with medical needs in deciding what constitutes informed consent. This balance should be based on the anesthesiologist's best judgment. The anesthesiologist's conversation with the patient should be recorded as a separate note in the chart.

Drane JF: Competency to give an informed consent: A model for making clinical assessments. JAMA 1984;252:925.

IMMEDIATE PREOPERATIVE MANAGEMENT

Selection of Preoperative Medication

The principal goals of preoperative medication are (1) to relieve anxiety and provide sedation; (2) to induce amnesia; (3) to decrease secretion of saliva and gastric juices; (4) to elevate the gastric pH; and (5) to prevent allergic reactions to anesthetic drugs. Medication is usually given 1–2 hours before the induction of anesthesia. It is not necessary to give medication specifically to facilitate the induction of anesthesia. The selection of drugs is largely subjective. Sedation can be achieved by barbiturates, benzodiazepines, or narcotics. To avoid an intramuscular injection, diaze-

Table 11–3. Issues that should be discussed with patients preoperatively.

Preoperative medication (time, route of administration, and effect)
Anticipated time of transport to the operating room
Sequence of events prior to induction of anesthesia
Anticipated duration of surgery
Description of where awakening from anesthesia will occur
Presence of catheters (eg, tracheal, bladder, arterial) on awakening
Expected time of return to hospital ward room
Likelihood of postoperative nausea and vomiting
Magnitude of postoperative pain and methods for treatment
Whether they will receive blood transfusions, with associated risks

pam, 0.12 mg/kg, is especially effective for sedation when given orally 1–2 hours preoperatively. Midazolam is a benzodiazepine with powerful amnestic properties, but it cannot be given orally and so must be administered intramuscularly or intravenously. Gastric secretion can be decreased by H_2 receptor antagonists such as cimetidine. Anticholinergics such as atropine or scopolamine are rarely indicated. The traditional practice of prolonged fasting (eg, NPO after midnight or for 8 hours before induction of anesthesia) in patients without risk factors (eg, obesity, bowel obstruction, severe pain) is being reevaluated. The volume and pH of gastric contents are not affected by fluids ingested more than 2 hours previously. Although it is reasonable to allow clear fluids orally up to 2 hours before induction of anesthesia, this does not apply to patients with known risks for aspiration or those who have ingested solid food.

The anesthesiologist's explanation to the patient of what will occur can substantially alleviate fears about anesthesia and surgery. In fact, it has been shown that a thorough explanation has a calming effect comparable to that of medications given to relieve anxiety.

For some other conditions associated with surgery, it is better to give medication as the need arises. Cardiac vagal activity is best controlled with atropine given just before anticipated vagal stimulation. Postoperative analgesia is better achieved by giving narcotics intravenously just before they are needed, and antiemetics should be given just before postoperative nausea and vomiting are expected to occur.

Selection of Anesthesia

Many factors influence the choice of anesthesia for a given patient. The site of surgery and positioning of the patient on the operating table are obviously important factors. A regional nerve block may be contraindicated in a patient with neuropathy due to diabetes mellitus. Spinal anesthesia is inappropriate for thyroidectomy. Different types of anesthesia may be given for elective or emergency surgery, particularly if the patient requiring emergency surgery has a full stomach. Coexisting diseases (eg, hypertension, cardiac disease) must be considered. The age and preferences of the patient must also be taken into account.

Preparation for Administration of Anesthesia

Several important steps must be taken before anesthesia is administered. Upon arrival in the operating room, the patient should be identified and the scheduled operation reconfirmed. The nurses' notes from the preceding evening should be examined to determine whether there were any unexpected changes in the patient's condition. The administration of preoperative medication should be verified.

Anesthesia usually begins by starting an intravenous infusion and applying a blood pressure cuff. Monitors (eg, electrocardiographic leads), a peripheral nerve stimulator, and a chest stethoscope should be applied while the patient is awake, and vital signs should be recorded before anesthesia is begun.

The machine for administering anesthesia must be checked for proper functioning, and drugs and other necessary supplies must be at hand (eg, the apparatus needed to suction the pharynx and ventilate the lungs with oxygen via a cuffed endotracheal tube).

National standards are evolving for patient monitoring during anesthesia. In general, minimum monitoring dictates measurement of arterial blood pressure and heart rate every 5 minutes, and the ECG should be displayed continuously. A means of detecting disconnection of an automatic ventilator is mandatory. The oxygen concentration must be measured during general anesthesia, and a means of measuring temperature should be readily available. Increasingly, use of pulse oximetry is becoming a standard of care.

Positioning of the Patient on the Operating Table

It is important that the patient be positioned properly on the operating table to avoid physical or physiologic complications. Immediate complications (eg, decreased cardiac output) or long-term complications (eg, peripheral neuropathy) can result from improper positioning. Nerve damage can be caused by placing the patient in a position that stretches or applies pressure to a nerve. Pressure on a vulnerable area may lead to skin necrosis and ulceration, which in rare cases requires skin grafting. Damage to the toes or fingers may occur when positioning of equipment (eg, Mayo stand) is adjusted. Because anesthesia blunts the normal compensatory mechanisms, a sudden change in the patient's position can cause cardiovascular changes (eg, a shift from the supine to a sitting position may result in hypotension and cerebral hypoperfusion).

A. Common Nerve Injuries Due to Improper Positioning: Some peripheral nerves are at risk of trauma during anesthesia. Injury to the brachial plexus nerve is most common and usually results from extension of the arm more than 90 degrees while the patient is supine. The radial nerve may be injured if the patient's arm slips off the operating table or if pressure is applied to the nerve at the point where it traverses the spiral groove of the humerus. If the elbow is allowed to hang over the edge of the operating table, the ulnar nerve, which runs superficially along the medial aspect of the elbow, may be compressed between the medial epicondyle and the operating table.

The sciatic nerve may be damaged if the patient is in the lithotomy position with thighs and legs extended outward and rotated or if the knees are extended. The common peroneal nerve is typically damaged by compression between the fibula and the metal brace used in the lithotomy position.

B. Injuries Due to Improper Placement of Anesthetic Equipment: Complications can also occur from improper application of the anesthetic mask, mask strap, or tracheal tube connector. Necrosis of the bridge of the nose due to excessive pressure by the mask is the most common injury. This can be minimized if the mask is removed every 5 minutes and the bridge of the nose gently massaged. The outer third of the eyebrow may be lost, often permanently, owing to pressure from the mask strap; this can be avoided by putting a pad under the strap. Excessive pressure on the buccal branch of the facial nerve can cause loss of function of the orbicularis oris muscle or necrosis of the ear.

Alvine FG, Schurrer ME: Postoperative ulnar-nerve palsy: Are there predisposing factors? J Bone Joint Surg [Am] 1987;69:255.

Cote CJ: NPO after midnight for children: A reappraisal. Anesthesiology 1990;72:589.

Eichhorn JH et al: Standards for patient monitoring during anesthesia at Harvard Medical School. JAMA 1986; 256:1017.

Maltby JR et al: Gastric fluid Volume, pH, and emptying in elective inpatients: Influences of narcotic-atropine premedication, oral fluid, and ranitidine. Can J Anaesth 1988;35:562.

Manchikanti L et al: Preanesthetic cimetidine and metoclopramide for acid aspiration prophylaxis in elective surgery. Anesthesiology 1984;61:48.

Martin JT: The lawn chair (contoured spine) position. In: *Positioning in Anesthesia and Surgery,* 2nd ed. Martin JT (editor). Saunders, 1987.

MANAGEMENT OF ANESTHESIA DURING OPERATION

1. GENERAL ANESTHESIA

Induction of General Anesthesia

General anesthesia can be induced by giving drugs intravenously, by inhalation, or by a combination of both methods.

A. Rapid-Sequence Induction: Anesthesia is most commonly induced by the method of rapid-sequence induction, in which rapid administration of an ultra-short-acting barbiturate (eg, thiopental) is followed by a depolarizing muscle relaxant (eg, succinylcholine). While other drugs (eg, ketamine, propofol, etomidate) can be used for rapid-sequence induction of anesthesia, the combination of thiopental and succinylcholine is the standard against which others must be compared. This approach allows anesthesia to be induced within 30 seconds and the trachea to be intubated within 60–90 seconds. Oxygen is usually given by mask beforehand to allow maximum time for intubation while the patient is apneic. A nondepolarizing neuromuscular blocking drug (eg, vecuronium, atracurium, or pancuronium) can be substituted for succinylcholine, but the onset of paralysis is delayed by about 60 seconds.

Rapid-sequence induction minimizes the time during which the trachea is unprotected. Consequently, this method is often used in emergency surgery in patients who have eaten recently. The disadvantage of giving depressant drugs rapidly is that hypotension may occur in patients with questionable cardiovascular status or marginal circulatory volume.

B. Inhalation Induction: Inhalation of nitrous oxide plus a potent volatile anesthetic (eg, halothane, enflurane, desflurane, or isoflurane) can produce anesthesia within 3–5 minutes. After induction, a depolarizing or nondepolarizing neuromuscular blocking drug can be given intravenously to facilitate tracheal intubation. If there is some question about the difficulty of intubation, it can be attempted while the patient is breathing spontaneously, without giving a muscle relaxant. Although conditions for intubation may not be as good with this method, the patient will still be breathing if difficulties with intubation prolong the time before complete airway control is achieved.

The advantage of inhalation induction is that anesthetic drugs can be titrated according to the patient's needs. This allows for administration of more precise doses and minimizes the risk of an accidental overdose with resultant cardiovascular depression. The disadvantages are a slower induction time and lack of protection for the airway for a longer period of time.

C. Combined Intravenous-Inhalation Induction: Short-acting anesthetic drugs such as thiopental or midazolam are often administered intravenously before inhalation of a volatile anesthetic. This is done to minimize the discomfort of wearing the anesthetic mask and to facilitate inhalation of the anesthetic agent, which many people consider to have an offensive odor. This technique combines the advantages of both the intravenous and inhalation approaches. Anesthesia is induced rapidly, and anesthetic drug dosages can be titrated according to the patient's requirements.

Maintaining the Airway

Administering general anesthesia without endotracheal intubation is increasingly uncommon. While this approach avoids the complications of intubation, it has many disadvantages. If the patient vomits even a small amount, the airway is unprotected and aspiration will occur. Furthermore, the anesthesiologist must hold the mask with one hand during the entire procedure, and this hinders performance of the many other tasks required (eg, administration of other drugs or blood, record keeping, and monitoring).

A. Indications for Endotracheal Intubation: Endotracheal intubation is now almost routinely performed during general anesthesia (Table 11–4). Clearly, any patient who has recently eaten or has in-

Table 11–4. Indications for endotracheal intubation.

To provide a patent airway
To prevent aspiration of gastric contents
To provide tracheal or bronchial suctioning
To facilitate positive pressure ventilation
To provide adequate ventilation
    when the position of the patient is other than supine,
    when ventilation provided by mask is not sufficient,
    when disease of the upper airway is present

testinal obstruction should be managed by rapid intubation. Tracheal intubation is mandatory also for patients requiring positive pressure ventilation (eg, during thoracotomy or when neuromuscular blocking drugs are given). When the patient must be placed in a position other than supine, intubation is often required.

B. Complications of Endotracheal Intubation: The most important complication is failure to intubate the trachea, the most common cause of serious anesthesia-induced morbidity. The difficulty of tracheal intubation is related to body weight, head and neck movement, jaw movement, receding mandible, and buck teeth. A variety of techniques are available, including fiberoptic laryngoscopy, to facilitate intubation. Complications occurring during direct laryngoscopy and passage of the tube most often involve injuries to the teeth. The laryngoscope blade should not be used as a lever on the teeth. If a tooth is dislodged, it must be removed. If the tooth cannot be located, radiographs of the chest and abdomen should be obtained to ascertain that the tooth has not passed through the glottic opening.

Hypertension and tachycardia may be associated with endotracheal intubation, but they are usually transient and of no clinical significance. They can be minimized by ensuring that the depth of anesthesia is adequate and by giving lidocaine, 100 mg/70 kg intravenously, to susceptible patients. Administration of small doses of a potent opioid (eg, 150 μg/70 kg of fentanyl) during induction of anesthesia will attenuate the cardiovascular responses to tracheal intubation.

The endotracheal tube can be obstructed or accidentally removed. If it has been incorrectly placed (eg, into the bronchus or esophagus), hypoxemia will result. Auscultation of the lungs and stomach will determine whether the tube is in the esophagus. If too much pressure is applied by the balloon cuff to the tracheal wall, the tracheal mucosa may become ischemic. Previously, endotracheal tubes had "high-pressure cuffs" that required 80–250 mm Hg of pressure before they expanded enough to seal the tracheal lumen. The currently available "low-pressure cuffs" adapt to irregularities in the tracheal circumference and produce a seal at pressures of 15–30 mm Hg. With these cuffs, the incidence of tracheal ischemia is minimal. However, there is no way to entirely avoid laryngotracheal damage. For example, ciliary denu-

dation can occur over the tracheal rings with only 2 hours of intubation and tracheal pressures of less than 25 mm Hg.

The most common complications following extubation are laryngospasm, aspiration of gastric contents, pharyngitis (sore throat), laryngitis, and laryngeal or subglottic edema. Later complications include laryngeal ulceration with or without granuloma formation, tracheitis, tracheal stenosis, vocal cord paralysis, and arytenoid cartilage dislocation.

The incidence of many of these complications can be reduced by using low-pressure endotracheal tube cuffs to minimize tissue damage and by performing prompt extubation when clinically possible.

Maintaining General Anesthesia

The main objectives of general anesthesia are analgesia, unconsciousness, skeletal muscle relaxation, and control of sympathetic nervous system responses to noxious stimulation. Inhaled and intravenous anesthetics, narcotics, and muscle relaxants should be selected with specific pharmacologic goals in mind.

A. Nitrous Oxide, Volatile Anesthetics, and Narcotics: Since nitrous oxide does not provide total anesthesia, it is given in combination with a volatile anesthetic or narcotic. The main disadvantage of most volatile anesthetics is dose-dependent cardiac depression; when they are used in combination with nitrous oxide, which is relatively free of cardiovascular effects, their total dose can be decreased. Delivery of the highly potent volatile anesthetics is controlled by a machine that allows the anesthesiologist to titrate the dose to the needs of the patient.

Narcotics, which generally do not depress the cardiovascular system, are often combined with nitrous oxide. However, in patients with normal ventricular function, the lack of narcotic-induced cardiovascular depression in the face of unblocked sympathetic nervous system responses may produce hypertension. If this happens, the addition of low concentrations of a volatile anesthetic will usually control the blood pressure. With a combined narcotic-nitrous oxide anesthetic, muscle relaxants are more frequently needed to facilitate skeletal muscle relaxation.

B. Monitoring the Depth of Anesthesia: Signs for assessing the depth of anesthesia are listed in Table 11–5. Although paralysis by muscle relaxants simplifies exposure of the operative site and decreases the need for volatile anesthetics, many signs of anesthesia are absent in the paralyzed patient. It is essential that the anesthesiologist continuously assess the depth of anesthesia. Failure to do so may result in the patient being awake but paralyzed during the procedure.

C. Neuromuscular Blockade: One of the greatest challenges for the anesthesiologist is to administer the proper dosage of muscle relaxant—ie, a dosage high enough to facilitate the surgical procedures but not so high as to cover up inadequate doses of anes-

Table 11–5. Signs indicating depth of anesthesia.*

Anesthetic	Signs						
	Blood Pressure	Heart Rate	Respiration	Sweating	Muscle Relaxation	Pupil Size	Pupil Movement
Enflurane	++	++	+	0	++	+	±
Halothane	++	++	+	0	++	+	±
Isoflurane	++	+	0	++	+	±	±
N₂O-narcotic	+	+	+	+	0	0	0
N₂O-ketamine	0	0	+	0	0	0	+

*Usefulness of signs is graded as follows: ++ = very useful; + = moderately useful; ± = questionably useful; 0 = not useful.

thetic agents and thereby expose the patient to the risk of prolonged postoperative paralysis. A peripheral nerve stimulator is of help in gauging the extent of neuromuscular blockade intraoperatively. Usually, the ulnar nerve is stimulated, and adduction of the thumb is observed. If anesthesia is sufficient, obliteration of 90% of the response will in general result in adequate relaxation. The increasing need for profound muscular relaxation has increased the incidence of weakness causing inadequate ventilation in the recovery room. This can be partly ascribed to difficulties in reversing profound neuromuscular blockade. As a result, the surgical team should also take all other measures to aid in exposure (eg, correct positioning and adequate depth of anesthesia), so that the amount of muscle relaxant can be kept to a minimum. This decreases the incidence of prolonged paralysis and dependence on mechanical ventilation postoperatively.

Deliberate Hypotension

The role of deliberate hypotension for surgical procedures is controversial. Blood loss is less, but there is a risk of hypoperfusion of vital organs. Deliberate hypotension is occasionally used in neurosurgery, total hip arthroplasty, and operations for head and neck cancer. The brain can tolerate a mean arterial pressure of 55 mm Hg, but the lower limits and the influence of specific diseases have not been defined. Patients who have had strokes, transient ischemic attacks, myocardial infarction within the previous 3 years, renal disease (ie, increased serum creatinine levels), previous renal transplant, systolic blood pressure greater than 170 mm Hg, or diastolic blood pressure greater than 110 mm Hg should not be considered for deliberate hypotension.

Deliberate hypotension is induced by position of the patient (eg, head up), continuous intravenous infusion of a short-acting vasodilator (eg, sodium nitroprusside), use of a volatile anesthetic, or any combination of these.

With an increased emphasis on minimizing blood transfusions, there may be an increase in the use of deliberate hypotension in selected patients.

Bevan DR: Postoperative residual paralysis in the recovery room. In: *Neuromuscular Blocking Agents Past, Present and Future.* Bowman WC, Denissen PAF, Feldman S (editors). Excerpta Medica, 1990.

Finfer SR et al: Cardiovascular responses to tracheal intubation: A comparison of direct laryngoscopy and fiberoptic intubation. Anaesth Intens Care 1989;17:44.

O'Leary JJ, Pollard BJ, Ryan MJ: A method of detecting oesophageal intubation or confirming tracheal intubation. Anaesth Intens Care 1988;16:299.

Miller ED, Jr: Deliberate hypertension. In: *Anesthesia,* 3rd ed. Miller RD (editor). Churchill Livingstone, 1990.

Miller RD: How should residual neuromuscular blockage be detected? Anesthesiology 1989;70:379.

Thompson KD et al: Use of the Bain laryngeal mask airway in anticipation of difficult tracheal intubation. Br J Plast Surg 1989;42:478.

Wilson ME et al: Predicting difficult intubation. Br J Anaesth 1988;61:211.

2. REGIONAL ANESTHESIA

A regional anesthetic is used when it is desirable that the patient remain conscious during the operation. Skeletal muscle relaxation is usually excellent, especially with spinal and epidural anesthesia. Thus, muscle relaxants (eg, vecuronium) are unnecessary. Patients often have misconceptions about regional anesthesia that require detailed explanation of the safety of this technique. One disadvantage of regional anesthesia is the occasional failure to produce adequate anesthesia; another is hypotension due to sympathetic blockade. Regional anesthesia is used most often for surgery of the lower abdomen or lower extremities, since the effect of sympathetic blockade of these areas is minimal.

Despite its limitations, regional anesthesia does have many attractive features. Anesthetizing only the part of the body upon which surgery is being performed (eg, spinal anesthesia for lower abdominal surgery or brachial plexus nerve block for arm surgery) may decrease postoperative morbidity. Some examples are as follows:

(1) Blood loss from total hip arthroplasty or prostatectomy is decreased by spinal or epidural anesthesia.

(2) Thromboembolic complications after hip and prostate operations are less.

(3) Lung function may be less affected.

(4) Postoperative impairment of immune function is avoided.

(5) Convalescence may be shorter.

Spinal & Epidural Blocks

Spinal anesthesia is achieved by injecting a local anesthetic into the lumbar intrathecal space. This blocks the spinal nerve roots and dorsal root ganglia and probably also blocks the periphery of the spinal cord. Epidural anesthesia is accomplished by injecting a local anesthetic into the extradural (epidural) space. The epidural space is usually identified via the lumbar approach. The gastrointestinal tract is usually contracted with spinal and epidural anesthesia, facilitating exposure of the surgical site. A limitation not only of spinal and epidural anesthesia but of regional anesthesia generally is the need to provide some sedation. Proper selection will eliminate those patients who need excessive sedation. When enough sedatives are given, the result is a comfortable-appearing, sleep-like state in which there is no spontaneous verbalization. Excess sedation can produce respiratory insufficiency leading to cardiac arrest. Monitoring with a pulse oximeter should allow detection of more subtle degrees of respiratory insufficiency.

There are several complications of spinal anesthesia. Headache is the most common and is seen most frequently in young patients. The incidence is only 1% when a 25-gauge needle is used. For severe headache, a "blood-patch" epidural injection should be performed. This involves injecting 5–10 mL of the patient's blood into the epidural space at the site of the previous lumbar puncture. Pain relief is usually prompt, and headache usually does not recur. This technique is thought to plug the leak of cerebrospinal fluid, restoring pressure in the subarachnoid space to normal.

Because spinal anesthesia blocks innervation of the bladder, administration of large amounts of intravenous fluids may cause bladder distention, and a urethral catheter may be required. This usually occurs with minor operations such as inguinal hernia repairs and can be avoided by keeping fluids to a minimum. Nausea and vomiting may occur when a spinal anesthetic is begun, especially if hypotension is present. If nausea and vomiting persist despite successful treatment of hypotension, diazepam or droperidol may be effective. Peripheral nerve damage is rare, occurring in one out of 10,000 cases.

Complications from epidural anesthesia are the same as those for spinal anesthesia, with the exception of headache.

Nerve Blocks

Nerve blocks are most appropriate for surgery of the upper extremities. Intercostal nerve blocks are useful for postoperative pain relief. Overall, nerve blocks play a minor role in anesthesia because of the discomfort they cause the patient and the time they require. However, in a well-organized anesthesia department, nerve blocks can be performed with a minimum of turnaround time between cases, and patient comfort can be assured with adequate premedication.

3. MONITORED ANESTHETIC CARE (Standby Anesthesia)

Monitored (standby) anesthesia is the use of local anesthesia by the surgeon along with administration of sedative-hypnotics (eg, diazepam, midazolam) and narcotics (eg, morphine) by the anesthesiologist. In elderly or fragile patients—especially those with unprotected airways—these cases can become quite challenging. When unexpectedly large amounts of sedative-hypnotics are required, the decision to interrupt surgery and convert to a general anesthetic with endotracheal intubation is often difficult but obviously crucial.

Axelsson K et al: Bladder function in spinal anesthesia. Acta Anaesth Scand 1985;29:315.

Caplan RA et al: Unexpected cardiac arrest during spinal anesthesia: A closed claims analysis of predisposing factors. Anesthesiology 1988;68:5.

Lillie PE et al: Site of action of intravenous regional anesthesia. Anesthesiology 1984;61:507.

Mouren S et al: Normovolemic hemodilution and lumbar epidural anesthesia. Anesth Analg 1989;69:174.

Yeager MP et al: Epidural anesthesia and analgesia in high-risk surgical patients. Anesthesiology 1987,66:729.

Zelcer V, White PF: Monitored anesthesia care. In: *Anesthesia,* 3rd ed. Miller RD (editor). Churchill Livingstone, 1990.

POSTOPERATIVE PROCEDURES ASSOCIATED WITH ANESTHESIA

Recovery Room Procedures

The recovery room is designed for the monitoring and care of patients during the period immediately following anesthesia and surgery. The recovery room must be near the operating room, so that the physician is available for consultation and assistance. The size of the recovery room depends on the number and kind of operations performed, with approximately 1½ beds for each operating room.

Recovery from anesthesia begins in the operating room with the discontinuation of anesthetic drugs and extubation of the trachea. Volatile anesthetics are eliminated by the lungs and intravenous anesthetics by metabolism or renal excretion. Residual activity of muscle relaxants should be assessed with a peripheral nerve stimulator, and any residual blockade should be treated with antagonists.

Patients frequently enter the recovery room in a state of hypothermia. Rewarming is important to minimize the adverse effects of shivering on oxygen consumption. Surgeons could help keep their patients from becoming hypothermic by allowing operating room temperatures to be warmer.

The most common immediate postoperative complications are upper airway obstruction, arterial hypoxemia, alveolar hypoventilation, hypotension, hypertension, cardiac dysrhythmias, and agitation (delirium tremens).

The physician must make sure that the patient is breathing adequately before initiating the transfer from the recovery room to the ward, where monitoring is much less intense.

Nausea & Vomiting

Nausea and vomiting is a common problem in the immediate postoperative period. Most pharmacologic therapy (eg, small doses of droperidol) are reactive instead of preventive. Two new approaches may decrease the frequency of nausea and vomiting. The intraoperative use of narcotics augments the incidence of nausea and vomiting. Ketorolac tromethamine, a nonsteroidal, nonopioid anti-inflammatory drug, can produce postoperative analgesia (ie, equivalent to morphine) without respiratory depression and minimal nausea and vomiting. The second approach is the preoperative administration of ondansetron, a 5-HT$_3$ receptor antagonist. It is effective against chemotherapy-induced nausea and vomiting and possibly against anesthesia and surgery induced nausea and vomiting.

Pain Relief

Morphine is still the best narcotic for pain relief. In the recovery room, narcotics are first given intravenously and later intramuscularly. Regional anesthesia can also be used for postoperative pain relief. For example, after a cholecystectomy, intercostal nerve blocks with 0.5% bupivacaine will often provide 12–18 hours of pain relief.

Epidural administration of narcotics is an important advance in pain relief. Complete analgesia can be obtained for 12–24 hours with no interference with autonomic or motor function. If the epidural catheter remains in place postoperatively, the analgesia can be sustained for several days. Several complications can occur from epidural narcotics (Table 11–6). Pruritus is common but seldom bothersome. Although not caused by histamine release, antihistamines often provide symptomatic relief. Naloxone is reliably effective in doses that do not reverse the analgesia (eg, 0.05 mg/70 kg), but it may have to be repeated frequently or infused. These small doses of naloxone may reverse urinary retention, though some patients may require bladder catheterization. Nausea and vomiting can be relieved by antiemetics or transdermal scopolamine. Inadequate analgesia can be treated by administration of fentanyl, 50 µg, into the epidural catheter. Lastly, respiratory depression is always to be feared and can be detected by standard nursing

Table 11–6. Complications of epidural narcotics.

Complication	Estimated Occurrence (%)
Pruritus	15–20
Nausea	10–15
Urinary retention requiring catheterization	6–12
Inadequate pain relief	15–20
Severe respiratory depression	< 1

care, with specific monitoring orders, on the ward. Even smaller community hospitals that do not have continuous physician coverage are now using this technique.

The addition of clonidine, an α_2-adrenergic agonist, to epidural narcotics markedly reduces the required dose of narcotic. The ultimate role of clonidine has yet to be determined.

Patient-controlled analgesia is another technique used to control postoperative pain. With this technique, the patient can regulate his or her analgesic dose within limits that prevent excessive administration of narcotics. Devices are now available that allow the patient to self-administer small bolus doses of opiates. The dose is preset by the physician or nurse and is delivered when the patient presses a button at the bedside. After the dose is given, a preselected "lockout" interval must elapse before another dose can be administered. Another technique is intrapleural injection (ie, through a catheter) of local anesthetics.

Catley DM et al: Pronounced, episodic oxygen desaturation in the postoperative period: Its association with ventilatory pattern and analgesic regimen. Anesthesiology 1985;63:20.

Cross DA, Hunt JB: Feasibility of epidural morphine for postoperative analgesia in a small community hospital. Anesth Analg 1991;72:765.

Cuschieri RJ et al: Postoperative pain and pulmonary complications: Comparison of three analgesic regimens. Br J Surg 1985;72:495.

Dahl JB, Kehlet H: Non-steroidal anti-inflammatory drugs: Rationale for use in postoperative pain. Br J Anaesth 1991;66:703.

Moss G, Regal ME, Lichtig L: Reducing postoperative pain, narcotics, and length of hospitalization. Surgery 1986; 99:206.

Leeser J, Lip H: Prevention of postoperative nausea and vomiting using ondansetron, a new, selective, 5HT$_3$ receptor antagonist. Anesth Analg 1991;72:751.

Penon C, Ecoffey C, Cohen S: Ventilatory response to carbon dioxide after epidural clonidine injection. Anesth Analg 1991;72:761.

Ready LB et al: Acute postoperative pain. In: Anesthesia, 3rd ed. Miller RD (editor). Churchill Livingstone, 1990.

ANESTHESIA FOR AMBULATORY SURGERY

Increasingly, surgical procedures are being performed on an outpatient basis. An abbreviated form of inpatient care that involves overnight admission to the hospital following surgery ("come-and-stay" surgery) has the advantage of same-day admission but allows for better monitoring of immediate anesthetic or operative complications.

Patients who report to the hospital on the day of surgery must be given detailed instructions well in advance (Table 11–7). Local or general anesthesia is usually used in ambulatory surgical procedures. Peripheral nerve blocks are often ideal (especially intravenous Bier block) for superficial surgery of the extremities. Although epidural anesthesia can be used, spinal anesthesia is inadvisable because of the possibility of postanesthesia headache.

Recovery from anesthesia is accompanied by return of vital signs to normal, normal level of consciousness, and ability to walk without assistance. After regional anesthesia, it is important to document complete return of sensory and motor function. Nausea, vomiting, and vertigo should be absent, and the patient should not have excessive pain. The patient should be able to drink fluids. Hoarseness or stridor in a patient who was intubated must be watched carefully. Significant laryngeal edema, if present, typically becomes evident within the first hour following extubation of the trachea. Most patients with stridor improve and can be discharged without hospitalization.

The patient should be reminded that mental clarity and dexterity may remain impaired for 24–48 hours, despite an overall feeling of well-being. Driving motor vehicles or operating complex equipment should not be attempted during this period. The use of alcohol or depressant drugs should be avoided, since additive interactions with residual amounts of anesthetic are possible. Oral analgesics should be provided when appropriate. Lastly, the patient should be given the physician's telephone number and instructed to report any new symptoms or other concerns.

Carter JA, Dye AM, Cooper GM: Recovery from day-case anaesthesia: The effect of different inhalational anaesthetic agents. Anaesthesia 1985;40:545.

Ryan JA Jr et al: Outpatient inguinal herniorrhaphy with both regional and local anesthesia. Am J Surg 1984;148: 313.

Wyatt WJ, Reed DN Jr, Apelgren KN: Pitfalls in the role of standardized preadmission laboratory screening for ambulatory surgery. Am Surg 1989;55:343.

COMPLICATIONS

Aspiration Pneumonitis

A significant percentage of anesthesia-related deaths are the result of aspiration of food particles, foreign bodies, blood, gastric acid, oropharyngeal secretions, or bile during induction of anesthesia.

Aspiration pneumonitis usually takes one of two forms. Undigested food may be aspirated, producing airway obstruction and respiratory distress. Depending on the amount of material aspirated, respiratory distress can be severe, with cyanosis and cardiac arrest. Other cases may follow a milder, chronic course, leading to lobar pneumonia and lung abscess formation. Treatment involves removal of the particles by suction and bronchoscopy, followed by intensive care support. The second (more common) form of aspiration pneumonitis is caused by aspiration of gastric secretions with a pH below 2.50, producing sudden bronchospasm, tachypnea, labored respiration, diffuse rales, cyanosis, and hypotension. Cardiac arrest may occur in severe cases.

Prevention is obviously most desirable. Generally, any patient who has eaten solid food within 8 hours should be considered to have a full stomach and therefore at risk of vomiting during induction. However, it should be recognized that 8 hours of fasting does not guarantee a low gastric volume. In traumatized or pregnant patients, gastric emptying may be delayed, and the interval between eating and elective surgery should be lengthened to 12 hours. Premedication with H_2 receptor blockers such as cimetidine and other drugs such as metoclopramide is frequently recommended. Drinking sodium citrate will raise the gastric pH in most patients, but this must be done 45–75 minutes before induction. If time does not permit such a wait, either endotracheal intubation with the patient awake or rapid-sequence induction must be performed.

Malignant Hyperthermia

Malignant hyperthermia associated with anesthesia is an inherited disease manifested by a rapid in-

---

Table 11–7. Written instructions given to patients receiving anesthesia on an outpatient basis.

Complete all laboratory tests requested prior to surgery.
Notify the surgeon if your medical condition changes before surgery.
Do not eat or drink anything 8 hours before surgery.
Do not wear cosmetics or jewelry.
Report for surgery _____(where and when)_____ .
The estimated time of discharge will be _____(when)_____ .
You must be accompanied by an adult when you leave the hospital or clinic after surgery.
Following surgery, eat when hungry, starting with fluids and progressing to solid food.
Do not drive or make important decisions during the 24–48 hours following surgery.
Contact the physician in case of complications (phone number).

crease in body temperature, which is often lethal if not promptly treated. The caffeine-halothane contracture test, which measures the concentration of caffeine required to trigger contracture in freshly biopsied skeletal muscle, is the standard test used to establish susceptibility to malignant hyperthermia. A linkage has been established between the human gene for malignant hyperthermia and the ryanodine receptor gene. This receptor is a protein that comprises the calcium release channel of skeletal muscle sarcoplasmic reticulum. Genetic studies suggest that the caffeine-halothane contracture test may yield many false-positive results. In any event, the incidence during anesthesia is approximately 1:15,000 for pediatric patients and 1:50,000 for adult patients. This disease is due to a defect in excitation-contraction coupling in skeletal muscles and high calcium concentrations in the myoplasm. Exposure to a triggering drug such as a volatile anesthetic, succinylcholine, or an amide local anesthetic causes unusually high and sustained levels of calcium in the myoplasm and persistent skeletal muscle contraction. This results in hypermetabolism, including tachycardia, arterial hypoxemia, metabolic and respiratory acidosis, and profound hyperthermia. Dantrolene, up to 10 mg/kg intravenously, is the treatment of choice.

Patients who will require anesthesia and are susceptible to malignant hyperthermia should be pretreated with dantrolene, 5 mg/kg/d orally in four divided doses for 1–3 days; drugs known to trigger the syndrome should be avoided during anesthesia. No anesthetic approach is completely safe in these patients, though the drugs usually used are narcotics, barbiturates, nitrous oxide, and ester local anesthetics.

Recurrence of Myocardial Infarction

Patients with prior myocardial infarction are at more risk for perioperative reinfarction (5–8%) than those without prior myocardial infarction (0.1–0.7%) and have a reinfarction mortality rate of 36–70%. The more recent the previous myocardial infarction, the more likely is reinfarction. Within 3 months, the reinfarction rate exceeds 30%; at 3–6 months, it is 15%; and after 6 months, it is approximately 5%.

The incidence of myocardial infarction is increased in patients having intrathoracic or intra-abdominal operations lasting more than 3 hours. There is no correlation between risk and the site of previous infarction, the history of surgery for atherosclerosis of peripheral arteries, the site of operation if the duration of operation is less than 3 hours, or the drugs and techniques used in anesthesia. Close hemodynamic monitoring using intra-arterial and pulmonary artery catheters and prompt treatment of hypotension or hypertension decrease the risk of perioperative infarction in high-risk patients. Furthermore, early detection and treatment of intraoperative cardiac ischemia dictates monitoring with the V_5 lead (either uni- or bipolar) in patients with a risk of ischemia. The V_4 lead is more sensitive than lead II and should be considered as a second choice. However, lead II, superior for detection of atrial dysrhythmias, is more easily obtained with conventional monitors. The use of all three leads seems to be optimal in a patient at high risk.

In addition to a recent myocardial infarction (ie, < 6 months), existing congestive heart failure is the only preoperative predictor of perioperative cardiac morbidity. Both intraoperative hypotension and tachycardia are intraoperative predictors. Lastly, perioperative cardiac morbidity is also increased in emergency surgery, vascular surgery, and prolonged (> 3 hours) thoracic or upper abdominal surgery.

Hepatotoxicity

Halothane anesthesia has been shown to be unrelated to massive postoperative hepatic necrosis and is safe to use in hepatobiliary surgery. Repeated exposures to halothane over short periods, however, may cause mild hepatitis, though the incidence is extremely low. Hepatitis may be caused by an allergic reaction. It is associated with eosinophilia, and more severe liver dysfunction follows repeated exposure to halothane or one of its metabolites. Perhaps antigenicity of the hepatocytes is changed by halothane, leading to production of antibodies against the liver. Individual susceptibility to cell damage after exposure to electrophilic drug metabolites is probably one factor predisposing to halothane hepatitis.

More recent evidence indicates that patients with halothane hepatitis may generate antibodies toward a covalently bound metabolite of halothane. These antibodies are produced to a lesser extent after administration of enflurane and isoflurane. Perhaps antibody assays will allow detection of patients sensitized to volatile anesthetics. Furthermore, development of such a test would provide more definitive evidence for the influence of the anesthetic on postoperative hepatic dysfunction.

Farrell G, Prendergast D, Murray M: Halothane hepatitis: Detection of a constitutional susceptibility factor. N Engl J Med 1985;313:1310.

MacKenzie AE et al: A comparison of the caffeine halothane muscle contracture with the molecular genetic diagnosis of malignant hyperthermia. Anesthesiology 1991;75:4.

Mangano DT: Perioperative cardiac morbidity. Anesthesiology 1990;72:153.

Martin JL, Kenna JG, Pohl LR: Antibody assays for the detection of patients sensitized to halothane. Anesth Analg 1990;70:154.

RISKS OF EXPOSURE OF OPERATING ROOM PERSONNEL TO ANESTHETICS

Thousands of operating room personnel are chronically exposed to trace concentrations of inhaled anesthetics; this is a concern because of potential mutagenicity, teratogenicity, and carcinogenicity. However, there has been no demonstrated cause-and-effect relationship. The incidence of spontaneous abortion in female operating room personnel is 1½–2 times the normal rate, but whether this is due to inhalation of trace concentrations or to other aspects of their work is not known. Because of these concerns, however, anesthetics are evacuated from the operating room via vacuum tubes and other devices. These devices occasionally malfunction, causing increased pressures in the anesthetic machine and resulting in pneumothorax in patients in whom the machine is being used.

REFERENCES

Barash PG, Cullen BF, Stoelting RK: *Clinical Anesthesia.* Lippincott, Philadelphia 1989.

Miller RD (editor): *Anesthesia,* 3rd ed. Churchill Livingstone, 1990.

Stoelting RK, Miller RD (editors): *Basics of Anesthesia,* 2nd ed. Churchill Livingstone, 1989.

Shock & Acute Pulmonary Failure in Surgical Patients

James W. Holcroft, MD, & David H. Wisner, MD

I. SHOCK

Severe cardiovascular failure, or shock, can be caused by (1) depletion of the vascular volume, (2) compression of the heart or great veins, (3) intrinsic failure of the heart itself, (4) loss of autonomic control of the vasculature, (5) severe, untreated sepsis, and (6) severe but partially compensated sepsis. Depending on the type and severity of cardiovascular failure and on the success of initial management, shock can go on to compromise other organ systems. For discussion of gastrointestinal failure, see Chapter 3; for hepatic failure and psychiatric problems, see Chapter 4; for kidney failure, see Chapter 5; for problems of catabolism and the resulting musculoskeletal debility, see Chapter 10; and for infection in seriously ill surgical patients, see Chapter 8.

This chapter discusses the cardiovascular and pulmonary disorders in shock.

DIAGNOSIS & TREATMENT OF THE CARDIOVASCULAR CONSEQUENCES OF SHOCK

HYPOVOLEMIC SHOCK

Pathophysiology

Hypovolemic shock (shock caused by inadequate circulating blood volume) can arise from bleeding, protracted vomiting or diarrhea, sequestration of fluid in the gut lumen (eg, bowel obstruction), or loss of plasma into injured tissues (eg, burns or trauma). Depletion of vascular volume, which allows systemic venules and small veins to collapse, decreases the driving pressure for return of blood to the heart, decreases end-diastolic ventricular volumes, and decreases cardiac output.

In mild to moderate shock, the body compensates through discharge of the cardiovascular adrenergic nerves and release of vasopressin and angiotensin, which constrict venules and small veins throughout the body and selectively constrict arterioles to the skin, fat, connective tissue, bone, skeletal muscle, gut, pancreas, spleen, and liver (but not the brain or heart). Venular constriction displaces blood to the heart to help reestablish end-diastolic volumes and cardiac output; the selective arteriolar constriction diverts blood away from organs that withstand ischemia relatively well to those that withstand it poorly. In addition, aldosterone is released. It and vasopressin stimulate tubular reabsorption of water and sodium and thus minimize urinary losses of plasma constituents.

Diagnosis

Although compensatory responses to arrested **mild shock** (a deficit of < 20% of the blood volume) are almost always adequate to ensure survival even without treatment, recognition of an untreated cause early in mild shock can prevent fatal progression. The signs of early hypovolemic shock are postural hypotension, cutaneous vasoconstriction, sweat gland stimulation, collapse of the neck veins, concentration of the urine, oliguria, and a decreasing hematocrit with administration of fluids (Table 12–1). These are manifestations either of the shock itself (such as postural hypotension, neck vein collapse, and serial falling hematocrits) or represent compensatory responses to the shock (cutaneous vasoconstriction and sweat production and urine concentration and oliguria).

The blood pressure in a supine mildly hypovolemic patient is usually normal but will fall by at least 10 mm Hg when the patient sits up, and the lower level typically persists for several minutes. (The blood pressure in a euvolemic patient may fall transiently when the patient sits up rapidly but will return to normal levels within 1 minute.) Postural hypotension is a sensitive sign of hypovolemia and can be elicited by nonphysician personnel. It cannot be used in multiply injured patients, however, and its use is limited mostly to patients who are suspected of being

Table 12–1. Clinical classification of hypovolemia.

Mild hypovolemia (deficit < 20% of blood volume)
  Pathophysiology: Decreased perfusion of organs that withstand ischemia well (skin, fat, skeletal muscle, bone).
  Manifestations: Patient complains of feeling cold. Postural changes in blood pressure and pulse. Pale, cool, clammy skin. Flat neck veins. Concentrated urine.
Moderate hypovolemia (deficit = 20–40% of blood volume)
  Pathophysiology: Decreased perfusion of organs that withstand ischemia poorly (pancreas, spleen, kidneys).
  Manifestations: Patient complains of being thirsty. Occasionally, low blood pressure and rapid pulse in supine position. Oliguria.
Severe hypovolemia (deficit > 40% blood volume)
  Pathophysiology: Decreased perfusion of brain and heart.
  Manifestations: Patient is restless, agitated, confused, obtunded, or "drunk." Low blood pressure and sometimes rapid, weak, irregular pulse. Deep breaths at rapid rate. Cardiac arrest.

---

hypovolemic from either dehydration or occult internal blood loss (eg, in a patient who might have gastrointestinal bleeding).

The skin manifestations of adrenergic discharge are sensitive and can be noted in any patient, including one with multiple injuries. They are easiest to detect in the feet. The subcutaneous veins collapse, which causes difficulty in inserting venous cannulas as an early finding in shock, and the skin becomes pale, cold, and clammy, so that microvascular refilling is slow. Coldness and clamminess are usually obvious. Pallor is best detected on the plantar surfaces of the toes or in the nail beds, where color changes can be seen in all patients, including those with dark skin. Compressing the toe to produce blanching and then releasing the compression and watching for color return can usually resolve any uncertainty. In a normovolemic patient without peripheral vascular disease, the color should return within 2 seconds; refill takes longer than 2 seconds in hypovolemic patients. The test should be done with the foot of the bed at the level of the heart.

Although examination of the skin can help in diagnosis of hypovolemia, it can sometimes be misleading. Fright, exposure to a cold environment, and difficulty in deciding if the skin really is pale are potentially confusing factors.

Looking for collapsed neck veins—an index of low CVP—is best done with the patient's head, neck, and torso elevated 30 degrees. Whether or not pulsations are present in the internal jugular vein gives a clue to filling pressures of the right heart, as there are no valves between the internal jugular vein and the right atrium. A normal right atrial pressure will distend the neck veins to about 4 cm above the manubrium.

A urine specimen should be promptly obtained in any patient suspected of being hypovolemic, and a Foley catheter should be inserted. Even in mild hypovolemia, the urine will be concentrated and the patient oliguric. Oliguria is defined as urine output less than 0.5 mL/kg/h in adults; less than 1 mL/kg/h in children; or less than 2 mL/kg/h in infants. It is an early and specific sign of hypovolemia.

The initial hematocrit is of no value in diagnosing hypovolemia except in chronic bleeding, when vascular equilibration has had time to dilute the hematocrit. Acute hemorrhage does not immediately reduce the hematocrit, so repeated measurements are required.

The hematocrit will always fall as asanguineous fluids are administered. A fall of 3% or 4% indicates that the blood volume has been depleted by about 10%; a fall of 6–8% indicates a deficit of about 20% (or 1 L in an average adult). These calculations assume that the patient has been given enough fluid to correct the hypovolemia.

Additional manifestations in **moderate hypovolemia** (a deficit of 20–40% of the blood volume) include thirst and sometimes moderate hypotension with the patient supine (Table 12–1). **Severe hypovolemia** (a deficit of more than 40% of blood volume) can produce signs of inadequate cerebral and cardiac perfusion. The former includes changes in mental status, eg, restlessness, agitation, confusion, lethargy, or the appearance of inebriation; or inadequate cardiac perfusion, eg, an irregular heartbeat or electrocardiographic evidence of myocardial ischemia, such as ST-T segment depression or the appearance of Q waves. Patients in severe hypovolemic shock will almost always be hypotensive, even when supine (Table 12–1).

Although the heart rate in some species increases proportionally in response to graded hemorrhage, there is little correlation between severity of hypovolemia and heart rate in humans. For example, hypovolemic patients often have normal heart rates, and severe hypovolemia can even produce bradycardia as a preterminal event. Thus, tachycardia can be taken as weak confirmation of the presence of shock, but a normal rate is not evidence against hypovolemia.

If the patient is inebriated, hypovolemia may be difficult to diagnose (Table 12–2). High blood etha-

Table 12–2. Manifestations of cardiovascular disorders in critically ill patients.

Condition	Skin	Neck Veins
Hypovolemia	Cold, clammy	Flat
Cardiac compression	Cold, clammy	Distended[1]
Cardiogenic	Cold, clammy	Distended
Neurogenic	Warm[2]	Flat
Low output sepsis	Warm	Flat to normal
High output sepsis	Cold, clammy	Flat
Hypoglycemia	Cold, clammy	Flat to normal
Inebriation[3]	Warm	Normal

[1]May be flat if patient is also hypovolemic.
[2]In denervated areas.
[3]Listed only to emphasize that alcohol can mask signs of other conditions.

nol levels produce warm, flushed, and dry skin and promote a diuresis of dilute urine—ie, alcohol ablates two of the principal signs. Postural hypotension—if it can be elicited—will remain, however, and supine hypotension occurs with less severe hypovolemia in inebriation.

Like hypovolemia, insulin shock also stimulates adrenergic discharge and release of vasoactive hormones (Table 12–2). The cold, clammy, oliguric, and hypotensive insulin-dependent diabetic who has just been in an automobile accident could either be hypovolemic or hypoglycemic. Blood glucose levels should be measured in such patients, and an intravenous bolus of 50 mL of 50% glucose should be administered while the patient is being evaluated for hypovolemia.

Treatment

Resuscitation of patients in hemorrhagic shock should begin with establishment of an airway, which can usually be accomplished by hyperextending the neck and supporting the jaw. Many hypovolemic patients can breathe adequately, and they may even hyperventilate. Supplemental nasal oxygen is usually all that is needed. Some patients, however, require tracheal intubation and mechanical ventilation. Trauma victims may require insertion of chest tubes. External hemorrhage, if present, should be controlled, and preparations should be made to operate on patients bleeding internally.

Percutaneously placed venous catheters should be used for mild hypovolemia; large-bore intravenous catheters placed by cut-down, for severe hypovolemia. The saphenous veins at the ankles provide an accessible site unless the extremity is badly traumatized. Catheters in the saphenous vein should be removed within 24 hours to avoid phlebitis.

Percutaneously placed central venous catheters should not be used for initial resuscitation, because a central line is not required to administer fluids and because technical problems during placement could produce complications. Central venous catheters may be inserted later, when they can be used to measure right atrial pressures. Large-bore (14-gauge or larger) catheters should be used. The commonly used 16-gauge subclavian lines are too long and narrow to permit rapid infusion of fluids.

Crystalloid solution with a sodium concentration approximating that of plasma (eg, lactated Ringer's injection) should be used for initial resuscitation. The lactate buffers the metabolic acidemia of shock by absorbing hydrogen ion to form lactic acid. The lactic acid is then oxidized to carbon dioxide and water in the Krebs cycle. Although, in theory, shock-induced hepatic hypoperfusion might impair metabolism of lactic acid, metabolism is in fact rapid, probably because liver blood flow is quickly reestablished with the initial resuscitation. However, patients with cirrhosis should be given normal saline supplemented with sodium bicarbonate instead of lactated Ringer's injection. Glucose should not be used in initial resuscitation (except to treat hypoglycemia), because it may induce osmotic diuresis.

The severity of shock should determine the rate and amount of fluid given. Two liters of crystalloid should be given as fast as possible in patients in severe shock, followed by a third liter infused over 10 minutes. Three liters of fluid will resuscitate any patient in whom hemorrhage has been arrested. Incomplete resuscitation indicates continued bleeding and probably the need for laparotomy. Less severe shock requires proportionately less fluid.

Resuscitation should begin with a crystalloid solution even if blood is available—indeed, even if the patient is bleeding. By restoring peripheral perfusion, the initial fluid bolus flushes into the circulation products of anaerobic and catabolic metabolism, which can temporarily depress the myocardium. Cold, acidotic, hyperkalemic blood at this point would compromise the myocardium even further.

In general, blood should be withheld until bleeding has been controlled, to minimize loss of transfused red blood cells. Young patients without heart disease tolerate hemodilution well, as long as the plasma volume is fully expanded. Hematocrits as low as 15% are safe for the 20 minutes or so required to control major hemorrhage.

Blood should be started, however, in patients who remain unstable after the initial crystalloid infusion, even if bleeding has not yet been contained. In young patients with normal coronary arteries, the hematocrit should be brought into the mid 20s. If bleeding is liable to continue, the objective should be a hematocrit in the low 30s. If the patient has coronary artery disease or shows signs of myocardial ischemia on electrocardiography, the hematocrit should be increased to the mid 30s. The heart is the first organ to show the ill effects of a too-low hematocrit.

The freshest possible blood should be used, especially if more than a few units will be necessary. Fresh blood minimizes coagulation abnormalities. If blood must be given before it can be cross-matched, type-specific non-cross-matched blood, which can usually be obtained within 10 minutes, should be used. The risk of a transfusion reaction is negligible compared with the risks of inadequate oxygen delivery to the tissues. If type-specific blood is not available, Rh-negative type O blood may be used. Whole blood should be given to resuscitate severely bleeding patients because of the time required to administer packed cells.

Albumin-containing solutions (other than blood) should not be used, since, during shock, they have little effect on plasma oncotic pressure and do not retain fluids within the vascular space, as was once thought. Instead, the protein extravasates into the interstitial space. Dextran, starch solutions, fluorocarbons, and stroma-free hemoglobin solutions have not been adequately evaluated, and their role in resuscitation is undefined.

In some cases, the total amount of fluid required for resuscitation is 20–30 L, especially in the presence of massive injuries. Much of this fluid ends up in the interstitium because of trauma-induced microvascular endothelial disruption. To minimize the increase in endothelial permeability, every effort should be made to rapidly control bleeding, immobilize fractures, and debride necrotic tissue. The combination of shock and tissue trauma stimulates coagulation and inflammation, which is manifested by generalized edema.

Elevation of the lower extremities above the level of the heart (Trendelenburg's position) may shift some blood to the right heart, but there is little lasting benefit, and the left ventricle must work harder to pump blood back to the elevated extremities. This time-honored procedure is best abandoned for treatment of hypovolemia. Neither is the pneumatic antishock garment, an inflatable overall enclosing the lower extremities and abdomen, useful in reversing the cardiovascular changes in shock, because it hinders blood return by compressing the inferior vena cava and perhaps the renal and hepatic veins, and it makes left ventricular emptying more difficult by compressing the arterioles in the lower body. Although in normovolemic subjects the garment displaces blood from subdiaphragmatic to supradiaphragmatic organs, this shift will already have been accomplished by adrenergic mechanisms in hypovolemic patients, and some residual blood flow to splanchnic viscera may be essential to prevent late organ failure. The garment precludes use of the saphenous vein as a site for venous access, and it may push the diaphragm into the thorax and interfere with ventilation. It may be effective, however, in splinting fractures and in tamponading bleeding in the parts of the body that it encloses. Its use should be restricted to these indications.

Treatment of nonhemorrhagic hypovolemic shock is similar to that of hemorrhagic shock. Blood is unnecessary, and in some cases, such as severe burns, one goal of therapy is to decrease the hematocrit. Asanguineous fluids should be given to eliminate postural hypotension, restore peripheral perfusion, and reestablish urine output. For hypovolemia caused by protracted vomiting or loss of fluid into the gut, volume replenishment should also take into account the need to correct electrolyte abnormalities. (See Chapter 9.)

CARDIAC COMPRESSIVE SHOCK

Pathophysiology

Shock can arise from any condition that compresses the heart or great veins, including pericardial tamponade; positive-pressure ventilation; tension pneumothorax; distention of the abdomen with compression of the inferior vena cava and elevation of the diaphragm into the chest; and rupture of the diaphragm with displacement of abdominal viscera into the chest. Compression of the inferior or superior vena cava or the pulmonary veins retards blood return to the heart; compression of the heart itself, especially the thin-walled atria and right ventricle, prevents adequate chamber filling.

Diagnosis

The signs of shock are present—ie, postural hypotension, poor cutaneous perfusion, oliguria, hypotension, mental status changes, or electrocardiographic signs of myocardial ischemia—combined with distended neck veins (Table 12–2). The only other condition that can produce this pattern is cardiogenic shock, which rarely poses a problem in differential diagnosis because cardiac compression usually follows trauma or occurs in a setting where mechanical compromise of the heart or great veins is a known risk, such as mechanical ventilation or massive ascites. Cardiogenic shock usually develops in a background of evident disease that predisposes to primary myocardial dysfunction (see below, in section on cardiogenic shock).

Confirmation of cardiac compression can be made by observing the neck veins and measuring the systolic blood pressure while the patient takes a deep breath. Inspiration in a normovolemic patient without cardiac compression decreases right atrial pressure, which can be detected by observing the neck veins. The decrease in pressure arises from the balance of three different influences: First, as the lungs pull away from the extrapericardial great veins, blood tends to surge into the right atrium and increase the pressure within the chamber. Second, the pressure inside the atrium tends to increase with a deep breath because a fully expanded lung compresses the interalveolar pulmonary vasculature and makes it difficult for the right ventricle to contract; blood tends to back up in the right heart and increase right atrial pressure. Third, the lungs pull away from the pericardium and from the enclosed thin-walled right heart chambers, which tends to decrease right atrial pressure. Under normal conditions, this last effect predominates.

In the presence of cardiac compression, however, the effect of the lungs pulling away from the heart is lost. An engorged pericardium acts as a barrier so that decreased pressure on the outside of the pericardium is no longer reflected by pressure changes on the heart. The effects of inspiration on the extrapericardial great veins and pulmonary vasculature, however, are not influenced by the tamponade. The overall result is increased right atrial pressure and further distention of the neck veins. This **Kussmaul sign** is pathognomonic of pericardial tamponade.

The so-called **paradoxic pulse** can also be helpful in diagnosis. A spontaneous breath in a normovolemic patient without cardiac compression produces little effect on systemic blood pressure. A fall in systolic pressure of more than 10 mm Hg ("pulsus paradoxus") supports the diagnosis of pericardial tamponade. As the lungs expand, the walls of the extra-alveolar pulmonary capacitance vessels are pulled apart, and blood pools within the vasculature. This transient pulmonary sequestration of blood decreases left atrial filling, reduces stretching of the atrial myocardium and the effectiveness of atrial contraction, and reduces the amount of blood delivered into the left ventricle. Left ventricular end-diastolic volume and stroke volume decrease. On the other hand, a spontaneous inspiration tends to increase stretching of the atrial myocardial fibers as the lungs pull away from the heart, which tends to increase left heart filling and left ventricular stroke volume.

These two opposing effects usually cancel out, and the stroke volumes associated with inspiration and expiration—and the corresponding blood pressures—are about the same. In the presence of pericardial tamponade, however, blood pressure can fall considerably because tamponade leaves unopposed the inspiration-induced pooling of blood in the pulmonary vasculature.

The diagnosis of cardiac compression is facilitated if the patient can be monitored in an intensive care unit with a Swan-Ganz catheter (see section on Swan-Ganz catheter), where a low cardiac output in the face of high filling pressures can be documented by direct measurement. In addition, the catheter can be used to compare pressures in the left and right atria. Under normal circumstances, the pressure in the left atrium is about 5 mm Hg higher than in the right. In tamponade, the pressures are identical, because cardiac compression dominates all other influences. This finding is sensitive but not specific, especially if the patient is being mechanically ventilated.

Positive-pressure ventilation has three potential adverse effects on cardiac output: (1) Inflation of the lungs compresses the superior and inferior vena cava and impedes filling of the right heart (in contrast, a spontaneous inspiration augments filling); (2) lung inflation compresses the thin-walled atria and right ventricle, decreases end-diastolic myocardial stretch, and decreases stroke volumes (again in contrast to a spontaneous inspiration); and (3) expansion of the lung compresses the interalveolar vessels and hinders right ventricular emptying. In extreme cases, these three effects can decrease cardiac output to the point that it can no longer meet metabolic needs, especially if the patient is hypovolemic.

Tension pneumothorax produces shock by kinking the great veins and by compressing the atria and right ventricle. Ascites, intra-abdominal bleeding, or distention of the gut compresses the inferior vena cava and pushes the diaphragm directly against the heart. Rupture of the diaphragm with displacement of abdominal viscera into the chest also directly compresses the heart. The clinical diagnosis of these conditions is discussed in the chapter on trauma; the hemodynamic changes that help make the diagnosis are shock in the presence of distended neck veins, sometimes with a Kussmaul sign or a paradoxic pulse.

Treatment

Infusion of fluid can transiently overcome some of the ill effects of cardiac compression, but the cause of shock in these patients is mechanical, and definitive treatment must correct the mechanical abnormality. Pericardial tamponade, tension pneumothorax, and ruptured diaphragm are discussed in Chapter 13; bowel obstruction in Chapter 30. Treatment of compressive shock caused by large-volume mechanical ventilation is discussed later in this chapter in the section on mechanical ventilation.

CARDIOGENIC SHOCK

Pathophysiology

Cardiogenic shock can arise from an arrhythmia, ischemia-induced myocardial failure, valvular or septal defects, systemic or pulmonary hypertension, myocarditis, or myocardiopathies. The diagnosis is usually made on the basis of a known history of cardiovascular disease in conjunction with an abnormal ECG in a patient in shock with distended neck veins (Table 12–2).

A slow heart rate (less than 50 beats/min in an adult) can cause inadequate cardiac output, because cardiac output is the product of stroke volume and heart rate. A rapid heart rate—one that exceeds the maximum aerobic limit of 230 minus the patient's age in years—can cause inadequate output because the ventricles have inadequate time to fill and the coronary arteries receive too little blood during diastole. Myocardial ischemia can cause shock because the myocardium lacks adequate oxygen; anatomic defects, because of wasted pumping; hypertension, because of an excessive load on the ventricles and because of superimposed abnormalities that develop in the myocardium with hypertrophy or dilation; and myocardial disease, because of intrinsic failure of the heart muscle.

Diagnosis

The diagnosis of cardiogenic shock usually depends on recognition of the underlying medical condition. Shock, distended neck veins, peripheral edema, an enlarged and tender liver, a third heart sound, rales, electrocardiographic signs of ischemia, and an enlarged heart on x-ray can all be helpful. The diagnosis is usually easy, but two common situations may pose a problem.

The first is a ruptured abdominal aortic aneurysm in a patient with coronary artery disease. The patient might have abdominal pain consistent with a myocardial infarction and electrocardiographic signs of ischemia, the ischemia caused by hypovolemia and severe shock. The key is to observe the neck veins.

The second is to ascribe shock to myocardial contusion in a patient who has just suffered a major chest injury. Although blunt chest trauma can damage the heart, damage of this kind is usually fatal at the scene of the injury. A contusion that produces failure but not death is rare. Shock after blunt trauma in a patient who survives to reach the hospital is almost never caused by contusion—it is far more likely to be caused by hypovolemia or cardiac compression.

Treatment

A. Opioids: Opioids relieve pain, provide sedation, block adrenergic discharge, decrease right ventricular filling, and lessen stress on the heart. They can be especially effective in treating cardiac failure after myocardial infarction.

B. Diuretics: By decreasing vascular volume, diuretics decrease right and left atrial pressures and alleviate peripheral and pulmonary edema. Pulmonary vascular pressures and volumes decrease; effectiveness of right ventricular contraction may increase. Coronary blood flow increases as coronary sinus pressure drops. Diuretics are ideal therapy in congestive heart failure with expanded vascular volumes; they are obviously contraindicated in cardiovascular disorders caused by hypovolemia, trauma, cardiac compression, sepsis, or loss of microvascular tone, even though these forms of shock are frequently associated with oliguria.

C. Chronotropic Agents: Patients in cardiac failure with bradycardia may on rare occasion temporarily benefit from administration of a chronotropic agent such as atropine or isoproterenol. Isoproterenol increases heart rate, augments myocardial contractility, and dilates the systemic arterioles. Chronotropic agents should be used to increase the heart rate only to levels that can be tolerated comfortably. A 60-year-old patient with normal coronary arteries should be able to tolerate a heart rate of 120/min; the limit is about 90/min in the presence of coronary artery disease.

Chronotropic agents increase myocardial work and shorten the time during diastole for coronary blood flow and ventricular filling and usually should not be used except as a temporary expedient. If they are used for more than 30 minutes, a Swan-Ganz catheter should be inserted. The goal of therapy is a normal or supranormal cardiac index. Cardiac indices should be determined at different heart rates produced by different doses of drug and the results compared with timing of chest pain and electrocardiographic signs of myocardial ischemia.

D. Inotropic Agents: Many patients in cardiac failure benefit from administration of an inotropic agent such as dopamine or dobutamine. In low doses, these drugs increase myocardial contractility. In addition, dopamine is said to dilate the renal vasculature, increasing renal blood flow and urine output. The principal use of these drugs is to increase flow in the cardiovascular system; rarely, they are used for vasoconstriction or diuresis. Dopamine frequently increases the heart rate excessively; dobutamine usually does not.

Dopamine and dobutamine must be used with caution, and the patient should be monitored in an intensive care unit. At doses of 10 µg/kg/min or greater, the drugs constrict the systemic arterioles, and in hypovolemic patients, even low doses (eg, dopamine in a dosage of 5 µg/kg/min) can cause ischemic necrosis of the digits.

If it is necessary to use inotropic agents for more than 1 hour, a Swan-Ganz catheter should be inserted. Filling pressures and cardiac indices should be determined at different infusion rates. If any question remains about the adequacy of volume resuscitation, filling pressures and cardiac indices should be measured before and after a fluid bolus is given.

Digitalis compounds should not be used in acute cardiac failure except to control dysrhythmias. Toxicity may develop, especially when pH and electrolyte changes are unpredictable. The inotropic actions of digitalis are no different from those of dopamine and dobutamine.

E. Vasodilators: The most useful vasodilating agents in surgical patients with cardiac failure are morphine sulfate, nitroprusside, and nitroglycerin, all of which are either easily reversible or short-acting. These drugs should be used as primary vasodilators only if systemic vascular resistance is known to be elevated (ie, only if a Swan-Ganz catheter is in place). They are usually used in patients with high mean systemic arterial pressures but can occasionally be used (with caution) in patients with normal arterial pressures as long as the systemic vascular resistance is high.

Vasodilators decrease systemic vascular resistance, allowing the left heart to pump more efficiently. These agents may also reduce pulmonary vascular resistance and increase pulmonary vascular compliance, improving right heart performance. Nitroglycerin and, to a lesser extent, nitroprusside dilate the systemic venules and small veins and decrease right heart filling.

All of these effects decrease myocardial work and oxygen demands. In some patients, however, excessive venous dilatation can decrease cardiac filling enough that cardiac output falls. Cardiac filling pressures and cardiac output should be measured before and after starting treatment. Excessive arteriolar dilatation may lead to inadequate perfusion pressures for the coronary arteries and myocardial ischemia. The patient should be monitored for chest pain and electrocardiographic evidence of myocardial ischemia while the drugs are being given.

F. Beta-Blocking Agents: An occasional patient in cardiac failure with ischemia and a rapid heart rate will benefit from a beta-adrenergic blocking agent (eg, esmolol or propranolol), which may reduce myocardial oxygen consumption and salvage marginal myocardium.

G. Vasoconstrictors: Vasoconstrictors are occasionally useful to increase perfusion pressures for atherosclerotic coronary arteries, although endogenous adrenergic mechanisms usually bring forth a maximum response. Because vasoconstrictors can decrease the efficiency of left ventricular pumping and produce ischemic necrosis of digits or extremities, they should be used only when absolutely necessary and not for more than 60 minutes unless a pulmonary arterial catheter is in place.

H. Transaortic Balloon Pump: The transaortic balloon pump is effective in resuscitating selected patients with severe reversible left ventricular dysfunction (eg, after cardiopulmonary bypass or acute myocardial infarction). It should only be used if a Swan-Ganz catheter is in place.

NEUROGENIC SHOCK

Shock caused by failure of the autonomic nervous system can arise from regional anesthetics, injuries to the spinal cord, or administration of autonomic blocking agents. The cardiac output decreases because the venules and small veins lose tone. Blood pools in the periphery, ventricular end-diastolic volumes decrease, and stroke volumes fall. The adrenergic nervous system above the level of denervation is activated, increasing heart rate and contractility to compensate for peripheral pooling of blood if the lesion is below the midthoracic sympathetic outflow. If the sympathetic nerves to the heart are also blocked, the patient may develop an absolute or relative bradycardia. If the lesion is associated with paralysis of the skeletal musculature, loss of perivenular support by skeletal muscle tone can aggravate venous pooling. The blood pressure in neurogenic shock can plummet to very low levels because arteriolar as well as venular tone will also be lost.

The diagnosis rests on knowledge of the circumstances preceding the onset of shock and on the physical examination. The patient will always be hypotensive, and the skin will be warm and flushed in the denervated areas (Table 12–2). The cause is usually obvious.

Head injury, as opposed to spinal cord injury, does not produce neurogenic shock or any other kind of shock. In fact, increased intracranial pressure typically increases blood pressure and slows heart rate (the Cushing reflex). Hypotension and tachycardia should never be attributed to head injury—even severe head injury with cerebral dysfunction—until concomitant hypovolemia has been ruled out.

Neurogenic shock is the only type in which vasoconstrictors are usually useful. The goal is to restore tone in the venules and small veins and to increase blood pressure to the point that coronary perfusion is sustained, as judged by normal ST–T segments on electrocardiography and absence of chest pain. Either norepinephrine or phenylephrine can be used. If vasoconstrictors are expected to be needed for more than 1 hour, the patient should be placed in an intensive care unit with Swan-Ganz monitoring. Trendelenburg's position can also be temporarily useful. Short-term steroids should be given if the patient has suffered an injury to the spinal cord, to optimize recovery of neurologic function.

HIGH-OUTPUT SEPTIC SHOCK

Bowel perforation, necrotic intestine, abscesses, gangrene, and soft tissue infections can produce high-output septic shock. Early or adequately treated sepsis presents with fever and compensatory cutaneous vasodilatation. Systemic vascular resistance and arterial blood pressure fall, but cardiac output increases because the left ventricle has little resistance to pump against. Although adrenergic activity increases somewhat, the need to decrease core temperature predominates, and flow to the skin remains high. Cardiac output remains elevated as long as the blood volume is maintained. This high-output septic state is frequently associated with deranged metabolism, so that the tissue's metabolic needs are not met even though the circulation is hyperdynamic.

Early sepsis is manifested by fever and hypotension in a patient who appears pink and well perfused (Table 12–2). If vascular volume is maintained, the cutaneous veins will be full, urine output will be adequate, and the pulse rate will be high. The patient is often anxious and confused. Intermittent chills and fever are common.

Treatment consists of administration of intravenous fluids and antibiotics, correction of gastrointestinal leaks, debridement of dead tissue, and drainage of pus. If the vascular volume can be maintained, the patient will remain well perfused; if treatment is delayed or if the infection cannot be controlled, late sepsis will develop. In the near future, monoclonal antibodies against endotoxin will in all likelihood be approved by the Food and Drug Administration for use in septic shock. They should be administered as soon as the diagnosis of sepsis and gram-negative bacteremia is made.

LOW-OUTPUT SEPTIC SHOCK

Untreated or late systemic sepsis, from either Gram-positive or Gram-negative bacteria, can disrupt the microvascular endothelium, prompt the loss of plasma into the interstitium, and produce shock similar to that associated with hypovolemia (Table 12–2). Pulmonary vascular resistance increases and hinders right ventricular emptying. In addition, in some patients, circulating plasma factors might depress myocardial contractility. (It is unlikely that myocardial depression plays any role in hypovolemic, cardiac compressive, or neurogenic shock.) The cardiovascular findings of low-output sepsis are identical to those of hypovolemic shock. The diagnosis is usually clear from the clinical circumstances. The initial cardiovascular resuscitation for low-output septic and hypovolemic shock is the same.

Abel FL: Myocardial function in sepsis and endotoxin shock. Am J Physiol 1989;257:R1265.

Anderson ID et al: An effect of trauma on human cardiovascular control: Baroreflex suppression. J Trauma 1990; 30:9742.

Braken MB et al: A randomized, controlled trial of methylprednisolone or naloxone in the treatment of acute spinal-cord injury. N Engl J Med 1990;322:1405.

Conrad SA et al: Effect of red cell transfusion on oxygen consumption following fluid resuscitation in septic shock. Circ Shock 1990;31:419.

Foley EF et al: Albumin supplementation in the critically ill: A prospective, randomized trial. Arch Surg 1990; 125:739.

Rackow EC et al: Cellular oxygen metabolism during sepsis and shock: The relationship of oxygen consumption to oxygen delivery. JAMA 1988;259:1989.

Velanovich V: Crystalloid versus colloid fluid resuscitation: A meta-analysis of mortality. Surgery 1989;105:65.

Wisner DH et al: Suspected myocardial contusion: Triage and indications for monitoring. Ann Surg 1990;212:82.

Zeigler EJ et al: Treatment of gram-negative bacteremia and septic shock with HA-1A human monoclonal antibody against endotoxin: A randomized, double-blind, placebo-controlled trial. N Engl J Med 1991;324:429.

NEUROHUMORAL & CELLULAR RESPONSES TO SHOCK

The neurohumoral responses to shock include discharge of the cardiovascular nerves and release of vasoactive, metabolically active, and volume-conserving hormones. The responses can be life-saving before therapy begins and serve to maintain homeostasis once therapy has started. The responses, however, can also contribute to postshock organ failure.

CARDIOVASCULAR ADRENERGIC DISCHARGE

Adrenergic discharge constricts the venules and small veins, constricts arterioles in all parts of the body except the brain and heart, and increases cardiac contractility. The result is increased cardiac output and blood pressure and diversion of flow to the brain and heart.

RELEASE OF VASOACTIVE HORMONES

The vasoactive hormones, angiotensin II and vasopressin, act in concert with discharge of the cardiovascular adrenergic nerves. Activation of angiotensin II begins with release of renin from the kidneys. Renin stimulates the liver to synthesize and release angiotensinogen, which is converted to angiotensin I; enzymes in the pulmonary endothelium convert angiotensin I to angiotensin II. Angiotensin II constricts the vasculature in the skin, kidneys, and splanchnic organs and diverts blood flow to the heart and brain.

Systemic hypotension and hyperosmolality (see below) stimulate the posterior pituitary to release vasopressin. Vasopressin, like adrenergic discharge and angiotensin II, constricts the vascular sphincters in the skin and splanchnic organs (it does not constrict the renal vasculature) and diverts blood flow to the heart and brain.

RELEASE OF METABOLICALLY ACTIVE HORMONES

Hypovolemia, hypotension, pain, and other stresses of critical illness stimulate the release of three metabolically active hormones—cortisol, glucagon, and epinephrine—all of which increase extracellular glucose concentrations. The glucose provides fuel for nervous system function, metabolism of blood cells, and wound healing; the increased extracellular osmolality helps to replenish vascular volume (see below).

Cortisol, glucagon, and epinephrine increase the extracellular glucose concentration by several mechanisms. All three hormones induce breakdown of hepatic glycogen into glucose, which is released into the hepatic veins and made available to the rest of the body. Cortisol and epinephrine induce breakdown of muscle glycogen into glucose, which is metabolized to lactate. Lactate is then carried to the liver, where it is converted into glucose (via the Cori cycle). Cortisol and epinephrine also induce breakdown of skeletal muscle protein into its constituent amino acids; the amino acids then lose their amino groups and form keto acids and alanine, which are carried to the liver, where they are converted into glucose by gluconeogenesis. To a certain extent, depending on perfusion of the adipose tissue, cortisol and epinephrine induce the breakdown of triglycerides in fat into glycerol and free fatty acids. Glycerol is carried to the liver, where it is converted into glucose, and the free fatty acids serve as an energy source for muscle and viscera.

The result is to increase blood glucose levels at the expense of liver glycogen, muscle glycogen, and muscle protein. If the illness persists, the patient will become debilitated. If the illness does not become too severe and if resuscitation proceeds well, metabolic priorities will be restored to normal. Oxygen consumption and energy expenditure will increase, and the augmented glucose levels will support wound healing and fight infection.

Other hormones with potential metabolic actions, including insulin and growth hormone, are also released during critical illnesses. They have little effect, however, compared with cortisol, glucagon, and epinephrine. Indeed, infusion of cortisol, glucagon, and epinephrine in normal subjects can produce most of the metabolic changes of critical illness.

RELEASE OF VOLUME-CONSERVING HORMONES

Vasopressin, besides being a selective vasopressor, potentiates reabsorption of water by the kidneys. Aldosterone, which is released in response to angiotensin II and corticotropin, stimulates tubular reabsorption of sodium and bicarbonate. These two hormones compensate for hypovolemia in critically ill patients by conserving (but not replenishing) vascular volume.

REPLENISHMENT OF VASCULAR VOLUME

Vascular volume is replenished in hypovolemic patients by the influx of fluid from the cells and interstitium. These fluid shifts are mediated by two mechanisms. The first—and probably the more effective—is initiated by the increased extracellular glucose concentrations of shock. Extracellular hyperosmolality draws water out of the cells, increases interstitial hydrostatic pressure, and drives interstitial protein into the lymphatics and from there into the vascular space. Interstitial oncotic pressure falls, and plasma oncotic pressure rises. The augmented oncotic gradient between the vascular and interstitial spaces draws water, sodium, and chloride into the vascular space. Vascular volume is replenished. This replenishment will continue as long as interstitial hydrostatic pressures are maintained and as long as interstitial protein stores, which constitute more than one-half of the total extracellular protein content, can be recruited.

A second, probably less important mechanism for replenishment of vascular volume arises from arteri-olar constriction and the low-flow state of many types of shock. Capillary hydrostatic pressure falls, and water, sodium, and chloride are drawn into the vascular space. The amount of fluid recovered by this mechanism is limited, however. The shift of protein-free fluid from the interstitium to the plasma increases interstitial oncotic pressure and decreases plasma oncotic pressure. The resultant unfavorable oncotic gradient opposes further recovery of fluid.

DILATATION OF SYSTEMIC ARTERIOLES

In severely ill patients, three responses—dilatation of systemic arterioles, failure of cell membrane function, and disruption of the vascular endothelium—serve to worsen the patient's condition. In decompensated shock, the systemic arterioles lose their ability to constrict, while the postcapillary sphincters remain constricted. Capillary hydrostatic pressure rises. Water, sodium, and chloride are driven out of the vascular space and into the interstitium. The process is limited, however, because the oncotic gradient, which increases as fluid is lost from plasma, prevents further fluid losses.

FAILURE OF CELL MEMBRANE FUNCTION

Cell membrane potentials deteriorate in severely ill patients, and water, sodium, and chloride shift from the extracellular space into the cells even in the face of high extracellular glucose concentrations. This membrane failure accounts for the loss of perhaps 2 L of interstitial fluid, which can be critical because it decreases interstitial hydrostatic pressure, the driving pressure that normally would force interstitial protein back into the vascular space. Membrane failure can thus eliminate the most effective mechanism for replenishment of vascular volume.

DISRUPTION OF VASCULAR ENDOTHELIUM

Trauma and sepsis activate coagulation and inflammation, which can disrupt endothelial integrity in severely ill patients. Platelet and white cell microaggregates that form in injured or infected tissues embolize to the lungs or liver, where they lodge in the capillaries. The microaggregates, endothelium, and plasma in the regions of embolization release kinins, fibrin degradation products, thromboxanes, prostacyclin, prostaglandins, complement, leukotrienes, lysosomal enzymes, oxygen radicals, and other toxic factors, which damage the endothelium and dilate the vasculature in the region of the emboli and distally. Protein, water, sodium, and chloride extravasate into the interstitium. The amount of extravasation is unlimited: As long as the endothelium is damaged, protein will extravasate, and water and electrolytes will follow. The edema that results can be massive and can involve any tissue in the body.

Gann DS, Lilly MP: The neuroendocrine response to multiple trauma. World J Surg 1983;7:101.
Meakins JL: Etiology of multiple organ failure. J Trauma 1990;30:S165.

II. ACUTE PULMONARY FAILURE

CAUSES OF PULMONARY FAILURE IN SURGICAL PATIENTS

There are nine causes of severe pulmonary failure in the surgical patient: the adult respiratory distress syndrome, inability to effectively expand the lungs because of mechanical abnormalities, atelectasis, aspiration, pulmonary contusion, pneumonia, pulmonary embolus, cardiogenic pulmonary edema, and, rarely, neurogenic pulmonary edema.

ADULT RESPIRATORY DISTRESS SYNDROME

Adult respiratory distress syndrome (ARDS) typically follows shock and either trauma or sepsis, which activate coagulation and inflammation in the injured or infected tissues and release coagulative and inflammatory mediators into the circulation. The lungs bear the brunt of the insult from any process that involves the nonsplanchnic portions of the body because they receive all the venous blood that returns to the heart and because they contain the first microvasculature encountered by the mediators. (The liver bears the initial brunt for mediators released into the portal venous system.) The mediators disrupt the microvascular endothelium, and plasma extravasates into the interstitium and alveoli. The resultant pulmonary edema impairs both ventilation and oxygenation; the embolization to the lungs impairs perfusion. Arterial oxygen saturation decreases and carbon dioxide content increases, assuming that no compensatory mechanisms come into play.

A number of different mediators of coagulation and inflammation have been implicated as causes of the increased permeability. Platelet and white cell aggregates formed in response to injury or infection are trapped in the lungs, where they engender an inflam-matory response. Proteases, kinins, complement, oxygen radicals, prostaglandins, thromboxanes, leukotrienes, lysosomal enzymes, and other mediators are released from the aggregates or from the endothelium or plasma as a consequence of the interaction between the aggregates and the vessel wall. Some of these substances are chemoattractants of more platelets and white blood cells, and a vicious cycle of inflammation develops that worsens the disruption of the vascular endothelium. Infection, disease, injury, and ischemia in nonpulmonary tissues thus lead to damage and dysfunction in previously healthy lungs.

The diagnosis is made by the development of hypoxemia approximately 24 hours after resuscitation from shock and either trauma or sepsis in the absence of other common causes of hypoxemia under these conditions—mechanical failure, atelectasis, aspiration, and pulmonary contusion. The chest x-ray usually shows a diffuse infiltrate. Pathologically, the lungs develop a nonspecific inflammatory reaction. Interstitial edema appears within a few hours after injury or sepsis; alveolar flooding is florid within 1 day. Monocytes and neutrophils invade the interstitium, and scar tissue begins to form within a week. If the process is unchecked, the lungs become sodden and resemble liver tissue on gross inspection; they eventually may become fibrosed. If treatment is effective, the lungs can return to normal, both grossly and microscopically. The process of diagnosis and the pathologic features of ARDS are identical to those of the so-called **fat embolism syndrome,** which is, for practical purposes, merely a special case of ARDS in which the release of marrow fat into the blood contributes to the development of pulmonary microvascular damage. Nothing is gained by making a distinction between the two entities.

MECHANICAL FAILURE

Mechanical failure can arise from chest wall trauma, pain and weakness after surgery and anesthesia, debility caused by the catabolic metabolism of long-term illness, or bronchopleural fistula. Massive trauma to the chest with multiple fractures of multiple ribs or bilateral disruption of the costochondral junctions can result in a free-floating segment of chest wall known as a **flail chest:** Expansion and relaxation of the rest of the chest wall with spontaneous breathing results in paradoxic motion of the free segment in response to changes in intrathoracic pressure; ventilation becomes compromised; and the arterial P_{CO_2} increases. Lesser degrees of chest wall injury can lead to hypoventilation because of pain associated with breathing. Prolonged mechanical ventilation with loss of muscle mass and power in the diaphragm and the accessory muscles of respiration can require ventilatory support until muscle function returns to normal. A bronchopleural fistula—a communication from the airway to the pleural cavity to the atmosphere, either through a chest tube or through a hole in the chest wall—can develop after pulmonary surgery, trauma, or infection. Large air leaks can compromise ventilation to the uninvolved lung as well as to the diseased side because insufflated air preferentially goes to the side with the fistula.

ATELECTASIS

Atelectasis, or localized collapse of alveoli, can develop with prolonged immobilization, as during anesthesia or in association with bed rest. The problem is usually full-blown within a few hours after the initiating event. Only mechanical failure (to which it is related), aspiration, and cardiogenic pulmonary edema can produce equivalent levels of hypoxemia so soon. The diagnosis is supported by auscultation of bronchial breath sounds at the dependent portions of the lung and occasionally, if severe enough, by x-ray confirmation of platelike collapse of pulmonary parenchyma. The most reliable confirmation of the diagnosis, however, comes with response to therapy, which can include encouragement of deep breathing and coughing, ambulation, bronchoscopy, and intubation and mechanical ventilation. Atelectasis should respond within a few hours. No other form of pulmonary insufficiency responds as quickly.

ASPIRATION

Aspiration of gastric contents or blood can occur in any patient who cannot protect the airway, eg, one who has just been injured or anesthetized or who is debilitated or obtunded for any reason. Gastric acid or particulate matter in the airways leads to disruption of the alveolar and microvascular membranes, causing interstitial and alveolar edema. The resultant hypoxemia is usually evident within a few hours and is associated with a localized infiltrate on x-ray. Recovery of gastric contents by suctioning from the endotracheal tree confirms the diagnosis.

PULMONARY CONTUSION

Pulmonary contusion arises from direct trauma to the chest wall and the underlying lung parenchyma. Hypoxemia associated with a localized infiltrate on x-ray develops over 24 hours as the injured lung becomes edematous.

PNEUMONIA

Pneumonias can arise primarily or can be superimposed on aspiration, pulmonary contusion, or ARDS. The diagnosis is made by recovery of bacteria and purulent material from the endotracheal tree, hypoxemia, signs of systemic sepsis, and a localized infiltrate on x-ray.

PULMONARY EMBOLISM
(See also Chapter 37.)

Sudden deterioration of pulmonary function 5 days or more after an event—such as an operation, injury, or the beginning of immobilization—that can stimulate deposition of clot in a large systemic vein should suggest the possibility of pulmonary embolism. Patients with cancer are at particularly high risk, and in any patient the greater the magnitude of operation or injury, the greater the chance of venous thrombosis and embolization. The chest film is usually nonspecific. Definitive diagnosis can on rare occasions be made by a radionuclide perfusion scan, but this approach can only be successful in the face of a completely normal chest x-ray—an unusual occurrence after a major procedure. Pulmonary angiography is necessary for diagnosis in most hospitalized surgical patients.

Clot emboli must be organized to be clinically significant; embolism to the lung of fresh soft clot rarely causes any difficulty. The pulmonary endothelium contains potent fibrinolysins that can break up any poorly organized embolus. Sudden deterioration in pulmonary function less than 5 days after an event that stimulates clot formation is only rarely caused by an embolus; the deterioration is more likely to be caused by mechanical failure, atelectasis, aspiration, or pneumonia.

CARDIOGENIC PULMONARY EDEMA

Cardiogenic pulmonary edema arises from high left atrial and pulmonary microvascular hydrostatic pressures. Patients who have suffered an acute myocardial infarction can present this way, as can patients with underlying myocardial or coronary artery disease when faced with fluid shifts and surgical stress. Occasionally, the rapid administration of intravenous fluid—especially in elderly patients with poor myocardial performance—will outstrip the heart's ability to pump, and pulmonary edema will result. Acute valvular disease, though quite rare after injury or cardiac surgery, is another possible cause of inability of the left heart to pump effectively. The diagnosis is made on the basis of hypoxemia, rales, a third heart sound, perihilar infiltrates, Kerley's lines, and cephalization of blood flow on x-ray along with elevated pulmonary arterial wedge pressures on Swan-Ganz catheterization.

NEUROGENIC PULMONARY EDEMA

Neurogenic pulmonary edema is associated both experimentally and clinically with head injury and increased intracranial pressure. The exact mechanism by which this occurs is unknown, but it is probably related to sympathetic discharge with postmicrovascular vasoconstriction in the lungs and a resultant increase in pulmonary microvascular hydrostatic pressure. This form of pulmonary edema and oxygenation defect is rare, and other causes should be also considered in patients with head injury.

Demling RH: Current concepts on the adult respiratory distress syndrome. Circ Shock 1990;30:297.
Sturm JA et al: Increased lung capillary permeability after trauma: A prospective clinical study. J Trauma 1986;26:409.

USE OF THE MECHANICAL VENTILATOR

INDICATIONS

Intubation of the airway and mechanical ventilation are indicated for treatment of established pulmonary failure, prophylaxis against potential failure, airway protection, and pulmonary toilet. Pulmonary insufficiency will usually require mechanical ventilation if on room air the patient has a Pa_{CO_2} of 45 mm Hg or more or a Pa_{O_2} of 60 mm Hg or less, but these guidelines should be related to the clinical status of the patient. A Pa_{CO_2} of 40 mm Hg in a patient breathing 40 times per minute is as alarming as a Pa_{CO_2} of 60 mm Hg in a patient with a respiratory rate of 10/min. A Pa_{O_2} of 60 mm Hg on room air in an elderly patient with chronic lung disease may be acceptable; the same value in a young patient who is tensing the sternocleidomastoid and intercostal muscles with each breath and who seems to be struggling to draw in enough air, making excessive or dyscoordinated use of the abdominal musculature, would mandate immediate intubation. A postoperative patient after debridement of necrotizing fasciitis should remain ventilated until it is clear that the overall clinical status is improving even if the patient is capable of independent oxygenation and ventilation in the immediate postoperative period. A patient with stridor or with maxillofacial trauma or pharyngeal edema may need intubation to maintain the airway. A patient

with a severe head injury and depressed mental status may require intubation to protect the airway from aspiration. Intubation may also be indicated for repeated suctioning of the tracheobronchial tree in a patient with a weak gag reflex or inability to cough and clear secretions.

In contrast to the usual medical patient, the indications for intubation in the surgical patient should be liberal. The medical patient with an exacerbation of chronic obstructive lung disease can be poorly served by placement of a foreign body in his trachea. Airway resistance increases, coughing effectiveness decreases, and opportunistic organisms obtain a foothold on and near the tube. Benefit from intubation may be minimal in that the patient may respond to treatment without mechanical ventilation.

Circumstances for the seriously ill surgical patient are usually different. The patient who has multiple injuries, for example, can temporarily tolerate the increased airway resistance, loss of cough, and increased likelihood of tracheobronchial infection. What cannot be tolerated is respiratory arrest during trauma resuscitation. Furthermore, in all likelihood, such patients will eventually require mechanical ventilation anyway. ARDS strikes the lungs 2 days after the injury, not initially. It is safest to secure the airway early; the tube can be removed later if the patient's condition improves faster than expected.

TYPES OF INTUBATION

The trachea can be intubated via the mouth, the nose, the cricothyroid membrane (cricothyroidostomy), or directly (tracheostomy). Orotracheal and nasotracheal intubation involve passage of a tube through the oropharynx and nasopharynx, respectively; cricothyroidostomy and tracheostomy are surgical procedures requiring a neck incision.

The orotracheal route allows for passage of a larger tube than the nasotracheal route. Nasotracheal intubation requires the presence of spontaneous ventilation in order to guide tube placement and therefore cannot be accomplished in many situations. Conversely, nasotracheal intubation is more comfortable for the awake patient and avoids any need for paralysis and heavy sedation. Nasotracheal tubes can lead to sinusitis by interfering with normal sinus drainage, a complication not seen with orotracheal intubation. Nasotracheal tubes can lead to pressure necrosis of the skin of the nares. Pressure necrosis can also occur in the corner of the mouth with orotracheal tubes but is less common than with nasotracheal intubation, because moving the tube from one side of the mouth to the other is possible. Nasotracheal intubation requires no neck extension and may be preferable to orotracheal intubation in patients with suspected cervical spine fractures. Under no circumstances, however, should concern about the cervical spine lead to prolonged unsuccessful attempts at nasotracheal intubation in critically injured patients. The risk of respiratory arrest outweighs the risk of exacerbating cervical spine injury in such situations. The limited neck extension required for orotracheal intubation is safe even in most cases of unstable cervical spine fracture. Flexion and rotation of the neck, on the other hand, put the unstable cervical spine at risk for increased neurologic damage. Axial traction should be maintained during intubation to guard against flexion and rotation.

Cricothyroidostomy is indicated when an emergent surgical airway is necessary. Tracheostomy is more difficult than cricothyroidostomy and should not be done in such situations. Patients with extensive maxillofacial trauma can be impossible to intubate by the orotracheal or nasotracheal route. Intubation can also be difficult because of poor patient cooperation, altered anatomy, or airway or laryngeal swelling—or because of inexperience on the part of the person trying to do the intubating. When the patient is in extremis and respiratory collapse is imminent, prolonged attempts at orotracheal or nasotracheal intubation should be avoided. If orotracheal intubation is not successful after one or two attempts, cricothyroidostomy should be done. The cricothyroid membrane in the midline is bounded superiorly by the lower border of the thyroid membrane and inferiorly by the cricoid cartilage. It is easily located by palpation and is incised by a stab incision. After the hole has been enlarged with the knife handle, a No. 4 or No. 6 tracheostomy tube should be inserted into the trachea. The patient can then be supported with mechanical ventilation and supplemental oxygen as necessary. Cricothyroidostomies maintained for longer than 2 or 3 days may produce glottic and subglottic stenosis; therefore, cricothyroidostomies should be converted to tracheostomies as soon as is safe and practical when intubation beyond 2–3 days is necessary.

Tracheostomies have several advantages over translaryngeal (orotracheal or nasotracheal) intubation: Airway resistance is lower; nursing care is simpler; accidental extubation is less serious—a well-established tracheostomy tract can usually be easily reintubated, and the patient can usually breath through the stoma while the tube is being replaced; suctioning is more direct; and the tubes do not damage the vocal cords or larynx.

Tracheostomy is also of benefit when weaning from mechanical ventilation is very slow and the patient has been on and off the ventilator a number of times. The presence of a tracheostomy allows for prolonged periods off the ventilator without the requirement for extubation. If the patient develops respiratory distress off the ventilator and a tracheostomy is present, the ventilator can simply be reconnected to the tracheostomy tube.

Translaryngeal intubation, however, has three major advantages over tracheostomies: First, because the tube can be repositioned, the balloon on the end of the tube does not always compress the same area of tracheal mucosa; the tube moves up and down with tracheal motion, minimizing axial friction by the balloon. The result is a much lower incidence of late tracheal stenosis and tracheo-innominate artery and tracheoesophageal fistulas. Second, because the opening of the tube is well away from the neck and chest, intravenous catheters in these areas can be kept sterile. Third, in patients with poor pulmonary compliance and high inspiratory pressures, maintenance of intrapulmonary volume and avoidance of volume leak around the tube cuff is minimized with translaryngeal intubation.

The timing of conversion from a translaryngeal intubation to a tracheostomy is controversial. Recommendations as short as 3 days have been made, but large numbers of patients have been intubated for months by the orotracheal or nasotracheal route without serious sequelae. Patients should be converted when airway protection, pulmonary toilet, or any of the other indications outlined above are present. If, in addition, the need for more than 2–3 weeks of intubation is obvious, the threshold for performing tracheostomy should be lowered. Conversion to tracheostomy should only be done as an elective procedure under controlled conditions. A transverse incision overlying the upper trachea is developed by separating the strap muscles of the neck in the midline. After exposure of the anterior surface of the trachea, a tracheostomy tube is placed through the second or third tracheal ring. Often the thyroid isthmus must be either retracted upward or divided to allow for adequate exposure of the trachea in the proper location.

Endotracheal tubes of all types come with either of two different types of cuffs. High-pressure, low-volume cuffs are useful for short-term intubation and ventilation. Because of the high cuff pressure, however, they interfere with tracheal blood supply and can lead to tracheomalacia, erosion into the innominate artery (tracheo-innominate fistula), erosion into the esophagus (tracheoesophageal fistula), or airway stenosis. They should not be used for long-term intubation; low-pressure, high-volume cuffs are preferable in this circumstance.

VOLUME VENTILATORS

Ventilators can be constructed either to deliver a preset volume (volume ventilators) or to deliver flow continuously until a preset pressure is reached (pressure ventilators). Volume ventilators are more commonly used in adults. The four main parameters that need to be set on volume ventilators are the rate of ventilation, the tidal volume of each ventilation, the inspired oxygen concentration (F_{IO_2}), and the level of positive end-expiratory pressure (PEEP). Although an oversimplification, ventilator management can be easily understood by dividing these parameters into those concerned primarily with ventilation (rate and tidal volume) and those concerned primarily with oxygenation (FIO_2 and PEEP).

Setting the ventilatory rate tells the ventilator how many times it should cycle per minute. Doubling the rate doubles the minute volume, or the amount of volume delivered by the ventilator each minute. It can be turned up or down, depending on the patient's needs. In patients who do not breathe spontaneously, the ventilator rate will equal the total respiratory rate; in patients with spontaneous breaths, the ventilator rate will ensure a certain number of machine-delivered breaths per minute, but the respiratory rate will be greater than the machine rate because of spontaneous breaths. The ventilator rate should be set between 12 and 15 breaths per minute in most patients beginning mechanical ventilation. The rate can be increased or decreased as necessary based on analysis of arterial blood gases. The PCO_2 should be kept close to 40 mm Hg unless hyperventilation is desired, as in patients with increased intracranial pressure.

Setting the tidal volume dictates how much volume will be delivered with each machine ventilation. The normal tidal volume during resting spontaneous ventilation is 7 mL/kg; the tidal volume in a ventilated patient should be set at 10–15 mL/kg. The increase above spontaneous tidal volume compensates for the dead space of the ventilator tubing and helps to minimize atelectasis. Tidal volumes above 15 mL/kg are usually not necessary and are associated with increased barotrauma. If more ventilation is needed, it is preferable to increase the other determinant of ventilation, the ventilatory rate. Occasionally, very high tidal volumes are necessary when a bronchopleural fistula is present. To compensate for the volume lost through the fistula, tidal volume as well as ventilatory rate must be increased.

Inspired oxygen concentration is set by adjusting the oxygen percentage of inspired gas. Oxygen leads to chronic pulmonary fibrosis when administered in concentrations above 50% for prolonged periods, and the FIO_2 should be kept as low as possible consistent with adequate oxygenation. All of the nonoxygen volume of ventilator gas is made up of nitrogen, which, unlike oxygen, is not absorbed from alveoli. When nitrogen is replaced by increasing concentrations of oxygen, increased atelectasis caused by oxygen absorption can occur. For this reason, ventilation with 80–100% oxygen for periods of greater than 1–2 hours should be avoided.

Positive end-expiratory pressure is the other primary determinant of arterial oxygenation. A valve placed in the expiratory circuit of the ventilator ensures that the airway pressure remains above a preset level even at the end of expiration. This keeps the airway pressure above the closing pressure of small airways and minimizes alveolar collapse at end-expiration.

Positive end-expiratory pressure, however, can decrease cardiac output, as described in the section on cardiac compressive shock, and can rupture the lungs. The remedy for decreased cardiac output is usually fluid infusion; the remedy for lung rupture is more of a problem. The ruptures are associated more with peak inspiratory airway pressures than with mean pressures. The patient may develop tension pneumothorax or mediastinal or subcutaneous emphysema, caused by rupture of a bronchus with decompression into the mediastinum. Occasionally, PEEP can even decrease the peak inspiratory pressure by improving oxygenation and ventilation and allowing a decrease in the tidal volume. In most cases, however, the PEEP increases the peak airway pressure by an amount equivalent to the level of the PEEP. This increase in the peak pressure is usually proportionately small, and, fortunately, rupture of the lung caused by PEEP is uncommon in surgical patients, who are likely to have the consolidated lungs of ARDS and not likely to have many pulmonary blebs. Medical patients with emphysema are at much greater risk.

Placement of an endotracheal tube bypasses the normal physiologic PEEP present during spontaneous ventilation from closure of the glottis at the end of expiration. Low levels of "physiologic" PEEP (5 cm H_2O) should probably be used in most intubated patients with severe pulmonary dysfunction to maintain arterial oxygen saturation and to keep the inspired oxygen concentration below 50%. Balancing the complications of high inspired oxygen concentration and high PEEP can be difficult in patients with major defects in oxygenation, but if possible the inspired oxygen concentration should be kept below 50% and the level of PEEP below 20 cm H_2O. The goal should be to maximize oxygen delivery.

The oxygen saturation of arterial blood should be kept above 90% in most cases. Patients with chronic obstructive pulmonary disease and long-standing CO_2 retention are an exception. Such patients have lost the ability to increase their respiratory drive in response to increases in PCO_2 and rely instead on their response to hypoxemia. Increasing the arterial oxygen saturation by adding exogenous oxygen takes away this hypoxic ventilatory stimulus and makes weaning from ventilatory support more difficult.

The two basic modes available on most volume ventilators are assist or control mode ventilation (assist-control ventilation) and intermittent mandatory ventilation (IMV). Assist-control ventilation is designed to assist any ventilatory efforts made by the patient by delivering a machine breath. Whenever the patient begins to inspire, the ventilator is triggered and the preset machine tidal volume is given. A machine backup rate is also set to ensure a minimal number of machine breaths in the absence of spontaneous ventilatory efforts. Assist-control mode ventilation requires minimal ventilatory effort from the patient and minimizes the work of breathing. It is useful in patients recovering from anesthesia and in patients with flail chest. Assist-control mode ventilation, by assisting all of the patient's ventilatory efforts, minimizes pain and paradoxic motion of the flail segment and encourages earlier recovery of chest wall stability. A disadvantage of assist-control ventilation is that hyperventilation can occur if the patient's respiratory rate increases. It is also difficult to wean a patient from ventilatory support when assist-control ventilation is being used because the ventilator continually compensates for weak or absent spontaneous ventilatory efforts.

Intermittent mandatory ventilation was designed to overcome the limitations of the assist-control mode. Intermittent machine breaths are delivered at a predetermined rate and—unlike assist-control—are given to the patient regardless of the spontaneous respiratory rate. Between the intermittent mandatory ventilations, however, the patient's spontaneous respiratory efforts are not assisted, and the patient thus generates his or her own tidal volume. Synchronized intermittent mandatory ventilation (SIMV) is a modification of IMV designed to deliver the preset number of machine breaths in synchrony with some of the patient's own ventilatory efforts, but the principle of spontaneously generated tidal volumes between machine breaths is the same as with IMV. Intermittent mandatory ventilation requires increased work of breathing by the patient as compared with assist-control, and the rate of machine breaths can be varied to increase or decrease the patient's contribution to ventilation. At very high IMV rates, all ventilation is done by the ventilator, and the patient's contribution is minimal. As the rate is gradually decreased, the patient must increasingly ventilate himself to maintain minute volume. Incrementally decreasing the IMV rate can be used as a means of weaning from the ventilator. Clinical status, respiratory rate, and the arterial P_{CO_2} are used to guide the weaning process.

The four basic parameters to be set on a volume ventilator—ventilatory rate, tidal volume, F_{IO_2}, and PEEP—and the two basic modes of ventilation—assist-control and IMV—thus need to be adjusted in relation to each other and in response to the patient's blood gases and clinical condition. As an example, the typical patient who requires mechanical ventilation after a major injury should be started on assist-control with a backup rate of 15 breaths/min and a tidal volume of 12 mL/kg. The F_{IO_2} should initially be set at 1.00, and no PEEP should be used. As blood gas measurements become available, the tidal volume can be varied between 10 and 15 mL/kg to generate a Pa_{CO_2} of 40 mm Hg; the F_{IO_2} can be lowered to bring an excessively high Pa_{O_2} down, but the value should be kept between 90 and 120 mm Hg until the patient is hemodynamically stable. Once stability is achieved and once the patient is in an ICU, the F_{IO_2} should be lowered to bring the Pa_{O_2} into the range of

65 to 90 mm Hg. PEEP should be added as full monitoring becomes available and increased to levels as high as 20 cm H_2O, if necessary, to bring the F_{IO_2} to less than 0.50. When the patient becomes a candidate for weaning, he or she can be switched to IMV.

PRESSURE VENTILATORS

Pressure ventilators are commonly used in neonates, in whom it is critical to avoid high airway pressures and minimize barotrauma. Newer modes of ventilation that can be used with ventilators with pressure mode capabilities have been found useful in selected adult patients as well. Pressure support ventilation and pressure control with inverse ratio ventilation (IRV) are two of these newer modes. Pressure support is usually used with IMV and provides the patient with a constant predetermined level of airway pressure during spontaneous inspiration. Machine IMV breaths are unaffected. The pressure support is typically supplied for approximately 90% of the time during which the patient inspires. The interval is determined by analog circuits within the ventilator and usually cannot be adjusted by the physician. Providing pressure support by assisting the patient during spontaneous breathing increases spontaneous tidal volumes and decreases the work of breathing. It also helps overcome resistance to inspiratory flow in the endotracheal tube and the ventilatory apparatus. Although its role is still being defined, pressure support seems to be useful in managing patients who have been difficult to wean from the ventilator. Arbitrary levels of pressure support between 5 and 25 cm H_2O can be provided, or the amount of pressure support necessary can be set by determining a desired level of spontaneous tidal volume and then gradually adjusting the pressure support until that tidal volume is reached.

Pressure control ventilation is similar conceptually to pressure support ventilation but provides a constant inspiratory pressure during machine breaths and for the entirety of the breath. It is generally used in conjunction with IRV, another recent development. In addition to ventilatory rate and tidal volume, the relative amounts of time in the ventilatory cycle spent in inspiration and expiration (I:E) must be set. In standard modes of ventilation, this ratio is set at 1:2 to approximate spontaneous ventilation. Inverse ratio ventilation increases the proportion of the ventilatory cycle spent in inspiration and changes this relationship to anywhere between 1:1 and 4:1. Pressure control ventilation is used with IRV in order to maintain a constant inspiratory airway pressure and safely allow initiation of a new inspiration before expiratory flow from the previous ventilatory cycle has reached zero. The resultant air trapping with each ventilatory cycle is thought to minimize alveolar collapse and improve the distribution of inspired volume. Pressure control and IRV are still being investigated but seem to be primarily useful in patients with profound oxygenation defects and poor compliance. Paralysis is usually required to tolerate IRV, and care must be taken to ensure that uncontrolled air trapping does not lead to barotrauma.

WEANING FROM MECHANICAL VENTILATION

Weaning from mechanical ventilation depends on the type of ventilatory support being provided. When the patient is on IMV, weaning is accomplished by gradually decreasing the IMV rate. Decreasing the rate with the object of removing the patient from the ventilator is generally not appropriate until oxygen requirements are at or below an FIO_2 of 40% and a PEEP of 5 cm H_2O. When these requirements have been met, the weaning process can begin and the IMV rate can be reduced. As outlined above, this requires the patient to contribute increasingly to the maintenance of adequate minute ventilation. The patient's overall clinical status, respiratory rate, and arterial PCO_2 should be used as guidelines to determine the rate of weaning. When an IMV of 4/min or less is well tolerated for long periods, a trial of spontaneous ventilation without any machine support should be carried out. This is done by putting the patient on a T-piece trial in which the endotracheal tube forms the long arm of the T and is connected to a blow-by oxygen source. All ventilation must be done by the patient and if well tolerated for 30 miunutes is usually an indication that the patient is extubatable. The patient should not be stressed excessively during trials of spontaneous ventilation. The ventilatory rate should not exceed 25/min, and breathing should not be allowed to become labored. T-piece trials lasting longer than 30 minutes should be supplemented with continuous positive airway pressure (CPAP) of 5 cm H_2O in order to prevent an end-expiratory pressure of zero and associated progressive atelectasis.

"Wind sprints" are another method for weaning patients who have required extended periods of mechanical ventilation. The patient is managed with intermittent periods on a T-piece alternating with periods of assist-control ventilation or IMV. The length and frequency of the T-piece periods are gradually increased as the patient's ability to ventilate spontaneously improves. When extended periods on a T-piece with CPAP are well tolerated, the patient can be extubated.

Pressure support is useful in weaning patients who have required mechanical ventilation for a long time. After it has been instituted, pressure support should be maintained while the IMV rate is gradually decreased. When the IMV rate has been reduced to 4/min or less, gradual decreases in the level of pressure support can be started. The patient can be tried on a T-piece when the pressure support is minimal or has been completely discontinued. As with weaning from IMV without pressure support, the patient's clinical status, respiratory rate, degree of dyspnea, and PCO_2 are the guidelines used during the weaning process.

Patients who seem to be doing well and who have required mechanical ventilation for less than 24 hours can frequently be extubated quickly after going straight to a single T-piece trial. Patients on IRV are not candidates for weaning from the ventilator until they improve enough to allow for their return to one of the standard modes of ventilation.

EXTUBATION

Both objective and subjective criteria are used to determine if a patient is ready for extubation. Objective measures of pulmonary function include the respiratory rate, the arterial PCO_2, and the patient's ability to oxygenate. The respiratory rate on a T-piece should be less than 25/min if extubation is being considered and in ideal circumstances should be below 20/min. In most instances, the PCO_2 should be 42 mm Hg or less with an acceptably low respiratory rate. In patients with chronic CO_2 retention or metabolic alkalosis with respiratory compensation, higher PCO_2 levels are acceptable as long as the arterial pH is 7.34 or greater. A pH lower than this indicates that the elevation in PCO_2 is acute and poorly tolerated. The patient should have an arterial oxygen saturation of greater than 90% on an FIO_2 of 40% or less and a PEEP of 5 cm H_2O or less. The vital capacity and most negative inspiratory pressure are other objective weaning parameters that can be measured at the bedside. The vital capacity should be at least 10 mL/kg and the most negative inspiratory pressure should be more negative than 20 cm H_2O before extubation is considered.

Subjective criteria for extubation are also important. The patient's underlying disease process will often dictate whether extubation is appropriate. A critically ill patient requiring further operative procedures and with a guarded prognosis may require continued intubation and mechanical ventilatory support in spite of current fairly good pulmonary function. Inability to protect the airway is another indication for continued intubation even when the patient's ability to oxygenate and ventilate are adequate. Finally, there is a gestalt determination of a patient's ability to tolerate extubation and spontaneous ventilation. A patient who can lift his head off the pillow, has a sparkle in his eye, and obviously wants the endotracheal tube removed is a good candidate for extubation; a lethargic, diaphoretic patient is not.

Brochard L et al: Inspiratory pressure support prevents diaphragmatic fatigue during weaning from mechanical ventilation. Am Rev Respir Dis 1989;139:513.

Colice GL: Prolonged intubation versus tracheostomy in the adult. J Intensive Care Med 1987;2:85.

Demling RH et al: Incidence and morbidity of extubation failure in surgical intensive care patients. Crit Care Med 1988;16:573.

Dupuis YG: *Ventilators: Theory and Clinical Application.* Mosby, 1986.

Fiastro JF et al: Pressure support compensation for inspiratory work due to endotracheal tubes and demand continuous positive airway pressure. Chest 1988;93:499.

Heffner JE: Tracheal intubation in mechanically ventilated patients. Clin Chest Med 1988;9:23.

Hurst JM et al: Comparison of blood gases during transport using two methods of ventilatory support. J Trauma 1989; 29:1637.

Hurst JM et al: Comparison of conventional mechanical ventilation and high-frequency ventilation. Ann Surg 1990;211:486.

Kreit JW, Eschenbacher WL: The physiology of spontaneous and mechanical ventilation. Clin Chest Med 1988; 9:11.

Lain DC et al: Pressure control inverse ratio ventilation as a method to reduce peak inspiratory pressure and provide adequate ventilation and oxygenation. Chest 1989; 95:1081.

Lee PC et al: Are low tidal volumes safe? Chest 1990; 97:425.

MacIntyre NR: New forms of mechanical ventilation in the adult. Clin Chest Med 1988;9:47.

Rodriguez JL et al: Early tracheostomy for primary airway management in the surgical critical care setting. Surgery 1990;108:655.

Saito S et al: Efficacy of flow-by during continuous positive airway pressure ventilation. Crit Care Med 1990;18:654.

Sassoon CSH et al: Inspiratory work of breathing on flowby and demand-flow continuous positive airway pressure. Crit Care Med 1989;17:1108.

Tharratt RS et al: Pressure controlled inverse ratio ventilation in severe adult respiratory failure. Chest 1988; 94:755.

Viale JP et al: Oxygen cost of breathing in postoperative patients: Pressure support ventilation vs continuous positive airway pressure. Chest 1988;93:506.

Yang KL, Tobin MJ: A prospective study of indexes predicting the outcome of trials of weaning from mechanical ventilation. N Engl J Med 1991;324:1445.

ADJUVANT TREATMENT OF PULMONARY INSUFFICIENCY

Mechanical ventilation is the mainstay of therapy for treatment of severe pulmonary insufficiency in the surgical patient. Mechanical ventilation, however, introduces problems, such as bacterial colonization of the tracheobronchial tree, that may require adjuvant treatment. The underlying disease process may also require adjuvant treatment.

ANTIBIOTICS

Bacteria can be recovered from tracheal secretions of any patient who has been intubated and on mechanical ventilation for several days. The question is when to treat with antibiotics. Indications include purulent sputum associated with abundant white cells on Gram-stained smears; pathogenic organisms recovered from suctioning; signs of systemic sepsis with increasing fluid requirements and increasing blood glucose concentrations; worsening pulmonary function, as judged by the need to increase inspired oxygen concentrations or end-expiratory pressure; and worsening signs on chest x-ray. If all of these are present, antibiotics should be started. If only one or two are present, antibiotics are probably best withheld to avoid overgrowth of resistant organisms that could later cause fatal pneumonia.

Older patients may have only one chance to survive a critical period of illness and should probably be given antibiotics sooner than younger patients, who are better able to recover after prolonged illness. Thus, an 80-year-old patient with flail chest should probably be given antibiotics early; a 20-year-old patient who was hospitalized for a gunshot wound involving the colon and who develops questionable pneumonia 2 weeks later should probably be given antibiotics only when infection is definitely confirmed and the causative organisms are identified.

ADRENAL CORTICOSTEROIDS

Adrenal corticosteroids inhibit the metabolism of arachidonic acid and production of oxygen radicals, lysosomal enzymes, leukotrienes, thromboxanes, prostacyclin, and prostaglandins and thus could inhibit the inflammatory response and protect the lungs. The inflammatory response is blocked throughout the body, however—peripherally as well as in the lungs. Since the initiating problem in patients with adult respiratory distress syndrome is peripheral trauma or sepsis, prolonged administration of corticosteroids is probably dangerous. Corticosteroids should be reserved for patients thought to have adrenal insufficiency, and they should be administered in physiologic rather than pharmacologic doses.

CLOTTING FACTORS

After severe trauma or major sepsis, many patients will demonstrate signs of intravascular coagulation, with prolonged clotting times, low platelet counts, decreased fibrinogen levels, and production of fibrin degradation products or fibrin monomers. Nevertheless, if the patient is not bleeding, fresh-frozen plasma and platelets should not be given; they will only add fuel to the fire of systemic inflammation and coagulation. They should, however, be given to patients who are bleeding and to those with severe head injuries who could develop a sudden, irretrievable and devastating hemorrhage.

MUSCLE RELAXANTS

Muscle relaxants sometimes greatly simplify ventilatory management in patients with severe pulmonary insufficiency, particularly those with recent injuries or sepsis. Because struggling against the ventilator can compromise ventilatory and cardiovascular function, it may be necessary to paralyze the patient when mechanical ventilation is being instituted. Muscle relaxants are dangerous, however, and should only be used when absolutely necessary and for the shortest possible time. Undetected malfunction of a ventilator may mean death for the paralyzed patient.

CHEST X-RAYS

Chest x-rays should be obtained daily in patients being treated with mechanical ventilation. Films are unreliable in differentiating cardiogenic from noncardiogenic edema, however, and visible changes lag behind clinical changes. Films are helpful in diagnosing contusion, aspiration, and pneumonia and may demonstrate a small pneumothorax or mediastinal emphysema. They show positioning of endotracheal tubes, nasogastric tubes, feeding tubes, central venous catheters, and pulmonary arterial catheters. They may show dilatation of the trachea at the site of the balloon on the end of the endotracheal tube.

Indeck M et al: Risk, cost, and benefit of transporting ICU patients for special studies. J Trauma 1988;28:1020.
Maier RV, Carrico CJ: Developments in the resuscitation of critically ill surgical patients. Adv Surg 1986;19:271.

EVALUATION OF SHOCK & PULMONARY FAILURE IN THE ICU

Serious pulmonary failure in the surgical patient can be associated with concomitant cardiac dysfunction and is almost always associated with hypoxemia, hypercapnia, or acidemia. The Swan-Ganz catheter can be very useful in evaluating cardiac function; an understanding of hypoxemia, hypercapnia, and acidemia rests on an understanding of (1) the relationship between the Po_2, the oxygen saturation of hemoglobin, and the oxygen content of blood; (2) the relationship between the Pco_2 in systemic arterial blood and the concept of alveolar ventilation; (3) the causes of hypoxemia; and (4) the relationship between hydrogen ion concentration ($[H^+]$), Pco_2, and bicarbonate concentration ($[HCO_3^-]$).

SWAN-GANZ CATHETER

The balloon- and thermistor-tipped pulmonary arterial catheter permits measurement of the cardiac output; right atrial, pulmonary arterial and pulmonary arterial wedge pressures; and mixed venous oxygen contents. Knowledge of the cardiac index (cardiac output divided by body surface area) and filling pressures can be used to assess ventricular function as fluid is administered or withheld. Knowledge of pulmonary and systemic vascular resistance indices (calculated as the cardiac index divided into the difference between the mean pulmonary arterial and wedge pressures or between the mean systemic arterial and right atrial pressures) can help in deciding whether vasodilators should be administered to unload the ventricles and, if so, how much dilatation is desirable. The mixed venous partial pressure of oxygen reflects the adequacy of oxygen delivery to the periphery; a value less than 30 mm Hg indicates inadequate peripheral oxygenation and can be used to evaluate adequacy of the cardiac index and of systemic arterial oxygen content. It can also be used to determine oxygen consumption, which is calculated as the cardiac index multiplied by the difference of the oxygen contents of blood in the systemic and pulmonary arteries. Oxygen consumption can fall in severely ill patients, and measurements of consumption can help assess the patient's response to resuscitation (Table 12–3).

The catheter is particularly useful when treatment of one organ system might harm another. For example, fluid administration might be needed to treat septic shock, but excess fluid might contribute to pulmonary failure; a diuretic might be indicated in an oliguric patient in congestive heart failure, but excessive diuresis might decrease the cardiac output to the point that the kidneys fail; and fluid might be needed for cardiovascular resuscitation in a patient with multiple injuries, but too much fluid might exacerbate cerebral edema. The pulmonary arterial catheter can be extremely helpful in these situations.

Data obtained from the Swan-Ganz catheter can be misleading, however, if mistakes are made in performing the measurements. The cardiac output, as measured by thermodilution, is obtained by injecting a known volume of a solution cooler than blood into the right atrium and measuring the temperature drop in the blood as it flows past a thermistor on the end of

Table 12–3. Normal values obtained from commonly used monitors.[1]

Variable	Abbreviation or Deviation	Normal Value	Units
Partial pressure of oxygen in systemic arterial blood	Pao_2	Varies (eg, 95 for young adult, 80 for elderly)	mm Hg
Partial pressure of carbon dioxide in arterial blood	$Paco_2$	40; does not vary with age	mm Hg
Oxygen saturation in arterial blood	Sao_2	97%	Dimensionless
Oxygen content in arterial blood	Cao_2[2] $4/3 \times [Hb] \times Sao_2$	20	mL O_2/dL blood, or vol %
Partial pressure of oxygen in mixed venous blood	$Pmvo_2$	40	mm Hg
Partial pressure of carbon in mixed venous blood	$Pmvco_2$	46	mm Hg
Oxygen saturation in mixed venous blood	$Smvo_2$	75%	Dimensionless
Oxygen content in mixed venous blood	$Cmvo_2$[2] $4/3 \times [Hb] \times Smvo_2$	15	mL O_2/dL blood, or vol %
pH	. . .	7.4	Dimensionless
Hydrogen ion concentration	See Table 5	40	nmol/L
Bicarbonate ion concentration	$(24 \times Pco_2) \div [H^+]$	24	mmol/L
Cardiac index	CI	3	$L \cdot min^{-1} \cdot min^{-2}$
Mean systemic arterial pressure	Pa	93	mm Hg
Mean right atrial pressure	P_{RA}	3[3]	mm Hg
Mean pulmonary arterial pressure	P_{RA}	15[3]	mm Hg
Mean wedge pressure	P_{wedge}	8[3]	mm Hg
Systemic vascular resistance index	$(Pa - P_{RA}) \div CI$	30	mm Hg $\cdot L^{-1} \cdot min \cdot m^2$
Pulmonary vascular resistance index	$(P_{PA} - P_{wedge}) \div CI$	2	mm Hg $\cdot L^{-1} \cdot min \cdot m^2$
Oxygen transport	$CI \times Cao_2$	600	mL $O_2 \cdot min^{-1} \cdot m^{-2}$
Oxygen return	$CI \times Cmvo_2$	450	mL $O_2 \cdot min^{-1} \cdot m^{-2}$
Oxygen consumption	$CI \times (Cao_2 - Cmvo_2)$	150	mL $O_2 \cdot min^{-1} \cdot m^{-2}$

[1]Reproduced, with permission, from Abrams JH, Cerra F, Holcroft JW: Cardiopulmonary monitoring, in: *Care of the Surgical Patient.* Vol 1. Critical Care, Section II. Care in the ICU. Wilmore DW et al (editors). Scientific American, 1989.
[2]Oxygen contents calculated on the assumption that [Hb] equals 15 g % and that O_2 consumption and cardiac index are normal.
[3]Values given are for when the patient is breathing spontaneously. Pressures, on average, will be 5 mm Hg higher if the patient is being mechanically ventilated.

the pulmonary arterial catheter. The greater the area under the temperature curve, the less the amount of flow through the right heart. Injections should be made at the same time in the ventilatory cycle, because flow through the right heart varies with the phase of ventilation. Calculations of the cardiac output are made by computer.

When one is obtaining pulmonary arterial or mixed venous blood, the balloon on the end of the catheter should be deflated, and the blood should be withdrawn slowly. If the blood is withdrawn too quickly, the walls of the pulmonary artery will collapse around the end of the catheter, and the specimen will be contaminated by blood that is pulled back, in a ret-

rograde manner, past ventilated and nonperfused alveoli.

All pressures measured with the pulmonary arterial catheter should be recorded from tracings displayed on an oscilloscope. The number recorded should be the pressure at end-expiration regardless of the patient's ventilatory mode.

Of the five pressures obtained from the catheter, only two, the right atrial and the mean pulmonary arterial pressures, can be taken at face value; the other three, the pulmonary arterial systolic, diastolic, and wedge pressures, are subject to errors of measurement and interpretation. The pulmonary arterial wedge pressure usually is the same as the left atrial pressure. The wedge pressure will not reflect left atrial pressure, however, if the catheter is in a portion of the vasculature occluded by inflated alveoli. If it is important to know whether the wedge pressure accurately reflects the left atrial pressure, it is best to obtain a lateral chest x-ray. The tip of the catheter should be in the mid or dorsal portion of the lung.

OXYHEMOGLOBIN DISSOCIATION

The concentration of oxygen in the blood, or oxygen content (C_{O_2}), is expressed as milliliters of O_2/dL of blood, or vol%. This quantity is the most important of the three different measures of oxygenation of the blood. The C_{O_2} can be measured directly, but the measurement is time-consuming, and the content is usually calculated on the basis of the other two measures of blood oxygenation, the oxygen saturation (S_{O_2}) and the P_{O_2}. The C_{O_2} is related to these other quantities by the following formula:

$$C_{O_2} = 1.34 \times [Hb] \times S_{O_2} + 0.0031 \times P_{O_2}$$

where [Hb] is expressed as g/dL and the P_{O_2} as mm Hg. Thus, for example, the C_{O_2} of a blood specimen with a [Hb] of 12 g/dL, a S_{O_2} of 90%, and a P_{O_2} of 60 mm Hg is 14.7 vol%.

The first term in the equation represents the O_2 carried by the hemoglobin molecule; the second, the O_2 dissolved in the blood water. This second term is small compared with the first as long as the [Hb] is greater than (say) 7 g/dL and the P_{O_2} is less than (say) 100 mm Hg. Omitting the second term then simplifies the formula to read as follows:

$$C_{O_2} = 1.34 \times [Hb] \times S_{O_2}$$

For the previous set of blood gases, this would give a C_{O_2} of 14.5 vol%.

The formula can be made even simpler by substituting the fraction $4/3$ for the decimal 1.34:

$$C_{O_2} = 4/3 \times [Hb] \times S_{O_2} \qquad \ldots (1)$$

Because [Hb] and the S_{O_2} can usually be approximated by integers with little loss of accuracy, the calculation frequently allows cancellation of the three and can be done mentally. For the previous example, the C_{O_2} would be 14.4 vol%.

Calculation of the C_{O_2} requires knowledge of the S_{O_2}. The S_{O_2} can be easily measured by an instrument known as a co-oximeter, but most laboratories only make this measurement by specific request. More commonly, the laboratories use the P_{O_2} as their primary measure of oxygenation and then calculate the S_{O_2} from the P_{O_2}.

This calculation, which is usually quite accurate, is made from equations that are based on the oxyhemo-

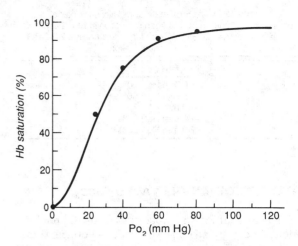

Figure 12–1. Oxyhemoglobin dissociation curve for human blood at 37 °C (98.6 °F) with a P_{CO_2} of 40 mm Hg, a pH of 7.40, and a normal 2,3-DPG red cell concentration. Approximate values from Table 12–4 fall close to the idealized curve.

globin dissociation curve (Figure 12–1), an empirically derived relationship between the S_{O_2} of human blood and its P_{O_2}. The saturation for a given P_{O_2} depends on blood temperature, [H^+], and P_{CO_2} and on the red cell concentration of 2,3-diphosphoglycerate (2,3-DPG). The laboratory should be told the temperature, and it will measure the [H^+] and P_{CO_2}. It will then calculate the S_{O_2} from the P_{O_2} with the assumption that the 2,3-DPG concentration is normal.

It is helpful, however, to have some guidelines for converting back and forth between S_{O_2} and P_{O_2}. Five approximations for points on the dissociation curve, for a patient with normal temperature, [H^+], P_{CO_2}, and 2,3-DPG level are given in Table 12–4. The P_{50} of human hemoglobin—the P_{O_2} at which the molecule is half-saturated—is 27 mm Hg (approximated as 25 mm Hg in the table). The P_{O_2} and S_{O_2} for mixed venous blood in a person with a [Hb] of 15 g/dL and a normal O_2 consumption and cardiac output are 40 mm Hg and 75%, respectively. A P_{O_2} of 60 mm Hg— a value that should be exceeded by most patients in an ICU—corresponds to a S_{O_2} of 89%. A P_{O_2} of 80 mm Hg corresponds to a S_{O_2} of 96%. Remembering the values in the table allows construction of a dissociation curve and facilitates conversion from one measure of oxygenation to the other. For example in a patient with a normal temperature, [H^+], P_{CO_2}, and 2,3-DPG and a [Hb] of 10 g/dL, a P_{O_2} of 60 mm Hg in the systemic arterial blood would create a C_{O_2} of 12 vol% (from Equation 1), a value that would be adequate if the patient had normal coronary arteries and a good heart. Such a value would be inadequate, however, in the face of underlying heart disease.

Table 12–4. Approximate correlations for partial pressures of oxygen and oxygen saturation in blood at 37° C with a pH of 7.4, a P_2 of 40 mm Hg, and a normal 2,3-DPG red cell concentration.

Po_2	So_2
0 mm Hg	0%
25 mm Hg	50%
40 mm Hg	75%
60 mm Hg	90%
80 mm Hg	95%

CAUSES OF AN ELEVATED $PaCO_2$

The arterial Pco_2 is proportionate to CO_2 production divided by alveolar ventilation—defined as the volume of air exchanged per unit time in functioning alveoli. Since CO_2 production is usually fairly constant in adequately perfused patients, the Pco_2 comes to be inversely proportionate to alveolar ventilation. An elevated Pco_2 in the presence of normal CO_2 production means inadequate alveolar ventilation. Ventilation should be assessed with respect to how much work is required to generate the Pco_2. In the case of spontaneous ventilation, this assessment involves the frequency and depth of breathing; in the case of mechanical ventilation, the frequency of the machine-generated breaths and the tidal volume of those breaths.

The Pco_2 also gives an indication of dead space ventilation—the ventilation of nonperfused airways. Since minute or total ventilation is dead space ventilation plus alveolar ventilation, a normal Pco_2 combined with a normal minute ventilation implies a normal dead space ventilation. A normal Pco_2 that must be generated by a supranormal minute ventilation implies increased dead space ventilation. Normal dead space ventilation is one-third of total ventilation, but many critically ill surgical patients will have a dead space ventilation that is up to two-thirds of total ventilation. Increased dead space ventilation can be caused by hypovolemia with poor perfusion of nondependent alveoli, ARDS, pulmonary emboli, pulmonary vasoconstriction, and mechanical ventilation-induced compression of the pulmonary vasculature. Hypovolemia should be treated by expansion of the vascular volume. Emboli should be treated by anticoagulation or by elimination of their source. Dead space generated by mechanical ventilation should be minimized by adjustment of the ventilator, usually by decreasing tidal volumes or end-expiratory pressures, while at the same time maintaining enough mechanical support to generate a normal Pco_2 and alveolar ventilation.

CAUSES OF A LOW PaO_2

There are five causes of arterial hypoxemia: low inspired O_2 concentration, diffusion block between alveolar gas and capillary blood, subnormal alveolar ventilation, shunting of blood through completely nonventilated portions of the lung or bypassing of blood past the lung, and perfusion of parts of the lung that have low ventilation/perfusion ratios. In addition, any process that decreases the mixed venous Co_2 in the presence of any of the above can lower the arterial Po_2 even further. Low mixed venous Po_2 can be caused by a low arterial Co_2, low cardiac output, or high O_2 consumption.

Arterial hypoxemia in the surgical patient is usually caused by shunting, low ventilation/perfusion ratios, low mixed venous Co_2, or a combination of these factors. Low inspired O_2 concentrations at sea level are impossible so long as the ventilator is functioning properly. (This must be checked, however, as the first step in diagnosing and correcting the cause of a low Po_2.) Diffusion block is exceedingly rare in surgical patients. Subnormal alveolar ventilation can be ruled out with a normal arterial Pco_2 assuming Co_2 production is not depressed. Thus, shunting and areas of low ventilation/perfusion ratios, along with low mixed venous Co_2, remain as causes for almost all cases of hypoxemia in the surgical patient. Shunting and low ventilation/perfusion ratios do not need to be distinguished from each other very often, but the distinction can be made by increasing the inspired O_2 concentration to 100%: Hypoxemia caused by areas of low ventilation/perfusion ratios will be corrected by 100% O_2; hypoxemia caused by shunting will not. The mixed venous Co_2 can be measured with the Swan-Ganz catheter. The causes of a low value can be evaluated by measuring the blood hemoglobin concentration, the cardiac output, and the O_2 consumption.

ACID-BASE BALANCE

Hypercapnia represents inadequate alveolar ventilation assuming a normal Co_2 production and, as such, should be a cause for concern, but the elevated Pco_2 by itself actually does no harm. It is the acidemia that usually accompanies the hypercapnia that disrupts vital metabolic processes. Thus, it is important to normalize not only the Pco_2 and Po_2 in the critically ill patient but also the $[H^+]$.

The $[H^+]$, Pco_2, and $[HCO_3^-]$ equilibrate with one another in the plasma water, and if two of the quantities are known, the third can be calculated. In practice the Pco_2 and $[H^+]$ are measured directly, and the $[HCO_3^-]$ is calculated by the Henderson-Hasselbalch equation, which can be written in the following form (see Chapter 9):

$$[HCO_3^-] = \frac{24 \times P_{CO_2}}{[H^+]} \quad \ldots (2)$$

where $[HCO_3^-]$ is expressed as mmol/L, P_{CO_2} as mm Hg, and $[H^+]$ as nmol/L. This form of the equation requires conversion of pH, the more common expression of $[H^+]$, into nmol/L, the more logical expression, but the conversion is not difficult (Table 12–5). The values in the table are easy to remember if one notes that each value in the column under $[H^+]$ is 80% of the value immediately above, with the exception of 80 and 63, which is off by 1. Thus, by Equation 2, if the P_{CO_2} is 60 mm Hg and the pH is 7.30, the $[HCO_3^-]$ is 29 mmol/L.

The $[HCO_3^-]$ calculated by this equation is the actual amount of bicarbonate ion dissolved in the plasma water and can be obtained only from a specimen of blood that is obtained and processed without exposure to the atmosphere. The "CO_2 combining power" that is typically measured along with electrolyte concentrations in blood that is not processed anaerobically includes not only the $[HCO_3^-]$ but any CO_2 gas and carbonic acid that is dissolved in the plasma as well. The CO_2 combining power is usually about 2 mmol/L greater than the calculated (and actual) $[HCO_3^-]$.

The base deficit or excess is determined by comparing the calculated $[HCO_3^-]$ with the $[HCO_3^-]$ that might be expected in a patient with a given P_{CO_2} and $[H^+]$. These expected values have been determined by analyzing blood obtained from patients with a wide variety of pulmonary disorders. For example, the kidneys in a patient with chronic respiratory acidemia can usually compensate to the extent that a chronic elevation in P_{CO_2} of 10 mm Hg will generate an increase in $[HCO_3^-]$ of 3 mmol/L. A patient with chronic obstructive lung disease and a chronically elevated P_{CO_2} of 60 mm Hg would be expected to have a $[HCO_3^-]$ of 30 mmol/L—6 mmol/L more than a normal value of 24. If such a patient had a pH of 7.30, the actual $[HCO_3^-]$ would be 29 mmol/L (from Equation 2; see the example in the preceding paragraph). That is, the observed value would be 1 mmol/L less

than predicted, and the patient would be said to have a base deficit of 1 mmol/L.

The difficulty with the concept of base deficit and excess is that it rests on historically determined values, which may not be applicable to the patient at hand. For example, if a surgical patient with previously normal lungs lost his or her airway after an operation and began to hypoventilate, one would expect the $[HCO_3^-]$ to be normal—24 mmol/L—because the kidneys would not have had time to compensate for the hypercapnia. If the P_{CO_2} were 60 mm Hg and the pH 7.30, the physician should be concerned because the $[HCO_3^-]$ is 29 mmol/L (these values are the same as in the preceding paragraphs). A value of 29 mmol/L should alert the physician to the fact that the $[HCO_3^-]$ is too high, perhaps because $NaHCO_3$ had been given unnecessarily. The base deficit, however, would be 1 mmol/L, suggesting that the patient's $[HCO_3^-]$ was appropriate. The base deficit would be misleading.

The use of base deficit and excess should probably be abandoned in surgical patients. Errors in patient evaluation are more likely to be minimized if the physician concentrates on the $[HCO_3^-]$ and interprets that value in the light of a particular patient's situation. If a chronically ill patient in the ICU has severe ARDS and a P_{CO_2} of 60 mm Hg with a pH of 7.30, no attempt should be made to change the accompanying $[HCO_3^-]$ of 29 mmol/L—that value represents the expected renal compensation for such a chronic hypercapnia (though the impaired alveolar ventilation should be of concern). On the other hand, if the patient's P_{CO_2} is 60 mm Hg and the pH is 7.45, the patient has an inappropriately high $[HCO_3^-]$ of approximately 40 mmol/L (calculated from Equation 2), perhaps because of unreplaced losses of hydrogen ion from the stomach, chronic use of a loop diuretic, or administration of excessive amounts of acetate in the patient's parenteral nutrition. In this situation, the $[HCO_3^-]$ should be brought down into the low 30s. The excessively high $[HCO_3^-]$ and its resultant alkalemia may be blunting the patient's ventilatory drive.

RISK ASSESSMENT

Predicting the likelihood of survival in critically ill surgical patients is best accomplished by evaluating clinical and laboratory findings. Computation of a severity of illness score is usually unnecessary. Nonetheless, several scoring systems have been developed with the intention of increasing the precision of the estimate. All such systems assign a mathematical probability for survival in groups of patients, and many are useful for research purposes because they allow comparisons of patients between different institutions. None of them are accurate enough to predict survival for an individual patient, however,

Table 12–5. Conversion of pH to hydrogen ion concentration.

pH		Hydrogen Ion Concentration (nmol/L)
7.0		100
7.1	$100 \times 0.8 =$	80
7.2	$80 \times 0.8 =$	63
7.3	$63 \times 0.8 =$	50
7.4	$50 \times 0.8 =$	40
7.5	$40 \times 0.8 =$	32
7.6	$32 \times 0.8 =$	25

Note: Values not indicated in the table can be derived by interpolation. For example, a pH of 7.35 corresponds to a hydrogen ion concentration of approximately 45.

though some are still clinically useful for assessing the effects of therapy.

One of the goals of treatment is to determine whether therapy is effective. Effective therapy should usually be left unchanged; ineffective therapy should be modified if possible. A scoring system that substantiates a clinical suspicion of failing therapy may cause changes to be made faster than might be done when responding to clinical impressions alone.

The best of the mathematically based scoring systems is the APACHE II, in which clinical data and 14 measured variables are entered into a formula to calculate probability of survival. The APACHE II score takes about 20 minutes to calculate by hand—less by computer. The score can predict survival in critically ill medical patients; it has not been found to be of value in the usual surgical patient, and in any case it is too cumbersome unless one has a particular interest in this kind of methodology.

Methods for predicting survival in trauma patients are well established, though most trauma systems are designed to evaluate all trauma patients and not the specific subset of critically ill trauma patients. The Injury Severity Score, the Revised Trauma Score, and the newer ASCOT score have proved to be most reliable. The Glasgow Coma Score is quite accurate for predicting survival in patients with head injuries. Combining the Glasgow Coma Score with a simple measurement of fluid requirement has also proved to be accurate in critically injured trauma patients.

Borlase BC et al: Surgical intensive care unit resource use in a specialty referral hospital: I. Predictors of early death and cost implications. Surgery 1990;109:687.

Celoria G, Steingrub JS et al: Clinical assessment of hemodynamic values in two surgical intensive care units. Arch Surg 1990;125:1036.

Cerra FB, Negro F et al: APACHE II score does not predict multiple organ failure or mortality in postoperative surgical patients. Arch Surg 1990;125:519.

Champion HR, Copes WS et al: A new characterization of injury severity. J Trauma 1990;30:539.

Civetta JM, Hudson-Civetta JA et al: Evaluation of APACHE II for cost containment and quality assurance. Ann Surg 1990;212:266.

Copes WS, Champion HR et al: Progress in characterizing anatomic injury. J Trauma 1990;30:1200.

Dellinger EP: Use of scoring systems to assess patients with surgical sepsis. Surg Clin North Am 1988;68:123.

Haber RJ: A practical approach to acid-base disorders. West J Med 1991;155:146.

Kaufmann CR, Maier RV et al: Evaluation of the pediatric trauma score. JAMA 1990;263:69.

Kelleher JF: Pulse oximetry. J Clin Monit 1989;5:37.

O'Quin R, Marini JJ: Pulmonary artery occlusion pressure: Clinical physiology, measurement, and interpretation. Am Rev Respir Dis 1983;128:319.

Poenaru D, Christou NV: Clinical outcome of seriously ill surgical patients with intra-abdominal infection depends on both physiologic (APACHE II score) and immunologic (DTH score) alterations. Ann Surg 1991;213:130.

Scalea TM, Simon HM et al: Geriatric blunt multiple trauma: Improved survival with early invasive monitoring. J Trauma 1990;30:129.

Stevens JH et al: Thermodilution cardiac output measurement. JAMA 1985;253:2240.

Vassar MJ et al: Early fluid requirements in trauma patients. Arch Surg 1988;123:1149.

Wiedemann HP, McCarthy K: Noninvasive monitoring of oxygen and carbon dioxide. Clin Chest Med 1989;10:239.

III. CASE EXAMPLES

Case No. 1: Acute Trauma

A 20-year-old man is involved in a motor vehicle accident. He was the unrestrained driver of a car that hit a tree. On arrival in the emergency room, he has evidence of maxillofacial trauma and is agitated and cyanotic.

Question: *Does this patient need intubation? What intubation route should be used?*

Agitation and cyanosis indicate the need for an airway. Nasotracheal intubation is difficult in an uncooperative patient with poor respiratory effort and is contraindicated in the presence of maxillofacial trauma because of concern that the nasotracheal tube might inadvertently pass backward into the cranial vault. Depending on the severity of facial trauma, one or two attempts at orotracheal intubation might be justified. Severe maxillofacial trauma or difficulties in passing an orotracheal tube should prompt the rapid placement of a surgical airway. Cricothyroidostomy is the procedure of choice because of its simplicity and the rapidity with which it can be done.

A cricothyroidostomy is done, and the patient's agitation and cyanosis improve. He will not follow commands but does respond to pain, and his abdomen is distended. The blood pressure is 90/60 mm Hg, and both femurs are broken.

Question: *Should the patient be mechanically ventilated? What type of ventilator and what settings should be used?*

The patient is hypotensive and has evidence of head, abdominal, and orthopedic injuries. He requires mechanical ventilation with a volume ventilator. An FIO_2 of 100% should be used to ensure maximal oxygen delivery in the face of shock and a head injury. The benefits of maximal oxygenation outweigh the risks of short-term administration of 100% oxygen. Because it may increase intracranial pressure by increasing central venous back pressure, PEEP should not be used. A tidal volume of 10–15 mL/kg should be used. Hyperventilation is effective in reducing intracranial pressure and should be used in this case until the status of the head injury is clarified. Hyperventilation can be effected by setting the ventilatory rate between 25/min and 30/min. Because there is little difference between assist-control and IMV at high ventilatory rates, either mode can be used.

The patient is placed on mechanical ventilation using the settings described above. Shortly thereafter, his systolic blood pressure drops to 60 mm Hg and his trachea is deviated to the right. There are no breath sounds over the left chest.

Question: *What is the problem and how should it be treated?*

The patient has a tension pneumothorax on the left. The initiation of positive-pressure mechanical ventilation has rapidly increased the size of the pneumothorax and resulted in high intrathoracic pressure and deviation of the trachea away from the side of the pneumothorax. This in turn interferes with venous return and leads to worsening of the patient's shock. The pneumothorax should be relieved with needle decompression of the left chest followed by a chest tube.

The patient is taken to the operating room for exploratory celiotomy and removal of a ruptured spleen. His leg fractures are treated with open reduction and internal fixation. No abnormalities are seen on CT scan of the head. His mental status clears rapidly, and no intracranial pressure monitoring is necessary. He is taken to the intensive care unit.

Question: *What ventilator settings should now be used? When and how should he be weaned from the ventilator?*

All of the injuries have been repaired, and rapid recovery is expected. The patient's mental status has cleared, and there is minimal evidence of head injury. The patient should be placed on IMV, and weaning from the ventilator should be started. Hyperventilation and a high FIO_2 are no longer necessary, and both the IMV and the FIO_2 should be reduced gradually. Arterial PO_2 and PCO_2 as well as the patient's clinical status should be used to guide the rapidity with which weaning is carried out. When an IMV rate of 4/min is reached and the patient is receiving an FIO_2 of 40% or less, a T-piece trial should be done for 30 minutes. If the patient tolerates the T-piece trial well, the prognosis for recovery remains good, and if the mental status is completely normal, the patient is ready for extubation. Weaning parameters can be obtained if desired to document the appropriateness of extubation.

Case No. 2: Intra-abdominal Sepsis

A 50-year-old man develops gallstone pancreatitis. He receives supportive care, but his condition worsens during his first 24 hours of hospitalization. He becomes increasingly tachypneic, and his respiratory rate reaches 35/min. His breathing is shallow, and he is using his accessory muscles of respiration. Because of concern about his respiratory status, an arterial blood gas measurement is obtained. His PO_2 on 70% oxygen by mask is 40 mm Hg (75% saturated). The PCO_2 is 40 mm Hg and the pH is 7.34.

Question: *Does this patient require intubation and ventilatory support? What mode of ventilation should be used, and what should his ventilator settings be? When and how should he be weaned from the ventilator?*

The patient requires intubation and mechanical ventilation for several reasons. The PO_2 of only 40 mm Hg on 70% oxygen by mask indicates a large pulmonary shunt. A PCO_2 of 40 mm Hg, though it would be normal if the respiratory rate were normal, is a sign of impending respiratory arrest at a respiratory rate of 35/min. The rate of 35/min cannot be maintained indefinitely and is itself a sign of impending collapse. Furthermore, the patient's disease process and the prognosis are unclear, and the subjective impression that he is clearly getting worse argues for intubation. Intermittent mandatory ventilation is appropriate, and the tidal volume should be set at 10–15 mL/kg. The initial ventilatory rate should be set between 15/min and 20/min and adjusted based on patient comfort and the PCO_2. The FIO_2 should initially be set between 70% and 100%, and PEEP should be instituted at 5 cm H_2O. Using the PO_2 as a guide, the inspired oxygen concentration should then be decreased to as low a level as possible compatible with an oxygen saturation above 90%. If necessary, PEEP should be increased in an attempt to lower the inspired oxygen concentration to at least 50%.

The patient is intubated and mechanical ventilation begun with a tidal volume of 15 mL/kg at a rate of 18/min, an FIO_2 of 90% and a PEEP of 5 cm H_2O. He is more comfortable and over the next several hours it is possible to decrease the inspired oxygen concentration to 50%. The PEEP is increased to 10 cm H_2O. A diagnosis of necrotizing pancreatitis is made, which requires operative debridement. On the first postoperative day, the FIO_2 is decreased to 40% and the oxygen saturation is 95%. PEEP remains at 10 cm H_2O. Rate and tidal volume are unchanged.

Question: *Is the patient ready for weaning and extubation?*

The prognosis for this patient is still guarded, and he may well require further operative debridement. Although the decrease in inspired oxygen concentration is encouraging, he remains on a PEEP of 10 cm H_2O. Prior to weaning, an attempt should be made to reduce the level of PEEP. Weaning should await further improvements in the patient's overall status.

Attempts to decrease the level of PEEP over the next several days are unsuccessful. Bilateral pulmonary infiltrates develop within 12 hours after his operation. Multiple further operative debridements of the pancreas and drainage procedures for intra-abdominal abscess are required, and the patient continues to require ventilatory support for the next 3 weeks. He receives several courses of antibiotics and is treated for pneumonia on two occasions. His intra-abdominal sepsis is ultimately controlled, and no further operations are planned. He is off of antibiotics. He is awake and is writing notes. The FIO_2 is 40%, and the PEEP is 5 cm H_2O. Tidal volume is unchanged, and the respiratory rate is 16/min.

Question: *Is the patient now ready for weaning? If so, how should it be done?*

Weaning is now appropriate. The patient is awake and alert, and his prognosis for recovery is good. He is on acceptably low levels of inspired oxygen and PEEP. The IMV rate should be gradually decreased, and his clinical status and PCO_2 should be monitored. If the patient tolerates decreases in the IMV rate to 4/min, a T-piece trial should be initiated. If this is well tolerated, the patient should be extubated.

The IMV rate is successfully decreased to 10/min. Further decreases, however, are tolerated poorly, with CO_2 retention and respiratory distress.

Question: *What are the alternatives for further weaning?*

Simply supporting the patient on an IMV of 10/min until further improvement in ventilatory capability occurs is one alternative. The addition of pressure support to allow for further decreases in IMV followed by weaning of the pressure support is another alternative. A third option would be a regimen of T-piece wind sprints of gradually increasing duration. Regardless of the weaning method chosen, a tracheostomy should be considered if it is anticipated that the patient will remain intubated for 2–3 more weeks.

A tracheostomy is done and a wind sprint regimen begun. The length of the wind sprints is gradually increased over the next 2 weeks until the patient can easily tolerate T-piece with CPAP for a 12-hour period. He is then successfully removed from the ventilator. The tracheostomy is removed 5 days later.

Case No. 3: Hypovolemic/Cardiogenic Shock

A 60-year-old man with a history of coronary artery disease and peptic ulcer disease presents to the emergency department with a 24-hour history of abdominal pain. The pain was sudden in onset and has become progressively more severe. He has had nothing by mouth for the past 24 hours. There is free air under the diaphragm on admission x-ray, and a presumptive diagnosis of perforated duodenal ulcer is

made. On admission, the patient is cool and capillary refill in the toes is 3 seconds. The blood pressure is 80/40 mm Hg. The pulse is thready and 130/min in the supine position. The neck veins are flat, and mentation is poor. A urinary catheter is placed, and only 5 mL of urine are initially drained from the bladder.

Question: *Is the patient in shock? What is the most likely cause of the shock and how should it be treated?*

There are several indications of shock in this patient. Peripheral perfusion is poor. He is hypotensive, tachycardiac, and his neck veins are flat. His mental status is depressed, and there is minimal urine output. Treatment at this point should be directed toward repletion of the intravascular volume with a balanced salt solution such as lactated Ringer's injection to replace fluid lost into the peritoneal cavity in response to peritonitis. Although the patient will require surgery, it is important to restore intravascular volume before induction of anesthesia.

The admission hematocrit comes back from the laboratory and is 50%. Two large intravenous catheters are placed, and the patient is given 4 L of lactated Ringer's injection over the next 2 hours. The blood pressure increases to 120/80 mm Hg, and the pulse decreases to 100/min. The toes are somewhat warmer to the touch, and capillary refill time decreases to 2 seconds. The patient undergoes exploratory laparotomy, and a duodenal ulcer is oversewn. Postoperatively, he is taken to the intensive care unit and is extubated the following day.

Question: *Why was the admission hematocrit 50%? How should the patient's volume status be followed in the postoperative period?*

The blood is hemoconcentrated because of the loss of plasma into the peritoneal cavity. In the postoperative period, as in the initial evaluation, blood pressure, pulse, capillary refill, temperature, and neck vein examination can be used to follow the patient. One of the best measures of perfusion, assuming there is no underlying renal disease, is the urinary output.

Initially, the patient does quite well. On the second postoperative day, however, he complains of substernal chest pain and shortness of breath. The blood pressure falls to 90/60 mm Hg, and the pulse increases to 120/min. The neck veins are distended. The arterial PO_2 is 50 mm Hg with the patient on 40% oxygen by face mask.

Question: *What is the most likely cause for this patient's deterioration? How should it be treated?*

The presence of chest pain associated with hypotension and respiratory distress suggests cardiogenic shock, as do the distended neck veins. The patient should initially be treated with increased oxygen and limitation of intravenous fluids. The diagnosis should be confirmed with placement of a Swan-Ganz catheter and determination of the pulmonary arterial wedge pressure and cardiac index. A high wedge pressure and low cardiac index should be treated with diuresis and inotropic support as needed. The diagnosis should be further confirmed with serial ECGs and cardiac enzymes, looking for signs of myocardial infarction as a cause of cardiogenic shock.

The oxygen concentration is increased to 100% by mask, and a Swan-Ganz catheter is placed. The pulmonary arterial wedge pressure is 40 mm Hg, and the cardiac index is 1.8 L/min/m^2. The patient is given diuretics to a wedge pressure of 15 mm Hg and dobutamine at a dose of 6 µg/kg/min. The blood pressure increases to 120/80 mm Hg, and the pulse decreases to 80/min. The cardiac index increases to 3.2 L/min/m^2. Myocardial infarction is confirmed by ECG and cardiac enzymes. The patient continues to improve, recovers completely except for occasional continued angina pectoris, and is discharged home on the 18th postoperative day. Three months later, he undergoes coronary angiography and coronary artery bypass grafting.

Case No. 4: Trauma & Sepsis

A 25-year-old man is shot once in the abdomen. On arrival in the emergency department, he is unresponsive, and his respirations are rapid and shallow. His blood pressure is 80/40 mm Hg, and his abdomen is distended. He is pale and cool to the touch, and there is minimal capillary refill. The neck veins are flat.

Question: *Is the patient in shock? What is the most likely cause, and how should it be treated?*

Hypotension, pallor, coolness, poor capillary refill, and decreased mental status indicate shock. The gunshot wound, abdominal distention, and flat neck veins point to hemorrhage as the likely cause. The patient requires immediate surgery for control of hemorrhage as the best means for correcting his shock.

The patient is intubated and ventilated. Several large intravenous catheters are placed, lactated Ringer's injection is infused as rapidly as possible, and an exploratory laparotomy is done. Two liters of blood are found on entry to the abdomen, and there is an injury to the infrarenal abdominal aorta. There are also several large holes in the transverse colon, with gross fecal contamination of the abdomen. The aorta is repaired and the right and transverse colon are resected, with creation of a diverting ileostomy. The peritoneal cavity is irrigated, and the abdomen is closed. Ten units of blood are transfused intraoperatively, and at the conclusion of the operation the hematocrit is 30%.

Question: *What should be done about the hematocrit of 30%?*

Nothing should be done about the hematocrit. A level of 30% is adequate for a young, otherwise healthy patient such as this one and may even improve perfusion because of decreased blood viscosity.

On the eighth postoperative day, the patient develops ileus, and large volumes of intravenous fluid are needed to maintain urine output and blood pressure. Whenever fluid rates are decreased, hypotension and decreased urine output recur. There is increasing respiratory distress and hypoxemia that requires intubation and mechanical ventilation on an inspired oxygen concentration of 60%. There are diffuse bilateral infiltrates on chest x-ray. The digits are warm, and capillary refill is normal. There are signs of glucose intolerance.

Question: *What kind of shock is this patient suffering from, and how should it be treated?*

This is a case of septic shock. Vigorous fluid administration to compensate for hypotension and decreased urine output has prevented low-output septic shock and resulted in high-output septic shock instead. Aggressive monitoring is indicated, and both an arterial catheter and a pulmonary arterial catheter should be placed. The pulmonary arterial catheter is helpful both in confirming the diagnosis and in monitoring subsequent therapy. In addition, a source of sepsis should be sought.

The pulmonary arterial wedge pressure is 15 mm Hg, and the cardiac index is 3.5 L/min/m^2. Intravenous fluid administration is continued, and the wedge pressure increases to 20 mm Hg. The cardiac index increases to 4.5 L/min/m^2. Positive end-expiratory pressure of 10 cm H$_2$O is added, and the inspired oxygen concentration is decreased to 50%. CT scan of the abdomen reveals a large subhepatic abscess, and the patient is taken to the operating room for drainage. He does well afterward, and his pulmonary function improves. Fluid requirements remain high for 2 days postoperatively, but spontaneous diuresis begins on postoperative day 3. The patient recovers completely and is discharged home 2 weeks later.

IV. NEW DEVELOPMENTS

Current research suggests there will be many new developments in the care of the critically ill surgical patient in the next few years. Human growth hormone, which can now be prepared in pure form, can augment nitrogen retention and skeletal muscle strength even in the face of surgical stress and hypocaloric feeding. Administration of such an agent to the critically ill patient on mechanical ventilation who is too weak to breath spontaneously might make possible successful weaning. The use of blockers of tumor necrosis factor or interleukin-1 might prevent metabolic wasting associated with sepsis. Administration of glutamine with total parenteral nutrition might promote recovery of the gut mucosa after shock and limit bacterial translocation. Use of hypertonic solutions might permit resuscitation of injured patients while they are still in the field, before they reach definitive care.

Nevertheless, the basic principles for care of the critically ill surgical patient will remain the same. The primary goal should be to prevent shock and sepsis, which in the surgical patient usually requires an operation. Blood loss should be controlled promptly. Pus should be drained. Dead tissue should be debrided. Damaged portions of the gastrointestinal tract should be resected, bypassed, or both. In the enthusiasm over new methods, these basic principles must not be forgotten.

REFERENCES

Wilmore DW et al (editors): Care of the Surgical Patient. Vol 1: Critical Care. Section 2. Care in the ICU. Scientific American Medicine, 1991.

Deitch EA: Bacterial translocation of the gut flora. J Trauma 1990;30:S184.

Demling RH et al: Effect of ibuprofen on the pulmonary and systemic response to repeated doses of endotoxin. Surgery 1989;105:421.

Mainous MR et al: Studies of the route, magnitude, and time course of bacterial translocation in a model of systemic inflammation. Arch Surg 1991;126:33.

Michie HR et al: Detection of circulating tumor necrosis factor after endotoxin administration. N Engl J Med 1988;318:1481.

Michie HR et al: Tumor necrosis factor and bacterial sepsis. Br J Surg 1989;76:670.

Michie HR, Wilmore DW: Sepsis, signals, and surgical sequelae. Arch Surg 1990;125:531.

Moore FA, Moore EE et al: Gut bacterial translocation via the portal vein: A clinical perspective with major torso trauma. J Trauma 1991;31:629.

Old LJ: Tumor necrosis factor. Sci Am 1988;258:59-60, 69-75.

Rudman D et al: Effects of human growth hormone in men over 60 years old. N Engl J Med 1990;323:1.

Souba WW et al: The effects of sepsis and endotoxemia on gut glutamine metabolism. Ann Surg 1990;211:543.

Management of the Injured Patient **13**

James R. Macho, MD, Frank R. Lewis, Jr., MD, & William C. Krupski, MD

EPIDEMIOLOGY OF TRAUMA

Injury can be defined as the damage to the body caused by acute exposure to energy. Trauma is the medical term used to describe injury and usually refers to life-threatening or serious injuries that require specialized surgical care if the patient is to survive without disability. As a "disease," trauma represents a major public health problem. It is the principal cause of death during the first half of the normal human life span and the fourth leading cause of death for all age groups. In persons under age 34, trauma is responsible for more deaths than all other diseases put together. In the USA, about 160,000 lives are lost per year because of injuries, and an additional 500,000 injured persons suffer some form of permanent disability. Because trauma affects mainly a young population, it results in the loss of more working years than all other causes. The financial costs of injury exceed $133 billion annually. What is most tragic is that as many as 40% of all trauma deaths are avoidable by preventive measures and by the establishment of regional trauma systems.

Trauma deaths have a trimodal distribution, with peaks that correspond to the types of intervention that would be most effective in reducing mortality. The first peak, the *immediate deaths,* represents patients who die of their injuries before reaching the hospital. The injuries accounting for these deaths include major brain or spinal cord injuries and lacerations of the heart or great vessels. Few of these patients would have any chance of survival even with access to immediate care. Prevention remains the major strategy to reduce these deaths.

The second peak, the *early deaths,* are those that occur within the first few hours after injury. They are mainly caused by internal hemorrhage, and almost all are treatable. However, in most cases salvage requires prompt and definitive operative care of the sort available at a **trauma center,** ie, a specialized institution that can provide immediate resuscitation and access to a prepared operating room 24 hours a day.

The third peak, the *late deaths,* consists of patients who die days or weeks after injury. Eighty percent are caused by sepsis and multiple organ failure. The critical care phase of trauma care is important in reducing these deaths. Evidence suggests that at present

about 50% of late deaths could be prevented by better critical care management. It is essential that surgeons caring for trauma patients have genuine expertise in surgical critical care.

PREVENTION OF TRAUMA

Prevention of injury has received much less scientific attention than has the treatment of diseases of far less consequence. Unfortunately, prevention programs aimed at altering human behavior have been largely unsuccessful because the programs do not reach the populations most at risk and because they often raise controversial social questions, including the right of individuals to engage in high-risk behavior. Programs mandated by law or official policies have met with greater success. It is estimated that 50–60% of all fatal motor vehicle accidents are caused by drunk drivers. Evidence suggests that stringent measures such as mandatory jail terms and revocation or suspension of a driver's license after a drunk driving conviction decrease the rate of drunk driving (and drunk driving arrests).

Experience with laws requiring the use of seatbelts and motorcycle helmets have demonstrated a clearcut survival benefit. In Australia, after seat belt use was required by law, deaths of automobile occupants decreased 25%. Initial experience suggests that the use of airbags as a form of passive restraint may decrease the number of deaths from certain kinds of accidents, such as head-on collisions. Laws mandating the use of motorcycle helmets have generated controversy, but data indicate that they reduce injury severity. After federal highway safety standards required the use of helmets by motorcycle riders, deaths from this activity decreased by 50%. Where such laws have been repealed or weakened, the mortality rate has increased by as much as 40%. Helmets provide even greater protection for bicycle riders, since nearly all fatal injuries are head injuries.

In penetrating trauma due to handguns and knives, the predisposing factors are less clear, but it is known that most are associated with use of alcohol or drugs or with assaults in which thefts of goods for the purpose of purchasing drugs is the object. Although controversial, decriminalization of drug use, particularly of narcotics, and registration of addicts would probably decrease this source of trauma. Gun control legislation and mandatory jail sentences for crimes committed with firearms are other proposed but largely untested options.

The possibilities of preventing injury by modifying the environment have been largely ignored. The record suggests that the nation's health might benefit more by increased emphasis on environmental factors. The few efforts at environmental modification have produced significant results. The national 55-mph speed limit in the USA reduced the death rate per 100 million vehicle miles from 4.3 in 1973 to 3.5 in 1974—a 19% decline, equal to a yearly saving of 10,000 lives. The effect of highway design is shown by the fact that death rates per vehicle mile on interstate highways are one-third those on other roads. Future efforts at injury prevention are more likely to be effective if they are directed toward environmental factors.

TRAUMA SYSTEMS

The goal of a trauma system is to provide timely, organized care in order to prevent avoidable death following injury. The system includes pre hospital care designed to identify, treat and transport victims with serious injuries. Criteria for staging patients with major trauma consist of standardized scoring systems based on readily obtainable anatomic and physiologic variables. The criteria are designed to identify not only the more severe and complex single injuries but also combinations of injuries that require tertiary care. Patients are transported to a trauma center designed to provide the highest possible level of care to patients with major injuries. When a patient arrives in the Trauma Center, additional triage occurs. The most severely injured patients are identified and receive more intense care. By the most optimistic estimates, only 25% of the US population is covered by regional trauma systems even though there is no disagreement that such systems decrease death and disability. The issue is highlighted by a recent study in which it was found that the percentage of preventable deaths in a California county dropped from 11% to 1% after the institution of regionalized trauma care. Similar data are available for other areas of the country.

The American College of Surgeons has defined three levels of institutional trauma care. Trauma centers designated as level I provide immediately available care 24 hours a day by in-hospital surgeons. Specialty care is provided by on-call physicians. The level I trauma center includes a research and teaching commitment. level II Trauma Centers provide 24-hour care by in-hospital and on-call physicians. They are able to deliver the same care as a level I center, but without the teaching and research obligations of a

level I center. Immediate operating room capability should be maintained 24 hours a day in level I and II centers. The level III hospital provides prompt assessment, resuscitation and stabilization followed by surgical treatment or inter hospital transfer as appropriate. Although it may not be able to provide definitive care in all circumstances, level III centers serve a valuable function in less populated areas where resuscitation and stabilization before transport may be lifesaving.

PREHOSPITAL CARE & TRIAGE

The effectiveness of paramedics in the treatment of trauma victims remains controversial owing to a lack of data regarding the success of specific prehospital treatments. Evidence of improved survival of cardiac arrest victims treated by well-trained paramedic teams have been inappropriately extrapolated to trauma victims. In the urban setting, where transportation from the scene of an accident to the hospital is typically 5–10 minutes, it is questionable whether any treatment by paramedics other than airway management, simple first aid, and splinting is beneficial. The principal causes of immediate death from trauma are head injury (50%), exsanguination (35%), and airway or pulmonary problems (15%). Only the last of these can treated in the field. Patients with head injury or airway and pulmonary problems benefit from endotracheal intubation to maintain effective ventilation and prevent aspiration and hypercapnia. Most life-threatening injuries require hospital facilities and a well-organized team that can provide immediate treatment, including surgery, and any delay in the field usually worsens outcome. One study showed that trauma victims with cardiac wounds who were treated by paramedics had longer delays in transportation and lower survival rates compared with victims treated by emergency medical technicians (EMTs) or nonmedical persons. However, recent information shows that well-trained paramedics can prepare patients for transport quickly and then perform life-support procedures en route with a high rate of patient survival. Further studies are required to identify the procedures other than intubation that would improve the survival of these patients.

IMMEDIATE MEASURES AT THE SCENE OF AN ACCIDENT

When first seen, the victim of an accident may not appear to be badly injured. There may be little external evidence of injury, so when the mechanism of trauma is sufficient to produce severe injury, the victim must be handled as if severe injury has occurred.

The injured person must be protected from further trauma. First aid at the scene of an accident should be administered by trained personnel whenever possible. The simple act of moving a victim from one position to another, if done improperly, may compress or lacerate the spinal cord, puncture a lung, sever a major blood vessel or compound a fracture, thereby converting a simple injury into a major one.

Whether the patient is first seen on the battlefield, beside a road, in the emergency ward, or in the hospital, the basic principles of initial management are the same:

(1) Is the victim breathing? If not, provide an airway and maintain respiratory exchange.

(2) Is there a pulse or heartbeat? If not, begin closed chest compression.

(3) Is there gross external bleeding? If so, elevate the part if possible and apply enough external pressure over the feeding artery to stop the bleeding. A tourniquet is rarely needed.

(4) Is there any question of injury to the spine? If so, protect the neck and spine before moving the patient.

(5) Splint obvious fractures.

As soon as these steps have been taken, the patient can be safely transported.

Specific details of prehospital management are considered in the following paragraphs.

1. AIRWAY MANAGEMENT

The most important therapy that can be provided before the patient gets to the hospital is airway management. Simple measures, such as clearing the airway, positioning the mandible and the use of oral airways, may be all that is necessary to insure adequate ventilation. This can often be done by simple manipulation of the mandible or traction on the tongue, particularly in unconscious or semiconscious patients. After the mouth is forced open, the tongue can be grasped between the thumb and forefinger covered with a handkerchief or gauze bandage. The tip of the tongue should be pulled forward beyond the front teeth. The mandible should be manipulated either by pulling forward the angles of the lower jaw or by inserting the thumb between the teeth, grasping the mandible in the midline, and drawing it forward until the lower teeth are leading (Figure 13–1).

Suctioning the mouth and pharynx may clear them of blood, mucus, or vomitus so as to permit normal respiration. Repeated suctioning may be required to maintain an adequate airway at the scene of the accident and during transit to a medical facility. Aspiration of vomitus, a frequent cause of sudden death, must be prevented at all costs. A lateral and slightly head-down position is best for patients who are liable to vomit. In respiratory arrest, a clear airway must be provided and mouth-to-mouth breathing instituted if other means of ventilation are not available. In extreme situations, where the upper airway is occluded and the foreign body cannot be removed, it can be lifesaving to insert one or two large-bore needles (14-gauge) through the cricothyroid membrane (Figure 13–2). Emergency tracheotomy should never be attempted at the scene of the accident or in the ambulance. Whenever possible, patients who are unconscious or in profound shock should have the airway controlled with an endotracheal tube (Figure 13–3). Although endotracheal intubation is the only pre hospital treatment proven to benefit trauma victims with potentially lethal injuries, few paramedics are trained or proficient in this skill. Extensive evaluation of the field use of endotracheal intubation by paramedics in the Pittsburgh emergency care system has shown that relatively limited training is needed, that intubation is successful in 85–95% of cases, and that paramedics retain their skill in this technique even when the frequency of field use is only moderate. If these results can be widely duplicated, endotracheal intubation should be taught to all paramedics.

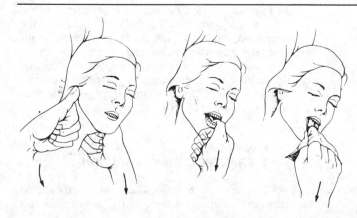

Figure 13–1. Relief of airway obstruction.

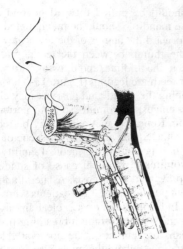

Figure 13–2. Needle in trachea to establish temporary airway.

2. INTRAVENOUS LINES

Starting intravenous lines is probably counterproductive, because the amount of fluid given during a brief trip to the hospital rarely compensates for the loss of blood that occurs during the time it takes. When long delays to definitive treatment are inevitable because of difficulty in evaluation, intravenous infusions are more apt to be a benefit. The infusion should be started after the patient is en route whenever possible. The administration of hypertonic saline may be preferable to conventional isotonic solu-

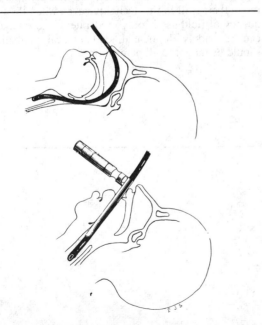

Figure 13–3. *Top:* Nasotracheal intubation. *Bottom:* Orotracheal intubation.

tions when transport time is long. However, no benefit of hypertonic saline has been demonstrated with short transport times or for in-hospital resuscitations.

3. PREHOSPITAL CARDIAC ARREST

Cardiac arrest following trauma, when encountered at the scene of an accident, is usually fatal unless a cause, such as airway obstruction, can be immediately identified and corrected. If blunt trauma is the cause of the prehospital arrest, the salvage rate almost is nil. If the cause is penetrating trauma, particularly stab wounds, the salvage rate is highest if the patient can be rapidly delivered to a trauma center. In such cases, ventilation by mouth-to-mouth resuscitation or a manual device should be initiated during transport, and closed chest cardiac compression should be performed.

4. MAST SUIT

Use of the MAST suit for field treatment of hypovolemia has been advocated increasingly since the Vietnam war. Originally, it was felt that autotransfused blood from the legs and pelvis to the circulation of the upper half of the body. This has been shown to be incorrect, for the augmentation of circulating volume is only 200–250 mL. The garment works instead by reducing perfusion to the lower half of the body and markedly increasing peripheral resistance, so that available cardiac output is directed to more important organs. Although this might seem worthwhile, there are two drawbacks. First, movement of the rib cage is markedly restricted by the abdominal portion of the garment. Direct compression of abdominal contents, elevation of the diaphragm, and restriction of rib cage motion all reduce vital capacity. In the patient with respiratory compromise or rib fractures, this may be of major importance. The second problem is the possibility of increased blood pressure that may lead to increased bleeding above the level of the MAST suit. Randomized studies on pre hospital use have not demonstrated survival benefits and they should not be applied routinely. On the other hand, the MAST suit is of proved value for in-hospital tamponade of bleeding in patients with severe pelvic fractures and massive pelvic bleeding. This gains time for angiography and embolization of the bleeding site. This is the only documented indication for use of the MAST suit.

5. NECK, SPINE & FRACTURE IMMOBILIZATION

All patients with major blunt trauma should be suspected of having spinal injury, and precautions should be taken to immobilize the spine and prevent further injury. Recognition and splinting of major fractures and immobilization of all injured parts before transportation are essential features of early management. Improper handling of the injured, patient may increase or prolong shock and aggravate existing trauma beyond the possibility of definitive repair. "Splint'em where they lie" is a time-honored rule of emergency care of fractures that has only a few exception eg, when it is necessary to remove an injured patient from imminent danger of fire, explosion, escaping gas, etc). Immobilization should be achieved rapidly and should not delay transfer to the hospital.

6. TRIAGE

Triage at the accident scene seeks to identify the patients who are most at risk of dying from their injuries and thus would benefit most from a trauma center. The American College of Surgeons has published guidelines for the triage of trauma victims (Figure 13–4). Whenever in doubt, the patient should be transported to a trauma center.

7. PREHOSPITAL TRANSPORT

Transportation by ground or air ambulance is preferable when feasible. The choice of helicopter or ambulance depends upon time and distance and the level of care that must be provided enrol. Ideally, transport should not exceed 15 minutes and the total pre hospital time should not exceed 30 minutes. Resuscitation of the seriously injured patient should be continued during transportation, and a constant effort must be made to avoid airway obstruction and aspiration if the patient is vomiting.

If no ambulance is available, a station wagon or truck is preferable to a passenger car. The manipulation necessary to load a seriously injured person into a passenger car may be more harmful than the time lost in waiting for proper transportation. Except in unusual circumstances, injured patients should be transported in the supine position.

EVALUATION OF THE TRAUMA PATIENT

HISTORY

In most cases the history is obtained from the prehospital personnel via radio communication or when the patient arrives at the hospital. It is important to determine the circumstances of the injury, including the speed of impact, the condition of the vehicle, the position of the patient at the scene, evidence of blood loss and the condition of other passengers. Record the time the injury occurred and the treatment rendered while enrol. Everyone who may have information about the circumstances of the injury should be questioned. Knowing the mechanism of the injury often gives a clue to concealed trauma. Information regarding serious underlying medical problems should be sought from Medic-alert bracelets or wallet cards. If the patient is conscious and stable, the examiner should obtain a complete history and use this information to direct the examination in order to avoid unnecessary tests.

Only a few trauma victims require a precise, rapid, systematic approach to initial evaluation in order to assure their survival. The Advanced Trauma Lifesupport system developed by the American College of Surgeons Committee on Trauma represents the best current approach to the severely injured patient. The sequence of evaluation includes primary survey, resuscitation, secondary survey, and definitive management. The **primary survey** attempts to identify and treat immediate life-threatening conditions. Resuscitation is performed, and the response to therapy is evaluated. The **secondary survey** includes a comprehensive physical examination designed to detect all injuries and set a treatment priority for potentially life-threatening ones. During this phase, appropriate laboratory and radiologic studies, such as diagnostic peritoneal lavage, CT scan, or angiography, are performed to prepare the patient for **definitive care.**

PRIMARY SURVEY

AIRWAY

The establishment of an adequate airway has the highest priority in the primary survey. The maneuvers used in the trauma patient must consider a possible cervical spine injury. Orotracheal intubation can be attempted with cervical spine precautions if a second person maintains axial traction on the head to prevent destabilization of the spine. When circumstances allow, a lateral film of the cervical spine can be obtained to rule out injury before attempting intubation. An adequate radiographic study to exclude injury requires that all seven vertebrae be clearly seen. Additional views are required frequently. If ventilatory failure occurs and an adequate airway cannot be obtained by conventional means, a surgical cricothy-

Surgery 13.4

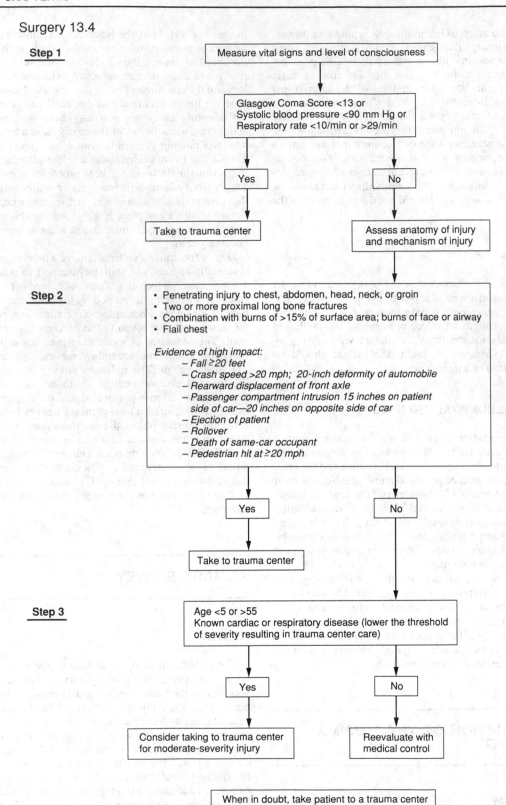

Figure 13–4. Triage scheme for trauma victims as published by the American College of Surgeons Committee on Trauma.

roidotomy should be performed as rapidly as possible (Figure 13–5).

BREATHING

Once the airway has been established, it is necessary to insure that ventilation is adequate. Examine the patient to determine the degree of chest expansion, breath sounds, tachypnea, crepitus from rib fractures, subcutaneous emphysema, and the presence of penetrating or open wounds. The immediately life-threatening pulmonary conditions are tension pneumothorax, open pneumothorax, flail chest, and occasionally a massive hemothorax. Chest injury is the second most common cause of asphyxia. The following are the chief examples.

(1) Tension penumothorax occurs from air in the pleural space under pressure. The harmful effects result more from shift of the mediastinum and impairment of venous return rather than from ventilatory failure. Tension pneumothorax is difficult to diagnose, even when the patient reaches hospital. The clinical findings consist of hypotension in the presence of distended neck veins, decreased or absent breath sounds on the affected side, hyperresonance to percussion, and tracheal shift. Cyanosis may be a late manifestation. Emergency treatment consists of insertion of a large-bore needle or plastic intravenous cannula to relieve the pressure and convert the tension pneumothorax to a simple pneumothorax. The needle or cannula may be left in place while a chest tube is inserted for definitive management (Figure 13–6).

(2) Open pneumothorax results from an open wound of the chest wall with free communication be-

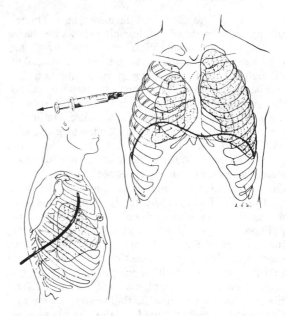

Figure 13–6. Relief of pneumothorax. Tension pneumothorax must be immediately decompressed by a needle introduced through the second anterior intercostal space. A chest tube is usually inserted in the midaxillary line at the level of the nipple and is directed posteriorly and superiorly toward the apex of the thorax. The tube is attached to a "three-bottle" suction device, and the rate of escape of air is indicated by the appearance of bubbles in the second of the three bottles. When bubbling ceases, this suggests that the air leak has become sealed.

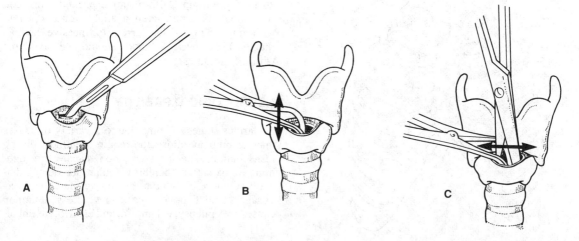

Figure 13–5. Surgical cricothyroidotomy.

tween the pleural space and the atmosphere. The resulting impairment of the thoracic bellows results in ineffectual ventilation. With ventilatory efforts, air moves in and out of the chest wall opening instead of through the trachea, producing hypoventilation that can be rapidly fatal. Emergency treatment is to seal the wound with a sterile dressing if possible, or with any material if nothing sterile is available. Definitive treatment requires placement of a chest tube and surgical closure of the defect.

(3) Flail chest: Multiple rib fractures, resulting in a free floating segment, may produce instability of the chest wall so that paradoxical motion occurs with ventilatory efforts. (Figure 13–7) However, this does not fully explain the pathophysiology. Associated pulmonary contusion is common and may be the major cause of the ventilatory failure. The injury is identified with careful inspection and palpation. Patients with large flail segments always, require prompt endotracheal intubation and mechanical ventilation, both to stabilize the flail segment and to optimize gas exchange. Smaller flail segments may be well tolerated if supplemental oxygen and adequate analgesia are provided. The work or breathing is increased considerably, however, and elderly patients who initially appear to be compensating well may suddenly deteriorate a few hours later.

CIRCULATION

Hemorrhage

Gross hemorrhage from accessible surface wounds is usually obvious and can be controlled in most cases by local pressure and elevation of the part. Firm pressure on the major artery in the axilla, antecubital space, wrist, groin, popliteal space, or at the ankle

may suffice for temporary control of arterial hemorrhage distal to these points. When other measures have failed, a tourniquet may rarely be necessary to control major hemorrhage from extensive wounds or major vessels in an extremity. Failure to release it periodically may cause irreparable vascular or neurologic damage, however, so the tourniquet must be kept exposed and loosened at least every 20 minutes for 1 or 2 minutes while the patient is in transit and permanently as soon as definitive care is given. It is wise to write the letters TK on the patient's forehead with a skin-marking pencil or adhesive tape.

Vascular Access

All patients with significant trauma should have a large-caliber intravenous catheter inserted immediately for administration of drugs and fluids as needed. If any degree of shock is present, two intravenous lines should be inserted, one of which should be a large-bore catheter placed through a venous cutdown. A No. 8F or 10F feeding tube with the tip cut off works well. An intravenous extension tube with its tip cut off is also useful. If severe shock, hypovolemic cardiac arrest, or major vascular lesions are present, three intravenous lines are necessary, two being large-bore catheters placed by cutdown. With any degree of shock, one of the venous lines should be placed so that central venous pressure can be measured as fluids are administered.

After the intravenous lines are inserted, crystalloid infusion should begin.* Adult patients should be given 2 L of normal saline or Ringer's lactate solution. An additional 2 L of crystalloid may be administered if there is no change in blood pressure or only a transient response. Beyond this amount, whole blood must also be given in combination with crystalloid solutions to avoid excessive hemodilution. Protein-containing solutions are unnecessary in shock or resuscitation and should generally be avoided. For children, the initial administered volume should be 20 mL/kg. Group O Rh-negative packed red blood cells should be immediately available for any patient with impending cardiac arrest or massive hemorrhage. Type-specific blood should be available within 15 minutes.

NEUROLOGIC DISABILITY

Various stages of coma due to a variety of causes may accompany injury and require treatment during resuscitation. The most common, causes are alcoholic intoxication, cerebrovascular accidents, diabetic acidosis, barbiturate poisoning, narcotic overdosage, and hypovolemic shock. Less common causes are epilepsy, eclampsia, and electrolyte imbal-

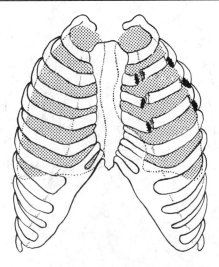

Figure 13–7. Flail chest.

---

*The treatment of shock is discussed in Chapter 12.

ances associated with metabolic and systemic diseases. Other causes include anaphylaxis, heavy metal poisoning, electric shock, tumors, severe systemic infections, hypercalcemia, asphyxia, heat stroke, severe heart failure, and hysteria.

The differential diagnosis depends upon (1) a careful history from available informants; (2) a careful and complete physical examination, with particular attention to the neurologic examination; and (3) laboratory tests such as urinalysis, blood counts, blood cultures, blood glucose, urea, ammonia, electrolytes, and alcohol, and cerebrospinal fluid examination; and (4) skull x-rays.

Laboratory studies may be helpful in ruling out the following: blood alcohol levels in acute alcoholism; blood and urine glucose levels in diabetic coma and hypoglycemic shock; and serum potassium, blood urea nitrogen, and creatinine in uremia.

EXPOSURE

All clothing should be removed at once (cut off, if necessary) from the seriously injured patient, with great care being taken to avoid unnecessary movement. The removal of helmets or other protective clothing may require additional personnel to stabilize the patient and prevent further injury. All surfaces should be examined to identify injuries that may not be readily apparent, such as posterior penetrating trauma or open fractures.

EMERGENCY ROOM THORACOTOMY

Certain injuries are so critical that operative treatment must be undertaken as soon as the diagnosis is made. In these cases, resuscitation is continued as the patient is being operated on. For cardiopulmonary arrest that occurs in the emergency room as a direct result of trauma, external cardiac compression is rarely successful in maintaining effective perfusion of vital organs. An emergency left anterolateral thoracotomy should be performed in the fourth or fifth intercostal space, and the pericardium should be opened anterior to the phrenic nerve (Figure 13–8). Open cardiac massage, cross-clamping of the descending thoracic aorta, repair of cardiac injuries, and internal defibrillation can be performed as appropriate. Wounds of the lung producing severe hemorrhage or systemic air embolus may require hilar cross-clamping. This extreme procedure is most useful for cardiac arrest due to penetrating thoracic trauma. Emergency room thoracotomy is ineffective for patients without detectable vital signs in the field. If vital signs are present but arrest appears imminent, the patient should be transferred to the operating room, since the conditions there for surgical intervention including light, equipment, and personnel are optimal.

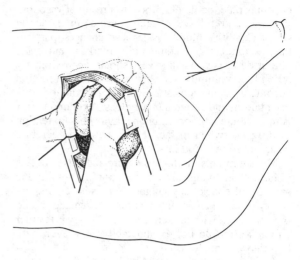

Figure 13–8. Emergency thoracotomy and open cardiac massage.

RESUSCITATION PHASE

Shock

Some degree of shock accompanies most severe injuries and is manifested initially by pallor, cold sweat, weakness, lightheadedness, hypotension, tachycardia, thirst, air hunger, and, eventually, loss of consciousness.

A. Primary or Neurogenic Shock (Syncope or Fainting): Primary shock is due to the rapid pooling of blood in the splanchnic vascular bed and voluntary muscles and is usually caused by psychic or nervous stimuli such as fright, sudden pain, or anxiety. It is self-limited and can be relieved by rest in the recumbent or Trendelenburg position. If the patient does not improve quickly, other kinds of shock must be considered.

B. Hypovolemic or Oligemic Shock: Hypovolemic shock is due to loss of whole blood or plasma. Blood pressure may be maintained initially by vasoconstriction. Tissue hypoxia increases when hypotension ensues, and shock may become irreversible if irreparable damage occurs to the vital centers. Massive or prolonged hemorrhage, severe crushing injuries, major fractures, and extensive burns are the most common causes. The presence of any of these conditions is an indication for prompt intravenous fluid infusions.

The patient must be kept recumbent and given reassurance and analgesics as necessary. If opioids are necessary for pain, they are best administered intravenously in small doses. Subcutaneous injections are poorly absorbed in these circumstances.

The most reliable clinical guide in assessing hypovolemic shock is skin perfusion. In mild shock (approximately 10–20% blood volume loss), the skin becomes pale, cool, and moist as a result of vasocon-striction and release of epinephrine. In moderate shock (20–30% blood loss), these changes, particularly diaphoresis, become more marked, and urine output decreases. With severe shock (approximately 30% blood volume loss), changes in cerebral function become evident, consisting chiefly of agitation, disorientation, and recent memory loss. A common error is to attribute uncooperative behavior to intoxication or drug use when in fact it may be due to cerebral ischemia from blood loss.

Measurements of blood pressure and pulse are less reliable than changes in urine output in assessing the severity of shock, as younger patients have compensatory mechanisms that maintain adequate blood pressure even with moderate volume loss, while older patients often do not exhibit tachycardia even with extreme volume loss.

A urinary catheter should be inserted for monitoring urine output in any patient with major injuries or shock. Oliguria is the most reliable sign of moderate shock, and successful resuscitation is indicated by a return of urine output to 0.5–1 mL/kg/h.

With significant hypovolemia or any degree of shock, balanced salt solution (eg, lactated Ringer's solution) should be given rapidly intravenously until the signs of shock abate and urine output returns to normal. Central venous pressure should be monitored to avoid fluid overload. Two to 4 L of crystalloid solution can be given rapidly if needed to resuscitate the patient in severe shock. Successful resuscitation is indicated by warm, dry, well-perfused skin, a urine output of 30–60 mL/h, and an alert sensorium.

Laboratory Studies

Immediately after intravenous catheters are placed, blood should be drawn for hematocrit, white blood count, creatinine, blood urea nitrogen, and whole blood typing and cross-matching. If the patient has a history of renal or cardiac disease or is taking diuretics, serum electrolytes should be measured. If there is any indication of liver disease, a liver panel is indicated. If the patient has a thoracic injury, any sign of respiratory compromise or distress, or any degree of shock, arterial blood gases should be measured (pH, PO_2, PCO_2). Urinalysis should be obtained, checking especially for hematuria. Even mild hematuria indicates the need for intravenous urography and, in selected cases, a cystogram and urethrogram.

Imaging Studies

Films of the chest and abdomen are required in all major injuries. An intravenous urogram is critical in abdominal injuries and pelvic fractures.

X-rays of the skull and long bones can usually be deferred until the more critical injuries of the thorax and abdomen have been cared for.

SECONDARY SURVEY & TREATMENT PRIORITIES

A rapid and complete history and physical examination (with a written record of the findings) are essential for patients with serious or multiple injuries. Progressive changes in clinical findings are often the key to correct diagnosis, and negative findings that change to positive may be of great importance in revising an initial clinical evaluation. This is particularly true in intra-abdominal, intrathoracic, and head injuries, which frequently do not become manifest until hours after the trauma.

Certain kinds of trauma are apt to cause more than one injury. Fractures of the calcaneus resulting from a fall from a great height are often associated with central dislocation of the hip and fractures of the spine and the base of the skull. A crushed pelvis is often combined with rupture of the posterior urethra or bladder. Crush injuries of the chest are often associated with lacerations or rupture of the spleen, liver, or diaphragm. Penetrating wounds of the chest may involve not only the thoracic contents but also the abdominal viscera. These combinations occur frequently and should always be suspected.

TREATMENT PRIORITIES

In all cases of multiple injury, there must be a "captain of the team" who directs the resuscitation, decides which x-rays or special diagnostic tests should be obtained, and establishes priority for care by continuous consultation with other surgical specialists and anesthesiologists. A general surgeon experienced in the care of the injured patient usually has this role.

If the injuries are extensive and there are signs of hypovolemic shock, coma is apt to be the result of cerebral ischemia. Resuscitation and blood volume replacement have first priority. If there are no signs of shock, coma is probably due to a head injury (see Chapter 38).

Deepening stupor in patients under observation should arouse suspicion of an expanding intracranial lesion requiring repeated and thorough neurologic examinations. Too often, obvious signs of acute alcoholism have been assumed to be the cause of unconsciousness, and intracranial hemorrhage has been overlooked.

Cerebral injuries take precedence in care only when there is rapidly deepening coma. Extradural bleeding is a critical emergency, requiring operation for control and cerebral decompression. Subdural bleeding may produce a similar emergency. If the patient's condition permits, arteriography or CT scanning should be performed for localization of the bleeding. In many cases of combined cerebral and abdominal injury with massive bleeding, laparotomy and craniotomy should be performed simultaneously.

In most cases, however, fractures of the skull have a low priority and can be dealt with after more critical abdominal or thoracic injuries have been treated.

Most urologic injuries are managed at the same time as associated intra-abdominal injuries. Pelvic fractures present special problems discussed in Chapters 41 and 43.

Unless there is associated vascular injury with threatened ischemia of the limb, fractures of the long bones can be splinted and treated on a semi-emergency basis. Open contaminated fractures should be cleansed and debrided as soon as possible.

Injuries of the hand run the risk of infection that, if not treated early, may result in a lifelong handicap. Early treatment of the hand at the same time as any life-threatening injuries avoids infection and preserves the means of livelihood.

Tetanus prophylaxis (see Chapter 8) should be given in all instances of open contaminated wounds, puncture wounds, and burns.

Details of definitive management of injuries are discussed in the sections on trauma that follow and in the various organ system chapters.

NECK INJURIES

All injuries to the neck are potentially life-threatening because of the many vital structures in this area. Injuries to the neck are classified as blunt or penetrating, and the treatment is different for each

Penetrating injuries of the neck are divided into three anatomic zones (Figure 13–9). Zone I injuries occur at the thoracic outlet, which extends from the level of the cricoid cartilage to the clavicles. Included in this area are the proximal carotid arteries, the subclavian vessels, and the major vessels in the chest. Proximal control of injuries to vascular structures in this zone requires thoracotomy. Zone II injuries occur in the area between the cricoid and the angle of the mandible. Injuries here are the easiest to expose and evaluate. Zone III injuries are between the angle of the mandible and the base of the skull. Exposure is much more difficult in this zone and in some cases may require disarticulation of the mandible. High injuries can be inaccessible, and control of hemorrhage may require ligation of major proximal vessels. Penetrating trauma to the posterior neck may injure the vertebral column, the cervical spinal cord, the interosseous portion of the vertebral artery, and the neck

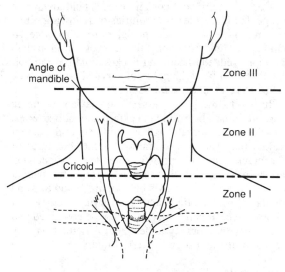

Figure 13–9. Zones of the neck.

musculature. Penetrating trauma to the anterior and lateral neck may injure the larynx, trachea, esophagus, thyroid, carotid arteries, subclavian arteries, jugular veins, and subclavian veins.

Blunt cervical trauma may cause fracture or dislocation of the cervical vertebrae (with the risk of spinal cord injury), traumatic occlusion of the carotid arteries, cerebrospinal fluid cysts, or laryngeal and tracheal injuries complicated by hemorrhage and airway obstruction.

The patient must be examined closely for associated head and chest injuries. The initial level of consciousness is of paramount importance; progressive depression of the sensorium signifies intracranial bleeding and requires craniotomy. Injuries of the base of the neck may lacerate major blood vessels. Hemorrhage into the pleural cavity may occur suddenly as contained hematomas rupture.

Clinical Findings

Injuries to the larynx and trachea may be asymptomatic or may cause hoarseness, laryngeal stridor, or dyspnea secondary to airway compression or aspiration of blood. Subcutaneous emphysema may appear if the wall of the larynx or trachea has been disrupted.

Esophageal injuries are rarely isolated and by themselves may not cause immediate symptoms. Severe chest pain and dysphagia are characteristic of esophageal perforation. Hours later, as mediastinitis develops, progressive sepsis may become manifest. Mediastinitis results because the deep cervical space is in direct continuity with the mediastinum. Esophageal injuries can be recognized promptly if the physician is alert to the possibility. Exploration of the neck or radiographic examination of the esophagus with contrast medium confirms the diagnosis.

Cervical spine and cord injuries should always be suspected in deceleration injuries or following direct trauma to the neck. If the patient complains of cervical pain or tenderness or if the level of consciousness is depressed, the head and neck should be immobilized (eg, with sandbags) until cervical x-rays can be taken to rule out cervical fracture.

Injury to the great vessels (subclavian, common carotid, internal carotid, and external carotid arteries; subclavian, internal jugular, and external jugular veins) may follow penetrating trauma. Fractures of the clavicle or first rib may lacerate the subclavian artery and vein. With vascular injuries, the patient typically presents with visible external blood loss and hematoma formation and in varying degrees of shock. Occasionally, bleeding may be contained and the injury temporarily undetected. Auscultation may reveal bruits that suggest arterial injury.

Diagnosis

With any penetrating cervical trauma, the likelihood of significant injury is high, because there are so many vital structures in such a small space. Any patient with shock, expanding hematoma, or uncontrolled hemorrhage should be taken to the operating room for emergency exploration. The location of the injury suggests which structures may be involved. Vascular injuries at the base of the neck require thoracotomy to obtain proximal control of injured blood vessels before the site of probable injury is exposed. If the patient is stable after resuscitation, additional diagnostic testing may be considered. Arteriography is usually recommended for patients with injuries in zones I and III because precise identification of the location and extent of injury may alter the operative approach. Arteriography should be performed, if possible, before exploration of any injury in which blood vessels may be damaged below the level of the cricoid cartilage or above a line connecting the mastoid process with the angle of the jaw. Arterial injuries above this line are practically inaccessible. If injury to the carotid artery at the base of the skull is confirmed by arteriography, repair may not be possible and ligation may be required to control bleeding. In addition, injured carotid arteries that have produced a neurologic deficit should be ligated. Since exposure of injuries in zone II is relatively easy to obtain, a policy of mandatory exploration has been proposed for all injuries penetrating the platysma in this area. Although this approach is safe, reliable, and time-tested, recent studies suggest that a selective approach is safe provided that invasive diagnostic testing does not detect a major injury. In the absence of an obvious vascular injury on clinical examination, arteriography may rule out carotid injury and perhaps identify an unsuspected vertebral artery injury. Rigid endoscopy can be used to evaluate the trachea and esophagus. A contrast study of the upper esophagus should be performed to identify esophageal injuries that might not

be readily apparent on endoscopy. These injuries can be difficult to detect and are occasionally missed on surgical exploration. In either case, repeated, careful examination should be performed.

Vertebral artery injuries should also be suspected when bleeding from a posterior or lateral neck wound cannot be controlled by pressure on the carotid artery or when there is bleeding from a posterolateral wound associated with fracture of a cervical transverse process.

X-rays of the soft tissues and cervical spine should be taken routinely. Fractures of the cervical spine can be confirmed by x-ray. X-rays of the soft tissues can locate opaque foreign bodies if present and help determine the route of the missile.

The most important injuries resulting from blunt cervical trauma are (1) cervical fracture, (2) cervical spinal cord injury, (3) vascular injury, and (4) laryngeal and tracheal injury. X-rays of the cervical spine and soft tissues are essential. Careful neurologic examination can differentiate between injuries to the cord, brachial plexus, and brain.

Complications

The complications of untreated neck injuries are related to the individual structures injured. Injuries to the larynx and trachea can result in acute airway obstruction, late tracheal stenosis, and sepsis. Cervicomediastinal sepsis can result from esophageal injuries. Carotid artery injuries can produce death from hemorrhage, brain damage, and arteriovenous fistula with cardiac decompensation. Major venous injury can result in exsanguination, air embolism, and arteriovenous fistula if there is concomitant arterial injury. Cervical fracture can result in paraplegia, quadriplegia, or death.

Prevention of these complications depends upon immediate resuscitation by intubation of the airway, prompt control of external hemorrhage and blood replacement, protection of the head and neck when cervical fracture is possible, accurate and rapid diagnosis, and prompt operative treatment when indicated.

Treatment

Any wound of the neck that penetrates the platysma requires prompt surgical exploration or angiography to rule out major vascular injury. If the patient presents with a neurologic deficit that is clearly not due to head injury, primary repair of the artery and reestablishment of blood flow to the brain will make the neurologic deficit worse, since an ischemic area of infarction in the brain is thus converted into a more lethal hemorrhagic infarction; in such cases, the carotid artery should be ligated. Arteries damaged by high-velocity missiles require debridement. End-to-end anastomosis of the mobilized vessels is preferred, but if a significant segment is lost, an autogenous vein graft can be used. Vertebral artery injury presents formidable technical problems, because of the interosseous course of the artery shortly after it arises from the subclavian artery. Although unilateral vertebral artery ligation has been followed by fatal midbrain or cerebellar necrosis, because of inadequate communication to the basilar artery, only 3% of patients with left vertebral ligation and 2% of patients with right vertebral ligation develop these complications. Therefore, in the face of massive hemorrhage from a partially severed vertebral artery, the risks of immediate ligation must be accepted.

Subclavian artery injuries are best approached through a combined cervicothoracic incision. Proper exposure is the key to success in the management of these difficult and too often fatal injuries. Ligation of the subclavian artery is relatively safe, but primary repair is preferable.

Venous injuries are best managed by ligation. The possibility of air embolism must be kept constantly in mind. A simple means of preventing this complication is to lower the patient's head until bleeding is controlled.

Esophageal injuries should be sutured and drained. Drainage is the hallmark of treatment. Extensive injury to the esophagus is often immediately fatal, because of associated injuries to the spinal cord. Systemic antibiotics should be administered routinely in esophageal injuries.

Minor laryngeal and tracheal injuries do not require treatment, but immediate tracheotomy should be performed when airway obstruction exists. If there has been significant injury to the thyroid cartilage, a temporary laryngeal stent (Silastic) should be employed to provide support. Mucosal lacerations should be approximated before insertion of the stent. Conveniently located small perforations of the trachea can be utilized for tracheotomy. Otherwise, the wounds can be closed after they are debrided and a distal tracheotomy performed. Extensive circumferential tracheal injuries may require resection and anastomosis or reconstruction using synthetic materials.

Primary neurorrhaphy should be attempted for nerve injury. Bilateral vagal nerve injury results in hoarseness and dysphagia. Cervical spinal cord injury should be managed in such a way as to prevent further damage. When there is cervical cord compression from hematoma formation, vertebral fractures, or foreign bodies, decompression laminectomy is necessary.

Blunt trauma to the neck rarely requires direct surgical treatment. More commonly, the soft tissues are contused, and hematomas develop that may cause tracheal compression and respiratory insufficiency. Tracheotomy is indicated in this instance. Cervical fractures are managed with skull tongs and traction. Surgical stabilization of cervical fractures is rarely indicated before 3 weeks after injury unless there is progressive paraplegia. The common or internal carotid arteries can be torn or can undergo disruption of the intima and require vascular reconstruction. Carotid arteriograms are essential to the diagnosis.

Prognosis

The prognosis after neck trauma varies with the extent of injury and the structures involved. Severance of the cervical spinal cord results in paralysis. Injuries to the soft tissues of the neck, trachea, and esophagus have a good to excellent prognosis if promptly treated. Major vascular injuries have a good prognosis if promptly treated before the onset of irreversible shock or neurologic deficit. The overall death rate for cervical injuries is about 10%.

Asensio J et al: Management of penetrating neck injuries: The controversy surrounding zone II injuries. Surg Clin North Am 1991;71:267.

Gerst P, Sharma S, Sharma P: Selective management of penetrating neck trauma. Am Surg 1990;56:553.

Khoury G et al: Penetrating trauma to the carotid vessels. Eur J Vasc Surg 1990;4:607.

Ngakane H, Muckart D, Luvuno F: Penetrating visceral injuries of the neck: Results of a conservative management policy. Br J Surg 1990;77:908.

Wood J, Fabian T, Mangiante E: Penetrating neck injuries: Recommendations for selective management. J Trauma 1989;29:602.

THORACIC INJURIES

Thoracic trauma accounts directly for or is a contributing factor in 50% of deaths due to trauma. Early deaths are commonly due to (1) airway obstruction, (2) flail chest, (3) open pneumothorax, (4) massive hemothorax, (5) tension pneumothorax, and (6) cardiac tamponade. Later deaths are due to respiratory failure, sepsis, and unrecognized injuries. Eighty percent of blunt thoracic injuries are caused by automobile accidents. Penetrating chest injuries from knives, bullets, etc, are almost as frequent as those from blunt trauma and increase annually as the level of civilian violence escalates. The death rate in hospitalized patients with isolated chest injury is 4–8%; it is 10–15% when one other organ system is involved and rises to 35% if multiple additional organs are injured.

Combined injuries of multiple intrathoracic structures are usual. There are often other injuries to the abdomen, head, or skeletal system. Eighty-five percent of chest injuries do not require open thoracotomy, but immediate use of lifesaving measures is often necessary and should be within the competence of all physicians.

When the physician is confronted with a patient who has sustained thoracic injuries, a rapid estimate of cardiorespiratory status and possible associated injuries gives a valuable overview. For example, patients with upper airway obstruction appear cyanotic, ashen, or gray; examination reveals stridor or gurgling sounds, ineffective respiratory excursion, constriction of cervical muscles, and retraction of the suprasternal, supraclavicular, intercostal, or epigastric regions. The character of chest wall excursions and the presence or absence of penetrating wounds can be observed. If respiratory excursions are not visible, ventilation is probably inadequate. Severe paradoxic chest wall movement in flail chest is usually located anteriorly and can be seen immediately. Sucking wounds of the chest wall should be obvious. A large hemothorax can usually be detected by percussion, and subcutaneous emphysema is easily detected. Both massive hemothorax and tension pneumothorax may produce absent or diminished breath sounds and a shift of the trachea to the opposite side, but in massive hemothorax, the neck veins are usually collapsed. If the patient has a thready or absent pulse and distended neck veins, the main differential diagnosis is between cardiac tamponade and tension pneumothorax. In moribund patients, diagnosis must be immediate, and treatment may require chest tube placement, pericardiocentesis, or thoracotomy in the emergency room. The first priority of management should be to provide an airway and restore circulation. One can then reassess the patient and outline definitive measures. A cuffed endotracheal tube and assisted ventilation are required for apnea, ineffectual breathing, severe shock, deep coma, airway obstruction, flail chest, or open sucking chest wounds. Persistent shock or hypoxia may be due to massive hemorrhage, cardiac tamponade, or tension pneumothorax. Shock due to thoracic trauma may be caused by any of the following: massive hemopneumothorax, cardiac tamponade, tension pneumothorax or massive air leak, or air embolism. If hemorrhage shock is not explained readily by findings on chest x-ray or external losses, it is almost certainly due to intra-abdominal bleeding.

Types of Injuries

A. Chest Wall: Rib fracture, the most common chest injury, varies from simple fracture, to fracture with hemopneumothorax, to severe multiple fractures with flail chest and internal injuries. With simple fractures, pain on inspiration is the principal symptom. Treatment of simple fractures consists of providing adequate analgesia. In cases of multiple fractures, intercostal nerve blocks or epidural analgesia may be required to ensure adequate ventilation. Measures such as strapping the chest wall with adhesive tape or the placement of elastic binders will interfere with adequate ventilation and lead to the development of atelectasis. They have no place in the modern management of rib fractures. Particularly in the elderly, multiple fractures may be associated with vol-

untarily decreased ventilation and subsequent pneumonitis.

Flail chest occurs when a portion of the chest wall becomes isolated by multiple fractures and moves in and out with inspiration and expiration with a potentially severe reduction in ventilatory efficiency. The magnitude of the effect is determined by the size of the flail segment and the amount of pain with breathing. Usually the rib fractures are anterior and there are at least two fractures of the same rib. Bilateral costochondral separation and the sternal fractures can also cause a flail segment. Often an associated lung contusion is present that 24–48 hours later produces a drop in lung compliance. Increased negative intrapleural pressure is then required for ventilation, and chest wall instability becomes apparent. If ventilation becomes inadequate, atelectasis, hypercapnia, hypoxia, accumulation of secretions, and ineffective cough occur. Arterial Po_2 is often low before clinical findings appear. Serial blood gas determination is the best way to determine if a treatment regimen is adequate. For less severe cases, intercostal nerve block or continuous epidural analgesia may be adequate treatment. However, most cases require ventilatory assistance for 2–3 weeks with a cuffed endotracheal tube and a mechanical ventilator. External fixation of the chest wall is less reliable than positive-pressure ventilation for the average case but may be useful for severe sternal flail or other extensive injuries with chest wall instability.

B. Trachea and Bronchus: Blunt tracheobronchial injuries are often due to compression of the airway between the sternum and the vertebral column in decelerating steering wheel accidents. The distal trachea or main stem bronchi are usually involved. Penetrating tracheobronchial injuries may occur anywhere. Most patients have pneumothorax, subcutaneous emphysema, pneumomediastinum, and hemoptysis. Cervicofacial emphysema may be dramatic. Tracheobronchial injury should be suspected when there is a massive air leak or when the lung does not readily reexpand after chest tube placement. In penetrating injuries of the trachea or main bronchi, there is usually massive hemorrhage and hemoptysis. Systemic air embolism resulting in cardiopulmonary arrest may occur if a bronchovenous fistula is present. If air embolism is suspected, emergency thoracotomy should be performed with cross-clamping of the hilum on the affected side. The diagnosis is confirmed by the aspiration of air from the heart. In blunt injuries, the tracheobronchial injury may not be obvious and may be suspected only after major atelectasis develops several days later. Diagnosis may require tracheobronchoscopy.

Primary repair is indicated for tracheobronchial lacerations.

C. Pleural Space: Hemothorax (blood within the pleural cavity) is classified according to the amount of blood: minimal, 350 mL; moderate, 350–

1500 mL; or massive, 1500 mL or more. The rate of bleeding after evacuation of the hemothorax is clinically even more important. If air is also present, the condition is called hemopneumothorax.

Hemothorax should be suspected with penetrating or severe blunt thoracic injury. There may be decreased breath sounds and dullness to percussion, but a chest x-ray (upright or semiupright, if possible) should be promptly obtained (Figure 13–10). Tube thoracostomy using one or two large-bore pleural catheters should be performed promptly. Needle aspiration is never adequate. In 85% of cases, tube thoracostomy is the only treatment required. If bleeding is persistent, as noted by continued output from the chest tubes, it is more likely to be from a systemic (eg, intercostal) rather than a pulmonary artery. When the rate of bleeding is 100–200 mL/h or the total hemorrhagic output exceeds 1000 mL, thoracotomy should usually be performed. In most cases, the chest wall is the source of hemorrhage, but the lung, heart, pericardium, and great vessels account for 15–25%.

Pneumothorax occurs in lacerations of the lung or chest wall following penetrating or blunt chest trauma. Hyperinflation (eg, blast injuries, diving accidents) can also rupture the lungs. After penetrating injury, 80% of patients with pneumothorax also have blood in the pleural cavity. Tension pneumothorax develops when a flap-valve leak allows air to enter the pleural space but prevents its escape; intrapleural pressure rises, causing total collapse of the lung and a shift of the mediastinal viscera to the opposite side. It must be relieved immediately to avoid interference with ventilation in the opposite lung and impairment of cardiac function. Sucking chest wounds, which allow air to pass in and out of the pleural cavity, should be promptly treated by an occlusive dressing and tube thoracostomy. The pathologic physiology resembles flail chest except that the extent of associated lung injury is usually less. After emergency measures have been instituted, traumatic pneumothorax should be treated by tube thoracostomy.

D. Lung Injury: Pulmonary contusion due to sudden parenchymal concussion occurs after blunt trauma or wounding with a high-velocity missile. Pulmonary contusion occurs in 75% of patients with flail chest but can also occur following blunt trauma without rib fracture. Alveolar rupture with fluid transudation and extravasation of blood are early findings. Fluid and blood from ruptured alveoli enter alveolar spaces and bronchi and produce localized airway obstruction and atelectasis. Increased mucous secretions and overzealous intravenous fluid therapy may combine to produce copious secretions (wet lung) and further atelectasis. The patient's ability to cough and clear secretions effectively is weakened because of chest wall pain or mechanical inefficiency from fractures. Elasticity of the lungs is decreased, resistance to air flow increases, and, as the work of breathing increases, blood oxygenation and pH drop and PCO_2 rises. The cardiac compensatory response may be compromised, because as many as 35% of these patients have an associated myocardial contusion.

Treatment is often delayed because clinical and x-ray findings may not appear until 12–24 hours after

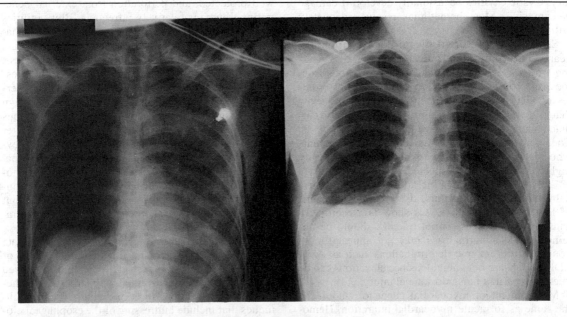

Figure 13–10. Hemopneumothorax. Supine *(left)* and upright films (on different patients).

injury. The clinical findings are loose, copious, blood-tinged secretions, chest pain, restlessness, apprehensiveness, and labored respirations. Eventually, dyspnea, cyanosis, tachypnea, and tachycardia develop. X-ray changes consist of patchy parenchymal opacification or diffuse linear peribronchial densities that may progress to diffuse opacification ("whiteout").

Mechanical ventilatory support permits adequate alveolar ventilation and the use of enriched oxygen mixtures and thus reduces the work of breathing. Blood gases should be monitored frequently and arterial saturation adequately maintained. There is some controversy over the best regimen for fluid management, but excessive hydration or blood transfusion should be avoided. Optimal management requires placement of a Swan-Ganz catheter in the pulmonary artery, preferably with a thermistor tip for measurement of cardiac output by thermodilution. Serial measurement of central venous pressure, pulmonary arterial pressure, wedge pressures, mixed venous oxygen saturation, and cardiac output help to avoid either under- or overtransfusion. Despite optimal therapy, about 15% of patients with pulmonary contusion die.

Most lung lacerations are caused by penetrating injuries, and hemopneumothorax is usually present. Tube thoracostomy is indicated to evacuate pleural air or blood and to monitor continuing leaks. Since expansion of the lung tamponades the laceration, most lung lacerations do not produce massive hemorrhage or persistent air leaks.

Lung hematomas are the result of local parenchymal destruction and hemorrhage. The x-ray appearance is initially a poorly defined density that becomes more circumscribed a few days to 2 weeks after injury. Cystic cavities occasionally develop if damage is extensive. Most hematomas resolve adequately with expectant treatment.

E. Heart and Pericardium: Blunt injury to the heart occurs most often from compression by a steering wheel in auto accidents. The injury varies from localized contusion to cardiac rupture. Autopsy studies of victims of immediately fatal accidents show that as many as 65% have rupture of one or more cardiac chambers and 45% have pericardial lacerations. The incidence of myocardial contusion in patients who reach the hospital is unknown but is probably higher than generally suspected.

Early clinical findings include friction rubs, chest pain, tachycardia, murmurs, dysrhythmias, or signs of low cardiac output. ECGs show nonspecific ST and T wave changes. Serial tracings should be obtained, since abnormalities may not appear for 24 hours. Serum enzyme determinations such as AST, LDH, or CK are not valuable, since elevations can be due to associated musculoskeletal injury.

Management of myocardial contusion should be the same as for acute myocardial infarction. Hemopericardium may occur without tamponade and can be treated by pericardiocentesis. Tamponade in blunt cardiac trauma is often due to myocardial rupture or coronary artery laceration. Tamponade produces distended neck veins, shock, and cyanosis. Immediate thoracotomy and control of the injury are indicated. If cardiopulmonary arrest occurs before the patient can be transported to the operating room, emergency room thoracotomy with relief of tamponade should be performed. Treatment of injuries to the valves, papillary muscles, and septum must be individualized; when tolerated, delayed repair is usually recommended.

Pericardial lacerations from stab wounds tend to seal and cause tamponade, whereas gunshot wounds leave a sufficient pericardial opening for drainage. Gunshot wounds produce more extensive myocardial damage, multiple perforations, and massive bleeding into the pleural space. Hemothorax, shock, and exsanguination occur in nearly all cases of cardiac gunshot wounds. The clinical findings are those of tamponade or blood loss.

Treatment of penetrating cardiac injuries has gradually changed from initial management by pericardiocentesis to prompt thoracotomy and pericardial decompression. Pericardiocentesis is reserved for selected cases when the diagnosis is uncertain or in preparation for thoracotomy. The myocardial laceration is closed with sutures placed to avoid injury to coronary arteries. Most patients do not require cardiopulmonary bypass. In approximately 75% of cases of stab wounds and 35% of cases of gunshot cardiac wounds, the patient survives the operation. However, it is estimated that 80–90% of patients with gunshot wounds of the heart do not reach the hospital.

F. Esophagus: Anatomically, the esophagus is well protected, and perforation from external penetrating trauma is relatively infrequent. Blunt injuries are very rare. The most common symptom of esophageal perforation is pain; fever develops within hours in most patients. Regurgitation of blood, hoarseness, dysphagia, or respiratory distress may also be present. Physical findings include shock, local tenderness, subcutaneous emphysema, or Hamman's sign (ie, pericardial or mediastinal "crunch" synchronous with cardiac sounds). Leukocytosis occurs soon after injury. X-ray findings on plain chest films include evidence of a foreign body or missile and mediastinal air or widening. Pleural effusion or hydropneumothorax is frequently seen, usually on the left side. Contrast x-rays of the esophagus should be performed but are positive in only about 70% of proved perforations.

A nasogastric tube should be passed to evacuate gastric contents. If recognized within 24–48 hours of injury, the esophageal perforation should be closed and pleural drainage instituted with large-bore catheters. Long-standing perforations require special techniques that include buttressing of the esophageal closure with pleural or pericardial flaps; pedicles of intercostal, diaphragmatic, or cervical strap muscles; and serosal patches from stomach or jejunum. Illness and death are due to mediastinal and pleural infection.

G. Thoracic Duct: Chylothorax and chylopericardium are rare complications of trauma but, when they occur, are difficult to manage. Penetrating injuries of the neck, thorax, or upper abdomen can injure the thoracic duct or its major tributaries. The occurrence of chylothorax after a trivial injury should lead one to suspect underlying cancer.

Symptoms are due to mechanical effects of the accumulations, eg, shortness of breath from lung collapse or low cardiac output from tamponade. The diagnosis is established when the fluid is shown to have characteristics of chyle or by special tests such as feeding the patient fat and a lipophilic dye.

The patient should be maintained on a fat-free, high-carbohydrate, high-protein diet and the effusion aspirated. Chest tube drainage should be instituted if the effusion recurs. Intravenous hyperalimentation with no oral intake may be effective in persistent leaks. Three or 4 weeks of conservative treatment usually are curative. If daily chyle loss exceeds 1500 mL for 5 successive days or persists after 2–3 weeks of conservative treatment, the thoracic duct should be ligated via a right thoracotomy. Intraoperative identification of the leak may be facilitated by preoperative administration of fat containing a lipophilic dye.

H. Diaphragm: Penetrating injuries of the diaphragm outnumber blunt diaphragmatic injuries by at least 4:1. Diaphragmatic lacerations occur in 10–15% of cases of penetrating wounds to the chest. The injury is rarely obvious. Wounds of the diaphragm must not be overlooked, because they rarely heal spontaneously and because herniation of abdominal viscera into the chest can occur either immediately or years after the injuries.

Associated injuries are usually present, and as many as 25% of patients are in shock when first seen. There may be abdominal tenderness, dyspnea, shoulder pain, or unilateral breath sounds. The diagnosis is often missed. Although chest radiography is the most sensitive diagnostic tool, it is entirely normal in about 20% of cases. The most common finding is ipsilateral hemothorax. Occasionally, a distended, herniated stomach is confused with a pneumothorax. Passage of a nasogastric tube before x-rays will help identify an intrathoracic stomach.

Once the diagnosis is made, the diaphragm should be sutured with closely placed, heavy nonabsorbable sutures. Because pulmonary complications are frequent, diaphragmatic injury should be approached through the abdomen when there is no other injury requiring thoracotomy.

Bishop M et al: Evaluation of a comprehensive algorithm for blunt and penetrating thoracic and abdominal trauma. Am Surg 1991;57:737.

Bladergroen M et al: A twelve year survey of cervicothoracic vascular injuries. Am J Surg 1989;157:483.

Brown PF, Larsen CP, Symbas PN: Management of the asymptomatic patient with a stab wound to the chest. South Med J 1991;84:591.

Capizzi FD et al: Pneumomediastinum not associated with lesion of mediastinal organs. Acta Chir Scand 1989;155:159.

Demetriades D et al: Penetrating injuries of the diaphragm. Br J Surg 1988;75:824.

Esposito TJ et al: Reappraisal of emergency room thoracotomy in a changing environment. J Trauma 1991;31:881.

Garcia VF, Eichelberger MR, Bowman LM: Rib fractures in children: A marker of severe trauma. J Trauma 1990;30:695.

Garramone R, Jacobs LM, Sahdev P: An objective method to measure and manage occult pneumothorax. Surg Gynecol Obstet 1991;173:257.

Gunnar WP et al: The utility of cardiac evaluation in the hemodynamically stable patient with suspected myocardial contusion. Am Surg 1991;57:373.

Helling TS et al: Complications following blunt and penetrating injuries in 216 victims. J Trauma 1989;29:1367.

Holm A, Bessey P, Aldrete J: Diaphragmatic rupture due to blunt trauma: Morbidity and mortality in 42 cases. South Med J 1988;81:956.

Mattox KL et al: Prospective MAST study in 911 patients. J Trauma 1989;29:1104.

Mattox KL: Indications for thoracotomy: Deciding to operate. Surg Clin North Am 1989;69:47.

Millham FH et al: Carinal injury: Diagnosis and treatment: Case report. J Trauma 1991;31:1420.

Shkrum MJ, Green RN, Shum DT: Azygos vein laceration due to blunt trauma. J Forensic Sci 1991;36:410.

Shorr R et al: Blunt chest trauma in the elderly. J Trauma 1989;29:234.

Smithers BM, O'Loughlin B, Strong RW: Diagnosis of ruptured diaphragm following blunt trauma: Results from 85 cases. Aust N Z J Surg 1991;61:737.

Stellin G: Survival in trauma victims with pulmonary contusion. Am Surg 1991;57:780.

ABDOMINAL INJURIES

Twenty percent of all trauma operations are performed for the management of abdominal injury. The distribution of blunt and penetrating injury in a given population is highly dependent upon geographic location. Blunt injuries predominate in rural areas, while penetrating injuries are more common in urban areas. The specific type of injury varies according to whether the trauma is penetrating or blunt. The mechanism of injury in blunt trauma is rapid deceleration, and noncompliant organs such as the liver, spleen, pancreas, and kidneys are at greater risk of injury due to parenchymal fracture. Occasionally, hollow organs may be injured, with the duodenum and urinary bladder being particularly susceptible. The intestines occupy a large portion of the total abdominal volume, and they are more likely to be injured by penetrating trauma. Most blunt abdominal injuries are related to motor vehicle accidents. Although the use of restraints has been associated with a decrease in the incidence of head, chest, and solid organ injuries, their use may be associated with pancreatic, mesenteric, and intestinal injuries due to compression against the spinal column. These injuries should be considered in the evaluation of patients who have signs of seat belt-related abrasions or hematomas. Internal injury may be present in as many as 30% of these cases.

As many as 30% of patents with significant hemoperitoneum may not manifest clinical signs of peritoneal irritation. Retroperitoneal injury may be more subtle and difficult to diagnose during the initial evaluation.

Deaths from abdominal trauma result principally from sepsis or hemorrhage. Most deaths from abdominal trauma are preventable. Patients at risk of abdominal injury should undergo prompt and thorough evaluation. In some cases, dramatic physical findings may be due to abdominal wall injury in the absence of intraperitoneal injury. If the results of diagnostic studies are equivocal, exploratory laparotomy should be considered, since it may be lifesaving and because it is a relatively benign procedure in the absence of positive findings.

Types of Injuries

If the abdomen is the probable source of exsanguinating hemorrhage, the patient should be transferred to the operating room for immediate laparotomy. The hemodynamically stable patent can be more thoroughly assessed within the framework of the secondary survey. Evaluation always includes comprehensive physical examination with pelvic and rectal examinations and may require peritoneal lavage and specific laboratory and radiologic tests. Serially performed examinations may be necessary to detect subtle findings.

A. Penetrating Trauma: Penetrating injuries may cause sepsis if they perforate a hollow viscus. When a full bowel is injured, the contents are evacuated into the peritoneal cavity, and clinical signs of injury are obvious. When an empty bowel is injured or when the retroperitoneal portion of the bowel is penetrated, spillage of bowel contents may be negligible initially, and findings may be minimal. Increasing abdominal tenderness demands surgical exploration. An elevated white blood cell count or fever appearing several hours following injury are keys to early diagnosis.

Penetrating injuries cause severe and early shock if they involve a major vessel or the liver. Penetrating injuries of the spleen, pancreas, or kidneys usually do not bleed massively unless a major vessel to the organ (eg, the renal artery) is damaged. Bleeding

must be controlled promptly. A patient in shock with a penetrating injury of the abdomen who does not respond to 4 L of fluid resuscitation should be operated on immediately following chest x-ray.

The treatment of hemodynamically stable patients with penetrating injuries to the lower chest or abdomen varies. All surgeons agree that patients with signs of peritonitis or hypovolemia should undergo surgical exploration, but treatment is less certain for patients with no signs of sepsis who are hemodynamically stable.

Most stab wounds of the lower chest or abdomen should be explored, since a delay in treatment of a hollow viscus perforation can result in severe sepsis. Some surgeons have recommended a selective policy in the management of these patients. When the depth of injury is in doubt, local wound exploration may rule out peritoneal penetration. Laparoscopy may ultimately have a role in the evaluation of penetrating injuries. All gunshot wounds of the lower chest and abdomen should be explored, because the incidence of injury to major intra-abdominal structures exceeds 90% in such cases.

B. Blunt Trauma: Although numerous algorithms for the management of blunt trauma have been described in recent years, peritoneal lavage and CT scanning are the diagnostic procedures most commonly used in patients without obvious indications for laparotomy.

Diagnostic Peritoneal Lavage

Diagnostic peritoneal lavage is designed to detect the presence of intraperitoneal blood and is still considered to be the standard procedure because of its high sensitivity and specificity. Additional determination of leukocytes, particulate matter, or amylase in the lavage fluid may indicate the presence of a bowel injury. Drainage of the lavage fluid from a chest tube or urinary catheter may indicate a lacerated diaphragm or bladder. Lavage can be performed easily and rapidly, with minimal cost and morbidity. It is an invasive procedure that will affect the findings on physical examination, and it should be performed by a surgeon. The procedure is neither qualitative nor quantitative. It cannot identify the source of hemorrhage, and relatively small amounts of intraperitoneal bleeding may result in a positive study. It may not detect small and large injuries to the diaphragm and cannot rule out injury to bowel or retroperitoneal organs. The indications for diagnostic peritoneal lavage include abdominal pain or tenderness, low abdominal rib fractures, unexplained hypotension, spinal or pelvic fractures, paraplegia or quadriplegia, and assessment hampered by altered mental status due to neurologic injury or intoxication. The only real contraindication is need for emergency laparotomy. The procedure may be performed with careful technique on patients with prior surgery and in the pregnant patient. It should usually be performed through a small infra-umbilical incision with placement of the catheter under direct vision (Figure 13–11). Closed techniques of catheter placement utilizing trocars or guidewires have been associated with high rates of complications and should be avoided. One liter of normal saline is instilled into the peritoneal cavity and then allowed to drain by gravity. At least 200 mL of lavage fluid should be recovered to allow for accurate interpretation. A portion of the recovered fluid is sent for laboratory analysis of cell counts, presence of particulate matter, and amylase. Criteria for evaluation of results are summarized in Table 13–1.

Computed Tomography

CT is qualitative, sensitive, and accurate for the diagnosis of intra-abdominal injury and is useful in the hemodynamically stable patient. Although CT is noninvasive, it is expensive and time-consuming and depends on an experienced radiologist for proper interpretation. It requires transport of the patient from the acute care area and should not be attempted in the unstable patient. It has a primary role in defining the location and magnitude of intra-abdominal injuries related to blunt trauma. CT has the advantage of detecting most retroperitoneal injuries, but it frequently misses small gastrointestinal perforations. The information provided on the magnitude of injury may allow nonoperative management of selected patients without evidence of active hemorrhage. In some cases, both CT and diagnostic peritoneal lavage may be performed in the same patient and used in a complementary fashion.

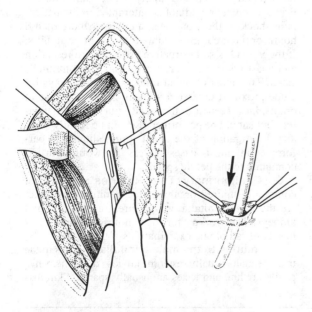

Figure 13–11. Diagnostic peritoneal lavage.

Table 13–1. Criteria for evaluation of peritoneal lavage fluid.

Positive	20 mL gross blood on free aspiration (10 mL in children) ≥ 100,000 RBC/µL ≥ 500 WBC/µL (if obtained ≥ 3 hours after the injury) ≥ 175 units amylase/dL Bacteria on Gram stain Bile (by inspection or chemical determination of bilirubin content) Food particles (microscopic analysis of strained or spun specimen)
Intermediate	Pink fluid on free aspiration 50,000–100,000 RBC/µL in blunt trauma 100–500 WBC/µL 75–175 units amylase/dL
Negative	Clear aspirate ≤ 100 WBC/µL ≤ 75 units amylase/dL

Exploratory Laparotomy

The three main indications for exploration of the abdomen following blunt trauma are peritonitis, hypovolemia, or the presence of other injuries known to be frequently associated with intra-abdominal injuries. Peritonitis after blunt abdominal trauma is rare but always requires exploration. Signs of peritonitis can arise from rupture of a hollow organ, such as the duodenum, bladder, intestine, or gallbladder; from pancreatic injury; or occasionally from the presence of retroperitoneal blood.

Hypovolemia in patients with a normal chest x-ray is also an indication for abdominal exploration unless intra-abdominal bleeding is ruled out by peritoneal lavage or CT scan of the abdomen or unless extra-abdominal blood loss is sufficient to account for the hypovolemia. Patients with blunt trauma and hypovolemia should be examined first for intra-abdominal bleeding even if there is no overt evidence of abdominal trauma. For example, hypovolemia may be due to loss of blood from a large scalp laceration, but it may also be due to unsuspected rupture of the spleen. Hemoperitoneum may present with no signs except for hypovolemia. The abdomen may be flat and nontender. Patients whose extra-abdominal bleeding has been controlled should respond to initial fluid resuscitation with an adequate urine output and stabilization of vital signs. If hypovolemia recurs, intra-abdominal bleeding must be considered to be the cause.

Injuries frequently associated with abdominal injuries are rib fractures, pelvic fractures, abdominal wall injuries, and fractures of the thoracolumbar spine (eg, 20% of patients with fractures of the left lower ribs have a ruptured spleen).

Treatment

A. Abdominal Wall Injuries: Abdominal wall injuries from blunt trauma are most often due to shear forces, such as being run over by the wheels of a tractor or bus. The shearing often devitalizes the subcutaneous tissue and skin, and if debridement is delayed, a serious necrotizing anaerobic infection may develop. The management of penetrating abdominal wall injuries is usually straightforward. Debridement and irrigation are appropriate surgical treatment. Every effort must be made to remove foreign material, shreds of clothing, necrotic muscle, and soft tissue. Abdominal wall defects may require insertion of prosthetic material (eg, Marlex mesh) or coverage with a myocutaneous flap.

B. Liver Injuries: Seventy percent of liver injuries are so small that they do not even require drainage. They are discovered incidentally during laparotomy for other more serious injuries. Bleeding is a problem in 25% of liver injuries and is best controlled by suture ligation or application of stainless steel clips directly to the bleeding vessels. Sutures can also be used to control leaking biliary ducts. In 5% of patients with hepatic injuries, bleeding is severe and requires special procedures for control. When injury has already resulted in massive blood loss, packing of the abdomen with laparotomy pads and planned reexploration should be considered. At the time of reexploration in 24–48 hours, hemorrhage is usually well controlled and can be managed with individual vessel ligation and debridement. Evidence of persistent hemorrhage should prompt earlier reexploration. Rarely, selective hepatic artery ligation, resectional debridement, or hepatic lobectomy may be required to control hemorrhage. Vascular control during resection is best achieved by the Pringle maneuver or compression of the parenchyma. The raw surface of the liver may then be covered with omentum. Drains should be used. Decompression of the biliary system is contraindicated.

Hepatic vein injuries frequently bleed massively. Isolation of the intrahepatic cava is useful in repair of these injuries or in resection.

Diagnosis and management of liver injuries are discussed in detail in Chapter 24.

C. Biliary Tract Injuries: Injury to the gallbladder should be treated in most cases by cholecystectomy, but minor lacerations may be closed with absorbable suture material.

Most injuries to the common bile duct can be treated by suture closure and insertion of a T tube. Avulsion of the common duct due to duodenal or ampullary trauma may require choledochojejunostomy in conjunction with total or partial pancreatectomy, duodenectomy, or some other diversion procedures. Segmental loss of the common bile duct may be treated by mobilization and end-to-end anastomosis. Occasionally, this may require choledochojejunostomy.

D. Splenic Injuries: The spleen is the most commonly injured organ in blunt abdominal trauma. Diagnosis and management are covered in detail in Chapter 28.

E. Pancreatic Injuries: Pancreatic injuries may present with few clinical manifestations. Pancreatic injury should be suspected whenever the upper abdomen has been traumatized, especially when serum amylase levels remain persistently elevated. The best diagnostic study for pancreatic injury (other than exploratory celiotomy) is CT scan of the abdomen. Peritoneal lavage may be helpful but usually is not. Upper gastrointestinal studies with water-soluble contrast material help delineate retroperitoneal injuries.

F. Gastrointestinal Tract Injuries: Most injuries of the stomach can be repaired. Large injuries, such as those from shotgun blasts, may require subtotal or total resection.

Most duodenal injuries can be treated with lateral repair, but some may require resection with end-to-end anastomosis depending on how well preserved the duodenal blood supply is. Occasionally, total duodenectomy plus pancreatectomy is required to manage a severe injury. Duodenostomy is useful in decompressing the duodenum and can be used to control a fistula caused by suture line leak. Jejunal or omental patches may also aid in preventing suture line leak.

Most small bowel injuries can be treated with bilayer closure, though devascularizing injuries to the mesentery or small bowel require resection. The underlying principle is to preserve as much small bowel as possible.

For injuries to the colon, the standard approach has been to divert the fecal stream or exteriorize the injury. Recent studies suggest that primary repair of colon injuries can be performed safely in certain circumstances. Wounds that involve less than one-third of the bowel circumference and are located on the antimesenteric surface should be considered for primary repair if the blood supply is not compromised. Primary repair should not be attempted in the patient is in shock, if there has been a delay of more than 8 hours, or if there is gross contamination or peritonitis. If the wound is so destructive as to require resection and anastomosis, primary repair may be contraindicated. Treatment of rectal injuries should always include proximal diversion with insertion of presacral drains. Direct repair of the rectal injury is not mandatory but should be performed if it can be readily visualized. Irrigation of the distal stump should be performed in most cases unless it would further contaminate the pelvic space.

G. Genitourinary Tract Injuries*: The most commonly injured organs of the genitourinary tract are the male genitalia, uterus, urethra, bladder, and kidneys. The workup for these injuries consists primarily of radiologic examinations.

1. Injuries to the male genitalia–Injuries to the male genitalia usually result in skin loss only; the penis, penile urethra, and testes are usually spared. Skin loss

---

*Also see Chapter 41

from the penis should be treated with a primary skin graft. Scrotal skin loss should be treated by delayed reconstruction; an exposed testis can be temporarily protected by placing it subcutaneously in the thigh.

2. Uterine injuries–Injuries of the female reproductive organs are infrequent except in combination with genitourinary or rectal trauma. Injuries to the uterine fundus can usually be repaired by chromic catgut sutures; drainage is not necessary. In more extensive injuries, hysterectomy may be preferable. The vaginal cuff may be left open for drainage, particularly if there is associated urinary tract or rectal injury. Injuries involving the uterus in a pregnant woman usually result in death of the fetus. Bleeding may be massive in such patients, particularly in women approaching parturition. Cesarean section plus hysterectomy may be the only alternative.

3. Urethral injuries–Prostatomembranous urethral disruption is usually associated with pelvic fracture. The prostate may be elevated superiorly by the pelvic hematoma and will be free-riding and high on rectal examination. Urethrography will demonstrate free extravasation of blood in the pelvis.

Initial management is by suprapubic bladder drainage. Urethral alignment is delayed for approximately 3 months, at which time a urethroplasty can be performed by a perineal suprapubic approach, with removal of the pubic symphysis. The incidence of impotence, incontinence, and stricture after reconstruction is low.

Major injuries to the bulbous or penile urethra should be managed by suprapubic urinary diversion. A voiding cystourethrogram may later reveal a stricture, but operative correction or dilation is usually unnecessary.

4. Bladder injuries–Rupture of the bladder, like urethral disruption, is frequently associated with pelvic fractures. Seventy-five percent of ruptures are extraperitoneal and 25% intraperitoneal. A ruptured bladder should be repaired through a midline abdominal incision. Rupture of the anterior wall of the bladder can be repaired by direct suture; rupture of the posterior wall can be repaired from inside the bladder after an opening has been made in the anterior wall, care being taken to avoid entering a pelvic hematoma. Postoperatively, urine should be diverted for 10 days by a suprapubic cystostomy.

5. Kidney injuries–All penetrating renal injuries require operative exploration unless preoperative studies have eliminated the possibility of significant damage. Operation is required for approximately 15% of blunt injuries. Indications for operation include persistent retroperitoneal bleeding and extensive urinary extravasation, or nonviable parenchyma on the renogram. A midline transabdominal approach is preferred. The renal artery and vein are secured before Gerota's fascia is opened. The injury should be managed by partial nephrectomy, suture repair, or, if necessary, total nephrectomy. Pedicle grafts of omen-

tum or free peritoneal patch grafts can be used to cover defects. Renal vascular injuries require immediate operation to save the kidney.

Perirenal hematomas found incidentally at celiotomy should be explored if they are expanding, pulsatile, or not contained by retroperitoneal tissues or if a preexploration urogram shows extensive urinary extravasation.

Berne T: Management of penetrating back trauma. Surg Clin North Am 1990;70: 71.

Bishop M et al: Evaluation of a blunt and penetrating trauma algorithm for truncal injury. Crit Care Clin 1991;7:383.

Cue J et al: Packing and planned reexploration for hepatic and retroperitoneal hemorrhage: Critical refinements of a useful technique. J Trauma 1990;30:1007.

Feliciano D: Diagnostic modalities in abdominal trauma: Peritoneal lavage, ultrasonography, computed tomography scanning, and arteriography. Surg Clin North Am 1991;71:241.

Henneman PL: Penetrating abdominal trauma. Emerg Med Clin North Am 1989;7:647.

Lopez VMA, Mickel TJ, Weigelt JA: Open versus closed diagnostic peritoneal lavage in the evaluation of abdominal trauma. Am J Surg 1990;160: 594.

McAnena O, Marx J, Moore E: Peritoneal lavage enzyme determinations following blunt and penetrating abdominal trauma. J Trauma 1991;31:1161.

McCarthy MC et al: Prediction of injury caused by penetrating wounds to the abdomen, flank, and back. Arch Surg 1991;126:962.

McConnell D, Trunkey D: Nonoperative management of abdominal trauma. Surg Clin North Am 1990;70:677.

Miller F et al: Negative findings on laparotomy for trauma. South Med J 1989;82:1231.

Willsher P, Cade R: Traumatic diaphragmatic rupture. Aust N Z J Surg 1991;61:207.

ARTERIAL INJURIES

William Krupski, MD

During World War II, only 33% of arterial injuries were repaired. The amputation rate was 49% following arterial ligation and 36% following arterial repair. In the Korean War, 304 major arterial repairs were followed by amputation in only 13% of cases. The amputation rate associated with arterial injuries during the Vietnam War fell to 8%. Amputation rates have dropped to 2% for arterial injuries of the extremities. This is a result of more rapid transport of injured people, improved blood volume replacement, selective use of arteriography, and better operative techniques.

Types of Injuries

A. Penetrating Trauma: Penetrating wounds

are the most common cause of arterial injury. Stab wounds, low-velocity (< 2000 ft/s) bullet wounds, iatrogenic injuries from percutaneous catheterization, and inadvertent intra-arterial injection of drugs are the principal causes of civilian arterial injuries. The high-velocity missiles responsible for war wounds produce more extensive vascular injuries, which involve massive destruction and contamination of surrounding tissues. The temporary cavitational effect of high-velocity missiles causes additional trauma to the ends of severed arteries and may produce arterial thrombosis due to disrupted intima even when the artery has not been directly hit. This blast effect can also draw material such as clothing, dirt, or pieces of skin along the wound tract, which contributes to the risk of infection. Associated injuries are often major determinants of the eventual outcome.

Shotgun blasts present special problems. Although muzzle velocity is low ($\approx$ 1200 ft/s), the multiple pellets produce widespread damage, and shotgun wadding entering the wound enhances the likelihood of infection. Similar to high-velocity injuries, the damage is often much greater than might be anticipated from inspection of the entry wound.

B. Blunt Trauma: Motor vehicle accidents continue to increase in frequency and severity and are a major cause of blunt vascular trauma. Commonly, multiple injuries occur that include fractures and dislocations; and while direct vascular injury may occur, in most instances the damage is indirect due to fractures. This is especially likely to occur with fractures near joints, where vessels are relatively fixed and vulnerable to shear forces. For example, the popliteal artery and vein are frequently injured in association with posterior dislocation of the knee. Fractures of large heavy bones such as the femur or tibia transmit forces that have cavitation effects similar to those caused by high-velocity bullets. There is extensive damage of soft tissues and neurovascular structures, and edema formation interferes with evaluation of pulses. Delay in diagnosis and the presence of associated injuries decrease the chances of limb salvage. Contusions or crush injuries may result in complete or partial disruption of arteries, producing intimal flaps or intramural hematomas that impede blood flow.

Almost any vessel can be injured by blunt trauma, including the extracranial cerebral and visceral arteries. The brachial and popliteal arteries, which cross joints and are exposed to direct trauma, are particularly susceptible to injury as a result of fractures and dislocations.

Clinical Findings

A. Hemorrhage: The possibility of arterial injury should be considered whenever a penetrating wound occurs near a major blood vessel. When pulsatile external hemorrhage is present, the diagnosis is obvious, but when blood accumulates in deep tissues

or the thorax, abdomen, or retroperitoneum, the only manifestation may be shock. Peripheral vasoconstriction may make evaluation of peripheral pulses difficult until blood volume is restored. If the artery is completely severed, thrombus may form at the contracted vessel ends and a major vascular injury may not be suspected. The presence of arterial pulses distal to a penetrating wound does not preclude arterial injury; as many as 20% of patients with injuries of major arteries in an extremity have palpable pulses distal to the injury, either because the vessel has not thrombosed or because pulse waves are transmitted through soft clot.

B. Ischemia: Acute arterial insufficiency must be diagnosed promptly to prevent tissue loss. Ischemia should be suspected when the patient has one or more of the "five Ps": pain, pallor, paralysis, paresthesia, or pulselessness. The susceptibility of different cells to hypoxia varies (eg, sudden occlusion of the carotid artery results in brain damage within minutes unless collateral circulation can maintain adequate perfusion, but a kidney can survive severe ischemia for several hours). Peripheral nerves and muscles are less resistant to ischemia than is skin, and they develop irreversible changes after 4–6 hours. With ischemia, the sodium pump fails, cells swell, and the integrity of cellular membranes is lost; intracellular water production increases owing to a shift to anaerobic metabolism; and blood viscosity increases and red blood cells sludge within capillaries. At this stage, restoration of perfusion may increase swelling (reperfusion edema), sometimes causing tissue necrosis.

C. False Aneurysm: Disruption of an arterial wall as a result of trauma may lead to formation of a false aneurysm. The wall of a false aneurysm is composed primarily of fibrous tissue derived from nearby tissues, not arterial tissue. Because blood continues to flow past the fistulous opening, the extremity is seldom ischemic. False aneurysms may rupture at any time. They continue to expand because they lack elastic fibers. Spontaneous resolution is unlikely, and operative repair becomes increasingly more difficult as the aneurysms increase in size and complexity with time. Symptoms gradually appear as a result of compression of adjacent nerves of collateral vessels or from rupture of the aneurysm, or as a result of thrombosis with ischemic symptoms. Iatrogenic false aneurysms after atrial puncture may thrombose with ultrasound-directed compression.

D. Arteriovenous Fistula: With simultaneous injury of an adjacent artery and vein, a fistula may form that allows blood from the artery to enter the vein. Because venous pressure is lower than arterial pressure, flow through an arteriovenous fistula is continuous; accentuation of the bruit and thrill can be detected over the fistula during systole. Traumatic arteriovenous fistulas may occur as operative complications (eg, aortocaval fistula following removal of a herniated intervertebral disk). Iatrogenic femoral arteriovenous fistulas after arteriograms and cardiac catheterization are seen with increasing frequency. Long-standing arteriovenous fistulas may result in cardiac failure. Repair should be performed as soon as possible, since progressive dilatation of arteries and veins occurs, increasing the technical difficulty of operation.

Diagnosis

A high index of suspicion of arterial injury must be maintained in any injured patient. Patients who present in shock following penetrating injury or blunt trauma should be considered to have vascular injury until proved otherwise. Any injury near a major artery should arouse suspicion. A plain film may be helpful in demonstrating a fracture whose fragments could jeopardize an adjacent vessel or a bullet fragment that could have passed near to a major vessel. Before the x-ray is taken, entrance and exit wounds should be marked with radiopaque objects, such as safety pins.

Diagnosis is usually suspected on the basis of physical examination. In addition to checking for obvious hemorrhage and the "five Ps," the physician should listen for a bruit (eg, of an arteriovenous fistula) and look for an expanding hematoma (eg, of a false aneurysm). Secondary hemorrhage from a wound is an ominous sign that may herald massive hemorrhage.

Doppler flow studies may be of some assistance in the diagnosis of arterial injury. A decrease in velocity of flow, loss of normal biphasic arterial flow signals, and diminished distal pressures suggest a proximal arterial injury (assuming the patient has no preexisting arterial disease). A systolic pressure of 60 mm Hg usually means that flow is sufficient to maintain viability of the extremity, and this knowledge may help determine the priority of arterial repair in patients with multiple injuries. Doppler measurement of normal pressures in the artery distal to the wound reliably excludes significant injury. Doppler studies are also useful for assessing pulses postoperatively, when edema makes palpation of pulses difficult.

Arteriography is the most accurate diagnostic procedure for identifying vascular injuries. Patients with unequivocal signs of arterial injury on physical examination or plain films should have urgent operation. Stable patients with equivocal physical signs and multiple injuries should first have arteriograms. Since the false-negative rate of arteriography is low, a normal arteriogram usually precludes the need for surgical exploration. Technical considerations in performing arteriography include the following: (1) entrance and exit wounds should be marked with a radiopaque marker; (2) the injection site should not be near the suspected injury; (3) an area 10–15 cm proximal and distal to the suspected injury should be included in the arteriographic field; (4) sequential films

should be obtained to detect early venous filling; (5) any abnormality should be considered an indication of arterial injury unless it is obviously the result of preexisting disease; and (6) two different projections should be obtained. Arteriography may be particularly useful in differentiating arterial injury from spasm. In general, it is risky to attribute abnormal physical findings in an injured patient to arterial spasm; an arteriogram is indicated in such patients.

Screening isotope angiography has little value in patients with arterial trauma. The technique cannot detect subtle arterial injuries, such as intimal fractures, and often causes unnecessary delay and confusion in interpretation of results. Venography also has little usefulness; if surgical exploration is planned, the vein can be directly inspected. CT scans may reveal intra-abdominal or thoracic hematomas or organ displacement, suggesting the presence of a hematoma. This suggests the need for arteriography or immediate surgery.

Treatment

A. Initial Treatment: A rapid but thorough examination should be performed to determine the complete extent of injury. The physician must establish the priority of arterial injury in the overall management of the patient and should keep in mind that delay in arterial repair decreases chances of a favorable outcome. When repair is performed within 12 hours of injury, amputation is rarely necessary; if repair is performed later, the incidence of amputation is about 50%. Depending on the degree of ischemia, delay in arterial repair will lead to lasting neuromuscular damage after as short a period as 8 hours.

Restoration of blood volume and control of hemorrhage are carried out simultaneously. If exsanguinating hemorrhage precludes resuscitation in the emergency room, the patient should be moved directly to the operating room. External bleeding is best controlled by firm direct pressure or packing. Probes or fingers should not be inserted into the wound, because a clot may be dislodged, causing profuse bleeding. Tourniquets occlude venous return, disturb collateral flow, and further compromise circulation and should not be employed. Atraumatic vascular clamps may be applied to accessible vessels, but blind clamping can increase damage and injure adjacent nerves and veins.

After hemorrhage has been controlled and general resuscitation accomplished, further assessment is possible. The extent of associated injuries is determined and a plan of management made. Large-bore intravenous catheters should be placed in extremities with no potential venous injuries. It is prudent to preserve the saphenous or cephalic vein in an uninjured extremity for use as a venous autograft for vascular repair.

B. Surgical Treatment: General anesthesia is preferable to spinal or regional anesthesia. When vascular injuries involve the neck or thoracic outlet, endotracheal intubation must be performed carefully to avoid dislodging a clot. Moreover, care is necessary to avoid neurologic damage in patients with associated cervical spine injuries. At least one uninjured extremity should also be prepared for surgery, so that a saphenous or cephalic vein may be obtained if a vein graft is required. Provision should also be made for operative arteriography.

Incisions should be generous and parallel to the injured vessel. Meticulous care in handling incisions is essential to avoid secondary infections; all undamaged tissue should be conserved for use in covering repaired vessels. Preservation of all arterial branches is important in order to maintain collateral circulation. Control of the vessel should be achieved proximal and distal to the injury, so that the injured area may be dissected free of other tissues and inspected without risk of further bleeding. When large hematomas and multiple wounds make exposure and clamping of vessels difficult, it is wise to place an orthopedic tourniquet proximal to the injury that can be inflated temporarily if needed.

The extent of arterial injury must be accurately determined. Arterial spasm generally responds to gentle hydraulic or mechanical dilatation. Local application of warm saline or drugs such as papaverine, tolazoline, or lidocaine is occasionally effective in relieving spasm. Intra-arterial injection of nitroglycerin is also very effective in alleviating spasm. If spasm persists, however, it is best to assume that it is caused by an intramural injury, and the vessel should be opened for direct inspection.

All devitalized tissue, including damaged portions of the artery, must be debrided. Resect only the grossly injured portion of the vessel (ie, margins of healthy vessel do not need to be removed, as was once recommended). The method of reconstruction depends on the degree of arterial damage. In some instances, the ends of injured vessels can be approximated and an end-to-end anastomosis performed. If the vessels cannot be mobilized well enough to provide a tension-free anastomosis, an interposition graft should be used. Early experience with prosthetic interposition grafts was disappointing, since postoperative infection, thrombosis, and anastomotic disruption were common. These problems have decreased considerably with the use of grafts made of expanded polytetrafluoroethylene (PTFE). Nevertheless, most surgeons still prefer to use an autogenous graft (ie, vein or artery) in contaminated wounds. Saphenous vein grafts should be obtained from the noninjured leg to avoid impairment of venous return on the side of the injury. Patch angioplasty using saphenous vein is performed when closure of a partially transected vessel would result in narrowing. Suturing should be done with fine monofilament suture material.

In the unusual circumstance of isolated vascular injury, 5000–10,000 units of intravenous heparin should be given to prevent thrombosis. Otherwise, a small amount of dilute heparin solution (100 units/mL) may be gently injected into the lumen of the injured vessel before clamps are applied. Proximal and distal thrombi are removed with a Fogarty embolectomy catheter. Back-bleeding from the distal artery is not a sure indication that thrombus is absent. An operative arteriogram is indicated to determine distal patency and to check on the adequacy of the reconstruction—even when distal pulses are palpable.

In the past, it was taught that fractures should be stabilized before vascular injuries were repaired, so that manipulation of bones would not jeopardize vascular repair. The disadvantages of this sequence include delay in restoration of flow to ischemic tissue and interference with vascular reconstruction and subsequent arteriographic study of the completed repair by the fixation device. Currently, it is recommended that vascular repair be performed first, followed by careful application of external traction devices that allow easy access to the wound for observation and dressing changes. Another alternative is to place an intraluminal shunt temporarily across the vascular injury to decrease ischemia while fractures or other injuries are treated. There is controversy about the best time to repair injured peripheral nerves; the trend favors concomitant repair except for high-velocity or complicated injuries. Likewise, there is disagreement concerning the necessity for performing venous repair versus ligation. Most surgeons feel that venous injuries should be repaired to prevent late venous thrombosis and protect the arterial repair, particularly with popliteal, common femoral, portal, or mesenteric venous injuries. The technical principles of venous repair are the same as those for arterial repair.

Repaired vessels must be covered with healthy tissue. If left exposed, they invariably desiccate and rupture. Skin alone is inadequate, because subsequent necrosis of the skin would leave the vessels exposed, greatly endangering the reconstruction. Generally, an adjacent muscle (eg, sartorius muscle for coverage of the common femoral artery) can be mobilized and placed over the repair. Musculocutaneous flaps can be constructed by plastic surgeons to cover almost any site. In an extensive or severely contaminated wound, a remote bypass may be routed through clean tissue planes to circumvent difficult soft tissue coverage problems.

Fasciotomy is an important adjunctive treatment in many cases of arterial trauma. Indications include the following: (1) combined arterial and venous injury, (2) massive soft tissue damage, (3) delay between injury and repair (4–6 hours), (4) prolonged hypotension, or (5) excessive swelling or high tissue pressure measured by one of several techniques. Whenever compartment pressures (measured with a needle and manometer) approach diastolic pressure, fasciotomy should be performed promptly. Fasciotomies must be performed through adequate skin incisions because when edema is massive the skin envelope itself can compromise neurovascular function.

When destruction of soft tissues, bones, blood vessels, and nerves is extensive, amputation is preferable to a useless limb, and in some cases, amputation may be required as a lifesaving procedure. Likewise, ligation of injured arteries and veins is indicated if the injured vessel is small and expendable or when the patient is rapidly deteriorating from the consequences of other injuries.

Anderson RJ et al: Penetrating extremity trauma: Identification of patients at high-risk requiring arteriography. J Vasc Surg 1990;11:544.

Bladergroen M et al: A twelve-year survey of cervicothoracic vascular injuries. Am J Surg 1989;157:483.

Bongard FS, Klein SR: The problem of vascular shotgun injuries: Diagnostic and management strategy. Ann Vasc Surg 1989;3:299.

Bongard FS, White GH, Klein SR: Management strategy of complex extremity injuries. Am J Surg 1989;158:151.

Cass AS: Renovascular injuries from external trauma: Diagnosis, treatment, and outcome. Urol Clin North Am 1989;16:213.

Chervu A, Quinones-Baldrich WJ: Vascular complications in orthopedic surgery. Clin Orthop Rel Res 1988;235:275.

Cone JB: Vascular injury associated with fracture-dislocations of the lower extremity. Clin Orthop Rel Res 1989;243:30.

Demetriades D et al: Carotid artery injuries: Experience with 124 cases. J Trauma 1989;29:91.

Dennis JW et al: New perspectives on the management of penetrating trauma in proximity to major limb arteries. J Vasc Surg 1990;11:84.

Fabian TC et al: Carotid artery trauma: Management based on mechanism of injury. J Trauma 1990;30:953.

Feliciano DV: Abdominal vascular injuries. Surg Clin North Am 1988;68:741.

Frykberg ER et al: A reassessment of the role of arteriography in penetrating proximity extremity trauma: A prospective study. J Trauma 1989;29:1041.

Frykberg ER, Vines FS, Alexander RH: The natural history of clinically occult arterial injuries: A prospective evaluation. J Trauma 1989;29:577.

Hetz SP et al: Penetrating injury of the vertebral artery: A unique management approach. South Med J 1989;82:1037.

Jebara VA et al: Penetrating carotid injuries: A wartime experience. J Vasc Surg 1991;14:117.

Johns JP, Pupa LE Jr, Bailey SR: Spontaneous thrombosis of iatrogenic femoral artery pseudoaneurysms: Documentation with color Doppler and two-dimensional ultrasonography. J Vasc Surg 1991;14:24.

Kram HB et al: Diagnosis of traumatic aortic rupture: A 10-year retrospective analysis. Ann Thorac Surg 1989;47:282.

Martin RF et al: Blunt trauma to the carotid arteries. J Vasc Surg 1991;14:789.

Mattox KL: Approaches to trauma involving the major vessels of the thorax. Surg Clin North Am 1989;69:77.

McCrosky BL et al: Traumatic injuries of the brachial artery. Am J Surg 1988;156:553.

Michell FL III, Thal ER: Results of venous interposition grafts in arterial injuries. J Trauma 1990;30:336.

Myers SI et al: Complex upper extremity trauma in an urban population. J Vasc Surg 1990;12:305.

Neville RF Jr et al: Endovascular management of arterial intimal defects: An experimental comparison by arteriography, angioscopy, and intravascular ultrasonography. J Vasc Surg 1991;13:496.

Nichols JS, Lillehei KO: Nerve injury associated with acute vascular trauma. Surg Clin North Am 1988;68:837.

Patel KR et al: Subclavian artery to innominate vein fistula after insertion of a hemodialysis catheter. J Vasc Surg 1991;13:382.

Poole GV: Fracture of the upper ribs and injury to the great vessels. Surg Gynecol Obstet 1989;169:275.

Reid JD et al: Wounds of the extremities in proximity to major arteries: Value of angiography in the detection of arterial injury. AJR 1988;151:1035.

Richardson JD, Simpson C, Miller FB: Management of carotid artery trauma. Surgery 1988;104:673.

Richardson JD, Wilson ME, Miller FB: The widened mediastinum: Diagnostic and therapeutic priorities. Ann Surg 1990;211:731.

Rutherford RB: Diagnostic evaluation of extremity vascular injuries. Surg Clin North Am 1988;68:683.

Shah PM et al: Compartment syndrome in combined arterial and venous injuries of the lower extremities. Am J Surg 1989;158:136.

Snyder WH III: Popliteal and shank arterial injury. Surg Clin North Am 1988;68:787.

Varnell RM et al: Arterial injury complicating knee disruption. Am Surg 1989;55:699.

Wood J, Fabian TC, Mangiante EC: Penetrating neck injuries: Recommendations for selective management. J Trauma 1989;29:602.

Young JN et al: Surgical management of traumatic disruption of the descending aorta. West J Med 1989;150:662.

BLAST INJURY

Blast injuries in civilian populations occur as a result of fireworks, household explosions, or industrial accidents. Urban guerrilla warfare tactics may take the form of letter bombs, car bombs, or satchel-suitcase bombs. Injuries occur from the effects of the blast itself, propelled foreign bodies, or, in large blasts, from objects falling from buildings. Military blast injuries may also involve personnel submerged in water. Water increases energy transmission and the possibility of injury to the viscera of the thorax or abdomen. The pathophysiology of blast injuries involves two mechanisms. **Crush injury** results from rapid displacement of the body wall and may result in laceration and contusion of underlying structures. Minor displacements may produce serious injury if the body wall velocity is high. In addition, the motion of the body wall generates waves that propagate within the body and transfer energy to internal sites.

Clinical Findings

A. Symptoms and Signs: The injury is dependent upon proximity to the blast, space confinement, and detonation size. Large explosions cause multiple foreign body impregnations, bruises, abrasions, and lacerations. Gross soilage of wounds from clothing, flying debris, or explosive powder is usual. About 10% of all casualties have deep injuries to the chest or abdomen. Lung damage usually involves rupture of the alveolus with hemorrhage. Air embolism from bronchovenous fistula may cause sudden death. The mechanisms of lung injury are thought to be due to spalling effects (splintering forces produced when a pressure wave hits a fluid-air interface), implosion effects, and pressure differentials. Blast injury causing pneumatic disruption of the esophagus or bowel has been reported. Letter bombs cause predominantly hand, face, eye, and ear injuries. Energy transmission within the fluid media of the eye can cause globe rupture, dialysis of the iris, hyphema of the anterior chamber, lens capsule tears, retinal rupture, or macular pucker. Ear injuries may be drum rupture or cochlear damage. There may be nerve or conduction hearing deficit or deafness. Tinnitus, vertigo, and anosmia are also seen in letter bomb casualties. Patients with pulmonary injury may die despite intensive respiratory support.

B. Imaging Studies: Chest x-ray may initially be normal or may show pneumothorax, pneumomediastinum, or parenchymal infiltrates.

Treatment

Severe injuries with shock from blood loss or hypoxia require resuscitative measures to restore perfusion and oxygenation. Surgical treatment of extremity injuries requires wide debridement of devitalized muscle, thorough cleansing of wounds, and removal of foreign materials. The usual criteria for exploring penetrating wounds of the thorax or abdomen are employed. Perforation of hollow organs should be suspected in patients with appropriate mechanisms, particularly those that were submerged at the time of injury. Eye injuries may require immediate repair. Ear injuries are usually treated expectantly. Respiratory insufficiency may result from pulmonary injury or may be secondary to shock, fat embolism, or other causes. Tracheal intubation and prolonged respiratory care with mechanical ventilation may be necessary. The possibility of gas gangrene in contaminated muscle injuries may warrant open treatment.

Cooper GJ, Taylor DE: Biophysics of impact injury to the chest and abdomen. J R Army Med Corps 1989;135:58.

Cooper GJ et al: The role of stress waves in thoracic visceral injury from blast loading: Modification of stress transmission by foams and high-density materials. J Biomech 1991;24:273.

Guth AA, Gouge TH, Depan HJ: Blast injury to the thoracic esophagus. Ann Thorac Surg 1991;51:837.

Haywood I, Skinner D: ABC of major trauma: Blast and gunshot injuries. Br Med J 1990;301:1040.

Knapp JF et al: Blast trauma in a child. Pediatr Emerg Care 1990;6:122.

Logan SE, Bunkis J, Walton RL: Optimum management of hand blast injuries. Int Surg 1990;75:109.

Rignault DP, Deligny MC: The 1986 terrorist bombing experience in Paris. Ann Surg 1989;209:368.

Stigall KE, Dorsey JS: Transection of the first portion of jejunum from blast injury in accidental discharge of a (2.75-inch aircraft) rocket from an F-15. Mil Med 1989;154:431.

DROWNING

Drowning is a major cause of accidental death in the USA, resulting in 5500 deaths yearly for the last 3 decades. During summer vacation weekends, the number of deaths may rise to 50 per day. Approximately 25% of all drowning victims are teenagers; 20% are less than 10 years of age; and 10% occur in each decade of life from age 20 to age 70. Drowning victims are males in 85% of cases. In the USA, most cases of drowning occur in lakes, rivers, canals, swimming pools, or spas; only about one-fourth occur in seawater. Alcohol ingestion is a factor in as many as 38% of the cases of adult drowning. Inadequate supervision and improperly covered pools or spas are the chief causes of childhood drownings.

The effects of drowning or near drowning are principally due to hypoxemia and aspiration. The physiologic effects of aspiration differ, depending on whether the drowning medium is fresh water or salt water, which are hypo- and hypertonic, respectively, compared with plasma. It is possible for a drowning victim to die of hypoxemia without aspiration, but this occurs rarely. In animal studies, arterial Po_2 falls rapidly after tracheal obstruction, reaching a Po_2 of 10 mm Hg within 3 minutes. In human volunteers who hyperventilated, then held their breath as long as possible, Po_2 declined to 58 mm Hg after 146 seconds of breath holding without exercise but reached 43 mm Hg at 85 seconds if the subject was exercising. Within 3–5 minutes after total immersion in water, the degree of hypoxemia would be enough to cause loss of consciousness in all victims.

If fresh water is aspirated, the fluid is rapidly absorbed from the alveoli, producing intravascular hypervolemia, hypotonicity, dilution of serum electrolytes, and intravascular hemolysis. Animal studies show that the intravascular volume may increase 50% within 3 minutes after fresh water aspiration. In addition, direct injury to pulmonary surfactant results in increased surface tension and damage to the pulmonary capillary membrane. Debris and microorganisms are deposited in the alveoli, setting the stage for later infectious complications if the victim survives.

Salt water aspiration produces opposite effects because water is drawn into the alveoli from the vascular space, producing hypovolemia, hemoconcentration, and hypertonicity. Hemolysis is not significant after salt water drowning. Treatment of the near drowning victim should be directed at immediate restoration of ventilation, as the degree of hypoxemia and resulting damage increases rapidly. Time should not be wasted in trying to drain the victim's lungs of water, since the actual amount of water aspirated is not large, and in fresh water drowning it is rapidly absorbed from the alveoli anyway.

After restoration of ventilation, the major goals of treatment are to evaluate and correct residual hypoxemia or acidosis and electrolyte abnormalities. If the patient has aspirated significant quantities of fluid, endotracheal intubation and ventilation will usually be necessary. Metabolic acidosis will be self-correcting if the circulation can be restored; in extreme cases, sodium bicarbonate may be given intravenously if the pH is below 7.2. No specific drugs appear to be useful other than those normally used in cardiopulmonary resuscitation. Prophylactic antibiotics and corticosteroids have specifically been shown not to be beneficial.

If immediate resuscitation is successful, the victim is still at high risk of acute pulmonary insufficiency if aspiration occurred. This is the major cause of late fatalities. Treatment is identical to that for acute respiratory failure of any cause (see Chapter 12).

Neurologic damage is the next most common sequela of near drowning and results from the period of hypoxemia. If the victim never lost consciousness during the drowning episode, the chance of neurologic damage is negligible. In patients who sustain neurologic damage, the neurologic changes and the prognosis are similar to those after cerebral damage from other forms of cardiopulmonary arrest.

The kidney may also be affected if significant intravascular hemolysis has occurred. Hemoglobinuria is treated initially by osmotic diuretics and alkalinization of the urine. If acute renal failure occurs, dialysis may be necessary.

Biggart MJ, Bone DJ: Effect of hypothermia and cardiac arrest on outcome of near-drowning accidents in children. J Pediatr 1990;117:179.

Cass D, Ross F, Grattan-Smith T: Child drownings: A changing pattern. Med J Aust 1991;154:163.

Edwards N et al: Survival in adults after cardiac arrest due to drowning. Intensive Care Med 1990;16:336.

Howland J et al: A pilot survey of aquatic activities and related consumption of alcohol, with implications for drowning. Public Health Rep 1990;105:415.

Kibel S et al: Childhood near-drowning: A 12-year retrospective review. S Afr Med J 190;78:418.

Nagel F, Kibel S, Beatty D: Childhood near-drowning: Factors associated with poor outcome. S Afr Med J 190;78:422.

O'Shea JS: House-fire and drowning deaths among children and young adults. Am J Forensic Med Pathol 1991;12:33.

Press E: The health hazards of saunas and spas and how to minimize them. Am J Public Health 1991;81:1034.

Tipton MJ, Stubbs DA, Elliott DH: Human initial responses to immersion in cold water at three temperatures and after hyperventilation. J Appl Physiol 1991;70:317.

Walpoth B et al:: Accidental deep hypothermia with cardiopulmonary arrest: Extracorporeal blood rewarming in 11 patients. Eur J Cardiothorac Surg 1990;4:390.

Wintemute G et al: Alcohol and drowning: An analysis of contributing factors and a discussion of criteria for case selection. Accid Anal Prev 1990;22:291.

Wood SC: Interactions between hypoxia and hypothermia. Annu Rev Physiol 1991;53:71.

REFERENCES

Cobb AB: Trauma. J Miss State Med Assoc 1991;32:87.

Davis JW et al: Complications in evaluating abdominal trauma: Diagnostic peritoneal lavage versus computerized axial tomography. J Trauma 1991;30:1506.

Davis JW et al: The significance of critical care errors in causing preventable death in trauma patients in a trauma system. J Trauma 1991;31:813.

Deane SA et al: Interhospital transfer in the management of acute trauma. Aust N Z J Surg 1990;60:441.

Fischer RP et al: Academic consequences of a trauma system failure. J Trauma 1990;30:784.

Gillott AR, Thomas JM, Forrester C: Development of a statewide trauma registry. J Trauma 1989;29:1667.

Goins WA et al: Outcome following prolonged intensive care unit stay in multiple trauma patients. Crit Care Med 1991;19:339.

Guss DA et al: The impact of a regionalized trauma system on trauma care in San Diego County. Ann Emerg Med 1989;18:1141.

Hammond J, Gomez G, Eckes J: Trauma systems: Economic and political considerations. J Fla Med Assoc 1990;77:603.

Harris BH: Creating pediatric trauma systems. J Pediatr Surg 1989;24:149.

Higgins B, Popil V: Air transport of the trauma patient. AACN Clin Issues Crit Care Nurs 1991;1:451.

Honigman B et al: Prehospital advanced trauma life support

for penetrating cardiac wounds. Ann Emerg Med 1990;19:145.

Kreis DJ Jr: Trauma systems: An interdisciplinary approach to prevention, treatment, and education. Bull N Y Acad Med 1988;64:835.

Mendeloff JM, Cayten CG: Trauma systems and public policy. Annu Rev Public Health 1991;12:401.

Morris JA Jr et al: Trauma patients return to productivity. J Trauma 1991;:6.

Rowlands BJ: Are we ready for the next disaster? Injury 1990;21:61.

Schiowitz M, Stanovich H: The impact of volume on out-come in seriously injured trauma patients: Two years' experience of the Chicago trauma system. J Trauma 1991;31:1125.

Sloan EP et al: The effect of urban trauma system hospital bypass on prehospital transport times and level 1 trauma patient survival. Ann Emerg Med 1989;18:1146.

Smith RF et al: The impact of volume on outcome in seriously injured trauma patients: Two years' experience of the Chicago Trauma System. J Trauma 1990;30:1075.

Young WW et al: Defining the major trauma patient and trauma severity. J Trauma 1991;31:1125.

Burns & Other Thermal Injuries 14

Robert H. Demling, MD, & Lawrence W. Way, MD

BURNS

A severe thermal injury is one of the most devastating physical and psychologic injuries a person can suffer. Recent statistics indicate that over 2 million burns require medical attention each year in the USA, with 14,000 deaths resulting. Fires in the home are responsible for only 5% of burn injuries but 50% of burn deaths—most due to smoke inhalation. The fire death rate in the USA (57.1 deaths per million population in 1988) is the second highest in the world and the highest of all industrialized countries—almost twice that of second-ranking Canada (29.7 deaths per million in the same year). Fifty thousand burn patients annually remain hospitalized for over 2 months each year, indicating the severity of illness associated with this injury.

ANATOMY & PHYSIOLOGY OF THE SKIN

The skin is the largest organ of the body, ranging in area from 0.25 m^2 in the newborn to 1.8 m^2 in the adult. It consists of two layers: the epidermis and the dermis (corium). The outermost cells of the epidermis are dead cornified cells that act as a tough protective barrier against the environment. The second, thicker layer, the corium (0.06–0.12 mm), is composed chiefly of fibrous connective tissue. The corium contains the blood vessels and nerves to the skin and the epithelial appendages of specialized function. Since the nerve endings that mediate pain are found only in the corium, partial-thickness injuries may be extremely painful, whereas full-thickness burns are usually anesthetic.

The corium is a barrier that prevents loss of body fluids by evaporation and loss of excess body heat. Sweat glands help maintain body temperature by controlling the amount of water evaporated. They also excrete small amounts of sodium chloride and cholesterol and traces of albumin and urea. The corium is interlaced with sensory nerve endings that identify the sensations of touch, pressure, pain, heat,

and cold. This is a protective mechanism that allows an individual to adapt to changes in the physical environment.

The skin produces vitamin D, which is synthesized by the action of sunlight on certain intradermal cholesterol compounds. The skin also acts as a protective barrier against infection by preventing penetration of the subdermal tissue by microorganisms.

DEPTH OF BURNS
(Figure 14–1)

The depth of the burn significantly affects all subsequent clinical events. The depth may be difficult to determine and in some cases is not known until after spontaneous healing has occurred or when the eschar is removed and granulation tissue is seen.

Traditionally, burns have been classified as first-, second-, and third-degree, but the current emphasis on burn healing has led to classification as partial-thickness burns, which heal spontaneously, and full-thickness burns, which require skin grafting.

A **first-degree burn** involves only the epidermis and is characterized by erythema and minor microscopic changes; tissue damage is minimal, protective functions of the skin are intact, skin edema is minimal, and systemic effects are rare. Pain, the chief symptom, usually resolves in 48–72 hours, and healing takes place uneventfully. In 5–10 days, the damaged epithelium peels off in small scales, leaving no residual scarring. The most common causes of first-degree burns are overexposure to sunlight and brief scalding.

Second-degree burns are deeper, involving all of the epidermis and some of the corium. The systemic severity of the burn and the quality of subsequent healing are directly related to the amount of undamaged corium. Superficial burns are often characterized by blister formation, while deeper partial-thickness burns have a reddish appearance or a layer of whitish nonviable dermis firmly adherent to the remaining viable tissue. Blisters, when present, continue to increase in size in the postburn period as the osmotically active particles in the blister fluid attract water. Complications are rare from superficial sec-

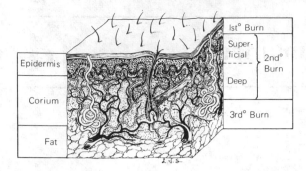

Figure 14–1. Layers of the skin showing depth of first-degree, second-degree, and third-degree burns.

ond-degree burns, which usually heal with minimal scarring in 10–14 days unless they become infected.

Deep dermal burns heal over a period of 25–35 days with a fragile epithelial covering that arises from the residual uninjured epithelium of the deep dermal sweat glands and hair follicles. Severe hypertrophic scarring occurs when such an injury heals; the resulting epithelial covering is prone to blistering and breakdown. Evaporative losses after healing remain high compared to losses in normal skin. Conversion to a full-thickness burn by bacteria is common. Skin grafting of deep dermal burns, when feasible, improves the physiologic quality and appearance of the skin cover.

Full-thickness, or **third-degree burns,** have a characteristic white, waxy appearance and may be misdiagnosed by the untrained eye as unburned skin. Burns caused by prolonged exposure, with involvement of fat and underlying tissue, may be brown, dark red, or black. The diagnostic findings of full-thickness burns are lack of sensation in the burned skin, lack of capillary refill, and a leathery texture that is unlike normal skin. All epithelial elements are destroyed, leaving no potential for reepithelialization.

DETERMINATION OF SEVERITY
OF INJURY

Illness and death are related to the size (surface area) and depth of the burn, the age and prior state of health of the victim, the location of the burn wound, and the severity of associated injuries (if any)—particularly lung injury.

The total body surface area involved in the burn is most accurately determined by using the age-related charts designed by Lund and Browder (Figure 14–2). A set of these charts should be filled out for every burn patient on admission and when resuscitation is begun.

A careful calculation of the percentage of total body burn is useful for several reasons. First, there is a general tendency to underestimate clinically the size of the burn and thus its severity. The American Burn Association has adopted a severity index for burn injury (Table 14–1). Second, prognosis is directly related to the extent of injury. Third, the decision about who should be treated in a specialized burn facility or managed as an outpatient is based in part on the estimate of burn size.

Patients under age 2 years and over age 60 years have a significantly higher death rate for any given extent of burn. The higher death rate in infants results from a number of factors. First, the body surface area in children relative to body weight is much greater than in adults. Therefore, a burn of comparable surface area has a greater physiologic impact on a child. Second, immature kidneys and liver do not allow for removal of a high solute load from injured tissue or the rapid restoration of adequate nutritional support. Third, the incompletely developed immune system increases susceptibility to infection. Associated conditions such as cardiac disease, diabetes, or chronic obstructive pulmonary disease significantly worsen the prognosis in elderly patients.

Burns involving the hands, face, feet, or perineum will result in permanent disability if not properly treated. Patients with such burns should always be admitted to the hospital, preferably to a burn center. Chemical and electrical burns or those involving the respiratory tract are invariably far more extensive than is evident on initial inspection. Therefore, hospital admission is necessary in these cases also.

PATHOLOGY & PATHOPHYSIOLOGY
OF THERMAL INJURIES

The microscopic pathologic feature of the burn wound is principally coagulation necrosis. Beneath any obviously charred tissue there are three distinct zones. The first is the zone of "coagulation," with irreversible vessel coagulation and no capillary blood flow. The depth of this most severely damaged zone is determined by the temperature and duration of exposure. Surrounding this is a zone of stasis, characterized by sluggish capillary blood flow. Although damaged, the tissue has not been coagulated. Stasis can occur early or late. Avoiding additional injury from rubbing or dehydration may prevent stasis changes from developing and thereby prevent extension of the depth of the burn. Prevention of venous occlusion is important because it may lead to thrombosis and infarction in this zone. The third zone is that of "hyperemia," which is the usual inflammatory response of healthy tissue to nonlethal injury.

A rapid loss of intravascular fluid and protein occurs through the heat-injured capillaries. The volume loss is greatest in the first 6–8 hours, with capillary integrity returning toward normal by 18–24 hours. A

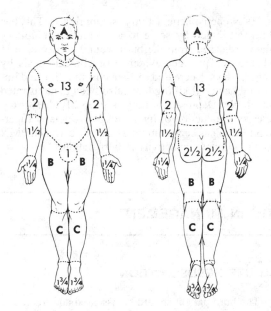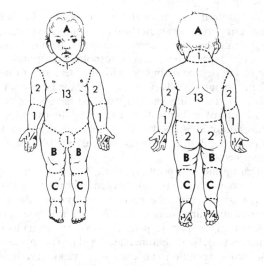

Relative Percentages of Areas Affected by Growth

Area	Age		
	10	15	Adult
A = half of head	5 ½	4 ½	3 ½
B = half of one thigh	4 ¼	4 ½	4 ¾
C = half of one leg	3	3 ¼	3 ½

Relative Percentages of Areas Affected by Growth

Area	Age		
	0	1	5
A = half of head	9 ½	8 ½	6 ½
B = half of one thigh	2 ¾	3 ¼	4
C = half of one leg	2 ½	2 ½	2 ¾

Figure 14–2. Table for estimating extent of burns. In adults, a reasonable system for calculating the percentage of body surface burned is the "rule of nines": each arm equals 9%, the head equals 9%, the anterior and posterior trunk each equal 18%, and each leg equals 18%; the sum of these percentages is 99%.

Table 14–1. Summary of American Burn Association burn severity categorization.

Major burn injury
    Second-degree burn of >25% body surface area in adults.
    Second-degree burn of >25% body surface area in children.
    Third-degree burn of >10% body surface area.
    Most burns involving hands, face, eyes, ears, feet, or perineum.
    Most patients with the following:
        Inhalation injury.
        Electrical injury.
        Burn injury complicated by other major trauma.
    Poor-risk patients with burns.
Moderate uncomplicated burn injury
    Second-degree burn of 15–25% body surface area in adults.
    Second-degree burn of 10–20% body surface area in children.
    Third-degree burn of <10% body surface area.
Minor burn injury
    Second-degree burn of <15% body surface area in adults.
    Second-degree burn of <10% body surface area in children.
    Third-degree burn of <2% body surface area.

transient increase in vascular permeability also occurs in nonburned tissues, probably as a result of the initial release of vasoactive mediators. However, the edema that develops in nonburned tissues during resuscitation appears to be due in large part to the marked hypoproteinemia caused by protein loss into the burn itself. A generalized decrease in cell ATPase activity and membrane potential occurs as a result of the early decrease in tissue perfusion. This leads to a shift of extracellular sodium and water into the intracellular space, which, in turn, increases fluid requirements. This process is also corrected as hemodynamic stability is restored, beginning at about 24 hours after injury.

METABOLIC RESPONSE TO BURNS & METABOLIC SUPPORT

As with any major injury, the body increases the secretion of catecholamines, cortisol, glucagon, renin-angiotensin, antidiuretic hormone, and aldosterone. The consequence is a tendency toward retention of sodium and water and excretion of potassium by the kidneys. Early in the response, energy is supplied by the breakdown of stored glycogen and via anaerobic glycolysis.

A profound hypermetabolism occurs in the postburn period, characterized by an increase in metabolic rate that approaches doubling of the basal rate in severe burns. The degree of response is proportionate to the degree of injury, with a plateau occurring when the burn involves about 70% of total body surface. The initiating and perpetuating factors are the mediators of inflammation, especially the cytokines and endotoxin. Added environmental stresses, such as pain, cooling, and sepsis, increase the obligatory hypermetabolism.

During the first postburn week, the metabolic rate (or heat production) and oxygen consumption rise progressively from the normal level present during resuscitation and remain elevated until the wound is covered. The specific pathophysiologic mechanism remains undefined, but increased and persistent catecholamine secretion and excessive evaporative heat loss from the burn wound are major factors, as is increased circulating endotoxin from wound or gut.

The evaporative water loss from the wound may reach 300 $mL/m^2/h$ (normal is about 15 $mL/m^2/h$). This produces a heat loss of about 580 kcal/L of water evaporated. Covering the burn with an impermeable membrane, such as skin substitute, reduces the hypermetabolism. Similarly, placing the burn patient in a warm environment, where convection and radiant loss of heat are minimized, also modestly reduces the metabolic rate. Placing the burn patient in an unwarmed environment (room temperature at or below 27 °C [80 °F]) accentuates heat loss and markedly increases the hypermetabolic state. The persistently elevated circulating levels of catecholamines stimulate an exaggerated degree of gluconeogenesis and protein breakdown. Protein catabolism, glucose intolerance, and marked total body weight loss result.

Aggressive nutritional support along with rapid wound closure and control of pain, stress, and sepsis are the only means available to decrease the hypermetabolic state. The use of selective antiinflammatory agents may be of some benefit in the future.

IMMUNOLOGIC FACTORS IN BURNS

A number of immunologic abnormalities in burn patients predispose to infection. Serum IgA, IgM, and IgG are frequently depressed, reflecting depressed B cell function. Cell-mediated immunity or T cell function is also impaired, as demonstrated by prolonged survival of homografts and xenografts. A decrease in interleukin-2 production due to circulating mediators may be responsible. An excess of suppressor T cell activity is seen in severely burned patients, and the degree of activity has been found to be a good predictor of sepsis and eventual fatality.

PMN chemotactic activity is suppressed. This has been attributed by some to a circulating inhibitory factor released from the burn wound. A decrease in chemotaxis predates evidence of clinical sepsis by several days. Decreased oxygen consumption and impaired bacterial killing have also been demonstrated in PMNs. Depressed killing is probably due to decreased production of hydrogen peroxide and superoxide; this has been demonstrated by decreased PMN chemiluminescent activity in burn patients.

BURN MANAGEMENT

ACUTE RESUSCITATION

The burn patient should be assessed and treated as any patient with major trauma. The first priority is to ensure an adequate airway. If there is a possibility that smoke inhalation has occurred—as suggested by exposure to a fire in an enclosed space or burns of the face, nares, or upper torso—arterial blood gases and arterial oxygen saturation of hemoglobin and carboxyhemoglobin levels should be measured and oxygen should be administered.

Endotracheal intubation is indicated if the patient is semicomatose, has deep burns to the face and neck, or is otherwise critically injured. Intubation should be done early in all doubtful cases, because delayed intubation will be difficult to achieve in cases associated with pharyngeal edema or upper airway injury, and an emergency tracheostomy may become necessary later under difficult circumstances. If the burn exceeds 20% of body surface area, a urinary catheter should be inserted to monitor urine output. A large-bore intravenous catheter should be inserted, preferably into a large peripheral vein. There is a significant complication rate with the use of central lines in burn patients owing to the increased risk of infection.

Severe burns are characterized by large losses of intravascular fluid, which are greatest during the first 8–12 hours. Fluid loss occurs as a result of the altered capillary permeability, severe hypoproteinemia, and also the shift of sodium into the cells. Both fluid shifts are significantly diminished by 24 hours postburn. The lung appears to be reasonably well protected from the early edema process, and pulmonary edema is uncommon during the resuscitation period unless there is a superimposed inhalation injury.

Initially, an isotonic crystalloid salt solution is infused to counterbalance the loss of plasma volume into the extravascular space and the further loss of extracellular fluid into the intracellular space. Lactated Ringer's is commonly used, the rate being dictated by urine output, pulse (character and rate), state of consciousness, and, to a lesser extent, blood pressure. Urine output should be maintained at 0.5 mL/kg/h and the pulse at 120 beats/min or slower.

Swan-Ganz catheters and central venous pressure lines are seldom needed unless a patient has sufficient cardiopulmonary disease so that accurate monitoring of volume status would be difficult without measurement of filling pressures or a persistent base deficit is present, indicating continued impaired perfusion. It has been estimated that the amount of lactated Ringer's necessary in the first 24 hours for adequate resuscitation is approximately 3–4 mL/kg of body weight per percent of body burn. This is the amount of fluid needed to restore the estimated sodium deficit. At least half of the fluid is given in the first 8 hours because of the greater initial volume loss. It has been demonstrated that patients can be adequately resuscitated with less fluid and in turn less edema if a hypertonic salt solution is used instead of lactated Ringer's solution. The main concern with hypertonic salt solutions has been the ease with which an excessive salt load can be administered. Serum sodium must be carefully monitored to avoid exceeding a value of 160 meq/L. Discontinuation of the hypertonic salt solution and a return to Ringer's lactate are required if this occurs. Dextrose-containing solutions are not used initially, because of early stress-induced glucose intolerance.

Although the importance of restoring colloid osmotic pressure and plasma proteins is well recognized, the timing of colloid infusion remains somewhat varied. Plasma proteins are ordinarily not infused until after the initial severe plasma leak in burned tissues begins to decrease. This usually occurs about 8–12 hours postburn. The addition of a protein infusion to the treatment regimen after this period will decrease the fluid requirements and, in very young or elderly patients and in patients with massive burns (in excess of 50% of body surface), will improve hemodynamic stability.

After intravenous fluids are started and vital signs stabilized, the wound should be debrided of all loose skin and dirt. To avoid severe hypothermia, debridement is best done by completing one body area before exposing a second. An alternative is to use an overhead radiant heater, which will decrease heat loss. Cool water is a very good analgesic on a small superficial burn; however, it should not be used for larger burns, because of the risk of hypothermia. Pain is best controlled with the use of intravenous rather than intramuscular narcotics. Tetanus toxoid, 0.5 mL, should be administered to all patients with any significant burn.

POSTRESUSCITATION PERIOD

Intravenous fluid therapy during the second 24 hours should consist of glucose in water or hypotonic salt solution to replace evaporative losses and of plasma proteins to maintain adequate circulating volume. Evaporative losses are considerable and will continue until the wound is healed or has been grafted. An estimate of these losses in milliliters per hour is arrived at as follows:

$$(25 \times \% \text{ burn}) \times m^2 \text{ body surface}$$

Treatment should aim to decrease excessive catecholamine stimulation and provide enough calories to offset the effects of the hypermetabolism. Hypovolemia should be prevented by giving enough fluid to make up for the body losses.

Nutritional support should begin as early as possible in the postburn period to maximize wound healing and minimize immune deficiency. Patients with moderate body burns may be able to meet nutritional needs by voluntary oral intake. Patients with large burns invariably require calorie and protein supplementation. This can usually be accomplished by administering a formula diet through a small feeding tube. Parenteral nutrition is also occasionally required, but the intestinal route is preferred if needs can be met this way. Early restoration of gut function will also decrease gut bacterial translocation and endotoxin leak. The reader should consult Chapter 10 for detailed information on nutrition.

The use of antibiotics (eg, penicillin) during the first few days following the occurrence of a burn is a controversial subject. It is probably better to treat streptococcal infections in the few patients who acquire them than to cover all patients prophylactically. Broad-spectrum antibiotics should never be given for prophylaxis.

Vitamins A and C and zinc should be given until the burn wound is closed. Low-dose heparin therapy may have some benefit, as with other immobilized patients with soft tissue injury.

CARE OF THE BURN WOUND

In the management of first- and second-degree burns, one must provide as aseptic an environment as possible to prevent infection. However, superficial burns generally do not require the use of topical antibiotics. Occlusive dressings to minimize exposure to air have been shown to increase the rate of reepithelialization and to decrease pain. If there is no infection, burns will heal spontaneously.

The goals in managing full-thickness (third-degree) burns are to prevent invasive infection (ie, burn wound sepsis), to remove dead tissue, and to cover the wound with skin as soon as possible.

All topical antibiotics retard wound healing to some degree and therefore should be used only on deep second- or third-degree burns or wounds with a high risk of infection.

Topical Antibacterial Agents

Topical agents have definitely advanced the care of burn patients. Although burn wound sepsis is still a major problem, the incidence is lower and the death rate has been reduced, particularly in burns of less than 50% of body surface area. Silver sulfadiazine is the most widely used preparation today. Mafenide, silver nitrate, povidone-iodine, and gentamicin ointments are also used.

Silver sulfadiazine is effective against a wide spectrum of gram-negative organisms and is moderately effective in penetrating the burn eschar. A transient leukopenia secondary to bone marrow suppression often occurs with use of silver sulfadiazine in large burns, but the process is usually self-limiting, and the agent does not have to be discontinued.

Mafenide penetrates the burn eschar and is a more potent antibiotic, but there are more complications with its use. The agent produces considerable pain upon application in over half of patients. Mafenide is also a carbonic anhydrase inhibitor, and metabolic acidosis can result if it is used over a large surface area, particularly in children or the elderly. The patient can usually eliminate excess CO_2 through the lungs if respiratory complications do not supervene, but patients with pulmonary insufficiency may not be able to tolerate mafenide. This agent is used chiefly on burns already infected or when silver sulfadiazine is no longer controlling bacterial growth.

Exposure Versus Closed Management

There are two methods of management of the burn wound with topical agents. In **exposure therapy,** no dressings are applied over the wound after application of the agent to the wound twice or three times daily. The advantages of this method are that bacterial growth is not enhanced, as may be the case under a closed dressing, and the wound remains visible and readily accessible. This approach is typically used on the face and head. Disadvantages are increased pain and heat loss as a result of the exposed wound.

In the **closed method,** an occlusive dressing is applied over the agent and is usually changed twice daily. The disadvantage of this method is the potential increase in bacterial growth if the dressing is not changed twice daily, particularly when thick eschar is present. The advantages are less pain and less heat loss. The closed method is generally preferred.

Temporary Skin Substitutes

Skin substitutes are another alternative to topical agents for the partial-thickness burn or the clean excised wound. Split-thickness **porcine xenografts** are commercially available and have gained popularity as a biologic dressing that can be applied to clean partial thickness wounds and to cover primarily excised areas when grafting must be delayed or when autografts are not available. **Homografts (human skin)** work better for this purpose but are difficult to obtain.

Other alternatives include a number of synthetic skin substitutes such as Biobrane, a thin plastic membrane that reduces water evaporative loss.

These agents are particularly effective on second-degree burns. After the initial cleansing and removal of blisters, immediate application prevents fluid loss, protects against infection, and stops pain. The patient can walk about in comfort immediately. The resultant healing has minimal scarring.

Hydrotherapy

The use of hydrotherapy for wound management remains controversial. A number of studies have shown that the infection rate is actually increased when patients are immersed in a tub because of the generalized inoculation of burn wounds with bacteria from what was previously a localized infection. Hydrotherapy, however, is a very useful form of physical therapy once the wounds are in the process of being debrided and closed. Showering is also effective for wound cleansing in the more stable patient.

Debridement & Grafting

Burn wound inflammation, even in the absence of infection, can result in organ dysfunction and perpetuation of the hypermetabolic state. Early wound closure would be expected to better control this process. Surgical management of burn wounds has now become much more aggressive, with operative debridement beginning within the first several days postburn rather than after eschar has sloughed. More rapid closure of burn wounds clearly decreases the rate of sepsis and, in full-thickness burn injuries in excess of 60% of body surface, significantly decreases the death rate. The approach to operative debridement varies from an extensive burn excision and grafting within several days of injury to a more moderate approach of limiting debridements to less than 15% of the burned area and no more than four units of blood loss per procedure. Excision can be carried down to fascia or to viable remaining dermis or fat. Excision to fascia has the advantage of allowing for nearly a 100% graft take and also allows the use of wide-meshed grafts if necessary. The procedure can be performed on an extremity, using a tourniquet to decrease blood loss. The mesh can be covered with a biologic dressing to avoid desiccation of the uncovered wound. Excision to viable tissue, referred to as tangential excision, is advantageous because it provides a vascular base for grafting while preserving remaining viable tissue, especially dermis. Blood loss is substantial in view of the vascularity of the dermis.

A number of **permanent skin substitutes** are being tested that could further facilitate wound closure, particularly in massive burns with insufficient donor sites. Autologous cultures of epithelium have been applied with some success. Permanent skin substitutes composed of both dermis and epidermis have been designed in order to maintain coverage and improve skin function.

Maintenance of Function

The maintenance of functional motion during evolution of the burn wound is especially desirable to avoid loss of motion at joints. Wound contraction, a normal event during healing, may result in extremity contracture. Immobilization may produce joint stiffness, which at one time was thought to be caused by edema but probably is more a result of pain, disuse, or immobilizing dressings. Contracture of the scar, muscles, and tendons across a joint also causes loss of motion and can be diminished by traction, early motion, and pressure distributed directly over the wound to decrease the hypertrophic scar formation.

The scar is a metabolically active tissue, continually undergoing reorganization. The extensive scarring that frequently occurs after burns can lead to disfiguring and disabling contractures, but it may be avoided by the use of splints and elevation to maintain a functional position before grafting. Following application of the skin graft, maintenance of proper positioning with splints is indicated. In the convalescent period, application of a pressure dressing and pressure and isoprene splints will result in less hypertrophic scarring and contracture. The pressure should be maintained with elastic garments for at least 6 months and in some cases may be necessary for as long as a year. Early burn contractures can usually be stretched by constant light force.

If reinjury does not occur, the amount of collagen in the scar tends to decrease with time. Stiff collagen becomes softer, and on flat surfaces of the body, where reinjury and inflammation are prevented, remodeling may totally eliminate contracture. However, around joints or the neck, contractures usually persist and plastic surgical reconstruction is often necessary. The sooner granulation tissue can be covered with skin grafts, the less likely is contracture.

MANAGEMENT OF COMPLICATIONS

Infection remains a critical problem in burns, though the incidence has been reduced by modern therapy with topical antibacterial agents. Sequential quantitative cultures of the burn will show when a concentration of 10^5 organisms—the level defining invasive infection—is present. The cultures also show the sensitivity of the bacteria, and when the bacterial concentration passes 10^5 organisms per gram, specific systemic antibiotics should be instituted (Tables 14–2 and 14–3).

Sepsis can be difficult to diagnose, since fever and leukocytosis are often present with a burn alone. Hemodynamic instability is a late sign. The temperature may fall below normal, the appearance of the wound may deteriorate, and the white count may fall,

Table 14–2. Diagnosis of burn wound infection.

Systemic Changes	Colonized or Clean	Wound Infection
Body temperature	Increased	Variable
White blood cell count	Increased Mild left shift	High or low Severe left shift
Wound appearance	Variable—may appear purulent or benign	Purulence may be present, or wound surface may appear dry and pale
Bacterial content Surface Quantitative Biopsy	Scant to large amount Usually <10^5/g No invasion of normal tissue	Variable Usually >10^5/g Invasion of normal tissue by organisms

ending finally with septic shock. Aggressive antibiotic therapy must be initiated and an attempt made to identify the source of the infection. Pneumonitis, urinary tract infection, and intravenous catheter sepsis should be considered in the differential diagnosis. If other causes are not found, the wound is usually the septic focus and will have to be debrided. Blood volume, nutrition, and oxygenation must be assessed. Steroids should not be given, because they depress already weakened immune defenses.

Circumferential burns of an extremity or of the trunk pose special problems. Swelling beneath the unyielding eschar may act as a tourniquet to blood and lymph flow, and the distal extremity may become swollen and tense. More extensive swelling may compromise the arterial supply. escharotomy or excision of the eschar may be required. To avoid permanent damage, escharotomy must be performed before arterial ischemia develops. Constriction involving the chest or abdomen may severely restrict ventilation and may require longitudinal escharotomies. Anesthetics are rarely required, and the procedure can usually be performed in the patient's room.

Acute gastroduodenal (Curling's) ulcers used to be a frequent complication of severe burns, but the incidence is now decreasing, largely as a result of the early and routine institution of antacid and nutritional therapy and the decrease in the rate of sepsis. Management of Curling's ulcers is discussed in Chapter 23.

A complication unique to children is seizures, which may result from electrolyte imbalance, hypoxemia, infection, or drugs; in one-third of cases, the cause is unknown. Hyponatremia, the most frequent cause, is becoming less common with the diminishing use of topical silver nitrate. Drugs that have been implicated include penicillin, phenothiazine, diphenhydramine, and aminophylline.

Acute gastric dilatation, which occurs in the first

Table 14–3. Most common organisms in burn infections.

	S aureus	P aeruginosa	C albicans
Wound appearance	Loss of wound granulation	Surface necrosis; patchy, black.	Minimal exudate
Course	Slow onset over 2–5 days	Rapid onset over 12–36 hours	Slow (days)
CNS signs	Disorientation	Modest changes	Often no change
Temperature	Marked increase	High or low	Modest changes
White blood count	Marked increase	High or low	Modest changes
Hypotension	Modest	Often severe	Minimal change
Mortality rate	5%	20–30%	30–50%

week after injury, should be suspected when the patient repeatedly vomits small quantities of food. Fecal impaction resulting from immobilization, dehydration, and narcotic analgesics is a fairly common occurrence. Systemic hypertension occurs in about 10% of cases in the postresuscitation period.

RESPIRATORY TRACT INJURY IN BURNS

Today the major cause of death after burns is injury or complications in the respiratory tract. The problems include inhalation injury, aspiration in unconscious patients, bacterial pneumonia, pulmonary edema, pulmonary embolism, and posttraumatic pulmonary insufficiency.

Direct inhalation injuries, which predispose to other complications, are divided into three categories: carbon monoxide poisoning (Table 14–4), heat injury to the airway, and inhalation of noxious gases (Table 14–5).

Direct inhalation of dry heat is a rare cause of damage below the vocal cords, because in most cases the upper airway effectively cools the inspired gases before they reach the trachea, and reflex closure of the cords and laryngeal spasm halt full inhalation of the hot gas. Direct burns to the upper airway are associated with burns of the face, lips, and nasal hairs and necrosis or swelling of the pharyngeal mucosa. Acute edema of the upper tract may cause airway obstruc-

tion and asphyxiation without lung damage. Laryngeal edema must be anticipated in patients with airway burns, and endotracheal intubation should be performed well before manifestations of airway obstruction appear. The endotracheal tube should be large enough to allow removal of thick copious secretions during subsequent care. Tracheostomies performed through burned tissue are associated with a prohibitively high complication rate and should only be done if endotracheal intubation is impossible.

Treatment is primarily supportive, including maintenance of pulmonary toilet, mechanical ventilation (when indicated), and antibiotics.

Carbon monoxide poisoning must be considered in every patient suspected of having inhalation injury on the basis of having been burned in a closed space, physical evidence of inhalation, or dyspnea. Arterial blood gases and carboxyhemoglobin levels must be determined. Levels of carboxyhemoglobin above 5% in nonsmokers and above 10% in smokers indicate carbon monoxide poisoning. Carbon monoxide has an affinity for hemoglobin 200 times that of oxygen, displaces oxygen, and produces a leftward shift in the oxyhemoglobin dissociation curve (P-50, the oxygen tension at which half the hemoglobin is saturated with oxygen, is lowered). Measurements of oxyhemoglobin saturation may be misleading, because the hemoglobin combined with carbon monoxide is not detected and the percentage saturation of oxyhemoglobin may appear normal.

Mild carbon monoxide poisoning (less than 20% carboxyhemoglobin) is manifested by headache, slight dyspnea, mild confusion, and diminished visual acuity. Moderate poisoning (20–40% car-

Table 14–4. Carbon monoxide poisoning.

Carboxyhemoglobin Level	Severity	Symptoms
<20%	Mild	Headache, mild dyspnea, visual changes, confusion
20–40%	Moderate	Irritability, diminished judgment, dim vision, nausea, easy fatigability
40–60%	Severe	Hallucinations, confusion, ataxia, collapse, coma
>60%	Fatal	

Table 14–5. Sources of noxious chemicals in smoke.

Polyethylene, polypropylene	Clean burning combustion to CO_2 and H_2O
Polystyrene	Copious black smoke and soot—CO_2, H_2O, some CO
Wood, cotton	Aldehydes (acrolein)
Polyvinylchloride	Hydrochloric acid
Acrylonitrile, polyurethane, nitrogeneous compounds	Hydrogen cyanide
Fire retardants may produce toxic fumes	Halogens (F_2, Cl_2, Br_2), ammonia

boxyhemoglobin) leads to irritability, impairment of judgment, dim vision, nausea, and fatigability. Severe poisoning (40–60% carboxyhemoglobin) produces hallucinations, confusion, ataxia, collapse, and coma. Levels in excess of 60% carboxyhemoglobin are usually fatal.

Various **toxic chemicals** in inspired smoke produce specific respiratory injuries. Inhalation of kerosene smoke, for example, is relatively innocuous. Smoke from a wood fire is extremely irritating because it contains aldehyde gases, particularly acrolein. Direct inhalation of acrolein, even in low concentrations, irritates mucous membranes and produces an outpouring of fluid. A concentration of 10 ppm will cause pulmonary edema. Smoke from some of the newer plastic compounds, such as polyurethane, is the most serious type of toxic irritant. Poisonous gases such as chlorine, sulfuric acid, or cyanides are given off. Cyanide absorption can be lethal.

Inhalation injury causes severe mucosal edema followed soon by sloughing of the mucosa. The destroyed mucosa in the larger airways is replaced by a mucopurulent membrane. The edema fluid enters the airway and, when mixed with the pus in the lumen, may form casts and plugs in the smaller bronchioles. Terminal bronchioles and alveoli may contain carbonaceous material. Acute bronchiolitis and bronchopneumonia commonly develop within a few days. Daily sputum smears to detect early bacterial tracheobronchial infection are indicated.

When inhalation injury is suspected, early endoscopic examination of the airway with either fiberoptic or standard bronchoscopy is helpful in determining the area of injury, ie, whether just the upper airway is involved or the lower airway as well. Unfortunately, the severity of the injury cannot be accurately quantitated by bronchoscopy—it can only be shown that an injury is present. Recent evidence indicates that direct laryngoscopy may give as much information. Xenon lung scanning can also be used to detect lung injury, particularly to the lower airways. Delayed xenon washout from the airways and parenchyma indicates bronchiolar edema and spasm.

Less common causes of respiratory failure are pulmonary embolus and "overload" pulmonary edema. Emboli usually occur later in the course of treatment after prolonged bed rest and should be suspected if respiratory function suddenly deteriorates. When a pulmonary embolus is diagnosed, heparin anticoagulation is indicated (see Chapter 37). Pulmonary edema from fluid overload during resuscitation usually occurs only in patients with preexisting heart disease. The inhalation-injured lung is very susceptible to edema, which is difficult to manage, since systemic hypoperfusion must be avoided by attempts at diuresis.

Probably the most common cause of respiratory failure is bacterial pneumonia due to either inhalation injury, contamination of the lungs through a tracheostomy or endotracheal tube, airborne infection, or hematogenous spread of bacteria from the burn wound. Alteration of oropharyngeal normal flora with colonization by pathogens and subsequent aspiration of infected secretions is the most common cause of the lung infections.

Pulmonary insufficiency may develop, which is associated with systemic sepsis. Differentiating this condition, known as adult respiratory distress syndrome (ARDS), from bacterial pneumonia may be difficult. There is damage to the pulmonary capillaries and leakage of fluid and protein into the interstitial spaces of the lung. Loss of compliance and difficulty in oxygenating the blood are progressive. Modern methods of ventilatory support and vigorous pulmonary toilet have significantly reduced the death rate in recent years.

Treatment

Management of a burn patient should include frequent evaluation of the lungs throughout the hospital course. All patients who initially have evidence of smoke inhalation should receive humidified oxygen in high concentrations. If carbon monoxide poisoning has occurred, 100% oxygen should be given until the carboxyhemoglobin content returns to normal levels and until symptoms of carbon monoxide toxicity resolve. With severe exposures, carbon monoxide may still be bound to the cytochrome enzymes, leading to cell hypoxia after carboxyhemoglobin levels are returning to near normal. Continued oxygen administration will also reverse this process.

The use of corticosteroids for inhalation injuries is no longer controversial and is clearly contraindicated.

Bronchodilators by aerosol or aminophylline intravenously may help if wheezing is due to reflex bronchospasm. Chest physical therapy with postural drainage is also required.

When endotracheal intubation is used without mechanical ventilation (eg, for upper airway obstruction), mist and continuous positive pressure ventilatory assistance should be included. The humidity will help loosen the secretions and prevent drying of the airway; the continuous positive pressure will help prevent atelectasis and closure of lung units distal to the swollen airways. Tracheostomy is indicated in the first several days for patients who are expected to require ventilatory support for a few weeks or more. If the neck is burned, excision and grafting followed by tracheostomy is indicated in order to improve pulmonary toilet.

Mechanical ventilation should be instituted early if a significant pulmonary injury is anticipated. A large body burn with chest wall involvement will result in decreased chest wall compliance, increased work of breathing, and subsequent atelectasis. Tracheobronchial injury from inhaled chemicals is accentuated by the presence of a body burn, with a resultant increase in the potential for atelectasis and infection. Controlled ventilation along with sedation will diminish the degree of injury and also conserve energy expenditure. A discussion of ventilatory support is presented in Chapters 3 and 13. Early excision of the deep chest wall burn and wound closure will help remove the constricting component. Wound closure in general will decrease the excessive CO_2 production caused by the hypermetabolic state.

REHABILITATION

Plastic surgical revisions of scars are often necessary after the initial grafting, particularly to release contractures over joints and for cosmetic reasons. The physician must be realistic in defining an acceptable result, and the patient should be told that it may require years to achieve. Burn scars are often unsightly, and although hope should be extended that improvement can be made, total resolution is not possible in many cases.

The recent introduction of skin expansion techniques utilizing a subdermal Silastic bag that is gradually expanded has greatly improved scar revision techniques. The ability to enlarge the available skin to be used for replacement of scar improves both cosmesis and function. Advances in microvascular flap surgery have also resulted in substantial improvements in outcome.

The patient must take special care of the skin of the burn scar. Prolonged exposure to sunlight should be avoided, and when the wound involves areas such as the face and hands, which are frequently exposed to the sun, ultraviolet screening agents should be used. Hypertrophic scars and keloids are particularly bothersome and can be diminished with the use of pressure garments, which must be worn until the scar matures, or approximately 12 months. Since the skin appendages are often destroyed by full-thickness burns, use of creams and lotions is required to prevent drying and cracking and to reduce itching. Substances such as lanolin, A and D ointment, and Eucerin cream have all proved effective.

Alexander J: Mechanism of immunologic suppression in burn injury. J Trauma 1990;30:70.

Alsbjorn BF: Biologic wound coverings in burn treatment. World J Surg 1992;16:43.

Becker WK et al: Fungal burn wound infection: A 10-year experience. Arch Surg 1991;126:44.

Blank IH: What are the functions of skin lost in burn injury that affect short- and long-term recovery? J Trauma 1984;24:S10.

Brown G et al: Enhancement of wound healing by topical treatment with epidermal growth factor. N Engl J Med 1989;321:76.

Burke JF: From desperation to skin regeneration: Progress in burn treatment. J Trauma 1990;30:S36.

Cioffi WG Jr et al: Prophylactic use of high-frequency percussive ventilation in patients with inhalation injury. Ann Surg 1991;213:575.

Clark CJ et al: Mortality probability in victims of fire trauma: Revised equation to include inhalation injury. Br Med J 1986;292:1303.

Clark WR Jr: Smoke inhalation: Diagnosis and treatment. World J Surg 1992;16:24.

Crum RL et al: Cardiovascular and neurohumoral responses following burn injury. Arch Surg 1990;125:1065.

Curreri PW: Assessing nutritional needs for the burned patient. J Trauma 1990;30:S20.

Decamp M, Demling R: Posttraumatic multisystem organ failure. JAMA 1988;260:530.

Deitch EA: Intestinal permeability is increased in burn patients after injury. Surgery 1990;107:411.

Deitch EA: The management of burns. N Engl J Med 1990;323:1249.

Demling RH et al: Identification and modifications of the pulmonary and systemic inflammatory and biochemical changes caused by a skin burn. J Trauma 1990;30:60.

Demling RH, Frye E, Read T: Effect of sequential early burn wound excision and closure on postburn oxygen consumption. Crit Care Med 1991;19:861.

Demling RH: Burn care in the immediate resuscitation period. In: Care of the Surgical Patient. Wilmore D (editor). Scientific American, 1989.

Desai MH et al: Early burn wound excision significantly reduces blood loss. Ann Surg 1990;211:753.

Desai MH et al: Ischemic intestinal complications in patients with burns. Surg Gynecol Obstet 1991;172:257.

Dries DJ, Waxman K: Adequate resuscitation of burn patients may not be measured by urine output and vital signs. Crit Care Med 1991;19:327.

Hanborough J: Current status of skin replacements for coverage of extensive burns. J Trauma 1990;30:156.

Heimbach D et al: Burn depth. World J Surg 1992;16:10.

Heimbach DM et al: Burn depth estimation: Man or machine. J Trauma 1984;24:373.

Herndon DN et al: The effect of resuscitation on inhalation injury. Surgery 1986;100:248.

Lalonde C, Demling RH: Effect of complete burn wound closure on postburn oxygen consumption. Surgery 1987;102:862.

Lewis W, Sun K: Hypertrophic scar: A genetic hypothesis. Burns 1990;16:176.

Libber SM, Stayton DJ: Childhood burns reconsidered: The child, the family, the burn injury. J Trauma 1984;24:245.

Lund T, Onarheim H, Reed RK: Pathogenesis of edema formation in burn injuries. World J Surg 1992;16:2.

Mazingo D et al: Chemical burns. J Trauma 1988;28:642.

McDonald WS, Sharp CW Jr, Deitch EA: Immediate enteral feeding in burn patients is safe and effective. Ann Surg 1991;213:177.

Monafo WW, Bessey PQ: Benefits and limitations of burn wound excision. World J Surg 1992;16:37.

Neurohumoral responses to thermal injury. Lancet 1990;336:1221.

Pruitt BA Jr et al: Evaluation and management of patients with inhalation injury. J Trauma 1990;30:S63.

Pruitt BA Jr: Infection and the burn patient. Br J Surg 1990;77:1081.

Purdue GR, Hunt JL: inhalation injuries and burns in the inner city. Surg Clin North Am 1991;71:385.

Robson MC et al: Prevention and treatment of postburn scars and contracture. World J Surg 1992;16:87.

Saffle JR et al: The continuing challenge of burn care in the elderly. Surgery 1990;108:534.

Shimazaki S, Yukioka T, Matuda H: Fluid distribution and pulmonary dysfunction following burn shock. J Trauma 1990;31:623.

Tompkins RG, Burke JF: Burn wound closure using permanent skin replacement materials. World J Surg 1992;16:47.

Tredget EE et al: The role of inhalation injury in burn trauma. Ann Surg 1990;212:720.

Tredget EE, Yu UM: The metabolic effects of thermal injury. World J Surg 1992;16:68.

Warden GD: Burn shock resuscitation. World J Surg 1992;16:16.

Waymack JP, Herndon DN: Nutritional support of the burned patient. World J Surg 1992;16:80.

Wilmore DW: Pathophysiology of the hypermetabolic response to burn injury. J Trauma 1990;30:S4.

Wolfe R et al: Substrate cycling in thermogenesis and amplification of net substrate flux in burned patients. J Trauma 1990;30:6.

Youn YK, Lalonde C, Demling R: The role of mediators in the response to thermal injury. World J Surg 1992;16:30.

ELECTRICAL INJURY

There are three kinds of electrical injuries: electrical current injury, electrothermal burns from arcing current, and flame burns caused by ignition of clothing. Occasionally, all three will be present in the same victim.

Flash or arc burns are thermal injuries to the skin caused by a high-tension electrical current reaching the skin from the conductor. The thermal injury to the skin is intense and deep, because the electrical arc has a temperature of about 2500 °C (high enough to melt bone). Flame burns from ignited clothing are often the most serious part of the injury. Treatment is the same as for any thermal injury.

The damage from electrical current is directly proportionate to its intensity as governed by Ohm's law:

$$\frac{\text{Amperage}}{\text{(intensity of current)}} = \frac{\text{Voltage (tension or potential)}}{\text{Resistance}}$$

Thus, the amperage depends on the voltage and on the resistance provided by various parts of the body. Voltages above 40 V are considered dangerous.

Once current has entered the body, its pathway depends on the resistances it encounters in the various organs. The following are listed in descending order of resistance: bone, fat, tendon, skin, muscle, blood, and nerve. The pathway of the current determines immediate survival; for example, if it passes through the heart or the brain stem, death may be immediate from ventricular fibrillation or apnea. Current passing through muscles may cause spasms severe enough to produce long-bone fractures or dislocations.

The type of current is also related to the severity of injury. The usual 60-cycle alternating current that causes most injuries in the home is particularly severe. Alternating current causes tetanic contractions, and the patient may become "locked" to the contact. Cardiac arrest is common from contact with house current.

Electrical current injuries are more than just burns. Focal burns occur at the points of entrance and exit through the skin. Once inside the body, the current travels through muscles, causing an injury more like a crush than a thermal burn. Thrombosis frequently occurs in vessels deep in an extremity, causing a greater depth of tissue necrosis than is evident at the initial examination. The treatment of electrical injuries depends on the extent of deep muscle and nerve destruction more than any other factor.

Myoglobinuria may develop with the risk of acute tubular necrosis. The urine output must be kept two to three times normal with intravenous fluids. Alkalinization of the urine and osmotic diuretics may be indicated if myoglobinuria is present.

A rapid drop in hematocrit sometimes follows sudden destruction of red blood cells by the electrical energy. Bleeding into deep tissues may occur as a result of disruption of blood vessels and tissue planes. In some cases, thrombosed vessels disintegrate later and cause massive interstitial hemorrhage.

The skin burn at the entrance and exit sites is usually a depressed gray or yellow area of full-thickness destruction surrounded by a sharply defined zone of hyperemia. Charring may be present if an arc burn coexists. The lesion should be debrided to underlying healthy tissue. Frequently there is deep destruction not initially evident. This dead and devitalized tissue must also be excised. A second debridement is usually indicated 24–48 hours after the injury, because the necrosis is found to be more extensive than originally thought. The strategy of obtaining skin covering for these burns can tax ingenuity, because of the extent and depth of the wounds. Microvascular flaps are now used routinely to replace large tissue losses.

In general, the treatment of electrical injuries is complex at every step, and after the initial resuscitation these patients should be referred to specialized centers.

Craig SR et al: When lightning strikes: Pathophysiology and treatment of lightning injuries. Postgrad Med 1986;79:109.

Eriksson A, Ornehult L: Death by lightning. Am J Forensic Med Pathol 1988;9:295.

Finkelstein JL et al: Management of electrical injuries. Infect Surg 1990;43.

Haberal M et al: Electrical burns: A five-year experience. J Trauma 1986;26:103.

Ku CS et al: Myocardial damage associated with electrical injury. Am Heart J 1989;118:621.

Rosenberg DB, Nelson M: Rehabilitation concerns in electrical burn patients. J Trauma 1988;28:808.

Wang XW, Bartle EJ, Roberts BB: Early vascular grafting to prevent upper extremity necrosis after electric burns: Additional commentary on indications for surgery. J Burn Care Rehabil 1987;8:391.

Zachary LM, Lee RC, Gottlieb LJ: Evolving clinical and scientific concepts of upper extremity electrical trauma. Hand Clin 1990;6:243.

HEAT STROKE

Heat stroke occurs when core body temperature exceeds 40 °C (104 °F) and produces severe central nervous system dysfunction. Two other related syndromes induced by exposure to heat are heat cramps and heat exhaustion.

Heat cramps, painful muscles after exertion in a hot environment, have usually been attributed to salt deficit. It is probable, however, that many cases are really examples of exertional rhabdomyolysis. The latter condition, which may also be a complicating factor in heat stroke, involves acute muscle injury due to severe exertional efforts beyond the limits for which the individual has trained. It often produces myoglobinuria, which rarely affects kidney function except when it occurs in patients also suffering from heat stroke. Complete recovery is the rule after uncomplicated heat cramps.

Heat exhaustion consists of fatigue, muscular weakness, tachycardia, postural syncope, nausea, vomiting, and an urge to defecate caused by dehydration and hypovolemia from heat stress. Although body temperature is normal in heat exhaustion, there is a continuum between this syndrome and heat stroke.

Heat stroke, a result of imbalance between heat production and heat dissipation, kills about 4000 persons yearly in the USA. Exercise-induced heat stroke most often affects young people (eg, athletes, military recruits, laborers) who are exercising strenuously in a hot environment, usually without adequate training. Sedentary heat stroke is a disease of elderly or infirm people whose cardiovascular systems are unable to adapt to the stress of a hot environment. Epidemics of heat stroke in elderly people can be predicted when the ambient temperature surpasses 32.2 °C (90 °F) and the relative humidity reaches 50–76%.

In humans, heat is dissipated from the skin by radiation, conduction, convection, and evaporation. When the ambient temperature rises, heat loss by the first 3 is impaired; loss by evaporation is hindered by a high relative humidity. Predisposing factors to heat accumulation are dermatitis; use of phenothiazines, beta-blockers, diuretics, or anticholinergics; intercurrent fever from other disease; obesity; alcoholism; and heavy clothing. Cocaine and amphetamines may increase metabolic heat production.

The mechanism of injury is direct damage by heat to the parenchyma and vasculature of the organs. The central nervous system is particularly vulnerable, and cellular necrosis is found in the brains of those who die of heat stroke. Hepatocellular and renal tubular damage are apparent in severe cases. Subendocardial damage and occasionally transmural infarcts are discovered in fatal cases even in young persons without previous cardiac disease. Disseminated intravascular coagulation may develop, aggravating injury in all organ systems and predisposing to bleeding complications.

Clinical Findings

A. Symptoms and Signs: Heat stroke should be suspected in anyone who develops sudden coma in a hot environment. If the patient's temperature is above 40 °C (104 °F) (range: 40–43 °C [104–109.4 °F]), the diagnosis of heat stroke is definite. Measurements of body temperature must be made rectally. A prodrome including dizziness, headache, nausea, chills, and gooseflesh of the chest and arms is seen occasionally but is not common. In most cases, the patient recalls having experienced no warning symptoms except weakness, tiredness, or dizziness. Confusion, belligerent behavior, or stupor may precede coma. Convulsions may occur after admission to the hospital.

The skin is pink or ashen and sometimes, paradoxically, dry and hot; dry skin is virtually pathognomonic in the presence of hyperpyrexia. Profuse sweating is usually present in runners and other athletes who have heat stroke. The heart rate ranges from 140 to 170/min, central venous or pulmonary wedge pressure is high, and in some cases the blood pressure is low. Hyperventilation may reach 60/min and may give rise to a respiratory alkalosis. Pulmonary edema and bloody sputum may develop in severe cases. Jaundice is frequent within the first few days after onset of symptoms.

Dehydration, which may produce the same central nervous system symptoms as heat stroke, is an aggravating factor in about 15% of cases.

B. Laboratory Findings: There is no characteristic pattern to the electrolyte changes: The serum sodium concentration may be normal or high; the potassium concentration is usually low on admission or at some point during resuscitation. Hypocalcemia is common, and hypophosphatemia may occur. In the first few days, the AST, LDH, and CK may be elevated, especially in exertional heat stroke. Alkalosis may follow hyperventilation; acidosis can result from lactic acidosis or acute renal failure. Proteinuria and granular and red cell casts are seen in urine specimens collected immediately after diagnosis. If the urine is dark red or brown, it probably contains myoglobin. The blood urea nitrogen and serum creatinine rise transiently in most patients, and they continue to climb if renal failure develops. The hematologic findings may be normal or may be typical of disseminated intravascular coagulation (ie, low fibrinogen, increased fibrin split products, low prothrombin and partial thromboplastin times, and decreased platelet count).

Prevention

For the most part, heat stroke in military recruits and athletes in training is preventable by adhering to a graduated schedule of increasing performance requirements that allows acclimatization over 2–3 weeks. Heat produced by exercise is dissipated by increased cardiac output, vasodilatation in the skin, and increased sweating. With acclimatization there is increased efficiency for muscular work, increased myocardial performance, expanded extracellular fluid volume, greater output of sweat for a given amount of work, a lower salt content of sweat, and a lower central temperature for a given amount of work.

Access to drinking water should be unrestricted during vigorous physical activity in a hot environment. Free water is preferable to electrolyte-containing solutions. Most training regimens should not include the use of supplemental salt tablets, since enough salt (10–15 g/d) will be consumed with food to meet the electrolyte losses in sweat and since hypernatremia can develop if ingested salt tablets are not taken with enough water. Clothing and protective gear should be lightened as heat production and air temperature rise, and heavy exercise should not be scheduled at the hottest times of day, especially at the beginning of a training schedule. Long-distance runs with open competition, which attract novice runners, should be held in late summer or fall, when heat acclimatization is more apt to have occurred, and should be started before 8 AM or after 6 PM.

Treatment

The patient should be cooled rapidly. The most efficient method is to induce evaporative heat loss by spraying the patient with water at 15 °C (59 °F) and fanning with warm air. Immersion in an ice water bath or use of ice packs is also effective but causes cutaneous vasoconstriction and shivering and makes patient monitoring more difficult. Monitor the rectal temperature frequently. To avoid overshooting the end point, vigorous cooling should be stopped when the temperature reaches 38.9 °C (102 °F). Shivering should be controlled with parenteral phenothiazines. Oxygen should be administered, and if the Pao_2 drops below 65 mm Hg, tracheal intubation should be performed to control ventilation. Fluid, electrolyte, and acid-base balance must be controlled by frequent

monitoring. Intravenous fluid administration should be based on the central venous or pulmonary artery wedge pressure, blood pressure, and urine output; overhydration must be avoided. On the average, about 1400 mL of fluid is required in the first 4 hours of resuscitation. Intravenous mannitol (12.5 g) may be given early if myoglobinuria is present. Renal failure may require hemodialysis. Disseminated intravascular coagulation may require treatment with heparin. Digitalis and occasionally inotropic agents (eg, isoproterenol, dopamine) may be indicated for cardiac insufficiency, which should be suspected if hypotension persists after hypovolemia has been corrected.

Prognosis

Bad prognostic signs are temperature of 42.2 °C (108 °F) or more, coma lasting over 2 hours, shock, hyperkalemia, and an AST greater than 1000 Karman units during the first 24 hours. The death rate is about 10% in patients who are correctly diagnosed and treated promptly. Deaths in the first few days are usually due to cerebral damage; later deaths may be from bleeding or cardiac, renal, or hepatic failure.

Anderson RJ et al: Heatstroke. Adv Intern Med 1983; 28:115.

Khogali M, Weiner JS: Heat stroke. Lancet 1980;2:276.

Kilbourne ED et al: Risk factors for heatstroke: A case-control study. JAMA 1982;247:3332.

Knochel JP: Heat stroke and related heat stress disorders. DM 1989;35:301.

Management of heatstroke. (Editorial.) Lancet 1982;2:910.

Sprung CL et al: The metabolic and respiratory alterations of heat stroke. Arch Intern Med 1980;140:665.

Tucker LE et al: Classical heatstroke: Clinical and laboratory assessment. South Med J 1985;78:20.

Vicario SJ et al: Rapid cooling in classic heatstroke: Effect on mortality rates. Am J Emerg Med 1986;4:394.

Yaqub BA et al: Heat stroke at the Mekkah Pilgrimage: Clinical characteristics and course of 30 patients. J Med 1986;59:523.

FROSTBITE

Frostbite involves freezing of tissues. Ice crystals form between the cells and grow at the expense of intracellular water. The resulting cellular dehydration coupled with ischemia due to vasoconstriction and increased blood viscosity are the mechanisms of tissue injury. Skin and muscle are considerably more susceptible to freezing damage than tendons and bones, which explains why the patient may still be able to move severely frostbitten digits.

Frostbite is caused by cold exposure, the effects of

which can be magnified by moisture or wind. For example, the chilling effects on skin are the same with an air temperature of +6.7 °C (+44 °F) and a 40-mile-per-hour wind as with an air temperature of –40 °C (–40 °F) and only a 2-mile-per-hour wind. Contact with metal or gasoline in very cold weather can cause virtually instantaneous freezing; skin will often stick to metal and be lost. The risk of frostbite is increased by generalized hypothermia, which produces peripheral vasoconstriction as the organism attempts to preserve the core body temperature.

Two related injuries, trench foot and immersion foot, involve prolonged exposure to wet cold above freezing (eg, 10 °C [50 °F]). The resulting tissue damage is produced by ischemia.

Clinical Findings

Frostnip, a minor variant of this syndrome, is a transient blanching and numbness of exposed parts that may progress to frostbite if not immediately detected and treated. It often appears on the tips of fingers, ears, nose, chin, or cheeks and should be managed by rewarming through contact with warm parts of the body or warm air.

Frostbitten parts are numb, painless, and of a white or waxy appearance. With **superficial frostbite,** only the skin and subcutaneous tissues are frozen, so the tissues beneath are still compressible with pressure. **Deep frostbite** involves freezing of underlying tissues, which imparts a wooden consistency to the extremity.

After rewarming, the frostbitten area becomes mottled blue or purple and painful and tender. Blisters appear that may take several weeks to resolve. The part becomes edematous and to a varying degree painful.

Treatment

The frostbitten part should be rewarmed (thawed) in a water bath at 40–42.2 °C (104–108 °F) for 20–30 minutes. Thawing should not be attempted until the victim can be kept permanently warm and at rest. It is far better to continue walking on frostbitten feet even for many hours than to thaw them in a remote cold area where definitive care cannot be provided. If a thermometer is unavailable, the temperature of the water should be adjusted to be warm but not hot to a normal hand. Never use the frozen part to test the water temperature or expose it to a source of direct heat such as a fire. The risk of seriously compounding the injury is great with any method of thawing other than immersion in warm water.

After thawing has been completed, the patient should be kept recumbent and the injured part left open to the air, protected from direct contact with sheets, clothing, etc. Blisters should be left intact and the skin gently debrided by immersing the part in a whirlpool bath for about 20 minutes twice daily. No scrubbing or massaging of the injured part should be

allowed, and topical ointments, antiseptics, etc, are of no value. Vasodilating agents and surgical sympathectomy do not appear to improve healing.

The tissues will heal gradually, and any dead tissue will become demarcated and will usually slough spontaneously. Early in the course, it is nearly impossible, even for someone with considerable experience in the treatment of frostbite, to judge the depth of injury; most early assessments tend to overestimate the extent of permanent damage. Therefore, expectant treatment is the rule, and surgical debridement should be avoided even if evolution of the injury requires many months. Surgery may be indicated to release constricting circumferential eschars, but rarely should the process of spontaneous separation of gangrenous tissue be surgically facilitated. Even in severe injuries, amputation is rarely indicated before 2 months unless invasive infection supervenes.

Concomitant fractures or dislocations create challenging and complex problems. Dislocations should be reduced immediately after thawing. Open fractures require operative reduction, but closed fractures should be managed with a posterior plastic splint. An anterior tibial compartment syndrome, which may develop in patients with associated fractures, may be diagnosed by arteriography and treated by fasciotomy.

After the eschar separates, the skin is noted to be thin, shiny, tender, and sensitive to cold; occasionally it exhibits a tendency to perspire more readily. Gradually it returns toward normal, but pain on exposure to cold may persist indefinitely.

Prognosis

The prognosis for normal function is excellent if treatment is appropriate. Individuals who have recovered from frostbite have increased susceptibility to another frostbite injury on exposure to cold.

Fritz RL, Perrin DH: Cold exposure injuries: Prevention and treatment. Clin Sports Med 1989;8:111.

Grace TG: Cold exposure injuries and the winter athlete. Clin Orthop (March) 1987;55.

Heggers JP et al: Experimental and clinical observations on frostbite. Ann Emerg Med 1987;16:1056.

Vogel JE, Dellon AL: Frostbite injuries of the hand. Clin Plast Surg 1989;16:575.

Zhang ZX, Li FZ: Experimental studies of combined therapy of severe frostbite. Cryobiology 1989;26:378.

ACCIDENTAL HYPOTHERMIA

Accidental hypothermia (in contrast with deliberate iatrogenic hypothermia used as an adjunct to anesthesia, etc) consists of the uncontrolled lowering of core body temperature below 35 °C (95 °F) by exposure to cold. In Britain, hypothermia largely affects elderly people living alone in inadequately heated homes. In the USA, most patients are alcoholics who have experienced excessive cold exposure during a binge. Alcohol facilitates the induction of hypothermia by producing sedation (inhibiting shivering) and cutaneous dilatation. Other sedatives, tranquilizers, and antidepressants are occasionally implicated. Diseases that predispose to hypothermia are myxedema, hypopituitarism, cerebral vascular insufficiency, mental impairment, and cardiovascular disorders.

Accidental hypothermia differs from controlled hypothermia principally by its longer duration. The heart is the organ most sensitive to cooling and is subject to ventricular fibrillation or asystole when the temperature drops to 21–23.9 °C (70–75 °F). Cardiac standstill may cause death in less than 1 hour in shipwreck victims immersed in cold (< 6.7 °C [< 44 °F]) water. Increased capillary permeability, manifested by generalized edema and pulmonary, hepatic, and renal dysfunction, may develop as the patient is rewarmed. Disseminated intravascular coagulation is seen occasionally. Pancreatitis and acute renal failure are common in patients whose temperature on admission is below 32.2 °C (90 °F).

Clinical Findings

A. Symptoms and Signs: The patient is mentally depressed (somnolent, stuporous, or comatose), cold, and pale to cyanotic. The clinical findings are not always striking and may be mistaken for the effects of alcohol. The core temperature ranges from 21 to 35 °C (70–95 °F). Shivering is absent when the temperature is below 32 °C (90 °F). Respirations are slow and shallow. Many patients have bronchopneumonia. The blood pressure is usually normal and the heart rate slow. When the core temperature drops below 32 °C (90 °F), the patient may appear to be dead.

B. Laboratory Findings: Dehydration may increase the concentration of various blood constituents. Severe hypoglycemia is common, and unless detected and treated immediately, it may become dangerously worse as rewarming produces shivering. The serum amylase is elevated in about half of cases, but autopsy studies show that it does not always reflect pancreatitis. Diabetic ketoacidosis becomes a management problem in some of the patients whose amylase values are elevated on entry. The AST, LDH, and CK enzymes are usually elevated but are of no predictive significance. The ECG shows lengthening of the PR interval, delay in interventricular conduction, and a pathognomonic J wave at the junction of the QRS complex and ST segment.

Treatment

For severe cases, rewarming should be performed with a warm (40–42 °C [104–108 °F]) water bath at a rate of 1–2 degrees per hour. Hypothermic patients should never be considered dead until all measures for resuscitation have failed—prolonged cardiopulmonary arrest in severe hypothermia is compatible with complete recovery. Mild cases (body temperature 32.2–35 °C [90–95 °F])—especially shivering patients—may need nothing more than wool blankets (passive rewarming) for a few hours. The patient's temperature should be constantly monitored with a rectal or esophageal probe until normal body temperature has been reached. Core rewarming with partial cardiopulmonary bypass is indicated for patients with ventricular fibrillation and severe hypothermia. In the absence of cardiac complications, peritoneal dialysis (dialysate at 43.5 °C [113.5 °F]) may be used to hasten rewarming in severe hypothermia (core temperature below 29.4 °C [85 °F]).

In severe cases, endotracheal intubation should be used for better management of ventilation and protection against aspiration, a common lethal complication. Arterial blood gases should be monitored frequently. Antibiotics are often indicated for coexisting pneumonitis. Serious infections are often unsuspected upon admission, and delay in appropriate therapy may contribute to severity of illness. Hypoglycemia calls for intravenous administration of 50% glucose solution. Fluid administration must be gauged by central venous or pulmonary artery wedge pressures, urine output, and other circulatory parameters. Increased capillary permeability following rewarming predisposes to the development of pulmonary edema. To avoid this complication, the central venous or wedge pressure should be kept below 12–14 cm water. Drugs should not be injected into peripheral tissues, because absorption will not take place while the patient is cold and because drugs may accumulate to produce serious toxicity as rewarming occurs.

As rewarming proceeds, the patient should be continually reassessed for signs of concomitant disease that may have been masked by hypothermia, especially myxedema and hypoglycemia.

Prognosis

Survival can be expected in only 50% of patients whose core temperature drops below 32.2 °C (90 °F). Coexisting diseases (eg, stroke, neoplasm, myocardial infarction) are common and increase the death rate to 75% or more. Survival does not correlate closely with the lowest absolute temperature reached. Death may result from pneumonitis, heart failure, or renal insufficiency.

Celestino FS, Van-Noord GR, Miraglia CP: Accidental hypothermia in the elderly. J Fam Pract 1988;26:259.

Danzl DF et al: Multicenter hypothermia survey. Ann Emerg Med 1987;16:1-42.

Gentilello LM, Rifley WJ: Continuous arteriovenous re-

warming: Report of a new technique for treating hypothermia. J Trauma 1991;31:1151.
Hauty MG et al: Prognostic factors in severe accidental
hypothermia: Experience from the Mt. Hood tragedy. J
Trauma 1987;27:1107.

Keatinge WR: Hypothermia. Br Med J 1991;302:3.
Moss J et al: Accidental severe hypothermia. Surg Gynecol
Obstet 1986;162:501.
Swain JA: Hypothermia and blood pH: A review. Arch In-
tern Med 1988;148:1643.

Head & Neck Tumors

15

Marshall M. Urist, MD, Samuel W. Beenken, MD, & Christopher J. O'Brien, FRACS

In 1991, 21,400 patients in the USA were diagnosed as having carcinoma of the oral cavity and 9400 as having carcinoma of the pharynx. The incidence of tumors of these sites would decline substantially if the use of tobacco were decreased. When detected and treated at an early stage, head and neck tumors are curable in 80% of cases. For a variety of reasons, many patients present with locally advanced primaries, involved regional lymph nodes, or distant metastases. Accurate staging is essential to determine the best therapy and to permit comparison of treatment results. In addition to surgery, therapy often involves collaboration with workers in other disciplines such as radiation oncology, medical oncology, maxillofacial prosthodontics, and speech therapy. The first priority is to treat the cancer adequately, then to maintain function, and finally to preserve appearance.

ETIOLOGY OF HEAD & NECK CANCER

A carcinogen is an agent that initiates a cancer. Examples include tobacco, ionizing radiation, and certain viruses. Initiating agents may require cofactors to achieve or hasten carcinogenesis. The process is affected by the intensity and duration of exposure to initiating and promoting factors as well as by host factors such as genetic susceptibility and immune status.

A number of factors have been implicated as causes of squamous cell carcinomas of the oral and nasal passages. The vermilion surfaces of the lips are susceptible to ultraviolet irradiation and tobacco. Over 90% of squamous cell carcinomas of the lips involve the more exposed lower lip, and 70% of lip cancers occur in elderly, fair-skinned men with a history of prolonged sun exposure. Women and blacks are rarely affected. Sunlight is not the sole cause of carcinoma of the lip, however, because there is a poor correlation between the incidence of lip cancer and other sun-related skin cancers. Tobacco is probably the other main etiologic agent, since about 80% of patients with lip cancer are smokers. Neoplasia could be initiated by chemical damage from the tobacco or thermal damage from the heat of the cigarette or pipe stem.

Tobacco is the principal carcinogen responsible for oral and oropharyngeal cancer, but alcohol consumption is also important. The increasing incidence of oral and lung cancers among women in the USA is directly attributable to increasing cigarette consumption. The geographic and anatomic incidence of oral and oropharyngeal squamous carcinomas varies according to local customs and patterns of tobacco use. Alcohol may contribute by directly damaging the oral mucosa or by causing nutritional deficiencies that destabilize the squamous mucosa and promote the carcinogenic effects of tobacco condensates in saliva. Alcohol may also be carcinogenic independently of tobacco, but this is difficult to prove, because most alcoholics are smokers. For a given level of tobacco exposure, however, the risk of oral cancer increases with increasing alcohol consumption.

The dominant associations of tobacco and alcohol use with cancer have made it difficult to identify other independent risk factors. Poor oral hygiene is common among patients with oral cancer, but it is not clear whether this is a causative or only an associated factor. Chronic irritation from sharp teeth and ill-fitting dentures has also been implicated but in the absence of other risk factors is unlikely to cause cancer.

The incidence of Plummer-Vinson syndrome, an uncommon condition consisting of iron deficiency anemia, atrophic glossitis, hypochlorhydria, pharyngeal webs, and postcricoid carcinoma of the hypopharynx, has decreased as a result of improved nutrition and health services.

Certain occupations are associated with an increased risk of head and neck cancer. Wood workers in the furniture industry of Oxfordshire, England, have a high incidence of adenocarcinomas of the nasal cavity and paranasal sinuses. The same is true of workers in the shoe industry, although a definite carcinogen has not been identified.

Many factors have been implicated in the etiology of carcinoma of the nasopharynx, a rare disease among blacks and Caucasians but among the most common cancers affecting people from Kwangtung Province in China. The major causative factors appear to be genetic and viral. Chinese who emigrate to the United States have a diminished risk, but the incidence is still almost 20 times higher than among native-born Americans. Epstein-Barr virus (EBV) is believed to be a promoting factor—if not the actual cause—of some nasopharyngeal carcinomas. Most patients have elevated antibody titers to EBV that roughly correlate with the stage or volume of disease.

Radiation therapy has been shown to increase the incidence of thyroid, salivary gland, and some mucosal carcinomas. The latent period varies from a few years to many years. Irradiation was used in the past to treat benign head and neck conditions, but this practice has now been stopped. Nonetheless, patients still present with thyroid carcinomas who had radiotherapy for acne or benign lymphoid enlargement during childhood. A few patients develop radiation-induced mucosal carcinomas and sarcomas many years after radiotherapy for other head and neck cancers.

The *INT*-2 gene is frequently amplified in squamous cell carcinoma of the head and neck, and *INT*-2 amplification may correlate with rapid spread and a poor diagnosis.

Blott WJ et al: Smoking and drinking in relation to oral and pharyngeal cancer. Cancer Res 1988;48:3282.

Luka J et al: Detection of antigens associated with Epstein-Barr virus replication in extracts from biopsy specimens of nasopharyngeal carcinomas. J Natl Cancer Inst 1988;80:1164.

McLaughlin JK et al: Dietary factors in oral and pharyngeal cancer. J Natl Cancer Inst 1988;80:1237.

Somers KD, Cartwright SL, Schecter GL: Amplifications of the INT-gene in human head and neck squamous cell carcinomas. Oncogene 1990;5:915.

DIAGNOSIS

The evaluation of a patient with a tumor of the head or neck begins with a complete history and physical examination.

History

Common presenting symptoms are pain, bleeding, obstruction, and a mass. Pain should be characterized as to frequency, duration, severity, location, and radiation. It is difficult to quantify pain, so it may be more helpful to inquire about the amount and type of analgesics used. Several specific patterns are important. Pain around the orbits and at the skull base can be referred from the nasopharynx. Otalgia can be caused by tumors of the base of the tongue, tonsil, or hypopharynx because of involvement of cranial nerves V, IX, and X. Odynophagia may result from deep penetration by tumors of the base of the tongue or hypopharynx or from extensive cervical lymph node metastases. Bleeding is usually mild and intermittent and is most commonly associated with tumors of the nasal cavity, nasopharynx, and oral cavity. Obstruction causing alterations of phonation, breathing, swallowing, or hearing may be a manifestation of either early or advanced disease. Hoarseness is often an early finding in tumors of the glottis, whereas cancers only a few millimeters away on the false vocal cord can grow and metastasize before causing a change in voice. Trismus usually indicates extension of tumor into the pterygoid muscles. Dysphagia is often a late symptom of obstruction at the base of the tongue, hypopharynx, or cervical esophagus. Loss of hearing may be the first symptom of tumors arising in or invading the auditory tract from the external auditory canal or nasopharynx.

A history of cancer in the region is common, and accurate documentation of its histologic type, stage, and date is vital. Squamous cell tumors arising in the same general area after more than 3 years are usually new primaries. The late appearance of lymph node metastases may be from the original tumor or from a new primary lesion. Lung lesions following treatment of squamous cell cancer of the head and neck are just as likely to be new pulmonary tumors as metastases.

The medical, social, occupational, and family history should be reviewed. Information should be obtained about the use of tobacco and alcohol and exposure to ionizing radiation and chemical carcinogens. A nutritional history, noting diet and weight loss, is important in planning treatment and in identifying patients who will require aggressive nutritional therapy. Patients with tumors of the head or neck are often noncompliant and of low socioeconomic status. A full family and psychosocial history will also be helpful in assessing the need for postoperative support. It is important to obtain a detailed family history in patients with enlarged cervical nodes or thyroid nodules, because of the possibility of multiple endocrine neoplasia syndromes.

Physical Examination

The examination must be conducted in a well-lighted area with all necessary instruments and supplies close at hand. The examiner should use the same sequence of examinations with each patient, but it is often best to delay palpation of tender areas until the end of the session. The head and neck area should be observed while taking the history. It may be easier to note facial weakness or areas of asymmetry and hear changes in voice during the interview.

The examination should start with inspection. Small squamous cell carcinomas of the skin and melanomas are common causes of enlarged regional nodes. Each subsite of the upper aerodigestive tract must be carefully inspected. Dentures must be removed and the lips and tongue retracted to obtain a clear view of the oral cavity. The dimensions of a mass or ulcer can be estimated by placing a tongue blade (2 cm wide) over the area. Careful inspection is required to see changes of erythroplasia and leukoplakia, which may be limited to small areas in users of smokeless tobacco. A bimanual technique should be used to examine the floor of the mouth. Palpation is also useful to detect tumors in all areas of the oropharynx, especially the base of the tongue. Parapharyngeal tumors arising from the retromandibular extension of the parotid gland, nerves, lymph nodes, and carotid body may present as masses in the tonsillar area. Complete examination of the nasopharynx, larynx, and hypopharynx may require the use of a topical anesthetic spray. Although most sites are well seen with a head light and laryngeal mirror, flexible fiberoptic endoscopes often provide a better view with less patient discomfort, particularly of the nasopharynx and hypopharynx.

A detailed neurologic examination may reveal localizing signs when no other findings are present. Hyposmia may be caused by primary tumors of the olfactory bulb or tumors of the nasal cavity and paranasal sinuses. Sensory loss in the distribution of the infraorbital nerve is more often a manifestation of maxillary sinus tumors than of inflammation. Dysfunction of cranial nerves III–VII and IX–XII may occur with nasopharyngeal carcinoma. Horner's syndrome suggests metastases or a simultaneous lung primary.

Lymph nodes along the jugular chain, which lie medial to the sternocleidomastoid muscle, are best examined by grasping around the muscle and feeling the nodes between the thumb and first two fingers. Nevertheless, physical examination of lymph nodes is not very accurate. Thirty percent of patients with clinically negative nodes have metastases on pathologic staging, and 20% of those with clinically suspicious nodes will be histologically free of tumor. Tumor in lymph nodes above the clavicles originates from primary lesions above the clavicles in 85% of cases (Figure 15–1).

Biopsy

Definitive diagnosis can usually be made with biopsy at the time of the initial examination. For mucosal lesions, pinch or punch biopsy is obtained at the margin away from areas of obvious necrosis. One important exception is the small lesion that would be completely removed by a biopsy. It is important that the responsible surgeon perform the biopsy, because knowledge of the original findings is crucial when planning treatment. Another exception is tumors in the area of the parotid gland (see salivary gland tumors), which are best managed by exploration and appropriate resection rather than incisional or excisional biopsy.

The diagnosis of masses elsewhere in the neck should be made by aspiration needle biopsy when feasible. Incisions for open biopsies should be chosen to facilitate later resections. Lymph node specimens may require special handling for cultures, lymphocyte markers, and immunohistochemical stains.

Additional Studies

Examination under anesthesia is often indicated. In addition to palpation of the oral cavity and neck, direct laryngoscopy, rigid esophagoscopy, nasopharyngoscopy, and bronchoscopy are often appropriate. A search should always be made for a second primary lesion. The location and extent of the tumor should be defined in detail in order to plan therapy and assess its effects.

A chest x-ray is routine. Barium swallow examination of the hypopharynx and esophagus is sometimes useful, but it does not replace a good endoscopic examination. Mandible x-rays may identify bony invasion from an oral or oropharyngeal tumor, but they are not very accurate. Axial and coronal CT scanning of the head and neck is the imaging study of choice for most advanced head and neck lesions. Cross-sectional views image such important areas as the paranasal sinuses, the parapharyngeal and pterygomaxillary spaces, the orbits, and the anterior skull base. The role of MRI is still being defined. Soft tissue resolution is good—including that of the tumor-tissue interface—but bone delineation is poor. At present, MRI is most useful for imaging the extent of tumors at the skull base, the parapharyngeal space, and the orbits.

AMA Council on Scientific Affairs: Magnetic resonance imaging of the head and neck region: Present status and future potential. JAMA 1988;260:3313.

Jacobs CD, Goffinet DR, Fee WE Jr.: Head and neck squamous cancers. Curr Probl Cancer 1990;14:1.

Shaha AM et al: Synchronicity, multicentricity and metachronicity of head and neck cancer. Head Neck Surg 1988;10:225.

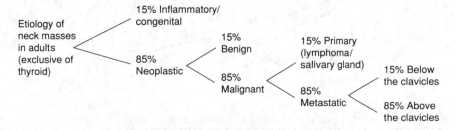

Figure 15–1. Differential diagnosis of neck masses.

Shuman WP, Moss AA: Imaging studies in head and neck cancers. In: *Radiation Therapy of Head and Neck Cancer.* Laramore GE (editor). Springer-Verlag, 1989.

LYMPHATIC ANATOMY OF THE HEAD & NECK

Since the majority of head and neck tumors are squamous cell carcinomas, metastases most often involve regional lymph nodes. Salivary gland tumors, papillary carcinoma of the thyroid, and melanoma also spread principally via lymphatics. There are three main groups of lymphatic tissue in the head and neck. The first contains the structures of Waldeyer's ring (palatine tonsils, lingual tonsils, adenoids, and adjacent submucosal lymphatics); the second comprises transitional lymphatics (submental, submandibular, parotid, retroauricular, and occipital nodes); and the third includes the cervical lymph nodes (internal jugular chain, spinal accessory chain, supraclavicular area). The lymph nodes are also categorized by level within the neck, and clinicians and pathologists should report findings in these terms (Figure 15–2). An accurate prediction of the origin of a metastasis can often be made just by knowing the site of the involved node. Table 15–1 summarizes the anatomic sites that drain to each lymph node group.

The pattern of flow within the lymphatics is predictable unless it has been distorted by a tumor, previous surgery, or irradiation. The jugular chain and transverse cervical lymphatics drain into the thoracic duct on the left side of the neck. In 15% of individuals, there is also a thoracic duct on the right side. The thoracic duct empties into the great vessels near the junction of the internal jugular and subclavian veins in Waldeyer's triangle. Care must be taken to avoid injury to the duct during neck dissections and supraclavicular lymph node biopsies.

Virchow's node, located at the terminus of the thoracic duct in the left supraclavicular region, may contain lymph node metastases from distant primary sites via the retroperitoneal and posterior mediastinal lymph channels.

Table 15–1. Primary sites of lymph node metastases.

Lymph Node Level	Primary Site
Level I	Lip, oral cavity, skin
Level II	Oral cavity, oropharynx, nasopharynx, hypopharynx, larynx
Level III	Oral cavity, oropharynx, hypopharynx, larynx, thyroid
Level IV	Oropharynx, hypopharynx, larynx, cervical esophagus, thyroid

Level V
  Accessory nerve chain
  Supraclavicular
  Occipital
	
	Nasopharynx, scalp
	Breast, lung, gastrointestinal tract
	Scalp

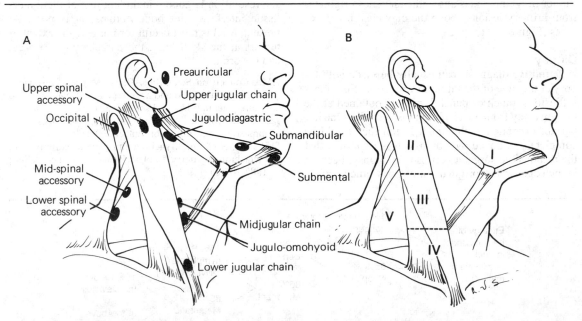

Figure 15–2. **A:** Major lymph node areas of the head and neck. **B:** Levels of cervical lymph nodes used in descriptions of clinical findings, operations, and pathology specimens. (I, submandibular; II, upper jugular chain; III, midjugular chain; IV, lower jugular chain; V, posterior cervical triangle.)

STAGING OF HEAD & NECK CANCER

Head and neck cancer should be staged in order to classify the tumor, estimate the prognosis, and plan treatment. This entails an accurate description of the location and size of the primary, the status of the cervical lymph nodes, and the presence or absence of distant metastases. A chart should be made containing a drawing and a written description of the findings. The TNM staging system has done much to standardize the reporting of results of treatment. In the oral cavity, oropharynx, and major salivary glands, T stage is defined primarily by tumor size; while in the larynx, hypopharynx, and nasopharynx, definition of T stage depends on the extent of local involvement. The following summarizes the TNM system as it applies to head and neck cancer. The specifics of the T (tumor) category differ for each primary site.

Definitions of T (tumor) categories:

T_x: No available information on primary tumor.

T_0: No evidence of primary tumor.

T_{is}: Carcinoma in-situ.

T_1: Greatest diameter 2 cm or less, or confined to the anatomic site of origin.

T_2: Greatest diameter 2–4 cm, or extending into an adjacent site.

T_3: Greatest diameter more than 4 cm, or tumor extending into adjacent region, or with fixation of the vocal cord.

T_4: Massive tumor with invasion of surrounding structures (soft tissue, bone, cartilage, facial nerve).

Definitions of N (lymph node) categories:

N_x: Nodes cannot be assessed.

N_0: No clinically positive nodes

N_1: Single ipsilateral clinically positive node, 3 cm or less in diameter

N_2:

   A: Single ipsilateral node 3–6 cm in diameter

   B: Multiple ipsilateral nodes less than 6 cm in diameter

N_3:

   A: Ipsilateral node greater than 6 cm in diameter

   B: Bilateral clinically positive nodes

   C: Contralateral clinically positive node only

Definition of M (metastasis) categories:

M_x: Not assessed.

M_0: No distant metastases

M_1: Distant metastases present.

Once the TNM classification is established, the tumor stage, ie, stage I, II, III, or IV, is defined by the following scheme:

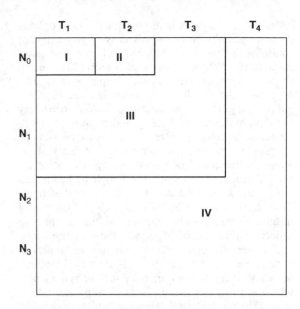

The prognosis for each stage at different sites is not the same, although it is roughly equivalent. The approximate 5-year survival is as follows: stage I, 75–95%; stage II, 50–75%; stage III, 25–50%; and stage IV, less than 25%. Additional factors, including a past history of cancer, medical illnesses, nutrition, and activity status, have a great bearing on outcome. This pattern applies to patients with squamous cell carcinomas and minor salivary cancers arising from the mucous membranes. Cancers from the skin and thyroid gland, melanoma, and lymphoma are classified differently.

CANCER OF THE ORAL CAVITY

Anatomy

The oral cavity is bounded anteriorly by the vermilion border of the lips and posteriorly by the anterior tonsillar pillars, the posterior aspect of the hard palate, and the circumvallate papillae of the tongue. Subsites are (1) the vermilion surfaces of the lips; (2) the alveolar process of the mandible; (3) the alveolar process of the maxilla; (4) the retromolar trigone, which overlies the ascending ramus of the mandible behind the last lower molar tooth; (5) the hard palate; (6) the buccal mucosa, which lines the cheeks and inner aspects of the lips and includes the upper and lower buccoalveolar gutters; (7) the floor of the mouth; and (8) the anterior two-thirds of the tongue (oral tongue), which is limited posteriorly by the circumvallate papillae and includes the tip, dorsum, lateral borders, and undersurface of the mobile tongue.

Pathology

Over 95% of cancers of the oral cavity are squamous cell carcinomas. They are predominantly well and moderately well differentiated and can be preceded by leukoplakia or erythroplakia. Leukoplakia ("white patch") is not necessarily a premalignant condition, although it is induced by factors that cause carcinomas. When a biopsy of a leukoplakic patch shows severe cellular atypia, dysplasia, and dyskeratosis, the condition is premalignant. Erythroplakia (red granular patches of mucosa) is more likely to be premalignant or frankly malignant than is leukoplakia. Macroscopically, oral cavity cancers can be exophytic growths, flat tumors with central ulceration and indurated edges, or deeply infiltrating ulcers. Verrucous carcinoma is an exophytic lesion that is usually white because of surface hyperkeratosis. This tumor is histologically well differentiated throughout and has a better prognosis than infiltrating lesions. Oral cancers, especially those of the upper and lower alveolar mucosa, often invade nearby bone. The mandible is most frequently involved. Minor salivary tumors arise in submucosal glands, which are most abundant in the hard palate. Ulceration is a late feature. Melanoma, which may affect the mucosa of the mouth, has a very poor prognosis.

Cancers of the upper lip drain to parotid and submandibular nodes, while those of the lower lip drain to submental and submandibular nodes. Lateral tongue, floor of mouth, and buccal cancers drain to the ipsilateral submandibular and upper and mid jugular chain nodes, but they may also drain to lower jugular nodes. Midline tumors of the lip, tongue, and floor of mouth may drain bilaterally.

The incidence of lymph node involvement from squamous cancers of the oral cavity is related to the site and size of the primary lesion. Cancers of the oral tongue and floor of mouth have a higher incidence of nodal involvement than do cancers of the lip, hard palate, or buccal mucosa.

Clinical Features

Patients with squamous carcinoma of the oral cavity usually present with ulcerated tumors that have been present for weeks or months. They are typically men aged 50–70 years with a history of heavy tobacco and alcohol use. Dental hygiene is frequently poor, and areas of surrounding erythroplakia and leukoplakia may be seen adjacent to the lesion. Submandibular or jugular chain nodes are palpable in about 30% of patients. Clinical assessment of both normal and enlarged lymph nodes tends to be wrong in one-third of patients (false-negatives and false-positives). Pain is usually not a prominent feature in the absence of deep invasion.

Treatment

A. Primary Tumor: The site and size of the tumor determine the choice of therapy. Squamous carcinomas of the vermilion surface of the lip are best excised and the defect primarily closed as long as no more than 30% of the lip must be removed. With lesions requiring removal of more than one-third of the lip, closure can usually be achieved by transposition of a segment of the opposite lip on a vascular pedicle. When the entire vermilion border has been damaged, vermilionectomy may be performed along with excision of the tumor, and a new vermilion surface can be created by advancing the buccal mucosa.

Within the oral cavity, small tumors can usually be excised through the open mouth. Small defects may be closed by direct suture or split-thickness skin grafts. Tumors larger than 2 cm in diameter require more extensive excision, aiming for at least 1- to 2-cm margins from macroscopic disease. The resulting defect requires reconstruction to replace the oral lining and to maintain oral function. For squamous carcinomas involving bone, it is necessary to remove bone deep to the tumor. If the bone is invaded clinically or by x-ray, segmental resection of the mandible should be performed.

An operation for removal of an oral tumor that includes segmental resection of the mandible and a neck dissection is termed a composite resection.

Radiotherapy is an alternative to surgery for oral cavity cancers smaller than 4 cm in diameter (T_1 and T_2 tumors). The potential side effects of mucositis, xerostomia, and osteoradionecrosis of the mandible must be balanced against potential advantages. Large tumors are better treated with combined surgery and postoperative radiotherapy, because this improves the chances of local control. It has been suggested that radiotherapy may induce anaplastic changes in verrucous carcinomas, but there is no evidence to support this claim.

B. The Neck: Clinically palpable lymph nodes are usually treated by radical neck dissection, which involves removal of all the lymphatic tissue of the neck along with the sternocleidomastoid muscle, internal jugular vein, and spinal accessory nerve. To save structures not directly involved, modified neck dissections are sometimes feasible. A "modified radical neck dissection" preserves the spinal accessory nerve; a "functional neck dissection" preserves the sternocleidomastoid muscle, the internal jugular vein, and the spinal accessory nerve. It may be unnecessary to remove tissue from all the nodal levels of the neck. Node levels II, III, V, and possibly I are removed with a "supraomohyoid neck dissection" while preserving the sternocleidomastoid muscle, the internal jugular vein, and the spinal accessory nerve (Table 15–2).

Since lymph nodes are histologically involved in 30% of patients with oral cavity cancers when the neck is clinically normal, prophylactic neck dissection is sometimes recommended. There is no evidence, however, that this improves survival. When the specimen contains multiple involved lymph nodes or extracapsular invasion of lymph nodes, postoperative adjuvant radiotherapy decreases the chance of local recurrence.

Table 15–2. Classification of neck dissections.

Type of Neck Dissection	Node Level of Dissection	Structures Preserved
Radical	I–V	None
Modified radical	I–V	SAN
Functional	II–V (± I)	SCM, IJV, SAN
Anterior	II–IV	SCM, IJV, SAN
Posterior	V	SCM, IJV, SAN
Supramyohyoid	II, III (± I)	SCM, IJV, SAN

Key:
SCM = Sternocleidomastoid muscle
IJV = Internal jugular vein
SAN = Spinal accessory nerve

Prognosis

For T_1, T_2, T_3, and T_4 tumors, the 5-year survival rates are 80%, 60%, 40%, and 20%, respectively. The presence of lymph node metastases halves the prognosis for any given T stage.

Byers BM, Wolf PF, Ballantyne AJ: Rationale for elective modified neck dissection. Head Neck Surg 1988;1:160.

Cusumano RJ, Persky MS: Squamous cell carcinoma of the oral cavity and oropharynx in young adults. Head Neck Surg 1988;10:229.

Maddox WA, Urist MM: Histopathological prognostic factors of certain primary oral cancers. Oncology 1990;4 (12):39.

Mashberg A, Samit AM: Early detection, diagnosis, and management of oral and oropharyngeal cancer. CA 1989;39:67.

Shah JP, Candela FC, Poddar AK: The patterns of cervical lymph node metastases from squamous carcinoma of the oral cavity. Cancer 1990;66:109.

Soo KC et al: Squamous carcinoma of the gums. Am J Surg 1988;156:281.

Suen JY, Goepfert H: Standardization of neck dissection nomenclature. Head Neck Surg 1987;6:75.

Urist MM, Beenken SW: Carcinoma of the tongue. Postgrad Gen Surg 1990;2:227.

CANCER OF THE OROPHARYNX

Anatomy

The oropharynx extends from the hard palate superiorly to the hyoid bone inferiorly (Figure 15–3). The subsites of the oropharynx are (1) the inferior surface of the soft palate, including the uvula; (2) the posterior pharyngeal wall; (3) the anterior and posterior tonsillar pillars; (4) the tonsils and tonsillar fossae; and (5) the posterior one-third of the tongue, which lies between the circumvallate papillae and the valleculae. The lingual surface of the epiglottis is part of the supraglottic larynx.

Pathology

Most oropharyngeal tumors are squamous carcinomas, but they tend to be less well differentiated than oral cavity lesions, and deep infiltration is common. Minor salivary gland neoplasms and lymphomas—particularly non-Hodgkin's lymphoma involving the tonsil and other parts of Waldeyer's ring—arise in this area. Tumors of the parapharyngeal space may also present as oropharyngeal swellings, causing the mucosa of the lateral pharyngeal wall or soft palate to bulge. These are most often retromandibular parotid tumors, neurogenic tumors (eg, neurilemmoma, neurofibroma), or carotid body tumors.

The oropharynx is richly supplied with lymphatics.

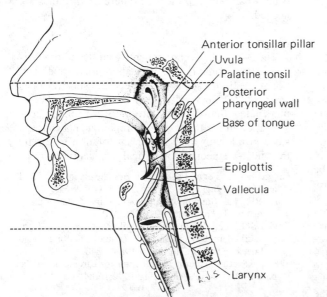

Figure 15–3. Anatomy of the oropharynx.

Posterior pharyngeal wall tumors drain bilaterally to jugular chain nodes and retropharyngeal nodes of Ranvier. Tumors of the tonsillar region drain primarily to the upper and mid jugular chain nodes and also to spinal accessory nodes in the posterior triangle after involvement of the jugular chain nodes.

The overall incidence of nodal involvement from oropharyngeal cancers is approximately 70% and correlates with tumor size. Even small lesions of the tonsillar region or tongue base are likely to have nodal metastases.

Clinical Features

Patients usually present with ulcerating tumors, and about 60% have nodal involvement. Tumors of the base of the tongue tend to be diagnosed at an advanced stage, and presentation with a neck mass and no obvious primary is common with these lesions. The poorer prognosis of tongue base cancers is due to larger size at diagnosis and an increased incidence of nodal metastases at the time of diagnosis. Approximately 70% of patients with tongue base tumors present with advanced disease (stage III or IV), compared with only 30% of patients with carcinoma of the oral tongue.

Tumors of the tonsillar region readily extend to the mandible and may invade the bone. Large tumors in this region may also invade the medial pterygoid muscle, producing trismus. This is an important presenting symptom, and it may limit access for examination. Referred otalgia is also common with deeply infiltrating cancers. Tongue base cancers may spread laterally to involve the mandible, anteriorly to involve the oral tongue, and inferiorly to involve the preepiglottic space and supraglottic larynx. The diagnosis of a parapharyngeal mass presenting as an oropharyngeal swelling is usually not difficult; bimanual palpation is useful.

Treatment

A. The Primary: The best treatment for oropharyngeal cancer remains controversial. For small tumors (T_1 and T_2), surgery or radiotherapy gives similar results, and treatment must be individualized. Small cancers of the tonsillar region respond well to radiotherapy (ie, 75% local control at 3 years). While tongue base cancers are less radioresponsive, irradiation is often the best initial treatment, since resection of this area produces so much morbidity. For early oropharyngeal cancers, surgical access may be achieved by splitting the lower lip and jaw and retracting the mandible laterally. Larger tumors pose a greater problem, and the choices for therapy are (1) surgery combined with postoperative radiation therapy versus (2) initial radiotherapy followed by surgery in the event of recurrence. Overall, combined therapy offers the best chance of disease control and prolonged survival. In this region, resection must be radical and often entails removal of a segment of the

mandible with the primary tumor. This is necessary even when the mandible is not invaded, since it allows wide removal of the nearby pterygoid muscles, which are frequently invaded. Total glossectomy may be necessary to encompass large tumors of the tongue base, but this creates a substantial functional loss. Total glossectomy must often be accompanied by laryngectomy to remove the tumor completely or to prevent subsequent aspiration pneumonia. Operative defects may be repaired with skin grafts, pedicled myocutaneous flaps, or microvascular free flaps. Tracheotomy is mandatory to protect the airway after most oropharyngeal resections.

Excision of a soft palate cancer is relatively straightforward but leads to regurgitation of food into the nasal cavity upon swallowing. Therefore, small lesions may be treated with radiation therapy and surgical salvage if necessary.

B. The Neck: Clinically palpable nodes should be treated by radical neck dissection. If the neck is clinically clear, surgery or radiotherapy to at least the upper neck nodes (levels 2 and 3) (Figure 15–2) is appropriate for all but the earliest tumors. If the primary lesion is treated by irradiation, the upper level neck nodes should be included in the radiation fields. If the primary is treated surgically, an elective modified neck dissection is appropriate, since the resection or reconstruction usually entails entering the neck. If the neck is not entered in the course of resecting an oropharyngeal tumor and postoperative radiotherapy is planned for the primary site, it is reasonable to include the area at risk in the radiation field instead of performing an elective neck dissection.

Initial (induction) chemotherapy gives response rates of 80%, and induction chemotherapy followed by radiotherapy can render stage III and stage IV patients clinically free of disease. No overall survival benefit has been reported, so randomized studies are needed.

Prognosis

The 5-year survival of patients with stage I oropharyngeal carcinoma is 75% with appropriate treatment. For stage II and stage III cancers, the survival rates are 45–70%. Survival of patients with stage IV tumors is less than 30%. Quality of life is a major consideration in the treatment of oropharyngeal cancers, since swallowing and speech are often affected by treatment—especially by radical surgical resection.

Guggenheimer J et al: Factors delaying the diagnosis of oral and oropharyngeal carcinomas. Cancer 1989;64:932.
Spiro RH et al: Squamous carcinoma of the posterior pharyngeal wall. Am J Surg 1990;160:420.
Taylor SG IV et al: Combined simultaneous cisplatin/fluorouracil chemotherapy and split course radiation in head and neck cancer. J Clin Oncol 1989;7:846.
Weber RS et al: Treatment selection for carcinoma of the base of the tongue. Am J Surg 1990;160:415.

CANCER OF THE HYPOPHARYNX

Anatomy

The hypopharynx extends from the hyoid bones superiorly to the lower border of the cricoid cartilage inferiorly. It comprises four subsites: (1) the piriform sinuses (one on each side of the larynx); (2) the postcricoid area (immediately behind the larynx); (3) the posterior pharyngeal wall; and (4) the marginal area, where the medial wall of the piriform sinus and the false vocal cord meet superiorly at the aryepiglottic fold. Laterally, the piriform sinuses are bounded by the ala of thyroid cartilage and the thyrohyoid membrane. The hypopharynx, lined by stratified squamous epithelium, has a muscular wall consisting of the middle and inferior constrictor muscles. The retropharyngeal space posterior to the hypopharynx, which contains lymphatics and loose areolar tissue, separates the visceral compartment of the neck from the prevertebral muscles with their overlying prevertebral fascia.

Pathology

Over 95% of hypopharyngeal cancers are squamous carcinomas, which usually present as infiltrating ulcers with indurated borders. The incidence of poorly differentiated lesions is higher in the hypopharynx than in other regions. The size of these cancers can be deceptive on clinical evaluation because of submucosal lymphatic extension. Minor salivary tumors and lymphomas occasionally occur in the hypopharynx, where they are usually submucosal. Benign hypopharyngeal lesions include webs, strictures, and pharyngoesophageal (Zenker's) diverticula.

Squamous carcinomas of the hypopharynx have a great propensity for lymphatic invasion. Many patients have positive lymph nodes at the time of initial presentation, and the hypopharynx—especially the piriform sinus—must be examined in any adult with metastatic cancer in a cervical node and no obvious primary tumor. Occult node metastases (ie, clinically negative but histologically positive) are also common, making the overall incidence of nodal involvement with hypopharyngeal cancer about 70%. The principal nodal groups involved are the upper, mid, and lower jugular chain nodes; the retropharyngeal nodes of Ranvier; and, less frequently, the nodes along the spinal accessory nerve in the posterior triangle.

Clinical Features

The most common site for hypopharyngeal carcinoma is the piriform sinus, accounting for 60% of cases. The postcricoid region is affected in 25% of patients and the posterior pharyngeal wall in 15%. Postcricoid lesions are frequently circumferential and cause dysphagia, while piriform sinus lesions tend to be silent for a longer time. Patients with this disease are typically men in their fifth to eighth decades who have a history of excessive alcohol and tobacco use. Plummer-Vinson syndrome, the main exception, is seen principally in Scandinavian women with iron deficiency anemia.

The chief symptoms are pain, dysphagia, and weight loss. Pain may be localized to the site of the tumor or may be referred to the ipsilateral ear. About 25% of patients, especially those with lesions of the piriform sinus, present with a palpable neck node and no other symptoms. Advanced tumors may invade the larynx and cause vocal cord paralysis and hoarseness. A barium swallow may aid in the diagnosis of hypopharyngeal cancer, but direct laryngopharyngoscopy and biopsy are necessary to confirm the diagnosis and assess the extent of disease.

Treatment

The objectives of treatment are to cure the disease and maintain continuity of the upper digestive tract. Intensive nutritional therapy may be necessary before treatment if long-standing dysphagia has resulted in cachexia. These patients also commonly have pulmonary disease that must be assessed preoperatively.

A. The Primary: Hypopharyngeal tumors are usually best treated by surgery. Elderly or medically unfit patients with small tumors may be treated with radiotherapy, but local mucositis and swallowing difficulties can be major problems during therapy. Even for small lesions, surgery often must be extensive, usually entailing total laryngectomy and at least partial pharyngectomy. For larger lesions, total pharyngolaryngectomy is usually required, which necessitates pharyngeal reconstruction. Some surgeons recommend that the entire esophagus be removed along with the larynx and pharynx, which decreases the likelihood of local recurrence at the inferior suture line and facilitates reconstruction by the gastric pull-up technique. However, not all patients require total laryngopharyngoesophagectomy. When laryngopharyngectomy has been performed and the pharynx cannot be closed primarily, pharyngeal reconstruction is best done as a one-stage procedure using either a microvascular free jejunal graft or a myocutaneous flap using the pectoralis major muscle and overlying skin.

If surgical treatment is followed by postoperative radiotherapy to the primary site and neck, the locoregional control rate may be improved.

B. The Neck: The incidence of metastases is so high that some form of neck treatment is appropriate for all patients. Radical neck dissection is indicated for palpable node disease. For clinically negative nodes, when the primary site is treated by radiotherapy, the neck should also be irradiated. If the primary is treated surgically, modified neck dissection should be performed. If postoperative radiotherapy is given to the area of the primary, radiotherapy should also encompass the neck, and neck dissection can be avoided.

Prognosis

Recurrence is most common at the primary site or neck, usually within 2 years after treatment. Distant metastases appear in 25% of patients—higher than with cancers of the oral cavity and oropharynx. The overall 5-year survival rate for patients with carcinoma of the hypopharynx is 25%. The survival rate is moderately good for early lesions but dismal for advanced tumors. The role of adjuvant chemotherapy is unclear, because clinical trials have so far failed to show better results.

Candela FC, Kothari K, Shah JP: Patterns of cervical node metastases from squamous carcinoma of the oropharynx and hypopharynx. Head Neck Surg 1990;12:197.

Flynn MB, Barris J, Acland R: Reconstruction with free bowel autographs after pharyngoesophageal or laryngoesophageal resection. Am J Surg 1989;158:333.

Kajanti M, Montula M: Carcinoma of the hypopharynx. A retrospective analysis of the treatment results over a 25-year period. Acta Oncol 1990;29:903.

Maddox WA et al: Total pharyngeal reconstruction using a pectoralis major myocutaneous tunnel. Arch Surg 1988;123:391.

Mansour KA, Picone AL, Coleman JJ: Surgery for high cervical esophageal carcinoma: Experience with 11 patients. Ann Thorac Surg 1990;49:597.

CANCER OF THE NASAL CAVITY, NASOPHARYNX, & SINUSES

Anatomy

The nasal cavity is divided into right and left nasal fossae by the nasal septum. Each fossa has an anterior opening (naris, or nostril), a posterior opening (choana), and bony projections called conchae, or turbinates, protruding from the lateral walls. Posterior to the nasal cavity is the nasopharynx. Its roof is formed by the skull base, which slopes downward and backward, while the inferior limit is level with the plane of the hard palate. The lateral wall is composed of the torus tubularis, the auditory tube orifice, and the lateral wall of Rosenmuller's fossa. The paranasal sinuses consist of the maxillary and ethmoid sinuses bilaterally, the frontal sinus, and the sphenoid sinus. Each maxillary sinus shares a common wall with the orbit above, the nasal cavity medially, the oral cavity inferiorly, and the infratemporal fossa posteriorly.

The mucosa of the nasal cavity consists of ciliated pseudostratified columnar epithelium (respiratory mucosa) except in the region of the superior turbinate and the adjacent lateral wall and septum, which is lined by specialized nonciliated epithelium (olfactory mucosa). The sinuses are lined by respiratory epithelium, and melanocytes are scattered throughout the region. The nasopharynx is lined by respiratory epithelium in early life, but squamous metaplasia occurs with aging, so that about 60% of the respiratory mucosa is replaced by squamous epithelium in the first decade of life. Initially, this squamous epithelium is nonkeratinizing, but after age 50 more keratinization occurs.

Pathology

The most common tumor of the nasal cavity and paranasal sinuses is squamous cell carcinoma. The maxillary antrum is the most common site, while primary malignant neoplasms of the nasal cavity are rare. Adenocarcinoma, sarcoma, melanoma, lymphoma, and minor salivary gland tumors also occur. Esthesioneuroblastoma is an uncommon malignant neoplasm that arises from olfactory mucosa at the superior aspect of the nasal cavity. It readily invades the ethmoid sinuses and may involve the orbit. In the nasopharynx, squamous carcinomas, 80% of which are nonkeratinizing, also predominate. Lymphoepithelioma, a subgroup of nonkeratinizing squamous carcinoma, is poorly differentiated, lacks squamous or glandular differentiation, and has an accompanying lymphocyte component. It is quite radiosensitive.

Tumors of the skin of the vestibule of the nose may drain to parotid, submandibular, or upper jugular nodes. Otherwise, nasal cavity and antral cancers tend not to have nodal metastases unless they are advanced and have invaded surrounding skin, muscle, oral cavity, or pharynx. The nasopharynx is richly supplied with lymphatics, and tumors in this region readily drain bilaterally to upper and midjugular chain nodes and to posterior triangle nodes. Nodal metastases occur in 80% of patients with nasopharyngeal cancers, and a neck mass is the initial manifestation of 50% of patients with this tumor. Unlike nearly all other head and neck sites, tumors of the nasopharynx may metastasize to the posterior triangle in the absence of jugular chain lymph nodes.

Clinical Features

Tumors of the nasal cavity, paranasal sinuses, and nasopharynx are frequently advanced at presentation. Early symptoms, such as nasal obstruction, nasal discharge, and sinus congestion, are so commonly associated with benign conditions that they are frequently neglected until the disease is advanced. Bleeding may occur. Bone invasion and involvement of adjacent structures are common. Cancers of the maxillary sinus may invade the hard palate and enter the oral cavity or the orbital floor, causing visual symptoms and proptosis. Anterior invasion through the skin may also occur. In advanced disease, metastases in the neck may be the initial manifestation. Cranial nerve symptoms may result from invasion of the skull by tumor. Along with the tonsillar fossa, the tongue base, and the piriform sinus, the nasopharynx is an important site of clinically occult primary cancer.

Treatment

The diagnosis and assessment of extent of disease are more difficult with tumors in this area than elsewhere in the head and neck and require histologic examination of a good biopsy specimen. CT scanning should be performed to delineate the extent of disease, although it is sometimes difficult to differentiate between tumor and edematous mucosa in a sinus. MRI can be helpful in making this differentiation.

Radiotherapy is the principal treatment for carcinoma of the nasopharynx. Undifferentiated tumors respond better than well-differentiated ones, and treatment is more successful in younger patients. A dose of 7000 cGy is usually required for the primary site. Both sides of the neck should be treated because of the very high incidence of nodal metastases. Five-year survival rates for stages I, II, III, and IV disease, respectively, are 85%, 75%, 45%, and 10%. One-third of patients die of distant metastatic disease, most often located in bones, lung, and liver.

Although either surgery or radiotherapy may be used to treat early-stage tumors of the paranasal sinuses, combined therapy is best for advanced disease. Small cancers of the maxillary sinus may be treated by partial maxillectomy, but if radiotherapy is to be used, antrostomy will be required to allow drainage of the cavity. Surgery has advantages. The presence of early bone involvement decreases curability with radiotherapy, and salvage surgery is often required. Furthermore, it is difficult to detect recurrent disease following radiotherapy. For advanced tumors, radiotherapy may improve operability, but the subsequent resection should encompass the original extent of disease. Orbital exenteration is necessary for maxillary tumors that invade the periorbital tissues. Resectable cancers of the upper nasal cavity and ethmoid sinuses often require craniofacial excision, which entails frontal craniotomy to assess the extent of intracranial extension. Invasion of the anterior cranial fossa with dural involvement or posterior extension through the orbital apex makes tumors in this region incurable by surgery. Because the incidence of neck metastases is low with cancers of the paranasal sinuses, prophylactic neck dissection or irradiation is unnecessary.

Survival varies according to the stage of disease, and the 5-year survival rate averages 30%.

Fearon B, Forte V, Brama I: Malignant nasopharyngeal tumors in children. Laryngoscope 1990;100:470.

Harrison LB, Pfister DG, Bosl GJ: Chemotherapy as part of the initial treatment for nasopharyngeal cancer. Oncology 1991;5:67.

Levendag PC, Pomp J: Radiation therapy of squamous cell carcinoma of the nasal vestibule. Int J Radiat Oncol Biol Phys 1990;19:1363.

Myers EN et al: Management of inverted papilloma. Laryngoscope 1990;100:481.

Sham JS, Choy D: Prognostic factors of nasopharyngeal carcinoma: A review of 759 patients. Br J Radiol 1990; 63:51.

Wang DC et al: Long-term survival of 1035 cases of nasopharyngeal carcinoma. Cancer 1988;61:2338.

Zamora RL et al: Clinical classification and staging for primary malignancies of the maxillary antrum. Laryngoscope 1990;100:1106.

UNKNOWN PRIMARY CANCERS IN THE HEAD & NECK

In about 5% of cases of metastatic tumor in the neck, the primary is clinically occult. One-third of patients who have an unknown primary after the initial examination will have the site identified on subsequent workup. The site of the metastasis often suggests the location of the primary because of specific lymphatic flow patterns in the neck (Table 15–1). Fiberoptic examinations of the nasopharynx and hypopharynx can be performed under topical anesthesia in the office. Fine-needle aspiration of a mass can be performed at the initial examination. CT scans show the primary site in 15% of cases, but in most cases the primary is evident from clinical findings. Examination under anesthesia is required to thoroughly inspect all regions. Any abnormal areas should be biopsied. The most common sites of occult tumors are the nasopharynx, hypopharynx (piriform sinus), and oropharynx (tonsillar fossa and base of tongue), but lung and esophagus occasionally are implicated. Treatment is based on the extent and location of disease in the neck. When nodes are confined to the parotid area, an appropriate parotidectomy is performed (see salivary gland tumors). Cervical metastases should be treated by radical neck dissection, although a modified neck dissection may be used for minimal disease not close to the spinal accessory nerve. Postoperative radiation is recommended when there are multiple involved nodes or any node with extracapsular extension. Bilateral neck irradiation is used only for bilateral metastases. Prophylactic irradiation of all potential primary sites is not recommended. When the primary is not found initially and treatment is limited to the involved neck, only 20% of patients ever have the primary tumor identified. The cure rate is about 40% in the presence of lymph node metastases above the supraclavicular fossa. Involved nodes lower in the neck are associated with 5% survival at 5 years. All of the above statistics refer to patients with squamous cell carcinoma. Other histologic types have different prognoses.

Beenken SW, Urist MM: Solitary neck mass. In: *Current Surgical Therapy–4.* Cameron JL (editor). BC Decker, 1991.

Shah JP: Cervical lymph node metastases: Diagnostic, therapeutic, and prognostic implications. Oncology 1990; 4(10):61.

NECK METASTASES FROM PRIMARIES OUTSIDE THE HEAD & NECK

Only 15% of lymph node metastases in the neck come from primaries below the clavicles (see Figure 15–1). Most of these metastases arise in lower jugular chain and supraclavicular nodes, particularly on the left side. This is because lymphatic drainage terminates on the left side of the neck from (1) all areas below the diaphragm, (2) the left upper extremity, and (3) the left lung. The most common primary site is the lung; other sites include the pancreas, esophagus, stomach, breast, ovary, and prostate. Involved lymph nodes in the lower jugular chain on either side are particularly difficult to detect unless one palpates them between the index finger and thumb in the area medial to the sternocleidomastoid muscle. Aspiration needle biopsy is useful for differentiating adenocarcinoma from squamous cell tumors. CT scans of the chest and abdomen should be performed, but they reveal the primary in only 25% of cases. While most lesions that present this way have no effective treatment, it is important to diagnose breast, prostate, and genital cancers, which often do respond to specific therapy.

SALIVARY GLAND TUMORS

Salivary tissue consists of glands divided according to size into major and minor glands. The paired major salivary glands consist of the parotid and submandibular glands. The minor salivary glands are widely distributed in the mucosa of the lips, cheeks, hard and soft palate, uvula, floor of mouth, tongue, and peritonsillar region; a few are found in the nasopharynx, paranasal sinuses, larynx, trachea, bronchi, and lacrimal glands. Most salivary tumors occur in the parotid.

Tumors of salivary tissue constitute about 5% of head and neck tumors and affect major salivary glands five times more often than minor salivary glands. The incidence of malignancy among salivary gland tumors varies inversely with the size of the gland. About 25% of parotid tumors, 40% of submandibular gland tumors, and 70% of sublingual and minor salivary gland tumors are malignant. Since 70% of salivary gland tumors occur in the parotid and three-fourths of these are benign, the majority of salivary gland neoplasms are benign.

Salivary gland tumors are thought to originate from two cell types: intercalated and excretory duct reserve cells. Myoepithelial cells are present in many salivary tumors but rarely as the principal malignant cell type. A classification of salivary tumors is given in Table 15–3.

Benign Salivary Gland Tumors

The commonest benign tumor is the mixed salivary

Table 15–3. Classification of primary epithelial salivary gland tumors.

I. **Benign**
  Mixed tumor (pleomorphic adenoma)
  Warthin's tumor (papillary cystadenoma lymphomatosum)
  Oncocytoma
  Monomorphic tumor
  Sebaceous tumor
  Benign lymphoepithelial lesion
  Papillary ductal adenoma (papilloma)

II. **Malignant**
  Mucoepidermoid carcinoma: low-grade, intermediate-grade, high-grade
  Adenoid cystic carcinoma
  Acinic cell carcinoma
  Adenocarcinoma
  Clear cell carcinoma
  Malignant oncocytoma
  Carcinoma ex pleomorphic adenoma
  True malignant mixed carcinoma (biphasic malignancy)
  Primary squamous cell carcinoma
  Epithelial-myoepithelial carcinoma
  Undifferentiated carcinoma

gland tumor, or pleomorphic adenoma, which accounts for 70% of parotid tumors and 50% of all salivary gland tumors. Pleomorphic adenomas are more common in women than in men, and the peak incidence is the fifth decade. They are slow-growing, lobular, and not well encapsulated. They may become very large without interfering with facial nerve function. Although mixed tumors are benign, they recur unless completely removed. Enucleation is inadequate. When tumor recurs in the parotid region, the facial nerve is at greater risk from damage during reoperation than it was during the initial procedure. Malignant transformation in a benign tumor is uncommon.

Warthin's tumor (papillary cystadenoma lymphomatosum), the next most common benign tumor, accounts for about 5% of parotid neoplasms. It is believed to arise from ectopic epithelial salivary tissue within lymph nodes external to or within the parotid gland. Warthin's tumors are usually cystic, typically occur in men in the sixth and seventh decades, and are bilateral in about 10% of cases. They occur almost exclusively in the parotid gland and have a typical histologic appearance, consisting of a papillary-cystic pattern with a marked lymphoid component. The latter is not part of the neoplastic process.

Oncocytomas are benign tumors composed of large oxyphilic cells called oncocytes. On electron microscopy, the cytoplasm of the oxyphilic cells is packed with mitochondria.

Monomorphic tumors are rare benign salivary gland tumors that are usually epithelial (but occasionally myoepithelial) in origin. They may be related to benign mixed tumor and are most commonly seen in minor salivary glands of the lip.

The differential diagnosis of a swelling in the parotid region includes parotitis, primary salivary neoplasm, upper jugular chain node enlargement, tumor of the tail of the submandibular gland, enlarged preauricular or parotid lymph node, branchial cleft cyst, epithelial inclusion cyst, or any mesenchymal neoplasm.

Treatment

Benign salivary tumors should be excised. Adequate exposure of the parotid gland requires a preauricular incision carried into the neck to allow adequate exposure of the gland and facial nerve. The aim of the operation is to completely excise the tumor with an adequate margin of normal tissue. In the parotid, the minimum adequate operation is superficial parotidectomy, which entails removal of the salivary tissue superficial to the facial nerve. Enucleation should be avoided because it greatly increases the likelihood of recurrence and nerve damage. When a tumor arises in the gland deep to the facial nerve, a superficial parotidectomy is performed, the facial nerve is preserved, and the tumor deep to the nerve is removed.

Benign tumors of the submandibular gland require total removal of the gland for diagnosis and treatment. Aspiration biopsy may be helpful if cancer is suspected. The entire contents of the submandibular triangle should be removed.

Since tumors of minor salivary tissue have a higher likelihood of being malignant, they should be initially biopsied (aspiration biopsy) so that appropriate definitive treatment can be planned. If a preoperative diagnosis of cancer has not been made, frozen section should be done during surgery so that an appropriately radical procedure can be performed as indicated.

Malignant Salivary Tumors

Mucoepidermoid carcinoma is the most common parotid cancer. Acinic cell carcinomas are derived from serous acinar cells and thus are found almost exclusively in the parotid gland. Adenoid cystic carcinomas, which are uncommon in the parotid, have a great propensity for local recurrence and perineural invasion. Patients with this tumor tend to have a protracted illness, with recurrences appearing 15 years or more after treatment. Patients with distant metastases from adenoid cystic carcinoma may survive for 5 or more years. In the parotid region, the presence of pain, rapid recent enlargement of a preexisting nodule, skin involvement, or facial nerve paralysis suggests cancer. Enlarged lymph nodes in association with a salivary gland mass should always be considered a manifestation of cancer until proved otherwise. Less common tumors include carcinoma arising in a pleomorphic adenoma and primary squamous cell carcinoma. The former is typically an adenocarcinoma for which the synonym "malignant mixed tumor" should be avoided, since it implies cancer of both the epithelial and the myoepithelial components, which is exceedingly rare. Primary squamous carcinomas—approximately 1% of salivary cancers—must be differentiated from mucoepidermoid carcinoma and metastatic squamous carcinoma in a parotid lymph node.

Among minor salivary cancers, adenoid cystic carcinoma is the most common, followed by adenocarcinoma and mucoepidermoid carcinoma. Approximately 70% of all minor salivary tumors occur in the oral cavity, principally in the hard palate. The prognosis varies according to the site of origin, with tumors of the nasal cavity and sinuses having the worst prognosis. They often present at an advanced stage with local destruction. Neither the symptoms nor the gross appearance helps predict the histology, so biopsy is necessary.

Treatment

The diagnosis of cancer may be obvious when facial nerve paralysis or other evidence of local nodal invasion is present: under such circumstances, aggressive treatment can be planned. In general, complete local excision with a margin of normal tissue is the appropriate form of biopsy, which in the parotid region means superficial parotidectomy. For submandibular tumors, the entire submandibular triangle should be cleared. In contrast, minor salivary tumors are better biopsied using an incisional or punch technique, so the surgeon who will carry out definitive treatment can assess the site and extent of the lesion. Frozen section examination is adequate to confirm the diagnosis.

Surgical treatment depends on the extent of disease. Unless the facial nerve is paralyzed or found to be directly invaded by tumor at surgery, it should be preserved. Extensive invasion of parotid or submandibular tumors beyond the gland requires a radical resection designed to completely remove the lesion. For localized low-grade tumors, complete excision is usually sufficient. For high-grade malignancy or incomplete excision, postoperative radiotherapy is indicated for the primary site and draining lymph nodes. Postoperative radiotherapy is also appropriate following extensive resections for advanced tumors. Clinically involved lymph nodes should be removed by an appropriate neck dissection, but prophylactic neck dissection is unnecessary except perhaps for submandibular gland cancers, where this would facilitate radical excision of the primary. Radical surgery is usually not performed when distant metastases are present, except for adenoid cystic carcinoma.

When the facial nerve must be divided, it should be repaired (if functioning) prior to surgery. After planned surgical excision, the facial nerve can be reconstructed using a nerve graft, eg, the sural nerve. Complete recovery may take up to 2 years.

Prognosis

Prognosis depends on the clinical stage, the histologic grade, the tumor site, the patient's age, and the completeness of removal. The most important is the clinical stage of the disease. The prognosis for patients with stage I and stage II disease is good after adequate treatment. The prognosis is poor regardless of treatment in the face of local extension or lymph node or distant metastases.

The next most important factor is the histologic grade of the tumor. Low-grade tumors, such as acinic cell carcinomas and low-grade mucoepidermoid tumors, have an excellent prognosis; survival rates at 10 years are about 80%. The 10-year survival rate after treatment of high-grade lesions, such as malignant pleomorphic adenoma (adenocarcinoma), squamous cell carcinoma, and high-grade mucoepidermoid carcinoma, is about 30%.

Armstrong JG et al: Observations on the natural history and treatment of recurrent major salivary gland cancer. J Surg Oncol 1990;44:138.

Armstrong JG et al: Malignant tumors of major salivary gland origin: A matched-pair analysis of the role of combined surgery and post-operative radiotherapy. Arch Otolaryngol Head Neck Surg 1990;116:290.

Batsakis JG, Luna MA: Undifferentiated carcinomas of salivary glands. Ann Otol Rhinol Laryngol 1991;100:82.

Lewis JE, Olsen KD, Weiland LH: Acinic cell carcinoma: Clinicopathologic review. Cancer 1991;67:172.

Rodriguez-Bigas MA et al: Benign parotid tumors: A 24-year experience. J Surg Oncol 1991;46:159.

Shaha AR et al: Needle aspiration biopsy in salivary gland lesions. Am J Surg 1990;160:373.

Spiro RH et al: Carcinoma of major salivary glands: Recent trends. Arch Otolaryngol Head Neck Surg 1989;115:316.

Weber RS et al: Minor salivary gland tumors of the lip and buccal mucosa. Laryngoscope 1989;99:6.

Weber RS et al: Submandibular gland tumors. Adverse histologic factors and therapeutic implications. Arch Otolaryngol Head Neck Surg 1990;116:1055.

RECONSTRUCTION FOLLOWING HEAD & NECK SURGERY

The primary aim of head and neck surgery is complete eradication of disease. This is most likely to be achieved at the initial attempt, since treatment of recurrences is less successful. The dilemma is that surgery which achieves a good therapeutic result may be cosmetically and functionally unacceptable.

Surgical defects can be repaired by direct closure, skin grafting, or tissue transfer. Direct closure is ideal for small lesions of the skin and for mucosa of the oral cavity and oropharynx. Direct closure of large defects in the oral cavity and oropharynx can create distortion, with tongue tethering and so forth, and should be avoided. Skin grafts may be used for defects of the skin or mucosa of the mouth and oropharynx. The advantage is that skin grafting can be done quickly and avoids a lengthy reconstructive operation. Recurrences can be recognized earlier when a skin graft is used compared with a flap.

New tissue to close surgical defects may be obtained in several ways, including local rotation or transposition skin flaps for the skin of the face and neck and local flaps of buccal or tongue mucosa for small defects in the oral cavity. To close larger defects, tissue can be transferred from more distant sites using skin flaps (deltopectoral flap and forehead flap); myocutaneous flaps (pectoralis major flap and latissimus dorsi flap); and vascularized free tissue transfers, also called free flaps (radial forearm flap). Each of these techniques has advantages and disadvantages, and the reconstructive procedure must be tailored to the patient and the site and extent of operative defect.

Jaw reconstruction poses technical difficulties, but vascularized free compound flaps such as the deep circumflex iliac artery osteomyocutaneous flap appear to be most reliable. Most surgeons try to preserve the mandible when it is not invaded by tumor; but when a segmental resection is required, the continuity of the mandibular arch is disturbed, which leads to deformity. If part of the horizontal or vertical ramus of the mandible is resected, the resulting cosmetic and functional disturbance is usually acceptable. Removal of the anterior part of the mandibular arch destroys the contour of the chin and creates the so called "Andy Gump" deformity, which severely affects eating, speech, and appearance. Such defects should be reconstructed when operative risk is acceptable.

Prostheses are especially useful following amputation of the nose or ear or after orbital exenteration. A good facsimile of the lost part can usually be attached to a pair of glasses. Excellent function can be attained with dental obturators for patients with defects in the hard palate and upper alveolar ridges.

Argerakis GP: Psychosocial considerations of the post-treatment of head and neck cancer patients. Dent Clin North Am 1990;34:285.

de Vries EJ et al: Jejunal interposition for repair of stricture or fistula after laryngectomy. Ann Otol Rhinol Laryngol 1990;99:496.

Gahhos FN, Cuono CB: Double-Z rhombic technique for reconstruction of facial wounds. Plast Reconstr Surg 1990;85:869.

Goodman AL, Donald PJ: Use of the levator scapulae muscle flap in head and neck reconstruction. Arch Otolaryngol Head Neck Surg 1990;116:1440.

Kroll SS et al: Analysis of complications in 168 pectoralis major myocutaneous flaps used for head and neck reconstruction. Ann Plast Surg 1990;25:93.

Salibian AH et al: Total and subtotal glossectomy: Function after microvascular reconstruction. Plast Reconstr Surg 1990;85:513.

RADIATION THERAPY

Radiotherapy may be used as definitive treatment with curative intent, as a postoperative adjunct to surgery, or for palliation.

Definitive Radiotherapy

Mucosal squamous carcinomas are sensitive to irradiation, especially if they are small and only superficially invasive. Tumors of the oral cavity and oropharynx stage T_1 and T_2 (ie, 4 cm in diameter) may be equally well treated with surgery or radiotherapy. In some cases, radiotherapy has the advantage of avoiding the disfiguring side effects of surgery while being equally effective. However, mucositis, subsequent xerostomia, the possibility of osteoradionecrosis, and logistic problems associated with radiotherapy must be considered. Local control rates are about 70%, and 5-year cure rates are about 50% for early oral cancers, so radiotherapy is an acceptable alternative to surgery in many cases. Large oral cavity tumors respond poorly to radiotherapy, and surgery is most often the best treatment for these lesions, sometimes followed by local radiotherapy. In the oropharynx, especially for the tonsil, radiotherapy is best for small tumors, because the response rate is good and the neck can be irradiated simultaneously to treat occult metastatic disease. Large tumors of the tonsil require surgery combined with radiotherapy. The surgical treatment of tongue base cancers larger than about 3 cm usually entails total glossectomy and laryngectomy—a procedure with considerable morbidity. Radiotherapy is often the best initial treatment for these lesions, with surgery reserved for treatment failures.

Nasopharyngeal tumors are usually responsive to radiotherapy, and resection is usually not possible. A common side effect is occlusion of the auditory tube and subsequent otitis media. Irradiation may be used to treat nasal and paranasal sinus cancers, but current evidence suggests that surgery followed by radiation therapy gives better results. Radiotherapy is excellent for early (T_1 or T_2) laryngeal cancers and has the advantage that speech is preserved. Five-year survival rates range from 70% to 90% depending on the extent of disease.

Palpable neck metastases are sometimes treated by radiotherapy alone if they are small (ie, < 3 cm in diameter). If nodes remain palpable after treatment, neck dissection is necessary. In general, however, overt metastatic disease in the neck is best treated initially by neck dissection.

In most of these situations, treatment is given in fractions of 180–200 cGy, 5 days a week for approximately 6 weeks. Doses of 6000–7000 cGy are delivered to the primary site. When lymph nodes are not palpable but there is a high likelihood that they harbor occult cancer, elective irradiation to the neck to a dose of 5000 cGy is often added.

Changes in fraction size and timing have been used to decrease tumor cell regeneration during treatment. Current radiotherapy protocols involve (1) accelerated fractionation, giving two or three fractions per day and shortening the overall duration of treatment; (2) hyperfractionation, giving two or three smaller fractions per day but maintaining the overall treatment duration; (3) accelerated hyperfractionation, reducing overall treatment time through a combination of greater fraction number and smaller fraction size; and (4) concomitant boost, giving a second daily dose radiation to a reduced "field within a field" during the course of conventional radiotherapy. It is as yet unclear whether these techniques improve local-regional control.

Adjuvant Radiotherapy

Surgery is often combined with radiotherapy to improve tumor control. Preoperative radiotherapy has been used, but it has two disadvantages: It produces edema and increased vascularity of the operative field, and it alters the lesion so that accurate histologic assessment is impossible. Therefore, postoperative radiotherapy is more popular. Treatment can be more selective, since it is reserved for patients known from clinical or histologic findings to be at high risk of recurrence. Examples include a large primary lesion (T_3 or T_4), tumors of high histologic grade or poor differentiation, histologically positive surgical margins, macroscopic residual disease, and perineural invasion.

Treatment is usually started after the wound has healed. After a neck dissection in which positive lymph nodes have been found, adjuvant radiotherapy improves control when multiple lymph nodes are positive and when disease has spread beyond the node capsule.

When radiotherapy is given preoperatively, the dose is usually 4500 or 5000 cGy; when given postoperatively, the dose is 5000–6000 cGy, sometimes with a boost to an area of high risk.

Palliative Radiotherapy

In some instances, where the primary tumor is very large and not surgically resectable or metastatic neck disease is fixed, radiotherapy may be given in high doses (eg, 6000 cGy or more), but with palliation as the most realistic goal. Occasionally the response is good, and previously unresectable disease is sometimes rendered resectable. Nonetheless, the prognosis still depends on the original extent of disease, and the chances of cure are low.

The effects of radiotherapy are additive; once a full course of treatment has been given to an area, the tissue can tolerate no more without risking major complications. Surgical procedures in a previously irradiated field are more difficult, and tumors previously treated by radiotherapy tend to respond poorly to later chemotherapy. The main acute complications of radiotherapy are dermatitis and mucositis, which, if severe, may require treatment to be suspended temporarily or terminated. Long-term complications include fibrosis and vascular sclerosis, severe xerostomia, and osteoradionecrosis. Patients with bad teeth should have them extracted before radiotherapy. Those who retain their teeth must maintain excellent dental hygiene.

Ang KK, Peters LJ: Concomitant boost radiotherapy schedules in the treatment of carcinoma of the oropharynx and nasopharynx. Int J Radiation Oncol Biol Phys 1990;19:1339.

Datta NR et al: Twice a day versus once a day radiation therapy in head and neck cancer. Int J Radiation Oncol Biol Phys 1989;17(Suppl 1):132.

Friedman M et al: Effects of therapeutic radiation on the development of multiple primary tumors of the head and neck. Head Neck Surg 1988;10(Suppl 1):S48.

Marcial VA et al: Radiation Therapy Oncology Group (RTOG) studies in head and neck cancer. Semin Oncol 1988;15:39.

Parsons JT et al: Hyperfractionation for head and neck cancer. Int J Radiation Oncol Biol 1988;14:649.

Wang CC: Local control of oropharyngeal carcinoma after two accelerated hyperfractionation radiation therapy schemes. Int J Radiation Oncol Biol Phys 1988;14:1143.

ANTITUMOR CHEMOTHERAPY

For patients with locoregionally advanced head and neck cancer (stage III or IV), surgery and radiotherapy have generally been used sequentially for maximum control. Nevertheless, few patients are cured, so concomitant chemoradiotherapy regimens are now being studied.

Induction Chemotherapy

Untreated patients with advanced head and neck cancer who respond to chemotherapy live longer, and they also tend to respond to radiotherapy. This suggests that if those who respond to induction chemotherapy were subsequently given radiotherapy, surgery might be unnecessary. In one prospective, randomized trial, patients with stage III or stage IV laryngeal cancer received either induction chemotherapy using fluorouracil and cisplatin with subsequent radiotherapy or surgery followed by radiotherapy. Patients not responding to chemotherapy were crossed over to the surgery plus radiotherapy arm. The results showed no difference in survival between the two groups, but about 60% of patients treated with induction chemotherapy and subsequent radiotherapy avoided surgery and maintained laryngeal function. A second trial is being conducted that will investigate the potential of induction chemotherapy and subsequent radiotherapy for stage III and stage IV disease in the oropharynx and hypopharynx. At this time, induction chemotherapy is investigational—not standard therapy—and should not be used outside of clinical trials.

Concomitant Chemotherapy

Another strategy under investigation is whether simultaneous chemotherapy and radiotherapy can control micrometastatic systemic disease while enhancing the locoregional effects of radiotherapy. Several single agents have been shown to improve disease-free survival (bleomycin, mitocycin, fluorouracil) when used with concomitant radiotherapy, though the differences are small and are offset by the toxicity of the regimen.

Toxicity is even more severe when more than one drug is used in combination with radiotherapy. Therefore, combination chemotherapy may be used with protracted (split-course) radiotherapy, where scheduled interruptions of all therapy allow normal tissue to recover. Phase I and phase II studies using infusional fluorouracil with cisplatin or hydroxyurea—or cisplatin with fluorouracil or leucovorin plus hyperfractionated radiotherapy—have given encouraging results. To date, none of these regimens have been compared with standard therapy in a randomized trial.

Chemoprevention

Chemoprevention consists of pharmacologic inhibition of carcinogenesis or the reversal of premalignant changes. To be worthwhile, a chemopreventive agent requires the identification of individuals at high risk for development of head and neck cancer.

Data from in vitro animal and epidemiologic studies show that retinoic acid (vitamin A) can prevent epithelial carcinogenesis in the epithelium of the trachea, lung, and oral cavity. A randomized placebo-controlled trial of isotretinoin (13-cis-retinoic acid) in the treatment of oral leukoplakia showed a clinical response rate of 67%. Relapse was common after treatment was stopped. This and other studies indicate that isotretinoin is effective maintenance treatment in oral premalignancy. More work is needed to define the molecular events involved.

Demard F et al: Response to chemotherapy as a justification for modification of the therapeutic strategy for pharyngolaryngeal carcinomas. Head Neck Surg 1990;12:225.

Hong WK et al: 13-cis-Retinoic acid in the treatment of oral leukoplakia. N Engl J Med 1986;315:1501.

Hong WK et al: Prevention of second primary tumors with isotretinoin in squamous-cell carcinoma of the head and neck. N Engl J Med 1990;323:795.

Spaulding MB, Lore JM, Sundquist N: Long-term follow-up of chemotherapy in advanced head and neck cancer. Arch Otolaryngol Head Neck Surg 1989;115:68.

Stitch HF et al: Remission of oral leukoplakias and micronuclei in tobacco/betel quid chewers treated with beta-carotene and with beta-carotene plus vitamin A. Int J Cancer 1988;42:195.

Vokes EE et al: Cisplatin, fluorouracil, and high-dose leucovorin for recurrent or metastatic head and neck cancer. J Clin Oncol 1988;6:618.

Vokes EE et al: Induction chemotherapy with cisplatin, fluorouracil and high dose leukovorin for locally advanced head and neck cancer: A clinical and pharmacologic analysis. J Clin Oncol 1990;8:241.

Vokes EE et al: Neoadjuvant and adjuvant methotrexate, cisplatin, and fluorouracil in multimodal therapy of head and neck cancer. J Clin Oncol 1989;7:838.

REFERENCES

American Joint Committee for Cancer Staging and End Results Reporting: *Manual for Staging of Cancer,* 3rd ed. Lippincott, 1988.

Batsakis JG: *Tumors of the Head and Neck: Clinical and Pathological Considerations,* 2nd ed. Williams and Wilkins, 1979.

Jacobs CD, Goffinet DR, Free WE Jr: Head and neck squamous cancers. Curr Probl Cancer 1990;14(1):1.

Kagan AR, Miles J (editors): *Head and Neck Oncology: Clinical Management.* Pergamon 1989.

Lore JM: *An Atlas of Head and Neck Surgery,* vols 1 and 2. Saunders, 1988.

Million RR, Cassissi NJ, Clark Jr: Cancer of the head and neck. In: *Cancer: Principles and Practice of Oncology.* DeVita VT Jr (editor). Lippincott, 1991.

Myers EN, Suen JY (editors). *Cancer of the Head and Neck.* Churchill Livingstone, 1989.

Taramore GE (editor). *Radiation Therapy of Head and Neck Cancer.* Springer-Verlag, 1989.

16 Thyroid & Parathyroid

Orlo H. Clark, MD

I. THE THYROID GLAND

EMBRYOLOGY & ANATOMY
(Figure 16–1)

The main anlage of the thyroid gland develops as a median entodermal downgrowth from the first and second pharyngeal pouches. During its migration caudally, it contacts the ultimobranchial bodies developing from the fourth pharyngeal pouches. When it reaches the position it occupies in the adult, just below the cricoid cartilage, the thyroid divides into two lobes. The site from which it originated persists as the foramen cecum at the base of the tongue. The path the gland follows may result in thyroglossal remnants (cysts) or ectopic thyroid tissue (lingual thyroid). A pyramidal lobe is frequently present. Agenesis of one thyroid lobe may occur.

The normal thyroid weighs 15–25 g and is attached to the trachea by loose connective tissue. It is a highly vascularized organ that derives its blood supply principally from the superior and inferior thyroid arteries. A thyroid ima artery may also be present.

PHYSIOLOGY

The function of the thyroid gland is to synthesize, store, and secrete the hormones thyroxine (T_4) and triiodothyronine (T_3). Iodide is absorbed from the gastrointestinal tract and actively trapped by the acinar cells of the thyroid gland. It is then oxidized and combined with tyrosine in thyroglobulin to form monoiodotyrosine (MIT) and diiodotyrosine (DIT). These are coupled to form the active hormones T_4 and T_3, which initially are stored in the colloid of the gland. Following hydrolysis of the thyroglobulin, T_4 and T_3 are secreted into the plasma, becoming almost instantaneously bound to plasma proteins. Most T_3 in euthyroid individuals, however, is produced by extrathyroidal conversion of T_4 to T_3.

The function of the thyroid gland is regulated by a feedback mechanism that involves the hypothalamus and pituitary. Thyrotropin-releasing factor (TRF), a tripeptide amide, is formed in the hypothalamus and stimulates the release of thyrotropin (TSH), a glycoprotein, from the pituitary. Thyrotropin binds to TSH receptors on the thyroid plasma membrane, stimulating increased adenylyl cyclase activity; this increases cAMP production and thyroid cellular function. Thyrotropin also stimulates the phosphoinositide pathway and—along with cAMP—may stimulate thyroid growth.

Baxter JD: Advances in molecular biology: Potential impact on diagnosis and treatment of disorders of the thyroid. Med Clin North Am 1991;75:41.

Cavalieri RR: The effects of nonthyroid disease and drugs on thyroid function tests. Med Clin North Am 1991;75:27.

Clark OH: Surgical anatomy. In: *Werner and Ingbar's The Thyroid.* Braverman LE, Utiger RD (editors). Lippincott, 1991.

Nicoloff J, Spencer CA: The use and misuse of the sensitive thyrotropin assays. J Clin Endocrinol Metab 1991;71:553.

EVALUATION OF THE THYROID

In a patient with enlargement of the thyroid (goiter), the history and examination of the gland are most important and are complemented by the selective use of thyroid function tests. The surgeon must develop a systematic method of palpating the gland to determine its size, contour, consistency, nodularity, and fixation and to examine for displacement of the trachea and the presence of palpable cervical lymph nodes.

Thyroid function is assessed by highly sensitive TSH assays that can differentiate between patients with hypothyroidism (increased TSH levels), euthyroidism, and hyperthyroidism (increased TSH levels). In most cases, therefore, serum T_3, T_4, and other variables do not need to be measured. A free T_4 level is helpful in some patients with suspected hyper- or hypothyroidism, and free T_4 along with the TSH level can identify the occasional patient with low TSH and low free T_4 level. A serum T_3 level is useful for diagnosing T_3 toxicosis (high T_3 and low TSH), or the euthyroid sick, low T_3 syndrome (low T_3 and normal or slightly increased TSH).

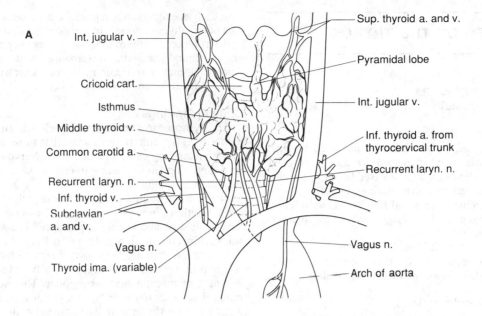

A

Int. jugular v.

Cricoid cart.

Isthmus

Middle thyroid v.

Common carotid a.

Recurrent laryn. n.

Inf. thyroid v.

Subclavian a. and v.

Vagus n.

Thyroid ima. (variable)

Sup. thyroid a. and v.

Pyramidal lobe

Int. jugular v.

Inf. thyroid a. from thyrocervical trunk

Recurrent laryn. n.

Vagus n.

Arch of aorta

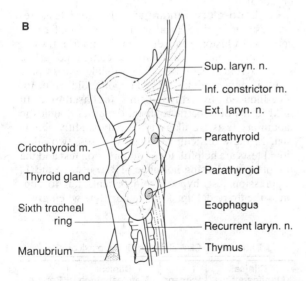

B

Sup. laryn. n.

Inf. constrictor m.

Ext. laryn. n.

Parathyroid

Parathyroid

Esophagus

Recurrent laryn. n.

Thymus

Cricothyroid m.

Thyroid gland

Sixth tracheal ring

Manubrium

Figure 16–1. Thyroid anatomy.

Radioactive iodine (RAI) uptake is useful for differentiating between hyperthyroidism and increased secretion of thyroid hormone (low TSH and increased radioactive iodine uptake) on the one hand and subacute thyroiditis (low TSH and low radioactive iodine uptake) on the other. Patients with the latter "leak" thyroid hormone from the gland which suppresses serum TSH levels and, consequently, iodine uptake by the thyroid. Patients with Graves' disease have increased levels of thyroid-stimulating immunoglobulins that increase iodine uptake despite low TSH levels.

DISEASES OF THE THYROID

HYPERTHYROIDISM
(Thyrotoxicosis)

Essentials of Diagnosis

- Nervousness, weight loss with increased appetite, heat intolerance, increased sweating, muscular weakness and fatigue, increased bowel frequency, polyuria, menstrual irregularities, infertility.
- Goiter, tachycardia, atrial fibrillation, warm moist skin, thyroid thrill and bruit, cardiac flow murmur; gynecomastia.
- Eye signs: stare, lid lag, exophthalmos.
- TSH low or absent; TSI, iodine uptake, T_3, and T_4 increased; T_3 suppression test abnormal.

General Considerations

Hyperthyroidism is caused by the increased secretion of thyroid hormone (**Graves' disease, Plummer's disease,** iodine **[jodbasedow],** amiodarone toxicity, TSH-secreting pituitary tumors, hCG-secreting tumors) or by other disorders that increase thyroid hormone levels without increasing thyroid gland secretion (factitious hyperthyroidism, subacute thyroiditis, struma ovarii, and, rarely, metastatic thyroid cancers that secrete excess thyroid hormone). The most common causes of hyperthyroidism are diffusely hypersecretory goiter (Graves' disease) and nodular toxic goiter (Plummer's disease).

In all forms, the symptoms of hyperthyroidism are due to increased levels of thyroid hormone in the bloodstream. The clinical manifestations of thyrotoxicosis may be subtle or marked and tend to go through periods of exacerbation and remission. Some patients ultimately develop hypothyroidism spontaneously or as a result of treatment. Graves' disease is an autoimmune disease, whereas the etiology of Plummer's disease is unknown. Most cases of hyperthyroidism are easily diagnosed on the basis of the signs and symptoms; others (eg, mild or **apathetic hyperthyroidism**) may be recognized only with difficulty.

Thyrotoxicosis has been described with a normal T_4 concentration, normal or elevated radioiodine uptake, and normal protein binding, but with increased serum T_3 by RIA (**T_3 toxicosis**). **T_4 pseudothyrotoxicosis** is occasionally seen in critically ill patients and is characterized by increased levels of T_4 and decreased levels of T_3 due to failure to convert T_4 to T_3. Thyrotoxicosis associated with toxic nodular goiter is usually less severe than that associated with Graves' disease and is only rarely if ever associated with the extrathyroidal manifestations of Graves' disease such as exophthalmos, pretibial myxedema, thyroid acropathy, or periodic hypocalcemic paralysis.

If left untreated, thyrotoxicosis causes progressive and profound catabolic disturbances and cardiac damage. Death may occur in thyroid storm or because of heart failure or severe cachexia.

Clinical Findings

A. Symptoms and Signs: The clinical findings are those of hyperthyroidism as well as those related to the underlying cause (Table 16–1). Nervousness, increased diaphoresis, heat intolerance, tachycardia, palpitations, fatigue, and weight loss in association with a nodular, multinodular, or diffuse goiter are the classic findings in hyperthyroidism. The patient may have a flushed and staring appearance. The skin is warm, thin, and moist, and the hair is fine.

In Graves' disease, there may be exophthalmos, pretibial myxedema, or vitiligo, virtually never seen in single or multinodular toxic goiter. The Achilles reflex time is shortened in hyperthyroidism and prolonged in hypothyroidism. The patient on the verge of thyroid storm has accentuated symptoms and signs of thyrotoxicosis, with hyperpyrexia, tachycardia, cardiac failure, neuromuscular excitation, delirium, or jaundice.

B. Laboratory Findings: Laboratory tests reveal a suppressed TSH and an elevation of T_3, free T_4, and RAI. A history of medications is important, since certain drugs and organic iodinated compounds affect some thyroid function tests, and iodide excess may result in either iodide-induced hypothyroidism or iodine-induced hyperthyroidism (**jodbasedow**). In mild forms of hyperthyroidism, the usual diagnostic laboratory tests are likely to be only slightly abnormal. In these difficult to diagnose cases, two additional tests are helpful: the T_3 suppression test and the thyrotropin-releasing hormone (TRH) test. In the T_3 suppression test, hyperthyroid patients fail to suppress the thyroidal uptake of radioiodine when given

Table 16–1. Clinical findings in thyrotoxicosis.*

Clinical Manifestations	Percent	Clinical Manifestations	Percent
Tachycardia	100	Weakness	70
Goiter	98	Increased appetite	65
Nervousness	99	Eye complaints	54
Skin changes	97	Leg swelling	35
Tremor	97	Hyperdefecation (without diarrhea)	33
Increased sweating	91		
Hypersensitivity to heat	89	Diarrhea	23
		Atrial fibrillation	10
Palpitations	89	Splenomegaly	10
Fatigue	88	Gynecomastia	10
Weight loss	85	Anorexia	9
Bruit over thyroid	77	Liver palms	8
Dyspnea	75	Constipation	4
Eye signs	71	Weight gain	2

*Data from Williams RH: *J Clin Endocrinol Metab* 1946:**6**:1.

exogenous T_3. In the TRH test, serum TSH levels fail to rise in response to administration of TRH in hyperthyroid patients.

Other findings include a high thyroid-stimulating immunoglobulin (TSI) level, low serum cholesterol, lymphocytosis, and occasionally hypercalcemia, hypercalciuria, or glycosuria.

Differential Diagnosis

Anxiety neurosis, heart disease, anemia, gastrointestinal disease, cirrhosis, tuberculosis, myasthenia and other muscular disorders, menopausal syndrome, pheochromocytoma, primary ophthalmopathy, and thyrotoxicosis factitia may be clinically difficult to differentiate from hyperthyroidism. Differentiation is especially difficult when the thyrotoxic patient presents with minimal or no thyroid enlargement. Patients may also have painless or spontaneously resolving thyroiditis and are hyperthyroid because of increased release of thyroid hormone from the thyroid gland. This condition, however, is self-limited, and definitive treatment with antithyroid drugs, radioactive iodine, or surgery is not necessary.

Anxiety neurosis is perhaps the condition most frequently confused with hyperthyroidism. Anxiety is characterized by persistent fatigue usually unrelieved by rest, clammy palms, a normal sleeping pulse rate, and normal laboratory tests of thyroid function. The fatigue of hyperthyroidism is often relieved by rest, the palms are warm and moist, tachycardia persists during sleep, and thyroid function tests are abnormal.

Organic disease of nonthyroidal origin that may be confused with hyperthyroidism must be differentiated largely on the basis of evidence of specific organ system involvement and normal thyroid function tests.

Other causes of exophthalmos (eg, orbital tumors) or ophthalmoplegia (eg, myasthenia) must be ruled out by ophthalmologic, ultrasonographic, CT or MRI scans, and neurologic examinations.

Treatment

Hyperthyroidism may be effectively treated by antithyroid drugs, radioactive iodine, or thyroidectomy. Treatment must be individualized and depends on the patient's age and general state of health, the size of the goiter, the underlying pathologic process, and the patient's ability to obtain follow-up care.

A. Antithyroid Drugs: The principal antithyroid drugs used in the USA are propylthiouracil (PTU), 300–1000 mg orally daily, and methimazole, 30–100 mg orally daily. These agents interfere with organic binding of iodine and prevent coupling of iodotyrosines in the thyroid gland. One advantage over thyroidectomy and radioiodine in the treatment of Graves' disease is that drugs inhibit the function of the gland without destroying tissue; therefore, there is a lower incidence of subsequent hypothyroidism. This form of treatment may be used either as definitive treatment or in preparation for surgery or radioactive iodine treatment. When propylthiouracil is given as definitive treatment, the goal is to maintain the patient in a euthyroid state until a natural remission occurs. Reliable patients with small goiters are good candidates for this regimen. A prolonged remission after 18 months of treatment occurs in 30% of patients, some of whom eventually become hypothyroid. Side effects include rashes and fever (3–4%) and agranulocytosis (0.1–0.4%). Patients must be warned to stop the drug and see the physician if sore throat or fever develops.

B. Radioiodine: Radioiodine (^{131}I) may be given safely after the patient has been treated with antithyroid medications and has become euthyroid. Radioiodine is indicated for patients who are over 40 or are poor risks for surgery and for patients with recurrent hyperthyroidism. It is less expensive than operative treatment and is effective. To date, radioiodine treatment at doses necessary to treat hyperthyroidism has not been associated with an increase in leukemia, thyroid cancer, or the induction of congenital anomalies. However, an increased incidence of benign thyroid tumors has been noted to follow treatment of hyperthyroidism with radioiodine. In young patients, the radiation hazard is certainly increased, and the chance of developing hypothyroidism is virtually 100%. After the first year of treatment with radioiodine, the incidence of hypothyroidism increases about 3% per year.

Hyperthyroid children and pregnant women should not be treated with radioiodine.

C. Surgery:

1. Indications for subtotal thyroidectomy– The main advantages of subtotal thyroidectomy are rapid control of the disease and a lower incidence of hypothyroidism than can be achieved with radioiodine treatment. Surgery is often the preferred treatment (1) in the presence of a very large goiter or a multinodular goiter with relatively low radioactive iodine uptake; (2) if there is a thyroid nodule that may be malignant; (3) for the treatment of pregnant patients or children; (4) for the treatment of women who wish to become pregnant within 1 year after treatment; (5) for patients with amiodarone-induced hyperparathyroidism; and (6) for the treatment of psychologically or mentally incompetent patients or patients who are for any reason unable to maintain adequate long-term follow-up evaluation.

2. Preparation for surgery–The risk of thyroidectomy for toxic goiter has become negligible since the introduction of the combined preoperative use of iodides and antithyroid drugs. Propylthiouracil or another antithyroid drug is administered until the patient becomes euthyroid and is continued until the time of operation. Two to 5 drops of potassium iodide solution or Lugol's iodine solution are then given for 10–15 days before surgery in conjunction with the propylthiouracil to decrease the friability and vascularity of the thyroid, thereby technically facilitating thyroidectomy.

An occasional untreated or inadequately treated hyperthyroid patient may require an emergency operation for some unrelated problem such as acute appendicitis and thus require immediate control of the hyperthyroidism. Such a patient should be treated in a manner similar to one in thyroid storm, since **thyroid storm** or hyperthyroid crises may be precipitated by surgical stress or trauma. Treatment of hyperthyroid patients requiring emergency operation or those in thyroid storm is as follows: Prevent release of preformed thyroid hormone by administration of Lugol's iodine solution or with ipodate sodium; give the β-adrenergic blocking agent propranolol to antagonize the peripheral manifestations of thyrotoxicosis; and decrease thyroid hormone production and extrathyroidal conversion of T_4 to T_3 by giving propylthiouracil. The combined use of propranolol and iodide has been demonstrated to lower serum thyroid hormone levels. Other important considerations are to treat precipitating causes (eg, infection, drug reactions); to support vital functions by giving oxygen, sedatives, intravenous fluids, and corticosteroids; and to reduce fever. Reserpine may be useful in the patient in whom nervousness is a prominent symptom, and a cooling blanket should be used in patients requiring operation.

3. Subtotal thyroidectomy—The treatment of hyperthyroidism by subtotal thyroidectomy eliminates both the hyperthyroidism and the goiter. As a rule, all but 3–8 g of thyroid are removed, sparing the parathyroid glands and the recurrent laryngeal nerves.

The death rate associated with the procedure is extremely low—less than 0.1% in a recent collected review. Subtotal thyroidectomy thus provides safe and rapid correction of the thyrotoxic state. The frequency of recurrent hyperthyroidism and hypothyroidism depends on the amount of thyroid removed and on the natural history of the hyperthyroidism. Given an accomplished surgeon and good preoperative preparation, injuries to the recurrent laryngeal nerves and parathyroid glands occur in less than 2% of cases. Adequate exposure and precise identification of the vasculature, recurrent laryngeal nerves, and parathyroid glands are essential.

Ocular Manifestations of Graves' Disease

The pathogenesis of the ocular problems in Graves' disease remains unclear. Evidence originally supporting the role of either long-acting thyroid stimulator (LATS) or exophthalmos-producing substance (EPS) has not been authenticated.

The eye complications of Graves' disease may begin before there is any evidence of thyroid dysfunction or after the hyperthyroidism has been appropriately treated. Usually, however, the ocular manifestations develop concomitantly with the hyperthyroidism. Relief of the eye problems is often difficult to accomplish until coexisting hyperthyroidism or hypothyroidism is controlled.

The eye changes of Graves' disease vary from no signs or symptoms to loss of sight. Mild cases are characterized by upper lid retraction and stare with or without lid lag or proptosis. These cases present only minor cosmetic problems and require no treatment. When moderate to severe eye changes occur, there is soft tissue involvement with proptosis, extraocular muscle involvement, and finally optic nerve involvement. Some cases may have marked chemosis, periorbital edema, conjunctivitis, keratitis, diplopia, ophthalmoplegia, and impaired vision. Ophthalmologic consultation is required.

Treatment of the ocular problems of Graves' disease includes maintaining the patient in a euthyroid state without increase in TSH secretion, protecting the eyes from light and dust with dark glasses and eye shields, elevating the head of the bed, using diuretics to decrease periorbital and retrobulbar edema, and giving methylcellulose or guanethidine eye drops. High doses of glucocorticoids are beneficial in certain patients, but their effectiveness is variable and unpredictable. If exophthalmos progresses despite medical treatment, lateral tarsorrhaphy, retrobulbar irradiation, or surgical decompression of the orbit may be necessary. Total thyroid ablation has been recommended, but whether it has a beneficial effect is controversial. It is important that patients with ophthalmopathy be made aware of the natural history of the disease and also that they be kept euthyroid, since hyper- and hypothyroidism may produce visual deterioration. Operations to correct diplopia should be deferred until after the ophthalmopathy has stabilized.

DeGroot LJ, Quintans J: The causes of autoimmune thyroid disease. Endocr Rev 1989;10:537.

Goldstein R, Hart IR: Follow-up of solitary autonomous thyroid nodules treated with [131]I. N Engl J Med 1983;309:1473.

Lennquist S et al: Beta blockers compared with antithyroid drugs as preoperative treatment in hyperthyroidism: Drug tolerance, complications and postoperative thyroid function. Surgery 1985;98:1141.

McDougal IR: Graves' disease: Current concepts. Med Clin North Am 1991;75:79.

Nicoloff JT: Thyroid storm and myxedema coma. Med Clin North Am 1985;69:1005.

Solomon G et al: Current trends in the management of Graves' disease. J Clin Endocrinol Metab 1990;70:1518.

Sridama V et al: Long-term follow-up study of compensated low-dose ^{131}I therapy for Graves' disease. N Engl J Med 1984;311:426.

Zakarija M, McKenzie JM: Do thyroid growth-promoting immunoglobulins exist? J Clin Endocrinol Metab 1990; 70:308.

EVALUATION OF THYROID NODULES & GOITERS

Thyroid Nodules

The problems facing the clinician when confronted by a patient with a nodular goiter or thyroid nodule are whether the lesion is symptomatic and whether it is benign or malignant. The differential diagnosis includes benign goiter, intrathyroidal cysts, thyroiditis, and benign and malignant tumors. The history should specifically emphasize the duration of swelling, recent growth, local symptoms (dysphagia, pain, or voice changes), and systemic symptoms (hyperthyroidism, hypothyroidism, or those from possible tumors metastatic to the thyroid). The patient's age, sex, place of birth, family history, and history of radiation to the neck are most important. Low-dose therapeutic radiation (6.5–2000 cGy) in infancy or childhood is associated with an increased incidence of thyroid cancer in later life. A thyroid nodule is more likely to be a cancer in a man than in a woman and in a young patient than in an old one. In certain geographic areas, endemic goiter is common, making benign nodules more common. Thyroid cancer has also been described in families with multiple endocrine neoplasia type II (medullary thyroid cancer), Cowden's disease, and Gardner's syndrome (papillary cancer).

The clinician must systematically palpate the thyroid to determine whether there is a solitary thyroid nodule or if it is a multinodular gland and whether there are palpable lymph nodes. A solitary hard thyroid nodule is likely to be malignant, whereas most multinodular goiters are benign.

In many patients, the possibility of cancer is difficult to exclude without microscopic examination of the gland itself. Percutaneous needle biopsy is very helpful if a skilled endocrine cytologist is available. Cytologic results are classified as malignant, benign, indeterminate or suspicious, and inadequate specimen (Figure 16–2). False positive diagnoses of cancer are rare, but about 20% of biopsy specimens reported as indeterminate and 5% of those reported as benign are actually malignant. If the specimen is reported as inadequate, biopsy should be repeated. Needle biopsy should not be performed in patients with a history of irradiation to the neck, because radiation-induced tumors are often multifocal, and a negative biopsy may therefore be unreliable. If an experienced cytologist is not available, radionuclide scanning and ultrasound are helpful. The radioiodine scan is helpful in determining whether the lesion is single or multiple and whether it is functioning (warm or hot) or nonfunctioning (cold). Hot solitary thyroid nodules may cause hyperthyroidism but are rarely malignant, whereas cold solitary thyroid nodules have an incidence of cancer of about 20% and should be removed. Thyroid carcinoma is uncommon (1%) in multinodular goiters, but if there is a domi-

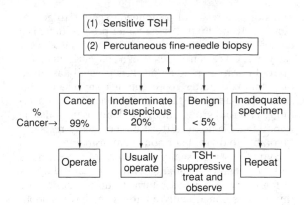

Figure 16–2. Evaluation of thyroid nodule.

nant nodule or one that enlarges, it should be biopsied or removed. Patients with thyroid nodules who received x-ray treatments to the head and neck in infancy and childhood have a 40% chance of having thyroid cancer. Thyroid cancer occurs in nearly 50% of the children with solitary cold thyroid nodules; therefore, thyroidectomy is usually indicated. Ultrasound differentiates solid and cystic lesions; purely cystic lesions less than 4 cm in diameter are almost never malignant. About 10–20% of cold solitary lesions are cystic. Fluorescent scanning using a collimated source of americium Am 241 is also used to differentiate benign from malignant thyroid nodules. This procedure is advantageous because no radioactive materials are introduced into the body and total radiation to the neck is only 0.05 cGy. A chest x-ray including the neck is helpful in demonstrating tracheal displacement, calcification of the thyroid nodule, or the presence of pulmonary metastases. CT or MRI scans are usually not necessary but are helpful when the limits of the tumor cannot be defined, such as in patient with large, invasive, or substernal goiters or tumors.

The principal indications for surgical removal of a nodular goiter are (1) suspicion of cancer, (2) symptoms of pressure, (3) hyperthyroidism, (4) substernal extension, and (5) cosmetic deformity. Solitary hard thyroid nodules or nodules that are cold on radioiodine scan and solid by ultrasound or are suspicious for cancer on aspiration biopsy cytology should be removed. Nonoperative treatment is indicated in patients with multinodular goiters and Hashimoto's thyroiditis unless there is a clinically suspicious area that is growing or if the patient was exposed to radiation or has a family history of medullary carcinoma.

Simple or Nontoxic Goiter (Diffuse & Multinodular Goiter)

Simple goiter may be physiologic, occurring during puberty or the menses or during pregnancy; or it may occur in patients from endemic (iodine-poor) regions or as a result of prolonged exposure to goitro-genic foods or drugs. As the goiter persists, there is a tendency to form nodules. Goiter may also occur early in life as a consequence of a congenital defect in thyroid hormone production. It is generally assumed that nontoxic goiter represents a compensatory response to inadequate thyroid hormone production, although thyroid growth immunoglobulins may also be important. Nontoxic diffuse goiter usually responds favorably to thyroid hormone administration.

Symptoms are usually awareness of a neck mass and dyspnea, dysphagia, or symptoms caused by interference with venous return. In diffuse goiter, the thyroid is symmetrically enlarged and has a smooth surface without areas of encapsulation. However, most patients have multinodular glands by the time they seek medical care. Thyroid function is usually normal, though the sensitive TSH may be suppressed and the radioiodine uptake increased. Surgery is indicated to relieve the pressure symptoms of a large goiter for substernal goiter or to rule out cancer when there are localized areas of hardness or rapid growth. Aspiration biopsy cytology is helpful in these patients.

Berghout A et al: The long-term outcome of thyroidectomy for sporadic non-toxic goiter. Clin Endocrinol 1989; 31:193.

Clark OH et al: TSH suppression in the management of thyroid nodules and thyroid cancer. World J Surg 1981; 5:39.

Gharib H: Fine-needle aspiration biopsy of the thyroid. Ann Intern Med 1984;101:25.

Greenspan FS: The problem of the nodular goiter. Med Clin North Am 1991;75:195.

Schneider AS: Radiation induced thyroid tumors. Endocrinol Metab Clin North Am 1990;19:495.

Utiger RD: Vanishing hypothyroidism. N Engl J Med 1992;326:562.

Takasu N et al: Disappearance of thyrotropin-blocking antibodies and spontaneous recovery from hypothyroidism in autoimmune thyroiditis. N Engl J Med 1992;326:513.

INFLAMMATORY THYROID DISEASE

The inflammatory diseases of the thyroid are termed acute, subacute, or chronic thyroiditis, which can be either suppurative or nonsuppurative.

Acute suppurative thyroiditis is uncommon and is characterized by the sudden onset of severe neck pain accompanied by dysphagia, fever, and chills. It usually follows an acute upper respiratory tract infection; can be diagnosed by percutaneous aspiration, smear, and culture; and is treated by surgical drainage. The organisms are most often streptococci, staphylococci, pneumococci, or coliforms. It may also be associated with a piriform sinus fistula. A barium swallow is recommended in persistent or recurrent cases.

Subacute thyroiditis, a noninfectious disorder, is characterized by thyroid swelling, head and chest pain, fever, weakness, malaise, palpitations, and weight loss. Some patients with subacute thyroiditis have no pain, in which case the condition must be distinguished from Graves' disease. In subacute thyroiditis, the erythrocyte sedimentation rate and serum gamma globulin are almost always elevated, and radioiodine uptake is very low or absent with increased or normal thyroid hormone levels. The illness is usually self-limited, and aspirin and corticosteroids relieve symptoms. These patients eventually become euthyroid.

Hashimoto's thyroiditis, the most common form of thyroiditis, is usually characterized by enlargement of the thyroid with or without pain and tenderness. It is much more common in women and occasionally causes dysphagia.

Hashimoto's thyroiditis is an autoimmune disease. Serum titers of antimicrosomal and antithyroglobulin antibodies are elevated. Appropriate treatment for most patients consists of giving suppressive doses of thyroid hormone. Operation is indicated for marked pressure symptoms, for suspected malignant tumor, and for cosmetic reasons. In patients with pressure or choking symptoms, surgical division of the isthmus provides relief. If the thyroid is large or asymmetric and fails to regress after treatment with exogenous thyroid hormone, or if it contains a discrete nodule, percutaneous needle biopsy or thyroidectomy is recommended. Needle biopsy is helpful in confirming the diagnosis.

Riedel's thyroiditis is a rare condition that presents as a hard woody mass in the thyroid region with marked fibrosis and chronic inflammation in and around the gland. The inflammatory process infiltrates muscles and causes symptoms of tracheal compression. Hypothyroidism is usually present, and surgical treatment is required to relieve tracheal or esophageal obstruction.

Clark OH et al: Hashimoto's thyroiditis and thyroid cancer. Am J Surg 1980;140:65.

Iitaka M et al: Studies on the effect of suppressor T lymphocytes on the induction of antithyroid microsomal antibody secretory cells in autoimmune thyroid disease. J Clin Endocrinol Metab 1988;66;708.

Miyauchi A et al: Piriform sinus fistula: An underlying abnormality common in patients with autosuppurative thyroiditis. World J Surg 1990;14:400.

Singer PA: Thyroiditis: Acute, subacute and chronic. Med Clin North Am 1991;75:61.

Sheigmasa C et al: Chronic thyroiditis with painful tender thyroid enlargement and transient thyrotoxicosis. J Clin Endocrinol Metab 1990;70:385.

BENIGN TUMORS OF THE THYROID

Benign thyroid tumors are adenomas, involutionary nodules, cysts, or localized thyroiditis. Most adenomas are of the follicular type. Adenomas are usually solitary and encapsulated and compress the adjacent thyroid. The major reasons for removal are a suspicion of cancer, functional overactivity producing hyperthyroidism, and cosmetic disfigurement.

MALIGNANT TUMORS OF THE THYROID

Essentials of Diagnosis

* History of irradiation to the neck in some patients.
* Painless or enlarging nodule, dysphagia, or hoarseness.
* Firm or hard, fixed thyroid nodule; cervical lymphadenopathy.
* Normal thyroid function; nodule stippled with calcium (x-ray), cold (radioiodine scan), solid (ultrasound); positive or suspicious cytology.

General Considerations

An appreciation of the classification of malignant tumors of the thyroid is important, because thyroid tumors demonstrate a wide range of growth and malignant behavior. At one end of the spectrum is **papillary adenocarcinoma,** which usually occurs in young adults, grows very slowly, metastasizes through lymphatics, and is compatible with long life even in the presence of metastases (Figure 16–3). At the other extreme is **undifferentiated carcinoma,** which appears late in life and is nonencapsulated and invasive, forming large infiltrating tumors composed of small or large anaplastic cells. Most patients with anaplastic thyroid carcinoma succumb as a consequence of local recurrence, pulmonary metastasis, or both. Between these two extremes are follicular and medullary carcinomas, sarcomas, lymphomas, and metastatic tumors. The prognosis depends on the histologic pattern, the age and sex of the patient, the extent of tumor spread at the time of diagnosis, and the DNA ploidy of the tumor.

The cause of most cases of thyroid carcinoma is unknown, although persons who received low-dose (6.5–2000 cGy) therapeutic radiation to the thymus, tonsils, scalp, and skin in infancy, childhood, and adolescence have an increased risk of developing thyroid tumors. Both children and adults up to 50 years of age who were exposed to the atomic blast at Hiroshima had an increased incidence of benign and malignant thyroid tumors. The incidence of thyroid cancer increases for at least 30 years after irradiation.

Types of Thyroid Cancer

A. Papillary Adenocarcinoma: Papillary adenocarcinoma accounts for 85% of cancers of the thyroid gland. The tumor usually appears in early adult

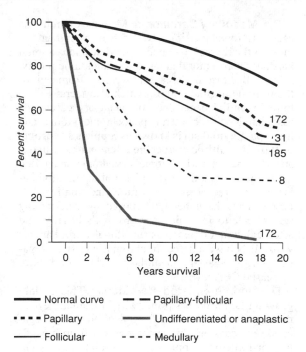

Figure 16–3. Survival rates after thyroidectomy for papillary, mixed papillary-follicular, follicular, medullary, and undifferentiated thyroid cancer.

life and presents as a solitary nodule. It then spreads via intraglandular lymphatics within the thyroid gland and then to the subcapsular and pericapsular lymph nodes. Eighty percent of children and 20% of adults present with palpable lymph nodes. The tumor may metastasize to lungs or bone. Microscopically, it is composed of papillary projections of columnar epithelium. Psammoma bodies are present in about 60% of cases. A mixed papillary-follicular or a follicular variant of papillary carcinoma is sometimes found. The rate of growth may be stimulated by TSH.

B. Follicular Adenocarcinoma: Follicular adenocarcinoma accounts for approximately 10% of malignant thyroid tumors. It appears later in life than the papillary form and may be rubbery or even soft on palpation. It may appear to be encapsulated and to contain colloid on gross examination. Microscopically, follicular carcinoma may be difficult to distinguish from normal thyroid tissue. Capsular and vascular invasion distinguish follicular carcinomas from follicular adenomas. Follicular thyroid cancers only occasionally (7%) metastasize to the regional lymph nodes, but they have a greater tendency to spread by the hematogenous route to the lungs, skeleton, and liver. Metastases from this tumor often demonstrate an avidity for radioactive iodine after total thyroidectomy. Skeletal metastases from follicular carcinomas may appear 10–20 years after resection of the primary lesion. The prognosis is not as good as with the papillary type (Figure 16–3).

C. Medullary Carcinoma: Medullary carcinoma accounts for approximately 2–5% of malignant tumors of the thyroid. It contains amyloid and is a solid, hard, nodular tumor that takes up radioiodine poorly. It is felt that medullary carcinomas arise from cells of the ultimobranchial bodies, which also secrete calcitonin. Familial occurrence of medullary carcinoma associated with bilateral pheochromocytoma and hyperparathyroidism is known as **Sipple's syndrome** or **type II multiple endocrine adenomatosis.** In relatives of patients with Sipple's syndrome or familial medullary carcinoma, hyperplasia of the parafollicular cells (a precancerous condition) and small medullary cancers have been diagnosed by determining serum calcitonin concentrations both basally and after calcium or pentagastrin stimulation. Patients with MEN have a defect in chromosome 10, and patients with metastatic medullary thyroid cancer have increased CEA levels.

D. Undifferentiated Carcinoma: This rapidly growing tumor occurs principally in women beyond middle life and accounts for 3% of all thyroid cancers. On occasion, this lesion evolves from a papillary or follicular neoplasm. It is a solid, quickly enlarging, hard, irregular mass diffusely involving the gland and invading the trachea, muscles, and neurovascular structures early. The tumor may be painful and somewhat tender, may be fixed on swallowing, and may cause laryngeal or esophageal obstructive symptoms. Microscopically, there are three major types: giant cell, spindle cell, and small cell. Mitoses are frequent. Cervical lymphadenopathy and pulmonary metastases are common. Local recurrence after surgical treatment is the rule. External radiation therapy and chemotherapy offer palliation to some patients, but radioiodine is ineffective. The prognosis is poor (Figure 16–3).

Treatment

The treatment of differentiated thyroid carcinoma is operative removal. For papillary carcinoma, total lobectomy with isthmectomy, near total thyroidectomy, or total thyroidectomy are acceptable operations and are followed by a 10-year survival rate of over 80%. Subtotal or partial lobectomy is contraindicated, because the incidence of tumor recurrence is greater and survival is shorter. Total thyroidectomy is recommended by the author for papillary (> 1.5 cm), follicular, Hürthle cell, and medullary carcinomas if the operation can be done without producing permanent hypoparathyroidism or injury to the recurrent laryngeal nerves. Total is preferred over other operations because of the high incidence of multifocal tumor within the gland, a clinical recurrence rate of about 7% in the contralateral lobe if it is spared, and the ease of assessment for recurrence by serum thyroglobulin assay or radioiodine scan during follow-up examinations.

A conservative modified radical neck dissection preserving the sternocleidomastoid muscle and spinal accessory nerve is performed if lymph nodes are grossly involved.

Medullary carcinoma has such a high incidence of nodal involvement that a central neck node clean-out should be done in all patients as well as a concomitant or interval prophylactic neck dissection, especially if serum calcitonin or CEA levels remain elevated after thyroidectomy.

Metastatic deposits of follicular and papillary carcinoma should be treated with ^{131}I after total thyroidectomy or thyroid ablation with radioactive iodine. All patients with thyroid cancer should be maintained indefinitely on suppressive doses of thyroid hormone. For follow-up, it is helpful to measure serum levels of thyroglobulin (a tumor marker for differentiated thyroid cancer), which are usually increased in patients with residual tumor after total thyroidectomy. For **undifferentiated carcinoma, malignant lymphoma,** or **sarcoma,** the tumor should be excised as completely as possible and then treated by radiation and chemotherapy. Doxorubicin (Adriamycin), vincristine, and chlorambucil are the most effective agents. Carcinomas of the kidney, breast, and lung and other tumors sometimes metastasize to the thyroid, but they rarely present as a solitary nodule.

Clark OH, Duh QY: Thyroid cancer. Med Clin North Am 1991;75;211.

Demeure MJ, Clark OH: Surgery in the treatment of thyroid cancer. Endocrinol Metab Clin North Am 1990;19:663.

Duh QY et al: Medullary thyroid carcinoma: The need for early diagnosis and total thyroidectomy. Arch Surg 1989;124:1206.

Grant CS: Long-term course of patients with persistent hypercalcitoninemia after apparent curative primary surgery for medullary thyroid carcinoma. Ann Surg 1990;212:395.

Hay ID: Papillary thyroid carcinoma. Endocrinol Metab Clin North Am 1990;19:545.

Maxon HR, Smith HS: Radioiodine-131 in the diagnosis and treatment of metastatic well differentiated thyroid cancer. Endocrinol Metab Clin North Am 1990;19:685.

McHenry CR et al: Prospective management of nodal metastasis in differentiated thyroid cancer. Am J Surg 1991;162:353.

Ordonez NG et al: Anaplastic thyroid carcinoma. Am J Clin Pathol 1991;96:15.

Robbins J et al: Thyroid cancer: A lethal endocrine neoplasm. Ann Intern Med 1991;115:133. Wong JB et al: Ablative radioactive iodine therapy for apparently localized thyroid carcinoma. Endocrinol Metab Clin North Am 1990;19:741.

II. THE PARATHYROID GLANDS

EMBRYOLOGY & ANATOMY

Phylogenetically, the parathyroids appear rather late, being first seen in amphibia. They arise from pharyngeal pouches III and IV and may be arrested as high as the level of the hyoid bone during their descent to the posterior capsule of the thyroid gland. Four parathyroid glands are present in 85% of the population, and about 15% have more than four glands. Occasionally, one or more may be incorporated into the thyroid gland or thymus and hence are intrathyroidal or mediastinal in location. Parathyroid III, which normally assumes the inferior position, may be found in the anterior mediastinum, usually in the thymus. The upper parathyroids (parathyroid IV) usually remain in close association with the upper portion of the lateral thyroid lobes but may be loosely attached by a long vascular pedicle and migrate caudally along the esophagus into the posterior mediastinum. The parathyroid glands may be separated from the thyroid gland, lying in front of or behind the internal jugular vein and common carotid artery.

The normal parathyroid gland has a distinct yellowish-brown color, is ovoid, tongue-shaped, polypoid, or spherical, and averages $2 \times 3 \times 7$ mm. The total mean weight of four normal parathyroids is about 150 mg. These encapsulated glands are usually supplied by a branch of the inferior thyroid artery but may be supplied by the superior thyroid or, rarely, the thyroid ima arteries. The vessels can be seen entering a hilum-like structure, a feature that differentiates parathyroid glands from fat.

Akerstom G et al: Surgical anatomy of human parathyroid glands. Surgery 1984;95:14,

Fraker DL et al: Undescended parathyroid adenoma: An important etiology for failed operations for primary hyperparathyroidism. World J Surg 1990;14:406.

PHYSIOLOGY

Parathyroid hormone (PTH), vitamin D, and probably calcitonin play vital roles in calcium and phosphorus metabolism in bone, kidney, and gut. Specific radioimmunoassays are available to measure PTH, vitamin D, and calcitonin. Ionized calcium, the physiologically important fraction, can now be measured, but most laboratories are only equipped at present to measure total serum calcium concentration, which is composed of approximately 48% ionized calcium, 46% protein-bound calcium, and 6% calcium complexed to organic anions. Total serum calcium varies directly with plasma protein concentrations, but calcium ion concentrations are unaffected.

PTH and calcitonin work in concert to modulate fluctuations in plasma levels of ionized calcium. When the ionized calcium level falls, the parathyroids secrete more PTH and the parafollicular cells within the thyroid secrete less calcitonin. The rise in PTH and fall in calcitonin produce increased bone resorption and increased resorption of calcium in the renal tubules. More calcium enters the blood, and ionized calcium levels return to normal.

In the circulation, immunoreactive PTH is heterogeneous, consisting of the intact hormone and several hormonal fragments. The amino terminal (N-terminal) fragment is biologically active, whereas the carboxyl terminal (C-terminal) fragment is biologically inert. Measurement of the fragments or intact PTH by immunoassay is best for screening for hyperparathyroidism and for selective venous catheterization to localize the source of PTH production. PTH-related peptide that is secreted by parathyroid tumors does not cross-react with this PTH assay.

Because PTH levels rise in normal subjects if ionized calcium levels are low, calcium and PTH must be determined from samples drawn simultaneously to diagnose hyperparathyroidism. The combination of increased PTH levels and hypercalcemia is almost always pathognomonic of hyperparathyroidism (Figure 16–4).

Brown RC et al: Circulating intact parathyroid hormone measured by a two-site immunochemoluminometric assay. J Clin Endocrinol Metab 1987;65:407.

Lunghall S et al: Disturbances of basal and stimulated serum levels of intact parathyroid hormone in primary hyperparathyroidism. Surgery 1991;110:47.

Picotte SL et al: Regulation of parathyroid hormone secretion. Endocr Rev 1991;12:291.

DISEASES OF THE PARATHYROIDS

PRIMARY HYPERPARATHYROIDISM

Essentials of Diagnosis

- Increased muscular fatigability, arthralgias, nausea, vomiting, constipation, polydipsia, polyuria, psychiatric disturbances, renal colic, bone, and joint pain. ("Stones, bones, abdominal groans, psychic moans, and fatigue overtones.") Some patients are asymptomatic.
- Nephrolithiasis and nephrocalcinosis, peptic ulcer disease, gout, chondrocalcinosis, pancreatitis.
- Hypertension, kyphosis, clubbing, band keratopathy.

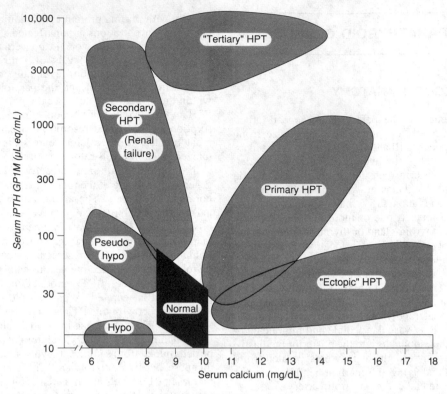

Figure 16–4. PTH assay.

- Serum calcium, PTH, chloride, uric acid increased; serum phosphate low or normal; urine calcium increased, normal, or, rarely, decreased; urine phosphate increased; TRP decreased.
- X-rays: subperiosteal resorption of phalanges, demineralization of the skeleton, bone cysts, and nephrocalcinosis or nephrolithiasis.

General Considerations

Primary hyperparathyroidism is due to excess PTH secretion from a single parathyroid adenoma (83%), multiple adenomas (4%), hyperplasia (12%), or carcinoma (1%). Once thought to be rare, primary hyperparathyroidism is now found in 0.1–0.3% of the general population and is the most common cause of hypercalcemia in unselected patients. It is uncommon before puberty; its peak incidence is between the third and fifth decades, and it is two to three times more common in women than in men.

Overproduction of parathyroid hormone results in mobilization of calcium from bone and inhibition of the renal reabsorption of phosphate, thereby producing hypercalcemia and hypophosphatemia. This causes a wasting of calcium and phosphorus, with osseous mineral loss and **osteoporosis.** Other associated or related conditions that offer clues to the diagnosis of hyperparathyroidism are nephrolithiasis, nephrocalcinosis, osteitis fibrosa cystica, peptic ulcer, pancreatitis, hypertension, and gout or pseudogout. Hyperparathyroidism also occurs in both multiple endocrine adenomatosis (MEN) type I, known as **Werner's syndrome,** and MEN type II, known as **Sipple's syndrome.** The former is characterized by tumors of the parathyroid, pituitary, and pancreas (hyperparathyroidism, pituitary tumors, Zollinger-Ellison syndrome, adrenocortical tumor, carcinoid tumor, and insulinoma); the latter consists of hyperparathyroidism in association with medullary carcinoma of the thyroid and pheochromocytoma.

Parathyroid adenomas range in weight from 65 mg to over 35 g, and the size usually parallels the degree of hypercalcemia. Microscopically, these tumors may be of chief cell, water cell, or, rarely, oxyphil cell type.

Primary parathyroid hyperplasia involves all of the parathyroid glands. Microscopically, there are two types: chief cell hyperplasia and water-clear cell (wasserhelle) hyperplasia. Hyperplastic glands vary considerably in size but are usually larger than normal (65 mg).

Parathyroid carcinoma is rare but is more common in patients with profound hypercalcemia. Parathyroid cancers are palpable in half the patients and should be suspected in patients at operation when the parathyroid gland is hard, has a whitish or irregular capsule, or is invasive.

Clinical Findings

A. Symptoms and Signs: Historically, the clinical manifestations of hyperparathyroidism have changed. Thirty years ago, the diagnosis was based on bone pain and deformity (osteitis fibrosa cystica), and in later years on the renal complications (nephrolithiasis and nephrocalcinosis). At present, over two-thirds of patients are detected by routine screening, and some are asymptomatic. After successful surgical treatment, many patients thought to be asymptomatic become aware of improvement in unrecognized preoperative symptoms such as muscle fatigability, weakness, psychiatric disturbances, constipation, polydipsia and polyuria, and bone and joint pain. Hyperparathyroidism should be suspected in all patients with hypercalcemia and the above symptoms, especially if associated with nephrolithiasis, nephrocalcinosis, hypertension, peptic ulcer, pancreatitis, or gout.

B. Laboratory Findings, Imaging Studies, and Differential Diagnosis (Approach to the Hypercalcemic Patient): See Table 16–2.

1. Laboratory findings–Hyperparathyroidism and cancer are responsible for about 90% of all cases of hypercalcemia. Hyperparathyroidism is the most common cause of hypercalcemia detected by undirected methods such as routine screening, whereas cancer is the most common cause of hypercalcemia in hospitalized patients. Other causes of hypercalcemia are listed in Table 16–3. In many patients the diagnosis is obvious, while in others it may be exceedingly difficult. At times, more than one reason for hypercalcemia may exist in the same patient, such as cancer or sarcoidosis plus hyperparathyroidism. A careful history must be obtained documenting (1) the

Table 16–3. Causes of hypercalcemia.

	Approximate Frequency (%)
Cancer	45
Breast cancer	
Metastatic	
PTH-related peptide secreting (lung, kidney)	
Multiple myeloma	
Leukemias	
Others	
Endocrine disorders	46
Hyperparathyroidism	
Hyperthyroidism	
Addison's disease, pheochromocytoma	
Hypothyroidism, VIPoma	
Increased Intake	4
Milk-alkali syndrome	
Vitamin D and A overdosage	
Thiazides, lithium, aluminum	
Granulomatous diseases	3
Sarcoidosis, tuberculosis, etc	
Benign familial hypocalciuric hypercalcemia and other disorders	2
Paget's disease	
Immobilization	
Idiopathic hypercalcemia of infancy	
Aluminum intoxication	
Dysproteinemias	
Rhabdomyolysis	

duration of any symptoms possibly related to hypercalcemia; (2) symptoms related to malignant disease; (3) conditions associated with hyperparathyroidism, such as renal colic, peptic ulcer disease, pancreatitis, hypertension, or gout; or (4) possible excess use of milk products, antacids, baking soda, or vitamins. In patients with a recent cough, wheeze, or hemoptysis, epidermoid carcinoma of the lung should be considered. Hematuria might suggest hypernephroma, bladder tumor, or renal lithiasis. Chest roentgenograms and intravenous urograms should be performed as appropriate. A long history of renal stones or peptic ulcer disease suggests that hyperparathyroidism is likely.

The most important tests for the evaluation of hypercalcemia are, in order of importance, serum calcium, parathyroid hormone, phosphate, chloride, protein electrophorectic pattern, alkaline phosphatase, creatinine; uric acid, and urea nitrogen; urinary calcium; blood hematocrit and pH; serum magnesium; and erythrocyte sedimentation rate. Measurement of nephrogenous cAMP, 1,25-hydroxy vitamin D levels, and tubular reabsorption of phosphate are helpful in selected patients when other tests are equivocal.

A high serum calcium and a low serum phosphate suggest hyperparathyroidism, but about half of patients with hyperparathyroidism have normal serum phosphate concentrations. Patients with vitamin D intoxication, sarcoidosis, malignant disease without

Table 16–2. Laboratory evaluation of hypercalcemia.[1]

Blood tests
Calcium
Phosphate
Chloride
Protein electrophoresis or albumin/globulin ratio
Parathyroid hormone (intact or two-site assay)
Alkaline phosphatase
Creatinine and BUN
Uric acid
Hematocrit
pH
X-rays
Chest x-ray
Abdominal plain films
Other
Bone densitometry
Urinalysis
Deoxypyridinoline cross-links
Osteocalcin

---

[1]With few exceptions, every patient with hypercalcemia should receive the entire battery of tests before an attempt is made to make a final diagnosis. If the diagnosis is still unclear at this point, special tests described in the text may be indicated.

metastasis, and hyperthyroidism may also be hypophosphatemic, but patients with breast cancer and hypercalcemia are only rarely so. In fact, if hypophosphatemia and hypercalcemia are present in association with breast cancer, concomitant hyperparathyroidism is probable. Measurement of **serum parathyroid hormone** has its greatest value in this situation, since the PTH level is low or nil in patients with hypercalcemia due to *all* causes other than primary or ectopic hyperparathyroidism. In general, serum PTH levels should be measured in all cases of persistent hypercalcemia without an obvious cause other than hyperparathyroidism and in normocalcemic patients who are suspected of having hyperparathyroidism. Determination of intact serum PTH levels using the new two-site assays is the best PTH assay since it is sensitive and is not influenced by tumors that secrete parathyroid-related peptide. Parathyroid tumors that secrete pure PTH are now rare.

An elevated serum chloride concentration is a useful diagnostic clue found in about 40% of hyperparathyroid patients. PTH acts directly on the proximal renal tubule to decrease the resorption of bicarbonate, which leads to increased resorption of chloride and a mild hyperchloremic renal tubular acidosis. Other causes of hypercalcemia do not give increased serum chloride concentrations. Calculation of the **serum chloride to phosphate ratio** takes advantage of slight increases in serum chloride and slight decreases in serum phosphate concentrations. A ratio above 33 suggests hyperparathyroidism.

Serum protein electrophoretic patterns should always be measured to exclude multiple myeloma and sarcoidosis. Hypergammaglobulinemia is rare in hyperparathyroidism but is not uncommon in patients with multiple myeloma and sarcoidosis. Roentgenograms of the skull or site of bone pain will often reveal typical "punched-out" bony lesions, and the diagnosis of myeloma can be firmly established by bone marrow examination. Sarcoidosis can be difficult to diagnose, because it may exist for several years with few clinical findings. A chest x-ray revealing a diffuse fibronodular infiltrate and prominent hilar adenopathy is suggestive, and the demonstration of noncaseating granuloma in lymph nodes is diagnostic. The **hydrocortisone suppression test** (150 mg of hydrocortisone per day for 10 days) reduces the serum calcium concentration in most cases of sarcoidosis and vitamin D intoxication and in many patients with carcinoma and multiple myeloma but only rarely in patients with hyperparathyroidism. It is therefore a useful diagnostic maneuver if these conditions are considered. Hydrocortisone suppression is used to treat the hypercalcemic crises that may occur with these disorders.

Serum alkaline phosphate levels are elevated in about 15% of patients with primary hyperparathyroidism and may also be increased in patients with Paget's disease and cancer. When the serum alkaline phosphatase level is elevated, serum 5'-nucleotidase, which parallels liver alkaline phosphatase, should be measured to determine if the increase is from bone, which suggests parathyroid disease, or liver. A 24-hour urine calcium level is helpful for diagnosing hypercalcemic patients who have low urinary calcium levels resulting from benign familial hypocalciuric hypercalcemia. These patients do not benefit from parathyroidectomy.

2. Bone studies–Radiographic examination of bone frequently reveals osteopenia, but overt skeletal changes are found in only 10% of patients with hyperparathyroidism. Dual photon bone density studies of the femur, lumbar spine, and radius help document osteopenia that occurs in about 70% of female patients with hyperparathyroidism. Bone changes of osteitis fibrosa cystica are rare on x-ray unless the serum alkaline phosphatase concentration is increased. Primary and secondary hyperparathyroidism produce subperiosteal resorption of the phalanges and bone cysts (Figure 16–5). A ground-glass appearance of the skull with loss of definition of the tables and demineralization of the outer aspects of the clavicles are less frequently seen. In patients with markedly elevated serum alkaline phosphatase levels without subperiosteal resorption on x-ray, Paget's disease or cancer must be suspected. A 24-hour urine test for deoxypyridinoline cross-link assay or osteocalcin detects increased bone loss.

3. Differential diagnosis–The differentiation between hyperparathyroidism due to primary parathyroid disease and that due to ectopic hyperparathyroidism or nonparathyroid cancer is often difficult. The most common tumors causing ectopic hyperparathyroidism are squamous cell carcinoma of the lung, hypernephroma, and bladder cancer. Less commonly it is due to hepatoma or to cancer of the

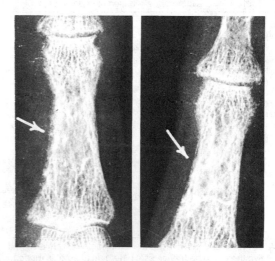

Figure 16–5. Subperiosteal resorption of radial side of second phalanges.

ovary, stomach, pancreas, parotid gland, or colon. Recent onset of symptoms, increased sedimentation rate, anemia, serum calcium greater than 14 mg/dL, and increased alkaline phosphatase activity without osteitis fibrosa cystica suggest **ectopic hyperparathyroidism;** mild hypercalcemia with a long history of nephrolithiasis or peptic ulcer suggests primary hyperthyroidism. Documented hypercalcemia of 6 months or longer essentially rules out malignancy-associated hypercalcemia. Specific radioimmunoassays for PTH-related peptide have been developed and are helpful in differentiating between primary and ectopic hyperparathyroidism.

In **milk-alkali syndrome,** a history of excessive ingestion of milk products, calcium-containing antacids, and baking soda is often obtained. These patients become normocalcemic after discontinuing these habits. Patients with milk-alkali syndrome usually have renal insufficiency and low urinary calcium concentrations and are usually alkalotic rather than acidotic. Because of the high incidence of ulcer disease in hyperparathyroidism, it should be kept in mind that milk-alkali syndrome may coexist with hyperparathyroidism.

Hyperthyroidism, another cause of hypercalcemia and hypercalciuria, can usually be differentiated because manifestations of thyrotoxicosis rather than hypercalcemia bring the patient to the physician. Occasionally, an elderly patient with apathetic hyperthyroidism may be hypercalcemic, so that a sensitive TSH test should be evaluated in all hypercalcemic patients. Treatment of hyperthyroidism with antithyroid medications causes serum calcium to return to normal levels within 8 weeks.

Normal subjects who are given **thiazides** may develop a transient increase in serum calcium levels, usually less than 1 mg/dL. Larger rises in serum calcium induced by thiazides have been reported in patients with primary hyperparathyroidism and idiopathic juvenile osteoporosis. The best way to evaluate these patients is to switch them to a nonthiazide antihypertensive agent or diuretic and to measure the PTH level. Thiazide-induced hypercalcemia is not associated with increased serum PTH in patients without hyperparathyroidism.

Benign familial hypocalciuric hypercalcemia is one of the few conditions that causes chronic hypercalcemia. It can be difficult to distinguish from primary hyperparathyroidism. The best way to diagnose this disorder is to document a low urinary calcium and a family history of hypercalcemia, especially in children.

Other miscellaneous causes of hypercalcemia are Paget's disease, immobilization (especially in Paget's disease or in young patients), dysproteinemias, idiopathic hypercalcemia of infancy, aluminum intoxication, and rhabdomyolysis (Table 16–3).

Other tests (seldom necessary) include bone bi-

opsy, urinary cAMP and hydroxyproline, and PTH by bioassay.

C. Approach to the Normocalcemic Patient With Possible Hyperparathyroidism: Renal failure, hypoalbuminemia, pancreatitis, deficiency of vitamin D or magnesium, and excess phosphate intake may cause serum calcium levels to be normal in hyperparathyroidism. Correction of these disorders results in hypercalcemia if hyperparathyroidism is present. The incidence of normocalcemic hyperparathyroidism in patients with hypercalciuria and recurrent nephrolithiasis (idiopathic hypercalciuria) is not known. Because the serum calcium concentration may fluctuate, it should be measured on more than three separate occasions. The serum should be analyzed the day it is obtained, because the calcium level decreases with refrigeration or freezing. Determination of serum ionized calcium is also useful, since it may be increased in patients with normal total serum calcium levels.

If a patient has elevated serum levels of ionized calcium and PTH, the diagnosis of normocalcemic hyperparathyroidism has been confirmed. There are three major causes of hypercalciuria and nephrolithiasis: (1) increased absorption of calcium from the gastrointestinal tract (absorptive hypercalciuria), (2) increased renal leakage of calcium (renal hypercalciuria), and (3) primary hyperparathyroidism. Patients with absorptive hypercalcemia absorb too much calcium from the gastrointestinal tract and therefore have low serum PTH levels. Patients with renal hypercalciuria lose calcium from leaky renal tubules and have increased PTH levels. They can be distinguished from patients with normocalcemic hyperparathyroidism by their response to treatment with thiazides. In the former condition, serum PTH levels become normal, because thiazides correct the excessive loss of calcium, whereas in the latter, increased serum PTH levels persist and the patient often becomes hypercalcemic.

Natural History of Untreated & Treated Hyperparathyroidism

Patients with untreated hyperparathyroidism have an increased risk of dying prematurely, mainly from cardiovascular and malignant disease. There is decreased respiratory muscular capacity and increased frequency of hypertrophic cardiomyopathy even in hyperparathyroid patients without hypertension. Hyperparathyroid patients have more hypertension, nephrolithiasis, osteopenia, peptic ulcer disease, gout, renal dysfunction, and pancreatitis. After successful parathyroidectomy, previously hyperparathyroid patients still have an increased risk of premature death. Younger patients and those with less severe disease, however, return to a normal survival curve sooner than do older patients or those with more severe hyperparathyroidism. Most patients with hyperparathyroidism—even those with normocalcemic hyperparathyroidism—have symptoms and associated conditions. In 80% of patients, these clinical manifestations improve or disappear after parathyroidectomy.

Treatment

The only successful treatment of primary hyperparathyroidism is parathyroidectomy. The author feels that virtually all patients with either asymptomatic or symptomatic hyperparathyroidism benefit from the operation both symptomatically and metabolically. There are no data to support a plan of medical observation, and considerable data support an active surgical approach. Once associated conditions such as hypertension and renal dysfunction become well-established, they seem to progress despite correction of the primary hyperparathyroidism. Thus, it is better to intervene early while it is still possible to correct these problems. In all patients, however, the diagnosis should be established, and short delays to clarify the diagnosis are justified.

A. Marked Hypercalcemia (Hypercalcemic Crisis): The initial treatment in patients with marked hypercalcemia and acute symptoms is hydration and correction of hypokalemia and hyponatremia. While the patient is being hydrated, assessment of the underlying problem is essential so that more specific therapy may be started. Milk and alkaline products, estrogens, thiazides, and vitamins A and D should be immediately discontinued. Furosemide is useful to increase calcium excretion in the rehydrated patient. Etidronate, plicamycin (mithramycin), and calcitonin are usually effective for short periods in treating hypercalcemia regardless of cause. Glucocorticoids are very effective in vitamin D intoxication and sarcoidosis and in many patients with cancer, including those with peptide-secreting tumors, but are less effective when there is extensive bone disease. As mentioned previously, hyperparathyroid patients only occasionally respond to glucocorticoid administration.

In patients with marked hypercalcemia, once the diagnosis of hyperparathyroidism is established, cervical exploration and parathyroidectomy should be performed in a vigorously hydrated patient, since this is the most rapid and effective method of reducing serum calcium.

B. Localization: Preoperative localization of parathyroid tumors can now be accomplished in about 75% of patients with ultrasonography, CT scan, and thallium 201-technetium Tc 99m subtraction scan. These studies, however, are only occasionally helpful in patient with parathyroid hyperplasia. Localization studies are essential in patients with persistent or recurrent hyperparathyroidism. An experienced surgeon can find the tumors in about 95% of patients who have not had previous parathyroid or thyroid surgery without preoperative tests. Selective venous catheterization with parathyroid hormone immunoassay is also recommended for patients who

have had an unsuccessful previous operation when the noninvasive localization tests are negative or equivocal. This study helps localize the tumor in about 80% of patients. Digital subtraction angiography is useful for mapping the venous pattern. Arteriography is now rarely used.

C. Operation: The approach is similar to that for thyroidectomy. In over 80% of cases, the parathyroid tumor is found attached to the posterior capsule of the thyroid gland. The parathyroid glands are usually symmetrically placed, and lower parathyroid glands are situated anterior to the recurrent laryngeal nerve, whereas the upper parathyroid glands lie posterior to the recurrent laryngeal nerve, where it enters the cricothyroid muscle. Parathyroid tumors may also lie cephalad to the superior pole of the thyroid gland, along the great vessels of the neck in the tracheoesophageal area, in thymic tissue, in the substance of the thyroid gland itself, or in the mediastinum. Care must be taken not to traumatize the parathyroid gland or tumors, since color is useful in distinguishing them from surrounding thyroid, thymus, lymph node, and fat. Two helpful maneuvers for localizing parathyroid tumors at operation are following the course of a branch of the inferior thyroid artery and gently palpating for the parathyroid tumor. One should attempt to identify four parathyroid glands, although there may be more or fewer than four.

If a probable parathyroid adenoma is found, it is removed and the diagnosis confirmed by frozen section. It seems unwise to remove a grossly normal parathyroid gland intentionally, both because this has no beneficial effect and because the gland may be needed to maintain normal function after all the hyperfunctioning tissue is removed. If two adenomas are found, both are removed, and both normal glands are marked and biopsied but not removed.

The presence of a normal parathyroid gland at operation indicates that the tumor removed is an adenoma rather than parathyroid hyperplasia, since in hyperplasia all the parathyroid glands are involved. A compressed rim of normal parathyroid tissue is also suggestive of an adenoma. When all parathyroid glands are hyperplastic, the most normal gland should be subtotally resected, leaving a 50 mg remnant, and confirmed histologically before removal of the remaining gland. The upper thymus and perithymic tract should be removed in patients with hyperplasia, because a fifth parathyroid gland is present in 15% of cases.

If exploration fails to reveal a parathyroid tumor, perform a thymectomy, thyroid lobectomy, or partial thyroidectomy on the side that has only one parathyroid gland, since tumors may be found within the thymus or intrathyroidally. If thyroid nodules are present, they should be treated as nodular goiter and possible thyroid cancer. Differentiated thyroid carcinoma occurs in 3% of patients with hyperparathyroidism.

The recurrence rate of hyperparathyroidism after the removal of a single adenoma in most medical centers is 5% or less, so that the removal of normal-appearing parathyroid glands is unwarranted. In patients with multiple endocrine adenopathy and familial hyperparathyroidism, recurrent hyperparathyroidism is more common; therefore, extra care should be taken to remove all abnormal parathyroid tissue and to carefully mark the remaining parathyroid tissue. These hyperthyroid patients are candidates for possible prophylactic subtotal parathyroidectomy. Total parathyroidectomy with autotransplantation to the forearm is recommended by some surgeons for patients with multiple endocrine adenopathy or familial hyperparathyroidism. I prefer subtotal parathyroidectomy leaving a well-marked parathyroid remnant because not all parathyroid transplants function effectively.

Exploration of the mediastinum via a sternal split is necessary in only 1–2% of cases and is only recommended in patients with a serum calcium level above 13.5 mg/dL. If cervical exploration was nonproductive or if localization studies suggest a mediastinal tumor, the patient should be allowed to recover from the initial operation and return in 6–8 weeks for mediastinal exploration.

D. Postoperative Care: Following removal of a parathyroid adenoma or hyperplastic glands, the serum calcium concentration falls to normal or below normal in 24–48 hours. Patients with severe skeletal depletion ("hungry bones"), long-standing hyperparathyroidism, or high calcium levels may develop paresthesias, carpopedal spasm, or even seizures. If the symptoms are mild and serum calcium falls slowly, oral supplementation with calcium is all that is required. When marked symptoms develop, it is necessary to give calcium chloride slowly intravenously, avoiding infiltration outside the vein, as it causes tissue necrosis. If the response is not rapid, the serum magnesium concentration should be determined and magnesium given. (See section on Hypoparathyroidism, below.)

E. Reoperation: Reexploration for persistent or recurrent hyperparathyroidism or after a previous thyroidectomy presents formidable problems and an increased risk of complications. First ascertain that the diagnosis is correct and that the patient does not have benign familial hypocalciuric hypercalcemia or hypercalcemia due to another cause such as a malignant tumor. Ultrasound, CT or MRI scan, and thallium 201-technetium Tc 99m subtraction scan should be done first. If these studies are unsuccessful or equivocal, digital subtraction angiography and highly selective venous catheterization with parathyroid hormone immunoassay are recommended. Most such patients have a parathyroid tumor that can be removed through a cervical incision, making mediastinal exploration unnecessary. The success rate of parathyroidectomy performed by experienced surgeons is 95% or better versus a success rate of about 75% with less experienced surgeons.

Clark OH: Hyperparathyroidism. In: *Endocrine Surgery of the Thyroid and Parathyroid Glands.* Clark OH (editor). Mosby, 1985.

Clark OH et al: Diagnosis and management of asymptomatic hyperparathyroidism: Safety, efficacy and deficiencies in our knowledge. J Bone Miner Res 1991;6:135.

Doherty GM et al: Results of multidisciplinary strategy for management of mediastinal parathyroid adenoma or a cause of persistent primary hyperparathyroidism. Ann Surg 1992;215:101.

Heath H III: Clinical spectrum of primary hyperparathyroidism evolution with changes in medical practice and technology. J Bone Miner Res 1991;6:563.

Hedbeck G et al: The influence of surgery on the risk of death in patients with hyperparathyroidism. World J Surg 1991;15:399.

Hedbeck G et al: Premature death in patients operated on for primary hyperparathyroidism. World J Surg 1991;14:829.

Kaplan RA et al: Metabolic effects of parathyroidectomy in asymptomatic primary hyperparathyroidism. J Clin Endocrinol Metab 1976;42;415.

Kristoffersson A et al: Pre and postoperative respiratory muscle strength in primary hyperparathyroidism. Acta Chir Scand 1988;154:415.

Levin KE, Clark OJ: The reasons for failures in parathyroid operations. Arch Surg 1989;124:911.

Levin KE et al: Advances in localizing studies (MRI, ultrasound, CT, thallium-technetium scanning) in patients with persistent and recurrent hyperparathyroidism. Surgery 1987;1025:917.

Ljunghall S et al: Longitudinal studies of mild primary hyperparathyroidism. J Bone Miner Res 1991;6:111.

Madvic P et al: Assessment of adenosine 3′,5′-monophosphate excretion and an oral calcium tolerance test in the diagnosis of mild primary hyperparathyroidism. J Clin Endocrinol Metab 1984;58:480.

Marx SJ: Familial hypocalciuric hypercalcemia. N Engl J Med 1980;303:810.

Palmer M et al: Survival and renal function in persons with untreated hypercalcemia: A population-based cohort study with 14 years follow-up. Lancet 1987;1:59.

Pang PKT, Benishin CG, Lewanczuk RZ: Parathyroid hypertensive factor, a circulating factor in animal and human hypertension. Am J Hypertens 1991;4:472.

Scholz DA, Purnell DC: Asymptomatic primary hyperparathyroidism. Mayo Clin Proc 1981;56:473.

Seibel MJ et al: Urinary hydroxypyridinium cross-links of collagen in primary hyperparathyroidism. J Clin Endocrinol Metab 1992;74:481.

Symons C et al: Cardiac hypertrophy, hypertrophic cardiomyopathy, and hyperparathyroidism—an association. Br Heart J 1985;54:539.

Wagner PK et al: Replantation of cryopreserved human parathyroid tissue. World J Surg 1991;6:751.

SECONDARY & TERTIARY HYPERPARATHYROIDISM

In secondary hyperparathyroidism, there is an increase in parathyroid hormone secretion in response to low plasma concentrations of ionized calcium, usually owing to renal disease and malabsorption. This results in chief cell hyperplasia. When secondary hyperparathyroidism occurs as a complication of renal disease, the serum phosphorus level is usually high, whereas in malabsorption, osteomalacia, or rickets it is frequently low or normal. Secondary hyperparathyroidism with renal osteodystrophy is a frequent if not universal complication of hemodialysis. Factors that play a role in renal osteodystrophy are (1) phosphate retention secondary to a decrease in the number of nephrons; (2) failure of the diseased or absent kidneys to hydroxylate 25-dihydroxyvitamin D to the biologically active metabolite 1,25-dihydroxyvitamin D, with decreased intestinal absorption of calcium; (3) resistance of the bone to the action of parathyroid hormone; and (4) increased serum calcitonin concentrations. The resulting skeletal changes are identical with those of primary hyperparathyroidism but are often more severe.

Most patients with secondary hyperparathyroidism may be treated medically. Maintaining relatively normal serum concentrations of calcium and phosphorus during hemodialysis and treatment with vitamin D have decreased the incidence of bone disease dramatically.

Occasionally, a patient with secondary hyperparathyroidism develops relatively autonomous hyperplastic parathyroid glands (tertiary hyperparathyroidism). In most patients after successful renal transplantation, the serum calcium concentration returns to normal, and one should wait at least 6 months after surgery before considering parathyroidectomy for persistent mild hypercalcemia. In some patients, however, profound hypercalcemia develops. In general, surgical therapy for so-called tertiary hyperparathyroidism should be withheld until all medical approaches, including treatment with vitamin D, calcium supplementation, and phosphate binders, have been exhausted. Indications for operation include (1) a calcium × phosphate product > 70, (2) severe bone disease and pain, (3) pruritus, and (4) extensive soft tissue calcification and calciphylaxis. Most patients with secondary hyperparathyroidism requiring parathyroidectomy have very high serum PTH levels, whereas patients with aluminum bone disease may be hypercalcemic with bone pain but PTH levels are normal or only slightly increased. In the rare patient in whom subtotal parathyroidectomy or total parathyroidectomy with autotransplantation is indicated, all but about 50 mg of parathyroid tissue should be removed, or fifteen 1-mm slices of parathyroid tissue should be transplanted into individual muscle pockets in the forearm. Some parathyroid tissue should also be cryopreserved in case the transplanted tissue does not function. These patients usually respond with dramatic relief of symptoms. A few patients may continue to have bone pain due to osteomalacia thought to be secondary to aluminum toxicity. Profound hypocalcemia frequently results following subtotal parathyroidectomy for renal osteodystrophy, both because of "hungry bones" and because of decreased parathyroid hormone secretion.

Clark OH; Secondary hyperparathyroidism. In: *Endocrine Surgery of the Thyroid and Parathyroid Glands.* Clark OH (editor). Mosby, 1985.

Delmez JA, Slatoplosky E: Recent advances in the pathogenesis and therapy of uremic secondary hyperparathyroidism. J Clin Endocrinol Metab 1991;72:735.

Demeure MJ et al: Results of surgical treatment for hyperparathyroidism associated with renal disease. Am J Surg 1990;160:337.

Denizot A et al: Results of reoperation for persistent or recurrent secondary hyperparathyroidism in hemodialysis patients. World J Surg 1990;14:303.

Dubost C, Dureke T: Comparison of subtotal parathyroidectomy with total parathyroidectomy and autotransplantation. *Surgery of the Thyroid and Parathyroid Glands.* Churchill Livingstone, 1983.

Duh QY et al: Calciphylaxis in secondary hyperparathyroidism. Arch Surg 1991;126:1213.

Llach F, Massry SG: On the mechanism of secondary hyperparathyroidism in moderate renal insufficiency. J Clin Endocrinol Metab 1985:61:601.

HYPOPARATHYROIDISM

Essentials of Diagnosis

- Paresthesias, muscle cramps, carpopedal spasm, laryngeal stridor, convulsions, malaise, muscle and abdominal cramps, tetany, urinary frequency, lethargy, anxiety, psychoneurosis, depression, and psychosis.
- Surgical neck scar. Positive Chvostek and Trousseau signs.
- Brittle and atrophied nails, defective teeth, cataracts.
- Hypocalcemia and hyperphosphatemia, low or absent urinary calcium, low or absent circulating parathyroid hormone.
- Calcification of basal ganglia, cartilage, and arteries as seen on x-ray.

General Considerations

Hypoparathyroidism, although uncommon, occurs most often as a complication of thyroidectomy, especially when performed for carcinoma or recurrent goiter. Idiopathic hypoparathyroidism, an autoimmune process associated with autoimmune adrenocortical insufficiency, is also unusual, and hypoparathyroidism after ^{131}I therapy for Graves' disease is rare. Neonatal tetany may be associated with maternal hyperparathyroidism.

Clinical Findings

A. Symptoms and Signs: The manifestations of acute hypoparathyroidism are due to hypocalcemia. Low serum calcium levels precipitate tetany. Latent tetany may be indicated by mild or moderate paresthesias with a positive Chvostek or Trousseau sign. The initial manifestations are paresthesias, circumoral numbness, muscle cramps, irritability, carpopedal spasm, convulsions, opisthotonos, and marked anxiety. Dry skin, brittleness of the nails, and spotty alopecia including loss of the eyebrows are common. Since primary hypoparathyroidism is rare, a history of thyroidectomy is almost always present. Generally speaking, the sooner the clinical manifestations appear postoperatively, the more serious the prognosis. After many years, some patients become adapted to a low serum calcium concentration, so that tetany is no longer evident.

B. Laboratory Findings: Hypocalcemia and hyperphosphatemia are demonstrable. The urine phosphate is low or absent, tubular resorption of phosphate is high, and the urine calcium is low.

C. Imaging Studies: In chronic hypoparathyroidism, x-rays may show calcification of the basal ganglia, arteries, and external ear.

Differential Diagnosis

A good history is most important in the differential diagnosis of hypocalcemic tetany. Occasionally, tetany occurs with alkalosis and hyperventilation. Symptomatic hypocalcemia occurring after thyroid or parathyroid surgery is due to parathyroid removal or injury by trauma or devascularization or is secondary to "hungry bones." Other major causes of hypocalcemic tetany are intestinal malabsorption and renal insufficiency. These conditions may also be suggested by a history of diarrhea, pancreatitis, steatorrhea, or renal disease. Laboratory abnormalities include decreased concentrations of serum proteins, cholesterol, and carotene and increased concentrations of stool fat in malabsorption and an increased blood urea nitrogen and creatinine in renal failure. Serum parathyroid hormone concentrations are low in hypocalcemia secondary to idiopathic or iatrogenic hypoparathyroidism. Consequently, serum calcium concentrations and urinary calcium, phosphorus, and hydroxyproline levels are decreased, whereas serum phosphate concentrations are increased. In hypocalcemia secondary to malabsorption and renal failure, serum PTH concentrations are elevated and the serum alkaline phosphatase concentration is normal or increased.

Treatment

The aim of treatment is to raise the serum calcium concentration, to bring the patient out of tetany, and to lower the serum phosphate level so as to prevent metastatic calcification. Most postoperative hypocalcemia is transient; if it persists longer than 2–3 weeks, it is apt to require chronic treatment.

A. Acute Hypoparathyroid Tetany: Acute hypoparathyroid tetany requires emergency treatment. Make certain an adequate airway exists. Reassure the anxious patient to avoid hyperventilation and resulting alkalosis. Give calcium chloride, 10–20 mL of 10% solution slowly intravenously, until tetany disappears. Ten to 50 mL of 10% calcium chloride may then be added to 1 L or saline or 5% dextrose solution and administered by slow intravenous drip. Adjust the rate of infusion so that hourly determinations of serum calcium are normal. Calcitriol (1,25-dihydroxyvitamin D) is very helpful for managing acute hypocalcemia because of its rapid onset of action (compared to other vitamin D preparations) and its short duration of action. Occasionally, hypomagnesemia may be found in some cases of tetany not responding to calcium treatment. In such cases, magnesium (as magnesium sulfate) should be given in a dosage of 4–8 g/d intramuscularly or 2–4 g/d intravenously.

B. Chronic Hypoparathyroidism: Once tetany has responded to intravenous calcium, change to oral calcium (gluconate, lactate, or carbonate) three times daily or as necessary. The management of the hypoparathyroid patient is difficult, because the difference between the controlling and intoxicating dose of vitamin D may be quite small. Episodes of hypercalcemia in treated patients are often unpredictable and may occur in the absence of symptoms. Vitamin D intoxication may develop after months or years of good control on a given therapeutic regimen. Dihydrotachysterol is useful in the exceptional case when the usual measures fail to control the hypocalcemia. Frequent serum calcium determinations are necessary to regulate the proper dosage of vitamin D and to avoid vitamin D intoxication. The dose of vitamin D required to correct hypocalcemia may vary from 25,000 to 200,000 IU/d. Phosphorus should also be limited in the diet; in most patients, simple elimination of dairy products is sufficient. In some patients, aluminum hydroxide gel may be necessary to bind phosphorus in the gut to increase fecal losses.

PSEUDOHYPOPARATHYROIDISM & PSEUDOPSEUDOHYPO-PARATHYROIDISM

Pseudohypoparathyroidism is an X-linked autosomal syndrome due to a defective renal adenylyl cyclase system. It is characterized by the clinical and chemical features of hypoparathyroidism associated with a round face; a short, thick body; stubby fingers with short metacarpal and metatarsal bones; mental deficiency; and x-ray evidence of calcification. It is also associated with thyroid and ovarian dysfunction. There is evidence of increased bone resorption and osteitis fibrosa cystica despite the hypocalcemia that accompanies the syndrome. Patients with pseudohypoparathyroidism do not respond to intravenous administration of 200 units of parathyroid hormone with phosphaturia (Ellsworth-Howard test) and have increased serum concentrations of PTH. This condition is usually controlled with smaller amounts of vitamin D than idiopathic hypoparathyroidism, and resistance to therapy is uncommon.

Pseudopseudohypoparathyroidism is also a genetically transmitted disease with the same physical findings of pseudohypoparathyroidism but with normal serum calcium and phosphorus concentrations. Patients with this condition may become hypocalcemic during periods of stress, such as pregnancy and rapid growth; this suggests that a genetic defect is common with pseudohypoparathyroidism.

Faull CM, et al: Pseudohypoparathyroidism: Its phenotypic variability and associated disorders in a large family. J Med 1991;78:251.

Lebowitz MR, Moses AM: Hypocalcemia. Semin Nephrol 1992;12:146.

Lin CK et al: Prevalence of three mutations in the Gs alpha gene among 24 families with pseudohypoparathyroidism type Ia. Biochem Biophys Res Com 1992;189:343.

Murray TM et al: Pseudohypoparathyroidism with osteitis fibrosa cystica: Direct demonstration of skeletal responsiveness to parathyroid hormone in cells cultured from bone. J Bone Min Res 1993;8:83.

Spiegel AM: Albright's hereditary osteodystrophy and defective G proteins. N Engl J Med 1990;322:1461.

Stirling HF, Darling JA, Barr DG: Plasma cyclic AMP response to intravenous parathyroid hormone in pseudohypoparathyroidism. Acta Paed Scand 1991;80:333.

REFERENCES

Braverman LE, Utiger RD (editors): *Werner & Ingbar's The Thyroid,* 6th ed. Lippincott, 1991.

Cady B, Rossi FL: *Surgery of the Thyroid and Parathyroid Glands,* 3rd ed. Saunders, 1991.

Clark OH: *Surgery of the Thyroid and Parathyroid Glands.* Mosby, 1985.

Clark OH, Weber C: Endocrine surgery. Surg Clin North Am 1987;67:1.

Degroot LJ (editor): *Endocrinology,* vol 1, 2nd ed. Saunders, 1989.

Degroot LJ, Stanburg JB: *The Thyroid and Its Diseases,* 4th ed. Wiley, 1975.

Greenspan FS, Forsham PH (editors): *Basic and Clinical Endocrinology,* 3rd ed. Appleton & Lange, 1991.

Greenspan FS: Thyroid disease. Med Clin North Am 1991;75:1.

Greer MA (editor): *The Thyroid Gland–Comprehensive Endocrinology* (Rev Series). Raven Press, 1990.

Kaplan MM: Thyroid carcinoma. Endocrinol Metab Clin North Am 1990;19:1.

Lanvin N: *Manual of Endocrinology and Metabolism.* Little, Brown 1986.

LiVolsi VA: *Surgical Pathology of the Thyroid.* Saunders, 1990.

Najarian JS, Delaney JP: *Advances in Breast and Endocrine Surgery.* Year Book, 1986.

Rocher HD, Clark OH: Thyroid tumors. Prog Surg 1988;19:205.

Thompson NW, Vinik AI (editors): *Endocrine Surgery Update.* Grune & Stratton, 1983.

Williams RH (editor): *Textbook of Endocrinology,* 6th ed. Saunders. 1981.

Breast

17

Armando E. Giuliano, MD

CARCINOMA OF THE FEMALE BREAST

Essentials of Diagnosis

- Higher incidence in women who have delayed childbearing, the with a family history of breast cancer, and those with a personal history of breast cancer or some types of mammary dysplasia.
- Early findings: Single, nontender, firm to hard mass with ill-defined margins; mammographic abnormalities and no palpable mass.
- Later findings: Skin or nipple retraction; axillary lymphadenopathy; breast enlargement, redness, edema, pain; fixation of mass to skin or chest wall.
- Late findings: Ulceration; supraclavicular lymphadenopathy; edema of arm; bone, lung, liver, brain, or other distant metastases.

COMMON SIGNS & SYMPTOMS

The most common sign and symptom of breast disease is a palpable mass. This is usually found by the patient and may lead to the diagnosis of either benign or malignant disease. A palpable mass may be smooth and rubbery (fibroadenoma, tense cyst) or firm and irregular (carcinoma). While many patients complain of breast pain, this is not commonly associated with a serious disease and usually is due to underlying fibrocystic changes in a premenopausal woman. However, some patients who complain of pain are found to have a malignancy. Most commonly, patients have diffuse nodularity associated with pain leading to the clinical diagnosis of fibrocystic disease. Benign and malignant breast disease may present as nipple discharge or even erosion or an eczema-like rash of the nipple. Most nipple discharge is associated with benign duct ectasia or cysts. A bloody discharge can be a sign of a malignancy but is usually a sign of a benign intraductal papilloma. Nipple erosion or even an eczema-like rash can be related to an underlying malignancy, as in Paget's disease. More diffuse skin changes can also be seen in benign and malignant conditions. Erythema and edema may signify underlying mastitis or advanced or inflammatory carcinoma. Breast tenderness is associated most commonly with fibrocystic disease, but when accompanied by erythema and edema it signifies mastitis. Local skin dimpling (indentation) or nipple retraction may be a sign of benign fibrocystic disease or a past mastitis but may signify an underlying malignancy. Rarely, a malignancy may present with palpable adenopathy and no abnormality within the breast itself.

A malignancy may be very obvious, presenting with a mass, adenopathy, and skin involvement, or may be a subtle thickening in a portion of the breast with no other identifiable abnormality. While the overwhelming majority of patients with complaints related to their breasts will have benign conditions, most breast symptoms and signs may be due to an associated or underlying malignancy and warrant workup and follow-up care.

DIAGNOSTIC TESTS

The most reliable diagnostic test for breast cancer is **open excisional biopsy.** When the sample is properly taken by the surgeon and examined by the pathologist, such a test should give no false-negative and no false-positive results.

Large-needle (core needle) biopsy is an accepted diagnostic technique in which a core of tissue is removed with a large cutting needle. As in the case of any needle biopsy, the main problem is sampling error due to improper positioning of the needle, giving rise to a false-negative test result.

Fine-needle aspiration cytology is a useful technique whereby cells from a breast tumor are aspirated with a small (usually 22-gauge) needle and examined by the pathologist. This technique can be performed easily with no morbidity and is much less expensive than excisional or open biopsy. The main disadvantages are that it requires a pathologist skilled in the cytologic diagnosis of breast cancer and that it is subject to sampling problems, particularly because deep lesions may be missed. The incidence of false-positive diagnoses is extremely low, perhaps 1–2%. The rate of false-negative diagnoses with fine-needle aspiration biopsy is as high as 10% in some series. Most experienced clinicians would not leave a dominant mass in the breast even when fine-needle aspiration cytology is negative unless the clinical diagnosis, breast imaging studies, and cytologic studies were all in agreement.

Ultrasonography is performed chiefly to differentiate cystic from solid lesions and is not diagnostic of malignancy. Ultrasonography may show an irregular mass within a cyst in the rare case of intracystic carcinoma. If a tumor is palpable and clinically feels like a cyst, an 18-gauge needle can be used to aspirate the fluid and make the diagnosis of cyst. If a cyst is aspirated and the fluid is nonbloody, it does not have to be examined cytologically. If the mass does not recur, no further diagnostic test is necessary. Nonpalpable mammographic densities that appear benign should be investigated with ultrasound to determine whether the lesion is cystic or solid.

When a suspicious abnormality is identified by mammography alone and cannot be palpated by the clinician, the patient should undergo **mammographic localization biopsy.** This is performed by obtaining a mammogram in two perpendicular views and placing a needle or hook-wire near the abnormality so that the surgeon can use the metal needle or wire as a guide during operation to locate the lesion. After mammography confirms the position of the needle in relation to the lesion, an incision is made and the subcutaneous tissue is dissected until the needle is identified. Using the films as a guide, the abnormality can then be localized and excised. It often happens that the abnormality cannot even be palpated through the incision—this is the case with microcalcifications—and it is thus essential to obtain a mammogram of the specimen to document that the lesion was excised. At that time, a second marker needle can further localize the lesion for the pathologist.

Computerized stereotactic modifications have recently been added to mammographic units in order to localize abnormalities and perform needle biopsy without surgery. Under mammographic guidance, a biopsy needle can be inserted into the lesion in the mammographer's suite, and a core of tissue for histologic examination or cells for cytology can be examined. Some studies suggest that the false-negative rate may be too high to justify this technique. However, continued trials of new stereotactic equipment may permit mammographic localization biopsies to be done accurately without surgical excision.

INCIDENCE & RISK FACTORS

The breast is the most common site of cancer in women, and cancer of the breast is second only to lung cancer as a cause of death from cancer among women. The probability of developing breast cancer increases throughout life. The mean and the median age of women with breast cancer is between 60 and 61 years.

There will be about 182,000 new cases of breast cancer and about 46,000 deaths from this disease in women in the USA in 1994. At the present rate of incidence, the American Cancer Society predicts that one of every eight or nine American women will develop breast cancer during her lifetime. Women whose mothers or sisters had breast cancer are more likely to develop the disease than others. Risk is increased in patients whose mothers' or sisters' breast cancers occurred before menopause or was bilateral and in those with a family history of breast cancer in two or more first-degree relatives. However, there is no history of breast cancer among female relatives in over 90% of breast cancer patients. Nulliparous women and women whose first full-term pregnancy was after age 35 have a slightly higher incidence of breast cancer than multiparous women. Late menarche and artificial menopause are associated with a lower incidence of breast cancer, whereas early menarche (under age 12) and late natural menopause (after age 50) are associated with a slight increase in risk of developing breast cancer. Mammary dysplasia (fibrocystic disease of the breast), when accompanied by proliferative changes, papillomatosis, or atypical epithelial hyperplasia, is associated with an increased incidence of cancer. A woman who has had cancer in one breast is at increased risk of developing cancer in the other breast. Women with cancer of the uterine corpus have a breast cancer risk significantly higher than that of the general population, and women with breast cancer have a comparably increased endometrial cancer risk. In the USA, breast cancer is more common in whites than in nonwhites. The incidence of the disease among nonwhites (mostly blacks), however, is increasing, especially in younger women. In general, rates reported from developing countries are low, whereas rates are high in developed countries, with the notable exception of Japan. Some of the variability may be due to underreporting in the developing countries, but a real difference probably exists. Dietary factors, particularly increased fat content, may account for some differences in incidence. Oral contraceptives do not appear to increase the risk of breast cancer. There is some evidence that administration of estrogens to postmenopausal women may result in a slightly increased risk of breast cancer, but only with higher, long-term doses of estrogens. Other studies suggest that women with a family history of breast cancer who take postmenopausal estrogens or those who take estradiol or unconjugated estrogens do slightly increase their risk of breast cancer. Alcohol consumption may increase the risk of breast cancer slightly.

Women who are at greater than normal risk of developing breast cancer (Table 17–1) should be identified by their physicians, taught the techniques of

Table 17–1. Factors associated with increased risk of breast cancer.[1]

Race	White
Age	Older
Family History	Breast cancer in mother or sister (especially bilateral or pre-menopausal)
Previous medical history	Endometrial cancer Some forms of mammary dysplasia Cancer in other breast
Menstrual history	Early menarche (under age 12) Late menopause (after age 50)
Pregnancy	Late first pregnancy

[1] Normal lifetime risk in white women = 1 in 8 or 9.

breast self-examination, and followed carefully. Screening programs involving periodic physical examination and mammography of asymptomatic high-risk women increase the detection rate of breast cancer and improve the survival rate by as much as 30%. Unfortunately, most women who develop breast cancer do not have significant identifiable risk factors, and analysis of epidemiologic data has failed to identify women who are not at significant risk and would not benefit from screening. Therefore, virtually all women over about age 35 are at sufficient risk of breast cancer so that they could benefit from screening. The cost-benefit ratio of screening programs to society as a whole is unclear. Less expensive screening techniques such as single-view mammography and the use of mobile vans are being investigated in an attempt to reduce the cost of widespread screenings. Recently, the NSAB began actually comparing tamoxifen with placebo for patients who show no evidence of breast cancer but who are at high risk for its occurrence. This controversial trial may identify a pharmacologic means of preventing the disease in young women.

EARLY DETECTION OF BREAST CANCER

Screening Programs

A number of mass screening programs consisting of physical and mammographic examination of the breasts of asymptomatic women have been conducted. Such programs frequently identify more than six cancers per 1000 women. About 80% of these women have negative axillary lymph nodes at the time of surgery, whereas only 45% of patients found in the course of usual medical practice have uninvolved axillary nodes. Detecting breast cancer before it has spread to the axillary nodes greatly increases the chance of survival, and about 85% of such women will survive at least 5 years.

Both physical examination and mammography are necessary for maximum yield in screening programs, since about 35–50% of early breast cancers can be discovered only by mammography and another 40% can be detected only by palpation. About one-third of the abnormalities detected on screening mammograms will be found to be malignant when biopsy is performed. Women 20–40 years of age should have a breast examination as part of routine medical care every 2–3 years. Women over age 40 should have yearly breast examinations. The sensitivity of mammography varies from approximately 60% to 90%. This sensitivity depends on several factors, including patient age (breast density), tumor size, location, and mammographic appearance. In young women with dense breasts, mammography is less sensitive than in older woman with fatty breasts, in whom mammography can detect nearly 90% of malignancies. Smaller tumors, particularly those without calcifications, are more difficult to detect, especially in dense breasts. The lack of sensitivity in young women is leading to questions concerning the value of mammography for screening in women 40–50 years of age. The specificity of mammography varies from about 30% to 40% for nonpalpable mammographic abnormalities to 85% to 90% for clinically evident malignancies.

The American College of Radiology and the American Cancer Society have published guidelines regarding use of mammography in asymptomatic women. A baseline mammogram should be performed on all women between ages 35 and 40 years. Women aged 40–49 years should have a mammogram every 1–2 years. Annual mammograms are indicated for women age 50 years or older. The US Preventive Services Task Force recommends mammography screening every 1 or 2 years for women aged 50–75 and physical examination annually for women over age 40. High-risk women—those whose mothers or sisters had bilateral or premenopausal breast cancer, those who have had cancer of one breast, and those with histologic abnormalities associated with subsequent cancer (eg, atypical epithelial hyperplasia, papillomatosis, lobular carcinoma in situ)—should have a yearly mammogram and twice-yearly physical examinations. The usefulness of screening mammography in young women without identifiable risk factors is not yet of proved value. However, in a recent large study of women under age 50, nearly half of all cancers were detected by mammography alone. Critics of screening question whether early detection actually improves survival sufficiently to justify its cost. Mammographic parenchymal patterns are not a reliable predictor of the risk of developing breast cancer.

Ductography is useful to evaluate the cause of nipple discharge. In this study, the radiologist injects contrast medium into the discharging duct and obtains a mammogram. The injected duct may contain a filling defect (most commonly an intraductal papilloma) or may have a dilated or cystic appearance in patients with duct ectasia or fibrocystic disease. Malignancy may appear as an abrupt obstruction or filling defect.

Other modalities of breast imaging have been investigated. Automated breast ultrasonography is very useful in distinguishing cystic from solid lesions but should be used only as a supplement to physical examination and mammography in screening for breast cancer. Diaphanography (transillumination of the breasts) and thermography are of no proved screening value.

Self-Examination

All women over age 20 should be advised to examine their breasts monthly. Premenopausal women should perform the examination 7–8 days after the menstrual period. The breasts should be inspected initially while standing before a mirror with the hands at the sides, overhead, and pressed firmly on the hips to contract the pectoralis muscles. Masses, asymmetry of breasts, and slight dimpling of the skin may become apparent as a result of these maneuvers. Next, in a supine position, each breast should be carefully palpated with the fingers of the opposite hand. Physicians should instruct women in the technique of self-examination and advise them to report at once for medical evaluation if a mass or other abnormality is noted.

Some women discover small breast lumps more readily when their skin is moist while bathing or showering.

Most women do not practice self-examination, and its value is controversial. Clearly, however, it is not harmful and may be beneficial.

Mammography

Mammography is the most useful technique for the detection of early breast cancer. The two methods of mammography in common use are ordinary film screen radiography and xeroradiography. From the standpoint of diagnosing breast cancer, the two methods give comparable results. Using film screen techniques, it is now possible to perform a high-quality mammogram while delivering less than 0.4 cGy to the mid breast per view, and for this reason film screen mammography has largely replaced the xeromammographic technique, which delivers more radiation.

Mammography is the only reliable means of detecting breast cancer before a mass can be palpated in the breast. Slowly growing breast cancers can be identified by mammography at least 2 years before reaching a size detectable by palpation.

Calcifications are the most easily recognized mammographic abnormality. The most common mammographic abnormalities associated with carcinoma of the breast are clustered polymorphic microcalcifications. Such calcifications are usually at least five to eight in number, aggregated in one part of the breast and differing from each other in size and shape, often including branched or V- or Y-shaped configurations. There may be an associated mammographic mass density or, at time, only a mass density with no calcifications. Such a density usually has irregular or ill-defined borders and may lead to architectural distortion within the breast. A small mass or architectural distortion, particularly in a dense breast, may be subtle and difficult to detect.

Indications for mammography are as follows: (1) to evaluate each breast when a diagnosis of potentially curable breast cancer has been made, and at yearly intervals thereafter; (2) to evaluate a questionable or ill-defined breast mass or other suspicious change in the breast; (3) to search for an occult breast cancer in a woman with metastatic disease in axillary nodes or elsewhere from an unknown primary; (4) to screen women prior to cosmetic operations or prior to biopsy of a mass, to examine for an unsuspected cancer; (5) to screen at regular intervals a selected group of women who are at high risk for developing breast cancer (see below); and (6) to follow those women with breast cancer who have been treated with breast-conserving surgery and radiation.

Patients with a dominant or suspicious mass must undergo biopsy despite mammographic findings. The mammogram should be obtained prior to biopsy so that other suspicious areas can be noted and the contralateral breast can be checked. Mammography is never a substitute for biopsy, because it may not reveal clinical cancer in a very dense breast, as may be seen in young women with mammary dysplasia, and may not reveal medullary type cancers.

CLINICAL FINDINGS & DIAGNOSIS

The patient with breast cancer usually presents with a lump in the breast. When the history is taken, special note should be made of breast cancer risk factors, the temporal relationship of mass to menstrual cycle, and previous breast problems. Clinical evaluation should include assessment of the local lesion and a search for evidence of metastases in regional nodes or distant sites. After the diagnosis of breast cancer has been confirmed by biopsy, additional studies are often needed to complete the search for distant metastases or an occult primary in the other breast. Then, before any decision is made about treatment, all the available clinical data are used to determine the extent or stage of the patient's disease.

Symptoms

The presenting complaint in about 70% of patients with breast cancer is a lump (usually painless) in the breast. About 90% of breast masses are discovered by the patient herself. Less frequent symptoms are breast pain; nipple discharge; erosion, retraction, enlargement, or itching of the nipple; and redness, generalized hardness, enlargement, or shrinking of the breast. Rarely, an axillary mass or swelling of the arm may be the first symptom. Back or bone pain, jaundice, or weight loss may be the result of systemic metastases, but these symptoms are rarely seen on initial presentation.

Signs

The relative frequency of carcinoma in various anatomic sites in the breast is shown in Figure 17–1.

Inspection of the breast is the first step in physical examination and should be carried out with the patient sitting, arms at sides and then overhead. Abnormal variations in breast size and contour, minimal nipple retraction, and slight edema, redness, or retraction of the skin can be identified. Asymmetry of the breasts and retraction or dimpling of the skin can often be accentuated by having the patient raise her arms overhead or press her hands on her hips in order to contract the pectoralis muscles. Axillary and supraclavicular areas should be thoroughly palpated for enlarged nodes with the patient sitting (Figure 17–2). Palpation of the breast for masses or other changes should be performed with the patient both seated and supine with the arm abducted (Figure 17–3). Some authorities recommend palpation with a rotary motion of the examiner's fingers as well as a horizontal stripping motion.

Breast cancer usually consists of a nontender, firm or hard lump with poorly delineated margins (caused by local infiltration). Slight skin or nipple retraction is an important sign. Minimal asymmetry of the breast may be noted. Very small (1–2 mm) erosions of the nipple epithelium may be the only manifestation of Paget's carcinoma. Watery, serous, or bloody

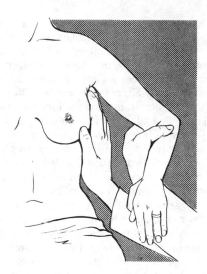

Figure 17–2. Palpation of axillary region for enlarged lymph nodes.

discharge from the nipple is an occasional early sign but is more often associated with benign disease.

A lesion smaller than 1 cm in diameter may be difficult or impossible for the examiner to feel and yet may be discovered by the patient. She should always be asked to demonstrate the location of the mass; if the physician fails to confirm the patient's suspicions, the examination should be repeated in 1 month, preferably 1–2 weeks after the onset of menses. During the premenstrual phase of the cycle, increased innocuous nodularity may suggest neoplasm or may obscure an underlying lesion. If there is any question regarding the nature of an abnormality under these circumstances, the patient should be asked to return after her period. Thirty-five to 50 percent of women with cancers detected during organ-

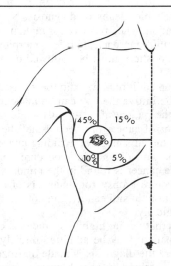

Figure 17–1. Frequency of breast carcinoma at various anatomic sites.

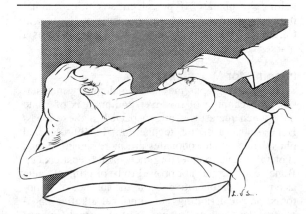

Figure 17–3. Palpation of breasts. Palpation is performed with the patient supine and arm abducted.

ized screening programs have them detected by mammography only and not physical examination.

The following are characteristic of advanced carcinoma: edema, redness, nodularity, or ulceration of the skin; the presence of a large primary tumor; fixation to the chest wall; enlargement, shrinkage, or retraction of the breast; marked axillary lymphadenopathy; supraclavicular lymphadenopathy; edema of the ipsilateral arm; and distant metastases.

Metastases tend to involve regional lymph nodes, which may be clinically palpable. With regard to the axilla, one or two movable, nontender, not particularly firm lymph nodes 5 mm or less in diameter are frequently present and are generally of no significance. Firm or hard nodes larger than 5 mm in diameter usually contain metastases. Axillary nodes that are matted or fixed to skin or deep structures indicate advanced disease (at least stage III). Histologic studies show that microscopic metastases are present in about 30% of patients with clinically negative nodes. On the other hand, if the examiner thinks that the axillary nodes are involved, that impression will be borne out by histologic section in about 85% of cases. The incidence of positive axillary nodes increases with the size of the primary tumor and with the local invasiveness of the neoplasm.

In most cases no nodes are palpable in the supraclavicular fossa. Firm or hard nodes of any size in this location or just beneath the clavicle (infraclavicular nodes) are suggestive of metastatic cancer and should be biopsied. Ipsilateral supraclavicular or infraclavicular nodes containing cancer indicate that the tumor is in an advanced stage (stage IV). Edema of the ipsilateral arm, commonly caused by metastatic infiltration of regional lymphatics, is also a sign of advanced (stage IV) cancer.

Laboratory Findings

A consistently elevated sedimentation rate may be the result of disseminated cancer. Liver or bone metastases may be associated with elevation of serum alkaline phosphatase. Hypercalcemia is an occasional important finding in advanced cancer of the breast. Carcinoembryonic antigen (CEA) may be used as a marker for recurrent breast cancer.

Imaging for Metastases

Chest radiographs may show pulmonary metastases. CT scanning of the liver and brain is of value only when metastases are suspected in these areas. Bone scans utilizing technetium Tc 99m-labeled phosphates or phosphonates are more sensitive than skeletal x-rays in detecting metastatic breast cancer. Bone scanning has not proved to be of clinical value as a routine preoperative test in the absence of symptoms, physical findings, or abnormal alkaline phosphatase levels. The frequency of abnormal findings on bone scan parallels the status of the axillary lymph nodes on pathologic examination. Bone scan should be performed for patients with symptoms and for those with elevated calcium or alkaline phosphatase levels.

Biopsy

The diagnosis of breast cancer depends ultimately upon examination of tissue removed by biopsy. Treatment should never be undertaken without an unequivocal histologic diagnosis of cancer. The safest course is biopsy examination of all suspicious masses found on physical examination and, in the absence of a mass, of suspicious lesions demonstrated by mammography. About 30% of lesions thought to be definitely cancer prove on biopsy to be benign, and about 15% of lesions believed to be benign are found to be malignant. These findings demonstrate the fallibility of clinical judgment and the necessity for biopsy. Dominant masses or suspicious nonpalpable mammographic findings must be biopsied. A breast mass should not be followed without histologic diagnosis, except perhaps in the premenopausal woman with a nonsuspicious mass presumed to be fibrocystic disease. A lesion such as this could be observed through one or two menstrual cycles. However, if the mass does not completely resolve during this time, it must be biopsied. Figures 17–4 and 17–5 present algorithms for management of breast masses in pre- and postmenopausal patients.

The simplest method is needle biopsy, either by aspiration of tumor cells (fine-needle aspiration cytology) or by obtaining a small core of tissue with a Vim-Silverman or other special needle. A nondiagnostic needle biopsy or fine-needle aspiration should be followed by open biopsy, because false-negative needle biopsies may occur in 5–10% of cancers. False-positive results occur rarely (< 1%).

Open biopsy under local anesthesia as a separate procedure prior to deciding upon definitive treatment is the most reliable means of diagnosis. Needle biopsy or aspiration, when positive for malignancy, offers a more rapid approach with less morbidity, but when nondiagnostic it must be followed by excisional biopsy.

Decisions on additional workup for metastatic disease and on definitive therapy can be made and discussed with the patient after the histologic or cytologic diagnosis of cancer has been established. This approach has the advantage of avoiding unnecessary hospitalization and diagnostic procedures in many patients, since cancer is found in the minority of patients who require biopsy for diagnosis of a breast lump. In addition, in situ cancers are not easily diagnosed cytologically.

As an alternative in highly suspicious circumstances, the patient may be admitted directly to the hospital, where the diagnosis is made on frozen section of tissue obtained by open biopsy under general anesthesia. If the frozen section is positive, the surgeon could proceed immediately with operation. This

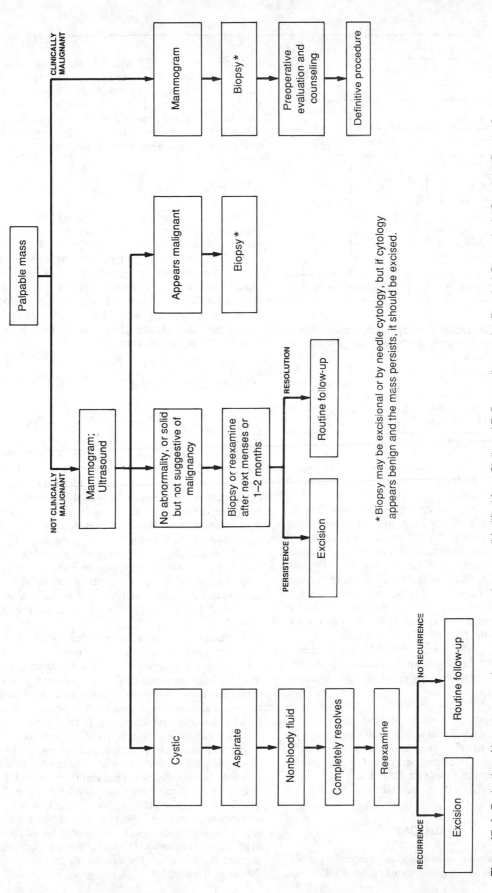

Figure 17-4. Evaluation of breast masses in premenopausal women. (Modified from Giuliano AE: Breast disease. In: *Practical Gynecologic Oncology*. Berek JS, Hacker NF [editors]. Williams & Wilkins, 1989.)

Palpable mass

NOT CLINICALLY MALIGNANT

CLINICALLY MALIGNANT

Mammogram; Ultrasound

Mammogram → Biopsy* → Preoperative evaluation and counseling → Definitive procedure

Appears malignant → Biopsy *

No abnormality, or solid but not suggestive of malignancy → Biopsy or reexamine after next menses or 1–2 months

RESOLUTION → Routine follow-up

PERSISTENCE → Excision

Cystic → Aspirate → Nonbloody fluid → Completely resolves → Reexamine

NO RECURRENCE → Routine follow-up

RECURRENCE → Excision

*Biopsy may be excisional or by needle cytology, but if cytology appears benign and the mass persists, it should be excised.

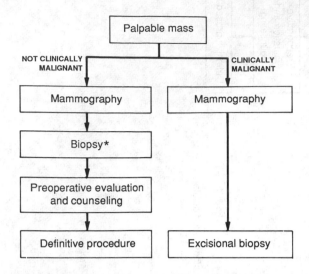

* Biopsy may be excisional or by needle cytology, but if cytology appears benign and the mass persists, it should be excised.

Figure 17–5. Evaluation of breast masses in postmenopausal women. (Modified from Giuliano AE: Breast disease. In: *Practical Gynecologic Oncology.* Berek JS, Hacker NF [editors]. Williams & Wilkins, 1989.)

one-step method should rarely be used today except perhaps when cytologic study has already suggested the presence of cancer.

In general, the two-step approach—outpatient biopsy followed by definitive operation at a later date—is preferred in the diagnosis and treatment of breast cancer, because patients can be given time to adjust to the diagnosis of cancer, can carefully consider alternative forms of therapy, and can seek a second opinion if they wish. Studies have shown no adverse effect from the short (1–2 weeks) delay of the two-step procedure, and this is the current recommendation of the National Cancer Institute.

At the time of the initial biopsy of breast cancer, it is important for the physician to preserve a portion of the specimen for determination of estrogen and progesterone receptors.

Other Cytology

Cytologic examination of nipple discharge or cyst fluid may be helpful on rare occasions. As a rule, mammography (or ductography) and breast biopsy are required when nipple discharge or cyst fluid is bloody or cytologically questionable.

DIFFERENTIAL DIAGNOSIS

The lesions to be considered most often in the differential diagnosis of breast cancer are the following,

in descending order of frequency: mammary dysplasia (cystic disease of the breast), fibroadenoma, intraductal papilloma, lipoma, and fat necrosis. The differential diagnosis of a breast lump should be established without delay by biopsy, by aspiration of a cyst, or by observing the patient until disappearance of the lump within a period of a few weeks.

STAGING

The extent of disease evident from physical findings and special preoperative studies is used to determine its clinical stage. Currently, the American Joint Committee on Cancer and the International Union Against Cancer have agreed on a TNM (Tumor, Regional Lymph Nodes, Distant Metastases) staging system for breast cancer. The use of this uniform TNM staging system will enhance communication among investigators and clinicians. Table 17–2 sets forth the TNM classification.

PATHOLOGIC TYPES

Numerous pathologic subtypes of breast cancer can be identified histologically (Table 17–3). These types are distinguished by the histologic appearance and growth pattern of the tumor. In general, breast cancer arises either from the epithelial lining of the large or intermediate-sized ducts (ductal) or from the epithelium of the terminal ducts of the lobules (lobular). The cancer may be invasive or in situ. Most breast cancers arise from the intermediate ducts and are invasive (invasive ductal, infiltrating ductal), and most histologic types are merely subtypes of invasive ductal cancer with unusual growth patterns (colloid, medullary, scirrhous, etc). Ductal carcinoma that has not invaded the extraductal tissue is intraductal or in situ ductal. Lobular carcinoma may be either invasive or in situ.

Except for the in situ cancers, the histologic subtypes have only a slight bearing on prognosis when outcomes are compared after accurate staging. Various histologic parameters, such as invasion of blood vessels, tumor differentiation, invasion of breast lymphatics, and tumor necrosis have been examined, but they too seem to have little prognostic value.

The noninvasive cancers by definition lack the ability to spread. However, in patients whose biopsies show noninvasive intraductal cancer, associated invasive ductal cancers are present in about 1–3% of cases. Some clinicians consider lobular carcinoma in situ (LCIS) to be a premalignant lesion that is not a true cancer. It lacks the ability to spread but is associated with subsequent development of invasive cancer in at least 20% of cases. In LCIS, the subsequent cancer may occur in either breast regardless of the side of the original biopsy.

Table 17–2. TNM staging for breast cancer.[1]

Stage	T	N	M
0	Tis	N0	M0
I	T1	N0	M0
IIA	T0	N1	M0
	T1	N1	M0
	T2	N0	M0
IIB	T2	N1	M0
	T3	N0	M0
IIIA	T0	N2	M0
	T1	N2	M0
	T2	N2	M0
	T3	N1, N2	M0
IIIB	T4	Any N	M0
	Any T	N3	M0
IV	Any T	Any N	M1

Tumor Size (T)	
TX	Primary tumor cannot be assessed.
T0	No evidence of primary tumor.
Tis	Carcinoma in situ; intraductal carcinoma, lobular carcinoma in situ, or Paget's disease of the nipple with no tumor.
T1	Tumor 2 cm or less in greatest dimension. T1a 0.5 cm or less in greatest dimension. T1b More than 0.5 cm but not more than 1 cm in greatest dimension. T1c More than 1 cm but not more than 2 cm in greatest dimension.
T2	Tumor more than 2 cm but not more than 5 cm in greatest dimension.
T3	Tumor more than 5 cm in greatest dimension.
T4	Tumor of any size with direct extension to chest wall or skin.

Regional Lymph Nodes (N)	
NX	Regional lymph nodes cannot be assessed (eg, previously removed).
N0	No regional lymph node metastases.
N1	Metastasis to movable ipsilateral lymph node(s).
N2	Metastasis to ipsilateral axillary lymph node(s) fixed to one another or to other structures.
N3	Metastasis to ipsilateral internal mammary lymph node(s).

Distant Metastases (M)	
MX	Presence of distant metastasis cannot be assessed.
M0	No distant metastasis.
M1	Distant metastasis (includes metastasis to ipsilateral supraclavicular lymph node[s]).

[1]American Joint Committee on Cancer: *Manual for Staging of Cancer*, 3rd ed. Lippincott, 1988.

Table 17–3. Histologic types of breast cancer.

	Percent Occurrence
Infiltrating ductal (not otherwise specified)	70–80
Medullary	5–8
Colloid (mucinous)	2–4
Tubular	1–2
Papillary	1–2
Invasive lobular	6–8
Noninvasive	4–6
Intraductal	2–3
Lobular in situ	2–3
Rare cancers	<1
Juvenile (secretory)	…
Adenoid cystic	…
Epidermoid	…
Sudoriferous	…

SPECIAL CLINICAL FORMS OF BREAST CANCER

Paget's Carcinoma

The basic lesion is usually an infiltrating ductal carcinoma, usually well differentiated. The nipple epithelium is infiltrated, but gross nipple changes are often minimal, and a tumor mass may not be palpable. The first symptom is often itching or burning of the nipple, with superficial erosion or ulceration. The diagnosis is established by biopsy of the erosion.

Paget's carcinoma is not common (about 1% of all breast cancers), but it is important because it appears innocuous. It is frequently diagnosed and treated as dermatitis or bacterial infection, leading to unfortunate delay in detection. When the lesion consists of nipple changes only, the incidence of axillary metastases is about 5%, and the prognosis is excellent. When a breast tumor is also present, the incidence of axillary metastases rises, with an associated marked decrease in prospects for cure by surgical or other treatment.

Inflammatory Carcinoma

This is the most malignant form of breast cancer and constitutes less than 3% of all cases. The clinical findings consist of a rapidly growing, sometimes painful mass that enlarges the breast. The overlying skin becomes erythematous, edematous, and warm. Often there is no distinct mass, since the tumor infiltrates the involved breast diffusely. The diagnosis should be made when the redness involves more than one-third of the skin over the breast and biopsy shows invasion of the subdermal lymphatics. The inflammatory changes, often mistaken for an infectious process, are caused by carcinomatous invasion of the dermal lymphatics, with resulting edema and hyperemia. If the physician suspects infection but the lesion does not respond rapidly (1–2 weeks) to antibiotics, biopsy examination must be performed. Metastases tend to occur early and widely, and for this reason inflammatory carcinoma is rarely curable. Mastectomy is seldom, if ever, indicated. Radiation, hormone therapy, and anticancer chemotherapy are the measures most likely to be of value.

Breast Cancer Occurring During Pregnancy or Lactation

Only 1–2% of breast cancers occur during pregnancy or lactation. Breast cancer complicates approximately one in 3000 pregnancies. The diagnosis is frequently delayed, because physiologic changes in the breast may obscure the true nature of the lesion. This results in a tendency of both patients and physicians to misinterpret the findings and to procrastinate in deciding on biopsy. When the neoplasm is confined to the breast, the 5-year survival rate after mastectomy is about 70%. Axillary metastases are already present in 60–70% of patients, and for them the 5-year survival rate after mastectomy is only 30–40%. Pregnancy (or lactation) is not a contraindication to operation, and treatment should be based on the stage of the disease as in the nonpregnant (or nonlactating) woman. Overall survival rates have improved, since cancers are now diagnosed in pregnant women earlier than in the past.

Bilateral Breast Cancer

Clinically evident simultaneous bilateral breast cancer occurs in less than 1% of cases, but there is a 5–8% incidence of later occurrence of cancer in the second breast. Bilaterality occurs more often in women under age 50 and is more frequent when the tumor in the primary breast is lobular. The incidence of second breast cancers increases directly with the length of time the patient is alive after her first cancer—about 0.5% per year.

In patients with breast cancer, mammography should be performed before primary treatment and at regular intervals thereafter, to search for occult cancer in the opposite breast. Routine biopsy of the opposite breast is usually not warranted.

Noninvasive Cancer

Noninvasive cancer can occur within the ducts (ductal carcinoma in situ) or lobules (lobular carcinoma in situ). While ductal carcinoma in situ behaves as an early malignancy, lobular carcinoma in situ would perhaps be better called lobular neoplasia. Ductal carcinoma in situ tends to be unilateral and most likely progresses to invasive cancer. Approximately 40–60% of women who have ductal carcinoma in situ treated with biopsy alone will develop invasive cancer within the same breast. Lobular carcinoma in situ, however, appears to be more of a risk factor calling attention to the probability of developing invasive cancer in either breast. Approximately 20% of women with lobular carcinoma in situ will develop invasive cancer (usually ductal). This invasive cancer occurs with equal frequency in either breast.

The treatment of intraductal lesions is controversial. Ductal carcinoma can be treated with total mastectomy or breast conservation with wide excision with or without radiation therapy. Lobular carcinoma in situ is probably best managed with careful observation. However, patients who are unwilling to accept the increased risk of breast cancer may be offered bilateral total mastectomy. Axillary metastases are rare.

HORMONE RECEPTOR SITES

The presence or absence of estrogen and progesterone receptors in the cytoplasm of tumor cells is of paramount importance in managing all patients with breast cancer, especially those with recurrent or metastatic disease. They are of proved value in determining adjuvant therapy and therapy for patients with advanced disease. Up to 60% of patients with metastatic breast cancer will respond to hormonal manipulation if their tumors contain estrogen receptors. However, fewer than 5% of patients with metastatic, ER-negative tumors can be successfully treated with hormonal manipulation.

Progesterone receptors may be an even more sensitive indicator than estrogen receptors of patients who may respond to hormonal manipulation. Up to 80% of patients with metastatic progesterone receptor-positive tumors seem to respond to hormonal manipulation. Receptors probably have no relationship to response to chemotherapy.

Some studies suggest that estrogen receptors are of prognostic significance. Patients whose primary tumors are receptor-positive have a more favorable course than those whose tumors are receptor-negative.

Receptor status is not only valuable for the management of metastatic disease but may help in the selection of patients for adjuvant therapy. Some studies suggest that adjuvant hormonal therapy (tamoxifen) for patients with receptor-positive tumors and adjuvant chemotherapy for patients with receptor-negative tumors may improve survival rates even in the absence of lymph node metastases (see Adjuvant Therapy).

Estrogen and progesterone receptor assays should be done routinely for every breast cancer at the time of initial diagnosis. Small tumors with insufficient tissue volume for quantitative assay may be examined by immunohistochemistry. The value of this assay technique remains to be proved. Receptor status may change after hormonal therapy, radiotherapy, or chemotherapy. The specimen requires special handling, and the laboratory should be prepared to process the specimen correctly.

CURATIVE TREATMENT

Treatment may be curative or palliative. Curative treatment is advised for clinical stage I and stage II disease (Table 17–2). Patients with locally advanced (stage III) tumors may be cured with multimodality therapy, but in most cases palliation is all that can be expected. Palliative treatment is appropriate for all patients with stage IV disease and for previously treated patients who develop distant metastases or who have unresectable local cancers.

The growth potential of tumors and host resistance factors vary over a wide range from patient to patient and may be altered during the course of the disease. The doubling time of breast cancer cells ranges from several weeks in a rapidly growing lesion to nearly a year in a slowly growing one. Assuming that the rate of doubling is constant and that the neoplasm originates in one cell, a carcinoma with a doubling time of 100 days may not reach clinically detectable size (1 cm) for about 8 years. On the other hand, rapidly growing cancers have a much shorter preclinical course and a greater tendency to metastasize to regional nodes or more distant sites by the time a breast mass is discovered.

The relatively long preclinical growth phase and the tendency of breast cancers to metastasize have led many clinicians to believe that breast cancer is a systemic disease at the time of diagnosis. Although it may be true that breast cancer cells are released from the tumor prior to diagnosis, variations in the host-tumor relationship may prohibit the growth of disseminated disease in many patients. For this reason, a pessimistic attitude concerning the management of localized breast cancer is not warranted, and many patients can be cured with proper treatment.

Choice of Primary Therapy

The extent of disease and its biologic aggressiveness are the principal determinants of the outcome of primary therapy. Clinical and pathologic staging help in assessing extent of disease (Table 17–2), but each is to some extent imprecise. Other factors such as DNA flow cytometry, tumor grade, hormone receptor assays, and oncogene amplification may be of prognostic value but are not important in determining the type of local therapy. Since about two-thirds of patients eventually manifest distant disease regardless of the form of primary therapy, there is a tendency to think of breast carcinoma as being systemic in most patients at the time they first present for treatment.

There is a great deal of controversy regarding the optimal method of primary therapy of stage I, II, and III breast carcinoma, and opinions on this subject have changed considerably in the past decade. Legislation initiated in California and Massachusetts and now adopted in numerous states requires physicians to inform patients of alternative treatment methods in the management of breast cancer.

Breast-Conserving Therapy

The results of the Milan trial and a large randomized trial conducted by the National Surgical Adjuvant Breast Project (NSABP) in the USA showed that disease-free survival rates were similar for patients treated by partial mastectomy plus axillary dissection followed by radiation therapy and for those treated by modified radical mastectomy (total mastectomy plus axillary dissection). All patients whose axillary nodes contained tumor received adjuvant chemotherapy.

In the NSABP trial, patients were randomized to three treatment types: (1) "lumpectomy" (removal of the tumor with *confirmed* tumor-free margins) plus whole breast irradiation, (2) lumpectomy alone, and (3) total mastectomy. All patients underwent axillary lymph node dissection. Some patients in this study had tumors as large as 4 cm with (or without) palpable axillary lymph nodes. The lowest local recurrence rate was among patients treated with lumpectomy and postoperative irradiation; the highest was among patients treated with lumpectomy alone. However, no statistically significant differences were observed in overall or disease-free survival among the three treatment groups. This study shows that lumpectomy and axillary dissection with postoperative radiation therapy is as effective as modified radical mastectomy for the management of patients with stage I and stage II breast cancer. A high local failure rate (nearly 40% at 8 years) was seen for lumpectomy without radiation therapy.

The results of these and other trials have demonstrated that much less aggressive surgical treatment of the primary lesion than has previously been thought necessary gives equivalent therapeutic results and may preserve an acceptable cosmetic appearance.

Tumor size is a major consideration in determining the feasibility of breast conservation. The lumpectomy trial of the NSABP randomized patients with tumors as large as 4 cm. To achieve an acceptable cosmetic result, the patient must have a breast of sufficient size to enable excision of a 4 cm tumor without considerable deformity. Therefore, large size is only a relative contraindication. Subareolar tumors are also difficult to excise without considerable deformity. Clinically detectable multifocality is a relative contraindication to breast-conserving surgery, as is fixation to the chest wall or skin or involvement of the nipple or overlying skin. However, the patient and not the surgeon should be the judge of what is cosmetically acceptable; some patients would prefer breast deformity rather than complete absence of the breast or even reconstruction.

It is important to recognize that axillary dissection is valuable both in planning therapy and in staging cancer. Operation is extremely effective in preventing axillary recurrences. In addition, lymph nodes removed during the procedure can be pathologically assessed. This assessment is essential for the planning of adjuvant therapy, which is often recommended.

Current Recommendations

A recent NIH consensus statement argues that breast-conserving surgery with radiation is the preferred form of treatment for patients with early-stage breast cancer. However, this technique has still not gained wide acceptance by physicians or patients. Despite the numerous randomized trials comparing breast conserving surgery and radiation therapy to mastectomy, breast-conserving surgery appears underutilized and mastectomy remains the more common treatment. In a recent survey, only 25% of patients in the United States with stage I or II breast cancer were treated with breast-conserving surgery and radiation therapy, compared with 75% treated with mastectomy. This seems to vary by region of the country, ranging from 15% in the South Central United States to approximately 30% in the Pacific Region.

Modified radical mastectomy (total mastectomy plus axillary lymph node dissection) has been the standard therapy for most patients with breast cancer. This operation removes the entire breast, overlying skin, nipple, and areolar complex as well as the underlying pectoralis fascia with the axillary lymph nodes in continuity. It offers the same overall survival and local control rates as does lumpectomy with axillary dissection and postoperative radiation therapy. The major advantage of modified radical mastectomy is that radiation therapy is usually not necessary. The disadvantage, of course, is the psychologic trauma associated with breast loss. Radical mastectomy, which removes the underlying pectoralis muscle, should be performed rarely if at all. Axillary node dissection is not indicated for noninfiltrating cancers, because nodal metastases are rarely present.

Preoperatively, full discussion with the patient regarding the rationale for operation and various alternative forms of treatment is essential. Breast-conserving surgery and radiation should be offered whenever possible, since most patients would prefer to save the breast. Breast reconstruction should be discussed with patients who choose or require mastectomy, and the option of simultaneous mastectomy with immediate reconstruction should be discussed. Time spent preoperatively in educating the patient and her family about these matters is time well spent.

Adjuvant Therapy

Chemotherapy or hormonal therapy is advocated for most patients with curable breast cancer. The objective of adjuvant therapy is to eliminate the occult metastases responsible for late recurrences while they are microscopic and theoretically most vulnerable to anticancer agents.

Numerous clinical trials with various adjuvant chemotherapeutic regimens have been completed. The most extensive clinical experience to date is with the CMF regimen (cyclophosphamide, methotrexate, and fluorouracil). Cyclophosphamide can be given either orally, in a dose of 100 mg/m^2 daily for 14 days; or intravenously, in a dose of 600 mg/m^2 on days 1 and 8. Methotrexate is given intravenously, 40 mg/m^2 on days 1 and 8; and fluorouracil is given intravenously, 600 mg/m^2 on days 1 and 8. This cycle is repeated every 4 weeks. Some clinicians prefer to give the drugs on 1 day only every 3 weeks. There appears to be no obvious advantage except that patient compliance is assured when the cyclophosphamide is give intravenously. The regimen should be continued for 6 months in patients with axillary metastases. Premenopausal women with positive axillary nodes definitely benefit from adjuvant chemotherapy. The recurrence rate in premenopausal patients who received no adjuvant chemotherapy was more than 1½ times that of those who received such therapy. No therapeutic effect with CMF has been shown in postmenopausal women with positive nodes, perhaps because therapy was modified so often in response to side effects that the total amount of drugs administered was less than planned. Other trials with different agents support the value of adjuvant chemotherapy; in some studies, postmenopausal women benefit as well.

Adjuvant chemotherapy can be offered confidently to premenopausal women with metastases in axillary lymph nodes, but the use of adjuvant chemotherapy in postmenopausal women and patients with negative axillary lymph nodes is more controversial. While postmenopausal women benefit from chemotherapy, selection of patients must take into account other common health problems that older women may have and the effects of chemotherapy on the patient's overall health. Tamoxifen can be given with few side effects even in the elderly. Tamoxifen appears to increase bone density and favorably affect lipid and lipoprotein profiles, which may explain the observed decreased mortality rate from coronary artery disease seen in patients taking tamoxifen.

The addition of hormones may improve the results of adjuvant therapy. For example, tamoxifen has been shown to enhance the beneficial effects of melphalan and fluorouracil in postmenopausal women whose tumors are ER-positive. Tamoxifen alone in a dosage of 10 mg orally twice a day has been the recommended treatment for postmenopausal women with ER-positive tumors. However, a recent NSABP trial showed that tamoxifen plus chemotherapy (Adriamycin [doxorubicin] plus cyclophosphamide [AC] or prednisone plus Adriamycin plus fluorouracil [PAF]) lowered recurrence rates more than tamoxifen alone in postmenopausal women with ER-positive tumors.

The length of time adjuvant therapy must be administered remains uncertain. Several studies suggest that shorter treatment periods may be as effective as longer ones. For example, one study compared 6 versus 12 cycles of postoperative CMF and found 5-year disease-free survival rates to be comparable. One of the earliest adjuvant trials used a 6-day perioperative regimen of intravenous cyclophosphamide alone; follow-up at 15 years shows a 15% improvement in disease-free survival rates for treated patients, suggesting that short-term therapy may be effective.

Patients with negative nodes have not been treated with adjuvant therapy until recently. Several studies of adjuvant therapy in node-negative women have now been published and show a beneficial effect of adjuvant chemotherapy or tamoxifen in delaying recurrence, but as of yet no effect has been seen on survival. A number of protocols, including CMF—cyclophosphamide, methotrexate, and fluorouracil—with leucovorin rescue as well as tamoxifen alone have increased disease-free survival times. The magnitude of this improvement is about one-third, ie, a group of women with an estimated 30% recurrence rate would have a 20% recurrence rate after adjuvant systemic therapy. Quality of life while receiving chemotherapy does not appear to be greatly altered.

The current recommendations for adjuvant chemotherapy can be summarized as follows (Tables 17–4 and 17–5):

(1) Premenopausal women with positive lymph nodes and either ER-positive or ER-negative tumors should be treated with adjuvant combination chemotherapy.

(2) Premenopausal women with negative nodes whose tumors are ER-positive benefit from tamoxifen; premenopausal women with negative axillary nodes whose tumors are ER-negative benefit from combination chemotherapy.

(3) Postmenopausal patients with positive lymph nodes and positive hormone receptor tumors should receive tamoxifen.

(4) Postmenopausal patients with positive lymph nodes whose tumors are ER-negative benefit from adjuvant combination chemotherapy.

(5) Postmenopausal women with negative ax-

illary nodes whose tumors are ER-positive may benefit from adjuvant tamoxifen; postmenopausal women with negative axillary lymph nodes whose tumors are ER-negative may benefit from adjuvant chemotherapy.

A 1990 consensus statement from the NIH on early-stage breast cancer recommends (1) that all patients who are candidates for clinical trials be offered the opportunity to participate, and (2) that node-negative patients who are not candidates for clinical trials ". . . should be made aware of the benefits and risks of adjuvant systemic therapy. The decision to use adjuvant treatment should follow a thorough discussion with the patient regarding the likely risk of recurrence without adjuvant therapy, the expected reduction in risk with adjuvant therapy, toxicities of therapy, and its impact on quality of life." In practice, most medical oncologists are currently using systemic adjuvant therapy for patients with early-stage breast cancer. Other prognostic factors being used to determine the patient's risks are tumor size, estrogen and progesterone receptor status, nuclear grade, histologic type, proliferative rate, and oncogene expression. Table 17–6 summarizes these prognostic factors. The assumption is made that patients with node-negative aggressive tumors should receive ad-

Table 17–4. Adjuvant chemotherapy for premenopausal women. (Summary of NIH Consensus Conference June 18–21, 1990.)

Nodal Involvement	Estrogen Receptors	Adjuvant Systemic Therapy
Yes	Positive	Combination chemotherapy
Yes	Negative	Combination chemotherapy
No	Positive	Tamoxifen[1]
No	Negative	Combination chemotherapy[1]

[1]Effect on overall survival not yet clearly demonstrated.

Table 17–5. Adjuvant chemotherapy for postmenopausal women. (Summary of NIH Consensus Conference June 18–21, 1990.)

Nodal Involvement	Estrogen Receptors	Adjuvant Systemic Therapy
Yes	Positive	Tamoxifen
Yes	Negative	Combination chemotherapy[1]
No	Positive	Tamoxifen[1]
No	Negative	Combination chemotherapy[1]

[1]Effect on overall survival not yet clearly demonstrated.

Table 17–6. Prognostic factors in node-negative breast cancer.

Prognostic Factor	Increased Recurrence	Decreased Recurrence
Size	T3 T2	T1 T0
Hormone receptors	Negative	Positive
DNA flow cytometry	Aneuploid	Diploid
Histologic grade	High	Low
Tumor labeling index	<3%	>3%
S phase fraction	>5%	<5%
Lymphatic or vascular invasion	Present	Absent
Cathepsin D	High	Low
HER—*neu* oncogene	High	Low
Epidermal growth factor receptor	High	Low

juvant therapy. However, the role of adjuvant therapy for these patients is still unclear because of the short follow-up in the node-negative studies and the lack of an observed effect on survival to date.

Important questions remaining to be answered are the timing and duration of adjuvant chemotherapy, which chemotherapeutic agents should be applied for which subgroups of patients, how best to coordinate adjuvant chemotherapy with postoperative radiation therapy, the use of combinations of hormonal therapy and chemotherapy, and the value of prognostic factors other than hormone receptors in predicting response to adjuvant therapy. Adjuvant systemic therapy is not currently indicated for patients with small nonpalpable tumors (ie, tumors that cannot be quantitatively tested for hormonal receptors) and those with negative lymph nodes who have had favorable DNA studies.

PALLIATIVE TREATMENT

This section covers palliative therapy of disseminated disease incurable by surgery (stage IV).

Radiotherapy

Palliative radiotherapy may be advised for locally advanced cancers with distant metastases in order to control ulceration, pain, and other manifestations in the breast and regional nodes. Irradiation of the breast and chest wall and the axillary, internal mammary, and supraclavicular nodes should be undertaken in an attempt to cure locally advanced and inoperable lesions when there is no evidence of distant metastases. A small number of patients in this group are cured in spite of extensive breast and regional node involvement. Adjuvant chemotherapy should be considered for such patients.

Palliative irradiation is of value also in the treatment of certain bone or soft tissue metastases to control pain or avoid fracture. Radiotherapy is especially useful in the treatment of isolated bony metastasis and chest wall recurrences.

Hormone Therapy

Disseminated disease may respond to prolonged endocrine therapy such as administration of hormones (eg, estrogens, androgens, progestins; see Table 17–7); ablation of the ovaries, adrenals, or pituitary; or administration of drugs that block hormone receptor sites (eg, antiestrogens) or drugs that block the synthesis of hormones (eg, aminoglutethimide). Hormonal manipulation is usually more successful in postmenopausal women. If treatment is based on the presence of estrogen receptor protein in the primary tumor or metastases, however, the rate of response is nearly equal in premenopausal and postmenopausal women. A favorable response to hormonal manipulation occurs in about one-third of patients with metastatic breast cancer. Of those whose tumors contain estrogen receptors, the response is about 60% and perhaps as high as 80% for patients whose tumors contain progesterone receptors as well. Because only 5–10% of women whose tumors do not contain estrogen receptors respond, they should not receive hormonal therapy except in unusual circumstances such as an elderly patient who could not tolerate chemotherapy.

Since the quality of life during a remission induced by endocrine manipulation is usually superior to a remission following cytotoxic chemotherapy, it is usually best to try endocrine manipulation first in cases where the estrogen receptor status of the tumor is unknown. However, if the estrogen receptor status is unknown but the disease is progressing rapidly or involves visceral organs, endocrine therapy is rarely successful, and introducing it may waste valuable time.

In general, only one type of systemic therapy should be given at a time unless it is necessary to irradiate a destructive lesion of weight-bearing bone while the patient is on another regimen. The regimen should be changed only if the disease is clearly progressing but not if it appears to be stable. This is especially important for patients with destructive bone metastases, since minor changes in the status of these lesions are difficult to determine radiographically. A plan of therapy that would simultaneously minimize

Table 17–7. Commonly used hormonal agents for management of metastatic breast cancer.

Drug	Action	Usual Oral Dose	Major Side Effects
Tamoxifen (Nolvadex)	Antiestrogen	10 mg twice daily	Hot flashes, uterine bleeding, thrombophlebitis, rash
Diethylstilbestrol (DES)	Estrogen	5 mg 3 times daily	Fluid retention, uterine bleeding, thrombophlebitis, nausea
Megestrol acetate (Megace)	Progestin	40 mg 4 times daily	Fluid retention
Aminoglutethimide (Cytadren)[1]	Aromatase inhibitor	250 mg 4 times daily	Adrenal suppression, skin rashes, neurologic reactions

[1]Used with hydrocortisone.

toxicity and maximize benefits is often best achieved by hormonal manipulation.

The choice of endocrine therapy depends on the menopausal status of the patient. Women within 1 year of their last menstrual period are considered to be premenopausal, while women whose menstruation ceased more than a year ago are postmenopausal. The initial choice of therapy is referred to as primary hormonal manipulation; subsequent endocrine treatment is called secondary or tertiary hormonal manipulation.

A. The Premenopausal Patient:

1. Primary hormonal therapy–The potent antiestrogen tamoxifen is the endocrine treatment of choice in the premenopausal patient. Tamoxifen is usually given orally in a dose of 10 mg twice a day. At least two randomized clinical trials have now shown no significant difference in survival or response between tamoxifen therapy and bilateral oophorectomy. Most physicians prefer to use tamoxifen rather than perform oophorectomy, since it can be given with little morbidity and few side effects. Controversy continues about whether a response to tamoxifen is predictive of probable success with other forms of endocrine manipulation.

Bilateral oophorectomy is a reasonable alternative for primary hormonal manipulation in premenopausal women. It can be achieved rapidly and safely by surgery or, if the patient is a poor operative risk, by irradiation of the ovaries. Ovarian radiation therapy should be avoided in otherwise healthy patients, however, because of the high rate of complications and the longer time necessary to achieve results. Oophorectomy presumably works by eliminating estrogens, progestins, and androgens, which stimulate growth of the tumor. The average remission is about 12 months.

2. Secondary or tertiary hormonal therapy–Although patients who do not respond to tamoxifen or oophorectomy should be treated with cytotoxic drugs, those who respond and then relapse may subsequently respond to another form of endocrine treatment (Table 17–7). The initial choice for secondary endocrine manipulation has not been clearly defined. Adrenalectomy or hypophysectomy induces regression in approximately 30–50% of patients who have previously responded to oophorectomy. However, these procedures are rarely performed now.

Patients who respond initially to oophorectomy but subsequently relapse should receive tamoxifen. If this treatment fails, use of aminoglutethimide or megestrol acetate should be considered. Aminoglutethimide is an inhibitor of adrenal hormone synthesis and, when combined with a corticosteroid, provides a therapeutically effective "medical adrenalectomy." Megestrol is a progestational agent. Both drugs cause less morbidity and mortality than surgical adrenalectomy; can be discontinued once the patient improves; and are not associated with the many problems of postsurgical hypoadrenalism, so that patients who require chemotherapy are more easily managed.

B. The Postmenopausal Patient:

1. Primary hormonal therapy–Tamoxifen, 10 mg twice daily, is now the initial therapy of choice for postmenopausal women with metastatic breast cancer amenable to endocrine manipulation. It has fewer side effects than diethylstilbestrol, the former therapy of choice, and is just as effective. The main side effects of tamoxifen are nausea, vomiting, and skin rash. Rarely, it may induce hypercalcemia.

2. Secondary or tertiary hormonal therapy–Postmenopausal patients who do not respond to primary endocrine manipulation should be given cytotoxic drugs such as cyclophosphamide, methotrexate, and fluorouracil (CMF) or Adriamycin (doxorubicin) and cyclophosphamide (AC). Postmenopausal women who respond initially to tamoxifen but later manifest progressive disease could be given diethylstilbestrol or megestrol acetate. Some authorities use aminoglutethimide. Megestrol has fewer side effects than either aminoglutethimide or diethylstilbestrol. Androgens have many side effects and should rarely be used. In general, hypophysectomy or adrenalectomy is rarely necessary.

Chemotherapy

Cytotoxic drugs should be considered for the treatment of metastatic breast cancer (1) if visceral metastases are present (especially brain or lymphangitic pulmonary); (2) if hormonal treatment is unsuccessful or the disease has progressed after an initial response to hormonal manipulation; or (3) if the tumor is ER-negative. The most useful single chemotherapeutic agent to date is doxorubicin (Adriamycin), with a response rate of 40–50%. Single agents are rarely used. The remissions tend to be brief, and in general, experience with single-agent chemotherapy in patients with disseminated disease has not been encouraging.

Combination chemotherapy using multiple agents has proved to be more effective, with objectively observed favorable responses achieved in 60–80% of patients with stage IV disease. Various combinations of drugs have been used, and clinical trials are continuing in an effort to improve results and reduce undesirable side effects. Doxorubicin (40 mg/m^2 intravenously on day 1) and cyclophosphamide (200 mg/m^2 orally on days 3–6) produce an objective response in about 85% of patients so treated. Other chemotherapeutic regimens have consisted of various combinations of drugs, including cyclophosphamide, vincristine, methotrexate, and fluorouracil, with response rates ranging up to 60–70%. Prior adjuvant chemotherapy does not seem to alter response rates in patients who relapse. Few new drugs or combinations of drugs have been sufficiently effective in breast cancer to warrant wide acceptance.

Recently, high-dose chemotherapy and autologous bone marrow transplantation have aroused widespread interest for the treatment of metastatic breast cancer. With this technique, the patient receives high doses of cytotoxic agents. These cause severe side effects, including bone marrow suppression, for which the patient subsequently undergoes autologous bone marrow transplantation. Reported complete response rates are as high as 30–35%—considerably better than what can be achieved with conventional chemotherapy. However, median survival times and overall survival rates do not appear to be significantly different from those reported with conventional chemotherapy. No randomized controlled clinical trial has been published that compares high-dose chemotherapy followed by bone marrow transplantation with conventional chemotherapy. A study is under way to evaluate these two options in a controlled prospective manner. High-dose chemotherapy with autologous bone marrow transplantation is an exciting modality with promise for the future, but the procedure is probably best regarded as experimental at present. Some studies are currently examining the technique in an adjuvant setting for patients at extremely high risk of recurrence of breast cancer.

Malignant Pleural Effusion

This condition develops at some time in almost half of patients with metastatic breast cancer (see Chapter 18).

PROGNOSIS

The stage of breast cancer is the single most reliable indicator of prognosis (Table 17–8). Patients with disease localized to the breast and no evidence of regional spread after microscopic examination of the lymph nodes have by far the most favorable prognosis. Estrogen and progesterone receptors appear to be an important prognostic variable, because patients with hormone receptor-negative tumors and no evidence of metastases to the axillary lymph nodes have a much higher recurrence rate than do patients with hormone receptor-positive tumors and no regional metastases. The histologic subtype of breast cancer (eg, medullary, lobular, comedo) seems to have little, if any, significance in prognosis once these tumors are truly invasive. Flow cytometry of tumor cells to analyze DNA index and S-phase frequency aid in prognosis. Tumors with marked aneuploidy have a poor prognosis (Table 17–6). Her 2-*neu* oncogene amplification growth factors and cathepsin D may have some prognostic value, but few data exist as to their usefulness.

Most patients who develop breast cancer will ultimately die of that disease. The mortality rate of breast cancer patients exceeds that of age-matched normal controls for nearly 20 years. Thereafter, the mortality rates are equal, although deaths that occur among breast cancer patients are often directly the result of tumor. Five-year statistics do not accurately reflect the final outcome of therapy.

When cancer is localized to the breast, with no evidence of regional spread after pathologic examination, the clinical cure rate with most accepted methods of therapy is 75–90%. Exceptions to this generalization may be related to the hormonal receptor content of the tumor, tumor size, host resistance, or associated illness. Patients with small estrogen and progesterone receptor-positive tumors and no evidence of axillary spread probably have a 5-year survival rate of nearly 90%. When the axillary lymph nodes are involved with tumor, the survival rate drops to 40–50% at 5 years and probably less than 25% at 10 years. In general, breast cancer appears to be somewhat more malignant in younger than in older women, and this may be related to the fact that fewer younger women have ER-positive tumors.

FOLLOW-UP CARE

After primary therapy, patients with breast cancer should be followed for life for at least two reasons: to detect recurrences and to observe the opposite breast for a second primary carcinoma. About 10% of patients will develop a contralateral primary malignancy. Local and distant metastases occur most frequently within the first 3 years. During this period, the patient is examined every 3–4 months. Thereafter, examination is done every 6 months until 5 years postoperatively and then every 6–12 months. Special attention is given to the remaining breast, because of the increased risk of developing a second primary. The patient should examine her own breast monthly, and a mammogram should be obtained annually. In some cases, metastases are dormant for long periods and may appear up to 10–15 years or longer after removal of the primary tumor. Estrogen and progestational agents are rarely used for a patient free of disease after treatment of primary breast cancer,

Table 17–8. Approximate survival (%) of patients with breast cancer by TNM stage.

TNM Stage	Five Years	Ten Years
0	95	90
I	85	70
IIA	75	50
IIB	70	40
IIIA	55	30
IIIB	30	30
IV	5	2
All	65	30

particularly if the tumor was hormone receptor-positive. However, studies have failed to show an adverse effect of hormonal agents in patients who are free of disease. Indeed, even pregnancy has not been clearly associated with shortened survival of patients rendered disease-free—yet most oncologists are reluctant to advise a young patient with breast cancer that she may become pregnant.

Local Recurrence

The incidence of local recurrence correlates with tumor size, the presence and number of involved axillary nodes, the histologic type of tumor, and the presence of skin edema or skin and fascia fixation with the primary. About 8% of patients develop local recurrence on the chest wall after total mastectomy and axillary dissection. When the axillary nodes are not involved, the local recurrence rate is 5%, but the rate is as high as 25% when they are involved. A similar difference in local recurrence rate was noted between small and large tumors. Factors that affect the rate of local recurrence in patients who had partial mastectomies are not yet determined. However, early studies show that such things as multifocal cancer, in situ tumors, positive resection margins, chemotherapy, and radiotherapy are important.

Chest wall recurrences usually appear within the first 2 years but may occur as late as 15 or more years after mastectomy. Suspect nodules should be biopsied. Local excision or localized radiotherapy may be feasible if an isolated nodule is present. If lesions are multiple or accompanied by evidence of regional involvement in the internal mammary or supraclavicular nodes, the disease is best managed by radiation treatment of the entire chest wall including the parasternal, supraclavicular, and axillary areas.

Local recurrence after mastectomy usually signals the presence of widespread disease and is an indication for bone and liver scans, posteroanterior and lateral chest x-rays, and other examinations as needed to search for evidence of metastases. Most patients with locally recurrent tumor will develop distant metastases within 2 years. When there is no evidence of metastases beyond the chest wall and regional nodes, irradiation for cure or complete local excision should be attempted. Patients with local recurrence may be cured with local resection or radiation. After partial mastectomy, however, local recurrence does not have as serious a prognostic significance. However, those patients who do develop a breast recurrence have a worse prognosis than those who do not. It is speculated that the ability of a cancer to recur locally after radiotherapy is a sign of aggressiveness associated with distant disease rather than a cause of it. Completion of the mastectomy should be done for local recurrence after partial mastectomy; overall survival does not appear to be altered. Systemic chemotherapy or hormonal treatment should be used for postmenopausal women who develop disseminated disease or

those in whom local recurrence occurs following total mastectomy.

Edema of the Arm

Significant edema of the arm occurs in about 5% after modified radical mastectomy and about 10–30% of patients after radical mastectomy. Edema of the arm is less frequent after modified radical mastectomy than after radical mastectomy and occurs more commonly if radiotherapy has been given or if there was postoperative infection. Early trials suggest that partial mastectomy with radiation to the axillary lymph nodes is followed by chronic edema of the arm in 10–20% of patients. To avoid this complication, many authorities advocate axillary lymph node sampling rather than complete axillary dissection. However, since axillary dissection is a more accurate staging operation than axillary sampling, we recommend axillary dissection, with removal of at least level I and II lymph nodes, in combination with partial mastectomy. Judicious use of radiotherapy, with treatment fields carefully planned to spare the axilla as much as possible, can greatly diminish the incidence of edema.

Late or secondary edema of the arm may develop years after treatment, as a result of axillary recurrence or of infection in the hand or arm, with obliteration of lymphatic channels. Infection in the arm or hand on the dissected side should be treated promptly with antibiotics, rest, and elevation. When edema develops, careful examination of the axilla should be done to detect a regional recurrence. If there is no sign of recurrence, the swollen extremity should be treated with rest and elevation. A mild diuretic may be helpful for a few weeks. If there is no improvement, a compressor pump should be used to decrease the swelling, and the patient should then be fitted with an elastic glove or sleeve. Most patients are not bothered enough by mild edema to wear an uncomfortable glove or sleeve and will treat themselves with elevation alone. Rarely, edema may be severe enough to interfere with use of the limb.

Breast Reconstruction

Breast reconstruction, with the implantation of a prosthesis, is usually feasible after standard or modified radical mastectomy. Reconstruction should probably be discussed with patients prior to mastectomy, because it offers an important psychologic focal point for recovery. However, most patients who are initially interested in reconstruction decide later that they no longer wish to undergo the procedure. Reconstruction is not an obstacle to the diagnosis of recurrent cancer. The most common breast reconstruction has been implantation of a silicone gel prosthesis in the subpectoral plane between the pectoralis minor and pectoralis major muscles. Recently, the Food and Drug Administration has placed a moratorium on the use of silicone gel implants because of possible leakage of silicone and associated autoimmune disorders. This remote possibility should not prevent the cancer patient from having a reconstruction. Most plastic surgeons currently would place a saline-filled prosthesis rather than a silicone gel implant. Alternatively, autologous tissue can be used for reconstruction. The most popular autologous technique currently is the trans-rectus abdominis muscle flap (TRAM flap), which is done by rotating the rectus abdominis muscle with attached fat and skin cephalad to make a breast mound. A latissimus dorsi flap can be swung from the back but offers less fullness than the TRAM flap and is therefore less acceptable cosmetically. All patients who undergo mastectomy should be offered the option of breast reconstruction.

Risks of Pregnancy

Data are insufficient to determine whether interruption of pregnancy improves the prognosis of patients who are discovered during pregnancy to have potentially curable breast cancer and who receive definitive treatment. Theoretically, the increasingly high levels of estrogen produced by the placenta as the pregnancy progresses could be detrimental to the patient with occult metastases of hormone-sensitive breast cancer. Moreover, occult metastases are present in most patients with positive axillary nodes, and treatment by adjuvant chemotherapy would be potentially harmful to the fetus. Under these circumstances, interruption of early pregnancy seems reasonable, with progressively less rationale for the procedure as term approaches. Obviously, the decision must be highly individualized and will be affected by many factors, including the patient's desire to have the baby and the generally poor prognosis when axillary nodes are involved.

Equally problematic and important is the advice regarding future pregnancy (or abortion in case of pregnancy) to be given to women of child-bearing age who have had a mastectomy or other definitive treatment for breast cancer. Under these circumstances, one must assume that pregnancy will be harmful if occult metastases are present, although this has not been demonstrated. Patients whose tumors are ER-negative probably would not be affected by pregnancy. A number of studies have shown no adverse effect of pregnancy on survival of pregnant women who have had breast cancer.

In patients with inoperable or metastatic cancer (stage IV disease), induced abortion is usually advisable because of the possible adverse effects of hormonal treatment, radiotherapy, or chemotherapy upon the fetus.

General

American College of Radiology et al: Standards for breast-conservation treatment. CA 1992;42:134.

Baines CJ: Breast self-examination. Cancer 1989;64: 2661.

Bassett LW et al: The prevalence of carcinoma in palpable vs. impalpable, mammographically detected lesions. Am J Roentgenol 1991;157:21.

Bassett LW, Giuliano AE, Gold RH: Staging for breast carcinoma. Am J Surg 1989;157:250.

Bornstein BA et al: Results of treating ductal carcinoma in situ of the breast with conservative surgery and radiation therapy. Cancer 1991;67:7.

Bulens P et al: Breast conserving treatment of Paget's disease. Radiother Oncol 1990;17:305.

Callahan R et al: Somatic mutations and human breast cancer: A status report. Cancer 1992;69;1582.

Clayton F, Hopkins CL: Pathologic correlates of prognosis in lymphnode-positive breast carcinomas. Cancer 1993;71:1780.

Donegan WL, Padrta B: Combined therapy for inflammatory breast cancer. Arch Surg 1990;125:578.

Donovan AJ: Bilateral breast cancer. Surg Clin North Am 1990;70:1141.

Dorr FA: Prognostic factors observed in current clinical trials. Cancer 1993;71:2163.

Dupont WD, Page DL: Menopausal estrogen replacement therapy and breast cancer. Arch Intern Med 1991;151;67.

Elliott RL et al: Steriotaxic needle localization and biopsy of occult breast lesions: first years experience. Amn Surg 1992;58:126.

Fisher B et al: DNA flow cytometric analysis of primary operable breast cancer: Relation of ploidy and S-phase fraction to outcome of patients in NSABP B 04. Cancer 1991;68:1465.

Fisher B et al: Eight-year results of a randomized clinical trial comparing total mastectomy and lumpectomy with or without irradiation in the treatment of breast cancer. N Engl J Med 1989;320:822.

Fisher B et al: Significance of ipsilateral breast tumour recurrence after lumpectomy. Lancet 1991;338:327.

Fisher ER et al: Pathologic findings from the National Surgical Adjuvant Breast Project (protocol 4): Discriminants for 15 year survival. Cancer 1993;71:2141.

Harris JR et al: Breast Cancer. (Three parts.) N Engl J Med 1992;327:319, 390, 473.

Harris JR et al: Conservative surgery and radiotherapy for early breast cancer. Cancer 1990;66:1427.

Henrich JB: The postmenopausal estrogen/breast cancer controversy. JAMA 1992;268:1900.

Henson DE, Ries LA: Progress in early breast cancer detection. Cancer 1990;65(9 Suppl):2155.

Holm LE et al: Treatment failure and dietary habits in women with breast cancer. J Natl Cancer Inst 1993; 85:32.

Isola J: Cathepsin D expression detected by immunohistochemistry has independent prognostic value in axillary node-negative breast cancer. J Clin Oncol 1993;11:36.

Kinne DW: Staging and follow-up of breast cancer patients. Cancer 1991;67(Suppl 4):1196.

Kopald KH et al: The pathology of nonpalpable breast cancer. Am Surg 1990;56:782.

Layfield LJ et al: Mammographically guided fine-needle aspiration biopsy of non-palpable breast lesions: Can it replace open biopsy? Cancer 1991;68:2007.

Lazovich D et al: Underutilization of breast-conserving

surgery with radiation therapy among women with stage I or II breast cancer. JAMA 1991;266:3433.

Leis HP Jr: Concepts regarding breast biopsies. Breast Dis 1991;4:223.

Lichter AS: Lumpectomy and radiation: Improving the outcome. J Clin Oncol 1992;10:349.

McDivitt RW et al: Histologic types of benign breast disease and the risk for breast cancer. Cancer 1992; 69:1408.

Mesko TW et al: Risk factors for breast cancer. Compr Ther 1990;16:3.

Moore MP et al: Inflammatory breast cancer. Arch Surg 1991;126:304.

Morrison AS: Review of evidence on the early detection and treatment of breast cancer. Cancer 1989;64(12 Suppl):2651.

Nattinger AB et al: Screening mammography for older women: a case of mixed messages. Arch Intern Med 1992;152:922.

Rosner D et al: Ductal carcinoma in situ with microinvasion: A curable entity using surgery alone without need for adjuvant therapy. Cancer 1991;67:1498.

Senie RT et al: Obesity at diagnosis of breast carcinoma influences duration of disease-free survival. Ann Intern Med 1992;116:26.

Stotter AT et al: The role of limited surgery with radiation and primary treatment of ductal in situ breast cancer. Int J Radiat Oncol Biol Phys 1990;18:283.

Vetrani A et al: Fine-needle aspiration biopsies of breast masses: An additional experience with 1153 cases (1985–1988) and a meta-analysis. Cancer 1992; 69:736.

Vicini FA et al: The optimal extent of resection for patients with stages I or II breast cancer treated with conservative surgery and radiotherapy. Ann Surg 1991;214:200.

Wazer DE et al: Factors influencing cosmetic outcome and complication risk after conservative surgery and radiotherapy for early-stage carcinoma. J Clin Oncol 1992;10:356.

Witzig TE et al: DNA ploidy and percent S-phase as prognostic factors in node-positive breast cancer: Results from patients enrolled in two prospective randomized trials. J Clin Oncol 1993;11:351.

Zavertnik JJ et al: Cost effective management of breast cancer. Cancer 1992;69:1979.

Mammography

Feig SA, Ehrlich SM: Estimation of radiation risks from screening mammography: Recent trends and comparison with expected benefits. Radiology 1990;174(3 Part 1):638.

Harris RP et al: Mammography and age: Are we targeting the wrong women? A community survey of women and physicians. Cancer 1991;67:2010.

Hindle WH: Screening mammography reports: toward clear concise clinical descriptions. West J Med 1992;157:152.

Holleb AI: Review of breast cancer screening guidelines. Cancer 1992;69:1911.

McLelland R: Screening mammography. Cancer 1991;67(4 Suppl)1129.

Nattinger AB et al: Geographic variation in the use of breast-conserving treatment for breast cancer. N Engl J Med 1992;326:1102.

Hormone Receptors

Ferno M et al: Estrogen and progesterone receptor analyses in more than 4000 human breast cancer samples: A study with special reference to age at diagnosis and stability of analyses. (From the Southern Swedish Breast Cancer Study Group.) Acta Oncol 1990; 29:129.

Hawkins RA et al: Does the estrogen receptor concentration of a breast cancer change during systemic therapy? Br J Cancer 1990;61:877.

Lerner LJ, Jordan CV: Development of antiestrogens and their use in breast cancer. Cancer Res 1990;50:4177.

Lundy J et al: The use of fine-needle aspirates of breast cancers to evaluate hormone-receptor status. Arch Surg 1990;125:174.

Pertschuk LP et al: Steroid hormone receptor immunohistochemistry and amplification of c-myc protooncogene. Cancer 1993;71:162.

Robertson JFR et al: Comparison of two oestrogen receptor assays in the prediction of the clinical course of patients with advanced breast cancer. Br J Cancer 1992;65:727.

Adjuvant Systemic Therapy

Bagdade JD et al: Effects of tamoxifen treatment on plasma lipids and lipoprotein lipid composition. J Clin Endocrinol Metab 1990;70:1132.

Buzdar AU et al: Is chemotherapy effective in reducing the local failure rate in patients with operable breast cancer? Cancer 1990;65:394.

Carbone PP: Breast cancer adjuvant therapy. Cancer 1990;66:1378.

Castiglione M et al: Adjuvant systematic therapy for breast cancer in the elderly: Competing causes of mortality. J Clin Oncol 1990;8:519.

Cooper MR: The role of chemotherapy for node-negative breast cancer. Cancer 1991;67:1744.

Davidson NE, Abeloff MD: Adjuvant systemic therapy in women with early-stage breast cancer at high risk for relapse. J Natl Cancer Inst 1992;84:301.

DeGregorio MW: Is tamoxifen chemo prevention worth the risk in healthy women? J NIH Res 1992;4:84.

DeVita VT Jr: Breast cancer therapy: Exercising all our options. (Editorial.) N Engl J Med 1989;320:527.

Early Breast Cancer Trialists' Collaborative Group: Systemic treatment of early breast cancer by hormonal cytotoxic or immune therapy: 133 randomized trials involving 31,000 recurrences and 24,000 deaths among 75,000 women. Lancet 1992;339:1, 71.

Fisher B et al: A randomized clinical trial evaluating sequential methotrexate and fluorouracil in the treatment of patients with node-negative breast cancer who have estrogen receptor-negative tumors. N Engl J Med 1989;320:473.

Fisher B et al: A randomized clinical trial evaluating tamoxifen in the treatment of patients with node-negative breast cancer who have estrogen receptor-positive tumors. N Engl J Med 1989;320:479.

Fisher ER et al: Pathologic findings from the National Surgical Adjuvant Breast and Bowel Projects (NSABP): Prognostic discriminants for 8-year survival for node-negative invasive cancer patients. Cancer 1990;65 (9 Suppl): 2121.

Fornander T et al: Long term adjuvant tamoxifen in early

breast cancer: Effect on bone mineral density in postmenopausal women. J Clin Oncol 1990;8:1019.

Levine MN et al: A bedside decision instrument to elicit a patient's preference concerning adjuvant chemotherapy for breast cancer. Ann Intern Med 1992; 17:53.

Ludwig Breast Cancer Study Group: Prolonged disease-free survival after one course of perioperative adjuvant chemotherapy for node-negative breast cancer. N Engl J Med 1989;320:491.

McGuire WL: Adjuvant therapy of node-negative breast cancer. (Editorial.) N Engl J Med 1989;320:525.

Mueller CB, Lesperance ML: NSABP trials of adjuvant chemotherapy for breast cancer: A further look at the evidence. Ann Surg 1991;214:206.

National Institutes of Health: Clinical Alert. National Institutes of Health Consensus Development Conference Statement: Adjuvant chemotherapy for breast cancer. Vol 8, No. 16, 1990.

Recht A et al: Integration of conservative surgery, radiotherapy, and chemotherapy for the treatment of early-stage, node-positive breast cancer: sequencing, timing, and outcome. J Clin Oncol 1991;9:1662.

Treatment of Advanced Breast Cancer

Buzdar AU: Current status of endocrine treatment of carcinoma of the breast. Semin Surg Oncol 1990;6:77.

Christman K et al: Chemotherapy of metastatic breast cancer in the elderly: The Piedmont Oncology Association Experience. JAMA 1992;268:57.

Eddy DM: High-dose chemotherapy with autologous bone marrow transplantation for the treatment of metastatic breast cancer. J Clin Oncol 1992;10:657.

Henderson IC et al: Comprehensive management of disseminated breast cancer. Cancer 1990;66:1439.

Hillner BE et al: Efficacy and cost-effectiveness of autologous bone marrow transplantation in metastatic breast cancer: Estimate using decision analysis while awaiting clinical trial results. JAMA 1992;267:2055.

Ingle JN: Principles of therapy in advanced breast cancer. Hematol Oncol Clin North Am 1989;3:743.

Nemoto T et al: Aminoglutethimide in patients with metastatic breast cancer. Cancer 1989;63:1673.

Perez DJ et al: A randomized comparison of single-agent doxorubicin and epirubicin as first-line cytotoxic therapy in advanced breast cancer. J Clin Oncol 1991; 9:2148.

Price JE: The biology of metastatic breast cancer. Cancer 1990;66(6 Suppl):1313.

Rose C, Mouridsen HT: Endocrine management of advanced breast cancer. Hormone Res 1989;32(Suppl 1):189.

Swain SM et al: Fluorouracil and high dose leucovorin in previously treated patients with metastatic breast cancer. J Clin Oncol 1989;7:890.

Turken S et al: Effects of tamoxifen on spinal bone density in women with breast cancer. J Natl Cancer Inst 1989;81:1086.

CARCINOMA OF THE MALE BREAST

Essentials of Diagnosis

- A painless lump beneath the areola in a man usually over 50 years of age.
- Nipple discharge, retraction, or ulceration may be present.

General Considerations

Breast cancer in men is a rare disease; the incidence is only about 1% of that in women. The average age at occurrence is about 60—somewhat older than the commonest presenting age in women. The prognosis, even in stage I cases, is worse in men than in women. Blood-borne metastases are commonly present when the male patient appears for initial treatment. These metastases may be latent and may not become manifest for many years. As in women, hormonal influences are probably related to the development of male breast cancer. There is a high incidence of both breast cancer and gynecomastia in Bantu men, theoretically owing to failure of estrogen inactivation by a damaged liver associated with vitamin B deficiency.

Clinical Findings

A painless lump, occasionally associated with nipple discharge, retraction, erosion, or ulceration, is the chief complaint. Examination usually shows a hard, ill-defined, nontender mass beneath the nipple or areola. Gynecomastia not uncommonly precedes or accompanies breast cancer in men. Nipple discharge is an uncommon presentation for breast cancer in men, as it is in women. However, nipple discharge in a man is an ominous finding associated with carcinoma in nearly 75% of cases.

Breast cancer staging is the same in men as in women. Gynecomastia and metastatic cancer from another site (eg, prostate) must be considered in the differential diagnosis of a breast lesion in a man. Biopsy settles the issue.

Treatment

Treatment consists of modified radical mastectomy in operable patients, who should be chosen by the same criteria as women with the disease. Irradiation is the first step in treating localized metastases in the skin, lymph nodes, or skeleton that are causing symptoms. Examination of the cancer for hormone receptor proteins may prove to be of value in predicting response to endocrine ablation. Adjuvant chemotherapy is used for the same indications as in breast cancer in women.

Since breast cancer in men is frequently a disseminated disease, endocrine therapy is of considerable importance in its management. Castration in advanced breast cancer is the most successful palliative measure and more beneficial than the same procedure in women. Objective evidence of regression may be seen in 60–70% of men who are castrated—approximately twice the proportion in women. The average duration of tumor growth remission is about 30 months, and life is prolonged. Bone is the most frequent site of metastases from breast cancer in men (as in women), and castration relieves bone pain in most patients so treated. The longer the interval between mastectomy and recurrence, the longer the tumor growth remission following castration. As in women, there is no correlation between the histologic type of the tumor and the likelihood of remission following castration.

Tamoxifen (10 mg orally twice daily) is becoming increasingly popular and should replace castration as the initial therapy for metastatic disease. However, little clinical experience is available with tamoxifen in male breast cancers. Aminoglutethimide (250 mg orally four times a day) should replace adrenalectomy in men as it has in women. Corticosteroid therapy alone has been considered to be efficacious but probably has no value when compared with major endocrine ablation.

Estrogen therapy—5 mg of diethylstilbestrol three times daily orally—may be effective as secondary hormonal manipulation after medical adrenalectomy (with aminoglutethimide). Androgen therapy may exacerbate bone pain. Castration and tamoxifen are the main therapeutic resources for advanced breast cancer in men at present. Chemotherapy should be administered for the same indications and using the same dosage schedules as for women with metastatic disease.

Prognosis

The prognosis of breast cancer is poorer in men than in women. The crude 5- and 10-year survival rates for clinical stage I breast cancer in men are about 58% and 38%, respectively. For clinical stage II disease, the 5- and 10-year survival rates are approximately 38% and 10%. The survival rates for all stages at 5 and 10 years are 36% and 17%.

Donegan WL: Cancer of the breast in men. CA 1991; 41:539.

Guinee VF et al: The prognosis of breast cancer in males. Cancer 1993;71:154.

Jaiyesimi IA et al: Carcinoma of the male breast. Annals Internal Medicine 1992;117:771.

Ribeiro G, Swindell R: Adjuvant tamoxifen for male breast cancer. British Journal of Cancer 1992;65:252.

OTHER BREAST DISORDERS

MAMMARY DYSPLASIA
(Fibrocystic Disease)

Essentials of Diagnosis

- Painful, often multiple, usually bilateral masses in the breast.
- Rapid fluctuation in the size of the masses is common.
- Frequently, pain occurs or increases and size increases during premenstrual phase of cycle.
- Most common age is 30–50. Rare in postmenopausal women.

General Considerations

This disorder, also known as fibrocystic disease or chronic cystic mastitis, is the most frequent lesion of the breast. It is common in women 30–50 years of age but rare in postmenopausal women; this suggests that it is related to ovarian activity. Estrogen hormone is considered a causative factor. The term "mammary dysplasia," or "fibrocystic disease," is imprecise and encompasses a wide variety of pathologic entities. These lesions are always associated with benign changes in the breast epithelium, some of which are found so commonly in normal breasts that they are probably variants of normal breast histology but have unfortunately been termed a "disease."

The microscopic findings of fibrocystic disease include cysts (gross and microscopic), papillomatosis, adenosis, fibrosis, and ductal epithelial hyperplasia. Although mammary dysplasia has generally been considered to increase the risk of subsequent breast cancer, only the variants in which proliferation of epithelial components is demonstrated represent true risk factors.

Clinical Findings

Mammary dysplasia may produce an asymptomatic lump in the breast that is discovered by accident, but pain or tenderness often calls attention to the mass. There may be discharge from the nipple. In many cases, discomfort occurs or is increased during the premenstrual phase of the cycle, at which time the cysts tend to enlarge. Fluctuation in size and rapid appearance or disappearance of a breast tumor are common in cystic disease. Multiple or bilateral masses are common, and many patients will give a history of a transient lump in the breast or cyclic breast pain.

Differential Diagnosis

Pain, fluctuation in size, and multiplicity of lesions are the features most helpful in differentiation from carcinoma. However, if a dominant mass is present, the diagnosis of cancer should be assumed until disproved by biopsy. Final diagnosis often depends on biopsy. Mammography may be helpful, but the breast tissue in these young women is usually too radiodense to permit a worthwhile study. Sonography is useful in differentiating a cystic from a solid mass.

Treatment

Because mammary dysplasia is frequently indistinguishable from carcinoma on the basis of clinical findings, suspicious lesions should be biopsied. Fine-needle aspiration cytology may be used, but if a suspicious mass that is nonmalignant on cytologic examination does not resolve over several months, it must be excised. Surgery should be conservative, since the primary objective is to exclude cancer. Simple mastectomy or extensive removal of breast tissue is rarely, if ever, indicated for mammary dysplasia.

When the diagnosis of mammary dysplasia has been established by previous biopsy or is practically certain because the history is classic, aspiration of a discrete mass suggestive of a cyst is indicated. The patient is reexamined at intervals thereafter. If no fluid is obtained or if fluid is bloody, if a mass persists after aspiration, or if at any time during follow-up a persistent lump is noted, biopsy examination should be performed.

Breast pain associated with generalized mammary dysplasia is best treated by avoiding trauma and by wearing (night and day) a brassiere that gives good support and protection. Hormone therapy is not advisable, because it does not cure the condition and has undesirable side effects. Danazol (100–200 mg twice daily orally), a synthetic androgen, has been used for patients with severe pain. This treatment suppresses pituitary gonadotropins, and androgenic effects (acne, edema, hirsutism) usually make this treatment intolerable; it should therefore be reserved for the unusual severe case.

The role of caffeine consumption in the development and treatment of fibrocystic disease is controversial. Some studies suggest that eliminating caffeine from the diet is associated with improvement. Many patients are aware of these studies and report relief of symptoms after giving up coffee, tea, and chocolate. Similarly, many women find vitamin E (400 IU daily) helpful. However, these observations have been difficult to confirm and are anecdotal.

Prognosis

Exacerbations of pain, tenderness, and cyst formation may occur at any time until the menopause, when symptoms usually subside, except in patients receiving estrogens. The patient should be advised to examine her own breasts each month just after menstruation and to inform her physician if a mass appears. The risk of breast cancer in women with mammary dysplasia showing proliferative or atypical changes in the epithelium is higher than that of women in general. Follow-up examinations at regular intervals should therefore be arranged.

Dogliotti L, Orlandi R, Angeli A: The endocrine basis of benign breast disorders. World J Surg 1989;13:674.

Dupont WD et al: Influence of exogenous estrogens, proliferative breast disease, and other variables on breast cancer risk. Cancer 1989;63:948.

London SJ et al: A prospective study of benign breast disease and the risk of breast cancer. JAMA 1992;267:941.

Maddox PR, Mansel RE: Management of breast pain and nodularity. World J Surg 1989;13:699.

McDivitt RW et al: Histologic types of benign breast disease and the risk for breast cancer. Cancer 1992;69:1408.

Page DL, Dupont WD: Anatomic markers of human premalignancy and risk of breast cancer. Cancer 1990;66(6 Suppl):1326.

FIBROADENOMA OF THE BREAST

This common benign neoplasm occurs most frequently in young women, usually within 20 years after puberty. It is somewhat more frequent and tends to occur at an earlier age in black than in white women. Multiple tumors in one or both breasts are found in 10–15% of patients.

The typical fibroadenoma is a round, firm, discrete, relatively movable, nontender mass 1–5 cm in diameter. The tumor is usually discovered accidentally. Clinical diagnosis in young patients is generally not difficult. In women over 30, cystic disease of the breast and carcinoma of the breast must be considered. Cysts can be identified by aspiration. Fibroadenoma does not normally occur after the menopause, but postmenopausal women may occasionally develop fibroadenoma after administration of estrogenic hormone.

Treatment is by excision under local anesthesia as an outpatient procedure, with pathologic examination of the specimen.

Cystosarcoma phyllodes is a type of fibroadenoma with cellular stroma that tends to grow rapidly. This tumor may reach a large size and if inadequately excised will recur locally. The lesion is rarely malignant. Treatment is by local excision of the mass with a margin of surrounding breast tissue. The treatment of malignant cystosarcoma phyllodes is more controversial. In general, complete removal of the tumor and a rim of normal tissue should avoid recurrence. Since these tumors may be large, simple mastectomy is sometimes necessary to achieve complete control.

Dent DM, Cant PJ: Fibroadenoma. World J Surg 1989; 13:706.

Hart J et al: Practical aspects in the diagnosis and management of cystosarcoma phyllodes. Arch Surg 1988;123: 1079.

Hindle WH, Alonzo LJ: Conservative management of breast fibroadenomas. Am J Obstet Gynecol 1991;164: 1647.

Yu H et al: Risk factors for fibroadenoma: A case-control study in Australia. Am J Epidemiol 1992;135:247.

NIPPLE DISCHARGE

In order of increasing frequency, the following are the commonest causes of nipple discharge in the non-lactating breast: carcinoma, intraductal papilloma, and mammary dysplasia with ectasia of the ducts. The important characteristics of the discharge and some other factors to be evaluated by history and physical examination are as follows:

(1) Nature of discharge (serous, bloody, or other).

(2) Association with a mass or not.

(3) Unilateral or bilateral.

(4) Single duct or multiple duct discharge.

(5) Discharge is spontaneous (persistent or intermittent) or must be expressed.

(6) Discharge produced by pressure at a single site or by general pressure on the breast.

(7) Relation to menses.

(8) Premenopausal or postmenopausal.

(9) Patient taking contraceptive pills, or estrogen for postmenopausal symptoms.

Unilateral, spontaneous serous or serosanguineous discharge from a single duct is usually caused by an intraductal papilloma or, rarely, by an intraductal cancer. In either case, a mass may not be palpable. The involved duct may be identified by pressure at different sites around the nipple at the margin of the areola. Bloody discharge is more suggestive of cancer but is usually caused by a benign papilloma in the duct. Cytologic examination may identify malignant cells, but negative findings do not rule out cancer, which is more likely in women over age 50. In any case, the involved duct—and a mass if present—should be excised. Ductography may identify a filling defect prior to excision of the duct system.

In premenopausal women, spontaneous multiple duct discharge, unilateral or bilateral, most marked just before menstruation, is often due to mammary dysplasia. Discharge may be green or brownish. Papillomatosis and ductal ectasia are usually seen on biopsy. If a mass is present, it should be removed.

Milky discharge from multiple ducts in the non-lactating breast may occur in certain syndromes (Chiari-Frommel, Argonz-Del Castillo [Forbes-Albright]), presumably as a result of increased secretion of pituitary prolactin. Serum prolactin and TSH levels should be obtained to search for a pituitary tumor or hypothyroidism. Drugs of the chlorpromazine type and contraceptive pills may also cause milky discharge that ceases on discontinuance of the medication.

Oral contraceptive agents may cause clear, serous, or milky discharge from a single duct, but multiple duct discharge is more common. The discharge is more evident just before menstruation and disappears on stopping the medication. If it does not and is from a single duct, exploration should be considered.

Purulent discharge may originate in a subareolar abscess and require excision of the abscess and related lactiferous sinus.

When localization is not possible and no mass is palpable, the patient should be reexamined every week for 1 month. When unilateral discharge persists, even without definite localization or tumor, exploration must be considered. The alternative is careful follow-up at intervals of 1–3 months. Mammography should be done. Cytologic examination of nipple discharge for exfoliated cancer cells may be helpful in diagnosis.

Chronic unilateral nipple discharge, especially if bloody, is an indication for resection of the involved ducts.

Leis HP Jr: Management of nipple discharge. World J Surg 1989;13:736.

Takeda T et al: Nipple discharge cytology and mass screening for breast cancer. Acta Cytol 1990;34:21.

FAT NECROSIS

Fat necrosis is a rare lesion of the breast but is of clinical importance because it produces a mass, often accompanied by skin or nipple retraction, that is indistinguishable from carcinoma. Trauma is presumed to be the cause, though only about half of patients give a history of injury to the breast. Ecchymosis is occasionally seen near the tumor. Tenderness may or may not be present. If untreated, the mass associated with fat necrosis gradually disappears. As a rule, the safest course is to obtain a biopsy. The entire mass should be excised, primarily to rule out carcinoma. Fat necrosis is common after segmental resection and radiation therapy.

BREAST ABSCESS

During nursing, an area of redness, tenderness, and induration not infrequently develops in the breast. The organism most commonly found in these abscesses is *Staphylococcus aureus.* In the early stages, the infection can often be reversed while nursing is continued from that breast by administering an antibiotic such as dicloxacillin or oxacillin, 250 mg four times daily for 7–10 days. If the lesion progresses to form a localized mass with local and systemic signs of infection, an abscess is present and should be drained, and nursing should be discontinued.

A subareolar abscess may develop (rarely) in young or middle-aged women who are not lactating. These infections tend to recur after incision and drainage unless the area is explored in a quiescent interval with excision of the involved lactiferous duct or ducts at the base of the nipple. Except for the sub-areolar type of abscess, infection in the breast is very rare unless the patient is lactating. In the nonlactating breast, inflammatory carcinoma must always be considered. Therefore, findings suggestive of abscess in the nonlactating breast are an indication for incision and biopsy of any indurated tissue.

Benson EA: Management of breast abscesses. World J Surg 1989;13:753.

Edmiston CE Jr et al: The nonpuerperal breast infection: Aerobic and anaerobic microbial recovery from acute and chronic disease. J Infect Dis 1990;162:695.

REFERENCES

Bland KI, Copeland EM III: *The Breast: Comprehensive Management of Benign and Malignant Diseases.* Saunders, 1991. Kopans DD: *Breast Imaging.* Lippincott, 1989.

Ragaz J, Ariel IM: *High Risk Breast Cancer.* Springer-Verlag, 1989.

Thoracic Wall, Pleura, Mediastinum, & Lung

18

Kevin Turley, MD

ANATOMY & PHYSIOLOGY

ANATOMY OF THE CHEST WALL & PLEURA

The chest wall is an airtight, expandable, cone-shaped cage. Lung ventilation occurs by the generation of negative pressure within the thorax by simultaneous expansion of the rib cage and downward diaphragmatic excursion.

The ventral wall of the bony thorax is the shortest dimension. It extends from the suprasternal notch to the xiphoid—a distance of approximately 18 cm. It is formed by the vertically aligned manubrium, sternum, and xiphoid and the costal cartilages of the first ten ribs. The sides of the chest wall consist of the upper ten ribs, which slope downward and forward from their posterior attachments. The posterior chest wall is formed by the 12 thoracic vertebrae, their transverse processes, and the 12 ribs (Figure 18–1). The upper ventral portion of the thoracic cage is covered by the clavicle and subclavian vessels. Laterally, it is covered by the shoulder and axillary nerves and vessels; dorsally, it is covered by the scapula.

The superior aperture of the thorax (also called either the thoracic inlet or the thoracic outlet) is a 5- × 10-cm kidney-shaped opening bounded by the first costal cartilages and ribs laterally, the manubrium anteriorly, and the body of the first thoracic vertebra posteriorly. The inferior aperture of the thorax is bounded by the 12th vertebra and ribs posteriorly and the cartilages of the seventh to 12th ribs and the xiphisternal joint anteriorly. It is much wider than the superior aperture and is occupied by the diaphragm.

The blood supply and innervation of the chest wall are via the intercostal vessels and nerves (Figures 18–2 and 18–3), and the upper thorax also receives vessels and nerves from the cervical and axillary regions.

The parietal pleura is the innermost lining of the chest wall and is divided into four parts: the cervical pleura (cupula), costal pleura, mediastinal pleura, and diaphragmatic pleura. The visceral pleura is the se-rous layer investing the lungs and is continuous with the parietal pleura, joining it at the hilum of the lung. The potential pleural space is a capillary gap that normally contains only a few drops of serous fluid. This space may be enlarged when fluid (hydrothorax), blood (hemothorax), pus (pyothorax or empyema), or air (pneumothorax) is present.

PHYSIOLOGY OF THE CHEST WALL & PLEURA

Mechanics of Respiration

Breathing entails expansion of thoracic volume by elevation of the rib cage and descent of the diaphragm. The former predominates in men and the latter in women. In infants, because the ribs have not yet assumed their oblique contour, diaphragmatic breathing is required to provide sufficient ventilation.

Expiration is mainly passive and depends upon elastic recoil of the lungs except with deep breathing, when the abdominal musculature contracts, pulling the rib cage downward and simultaneously elevating the diaphragm by compressing the abdominal viscera against it.

Physiology of the Pleural Space

A. Pressure: The pleural cavity pressure is normally negative, owing to the elastic recoil of the lung and chest wall. During quiet respiration, it varies from -15 cm H_2O with inspiration to $0-2$ cm H_2O during expiration. Deep breathing may cause large pressure changes (eg, -60 cm H_2O during forced inspiration to $+30$ cm H_2O during vigorous expiration). Because of gravity, pleural pressure at the apex is more negative when the body is erect and changes about 0.2 cm H_2O per centimeter of vertical height.

B. Fluid Formation and Reabsorption: Transudation and absorption of fluid within the pleural space normally follow the Starling equation, which depends on hydrostatic, colloid, and tissue pressures. In health, fluid is formed by the parietal pleura and absorbed by the visceral pleura (Figure 18–4). Systemic capillary hydrostatic pressure is 30 cm H_2O, and intrapleural negative pressure averages -5 cm

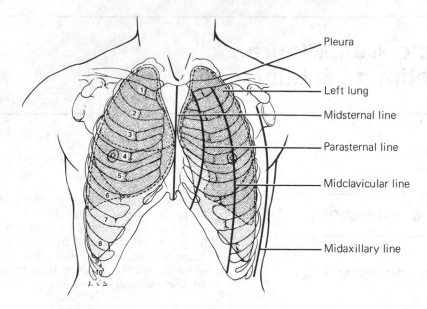

Figure 18–1. The thorax, showing rib cage, pleura, and lung fields.

H_2O. Together, these give a net hydrostatic pressure of 35 cm H_2O that causes fluid transudation from the parietal pleura. The colloid osmotic pressure of the systemic capillaries is 34 cm H_2O; this is opposed by 8 cm H_2O of pleural space osmotic pressure. Thus, a net 26 cm H_2O osmotic pressure draws fluid back into systemic capillaries. Systemic hydrostatic pressure (35 cm H_2O) exceeds osmotic capillary pressure (26 cm H_2O) by 9 cm H_2O; thus, there is a 9-cm H_2O net drive of fluid into the pleural space by systemic capillaries in the chest wall. Similar calculations for the visceral pleura involving the low-pressure pulmonary circulation will show that there is a resulting net drive of 10 cm H_2O that attracts pleural fluid into pulmonary capillaries.

In health, pleural fluid is low in protein (100

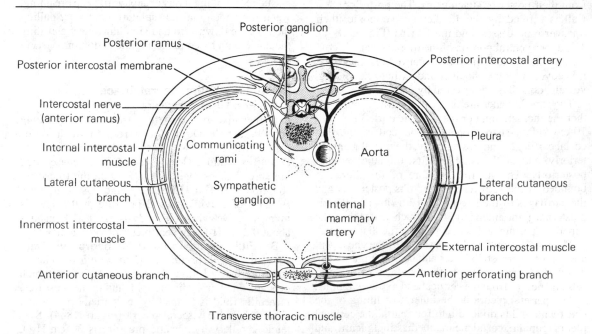

Figure 18–2. Transverse section of thorax.

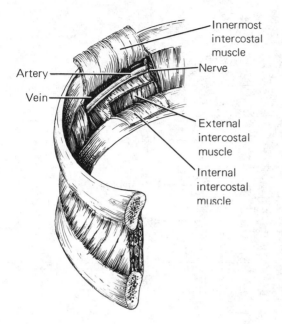

Figure 18–3. Intercostal muscles, vessels, and nerves.

mg/dL). When it increases in disease to about 1 g/dL, the net colloid osmotic pressure of the visceral pleural capillaries is equaled and pleural fluid reabsorption becomes dependent on lymphatic drainage. Thus, abnormal amounts of pleural fluid may accumulate (1) when hydrostatic pressure is increased, such as in heart failure; (2) when capillary permeability is increased, as in inflammatory or neoplastic disease; or (3) when colloid osmotic pressure is decreased.

ANATOMY OF THE MEDIASTINUM

The mediastinum is the compartment between the pleural cavities. It extends anteriorly from the suprasternal notch to the xiphoid process and posteriorly from the first to the 11th thoracic vertebrae. Superiorly, fascial planes in the neck are in direct communication; inferiorly, the mediastinum is limited by the diaphragm, although extensions through diaphragmatic apertures communicate with retroperitoneal fascial planes.

In Burkell's classification (Figure 18–5), the **anterior mediastinum** contains the thymus gland, the lymph nodes, the ascending and transverse aorta, the great vessels, and areolar tissue. The **middle mediastinum** contains the heart, the pericardium, the trachea, the hila of the lungs, the phrenic nerves, lymph nodes, and areolar tissue. The **posterior mediasti-**

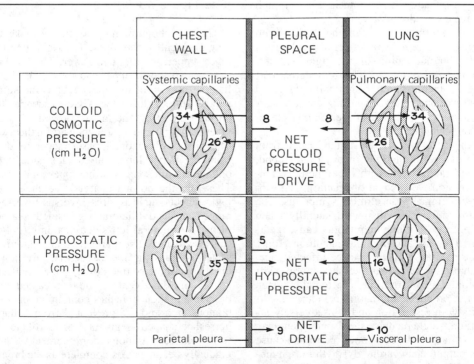

Figure 18–4. Movement of fluid across the pleural space, showing production and absorption of pleural fluid.

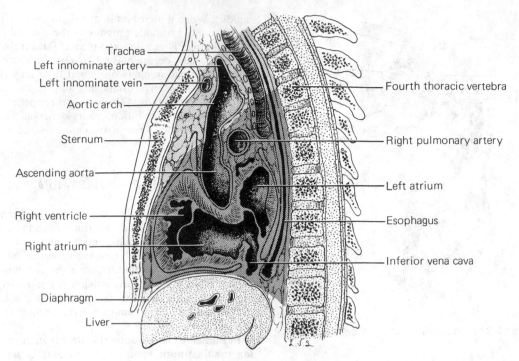

Figure 18–5. Divisions of the mediastinum (Burkell's classification). Upper mediastinum; light screening: anterior mediastinum; lower dark screening: middle mediastinum; dotted area at right: posterior mediastinum.

num contains the sympathetic chains, the vagus nerves, the esophagus, the thoracic duct, lymph nodes, and the descending aorta.

Congenital abnormalities within the mediastinum are numerous. A defect in the anterior mediastinal pleura with communication of the right and left hemithorax is rare in humans. This retrosternal part of the anterior mediastinum is normally thin, and overexpansion of one pleural space may cause "mediastinal herniation" or a bulge of mediastinal pleura toward the opposite side.

Displacements of the mediastinum occur from masses or from accumulations of air, fluid, blood, chyle, etc, and can interfere with vital functions. Tracheal compression, vena caval obstruction, and esophageal obstructions cause clinical symptoms. The mediastinum can also be displaced laterally when pathologic processes of one hemithorax cause mediastinal shift. Fibrosis and previous pneumonectomy can shift the mediastinum toward the affected side. Open pneumothorax and massive hemothorax shift the mediastinum away from the affected side. Open pneumothorax produces alternating paradoxic mediastinal shifts with respiration and will adversely affect ventilation. Acute mediastinal displacement may produce hypoxia or reduced venous return and cause low cardiac output, tachycardia, dysrhythmias, hypotension, or cardiac arrest.

ANATOMY OF THE LUNG
(See Figure 18–6.)

The bronchopulmonary segments make up large lung units called the lobes. The right lung has three lobes: upper, middle, and lower. The left lung consists of two lobes: upper and lower. On the left, the lingular portion of the upper lobe is the homolog of the right middle lobe. Two fissures separate the lobes on the right side. The major, or oblique, fissure divides the upper and middle lobes from the lower lobe. The minor, or horizontal, fissure separates the middle from the upper lobe. On the left side, the single oblique fissure separates the upper and lower lobes. These are the normal anatomic segments; embryologic defects such as situs inversus reverse this arrangement, and bilateral right-sided anatomy (asplenia) or bilateral left-sided anatomy (polysplenia) can also occur. The parenchymal anatomy can be seen by studying the sequential division of the bronchopulmonary tree down to the smallest unit of ventilation, the alveolus. The trachea and main stem bronchi and their branches contain an anterior membranous area and are prevented from collapsing by horseshoe-shaped segments of cartilage in their walls. The cartilaginous reinforcement of the airway gradually becomes less complete as the branches become smaller, and reinforcement ceases with bronchi

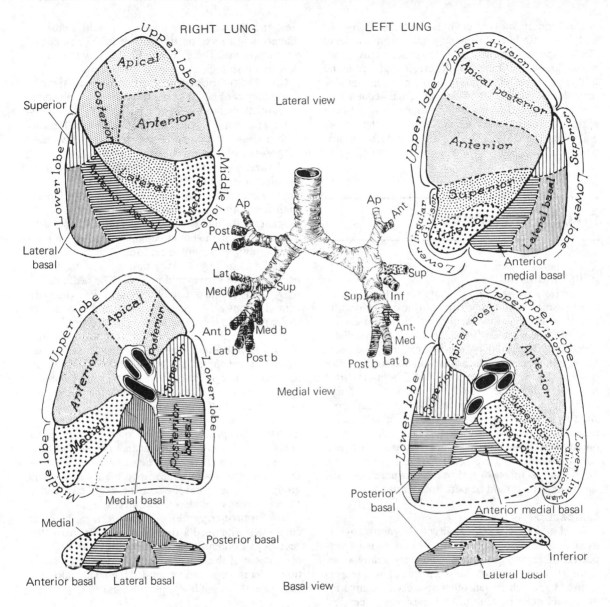

Figure 18–6. Segmental anatomy of the lungs.

of 1–2 mm. The bronchopulmonary segmental anatomy is designated by numbers (Boyden) or by name (Jackson and Huber).

The lungs have a dual blood supply: the pulmonary and the bronchial arterial systems. The pulmonary arteries transmit venous blood from the right ventricle for oxygenation. They closely accompany the bronchi. The bronchial arteries usually arise directly from the aorta or nearby intercostal arteries and are variable in number. They transmit oxygenated blood at systemic arterial pressure to the bronchial wall to the level of the terminal bronchioles.

The pulmonary veins travel in the interlobar septa and do not correspond to the distribution of the bronchi or the pulmonary arteries.

THE LYMPHATIC SYSTEM

The lymphatics travel in intersegmental septa centrally as well as to the parenchymal surface to form subpleural networks. Drainage continues toward the hilum in channels that follow the bronchi and pulmonary arteries. The lymphatics eventually enter lymph nodes in the major fissures of the lungs, the hilum, and the paratracheal regions.

The direction of lymphatic drainage—irrespective

of the primary site—is cephalad and usually ipsilateral, but contralateral flow may occur from any lobe. The lymphatics from the left lower lobe may be almost equally distributed to the left and right; from the left upper lobe, distribution is often to the anterior mediastinal group. Otherwise, the usual sequence of lymphatic spread of pulmonary cancer is first to the regional parabronchial nodes and then to the ipsilateral paratracheal, scalene, or inferior deep cervical nodes.

DIAGNOSTIC STUDIES

Skin Tests

Skin tests are used in the diagnosis of tuberculosis, histoplasmosis, and coccidioidomycosis. Tuberculin testing is usually done with purified protein derivative (PPD) injected intradermally. Intermediate-strength PPD should be used in patients who seem likely to have active disease. Induration of 10 mm or more at the injection site after 48–72 hours is called positive and indicates either active or arrested disease. Mumps antigen is usually placed on the opposite forearm to test for anergy. Because false-negative reactions are rare, a negative test fairly reliably rules out tuberculosis. Skin tests for histoplasmosis and coccidioidomycosis are performed in a similar way, but for fungal infections, skin tests are unreliable and serologic tests should be performed instead.

Endoscopy

A. Laryngoscopy: Indirect laryngoscopy is used to assess vocal cord mobility in patients suspected of having lung carcinoma, especially when there has been a voice change. It should also be performed to search for an otherwise occult source for malignant cells in sputum or metastases in cervical lymph nodes.

B. Bronchoscopy: Roentgenographic evidence of bronchial obstruction, unresolved pneumonia, foreign body, suspected carcinoma, undiagnosed hemoptysis, aspiration pneumonia, and lung abscess are only a few of the indications for bronchoscopy. The procedure can be done using either the standard hollow metal or the flexible fiberoptic bronchoscope and local or general anesthesia. Washings are usually obtained for bacterial or fungal culture and cytologic examination. Visible lesions are biopsied directly, and occasionally biopsies are taken of the carina even though it appears normal. Brush biopsies are obtained from specific bronchopulmonary segments. Occasionally, transcarinal needle biopsy of a subcarinal node is obtained. Thirty to 50% of lung tumors are visible bronchoscopically. Brushing, random biopsies, and sputum cytology may still yield a positive diagnosis of cancer or tuberculosis in the absence of a visible lesion. The yield is influenced by size, location, and histologic cell type of the lesion.

C. Mediastinoscopy: Mediastinoscopy permits direct biopsy of paratracheal and carinal lymph nodes without thoracotomy. Tumor is found by this technique in about 40% of cases of lung cancer. Persons with a negative biopsy have a relatively favorable prognosis with surgical treatment.

Mediastinoscopy is almost invariably accurate in the diagnosis of sarcoidosis. It is also useful to diagnose tuberculosis, histoplasmosis, silicosis, metastatic carcinoma, lymphoma, and carcinoma of the esophagus. It should not be used in primary mediastinal tumors, which should be approached by an incision permitting definitive excision.

Mediastinoscopy is done through a suprasternal, parasternal, or subxiphoid incision. The death rate is 0.09% and the rate of complication is 1.5%. The main complications are hemorrhage, pneumothorax, injury to the recurrent laryngeal nerve, and infection.

D. Anterior Parasternal Mediastinotomy (Chamberlain Procedure): This procedure is a useful alternative approach to inspection of the mediastinal nodes, especially the nodes of the anterior mediastinal chain on the left into which lymphatic drainage of the left upper lobe flows. A 2-cm incision is made, the costocartilage is resected, and the mediastinoscope is inserted to obtain nodal specimens from the anterior mediastinal chains and hilar nodes. This procedure is more extensive than mediastinoscopy, but it allows access to the anterior nodal group on the left, and the incision may be extended for wider biopsy or resection, if necessary.

E. Pleuroscopy: Pleuroscopy, either direct or combined with mediastinoscopy, may increase the accuracy of diagnosis of thoracic disease or improve assessment of the extent of cancer. In specific situations, pleuroscopy can be applied therapeutically (eg, intrapleural foreign body, pleurodesis).

Scalene Lymph Node Biopsy

Scalene lymph node biopsy has been largely replaced by mediastinoscopy in the evaluation of pulmonary disease, since it offers the same information but is less reliable and does not evaluate nodes within the mediastinum. In the evaluation of lung cancer, about 15% of scalene node biopsies are positive when the cervical nodes are not palpable compared with 85% when the nodes are palpable. The risk of major complications is about 5%. Deaths are rare.

Pleural Biopsy

A. Needle Biopsy: This procedure is indicated when the cause of a pleural effusion cannot be determined by analysis of the fluid or when tuberculosis is suspected. Any one of three needles can be used: the Vim-Silverman, Cope, or Abrams (Harefield) needle.

A positive diagnosis can be obtained in 60–80% of cases of tuberculosis or cancer. The principal complication is pneumothorax. Five to 10 percent of biopsy specimens are inadequate for diagnosis.

B. Open Biopsy: Open pleural biopsy is especially useful in those without pleural effusion, or when needle biopsy has failed. The quality of the specimen and the likelihood of its representing the pathology are better than with needle biopsy, but open biopsy is a more extensive procedure.

Lung Biopsy

A. Needle Biopsy: The indications for percutaneous needle biopsy are not well established. It may be indicated in diffuse parenchymal disease and in some patients with localized lesions. The diagnosis of interstitial pneumonia, carcinoma, sarcoidosis, hypersensitivity lung disease, lymphoma, pulmonary alveolar proteinosis, and miliary tuberculosis has been established by this method.

Needle biopsies are done by any of three techniques: by aspiration with a cutting needle, by trephine, or by air drill. Needle biopsy of the lung is also possible by a transbronchial technique in which a modified Vim-Silverman or ultra-thin needle is used.

There is controversy concerning the risks of spreading the tumor by needle biopsy in localized disease. Complications following percutaneous needle biopsy include pneumothorax (20–40%), hemothorax, hemoptysis, and air embolism. Pulmonary hypertension or cysts and bullae are contraindications. Several deaths have been reported. There is about a 60% chance of obtaining useful information.

B. Open Biopsy: A limited intercostal or anterior parasternal incision is used to remove a 3- to 4-cm wedge of lung tissue in diffuse parenchymal lung disease. The site of incision is selected for accessibility and potential diagnostic value. The incision is generally made at the fifth interspace on the right at the anterior axillary line to allow for access to all three lobes for biopsy, or at the lower lobes bilaterally. The middle lobe and lingula are selected in specific cases when pathology exists only in these areas, as they generally yield the poorest quality results. Open lung biopsy is associated with a lower death rate, fewer complications, and greater diagnostic yield than needle biopsy. It is especially useful in critically ill, immunosuppressed patients for differentiation of infectious infiltrative lesions from neoplastic infiltrative lesions. When a focal lesion is biopsied, a larger incision is used. Peripheral lesions are totally excised by wedge or segmental resection, and deeply placed lesions are removed by lobectomy in suitable candidates.

Sputum Analysis

Exfoliative sputum cytology is most valuable for detection of lung cancer. Specimens are obtained by deep coughing or by abrasion with a brush, or bronchial washings are obtained by either bronchoscopic or percutaneous transtracheal washing techniques. Specimens should be collected in the morning and delivered to the laboratory promptly. Centrifugation or filtration can be used to concentrate the cellular elements.

In primary lung cancer, sputum cytology is positive in 30–60% of cases. Repeated sputum examination improves the diagnostic return. Examination of the first bronchoscopic washing material yields a diagnosis in 60% of cases. Postbronchoscopy sputum analysis should always be made at 6–12 and 24 hours, as findings may be positive at these times when previous tests are negative.

Computed Tomography (CT Scan)

Computed tomography can accurately distinguish between aneurysmal dilatation of the aorta and other lesions as the cause of a mediastinal mass. It is helpful in delineating fluid collections within the thoracic cavity and can be used to differentiate between empyema and parenchymal abscess of the lung. Metastases to the lung are more readily demonstrated by CT scan than by other techniques. Pulmonary infarcts can be detected in some cases when plain films of the chest are equivocal. While CT scanning is of limited use in the staging of carcinoma, it has proved to be of great value in defining the extent of metastatic disease.

Magnetic Resonance Imaging (MRI)

Magnetic resonance imaging uses radio waves in a magnetic field to produce images that can distinguish between tumor, cyst, normal tissues and flowing blood. Although its major value in the thorax has been in cardiovascular imaging, it has been helpful in showing invasion of lung cancer into chest wall and mediastinal structures.

DISEASES OF THE CHEST WALL

Defects of development are described in Chapter 46. Neuromuscular syndromes of the inlet or shoulder are described in Chapter 35. Injuries to the chest wall are described in Chapter 13.

LUNG HERNIA (Pneumatocele)

A pneumatocele is a herniation of the lung resulting from a defect in the chest wall caused by abnormal development, trauma, or surgery. Most pneumatoceles are thoracic in location, but cervical (defects of Sibson's fascia) or diaphragmatic herniation may occur occasionally. Lung hernias are usually asymptomatic, but some patients experience local tenderness, pain, or mild dyspnea. Operative repair rather than external support produces optimal results if symptoms are present.

CHEST WALL INFECTIONS

Infections that appear to involve only the skin and soft tissues may actually represent outward extensions of deeper infection of the ribs, cartilage, sternum, or even the pleural space (empyema necessitatis). Inadequate drainage of superficial infection can lead to inward extension into the pleural space, causing empyema.

Subpectoral abscess is caused by suppurative adenitis of the axillary lymph nodes, rib or pleural infection, or posterior extension of a breast abscess, or it may occur as a complication of chest wall surgery (eg, mastectomy, pacemaker placement). Symptoms include systemic sepsis, erythema, induration of the pectoral region, and obliteration of the normal infraclavicular depression. Shoulder movement is painful. Organisms most commonly involved include hemolytic streptococci and Staphylococcus aureus. Treatment involves incisional drainage along the lateral border of the pectoralis major muscle and antibiotics.

Subscapular abscess may arise from osteomyelitis of the scapula but most commonly follows thoracic operations such as thoracotomy or thoracoplasty. Winging of the scapula or paravertebral induration of the trapezius muscle is usually present. A pleural communication is suggested if a cough impulse is present or if the size of the mass varies with position or direct pressure. The diagnosis is established by needle aspiration. Origin open drainage is indicated for pyogenic infections not involving the pleural space. Tubercular lesions should be treated by chemotherapy and needle aspiration, if possible.

Osteomyelitis of the Ribs

In the past, osteomyelitis of the ribs was often caused by typhoid fever and tuberculosis. Except in children, hematogenous osteomyelitis is a rare problem today. Thoracotomy incisions may result in osteomyelitis.

Sternal Osteomyelitis

Infection of the sternum most commonly follows sternotomy incisions and presents as a postoperative wound infection or mediastinitis. Treatment consists of either open drainage or a closed irrigation drainage system with antibiotics, as well as systemic antibiotics. Resection of the involved sternum and a margin of adjacent normal bone may be necessary.

Infection of the Costal Cartilages & Xiphoid

Costal cartilage infections are relatively unresponsive to antibiotic therapy, because once perichondral vascularity is interrupted, the cartilage dies and remains as a foreign body to perpetuate the infection and sinus tract formation. The infection may be established during the course of septicemia, but the most common cause is direct extension of other surgical infections (eg, wound infection, subphrenic abscess). Surgical division of costal cartilages, as in a thoracoabdominal incision, may predispose to cartilage infection postoperatively if local sepsis develops. A wide variety of organisms have been implicated.

Erythema and induration with fluctuance and often spontaneous drainage can occur. The course can be fulminant or may be indolent over months or years, with periodic exacerbations. Associated osteomyelitis of the sternum, ribs, or clavicle may occur.

The differential diagnosis includes local bone or cartilage tumors, Tietze's syndrome, chest wall metastasis, eroding aortic aneurysm, and bronchocutaneous fistula.

The treatment of choice includes resection of the involved cartilage and adjacent involved bony structures. Recurrence is due to underestimation of the extent of disease and inadequate resection.

Reconstruction of the Chest Wall

Chest wall reconstruction may be necessary following trauma, surgical resection, or infectious processes. Recent advances in the use of musculocutaneous flaps and the supportive use of methylcrylate and Marlex mesh to produce solidity below these muscular flaps have facilitated repairs. In massive chest wall defects, vascularization of the area is essential and can be accomplished by use of omental flaps as well as pectoralis, latissimus dorsi, and rectus flaps. Microsurgical techniques for repair of such defects have greatly expanded the ability of plastic surgeons to deal with extensive resectional and infective processes.

Adler BD, Padley SP, Muller NL: Tuberculosis of the chest wall: CT findings. J Comput Assist Tomogr 1993; 17:271.

Mansour KA, Anderson TM, Hester TR: Sternal resection and reconstruction. Ann Thorac Surg 1993;55:838.

Pairolero PC, Arnold PG, Harris JB: Long-term results of pectoralis major muscle transposition for infected sternotomy wounds. Ann Surg 1991;213:583.

Siegman-Igra Y et al: Serious infectious complications of midsternotomy: A review of bacteriology and antimicrobial therapy. Scand J Infect Dis 1990;22:633.

TIETZE'S SYNDROME

Tietze's syndrome is a painful nonsuppurative inflammation of the costochondral cartilages and is of unknown cause. Local swelling and tenderness are the only symptoms; they usually disappear without therapy. The syndrome may recur.

Treatment is symptomatic and may include analgesics and local or systemic corticosteroids. When symptoms persist longer than 3 weeks and tumefaction suggests neoplasm, excision of the involved cartilage may be indicated and is usually curative.

Aeschlimann A, Kahn MF: Tietze's syndrome: A critical review. Clin Exper Rheumatol 1990;8:407.

MONDOR'S DISEASE (Thrombophlebitis of the Thoracoepigastric Vein)

Mondor's disease consists of localized thrombophlebitis of the anterolateral chest wall. It is more prominent in women than in men and occasionally follows radical mastectomy. There are few symptoms other than the presence of a localized tender cord-like structure in the subcutaneous tissues of the abdomen, thorax, or axilla. The disease is self-limited and devoid of complications such as thromboembolism. The possibility of an infective origin or stasis of the interrupted venous return due to neoplasm must be ruled out.

Bejanga BI: Mondor's disease: analysis of 30 cases. J R Col Surg Edinburgh 1992;37.322.

CHEST WALL TUMORS

Chest wall tumors may be simulated by enlarged costal cartilages, chest wall infection, fractures, rickets, scurvy, hyperparathyroidism, and other conditions. Incisional biopsy or needle biopsy is rarely of benefit. Examination of the complete tumor tissue type is critical, and when cancer is present, wide excision is necessary.

Specific Neoplasms
A. Benign Soft Tissue Tumors:
1. Lipomas–Lipomas are the most common benign tumors of the chest wall. Occasionally, they are very large, lobulated, and may have dumbbell-shaped extensions that indent the endothoracic fascia beneath the sternum through a vertebral foramen. They may on occasion communicate with a large mediastinal or supraclavicular component.

2. Neurogenic tumors–These may arise from intercostal or superficial nerves. Solitary neurofibromas are most common, followed by neurolemmomas.

3. Cavernous hemangiomas–Hemangiomas of the thoracic wall are usually painful and occur in children. Tumors may be isolated or may involve

other tissues (eg, lung), as in Rendu-Osler-Weber syndrome.

4. Lymphangiomas–This rare lesion is seen most often in children. It may have poorly defined borders that make complete excision difficult.

B. Malignant Soft Tissue Tumors:
1. Fibrosarcomas–Fibrosarcoma is the most common primary soft tissue cancer of the chest wall. It occurs most frequently in young adults.

2. Liposarcomas–These tumors account for approximately one-third of all primary cancers of the chest wall. They occur more often in men.

3. Neurofibrosarcomas–These tumors involve the thoracic wall almost twice as often as other parts of the body. They often occur in patients with Recklinghausen's disease and usually originate from intercostal nerves.

C. Benign Skeletal Tumors:
1. Chondromas, osteochondromas, and myxochondromas–The combined frequency of these three cartilaginous tumors is nearly the same as that of fibrous dysplasia (ie, they comprise about 30–45% of all benign skeletal tumors). Cartilaginous tumors are usually single and occur with equal frequency in males and females between childhood and the fourth decade. The tumors are usually painless and tend to occur anteriorly along the costal margin or in the parasternal area. Wide local excision is curative.

2. Fibrous dysplasia–Fibrous dysplasia (bone cyst, osteofibroma, fibrous osteoma, fibrosis ossificans) accounts for a third or more of benign skeletal tumors of the chest wall. This cystic bone tumor can occur in any portion of the skeletal system, but approximately half involve the ribs. They may be clinically differentiated from cystic bone lesions associated with hyperparathyroidism. The tumor is usually single and may be related to trauma. Some patients complain of swelling, tenderness, or vague pain or discomfort, but the lesion is usually silent and is detected on routine chest x-ray. Treatment consists of local excision.

3. Eosinophilic granuloma–Eosinophilic granuloma may occur in the clavicle, the scapula, or (rarely) the sternum. Coexisting infiltrates of the lung are often present. This condition often represents a more benign form of Letterer-Siwe disease or Hand-Schüller-Christian syndrome. Fever, malaise, leukocytosis, eosinophilia, or bone pain may be present. Rib involvement presents as a swelling with cortical bone destruction and periosteal new growth. The clinical picture can resemble osteomyelitis or Ewing's sarcoma. When the disease is localized, excision will result in cure.

4. Hemangioma–Cavernous hemangioma of the ribs presents as a painful mass in infancy or childhood. The tumor appears on chest x-ray as either multiple radiolucent areas or a single trabeculated cyst.

5. Miscellaneous–Fibromas, lipomas, osteomas, and aneurysmal bone cysts are all relatively rare lesions of the skeletal chest wall. The diagnosis is established after excisional biopsy.

D. Malignant Skeletal Tumors:

1. Chondrosarcomas–Chondrosarcomas are the most common primary malignant tumors of the chest wall. About 15–20% of all skeletal chondrosarcomas occur in the ribs or sternum. Most appear in patients 20–40 years of age. They occur most commonly at the costochondral junction of the rib cage but may occur anywhere along the rib. Local involvement of pleura, adjacent ribs, muscle, diaphragm, or other soft tissue may develop. Pain is rare, however, and most patients complain only of the mass. Chest x-ray shows destroyed cortical bone, usually with diffuse mottled calcification, and the border of the tumor is indistinct. Treatment consists of wide radical excision. Only occasionally are regional lymph nodes involved. The 5-year survival rate is 10–30%, depending largely upon the adequacy of the initial excision.

2. Osteogenic sarcoma (osteosarcoma)–Osteosarcoma occurs in the second and third decades, and 60% of cases occur in men. It is more malignant than chondrosarcoma. X-ray findings consist of bone destruction and recalcification at right angles to the bony cortex, which gives the characteristic "sunburst" appearance. Hematogenous metastasis with pulmonary involvement is common. Treatment consists of radical local excision, but the prognosis is poor and survival beyond 5 years is rare.

3. Myeloma (solitary plasmacytoma)–These tumors are often found as a manifestation of systemic multiple myeloma, and patients with myeloma of the chest wall usually develop manifestations of systemic disease. The x-ray findings are punched-out, osteolytic lesions without evidence of new bone formation. The disease affects adults in the fifth to seventh decades and is seen nearly twice as often in men as in women. Solitary myeloma is quite rare, and systemic involvement eventually occurs in all cases. Treatment with antimetabolites relieves bone pain, although life is not prolonged. The 5-year survival rate is only about 5%.

4. Ewing's sarcoma (hemangioendothelioma, endothelioma)–Ewing's tumors are associated with systemic symptoms such as fever and malaise and, locally, a painful, warm chest wall mass. X-ray findings show a characteristic "onion skin" calcification. These tumors are highly malignant, and evidence of other skeletal lesions is present in 30–75% of patients when first seen. The diagnosis should be established by needle biopsy, since surgical excision does not improve survival time. X-ray irradiation is the only treatment available. Survival for as long as 5 years is rare.

5. Lymphoma–The diagnosis and treatment of chest wall lymphomas are essentially the same as for those lesions found elsewhere in the body.

E. Metastatic Chest Wall Tumors: Metastases to bones of the thorax are often multiple and are usually from tumors of the kidney, thyroid, lung, breast, prostate, stomach, uterus, or colon (Figure 18–7). Involvement by direct extension occurs in carcinoma of the breast and lung. Some cases of lung carcinoma involving the chest wall by direct extension have been cured by radical resection.

Brodsky JT et al: Desmoid tumors of the chest wall: A locally recurrent problem. J Thorac Cardiovasc Surg 1992;104:900.

Burt M et al: Primary bony and cartilaginous sarcomas of chest wall: Results of therapy. Ann Thorac Surg 1992; 54:226.

Perry RR et al: Survival after surgical resection for high-grade chest wall sarcomas. Ann Thorac Surg 1990; 49:363.

Ryan MB, McMurtrey MJ, Roth JA: Current management of chest-wall tumors. Surg Clin North Am 1989;69: 1061.

Schaefer PS, Burton BS: Radiographic evaluation of chest-wall lesions. Surg Clin North Am 1989;69:911.

DISEASES OF THE PLEURA

The most common symptom of pleural disease is **pleuritic pain,** chest pain associated with respiratory excursion that sometimes reflexively inhibits respiration. Pleural pain is mediated through the sympathetic nerves of the parietal pleura or diaphragm, since the visceral pleura does not contain sympathetic fibers. Referred pain often results from involvement of a visceral process with the parietal pleura. Pleuritic

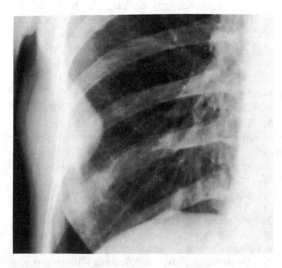

Figure 18–7. Rib metastasis and extrapleural mass from leiomyosarcoma of the uterus.

pain is felt in the shoulder over the distribution of the third through fifth cervical segments. Diseases involving the pleural surface can also produce an audible friction rub on auscultation. Both pleuritic pain and friction rubs may diminish if a pleural effusion forms.

PLEURAL EFFUSION

With pleural effusion, physical findings may be normal when there is less than 300 mL of fluid in the pleural space. Generally, more than 1000 mL of pleural fluid is required to cause a contralateral mediastinal shift. When contralateral mediastinal shift does not occur with the critical volume of fluid present, the cause may be carcinoma of the main stem bronchus with atelectasis of the ipsilateral lung; fixed mediastinum due to neoplastic lymph nodes; malignant mesothelioma; or pronounced infiltration of the ipsilateral lung, usually with tumor. Respiratory movement may lag on the affected side. Fullness or even bulging may occur, and with long-standing effusion, there may be contraction and immobility of the involved hemithorax. The intercostal spaces are narrowed, and the ribs have a shingled relationship. Acute inflammation of the pleura may be associated with tenderness of the intercostal spaces or, in advanced cases, with swelling, redness, and local warmth. Tactile fremitus is diminished with effusion, and there is dullness to percussion. Breath sounds may be exaggerated, bronchial, or amphoric in quality over a lung compressed by pleural effusion.

The term pleural effusion denotes endogenous fluid in the pleural space. A more exact terminology is used when the character of the fluid is known. **Hydrothorax** denotes serous effusion, either transudate or exudate. **Pyothorax (empyema), hemothorax,** and **chylothorax** are other categories.

Pleural effusions may occur with disease of the lungs, mediastinum, or chest wall. Identification of the specific type of effusion often depends on examination of fluid obtained by thoracentesis (Table 18–1). If this procedure is unsuccessful, either needle or open pleural biopsy must be considered.

Transudates have a specific gravity of less than 1.016 and a protein content of less than 3 g/dL. They contain only a few cells and are most often clear and yellow but occasionally are blood-tinged.

Abnormal amounts of pleural fluid accumulate when there is increased hydrostatic pressure (congestive heart failure), decreased colloidal osmotic pressure (severe hypoalbuminemia), increased capillary permeability (pneumonia), increased intrapleural negative pressure (atelectasis), and decreased lymphatic drainage (mediastinal carcinomatosis). Blood may directly enter the pleural space with trauma (vascular injury, tumor erosion of vessels), and chyle may accumulate with rupture of the thoracic duct or disruption of mediastinal parietal pleura with its lymphatics. Examination of centrifuged sediment may show tumor cells, bacteria, fungi, tubercle bacilli, amebas, or other pathogenic organisms.

1. PLEURAL EFFUSION FROM NONPULMONARY DISEASES

Immunologic Diseases

Systemic lupus erythematosus is associated with pleural effusion in about half of cases. Isolated pleural involvement occurs in only 10% of these cases; effusions are usually small. In about 30–50% of cases, the heart is enlarged on x-ray.

Pleural effusion may occur with rheumatoid arthritis, usually in middle-aged men. The effusions are usually unilateral and involve the right side somewhat more often than the left. There appears to be no relationship between the pulmonary manifestations of rheumatoid disease and pleural effusion.

Cardiovascular Diseases

Pleural effusion is seen in constrictive pericarditis and congestive heart failure (Figure 18–8). The right hemithorax alone is most often affected, though the effusion may be bilateral. Fluid occasionally localizes in interlobar fissures, simulating mass lesions that may spontaneously resolve (known as "phantom tumors" or "disappearing tumors"). When this fluid is hemorrhagic, the possibility of concomitant pulmonary infarction should be considered. Interlobar effusions involve the right horizontal fissure in most cases but may be bilateral.

Pancreatitis

Pleural effusion secondary to pancreatitis usually affects only the left side. The diagnosis is confirmed by finding an amylase concentration in the fluid substantially above that in the serum.

Meigs' Syndrome

Meigs' syndrome (ascites and hydrothorax) was first described in patients with fibroma of the ovary. It has also been noted with pelvic tumors such as thecomas, granulosa cell tumors, Brenner tumors, cystadenomas, adenocarcinomas, and fibromyomas of the uterus. Removal of the pelvic tumor is invariably followed by clearing of both effusions.

Cirrhosis of the Liver

Right-sided hydrothorax occurs in about 5% of patients with cirrhosis and ascites.

Renal Disease

Hydronephrosis, nephrotic syndrome, and acute glomerulonephritis are sometimes associated with hydrothorax.

Table 18–1. Differential diagnosis of pleural effusions.*

	Tuberculosis	Cancer	Congestive Heart Failure	Pneumonia and Other Non-tuberculous Infections	Rheumatoid Arthritis and Collagen Disease	Pulmonary Embolism
Clinical context	Younger patient with history of exposure to tuberculosis.	Older patient in poor general health.	Presence of congestive heart failure.	Presence of respiratory infection.	History of joint involvement; subcutaneous nodules.	Postoperative, immobilized, or venous disease.
Gross appearance	Usually serious; often sanguineous.	Often sanguineous.	Serous.	Serous.	Turbid or yellow-green.	Often sanguineous.
Microscopic examination	May be positive for acid-fast bacilli; cholesterol crystals.	Cytology positive in 50%.	...	May be positive for bacilli.	...	...
Cell count	Few have > 10,000 erythrocytes; most have > 1000 leukocytes, mostly lymphocytes.	Two-thirds bloody; 40% > 1000 leukocytes, mostly lymphocytes.	Few have > 10,000 erythrocytes or > 1000 leukocytes.	Polymorphonuclears predominate.	Lymphocytes predominate.	Erythrocytes predominate.
Culture	May have positive pleural effusion; few have positive sputum or gastric washings.	...	...	May be positive.	...	...
Specific gravity	Most > 1.016.	Most > 1.016.	Most < 1.016.	> 1.016.	> 1.016.	> 1.016.
Protein	90% 3 g/dL or more.	90% 3 g/dL or more.	75% > 3 g/dL.	3 g/dL or more.	3 g/dL or more.	3 g/dL or more.
Sugar	60% < 60 mg/dL.	Rarely < 60 mg/dL.	...	Occasionally 60 mg/dL.	5–17 gm/dL (rheumatoid arthritis).	...
Other	No mesothelial cells on cytology. Tuberculin test usually positive. Pleural biopsy positive.	If hemorrhagic fluid, 65% will be due to tumor; tends to recur after removal.	Right-sided in 55–70%.	Associated with infiltrate on x-ray.	Rapid clotting time; LE cell or rheumatoid factor may be present.	Source of emboli may be noted.

Other exudates: (Sr gr > 1.016.)
  Fungal infection: Exposure in endemic area. Source fluid. Microscopy and culture may be positive for fungi. Protein 3 g/dL or more. Skin and serologic tests may be helpful.
  Trauma: Serosanguineous fluid. Protein 3 g/dL or more.
  Chylothorax: History of injury or cancer. Chylous fluid with no protein but with fat droplets.

* Modified from: Therapy of pleural effusion: A statement by the Committee on Therapy of the American Thoracic Society. Am Rev Respir Dis 1968;97:479.

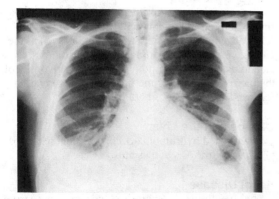

Figure 18–8. Pleural effusion secondary to heart failure (myocarditis).

Thromboembolic Disease

Pleural effusion following thromboembolism to the lungs is usually scrosanguineous but may be grossly bloody. These effusions are occasionally massive but usually are small and are associated with characteristic x-ray findings in the lung. Treatment of the pleural effusion is usually not necessary, and the fluid is reabsorbed in several days.

2. MALIGNANT PLEURAL EFFUSION

About half of all patients with carcinoma of the breast or lung develop pleural effusion during the course of their disease, and 25% of all effusions are the result of cancer. Cytologic examination of pleural fluid is positive in 70% and pleural biopsy in 80% of malignant effusions. About 10% of malignant effusions are due to pleural mesotheliomas and the rest to metastatic tumors. About half of bilateral effusions associated with normal heart size are due to cancer, and these are almost invariably associated with hepatic metastases.

Multiple methods have been used to treat malignant pleural effusions (Figure 18–9). The usual objective is full lung expansion and pleural symphysis so that effusion does not recur. The most commonly used regimens are closed tube drainage for 4–7 days, with or without instillation of a sclerosing agent such as tetracycline into the pleural space. Chemical pleurodesis is successful in 50–70% of cases, and although operative pleurodesis is successful in 95% of cases, operative intervention is avoided if possible in these patients. Multiple agents have been used for chemical pleurodesis, including nitrogen mustard, radioactive colloidal gold, doxorubicin, quinacrine, and *Corynebacterium parvum*. Increased efficacy over more benign agents has not been proved.

Thoracentesis or tube drainage may be complicated by pneumothorax, fever, fluid loculation, and infection. Early tube drainage avoids the problem of loculation produced by multiple attempts at needle aspiration. Recurrence of effusion is inevitable after needle aspiration alone but occurs in only 15% of patients treated with tube drainage. The average duration of life in patients with malignant effusion due to solid tumors is approximately 6 months and with lymphomas, approximately 16 months.

Escudero Bueno C et al: Cytologic and bacteriologic analysis of fluid and pleural biopsy specimens with Cope's needle: Study of 414 patients. Arch Intern Med 1990; 150:1190.

Henschke CI et al: The pathogenesis, radiologic evaluation, and therapy of pleural effusions. Radiol Clin North Am 1989;27:1241.

Keller SM: Current and future therapy for malignant pleural effusion. Chest 1993;103:63S.

McLoud TC, Flower CD: Imaging the pleura: sonography, CT, and MR imaging. AJR Am J Roentgenol 199 1;156: 1145.

Sahn SA: The pathophysiology of pleural effusions. Ann Rev Med 1990;41:7.

Yang PC et al: Value of sonography in determining the nature of pleural effusion: analysis of 320 cases. AJR Am J Roentgenol 1992;159:29.

3. EMPYEMA

Empyema denotes an infected effusive process within the pleural space. Findings may mimic simple pleural effusion. More commonly, there is chest pain, hemoptysis, shortness of breath, weakness with fever, and, in severe cases, toxemia. The effusion is an exudate. Empyema thoracis thus represents an acute or chronic suppurative pleural exudate and may be

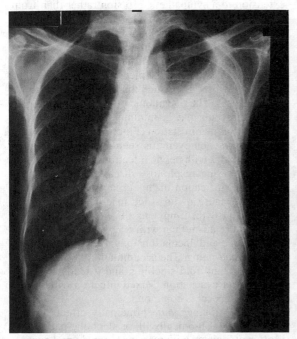
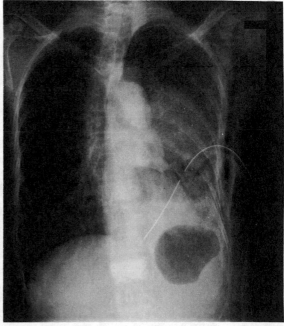

Figure 18–9. Malignant pleural effusion (carcinoma of lung). *Left:* Posteroanterior projection before treatment. *Right:* After chest tube drainage. Note left hilar mass and osteoblastic metastasis to the first lumbar vertebra.

caused by multiple organisms, including pneumo-cocci, streptococci, staphylococci, *Bacteroides, Escherichia coli, Proteus vulgaris,* tubercle bacilli, fungi, and amebas. Such infections extend into the pleural space in the following ways: (1) directly from pneumonic infiltrate; (2) by lymphatic spread from neighboring infections of the lungs, mediastinum, chest wall, or diaphragm; (3) by hematogenous spread from a remote infection; (4) by direct inoculation by penetrating trauma, surgical incisions, or attempted percutaneous needle or tube drainage of a pulmonary abscess (sterile pleural effusion) (Figure 18–10); (5) from ruptured thoracic viscera (eg, esophagus) or displaced abdominal viscera (eg, strangulated traumatic diaphragmatic hernia); or (6) by extension of subdiaphragmatic processes such as subdiaphragmatic abscesses, hepatic abscesses, or perinephric abscesses.

Clinical Findings

Signs and symptoms include chest pain, shortness of breath, fever, weakness, and hemoptysis, although some patients are severely systemically toxic or even comatose. They may be cyanotic, hypotensive, dehydrated, and oliguric. Temperatures may reach 40.6 °C (105 °F). Respirations may be grunting, and physical findings of pleural effusion are common (Table 18–2). In the absence of fever, empyema must be differ-

Table 18–2. Incidence of various complications of staphylococcal pneumonia in adults and children (in %).

	Adults	Children
Abscess	25	50
Empyema	15	15
Pneumatocele	1	35
Effusion	30	55
Bronchopleural fistula	2	5

entiated from pulmonary embolus with effusion. Laboratory findings include hematocrit in the low 30s, particularly after rehydration, and a white blood cell count in the range of 14,000–18,000/μL, with a shift to the left.

Staphylococcus aureus is the most common organism in all age groups, accounting for over 90% of cases in infants and children. It may lead to the formation of **pneumatoceles,** which are thin-walled cystic spaces that form as a result of a check-valve type of obstruction of small bronchi. This type of pneumatocele must be differentiated from the benign hernia of the chest wall of the same name, an unrelated condition. Pneumatoceles are commonly found in staphylococcal pneumonia. Staphylococcal abscess may also occur. Both pneumatoceles and abscesses may overexpand and rupture, leading to empyema formation.

Empyema due to *Streptococcus pyogenes* commonly follows streptococcal pneumonia. It is characterized by thick green pus that tends to become loculated within 2 or 3 days. The empyema results from extension to a sympathetic effusion rather than from rupture of an abscess. Streptococcal organisms can often be diagnosed by sputum culture (60%), but throat culture is negative in about 80% of cases and blood cultures are rarely positive. The diagnosis is best made by culture of the pleural effusion. The antistreptolysin titer is greater than 250 Todd units in 97% of cases. The pneumonic component of streptococcal empyema may be minimal, and empyema may be the initial manifestation (Figure 18–11).

Bacteroides empyema is seen most commonly in young females with pelvic infections and elderly men with underlying respiratory disease, alcoholism, or cancer. Identification of this organism is sometimes difficult because of its strict anaerobic requirement and slow growth. Empyema develops more rapidly with this organism than with *E coli* or *Pseudomonas aeruginosa,* and loculation may be present almost from the beginning. The accumulation of pus is massive, thick, and foul-smelling, and it tends to return rapidly after evacuation. Mixed infection with anaerobic streptococci is common.

Klebsiella pneumoniae principally affects debilitated, elderly, chronically ill, or alcoholic patients. It is often associated with massive parenchymal consolidation. Abscess and cavitation occur in about half of patients, and one-third of these develop empyema.

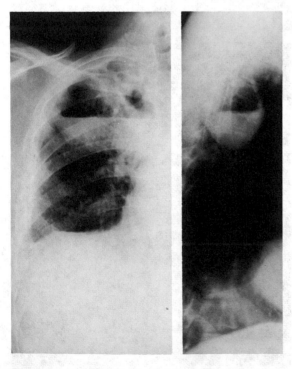

Figure 18–10. Postoperative loculated empyema with bronchopleural fistula. Left: Posteroanterior projection. Right: Lateral projection.

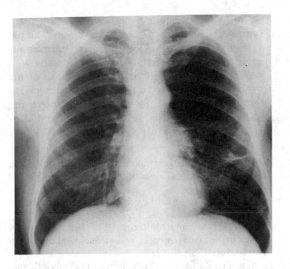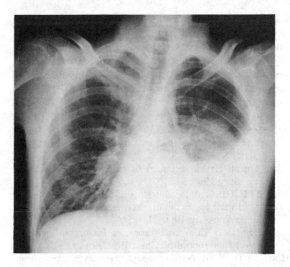

Figure 18–11. Streptococcal empyema. *Left:* Normal x-ray when patient was admitted with high fever. *Right:* Chest x-ray 3 days after admission.

Extensive parenchymal necrosis and the frequent development of a bronchopleural fistula with this organism demand early aggressive therapy.

Streptococcus pneumoniae is now less often a cause of empyema than it was in the preantibiotic era. Pleural involvement following pneumococcal pneumonia usually occurred 7–10 days after onset, and most patients now have received effective antibiotic therapy by this time.

E coli, Pseudomonas, and *Proteus* may cause empyema in patients with underlying systemic disease.

X-ray findings in all cases involve opacification of a portion of the pleural space, sometimes with a fluid level. A pneumonic infiltrate is usually present but may be obscured by the effusion.

Complications

The complications of empyema are **empyema necessitatis** (invasion of the chest wall), bronchopleural fistula, pericardial extension, mediastinal abscess, osteomyelitis of ribs or cartilage, septicemia, and chronicity. Formation of a bronchial fistula into an empyema requires emergency treatment to avoid flooding of the opposite lung with pus and subsequent fatal pneumonia.

Metastatic abscesses, particularly to the brain, are unusual when antibiotic coverage is adequate. Prolonged suppuration such as may occur in postpneumonectomy empyema can result in amyloid deposition, particularly in the liver and kidneys.

Treatment

Therapy of pyogenic empyema involves use of antibiotics, drainage of the pleural space, and rarely, more extensive surgical drainage. Aspiration will accomplish drainage of the pleural space in a small per-

centage of patients when pleural effusion is minimal and watery and a prompt response to antibiotic therapy is expected. However, even in favorable cases such as streptococcal empyema in young men, hospitalization time is almost 2 weeks longer when needle aspiration rather than closed tube drainage is used. In general, inadequate early drainage is the most frequent cause of subsequent therapeutic intractability secondary to loculations.

Prompt underwater-seal closed tube drainage of the pleural space is preferred in most cases that do not respond to simple drainage or where roentgenographic demonstration of multiple air-fluid levels indicates that loculation has already occurred. Insertion of the tube may be combined with local rib resection (2.5–5 cm) and limited thoracic exploration to remove necrotic material and break down loculations. The chest tube can be brought through the chest wall by a separate incision or through the same incision. The incision can be made airtight with layered absorbable sutures. Closed tube drainage with negative pressure minimizes the size of the residual air space.

When empyema is associated with parenchymal necrosis or lung trapping, the pleural space may not be obliterated by the above measures, and the residual space may require prolonged drainage to prevent sealing off and reactivation of the infection. By 5–7 days, the space communicating with the chest tube is usually isolated from the remaining pleural space, and the underwater seal is no longer necessary to prevent lung collapse. At this point, the chest tube can be cut, leaving a portion protruding from the chest wall to maintain a chronic draining tract. Later, if the space does not seem to be decreasing in size or if debridement is required, it can be managed by a larger chest wall and rib resection, known as an **Eloesser**

flap. This procedure consists of suturing a flap of skin to the pleura, creating an epithelium-lined sinus into the empyema cavity for simpler long-term care.

More aggressive surgical measures are reserved for unusual cases. Thoracoplasty, which involves collapsing the chest wall to obliterate pleural space, is rarely indicated.

Alfageme I et al: Empyema of the thorax in adults: Etiology, microbiologic findings, and management. Chest 1993;103:839.

Ali I, Unruh H: Management of empyema thoracis. Ann Thorac Surg 1990;50:355.

Arnold PG, Pairolero PC: Intrathoracic muscle flaps: An account of their use in the management of 100 consecutive patients. Ann Surg 1990;211:656.

Ashbaugh DG: Empyema thoracis. Factors influencing morbidity and mortality. Chest 1991;99:1162.

Horrigan TP, Snow NJ: Thoracoplasty: Current application to the infected pleural space. Ann Thorac Surg 1990;50:695.

Miller JI: Empyema thoracis. Ann Thorac Surg 1990;50:343.

Pairolero PC, Trastek VF: Surgical management of chronic empyema: The role of thoracoplasty. Ann Thorac Surg 1990;50:90.

Ridley PD, Braimbridge MV: Thoracoscopic debridement and pleural irrigation in the management of empyema thoracis. Ann Thorac Surg 1991;51:461.

Smith JA et al: Empyema thoracis: 14-year experience in a teaching center. Ann Thorac Surg 1991;51:39.

4. CHYLOTHORAX

Accumulation of chyle in the pleural space may be (1) congenital, (2) traumatic postoperative, (3) traumatic nonsurgical, or (4) nontraumatic.

Congenital chylothorax is relatively rare. It is due to congenital abnormalities of the lymphatic system, such as absence of the thoracic duct or a fistula between the thoracic duct and the pleural space. Traumatic postoperative chylothorax follows operations or diagnostic procedures that injure the thoracic duct, most commonly cardiovascular and esophageal operations, although percutaneous cannulations of the left subclavian and internal jugular veins have increasingly been associated with this problem. Traumatic nonsurgical chylothorax follows penetrating, blunt, or blast injuries. Fractures are not necessary for thoracic duct injury to occur. The usual mechanism is thought to be a shearing of the duct at the right crus of the diaphragm. This may occur with violent coughing or hyperextension of the spine. Nontraumatic chylothorax is generally regarded as ominous, since cancer is the most frequent cause. Other causes include hepatic cirrhosis, thoracic aortic aneurysm, and filariasis.

The treatment of nonmalignant chylothorax consists of removing enough fluid by needle or closed tube drainage to obtain full lung expansion. In many cases, the irritating nature of chyle will promote pleural symphysis and plug the leakage of chyle. The patient should be given a low-fat diet. Intravenous hyperalimentation has greatly improved results with this condition. Surgical division and ligation of the duct should be considered if drainage does not lead to prompt improvement. Instillation of sclerosing agents, such as those used in malignant pleural effusions, may be effective, especially in infants.

Dougenis D et al: Management of chylothorax complicating extensive esophageal resection. Surg Gynecol Obstet 1992;174:501.

Marts BC et al: Conservative versus surgical management of chylothorax. Am J Surg 1992;164:532.

Murphy MC, Newman BM, Rodgers BM: Pleuroperitoneal shunts in the management of persistent chylothorax. Ann Thorac Surg 1989;48:195.

Valentine VG, Raffin TA: The management of chylothorax. Chest 1992;102:586.

5. HEMOTHORAX

Accumulation of blood in the pleural space is most commonly due to trauma, pulmonary infarction, neoplasms, or tuberculosis. It may also occur as a complication of surgery or diagnostic procedures.

Treatment consists of closed tube drainage to evacuate the blood before clotting occurs. Since large amounts of blood clot are absorbed spontaneously from the pleural space without significant sequelae if secondary infection does not occur, a conservative approach to such accumulations is indicated. Occasionally, a persistent blood clot may result in fibrosis or impaired pulmonary function, in which case decortication should be considered.

PRIMARY PLEURAL TUMORS

Two types of primary pleural tumors have been identified: localized mesothelioma and diffuse malignant mesothelioma. **Localized mesothelioma** most often arises from the visceral pleura, may be either pedunculated or sessile, and may either protrude into the pleural cavity or be embedded within the lung. It may achieve a gigantic size. Microscopically, this tumor is composed mainly of spindle cells and appears quite malignant, but usually the tumor is well encapsulated. Local excision is the treatment of choice, since only about 30% of solitary mesotheliomas are malignant. Pleural effusion is present in 10–15% of cases. The presence of blood in the effusion does not indicate incurability. The roentgenographic findings consist of a peripheral, well-demarcated mass, often forming an obtuse angle with the chest wall. Bone and joint pain, swelling, and arthritis have been described in as many as two-thirds of localized mesotheliomas. Recurrence is often heralded by return of arthritic symptoms and may be benign or malignant. Malignant tumors have a poor prognosis; most patients die within 2 years.

Diffuse mesothelioma may arise anywhere within the pleura. From mesothelial cell origin, it may rapidly proliferate along the pleural surface to encase the lung. Pleural effusion is almost always present and is usually bloody. In cases without effusion, this lesion may present as diffuse pleural thickening. There is little evidence that these lesions arise from originally benign localized mesothelioma. Diffuse mesotheliomas occur in all age groups but are often seen in relatively young patients, especially men, between 40–50 years of age. Development of mesothelioma has been directly linked to previous exposure to certain mineral elements used in commercial asbestos products; these elements include crocidolite, tremolite, and, most pervasively, chrysotile. The mean interval between first exposure to chrysotile and manifestation of disease is about 40 years. Patients complain of pleural pain, malaise, weight loss, weakness, anemia, fever, irritative cough, or dyspnea. The physical findings are those of pleural thickening or effusion.

Treatment of diffuse mesothelioma is rarely surgical but consists principally of relief of symptoms and management of the pleural effusion, which may rapidly reaccumulate. Radiotherapy and intrapleural radioactive isotopes occasionally provide long-term remissions. The use of chemotherapeutic regimens containing doxorubicin (Adriamycin) appears to prolong survival of patients with epithelial type tumors.

Antman KH: Natural history and epidemiology of malignant mesothelioma. Chest 1993;103:373S.

Mossman BT, Gee JB: Asbestos-related diseases. N Engl J Med 1989;320:1721.

Patz EF Jr et al: Malignant pleural mesothelioma: Value of CT and MR imaging in predicting resectability. AJR Am J Roentgenol 1992;159:961.

Rusch VW, Piantadosi S, Holmes EC: The role of extrapleural pneumonectomy in malignant pleural mesothelioma: A Lung Cancer Study Group trial. J Thorac Cardiovasc Surg 1991;102:1.

Sridhar KS et al: New strategies are needed in diffuse malignant mesothelioma. Cancer 1992;70:2969.

Sugarbaker DJ et al: Extrapleural pneumonectomy, chemotherapy, and radiotherapy in the treatment of diffuse malignant pleural mesothelioma. J Thorac Cardiovasc Surg 1991;102:10.

Sugarbaker DJ, Mentzer SJ, Strauss G: Extrapleural pneumonectomy in the treatment of malignant pleural mesothelioma. Ann Thorac Surg 1992;54:941.

PNEUMOTHORAX

Air or gas in the pleural space (pneumothorax) may originate from rupture of the respiratory system, esophagus, or chest wall, or it may be generated by microorganisms in the pleural space. Pneumothorax may be classified as spontaneous, traumatic, or iatrogenic, depending on the cause. It is referred to as "closed" when the chest wall is intact or "open" when a breach in the chest wall exists. The magnitude of pneumothorax is expressed as an estimate of the percentage of collapse of the lung. Since the pleural space is a cone-shaped cage, a small rim of air may represent a 10–15% pneumothorax and relatively minimal compression of the lung a 50% pneumothorax, the volume loss decreasing from lateral to medial. When the visceral and parietal pleuras are not adherent, pressure in the pleural space may be sufficient to displace the mediastinum to the opposite side **(tension pneumothorax).** *Both open ("sucking") chest wounds and tension pneumothorax are surgical emergencies, since they seriously compromise ventilation and, because of shifts in the mediastinum, alter venous return.*

In trauma patients, pneumothorax is often associated with blood in the pleural space (hemopneumothorax). With esophageal rupture, the combination of pleural suppuration and air is known as pyopneumothorax.

Clinical Findings

Essentials in diagnosis include chest pain referred to the shoulder or arm of the involved side, dyspnea, hyperresonance, decreased chest wall motion, decreased breath sounds and voice sounds on the involved side, mediastinal shift away from the involved side in the case of tension pneumothorax, and a chest x-ray revealing retraction of the lung from the parietal pleura.

Iatrogenic pneumothorax may occur as a result of inadvertent introduction of air into the pleural space, puncture or rupture of the lung, or intentional introduction of air into the pleural space or mediastinum. Procedures often complicated by pneumothorax are thoracentesis; placement of a percutaneous vein catheter (subclavian, internal jugular) for central venous pressure monitoring or hyperalimentation; operations on the chest wall, neck, back, or upper abdomen; lung or pleural biopsy; brachial plexus block; arteriography; and intercostal nerve block. Inadvertent rupture of the lung may occur with assisted ventilation for anesthesia or respiratory support. Pneumothorax may intentionally be induced for diagnosis or treatment.

Spontaneous pneumothorax may occur in any age group but is most common in males 15–35 years of age (Figure 18–12). A high incidence is reported in patients with Marfan's syndrome. In newborn infants, spontaneous pneumothorax may be asymptomatic and discovered as an incidental finding on a chest x-ray, or it may cause respiratory distress. In young adults, spontaneous pneumothorax develops without known cause in localized emphysematous blebs near the apex of the upper lobe or along the superior seg-

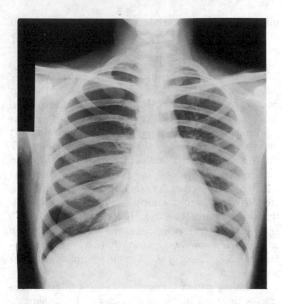

Figure 18–12. Spontaneous pneumothorax on right side.

ment of the lower lobe. In elderly patients, generalized emphysema, bullous emphysema, or some other predisposing cause is usual. The left and right sides are involved with approximately equal frequency. Bilateral involvement and tension pneumothorax are both uncommon. Males predominate over females 10:1. An associated effusion that may contain blood is present in 10% of cases.

About 30% of patients with spontaneous pneumothorax have chronic pulmonary disease, usually consisting of chronic bronchitis or emphysema. A history of smoking, pneumonia, recent upper respiratory infection, or asthma is often obtained. Secondary spontaneous pneumothorax (pneumothorax related to active disease) may occur in staphylococcal pneumonia, lung abscess, or a multitude of other less common pulmonary conditions, including sarcoidosis, endometriosis, and bronchogenic carcinoma.

Critical to definitive treatment is the nature of the pneumothorax. In the case of simple pneumothorax, if air only is introduced into the chest space and no dyspnea is noted, observation and symptomatic therapy are indicated. If simple pneumothorax is secondary to lacerations of the lung from iatrogenic cause or rupture of bleb disease, the severity of symptoms—chest pain, shortness of breath, nausea, vomiting, syncope, and shock—is evaluated to define the need for drainage.

Physical findings may include diminished ventilation of the affected lung and hyperresonance, but diagnosis may elude the examiner in minimal pneumothorax unless a chest x-ray is obtained. If the size of the pneumothorax increases in a patient who is being observed, a thoracostomy tube must be placed. Tension pneumothorax may produce mediastinal shift and tracheal displacement away from the affected side, with neck vein distention, cyanosis, and shock due to obstruction of venous return.

X-ray findings show the extent of pneumothorax (Figure 18–12). The main disorders that must be differentiated from tension pneumothorax are cardiac tamponade and acute congestive heart failure. The physical findings of tension pneumothorax are occasionally obscure, and the condition in such cases is first suspected only with a chest x-ray. The x-ray appearance of a giant lung cyst is similar to that of a distended stomach within the thorax after rupture of the diaphragm and should be differentiated. Placement of a nasogastric tube in the latter condition may be diagnostic.

Treatment

Treatment of pneumothorax involves reexpansion of the involved lung. With a simple, stable pneumothorax of minimal amount, reabsorption of air will achieve reexpansion. Occasionally, thoracentesis is used for diagnosis and, rarely, for reexpansion, as continuous observation for possible recurrence is necessary. Closed tube drainage is the most reliable treatment. The tube is inserted anteriorly via the second intercostal space into the apex of the pleural cavity. Air leaks that persist for 5–7 days and recurrent pneumothorax are usually treated by thoracotomy. The apical blebs are excised, and pleural symphysis is achieved through pleural scarification, pleurectomy, or the use of pleural irritants.

Prognosis

The prognosis in properly managed patients with primary spontaneous pneumothorax is excellent. In patients with spontaneous pneumothorax secondary to another condition, the prognosis is determined by the underlying disease.

Recurrence is the most common indication for operative treatment, and the probability of another recurrence increases geometrically with each attack. The average interval between attacks is 2–3 years, but pneumothorax can recur almost immediately or as long as 20 years later. Asynchronous bilateral involvement occurs in about 10% of patients. Definitive surgical therapy should be performed at the first occurrence in patients with Marfan's syndrome, because after more conservative therapy, there is a high recurrence rate whether or not pleurodesis is performed.

Baumann MH, Sahn SA: Tension pneumothorax: Diagnostic and therapeutic pitfalls. Crit Care Med 1993;21:177.

Hazelrigg SR et al: Thoracoscopic stapled resection for spontaneous pneumothorax. J Thorac Cardiovasc Surg 1993;105:389.

Inderbitzi RG et al: Thoracoscopic pleurectomy for treatment of complicated spontaneous pneumothorax. J Thorac Cardiovasc Surg 1993;105:84.

Tanaka F et al: Secondary spontaneous pneumothorax. Ann Thorac Surg 1993;55:372.

Wait MA, Estrera A: Changing clinical spectrum of spontaneous pneumothorax. Am J Surg 1992;164:528.

PLEURAL CALCIFICATION OR PLAQUES

Pleural calcification occasionally occurs after long-term pleural infections, in organized collections of pleural blood, following empyema, in tuberculosis, and in asbestosis or silicosis. The costal and diaphragmatic pleuras are involved more often than the visceral pleura.

Hyaline plaques may be seen at thoracotomy and may be confused with pleural metastatic implants. The cause of pleural plaques is not known, but the condition may follow tuberculosis or inhalation of asbestos fibers.

DISEASES OF THE MEDIASTINUM

MEDIASTINITIS

Mediastinitis may be acute or chronic. There are four sources of mediastinal infection: direct contamination; hematogenous or lymphatic spread; extension of infection from the neck or retroperitoneum; and extension from the lung or pleura. The most common direct contamination is esophageal perforation. Acute mediastinitis may follow esophageal, cardiac, and other mediastinal operations. Rarely, the mediastinum is directly infected by suppurative conditions involving the ribs or vertebrae. Most direct mediastinal infections are caused by pyogenic organisms. Most mediastinal infections that invade via the hematogenous and lymphatic routes are granulomas. Contiguous involvement of the mediastinum along fascial planes from cervical infection is frequent; this occurs less commonly from the retroperitoneum because of the influence of the diaphragm. Empyema often loculates to form a paramediastinal abscess, but extension to form a true mediastinal abscess is uncommon. Extension of mediastinal infections to involve the pleura is common.

1. ACUTE MEDIASTINITIS

Esophageal perforation, the source of 90% of acute mediastinal infections, can be caused by vomiting (Boerhaave's syndrome), iatrogenic trauma (endoscopy, dilatation, operation), external trauma (penetrating or blunt), cuffed endotracheal tubes, ingestion of corrosives, carcinoma, or other esophageal disease. Mediastinal infection secondary to cervical disease may follow oral surgery; cellulitis; external trauma involving the pharynx, esophagus, or trachea; and cervical operative procedures such as tracheostomy.

Clinical Findings

Emetogenic esophageal perforation is usually associated with a history of vomiting but in some cases is insidious in onset. Severe boring pain located in the substernal, left or right chest, or epigastric regions is the chief complaint in over 90% of cases. One-third of patients have radiation to the back, and in some cases, pain in the back may predominate. Low thoracic mediastinitis can sometimes be confused with acute abdominal diseases or pericarditis. Acute mediastinitis is often associated with chills, fever, or shock. If pleurisy develops, breathing may aggravate the pain or cause radiation to the shoulder. Swallowing increases the pain, and dysphagia may be present. The patient is febrile, and tachycardia is noted. About 60% of patients have subcutaneous emphysema or pneumomediastinum. A pericardial crunching sound with systole (Hamman's sign) is often a late sign. Fifty percent of patients with esophageal perforation have pleural effusion or hydropneumothorax. Neck tenderness and crepitation are more often found in cervical perforations.

The diagnosis may be confirmed by contrast x-ray examination of the esophagus, preferably using water-soluble media, or by endoscopic visualization of the perforation. Myocardial infarction is sometimes mistakenly diagnosed in patients with esophageal perforation when a predisposing cause of pneumomediastinum is not apparent.

Treatment

Treatment includes fluid resuscitation, broad-spectrum antibiotic coverage, and nasogastric suction. An emetogenic esophageal perforation usually results in a vertical tear located just proximal to the esophagogastric junction. These patients require thoracotomy, because gastric or esophageal contents are extravasated into the mediastinum. Instrumental perforation can occur in the cervical (80%), distal thoracic (15%), and, rarely, midthoracic esophagus (less than 5%). Wide drainage and closure of the perforation is required if the esophagus in not too friable. The amount of time lost before diagnosis and the degree of spillage are critical in determining whether such repair is possible. The mediastinum is drained via the pleural cavity using large-bore catheters. Postoperatively, nutritional needs are provided by either intravenous alimentation or feeding via nasogastric, gastrostomy, or jejunostomy tube. Gastrostomy may help to minimize reflux into the esophagus.

Following operative treatment for perforations of the esophagus, complications occur in about 40% of cases. The frequency of leaks may be reduced by buttressing the esophageal suture line. The death rate is about 10% in instrumental, 20% in emetogenic, 35% in postoperative, and 75–80% in corrosive perforation. Prompt drainage and repair are the most important factors in determining outcome. Delay beyond 24 hours results in a 90% death rate. The death rate after cervical perforation is less than after endothoracic perforation.

2. CHRONIC MEDIASTINITIS

Chronic mediastinitis usually involves specific granulomatous processes, with mediastinal fibrosis and cold abscesses of the mediastinum. Histoplasmosis, tuberculosis, actinomycosis, nocardiosis, blastomycosis, and syphilis have been incriminated. Amebic abscesses and parasitic disease such as echinococcal cysts are rare causes. Usually, the infectious process is due to histoplasmosis or tuberculosis and involves the mediastinal lymph nodes. Esophageal obstructions may occur. Adjacent mediastinal structures may become secondarily infected. It is thought that granulomatous mediastinitis and fibrosing mediastinitis are different manifestations of the same disease. Mediastinal fibrosis is a term used synonymously with idiopathic, fibrous, collagenous, or sclerosing mediastinitis. Eighty or more cases of mediastinal fibrosis have been reported, but the cause has been determined in only 16%, and of these over 90% were due to histoplasmosis. In only 25% of 103 cases of granulomatous mediastinitis has the cause been identified. Histoplasmosis was the most common known cause (60%) and tuberculosis the second most common (25%).

About 85% of patients with mediastinal fibrosis have symptoms from entrapment of mediastinal structures as follows: superior vena caval obstruction in 82%; tracheobronchial obstruction, 9%; pulmonary vein obstruction, 6%; pulmonary artery occlusion, 6%; and esophageal obstruction, 3%. Rarely, inferior vena caval obstruction or involvement of the thoracic duct, atrium, recurrent laryngeal nerve, or stellate ganglion is found. Multiple structures may be simultaneously involved.

Seventy-five percent of patients with granulomatous mediastinitis have no symptoms, and disease is discovered by chest x-ray, which shows a mediastinal mass. The mass is in the right paratracheal region in 75% of cases. In the 25% of patients with symptoms, about half have superior vena caval obstruction and a third have esophageal obstruction. Occasional patients have bronchial obstruction, bronchoesophageal fistula, or pulmonary venous obstruction.

A mediastinal tuberculous or fungal abscess occasionally dissects long distances to present on the chest wall paravertebrally or parasternally. Secondary rib or costal cartilage infections with multiple draining sinus tracts occur.

Clinical Findings

A. Symptoms and Signs: Granulomatous and fibrosing mediastinitis involves both sexes equally, and the average age is 35–40 years. Esophageal involvement results in dysphagia or hematemesis. Tracheobronchial involvement may cause severe cough, hemoptysis, dyspnea, wheezing, and episodes of obstructive pneumonitis. Pulmonary vein obstruction, the most common serious manifestation, produces congestive heart failure resembling advanced mitral stenosis and is usually fatal. Although not diagnostic, the respective skin tests in cases due to histoplasmosis or tuberculosis are strongly positive.

B. Imaging Studies: X-ray findings demonstrate a right paratracheal or anterior mediastinal mass. There may be spotty or subcapsular calcification. Calcification also can occur in thymoma or teratoma located in this region.

Treatment

Specific medical therapy is indicated when diagnosis of an infecting organism is noted. In general, however, mediastinal masses should be resected.

Prognosis

The prognosis following surgical excision of granulomatous mediastinal masses is good. Operative procedures do not appear to activate fibrosing mediastinitis, but success in treatment has been unpredictable. Most patients with fibrosing mediastinitis, whether treated or not, survive but have persistent symptoms.

Cherveniakov A, Cherveniakov P: Surgical treatment of acute purulent mediastinitis. Eur J Cardiothorac Surg 1992;6:407.

Doty DB, Doty JR, Jones KW: Bypass of superior vena cava: Fifteen years' experience with spiral vein graft for obstruction of superior vena cava caused by benign disease. J Thorac Cardiovasc Surg 1990;99:889.

Ehrenkranz NJ, Pfaff SJ: Mediastinitis complicating cardiac operations: evidence of postoperative causation. Rev Infect Dis 1991;13:803.

Kistler AM et al: Superior vena cava obstruction in fibrosing mediastinitis: Demonstration of right-to-left shunt and venous collaterals. Nucl Med Commun 1991;12:1067.

Loop FD et al: Sternal wound complications after isolated coronary artery bypass grafting: Early and late mortality, morbidity, and cost of care. Ann Thorac Surg 1990;49:179.

Urschel HC Jr et al: Sclerosing mediastinitis: Improved management with histoplasmosis titer and ketoconazole. Ann Thorac Surg 1990;50:215.

Wheatley MJ et al: Descending necrotizing mediastinitis: Transcervical drainage is not enough. Ann Thorac Surg 1990;49:780.

SUPERIOR VENA CAVAL SYNDROME

Superior vena caval obstruction produces a distinctive clinical syndrome. Malignant tumors are the cause in 80–90% of cases; lung cancer accounts for about 90%. The incidence of superior vena caval syndrome in lung cancer patients is 3–5%. The male/female ratio is about 5:1. Other primary mediastinal tumors that may cause superior vena caval obstruction include thymoma, Hodgkin's disease, and lymphosarcoma. Metastatic tumors from the breast or thyroid or from melanoma also occasionally cause superior vena caval obstruction. Benign tumors are an unusual cause, but substernal goiter, any large benign mediastinal masses, and atrial myxoma have been implicated. Thrombotic conditions, either idiopathic or associated with polycythemia, mediastinal infection, or indwelling catheters, are unusual causes. The association of superior vena caval obstruction with chronic mediastinitis is discussed in the preceding section. Trauma may produce acute venous obstruction (eg, traumatic asphyxia, mediastinal hematoma).

The clinical manifestations depend on the abruptness of onset, location of obstruction, completeness of occlusion, and availability of collateral pathways. Venous pressure measured in the arms or head varies from 200 to 500 mm H_2O, and severity of symptoms is correlated with the pressure. Fatal cerebral edema can occur within minutes of an acute complete obstruction, whereas a slowly evolving one permits development of collaterals and may be only mildly symptomatic. Symptoms are milder when the azygos vein is patent. Azygous blood flow, normally about 11% of the total venous return, can increase to 35% of the venous return from the head, neck, and upper extremities. Thus, the most severe cases occur when occlusion is complete and the azygos vein is involved. The thrombus may propagate proximally to occlude the innominate and axillary veins.

Clinical Findings

Symptoms include puffiness of the face, arms, and shoulders and a blue or purple discoloration of the skin. Central nervous system symptoms include headache, nausea, dizziness, vomiting, distortion of vision, drowsiness, stupor, and convulsions. Respiratory symptoms include cough, hoarseness, and dyspnea, often due to edema of the vocal cords or trachea. These symptoms are made worse when the patient lies flat or bends over. In long-standing cases, esophageal varices may develop and produce gastrointestinal bleeding. The veins of the neck and upper extremities are visibly distended, and in long-standing cases, there are marked collateral venous channels over the anterior chest and abdomen. Onset of symptoms in fibrosing mediastinitis may be insidious, consisting initially of early morning edema of the face and hands. Occasionally, symptoms and findings are localized to one side when the level of obstruction is

above the vena cava and only the innominate vein is blocked. In this situation, symptoms are mild, because communicating veins in the neck usually decompress the affected side.

The diagnosis is confirmed by measuring upper extremity venous pressure; in patients with severe symptoms, a pressure of 350 mm water or more is usual. The location and extent of obstruction are best determined by venography. When patients with malignant vena caval obstruction are studied by venography, 35% have thrombosis involving the innominate or axillary veins, 15% have complete caval obstruction without thrombosis, and 50% have partial superior vena caval obstruction. If patency of the azygos vein is in question, interosseous azygography may be useful. Chest x-ray may show a right upper lobe lung lesion or right paratracheal mass. Aortography is occasionally required to exclude aortic aneurysm, although CT scan with contrast enhancement for such lesions is increasingly diagnostic. The differential diagnosis may include angioneurotic edema, congestive heart failure, and constrictive pericarditis. Effort thrombosis of the axillary vein and innominate vein obstruction from elongation and buckling of the innominate artery can be considered in unilateral cases.

Complications

In patients with partial superior vena caval obstruction, thrombosis may suddenly change mild symptoms to marked venous distention, cyanotic swelling, vocal cord edema, and impaired cerebration. Bleeding from esophageal varices is rare except in severe long-standing cases.

Treatment

Superior vena caval obstruction caused by cancer should be treated with diuretics, fluid restriction, and prompt radiation therapy. Because of the possibility of thrombosis in malignant cases, anticoagulants or fibrinolytic agents have been suggested. Chemotherapy is sometimes used alone or with radiotherapy. Most cases of malignant superior vena caval obstruction are not remediable by operation.

In benign incomplete superior vena caval obstruction, surgical excision of the compressing mass can provide an excellent result. In total obstruction, such as occurs in fibrosing mediastinitis, most patients will gradually improve without treatment. There are numerous surgical procedures designed to bypass caval obstruction, replace the superior vena cava, or recanalize the vena caval lumen. The results following these procedures have been dramatically effective in some cases, but only recently have these procedures been of sufficient success to warrant consideration.

Prognosis

Radiotherapy is most effective when superior vena

caval obstruction is incomplete. Mean survival of patients with malignant caval obstruction from lung cancer is 6–8 months. The death rate from causes related to vena caval obstruction itself is only 1–2%.

Cherveniakov A, Cherveniakov P: Surgical treatment of acute purulent mediastinitis. Eur J Cardiothorac Surg 1992;6:407.

Doty DB, Doty JR, Jones KW: Bypass of superior vena cava: Fifteen years' experience with spiral vein graft for obstruction of superior vena cava caused by benign disease. J Thorac Cardiovasc Surg 1990;99:889.

Ehrenkranz NJ, Pfaff SJ: Mediastinitis complicating cardiac operations: evidence of postoperative causation. Rev Infect Dis 1991;13:803.

Kistler AM et al: Superior vena cava obstruction in fibrosing mediastinitis: Demonstration of right-to-left shunt and venous collaterals. Nucl Med Commun 1991;12:1067.

Loop FD et al: Sternal wound complications after isolated coronary artery bypass grafting: Early and late mortality, morbidity, and cost of care. Ann Thorac Surg 1990;49:179.

Urschel HC Jr et al: Sclerosing mediastinitis: Improved management with histoplasmosis titer and ketoconazole. Ann Thorac Surg 1990;50:215.

Wheatley MJ et al: Descending necrotizing mediastinitis: Transcervical drainage is not enough. Ann Thorac Surg 1990;49:780.

MEDIASTINAL MASS LESIONS

Mediastinal masses may be of congenital, traumatic, infectious, degenerative, or neoplastic origin. Thyroid goiters occasionally can be at least partially substernal; skeletal tumors may grow into the mediastinum; or diaphragmatic lesions may involve the mediastinum.

An extensive workup of a mediastinal lesion is usually not required for diagnosis, since surgery is usually required both to establish the diagnosis and provide effective treatment. Standard posteroanterior and lateral chest films will often provide all the information required. CT scan has become an important means of evaluating mediastinal lesions.

Oblique or overpenetrating x-rays are sometimes helpful. Fluoroscopy may show pulsation or variation of shape or location with change of position and respiration. Tomography may reveal calcification or air-fluid levels. Barium swallow is used to evaluate intrinsic esophageal lesions or esophageal displacement by extrinsic masses. Contrast studies of the intestinal tract may reveal the stomach, colon, or small bowel in a hernia. Myelography can be of crucial importance in neurogenic tumors to explain symptoms or plan operative management. Bronchography may be useful to differentiate lung tumors mimicking a mediastinal mass.

Venography is used to evaluate distortion, obstruction, or collateral channels. Angiocardiography and aortography help to identify aneurysms or displacement. Pulmonary arteriography may be useful to distinguish mediastinal and pulmonary tumors. Interosseous azygography may be useful in evaluation of vena caval obstruction, although the later angiographic approaches have been largely supplanted by contrast-enhanced CT scan.

Scintiscan is important in evaluating possible substernal goiter in anterior mediastinal lesions, since goiters can almost always be removed by a cervical approach. Skin tests and serologic studies may be used in suspected granuloma. Bone marrow examination, hormone assays, etc, are occasionally indicated.

Bronchoscopy and esophagoscopy are occasionally useful to identify primary lung lesions or lesions of the esophagus. Mediastinoscopy and mediastinal biopsy must be used cautiously in mediastinal tumors that are potentially curable. Excisional biopsy is preferable in lesions (eg, thymoma) that are histologically difficult to evaluate, since a curable cancer might be seeded. Mediastinoscopy is useful in sarcoidosis or disseminated lymphoma.

When substernal goiter is excluded, neurogenic tumors constitute 26%, cysts 21%, teratodermoids 16%, thymomas 12%, lymphomas 12%, and all other lesions 12% of mediastinal masses. About 25% are malignant. In children, the incidence of cancer is about the same, but teratodermoids and vascular tumors are more common.

The distribution of mediastinal tumors is as shown in Table 18–3.

Clinical Findings

Symptoms are much more frequent in malignant than benign lesions. About one-third of patients have no symptoms. Fifty percent of patients have respiratory symptoms such as cough, wheezing, dyspnea, and recurrent pneumonias. Hemoptysis and, rarely, expectoration of cyst contents may occur. Chest pain, weight loss, and dysphagia are found with equal frequency, each in about 10% of patients. Myasthenia, fever, and superior vena caval obstruction are each found in about 5% of patients.

Table 18–3. Distribution of tumors and other mass lesions in the mediastinum.

All parts of mediastinum	Anterior mediastinum
Lymph node lesions	Teratoma
Bronchogenic cysts	Lymphangioma
Middle mediastinum	Angiomas
Teratoma	Pericardial cysts
Thymoma	Esophageal lesions
Parathyroid adenoma	**Posterior mediastinum**
Aneurysms	Neurogenic tumors
Lipoma	Pheochromocytoma
Myxoma	Aneurysms
Goiter	Enterogenous cysts
	Spinal lesions
	Hiatal hernia

The following symptoms suggest cancer and thus have a poorer prognosis: hoarseness, Horner's syndrome, severe pain, and superior vena caval obstruction. Malignant tumors may produce chylothorax. Fever may be intermittent in Hodgkin's disease. Thymoma produces myasthenia, hypogammaglobulinemia, Whipple's disease, red blood cell aplasia, and Cushing's disease. Hypoglycemia is a rare complication of mesotheliomas, teratomas, and fibromas. Hypertension and diarrhea occur with pheochromocytoma and ganglioneuroma. Neurogenic tumors may produce specific neurologic findings from cord pressure or may be associated with hypertrophic osteoarthropathy and peptic ulcer disease.

A. Neurogenic Tumors: Neurogenic tumors almost always occur in the posterior mediastinum, often the superior portion, arising from intercostal or sympathetic nerves. Rarely, the vagus or phrenic nerve is involved. The most common variety of tumor arises from the nerve sheath (schwannoma) and is usually benign. Ten percent of neurogenic tumors are malignant. Malignant tumors occur more frequently in children. Most malignant tumors arise from the nerve cells. Neurogenic tumors may be multiple or dumbbell in type, with widening of the intervertebral foramen. In these cases, CT scan is necessary to determine if a portion of the growth is within the spinal canal. Myelography may also be necessary. Dumbbell tumors have been removed in the past by a two-stage approach, although a single-stage approach has recently been successful.

Pheochromocytomas of the middle mediastinum can be localized using ^{131}I meta-iodobenzylguanidine.

B. Mediastinal Cystic Lesions: Cysts of the mediastinum may arise from the pericardium, bronchi, esophagus, or thymus. Pericardial cysts are also called springwater or mesothelial cysts. Seventy-five percent are located near the cardiophrenic angles; of these 75% are on the right side. Ten percent are actually diverticula of the pericardial sac that communicate with the pericardial space. Bronchogenic cysts arise close to the main stem bronchus or trachea, often just below the carina. Histologically, they contain elements found in bronchi, such as cartilage, and are lined by respiratory epithelium. Enterogenous cysts are known by several names, including esophageal cyst, enteric cyst, or duplication of the alimentary tract. They arise along the surface of the esophagus and may be embedded within its wall. They may be lined by squamous epithelium similar to the esophagus or gastric mucosa. Enterogenous cysts are occasionally associated with congenital abnormalities of the vertebrae. About 10% of cysts in the mediastinum are nonspecific, without a recognizable lining.

C. Teratodermoid Tumors: Teratodermoid tumors are the most common mass lesion of the anterior mediastinum. They are both solid and cystic and may contain hair or teeth. Microscopically, ectodermal, endodermal, and mesodermal elements are present. Occasionally these tumors rupture into the pleural space, lung, pericardium, or vascular structures.

D. Lymphomas: Lymphomas are usually associated with disseminated disease metastatic to the mediastinum. Occasionally, lymphosarcoma, Hodgkin's disease, or reticulum cell sarcoma arises as a primary mediastinal lesion.

Treatment

Operation is usually indicated for an undiagnosed mediastinal mass to determine the histologic diagnosis and provide a chance for surgical cure. In malignant lesions, surgery is combined with radiotherapy or chemotherapy as indicated.

Prognosis

The postoperative death rate is 1–4%. About one-third of patients with malignant mediastinal tumors survive 5 years.

Cherveniakov A, Cherveniakov P: Surgical treatment of acute purulent mediastinitis. Eur J Cardiothorac Surg 1992;6:407.

Doty DB, Doty JR, Jones KW: Bypass of superior vena cava: Fifteen years' experience with spiral vein graft for obstruction of superior vena cava caused by benign disease. J Thorac Cardiovasc Surg 1990;99:889.

Ehrenkranz NJ, Pfaff SJ: Mediastinitis complicating cardiac operations: evidence of postoperative causation. Rev Infect Dis 1991;13:803.

Kistler AM et al: Superior vena cava obstruction in fibrosing mediastinitis: Demonstration of right-to-left shunt and venous collaterals. Nucl Med Commun 1991;12:1067.

Loop FD et al: Sternal wound complications after isolated coronary artery bypass grafting: Early and late mortality, morbidity, and cost of care. Ann Thorac Surg 1990;49:179.

Urschel HC Jr et al: Sclerosing mediastinitis: Improved management with histoplasmosis titer and ketoconazole. Ann Thorac Surg 1990;50:215.

Wheatley MJ et al: Descending necrotizing mediastinitis: Transcervical drainage is not enough. Ann Thorac Surg 1990;49:780.

TUMORS OF THE THYMUS & MYASTHENIA GRAVIS

The thymic gland is the site of many neoplasms, such as thymomas, lymphomas, Hodgkin's granulomas, and other less common neoplasms. Thymoma, the most common type, may be difficult to differentiate from lymphoma even with an adequate biopsy. About 30% of patients with thymoma have myasthenia gravis, and about 15% of patients with myasthenia develop a thymoma.

The relationship of myasthenia gravis to thymoma is interesting and incompletely understood. Myasthenia gravis is a neuromuscular disorder characterized by weakness and fatigability of voluntary muscles owing to decreased numbers of acetylcholine receptors at neuromuscular junctions. Because of the high incidence of thymic abnormalities, improvement after thymectomy, association with other autoimmune disorders, and presence in the serum of 90% of patients of an antibody against acetylcholine receptors, myasthenia gravis is thought to be the result of autoimmune processes. The disease has been produced in several species of laboratory animals by immunization with specific acetylcholine receptors. About 85% of patients with myasthenia gravis have thymic abnormalities, consisting of germinal center formation in 70% and thymoma in 15%.

Thymomas may be classified according to the predominant cell type into lymphocytic (25%), epithelial (45%), and lymphoepithelial (30%) varieties. Spindle cell tumors, which are sometimes associated with red cell aplasia, are considered among the epithelial tumors. Myasthenia gravis may occur in association with tumors of any cell type but is more common with the lymphocytic variety.

The presence of cancer cannot be determined by the histologic appearance of the tumor. The most reliable determinant of cancer is the extent of local spread. The lesions are categorized as follows: stage I, tumor confined within the capsule of the gland; stage II, tumor extending through the capsule into periglandular fat but not invading adjacent organs; and stage III, tumor extending through the capsule of the gland and invading nearby organs. Fifty percent of stage III tumors have metastatic deposits on the pleura. Metastases to lymph nodes are so rare from thymomas that this finding would suggest some other diagnosis.

Clinical Findings

Fifty percent of thymomas are first identified in an asymptomatic patient on a chest x-ray obtained for another purpose. Symptomatic patients may present with chest pain, dysphagia, myasthenia gravis, dyspnea, or superior vena caval syndrome.

In addition to the chest x-ray, CT scans are useful in making the diagnosis in equivocal cases and in assessing the extent of the lesion. A barium esophagogram may be obtained, and bronchoscopy and venous angiography should be performed in selected cases.

The diagnosis of myasthenia gravis can be made from the patient's easy fatigability and associated decremental response in muscular contraction to repeated stimulation of the motor nerve and from improvement in these abnormalities in response to edrophonium (Tensilon), a short-acting anticholinesterase drug.

Definitive diagnosis of thymoma is based on histologic study of a biopsy specimen.

Treatment

The treatment of choice for thymoma is total thymectomy. The operation is usually performed through a median sternotomy, which allows a more thorough dissection than the cervical incision favored by some surgeons. A careful but aggressive resection should be performed for stage III tumors when they can be removed without sacrificing vital structures. Postoperative radiotherapy is indicated for stage II and III lesions.

Anticholinesterase drugs (eg, neostigmine bromide) are given as initial treatment to patients with myasthenia gravis. Corticosteroids may be given in selected cases, but a high incidence of side effects makes them unsuitable for more liberal use. Thymectomy is now recommended for all patients with myasthenia gravis, whether or not a thymoma is present. The course of the disease is usually improved and subsequent development of a thymoma is obviated in those without a neoplasm. Thymectomy may be postponed in the occasional patient with mild disease well controlled on anticholinesterase therapy.

Prognosis

The rates of complication and death with thymectomy are low except for extensive tumors. Respiratory care of patients with myasthenia gravis in the immediate postoperative period now presents little difficulty because of the availability of anticholinesterase drugs.

The stage and histologic type of the tumor are the main determinants of survival after thymectomy, although the presence of myasthenia also has an adverse effect. Ten-year survival rates are about 65% for those with noninvasive tumors and 30% for those with invasive tumors. The prognosis for stage II lesions is not much different from that of stage I lesions. Ten-year survival rates are 75% for spindle cell and lymphocyte-rich tumors, 50% for differentiated epithelial cell tumors, and nil for undifferentiated tumors.

Following thymectomy, about 75% of patients with myasthenia gravis are improved and 30% achieve complete remission. Younger patients benefit more from thymectomy than do those over age 40 years, but a positive effect also occurs in the latter group.

Cherveniakov A, Cherveniakov P: Surgical treatment of acute purulent mediastinitis. Eur J Cardiothorac Surg 199 2;6:407.

Doty DB, Doty JR, Jones KW: Bypass of superior vena cava: Fifteen years' experience with spiral vein graft for obstruction of superior vena cava caused by benign disease. J Thorac Cardiovasc Surg 1990;99:889.

Ehrenkranz NJ, Pfaff SJ: Mediastinitis complicating cardiac operations: evidence of postoperative causation. Rev Infect Dis 1991;13:803.

Kistler AM et al: Superior vena cava obstruction in fibrosing mediastinitis: Demonstration of right-to-left shunt and venous collaterals. Nucl Med Commun 1991;12: 1067.

Loop FD et al: Sternal wound complications after isolated coronary artery bypass grafting: Early and late mortality, morbidity, and cost of care. Ann Thorac Surg 1990; 49:179.

Urschel HC Jr et al: Sclerosing mediastinitis: Improved management with histoplasmosis titer and ketoconazole. Ann Thorac Surg 1990;50:215.

Wheatley MJ et al: Descending necrotizing mediastinitis: Transcervical drainage is not enough. Ann Thorac Surg 1990;49:780.

DISEASES OF THE LUNGS

STRUCTURAL LESIONS OF THE LUNG

Structural lesions of the lung include the following:

(1) Bronchogenic cysts: Congenital epithelium-lined developmental abnormalities.

(2) Pneumatoceles: Nonepithelialized cavities in the parenchyma, often associated with staphylococcal pneumonia.

(3) Emphysematous bullae: Nonepithelialized lung cavities resulting from degenerative changes in emphysema (Figure 18–13).

(4) Cystic bronchiectasis: Cyst-like bronchial dilatation, which may be acquired or congenital.

(5) Lung cavities: Acquired lung spaces following destructive lung disease such as abscess, tuberculosis, fungal infection, cancer.

(6) Parasitic cysts.

(7) Diffuse cystic disease: Seen in mucoviscidosis and Letterer-Siwe disease.

CONGENITAL CYSTIC LESIONS

Congenital cystic disease of the lung is uncommon and usually not associated with cysts of other organs. Cysts that involve the lung arise in three areas: air passages, pulmonary lymphatics, or pleural surfaces. Four distinct types of congenital cysts arising from the air passages are recognized: (1) bronchogenic cysts, (2) sequestration of the lung, (3) congenital cystic adenomatoid malformation, and (4) infantile lobar emphysema. Except for the last, all can present at any age but are more common in children and young adults. These lesions must sometimes be distinguished from pneumatoceles, blebs, bullae, or tumors.

The lungs and the trachea develop from the ventral bud of the primitive foregut. Abnormalities of ventral budding cause various types of bronchogenic cysts and pulmonary sequestration. The ultimate location of the cyst or sequestration depends upon the extent of differentiation of the foregut. Early anomalies of budding lead to peripheral lung cysts or intralobar sequestration; later anomalies may cause cysts to remain extrapleural (bronchogenic) or sequestrations to be separate from the rest of the lung and to possess their own pleural coverings (extralobar sequestration). Abnormalities of development of the terminal bronchioles and alveolar ducts result in cystic adenomatoid formation. Alveoli develop by the 28th week of gestation, and abnormal alveolar development accounts for most cases of infantile lobar emphysema.

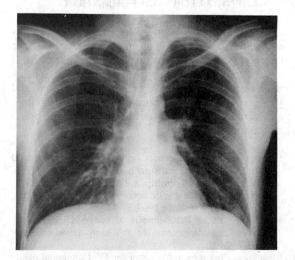 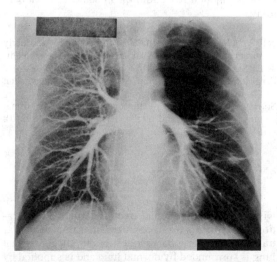

Figure 18–13. Emphysematous bullae of left lung. *Left:* Posteroanterior projection. *Right:* Pulmonary angiogram.

1. BRONCHOGENIC CYSTS

The term bronchogenic cyst includes both bronchial and lung cysts. They may be located in the mediastinum or hilum, but 50–70% are located in the lung. The more proximal cysts (bronchial) seldom have a bronchial communication and therefore are less likely to become secondarily infected. These cysts, usually considered mediastinal, are often in the right paratracheal, carinal, hilar, or paraesophageal locations. More peripheral bronchogenic cysts (congenital lung cysts) are thin-walled, often multiloculated or multiple, and usually have bronchial communications. They tend to become infected and to result in recurrent pneumonia, fever, sepsis, or other types of respiratory distress.

Clinical Findings

Congenital pulmonary cysts are manifested in infancy with respiratory embarrassment, pneumothorax, or compression atelectasis. If air trapping is the main feature, there will be dyspnea, cyanosis, and subcostal retraction. Less severe cases present as recurrent infection, hemoptysis, or an undiagnosed finding on chest roentgenogram.

Congenital lung cysts may occur anywhere in the lungs but involve the lower lobes twice as often as other sites. In adults, the lesion may be asymptomatic when detected by a chest roentgenogram. The mass may appear as a homogeneous density, a cavity with an air-fluid level, or an air cyst. It may be difficult to distinguish lung cysts from benign or malignant tumors, cavitary lesions due to fungi or tuberculosis, or pulmonary abscess. The occasional development of cancer in long-standing lung cysts has been reported.

Treatment

Treatment consists of local removal by enucleation, segmental resection, or, in some cases, lobectomy.

dell'Agnola CA et al: Prenatal ultrasonography and early surgery for congenital cystic disease of the lung. J Pediatr Surg 1992;27:1414

Ferguson TB Jr: Congenital lesions of the lungs. Ann Thorac Surg 1989;47:481.

Soosay GN et al: Symptomatic cysts in otherwise normal lungs of children and adults. Histopathology 1992;20:517.

2. SEQUESTRATION OF THE LUNG

Masses of lung tissue that have no communication with the tracheobronchial tree are termed sequestrations. Two types are recognized: intralobar and extralobar. In intralobar sequestration, the abnormal lung is surrounded by normal lung and is supplied by anomalous systemic arteries; the venous drainage is into the pulmonary veins. Bronchial communication may be acquired through infection (about 15% of cases), but it is difficult to demonstrate radiologically. Repeated infections frequently occur because of poor drainage. Eighty-five percent of sequestrations are of the intralobar type. Extralobar sequestration consists of a separate or accessory mass of lung tissue invested by its own pleura. Anatomic and physiologic separation from adjacent lung tissue is complete, but vascular supply is the same as with intralobar sequestration.

The diagnosis is verified in each type by arteriographic demonstration of a systemic arterial supply to the sequestered segment. Some cases are asymptomatic and are first discovered on chest x-rays, which usually reveal a mass lesion.

After infection is controlled, resection of the sequestration is indicated to prevent recurrent suppuration. Intralobar sequestration usually requires lobectomy; extralobar sequestrations can usually be excised locally. The main technical hazard is the aberrant blood supply.

Bailey PV et al: Congenital bronchopulmonary malformations: Diagnostic and therapeutic considerations. J Thorac Cardiovasc Surg 1990;99:597;

Dolkart LA et al: Antenatal diagnosis of pulmonary sequestration: A review. Obstet Gynecol Surv 1992;47:515.

Ellis K: Fleischner Lecture: Developmental abnormalities in the systemic blood supply to the lungs. AJR Am J Roentgenol 1991;156:669.

Felker RE, Tonkin IL: Imaging of pulmonary sequestration. AJR Am J Roentgenol 1990;154:241.

Gustafson RA et al: Intralobar sequestration: A missed diagnosis. Ann Thorac Surg 1989;47:841.

Kent M: Intralobar pulmonary sequestration. Prog Pediatr Surg 1991;27:84.

3. CONGENITAL CYSTIC ADENOMATOID MALFORMATION

Congenital cystic adenomatoid malformation presents with manifestations of air trapping, progressive distention of the abnormal lung, and multiple cysts. It may be found in stillborns with anasarca, in neonates with respiratory distress, or in older children and young adults as an asymptomatic chest x-ray finding, a recurrent infection, or a condition following pneumothorax.

Harrison MR et al: Antenatal intervention for congenital cystic adenomatoid malformation. Lancet 1990;336:965.

Mentzer SJ, Filler RM, Phillips J: Limited pulmonary resections for congenital cystic adenomatoid malformation of the lung. J Pediatr Surg 1992;27:1410.

Moerman P et al: Pathogenesis of congenital cystic adenomatoid malformation of the lung. Histopathology 1992;21:315.

Rosado-de-Christenson ML, Stocker JT: Congenital cystic adenomatoid malformation. Radiographics 1991;11:865.

4. INFANTILE LOBAR EMPHYSEMA

Infantile lobar emphysema with acute overinflation of the upper lobes or middle lobe is a cause of acute respiratory distress in infants. It is discussed in Chapter 46.

Kennedy CD et al: Lobar emphysema: Long-term imaging follow-up. Radiology 1991;180:189.

Markowitz RI et al: Congenital lobar emphysema. The roles of CT and V/Q scan. Clin Pediatr 1989;28:19.

Stigers KB, Woodring JH, Kanga JF: The clinical and imaging spectrum of findings in patients with congenital lobar emphysema. Pediatr Pulmonol 1992;14:160.

VASCULAR LESIONS OF THE LUNG

Pulmonary arteriovenous fistulas of the lung are either congenital or acquired. Angiography is useful to determine if the blood supply is from the pulmonary artery or from a systemic artery. Fistulas may be associated with syndromes involving multiple telangiectasia, or they may be isolated lesions.

INFECTIONS OF THE LUNGS

Surgical treatment of infections of the lungs involves treatment of complications of such infections. Complications of pleural involvement, parenchymal involvement, and endobronchial involvement are often specific to the organisms involved.

1. LUNG ABSCESS

Essentials of Diagnosis

- Development of pulmonary symptoms about 2 weeks after possible aspiration, bronchial obstruction, or pneumonia.
- Septic fever and sweats.
- Periodic sudden expectoration of large amounts of purulent sputum, foul-smelling or "musty."
- Hemoptysis may occur.
- X-ray density with central radiolucency and fluid level.

General Considerations

Lung abscess may result from a number of causes, the most common of which is aspiration with subsequent pneumonia (50%). Bronchial obstruction due to any cause may result in infection behind the obstruction and abscess formation. Approximately 20% of cases of necrotizing pneumonia will result in abscess. Parenchymal lesions such as cysts or bullae can become secondarily infected, resulting in abscess formation. Extensions of infection from the subdiaphragmatic spaces or liver, postembolic phenom-

ena, or posttraumatic abscesses can also cause lung abscess.

The cause of lung abscess often determines its location. In abscess secondary to aspiration, the patient's position at the time of aspiration is important. When the patient is supine, there is a tendency for aspirated material to enter the posterior segment of the right upper lobe or the superior segment of the right lower lobe. Carcinomatous abscess more frequently involves the anterior segments of the upper lobes. Embolic abscesses are often small and multiple and tend to involve the lower lobes. Basilar abscesses often occur secondary to pneumonia.

Certain predisposing factors to abscess formation have been identified, including a history of alcoholism, debilitation secondary to carcinoma, or chronic disease. Aspiration can follow anesthesia and surgery or may be associated with some predisposing process such as hiatal hernia, carcinoma of the esophagus, achalasia, or tracheoesophageal fistula. Diabetes, preexisting lung disease, dental caries, and epilepsy are all often predisposing factors. Pulmonary infarcts may become infected in patients with septic bacterial endocarditis or in drug addicts through use of an intravenous apparatus. It should be noted that lung abscesses following emboli are often near the pleural surfaces, and bronchopleural fistulas and emphysema may result in these cases.

Clinical Findings

A. Symptoms and Signs: The predisposing cause of lung abscess often contributes prominently to the clinical picture. During the development of an abscess, the clinical findings are indistinguishable from those of severe acute bronchopneumonia. The patient usually has fever, chills, pleuritic chest pain, and prostration. Sputum production may initially be minimal but can become putrid or fetid; this strongly suggests the diagnosis. Hemoptysis occasionally precedes the onset of productive cough. Physical findings may be indistinguishable from those of pneumonia.

B. Laboratory Findings: Leukocytosis is present.

C. Imaging Studies: Chest x-ray initially shows only collapse or consolidation. If a solid or dense infiltrate is present, the diagnosis of carcinoma or tuberculosis may be suggested. Air-fluid levels develop once bronchial communication is established (Figure 18–14).

Differential Diagnosis

An abscess differs from bronchiectasis in that in abscess, the infection is extrabronchial. The most common conditions causing abscess of the lung are tuberculosis, fungal infections, and carcinoma. Since carcinoma underlies 10–20% of lung abscesses, this should always be excluded. Bronchoscopy, sputum cytologic examination, and close follow-up are es-

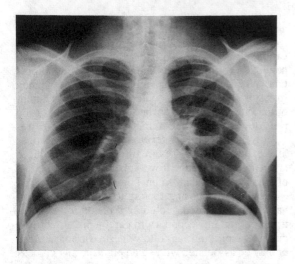

Figure 18–14. Lung abscess involving the superior segment of the left lower lobe.

Rasmussen aneurysms secondary to tuberculosis and lung abscess.

Prognosis

Medical therapy is successful in about 95% of cases. There is a 10–15% death rate in those who need operation because of an inadequate response to antibiotics.

Bartlett JG: Antibiotics in lung abscess. Semin Resp Infect 1991;6:103.

Groskin SA et al: Bacterial lung abscess: A review of the radiographic and clinical features of 50 cases. J Thorac Imaging 1991;6:62.

Lambiase RE et al: Percutaneous drainage of 335 consecutive abscesses: Results of primary drainage with 1-year follow-up. Radiology 1992;184:167.

Pennza PT: Aspiration pneumonia, necrotizing pneumonia, and lung abscess. Emerg Med Clin North Am 1999;7: 279.

vanSonnenberg E et al: Lung abscess: CT-guided drainage. Radiology 1991;178:347.

sential. The x-ray appearance may resemble lung cysts or blebs.

Complications

The complications of lung abscess are local spread, causing loss of additional parenchyma or even loss of an entire lobe; hemorrhage into the abscess, which can be massive; bronchopleural fistula; and emphysema, tension pneumothorax, pyopneumothorax, and pericarditis. Metastatic abscesses may occur, especially to the brain. Failure to heal, the most common complication, requires resection. Late complications are residual bronchiectasis, chronic abscess, chronic bronchopleural fistula, and recurrent pneumonitis.

Treatment

A. General Measures: Treatment of patients with lung abscess involves the general immediate resuscitative measures necessary for a patient in profound sepsis, including rehydration and control of fever. Sputum should be sent immediately for culture for aerobic and anaerobic organisms. Examination of stained smears of sputum or tracheal aspirates can suggest appropriate antibiotic therapy. Bronchoscopy may be repeated at regular intervals to maintain drainage.

B. Surgical Treatment: Occasionally, external closed drainage may be considered in severely ill patients with acute disease who are poor operative risks and have persistent sepsis because of inadequate bronchial drainage.

Fewer than 5% of patients require surgical therapy unless an underlying carcinoma exists. As long as improvement occurs on medical therapy, surgery is unnecessary. Rarely, emergency lobectomy may be required for massive hemoptysis, as in patients with

2. BRONCHIECTASIS

Bronchiectasis represents dilatation of the bronchial tree, often coexistent with chronic bronchitis. This process used to be considered irreversible, but this is now known to be false. Involvement is bilateral in 50% of cases, usually in the lower lobes, and in only 10% of cases is the lingular or middle lobe involved without ipsilateral lower lobe involvement. Although bronchiectasis was commonly treated with operative resection in the preantibiotic era, surgical therapy is now rare, because antimicrobial therapy of pulmonary infections has largely prevented this disease.

Fifty percent of patients have onset of symptoms before 3 years of age. Most cases begin with pneumonia complicating one of the childhood contagious diseases such as pertussis. Rarely, congenital defects such as mucoviscidosis and Kartagener's triad (situs inversus, sinusitis, and bronchiectasis) are involved in the pathogenesis. Bronchiectasis may be associated with preexisting pulmonary disease such as lung abscess or bronchial obstruction by tuberculosis, tumors, or foreign body. The common feature in many of these is long-standing destructive bronchial infection.

The diagnosis of bronchiectasis depends on radiologic demonstration by bronchography of the typical irregular cylindric or saccular bronchial dilatations.

Patients with bronchiectasis have cough, sputum production, and sometimes dyspnea; the symptoms are aggravated by frequent upper respiratory infections. Hemoptysis occurs in 50% of older patients. A few patients have little sputum ("dry bronchiectasis"). There may be associated pulmonary fibrosis or emphysema in advanced cases. Clubbing of the fingers is seen in about a third of cases.

Medical treatment consists of postural drainage, cessation of smoking, antibiotic therapy, and treatment of underlying conditions such as sinusitis. Humidification, bronchodilators, and expectorants may facilitate clearing of secretions. Upper respiratory infections may be treated with broad-spectrum antibiotics such as tetracyclines or ampicillin.

As previously noted, surgical therapy is reserved for patients with localized disease (ie, involving one lobe) who have failed to respond to a strict medical regimen. The presence of diffuse pulmonary emphysema may limit the feasibility of surgery. In well-selected cases, resection for bronchiectasis shows improvement in 95% with lobar disease. The quality of life in patients with chronic resistant disease confined to an isolated segment is markedly improved with surgical resection. Bilateral involvement—particularly if the middle lobe or lingula is involved—has a poor prognosis following surgery.

Dogan R et al: Surgical treatment of bronchiectasis: A collective review of 487 cases. Thorac Cardiovasc Surg 1989;37:183.

Ip M et al: Multivariate analysis of factors affecting pulmonary function in bronchiectasis. Respiration 1993;60:45.

Laros CE et al: Resection of more than ten lung segments: A 30-year survey of 30 bronchiectatic patients. J Thorac Cardiovasc Surg 1988;95:119.

McGuinness G et al: Bronchiectasis: CT evaluation. AJR Am J Roentgenol 199 3;160:253.

Trucksis M, Swartz MN: Bronchiectasis: A current view. Curr Clin Top Infect Dis 1991;11:170.

3. MIDDLE LOBE SYNDROME

The middle lobe syndrome consists of repeated infections in this lobe that usually respond to antibiotics. It is usually a manifestation of partial bronchial obstruction.

Broncholithiasis (see below) and middle lobe syndrome have been considered to be caused by compression or erosion of the bronchus by adjacent diseased lymph nodes. Other factors, such as poor natural drainage and lack of collateral ventilation, probably explain the frequency of middle lobe involvement and in some cases are sufficient to cause symptoms even though the bronchus is entirely patent. Bronchial obstruction may be demonstrable in as few as one-fourth of cases. The presence of complete fissures in the middle lobe limits collateral ventilation and favors the persistence of collapse, retained secretions, and infection.

Endobronchial tumors and foreign bodies must be ruled out by bronchoscopy or bronchography.

Most patients respond to intensive medical therapy, and surgery is rarely required. Indications for surgery, which usually involves middle lobectomy, include bronchiectasis, fibrosis (bronchostenosis), abscess, unresolved or intractable recurrent pneumonia, and suspicion of neoplasm.

Ring-Mrozik E et al: Clinical findings in middle lobe syndrome and other processes of pulmonary shrinkage in children (atelectasis syndrome). Eur J Pediatr Surg 1991;1:266.

4. BRONCHOLITHIASIS

In broncholithiasis, a calcified parabronchial lymph node erodes into the bronchial lumen and either is coughed up or lodges there. Rarely, inspissated and impacted mucoid material may undergo calcification and form a broncholith, or "lung stone." In Europe, 10% of operated patients had documented tuberculosis. Histoplasmosis is more commonly associated in the USA.

The criteria for diagnosis of broncholithiasis are (1) bronchoscopic evidence of peribronchial disease, (2) significant hilar calcifications, and (3) absence of associated pulmonary disease to explain the patient's symptoms.

Sudden unexpected hemoptysis in an otherwise healthy patient is the cardinal manifestation. The bleeding stops without specific measures and is only rarely massive.

Other symptoms are cough, fever and chills, and purulent sputum. There may be localized pleuritic pain or localized wheezing. A history of expectoration of stones is present in approximately one-third of cases. The chest roentgenogram invariably shows hilar calcification. One-third of cases have obstructive pneumonitis. Bronchoscopy demonstrates broncholiths in over 25%, and other endobronchial abnormalities occur in about 20% of cases.

The complications of broncholithiasis are suppurative lung disease, life-threatening hemoptysis, and bronchoesophageal fistula.

Treatment involves removal of the broncholith and medical therapy of associated lesions. Surgical intervention (most commonly lobectomy) may be required in 25% of patients. Bronchoesophageal fistula may require only fistula repair.

Conces DJ Jr, Tarver RD, Vix VA: Broncholithiasis: CT features in 15 patients. AJR Am J Roentgenol 1991; 157:249.

Galdermans D et al: Broncholithiasis: Present clinical spectrum. Respir Med 1990;84:155.

Igoe D, Lynch V, McNicholas WT: Broncholithiasis: Bronchoscopic vs. surgical management. Respir Med 1990; 84:163.

McLean TR, Beall AC Jr, Jones JW: Massive hemoptysis due to broncholithiasis. Ann Thorac Surg 1991;52:1173.

5. MUCOVISCIDOSIS & MUCOID IMPACTION OF THE BRONCHI

Mucoviscidosis is a serious pulmonary disorder of children that may lead to bronchitis, bronchiectasis, pulmonary fibrosis, emphysema, or lung abscess.

Mucoid impaction occurs in adults and is associated with asthma and bronchitis. The mucoid plugs are rubbery, semisolid, gray to greenish-yellow in color, and round, oval, or elongated in shape. There is often a history of recurrent upper respiratory infection, fever, and chest pain. Expectoration of hard mucous plugs or hemoptysis may occur.

Bronchogenic carcinoma, fungal disease, tuberculosis, bronchiectasis, abscess, bacterial pneumonia, lipoid pneumonia, pulmonary eosinophilic granuloma, Löffler's syndrome, and cystic fibrosis must be ruled out.

Treatment includes expectorants, detergents, bronchodilators, antibiotics, and aerosol inhalation therapy. The availability of acetylcysteine has largely converted this condition to a purely medical disease. Surgery is indicated when cancer cannot be ruled out, for destroyed lung, or in the treatment of abscess.

Fiel SB: Clinical management of pulmonary disease in cystic fibrosis. Lancet 1993;341:1070.

Kerem E et al: Prediction of mortality in patients with cystic fibrosis. N Engl J Med 1992;326:1187.

Kerem E et al: Wheezing in infants with cystic fibrosis: Clinical course, pulmonary function, and survival analysis. Pediatrics 1992;90:703.

Shennib H et al: Double-lung transplantation for cystic fibrosis. The Cystic Fibrosis Transplant Study Group. Ann Thorac Surg 1992;54:27.

Starnes VA et al: Cystic fibrosis. Target population for lung transplantation in North America in the 1990s. J Thorac Cardiovasc Surg 1992;103:1008.

6. TUBERCULOSIS

Essentials of Diagnosis

- Minimal symptoms: malaise, lassitude, easy fatigability, anorexia, mild weight loss, afternoon fever, cough, apical rales, and hemoptysis.
- Positive tuberculin skin test; especially, recent change from negative to positive.
- Apical lung infiltrates, often with cavities on chest films.
- *Mycobacterium tuberculosis* in sputum or in gastric or tracheal washings.

General Considerations

Tuberculosis is common in the USA but has markedly declined as a cause of death. However, a reservoir of about 5000–8000 clinical cases exist, and an additional 30,000 new cases occur annually. In the USA, less than 20% of the population is tuberculin-positive, but tuberculosis remains the most common infectious cause of death worldwide.

Several species of the genus *Mycobacterium* may cause lung disease, but 95% of cases of lung disease are due to *M tuberculosis*. *Mycobacterium bovis* and *Mycobacterium avium* are seldom found in humans. Several "atypical" species of *Mycobacterium* that are chiefly soil-dwellers have become clinically more important in recent years, because they are less responsive to preventive and therapeutic measures. Mycobacteria are nonmotile, nonsporulating, weakly gram-positive rods classified in the order Actinomycetales. Dormant organisms remain alive in the host for life.

The initial infection often involves pulmonary parenchyma in the midzone of the lung. When hypersensitivity develops after several weeks, the typical caseation appears. Regional hilar lymph nodes become enlarged. Most cases arrest spontaneously at this stage. If the infection progresses, caseation necrosis develops and giant cells produce a typical tubercle. A cause of latent disease in the elderly or debilitated patient is dormant reactivation tubercles. Sites in the apical and posterior segments of the upper lobes and superior segments of the lower lobes are the usual areas of infection.

Clinical Findings

A. Symptoms and Signs: Patients present with minimal symptoms, including fever, cough, anorexia, weight loss, night sweats, excessive perspiration, chest pain, lethargy, and dyspnea. Extrapulmonary disease may be associated with more severe symptoms, such as involvement of the pericardium, bones, joints, urinary tract, meninges, lymph nodes, or pleural space. Erythema nodosum is seen occasionally in patients with active disease.

B. Laboratory Findings: False-negative tests with intermediate-strength PPD are usually due to anergy, improper testing, or outdated tuberculin. Anergy is sometimes associated with disseminated tuberculosis, measles, sarcoidosis, lymphomas, or recent vaccination with live viruses (eg, poliomyelitis, measles, German measles, mumps, influenza, or yellow fever). Immunosuppressive drugs (eg, corticosteroids or azathioprine) may also cause false-negative responses. Mumps skin tests will be negative in patients taking immunosuppressive drugs.

Culture of sputum, gastric aspirate, and tracheal washings as well as pleural fluid and pleural and lung biopsies may establish the diagnosis.

C. Imaging Studies: X-ray findings include involvement of the apical and posterior segments of the upper lobes (85%) or the superior segments of the lower lobes (10%). Seldom is the anterior segment of the upper lobe solely involved, as in other granulomatous diseases such as histoplasmosis. Involvement of the basal segments of the lower lobes is uncommon except in women, blacks, and diabetics, but endobronchial disease usually involves the lower lobes, producing atelectasis or consolidation. Differing x-ray patterns correspond to the pathologic variations of the disease: the local exudative lesion, the local productive lesion, cavitation, acute tuberculous pneumonia, miliary tuberculosis, Rasmussen's aneurysm, bronchiectasis, bronchostenosis, and tuberculoma.

Differential Diagnosis

Critical in the differential diagnosis is the distinguishing of such lesions from bronchogenic carcinoma, particularly when there is tuberculoma without calcification.

Treatment

A. Medical Treatment: Active disease should be treated with one of the chemotherapeutic regimens that have recently been shown to shorten the period of treatment while maintaining their potency. Such drugs include isoniazid, streptomycin, rifampin, and ethambutol (Table 18–4). These multiple-drug regimens are designed to prevent the emergence of resistant strains and minimize toxicity.

B. Surgical Treatment: The role of surgery in treatment of tuberculosis has diminished dramatically since chemotherapy became available. It is now confined to the following indications: (1) failure of chemotherapy, (2) performance of diagnostic procedures, (3) destroyed lung, (4) postsurgical complications, (5) persistent bronchopleural fistula, and (6) intractable hemorrhage.

Surgical resection for diagnosis may be necessary

Table 18–4. Antituberculosis drugs and their side effects.*

Drug	Dosage (Adult Daily)	Side Effects (Usual)	Monitoring†	Remarks
Isoniazid (INH)	5–10 mg/kg; 300–600 mg.	Peripheral neuritis, hepatitis, hypersensitivity, convulsions.	SGOT (AST)/SGPT (ALT) (not as routine).	To prevent neuritis, give pyridoxine, 25–50 mg/d orally.
Ethambutol (EMB)	15–25 mg/kg/d for 60 days, then 15 mg/kg/d.	Optic neuritis (very rare at 15 mg/kg/d).	Visual acuity, red-green color discrimination.	Ocular history and funduscopic examination before use; contraindicated with optic neuritis.
Rifampin	600 mg once daily (children, 10–20 mg/kg to a maximum of 600 mg).	Hepatotoxicity (rare under age 20, 2.5% of cases over age 50). Occasionally, thrombocytopenia, anemia, nephritis.	SGOT (AST)/SGPT (ALT).	Harmless orange staining of urine, sweat, contact lenses, etc. "Flu syndrome" if rifampin given less than twice weekly.
Streptomycin (SM)	0.5–1.5 g/d IM (children, 20–40 mg/kg/d IM).	Ototoxicity, nephrotoxicity.	Gross hearing (ticking of watch); if abnormal audiograms, BUN and creatinine.	Used mainly in very ill patients as part of triple-drug regimen.
Aminosalicylic acid (PAS)	10–12 g/d.	Gastrointestinal intolerance, skin rashes, hypersensitivity.	SGOT (AST)/SGPT (ALT).	Because of poor tolerance, rarely used now.
Pyrazinamide† (PZA)	20–35 mg/kg/d, up to 3 g/d.	Hyperuricemia, hepatotoxicity, arthralgia.	Uric acid, SGOT (AST)/SGPT (ALT).	Sometimes given as first-line drug in short-course regimen (50 mg/kg twice weekly); inexpensive.
Ethionamide†	0.5–1 g/d.	Gastrointestinal, hepatotoxicity, hypersensitivity (rash).	SGOT (AST)/SGPT (ALT).	Temporarily stop or reduce dose with gastrointestinal irritation and hepatotoxicity.
Cycloserine†	0.5–1 g/d.	Psychosis, personality changes, convulsions, rash.	Drug blood levels if poor renal function.	CNS reactions sometimes controlled by phenytoin.
Capreomycin†	20 mg/kg/d, up to 1 g/d, IM.	Nephrotoxicity, ototoxicity, hepatotoxicity.	Same as streptomycin with SGOT (AST)/SGPT (ALT) in addition.	Sometimes given as 1 g 2 or 3 times weekly.
Viomycin†	1 g twice daily IM 2–3 times weekly.	Nephrotoxicity, ototoxicity.	As for streptomycin, plus urinalysis.	As for streptomycin.
Kanamycin†	0.5–1 glM.	See streptomycin.	As for streptomycin, plus urinalysis.	Used mainly for atypical mycobacterial infections.

* See also Jawetz E: Antimycobacterial drugs. Chap 46, pp 541–548, in: *Basic and Clinical Pharmacology*, 3rd ed. Katzung BG (editor). Lange, 1987.
† Used only as second-line drug in *M tuberculosis* infections, mainy for re-treatment or in drug-resistance cases. Used as first-line drug, in combinations, in atypical mycobacterial infections.

to rule out other diseases, such as cancer, or to obtain material for cultures. Patients with destroyed lobes (Figure 18–15) or cavitary tuberculosis of the right upper lobe (Figure 18–16) containing large infected foci may sometimes be candidates for resection.

The disease becomes reactivated in some patients who have had thoracoplasty, plombage, or resection, and a few will require reoperation. The most common indications for surgery after plombage therapy are pleural infection (pyogenic or tuberculous) and migration of the plombage material, causing pain or compression of other organs. Following pulmonary resection, tuberculous empyema may develop in the postpneumonectomy space, sometimes associated with a bronchopleural fistula or bony sequestration. Persistent bronchopleural fistula after chemotherapy and closed tube drainage may require direct operative closure.

Tuberculous empyema poses unique problems of management. Treatment depends upon whether the empyema is (1) associated with parenchymal disease, (2) mixed tuberculous and pyogenic or purely tuberculous, and (3) associated with bronchopleural fistula. The ultimate objective is complete expansion of the lung and obliteration of the empyema space. Pulmonary decortication or resection may be used for tuberculosis, but open or closed drainage is necessary when the process is complicated by pyogenic infection or bronchopleural fistula.

Prognosis

The prognosis is excellent in most cases treated medically; the death rate decreased from 25% in 1945 to less than 10% currently. The operative death rate in pulmonary resections for tuberculosis is about 10%

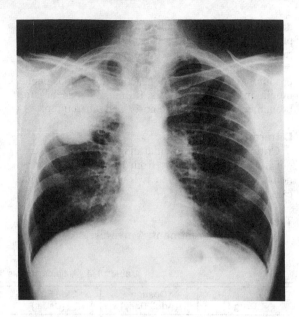

Figure 18–16. Cavitary tuberculosis of the right upper lobe.

for pneumonectomy, 3% for lobectomy, and 1% for segmentectomy and subsegmental resections.

The relapse rate following modern chemotherapy is about 4%.

Bloom BR, Murray CJ: Tuberculosis: Commentary on a re-emergent killer. Science 1992;257:1055.

Coker RJ et al: Clinical aspects of mycobacterial infections in HIV infection. Res Microbiol 1992;143:377.

Horowitz MD et al: Late complications of plombage. Ann Thorac Surg 1992;53:803.

Iceman MD et al: Surgical intervention in the treatment of pulmonary disease caused by drug-resistant *Mycobacterium tuberculosis.* Am Rev Resp Dis 1990;141:623.

Language LA et al: Tuberculosis and the surgeon. Am J Surg 1992;163:505.

Langston HT: Thoracoplasty: The how and the why. Ann Thorac Surg 1991;52:1351.

Misprision DA: The Garrod Lecture. Understanding the chemotherapy of tuberculosis: Current problems. J Antimicrob Chemother 1992;29:477.

Nolan CM: Failure of therapy for tuberculosis in human immunodeficiency virus infection. Amer J Med Sci 1992;304:168.

Pomerantz M et al: Surgical management of resistant mycobacterial tuberculosis and other mycobacterial pulmonary infections. Ann Thorac Surg 1991;52:1108.

Reed CE, Parker EF, Crawford FA Jr: Surgical resection for complications of pulmonary tuberculosis. Ann Thorac Surg 1989;48:165.

Salpeter S: Tuberculosis chemoprophylaxis. West J Med 1992;157:421.

Snider DE Jr: Recognition and elimination of tuberculosis. Adv Intern Med 1993;38:169.

Whyte RI et al: Recent surgical experience for pulmonary tuberculosis. Respir Med 1989;83:357.

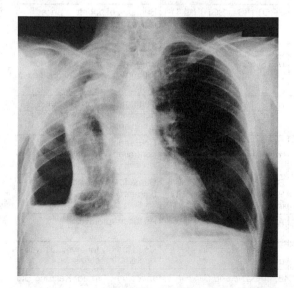

Figure 18–15. Tuberculosis of the right lung with empyema and bronchopleural fistula.

MYCOTIC INFECTIONS OF THE LUNGS

Fungal disease of the lung is related to the widespread use of broad-spectrum antibiotics, corticosteroids, and immunosuppressive drugs. The diseases include histoplasmosis (discussed here), coccidioidomycosis, blastomycosis, cryptococcosis, actinomycosis, nocardiosis, aspergillosis, and candidiasis. Several diseases are restricted to rather specific endemic areas.

Histoplasma capsulatum is a soil contaminant endemic to the Mississippi, Missouri, and Ohio River valleys. With use of data from histoplasmin skin tests, it has been estimated that approximately 30 million persons have been infected. Histoplasmosis has also been reported in South and Central America, India, Malaysia, and Cyprus. It is rare in Europe, Australia, England, and Japan.

The symptoms and roentgenographic findings of histoplasmosis resemble those of tuberculosis, although the disease appears to progress more slowly. There may be cough, malaise, hemoptysis, low-grade fever, and weight loss. As many as 30% of cases coexist with tuberculosis. Pulmonary fibrosis, bulla formation, and pulmonary insufficiency occur in advanced cases of histoplasmosis. Mediastinal involvement is quite frequent and may take the form of granuloma formation, fibrosis with superior vena caval syndrome, or dysphagia. Erosion of inflammatory lymph nodes into bronchi may cause expectoration of broncholiths, hemoptysis, wheezing, or bronchiectasis. Traction diverticula of the esophagus may lead to development of tracheoesophageal fistula. Pericardial involvement may lead to constrictive pericarditis.

In lesions that present as solitary pulmonary nodules, histoplasmosis is diagnosed in about 15–20% of cases. Radiologically, early infections appear as diffuse mottled parenchymal infiltrations surrounding the hila, with enlargement of hilar lymph nodes. Cavitation indicates advanced infection and is the complication for which the surgeon is most often consulted. The diagnosis rests upon finding a positive skin test or complement fixation test and culturing the fungus from sputum or a bronchial aspirate.

Medical therapy for histoplasmosis involves the use of amphotericin B. Surgical therapy is used to treat the complications of the cavitary phase or mediastinal involvement.

Boyars MC, Zwischenberger JB, Cox CS Jr: Clinical manifestations of pulmonary fungal infections. J Thorac Imaging 1992;7:12.

Davies SF: Histoplasmosis: Update 1989. Semin Resp Infect 1990;5:93.

Johnson P, Sarosi G: Current therapy of major fungal diseases of the lung. Infect Dis Clin North Am 1991;5:635.

Rubin SA, Winer-Muram HT: Thoracic histoplasmosis. J Thorac Imaging 1992;7:39.

PARASITIC DISEASES*

Pneumocystis carinii is an opportunistic protozoan organism afflicting patients with impaired immunity. Pulmonary involvement leads to progressive pneumonia and respiratory insufficiency. Disease has been seen with increasing frequency in recipients of organ transplants who are undergoing immunosuppressive therapy. Diagnosis is made by open lung biopsy. Without treatment with pentamidine isethionate, the course is one of relentless progression.

Golden JA, Sjoerdsma A, Santi DV: *Pneumocystis carinii* pneumonia treated with alpha-difluoromethylornithine: A prospective study among patients with the acquired immunodeficiency syndrome. West J Med 1984;141: 613.

Hughes WT: Natural mode of acquisition for de novo infection with *Pneumocystis carinii.* J Infect Dis 1982;145: 842.

Sterling RP et al: Comparison of biopsy-proven *Pneumocystis carinii* pneumonia in acquired immune deficiency syndrome patients and renal allograft recipients. Ann Thorac Surg 1984;38:494.

SARCOIDOSIS
(Boeck's Sarcoid, Benign Lymphogranulomatosis)

Sarcoidosis is a noncaseating granulomatous disease of unknown cause involving the lungs, liver, spleen, lymph nodes, skin, and bones. The highest incidence is reported in Scandinavia, England, and the USA. The incidence in blacks is 10–17 times that in whites. Half of patients are between ages 20 and 40 years, with women more frequently affected than men.

Clinical Findings

A. Symptoms and Signs: Sarcoidosis may present with symptoms of pulmonary infection, but usually these are insidious and nonspecific. Erythema nodosum may herald the onset, and weight loss, fatigue, weakness, and malaise may appear later. Fever occurs in approximately 15% of cases. Pulmonary symptoms occur in 20–30% and include dry cough and dyspnea. Hemoptysis is rare. One-fifth of patients with sarcoidosis have myocardial involvement, and heart block or failure may occur. Peripheral lymph nodes are enlarged in 75%; scalene lymph nodes are microscopically involved in 80% and mediastinal nodes in 90%; and cutaneous involvement is present in 30%. Hepatic and splenic involvement can be shown by biopsy in 70% of cases. There may be migratory or persistent polyarthritis, and central nervous involvement occurs in a few patients.

---

*Echinococcosis and amebiasis are discussed in Chapter 8.

NEOPLASMS OF THE LUNG

1. LUNG CANCER

Lung Cancer is a common problem in the United States. Each year, more than 150,000 new cases of lung cancer are diagnosed, and more than 100,000 individuals die of the disease. The incidence continues to increase, and lung cancer is now the commonest cause of cancer death in both men and women in the US.

Lung cancer typically manifests itself in the sixth decade. Smoking is the cause of 80% of cases, but asbestos exposure and atmospheric pollutants are also implicated. The patient who is at high risk for lung cancer started smoking at age 25 or before, smoked a pack a day for 20 years, and is over age 50. The highest risk is in a smoker working at or near asbestos.

Lung cancer is a lethal disease. Asymptomatic patients have the best prognosis, since once symptoms occur, 75% of patients are incurable. Those who have had symptoms for less than 3 months have a better prognosis than those with symptoms of longer duration. Once lung cancer is diagnosed, mean survival is 9 months. Of patients diagnosed with lung cancer, only 20% survive 1 year and 8% survive 5 years.

Classification

The classification of carcinoma of the lung, revised by the WHO in 1982, is shown in Table 18–5.

Pathologic Features

A. Squamous Cell Carcinoma: The major pathologic features of squamous cell carcinoma are keratinization, cellular stratification, and intercellular bridges. Squamous cell carcinomas account for about 30% of all cases of lung cancer. Two-thirds are located centrally near the hilum and one-third peripherally. The growth rate and the rate of metastasis tend to be slower than that of other lung tumors.

B. Adenocarcinoma: Adenocarcinomas, which constitute 30% of lung cancers, are characterized as acinar, papillary, and bronchoalveolar. Acinar adenocarcinoma is composed of glands lined by columnar

Table 18–5. WHO classification (1982) of malignant tumors of the lung.

Squamous cell
Adenocarcinoma
Small cell
Large cell
Adenosquamous
Carcinoid
Bronchial gland carcinoma

cells that secrete mucin. Bronchoalveolar carcinoma is characterized by intraluminal papillary fragments that appear in alveoli or small bronchioles. Bronchoalveolar carcinoma is a common "scar" carcinoma and may be spread by aerosol transmission. This incidence is increasing, perhaps as a consequence of the rise in lung cancer among women.

C. Small Cell: Small cell (oat cell) carcinomas have small, round nuclei with nuclear chromatin and cytoplasm. They are so biologically and clinically distinct from all other cell types that the term non-small cell lung cancer often is applied to all other cell types. Small cell carcinomas comprise 25% of all lung cancers. They occur centrally, metastasize early, and are the most resistant to combined-modality treatment.

D. Large Cell: Large cell carcinomas are composed of large polygonal spindle or oval cells arranged in sheets, nests or clusters. Multinucleated giant cells, intracellular hyalin droplets, glycogen, and acidophilic nuclear inclusions may be present. These tumors are seen peripherally and are less common and less malignant than small cell tumors.

E. Adenosquamous: These tumors show both squamous and adenocarcinomatous components. They account for less than 1% of lung cancers. Their behavior is similar to that of adenocarcinomas.

F. Carcinoid: Carcinoid tumors are derived from Kulchitsky type cells, are centrally located, and have a vascular stroma. They are sometimes classified as bronchial adenomas but are truly malignant, though they are slow-growing and slow to metastasize. Pulmonary carcinoids rarely produce the carcinoid syndrome.

G. Bronchial Gland Carcinomas: Bronchial gland carcinomas are of two types: adenoid cystic and mucoepidermoid. Adenoid cystic carcinomas are composed of epithelial cells that form small duct-like structures or larger masses with interspersed cystic spaces. These tumors were earlier referred to as cylindromas. They are more aggressive locally and tend to metastasize more frequently than carcinoids or mucoepidermoid carcinomas. The mucoepidermoid carcinomas are rare in the lung and are characterized by the presence of squamous cells, mucus-secreting cells, and cells of intermediate type. The cells have a much more bland appearance and are less aggressive than those of adenosquamous carcinomas.

At present, it is common to divide all lung cancer into two subgroups: small-cell lung cancer and non-small-cell lung cancer.

Clinical Findings

Clinical findings are related to the location and malignant potential of the tumor. In 5–10% of patients, no symptoms are present when the lung cancer is first diagnosed. The cancer is usually discovered on a chest x-ray or, rarely, a positive sputum cytologic examination. Most patients have symptoms, which may be designated as intrathoracic, extrathoracic, or nonspecific.

A. Intrathoracic Symptoms: Intrathoracic symptoms may be bronchopulmonary, resulting from irritation or obstruction of a bronchus, and include cough, hemoptysis, wheezing, and pneumonia. Intrathoracic symptoms may be extrapulmonary, resulting from extension of the tumor beyond the confines of the lung.Patients may have pain or pleural effusion due to extension to the pleura or chest wall, hoarseness due to involvement of the recurrent laryngeal nerve, neck or facial swelling due to obstruction of the superior vena cava, diaphragmatic paralysis due to involvement of the phrenic nerve, or pericardial effusion due to direct extension. A tumor in the apex of the lung or superior pulmonary sulcus may cause **Pancoast's syndrome** as a result of involvement of the bronchial plexus, the sympathetic ganglia, and the ribs and vertebral bodies. Symptoms are pain, upper arm weakness, and **Horner's syndrome** (ptosis, miosis, enophthalmos, and ipsilateral decreased sweating). Squamous cell carcinoma is the most frequent cause of a Pancoast tumor.

B. Extrathoracic Symptoms: Extrathoracic symptoms may be due to metastatic or nonmetastatic causes. The commonest sites of metastases (in decreasing order of frequency) are the liver, adrenal glands, brain, skeleton, and kidney. Extrathoracic nonmetastatic symptoms are caused by the secretion of endocrine or endocrine-like substances by the tumor. These paraneoplastic syndromes are classified as (1) metabolic (Cushing's syndrome, excessive antidiuretic hormone, hypercalcemia, ectopic gonadotropin); (2) neuromuscular (carcinomatous myopathy, peripheral neuropathy, subacute cerebellar degeneration, Eaton-Lambert myasthenic syndrome, polymyositis, encephalomyelopathy); (3) skeletal (clubbing, hypertrophic pulmonary osteoarthropathy); (4) dermatologic (acanthosis nigricans, scleredema, dermatomyositis); (5) vascular (migratory thrombophlebitis, nonbacterial verrucal endocarditis, arterial thrombosis); and (6) hematologic (anemia, fibrinoloytic purpura, nonspecific leukocytosis, polycythemia). Hypercalcemia due to a parathyroid hormone-like substance is most often associated with squamous cell carcinoma. Other paraneoplastic syndromes are most often associated with adenocarcinoma or small-cell carcinoma.

C. Nonspecific Symptoms: Nonspecific symptoms such as weight loss, anorexia, weakness, lassitude, and malaise may occur without other symptoms. In 10% of patients, these symptoms prompt the visit to a physician.

Diagnosis

Lung cancer is most often suspected when an abnormal chest x-ray is discovered in a patient presenting with symptoms or for a routine physical examination. The radiographic abnormalities are classified as hilar, pulmonary parenchymal, and intrathoracic extrapulmonary. The radiographic findings are often characteristic of the cell type. Approximately one-third of squamous cell cancers present as a peripheral mass, two-thirds of which are greater than 4 cm. Cavitation and obstructive pneumonitis are more common than in other cancers. Adenocarcinomas and large cell tumors present most often in the periphery and have a lesser incidence of hilar abnormality than squamous or small-cell lung cancer. Small-cell tumors appear primarily as hilar masses. Although chest x-ray remains the best method of detecting lung cancer—and although an asymptomatic patient who has a lung cancer discovered on routine chest x-ray has the best prognosis—several trials of routine chest x-ray screening for early detection of lung cancer have failed to demonstrate improved long-term survival.

Once a patient in the high-risk group is shown to have an abnormal chest x-ray, the primary objective should be to establish the diagnosis of lung cancer. Flexible fiberoptic bronchoscopy with biopsy or brushing—or fine needle aspiration with fluoroscopic or computed tomographic guidance—can establish the diagnosis in over 90% of cases. Mediastinoscopy for biopsy of hilar nodes or mediastinotomy for aortopulmonary nodes may be necessary. At present, it is rare to have to resort to exploratory thoracotomy to establish a histologic diagnosis.

Assessment for Surgery

The cure of lung cancer requires surgical resection of the primary tumor. Once the diagnosis is established, the next step is to determine whether the tumor is resectable for cure. Resectability is determined by answering the following questions: (1) Are there distant metastases? (2) Has the tumor spread beyond the confines of resection within the thorax? (3) Does the cell type preclude resection for cure? (4) Is there adequate pulmonary and cardiac reserve to allow safe resection of the involved lung?

In order to answer the first two questions, it is necessary to perform preoperative staging of the tumor. Anatomic staging is performed to provide prognostic information, aid in choice of treatment, and compare results from different treatments. The extent of disease is defined by the TNM criteria of the American Joint Committee for Cancer Staging and End Results Reporting. Tumor (T) is defined by size and location. Nodes (N) may be negative (N_0), ipsilateral hilar (N_1), ipsilateral mediastinal or subcarinal (N_2), or contralateral mediastinal, ipsilateral or contralateral scalene, or supraclavicular (N_3). Metastases may be absent (M_0) or present (M_1). (See Table 18–6.)

Stage grouping of TNM subsets is performed according to the revised International Clinical Staging System reported by Mountain in 1986 (see Table 18–6).

Table 18–6. Stage grouping of TNM subsets.

Primary tumors

T	Primary tumor.
T_0	No evidence of primary tumor.
T_x	Tumor proved by presence of malignant cells in bronchopulmonary secretions but not visualized bronchoscopically.
T_1S	Carcinoma in situ.
T_1	Tumor that is 3 cm or less in greatest diameter, or tumor of any size that invades the visceral pleura or is associated with atelectasis or obstructive pneumonitis and extends to the hilar region. At bronchoscopy, the proximal extent of demonstrable tumor must be within a lobar bronchus or at least 2 cm distal to the carina. Any associated atelectasis or obstructive pneumonitis must involve a main bronchus less than 2 cm distal to the carina; any tumor associated with atelectasis or obstructive pneumonitis of an entire lung or pleural effusion.
T_3	Tumor of any size with direct extension into an adjacent structure, such as a chest wall, diaphragm, or mediastinum, and its contents, or tumor demonstrated bronchoscopically to involve a main bronchus less than 2 cm distal to the carina; any tumor associated with atelectasis or obstructive pneumonitis of an entire lung or pleural effusion.
T_4	Tumor of any size with invasion of the mediastinum or involving the heart, great vessels, trachea, esophagus, vertebral body, or carina, or the presence of malignant pleural effusion.

Regional lymph nodes

N	Regional lymph nodes.
N_0	No demonstrable metastasis to regional lymph nodes.
N_1	Metastasis to lymph nodes in peribronchial or ipsilateral hilar region (or both) (including direct extension).
N_2	Metastasis to lymph nodes in the ipsilateral mediastinal or subcarinal nodes.
N_3	Metastasis to contralateral mediastinal nodes or scalene or supraclavicular nodes.

Distant metastases

M	Distant metastasis.
M_0	No distant metastasis.
M_1	Distant metastasis, such as in scalene, cervical, or contralateral hilar lymph nodes, brain, bones, lung, or liver.

Occult carcinoma (stage 0)

$T_xN_0M_0$	Occult carcinoma with bronchopulmonary secretions containing malignant cells but without other evidence of the primary tumor or evidence of metastasis.

Stage I

$T_1SN_0M_0$	Carcinoma in situ.
$T_1N_0M_0$	Tumor that can be classified T_1 without any metastasis to the regional lymph nodes.
$T_1N_1M_0$	Tumor that can be classified T_1 with metastasis to nodes or distant metastasis.
$T_2N_0M_0$	Tumor that can be classified T_2 without any metastasis to nodes or distant metastasis.
Note:	$T_xN_1M_0$ and $T_0N_1M_0$ are also theoretically possible, but such a clinical diagnosis would be difficult if not impossible to make. If it were made, it would be included in stage I.

Stage II

$T_1N_1M_0$	Tumor classified at T2 with metastasis to the lymph nodes in the ipsilateral hilar region only.

Stage IIIA

T_3N_0	Tumor classified as T_3 with no nodes.
T_3N_1	Tumor classified as T_3 with ipsilateral hilar nodes.
$T_{1-3}N_2$	Tumor classified as T1, T_2, or T_3 with metastasis to ipsilateral mediastinal nodes or subcarinal nodes.

Stage IIIB

Any T, N_3	Any size tumor with metastasis to contralateral, supraclavicular, or scalene nodes.
T_4, Any N	Tumor invading heart, great vessels, esophagus, or vertebral body or carina or presence of malignant pleural effusion.

Questions regarding resectability are examined sequentially below:

A. Distant Metastases: The best screening test for distant metastases is the history and physical examination. Patients with brain metastases will most often present with new neurologic symptoms. Skeletal metastases will be suspected on the basis of bone pain or tenderness. After the history and physical examination, the next best screening test is the serum alkaline phosphatase. If there are no new neurologic symptoms, no bone pain or tenderness, and the alkaline phosphatase is normal, routine CT or radionuclide scans of the brain, bone, and liver are not indicated, since it has been shown repeatedly that routine use of these scans is unrewarding. Some investigators have suggested that CT scans or MRI of the brain be performed in patients with adenocarcinoma, but to date the yield has been too low to validate their routine use. Although distant metastases (M_1) usually preclude resection, survival is improved if patients with a solitary cerebral metastasis have the metastasis and the primary tumor resected.

B. Intrathoracic Spread: Pleural effusion, recurrent laryngeal nerve involvement, phrenic nerve paralysis, and superior vena cava syndrome all denote spread of tumor beyond the confines of resection. Tumors that have invaded the chest wall and Pancoast tumors can be resected for cure. Spread to lymph nodes within the thorax must be investigated. In some institutions, mediastinal nodal involvement is routinely examined by mediastinoscopy. However, in most institutions, mediastinal involvement is first assessed by CT scan. If the nodes are less than 1 cm. in size, they will be positive for tumor in less than 5% of cases. If there are no nodes (N_0) or ipsilateral hilar nodes (N_1), the tumor is resectable for cure. If the nodes are only ipsilateral mediastinal or subcarinal (N_2), the tumor is potentially resectable (stage IIIA). If the nodes are contralateral or scalene or supraclavicular, they should be biopsied to prove there is disease outside the confines of resection. The CT scan for lung cancer staging routinely examines the upper abdomen, which will show involvement of the liver or adrenal glands. Although 10% of patients have an adrenal mass, all should be biopsied, since less than half are cancer.

C. Cell Type: Failure to obtain significant 5-year survival after surgical resection of small-cell lung cancer has led to a general attitude that this tumor is surgically incurable. However, it has been shown in a study of surgery for solitary pulmonary nodules that patients with small-cell lung cancer had a 35% 5-year survival rate. An aggressive approach with combination chemotherapy, radiation therapy, and surgery for stage I and II small-cell lung cancer is currently under investigation.

D. Pulmonary and Cardiac Reserve: The determination of adequate pulmonary reserve to undergo lung resection is often difficult. The decision is usually based on an assessment of the patient's preoperative exercise capacity. Clearly severe emphysema or pulmonary hypertension contraindicates resection. A PO_2 less than 50 mm Hg or a PCO_2 greater than 45 mm Hg indicates high risk. An exercise oxygen consumption (MVO_2) less than 10 mL/kg/min indicates high risk. An FEV_1 of 1 L should be present after the resection. For patients who will require pneumonectomy, a ventilation/perfusion lung scan will assign the percentage function to the lung that is to remain after resection. If this percentage is multiplied by the FEV_1, the results should be 1 L or greater

if the patient is to have adequate pulmonary reserve postoperatively.

Cardiac contraindications include recent myocardial infarction, uncontrollable heart failure, or arrhythmia. If the patient has angina or an abnormal ECG, exercise thallium testing is performed. If the exercise test is positive, cardiac catheterization should be performed. Potentially lethal coronary artery disease (left main or triple vessel disease) should be treated by revascularization first. Lesser degrees of coronary artery disease should be dealt with on an individual basis.

Treatment

A. Surgery: The surgical procedure has as its primary goal removal of the tumor and all involved lymph nodes. This is accomplished by lobectomy, bilobectomy on the right side, or pneumonectomy. In older patients or in patients with marginal pulmonary reserve, a segmental or wedge resection may be carried out. A secondary goal of the surgical procedure is to provide accurate anatomic staging. This requires sampling of N_1 nodes (hilar, interlobar, lobar, segmental), and N_2 nodes (superior mediastinal, aortic, inferior mediastinal). Two-year survival after surgery as the only therapy is as follows: stage I, 60%; stage II, 40%; stage IIIA, 20%; all stage III, 9%.

B. Radiation Therapy: Radiation therapy in lung cancer is employed for palliation of unresectable tumors, as adjuvant therapy in combination with surgery, and rarely for cure in medically inoperable patients. Curative radiation therapy in this latter group has a 5-year survival rate of 16%. Routine preoperative radiation therapy has been shown to provide no survival benefit. Preoperative radiation improves survival in patients with small-cell lung cancer and Pancoast tumors. Postoperative radiation therapy decreases the rate of local recurrence but does not affect distant recurrences or survival.

C. Chemotherapy: Numerous trials of single-drug postoperative chemotherapy have failed to show any benefit. The Lung Cancer Study Group has shown that in completely resected stage II and stage IIIA non-small-cell lung cancer, postoperative chemotherapy with cyclophosphamide, doxorubicin, and cisplatin results in fewer recurrences, delay in time to recurrence, and improved survival.

D. Neoadjuvant Therapy: There is currently interest in employing preoperative chemoradiotherapy in stage III and small-cell lung cancer in order to improve resectability. Tumor response has allowed for potentially curative resections, but the impact of this modality on long-term survival of large numbers of patients remains to be documented.

E. Brachytherapy: Brachytherapy is the operative implantation of radioactive seeds of iodine-125 directly into the tumor mass and the instillation of iridium-192 into mediastinal catheters postoperatively. Using this technique, the 5-year survival rate of medically unresectable patients with stage I and stage II lung cancer is 38%. Brachytherapy may also be used for palliation.

F. Immunotherapy: Passive immunotherapy with BCG vaccine and levamisole has been tried without success. Current interest is in focusing on the use of interferons, monoclonal antibodies against tumor growth factors, and interleukin-2 (IL-2) with or without lymphokine-activated killer (LAK) cells.

Dunn WF, Scanlon PD: Preoperative pulmonary function testing for patients with lung cancer. Mayo Clin Proc 1993;68:371.

Ginsberg RJ: Operation for small cell lung cancer: Where are we? Ann Thorac Surg 1990;49:692.

Hansen HH: Management of small-cell cancer of the lung. Lancet 1992;339:846.

Hara N et al: Influence of surgical resection before and after chemotherapy on survival in small cell lung cancer. J Surg Oncol 1991;47:53.

Icard P et al: Primary lung cancer in young patients: a study of 82 surgically treated patients. Ann Thorac Surg 1992; 54:99.

Ichinose Y et al: Comparison between resected and irradiated small cell lung cancer in patients in stages I through IIIa. Ann Thorac Surg 1992;53:95.

Ihde DC: Chemotherapy of lung cancer. N Engl J Med 1992;327:1434.

Kaiser D, Fritzsche A, Matthiesen W: Indication for surgery in small-cell carcinoma of the lung. Thorac Cardiovasc Surg 1992;40:185.

Karsell PR, McDougall JC: Diagnostic tests for lung cancer. Mayo Clin Proc 1993;68:288.

Macchiarini P et al: Surgery plus adjuvant chemotherapy for T13N0M0 small-cell lung cancer: Rationale for current approach. Am J Clin Oncol 1991;14:218.

Miller JD, Gorenstein LA, Patterson GA: Staging: the key to rational management of lung cancer. Ann Thorac Surg 1992;53:170.

Minna JD: The molecular biology of lung cancer pathogenesis. Chest 1993;103(4 Suppl):449S.

Patel AM, Davila DG, Peters SG: Paraneoplastic syndromes associated with lung cancer. Mayo Clin Proc 1993;68: 278.

Patel AM, Peters SG: Clinical manifestations of lung cancer. Mayo Clin Proc 1993;68:273.

Reilly JJ Jr, Mentzer SJ, Sugarbaker DJ: Preoperative assessment of patients undergoing pulmonary resection. Chest 1993;103(4 Suppl):342S.

Salzer GM et al: Operation for N2 small cell lung carcinoma. Ann Thorac Surg 1990;49:759.

Shepherd FA et al: Surgical treatment for limited small-cell lung cancer. J Thorac Cardiovasc Surg 1991;101:385.

Sugio K et al: Surgically resected lung cancer in young adults. Ann Thorac Surg 1992;53:127.

Ulsperger E, Karrer K, Denck H: Multimodality treatment for small cell bronchial carcinoma: Preliminary results of a prospective, multicenter trial. Eur J Cardiothorac Surg 1991;5:306.

Van Raemdonck DE, Schneider A, Ginsberg RJ: Surgical treatment for higher stage non-small cell lung cancer. Ann Thorac Surg 1992;54:999.

Zatopek NK et al: Resectability of small-cell lung cancer following induction chemotherapy in patients with limited disease (stage II–IIIb). Am J Clin Oncol 1991; 14:427.

2. SOLITARY PULMONARY NODULES ("Coin Lesions")

Solitary pulmonary nodules, or "coin lesions," are peripheral circumscribed pulmonary lesions that are due either to granulomatous diseases or to neoplasms. Diagnosis is by radiology. Nodules may be caused by infectious or neoplastic benign disease or malignant primary or secondary tumors. Many characteristics denote probable benignancy or malignancy, but often the diagnosis is not certain. Since 5-year survival following resection of a solitary nodule that turns out to be bronchogenic carcinoma may be as high as 90%, prompt surgical therapy is warranted when cancer cannot be excluded. In the average patient, the risk of thoracotomy is less than 1%, and if the chance of cancer is 5%, the probability of cure will outweigh the risk of thoracotomy.

The overall incidence of cancer in solitary nodular lesions seen on x-ray is about 5–10%. However, in patients ultimately selected for resection of the nodules, the probability of cancer is considerably higher. The breakdown is as follows: 35% primary carcinomas, 35% nonspecific granulomas, 20% tuberculous granulomas, about 5% mixed tumors (hamartomas), and 5% metastatic carcinomas. A small miscellaneous category includes adenomas, cysts, and other lesions. The overall incidence of solitary nodules is 3–9 times higher in males than females. Cancer is almost twice as frequent in males as in females.

Of special importance is the size of the lesions, since lesions greater than 1 cm in diameter have a significant probability of being malignant, and lesions of 4 cm or more in diameter have a very high likelihood of being malignant (Figures 18–17A and 18–17B), but lesions of 1 cm or less in diameter are probably granulomas.

Clinical Findings

A number of clinical, radiologic, and laboratory findings may influence the decision for operation.

A. Symptoms: Symptoms include cough, weight loss, chest pain, or hemoptysis. Symptoms are usually absent with a solitary pulmonary nodule.

B. History: A history of living in an endemic granuloma area and previous tuberculosis favor granuloma, whereas a history of smoking favors cancer. Ninety percent of patients with solitary metastatic lesions have a history of extrapulmonary cancer.

C. Signs: Physical findings are uncommon, with clubbing rarely seen in benign lesions and occasionally in malignant ones. Hypertrophic osteoarthropathy signifies an 80% or greater probability of cancer.

D. Laboratory Findings: Positive skin tests do

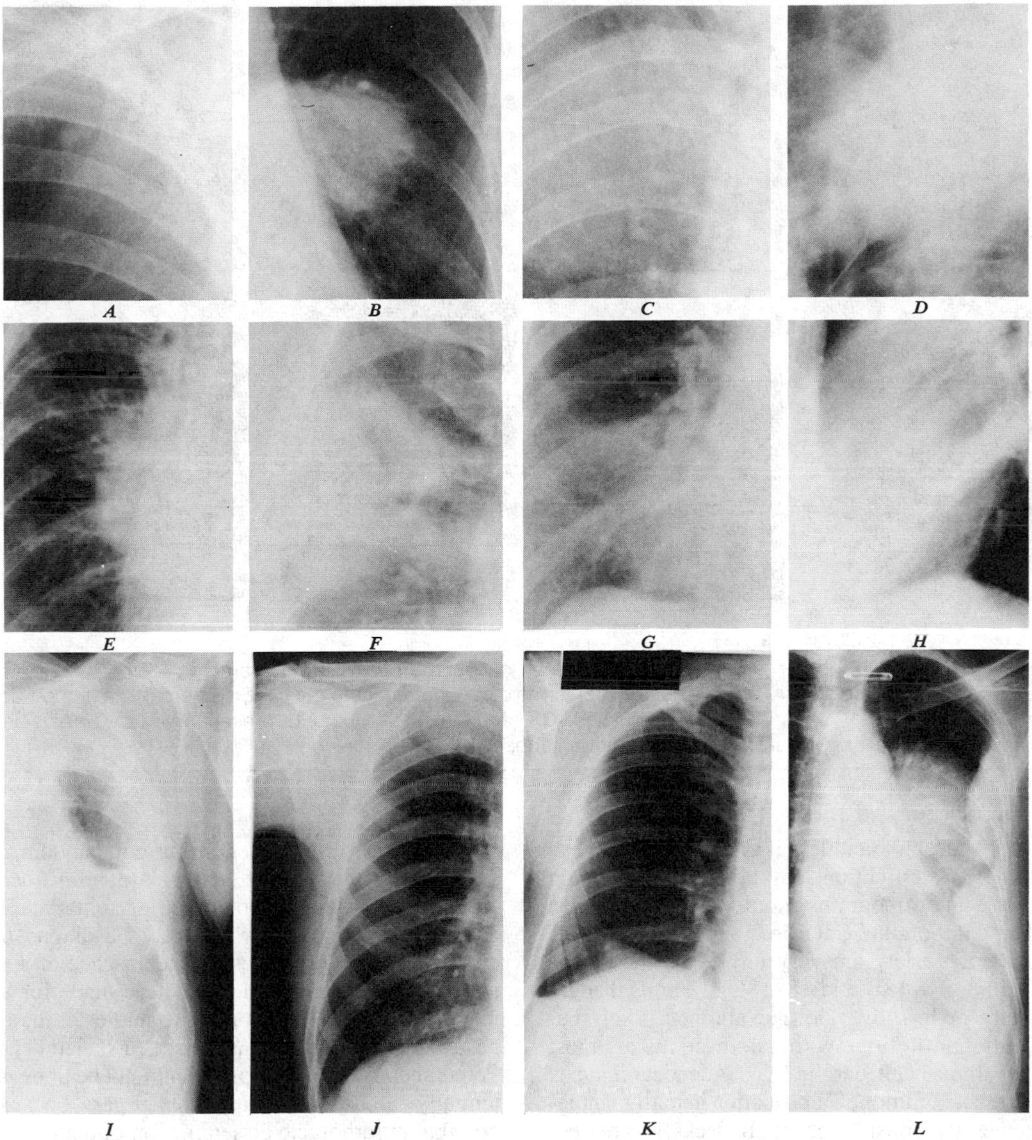

Figure 18–17. X-ray manifestations of lung cancer. ***A:*** Small epidermoid carcinoma in LUL (posteroanterior projection). ***B:*** Large coin lesions; adenocarcinoma in superior segment of LLL (lateral projection). ***C and D:*** Epidermoid carcinoma in RUL. ***E:*** Right hilar mass; oat cell carcinoma. ***F:*** Large cavitary epidermoid carcinoma in RUL. ***G*** (posteroanterior projection) and ***H*** (lateral projection): Middle lobe atelectasis from bronchial carcinoid (not visible). ***I:*** Opacification of left hemithorax; large cavitary epidermoid carcinoma. ***J:*** Pancoast's tumor; poorly differentiated epidermoid carcinoma with erosion of third rib and pathologic fracture of fourth rib. ***K:*** Right phrenic nerve paralysis caused by epidermoid carcinoma. ***L:*** Pleural metastasis caused by adenocarcinoma of LLL. (LUL = left upper lobe; LLL = left lower lobe, etc.)

not rule out cancer, but granulomatous disease is less likely when skin tests are negative. In granuloma of known cause, the skin test is positive in 90% of cases of tuberculosis, in 80% of cases of histoplasmosis, and in 70% of cases of coccidioidomycosis.

Sputum cultures are usually negative. Cytologic examination of sputum yields a diagnosis in only 5–20% of cases.

E. Imaging Studies: Coin lesions are diagnosed radiologically, but their benignity or malignancy can rarely be determined by this method (Figure 18–18). The most persuasive radiologic evidences of benignity are (1) calcification, especially if concentric or laminated; and (2) documented absence of growth for 1 year.

Calcification tends to favor granuloma but does

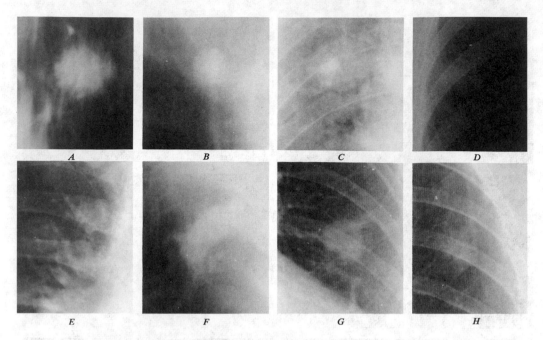

Figure 18–18. Coin lesions. **A:** Large-cell undifferentiated carcinoma in RUL (tomogram). **B:** Histoplasmosis (tomogram). **C:** Hamartoma. **D:** Solitary metastasis from epidermoid carcinoma of the cervix. **E:** Tuberculoma (tomogram). **F:** Foreign body granuloma in heroin addict (tomogram). **G:** Adenocarcinoma of LUL (present 6 years). **H:** Alveolar cell carcinoma of LUL (present 3 years). (RUL = right upper lobe; LUL = left upper lobe.)

not exclude carcinoma unless it appears as concentric laminations. Calcification may be misinterpreted on plain films, and tomograms should be obtained when considered important. Calcifications of the "target" or "popcorn" variety are very unlikely to be malignant (Figures 18–18B and 18–18C). Lesions that are completely or heavily calcified are most likely benign. Malignant lesions with calcifications are most often squamous cell carcinomas. Adenocarcinomas are next most common. Calcification in malignant lesions generally consists of small flecks located eccentrically or at the periphery of the nodule.

Density of lesions may be important, especially in lesions less than 3 cm in diameter; these lesions are often malignant (Figures 18–18D and 18–18E).

An irregular shape is often seen in inflammatory lesions and benign lung tumors (Figure 18–18F). A white rounded lesion with umbilication suggests cancer (Figure 18–18G). Indistinct margins favor cancer (Figure 18–18H), whereas discrete margins favor benignancy (Figure 18–18B), although circumscribed margins are seen in about 30% of malignant lesions.

Documented absence of growth for more than 1 year means that cancer is highly unlikely, but slow growth has been seen in malignant lesions followed for 6 years or more.

The presence of satellite densities favors a diagnosis of granuloma.

F. Other Studies: Probably the most useful study is a previous chest film for comparison. Other studies that may be of benefit are bronchoscopy, which is of value in about 10% of solitary lesions, and mediastinoscopy, which may be diagnostic of cancer in 6–15% of cases. In the absence of a pertinent history, a search should not be made for a primary lesion by roentgenographic studies of the upper gastrointestinal tract, urinary tract, or skeletal system. Percutaneous needle biopsy should not be done in potentially curable candidates for surgery because of possible intrathoracic dissemination of the tumor.

Treatment

Surgical diagnosis may be made by excisional biopsy in peripheral lesions and may constitute definitive therapy for benign lesions, for solitary metastasis, and for primary cancer in poor-risk patients. Centrally placed lesions or those suspected of being coccidioidomycosis should be treated by lobectomy. Primary cancers in good-risk patients are treated by lobectomy with regional node dissection. Pneumonectomy should not be done until a tissue diagnosis of cancer has been established.

Prognosis

The prognosis for malignant coin lesions is three to six times more favorable than that for lung cancer in general. The 5-year survival rate in patients with malignant coin lesions less than 2 cm in diameter is about 70%.

Caskey CI, Templeton PA, Zerhouni EA: Current evaluation of the solitary pulmonary nodule. Radiol Clin North Am 1990;28:511.

Midthun DE, Swensen SJ, Jett JR: Approach to the solitary pulmonary nodule. Mayo Clin Proc 1993;68:378.

Midthun DE, Swensen SJ, Jett JR: Clinical strategies for solitary pulmonary nodule. Annu Rev Med 1992;43:195.

Quoix E et al: Small cell lung cancer presenting as a solitary pulmonary nodule. Cancer 1990;66:577.

Swensen SJ et al: An integrated approach to evaluation of the solitary pulmonary nodule. Mayo Clinic Proceedings 1990;65:173.

Zwirewich CV et al: Solitary pulmonary nodule: High-resolution CT and radiologic-pathologic correlation. Radiology 1991;179:469.

3. SECONDARY MALIGNANT NEOPLASMS OF THE LUNG

Lung metastases occur in about 30% of all patients with cancer. Depending upon the primary lesion, the number of metastases may be limited, and a few of these patients may be surgically curable. The most frequent sources of solitary metastatic lesions are the colon, kidneys, uterus and ovaries, testes, malignant melanoma, pharynx, and bone. In coin lesions, solitary metastasis is the ultimate diagnosis in about 5%. Ten percent of malignant coin lesions are solitary metastases, and in 90% of these cases, a history of the primary is available.

Certain criteria for selection of patients suitable for resection have been developed: (1) The initial primary must be controlled, and no other metastases can be present. (2) When the initial primary is a squamous cell tumor, the lung lesion should be evaluated as a new primary. (3) When the initial lesion is an adenocarcinoma, other common sites of metastasis must be sought. (4) A waiting period of 3–6 months is advisable before thoracotomy if the primary lesion was treated within 2 years. (5) CT scan of the lung must be obtained to rule out additional metastases. (6) Synchronous appearance of a pulmonary metastasis and the primary lesion must be evaluated individually, but in general, the prognosis improves as the interval between control of the primary and the appearance of the lung metastasis increases. (7) Multiple lesions, particularly when bilateral or involving different lobes, usually indicate a poor prognosis. However, multiple resections for metastases from osteogenic sarcoma have been shown to be worthwhile.

About 80% of solitary metastases meeting the above criteria are found to be resectable. Eighty percent are carcinomas and 20% are sarcomas. The 5-year survival rate following removal of the carcinomas is 35%; for the sarcomas, 25%. However, multiple repeated resections may be effective. Only a few 5-year survivals following removal of lung cancers metastatic from malignant melanoma or the breasts have been reported.

Barr LC, Skene AI, Thomas JM: Metastasectomy. Br J Surg 1992;79:1268.

Davis SD: CT evaluation for pulmonary metastases in patients with extrathoracic malignancy. Radiology 1991;180:1.

Lejeune FJ et al: Surgical management of distant melanoma metastases. Semin Surg Oncol 1992;8:381.

McCormack P: Surgical resection of pulmonary metastases. Semin Surg Oncol 1990;6:297.

Mori M et al: Surgical resection of pulmonary metastases from colorectal adenocarcinoma: Special reference to repeated pulmonary resections. Arch Surg 1991;126:1297.

Murray KD: Excision of pulmonary metastasis of colorectal cancer. Semin Surg Oncol 1991;7:157.

Putnam JB Jr, Roth JA: Prognostic indicators in patients with pulmonary metastases. Semin Surg Oncol 1990;6:291.

Todd TR: Pulmonary metastectomy: Current indications for removing lung metastases. Chest 1993;103(4Suppl):401S.

4. BENIGN NEOPLASMS

Benign tumors of the lung are very uncommon and account for only 1–2% of all pulmonary neoplasms. Over half of cases included in this category are bronchial adenomas, which are in fact low-grade malignant tumors because about 15% metastasize. About 5–10% of coin lesions of the lung are benign neoplasms.

Most truly benign lesions of the lung are hamartomas (mixed tumors). Other types are fibrous mesotheliomas, xanthomatous and inflammatory pseudotumors, and miscellaneous rare lesions such as lipomas and benign granular cell myoblastomas.

Benign lung tumors may occur at almost any age. Hamartomas occur in men twice as often as in women. Symptoms are absent in 60% and nonspecific in many other cases. Bronchial obstruction by the lesion, pneumonitis, and hemoptysis are the most common symptoms. Clubbing or hypertrophic osteoarthropathy does not occur in benign tumors except in fibrous mesotheliomas. X-ray may show calcification.

Surgical excision should be conservative and enucleation or wedge excision done when possible. The prognosis is excellent.

Kobzik L: Benign pulmonary lesions that may be misdiagnosed as malignant. Semin Diag Pathol 1990;7:129.

Miller JI Jr: Benign tumors of the lung. Ann Thorac Surg 1992;53:179.

19   The Heart: I. Acquired Diseases

J. Scott Rankin, MD, Hani A. Hennein, MD, & Fraser M. Keith, MD

As the end of the 20th century approaches, acquired diseases of the heart continue to be the leading cause of morbidity and death in the Western world. Over one-third of the current United States population eventually will die from coronary artery disease; 1.5 million people annually experience myocardial infarction; and over 500,000 people die every year from coronary atherosclerosis.

The spectrum of valvular heart disease is changing as the population ages, increasing the incidence of degenerative valvular disorders and decreasing the incidence of rheumatic valvular diseases. Thoracic aortic diseases related to aging are now more common than formerly.

Epidemiologic models predict that as the baby-boom generation ages, the absolute prevalence, incidence, total mortality, and economic cost of cardiac disease will increase by 50% by the year 2010. Thus, the surgical significance of acquired cardiac disease and the number of patients presenting for operative management will no doubt increase in the coming decades.

ISCHEMIC HEART DISEASE
(Angina Pectoris)

ANGINA PECTORIS

The right and left coronary arteries arise from the sinuses of Valsalva as the first branches of the aorta. The right coronary artery passes deep in the right atrioventricular groove (Figure 19–1) and usually terminates as the posterior descending coronary artery in the posterior interventricular groove. The right coronary artery supplies multiple right ventricular branches and the right marginal artery. In 90% of patients, the right coronary artery gives rise to the posterior descending artery (right coronary dominance) and branches into an atrioventricular nodal artery and several terminal posterolateral left ventricular branches.

The left main coronary artery is usually about 1 cm long and gives rise to the left anterior descending and left circumflex coronary arteries (Figure 19–1). The left anterior descending artery provides several diagonal branches to the anterior wall of the left ventricle and a number of perforating branches to the interventricular septum. In most patients, the left anterior descending artery wraps the apex of the heart, anastomosing with the posterior descending artery. The left anterior descending artery usually is the largest and most important of the coronary arteries. The circumflex coronary artery lies in the left atrioventricular groove (Figure 19–1) and proceeds laterally and posteriorly around the lateral aspect of the left ventricle, usually terminating in several circumflex marginal arteries. In 10% of patients, the circumflex coronary artery provides the posterior descending coronary artery (left coronary dominance).

Coronary blood flow delivers oxygen and metabolic substrates to the myocardium and simultaneously removes carbon dioxide and metabolic byproducts via transcapillary exchange. Normal coronary blood flow approximates 1 mL per gram of myocardium per minute and delivers 0.1 mL of oxygen per gram per minute to the heart—a high rate of energy utilization compared with the rest of the body. The extraction of oxygen in the coronary bed averages 75% under normal conditions and increases to nearly 100% during stress. Coronary artery blood flow occurs primarily during diastole because systolic myocardial contraction increases intramyocardial vascular resistance. Normally, mean coronary resistance is three to six times the totally vasodilated value, implying an extreme vasodilator reserve. During stress, oxygen delivery increases as a result of vasodilation in response to the high baseline oxygen extraction. Assuming adequate perfusion pressure, total and regional myocardial blood flow under normal conditions is determined by autoregulation of regional arteriolar resistance modulated by local metabolic demand.

The metabolic activity of heart muscle converts the chemical energy from myocardial oxygen and substrate utilization into mechanical energy in the form of blood pressure and flow. With electrical depolarization of the myocardial cell membrane, chemomechanical alteration of the myosin cross-bridge produces sliding of myosin filaments relative to actin

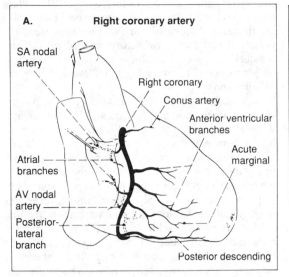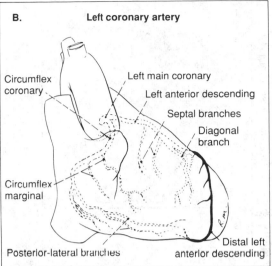

Figure 19–1. Anatomic representation of the right *(A)* and left *(B)* coronary arteries.

and shortening of the sarcomere. Over the physiologic range of sarcomere lengths (1.6–2.0 μm), the surface area of available cross-bridge interactions (and therefore the metabolic energy transferred into mechanical work during sarcomere contraction) is directly proportionate to end-diastolic sarcomere length. The ventricles seem to function as an integrated sum of their component sarcomeres. Mechanical energy production, in the form of pressure and flow (stroke work), is a direct linear function of end-diastolic volume (Figure 19–2) and is not influenced significantly by physiologic changes in afterload. Therefore, short-term alterations in ventricular performance can be assessed by the slope of the stroke work and end-diastolic volume relationship. This basic **Frank-Starling property** of the heart is probably a direct reflection of sarcomere and myosin cross-bridge dynamics. The clinical analogue of this principle allows cardiac function to be assessed as the product of cardiac output and mean arterial pressure (circulatory energy) at a given pulmonary capillary wedge pressure.

Pathology

Coronary atherosclerosis is a progressive disease whose earliest microscopic changes have been described in the newborn infant, and advanced lesions are present in half the hearts examined at autopsy during the second decade of life. Early lesions are characterized by intimal incorporation of lipid material, progressing to an expanding plaque surrounded by fibrosis and calcification. In the final stages, rupture of the intimal plaque appears to be a dominant mechanism of worsening symptoms, with deposition of platelets and thrombus progressing to thrombotic

occlusion and acute myocardial infarction. Subtotal occlusions by "dynamic" thrombotic plaques appear to be of major importance in the pathogenesis of unstable angina. The usual pattern of coronary atherosclerosis is one of multifocal lesions, characteristically involving more than one major trunk in the same heart. The stenoses tend to be short, and lesions in the left anterior descending artery and circumflex system are usually proximal. In the right coronary artery, the disease is more diffuse and involves chiefly the proximal and middle portions of the artery; however, the posterior descending artery and distal branches usually are spared.

When an atherosclerotic plaque decreases the coronary cross-sectional area by 75% (50% reduction in diameter), the resistance to flow becomes significant. The dominant point of coronary vascular resistance becomes the stenosis that limits myocardial perfusion to a fixed value. While flow may be adequate at rest, exercise or other factors that increase myocardial oxygen demand can produce relative ischemia, a fall in coronary pressure distal to the stenosis, and redistribution of blood flow away from the subendocardium. This appears to be the mechanism of exercise-induced angina pectoris. Coronary vasospasm or unstable thrombotic plaques can compound the obstructive physiology. Because of high metabolic demand and tight coupling between energy utilization and expenditure, acute coronary insufficiency, such as occurs with angina pectoris, produces an almost immediate decrement in myocardial segment shortening and work (Figure 19–3). Even when full reperfusion is accomplished after a 15-minute period of reversible ischemia, dysfunction can be prolonged, requiring 24–48 hours for complete recovery.

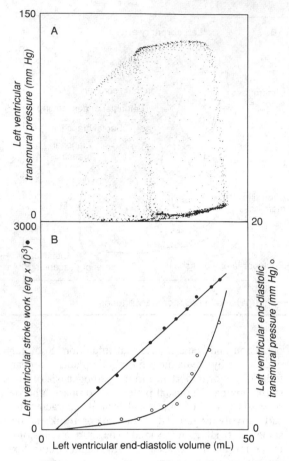

Figure 19–2. A: Left ventricular pressure-volume relationships in a normal conscious dog during a vena caval occlusion. The area of each pressure-volume loop is stroke work. **B:** Stroke work versus end-diastolic volume relationships for the pressure-volume loops shown above. The slope is a representation of the inotropic state.

Clinical Findings

A. Symptoms and Signs: The most common symptom of myocardial ischemia is retrosternal chest pain, or angina pectoris, produced by a reduction in coronary blood flow. The discomfort is often described by the patient as pressure, a choking sensation, or a feeling of tightness. Early in the symptomatic course, a variety of factors such as exercise, cold exposure, eating, and emotional stress can initiate the symptoms. The pain frequently radiates down the left arm and into the left neck and occasionally to the right arm, mandible, or ear. The severity of chest pain can be graded by the New York Heart Association (NYHA) classification, with class I indicating no symptoms; class II, symptoms with severe exertion; class III, chest pain with mild exertion; and class IV, pain at rest. While minimal anginal symptoms often are easily tolerated and compatible with a normal

life-style (stable angina), an increasing NYHA class over a short period of time (progressive angina) worsens the clinical prognosis. In the late stages, ischemia occurs at rest and is refractory to medical therapy (unstable angina). Unstable pain patterns imply a very poor outlook, with a high incidence of early infarction and death.

A large proportion of patients do not follow the classic symptomatic progression and present initially with acute myocardial infarction or sudden death. Still others experience *no symptoms at all* during ischemia (silent myocardial ischemia), and coronary artery disease is only discovered in the late stage of congestive heart failure after severe ventricular damage has occurred. The physical examination is frequently unremarkable. Cardiac enlargement may be evident in patients with advanced disease, but the chest radiograph is normal in the majority. While the ECG is normal in at least half of patients, abnormal findings consist of inverted T waves, ST segment abnormalities, or Q waves on the resting ECG. Transient ST segment and T wave changes may occur during an anginal episode or exercise stress test.

B. Imaging Studies: Cardiac catheterization and coronary arteriography are essential for determining the presence and extent of coronary atherosclerosis. In recent years, a trend has favored early angiography in most patients with suspected coronary disease in order to identify individual prognostic characteristics as precisely as possible. This approach has allowed a more objective application of medical therapy to low-risk subsets and selection of patients at high medical risk for elective coronary revascularization. The development of low-cost outpatient catheterization has facilitated this trend. At angiography, the major anatomic predictors of coronary death, such as the number of coronary vessels diseased and the resting left ventricular ejection fraction, are documented. While the extent of obstructive disease can be underestimated in up to 10% of patients, coronary arteriography has the highest sensitivity and specificity of any test available. Liberal utilization of coronary angiography, almost as a first-line study, is clearly more precise—and even perhaps more cost-effective—than other approaches. In patients with borderline anatomic indications for coronary revascularization, physiologic assessment with radionuclide exercise ventriculography or stress thallium scanning can be useful in making decisions about operative treatment.

Treatment

A. Medical Treatment: Hypertension should be controlled and smoking avoided. Lipid abnormalities should be treated with drugs or diet. After bypass grafting, risk factor modification and continued medical therapy are especially important, since atherosclerotic involvement of saphenous vein grafts is a major long-term risk. When making a choice between

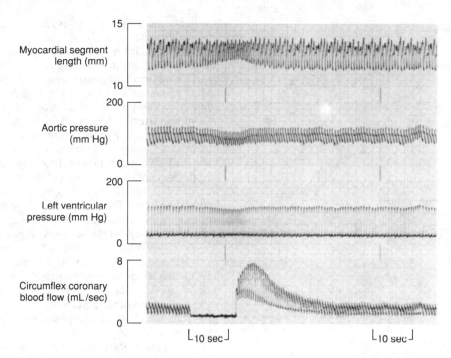

Figure 19–3. Myocardial dimension, pressure, and blood flow data obtained during a 12-second coronary occlusion in the conscious dog. Myocardial shortening begins to diminish rapidly after coronary occlusion, and vasodilation associated with postischemic reactive hyperemia increases coronary blood flow severalfold.

medical and surgical therapy, the natural history of angina pectoris should be reviewed. The annual coronary disease mortality rate is directly related to the number of vessels affected and the degree of impairment of left ventricular function (Figures 19–4 and 19–5). In current practice, adverse prognostic factors that might suggest referral for coronary revascularization include severe or progressive angina on medical therapy; refractory unstable angina; significant left main coronary disease; multivessel coronary obstruction (especially with proximal left anterior descending artery involvement); ventricular impairment with a reduced ejection fraction; and evidence of exercise-induced ischemia. Each of these factors, individually or in combination, significantly reduces survival with medical therapy and predicts an improved longevity after coronary bypass grafting.

In patients with low-risk clinical profiles, medical management is recommended if anginal symptoms and exercise capacity can be maintained satisfactorily. Sublingual nitroglycerin, long-acting nitrate preparations, and nitroglycerin ointment can be useful. Beta-adrenergic blocking agents such as propranolol, atenolol, and timolol are effective and safe. Calcium channel blocking agents such as nifedipine, diltiazem, and verapamil are also effective. Antiplatelet agents such as aspirin have a definite therapeutic role, and short-term heparinization has been effective in preventing coronary thrombosis and in-

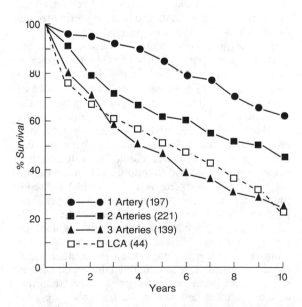

Figure 19–4. Survival in patients with significant lesions of one, two, and three coronary arteries and the left main coronary artery (LCA).

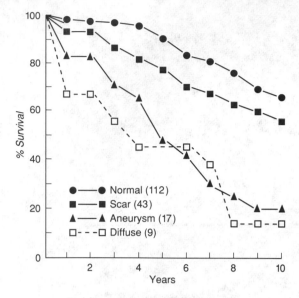

Figure 19–5. Survival according to ventriculographic estimates of resting left ventricular function in patients with ischemic heart disease.

farction in patients with unstable angina. Evidence exists, however, that the symptomatic efficacy of these drugs may not be directly associated with major improvement in ultimate outcome. Moreover, recent data indicate that long-term coronary morbidity and mortality are significantly reduced after contemporary coronary bypass in all forms of coronary disease, even single-vessel obstruction. This finding implies that coronary revascularization should be considered in the majority of patients and that long-term medical management should be discouraged.

B. Surgical Treatment: It is essential that the goals and anticipated results of coronary bypass be explained objectively and in detail to patient and family. Risks and possible complications should be discussed, and all aspects of the history, physical examination, and results of cardiac catheterization should be reviewed, with emphasis on imparting knowledge about cardiac anatomy and dynamics. The presence of carotid bruits should be evaluated, and respiratory status, renal function, and blood coagulation should be assessed. Aspirin should be discontinued, if possible, for 1–2 weeks prior to operation, because of an increased risk of postoperative bleeding. Antianginal agents should be continued until the day of operation. If further pharmacologic therapy is required for recurring angina, an intravenous nitroglycerin infusion can be employed. Intraortic balloon pumping is also effective for preoperative stabilization of unstable patients in the coronary care unit. Prophylactic broad-spectrum antibiotics are administered intravenously before anesthetic induction and for 24–48 hours postoperatively. Finally, excellent

cardiac anesthesia is essential for obtaining optimal surgical results.

The vast majority of procedures consist of simple bypass of the obstructed coronary vessels, using either the internal mammary artery or reversed segments of saphenous vein. In most cases, after a median sternotomy incision is made, the left internal mammary artery is dissected from the chest wall. Cardiopulmonary bypass is instituted, using aortic cannulation for arterial inflow and a single right atrial cannula for venous return to the pump. After clamping the ascending aorta, cold potassium cardioplegia solution is infused into the aortic root to arrest and protect the heart. The saphenous vein grafts or internal mammary arteries are then sutured to the coronary arteries beyond the stenoses (Figures 19–6 and 19–7), and additional volumes of cardioplegia solution are infused every 20–30 minutes to maintain myocardial temperature below 15 °C . After completion of the distal coronary anastomoses, the aorta is unclamped, proximal aorta-vein graft anastomoses are completed, and cardiopulmonary bypass is discontinued after adequate rewarming.

An average of three or four grafts are inserted, reflecting a philosophy of complete coronary revascularization together with the tendency to reserve surgical therapy for symptomatic patients with multivessel disease. In general, the internal mammary artery is the graft of choice owing to its superior long-term patency. At least one internal mammary artery graft is utilized in 95% of procedures, usually to the left anterior descending coronary artery, and adjunctive sa-

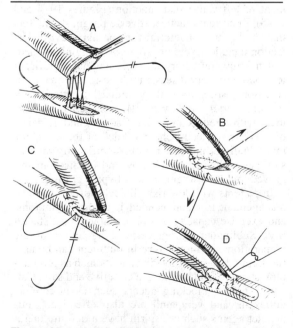

Figure 19–6. A standard method for distal vein graft anastomosis using a running suture technique.

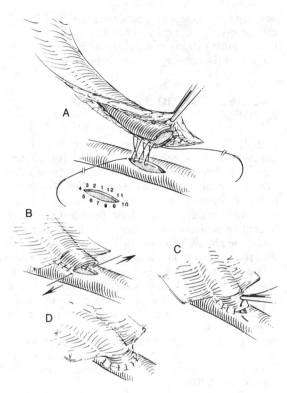

Figure 19–7. Technique of end-to-side internal mammary artery–coronary anastomosis.

phenous vein grafts are used for additional vessels. Multiple internal mammary artery procedures can be performed, using a combination of bilateral mammary artery pedicles, sequential mammary artery anastomoses, and free mammary artery grafts. At present, however, complex internal mammary artery grafting is reserved for patients with limited saphenous veins, younger patients with longer life expectancies, reoperative cases with previous vein graft failure, and patients with atherosclerotic calcification of the ascending aorta. Newer arterial conduits such as the inferior epigastric artery and the gastroepiploic artery are currently being investigated and hold promise for routine "all arterial" grafting.

Prognosis

Numerous risk factors are associated with increased early and late mortality rates after coronary revascularization. In a recent series of 1063 patients, 90% had left main or multivessel disease (Table 19–1), half required emergency surgery for refractory unstable angina or acute myocardial infarction, one-third were older than 65 years, and one-fourth had severe left ventricular dysfunction. Ninety-three percent of patients received at least one internal mammary artery graft, with an average of 3.6 grafts per patient. The overall operative mortality rate averaged 2%, with a 92% 4-year survival rate (Table 19–1). Better-risk patients with either elective operation, age under 65 years, or an ejection fraction greater than 0.4 experienced an operative mortality rate of approximately 1% with a 4-year survival rate exceeding 95%. Only 0.9% required reoperation after an average of 4 years of follow-up. Risk factors for long-term mortality included severe left ventricular dysfunction, advanced age, and emergency operation for acute myocardial infarction or unstable angina. Con-

Table 19–1. Results of operation for ischemic heart disease.

| Preoperative Data | | Survival Data | | | Multivariate Analysis of Risk Factors for Survival | | |
| | | | Survival | | | | |
Variable	Baseline Characteristics	Category	30-Day	4-Year	Variable	X^2	P
Left main, multi-vessel disease	90%	All patients Elective	0.98 0.99	0.92 0.96	Ejection fraction	14.6	<.001
Elective	53%	Unstable	0.96	0.89	Acute MI	7.1	<.008
Unstable angina	42%	Age ≥ 65 years	0.95	0.87	Acute MI	7.1	<.008
Acute MI	5%	Age < 65 years	0.99	0.95	Acute MI	7.1	<.008
Mean age (years)	60 ± 10	Ejection fraction ≥ 0.40			Age ≥ 65	6.7	<.009
Age >65 years	34%	Ejection fraction < 0.40	0.96	0.85	Unstable angina	4.8	<.03
Mean ejection fraction	50 ± 10	Ejection fraction < 0.40	0.96	0.85	Unstable angina	4.8	<.03
Ejection fraction <0.40	26%	Nondiabetics Diabetics	0.98 0.95	0.93 0.88			

sidering the serious baseline patient risk profiles, current long-term results of coronary bypass are remarkably good and serve as the standard with which other emerging therapies, such as coronary balloon angioplasty, must be compared. Performing one internal mammary artery graft independently reduces the probability of late cardiac death and reoperation, but consistent data demonstrating an additional survival advantage from multiple internal mammary artery grafting are not available at present.

Coronary bypass grafting significantly improves anginal symptoms in over 90% of patients long-term, and the incidence of myocardial infarction is likewise reduced. Successful revascularization improves resting left ventricular wall motion in a significant proportion of patients and enhances exercise ventricular performance. Most importantly, contemporary methods of coronary bypass grafting significantly improve survival in the population of patients with ischemic heart disease. Previous findings to the contrary, as in the CASS trial, were related to the selection of low-risk subsets for study and inadequate sample size. Moreover, surgical results have improved in the 15 years since the CASS study, further augmenting surgical survival benefit. By the mid 1980s, significant improvements in survival were evident in all patients with multivessel and left main disease (Figure 19–8); and more recently, infarction-free survival has been shown to be better for single-vessel disease. Worsening left ventricular function, severe symptoms, and

advanced age appear to enhance the benefits of surgical therapy. Thus, more recent data suggest that elective surgical therapy is appropriate for a larger percentage of the coronary disease population.

THE RELATIVE ROLES OF PTCA & CORONARY BYPASS

In 1977, Gruntzig introduced percutaneous transluminal coronary angioplasty (PTCA) for dilating stenotic coronary arterial lesions. Successful dilation rates per stenosis currently exceed 90%; complication rates have fallen to 4%; and procedure-related myocardial infarction and death remain uncommon. Recent enthusiasm for balloon dilation has been accompanied by its increasing application to more complex forms of coronary disease and a marked increase in the number of procedures performed annually. In many centers, PTCA now is the most commonly used invasive therapy for coronary disease. While the initial results of PTCA were considered acceptable, the major concern at present is long-term stability of revascularization. Significant restenosis occurs within the first year in up to 40% of lesions, and both symptomatic recurrence and reintervention rates have been high during follow-up.

Several retrospective analyses have examined the long-term results of PTCA versus surgical bypass. One representative study compared long-term results

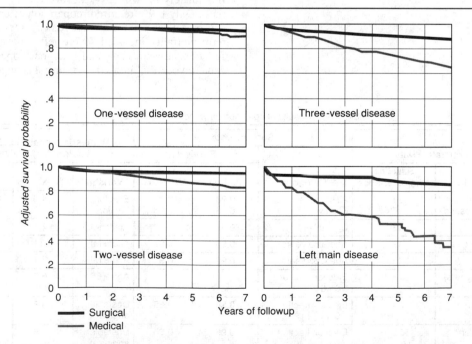

Figure 19–8. Survival of patients treated medically or surgically in 1984 with one-vessel disease, two-vessel disease, three-vessel disease, and left main coronary artery disease. The survival curves are adjusted for all known important baseline characteristics.

in 776 patients having successful PTCA with those observed in 146 patients requiring bypass for failed PTCA. Anginal recurrence and event-free survival rates were significantly better in the bypass group despite similar entry criteria (Figure 19–9). At present, a concept is emerging that the long-term results of primary PTCA are inferior to those achieved with contemporary coronary bypass. One might agree with Gruntzig that until further long-term data are available, the currently accelerating enthusiasm for PTCA in complex forms of coronary disease should be held in check and that its major application should be in patients at the prognostic ends of the spectrum. PTCA may be most useful (1) in patients with severe symptoms from low-risk obstructions (such as single-vessel and mild double-vessel disease) that do not warrant surgical intervention for prognostic reasons, and (2) in those at high-risk for operation, ie, patients with acute myocardial infarction, cardiogenic shock, etc.

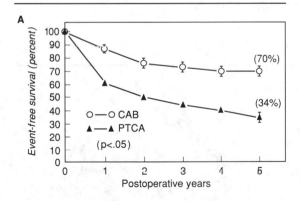

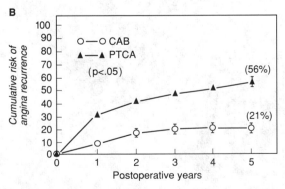

Figure 19–9. Event-free survival *(A)* and anginal recurrence *(B)* in patients having either percutaneous transluminal coronary angioplasty (PTCA) or coronary artery bypass (CAB) for coronary disease.

REOPERATION FOR CORONARY ARTERY DISEASE

Since the advent of coronary artery bypass, an increasing number of patients have presented for reoperation. Common reasons for reoperation include progression of atherosclerotic lesions in the native coronary arteries and atherosclerotic involvement of vein bypass grafts. Performing an internal mammary artery graft at the initial operation significantly reduces the need for reoperation. Control of postoperative hyperlipidemias should also reduce the incidence of reoperation.

The technical aspects of the second procedure are more difficult, but the operative mortality rate should be only slightly higher, generally in the range of 3%. Nevertheless, when appropriate clinical indications are present, reoperation should be undertaken with anticipation of excellent long-term results. In patients requiring reoperation for vein graft atherosclerosis and occlusion, mammary artery grafts offer the potential for a better long-term outcome.

POSTINFARCTION VENTRICULAR SEPTAL DEFECT

Infarction of the interventricular septum with subsequent formation of a ventricular septal defect occurs in less than 1% of patients with acute myocardial infarction. The interval between the acute infarct and septal rupture varies between 1 and 12 days and can be correlated with histologic findings of maximal cardiac muscle degeneration and weakening. Once rupture occurs, the prognosis is poor, with 24% of patients dying on the first day after rupture, 65% by the end of 2 weeks, and 81% by 2 months. The syndrome develops classically in a patient with myocardial infarction in whom shock or congestive heart failure suddenly appears.

Clinical Findings

A. Symptoms and Signs: A harsh holosystolic murmur is usually heard along the left sternal border, and two-thirds of patients demonstrate a palpable thrill.

B. Imaging Studies: Although clinical findings may be highly suggestive, the definitive diagnosis is made by Doppler echocardiography and cardiac catheterization. The defects are often irregular, ragged tracts through the anterior apical septum with occlusion of the left anterior descending artery or through the posterior basilar septum in cases of right coronary artery occlusion. In the latter, right ventricular infarction may compound the problem.

Differential Diagnosis

The differential diagnosis includes papillary muscle dysfunction, rupture of a papillary muscle with acute mitral insufficiency, and pericardial friction rub secondary to myocardial infarction.

Treatment

Surgical correction is indicated in nearly all cases, with the possible exception of elderly patients with advanced multiorgan failure. Intervention should not be delayed, and early or even emergency operation should be the rule. A preoperative intra-aortic balloon pump is placed in most patients, and patch closure of the septal defect along with coronary bypass should be performed early to prevent the consequences of acute right ventricular overload or multiorgan failure.

After institution of cardiopulmonary bypass and cardioplegic arrest, an incision is made in the area of infarction, and good exposure of both the left and right ventricles is obtained. A portion of the necrotic edge of the defect is resected, and a double patch technique is used for repair (Figure 19–10). Coronary bypass grafts are constructed to all diseased vessels, including the right coronary artery in cases of right ventricular infarction.

Prognosis

Fifty to 80 percent of patients should survive the operative procedure, depending on the severity of preoperative shock and multiorgan failure.

LEFT VENTRICULAR ANEURYSM

Left ventricular aneurysm occurs when a large myocardial infarction progresses to a thinned-out transmural scar that bulges paradoxically beyond the normal cavitary contours during systole. While aneurysms have occurred in 2–4% of myocardial infarctions, the incidence is probably decreasing with more aggressive infarct management. Ninety percent of aneurysms involve the anteroseptal left ventricle, and 10% are posterior. Over 50% contain mural thrombus.

Clinical Findings

Patients show signs and symptoms of congestive heart failure, angina, embolization, and ventricular dysrhythmias. Clinical manifestations include a prominent apical impulse, electrocardiographic evidence of an old Q wave myocardial infarction with persistent ST segment elevation, and a localized left ventricular bulge on chest x-ray.

Treatment

Surgical therapy should be considered in most cases, since the prognosis with medical management is poor. Treatment consists of aneurysm resection combined with complete coronary revascularization (Figure 19–11).

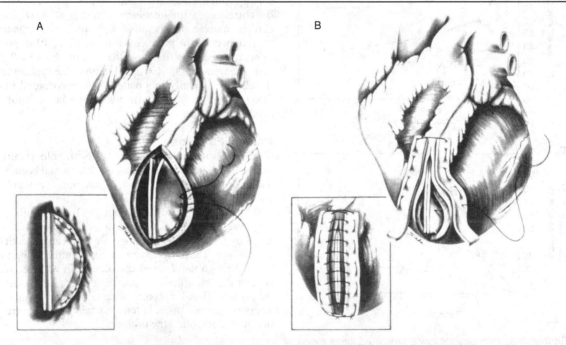

Figure 19–10. Double patch repair technique for anterior postinfarction ventricular septal defect. The ventricular septum is reconstructed by placing sheets of Teflon felt on each side of the septum **(A)** and then closing the ventricular walls to the septal patch **(B)**.

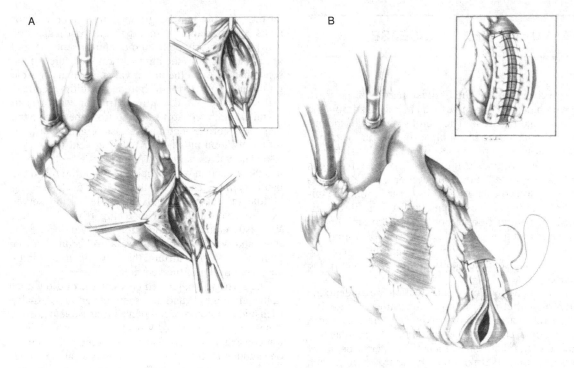

Figure 19–11. Technique of resection **(A)** and closure **(B)** of left ventricular aneurysm.

Prognosis

The prognosis without surgery is related to the acuity of symptoms, the degree of left ventricular dysfunction, and the extent of associated coronary artery disease.

Significant improvements in symptoms of congestive heart failure and angina are observed in 70–85% of surviving patients after operation, and left ventricular ejection fraction increases in the majority because of reduced end-diastolic volume. Long-term survival is improved significantly over medical therapy, with 70–80% of patients alive 5 years postoperatively. The operative mortality rate for elective cases is 5% and increases to 20% for emergency procedures. The hospital mortality rate associated with subendocardial resection for ventricular tachycardia has been 11%.

Barner HB et al: Use of the inferior epigastric artery as a free graft for myocardial revascularization. Ann Thorac Surg 1991;52:429.

Blankenhorn DH et al: Beneficial effects of combined colestipol-niacin therapy on coronary atherosclerosis and coronary venous bypass grafts. JAMA 1987;257:3233.

Callif RM et al: The evolution of medical and surgical therapy for coronary artery disease: A 15 year perspective. JAMA 1989;261:2077.

Connor AR et al: Early and late results of coronary artery bypass after failed angioplasty. J Thorac Cardiovasc Surg 1988;96:191.

Cosgrove DM et al: Predictors of reoperation after myocardial revascularization. J Thorac Cardiovasc Surg 1986;92:811.

Glower DD et al: Linearity of the Frank-Starling relationship in the intact heart: The concept of preload recruitable stroke work. Circulation 1985;71:994.

Loop FD et al: Influence of the internal mammary artery graft on 10-year survival and other cardiac events. N Engl J Med 1986;314:1.

Morris JJ et al: Clinical evaluation of single versus multiple mammary artery bypass. Circulation 1990;82:214.

Muhlbaier LH et al: Observational comparisons of event-free survival with medical and surgical therapy in patients with coronary artery disease: Twenty years of follow-up. Circulation 1991;84:1848.

Peyton RB et al: Eleven-year experience with the surgical management of left ventricular aneurysms. Circulation 1988;78(Suppl II):II-478.

Proudfit WL, Bruschke AVG, Sones FM Jr: Natural history of obstructive coronary artery disease: Ten-year study of 601 non-surgical cases. Progr Cardiovasc Dis 1987; 21:53.

Pryor DB et al: The changing survival benefits of coronary revascularization over time. Circulation 1987;76:V-13.

Rankin JS et al: The effects of coronary revascularization on left ventricular function in ischemic heart disease. J Thorac Cardiovasc Surg 1985;90:818.

Rankin JS et al: Clinical and angiographic assessment of complex mammary artery bypass grafting. J Thorac Cardiovasc Surg 1986;92:832.

VALVULAR HEART DISEASE

Developmentally, the fibrous skeleton of the heart, to which the cardiac valves attach, is derived from the endocardial cushions. The fibrous annulus of the mitral valve is a thin, incomplete ring of fibrous tissue, which is most apparent at two points: the right and left fibrous trigones (Figure 19–12). The left fibrous trigone is situated at the left anterior aspect of the mitral ring and consists of fibrous tissue joining the mitral ring to the base of the aorta. The right fibrous trigone, or central fibrous body, lies in the midline of the heart and represents the confluence of fibrous tissue from the mitral valve, the tricuspid valve, the membranous septum, and the posterior aspect of the base of the aorta.

In most patients, two mitral leaflets are evident: the anterior leaflet and the posterior leaflet (Figure 19–12). Both leaflets are approximately the shape of a trapezoid, each attaching by thin fibrous chordae tendineae to both the anterior and the posterior papillary muscles. Stated differently, the chordae from each papillary muscle fan out and attach to nearly half of both cusp margins. The edges of the leaflets have a slightly serrated appearance owing to the insertion of chordae tendineae on the ventricular surface; these serrations mark the line of closure of the normal valve.

The anatomy of the tricuspid valve apparatus is similar, except that three valve leaflets usually are evident: anterior, posterior, and septal (Figure 19–12). The anterior leaflet commonly is the largest of the three and the posterior leaflet the smallest, though many variations occur. The papillary muscles tend to

be multiple but can be grouped into three components: anterior (arising from the right ventricular free wall), inferior (arising from the inferior septum), and septal (arising from the high septum in the area of the septal band). As in the mitral valve, papillary muscle groups tend to contribute chordae to multiple leaflets.

The function of the atrioventricular valves is to permit uninhibited flow of blood from the atria to the ventricles during ventricular diastole and to prevent reflux of blood into the atria during ventricular systole. The valves achieve this objective by a coordinated contraction of ventricular myocardium and the papillary muscles during the cardiac cycle. During systole, the valve is closed, and the left atrium serves as a reservoir for blood returning from the lungs. With isovolumic relaxation, left ventricular pressure falls, and when ventricular pressure becomes lower than that of the full atrium, the valve opens and initiates rapid filling of the ventricle.

The aortic valve, located between the outflow tract of the left ventricle and the ascending aorta, is usually tricuspid and is composed of a fibrous skeleton, three cusps, and the sinuses of Valsalva. The fibrous skeleton consists of three U-shaped structures that adjoin one another at the valve commissures as at the points of a crown. Beneath each commissure is the pars membranacea. The skeleton is in fibrous continuity with the anterior leaflet of the mitral valve posterolaterally and with the membranous septum anteriorly. The cusps are delicate fibrous leaflets that insert into the outline of the valve skeleton. The free edge of each cusp is concave, is thicker than the rest of the leaflet, and has at its midpoint a fibrous node. At the beginning of systole, the three cusps rapidly retract to form a triangular orifice. Eddy currents within the sinuses of Valsalva cause a slow wave-like motion of the free edge and billowing of the base of each cusp, thus preventing occlusion of the coronary ostia. During ventricular diastole, the cusps fall passively into the center of the orifice and coapt over a considerable area. The closed valve supports the ejected column of blood and prevents regurgitation into the ventricle. In a healthy valve, approximation of the cusps during diastole is complete, and the three nodes come together near the center of the aortic lumen.

The three sinuses of Valsalva are slightly dilated pockets of the aortic root between the cusps and the aortic wall. The coronary arteries arise from two of the sinuses of Valsalva. Because the aortic valve lies in an oblique plane, the origin of the left coronary artery is posterior and slightly superior to that of the right coronary artery.

MITRAL STENOSIS

The most common cause of mitral stenosis is still rheumatic fever associated with group A streptococcal pharyngitis. The early valvular lesions of rheu-

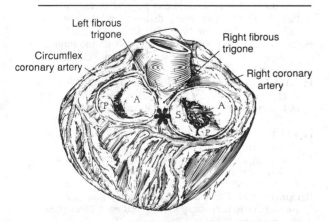

Figure 19–12. Anatomic interrelationships of the atrioventricular valves. (A, anterior leaflet; P, posterior leaflet; S, septal leaflet. The asterisk represents the area of the bundle of His.)

matic fever are characterized by an acute inflammatory infiltrate that gradually heals by organization with fibrous tissue. Chronically, the leaflets become fibrotic and thickened, so that pliability and surface area are reduced. Fusion of the anterior and posterior leaflets may be severe, and in many cases the commissures can no longer be identified. Calcification may occur in the leaflets or the fused commissures, being more common on the posteromedial aspect. The chordae are thickened, shortened, and fused by the same type of fibrosis, and occasionally the subvalvular apparatus may be calcified. The entire process transforms the mitral complex into a rigid funnel-shaped structure with a "fish-mouth" opening.

The most significant effects of mitral stenosis occur on the pulmonary vasculature and right ventricle. Congestion of the pulmonary vessels is characteristic, with distention and thickening of pulmonary capillaries. Intimal fibrosis of the pulmonary veins and arterioles also is observed, and in advanced cases, medial thickening and fibrosis are common. Pulmonary hypertension progresses with time and may increase to the point of producing systemic levels of systolic blood pressure in the right ventricle and inducing functional tricuspid valve regurgitation.

Clinical Findings

A. Symptoms and Signs: Pulmonary venous hypertension caused by valve obstruction produces the most prominent symptom in mitral stenosis, which is dyspnea. Initially, dyspnea is observed only with effort; but with time and progressive valve obstruction, dyspnea begins to occur at rest or at night and is worsened by lying flat (orthopnea). Atrial contraction augments transmitral flow significantly in mitral stenosis, so that development of atrial fibrillation increases mean left atrial pressure and reduces cardiac output by about 20%. In addition, a more rapid ventricular rate decreases diastolic filling time, further exacerbating the problem. Thus, it is common for the clinical status of a patient to deteriorate when atrial fibrillation develops. In clinically progressive cases, patients usually experience worsening cardiac disability or hemoptysis and eventually die from acute pulmonary edema.

On physical examination, the patient characteristically appears thin and cachectic, with a washed-out and sallow "mitral facies." Jugular venous pulsations may be prominent with fluid overload or with secondary tricuspid incompetence. If the cardiac rhythm is atrial fibrillation, irregularities in the jugular pulse and prominent V waves are observed. Peripheral edema and hepatic enlargement may be present as well as the classic "hepatojugular reflux." In the presence of pulmonary edema, respirations are rapid and shallow, the work of breathing is increased, and rales are present to varying degrees from the lung bases up the chest. A sternal heave indicates right ventricular enlargement and suggests pulmonary hypertension.

In severe cases of pulmonary hypertension, the pulmonary component of the second heart sound is often palpable in the second or third left intercostal space parasternally.

Auscultation of the heart reveals accentuation of the first heart sound (S_1) in the early stages, and with development of pulmonary hypertension the pulmonary component of the second heart sound (S_2) becomes accentuated. An opening snap of the mitral valve is common and appears to be due to sudden tensing of the valve leaflets by chordae after their opening excursion. The opening snap is best heard at the apex and is associated with pliability of the valve leaflets. The mitral opening snap follows S_2 by 40–120 ms, with a shorter interval indicating severe left atrial hypertension. The diastolic murmur of mitral stenosis has a low-pitched rumbling quality, best heard at the apex with the bell of the stethoscope. Because of its low frequency, the murmur can be difficult to detect. The murmur usually commences immediately after the opening snap, and its duration is directly related to the severity of valve obstruction. In sinus rhythm, a presystolic accentuation of the murmur is characteristic, as blood flow is accelerated across the valve by atrial contraction. Presystolic accentuation is lost with development of atrial fibrillation.

B. Electrocardiography: Ninety percent of patients in sinus rhythm exhibit a broad, notched P wave on the ECG, the so-called "P mitrale." In later stages, atrial fibrillation and right ventricular hypertrophy are cardinal electrocardiographic signs.

C. Imaging Studies: On x-ray, the overall cardiac silhouette may be normal, with the exception of left atrial enlargement. Pulmonary venous hypertension is accompanied by engorged, transversely oriented superior pulmonary veins. With pulmonary hypertension, the pulmonary arteries and right ventricle become enlarged, displacing the right ventricle toward the sternum on the lateral projection. Severe valvular obstruction is manifested by Kerley B lines and frank pulmonary edema.

Cardiac catheterization is performed in most patients but can be omitted in young patients with classic clinical and echocardiographic findings. Measurements of transvalvular gradients and calculations of valve area provide useful information about severity of the stenosis. The normal mitral orifice area is $3 \text{ cm}^2/\text{m}^2$ BSA, and significant mitral stenosis is suggested when the calculated area approaches $1 \text{ cm}^2/\text{m}^2$. Estimation of valve orifice area is subject to some error, however, particularly at low flow rates or in the presence of valvular regurgitation. Moreover, a well-diuresed patient with a contracted blood volume occasionally will exhibit a larger valve area and a lower left atrial pressure than suggested by the clinical evaluation. Thus, it should be emphasized that catheterization findings are only supplemental, and the entire clinical picture must be considered when making therapeutic decisions.

Treatment

A. Medical Treatment: Most would agree that asymptomatic patients should be treated medically and carefully observed.

B. Surgical Treatment: Mitral stenosis is second only to aortic stenosis in terms of mortality rate among the acquired valvular disease. Thus, available data would support the early election of surgical therapy for this disorder. To quote Wood's classic 1954 paper: "There can be little point in delaying mitral valvotomy long in anatomically suitable cases once unmistakable symptoms of stenosis have developed; to do so is to invite complications such as embolism and to deprive patients of good physical health at a time in life when they have the right to expect it." In the presence of clinically or hemodynamically significant valvular obstruction, firm indications for operation include NYHA class III or IV symptoms, the onset of atrial fibrillation (independent of symptoms), worsening pulmonary hypertension, an episode of systemic embolization, and infective endocarditis. Surgical therapy should be recommended also for class II patients who are over age 40, those who have severe reduction in valve area at catheterization, and those who experience unacceptable limitations on life-style.

Approximately 50% of stenotic mitral valves treated operatively can be managed with open commissurotomy. Absence of significant leaflet calcification, together with good leaflet mobility and surface area, increases the likelihood of successful repair. Complete incision of fused commissures is performed, together with Cavitron ultrasonic surgical aspirator (CUSA) debridement of localized calcium deposits when necessary. The submitral apparatus is inspected, and fused or thickened chordae are resected. The papillary muscle heads can be split to further improve submitral outflow. As the final step, a Carpentier mitral ring is inserted to lessen the incidence of early or late induced valve regurgitation. If significant leaflet calcification or fibrous retraction is evident, a standard prosthetic mitral valve replacement is performed, usually with the St. Jude valve (Figure 19–13).

Prognosis

The operative mortality rate for isolated primary mitral valve procedures ranges from 1% to 5%, depending on the severity of preoperative symptoms, the presence of severe pulmonary hypertension or right ventricular failure, and the need for mitral valve replacement. Contemporary operations significantly increase long-term survival and patient well-being. After open mitral commissurotomy or valve replacement, most patients experience improvement in

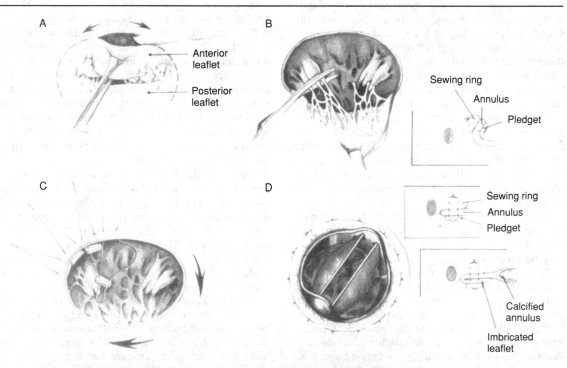

Figure 19–13. Technique for mitral valve replacement. Horizontal mattress sutures with supra-annular pledgets are used by many surgeons (top insert at right); the authors prefer subannular pledgets (middle insert). For cases with severely calcified annuli, a leaflet imbrication technique can be used (lower insert).

symptoms, though repeat operations are necessary at a rate of 2–4% per patient year after valve repair. The probabilities of systemic embolization and infective endocarditis are lessened significantly by surgical therapy, and patients experiencing atrial fibrillation for less than 1 year have an excellent chance of reverting to sinus rhythm with pharmacologic therapy or cardioversion or both.

MITRAL REGURGITATION

Competence of the mitral valve depends on an integrated function of the mitral annulus, the valve leaflets, the chordae tendineae, the papillary muscles, and the ventricular wall. Incompetence can be caused by abnormalities of any of these structures.

Rheumatic heart disease accounts for 35–45% of cases of mitral regurgitation. Involvement of the leaflets by the rheumatic process causes shortening, rigidity, and retraction of the cusps. The chordae tendineae also become fibrotic, fused, and shortened.

Idiopathic calcification of the mitral valve and annulus in the elderly can be an important cause of regurgitation and is associated with systemic hypertension, aortic stenosis, diabetes, and chronic renal failure. Calcification may involve the entire annulus and project into adjacent ventricular myocardium. Masses of calcium may protrude into the subvalvular region, immobilizing the valve or preventing leaflet coaptation, and calcium can invade the conduction system or adjacent coronary arteries.

Mitral valve prolapse is present in 3–4% of the general population and can be associated with a midsystolic click and late systolic murmur. Progressive and clinically significant mitral regurgitation develops in approximately 5% of these cases. The primary pathologic process is myxomatous degeneration of the fibrous layer of the valve leaflets and chordae tendineae, producing thinning, elongation, and redundancy. In many patients, rupture of weakened chordae can cause acute mitral regurgitation, the severity of which depends on the size of chordal rupture and the degree of regurgitation produced. In extreme cases, severe congestive heart failure and acute pulmonary edema may necessitate emergency treatment.

The final category of mitral incompetence is **ischemic mitral regurgitation,** defined as moderate to severe valve incompetence precipitated by acute myocardial infarction with no primary leaflet or chordal pathology. This disorder is observed to a significant degree in 3% of patients with coronary artery disease undergoing catheterization and is quite heterogeneous both from the pathophysiologic and the clinical viewpoints. Pathologically, the majority of patients exhibit posterior papillary-annular dysfunction in which regurgitation and congestive heart failure are coincident with the onset of a large posterior wall infarction. Combinations of posterior annular di-

lation, papillary muscle elongation, loss of papillary muscle shortening, and preexisting congenital leaflet defects produce valve incompetence at the posterior commissural region.

Postinfarction **papillary muscle rupture** occurs more rarely and is observed in only 0.1% of coronary disease patients undergoing catheterization. Congestive heart failure associated with a new murmur usually develops several days after infarction, and the majority have severe regurgitation requiring acute intervention. The infarction usually is posterior and often is small and localized; global ejection fraction is frequently maintained.

Physiologic derangements caused by mitral regurgitation are similar to those associated with mitral stenosis. Left atrial hypertension is transmitted to the pulmonary vasculature, causing dyspnea and pulmonary edema. Pulmonary arterial hypertension, right ventricular failure, and functional tricuspid regurgitation occur by similar mechanisms. However, unlike mitral stenosis, the left ventricle is subjected to a chronic volume overload, which ultimately causes myocardial failure.

Clinical Findings

A. Symptoms and Signs: Symptoms produced by mitral regurgitation are related to the level of pulmonary venous hypertension. Exertional dyspnea and orthopnea are common, and chronically reduced cardiac output produces easy fatigability and cardiac cachexia. Moderate to severe regurgitation can be tolerated for many years with relatively minor symptoms until irreversible left ventricular dysfunction develops. Therefore, the severity of symptoms cannot be used as the only criterion for intervention. Hemoptysis is rarely reported, and symptoms occasionally appear with the onset of atrial fibrillation, which complicates 75% of severe cases. Systemic emboli can occur in patients with atrial fibrillation but are not as common as in mitral stenosis. Infective endocarditis should be suspected if there are symptoms of malaise, fever, chills, or a new or worsening murmur, or when acute decompensation occurs in a previously stable patient. Angina secondary to mitral regurgitation is rare and should suggest coexisting coronary artery disease. Obviously, patients with ischemic mitral regurgitation usually manifest either acute or chronic myocardial ischemic syndromes.

The physical signs of congestive heart failure are similar to those of mitral stenosis. The apical impulse is displaced to the left in proportion to the degree of left ventricular enlargement, and an apical systolic thrill can be palpated. With significant right ventricular enlargement, a sternal heave is evident. On auscultation, the heart sounds usually are normal, with the exception of a third heart sound with congestive heart failure or an increased S_2 with pulmonary hypertension. The hallmark of mitral regurgitation is an apical, high-pitched, holosystolic murmur that radiates to the axilla and back. On occasion, the murmur will radiate to the base and have a musical quality. In the presence of infective endocarditis, peripheral signs such as splinter hemorrhages, Osler's nodes, clubbing, fever, and splenomegaly may be evident.

B. Electrocardiography: The ECG may show left ventricular hypertrophy from the chronic volume overload or biventricular hypertrophy with concomitant pulmonary arterial hypertension. In sinus rhythm, "P mitrale" may be present.

C. Imaging Studies: The chest radiograph illustrates left atrial enlargement in chronic cases, but because of the volume overload, the left ventricle also is dilated. Right ventricular enlargement, pulmonary vascular engorgement, and Kerley B lines are common. Cardiac catheterization documents prominent left atrial V waves, elevated left ventricular end-diastolic pressure and increased end-diastolic volume. Pulmonary hypertension in mitral incompetence has the same implications as in mitral stenosis. A reduction in cardiac index below 2 L/min/m^2 and a widened arteriovenous oxygen difference indicate severe hemodynamic impairment. Regurgitation is graded on the basis of the contrast left ventriculogram as 1–4+.

Treatment

A. Selection of Patients for Operation: The natural history of mitral regurgitation is more variable than that of mitral stenosis because of the greater number of etiologic factors. The clinical course can range from asymptomatic, with moderate mitral regurgitation remaining stable for many years, to a fulminant progression of overwhelming congestive heart failure. There are three determinants of clinical severity: (1) the degree of regurgitation, (2) the status of left ventricular function, and (3) the cause of the valve disease.

Significant symptoms are rare until the onset of heart failure, which usually appears late in the overall course. Interestingly, symptoms (NYHA functional class) and ejection fraction do not correlate with medical outcome using a multivariate analysis. This finding suggests that symptoms alone are an unreliable guide to the timing of operative treatment, and other factors, such as progressive cardiomegaly, need to be considered. This concept is further supported by the observation that the operative mortality rate is higher and long-term survival is depressed in patients with severe cardiomegaly or class IV symptoms. Thus, operation is recommended in chronic mitral regurgitation if symptoms significantly limit life-style or for NYHA class III or IV congestive heart failure. In class I or II patients, operation should be considered if pulmonary hypertension is progressing, if atrial fibrillation occurs, or if the left ventricle is dilating. Similar criteria for surgical selection are used in patients with mixed stenosis and regurgitation, mitral

valve calcification, or other forms of slowly progressive mitral incompetence.

B. Surgical Treatment: Mitral valve incompetence can be managed by mitral valve repair or replacement. Virtually all myxomatous valves with prolapse can be repaired. Fifty percent have isolated posterior leaflet prolapse or chordal rupture, and posterior leaflet reconstruction along with Carpentier ring annuloplasty (Figure 19–14) is highly effective. If primary chordae to the anterior leaflet are ruptured, artificial chords of 5-0 Gortex suture are inserted, again with Carpentier ring annuloplasty. In cases of ischemic papillary annular dysfunction, a simple commissural suture annuloplasty (Figure 19–15) combined with complete coronary revascularization is the procedure of choice. In cases of rheumatic leaflet retraction, valve calcification, or severe endocarditis, prosthetic valve replacement is in order (Figure 19–13).

Prognosis

Operative mortality rates for elective mitral valve procedures performed under stable conditions approximate 2–5%, and the quality and duration of life are improved. Occasionally, however, a more acute clinical course is observed, particularly with infective endocarditis, ruptured chordae tendineae, or ischemic mitral regurgitation. Under these conditions, emergency operations are required, and with extreme hemodynamic compromise, a preoperative intra-aortic balloon pump can produce clinical stabilization. Operative mortality rates in the emergency setting are higher, usually 10–20%. Long-term survival rates are reduced in patients with impaired preoperative ventricular function, in those requiring emergency operation, and in elderly patients with preexisting multiorgan failure.

TRICUSPID VALVE DISEASE

Pathologic disorders of the tricuspid valve can be either functional or organic. Tricuspid regurgitation is usually functional and is secondary to right ventricular dilation and enlargement of the free-wall tricuspid annulus. The annulus in the area of the septal leaflet is spared, and the valve leaflets and chordae generally are normal. Causes of functional tricuspid regurgitation include mitral valve disease, cor pulmonale, primary pulmonary hypertension, right ventricular infarction, and congenital heart disease. In most cases, valve incompetence reflects the presence of— and in turn further aggravates—severe right ventricular failure.

Tricuspid stenosis is almost always rheumatic, usually accompanies mitral valve involvement, and is clinically significant in about 5% of patients with rheumatic heart disease. Pathologic changes resemble those in the mitral valve, with thickening and fu-

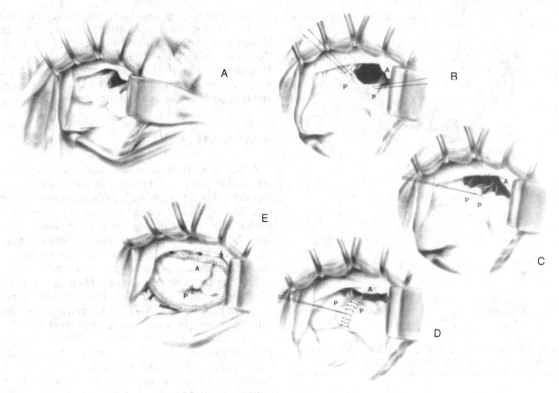

Figure 19–14. Panels *A–D* represent atrial views of posterior leaflet reconstruction for isolated posterior leaflet prolapse and insertion of Carpentier annuloplasty ring.

sion of the leaflets and chordae, producing a stenotic, fixed tricuspid orifice. Carcinoid involvement of the tricuspid valve is characterized by deposition of fibrous carcinoid plaques on the leaflets and ventricular attachments. Both tricuspid stenosis and tricuspid regurgitation produce right atrial hypertension, systemic venous engorgement, and hepatic congestion. Severe fluid retention, edema, and debility are characteristic. The process can progress to hepatic failure, cardiac cirrhosis, anasarca, and renal failure.

Clinical Findings

A. Symptoms and Signs: Symptoms in either tricuspid stenosis or regurgitation are related to the degree of systemic venous hypertension. Fatigue and weakness are common, usually without dyspnea or other signs of pulmonary congestion. Isolated tricuspid regurgitation is well tolerated in patients with normal pulmonary artery pressure, but when combined with mitral valve disease, pulmonary hypertension, and right ventricular failure, the clinical status deteriorates rapidly.

Tricuspid valve disease is easily overlooked unless the observer is alert to that diagnostic possibility. In sinus rhythm, contraction of the right atrium against a stenotic valve produces a prominent A wave in the jugular venous pulse; with regurgitant lesions, the jugular V wave is accentuated. The liver is often enlarged and may be pulsatile, but in congestive cirrhosis, the liver may be firm and fibrotic. While ascites and edema are common, the lung fields are clear despite engorged neck veins and other signs of congestive heart failure. A tricuspid opening snap may be present. Murmurs with tricuspid valve disease are similar to those observed in mitral disorders, and the two may be difficult to distinguish. Tricuspid murmurs usually are located more toward the left lower sternal border, and both the stenotic and the regurgitant varieties are augmented by inspiration. Both murmurs may be difficult to hear, even when the physiologic defects are severe.

B. Electrocardiography: In sinus rhythm, tricuspid valve disease is suggested if the lead II P wave amplitude exceeds 0.25 mV.

C. Imaging Studies: The key radiographic finding is cardiomegaly, with prominence of the right atrial shadow. At catheterization, tricuspid stenosis is confirmed by demonstrating a diastolic pressure gradient between the right atrium and right ventricle, utilizing simultaneous pressure measurements. A mean diastolic gradient of 5 mm Hg is significant in tricuspid stenosis, and values as low as 3 mm Hg may produce symptoms; the resting cardiac output is reduced. In tricuspid regurgitation, right atrial pressure is char-

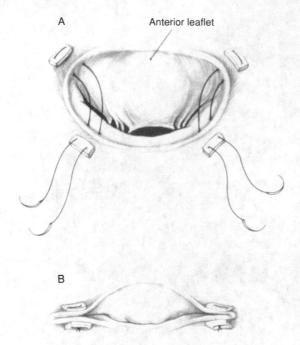

A
Anterior leaflet

B

Figure 19–15. Atrial view of commissural annuloplasty procedure for ischemic mitral regurgitation.

acterized by a prominent V wave, which in severe cases is described as "ventricularization" of atrial pressure. Occasionally, the atrial V wave may be normal despite severe regurgitation because of an enlarged, highly compliant venous system. Pulmonary arterial hypertension favors a functional cause in tricuspid regurgitation, whereas normal pulmonary pressures suggest organic disease.

Doppler echocardiography is the most quantitative and reliable method of assessing tricuspid valve incompetence, both preoperatively and intraoperatively.

Treatment

Rheumatic tricuspid stenosis is treated by either commissurotomy or valve replacement, depending on leaflet mobility, involvement of subvalvular structures, and the presence of regurgitation. Because residual gradients are tolerated poorly, valve replacement should be considered in significantly diseased valves. Bioprosthetic valves should be used exclusively for tricuspid valve replacement. Symptomatic cases of carcinoid valve disease require excision of the entire tricuspid apparatus and valve replacement.

Tricuspid endocarditis in drug addicts is a particularly difficult problem. For infections that cannot be eradicated with antibiotics, total excision of the valve has been recommended. Most patients tolerate loss of the tricuspid valve acutely, but valve replacement can be required at a later date. More recently, a variety of

reparative operations have been performed with good results. If possible, prosthetic valve replacement should be avoided because of the risk of late prosthetic endocarditis. Functional tricuspid regurgitation secondary to mitral valve disease usually is managed by Carpentier ring annuloplasty to obviate the early and late morbidity of residual tricuspid regurgitation.

AORTIC STENOSIS

Aortic stenosis causes obstruction to left ventricular outflow and can be subvalvular, valvular, or supravalvular. Aortic stenosis in the adult may be due to a congenitally unicuspid or bicuspid valve, congenital subvalvular or supravalvular stenosis, rheumatic heart disease, or, most frequently, degenerative fibrosis and calcification. The cause can often be surmised from the age of the patient—congenital lesions accounting for most cases in patients under 30 years of age, rheumatic heart disease or congenital bicuspid valves in patients aged 30–65 years, and degenerative calcific stenosis in patients over 65 years of age.

Resistance to left ventricular outflow produces a pressure overload on the left ventricle that compensates by the development of concentric left ventricular hypertrophy. Hypertrophy is associated with reduced left ventricular diastolic compliance, while systolic function—or ejection fraction—is well maintained. In this setting, atrial systole contributes significantly to left ventricular filling, and the development of atrial fibrillation may precipitate heart failure. Myocardial oxygen consumption is elevated in the hypertrophied ventricle, and the presence of concomitant coronary artery disease may be particularly deleterious by reducing myocardial oxygen delivery.

Clinical Findings

A. Symptoms and Signs: Most patients remain asymptomatic for many years. The classic triad of symptoms includes angina pectoris, syncope, and congestive heart failure and usually denotes an aortic valve gradient greater than 50 mm Hg or a valve area of less than 1.0 cm^2. Angina pectoris is due to the imbalance between myocardial oxygen demand and delivery caused by increased myocardial oxygen consumption, and in the 25–50% of patients with coronary artery disease it is aggravated by the superimposed reduced oxygen delivery. Syncope is typically exertional and most likely related to inability of the left ventricle to increase cardiac output in the face of a fixed, high-grade obstruction. Congestive heart failure usually occurs late and is an especially ominous sign.

The pulse pressure is often narrowed, with a decreased systolic arterial pressure. A harsh midsystolic murmur is heard best at the second intercostal space and along the left sternal border. The murmur may radiate to the carotid arteries, is generally audible at the apex, and typically does not radiate into the axilla. Approximately 25–50% of patients will also have a murmur of aortic regurgitation.

B. Electrocardiography: The ECG demonstrates left ventricular hypertrophy.

C. Imaging Studies: On chest roentgenography, the heart is usually of normal size, though moderate enlargement may exist in the presence of congestive heart failure. Poststenotic dilation of the ascending aorta or calcification in the area of the aortic valve can be observed. Doppler echocardiography can evaluate calcification and mobility of aortic valve leaflets, bicuspid aortic leaflet anatomy, left ventricular hypertrophy, left ventricular ejection fraction, transvalvular gradients, and the presence of aortic regurgitation. Cardiac catheterization yields important information on coronary anatomy, cardiac output, transvalvular pressure gradients, overall left ventricular function, and the presence of coexisting valvular lesions.

Treatment

A. Selection of Patients for Operation: Symptoms of angina pectoris, congestive heart failure, or syncope in a patient with aortic stenosis are associated with an average life expectancy of 1–3 years if left untreated and constitute the classic indication for aortic valve replacement. In addition, asymptomatic or minimally symptomatic patients in whom the aortic valve gradient is greater than 50 mm Hg or the aortic valve area is less than 1.0 cm^2 are also candidates for valve replacement, especially in the presence of left ventricular hypertrophy or coexisting coronary artery disease. Few clinical contraindications to aortic valve replacement exist in patients with hemodynamically significant aortic stenosis, and patient selection criteria should be liberal. Relief of the outflow tract gradient usually improves left ventricular pump function even in the presence of severe preoperative left ventricular dysfunction. Long-term survival and quality of life are significantly enhanced.

B. Surgical Treatment: Aortic valve repair for aortic stenosis is a surgical option in appropriately selected valves with minimal calcific leaflet infiltration and consists principally of Cavitron ultrasonic surgical aspirator (CUSA) decalcification of the valve, with or without commissurotomy.

Prognosis

Aortic valve replacement for elective isolated aortic stenosis is associated with a less than 5% operative mortality rate in all categories of patients. Advanced age, left ventricular dysfunction, and acute presentation increase surgical risk, but not as much as with mitral valve disease. Long-term survival approximates 85–90% at 5 years, and the outlook is adversely affected by preoperative left ventricular dysfunction, advanced age, and ventricular arrhythmias.

AORTIC INSUFFICIENCY

Aortic insufficiency is caused by abnormal coaptation of the aortic valve leaflets, allowing blood to return to the ventricle from the aorta during diastole. A common cause is rheumatic valvulitis, but varying degrees of annular dilation or annuloaortic ectasia also occur. Cystic medial necrosis, atherosclerosis, syphilitic degeneration, arthritic inflammatory diseases, and congenitally bicuspid valves are among some of the numerous causes of chronic insufficiency, while endocarditis and trauma account for the majority of cases of acute valve regurgitation.

Clinical Findings

A. Symptoms and Signs: Patients with chronic aortic regurgitation may be asymptomatic for many years but have a reduced life expectancy once symptoms of orthopnea, paroxysmal dyspnea, and congestive failure appear. On physical examination, the pulse pressure is widened and the diastolic pressure is low. The apical impulse is sustained and laterally and inferiorly displaced. Characteristically, a blowing high-pitched diastolic murmur is heard best along the left lower sternal border with the patient in full expiration. A third heart sound and a diastolic rumble (Austin Flint murmur) may be audible.

B. Electrocardiography: The ECG usually shows left ventricular hypertrophy with left axis deviation.

C. Imaging Studies: Chest roentgenography usually demonstrates left ventricular enlargement and may also show evidence of pulmonary congestion in symptomatic patients. Echocardiography is an important noninvasive examination, estimating left ventricular function and chamber size, while Doppler measurements can evaluate the degree of regurgitation. At cardiac catheterization, supravalvular aortography is performed to define the degree of aortic insufficiency. Catheterization also identifies the coronary anatomy along with any associated abnormalities of the aortic root and annulus.

Treatment

Aortic valve replacement is the standard operation and should be performed prior to the onset of irreversible left ventricular dilation, which not infrequently occurs prior to the onset of symptoms. The most accurate guide currently available for assessing progression toward irreversibility appears to be echocardiographic measurement of left ventricular dimensions, and significant ventricular dilation should be used as a guide to recommending valve replacement or repair.

In selected cases of aortic regurgitation due to simple annular dilation, valve repair with subcommissural annuloplasty has been effective. However, this is a new procedure, and more follow-up will be necessary to fully define its utility.

PROSTHETIC VALVE SELECTION

BIOPROSTHETIC VERSUS MECHANICAL VALVES

Bioprosthetic Valves

The modern era of tissue valves began in the early 1970s with the introduction of glutaraldehyde-fixed porcine heterografts for valve replacement. The incidence of thromboembolism is low (0.1–2% per patient year), so that warfarin anticoagulation is not required. Earlier reports recommending warfarin after mitral valve replacement in patients with atrial fibrillation have been superseded by the observation that aspirin anticoagulation is equally effective. Valve thrombosis is rare, but in smaller sizes, tissue valves may be distinctly stenotic. The incidence of postoperative prosthetic valve endocarditis is approximately the same as with mechanical valves (5–10% over the valve's lifetime).

The major concern with porcine valves is durability. Degeneration of leaflet tissue, calcification, and structural failure result in prosthetic valve dysfunction after an average of 7–10 years. The rate of valve failure is higher in the mitral than the aortic position because of higher stresses associated with valve closure. Virtually every tissue valve will require replacement if the patient lives long enough. The problem of tissue valve durability is significant and becomes even more evident with time, as increasing numbers of patients return with valve failure requiring reoperation.

Most surgeons have abandoned the routine use of bioprostheses except for specific indications.

Mechanical Valves

Current mechanical prostheses offer better predictability of performance and durability than tissue valves. However, all patients require warfarin therapy, and valve thrombosis or thromboembolism can occur despite adequate anticoagulation. Thromboembolic rates for most mechanical valves with adequate anticoagulation approximate 2–5% per patient year, though thromboembolism is less common with the St. Jude valve. The mortality rate attributable to warfarin therapy approaches 1% per year, but recent studies suggest that "modest" warfarin anticoagulation to a prothrombin time ratio of 1.3–1.5 will be effective in preventing thromboembolism but will reduce bleeding complications. The St. Jude valve has the best flow characteristics.

Because of its excellent durability, good flow characteristics, and low thromboembolic rates, the St. Jude valve is currently the prosthetic valve of choice in most centers.

SPECIFIC INDICATIONS

Young women desiring children may choose a porcine valve to reduce anticoagulation complications during pregnancy, with the understanding that the prosthesis eventually will require replacement. Patients with specific contraindications to anticoagulation also are candidates for tissue valves. Patients in the elderly age group generally should receive mechanical valves, since the return of an elderly patient 5–10 years later at an even older age with tissue valve failure is a difficult problem. Patients undergoing complicated valve procedures such as aortic and mitral valve replacement or valve replacement–coronary bypass combinations should receive mechanical valves because of the higher mortality rate associated with reoperation in these groups. In difficult technical cases, such as small left atria or calcified annuli, a low-profile valve, such as the St. Jude, is implanted because of its ease of insertion. Tricuspid valve replacement is performed exclusively with porcine valves because of a high incidence of mechanical valve thrombosis even with adequate anticoagulation. In the final analysis, however, the thromboembolic and anticoagulation complications of mechanical valves are roughly equivalent to the durability problems of bioprostheses, so that late results after mitral valve replacement are similar with both types of valves (Figure 19–16). This realization has led to the increasing application of valve reconstruction to an expanding range of cardiac valve disorders.

Antunes MJ: Valve replacement in the elderly. Is the mechanical valve a good alternative? J Thorac Cardiovasc Surg 1989;98:485.

Arom KV et al: Ten years' experience with the St. Jude Medical valve prosthesis. Ann Thorac Surg 1989;47:831.

Bortolotti U et al: Long-term durability of the Hancock porcine bioprosthesis following combined mitral and aortic valve replacement: An 11-year experience. Ann Thorac Surg 1987;44:130.

Carpentier A: Cardiac valve surgery: The "French correction." J Thorac Cardiovasc Surg 1983;86:323.

Cosgrove DM, Stewart WJ: Mitral valvuloplasty. Curr Probl Cardiol 1989;14(7):353.

Czer LS et al: Comparative clinical experience with porcine bioprosthetic and St. Jude valve replacement. Chest 1987;91:503.

Czer LS et al: The St. Jude valve: Analysis of thromboembolism, warfarin-related hemorrhage, and survival. Am Heart J 1987;114:389.

Duran CG et al: Indications and limitations of aortic valve reconstruction. Ann Thorac Surg 1991;52:447.

Duran CG et al: Stability of mitral reconstructive surgery at 10–12 years for predominantly rheumatic valvular disease. Circulation 1988;78(3 Part 2):191.

Galloway AC et al: A comparison of mitral valve reconstruction with mitral valve replacement: Intermediate-term results. Ann Thorac Surg 1989;47:655.

Hammermeister KE et al: Prediction of late survival in patients with mitral valve disease from clinical, hemodyna-

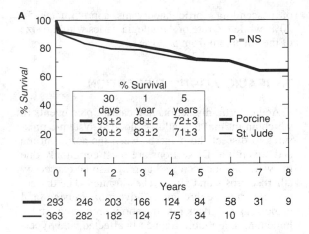

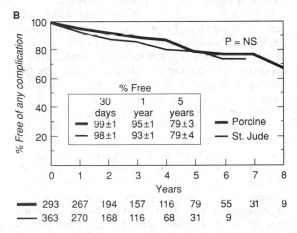

Figure 19–16. Overall survival *(A)* and complication rate *(B)* after valve replacement with St. Jude and porcine xenograft valves.

mic, and quantitative angiographic variables. Circulation 1978;57:341.

Jones EL et al: Complications from cardiac prostheses: I. Infection, thrombosis, and emboli associated with intracardiac prostheses. In: *Gibbon's Surgery of the Chest.* Sabiston DC Jr, Spencer FC (editors). Saunders, 1983.

Kay GL et al: Mitral valve repair for mitral regurgitation secondary to coronary artery disease. Circulation 1986;74:1.

Nunez L et al: Prevention of thromboembolism using aspirin after mitral valve replacement with porcine bioprosthesis. Ann Thorac Surg 1984;37:84.

Rankin JS et al: Trends in the surgical treatment of ischemic mitral regurgitation: Effects of mitral valve repair on hospital mortality. Semin Thorac Cardiovasc Surg 1989;1:149.

Sheikh KH et al: The utility of transesophageal echocardiography and Doppler color flow imaging in patients undergoing cardiac valve operations. J Am Coll Cardiol 1990;15:363.

Yee ES, Ullyot DJ: Reparative approach for right-sided en-

docarditis: Operative considerations and results of valvuloplasty. J Thorac Cardiovasc Surg 1988;96:133.

THORACIC AORTIC DISEASE

THORACIC AORTIC ANEURYSMS

The most common cause of thoracic aneurysms is arteriosclerosis, which causes a degenerative process in the aortic wall. Atherosclerotic aneurysms can be saccular or fusiform and occur in the ascending or descending thoracic aorta or in the arch. Another common pathophysiologic process, as seen in Marfan's syndrome, is cystic medial necrosis of the aortic wall, characterized by replacement of muscle cells and elastic lamina with mucoid-filled cystic spaces. Annuloaortic ectasia can occur in this setting and consists of enlargement of the entire aortic root, including the sinuses of Valsalva. Trauma and infection account for the remaining cases of thoracic aneurysms.

Clinical Findings

A. Symptoms and Signs: Thoracic aneurysms are more common in men, and a history of hypertension is usual. Symptoms, if present, are due to local pressure or obstruction of adjacent thoracic structures. In the ascending aorta, signs may include aortic regurgitation, superior vena cava obstruction, or chest pain with aneurysm expansion. In the arch of the aorta, tracheal compression may occur, while aneurysms of the descending aorta—the most common type—may be associated with recurrent laryngeal nerve compression, phrenic paralysis, dysphagia due to esophageal compression, or stridor due to tracheal compression.

B. Imaging Studies: The chest radiograph may show convexity of the right cardiac border in ascending aneurysms, a prominent aortic knob in transverse aneurysms, and posterior lateral thoracic masses in descending aneurysms. In the past, contrast thoracic aortography was the standard radiologic examination, though cine-MRI is now becoming the primary diagnostic procedure.

Treatment

Indications for operation in patients with thoracic aneurysms include symptomatic or enlarging aneurysms and aneurysms with a transverse diameter of 6 cm or greater. Dacron graft replacement is the standard operative procedure and is conducted in different ways depending on the location of the aneurysm.

A. Ascending Aorta and Aortic Arch Aneurysm: Ascending and arch aneurysms require cardiopulmonary bypass for graft replacement, most commonly via right atrial and femoral artery cannulation. The heart is protected during aortic cross-clamping with cold potassium cardioplegia. For aortic root aneurysms (annuloaortic ectasia), a composite prosthetic valve–ascending aortic graft conduit is utilized, with reimplantation of the coronary arteries into the graft (as in patients with Marfan's syndrome). More recently, aortic valve repair and reconstruction of the aortic root with a Dacron graft has been employed in this setting. For isolated ascending aortic aneurysms, Dacron graft replacement is utilized, again under cardiopulmonary bypass and hypothermic cardiac arrest.

Replacement of a transverse arch aortic aneurysm is more complex, since preservation of the central nervous system is a major concern. Profound hypothermia is induced with the cardiopulmonary bypass circuit to a core temperature of 15–20 °C , and the aneurysm is repaired via the inside of the aorta during transient circulatory arrest. The central nervous system is maintained at 15 °C during the repair. The brachycephalic vessels are excised from the native aorta and anastomosed to the Dacron graft as a single button. Great care is taken to remove all air from the grafts before cerebral reperfusion is instituted.

The operative mortality rate for ascending aortic or arch reconstructions has been reduced to about 10% because of advances in myocardial and cerebral protection.

B. Descending Aorta Aneurysm: Descending aorta aneurysms occur distal to the left subclavian artery. Operation is performed through a left thoracotomy incision with one-lung anesthesia. The aorta is clamped above and below the aneurysm, which is replaced with a Dacron tube graft. A major risk in descending thoracic aneurysm repair is spinal cord ischemia with resultant paraplegia. There is debate about the optimal method of protecting the spinal cord and lower body during thoracic aortic cross-clamping, and techniques vary from femorofemoral bypass with a pump oxygenator to simple cross-clamping without regard to distal blood flow. Currently, profound hypothermic cardiopulmonary bypass and distal hypothermic circulatory arrest are favored (with liberal reimplantation of spinal or intercostal arteries into the graft) as a means of decreasing spinal cord injury; however, further studies are required to clarify this issue.

Prognosis

Thoracic aortic aneurysms follow a natural history similar to that of abdominal aortic aneurysms—ie, the signs, symptoms, and prognosis are related to the size of the aneurysm. The 5-year survival rate of patients with thoracic aneurysms is 20–25%. Deaths are largely due to aneurysm rupture or complications of generalized atherosclerosis.

The operative mortality rate associated with repair of descending aortic aneurysms approximates 5–20%, while the rate of paraplegia varies with the size of the aneurysm from 5–30%.

THORACIC AORTIC DISSECTION

Acute aortic dissections are catastrophic events in which an intimal tear allows blood at systemic pressures to dissect the plane between the aortic intima and adventitia. Dissections are most commonly due to cystic medial necrosis but may also be caused by atherosclerosis and closed chest trauma. The dissection may rupture through the adventitia, causing fatal hemorrhage, or back into the aorta, producing a false lumen. Men are more frequently affected, and hypertension is a common predisposing condition.

DeBakey's classification in the most widely utilized. DeBakey type I dissections originate in the ascending aorta and extend (in 90% of cases) into the distal aorta beyond the left subclavian artery; type II dissections involve the ascending aorta only, are frequently chronic, and are associated with aortic valve incompetence; and type III dissections occur distal to the left subclavian artery and commonly extend into the abdominal aorta. This classification is a simplification, however, and the intimal tear can occur in any part of the aorta (even the arch and abdominal aorta). Moreover, the dissection may extend to any portion of the aorta (ascending involvement = Stanford type A; descending involvement only = Stanford type B). In practice, it is more useful to describe the dissection in terms of the location of the proximal intimal tear and the extent of aortic involvement.

Clinical Findings

A. Symptoms and Signs: The most common symptom is severe chest pain, which often signifies the onset of the intimal tear and formation of the false lumen. The chest pain often is described as a severe tearing sensation that is felt anteriorly in ascending dissections and posteriorly between the scapulas in descending dissections. Hypotension may accompany the pain as a result of loss of blood into the false lumen, free rupture into the mediastinum, or leak into the pericardium. Sudden death may occur from pericardial tamponade or from extension into the aortic root with occlusion of the right or left coronary arteries. Aortic root involvement also is associated with prolapse of the aortic valve commissures and leaflets, causing aortic insufficiency and congestive heart failure.

Other manifestations vary according to the degree of dissection and include stroke, asymmetric upper extremity pulses and pressures, paraplegia, renal failure, acute mesenteric occlusion, and lower extremity arterial occlusion.

B. Electrocardiography and Laboratory Findings: The ECG and cardiac enzyme determinations are helpful in excluding acute myocardial infarction, which may mimic many of the signs and symptoms of acute aortic dissection.

C. Imaging Studies: The chest radiograph may show a widened mediastinum but is normal in up to half of patients. Cardiomegaly may reflect congestive heart failure or pericardial effusion. With contained rupture, a left pleural effusion may be evident. Contrast aortography is the diagnostic procedure of choice and should demonstrate the location of the aortic tear along with delineating the proximal and distal extent of the dissection. Contrast-enhanced CT, MRI, and transesophageal echocardiography are also sensitive examinations and may be useful in certain clinical situations.

Treatment

A. Ascending Dissection: Descending aortic dissection is managed mainly by medical therapy; operation is indicated only for complications of vascular occlusion, expansion, or rupture. The patient is urgently admitted to the ICU, and complete hemodynamic monitoring is initiated. Arterial blood pressure is lowered with a primary vasodilator, most commonly sodium nitroprusside. As a routine, simul-

taneous beta blockade is instituted with esmolol or a longer-acting agent such as atenolol. It should be emphasized that medical therapy in uncomplicated descending dissections is associated with good long-term survival (Figure 19–17), and descending aortic graft replacement is indicated only for specific complications, such as expansion or vascular compromise.

B. Descending Dissection: In contrast, urgent surgical therapy is indicated for ascending aortic dissections, with the goals of segmental Dacron graft replacement of the ascending aorta and resuspension of the aortic valve. The major causes of early death, which are related to ascending aortic complications, are obviated, though continued patency of the distal false lumen is present in 90%. Over the first several postoperative years, the size of the distal aorta is monitored periodically with MRI, and further segmental aortic replacement is required if specific areas dilate.

C. Arch Dissection: Dissection of the aortic arch is a less common problem that until recently has been treated medically. Operative repair is now undertaken routinely and consists of ascending and arch aortic replacement, using deep hypothermia and cir-

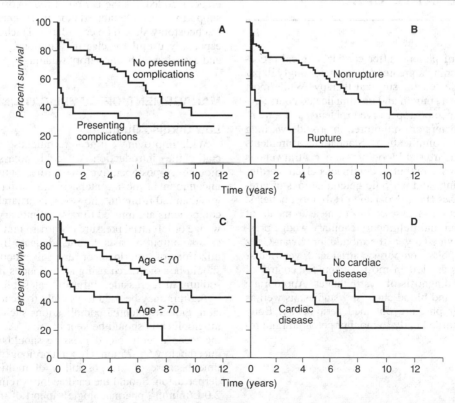

Figure 19–17. Plots of effects of presenting complications of aortic dissection *(A)*, pleural rupture *(B)*, age *(C)*, and cardiac disease *(D)* upon survival in group 1 patients with descending aortic dissection.

culatory arrest. Usually, a "hemi-arch" replacement is fashioned by beveling the distal anastomosis under the arch.

Prognosis

The operative mortality rate for ascending aortic and arch dissections is 10–20%, depending on age and on associated vascular problems such as stroke and bowel ischemia.

Fann JI et al: Preservation of the aortic valve in patients with type A aortic dissection complicated by aortic valvular regurgitation. J Thorac Cardiovasc Surg 1991; 102:62.

Glower DD et al: Comparison of medical and surgical therapy for uncomplicated descending aortic dissection. Circulation 1990;82(Suppl IV):IV-30.

Yun KL et al: Aortic dissection due to transverse arch tear: Is concomitant arch repair warranted? J Thorac Cardiovasc Surg 1991;102:355. (See also discussion on p 368.)

Kouchoukos NT et al: Elective hypothermic cardiopulmonary bypass and circulatory arrest for spinal cord protection during operations on the thoracoabdominal aorta. J Thorac Cardiovasc Surg 1990;99:659.

POSTOPERATIVE CARE

The care of patients after cardiac surgical procedures is assuming a greater role as increasingly ill patients are selected for surgical therapy. While most patients have a smooth and uncomplicated course, 5–10% experience postoperative problems, and a number of parameters are monitored to provide warning of developing complications. Standard measurements include radial arterial blood pressure, central venous pressure, urinary output, a continuous electrocardiographic tracing, and periodic determinations of arterial blood gases (Po_2, Pco_2) and pH. In most patients, cardiac function is assessed with measurements of cardiac output and pulmonary capillary wedge pressure, as provided by a thermodilution Swan-Ganz catheter. Bipolar temporary atrial and ventricular pacing wires are left in most patients for control of heart rate or diagnosis of dysrhythmias. Appropriate hematologic and blood chemistry studies, as well as chest radiographs, are obtained periodically. Body weight is recorded daily to monitor potential fluid retention.

ANTICOAGULATION

Postoperative anticoagulation with aspirin is used routinely for most coronary bypass, valve repair, or bioprosthetic valve replacement procedures. After mechanical valve replacement, all patients should have full warfarin anticoagulation, begun on the fourth postoperative day and continued indefinitely to maintain the prothrombin time ratio at approximately 1½ times control.

VENTILATORY SUPPORT

Following uncomplicated elective operations, most patients can be removed from ventilatory support and extubated within a few hours. After anesthetic recovery, criteria for early extubation include good pulmonary gas exchange, adequate ventilatory mechanics, a clear chest radiograph, absence of dysrhythmias and excess bleeding, and stable cardiac and neurologic function. Occasional patients exhibit prolonged pulmonary dysfunction, requiring controlled ventilation, positive end-expiratory pressure, diuresis, and transiently increased fractional inspired oxygen. If pulmonary infection is suggested by radiographic infiltrates, high white blood cell counts, or positive sputum cultures, appropriate antibiotic coverage is added. As the period of required ventilatory support via an endotracheal tube approaches 2 weeks, tracheostomy should be considered. Tracheostomy is especially useful for clearing pulmonary secretions and assisting with ventilatory weaning.

MANAGEMENT OF COMPLICATIONS

Low Cardiac Output

With improving surgical techniques—and especially the introduction of cold potassium cardioplegia—postoperative low cardiac output is now uncommon in most centers. If the cardiac index is less than 2.0 L/min/m², however, hetastarch or blood components are infused to raise pulmonary capillary wedge or left atrial pressure toward 15 mm Hg. If low cardiac output persists despite adequate filling, optimization of afterload or arterial blood pressure should be considered using a continuous infusion of sodium nitroprusside. Infusion rates of up to 10 µg/kg/min may be used transiently to treat hypertension, though potential complications such as methemoglobinemia should be kept in mind. Additionally, the mean arterial blood pressure should not be reduced below 65–75 mm Hg for a prolonged period of time because of the possibility of multiorgan underperfusion. Should the cardiac index remain below 2.0 L/min/m², pharmacologic support of the circulation is indicated. Dopamine is the first-line catecholamine chosen in most units owing to its simultaneous enhancement of myocardial contractility and renal blood flow. Continuous central venous infusion rates of 5–15 μg/kg/min are employed. For further support, second-line adrenergic agents, with varying degrees of mixed alpha and beta action, are selected, and the specific agent is chosen based on the desired peripheral physiologic effect. Epinephrine is used when mean arterial pressure is low because of vasoconstrictive properties, and dobutamine (a peripheral dilator) is chosen if arterial pressure is high. When circulatory insufficiency persists despite inotropic stimulation, placement of an intra-aortic balloon pump can be lifesaving.

Cardiac Tamponade

Cardiac tamponade can produce postoperative low cardiac output. The characteristic hemodynamic finding is elevated and equalized central venous and pulmonary wedge pressures, usually in the setting of excessive mediastinal bleeding. Low cardiac output is a sine qua non of tamponade. The chest radiograph may demonstrate mediastinal widening or blood collection, but if a significant question of tamponade exists, reoperation should be considered. Excessive mediastinal bleeding in the setting of stable hemodynamics is managed by correction of clotting defects using blood component therapy and by autotransfusion of shed mediastinal blood. Early reoperation is performed if bleeding remains excessive and is required in 2–3% of patients after cardiac procedures.

Atrial Dysrhythmias

Atrial dysrhythmias are common following coronary revascularization. Premature atrial contractions, atrial fibrillation, or atrial flutter reflect postoperative atrial irritability and occur in up to 40% of patients. Prophylactic treatment with beta-blocking agents such as atenolol significantly reduces the incidence of this complication and should be considered in most patients. If atrial tachycardia occurs, control of ventricular response is achieved with intravenous digoxin, followed by attempts at pharmacologic cardioversion using atenolol, procainamide, or calcium channel blocking agents. Rapid atrial pacing or direct-current cardioversion can sometimes be effective in atrial flutter after initial drug therapy. While transient atrial dysrhythmias are usually well tolerated, significant low cardiac output or systemic thromboembolism can occur rarely.

Ventricular Arrhythmias

Ventricular irritability manifested by frequent or multifocal premature ventricular contractions, ventricular tachycardia, or ventricular fibrillation is managed by intravenous lidocaine or procainamide, together with direct-current cardioversion when necessary. Short periods of closed-chest cardiac massage may be necessary, but early cardioversion should be emphasized. Serious ventricular dysrhythmias are usually a manifestation of significant myocardial ischemia, and problems with the quality of coronary revascularization should be considered. Beta-blocking agents, oral procainamide, or amiodarone can be used for long-term management of persistent ventricular ectopy.

Renal Dysfunction

Postoperative renal dysfunction can produce transient elevations in BUN and serum creatinine, progressing to oliguria or total renal shutdown. Ischemic renal injury can occur in the setting of low cardiac output or if excessively low perfusion pressures are encountered on cardiopulmonary bypass or perioperatively. Preexisting renal artery stenosis or arteriolar nephrosclerosis predisposes certain patients to renal hypoperfusion. In the appropriate clinical setting, developing sepsis must also be considered as a cause of worsening renal performance.

Therapy for renal dysfunction consists of maintaining a higher arterial perfusion pressure (especially in patients with preexisting hypertension), low-dose intravenous dopamine infusion, adequate free water hydration, and general support of cardiac output. Fluid balance and potassium intake are monitored carefully to prevent overhydration or hyperkalemia. If dialysis is required, peritoneal lavage is favored, since patient survival associated with a policy of aggressive hemodialysis has been disappointing.

Wound Infection

Sternal wound infection should occur in less than 1% of patients after cardiac surgery. Developing sternal instability, fever, leukocytosis, and wound drainage suggest the diagnosis. Severity varies from a superficial subcutaneous infection with a stable sternum to an isolated sternal infection with no mediastinal involvement to full-blown septic mediastinitis. At the first suspicion of a major wound infection, broad-spectrum antibiotics should be instituted and blood cultures obtained. The combination of diabetes and bilateral internal mammary artery harvesting may predispose some patients to sternal infection. Infections producing sternal disruption are treated with a brief course of open wound care followed by wound closure with pectoral or omental pedicle flaps. The mortality rate using this approach has been reduced to less than 10%, though morbidity remains high.

Myocardial Infarction

With improvements in myocardial protection and coronary grafting techniques, perioperative myocardial infarction should occur in only 1–2% of patients. The cause can vary from subclinical closure of an ungrafted small secondary coronary artery to failure of a major coronary bypass, leading to cardiogenic shock. Therefore, the cause should be carefully evaluated, and most cases produce little clinical morbidity or deterioration of global ventricular function. Conversely, the development of serious ventricular dysfunction or dysrhythmias might suggest early angiography or surgical reintervention if clinically feasible.

REFERENCES

Rankin JS: Hemodynamic management of the surgical patient. In: *American College of Surgeons: Care of the Surgical Patient.* 2 vols. Wilmore DW, Brennan MF, Harken AH (editors). Scientific American, 1988.

The Heart: II. Congenital Diseases   19

Edward D. Verrier, MD

DIAGNOSIS

A congenital heart lesion may produce different degrees of circulatory dysfunction and a wide spectrum of clinical manifestations. The various types of anatomic malformations vary widely, and few produce consistently recognizable sets of symptoms or signs. Many of these lesions change with age—eg, pulmonary stenosis becomes more severe; ventricular septal defect becomes smaller; and vascular resistance in the lungs decreases. Many newborns have obvious symptoms and signs of heart disease; others may have very complex lesions not detected for days to months.

Clearly, the most important feature in the diagnosis is recognition of an abnormal heart sound, murmur, or other symptom referable to the heart, such as feeding difficulty, lack of weight gain, frequent respiratory infections, fatigability, irritability, or cyanosis. Once a clinical abnormality is recognized, the investigation must be pursued until a definitive diagnosis is established.

Chest x-ray and electrocardiography should be done in all cases as part of the initial workup. For additional diagnostic screening and anatomic definition, a more specific noninvasive test such as echocardiography is essential. Two-dimensional color flow Doppler echocardiography has eliminated the need to perform cardiac catheterization on every child with suspected congenital heart disease. In infants particularly, cardiac catheterization may be difficult or hazardous, and electrocardiography has proved to give sufficient diagnostic information on which to base a decision to proceed directly to operation. However, in most cases of suspected congenital heart disease, cardiac catheterization and cineangiocardiography give the most accurate picture of the anatomic and physiologic status of the heart and great vessels. The procedures should be conducted meticulously, since the type (palliative versus corrective) and timing (early versus later) of operation are determined by the results. A finding of murmur with no significant cardiac anomaly is diagnostically useful, since it allows return to normal activity.

MANAGEMENT

Management of most congenital cardiac defects consists of surgical correction. Drugs, diet, and activity regulation are important in many forms of congenital heart disease, but the pediatrician should recognize the severity and type of lesion and recommend a treatment program leading to surgical repair at the optimal time. Careful observation should prevent development of irreversible complications such as pulmonary vascular disease, cerebral thrombosis, or infective endocarditis.

Operative Management

Few congenital heart lesions are completely cured by operation. Suture ligation of a patent ductus arteriosus and patch closure of a small atrial or ventricular septal defect are considered to be curative operations. In general, however, surgery for congenital heart lesions, though physiologically corrective, may not result in total repair or return to a normal status. Subsequent occurrence of dysrhythmias, ventricular dysfunction, and valve leakage prevent these operations from being considered totally corrective. Palliative operations are designed to reduce or increase the pulmonary blood flow; thus, banding of the pulmonary artery in an infant with ventricular septal defect may reduce pulmonary flow and allow the child to grow so that the defect can be closed with a lower operative risk when the child is larger. A shunt procedure to direct more blood to the lungs may be utilized in a child with pulmonary obstruction and some form of intraventricular communication in anticipation of later total correction with less risk. Most cardiac operations require cardiopulmonary bypass, which can be used in infants with about the same risks as in older patients. Thus, many corrective operations are being accomplished in infancy.

Total cardiopulmonary bypass is usually accomplished by draining blood through catheters placed in the right atrium or the venae cavae from the patient, through the heart-lung machine, and back to the patient through a small cannula in the aorta. The blood totally bypasses the heart, allowing cardiac standstill, so that operative repair may be performed within the cardiac chambers.

Hypothermia at the time of cardiopulmonary bypass reduces the rate of flow returning to the patient, since metabolism is lowered when body temperature is reduced. Thus, in order to perform a more precise operative repair, the amount of blood in the field can be reduced by adding hypothermia to the bypass system. In some small infants with lesions such as transposition of the great arteries or atrioventricular canal, or in situations where the entire operation is performed within the atrium, total circulatory arrest—in which the infant is maintained without any perfusion for 30–40 minutes—can be used. In most circumstances, the infant is core-cooled to 16 °C using the heart-lung machine prior to total circulatory arrest. The head is often packed in ice also to augment cerebral cooling. Neurologic sequelae due to total circulatory arrest are infrequent, and a much better surgical repair is achieved. Protection of the heart during operative repair is accomplished by a variety of techniques, including fibrillatory arrest, local or systemic hypothermia, and cold cardioplegic solutions (blood or crystalloid), which cause cardiac standstill usually at temperatures of 10–14 °C.

Postoperative Management

After open heart surgery, most patients are maintained with an endotracheal tube in place and controlled mechanical ventilation for 12–24 hours. Mechanical ventilation reduces tissue oxygen requirements since the effort of breathing is eliminated, though myocardial function may be improved with early extubation. Drainage catheters in the mediastinum for postoperative bleeding are usually removed the following morning. Arterial blood gases and pH are measured by intra-arterial monitoring. In most instances of complex repairs, small venous catheters are left in the major atria or pulmonary artery to accurately measure all major venous and arterial pressure changes.

The most common complication after open heart surgery is postoperative bleeding. This occurs because the patient is heparinized during bypass, and reversal with protamine, though efficient, is not always complete. About 5% of these patients have to be returned to the operating room because of uncontrolled bleeding. Postoperative bleeding is more frequent after repair of cyanotic heart lesions due to a relative lack of coagulation factors with polycythemia.

Problems such as dysrhythmia and poor cardiac performance are not as common after primary congenital defect repair as they are in patients with more severe acquired myocardial disease. Most patients receive antibiotics intravenously while lines are maintained, since denuded areas within the heart and prosthetic materials impose a major hazard of endocarditis or sepsis.

Castaneda AR et al: The neonate with critical congenital heart disease: Repair—a surgical challenge. J Thorac Cardiovasc Surg 1989;98:869.

Morris CD et al: 25-year mortality after surgical repair of congenital heart defect in childhood. A population based cohort study. JAMA 1991;266:3447.

Sam'anek M: Children with congenital heart disease: Probability of natural survival. Pediatr Cardiol 1992;13:152.

OBSTRUCTIVE CONGENITAL HEART LESIONS

Obstructive lesions impede the forward flow of blood and increase ventricular afterloads. In the absence of a ventricular septal defect, an obstructive lesion in the aortic or pulmonary valve causes the proximal ventricle to become hypertrophied. Sudden death is not uncommon in patients with aortic or pulmonary stenosis, and the degree of ventricular hypertrophy is of concern to cardiologists because of the high incidence of dysrhythmias, ischemic changes in the myocardium, and potential permanent muscle damage or replacement by fibrosis.

PULMONARY STENOSIS

Essentials of Diagnosis

- No symptoms in patients with mild or moderately severe lesions.
- Cyanosis and right-sided heart failure in patients with severe lesions.
- High-pitched systolic ejection murmur maximal in the second left interspace. S_2 delayed and soft. Ejection click often present. Increased right ventricular impulse.
- No ejection click and inaudible S_2 in severe cases.

General Considerations

Pulmonary stenosis with intact ventricular septum and a normal aortic root is a relatively common congenital heart lesion that occurs with equal frequency in males and females. Valvular pulmonary stenosis occurs in approximately 10% of patients with congenital heart disease. In most of these patients, the commissures are fused with a flexible tricuspid semilunar valve, producing a dome-like structure with a central opening of varying size (Figure 19–18A). Most patients with pulmonary stenosis have a patent foramen ovale; few have true atrial septal defects. In infants, severe valvular stenosis may be associated with a poorly developed right ventricle and can be an extremely serious condition requiring urgent operation. Isolated infundibular stenosis is extremely rare

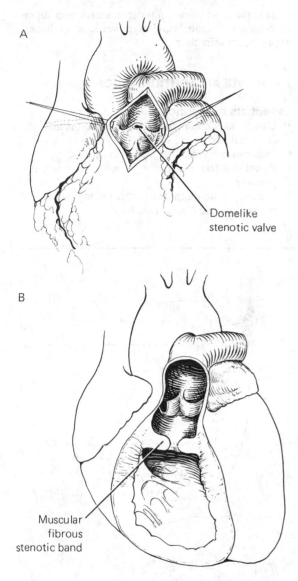

Figure 19–18. Pulmonary stenosis. **A:** Valvular pulmonary stenosis. **B:** Infundibular pulmonary stenosis.

and usually associated with less dramatic clinical findings, since the turbulence across the infundibular area is much less than across the tight stenotic pulmonary valve (Figure 19–18B).

Clinical Findings

Infants with more severe forms of pulmonary stenosis usually feed poorly and may have hypoxic spells. Sudden death has been reported. Older children with pulmonary stenosis and intact ventricular septa usually are asymptomatic and grow normally. A few may complain of fatigue and dyspnea on exertion. When the pulmonary stenosis physiologically

worsens as the child grows, shortness of breath, dizziness, and even angina may occur.

Approximately half of the deaths caused by pulmonary stenosis occur in infants under age 1 year. The remainder may be asymptomatic, but the murmurs of pulmonary stenosis are easily heard and usually do not go undetected. Complete evaluation is required; if the gradient between the right ventricle and the pulmonary artery is approximately 50 mm Hg, repair is usually recommended. The disease progresses slowly, and by adulthood it may result in a calcific pulmonary valve, which may still have a significant gradient—due to the stiffness of the valve—even though commissural fusion is not present.

Treatment

Infants with severe right ventricular failure or cyanotic spells require early operation. In critically ill neonates, prostaglandins (PGE_1) have proved effective in maintaining pulmonary blood flow through the ductus arteriosus until the pulmonary valve obstruction is relieved. The valve can be opened or can be excised without cardiopulmonary bypass using inflow occlusion (closed method), but most surgeons prefer open methods. The patient is placed on cardiopulmonary bypass, the valve is carefully inspected through the pulmonary artery, pulmonary valvotomy is done, and the patent foramen is closed. If the right ventricle is not fully developed and cannot sustain total circulation, the patent foramen is left open and a systemic to pulmonary shunt is created. It is hoped that relief of pulmonary stenosis will allow the ventricle to develop in a more normal fashion, so that the shunt can be obliterated and the patent foramen closed in about a year.

Most of these operations are performed through the pulmonary artery, with the valve opened by incising the commissures. In a few cases, marked infundibular hypertrophy may coexist, and this can usually be resected without difficulty through the pulmonary arteriotomy. If a hypoplastic pulmonary annulus is present—ie, if the valve is stenotic as well as the annulus—a patch should be placed across the annulus to guarantee right ventricular emptying into the pulmonary artery.

Percutaneous transventricular or transpulmonary artery balloon pulmonary valvuloplasty has recently been used more frequently with success for isolated pulmonary valve stenosis.

Prognosis

The hospital death rate for operations to correct pulmonary stenosis is 1–3%. The prognosis is generally good, though restenosis occurs in about 10% of patients. Restenosis may occur earlier after balloon valvuloplasty than after open surgical techniques. Right ventricular hypertrophy regresses after relief of the valvular stenosis.

Caspi J et al: Management of critical pulmonary stenosis in the balloon valvotomy era. Ann Thorac Surg 1990; 49:273.

O'Conner BK et al: Intermediate-term outcome after pulmonary balloon valvuloplasty: Comparison with a matched surgical control group. J Am Coll Cardiol 1992;20:169.

Rao PS: Transcatheter treatment of pulmonary outflow tract obstruction: A review. Prog Cardiovasc Dis 1992;35: 119.

AORTIC STENOSIS

Four types of congenital aortic stenosis are generally recognized (Figure 19–19). Valvular aortic stenosis is the most common type; subaortic and supravalvular aortic stenosis and asymmetric septal hypertrophy occur infrequently.

1. VALVULAR AORTIC STENOSIS

Essentials of Diagnosis

- Usually asymptomatic in children; angina and syncope indicate severe stenosis.
- May cause severe heart failure in infants.
- Prominent left ventricular impulse; narrow pulse pressure.
- Harsh systolic murmur and thrill along left sternal border; systolic ejection click.

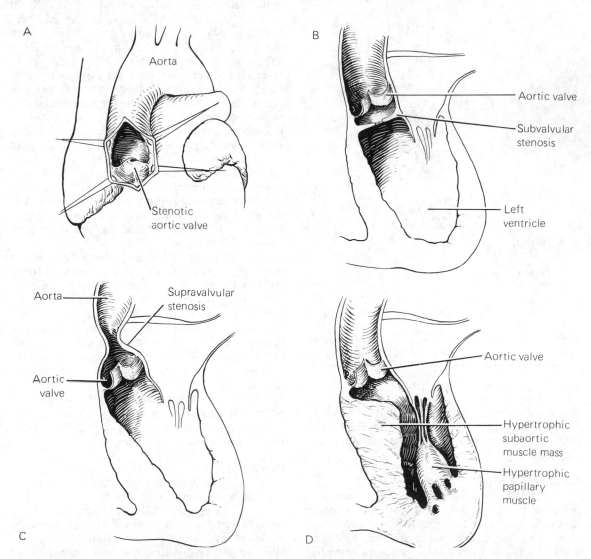

Figure 19–19. Types of congenital aortic stenosis. **A:** Valvular aortic stenosis. **B:** Subaortic stenosis (discrete fibrous band). **C:** Supravalvular aortic stenosis. **D:** Idiopathic hypertrophic subaortic stenosis.

General Considerations

Valvular aortic stenosis occurs predominantly in males, and in approximately 20% of the patients it is associated with other congenital heart defects. The aortic leaflets are often thickened, fibrotic, and malformed (Figure 19–19A). Three commissures can often be found, but frequently there are only two functioning aortic commissures. In the so-called bicuspid valve, the leaflets cannot completely move out of the way during systolic ejection, since they are attached 180 degrees across the diameter of the aorta. Thus, even though one may open the commissures completely, the geometric configuration of the leaflets does not permit adequate relief of stenosis. Newborns with valvular aortic stenosis often have very poor left ventricular function because of subendocardial ischemia and endocardial fibroelastosis. In many of these patients, the aorta and aortic annulus are small.

Clinical Findings

Most children with congenital valvular aortic stenosis are asymptomatic and grow normally. A few patients with severe stenosis develop dyspnea, angina, or syncope with effort. Newborns with aortic stenosis have severe heart failure and cyanosis and associated respiratory distress.

A harsh basilar systolic murmur with thrill along the left sternal border is a common finding. The murmur may at times be inaudible because of heart failure and low cardiac output. In most cases, chest x-rays are normal or show only left ventricular hypertrophy. The ascending aorta may be dilated. In the infant, the cardiac silhouette is usually large, and pulmonary venous congestion is present. After complete cardiovascular evaluation, operation is performed in children with symptoms of syncope, electrocardiographic changes due to ischemia, or pressure gradients of 50 mm Hg or greater between the left ventricle and ascending aorta. In many patients, the pressure gradient is not as important as the clinical symptoms or a change in the ECG. Sudden death has occurred in children with valvular aortic stenosis.

Treatment

In general, the first operation used is aortic valve commissurotomy (opening of the fused commissures). This can be accomplished by inflow occlusion (closed method) but usually is done with cardiopulmonary bypass and protection of the heart while the aorta is open and the aortic valve is inspected. Partial relief of aortic stenosis is often sufficient to significantly reduce the gradient. Balloon angioplasty of the stenotic aortic valve, either percutaneously or through the left ventricle on bypass, may be possible in some forms of congenital aortic stenosis. Unless aortic regurgitation is an associated feature, it is rarely necessary to insert a prosthesis in a child. Many surgical options are available for the older child or young adult requiring valve replacement, including bioprostheses (xenograft porcine-stented, xenograft pericardial-stented, aortic homografts, or pulmonary autografts [Ross procedure]) or mechanical prostheses (ball valve, monocusp, bileaflet)

Prognosis

In general, even after surgical correction, children with congenital aortic valve disease will have progressive thickening and, ultimately, calcification of the valve. The operation is not curative, and, although the death rate is fairly low, repeat operations can be anticipated. Most patients will someday require aortic valve replacement. Thus, follow-up is necessary to determine the rate and degree of restenosis if commissurotomy is the initial approach.

2. SUBAORTIC STENOSIS

Subaortic stenosis is usually due to a discrete fibromuscular ring of tissue located beneath the aortic valve. This causes a pressure difference between the body of the left ventricle and the aortic valve. The lesion is seldom seen in infants, and the symptoms and findings are similar to those observed in patients with valvular aortic stenosis. The turbulence from the subaortic membrane may cause thickening and damage to the aortic leaflets, leading to aortic valve insufficiency.

Patients with the discrete fibromuscular membrane have a very good prognosis, since operative resection of the membrane is possible and recurrence is uncommon. A diffuse type of subvalvular stenosis is sometimes seen—so-called tubular, or tunnel, type of left ventricular outflow tract obstruction—in which the entire left ventricular outflow tract is narrowed with no discrete area of obstruction. These patients have a more guarded prognosis, and one of two operative approaches is usually indicated: (1) a procedure in which the entire left ventricular outflow tract is enlarged with a prosthetic patch (Dacron) and aortic valve (Konno procedure); or (2) placement of a tubular graft and valve between the apex of the left ventricle and the descending aorta (apicoaortic conduit). This latter procedure is mostly of historical or salvage interest.

3. SUPRAVALVULAR AORTIC STENOSIS

In most patients, supravalvular aortic stenosis is an isolated, discrete lesion located just above the aortic valve that is due either to an hourglass constriction of the ascending aorta or to the presence of a thick, intraluminal fibromuscular ridge. Less commonly, supravalvular stenosis is found extending up to the transverse arch and involving its branches. In many cases, the proximal aorta between valve and stenosis can be very dilated. Approximately 20% of children with supravalvular aortic stenosis have a familial association characterized by mental retardation, "elfin facies," strabismus, dental anomalies, hypercalcemia, and peripheral pulmonary stenosis.

Symptoms and physical findings are similar to those of other forms of aortic stenosis. Operative repair for the common types of supravalvular stenosis consists of placing a wide prosthetic patch across the area of stenosis. The mortality rate of this operation is low, and the results are generally excellent.

4. ASYMMETRIC SEPTAL HYPERTROPHY

This genetically transmitted disease of cardiac muscle features disproportionate thickening of the ventricular septum when compared to the ventricular free wall. The myocardial sarcomeres are hypertrophied and arranged in a bizarre pattern. The asymmetric muscle mass may or may not cause obstruction of the left ventricular outflow tract (Figure 19–19D). Symptomatic patients nearly always have some degree of obstruction during systole. The severity of this obstruction increases during systole and is proportionate to the volume of the left ventricular cavity, the force of ventricular contraction, and the cross-sectional area of the left ventricular outflow tract during systole. Exercise or various pharmacologic agents such as digitalis, isoproterenol, epinephrine, and nitroglycerin may alter these relationships and change the degree of obstruction. The common symptoms are chronic fatigue, episodes of syncope and angina, and dyspnea on exertion.

This disease is quite variable, and the natural history is not entirely predictable. Some patients improve symptomatically with chronic beta-blockade therapy (propranolol); in other patients in whom discrete gradients can be identified between the body of the left ventricle and the aorta, operative repair by incising a wide or deep trough of this muscle bundle has been helpful. Left bundle branch block may be a complication of the operation, and complete relief of obstruction often cannot be accomplished because of diffusely diseased muscle. The other operative approach used either alone or in combination with myomectomy is mitral valve replacement. Valve replacement eliminates systolic anterior motion (SAM) of the anterior leaflet of the mitral valve, which accentuates the outflow tract obstruction.

Balaji S et al: Aortic valvotomy for critical aortic stenosis in neonates and infants aged less than one year. Br Heart J 1989;358.

Brown JW et al: Surgical spectrum of aortic stenosis in children: A thirty-year experience with 257 children. Ann Thorac Surg 1988;45:393.

Fleming WH, Sarafian LB: Aortic valve replacement with concomitant aortoventriculoplasty in children and young adults: Long term followup. Ann Thorac Surg 1987;43:575.

Gundry SR, Behrendt DM: Prognostic factors in valvotomy for critical aortic stenosis in infancy. J Thorac Cardiovasc Surg 1986;92:747.

Hammon JW et al: Predictors of operative mortality in critical valvular stenosis presenting in infancy. Ann Thorac Surg 1988;45:537.

Johnson RG et al: Reoperation in congenital aortic stenosis. Ann Thorac Surg 1985;40:156.

Lavee J et al: Myectomy versus myotomy as an adjunct to membranectomy in the surgical repair of discrete and tunnel subaortic stenosis. J Thorac Cardiovasc Surg 1986;92:944.

Messina LM et al: Successful aortic valvotomy for severe congenital valvular aortic stenosis in newborn infants. J Thorac Cardiovasc Surg 1984;88:92.

Penkoske PA et al: Subaortic stenosis in childhood: Frequency of associated anomalies and surgical options. J Thorac Cardiovasc Surg 1989;98:852.

Schaffer MS et al: Aortoventriculoplasty in children. J Thorac Cardiovasc Surg 1986;92:391. Stewart JR et al: Reappraisal of localized resection for subvalvular aortic stenosis. Ann Thorac Surg 1990;50:197.

Sweeney MS et al: Apicoaortic conduits for complex left ventricular outflow obstruction: 10 year experience. Ann Thorac Surg 1986;42:609.

Treter KJ et al: Long-term evaluation of aortic valvotomy for congenital aortic stenosis. Ann Surg 1987;206:496.

Wren C et al: Percutaneous balloon dilatation of aortic valve stenosis in neonates and infants. Br Heart J 1987;58:608.

Zeevi B et al: Neonatal critical valvular aortic stenosis: A comparison of surgical and balloon dilation therapy. Circulation 1989;80:831.

COARCTATION OF THE AORTA

Essentials of Diagnosis

- Infants may have severe heart failure; children are usually asymptomatic.
- Absent or weak femoral pulses.
- Systolic pressure higher in upper extremities than in lower extremities; diastolic pressures are similar.
- Harsh systolic murmur heard in the back.

General Considerations

Coarctation of the aorta is a relatively common congenital lesion that occurs twice as frequently in males as in females. Ninety-eight percent of all aortic coarctations are located at or near the aortic isthmus (the segment of aorta adjacent to the ligamentum arteriosum or ductus arteriosus). In approximately 40% of these patients, the aortic valve is bicuspid. The aortic constriction is usually well localized and produced by both external narrowing and an intraluminal membrane. The coarctation causes systolic and diastolic hypertension in the proximal aorta and upper extremities and stimulates the development of large collateral vessels that connect branches of the proximal aorta and the subclavian arteries to arteries originating from the aorta below the level of the coarctation. In most patients, blood flow to the lower body is not reduced, but pulse pressure distal to the aortic coarctation is decreased. The left ventricular work load is increased.

Clinical Findings

The hemodynamic consequences of coarctation of the aorta depend on the rate of ductus arteriosus closure, the severity of obstruction, the development of collaterals, and the presence and severity of associated anomalies. There appear to be two distinct clinical presentations: patients who present in early infancy and those who present in later childhood. Infants with coarctation may have severe congestive heart failure. Over half of these infants have an associated cardiac lesion such as patent ductus arteriosus, ventricular septal defect, or endocardial cushion defect. Some infants may actually be ductus-dependent for lower body blood flow; therefore, the ductus must be kept open with prostaglandin E until correction can be achieved. Rare forms of coarctation such as hypoplasia of the transverse arch or ascending aorta may also been seen in this group.

Infants with severe coarctation require immediate diagnosis and operative correction. The death rate in the first year of life without operation is approximately 75%. Operative repair in infancy can be accomplished with approximately a 5% death rate.

Many older children with coarctation are asymptomatic and well-developed. Complaints of headache, pains in the calves when running, or frequent nosebleeds are common. Most of these children have hypertension in the upper extremities, and many have electrocardiographic evidence of left ventricular hypertrophy.

Treatment

Operative repair of the aortic coarctation is recommended for nearly all patients. It is thought that the younger the patient when repair is done, the less serious the degree of hypertension. Options for coarctation repair include the following: (1) resection with end-to-end anastomosis, (2) subclavian flap or subclavian advancement aortoplasty, (3) patch aortoplasty with polytetrafluoroethylene (Gore-Tex) or Dacron, and (4) percutaneous balloon dilation. Controversy continues as to the optimal surgical approach, but any one of the techniques may be best depending on anatomy and patient stability.

Resection of the coarctation segment with end-to-end anastomosis may be done in infants but is usually reserved for older children with discrete coarctations. Some form of patch aortoplasty is preferred in infants. The left subclavian artery can be sacrificed, opened longitudinally, and placed over the top of the coarcted segment as a large patch. If a membrane is present within the aorta, it is carefully excised and the ductus is ligated. This technique has the advantage of using autogenous tissue, so that subsequent growth is not impaired, but it has the disadvantages of a fairly high recurrence rate and sacrifice of the subclavian artery.

The second aortoplasty technique is to patch the aorta with a synthetic material such as polytetrafluoroethylene or Dacron. With this technique, the left subclavian artery is not sacrificed and the prosthetic patch can be made somewhat larger then the aortic lumen, so that growth of the posterior wall of the aorta can be anticipated. Aneurysms at the patch remain a long-term concern. All three techniques continue to be commonly used, and controversy continues over which one is superior. With the reduced death rate of coarctation correction, an extensive trial of medical management is not indicated.

Prognosis

The results of coarctation repair have been good. Residual hypertension remains a problem, though operative repair makes hypertension more easily controllable by medication. The blood pressure may remain elevated, and the question of whether latent hypertension may be present years after resection of the coarctation is still unresolved.

The operative death rate is low (5–15%) even in infants, and the deaths that do occur are usually related to associated congenital heart lesions. Paraplegia or paraparesis is a rare but catastrophic complication probably related to the adequacy of collateral circulation and the duration of aortic cross-clamping during construction of the anastomosis. Necrotizing arteritis of mesenteric vessels has been recognized, as patients frequently develop abdominal pain 1–2 days after coarctation resection. Arteritis is thought to be due to increased pulse pressure. Sympatholytic drugs that lower blood pressure are indicated for patients with persistent hypertension in the early postoperative period or in those who develop abdominal pain.

Amato JJ et al: Role of extended aortoplasty related to the definition of coarctation of the aorta. Ann Thorac Surg 1991;52:615.

Dietl CA et al: Risk of recoarctation in neonates and infants after repair with patch aortoplasty, subclavian flap, and combination resection-flap procedure. J Thorac Cardiovasc Surg 1992;103:724.

Johnson MC et al: Repair of coarctation of the aorta in infancy: comparison of surgical and balloon angioplasty. Am Heart J 1993;125:464.

Kopf GS et al: Repair of aortic coarctation in the first three months of life: Immediate and long term results. Ann Thorac Surg 1986;41:425.

Korfer R et al: Early and late results after resection and end-to-end anastomosis of coarctation of the thoracic aorta in early infancy. J Thorac Cardiovasc Surg 1985;89:616.

Meier MA et al: A new technique for repair of aortic coarctation: Subclavian flap aortoplasty with preservation of arterial blood flow to the left arm. J Thorac Cardiovasc Surg 1986;92:1005.

Sharma BK et al: Coarctation repair in neonates with subclavian-sparing advancement flap. Ann Thorac Surg 1992;54:137.

Tynan M et al: Balloon angioplasty for the treatment of native coarctation: Results of Valvuloplasty and Angioplasty of Congenital Anomalies Registry. Am J Cardiol 1990;65:790.

INTERRUPTED AORTIC ARCH

Absence of the aortic arch distal to the left subclavian artery (type A, 50%), between the left carotid and left subclavian artery (type B, 45%), or between the innominate and left carotid arteries (type C, 5%) is an uncommon but severe form of developmental obstruction within the aorta. The distal aorta receives blood from the patent ductus that may constrict shortly after birth and thus limit flow to the lower extremities. This lesion is almost always accompanied by other intracardiac anomalies such as ventricular septal defect, truncus arteriosus, or endocardial cushion defect. Most of these patients are symptomatic in the first few days of life, require prostaglandin E for hemodynamic stabilization, and require early operation for correction. Operative repair may be done in one or more stages.

Fowler BN et al: Interruption of the aortic arch: Experience in 17 infants. Ann Thorac Surg 1984;37:28.

Galla JD et al: Primary reconstruction of interrupted aortic arch by total aortic outflow obstruction. J Thorac Cardiovasc Surg 1986;91:200.

Ilbawi MN et al: Surgical management of patients with interrupted aortic arch and severe subaortic stenosis. Ann Thorac Surg 1988;45:174.

Hammon JW et al: Repair of interrupted aortic arch and associated malformations in infancy: Indications for complete or partial repair. Ann Thorac Surg 1986;42:17.

Scott WA et al: Repair of interrupted aortic arch in infancy. J Thorac Cardiovasc Surg 1988;96:564.

Sell JE et al: The results of a surgical program for interrupted aortic arch. J Thorac Cardiovasc Surg 1988; 96:864.

Turley K, Yee ES, Ebert PA: The total repair of interrupted arch complex in infants: The anterior approach. Circulation 1984;70(3-Part 2):I-16.

AORTIC ATRESIA-HYPOPLASTIC LEFT HEART SYNDROME

Aortic valve atresia commonly occurs along with hypoplasia of the ascending aorta and hypoplasia or atresia of the left ventricle and associated mitral valve. The coronary arteries arise from the base of the hypoplastic ascending aorta. Most of these patients require a large patent ductus and an atrial septal defect to sustain life. Corrective operations are usually not possible in this group of patients, since the hypoplastic ascending aorta rarely grows. In the early 1980s, a complex two-stage palliative procedure was developed by Norwood and colleagues. An initial shunt procedure with reconstruction of the ascending aorta is followed by a Fontan-type physiology procedure in which the systemic venous flow is channeled from the right atrium to the pulmonary arteries and the systemic arterial flow is channeled through the right ventricle to the aorta. After a substantial learning curve by most surgeons attempting this procedure, more recent results have included many children now reaching the second stage of reconstruction. In addition, orthotopic cardiac transplantation has been done successfully for this complex congenital lesion in infancy. The short- and long-term results of both the Norwood procedure and neonatal transplantation are presently being investigated closely.

Austin EH et al: Aortic atresia with normal left ventricle. J Thorac Cardiovasc Surg 1989;97:392.

Bailey LL et al: Hypoplastic left heart syndrome. Pediatr Clin North Am 1990;37:137.

Helton JG et al: Analysis of potential anatomic or physiologic determinants of outcome of palliative surgery for hypoplastic left heart syndrome. Circulation 1986;74 (Suppl I):70.

Jonas RA: Intermediate procedures after first stage Norwood operation facilitate subsequent repair. Ann Thorac Surg 1991;52:696.

Mavroudis CA et al: Infant orthotopic cardiac transplantation. J Thorac Cardiovasc Surg 1988;96:912.

Norwood WI et al: Fontan procedure for hypoplastic heart syndrome. Ann Thorac Surg 1992;54:1025.

Pigott JD et al: Palliative reconstructive surgery for hypoplastic left heart syndrome. Ann Thorac Surg 1988;45: 122.

Starnes VA et al: Current approach to hypoplastic heart syndrome: Palliation, transplantation, or both? J Thorac Cardiovasc Surg 1992;104:189.

MITRAL ATRESIA & STENOSIS

Congenital mitral stenosis or atresia is often associated with hypoplasia of the left heart and aorta. Patients who have mitral atresia with a normal aortic valve often have a hypoplastic left ventricle that communicates with a large right ventricle through a ventricular septal defect. Other anomalies such as atrial septal defect are commonly present. Infants with mitral atresia and normal aortic valves seldom survive beyond infancy. In some forms of single ventricle, the mitral valve is atretic, and these patients have a longer life expectancy. Direct surgical corrections are rarely attempted in infancy.

Kadoba K et al: Mitral valve replacement in the first year of life. J Thorac Cardiovasc Surg 1990;100:762.

Zweng TN et al: Mitral valve replacement in the first 5 years of life. Ann Thorac Surg 1989;48:444.

COR TRIATRIATUM

In this rare anomaly, the pulmonary veins enter a small accessory left atrial chamber that communicates with the normal-sized true left atrium through a small opening. Pulmonary venous hypertension causes pulmonary congestion and may eventually result in pulmonary vascular disease. Patients are frequently symptomatic in infancy, with signs of pulmonary edema. Operation is usually successful, since the narrowed membrane separating the two atrial chambers can be excised and a patch used to enlarge the lateral wall of the left atrium and the chamber collecting the pulmonary veins.

Salomone G et al: Cor triatriatum: Clinical presentation and operative results. J Thorac Cardiovasc Surg 1991;101: 1088.

VALVE REPLACEMENT IN CHILDREN

Valve replacement may be required in children for a number of congenital and acquired problems. Both valvular stenotic lesions such as aortic stenosis or pulmonary stenosis and regurgitant lesions such as truncal valve insufficiency or mitral insufficiency with atrioventricular canal may not be amenable to reconstructive techniques and may therefore require valve replacement. Both mechanical and bioprosthetic valves have been used successfully in children, though there may be accelerated calcification and degeneration of bioprosthetic valves. Selected series have had good results with both warfarin and aspirin anticoagulation protocols. Autograft and homograft valve replacements have received recent renewed attention due to improved durability compared with stented xenografts.

Ahie F et al: Late results of mitral valve replacement with the Bjork-Shiley prosthesis in children under 16 years of age. J Thorac Cardiovasc Surg 1986;91:754.
Borkon AM et al: Five year follow-up after valve replacement with the Saint Jude medical valve in infants and children. Circulation 1987;74(Suppl 1):110.
Verrier ED et al: Aspirin anticoagulation in children with mechanical aortic valves. J Thorac Cardiovasc Surg 1986;92:1013.

CONGENITAL HEART LESIONS THAT INCREASE PULMONARY ARTERIAL BLOOD FLOW

Approximately 50% of all congenital heart lesions shunt blood from the systemic arterial circulation into the pulmonary circulation (left-to-right shunt). The most common lesions in this group are patent ductus arteriosus and defects of the atrial septum, atrioventricular canal, and ventricular septum. Rare lesions include ruptured sinus of Valsalva, aortopulmonary window, truncus arteriosus, some types of transposition of the great vessels, double outlet right ventricle, and other more complex lesions.

Because compliance of the thick-walled left ventricle is less than that of the right ventricle and because systemic vascular resistance is normal., about ten times higher than pulmonary vascular resistance, pressures in the left heart chambers and systemic arteries are higher than corresponding pressures in the right heart and pulmonary arteries. These higher pressures cause some of the oxygenated blood in the left heart and systemic arteries to shunt through abnormal anatomic communications and to recirculate through the lungs without passing through systemic capillaries. The excessive pulmonary circulation causes pulmonary vascular congestion, resulting in frequent respiratory infections, and places an additional burden on the involved ventricle (the right ventricle in atrial septal defects; the left ventricle in patent ductus arteriosus; and both ventricles in atrioventricular canal and ventricular septal defects). The increased "volume load," or "preload," increases the diastolic volume of the involved ventricle. As the ventricle dilates, end-diastolic pressure increases; eventually, the ventricle may fail (ie, at the point at which an increase in ventricular volume at end-diastole no longer causes an increase in ventricular stroke volume).

Increased pulmonary blood flow alone gradually increases pulmonary arterial blood pressure. Although pulmonary vessels are very distensible (and therefore compliant), pulmonary arterial pressure in the normal lung approximately doubles when pulmonary blood flow triples. Elevation of left atrial pressure from excessive flow or increased left ventricular end-diastolic pressure increases pulmonary arterial pressure, interstitial lung water, and probably pulmonary vascular resistance. If pulmonary arterioles also constrict in response to the increased blood flow, pulmonary vascular resistance increases (hyperkinetic pulmonary hypertension), and pulmonary arterial pressure may increase further unless flow decreases. Pulmonary vasoconstriction can be reversed by inhalation of oxygen or intravenous tolazoline, and this test is used to differentiate hyperkinetic pulmonary hypertension from fixed pulmonary vascular disease.

In some patients, increased pulmonary blood flow and increased pulmonary arterial pressure eventually cause muscular hypertrophy of the media of pulmonary arterioles (stage 1), proliferation of intima (stage 2), and, eventually, hyalinization and fibrosis of the media and adventitia (stage 3). These morphologic changes, termed pulmonary vascular disease, are acquired, but they are more likely to occur in congenital lesions producing both high pulmonary arterial pressure and large flows (ventricular septal defect, complete atrioventricular canal, truncus arteriosus) than in those producing increased pulmonary blood flow only (atrial septal defect, total anomalous pulmonary venous connection). Pulmonary venous hypertension and chronic hypoxemia from residence at high altitudes also favor the development of pulmonary vascular disease. As the cross-sectional area of the pulmonary vascular bed decreases as a result of the morphologic changes, pulmonary vascular resistance increases, and the ratio of pulmonary vascular resistance to systemic vascular resistance increases. The amount of blood shunted from left to right decreases. When pulmonary vascular resistance equals or exceeds systemic vascular resistance, left-to-right blood flow across the lesion ceases or reverses. In Eisenmenger's syndrome, obstruction of the pulmonary vasculature reduces pulmonary blood flow and causes blood to shunt from right to left. Patients who have advanced pulmonary vascular disease (stage 3) and balanced or reversed shunts (Eisenmenger's syndrome) cannot be helped by operation other than lung or heart-lung transplantation.

Pulmonary arterial banding is a palliative operation designed to reduce pulmonary arterial blood flow by placing an anatomically fixed resistance to blood flow across the lungs (Figure 19–20). The band constricts the main pulmonary artery downstream to the valve and adds a resistance in series to the vascular resistance of the lung. Ideally, total resistance of the band and the lungs should equal systemic vascular resistance. If vascular resistance in the lungs is already high, only a small resistance can be added by the band. Because of dynamic changes in cardiac output, pressures, and resistances within the circulation, addition of a fixed resistance (the band) cannot produce balanced pulmonary and systemic flows under all physiologic conditions. However, a good band can reduce pulmonary arterial blood flow sufficiently to alleviate ventricular failure and prevent rapid progression of pulmonary vascular disease. Unfortunately, preexisting pulmonary vascular disease may not regress after banding. Pulmonary artery banding is only palliative and is usually used only in very small infants when the risk of definitive repair is too high or for conditions for which no surgical correction is possible.

Horowitz MD et al: Pulmonary arterial binding: Analysis of a 25 year experience. Ann Thorac Surg 1989;48:444.
Kron IL: Pulmonary artery banding revisited. Ann Surg 1989;209:642.
Solis E et al: Percutaneously adjustable pulmonary artery band. Ann Thorac Surg 1986;41:65.

ATRIAL SEPTAL DEFECT, OSTIUM SECUNDUM TYPE

Essentials of Diagnosis
- Acyanotic, asymptomatic.
- Right ventricular lift.
- S_2 widely split and fixed.
- Grade 1–3/6 pulmonary systolic ejection murmur.
- Diastolic flow murmur at the lower left sternal border.

General Considerations
Ostium secundum defects occur in the region of the fossa ovalis and may be single or multiple. Secundum defects are the commonest and, usually, the largest of the atrial defects. Secundum defects high in the intra-atrial septum, often associated with partial anomalous pulmonary venous return, are referred to as sinus venosus defects. Anomalous venous returns associated with an atrial defect are really more of a physiologic consideration than an anatomic one at the time of surgical repair. The lateral wall of the atrial septum is often missing, and it is difficult to say whether the right pulmonary veins actually anatomically enter the right or left atrium. A patch is used in the repair of most of these atrial defects; it can be positioned so that the veins are not a major factor (Figure 19–21).

Heart failure from uncomplicated ostium secundum defects may occur in young children but is less common in adults. Pulmonary vascular disease is also rare, but atrial dysrhythmias are noted with increasing age. The average life expectancy in patients with untreated atrial septal defects is reduced because of right ventricular failure, dysrhythmias, and occasionally pulmonary vascular disease.

Treatment
Surgical closure is indicated for almost all ostium secundum defects. The death rate is quite low, and

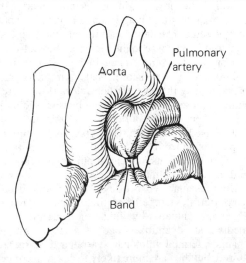

Figure 19–20. Pulmonary arterial banding.

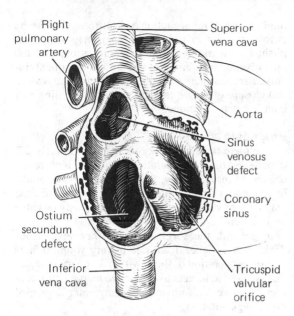

Figure 19–21. Sinus venosus and ostium secundum defects in the atrial septum as viewed from the opened right atrium.

Right pulmonary artery

Superior vena cava

Aorta

Sinus venosus defect

Coronary sinus

Ostium secundum defect

Inferior vena cava

Tricuspid valvular orifice

even small defects have the danger of paradoxic embolism or infective endocarditis. Thus, operative repair is recommended in almost all patients irrespective of the size of the shunts. A patch of pericardium, felt (Teflon), polytetrafluoroethylene (Gore-Tex), or Dacron is usually used for closure. The prognosis after operation is excellent.

Gustafson RA et al: Partial anomalous pulmonary venous connection to the right side of the heart. J Thorac Cardiovasc Surg 1989;43:861.

Murphy JG et al: Long-term outcome after repair of isolated atrial septal defect: Follow-up at 27–32 years. N Engl J Med 1990;323:1645.

Verrier ED: Secundum atrial defects. In: *Current Therapy in Cardiothoracic Surgery,* vol 1. Grillo HC et al (editors). Bryan Decker, 1989.

ATRIAL SEPTAL DEFECT, OSTIUM PRIMUM TYPE

Essentials of Diagnosis

- Acyanotic; asymptomatic, or dyspnea on exertion.
- Fixed, widely split second sound.
- Apical systolic murmur (often).
- ECG shows left axis deviation; QRS frontal vector is counterclockwise.

General Considerations

Ostium primum defects are part of a group of lesions that occur during development of the atrioventricular canal. These defects are occasionally called

incomplete atrioventricular canal and are located low in the atrial septum, adjacent to the coronary sinus and the orifice of the tricuspid valve. The aortic (anterior) leaflet of the mitral valve is usually cleft, and in occasional cases the septal leaflet of the tricuspid valve is also cleft. Most patients are asymptomatic, though mitral regurgitation may develop, and signs of heart failure are more common in ostium primum than in ostium secundum defects. Diagnosis is usually suggested by the ECG, which is characteristically abnormal in this lesion: the mean QRS axis is shifted to the left usually 0–60 degrees. The findings are suggestive but not pathognomonic of ostium primum defect.

Treatment

Surgical closure is usually recommended. When mitral regurgitation is present, the cleft in the mitral valve should be approximated and an attempt made to reduce the amount of regurgitation. Occasionally an annuloplasty may be necessary to reduce the valve orifice size. If no mitral regurgitation is present, the valve may be left alone and the ostial defect closed with a pericardium, polytetrafluoroethylene (Gore-Tex), felt (Teflon), or Dacron patch.

Prognosis

The operative death rate should be less than 2%. The most worrisome complication is injury to the conduction system during repair. The long-term prognosis depends on the growth and development of the mitral valve and whether mitral regurgitation will occur later in life.

King RM et al: Prognostic factors and surgical treatment of partial atrioventricular canal. Circulation 1986;74(Suppl 1):42.

Pillai R et al: Ostium primum atrioventricular septal defect: An anatomical and surgical review. Ann Thorac Surg 1986;41:458.

COMPLETE ATRIOVENTRICULAR CANAL

Essentials of Diagnosis

- Heart failure common in infancy.
- Cardiomegaly, blowing pansystolic murmur, other variable murmurs.
- Loud S_2 with fixed splitting.
- ECG shows left axis deviation and counterclockwise frontal QRS vector loop.

General Considerations

The atrioventricular canal defect is caused by deficiencies of both atrial and ventricular septal cushions and abnormalities of the mitral and tricuspid valves. In partial atrioventricular canal defects, the ventricular septum is formed and the atrioventricular valves may attach directly to the top of the ventricular septum, so that there is no communication beneath the atrioventricular valves between the right and left ventricles. In the complete form, there is a deficiency of mitral and tricuspid leaflet tissue, and the leaflets are not attached directly to the ventricular septa, so that a large defect is located between the top of the ventricular septum and the common leaflets of the mitral and tricuspid valves (Figure 19–22). The common physiologic abnormalities are shunting of blood at the ventricular level and at the atrial level, very often insufficiency of the mitral valve, and less often insufficiency of the tricuspid valve.

Clinical Findings

Many patients develop severe heart failure in early infancy and require early diagnosis and treatment. The cineangiogram usually shows the characteristic "gooseneck" deformity of the mitral valve and left ventricular outflow tract. Because of the large pulmonary shunt and mitral insufficiency, pulmonary vascular disease may develop early in childhood. Partial and complete atrioventricular canal defects frequently accompany Down's syndrome.

Treatment

Surgical correction should be undertaken early, before the development of severe congestive heart failure or pulmonary vascular disease. The success of operative repair usually depends on the amount of atrioventricular valve tissue present. In children with minimal mitral regurgitation or well-formed common atrioventricular valve leaflets, repair may be accomplished with minimal mitral regurgitation, and the operative results are good. Surgical treatment involves reconstruction of the atrioventricular valves and closure of the septal defects by either a single or double patch technique.

Prognosis

Complete heart block occurs in approximately 5% of patients surviving operation. Many will have residual mitral insufficiency, and those who reach adulthood without developing pulmonary vascular disease may require subsequent mitral valvuloplasty or valve replacement.

In general, the surgical success rate approaches 85%, with a higher death rate in very young infants requiring operation or those with pulmonary vascular disease. These infants usually have marked atrioventricular valve malformation and a greater degree of mitral regurgitation.

Anderson RH et al: Of clefts, commissures, and things. J Thorac Cardiovasc Surg 1985;90:605.

Ashraf MH et al: Atrioventricular canal defect: Two patch repair and tricuspidization of the mitral valve. Ann Thorac Surg 1993;55:347.

Capouya ER et al: Atrioventricular canal defects. Ann Thorac Surg 1991;51:860.

Pacifico AD et al: Corrective repair of complete atrioventricular canal defects and major associated cardiac anomalies. Ann Thorac Surg 1988;46:645.

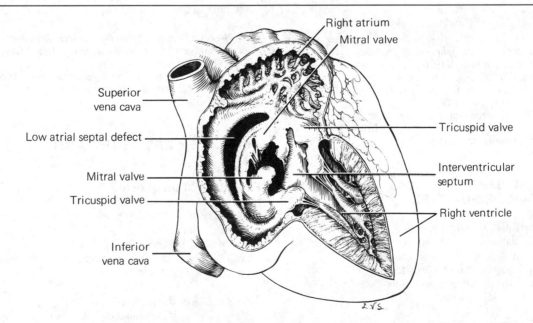

Figure 19–22. Complete atrioventricular canal. The most common type has a divided anterior common atrioventricular leaflet. Both the mitral and tricuspid portions are attached to the interventricular septum with long, nonfused chordae tendineae. The mitral and tricuspid portions of the common posterior atrioventricular leaflet are not separated. (Modified from Rastelli et al: J Thorac Cardiovasc Surg 1968;55:299.)

Ross DA et al: Atrioventricular canal defects: Results in the current era. J Cardiovasc Surg 1991;6:367.

VENTRICULAR SEPTAL DEFECT

Essentials of Diagnosis

- Asymptomatic if defect is small.
- Heart failure with dyspnea, frequent respiratory infections, and poor growth if the defect is large.
- Grade 2–6/6 pansystolic murmur maximal at the left sternal border.
- S_2 loud with apical diastolic flow murmur and biventricular enlargement if the defect is large.

General Considerations

Ventricular septal defects occur in four anatomic positions in the ventricular septum. About 85% of ventricular septal defects occur in the area of the membranous septum (Figure 19–23) (perimembranous). A few ventricular septal defects occur anterior to the crista supraventricularis (supracristal), some just beneath the septal leaflet of the tricuspid valve (canal) or in the muscular ventricular septum (muscular).

Ventricular septal defects are often one component of another more complex congenital heart lesion such as truncus arteriosus, atrioventricular canal defect, tetralogy of Fallot, or transposition of the great arteries.

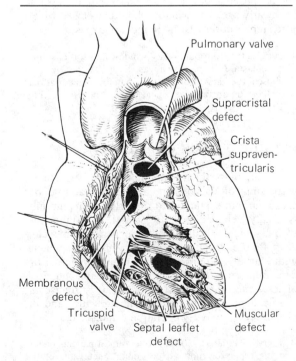

Pulmonary valve

Supracristal defect

Crista supraventricularis

Membranous defect

Tricuspid valve

Septal leaflet defect

Muscular defect

Figure 19–23. Anatomic locations of various ventricular septal defects. The wall of the right ventricle has been excised to expose the ventricular septum.

Patients with isolated perimembranous ventricular septal defects may have other associated lesions such as patent ductus arteriosus or coarctation of the aorta. Patients with supracristal ventricular septal defects occasionally have aortic valve regurgitation.

Clinical Findings

The clinical symptoms related to ventricular septal defect are usually those of a child with pulmonary overcirculation, ie, dyspnea on exertion, poor weight gain, and easy fatigability. Infants with large ventricular septal defects usually fail to grow and have chronic respiratory difficulties and poor feeding habits. In general, the heart is enlarged and the lung fields are overcirculated. Pulmonary vascular disease may develop as a result of the high pressure and large flow in the lungs. About one-third of all patients with isolated ventricular septal defect seen in the first year of life have small defects and, generally, no symptoms. Many of these defects will close spontaneously, usually by 7–8 years. About one-third of patients with large or multiple ventricular septal defects will be symptomatic in infancy and will require aggressive medical management, early diagnosis, and, usually, surgical correction.

Treatment

Optimal treatment consists of closure of the defect, which is done in most age groups with an acceptable death rate under 3%. In extremely small infants (< 3 kg), there may be a lower risk with banding of the pulmonary artery. Patients with symptomatic multiple defects in infancy may also do better with pulmonary artery banding, leaving correction for a later time. Almost all ventricular septal defects are patched with a prosthetic material of Dacron or Teflon. Most are approached through a right atriotomy (perimembranous, tetralogy, transposition) or ventriculostomy incision (truncus arteriosus), a left ventriculostomy incision (muscular ventricular septal defect), or through the pulmonary artery (supracristal ventricular septal defect). An aortic diastolic murmur is an indication for early closure of the supracristal defect; closure will in some cases stabilize the base of the aortic leaflet and may reduce—or at least not increase—the amount of aortic valve regurgitation.

Prognosis

Overall, improvement in symptoms is usually quite dramatic and the heart size reduces, but pulmonary vascular resistance probably does not change significantly from the time the defect is closed. Thus, earlier operation usually reduces the likelihood of significant pulmonary vascular disease.

McDaniel N et al: Repair of large muscular ventricular septal defects in infants employing left ventriculotomy. Ann Thorac Surg 1989;47:593.

Mehta AVB et al: Ventricular septal defect in the first year of life. Am J Cardiol 1992;70:364.

PATENT DUCTUS ARTERIOSUS

Essentials of Diagnosis

- Older patients with small or moderately large patent ductus are asymptomatic and have a continuous murmur over the pulmonary area, loud S_2, and bounding peripheral pulses.
- Poor feeding, respiratory distress, and frequent respiratory infections in infants with heart failure.
- Murmur usually systolic, sometimes continuous.
- Widened pulse pressure.

General Considerations

In most full-term infants, the ductus arteriosus closes in the first few days of life. The muscular component of the ductal wall contracts when exposed to higher levels of oxygen at the time of birth. For unknown reasons, closure does not always occur. If the ductus remains open and pulmonary vascular resistance decreases, pulmonary blood flow will increase, leading to heart failure and pulmonary congestion. In most term infants, the ductus is detected by the classic to-and-fro murmur in the left second intercostal space.

A persistent patent ductus arteriosus is much more common in premature infants, and most preterm infants with heart failure require ligation of the ductus.

Clinical Findings

Diagnosis is made by physical examination and confirmed by two-dimensional echocardiography. Cardiac catheterization is sometimes used to substantiate the presence of the open ductus, but most patients probably do not require this extensive workup unless associated lesions of the heart are suspected.

Approximately 5% of full-term infants with untreated patent ductus arteriosus die from heart failure and pulmonary complications in the first year of life. Another 5% have large shunts and ultimately develop pulmonary vascular disease. The remainder are usually asymptomatic, and the ductus is detected during routine examination.

Treatment

Surgical obliteration of the ductus by ligation, clipping, or division is the most efficient method of correction. Indomethacin, a prostaglandin E_1 inhibitor, will sometimes close a patent ductus arteriosus in both full-term and preterm infants. Its effectiveness is usually noted within 1 week, and surgical treatment should be undertaken if closure is not accomplished by this time. The operative death rate is less than 1% in elective cases and slightly higher in preterm infants, many of whom weigh less than 1 kg. Video-assisted endoscopic surgical techniques have recently been utilized successfully in this lesion, but their specific indications and uses remain to be clarified. Interventional cardiologic devices may also provide new therapeutic options.

Prognosis

In uncomplicated cases, the patient can be considered cured once obliteration of the ductus has been accomplished. Complications such as injury to the recurrent laryngeal nerve as it passes around the ductus are reported, but the results are generally excellent.

Coster DD et al: Surgical closure of the patent ductus arteriosus in the neonatal intensive care unit. Ann Thorac Surg 1989;48:386.

Hosking MC et al: Transcatheter occlusion of the persistently patent ductus arteriosus. Forty month followup and prevalence of residual shunting. Circulation 1991;84:2313.

Laborde F et al: A new video-assisted thoracoscopic surgical technique for interruption of patent ductus arteriosus in infants and children. J Thorac Cardiovasc Surg 1993;105:278.

AORTOPULMONARY WINDOW

A hole between the ascending aorta and the main pulmonary artery can produce a left-to-right shunt and physical findings very similar to those of patent ductus. Patients with large shunts have heart failure and are prone to develop pulmonary vascular disease at an early age. The window should be closed with a patch repair during cardiopulmonary bypass.

Tabak C et al: Aortopulmonary window and aortic isthmic hypoplasia. J Thorac Cardiovasc Surg 1983;86:273.

Tiraboschi R et al: Aortopulmonary window in the first year of life: Report on 11 surgical cases. Ann Thorac Surg 1988;46:438.

RUPTURED SINUS OF VALSALVA

Rupture of the thin membranous tissue between the aortic sinus of Valsalva and an intracardiac chamber causes an immediate left-to-right shunt. The murmur is usually well localized, parasternal, and continuous, with associated thrill. Most patients rapidly develop heart failure. Rupture is more common in patients with Marfan's syndrome or other autoimmune disorders. Rupture is into the right ventricle in about 70% of cases and into the right atrium in 20%. Precise anatomic diagnosis is by cardiac catheterization and angiocardiography Early operation is indicated.

Barragry TP et al: 15–30 year follow-up of patients undergoing repair of ruptured congenital aneurysms of the sinus of Valsalva. Ann Thorac Surg 1988;46:515.

Mayer ED et al: Ruptured aneurysms of the sinus of Valsalva. Ann Thorac Surg 1986;42:81.

Verghase M et al: Surgical treatment of ruptured aneurysms of the sinus of Valsalva. Ann Thorac Surg 1986;41:284.

LEFT VENTRICULAR–RIGHT ATRIAL SHUNT

A left ventricular-right atrial shunt is produced by a defect in the membranous septum near the annulus of the septal leaflet of the tricuspid valve or by a perforation or cleft of the septal leaflet. The lesion is uncommon, and the size of the shunt is variable. Symptoms of heart failure may be present in infancy or may not develop until late childhood. The systolic murmur is not diagnostic. At cardiac catheterization, blood oxygen saturation is increased in the right atrium, and on cineangiocardiograms the right atrium opacifies after injection of contrast material into the left ventricle.

In symptomatic patients, the defect is closed by direct sutures from the right atrium during cardiopulmonary bypass. The operative death rate is low.

CORONARY ARTERIAL FISTULA

A fistulous communication between the right (60%) or left (40%) coronary artery and the right ventricle (90%), right atrium, or coronary sinus produces a left-to-right shunt and increased pulmonary blood flow. The involved coronary vessels are dilated, and the fistulous openings may be multiple. Many patients are asymptomatic; some develop evidence of myocardial ischemia, and others have some degree of heart failure. A continuous murmur is usually present over the heart. Angiograms are required to determine the number and location of the fistulas.

The fistulous connections are ligated at operation without interrupting the coronary artery. Cardiopulmonary bypass is sometimes required. The operative death rate is less than 5%.

Turley K et al: Color flow doppler echocardiography in the diagnosis and treatment of congenital coronary artery anomalies. Circulation 1989;80:(Suppl II):68.

TOTAL ANOMALOUS PULMONARY VENOUS CONNECTION (TAPVC)

Essentials of Diagnosis

- Pulmonary congestion, tachypnea, cardiac failure, and variable cyanosis.
- Severe heart failure, cyanosis, poor pulses, acidosis in infants.
- Pulmonary midsystolic murmur present, with loud, fixed splitting of S_2 in some patients.
- Enlargement of right atrium and ventricle with severe pulmonary vascular congestion.
- Blood oxygen saturation similar in aorta and pulmonary artery.
- Pulmonary arterial and wedge pressures often elevated.

General Considerations

The term total anomalous pulmonary venous connection (TAPVC) indicates that the pulmonary veins do not make a direct connection with the left atrium. The blood reaches the left atrium only through an atrial septal defect or patent foramen ovale. Pulmonary and systemic venous blood is mixed in the right atrium; thus, except for streaming, the oxygen saturations in the aorta and pulmonary artery are similar. There are three basic types of total anomalous venous return (Figure 19–24), depending on the location of the pulmonary venous return to the systemic venous system: type 1, above the diaphragm (55%); type 2, coronary sinus (30%); and type 3, below the diaphragm (12%). Generally, in types 1 and 2, there is increased pulmonary blood flow and, less commonly, increased pulmonary vascular resistance. In type 3, there is frequently some obstruction to the pulmonary venous return through the long descending vein going down to the portal system. Type 3 patients, usually infants, frequently have elevated pulmonary vascular resistance. The remainder of patients belong to a fourth, miscellaneous group, in which the veins may enter any portion of the right venous side. Most patients with anomalous pulmonary venous return present with symptoms of increased pulmonary blood flow, cyanosis, and pulmonary congestion in infancy, many in the first days of life. The diagnosis is easy to make by cardiac catheterization and, more recently, by echocardiography. The amount of blood going to the systemic circulation is totally dependent on the size of the atrial septal defect. At the time of diagnostic catheterization, enlargement of the atrial defect with a balloon septostomy may result in temporary improvement.

Treatment

Treatment of all forms of TAPVC consists of operative repair. Correction of types 1 and 3 requires a direct anastomosis between the confluence of pulmonary veins and left atrium. Multiple operative approaches have been used, most commonly the internal approach through the right atrium, septum, and left atrium to perform the left atrial to common vein anastomosis, or the lateral approach on the left side with direct anastomosis between the left atrial appendage and the confluence. The persistent left vertical vein in type 1 and anomalous descending vein in type 3 are ligated. Type 2 TAPVC is usually repaired intra-atrially by baffling the coronary sinus into the left atrium. Operative repair is done on cardiopulmonary bypass and may require circulatory arrest.

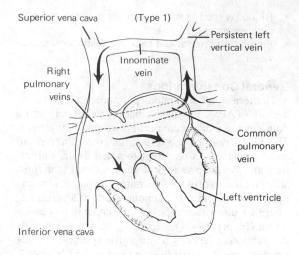

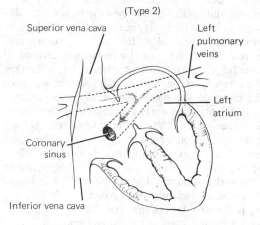

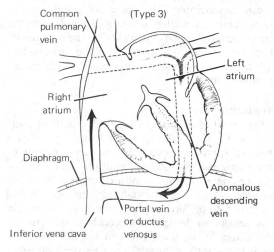

Figure 19–24. Common types of total anomalous pulmonary venous connection. ***Type 1:*** The pulmonary veins connect to a persistent left vertical vein, the innominate vein, and the right superior vena cava. ***Type 2:*** The pulmonary veins connect to the coronary sinus and the right atrium. ***Type 3:*** The pulmonary veins connect to an anomalous descending vein, a portal vein or persistent ductus venosus, and eventually the inferior vena cava.

Prognosis

Deaths and late complications occur most commonly in patients with the type 3 anomaly, because of the higher incidence of pulmonary venous obstruction and pulmonary vascular disease. Patients who survive—those with types 1 and 2—have good long-term prognoses and, usually, good cardiac performance with few symptoms.

Cobanaglu A et al: Total anomalous pulmonary venous connection in neonates and young infants: Repair in the current era. Ann Thorac Surg 1993;55:43.

Lincoln CR et al: Surgical risk factors in total anomalous pulmonary venous connection. Am J Cardiol 1988;61:608.

Pacifico AD et al: Repair of congenital pulmonary venous stenosis with living autologous atrial tissue. J Thorac Cardiovasc Surg 1985;89:604.

TRUNCUS ARTERIOSUS

In truncus arteriosus, a single large vessel overrides the ventricular septum and distributes all of the blood ejected from the heart. The pulmonary artery arises directly from the aorta and does not connect to the right ventricle. A large ventricular septal defect is present and is usually located directly beneath the truncal valve. In most cases, pulmonary blood flow is increased, and signs and symptoms of heart failure are present. Patients develop increased pulmonary vascular disease at a young age, and some form of palliative treatment should be undertaken before age 6 months.

The best form of palliation at present is a corrective operation in which a valved conduit is placed between the right ventricle and the pulmonary vessels and the ventricular septal defect is closed (Figure 19–25). The graft or conduit will have to be changed as the child grows, but the likelihood of development of pulmonary vascular disease is greatly reduced. Aortic homografts may be the conduit of choice, particularly at the time of the first conduit change. Long-term prognosis after correction is related to the presence or absence of pulmonary vascular disease or insufficiency of the truncal valve.

Bove EL et al: Repair of truncus arteriosus in the neonate and young infant. Ann Thorac Surg 1989;47:499.

Kay PH, Ross DN: Fifteen years' experience with the aortic homograft: The conduit of choice for right ventricular outflow tract reconstruction. Ann Thorac Surg 1985;40:360.

Pearl JM et al: Repair of truncus arteriosus in infancy. Ann Thorac Surg 1991;52:780.

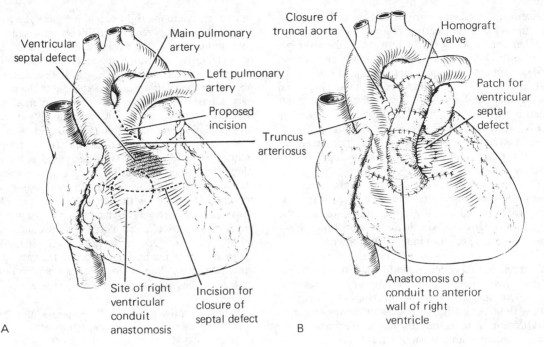

Figure 19–25. Type 1 truncus arteriosus. **A:** The main pulmonary artery arises from the truncus arteriosus downstream to the truncal semilunar valve. A ventricular septal defect is always present. **B:** The main pulmonary artery is incised from the truncus. The ventricular septal defect is closed with a patch. A conduit of Dacron that contains a homograft aortic valve is sutured to the anterior wall of the right ventricle and the distal pulmonary artery. A conduit between the right ventricle and pulmonary artery was successfully introduced by J. W. Kirklin in 1964 during correction of severe tetralogy of Fallot.

CONGENITAL HEART LESIONS THAT DECREASE PULMONARY ARTERIAL BLOOD FLOW

The combination of an obstructive lesion of the right heart and a septal defect reduces pulmonary arterial blood flow and causes some systemic venous blood to enter the systemic arterial circulation directly (right-to-left shunt). The degree of cyanosis is directly proportionate to the amount of the right-to-left shunt and inversely proportionate to the amount of pulmonary arterial blood flow. Tetralogy of Fallot is the most common lesion in this group, which also includes pulmonary atresia, tricuspid atresia, Ebstein's anomaly, and other complex malformations. Pulmonary vascular disease due to acquired hyperplasia of the intimal and medial layers of pulmonary arterioles develops in some patients who have lesions that initially produce excessive pulmonary blood flow. As pulmonary arterioles become obstructed, pulmonary blood flow decreases and causes blood to shunt from right to left (Eisenmenger's syndrome).

Severe cyanosis stimulates red cell production, which increases blood hematocrit and hemoglobin concentration. This improves oxygen transport, because blood that reaches the lungs will bind more oxygen per 100 milliliters. The elevated hematocrit, which may reach 80% or more, increases the viscosity of blood and may reduce certain clotting factors, particularly platelets and fibrinogen. Dehydration in patients with a very high hematocrit may cause systemic and pulmonary venous thrombosis in spite of the reduced concentration of clotting factors.

Variable cyanosis, hypoxic spells, squatting, and clubbing are frequently associated with lesions that reduce pulmonary blood flow. Several factors may alter the degree of cyanosis by altering the ratio of pulmonary and systemic resistances. Exercise decreases systemic vascular resistance, increases systemic blood flow, and, in tetralogy of Fallot, decreases pulmonary blood flow and arterial oxygen saturation. Increased catecholamines or acidosis can also reduce pulmonary blood flow in patients with tetralogy of Fallot.

Hypoxic spells indicate severe cerebral hypoxia and are due to acute reduction of pulmonary blood flow. Spasm of the infundibular muscle is the most likely cause of hypoxic spells, which can occur without warning. Infants and young children become unconscious for varying periods of time and occasionally die. The most effective treatment is to administer oxygen and small doses of morphine, place the patient in the knee-chest position with the head down, and correct the associated metabolic acidosis.

Children who have reduced pulmonary arterial blood flow and cyanotic heart disease squat frequently. In the squatting position (sitting on the heels), systemic vascular resistance increases. The increased systemic vascular resistance decreases right-to-left shunting and temporarily increases pulmonary arterial blood flow.

Clubbing of fingers and toes develops in late infancy and early childhood and is due to proliferation of capillaries and small arteriovenous fistulas in the distal phalanges. The mechanism and teleologic advantage (if any) of clubbing are not known.

Reduced pulmonary arterial blood flow stimulates enlargement of bronchial and mediastinal arteries. These vessels connect with pulmonary arteries and, in some cases, may provide most of the pulmonary blood flow. At birth, the ductus arteriosus is patent and provides substantial flow to the pulmonary arteries of patients with obstructive right ventricular outflow tract lesions. Unfortunately, this useful vessel (the patent ductus arteriosus) nearly always closes during the first few hours or days after birth. The intravenous administration of prostaglandin E_1 will maintain patency of this ductus for hours or days in some infants, thus allowing reversal of acidosis, reduction of cyanosis, and stabilization of the infant prior to operation.

Several palliative operations that shunt blood from the systemic to the pulmonary arterial circulation have been devised for infants and young children who have insufficient pulmonary arterial blood flow. The Blalock-Taussig operation connects the subclavian artery to the ipsilateral pulmonary artery with an end-to-side anastomosis (Figure 19–26A). The modified Blalock-Taussig shunt interposes a 4- to 6-mm tube graft usually of polytetrafluoroethylene (Gore-Tex) between the subclavian and pulmonary arteries. The Waterston aortic to right pulmonary arterial anastomosis connects the posterior portion of the ascending aorta to the anterior wall of the right pulmonary artery (Figure 19–26B). The Potts anastomosis joins the left pulmonary artery and the descending thoracic aorta by a side-to-side anastomosis (Figure 19–26C). The Waterston and Potts aortopulmonary shunts are mostly of historical interest because of the difficulty of regulating flow at the time of creation and of taking down the shunt at the time of later correction. In neonates, injection of the wall of the ductus arteriosus with 10% formalin has delayed closure of this valuable vessel for weeks or months. All of these connections increase pulmonary blood flow, because of the pressure difference between the systemic arterial and pulmonary circulations. The classic Glenn operation (Figure 19–26D) connects the superior vena cava to the right pulmonary artery in such a way that superior vena caval blood must enter the right pulmonary artery exclusively. The newer bidirectional Glenn operation connects the superior vena cava end-to-side, allowing flow to both lungs. Connection of the right atrium or ventricle to the pulmonary arteries either directly, with an internal atrial baffle, or with a conduit is now commonly used for both palliation and correction (Rastelli, Fontan).

Right ventricular to pulmonary artery conduits may be used for lesions with decreased pulmonary blood flow where the outflow tract cannot be reconstructed (pulmonary atresia, tetralogy of Fallot) or a few complex lesions with increased pulmonary blood flow (truncus arteriosus, transposition of the great arteries with ventricular septal defect). The conduits are usually made of Dacron or polytetrafluoroethylene and may or may not have an incorporated valve prosthesis. Recently, human aortic or pulmonary homograft tissue has been used more extensively.

Gold JP et al: A five year clinical experience with 112 Blalock-Taussig shunts. J Card Surg 1993;8:9.

Holman WL et al: the Blalock-Taussig shunt: An analysis of trends and techniques in the fourth decade. J Cardiac Surg 1989;4:113.

Kopf GS et al: Thirty year follow-up of superior vena cavapulmonary artery (Glenn) shunts. J Thorac Cardiovasc Surg 1990;100:662.

Larson JE et al: Combined prostaglandin therapy and ductal formalin infiltration in neonatal pulmonary oligemia. J Thorac Cardiovasc Surg 1985;90:907.

Opie JC et al: Experience with polytetrafluoroethylene grafts in children with cyanotic congenital heart disease. Ann Thorac Surg 1986;41:164.

Watterson KG et al: Very small pulmonary arteries: central end-to-side shunt. Ann Thorac Surg 1991;52:1132.

TETRALOGY OF FALLOT; PULMONARY ATRESIA WITH VENTRICULAR SEPTAL DEFECT

Essentials of Diagnosis

- History of hypoxic spells and squatting.
- Cyanosis and clubbing.
- Prominent right ventricular impulse, single S_2.
- Grade 1–3/6 ejection murmur in third left intercostal space.
- Systolic murmur softens or disappears during cyanotic spell.

General Considerations

Tetralogy of Fallot has four basic anatomic abnormalities (Figure 19–27): ventricular septal defect, pulmonary stenosis, overriding of the aorta over the ventricular septum, and right ventricular hypertrophy. The addition of an atrial septal defect falls in the category of pentalogy of Fallot. Pulmonary stenosis may be valvular or infundibular, but most cases have

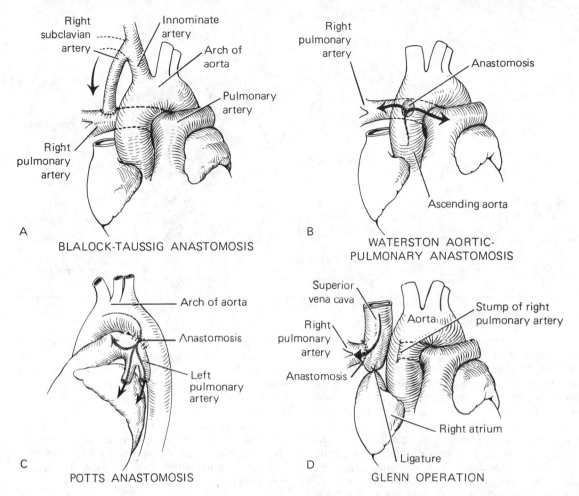

Figure 19–26. Palliative operations to increase pulmonary arterial blood flow. **A:** Blalock-Taussig subclavian-pulmonary arterial anastomosis. **B:** Waterston aortic to right pulmonary arterial anastomosis. **C:** Potts anastomosis between the left pulmonary artery and the descending thoracic aorta. **D:** The Glenn operation. The end of the right pulmonary artery is connected to the side of the superior vena cava, which is ligated caudad to the anastomosis.

some degree of hypertrophic muscle mass in the pulmonary outflow tract. In more severe forms, the pulmonary valve may be completely atretic. Focal stenotic lesions are also present occasionally in the distal pulmonary arteries as well as diffuse hypoplasia of all the pulmonary arterial trunks. Symptoms are directly related to the severity of right ventricular outflow obstruction and the amount of pulmonary blood flow. A patent ductus may mask the lesion and its symptoms in the early days of life. A systolic murmur is due to the pulmonary stenosis and is heard along the left sternal border. Because of the overriding aorta and the large size of the ventricular septal defect, the flow across the ventricular septal defect rarely causes enough turbulence to be heard. The hypoxic or cyanotic spell is the most serious symptom, since it can result in cerebral hypoxia, brain injury, and even death. The diagnosis can usually be made from the cyanosis, small heart size, and diminished pulmonary blood flow seen on chest x-ray. The ECG shows right ventricular hypertrophy. Cardiac catheterization is essential, and the degree of success of operative treatment (whether a definitive or palliative procedure can be performed on the small infant) correlates with the size of the pulmonary arteries. A successful correction is indicated by a ratio of right pulmonary artery size to ascending aorta size of 1:3. A lower ratio may indicate the need for an initial palliative operation.

Treatment

The selection of operation for tetralogy of Fallot remains controversial. If the main pulmonary artery and distal pulmonary vessels are of reasonable size, a corrective procedure is probably indicated irrespective of the patient's age. The outflow tract and pulmo-

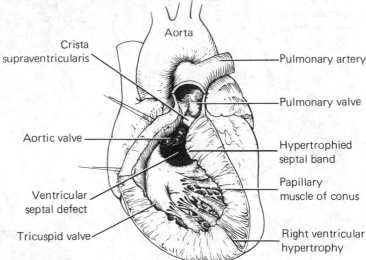

Figure 19–27. Tetralogy of Fallot. The aorta overrides the ventricular septum. A large ventricular septal defect is present, and the hypoplastic infundibulum with hypertrophied parietal and septal muscle bands obstructs blood to the pulmonary arteries.

nary annulus frequently require a small patch to adequately relieve the right ventricular outflow tract obstruction. The patch must not be so large that resultant pulmonary valve incompetence will be overwhelming. The pulmonary infundibular area is enlarged by resecting muscle and dividing many of the large muscle bands in the area. The ventricular septal defect can be closed with a patch of prosthetic material. Repairs are performed during total cardiopulmonary bypass to enhance visualization of the ventricular septal defect and the pulmonary outflow tract. Recently, total repairs have been accomplished through the right atrium, including closure of the ventricular septal defect and relief of the outflow tract obstruction. This operative approach avoids the need for ventriculostomy. After surgery, patients with tetralogy of Fallot usually have an elevated heart rate and mild degrees of right ventricular failure. In all tetralogy patients, more volume work is required of the heart after operation than before, because pulmonary flow is now normal or because pulmonary valve flow is increased owing to some incompetence of the pulmonary valve.

If the pulmonary arteries are small, an initial palliative procedure may be preferred. The outflow tract or annulus may be enlarged with a patch without closure of the ventricular septal defect. An alternative approach is a systemic to pulmonary shunt; the Blalock-Taussig subclavian-pulmonary artery anastomosis is probably the most popular (Figure 19–26A). Direct anastomosis between the ascending aorta and the right pulmonary artery, or Waterston technique (Figure 19–26B), is easier to construct, but selective flow to the right lung and subsequent injury to the right pulmonary artery can result. The Potts anastomosis (Figure 19–26C), between the descending aorta and

left pulmonary artery, is rarely used now because it is difficult to close during subsequent corrective operation. Both of these direct aorta-pulmonary artery anastomoses are likely to increase in size, resulting in increased pulmonary flow and increased vascular resistance.

In patients with complete pulmonary atresia (no connection between the right ventricle and pulmonary artery), a valved conduit may be used for correction, but an initial palliation shunt is usually required in infancy.

Prognosis

The overall success rate for surgical correction of tetralogy of Fallot is 90–95%. Currently, many patients undergo one-stage total correction in infancy, with better results than those who undergo a two-stage procedure.

Approximately 50% of the surviving patients have no exercise limitations and enjoy normal activity. The long-term outlook, though, for patients with residual pulmonary valve incompetence is uncertain. It may be that some of them will require subsequent pulmonary valve replacement, since pulmonary valve incompetence may not be tolerated as well over the long term as is anticipated now. Some patients will have recurrent pulmonary stenosis, and a few will have residual leaks in the ventricular septal closure. These defects usually can be corrected without difficulty.

Blackstone EH et al: Prediction of severe obstruction to right ventricular outflow after repair of tetralogy of Fallot and pulmonary atresia. J Thorac Cardiovasc Surg 1988;91:818.

Di-Donato RM et al: Neonatal repair of tetralogy of Fallot

with and without pulmonary atresia. J Thorac Cardiovasc Surg 1991;101:126.

Groh MA et al: Repair of Tetralogy of Fallot in infancy. Effect of pulmonary artery size on outcome. Circulation 1991;84(5 Suppl):III206.

Horneffer PJ et al: Long term results of total repair of Tetralogy of Fallot in childhood. Ann Thorac Surg 1990;50:179.

Kawashima Y et al: Ninety consecutive corrective operations for tetralogy of Fallot with or without minimal right ventriculotomy. J Thorac Cardiovasc Surg 1985;90:856.

Kirklin JW et al: Morphologic and surgical determinants of outcome events after repair of Tetralogy of Fallot and pulmonary stenosis. A two institution study. J Thorac Cardiovasc Surg 1992;103:692.

Lillehei CW et al: The first open heart corrections of tetralogy of Fallot: A 26–31 year follow-up of 106 patients. Ann Surg 1986;204:490.

Millikan JS et al: Staged surgical repair of pulmonary atresia, ventricular septal defect, and hypoplastic confluent pulmonary arteries. J Thorac Cardiovasc Surg 1986; 91:818.

Sullivan ID et al: Surgical unifocalization in pulmonary atresia and ventricular septal defect. Circulation 1988;78(Suppl III):5.

PULMONARY ATRESIA WITH INTACT VENTRICULAR SEPTUM

Pulmonary atresia with intact ventricular septum is a severe form of pulmonary stenosis. It is usually associated with a hypoplastic or rudimentary right ventricle. In a few situations, it does occur with a normal or dilated ventricle, and if correction is performed in early infancy, preservation of right ventricular performance may be possible. A patent ductus is mandatory for survival, and these infants are often at risk in the first days of life as the ductus attempts to close.

Cyanosis is usually present at birth, and the ECG shows left ventricular dominance. Tricuspid valve insufficiency or hypoplasia is often associated with the lesion. Coronary artery abnormalities are common with severe forms of pulmonary artery with intact ventricular septum, including coronary stenoses and ventriculocoronary corrections. In general, correction in infancy is impossible, so the combination of pulmonary stenosis relief (unloading the right ventricle) and systemic to pulmonary artery shunt is usually recommended. The shunt may subsequently be closed and the right ventricular outflow tract further enlarged if the right ventricle develops. All of these children have a patent foramen or an atrial septal defect, either of which would have to be closed at subsequent correction. The prognosis is poor and the death rate remains high.

Billingsley AM et al: Definitive repair in patients with pulmonary atresia and intact ventricular septum. J Thorac Cardiovasc Surg 1989;97:746.

Coles JG et al: Long-term results in neonates with pulmonary atresia and intact ventricular septum. Ann Thorac Surg 1989;47:213.

Hawkins JA et al: Early and late results in pulmonary atresia, and intact ventricular septum. J Thorac Cardiovasc Surg 1990;100:492.

Kirklin JW et al: Survival, functional status, and reoperations after repair of tetralogy of Fallot with pulmonary atresia. J Thorac Cardiovasc Surg 1988;96:102.

Steinberger J et al: Results of a right ventricular outflow tract patch for pulmonary atresia with intact ventricular septum. Circulation 1992;86(5 Suppl):II167.

TRICUSPID ATRESIA

The tricuspid valve is completely absent in about 2% of newborns with congenital heart disease. In most of these patients, the great vessels are in normal position, the right ventricle is hypoplastic, and a small muscular ventricular septal defect exists that provides flow to the pulmonary arteries. The blood passes from the right atrium through the patent foramen to the left atrium and into the large systemic ventricle. Infants with tricuspid atresia and reduced pulmonary flow develop cyanosis early in life and require some form of palliative shunt. In older children, if the pulmonary arteries are of reasonable size and pulmonary vascular resistance is normal, the so-called Fontan procedure or one of its modifications may be performed. This consists of either a direct connection or a conduit (either valved or nonvalved) between the right atrium and the pulmonary artery or the rudimentary right ventricle. Total cavopulmonary connection is gaining support as an alternative to the modified Fontan procedure. The superior vena cava is connected to the right pulmonary artery and a baffle is placed within the right atrium to direct inferior vena caval blood flow to the pulmonary arteries. Blood flow to the lungs is passive in all Fontan-type corrections and is dependent upon negative intrathoracic pressure during respiration, elevated systemic venous pressure, and right atrial contraction. The atrial septal defect is closed and the cyanosis eliminated. The long-term results are yet to be evaluated, but the modified Fontan procedure does eliminate any shunts in the heart and relieves cyanosis.

The therapeutic palliative alternatives to the Fontan procedure have been the use of a superior vena cava to right pulmonary artery anastomosis (Glenn) and a standard systemic to pulmonary artery shunt to increase pulmonary blood flow. The long-term outlook for children with tricuspid atresia is poor, and it is not yet known whether life is significantly extended by the Fontan type of bypass procedure.

Castaneda AR: From Glenn to Fontan: A continuing evolution. Circulation 1992;86(5 Suppl):II80.

deLeval MR et al: Total cavopulmonary connection: A logical alternative to atriopulmonary connection for complex Fontan operations. J Thorac Cardiovasc Surg 1988;96:682.

Driscoll DJ et al: Five to fifteen year follow-up after Fontan operation. Circulation 1992;85:469.

Franklin RC et al: Tricuspid atresia presenting in infancy: Survival and suitability for the Fontan operation. Circulation 1993;87:427.

Jonas RA, Castaneda AR: Modified Fontan procedure: Atrial baffle and systemic venous to pulmonary artery anastomotic techniques. J Cardiac Surg 1988;3;91.

Lee CN et al: Comparison of atriopulmonary versus atrioventricular connections for modified Fontan/Kreutzer repair of tricuspid valve atresia. J Thorac Cardiovasc Surg 1986; 92:1038.

Mair DD et al: Fontan operation in 176 patients with tricuspid atresia: Results and a proposed new index for patient selection. Circulation 1990;82(5 Suppl):IV164.

EBSTEIN'S ANOMALY

In this malformation, the septal and posterior leaflets of the tricuspid valve are small and deformed and usually displaced toward the right ventricular apex. A large piece of the right ventricle is quite thin and hypoplastic and becomes atrialized. Most patients have an associated atrial septal defect or patent foramen. Cyanosis and arrhythmias in infancy are common.

About half of these patients develop right heart failure, some degree of systemic desaturation, hepatomegaly, and dysrhythmias. Operative repair of this lesion without tricuspid valve replacement has been encouraging in approximately half of cases. In these cases, the atrialized portion of the ventricle may be oversewn and the tricuspid valve incompetence corrected. Newer surgical therapies are being developed to provide a functioning right ventricle and tricuspid valve. In others, tricuspid valve replacement is necessary, and sometimes the anatomic deformities are so extensive that effective surgical correction is impossible.

Danielson GK et al: Operative treatment of Ebstein's anomaly. J Thorac Cardiovasc Surg 1992;104:1497.

Gentles TL et al: Predictors of long term survival with Ebstein's anomaly of the tricuspid valve. Am J Cardiol 1992;69:377.

Starnes VA et al: Ebstein's anomaly appearing in the neonate: A new surgical approach. J Thorac Cardiovasc Surg 1991;101:1082.

HYPOPLASTIC RIGHT VENTRICLE

Underdevelopment of the right ventricle commonly occurs with pulmonary and tricuspid atresia and may occur with valvular pulmonary stenosis. The lesion has also been associated with atrial septal defect. It probably represents a spectrum of lesions due to pulmonary atresia and secondary intrauterine underdevelopment of the right heart. The degree of un-

derdevelopment will determine the clinical course. A Fontan operation after initial shunt palliation is apt to be the most productive treatment strategy.

TRANSPOSITION OF THE GREAT ARTERIES

Essentials of Diagnosis

- Situs solitus, levocardia.
- Cyanosis from birth; hypoxic spells sometimes present.
- Heart failure often present.
- Murmurs variable; often absent and not diagnostic.
- Cardiac enlargement and diminished pulmonary artery segment on x-ray.

General Considerations

Strictly defined, transposition of the great arteries shows the aorta originating from the morphologic right ventricle and the pulmonary artery originating from the left ventricle. The lesion is more common in males, and about 60% of patients with transposition of the great arteries have typical transposition with situs solitus and levocardia. The aorta arises from the normally placed anterior morphologic right ventricle (Figure 19–28). The atria and ventricles are concordant: the right atrium empties into the right ventricle and the left atrium into the left ventricle. The coronary arteries arise from the aorta.

Thus, transposition of the great arteries causes the systemic and pulmonary circulations to be independent. Some anatomic communication between the two systems must exist for the patient to survive. The common sites for mixing of blood are ventricular septal defect, atrial septal defect, and patent ductus arteriosus. The degree of cyanosis is proportionate to the relative amount of oxygenated venous blood that reaches the right ventricle and aorta. Approximately 30% of infants with transposition of the great arteries have coexisting ventricular septal defects, and about 5% have obstruction of the left ventricular outflow tract. The clinical symptoms are related to the degree of cyanosis, and many infants are dangerously cyanotic at birth, necessitating either emergency cardiac catheterization and balloon septostomy to enlarge the atrial septal defect and improve blood mixing or emergent surgery for arterial or atrial correction. The success of the balloon septostomy is related primarily to the compliance of the two ventricles. In some cases, a large atrial septal defect can be present but very little blood mixing occurs at the atrial level. This is thought to be due to equal compliance of the two ventricles: The left and right atrial filling pressures are so similar that mixing is minimal. Without treatment, about half of newborns with transposition of the great arteries die by age 1 month and 90% die within 1 year. Patients with intact ventricular septum and absent patent ductus have the worst initial prog-

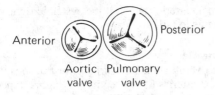

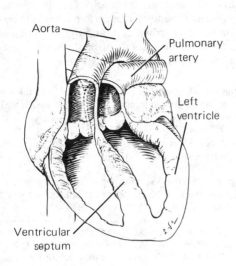

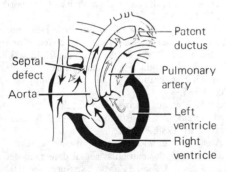

Figure 19–28. Typical transposition of the great arteries. The aorta arises from the morphologic right ventricle and is anterior to and slightly to the right of the pulmonary artery, which originates from the morphologic left ventricle. Inset at bottom illustrates the independent systemic and pulmonary circulations, which may be connected by a patent ductus arteriosus or atrial septal defect. Inset at top illustrates a common relationship of the two great arteries in typical transposition.

nosis, since the only area of mixing is at the atrial level. Patients with large ventricular septal defects and excessive pulmonary blood flow may die from severe heart failure or progressive pulmonary vascular disease.

Treatment

Most infants should have balloon septostomy and some type of intra-atrial baffle procedure or anatomic correction at the arterial level within the first 3 months of life. There is little place today for palliative atrial septectomy, since the risk of physiologic correction is less than that of palliative septectomy. An intra-atrial baffle procedure can be created using either the normal atrial septum (Senning procedure) or by using pericardium (Mustard procedure; Figure 19–29) to redirect blood from the vena cava through the mitral valve, into the left ventricle, and out the pulmonary artery. Blood returning through the pulmonary veins is redirected through the tricuspid valve, into the right ventricle, and out the aorta. In recent years, the Senning procedure has become favored because of fewer baffle complications and greater growth potential. The operative death rate for both of these procedures is about 5%, and the best candidates for correction are those without ventricular septal defects—the infants that are in difficulty at the earliest stages. Long-term complications of both procedures include atrial arrhythmias and long-term failure of the right ventricle to continue to perform as the systemic ventricle. Recently, anatomic correction at the arterial level (Jatene procedure) has become the preferred operative approach, with excellent intermediate-term results. The Jatene procedure involves switching the pulmonary artery and aorta and reimplanting the coronary arteries. Although the initial death rate approaches 15% in many series, the mortality rates now are less than 5% in the hands of experienced surgeons. The early complications have been also less, and it is hoped that the long-term complications will also be less. In infants with transposition of the great arteries and intact ventricular septum, the switch procedure must be done in the first days of life before the pulmonary vascular resistance decreases and the left ventricle adapts to the lowered resistance. The switch operation can be done at a later age in infants with ventricular septal defects as the left ventricle remains "prepared" to function as the systemic ventricle. The long-term benefits of the operation have not yet been substantiated; however, because of the excellent short-term results obtained at a number of centers, the arterial switch is presently the preferred definitive surgical procedure.

In some older children with transposition and ventricular septal defect, a valved conduit can be attached to the right ventricle, and the left ventricular blood can be redirected through the ventricular septal defect into the aorta (Rastelli procedure). Conduit replacement is usually necessary as the child grows. The Jatene procedure may be preferred in those patients with ventricular septal defect who have elevated left ventricular pressure, to ensure that the left ventricle can sustain systemic pressure after the great arteries have been switched. In these cases, the ventricular septal defect is also closed. The left ventricle must be capable of withstanding elevated pressure in order to sustain the increased work load required for systemic perfusion. Some patients with an initial atrial (Senning, Mustard) correction can be modified

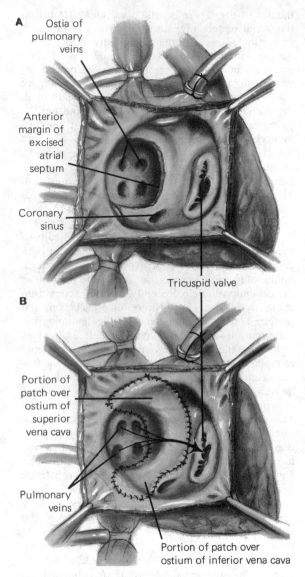

A:
- Ostia of pulmonary veins
- Anterior margin of excised atrial septum
- Coronary sinus
- Tricuspid valve

B:
- Portion of patch over ostium of superior vena cava
- Pulmonary veins
- Portion of patch over ostium of inferior vena cava

Figure 19–29. The Mustard operation. **A:** The atrial septum has been excised except for the anterior portion that contains the anterior intra-atrial conduction pathway. Pulmonary venous openings are visible at the posterior left atrial wall. **B:** A partition of pericardium or Dacron cloth is sutured around the left and right pulmonary venous openings, around the openings of the superior and inferior venae cavae, and to the anterior margin of the interatrial septum. Systemic venous blood then passes posterior to the partition toward the mitral valve. Pulmonary venous blood and blood from the coronary sinus pass anterior to the partition toward the tricuspid valve. A patch of Dacron or pericardium is often used to enlarge the right (now functional left) atrium when the atriotomy (not shown) is closed.

later to an arterial switch if the systemic right ventricle begins to fail.

Prognosis

The overall results of surgery for transposition of the great arteries have been improving. An operative death rate of less than 5% is reported in most series of intra-atrial and arterial repairs (Senning, Mustard). Long-term prognosis appears to relate to the development of atrial arrhythmias and right ventricular failure for atrial repairs and potential growth of the coronary arteries in arterial repairs.

Alonzo-de-Begona J et al: The Mustard procedure for correction of simple transposition of the great arteries before 1 month of age. J Thorac Cardiovasc Surg 1992;104:1218.

Castaneda AR et al: The early results of treatment of simple transposition in the current era. J Thorac Cardiovasc Surg 1988;95:14.

Ingram MT et al: Senning repair for transposition of the great without patch augmentation of the septum. J Thorac Cardiovasc Surg 1988;96:485.

Kirklin JW et al: Clinical outcomes after the arterial switch operation for transposition: Patient, support, procedural, and institutional risk factors. Circulation 1992;86:1501.

Kirklin JW et al: Complete transposition of the great arteries: Treatment in the current era. Pediatr Clin North Am 1990;37:171.

Lupinetti FM et al: Intermediate term survival and functional results after arterial repair for transposition of the great arteries. J Thorac Cardiovasc Surg 1992;103:421.

Mee RBB: Severe right ventricular failure after Mustard or Senning operation. J Thorac Cardiovasc Surg 1986;92:385.

Norwood WE et al: Intermediate results of the arterial switch repair: A 20-institution study. J Thorac Cardiovasc Surg 1988;96:854.

Serraf A et al: Anatomic correction of transposition of the great arteries with ventricular septal defect: Experience with 118 cases. J Thorac Cardiovasc Surg 1991;102:140.

Turley K et al: the Mustard procedure in infants (less than 100 days of age): Ten-year followup. J Thorac Cardiovasc Surg 1988;96:849.

CORRECTED TRANSPOSITION OF THE GREAT ARTERIES

Corrected transposition is a rare anomaly in which systemic venous blood reaches the lungs and pulmonary venous blood reaches the systemic arteries in spite of transposition or malposition of the great arteries. Pulmonary stenosis and ventricular septal defect are common associated lesions.

The clinical manifestations of corrected transposition vary according to the associated lesions. Asymptomatic patients without associated lesions elude diagnosis during life, with the anomaly only discovered at autopsy. Patients with large ventricular septal defects or tricuspid valvular incompetence, however, develop severe heart failure and present in infancy. The inverted positions of the great arteries make operation for relief of pulmonary stenosis difficult. The approach to the ventricular septal defect is controversial, but most surgeons feel that an approach through the systemic ventricle (in this case the anatomic right ventricle) can be used and that adequate closure can be accomplished. Since the tricuspid valve is subjected to systemic pressures of the anatomic right ventricle, incompetence of this tricuspid valve may occur. Operative management is similar to that of other patients with pulmonary stenosis and ventricular septal defect, and the indications for surgery usually relate to the symptoms caused by the associated defects.

Pederson RJ et al: Comparison of cardiac function in surgically corrected and congenitally corrected transposition of the great arteries. J Thorac Cardiovasc Surg 1988;96:227.

DOUBLE OUTLET RIGHT VENTRICLE

In double outlet right ventricle, both great arteries arise from the right ventricle. A ventricular septal defect is invariably present and is usually located either beneath the aorta or beneath the pulmonary artery.

Operative repair depends on whether blood flow from the left ventricle—which emerges through the ventricular septal defect—can be directed into the aorta. If flow can be directed into the aorta, an intraventricular baffle is all that is needed. If flow can only be directed into the pulmonary artery, some form of intra-atrial baffle to redirect venous inflow is necessary so that the pulmonary venous return will ultimately go to the aorta. The arterial switch operation or the Fontan procedure has been used successfully in some forms of double outlet right ventricle.

This is a rare and uncommon lesion, and pulmonary stenosis may be associated with it.

Musumeci F et al: Surgical treatment of double outlet right ventricle at the Brompton Hospital, 1973–1986. J Thorac Cardiovasc Surg 1988;96:278.

Pacifico AD et al: Intraventricular tunnel repair for Taussig-Bing heart and related cardiac anomalies. Circulation 1986;74(Suppl 1):52.

Russo P et al: Modified Fontan procedure for biventricular hearts with complex forms of double-outlet right ventricle. Circulation 1988;78(5 Part 2):III20.

Serraf A et al: Anatomic repair of Taussig-Bing hearts. Circulation 1991;84(5 Suppl):III200.

DOUBLE OUTLET LEFT VENTRICLE

This is an extremely rare form of congenital heart disease in which both great vessels arise from the left ventricle. In some cases, a ventricular septal defect and an adequate-sized right ventricle are present. The defect can be closed and a valved conduit placed between the right ventricle and the pulmonary artery. The ventricular septal defect usually cannot be closed without the use of a conduit to direct flow to the pulmonary arteries from the right ventricle.

SINGLE VENTRICLE

The term "single ventricle" denotes a heart with one ventricular chamber that receives blood from both the tricuspid and mitral valves or a common atrioventricular valve. The lesion is a feature of about 3% of congenital heart defects. Atypical or typical transposition of the great arteries occurs in approximately 85% of patients. Twenty-five to 35% of patients have a common atrioventricular valve, and another 25% have stenosis or regurgitation of one of the atrioventricular valves. One-third to one-half of patients have pulmonary stenosis or atresia, and another third have aortic stenosis. The lesion occurs in association with situs inversus, dextrocardia, and asplenia in approximately 20% of patients. Defects of the atrial septum, total anomalous pulmonary venous connection, and truncus arteriosus are occasionally seen with single ventricle.

Single ventricle has been subdivided into four anatomic groups on the basis of the morphology of the ventricle. In approximately 75% of patients, single predominant ventricle develops from the left ventricular portion of the ventricular canal and from the conus arteriosus and infundibulum of the right ventricle. The right ventricular contribution forms a small outflow chamber from which the great vessels originate. The diagnosis of single ventricle and specific associated lesions must be made by cardiac catheterization and cineangiocardiography. Demonstration of absence of the ventricular septum and information about the atrioventricular valves can be obtained by echocardiography.

Clinical findings and prognosis are related to the relative amounts of pulmonary and systemic arterial blood flow. Some patients have survived into their second decade, but most die in infancy. In infants, palliation may be achieved by pulmonary arterial banding or shunt operations. In older children with two atrioventricular valves, the ventricle can be partitioned using a thick prosthetic patch. A valved external conduit is often necessary to provide pulmonary blood flow. For some children, a modified Fontan procedure may provide palliation. Operative mapping of the ventricular conduction system is necessary to prevent heart block. The most suitable anatomic types for operation are patients with an anatomic left ventricle and outflow chamber and those with a common ventricle formed from both ventricular sinuses. Currently, any operation has a high hospital death rate.

De Leon SY et al: Fontan type operation for complex lesions. J Thorac Cardiovasc Surg 1986;92:1029.

Mayer JE et al: Factors associated with marked reduction in mortality for Fontan operations in patients with single ventricle. J Thorac Cardiovasc Surg 1992;103:444.

Stein DG et al: Results of total cavopulmonary connection in the treatment of patients with a functional single ventricle. J Thorac Cardiovasc Surg 1991;102:280.

CARDIAC MALPOSITION

Situs inversus totalis is a rare anomaly in which the stomach and other abdominal organs occupy positions that are the mirror images of normal (situs solitus). Except in asplenia and polysplenia (see below), the position of the viscera determines the location of the atrium; thus, in situs inversus, the atria are reversed and the heart is right-sided (dextrocardia). The morphologic left atrium is on the right. When the ventricles and atria are concordant, the right atrium (on the patient's left) empties into the anatomic right ventricle. If transposition is not present, the circulation is normal and the cardiac chambers and vessels are the mirror image of normal structures. If transposition is present, the aorta is anterior to the pulmonary artery in the right-sided heart.

Rather severe associated anomalies usually occur with situs inversus, dextrocardia, and malposition of the great arteries. If the atria and ventricles are discordant, transposition or malposition of the great arteries is always present and the lesion may be physiologically "corrected." In most cases, the aorta arises to the left of the pulmonary artery and severe associated anomalies are present.

Isolated levocardia is the remaining condition that occurs with situs inversus totalis. The heart is located in the left chest, and most patients have severe associated cardiac anomalies and agenesis of the left lung.

Isolated dextrocardia is the term used to designate mirror image position of the heart when the viscera are in normal position (situs solitus). Agenesis of the right lung is present in many of these patients.

Cardiac catheterization and cineangiocardiography are essential to understand the pathologic anatomy and physiology of these lesions. The diagnostic rules for locating the visceral situs, morphologic ventricles, and positions of the great vessels must be used to label each structure and chamber opacified by the contrast material.

Life expectancy depends upon the severity of the circulatory handicap. Some patients live to advanced age, and others can be helped by specific palliative operations to improve circulatory function. A few patients are candidates for totally corrective operations of less severe associated lesions.

ASPLENIA & POLYSPLENIA

Absence of the spleen, midline position of the stomach and liver (indeterminate situs), distinct middle lobes of both right and left lungs, and Howell-Jolly bodies within red cells are associated with severe cardiac anomalies. About a third of such patients have dextrocardia. Single atrium, single ventricle, atrioventricular canal, transposition, pulmonary atresia, and anomalies of systemic and pulmonary venous return may occur. These patients are abnormally susceptible to bacterial infections, particularly pneumococcal infections.

Many small spleens, interruption of the hepatic portion of the inferior vena cava, absence of middle pulmonary lobes in both lungs, and absence of the gallbladder are associated with the same severe cardiac anomalies listed above with the exception of transposition.

MISCELLANEOUS CONGENITAL HEART LESIONS

CONGENITAL HEART BLOCK

Complete atrioventricular dissociation occurs as an isolated lesion or in association with other congenital cardiac anomalies, particularly corrected transposition of the great vessels, atrial septal defect, and endocardial fibroelastosis. The cardiac rate is generally higher (40–80 beats/min) than that which occurs in adults or in children who have complete heart block as a result of intracardiac surgery. The diagnosis is made by electrocardiography. A few patients will develop Stokes-Adams syncopal attacks; others—particularly those with associated lesions—develop heart failure. Sudden death may occur in Stokes-Adams attacks. Digoxin is not recommended, but diuretics may help to control heart failure. Medical therapy also includes sublingual isoproterenol, but symptomatic patients are best treated with an implanted electrical pacemaker with epicardial electrodes.

CONGENITAL MITRAL INSUFFICIENCY

Isolated congenital mitral insufficiency is a rare lesion usually caused by deformed mitral leaflets. Most physicians attempt to control heart failure with medical management until the child reaches an age when an operative procedure can be done. A mitral prosthesis is required in most cases. The disadvantages of total valve replacement in childhood are the use of anticoagulants, emboli, and the need to change the valve as the child grows.

Chauvand S et al: Long-term results of valve repair in children with acquired mitral valve incompetence. Circulation 1986;74(Suppl 1):104.

ANOMALOUS LEFT CORONARY ARTERY

Origin of the left coronary artery from the pulmonary artery causes myocardial ischemia and heart failure in infancy. The right coronary artery is normal and supplies blood to the entire myocardium and intracoronary collaterals, resulting in blood flow in the anomalous left coronary artery going retrograde into the pulmonary artery. This large coronary steal results in myocardial ischemia, dilation of the heart, and in many cases, fibrosis. Myocardial infarction is not uncommon. The lesion is easily diagnosed by cineangiocardiography. The symptoms are usually pallor, sweating, tachycardia, and episodic chest pain that suggests angina pectoris. Repair is indicated at the time of diagnosis and may consist of either (1) ligation of the anomalous coronary artery to reduce the steal or shunt into the pulmonary artery or (2) graft attachment or direct anastomosis of the left coronary artery to the ascending aorta.

PULMONARY ARTERIOVENOUS FISTULA

In 50% of patients, this rare vascular anomaly is associated with multiple telangiectases (Rendu-Osler-Weber syndrome). One or more large arteriovenous fistulas that do not communicate with alveolar capillaries may occur anywhere in the lungs but are most commonly present in the lower lobes. Pulmonary arterial blood shunts through the fistula into the pulmonary veins to cause mild to moderate cyanosis. Pulmonary arterial and venous pressures are low. Occasional infants develop dyspnea, cyanosis, and right heart failure. Cyanosis, clubbing, and polycythemia are usually most pronounced in late childhood. A soft systolic or continuous murmur is occasionally present over the fistula. Chest x-rays show irregular opacified lesions in the peripheral lung fields at the site of the fistulas. The lesion is confirmed by cineangiocardiography after right ventricular or pulmonary arterial injection. Excision of the fistula is indicated in symptomatic patients and in patients with solitary lesions but is not generally recommended for patients with multiple lesions. Localized resection or lobectomy is most commonly performed.

PULMONARY ARTERIAL STENOSIS

Single or multiple stenoses of the pulmonary arteries occur commonly at the bifurcation of the main pulmonary artery but may occur anywhere between the pulmonary valve and the tertiary pulmonary arteries. About two-thirds of patients have pulmonary valvular stenosis, tetralogy of Fallot, ventricular septal defects, or patent ductus arteriosus. The stenotic lesions produce harsh systolic murmurs that are not well localized. The location of the stenotic areas is determined by observation of a pressure difference during catheterization of the main pulmonary arteries and by cineangiocardiograms after injection of contrast material into the right ventricle.

Patients without associated congenital heart lesions usually do not require operation. Supravalvular stenosis or hypoplasia of the main pulmonary artery of proximal portions of the right or left pulmonary artery is usually treated by balloon dilation angioplasty or enlargement with pericardium or Dacron patches during correction of associated intracardiac lesions.

PERSISTENT LEFT SUPERIOR VENA CAVA

Persistence of a left superior vena cava that connects the left jugular and subclavian veins to the coronary sinus causes no symptoms but is not uncommon. The anomaly is important to the surgeon, since a separate catheter must be inserted through the coronary sinus into the left superior vena cava to collect systemic venous blood during cardiopulmonary bypass. Rarely, the right superior vena cava is absent; in most cases, an innominate vein and both left and right cavae are present, and each cava is adequate to carry all of the systemic venous return from the upper body.

ENDOCARDIAL FIBROELASTOSIS

This lesion is not operable, but it may occur in association with operable lesions such as coarctation of the aorta, aortic stenosis, anomalous left coronary artery, and mitral valvular disease. Hyperplasia of subendocardial elastic and collagenous tissue and proliferation of capillaries cause marked thickening of the ventricular wall and a smooth, glistening lining of the left ventricle. Trabeculae are obliterated, and papillary muscles and chordae tendineae are contracted. The disease affects principally the left ventricle and left atrium; involvement of the right heart chambers is rare. There is some evidence that the disease results from subendocardial ischemia in utero.

Fibroelastosis affects 1–2% of patients with congenital heart disease and may occur primarily without other cardiac lesions. Nearly all infants die of left heart failure within the first year. No specific therapy is available.

CARDIAC TUMORS

Cardiac tumors are rare in infancy and childhood. Metastatic malignant sarcomas are the most common cardiac tumors. Most are inoperable, and none can be cured.

Benign tumors of the heart may cause cardiomegaly, heart failure, murmurs, dysrhythmias, and conduction disturbances. The heart silhouette may be irregular. Functional pathologic changes are directly related to the location and size of the intracardiac tumor mass.

Rhabdomyomas are most common in infants and are often associated with tuberous sclerosis. These tumors involve the ventricular wall, are often multiple, and to date have not been cured.

Fibromas and hamartomas usually present as intracavitary masses attached to the wall of a cardiac chamber. The left ventricle is most frequently involved. Intracavitary fibromas can be successfully excised; intramural tumors cannot.

Myxomas are unknown in infants and rare in children. Intracavitary myxomas are attached to either the atrial or ventricular septum, obstruct flow, and may shed peripheral emboli. Myxomas are usually easily excised but may recur if excision is incomplete.

Teratomas are often extracardiac and attached to the aortic root. Symptoms are produced by cardiac compression. Extracardiac teratomas are easily excised; intracardiac lesions may involve indispensable portions of the heart.

DIRECTIONS IN CONGENITAL HEART SURGERY—1993

Dramatic progress has occurred in the last decade in the treatment of complex congenital heart disease.

Probably the most striking surgical improvements have been (1) the ability to perform complex repairs in infants (anesthesia, extracorporeal circulation, nursing care); (2) applying the physiologic principles described by Fontan in the treatment of multiple lesions that lead to single ventricle physiology (tricuspid atresia, single ventricle, pulmonary atresia, hypoplastic heart syndrome); and (3) the emergence of durability of the anatomic arterial switch operation for the many forms of transposition of the great arteries.

New relationships between specialists in pediatric cardiology and surgery led to improvements in diagnostic and therapeutic decision-making processes. Many lesions no longer require invasive cardiac catheterization because of the improved quality of echocardiography. Handheld echo probes and transesophageal echocardiography have also assisted the surgeon intraoperatively, delineating the anatomy and assessing the quality of repair (residual shunts, valve repair) before the patient leaves the operating suite. Using interventional cardiology techniques it is now possible to close many residual defects after surgery and even some primary or recurrent (postoperative) defects, eg, atrial septal defects, patent ductus arteriosus, pulmonary stenosis, and coarctation of the aorta.

New understanding of fetal and neonatal physiology has led to improvements in myocardial protection and organ preservation. Assist devices and extracorporeal membrane oxygenation have supported critically ill children before and after cardiotomy. Transplantation has emerged as a therapeutic alternative in many complex congenital heart lesions (hypoplastic left heart syndrome) or primary or secondary cardiac or pulmonary failure (cardiomyopathy, cystic fibrosis, Eisenmenger's syndrome).

Treatment strategies have become more standardized for almost all congenital lesions, with higher standards of practice and improved results. Thus, the prognosis for children with congenital heart disease continues to improve.

REFERENCES

Arciniegas E (editor): *Pediatric Cardiac Surgery.* Year Book, 1985.

Fink B: *Congenital Heart Disease,* 2nd ed. Year Book, 1985.

Kirklin JW, Barret-Boyes B: *Cardiac Surgery.* Wiley, 1986.

Esophagus & Diaphragm

20

Carlos A Pellegrini, MD, & Lawrence W. Way, MD

I. THE ESOPHAGUS

With the recent advent of videoscopic techniques, surgery of the esophagus is currently undergoing another leap forward. In some cases, the difference in the postoperative course compared with conventional techniques is nothing short of dramatic. For example, within 24 hours after a videoscopic total esophagectomy, the patient may be fully ambulatory, disconnected from intravenous lines, and feeling well, whereas after the same operation performed by standard open surgery the patient would still be intubated and in need of continuous close monitoring in the intensive care unit. Although experience with this new surgical approach is still in its infancy, it appears likely that nearly all esophageal operations will eventually be feasible by minimally invasive methods. The future looks exceedingly bright and exciting.

ANATOMY
(Figure 20–1)

The esophagus is a muscular tube that serves as a conduit for the passage of food and fluids from the pharynx to the stomach. It originates at the level of the sixth cervical vertebra posterior to the cricoid cartilage. In the thorax, the esophagus passes behind the aortic arch and the left main stem bronchus, enters the abdomen through the esophageal hiatus of the diaphragm, and terminates in the fundus of the stomach. Its muscle fibers originate from the cricoid cartilage and pharynx above and interdigitate with those of the stomach below. About 2–4 cm of esophagus normally lie below the diaphragm. The junction between the esophagus and stomach is maintained in its normal intra-abdominal position by reflections of the peritoneum onto the stomach and of the phrenoesophageal ligament onto the esophagus. The latter is a fibroelastic membrane that lies beneath the peritoneum, on the inferior surface of the diaphragm. When it reaches the esophageal hiatus, the ligament is reflected orad onto the lower esophagus, where it in-

serts into the circular muscle layer above the gastroesophageal sphincter, 2–4 cm above the diaphragm.

Three anatomic areas of narrowing occur in the esophagus: (1) at the level of the cricoid cartilage (pharyngoesophageal sphincter); (2) in the mid thorax, from compression by the aortic arch and the left main stem bronchus; and (3) at the level of the esophageal hiatus of the diaphragm (gastroesophageal sphincter).

In the adult, the length of the esophagus as measured from the upper incisor teeth to the cricopharyngeus muscle is 15–20 cm; to the aortic arch, 20–25 cm; to the inferior pulmonary vein, 30–35 cm; and to the cardioesophageal junction, approximately 40–45 cm.

The musculature of the pharynx and upper third of the esophagus is skeletal in type; the remainder is smooth muscle. Physiologically, the entire organ behaves as a single functioning unit, so that no distinction can be made between the upper and lower esophagus from the standpoint of propulsive activity. As in the intestinal tract, the muscle fibers are arranged into inner circular and outer longitudinal layers.

The arterial supply to the esophagus is quite consistent. The upper end is supplied by branches from the inferior thyroid arteries. The thoracic portion receives elements from the bronchial arteries and from esophageal branches originating directly from the aorta. The intercostal arteries may also contribute. The diaphragmatic and abdominal segments are nourished by the left inferior phrenic artery and by the esophageal branches of the left gastric artery.

The venous drainage is more complex and variable. The most important veins are those that drain the lower esophagus. Blood from this region passes into the esophageal branches of the coronary vein, a tributary of the portal vein. This connection constitutes a direct communication between the portal circulation and the venous drainage of the lower esophagus and upper stomach. When the portal system is obstructed, as in cirrhosis of the liver, blood is shunted upward through the coronary vein and the esophageal venous plexus to eventually pass by way of the azygos vein into the superior vena cava. The esophageal veins may eventually form varices as they

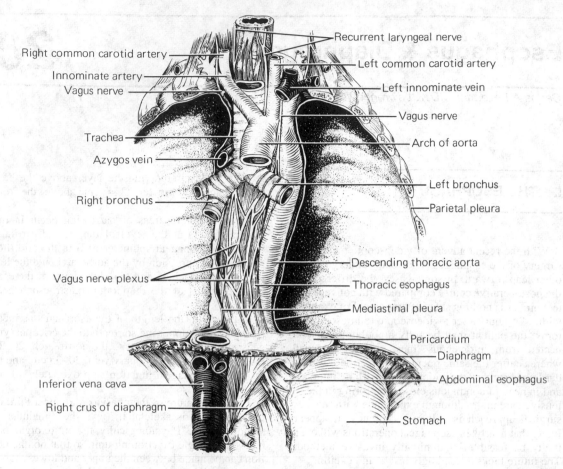

Figure 20–1. Anatomy of the esophagus.

become distended from the increased blood flow and pressure.

The mucosal lining of the esophagus consists of stratified squamous epithelium that contains scattered mucous glands throughout. The esophagus has no serosal layer and, for this reason, does not heal as readily after injury or surgical anastomosis as other portions of the gastrointestinal tract.

PHYSIOLOGY

The clinical physiology of the esophagus is best studied by measuring intraluminal pressure (manometry), pH, and transit time. Manometry is performed by passing into the esophagus and stomach a bundle of fine polyethylene catheters, each of which contains a small distal opening. Continuous perfusion of these tubes with small amounts of saline solution keeps the orifices open and offers a slight resistance to squeeze. The openings are situated 1–5 cm apart and oriented radially to face the esophageal lumen. Simultaneous recordings of pressure can be made at intervals over a segment of known length. Pressures are recorded within the stomach, the gastroesophageal sphincter, the body of the esophagus, and the upper esophageal sphincter during and after swallowing.

Esophageal pH is measured with a probe located 5 cm above the lower esophageal sphincter; a drop in pH reflects exposure to gastric juice. The number and duration of reflux episodes and the relationship of reflux to symptoms reflects the competency of the sphincter and the ability of the esophagus to clear gastric reflux.

Cineradiography is used to study the movement of liquids in relation to esophageal peristalsis. The transit time of radiolabeled food and liquid can be measured by gamma camera images.

The function of the esophagus is to transport food and fluids from the mouth to the stomach and occasionally in the reverse direction. The esophagus contains a sphincter at the junction of the pharynx and esophagus (pharyngoesophageal sphincter) and another between the esophagus and stomach (gastroesophageal sphincter). Pressures in the resting state as measured by manometry are higher in the region of these sphincters than on either side. Pressures in the mouth and pharynx are atmospheric; those within the body of the resting esophagus are slightly subatmospheric, a reflection of normal intrathoracic pressure. Pressure within the stomach is slightly greater than atmospheric.

The structures at the gastroesophageal junction normally function efficiently to prevent reflux of gastric acid and food from the stomach into the esophagus. The mechanism of gastroesophageal competence is complex and, despite intensive study, is incompletely understood at present.

The gastroesophageal sphincter comprises the lower 4 cm of esophagus, where resting pressure within the lumen normally exceeds intragastric pressure by 15–25 cm water owing to tonic contraction of the esophageal musculature. The high pressure is thought to be due mainly to thickening of the circular layer of the esophagus at this level and a special ability of these circular fibers to generate high pressures (due to different responses to neural and peptide stimulation). A small portion of the intraluminal pressure is due to the effects of extraesophageal structures (eg, diaphragmatic contraction).

Many activities transiently increase intra-abdominal pressure. Protection against reflux of gastric contents under these circumstances is aided by the presence of the intra-abdominal segment of esophagus, which is subjected to the same pressure increment, thus counterbalancing pressure increases within the stomach. Dislocation of the sphincter by a sliding hiatal hernia contributes to sphincter incompetence and gastroesophageal reflux.

Experimentally, the gastroesophageal sphincter is strengthened by gastrin and weakened by cholecystokinin, secretin, and glucagon. After a protein meal, contraction of the sphincter increases, and after a fat meal it becomes weaker; whether these effects reflect the actions of gastrin, cholecystokinin, or other hormones is unclear. Gastrin is no longer thought to be a major determinant of sphincter strength.

Cholinergic and alpha-adrenergic stimuli enhance and β-adrenergic stimuli inhibit contraction of the sphincter. A system of nonadrenergic inhibitory nerves involving vasoactive intestinal peptide (VIP) as a neurotransmitter may be responsible for sphincter relaxation.

When swallowing is begun, the tongue propels the bolus of food into the pharynx. Coordinated voluntary movement of the pharyngeal structures results in closure of the glottis and the nasopharynx. The glottis and pharynx rise during this maneuver, and the normal resting high-pressure zone at the pharyngoesophageal sphincter decreases, permitting entry of the food into the upper esophagus. After the food has traversed the pharynx and the pharyngoesophageal sphincter, the pharyngeal musculature re-

laxes and the high-pressure zone returns at the pharyngoesophageal sphincter. As the bolus of food enters the esophagus, a peristaltic wave begins that travels toward the stomach at a speed of 4–6 cm/s, propelling the food before it. The act of swallowing is a reflex response integrated in the medulla oblongata. The relative importance of neural and myogenic mechanisms in initiating and governing the strength, rate, and coordination of peristalsis is debated. When the subject is in the upright position, liquids and semisolid foods usually fall to the distal esophagus by gravity ahead of the slower peristaltic wave. The gastroesophageal sphincter relaxes in anticipation of the advancing food and peristalsis, thereby allowing the bolus to be transported into the stomach. After the food passes through, the sphincter regains its tone until another peristaltic wave arrives from above.

The term primary peristalsis denotes the wave of contraction initiated by swallowing that begins in the upper esophagus and travels the entire length of the organ (Figure 20–2). Local stimulation by distention at any point in the body of the esophagus will elicit a peristaltic wave from the point of stimulus. This is called secondary peristalsis and aids esophageal emptying when the primary wave has failed to clear the lumen of ingested food or when gastric contents reflux from the stomach. Tertiary waves are stationary nonpropulsive contractions that may occur in any portion of the esophagus. Tertiary waves are considered abnormal, but they are frequently present in elderly subjects who have no symptoms of esophageal disease.

Incompetence of the gastroesophageal sphincter takes place normally during vomiting. During this event, the gastroesophageal junction rises above the level of the diaphragmatic hiatus. Ascent is the result of contraction of the longitudinal musculature of the esophagus; an additional result is effacement of the

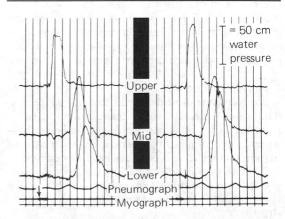

Figure 20–2. Deglutition. Normal esophageal peristaltic waves and pressures during consecutive swallows. Note the orderly downward progression of the waves.

mucosal rosette that ordinarily fills the lumen of the gastroesophageal junction. Expulsion of gastric contents by the violent contractions of the gastric antrum and abdominal wall then becomes possible. After vomiting has subsided, the structures resume their ordinary relationships, with the gastroesophageal junction below the level of the diaphragm.

The buccopharyngeal and esophageal structures engaged in swallowing and transmission of food to the stomach are innervated by motor fibers from the fifth, seventh, ninth, tenth, 11th, and 12th cranial nerves. Afferent sensory impulses are important in maintaining coordination of the motor activity.

ESOPHAGEAL MOTILITY DISORDERS

UPPER ESOPHAGEAL SPHINCTER DYSFUNCTION
(Cricopharyngeal Achalasia)

Essentials of Diagnosis
- Cervical dysphagia.
- Cricopharyngeal bar on barium swallow.
- Zenker's diverticulum in some patients.

General Considerations
Upper esophageal sphincter dysfunction—the term cricopharyngeal achalasia is too precise—may cause dysphagia in a variety of situations, most of which occur in patients over age 60. It may occur as an isolated abnormality or in association with Zenker's diverticulum.

A hereditary syndrome called oculopharyngeal muscular dystrophy, consisting of ptosis and dysphagia, has been described in patients of French-Canadian ancestry. The dysphagia is the result of weak pharyngeal musculature in the face of normal upper esophageal sphincter function; it is considerably improved by upper esophageal sphincter myotomy.

Clinical Findings
A. Symptoms and Signs: Cervical dysphagia, more pronounced for solids than for liquids, is the main symptom of upper esophageal sphincter dysfunction. A chronic cough develops in some patients from minor aspirations of saliva and ingested food.

B. Imaging Studies: Barium swallow nearly always shows a prominent cricopharyngeal bar, which is sometimes so striking as to suggest mechanical obstruction.

C. Endoscopy: The findings on endoscopy are of an extrinsic constriction that allows passage of the endoscope as it is advanced.

D. Manometry: Simultaneous determination of pharyngeal, cricopharyngeal, and upper esophageal pressures often reveals imperfect coordination of relaxation. Normally, the cricopharyngeal sphincter relaxes half a second before contraction of the pharyngeal musculature. In these patients, relaxation, though complete, occurs at or just after initiation of the pharyngeal contraction.

Differential Diagnosis
Esophageal neoplasms must be ruled out by endoscopy. Cervical dysphagia is occasionally the predominant complaint in reflux resulting from lower esophageal sphincter incompetence. In such cases, surgical correction of the reflux relieves the cervical dysphagia.

Treatment
Treatment consists of myotomy of the cricopharyngeus and upper 3–4 cm of the esophageal musculature. The esophagus is approached through an incision parallel to the anterior border of the sternomastoid muscle. The myotomy is made in the midline posteriorly, dividing all fibers of the muscle layers until the submucosa is reached.

Prognosis
Complications are uncommon, and relief of symptoms is usually complete and permanent postoperatively. The procedure should probably not be performed in patients with gastroesophageal reflux, because of the increased risk of aspiration.

Dantas RO et al: Biomechanics of cricopharyngeal bars. Gastroenterology 1990;99:1269.

Duranceau AC et al: Oropharyngeal dysphagia and oculopharyngeal muscular dystrophy. Surg Clin North Am 1983;63:825.

Ekberg O, Feinberg MJ: Altered swallowing function in elderly patients without dysphagia: Radiologic findings in 56 cases. AJR Am J Roentgenol 1991;156:1181.

Sears VW, Castell JA, Castell DO: Radial and longitudinal asymmetry of human pharyngeal pressures during swallowing. Gastroenterology 1991;101:1559.

DIFFUSE ESOPHAGEAL SPASM

Essentials of Diagnosis
- Dysphagia, substernal pain.
- Nervousness, intermittent symptoms.
- Fluoroscopic, cineradiographic, and manometric evidence of high-amplitude contractions.

General Considerations
Primary esophageal motility disorders are characterized by abnormal esophageal motor function, often associated with intermittent chest pain. The diagnosis is made by the characteristic findings on manometry and by eliciting the symptoms with provocative tests.

Although part of a spectrum, they can be broadly classified as follows: **achalasia,** described in the next section; **nutcracker esophagus,** a syndrome of high-amplitude peristaltic waves, seen in about half of patients with motility disorders; **diffuse esophageal spasm,** characterized by nonperistaltic contractions; and **hypertensive lower esophageal sphincter,** a less common disorder. About 35% of patients with primary motility disorders have manometric features of more than one of these conditions, in which case the disorder is called **nonspecific esophageal motor disorder.** The cause of these conditions is not known, though stress can induce similar manometric findings in normal subjects, so stress and psychologic disorders might play a role. Esophageal ischemia has also been postulated. Up to a third of patients with nutcracker esophagus have abnormal gastroesophageal reflux and respond favorably to medical therapy.

Clinical Findings

A. Symptoms and Signs: The most common symptom is intermittent chest pain, which varies from slight discomfort to severe spasmodic pain that simulates the pain of coronary artery disease. Most patients complain of dysphagia, but weight loss is uncommon.

B. Imaging Studies: The esophagogram is abnormal in 60% of patients. Fluoroscopic studies show segmental spasms, areas of narrowing, and irregular uncoordinated peristalsis described as "curling" or "corkscrew esophagus." A small hiatal hernia is frequently demonstrated; less commonly, an epiphrenic diverticulum is present.

C. Manometry: Manometry is the key to the diagnosis of these disorders. In patients with diffuse esophageal spasm, swallows induce repetitive, nonperistaltic (simultaneous) contractions instead of normal peristaltic waves. Some patients also exhibit abnormally strong nonperistaltic waves (140–200 mm Hg). In about 30% of patients, the lower esophageal sphincter fails to relax in response to swallows. In nutcracker esophagus, the primary abnormality is high-amplitude (about 200 mm Hg) peristalsis. Although pressure may be high, sphincter relaxation is normal with swallowing. Why these contractions feel like angina is not known. The hypertensive lower esophageal sphincter may represent a variant of achalasia, and some patients with this disorder have been seen to progress to typical achalasia.

Provocative testing during manometry is useful. The most commonly used drug is the anticholinesterase edrophonium (Tensilon), which can elicit strong esophageal contractions. Elicitation of pain similar to the spontaneous symptom means that the test is positive. Bethanechol and ergonovine may be used instead of edrophonium. If the diagnosis is doubtful, manometry and pH monitoring may be performed. Manometry gives data on esophageal motor activity and its relationship to symptoms, and pH monitoring may demonstrate reflux, a common associated problem.

Differential Diagnosis

The symptoms produced by these motility disorders must be distinguished from those produced by heart disease, mediastinal masses, benign and malignant esophageal tumors, and scleroderma. Although radiologic and pressure studies are diagnostically accurate, esophagoscopy should be performed to confirm the absence of intraluminal lesions such as esophagitis that often produce esophageal spasm.

Complications

Sliding hiatal hernia and epiphrenic diverticula may be secondary complications of the uncoordinated and severe contractions of the esophagus. Regurgitation and aspiration may occur, possibly leading to repeated pneumonic infections. In general, however, the condition is usually mild and does not lead to serious complications.

Treatment

In many patients, reassurance and symptomatic therapy are sufficient. Hydralazine, long-acting nitrates, or anticholinergic agents may give some relief. A soft diet taken in five or six small feedings per day may be required, especially when dysphagia is the most prominent symptom. Bougienage with mercury-weighted dilators is ineffective in diffuse spasm or nutcracker esophagus. Patients with severe pain and dysphagia refractory to medical therapy should have an esophageal myotomy extending from the gastroesophageal sphincter to the aortic arch or as high as the preoperative manometry shows abnormally elevated pressures. This procedure can be performed thoracoscopically or through a thoracotomy. The former is far easier on the patient, and the results are excellent. The open thoracotomy approach should be reserved for patients in whom thoracoscopic surgery is not feasible (eg, previous thoracotomy). Postoperative relief is associated with greatly reduced intraluminal pressures in the esophagus. Reflux esophagitis, the principal complication, may be avoided by preserving the lower esophageal sphincter. If the sphincter must be divided, a short (0.5 cm) Nissen fundoplication should also be performed. The operation is successful in 90% of cases. Persistent pain and dysphagia after surgical attempts to improve esophageal function may be treated by total thoracic esophagectomy and cervical esophagogastrostomy.

Browning TH et al: Diagnosis of chest pain of esophageal origin. Dig Dis Sci 1990;35:289.

Castell DO: Chest pain of undetermined origin: Overview of pathophysiology. Am J Med 1992;92:2S.

Chakkaphak S et al: Disorders of esophageal motility. Surg Gynecol Obstet 1991;172:325.

Eagle KA: Medical decision making in patients with chest pain. N Engl J Med 1991;321:1282.

Ghillebert G et al: Ambulatory 24 hour intraoesophageal pH and pressure recordings v provocation tests in the diagnosis of chest pain of oesophageal origin. Gut 1990;31:738.

Massey BT et al: Abnormal esophageal motility: An analysis of concurrent radiographic and manometric findings. Gastroenterology 1991;101:344.

Shimi SM, Nathanson LK, Cuschieri A: Thoracoscopic long oesophageal myotomy for nutcracker oesophagus: Initial experience of a new surgical approach. Br J Surg 1992;79:533.

Soffer EE, Scalabrini P, Wingate DL: Spontaneous noncardiac chest pain: Value of ambulatory esophageal pH and motility monitoring. Dig Dis Sci 1989;34:1651.

ACHALASIA

Essentials of Diagnosis

- Dysphagia.
- Retention of ingested food in the esophagus.
- Radiologic evidence of absent primary peristalsis, dilated body of the esophagus, and a conically narrowed cardioesophageal junction.
- Absent primary peristalsis by manometry and cineradiography.

General Considerations

Achalasia of the esophagus is a neuromuscular disorder in which esophageal dilatation and hypertrophy occur without organic stenosis. Primary peristalsis is absent and the cardioesophageal sphincter fails to relax in response to swallowing. The circular muscle layer hypertrophies, while the longitudinal coat retains its normal thickness. There is absence, atrophy, or disintegration of the ganglion cells of Auerbach's myenteric plexuses and a reduction in nerve fibers within the wall of the esophagus in most patients. Pharmacologic studies suggest that the cholinergic innervation of the sphincter is intact but the noncholinergic, nonadrenergic inhibitory innervation, which mediates sphincter relaxation through VIP and other peptides, has been lost. The cause is unknown, but two theories exist: (1) a degenerative disease of the neurons and (2) infection of neurons by a virus (eg, herpes zoster) or other infectious agent. The latter is supported by the fact that similar findings occur in patients with **Chagas' disease** (American trypanosomiasis), a condition in which the infective organism destroys parasympathetic ganglion cells throughout the body, including the heart and the gastrointestinal, urinary, and respiratory tracts.

Achalasia affects males more often than females and may develop at any age. The peak years are from 30 to 60.

Clinical Findings

A. Symptoms and Signs: Dysphagia is the dominant symptom, but weight loss is not usually marked despite the functional obstruction. The dilated esophagus is able to contain large quantities of food that only gradually pass into the stomach, largely by gravity. Pain is infrequent even though shallow ulcerations may be produced in the mucosa by the retention and disintegration of ingested food. Regurgitation of retained esophageal contents is common, especially during the night while the patient sleeps in a recumbent position. Aspiration may lead to repeated bouts of pneumonia.

A variant called **vigorous achalasia** is characterized by chest pain and esophageal spasms that generate nonpropulsive high-pressure waves in the body of the esophagus. Sphincteric dysfunction is the same as in ordinary achalasia. Diffuse esophageal spasm has been observed to progress to achalasia, and vigorous achalasia may be an intermediate step in this evolution.

During esophagoscopy, the instrument can be advanced through the narrow sphincter without increased force, a feature that distinguishes achalasia from carcinoma or benign peptic stricture.

B. Imaging Studies: Radiologic studies demonstrate the classic features even in early achalasia. The narrowing at the cardia has a characteristic contour. The dilated body of the esophagus blends into a smooth cone-shaped area of narrowing 3–6 cm long (Figure 20–3). On fluoroscopy the peristaltic waves are weak, simultaneous, irregular, uncoordinated, or absent. As the disease progresses, the esophagus dilates further and becomes tortuous and, in far-advanced cases, sigmoid in shape. The lowermost segment retains the classic long, linear narrowing

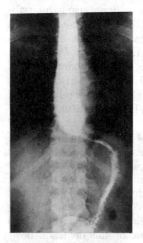 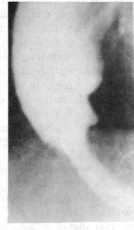

Figure 20–3. Achalasia of the esophagus. **Left:** Moderately advanced achalasia. Note dilated body of esophagus and smoothly tapered lower portion. **Right:** Widely patent cardioesophageal region following cardiomyotomy (Heller procedure).

even in the late stages of the disease. The column of barium is held up at the narrowed area because the sphincteric mechanism fails to relax normally.

C. Manometry: Manometric studies are of value in confirming the diagnosis. In the classic form of achalasia, the motility pattern is as follows: The pharyngoesophageal sphincter has a normal action; the body of the esophagus is devoid of primary peristaltic waves, but simultaneous disorganized muscular activity may be present. Occasionally, no peristalsis of any sort can be observed. The pressure in the gastroesophageal sphincter is about twice normal (40 mm Hg), and relaxation after swallowing is incomplete or absent. Since achalasia is one of several esophageal motor disorders and since there is considerable overlap between them, features of other disorders such as diffuse esophageal spasm, high-amplitude peristaltic waves, et, are occasionally seen in manometric studies. Transition from diffuse spasm or other nonspecific motility disorders into typical achalasia over time has been documented, reinforcing the notion that these represent a group of overlapping syndromes that may have a common pathogenesis. Provocative tests may also be useful in patients with unclear features. For example, subcutaneous administration of bethanechol results in a forceful sustained contraction of the lower two-thirds of the esophagus that is often briefly painful. This response is a manifestation of autonomic denervation of the organ and is absent in normal subjects. A positive response may also be noted in symptomatic diffuse spasm.

After successful forceful dilation or Heller myotomy of the sphincter, manometric evidence of peristalsis returns in a few patients.

Differential Diagnosis

Benign strictures of the lower esophagus and carcinoma at or near the cardioesophageal junction are important conditions to be distinguished from achalasia. Esophagoscopy should always be performed to aid in establishing the diagnosis and also to rule out other intraluminal lesions.

Rarely, an infiltrating intramural carcinoma at the cardia may produce a disorder with all of the pathophysiologic, radiologic, and clinical features of achalasia. The cause appears to be interference with neural control of esophageal motility by the neoplasm. The principal additional finding is marked weight loss.

Complications

Small mucosal ulcerations may develop from the irritation caused by retained food, but true peptic ulceration hemorrhage is rare in achalasia. Aspiration of regurgitated esophageal contents may lead to repeated episodes of pneumonitis, tracheobronchitis, and, rarely, asphyxiation. Malnutrition is usually mild to moderate, but it may be severe in neglected cases. Squamous cell carcinoma of the esophagus develops in 3–5% of patients with achalasia. The lesion occurs predominantly in the dilated portion of the esophagus, usually many years after the initial manifestations. Prolonged exposure to carcinogens from food retained in the esophagus is thought to cause inflammation and metaplasia with later development of dysplasia and cancer. There is no evidence that a Heller myotomy, pneumatic dilatation, or any other treatment reduces the risk of carcinoma.

Treatment

The aim of therapy is to relieve the functional obstruction at the cardia. This can be accomplished by either forceful dilation or direct surgical division of the muscle fibers of the lower esophageal sphincter. Calcium channel blockers also decrease pressure in the lower esophageal sphincter and may improve swallowing, but because of side effects they are not practical.

Forceful dilation involves rapid pneumatic expansion of an inflatable bag placed at the esophagogastric junction. It is accompanied by pain and is thought to disrupt some of the sphincteric musculature. Usually, three or four dilations with balloons of 3–4.2 cm are required to obtain the desired symptomatic and manometric result. A successful dilation is associated with about a 60% decrease in lower esophageal sphincter pressure. After dilation, most patients experience immediate relief of dysphagia, but long-term results are good in only 50%. Persistent dysphagia or reflux esophagitis develops in the remainder. Esophageal perforation, which complicates about 7% of cases, usually presents no clear-cut symptoms in the first few hours. Consequently, patients treated by dilation should routinely be examined by esophagography shortly thereafter and should remain overnight in the hospital for observation. Perforation, demonstrated by free flow of contrast into the mediastinum or pleural space, is a life-threatening problem that requires immediate operation. Dilation is contraindicated in advanced achalasia with megaesophagus because the risk of perforation is especially high in this situation.

An alternative approach—and the procedure of choice for those with advanced disease or failed dilation—is extramucosal cardiomyotomy (Heller myotomy). This procedure can be performed through a thoracoscopic or laparoscopic approach. Using electrocautery, the muscular layer of the esophagus is divided longitudinally for a distance of 6–8 cm, extending distally about 0.5 cm onto the stomach. All muscular fibers must be divided to avoid recurrent dysphagia. The patient may resume eating on the first postoperative day and can usually be discharged the next day. The results are good to excellent in 90% of patients. In the remainder, some dysphagia remains, usually as a result of the poor esophageal peristalsis.

Heller myotomy can also be performed through

open laparotomy or thoracotomy, but the videoscopic approach is technically straightforward and gives a much milder postoperative course. Some surgeons regularly add an antireflux procedure (eg, Nissen or Lind fundoplication) to a Heller myotomy. This can be done in conjunction with a laparoscopic but not a thoracoscopic myotomy. A definite need for this extra step has not been proved, and opinion is divided.

Perforation complicating forceful dilation is best managed by immediate operation, with closure of the perforation and a myotomy on the opposite side of the esophagus.

The results of therapy can be gauged by measuring the rate of esophageal passage of a technetium Tc 99m-labeled solid meal. The decrease in transit time postoperatively is proportionate to the reduction in lower esophageal sphincter pressure.

Prognosis

Relief of obstructive symptoms can be obtained by forceful dilation or by surgery in at least 85–90% of patients. A properly performed Heller procedure overcomes the functional obstruction and uncommonly leads to esophageal reflux. The addition of vagotomy and gastric drainage operations to the myotomy procedure is unnecessary. It may be wise to perform esophagoscopy periodically on all patients, since successful therapy for dysphagia does not lessen the increased risk of esophageal carcinoma seen in this disease.

Bonavina L et al: Primary treatment of esophageal achalasia. Arch Surg 1992;127:222.

Coccia C et al: Prospective clinical and manometric study comparing pneumatic dilatation and sublingual nifedipine in the treatment of oesophageal achalasia. Gut 1991;32:604.

Csendes A et al: Late results of a prospective randomized study comparing forceful dilatation and oesophagomyotomy in patients with achalasia. Gut 1989;30:299.

Ferguson MK: Achalasia: Current evaluation and therapy. Ann Thorac Surg 1991;52:336.

Goldenberg SP et al: Classic and vigorous achalasia: A comparison of manometric, radiographic, and clinical findings. Gastroenterology 1991;101:743.

Paricio JP et al: Achalasia of the cardia: Long-term results of oesophagomyotomy and posterior partial fundoplication. Br J Surg 1990;77:1371.

Pellegrini C, et al: Thoracoscopic esophagomyotomy. Initial experience with a new approach for the treatment of achalasia. Ann Surg 1992;216:291.

Pinotti HW et al: Surgical complications of Chagas' disease: Megaesophagus, achalasia of the pylorus, and cholelithiasis. World J Surg 1991;15:198.

Rosato EF et al: Transabdominal esophagomyotomy and partial fundoplication for treatment of achalasia. Surg Gynecol Obstet 1991;173:137.

Sauer L et al: The treatment of achalasia. Arch Surg 1989;124:929.

Shoenut J et al: Esophageal reflux before and after isolated myotomy for achalasia. Surgery 1990;108:876.

ESOPHAGEAL MANIFESTATIONS IN SCLERODERMA & OTHER SYSTEMIC DISEASES

Scleroderma and several other systemic diseases occasionally involve the esophagus, and when the esophageal symptoms overshadow other manifestations of the disease, the diagnosis may be difficult.

Esophageal dysfunction is common in patients with scleroderma. The initial symptoms are usually those of reflux: regurgitation, heartburn, and, occasionally, bleeding. Dysphagia may also occur but is a less common complaint until esophagitis progresses to stricture formation. The esophageal symptoms usually appear in patients with the characteristic skin changes and Raynaud's syndrome. However, the motility defects may antedate other findings of the disease.

The principal abnormality is atrophy and fibrosis of the esophageal musculature, resulting in progressively weakening function. The changes affect the smooth muscle portion of the esophagus and are most marked at the gastroesophageal sphincter. The motility disorder can be recognized by manometry and cineradiography. On manometry, the resting pressure of the lower esophageal sphincter is low (eg, 5 mm Hg), and primary peristaltic waves have low amplitude or are absent. The most noticeable radiographic abnormality is a patulous cardia with free reflux. A shortened esophagus and strictures can often be seen. pH monitoring shows substantial reflux and poor clearance of the refluxed material. Esophageal shortening may draw the sphincter above the diaphragmatic hiatus, producing a hiatal hernia. Gastric emptying of solids should be measured, even if an abnormality is not suspected from the patient's history, since delayed emptying commonly contributes to the severity of reflux. In about 40% of patients, associated intestinal involvement produces a form of pseudo-obstruction with malabsorption and delayed transit. Similar esophageal changes may also occur in rheumatoid arthritis, Sjögren's syndrome, Raynaud's disease, and systemic lupus erythematosus. Related motor abnormalities are occasionally seen in alcoholism, diabetes mellitus, myxedema, multiple sclerosis, and amyloidosis.

Medical management should always be tried first. It should include dietary (small, frequent, nonfatty meals), mechanical (elevation of the head of the bed), and behavioral (avoid smoking, etc) measures. The drug of choice for esophagitis in patients with scleroderma is omeprazole. Nothing has been found that will delay the deterioration of esophageal function in scleroderma, but in other diseases, specific treatment for the underlying disorder is often of benefit. Strictures can often be managed with repeated dilations. A Roux-en-Y gastrojejunostomy is the best means to correct markedly delayed gastric emptying. If intestinal function is good enough to sustain nutrition, esophageal reflux may be treated by a Nissen fundoplication or a Collis-Nissen procedure, which are at least temporarily successful in the majority of patients even in the face of stricture formation. The late results of these operations are less satisfactory, however, and esophageal replacement (eg, by a colon interposition) will be required in many cases.

Eckardt VF et al: Esophageal motor function in patients with muscular dystrophy. Gastroenterology 1986;90: 628.

Mansour KA, Malone CE: Surgery for scleroderma of the esophagus: A 12-year experience. Ann Thorac Surg 1988;46:513.

Soudah HC, Hasler WL, Owyang C: Effect of octreotide on intestinal motility and bacterial overgrowth in scleroderma. N Engl J Med 1991;325:1461.

Walton S, Bennett JR: Skin and gullet. Gut 1991;32:694.

Zamost BJ et al: Esophagitis in scleroderma: Prevalence and risk factors. Gastroenterology 1987;92:421.

ESOPHAGEAL DIVERTICULA

Diverticula of the esophagus are commonly associated with motor dysfunction. They are acquired lesions that result from the protrusion of mucosa and submucosa through a weakness or defect in the musculature (pulsion type) or from the pulling outward of the esophageal wall from inflamed and scarred peribronchial mediastinal lymph nodes (traction type). The latter are small incidental lesions of no clinical significance and will not be discussed further.

1. PHARYNGOESOPHAGEAL (ZENKER'S) DIVERTICULUM

Essentials of Diagnosis

- Dysphagia, pressure symptoms, and gurgling sounds in the neck.
- Regurgitation of undigested food, halitosis.
- Manual emptying of the diverticulum by the patient.

General Considerations

Pharyngoesophageal pulsion diverticulum is the most common of the esophageal diverticula and is three times more frequent in men than in women. It arises posteriorly in the midline of the neck—above the cricopharyngeus muscle and below the inferior constrictor of the pharynx. Between these two muscle groups is a weakened area through which the mucosa and submucosa gradually evaginate as a result of the high pressures generated during swallowing. Zenker's diverticulum is rarely seen in patients below age 30; most patients are over 60. Although its mouth is in the midline, the sac projects laterally, usually into the left paravertebral region. The body of the esophagus often shows abnormal motility patterns in patients with Zenker's diverticulum, and an associated hiatal hernia is common.

Clinical Findings

A. Symptoms and Signs: Dysphagia is the most common symptom and is related to the size of the diverticulum. Undigested food is regurgitated into the mouth, especially when the patient is in the recumbent position, and the patient may manually massage the neck after eating to empty the sac. Swelling of the neck, gurgling noises after eating, halitosis, and a sour metallic taste in the mouth are common symptoms.

B. Imaging Studies: Fluoroscopic examination demonstrates a smoothly rounded outpouching arising posteriorly in the midline of the neck (Figure 20–4).

C. Manometry and pH Studies: Esophageal manometry and pH measurements will show if the diverticulum is associated with an abnormal response of the cricopharyngeus muscle to swallowing (delayed opening of the sphincter) and the amount of gastroesophageal reflux. Abnormal reflux is present in about one-third of patients. Introduction of the probes is tricky, as they tend to enter the diverticulum, and care must be exercised to avoid a perforation.

Differential Diagnosis

The dysphagia produced by pharyngoesophageal diverticula must be distinguished from that produced by malignant lesions, although carcinoma at this level is uncommon. Achalasia of the cricopharyngeus muscle may produce symptoms similar to those of Zenker's diverticulum. Cervical esophageal webs must also be considered, and a web may occur in association with a diverticulum. The radiologic discovery of a smoothly rounded blind pouch is diagnostic of diverticulum. Esophagoscopy may be hazardous because the instrument may enter the ostium of the diverticulum instead of the true esophageal lumen. Since the diverticulum is composed only of mucosa and submucosa, it is easily perforated.

Regurgitation and aspiration may produce tracheobronchial irritation and pneumonitis. This usually occurs while the patient is in the recumbent position, as during sleep. Food may become trapped in the diverticulum and, rarely, may lead to perforation, mediastinitis, or a paraesophageal abscess. Retained food may ulcerate the mucosa and cause bleeding. Rarely, a fistula may form between the diverticulum and the trachea as a result of infection. Pulmonary infection is the most frequent serious complication, and many patients are first seen after experiencing repeated episodes of pneumonitis.

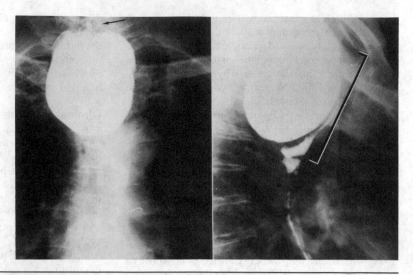

Figure 20–4. Large pharyngo-esophageal diverticulum. Note origin in midline *(arrow, left)* and compression of esophagus *(bracket, right)*.

Treatment

Surgical therapy is the treatment of choice. When done under general anesthesia, it is important to protect the airway immediately upon induction to prevent aspiration of contents that may have collected in the diverticulum. The operation consists of excision of the diverticulum and myotomy of the cricopharyngeal muscle (upper esophageal sphincter). Instead of excising the diverticulum, another option is to invert it into the esophageal lumen while closing the point of inversion so the change in position is permanent. For small diverticula (eg, 1–2 cm), myotomy alone is sufficient. For large diverticula, excision alone may be sufficient, but if myotomy is not performed, some patients still complain of dysphagia. If the patient also has significant gastroesophageal reflux, this should be corrected before the upper sphincter is divided, in order to avoid aspiration.

Prognosis

The prognosis is excellent. Complications are rare, and the patient is usually able to eat the day after the procedure.

Bowdler DA, Stell PM: Surgical management of posterior pharyngeal pulsion diverticula: Inversion versus one-stage excision. Br J Surg 1987;74:988.

Duranceau A, Rheault MJ, Jamieson GG: Physiologic response to cricopharyngeal myotomy and diverticulum suspension. Surgery 1983;94:655.

Ekberg O, Nylander G: Lateral diverticula from the pharyngoesophageal junction area. Radiology 1983;146:117.

Huang BS, Payne WS, Cameron AJ: Surgical management for recurrent pharyngoesophageal (Zenker's) diverticulum. Ann Thorac Surg 1984;37:189.

Low DE, Hill LD: Cervical esophageal web associated with Zenker's diverticulum. Am J Surg 1988;156:34.

2. EPIPHRENIC DIVERTICULUM

Essentials of Diagnosis

- Dysphagia and a sensation of pressure in the lower esophagus after eating.
- Intermittent vomiting, substernal pain.
- Typical radiologic contour.
- Disturbed motility of the lower esophagus.
- Associated hiatal hernia on occasion.

General Considerations

Epiphrenic pulsion diverticula are usually located just above the diaphragm but may occur as high as the mid thorax. They are usually associated with motility disturbances and are frequently larger than diverticula that arise elsewhere in the esophagus. Esophagitis may develop at the ostium. Peridiverticular localized mediastinitis may be seen, especially if ulceration of the mucosa occurs.

Dysphagia and regurgitation are the predominant symptoms, but aspiration and pulmonary symptoms are also seen. Manometric studies demonstrate simultaneous repetitive contractions (or sometimes high-amplitude, prolonged contractions) in the body of the esophagus and in many cases abnormal lower esophageal sphincter function (ie, high resting pressure, incomplete relaxation with swallowing, or an exaggerated postglutition pressure rise).

Diagnosis

The appearance on x-ray films and on fluoroscopy is so distinctive that a definitive diagnosis can usually be made. Associated conditions such as benign or malignant stenoses, webs, hiatal hernia, achalasia and other motility disorders must be ruled out. Esophageal manometry should be performed in every case.

Complications

Esophagitis, periesophagitis, and occasional bleeding from ulceration are the most frequent complications. Tracheobronchial aspiration of regurgitated esophageal contents is uncommon. Perforation occurs rarely.

Treatment

Most patients have minor symptoms that do not require surgery. Surgery is indicated when symptoms become severe. The operation should consist of thoracotomy (or thoracoscopy if feasible), diverticulectomy, and longitudinal myotomy placed opposite the diverticulum on the esophageal circumference. The myotomy should include the abnormal lower esophageal sphincter and should extend proximally to the level where esophageal function becomes manometrically normal. A Belsey or loose Nissen fundoplication is also performed to prevent reflux.

Prognosis

Surgery is successful in 80–90% of cases.

Evander A et al: Diverticula of the mid- and lower esophagus: Pathogenesis and surgical management. World J Surg 1986;10:820.

Mulder DG, Rosenkranz E, DenBesten L: Management of huge epiphrenic esophageal diverticula. Am J Surg 1989;157:303.

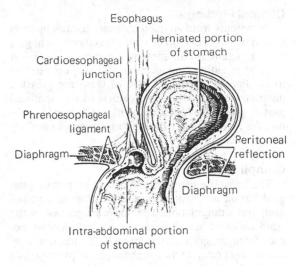

Figure 20–5. Paraesophageal hernia.

gastric contents is uncommon. Rarely, paraesophageal hernia occurs in association with the sliding type, and gastroesophageal reflux may occur along with other symptoms of an otherwise pure paraesophageal type. Paraesophageal hernia accounts for less than 10% of hernias of the esophageal hiatus.

HIATAL HERNIA & ESOPHAGEAL REFLUX

1. PARAESOPHAGEAL HIATAL HERNIA (Figures 20–5 and 20–6)

Essentials of Diagnosis

- Often asymptomatic.
- Symptoms from mechanical obstruction: dysphagia, incarceration, stasis gastric ulcer.

General Considerations

There are two types of esophageal hiatal hernia: paraesophageal and sliding. Sliding hiatal hernia is discussed below. Symptoms usually develop in adult life. Obesity, aging, and general weakening of the musculofascial structures set the stage for enlargement of the esophageal hiatus.

In the paraesophageal type of diaphragmatic hernia, all or part of the stomach herniates into the thorax immediately adjacent and to the left of an undisplaced gastroesophageal junction (Figure 20–6). Since the gastroesophageal sphincteric mechanism functions normally in most of these cases, reflux of

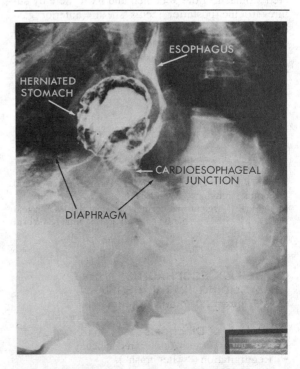

Figure 20–6. Paraesophageal hernia. Note that the cardioesophageal junction remains in its normal anatomic position below the diaphragm.

Clinical Findings

Symptoms from an uncomplicated paraesophageal hernia usually develop in adult life and consist of gaseous eructations, a sense of pressure in the lower chest after eating, and, occasionally, palpitations due to cardiac dysrhythmias. All of these are pressure phenomena caused by enlargement of the herniated gastric pouch by food displacing the fundic air bubble. As noted, heartburn due to gastroesophageal reflux is uncommon.

Complications

The most frequent complications of paraesophageal hernia are hemorrhage, incarceration, obstruction, and strangulation. The herniated portion of the stomach often becomes congested, and bleeding occurs from erosions of the mucosa. Obstruction may occur, most often at the esophagogastric junction as a result of torsion and angulation at this point—especially if a large portion (or all) of the stomach herniates into the chest. In paraesophageal hiatal hernia—in contrast to the sliding type—other viscera such as the small and large intestine and spleen may also enter the mediastinum along with the stomach.

Treatment

Since complications are frequent even in the absence of symptoms, operative repair is indicated in most cases. The usual method is to return the herniated stomach to the abdomen and fix it there by sutures to the posterior rectus sheath (anterior gastropexy). The enlarged hiatus is closed snugly around the gastroesophageal junction with interrupted sutures. It is unnecessary to excise the hernia sac. This operation can be performed with rare exceptions laparoscopically.

Prognosis

The results of surgical management are excellent.

Ellis FH Jr: Paraesophageal hiatus hernia: A surgical disease. Surg Rounds 1989;12:28.
Ellis FH Jr, Crozier RE, Shea JA: Paraesophageal hiatal hernia. Arch Surg 1986;121:416.
Menguy R: Surgical management of large paraesophageal hernia with complete intrathoracic stomach. World J Surg 12:415.

2. REFLUX ESOPHAGITIS & SLIDING HIATAL HERNIA (Figures 20–7 and 20–8)

Essentials of Diagnosis

- Heartburn, often worse on recumbency.
- Regurgitation ("water brash").
- Sliding hiatal hernia on upper gastrointestinal series.
- Endoscopic biopsy evidence of esophagitis.

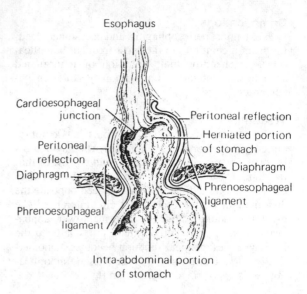

Figure 20–7. Sliding esophageal hernia.

- Decreased resting pressure in lower esophageal sphincter.
- Abnormal esophageal acid exposure on prolonged pH monitoring.

General Considerations

Small amounts of gastric contents reflux normally through the cardia, most commonly after meals and

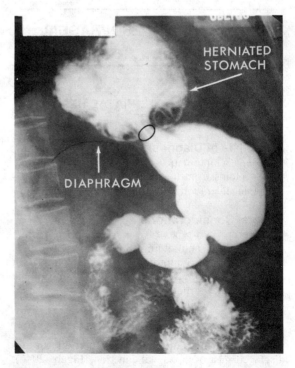

Figure 20–8. Large sliding hiatal hernia. Diaphragmatic hiatus is circled.

often in association with belching. The refluxed material triggers secondary peristalsis, which rapidly clears the esophagus. Esophagitis develops when the frequency of these episodes or the volume of reflux increases beyond a certain point or when the esophagus is unable to clear refluxed material readily. Inflammation worsens in direct relationship to the length of time the esophagus is exposed to refluxed material. Esophagitis, which is usually limited to the distal 7–10 cm of the esophagus, is caused primarily by acid and pepsin. The esophagus is particularly sensitive to bile acids, however, which may also play a role, especially in patients with previous gastric surgery.

The principal barrier to reflux is the lower esophageal sphincter. There is considerable overlap in the values for resting lower esophageal sphincter pressures in patients with reflux and normal subjects. The episodes of reflux that occur in normal persons follow transient relaxations of the sphincter. Three abnormalities of sphincter function allow reflux in patients with esophagitis: (1) transient relaxations of the sphincter in the presence of normal resting pressure; (2) spontaneous reflux in the presence of low resting pressure; and (3) transient increases in intra-abdominal pressure that overwhelm a low resting sphincter pressure. Three-fourths of the reflux episodes in patients with esophagitis follow a transient sphincteric relaxation. Most patients with esophagitis experience reflux at night while sleeping—an uncommon event in normal subjects. Nighttime reflux is related to increased frequency of transient relaxation of the sphincter and is associated with periodic bouts of increased gastric motility (phase III of the migrating motor complex). The chance of developing esophagitis is greater during the night because the refluxed material is primarily composed of acid and pepsin (no food in the stomach), esophageal peristalsis is decreased (delaying clearance), and there is less saliva available to neutralize the acid. As the inflammation of the esophageal wall worsens, peristalsis is further compromised, causing further esophageal acid exposure and damage.

Most patients (80%) with clinically significant reflux have a sliding hiatal hernia. In these patients, the cardioesophageal junction and the fundus of the stomach are displaced upward into the posterior mediastinum, exposing the lower esophageal sphincter to intrathoracic pressure. Normally, the intra-abdominal position of the lower esophagus causes it to be exposed to higher external pressures, and loss of this position accounts for the close association of reflux and hiatal hernia. In summary, sphincter competence is a function of sphincter pressure, sphincter length, and the length exposed to intra-abdominal pressure.

Clinical Findings

A. Symptoms and Signs: Retrosternal and epigastric burning pain—heartburn—occurs after eating and while sleeping or lying in a recumbent position. This distress is relieved partially or completely by drinking water or other liquids, by antacids, or, in many instances, by standing or sitting. The pain is sometimes similar to that of angina pectoris. Patients with severe regurgitation often report that bitter or sour-tasting fluid may regurgitate as far as the throat and mouth (water brash), especially when they are supine. Nausea and vomiting are uncommon in adults but are the most common symptoms in infants, who usually present with failure to thrive. This is the result of postprandial regurgitation leading to vomiting. Anemia is another common presentation in this age group. Pulmonary symptoms (eg, wheezing, dyspnea) may occur as the result of aspiration, and when heartburn is not prominent (especially in infants and children), esophageal reflux may be overlooked as a cause of the disease.

Dysphagia may be a prominent complaint and results from the inflammatory edema (stricture formation) in the lower esophagus. Dysphagia indicates a more advanced stage of the disease and a greater likelihood that complications will develop.

B. Imaging Studies: The diagnosis of sliding esophageal hiatal hernia is made by the radiographic demonstration of a portion of the stomach protruding upward through the esophageal hiatus (Figure 20–8). Fluoroscopic observations while the stomach is full of barium are insensitive (40%) but relatively specific (85%) for diagnosing reflux. Only the most severe cases of esophagitis produce changes in the wall of the esophagus that can be seen on x-ray. X-rays are also useful to evaluate peptic strictures of the esophagus and esophageal ulceration, two complications of reflux.

C. Special Examinations: Special examinations are needed (1) to diagnose abnormal reflux, (2) to quantify and characterize the amount of reflux, (3) to determine the extent of damage to the esophageal mucosa, and (4) to diagnose associated lesions and exclude cancer. Esophagoscopy (and biopsies) are particularly useful to determine the presence and degree of esophagitis and to diagnose associated upper gastrointestinal disease (eg, Barrett's epithelium, duodenal ulcer). One must be cautious, however, in interpreting the semiquantitative visual grading of esophagitis, for there is substantial inter-observer variation, particularly with the lower grades (Table 20–1).

Esophageal motility studies aid in the evaluation of gastroesophageal reflux by providing information on sphincter function and esophageal peristalsis. Mean resting pressure in the lower esophageal sphincter is lower in patients with reflux esophagitis (15 mm Hg) than in control subjects (30 mm Hg), but there is enough overlap so that abnormal reflux can only be diagnosed with certainty if resting pressure is below 6 mm Hg. Patients with more severe esophagitis have lower resting pressures than do those with less severe

Table 20–1. Endoscopic grading system for esophagitis.

Grade 1	Reddening of the mucosa without ulceration
Grade 2	Linear ulcerations lined with granulation tissue that bleeds easily when touched
Grade 3	Ulcerations have coalesced to leave islands of epithelium
Grade 4	Stricture

esophagitis. The normal amplitude of peristaltic contractions in the distal body of the esophagus averages 100 ± 40 mm Hg. Most patients with reflux have abnormal esophageal peristalsis: low amplitude and decreased velocity of propagation of the peristaltic wave. The defect is usually limited to the lower third of the esophagus, and it worsens with more severe esophagitis. Lack of peristalsis suggests the presence of another disease (eg, achalasia) or an associated condition (eg, scleroderma) that may require special treatment.

Prolonged monitoring of pH in the lower esophagus is the most sensitive method of establishing the presence of abnormal reflux. A pH probe is placed 5 cm above the manometrically identified lower esophageal sphincter, and a continuous recording of esophageal pH is stored in a small recorder attached to the patient's belt over a 24-hour period. The patient is asked to register any symptoms and is encouraged to live as normal a life as possible during the recording time. Computer analysis of the record provides a fairly accurate measurement of total esophageal acid exposure, frequency of reflux episodes, and time of day reflux occurred (Table 20–2). A relationship between reflux and symptoms can also be determined. This has virtually eliminated the need for the Bernstein test (infusion of acid in the esophagus to determine whether or not pain is elicited). Prolonged pH monitoring has demonstrated that most patients who have esophagitis reflux predominantly at night.

An accurate **scintigraphic technique** has been de-

Table 20–2. Normal values for ambulatory 24-hour pH monitoring.

Percentage of total time pH <4.0	4.5%
Percentage of upright time pH <4.0	8.4%
Percentage of supine time pH <4.0	3.5%
Number of episodes of reflux <4.0	47
Number of episodes >5 minutes	3½
Longest episode (minutes)	20
Composite score[1]	14.7

[1]The composite score indicates the extent to which the patient's values deviate from the normal means of the six variables. It allows one to express in a single figure the degree of the patient's abnormality. Calculation of the composite score is explained in Stein HJ et al: Outpatient physiologic testing and surgical management of foregut motility disorders. Curr Probl Surg 1992;24:495.

scribed for quantifying gastroesophageal reflux. It may be used for diagnosis or for assessing response to surgical therapy.

If sphincter function as measured manometrically seems good, the possibility of delayed gastric emptying should be suspected as a contributing factor. This should be assessed by measuring the rate of passage from the stomach of a technetium Tc 99m-labeled solid meal; symptoms are unreliable and barium x-rays and liquid emptying tests grossly insensitive.

Differential Diagnosis

Sliding esophageal hiatal hernia has been called the great masquerader of the upper abdomen. Other conditions may present symptoms that mimic those of hiatal hernia, and vice versa. The symptoms caused by a variety of abdominal and intrathoracic diseases are often difficult to differentiate from each other and from those of an uncomplicated sliding hernia. Cholelithiasis, diverticulitis, peptic ulcer, achalasia, and coronary artery disease are common examples. Since esophageal pain may be referred upward into the neck, shoulders, or arms, angina pectoris must be considered. The special examinations described above are particularly helpful in the differential diagnosis and in ascertaining the origin of symptoms in patients with associated diseases (cholelithiasis, angina pectoris, etc).

Complications

As indicated above, esophagitis due to reflux is the most common complication. Small, shallow ulcerations may develop. Areas of denuded epithelium at the cardia are occasionally replaced by columnar epithelium (Barrett's esophagus). This complication is associated with worse reflux and may lead to the development of adenocarcinoma. Aspiration of refluxed material may result in pneumonia, and rarely in pulmonary abscess. Aspiration of small amounts of regurgitated material or the presence of acid in the esophagus through reflex pathways has been thought to be responsible for the development of asthma.

Treatment

A. Medical Treatment: At least half of sliding esophageal hiatal hernias are asymptomatic and require no treatment. The great majority of patients with esophagitis can be managed by a conservative program.

Every effort must be made to enlist the aid of gravity in preventing reflux at night. The patient should not lie down after meals and should not eat a late meal before bedtime. The head of the patient's bed should be elevated on 4- to 6-inch blocks; attempting to sleep propped up on pillows almost never succeeds.

Frequent small meals keep gastric contents neutralized and avoid gastric distention. Meals low in fat and high in protein increase lower esophageal sphincter tone and decrease reflux. Prokinetic drugs such as cisapride and metoclopramide enhance healing of esophagitis, presumably by increasing sphincter tone and peristalsis of the esophagus and stomach.

Mild to moderate forms of esophagitis respond well to 8–12 weeks of treatment with H₂ receptor blockers. These drugs are less useful in severe esophagitis. Omeprazole is substantially better than cimetidine or ranitidine, achieving complete remission of symptoms and healing of esophagitis in 80–85% of patients. The problem with these drugs is that recurrences are the rule when they are discontinued, probably because neither sphincter pressure nor esophageal peristalsis is improved. The addition of a prokinetic agent does not appear to improve the outcome. Antacids do not add to the effects of H₂ blockers but may be used when side effects preclude their use. In this case, they should be used according to the principles outlined in Chapter 23.

B. Surgical Treatment: Surgery is indicated in the 15% of patients who have persistent or recurrent symptoms despite good medical therapy, in those with complete mechanical incompetence of the sphincter (pressure < 6 mm Hg), and in patients who present with or develop strictures during treatment. Antireflux operations can be performed laparoscopically or by open laparotomy or thoracotomy. Although experience is still somewhat limited, the same operations are feasible laparoscopically as by laparotomy but with a much simpler postoperative course. Laparotomy will soon be reserved for patients with contraindications (eg, extensive adhesions) to laparoscopy.

The objectives are to restore the gastroesophageal junction and lower 5 cm of the esophagus to their normal intra-abdominal position and to buttress the gastroesophageal sphincter. In addition, the hiatal opening is narrowed by several sutures posteriorly that approximate the crura. The most effective procedure is Nissen fundoplication (Figure 20–9A), which involves wrapping part of the fundus completely around the lower 3–4 cm of esophagus and suturing it in place so the gastroesophageal sphincter passes through a short tunnel of stomach (Figure 20–9B). The wrap should be made relatively loose with a No. 56F dilator in the esophagus. The top of the wrap should be sutured to the side of the esophagus to prevent axial slipping. Figure 20–10 shows the radiographic appearance of the esophagogastric junction before and after this operation. The Lind fundoplication is similar except that the fundus is wrapped only 270 degrees around the esophagus. It is useful when peristalsis in the body of the esophagus is weak.

Another approach tried for several years involved placing a doughnut-shaped silicone prosthesis (Angelchik prosthesis) around the intra-abdominal esophagus. After it was tied in place, the prosthesis prevented the hiatal hernia from recurring and mildly constricted the lower esophagus, increasing sphincter pressure. Although insertion of the prosthesis was

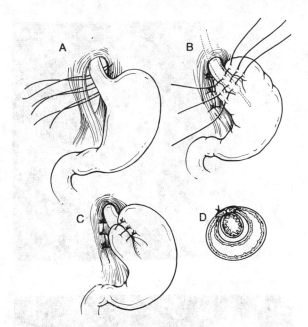

Figure 20–9. **A:** Dissection of the hiatus and lower mediastinum to mobilize the distal esophagus and restore about 6 cm to the abdominal position. **B:** Closure of the diaphragmatic crura behind the esophagus. **C:** Wrapping of the esophagus with the previously dissected fundus of the stomach. **D:** The transverse cut shows the gastric wrap around the distal esophagus. Note how increases in intragastric pressure would be transmitted to the esophagus, facilitating closure of the distal esophagus. The radius of this area of the esophagus is reduced, and the sphincter is prevented from dilating further because of the wrap.

easier than fundoplication, patients often required reoperation to remove the prosthesis (because of migration, esophageal compression, ulceration, etc), and this device is now rarely used. The Belsey fundoplication, performed via a thoracotomy, is less effective than the transabdominal repairs and has also fallen out of favor.

When the hernia cannot be reduced, the condition is called **acquired short esophagus.** Treatment involves constructing a tubular extension of the esophagus along the lesser curvature of the stomach (Collis procedure) with a GIA stapler. The resulting neofundus can be wrapped around the esophageal extension (Collis-Nissen). This is a rare operation. The alternative tactic of making a Nissen wrap in the chest has been associated with frequent complications unless the esophageal hiatus is surgically enlarged to prevent stasis in the thoracic portion of the stomach.

A procedure to reduce gastric acidity should not routinely be added to the hiatal hernia repair but should be reserved for patients with known peptic ulcer disease. A parietal cell vagotomy combined

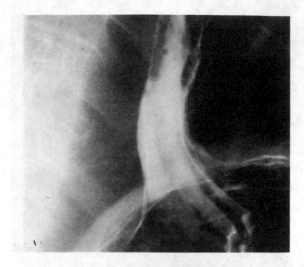

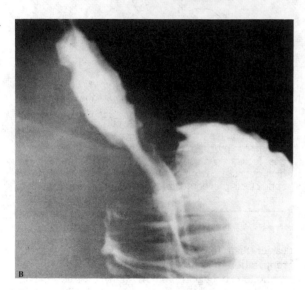

Figure 20–10. Esophagogram before and after Nissen fundoplication in the same patient. **A:** Wide-open reflux of barium occurs through an incompetent sphincter associated with a sliding hiatal hernia. **B:** Three months after surgery, the fundic wrap is evident. Note contrast passing through a small channel surrounded by the wrap. The slightly impregnated transverse folds around this channel represent fundal mucosa of the wrap.

with a Nissen fundoplication is probably best in such cases.

Mild strictures can be managed by dilations with orally passed bougies (eg, Hurst or Maloney dilators) and an intensive medical regimen for the esophagitis. If this approach fails to result in improvement, surgery should be considered. Hiatal hernia repair plus occasional dilations will provide relief in most cases. Rigid strictures that cannot be successfully dilated are best treated by excising the stricture and interposing a segment of colon between normal esophagus and the antrum of the stomach.

When there have been one or more complicated operations around the gastroesophageal junction that have failed, it may be impossible to perform a safe dissection in this area or to mobilize the tissues enough to accomplish fundoplication. Delayed gastric emptying is often found to be a major contributing factor to reflux in these cases, occasionally as a result of unintentional vagotomy from the previous operations. The best treatment for many of these patients is vagotomy, antrectomy, and a Roux-en-Y gastrojejunostomy, which decreases acid secretion, accelerates gastric emptying, and prevents bile and pancreatic juice from gaining access to the esophagus.

Prognosis

About 90% of patients experience a good result following surgery; the remaining 10% have persistent or recurrent reflux. Relief of symptoms is accompanied by an increase in resting pressure in the lower esophageal sphincter of about 10 mm Hg. Recurrence of symptoms is more frequent than an anatomic recurrence. The latter may be due to inadequate technical repair initially; to excessive tension on the point of fixation of the cardioesophageal junction due to shortening of the esophagus; or to weakening of the musculofascial structures by aging, atrophy, or obesity.

Bjerkeset T, Edna TH, Fjosne U: Long-term results after "floppy" Nissen/Rossetti fundoplication for gastroesophageal reflux disease. Scand J Gastroenterol 1992;27:707.

Bonavina L et al: Drug-induced esophageal strictures. Ann Surg 1987;206:173.

Bradpiece HA et al: Esophageal dilation as an outpatient procedure. Surg Gynecol Obstet 1988;167:45.

Bremner RM et al: Concentration of refluxed acid and esophageal mucosal injury. Am J Surg 1992;164:522.

Bytzer P, Havelund T, Hansen JM: Interobserver variation in the endoscopic diagnosis of reflux esophagitis. Scand J Gastroenterol 1993;28:119.

Csendes A et al: Late subjective and objective evaluations of antireflux surgery in patients with reflux esophagitis: Analysis of 215 patients. Surgery 1989;105:374. Dakkak M et al: Oesophagitis is as important as oesophageal stricture diameter in determining dysphagia. Gut 1993;34:152.

DeMeester TR et al: Indications, surgical technique and long-term functional results of colon interposition or bypass. Ann Surg 1988;208:460.

Fiorucci S et al: Gastric acidity and gastroesophageal reflux patterns in patients with esophagitis. Gastroenterology 1992;103:855.

Gotley DC et al: Composition of gastro-oesophageal refluxate. Gut 1991;32:1093.

Hirschowitz BI: A critical analysis, with appropriate controls, of gastric acid and pepsin secretion in clinical esophagitis. Gastroenterology 1991;101:1149.

Othersen HB et al: The surgical management of esophageal stricture in children. Ann Surg 1988;207:590.

Patterson DJ et al: Natural history of benign esophageal stricture treated by dilatation. Gastroenterology 1983;85: 346.

Patti MG, Debas HT, Pellegrini CA: Clinical and functional characterization of high gastroesophageal reflux. Am J Surg 1993;165:163.

Porro GB et al: Short-term treatment of refractory reflux esophagitis with different doses of omeprazole or ranitidine. J Clin Gastroenterol 1992;15:192.

Shaker R et al: Regional esophageal distribution and clearance of refluxed gastric acid. Gastroenterology 1991; 101:355.

Sontag SJ et al: Two doses of omeprazole versus placebo in symptomatic erosive esophagitis: The U.S. Multicenter Study. Gastroenterology 1992;102:109.

Spechler SJ: Comparison of medical and surgical therapy for complicated gastroesophageal reflux disease in veterans. N Engl J Med 1992;326:786.

Stein HJ et al: Complications of gastroesophageal reflux disease. Role of the lower esophageal sphincter, esophageal acid and acid/alkaline exposure, and duodenogastric reflux. Ann Surg 1992;216:35.

Streitz JM Jr, Glick ME, Ellis FH Jr: Selective use of myotomy for treatment of epiphrenic diverticula: Manometric and clinical analysis. Arch Surg 1992;127;585.

Stuart RC et al: A prospective randomized trial of Angelchik prosthesis versus Nissen fundoplication. Br J Surg 1989;76:86.

Tytgat GNJ: Dilation therapy of benign esophageal stenoses. World J Surg 1989;13:142. Vollan G et al: Long term results after Nissen fundoplication and Belsey Mark IV operation in patients with reflux oesophagitis and stricture. Eur J Surg 1992;158:357.

Watson A: Reflux stricture of the oesophagus. Br J Surg 1987;74:443.

Williams D et al: Identification of an abnormal esophageal clearance response to intraluminal distention in patients with esophagitis. Gastroenterology 1992;103:943.

Zaninotto G et al. Esophageal function in patients with reflux-induced strictures and its relevance to surgical treatment. Ann Thorac Surg 1989;47:362.

3. COLUMNAR-LINED LOWER ESOPHAGUS (Barrett's Esophagus)

This condition is the result of an acquired metaplasia that replaces the normal squamous epithelium of the distal esophagus. The change is thought to be induced by chronic gastroesophageal reflux, and its major clinical significance is its association with adenocarcinoma of the esophagus. Indeed, patients with Barrett's esophagus have a twofold increased risk of developing cancer; adenocarcinoma of the esophagus is found in 10% of patients with Barrett's epithelium at the time of first endoscopic examination. An increased incidence of other tumors (eg, colon cancer) has also been noted. The condition is more prevalent among men aged 50–70 years.

Barrett's esophagus is found in 10–15% of patients with reflux esophagitis, and it represents a more virulent form of gastroesophageal reflux. For example, lower esophageal sphincter pressure averages 5 mm Hg (compared with an average of 10 mm Hg for all patients with reflux); 24-hour pH monitoring reveals greater esophageal acid exposure than observed in uncomplicated esophagitis; and acid clearing of the distal esophagus is disproportionately impaired. As a result, damage to the esophagus is greater: ulcers and strictures are present in the majority of patients. In fact, 45% of patients with benign esophageal strictures have Barrett's esophagus. Ulcers in association with Barrett's epithelium are particularly worrisome because they have a tendency to penetrate adjacent organs, including the trachea, aorta, and heart. Barrett's esophagus in children is also associated with abnormal gastroesophageal reflux.

Limited extension of columnar epithelium above the gastroesophageal junction is relatively common in normal subjects. In order to qualify for the diagnosis of Barrett's, this epithelium must extend at least 3 cm above the gastroesophageal junction. The abnormal epithelium may be patchy when confined to the lower 10 cm of esophagus, but when it extends more proximally it is confluent from the gastroesophageal junction to the point of transition to squamous epithelium. Histologically, the epithelium may be one of three types: intestinal (the most common), junctional, or gastric fundic. The intestinal type does not absorb lipids, as does normal intestinal epithelium, and the gastric fundic type, although it contains parietal cells, is atrophic and not a source of significant amounts of acid.

Heartburn, regurgitation, and—with stricture formation—dysphagia are the most common symptoms. Heartburn is milder than in the absence of Barrett's changes, presumably because the metaplastic epithelium is less sensitive than squamous epithelium. The diagnosis is often suggested by the esophagoscopic finding of a pink epithelium in the lower esophagus instead of the shiny gray-pink squamous mucosa, but every case should be verified by biopsy. Radiographic findings consist of hiatal hernia, stricture, or ulcer or a reticular pattern to the mucosa—changes of low sensitivity and specificity.

Treatment is the same as for reflux esophagitis in general: antacids, H_2-blocking agents, elevation of the head of the bed, and avoidance of smoking and ulcerogenic beverages or drugs. Antireflux surgery (eg, Nissen fundoplication), is commonly indicated because of the severity of gastroesophageal reflux or the development of ulcers or strictures. Some strictures may require periodic postoperative dilatation. Resection is required on rare occasions to treat a nondilatable stricture or to control bleeding. The abnormal epithelium rarely regresses after medical or surgical therapy.

Because of the substantially increased risk of cancer, routine endoscopy and biopsy should be performed every 6–12 months, especially in patients with intestinal metaplasia. Biopsies should be obtained at multiple levels looking for carcinoma (which is not always identifiable by gross examination) and for dysplasia. High-grade dysplasia is clearly associated with carcinoma, but the histologic diagnosis is difficult. Flow cytometry can now identify abnormalities of DNA content, such as aneuploidy or increased G_2/tetraploid fractions, that are associated with high-grade dysplasia and increased risk of cancer. Transmission electron microscopy may detect abnormalities in cytoplasmic organelles that have similar implications. Patients who are found to have high-grade dysplasia or the abnormalities described should be considered for resection of the entire portion of esophagus lined with Barrett's mucosa.

Attwood SE et al: Role of intragastric and intraoesophageal alkalinisation in the genesis of complications in Barrett's columnar lined lower oesophagus. Gut 1993;34:11.

DeMeester TR: Barrett's esophagus. Surgery 1993;113:239.

Iftikhar SY et al: Length of Barrett's oesophagus: An important factor in the development of dysplasia and adenocarcinoma. Gut 1992;33:1155.

Jankowski J et al: Epidermal growth factor in the oesophagus. Gut 1992 33:1448.

Jankowski J et al: Epidermal growth factor receptors in the oesophagus. Gut 1992;33:439.

Pera M et al: Increasing incidence of adenocarcinoma of the esophagus and esophagogastric junction. Gastroenterol 1993;104:510.

Pera M et al: Barrett's esophagus with high-grade dysplasia: an indication for esophagectomy? Ann Thoracic Surgery 1992;54:199.

Stein HJ, Hoeft S, DeMeester TR: Functional foregut abnormalities in Barrett's esophagus. J Thorac Cardiovasc Surg 1993;105:107.

Streitz JM Jr, Andrews CW Jr, Ellis FH Jr: Endoscopic surveillance of Barrett's esophagus: Does it help? J Thorac Cardiovasc Surg 1993;105:383.

OTHER SURGICAL DISORDERS OF THE ESOPHAGUS

PERFORATION OF THE ESOPHAGUS

Essentials of Diagnosis

- History of recent instrumentation of the esophagus or severe vomiting.
- Pain in the neck, chest, or upper abdomen.
- Signs of mediastinal or thoracic sepsis within 24 hours.
- Contrast radiographic evidence of an esophageal leak.
- Crepitus and subcutaneous emphysema of the neck in some cases.

General Considerations

Esophageal perforations can result from iatrogenic instrumentation (eg, endoscopy, balloon dilatation), severe vomiting, external trauma, and other rare causes. The subsequent clinical manifestations are influenced by the site of the perforation (ie, cervical or thoracic) and, in the case of thoracic perforations, whether or not the mediastinal pleura has been ruptured. Morbidity resulting from esophageal perforation is principally due to cervical or mediastinal and thoracic infection. Immediately after injury, the tissues are contaminated by esophageal fluids, but infection has not become established; surgical closure of the defect will usually prevent the development of serious infection. If more than 24 hours have elapsed between injury and surgical treatment, infection will have occurred. At this time, the esophageal defect usually breaks down if it is surgically closed, and measures to treat mediastinitis and empyema may not be adequate to avoid a fatal outcome. Although serious infection usually occurs if surgical repair is delayed, a few cases of minor instrumental perforations can be managed by antibiotics without operation.

A. Instrumental Perforations: Instrumental perforations are most likely to occur in the cervical esophagus. The esophagoscope may press the posterior wall of the esophagus against osteoarthritic spurs of the cervical vertebrae, causing contusion or laceration. The cricopharyngeal area is the most common site of injury. Perforations of the thoracic esophagus may occur at any level but are most common at the natural sites of narrowing, ie, at the level of the left main stem bronchus and at the diaphragmatic hiatus.

B. Spontaneous (Emetogenic) Perforation (Boerhaave's Syndrome): Spontaneous perforation usually occurs in the absence of preexisting esophageal disease, but 10% of patients have reflux esophagitis, esophageal diverticulum, carcinoma, etc. Most cases follow a bout of heavy eating and drinking. The rupture usually involves all layers of the esophageal wall and most frequently occurs in the left posterolateral aspect 3–5 cm above the gastroesophageal junction. The tear results from excessive intraluminal pressure, usually caused by violent retching and vomiting. Cases have also been associated with childbirth, defecation, convulsions, heavy lifting, and forceful swallowing. The overlying pleura is also torn, so that the chest as well as the mediastinum is contaminated with esophageal contents. The second most common site of perforation is at the midthoracic esophagus on the right side at the level of the azygos vein.

Clinical Findings

A. Signs and Symptoms: The principal early manifestation is pain, which is felt in the neck with cervical perforations and in the chest or upper abdomen with thoracic perforations. The pain may radiate to the back. With cervical perforations, pain followed by crepitus in the neck, dysphagia, and gradually developing signs of infection is the extent of the syndrome. Thoracic perforations, which communicate with the pleural cavity in about 75% of cases, are usually accompanied by tachypnea, hyperpnea, dyspnea, and the early development of hypotension. With perforation into the chest, pneumothorax is produced followed by hydrothorax and, if not promptly treated, empyema. The left chest is involved in 70% and the right chest in 20%; involvement is bilateral in 10%. The rate of fluid accumulation in the chest may be as high a 1 L/h, which results in hypovolemia and a shift of the mediastinum to the right. Escape of air into the mediastinum may result in a "mediastinal crunch," which is produced by the heart beating against air-filled tissues (Hamman's sign). If the pleura remains intact, mediastinal emphysema appears more rapidly, and pleural effusion is slow to develop.

B. Imaging Studies: X-ray studies are important to demonstrate that perforation has occurred and to locate the site of the injury. In perforations of the cervical esophagus, x rays show air in the soft tissues, especially along the cervical spine. The trachea may be displaced anteriorly by air and fluid. Later, widening of the superior mediastinum may be seen. With thoracic perforations, mediastinal widening and pleural effusion with or without pneumothorax are the usual findings. Mediastinal emphysema, seen in about 40% of cases, takes at least an hour to develop.

An esophagogram using water-soluble contrast medium should be performed promptly in every patient suspected of having an esophageal perforation (Figure 20–11). The patient should be studied in the decubitus as well as the upright position. If a leak is not seen, the examination should be repeated using barium.

C. Special Studies: Thoracentesis will reveal cloudy or purulent fluid depending on how much time has passed since the contamination first occurred. The amylase content of the fluid is elevated, and serum amylase levels may also be high as a result of absorption of amylase from the pleural cavity.

Treatment

Antibiotics should be given immediately. Early surgery is appropriate for all but a few cases, and every effort should be made to operate before the perforation is 24 hours old. For lesions treated within this time limit, the operation should consist of closure of the perforation and external drainage. External drainage alone may suffice for small cervical perforations, which may be difficult to find. Patients with achalasia in whom perforation has resulted from balloon dilatation of the lower esophageal sphincter should have the tear in the esophagus repaired and a Heller myotomy performed on the opposite side of

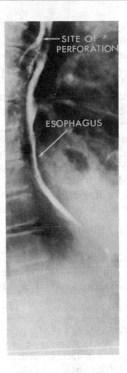

Figure 20–11. Extravasation of contrast material through instrumental perforation of upper thoracic esophagus. Note locules of air and fluid anterior to esophagus, indicating that mediastinitis has already developed.

the esophagus. Definitive therapy (eg, resection) should also be performed in patients with other surgical conditions, such as esophageal carcinoma.

Primary repair has a high failure rate if the perforation is older than 24 hours. The classic recommendation in this situation has been to isolate the perforation (ie, to minimize further contamination) by performing a temporary cervical esophagostomy, ligating the cardia, and constructing a feeding jejunostomy. Probably a better approach is to resect the site of the perforation, bringing the proximal end of esophagus out through the neck and closing the distal end. The mediastinum is drained and a feeding jejunostomy created. Later, the esophagostomy is taken down and colon interposed to bridge the gap at the site of resection. Blunt esophagectomy may be feasible as emergency treatment of instrumental perforation in a patient with lye stricture.

Spontaneous incomplete rupture of the esophagus is seen occasionally. This lesion may be the result of increased intraluminal pressure or may be idiopathic, but the tear is usually located in the mid esophagus. In incomplete rupture, the tear is confined to the mucosal layer; it dissects distally in the submucosal plane, often as far as the gastroesophageal junction. The manifestations consist of chest pain, dyspnea, odynophagia, and, sometimes, bleeding. An esophagogram demonstrates an intramural tract of barium (which may give a double-lumen appearance) and sometimes encroachment on the esophageal lumen by an intramural hematoma. Treatment is with antibiotics and total parenteral nutrition.

Nonoperative management consisting of antibiotics alone may be all that is necessary in a few selected cases of instrumental perforation. This approach should be confined to patients without thoracic involvement (eg, pneumothorax or hydrothorax) whose esophagogram demonstrates just a short extraluminal sinus tract without wide mediastinal spread (ie, the contamination is limited) and who have no systemic signs of sepsis (eg, hypotension and tachypnea).

Prognosis

The survival rate is 90% when surgical treatment is accomplished within 24 hours. The rate drops to about 50% when treatment is delayed.

Attar S et al: Esophageal perforation: A therapeutic challenge. Ann Thorac Surg 1990;50:45.

Chang CH et al: One-stage operation for treatment after delayed diagnosis of thoracic esophageal perforation. Ann Thorac Surg 1992;53:617.

Graeber GM, Murray GF: Injuries of the esophagus. Semin Thorac Cardiovasc Surg 1992;4:247.

Henderson JAM, Peloquin AJM: Boerhaave revisited: Spontaneous esophageal perforation as a diagnostic masquerader. Am J Med 1989;86:559.

Jones WG 2d, Ginsberg RJ: Esophageal perforation: A continuing challenge. Ann Thorac Surg 1992;53:534.

Tilanus HW et al: Treatment of oesophageal perforation: A multivariate analysis. Br J Surg 1991;78:582.

INGESTED FOREIGN OBJECTS

Most cases of ingested foreign objects occur in children who swallow coins or other small objects. In adults, the problem most often consists of esophageal meat impaction or, less commonly, lodged bones or toothpicks. Dentures, which interfere with the ability to judge the size and consistency of a food bolus, and esophageal disease, such as a benign stricture, are the principal predisposing factors in adults. Prisoners and mentally defective persons occasionally swallow foreign objects intentionally.

About 90% of swallowed foreign objects pass into the stomach and from there into the intestine and are eventually passed without incident. Ten percent hang up in the esophagus. If they traverse the esophagus, objects whose dimensions exceed 2 × 5 cm tend to remain in the stomach. Ten percent of ingested foreign objects require endoscopic removal, and 1% require surgery. About 10% of ingested foreign objects enter the tracheobronchial tree.

The history usually defines the problem adequately. The patient with a foreign object in the esophagus may or may not experience dysphagia or chest pain.

Specific Kinds of Ingested Foreign Objects

A. Coins: Pennies and dimes usually pass into the stomach, but larger coins will lodge in the esophagus at or just beyond the cricopharyngeus. It is important to know if a swallowed coin has remained in the esophagus, and whether or not the patient has symptoms is an unreliable basis for making the determination. Therefore, anteroposterior and lateral chest x-rays should be obtained to determine whether the coin is in the esophagus or trachea. Small children should be x-rayed from the base of the skull to the anus in order to find any additional coins in the gut.

Coins in the esophagus should be removed promptly, since serious complications (eg, esophagoaortic fistula) may occur if treatment delay exceeds 24 hours. The procedure is best accomplished with a grasping forceps passed through a flexible endoscope. Sedation is adequate for older children or adults, but general endotracheal anesthesia is required in order to protect the airway of infants and young children. A smooth foreign body too large to grasp with a forceps can be removed by passing a dilating balloon beyond it and then withdrawing the endoscope and balloon as a unit. If the object is small enough (< 20 mm), it may be pushed into the stomach.

Another popular technique for extracting coins is to pass a Foley catheter into the esophagus under radiologic control and withdraw the coin with the inflated balloon. Although usually successful, this method has the disadvantage of providing incomplete protection of the airway.

Once a coin has passed into the stomach, it can be observed by periodic x-rays for as long as a month before the conclusion is reached that spontaneous elimination is unlikely and endoscopic removal is indicated.

B. Meat Impaction: Meat is the most common foreign object that lodges in the esophagus of adults, and many affected patients have underlying esophageal disease. The site of meat impaction is usually at the cricopharyngeus muscle or cervical esophagus, where it may exert pressure anteriorly on the trachea and produce respiratory obstruction.

No x-rays (especially barium studies) are indicated, for they make the endoscopist's task more difficult. If obstruction is complete and the patient cannot handle saliva, endoscopy should be performed as an emergency to prevent aspiration. If the clinical findings are minor, however, endoscopy can be postponed for up to 12 hours (but no longer) to see whether the food will pass spontaneously.

Meat can usually be removed as a single piece using a polypectomy snare passed through a flexible endoscope. If the meat has begun to fragment, a rigid endoscope makes the job of piecemeal removal easier. In some cases, a meat bolus can be pushed into the stomach, which is safe so long as it passes with minimal pressure. After the esophagus has been cleared, it should be checked endoscopically for underlying disease. An esophageal stricture should be dilated if the esophageal wall is not acutely inflamed as a result of the meat impaction.

Attempts to digest meat in the esophagus with topical papain are not advised. The enzyme actually has little effect on the meat, and it may damage the esophageal wall. Gas-forming agents (which push the object) and glucagon (which relaxes the esophagus) have been recommended for this purpose, but these methods are less effective than flexible endoscopy.

C. Sharp and Pointed Objects: Bones, safety pins, hat pins, razor blades, toothpicks, nails, and many others constitute this group of foreign objects. The general principles of management are (1) to remove sharp or pointed objects endoscopically by grasping and pulling a blunt side (eg, the hinge of an open safety pin) if there is one with forceps; (2) to remove a piece of glass or a razor blade by pulling it into the lumen of a rigid esophagoscope; or (3) to operate if neither of these methods appears to be safe. Sharp or pointed objects in the stomach should be removed surgically, since 25% of them will perforate the intestine, usually near the ileocecal valve, if they exit the pylorus.

D. Button Batteries: These small batteries are swallowed by children, just like coins, but unlike coins they are highly corrosive and should be removed urgently before a serious complication such as an esophagotracheal or esophagoaortic fistula develops.

E. Cocaine Packets: Cocaine smugglers may swallow small packets of cocaine in balloons or condoms. Rupture of just one of these packets can be fatal, so attempts at endoscopic removal are unsafe. If it appears that the packets will pass spontaneously, the patient may be watched; otherwise, surgical removal is indicated.

F. Foreign Bodies in the Pharynx and Cricopharyngeus: Foreign objects at this level should be removed using sedation and direct laryngoscopy. Most are fish bones.

Complications:

Aspiration and esophageal ulceration are the most common complications. Perforation of the esophagus or other portions of the gut requires surgical repair. It is estimated that about 1500 people die in the USA each year from complications of ingested foreign bodies.

Bertoni G et al: Endoscopic protector hood for safe removal of sharp-pointed gastroesophageal foreign bodies. Surg Endosc 1992;6:255.

Brady PG: Esophageal foreign bodies. Gastroenterol Clin North Am 1991;20:691.

Litovitz T, Schmitz BF: Ingestion of cylindrical and button batteries: an analysis of 2382 cases. Pediatrics 1992; 89:747.

Rubin SZ, Mueller DL: Removal of esophageal foreign bodies with a Foley balloon catheter under fluoroscopic control. Can Med Assoc J 1987;137:125.

Stringer MD, Capps SN: Rationalising the management of swallowed coins in children. Br Med J 1991;302:1321.

Webb WA: Management of foreign bodies of the upper gastrointestinal tract. Gastroenterol 1988;94:204.

Zimmers TE et al: Use of gas-forming agents in esophageal food impactions. Ann Emerg Med 1988;17:693.

CORROSIVE ESOPHAGITIS

Essentials of Diagnosis

- History of ingestion of caustic liquids or solids.
- Burns of the lips, mouth, tongue, and oropharynx.
- Chest pain and dysphagia.

General Considerations

Ingestion of strong solutions of acid or alkali or of solid substances of similar nature produces extensive chemical burns, often leading to corrosive esophagitis. The injury usually represents a suicide attempt in adults and accidental ingestion in children. Strong alkali produces "liquefaction necrosis," which involves dissolution of protein and collagen, saponification of fats, dehydration of tissues, thrombosis of blood vessels, and deep penetrating injuries. Acids produce a "coagulation necrosis" involving eschar formation, which tends to shield the deeper tissues from injury. Depending upon the concentration and the length of time the irritant remains in contact with the mucosa, sloughing of the mucous membrane, edema and inflammation of the submucosa, infection, perforation, and mediastinitis may develop.

Ingested lye in solid form tends to adhere to the mucosa of the pharynx and proximal esophagus. Severe acute esophageal necrosis is rare, and the main clinical problems are early edema and late stricture formation, principally of the proximal esophagus. Liquid caustics commonly produce much more extensive esophageal necrosis, and occasionally even tracheoesophageal and esophagoaortic fistulas. If the patient survives the acute phase, a lengthy nondilatable stricture often develops.

Ingestion of strong acid characteristically produces greatest injury to the stomach, with the esophagus remaining intact in over 80% of cases. The result may be immediate gastric necrosis or late antral stenosis.

Nearly all severe injuries are caused by strong alkali. Weak alkali and acid are associated with less extensive lesions.

Clinical Findings

A. Symptoms and Signs: Systemic symptoms roughly parallel the severity of the caustic burn. The most common finding is inflammatory edema of the lips, mouth, tongue, and oropharynx; in the absence of visible injury in this area, severe esophageal damage is rare. Patients with serious esophageal burns often experience chest pain and dysphagia and drooling of large amounts of saliva. Pain on attempted swallowing may be intense. If the damage is severe, the patient often appears toxic, with high fever, prostration, and shock. The absence of toxicity does not rule out severe injury, however. Tracheobronchitis accompanied by coughing and increased bronchial secretions is frequently noted. Stridor may be present, and in a few patients respiratory obstruction progresses rapidly and requires tracheostomy for relief. Complete esophageal obstruction due to edema, inflammation, and mucosal sloughing may develop within the first few days.

B. Esophagoscopy: A determination of the extent of injury by esophagoscopy contributes substantially to therapeutic decisions. Esophagoscopic examination should be performed after the initial resuscitation, usually within 12 hours of admission. The scope is inserted far enough to gauge the most serious degree of burn, which is classified as first-, second-, or third-degree as defined in Table 20–3.

Treatment

Classic treatment for caustic injuries of the esophagus involved the administration of antibiotics and corticosteroids and observation for late stricture formation. The advent 20 years ago of strong liquid alkali in the marketplace, however, has resulted in more severe full-thickness injuries, which are too often fatal or cause lengthy nondilatable strictures when treated in this fashion. Furthermore, the evidence now indicates that corticosteroids really have little or no effect on stricture formation. Early surgery is now recommended for patients with second- and third-degree burns.

Patients with first-degree burns do not require aggressive therapy and may be discharged from the hospital after a short period of observation. Patients with second- or third-degree burns are best treated by early laparotomy, at which time the distal esophagus and stomach are inspected and a full-thickness biopsy of the gastric wall is taken to further grade the lesion. It is not possible to distinguish between a minor third-degree injury and extensive full-thickness third-degree necrosis from the esophagoscopic findings alone. This must be done from external appearances at laparotomy.

Second-degree and minor spotty third-degree injuries are treated by inserting an esophageal stent (a Silastic tube) and a jejunostomy feeding tube. If any question remains about the viability of the tissues, a second-look operation should be performed 36 hours later. Antibiotics and corticosteroids are given, and the stent is left in place for 3 weeks, at which time an esophagogram is performed. If barium passes freely alongside the stent, it is removed. If it does not, the stent is left in place for another week, and x-rays are repeated. Periodic esophagograms are obtained in late follow-up to look for stricture formation, which is treated early in its development by dilatations.

Third-degree burns involving extensive esophagogastric necrosis require emergency esophagogastrectomy, esophagostomy, and feeding jejunostomy. Esophagectomy is best performed by the blunt technique using a laparotomy and cervical incision. It is sometimes necessary to resect adjacent organs (eg, transverse colon) that have also been damaged. Reconstruction by substernal colon interposition is performed 6–8 weeks later.

Prognosis

Early and proper management of caustic burns provides satisfactory results in most cases. The ingestion of strong acid or alkaline solutions with extensive immediate destruction of the mucosa produces profound pathologic changes which may result in fibrous strictures that require dilatations and, in some cases, esophagectomy and colon interposition.

Table 20–3. Endoscopic grading of corrosive burns of esophagus and stomach.[1]

Grade	Definition	Endoscopic Findings
First-degree	Superficial mucosal injury	Mucosal hyperemia and edema; superficial mucosal desquamation.
Second-degree	Full-thickness mucosal involvement. No or partial-thickness muscular injury.	Sloughing of mucosa. Hemorrhage, exudate, ulceration, pseudomembrane formation, and granulation tissue when examined late.
Third-degree	Full-thickness esophageal or gastric injury with extension into adjacent tissues.	Sloughing of tissues with deep ulceration. Complete obliteration of esophageal lumen by edema; charring and eschar formation; full-thickness necrosis; perforation.

[1]Reproduced, with permission, from Estrera A et al: Corrosive burns of the esophagus and stomach: A recommendation for an aggressive surgical approach. Ann Thorac Surg 1986; 41:276.

Anderson KD, Rouse TM, Randolph JG: A controlled trial of corticosteroids in children with corrosive injury of the esophagus. N Engl J Med 1990;323:637.

Estrera A et al: Corrosive burns of the esophagus and stomach: A recommendation for an aggressive surgical approach. Ann Thorac Surg 1986;41:276.

Gorman RL et al: Initial symptoms as predictors of esophageal injury in alkaline corrosive ingestions. Am J Emerg Med 1982;10:189.

Graeber GM, Murray GF: Injuries of the esophagus. Semin Thorac Cardiovasc Surg 1992;4:247.

Horvath OP, Olah T, Zentai G: Emergency esophagogastrectomy for treatment of hydrochloric acid injury. Ann Thorac Surg 1991;52:98.

Howell JM et al: Steroids for the treatment of corrosive esophageal injury: A statistical analysis of past studies. Am J Emerg Med 1982;10:421.

Vergauwen P et al: Caustic burns of the upper digestive and respiratory tracts. Eur J Pediatr 1991;150:700.

Zargar SA et al: Ingestion of strong corrosive alkalis: Spectrum of injury to upper gastrointestinal tract and natural history. Am J Gastroenterol 1992;87:337.

TUMORS OF THE ESOPHAGUS

1. BENIGN TUMORS OF THE ESOPHAGUS

Essentials of Diagnosis

- Dysphagia often present but frequently mild.
- Sense of pressure in thorax or neck.
- Radiographic demonstration of intra- or extraluminal mass, smooth in outline.

General Considerations

Benign growths may arise in any layer of the esophagus. Inflammatory polyps or granulomas are occasionally associated with esophagitis and may be mistakenly interpreted as neoplastic lesions. Papillomas arising from the mucosa are either sessile or pedunculated; although they are usually small lesions, occasionally they become large enough to produce obstruction. They may slough off spontaneously into the esophageal lumen.

Leiomyoma is the most common benign lesion of the esophagus. Leiomyomas are benign tumors that originate in the smooth muscle of the esophagus. As they grow, they narrow the esophageal lumen. The mucosa overlying the tumor is generally intact, but occasionally it may become ulcerated as a result of pressure necrosis by an enlarging lesion. Leiomyomas are not associated with the development of cancer. Other tumors such as fibromas, lipomas, fibromyomas, and myxomas are rare.

Congenital cysts or reduplications of the esophagus (the second most common benign lesion after leiomyoma) may occur at any level, although they are most common in the lower esophagus.

Clinical Findings

Many benign lesions are asymptomatic and are discovered incidentally during upper gastrointestinal fluoroscopic examination. Cysts and leiomyomas may be large enough to appear as a density, usually round or ovoid, in the mediastinum on routine chest x-rays. Benign tumors or cysts grow slowly and become symptomatic only after enough encroachment of the esophageal lumen has occurred. Barium swallow in a patient with leiomyoma shows a smoothly rounded, often spherical mass that causes extrinsic narrowing of the esophageal lumen (Figure 20–12). The overlying mucosa is almost always intact. Peristalsis is not affected by leiomyomas but is often abnormal in the presence of cysts or reduplications. Spasm of the musculature adjacent to the cyst or duplication is the most common abnormality of peristalsis. Dilatation of the esophagus proximal to any of the benign lesions is rare. Intraluminal growths can be recognized at esophagoscopy, and a specific tissue diagnosis should always be obtained. Intramural lesions such as leiomyomas should not be biopsied, because (1) there is a risk of hemorrhage and (2) an adhesion develops between the tumor and the mucosa, making the lesion difficult to shell out during surgery and resulting in an otherwise avoidable mucosal opening.

Differential Diagnosis

Leiomyomas, cysts, and reduplications can be distinguished from cancerous growths by their classic radiographic appearance. Intraluminal papillomas, polyps, or granulomas may be indistinguishable radiographically from early carcinoma, so their exact nature must be confirmed histologically.

Complications

Cysts and duplications derive their arterial supply directly from the aorta. Hemorrhage into these lesions may occur, especially following infection, although this complication is uncommon. Adhesions that form between the cystic lesions and the adjacent esophagus often produce progressive dysphagia. Pedunculated intraluminal tumors may cause sudden obstruction by torsion of their pedicles, which is fol-

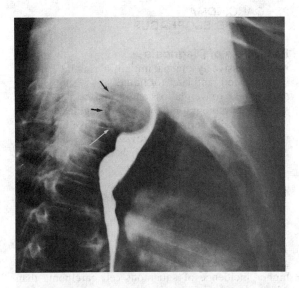

Figure 20–12. Leiomyoma of esophagus. Note smooth, rounded density causing extrinsic compression of esophageal lumen.

lowed by edema, infection, and bleeding. In the upper esophagus, pedunculated polypoid growths may be regurgitated upward into the hypopharynx and occasionally may fall into the glottic chink and produce laryngeal obstruction.

Bleeding may occur from ulcerations of the mucosa overlying a leiomyoma. Symptoms related to benign lesions of the esophagus are usually due to the presence of the lesion itself; the severity of the dysphagia is accentuated by the development of swelling, infection, hemorrhage, or obstruction.

Treatment

Small polypoid intraluminal lesions may be removed completely with biopsy forceps during esophagoscopy. Some intramural lesions can also be removed endoscopically or, in the cases of cysts, injected through the endoscope after endosonographic localization. However, most intramural lesions, such as leiomyomas, should be resected if symptomatic. This can be accomplished in most cases thoracoscopically. A cervical approach is used for lesions in the cervical esophagus.

Benedetti G et al: Fiberoptic endoscopic resection of symptomatic leiomyoma of the upper esophagus. Acta Chir Scand 1990;156:807.

Hoekstra HJ, Vermey A, Edens ET: Leiomyo(sarco)ma of the oesophagus. J Surg Oncol 1984;25:278.

Postlewait RW: Benign tumors and cysts of the esophagus. Surg Clin North Am 1983;63:925.

Rendina EA et al: Leiomyoma of the esophagus. Scand J Thorac Cardiovasc Surg 1990;24:79.

Yu TP et al: Endoscopic treatment of submucosal lesions of the gastrointestinal tract. Endoscopy 1992;24:190.

2. CARCINOMA OF THE ESOPHAGUS

Essentials of Diagnosis

- Progressive dysphagia, initially during ingestion of solid foods and later for liquids.
- Progressive weight loss and inanition.
- Classic radiographic outlines: irregular mucosal pattern with narrowing, with shelf-like upper border or concentrically narrowed esophageal lumen.
- Definitive diagnosis established by endoscopic biopsy or cytology.

General Considerations

Carcinoma of the esophagus constitutes about 1% of all malignant lesions and 4% of those of the gastrointestinal tract. In the USA, the annual incidence per 100,000 persons is 2.6 for squamous cell carcinoma and 0.4 for adenocarcinoma. Blacks have a fivefold higher incidence of squamous cell carcinoma than whites, but the incidence of adenocarcinoma among blacks is one-third that of whites. Both lesions are more common among men, with a male-to-female ratio of 7:10 for adenocarcinoma and 3:4 for squamous cell tumors. The peak incidence is between ages 50 and 60 years. Heavy alcohol or tobacco use is thought to predispose to esophageal carcinoma in the USA. Although some adenocarcinomas of the cardia represent an upward extension of a gastric tumor, true adenocarcinoma of the esophagus, primarily related to Barrett's epithelium, has been increasing in frequency in the USA and accounts for up to 40% of cases in some series. Twenty percent of esophageal tumors occur in the upper third, 30% in the middle third, and 50% in the lower esophagus. Squamous cell lesions predominate in the mid esophagus; adenocarcinomas are more common in the lower third.

The carcinoma usually appears as a fungating growth extending irregularly into the esophageal lumen and spanning a distance of 5 cm in the average case. Ulceration of its central portion is common. Annular lesions with extensive infiltration of the esophageal wall produce obstruction earlier than those that involve only a portion of the circumference of the esophagus. Regardless of cell type, the tumors disseminate by direct invasion into surrounding mediastinal structures, through the bloodstream by local vascular involvement, and by lymphatic dissemination. Direct intramural extension from the gross margin of the lesion is greater proximally than distally. It reaches 3 cm in 65% of cases; 6 cm in 20%; and 9 cm in 10%. In 15% of patients, there are additional islands of tumor within 5 cm of the gross margin of the lesion, suggesting a multicentric origin. Metastases to lymph nodes in the neck, mediastinum, or celiac area of the abdomen are present at the time of diagnosis in 80% of cases regardless of the site of the primary lesion. Lymph node metastases are present in 50% of cases with a primary tumor of less than 5 cm and in 90% of those with a larger tumor. Extramural extension of the tumor with involvement of other structures, such as the trachea, left main stem bronchus, or aorta is relatively common and carries an ominous prognosis. Lung, bone, liver, and adrenal glands are frequent sites of distant metastases. About 5% of patients have a second primary neoplasm of the stomach, oral cavity, pharynx, larynx, or skin. Flow cytometric analysis of nuclear DNA has shown that tumors with the aneuploid pattern have a higher frequency of lymph node metastasis and a higher recurrence rate after surgery. Other karyometric measurements, including total nuclear DNA content and nuclear area, also have prognostic significance. For example, the greater the area, the more likely it is that the tumor will have transmural penetration. Similarly, high levels of epidermal growth factor receptors are associated with a poor prognosis in patients with squamous cell carcinoma.

In certain well-circumscribed areas of the world (eg, Caspian littoral of Iran; Transkei, South Africa; and northern provinces of China), the incidence of esophageal carcinoma exceeds 100 cases per 100,000 population. The cause in these areas is still unknown. In northern China, silica particles have been detected in millet bran used in bread making and in the esophageal walls of affected patients. The presence of nitrosamines in drinking water, fungal contamination of food, and malnutrition are probably of etiologic importance in some regions of the world. Other premalignant states are chronic iron deficiency, esophageal stasis (eg, achalasia), Barrett's esophagus, reflux esophagitis, and congenital tylosis of the esophagus.

Clinical Findings

A. Symptoms and Signs: Dysphagia is the most prominent symptom, and as a result, loss of weight is often striking. Solid foods initially cause difficulty; later, even liquids may be difficult to swallow. Weight loss, weakness, anemia, and inanition are almost always present. Pain, a major complaint in 30% of patients at presentation, may be related to swallowing; if pain is constant, the tumor has probably invaded somatic structures. Regurgitation and aspiration are common, especially at night when the patient is recumbent. Coughing related to swallowing indicates either a high lesion or the presence of a tracheoesophageal fistula. Hoarseness most often reflects spread to the recurrent laryngeal nerves.

B. Imaging Studies: Chest x-rays may show pneumonitis, pleural effusion, or a lung abscess. A column of air in the esophageal lumen, absent in a normal esophagus, may be visible on plain films, or an air-fluid level may be present.

Barium swallow demonstrates narrowing of the esophageal lumen at the site of the lesion and dilatation proximally, although the magnitude of the dilatation is not as great as in benign conditions such as achalasia. The tumor appears as an irregular mass of variable size and length whose upper border is roughly horizontal and resembles a "shelf." Annular lesions appear as constricting bands with a narrowed lumen that contains an irregular mucosal outline (Figure 20–13). Angulation of the axis of the esophagus above and below the tumor may be seen, a finding that strongly suggests spread of the lesion to extraesophageal sites.

CT scans are useful to diagnose liver metastasis and, to a lesser degree, mediastinal and celiac axis nodal involvement. Esophageal endosonography is more accurate in the determination of wall penetration and mediastinal invasion.

C. Esophagoscopy and Bronchoscopy: Esophagoscopy with biopsy provides accurate tissue diagnosis in 95% of cases. However, the mucosa immediately proximal to a very stenotic lesion may be so redundant, edematous, and inflamed that the tumor may not be directly visible at esophagoscopy. In this case, cellular material should be obtained by esophageal washings or brushings.

Because lesions of the upper and mid esophagus

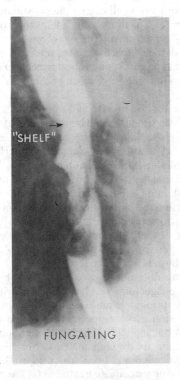

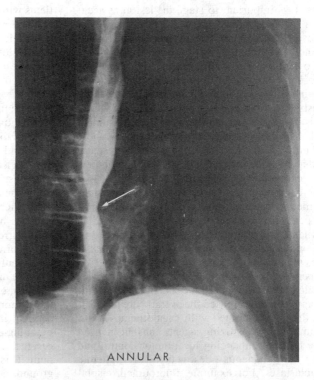

Figure 20–13. Two common types of esophageal carcinoma.

may invade the tracheobronchial tree, bronchoscopy is always indicated in the assessment of growths at these levels. Positive findings include distortion of the bronchial lumen, blunting of the carina, or intrabronchial tumor.

Differential Diagnosis

The fungating type of esophageal cancer presents a typical radiographic picture consisting of an irregular mucosal contour and the uppermost "shelf." Annular carcinomas may be mistaken for benign strictures, especially if most of the growth is intramural. Benign papillomas, polyps, or granulomatous masses can be distinguished from early carcinomas only on histologic examination.

Complications

Cancer of the esophagus rarely bleeds massively, although anemia due to occult bleeding is frequent. The most common complications result from invasion of important mediastinal structures such as the trachea, major bronchi, and pericardium. Fatal hemorrhage, tracheal obstruction, and cardiac dysrhythmias may result. A fistula may develop between the esophagus and the tracheobronchial tree and lead to aspiration pneumonitis, purulent bronchitis, and pulmonary abscess formation.

Treatment

Esophageal carcinoma is treated by surgery, radiotherapy, chemotherapy, or a combination of these methods. It is important to stage the lesion as accurately as possible before deciding on the treatment plan. Resectability of the primary lesion must first be determined. Nonresectability is suggested by direct spread to the tracheobronchial tree or aorta as seen on bronchoscopy or CT scans or by noting angulation of the esophageal axis. The presence of a tracheoesophageal fistula or hoarseness associated with vocal cord paralysis has a similar significance. Primary tumors larger than 10 cm are rarely resectable. Overall, about 50% of tumors are resectable at the time of presentation and about 75% following preoperative radiotherapy and chemotherapy. As long as the patient is a suitable candidate for major surgery and distant organ metastases are absent, the primary tumor should be resected if possible. If life expectancy is longer than a few months, resection is usually recommended regardless of the chance for cure, because it provides the best palliation.

Preoperative radiation therapy may convert an unresectable growth to a resectable one, but adjuvant radiotherapy has not increased the overall cure rate. Radiation therapy combined with chemotherapy, with or without radiosensitizing agents, has been used with the hope of enhancing local tumor control and effecting simultaneous destruction of systemic micrometastases. For example, fluorouracil, cisplatin, and mitomycin C or vincristine sulfate have been given in combination with 2500–3000 cGy directed at the primary lesion in several trials. This therapy produced complete remission in 20–35% of patients. In most trials, patients were subjected to esophagectomy following chemotherapy and radiation. Overall median survival was 18–24 months, with responders doing better than nonresponders. Even among those with complete responses, however, most tumors recurred, usually in distant sites. Because dysphagia was relieved in many patients by the combination of chemotherapy and radiation, some have proposed that esophagectomy adds little to the chemotherapy-radiation combination. The ultimate impact of these protocols on patient survival is unclear.

The patient must stop smoking, and respiratory therapy should be instituted to optimize pulmonary function. Patients who have lost more than 10% of their body weight are usually given total parenteral nutrition or supplemental enteral tube feedings before surgery, but evidence is lacking that this decreases complications.

For tumors of the lower third of the esophagus, most surgeons prefer to perform the resection through a laparotomy followed by a right thoracotomy. The limited access afforded by the left chest approach results in a less generous esophagectomy and a higher incidence of residual tumor at the esophageal margin. The resection should include the celiac lymph nodes and left gastric vessels, the stomach proximal to the left gastric artery, and the lower esophagus to a point above the azygos vein. The spleen is preserved in patients with squamous cell carcinoma but should probably be removed in those with adenocarcinoma. A pyloroplasty is performed. The site of gastric transection is closed, the stomach is pulled up into the chest, and an esophagogastrostomy is performed at a convenient spot on the anterior surface of the gastric remnant.

For tumors of the middle and upper thirds of the esophagus, less stomach need be resected, but the esophagectomy should extend to the cervical esophagus, and the anastomosis should be performed through a separate (third) incision in the neck. Whenever possible, at least 10 cm of grossly uninvolved esophagus should be resected proximal to an esophageal cancer, and the margins of transection should be checked by frozen sections during surgery. Patients with Barrett's esophagus are at high risk of developing recurrent cancer if any portion of the columnar-lined epithelium is left behind.

If the tumor does not involve the trachea, bronchi, or aorta, esophagectomy can be performed without a thoracotomy through simultaneous abdominal and cervical incisions. The esophagus is shelled out by blunt dissection, and the stomach is brought up to the cervical esophagus through the posterior mediastinum. This procedure has been criticized on theoretic grounds as being inadequate treatment for cancer, but the reported survival rates are similar to those achieved with more aggressive operations. Patients (especially those with chronic pulmonary disease) tolerate esophagectomy without thoracotomy better than other operations for removing the esophagus. Tumors of the lower esophagus lend themselves better to this operation than do those in the mid esophagus. The presence of any mediastinal extension beyond what can be directly controlled from the abdomen increases the chance of massive intraoperative bleeding or laceration of the membranous trachea.

If the lesion is unresectable, radiation therapy may be used. Radiotherapy relieves dysphagia in about two-thirds of the patients, but the relief is transient in half of those who do respond. Irradiation or chemotherapy should not be the initial therapy in patients with tracheobronchial involvement with or without a tracheoesophageal fistula, because patients without a fistula often develop one following treatment. Therefore, patients with an unresectable tumor who are able to withstand a major operation are best treated by a preliminary substernal gastric bypass with a cervical esophagogastrostomy. The esophagus is closed above and below the fistula or may be drained by a Roux-en-Y esophagojejunostomy. After the patient has recovered from the esophagogastrostomy, the primary tumor is treated by radiotherapy. Colon is rarely used to bypass an esophageal carcinoma, because the operation is more complex than gastric bypass and the death rate is higher.

The dose of x-ray should be between 4500 and 6000 cGy. Patients treated with doses at the higher end of this range are more likely to experience complications, such as pulmonary fibrosis, esophageal bleeding, or esophageal perforation.

Palliation may be attempted with intubation of the tumor in patients too weak to withstand a major operation. The tube is inserted by laparotomy (eg, Celestin tube, Mousseau-Barbin tube) or esophagoscopy (eg, Souttar tube). Unfortunately, the quality of palliation achieved with tube stents is generally very poor. The tube has a tendency to become dislodged or blocked with food, thus aggravating pain. Furthermore, concomitant radiotherapy increases the complications (eg, bleeding, perforation) of tubes. Therefore, intubation should be reserved for patients with extensive disease and a life expectancy limited to 1–2 months.

In some patients with unresectable tumors, dysphagia can be relieved by endoscopic laser therapy. With this technique, a core of tumor is vaporized, opening the lumen without perforating the esophagus. Treatment needs to be repeated every 6–8 weeks, and most patients are able to swallow only liquids and semiliquid diets. Success is greatest with lesions of the body of the esophagus 5 cm or less in length. Greatest technical difficulties are encountered with cervical lesions and angulated lesions at the cardioesophageal junction. When technically feasible, endoscopic laser therapy is preferable to Celestin tube intubation.

Patients with malignant tracheoesophageal fistulas cannot be cured, but palliation is a realistic goal. Aspiration of saliva and swallowed liquids produces incessant coughing, and dysphagia is usually pronounced. Nevertheless, the tumor is rarely widespread in these patients. The best treatment is probably substernal gastric bypass with a cervical esophagogastric anastomosis. Both ends of the thoracic esophagus are closed. The fistula is usually large enough to accommodate the small amount of esophageal secretion. Celestin tubes are of little value.

Prognosis

The operative death rate following resection or bypass averages 5–8%. After potentially curative resection, survival for 1 year is 70%; for 2 years, 30%; and for 5 years, 20%. About 50% of patients who have no lymph node involvement are cured. The 5-year survival rate after curative resection is about 30% for patients with squamous cell carcinoma and 10% for patients with adenocarcinoma. Surgery is much more successful in restoring and maintaining swallowing than is radiotherapy or intubation. Survival of patients following insertion of a Celestin tube averages 1 month.

Altorki NK et al: High-grade dysplasia in the columnar-lined esophagus. Am J Surg 1991;161:97.

Barbier PA et al: Quality of life and pattern of recurrence following transhiatal esophagectomy for cancer: Results of a prospective follow-up in 50 patients. World J Surg 1988;12:270.

Barr H et al: Prospective randomized trial of laser therapy only and laser therapy followed by endoscopic intubation for the palliation of malignant dysphagia. Gut 1990;31:252.

Botet JF et al: Preoperative staging of esophageal cancer: Comparison of endoscopic US and dynamic CT. Radiology 1991;181:419.

Bown SG: Palliation of malignant dysphagia: Surgery, radiotherapy, laser, intubation alone or in combination? Gut 1991;32:841.

Coia LR et al: Swallowing function in patients with esophageal cancer treated with concurrent radiation and chemotherapy. Cancer 1993;71:281.

DeMeester TR, Zaninotto G, Johansson K: Selective therapeutic approach to cancer of the lower esophagus and cardia. J Thorac Cardiovasc Surg 1988;95:42.

Fok M et al: Postoperative radiotherapy for carcinoma of the esophagus: A prospective, randomized controlled study. Surgery 1993;113:138.

Fok M et al: Pyloroplasty versus no drainage in gastric replacement of the esophagus. Am J Surg 1991;162:447.

Hankins JR et al: Carcinoma of the esophagus: A comparison of the results of transhiatal versus transthoracic resection. Ann Thorac Surg 1989;47:700.

Jacob P et al: Natural history and significance of esophageal squamous cell dysplasia. Cancer 1990;65:2731.

Lund O et al: Risk stratification and long-term results after surgical treatment of carcinomas of the thoracic esophagus and cardia: A 25-year retrospective study. J Thorac Cardiovasc Surg 1990;99:200.

Mannell A, Becker PJ: Evaluation of the results of oesophagectomy for oesophageal cancer. Br J Surg 1991;78:36.

Matgsuura H et al: Predicting recurrence time of esophageal carcinoma through assessment of histologic factors and DNA ploidy. Cancer 1991;67:1406.

Matsufuhi H et al: Preoperative hyperthermia combined with radiotherapy and chemotherapy for patients with incompletely resected carcinoma of the esophagus. Cancer 1988;62:889.

Mountain DF: Combined therapy for carcinoma of the esophagus: Panacea or puzzle? Ann Thorac Surg 1988;45:353.

Mukaida H et al: Clinical significance of the expression of epidermal growth factor and its receptor in esophageal cancer. Cancer 1991;68:142.

Nava HR et al: Endoscopic ablation of esophageal malignancies with neodymium-YAG laser and electrofulguration. Arch Surg 1989;124:225.

Orringer MB et al: Chemotherapy and radiation therapy before transhiatal esophagectomy for esophageal carcinoma. Ann Thorac Surg 1990;49:348.

Robaszkiewica M et al: Flow-cytometric DNA content analysis of esophageal squamous cell carcinomas. Gastroenterology 1991;101:1588.

Steiger Z: Perioperative multimodality management of esophageal cancer: Therapeutic or investigational? Ann Thorac Surg 1990;49:345.

Stewart FM et al: Cisplatin, 5-fluorouracil, mitomycin C, and concurrent radiation therapy with and without esophagectomy for esophageal carcinoma. Cancer 1989;64:622.

Teniere P et al: Postoperative radiation therapy does not increase survival after curative resection for squamous cell carcinoma of the middle and lower esophagus as shown by a multicenter controlled trial. Surg Gynecol Obstet 1991;173:123.

Tio TL et al: Esophagogastric carcinomas: Preoperative TNM classification with endosonography. Radiology 1989;173:411.

ESOPHAGEAL BANDS, WEBS, OR RINGS

Congenital bands or webs may develop at any level but are most frequent in the subcricoid region. Others form in the lower esophageal segment. These bands cause dysphagia and may be treated by endoscopic dilation in which the thin, web-like band is usually fractured, followed by complete relief of symptoms. Resection and primary anastomosis are occasionally necessary for the more fibrous unyielding concentric bands. The latter are more likely to be in the lower esophagus.

A narrow mucosal ring (**Schatzki's ring**) may develop at the lower end of the esophagus. Most patients are relatively free from symptoms unless the ring is less than 12 mm in diameter. Dysphagia may be severe, however. In most cases, the ring is located at the squamocolumnar junction and occurs in a pa-

tient with gastroesophageal reflux. Being confined to the mucosa, it differs from an inflammatory (peptic) stricture, which involves all layers of the esophagus. Endoscopy often fails to reveal the smooth concentric narrowing, since the overlying mucosa is intact. Esophagitis may be present but usually is not. Repair of an associated hiatal hernia is insufficient to control the dysphagia; the ring must be dilated or excised. In most cases, the ring can be ruptured by rapidly inflating a balloon in its lumen, as is done for achalasia. Afterward, the patient should be treated for esophagitis.

Eastridge CE, Pate JW, Mann JA: Lower esophageal ring: Experiences in treatment of 88 patients. Ann Thorac Surg 1984;37:103.

Low DE, Hill LD: Cervical esophageal web associated with Zenker's diverticulum. Am J Surg 1988;156:34.

Mohandas KM et al: Upper esophageal webs, iron deficiency anemia, and esophageal cancer. Am J Gastroenterol 1991;86:117.

Ott DJ et al: Esophagogastric region and its rings. AJR 1984;142:281.

Weaver JW, Kaude JV, Hamlin DJ: Webs of the lower esophagus: A complication of gastroesophageal reflux? AJR 1984;142:289.

II. THE DIAPHRAGM (Figure 20–14)

The diaphragm is a musculotendinous dome-shaped structure attached posteriorly to the first, second, and third lumbar vertebrae, anteriorly to the lower sternum, and laterally to the costal arches. It separates the abdominal and the thoracic cavities. The diaphragm allows the passage of various normal structures through anatomic foramens. The aortic hiatus lies posteriorly at the level of the 12th thoracic vertebra, and through it pass the aorta, the thoracic duct, and the azygos venous system. The esophageal hiatus lies immediately anteriorly and slightly to the left at the level of the tenth thoracic vertebra and is separated from the aortic hiatus by the decussation of the right crus of the diaphragm. Through this hiatus pass the esophagus and the vagus nerves. At the level of the ninth thoracic vertebra and slightly to the right of the esophageal hiatus is the vena caval foramen, which allows passage of the inferior vena cava and small branches of the phrenic nerve. The phrenic arteries arising directly from the aorta supply the diaphragm along with the lower intercostal arteries and the terminal branches of the internal mammary arteries.

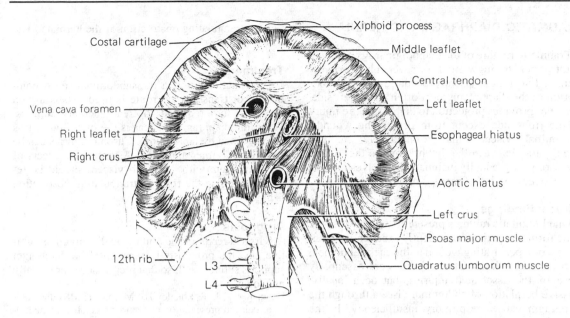

Xiphoid process

Costal cartilage

Middle leaflet

Central tendon

Vena cava foramen

Left leaflet

Right leaflet

Esophageal hiatus

Right crus

Aortic hiatus

Left crus

Psoas major muscle

12th rib

Quadratus lumborum muscle

L3

L4

Figure 20–14. Inferior surface of diaphragm.

PARASTERNAL OR RETROSTERNAL (FORAMEN OF MORGAGNI) HERNIA & PLEUROPERITONEAL (FORAMEN OF BOCHDALEK) HERNIA
(Figure 20–15)

Failure of fusion of the sternal and costal portions of the diaphragm anteriorly in the midline creates a defect (foramen of Morgagni) through which hernias can occur. Normally, the diaphragm becomes fused, allowing only the internal mammary arteries and their superior epigastric branches, along with lymphatics, to pass through this area. Posterolaterally, failure of fusion of the pleuroperitoneal canal creates a defect though which viscera may herniate to produce a foramen of Bochdalek hernia.

Although both types of hernia are congenital, symptoms in the Morgagni hernia usually do not develop until middle life or later. On the contrary, the Bochdalek hernia may cause severe respiratory distress at birth, requiring an emergency operation. In both types in the adult, complications are not common and many cases are asymptomatic. Routine chest films show a retrosternal solid mass, a retrosternal air-filled viscus, or similar findings in the posterolateral thorax if a Bochdalek hernia is present.

Elective surgical repair is indicated in most instances to prevent complications. An emergency operation may become necessary in the newborn infant who develops progressive cardiorespiratory insufficiency. Repair of the defect by a transabdominal approach is preferable, and the results are excellent.

Gale ME: Bochdalek hernia: Prevalence and CT characteristics. Radiology 1985;156:449.

Saha SP, Mayo P, Long GA: Surgical treatment of anterior diaphragmatic hernia. South Med J 1982;75:280.

Wiener ES: Congenital posterolateral diaphragmatic hernia: New dimensions in management. Surgery 1982;92:670.

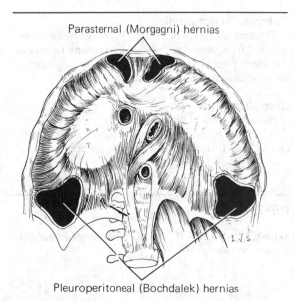

Parasternal (Morgagni) hernias

Pleuroperitoneal (Bochdalek) hernias

Figure 20–15. Sites of congenital diaphragmatic herniation.

TRAUMATIC DIAPHRAGMATIC HERNIA

Traumatic rupture of the diaphragm may occur as a result of penetrating wounds or severe blunt external trauma. Lacerations usually occur in the tendinous portion of the diaphragm, most often on the left side. The liver provides protection to diaphragmatic injury on the right side except from penetrating wounds. Abdominal viscera may immediately herniate through the defect in the diaphragm into the pleural cavity or may gradually insinuate themselves into the thorax over a period of months or years.

Clinical Findings

Diaphragmatic ruptures present in two ways. In the acute form, the patient has recently experienced blunt trauma or a penetrating wound to the chest, abdomen, or back. The clinical manifestations are essentially those of the associated injuries, but occasionally, massive herniation of abdominal viscera through the diaphragm causes respiratory insufficiency. In the chronic form, the diaphragmatic tear is unrecognized at the time of the original injury. Some time later, symptoms appear from herniation of viscera: pain, bowel obstruction, etc. Respiratory symptoms in such cases are rare.

Plain films of the chest may show a radiopaque area and occasionally an air-fluid level if hollow viscera have herniated. If the stomach has entered the chest, the abnormal path of a nasogastric tube may be diagnostic. Ultrasonography, CT scan, and MRI may demonstrate the diaphragmatic rent. Barium study of the colon may show irregular patches of barium in the colon above the diaphragm or a smooth colonic outline if the colon does not contain feces.

Differential Diagnosis

Traumatic rupture of the diaphragm must be differentiated from atelectasis, space-consuming tumors of the lower pleural space, pleural effusion, and intestinal obstruction due to other causes.

Complications

Hemorrhage and obstruction may occur. If herniation is massive, progressive cardiorespiratory insufficiency may threaten life. The most severe complication is strangulating obstruction of the herniated viscera.

Treatment

For acute ruptures, a transabdominal (most commonly) or transthoracic route is used depending on the procedure required to treat ancillary injuries. When the diaphragmatic tear is the only injury, it is usually fixed by laparotomy. Chronic injuries can be repaired by either approach. Asymptomatic tears of the diaphragm with herniated viscera should be repaired, because the risk of strangulating obstruction is high.

Prognosis

Surgical repair of the rent in the diaphragm is curative, and the prognosis is excellent. The diaphragm supports sutures well, so that recurrence is practically unknown.

Daum-Kowalski R, Shanley DJ, Murphy T: MRI diagnosis of delayed presentation of traumatic diaphragmatic hernia. Gastrointest Radiol 1991;16:298.

Falcone RE, Barnes FE, Hoogeboom JE: Blunt diaphragmatic rupture diagnosed by laparoscopy: Report of a case. J Laparoendosc Surg 1991;1:299.

Holland DG, Quint LE: Traumatic rupture of the diaphragm without visceral herniation: CT diagnosis AJR Am J Roentgenol 1991;157:17.

Smithers BM, O'Loughlin B, Strong RW: Diagnosis of ruptured diaphragm following blunt trauma: Results from 85 cases. Aust N Z J Surg 1991;61:737.

Sukul DM, Kats E, Johannes EJ: Sixty-three cases of traumatic injury of the diaphragm. Injury 1991;22:303.

TUMORS OF THE DIAPHRAGM

Primary tumors of the diaphragm are not common. The majority are benign lipomas. Pericardial cysts develop in the interval between the heart and the diaphragm and are usually unilocular and on the right side. Fibrosarcoma, the most common primary malignant diaphragmatic tumor, is extremely rare.

Benign tumors are usually asymptomatic. Since their benign nature cannot be established except by histologic study, all lesions of this type should be excised through an appropriate thoracotomy.

REFERENCES

Skinner DB, Belsey RH: *Management of Esophageal Disease*. Saunders, 1988.

Sleisenger M, Fordtran J: *Gastrointestinal Disease,* 5th ed. Saunders, 1993.

The Acute Abdomen

21

John H. Boey, MD

The term "an acute abdomen" denotes any sudden nontraumatic disorder whose chief manifestation is in the abdominal area and for which urgent operation may be necessary. Since there is frequently a progressive underlying intra-abdominal disorder, undue delay in diagnosis and treatment adversely affects outcome. The most common causes of the acute abdomen are listed in Table 21–1.

The approach to a patient with an acute abdomen must be orderly and thorough. An acute abdomen must be suspected even if the patient has only mild or atypical complaints. The history and physical examination should suggest the probable causes and guide the choice of diagnostic studies. The use of structured record forms (with or without computer programs) has consistently improved diagnostic accuracy by about 20%. The clinician must then decide if in-hospital observation is warranted; if additional tests are needed to clarify the situation; if early operation is needed; or if nonoperative treatment would be more suitable.

Other chapters in this book contain detailed descriptions of specific diseases and their management.

HISTORY

Abdominal Pain

Pain is usually the predominant and presenting feature of an acute abdomen. In order to elucidate its cause, the **location, mode of onset and progression,** and **character** of pain must be determined.

A. Location of Pain: Because of the complex dual visceral and parietal sensory network subserving the abdominal area, pain is not as precisely localized as in the extremities. Fortunately, some general patterns do emerge that provide clues to diagnosis. Visceral sensation is mediated primarily by afferent C fibers located in the walls of hollow viscera and in the capsule of solid organs. Unlike cutaneous pain, **visceral pain** is elicited either by distention, by inflammation or ischemia stimulating the receptor neurons, or by direct involvement (eg, malignant infiltration) of sensory nerves. The centrally perceived sensation is generally slow in onset, dull, poorly localized, and protracted. The different visceral structures are associated with different sensory levels in the spine

(Table 21–2). Because of this, increased wall tension due to luminal distention or forceful smooth muscle contraction (colic) leads to diffuse deep-seated pain felt in the mid epigastrium, periumbilical area, lower abdomen, or flank areas (Figure 21–1). Visceral pain is most often felt in the midline because of the bilateral sensory supply to the spinal cord.

By contrast, **parietal pain** is mediated by both C and A delta nerve fibers, the latter being responsible for the transmission of more acute, sharper, better-localized pain sensation. Direct irritation of the somatically innervated parietal peritoneum (especially the anterior and upper parts) by pus, bile, urine, or gastrointestinal secretions is associated with more exact localization of pain. The cutaneous distribution of parietal pain corresponds to the T6–L1 areas. Parietal pain is more easily localized than visceral pain because the somatic afferent fibers are directed to only one side of the nervous system. Abdominal parietal pain is conventionally described as occurring in one of the four abdominal quadrants or in the epigastric or central abdominal area.

Abdominal pain may be referred or may shift to sites far removed from the primarily affected organs (Figure 21–2). The term referred pain denotes noxious (usually cutaneous) sensations perceived at a site distant from the site of a strong primary stimulus. Distorted central perception of the site of pain is due to the confluence of afferent nerve fibers from widely different areas within the posterior horn of the spinal cord. For example, pain due to subdiaphragmatic irritation by air, peritoneal fluid, blood, or a mass lesion is referred to the shoulder via the C4-mediated (phrenic) nerve. Pain may also be referred to the shoulder from supradiaphragmatic lesions such as pleurisy or basal pneumonia, especially in young patients. Although more often perceived in the right scapular region, referred biliary pain may mimic angina pectoris if it is felt in the epigastric or left shoulder areas.

Spreading or shifting pain parallels the course of the underlying condition. The site of pain at onset should be distinguished from the site at presentation. Beginning classically in the epigastric or periumbilical region, the incipient visceral pain of acute appendicitis (due to distention of the appendix) later shifts to become sharper parietal pain in the right lower quadrant when the overlying peritoneum becomes in-

441

Table 21–1. Common causes of the acute abdomen. Conditions in italic type often require urgent operation.

Gastrointestinal tract disorders Nonspecific abdominal pain *Appendicitis* *Small and large bowel obstruction* *Incarcerated hernia* *Perforated peptic ulcer* *Bowel perforation* *Meckel's diverticulitis* *Boerhaave's syndrome* Diverticulitis Inflammatory bowel disorders Mallory-Weiss syndrome Gastroenteritis Acute gastritis Mesenteric adenitis **Liver, spleen, and biliary tract disorders** *Acute cholecystitis* *Acute cholangitis* *Hepatic abscess* *Ruptured hepatic tumor* *Spontaneous rupture of the spleen* Splenic infarct Biliary colic Acute hepatitis **Pancreatic disorders** Acute pancreatitis	**Urinary tract disorders** Ureteral or renal colic Acute pyelonephritis Acute cystitis Renal infarct **Gynecologic disorders** *Ruptured ectopic pregnancy* *Twisted ovarian tumor* *Ruptured ovarian follicle cyst* Acute salpingitis Dysmenorrhea Endometriosis **Vascular disorders** *Ruptured aortic and visceral aneurysms* *Acute ischemic colitis* *Mesenteric thrombosis* **Peritoneal disorders** *Intra-abdominal abscesses* Primary peritonitis Tuberculous peritonitis **Retroperitoneal disorders** Retroperitoneal hemorrhage

flamed (Figure 21–2). In perforated peptic ulcer, pain almost always begins in the epigastrium, but as the leaked gastric contents track down the right paracolic gutter, pain may migrate to the right lower quadrant.

The location of pain serves only as a rough guide to the diagnosis—"typical" descriptions are reported in only two-thirds of cases. This great variability is due to atypical pain patterns, a shift of maximum intensity away from the primary site, or advanced or severe disease. In cases presenting late with diffuse

Table 21–2. Sensory levels associated with visceral structures.

Structures	Nervous System Pathways	Sensory Level
Liver, spleen, and central part of diaphragm	Phrenic nerve	C3–5
Peripheral diaphragm, stomach, pancreas, gallbladder, and small bowel	Celiac plexus and greater splanchnic nerve	T6–9
Appendix, colon, and pelvic viscera	Mesenteric plexus and lesser splanchnic nerve	T10–11
Sigmoid colon, rectum, kidney, ureters, and testes	Lowest splanchnic nerve	T11–L1
Bladder and rectosigmoid	Hypogastric plexus	S2–4

peritonitis, generalized pain may completely obscure the precipitating event.

B. Mode of Onset and Progression of Pain: The mode of onset of pain reflects the nature and severity of the inciting process. Onset may be explosive (within seconds), rapidly progressive (within 1–2 hours), or gradual (over several hours). Unheralded, excruciating generalized pain suggests an intra-abdominal catastrophe such as a perforated viscus or rupture of an aneurysm, ectopic pregnancy, or abscess. Accompanying systemic signs (tachycardia, sweating, tachypnea, shock) soon supersede the abdominal disturbances and underscore the need for prompt resuscitation and laparotomy.

A less dramatic clinical picture is steady mild pain becoming intensely centered in a well-defined area within 1–2 hours. Any of the above conditions may present in this manner, but this mode of onset is more typical of acute cholecystitis, acute pancreatitis, strangulated bowel, mesenteric infarction, renal or ureteral colic, and high (proximal) small bowel obstruction.

Finally, some patients initially have slight—at times only vague—abdominal discomfort that is fleetingly present diffusely throughout the abdomen. It may be unclear whether these patients even have an acute abdomen or whether the illness is likely to be a matter for medical rather than surgical attention. Associated gastrointestinal symptoms are infrequent at first, and systemic symptoms are absent. Eventually, the pain and abdominal findings become more pronounced and steady and are localized to a smaller area. This pattern may reflect a slowly developing condition or the body's defensive efforts to cordon off an acute process. This broad category includes acute appendicitis, incarcerated hernias, low (distal) small bowel and large bowel obstructions, uncomplicated peptic ulcer disease, walled-off (often malignant) visceral perforations, some genitourinary and gynecologic conditions, and milder forms of the rapid-onset group mentioned in the first paragraph.

C. Character of Pain: The nature, severity, and periodicity of pain provide useful clues to the underlying cause (Figure 21–3). Steady pain is most common. Sharp superficial constant pain due to severe peritoneal irritation is typical of perforated ulcer and ruptured appendix. The gripping, mounting pain of small bowel obstruction (and occasionally early pancreatitis) is usually intermittent, vague, deep-seated, and crescendo at first but soon becomes sharper, unremitting, and better localized. Unlike the disquieting but bearable pain associated with bowel obstruction, pain caused by lesions occluding smaller conduits (bile ducts, uterine tubes, and ureters) rapidly becomes unbearably intense. Pain is appropriately referred to as colic if there are pain-free intervals that reflect intermittent smooth muscle contractions, as in ureteral colic. In the strict sense, the term "biliary colic" is a misnomer because biliary pain does not

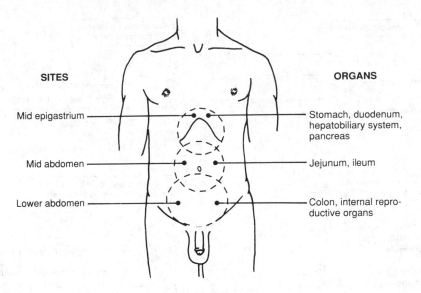

Figure 21–1. Visceral pain sites.

remit. The reason is that the gallbladder and bile duct, in contrast to the ureters and intestine, do not have peristaltic movements. The "aching discomfort" of ulcer pain, the "stabbing, breathtaking" pain of acute pancreatitis and mesenteric infarction, and the "searing" pain of ruptured aortic aneurysm remain apt descriptions. Despite the acceptance of such descriptive terms, however, the quality of visceral pain is not a reliable clue to its cause.

Agonizing pain denotes serious or advanced disease. Colicky pain is usually promptly alleviated by analgesics. Ischemic pain due to strangulated bowel

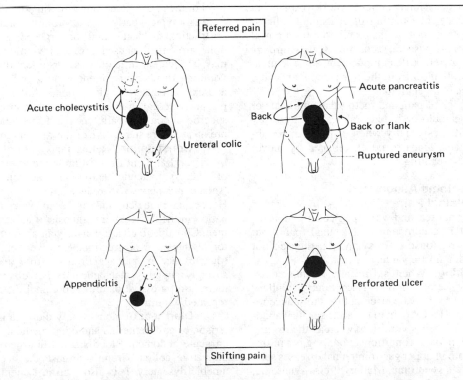

Figure 21–2. Referred pain and shifting pain in the acute abdomen. Solid circles indicate the site of maximum pain; dashed circles indicate sites of lesser pain.

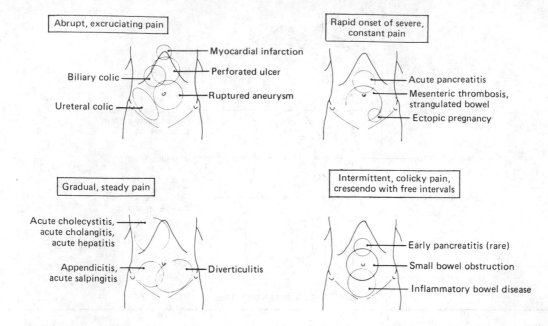

Figure 21–3. The location and character of pain are helpful in the differential diagnosis of the acute abdomen.

or mesenteric thrombosis is only slightly assuaged even by narcotics. Nonspecific abdominal pain is usually mild, but mild pain may also be found with perforated ulcers that are localized or mild acute pancreatitis. An occasional patient will deny pain but complain of a vague feeling of abdominal fullness that feels as though it might be relieved by a bowel movement. This visceral sensation (**gas stoppage sign**) is due to reflex ileus induced by an inflammatory lesion walled off from the free peritoneal cavity, as in retrocecal appendicitis.

Past episodes of pain and factors that aggravate or relieve pain should be noted. Pain caused by localized peritonitis, especially when it affects upper abdominal organs, tends to be exacerbated by movement or deep breathing.

Other Symptoms Associated
With Abdominal Pain

Anorexia, nausea and vomiting, constipation, or diarrhea often accompanies abdominal pain, but since these are nonspecific symptoms, they do not have much diagnostic value.

A. Vomiting: When sufficiently stimulated by secondary visceral afferent fibers, the medullary vomiting centers activate efferent fibers to induce reflex vomiting. Hence, pain in the acute surgical abdomen usually precedes vomiting, whereas the reverse holds true in medical conditions. Vomiting is a prominent symptom in upper gastrointestinal diseases such as Boerhaave's syndrome, Mallory-Weiss syndrome, acute gastritis, and acute pancreatitis. Severe uncontrollable retching provides temporary pain relief in

moderate attacks of pancreatitis. The absence of bile in the vomitus is a feature of pyloric stenosis. Where associated findings suggest bowel obstruction, the onset and character of vomiting may indicate the level of the lesion. Recurrent vomiting of bile-stained fluid is a typical early sign of proximal small bowel obstruction. In distal small or large bowel obstruction, prolonged nausea precedes vomiting, which may be feculent in late cases. Disorders that induce vomiting in younger patients may give rise only to anorexia or nausea in older patients. Although vomiting may present in either acute appendicitis or nonspecific abdominal pain, coexisting nausea and anorexia are more suggestive of the former condition.

B. Constipation: Reflex ileus is often induced by visceral afferent fibers stimulating efferent fibers of the sympathetic autonomic nervous system (splanchnic nerves) to reduce intestinal peristalsis. Hence, paralytic ileus undermines the value of constipation in the differential diagnosis of an acute abdomen. Constipation itself is hardly an absolute indicator of intestinal obstruction. However, **obstipation** (the absence of passage of both stool and flatus) strongly suggests mechanical bowel obstruction if there is progressive painful abdominal distention or repeated vomiting.

C. Diarrhea: Copious watery diarrhea is characteristic of gastroenteritis and other medical causes of an acute abdomen. Blood-stained diarrhea suggests ulcerative colitis, Crohn's disease, or bacillary or amebic dysentery. It is also seen in ischemic colitis but is often absent in intestinal infarction due to superior mesenteric artery occlusion.

D. Specific Gastrointestinal Symptoms: These are extremely helpful if present. **Jaundice** suggests hepatobiliary disorders; **hematochezia** or **hematemesis,** a gastroduodenal lesion or Mallory-Weiss syndrome; **hematuria,** ureteral colic or cystitis. The passage of blood clots or necrotic mucosal debris may be the sole evidence of advanced intestinal ischemia.

Other Relevant Aspects of History

Recent medications taken, travel, and previous illnesses and operations are also relevant to the diagnosis of an acute abdomen.

A. Menstrual History: The menstrual history is crucial to the diagnosis of ectopic pregnancy, mittelschmerz (due to a ruptured ovarian follicle), and endometriosis.

B. Drug History: The drug history is important not only in perioperative management but also because it may offer a diagnostic clue. Anticoagulants have been implicated in retroperitoneal and intramural duodenal and jejunal hematomas; oral contraceptives in the formation of benign hepatic adenomas and in mesenteric venous infarction. Corticosteroids, in particular, may mask the clinical signs of even advanced peritonitis.

C. Family History: The family history often provides the best information about medical causes of an acute abdomen (see below).

D. Travel History: A travel history may raise the possibility of amebic liver abscess or hydatid cyst, malarial spleen, tuberculosis, Salmonella typhi infection of the ileocecal area, or dysentery.

PHYSICAL EXAMINATION

The tendency to concentrate on the abdomen should be resisted in favor of a methodical and complete general physical examination. A systematic approach to the abdominal examination is outlined in Table 21–3. One should specifically search for signs that confirm or rule out differential diagnostic possibilities (Table 21–4).

(1) General observation: General observation affords a fairly reliable indication of the severity of the clinical situation. Most patients, although uncom-

Table 21–3. Steps in physical examination for acute abdomen.

(1) Inspection	(7) Punch tenderness
(2) Auscultation	Costal area
(3) Cough tenderness	Costovertebral area
(4) Percussion	(8) Special signs
(5) Guarding or rigidity	(9) External hernias and
(6) Palpation	male genitalia
One-finger	(10) Rectal and pelvic
Rebound tenderness	examination
Deep	

Table 21–4. Physical findings with various causes of acute abdomen.

Condition	Helpful Signs
Perforated viscus	Scaphoid, tense abdomen; diminished bowel sounds (late); loss of liver dullness; guarding or rigidity.
Peritonitis	Motionless; absent bowel sounds (late); cough and rebound tenderness; guarding or rigidity.
Inflamed mass or abscess	Tender mass (abdominal, rectal, or pelvic); punch tenderness; special signs (Murphy's, psoas, or obturator).
Intestinal obstruction	Distention; visible peristalsis (late); hyperperistalsis (early) or quiet abdomen (late); diffuse pain without rebound tenderness; hernia or rectal mass (some).
Paralytic ileus	Distention; minimal bowel sounds; no localized tenderness.
Ischemic or strangulated bowel	Not distended (until late); bowel sounds variable; severe pain but little tenderness; rectal bleeding (some).
Bleeding	Pallor, shock; distention; pulsatile (aneurysm) or tender (eg, ectopic pregnancy) mass; rectal bleeding (some).

fortable, remain calm. The writhing of patients with visceral pain (eg, intestinal or ureteral colic) contrasts with the rigidly motionless bearing of those with parietal pain (eg, acute appendicitis, generalized peritonitis).

(2) Systemic signs: Systemic signs usually accompany rapidly progressive or advanced disorders associated with an acute abdomen. Extreme pallor, hypothermia, tachycardia, tachypnea, and sweating suggest major intra-abdominal hemorrhage (eg, ruptured aortic aneurysm or tubal pregnancy). Extra-abdominal conditions must be rapidly excluded, but the precise nature of an intra-abdominal cause may be revealed only at laparotomy.

(3) Fever: Low-grade fever is common in inflammatory conditions such as diverticulitis, acute cholecystitis, and appendicitis. High fever with lower abdominal tenderness in a young woman without signs of systemic illness suggests acute salpingitis. Disorientation or extreme lethargy combined with a very high fever (39 °C) or swinging fever or with chills and rigors signifies impending septic shock. This is most often due to advanced peritonitis, acute cholangitis, or pyelonephritis. These rapid observations dictate the pace of the subsequent examination and diagnostic tests.

(4) Examination of the acute abdomen:

(a) Inspection: The abdomen should be carefully inspected before palpation. A tensely distended abdomen with an old surgical scar suggests both the presence and the cause (adhesions) of small bowel obstruction. A scaphoid contracted abdomen is seen with perforated ulcer; visible peristalsis occurs in thin patients with advanced bowel obstruction; and soft doughy fullness is seen in early paralytic ileus or mesenteric thrombosis.

(b) Auscultation: Auscultation of the abdomen should also precede palpation. Peristaltic rushes synchronous with colic are heard in mid small bowel obstruction and in early acute pancreatitis. They differ from the high-pitched hyperperistaltic sounds unrelated to the crampy pain of gastroenteritis, dysentery, and fulminant ulcerative colitis. An abdomen that is silent except for infrequent tinkly or squeaky sounds marks late bowel obstruction or diffuse peritonitis. Except for these more extreme patterns, the many auscultatory variants heard in paralytic ileus and other conditions render them largely useless for specific diagnosis.

(c) Coughing to elicit pain: The patient should be asked to cough and point to the area of maximal pain. Peritoneal irritation so demonstrated may be confirmed afterward without causing unnecessary pain by rigorous testing for rebound tenderness. Unlike the parietal pain of peritonitis, colic is visceral pain and is seldom aggravated by deep inspiration or coughing.

(d) Percussion: Percussion serves several purposes. Tenderness on percussion is akin to eliciting rebound tenderness; both reflect peritoneal irritation and parietal pain. With a perforated viscus, free air accumulating under the diaphragm may efface normal liver dullness. Tympany near the midline in a distended abdomen denotes air trapped within distended bowel loops. Free peritoneal fluid may be detected by demonstrating shifting dullness.

(e) Palpation: Palpation is performed with the patient resting in a comfortable supine position. Incisional and periumbilical hernias are noted. **Guarding** is assessed by placing both hands over the abdominal muscles and depressing them gently. Properly performed, this maneuver is comforting to the patient. If there is voluntary spasm, the muscle will be felt to relax when the patient inhales deeply through the mouth. With true involuntary spasm, however, the muscle will remain taut and rigid ("board-like") throughout respiration. Except for rare neurologic disorders—and, for unknown reasons, renal colic—only peritoneal inflammation (by reflex afferent stimulation of efferent motor fibers) produces rectus muscle rigidity. Unlike peritonitis, renal colic induces spasm confined to the ipsilateral rectus muscle.

Tenderness that connotes localized peritoneal inflammation is perhaps the most important finding in patients with an acute abdomen. Its extent and severity are determined first by one- or two-finger palpation, beginning away from the area of cough tenderness and gradually advancing toward it. Tenderness is usually well demarcated in acute cholecystitis, appendicitis, diverticulitis, and acute salpingitis. If there is diffuse tenderness unaccompanied by guarding, one should suspect gastroenteritis or some other inflammatory intestinal process without peritonitis. Compared with the degree of pain, unexpectedly little and only poorly localized tenderness is elicited in uncomplicated hollow viscus obstruction.

When the patient raises his or her head from the bed or examination table, the abdominal muscles will be tensed. Tenderness persists in abdominal wall conditions (eg, rectus hematoma), whereas deeper peritoneal pain due to intraperitoneal disease is lessened (Carnett's test). Hyperesthesia may be demonstrable in abdominal wall disorders or localized peritonitis, but it is more prominent in herpes zoster, spinal root compression, and other neuromuscular problems. Trigger point sensitivity, lateral costal rib tip tenderness, and pain exacerbated by spinal motion reflect parietal abdominal wall conditions that subside dramatically after infiltration with local anesthetic agents.

Abdominal masses. Abdominal masses are usually detected by deep palpation. Superficial lesions such as a distended gallbladder or appendiceal abscess are often tender and have discrete borders. If one suspects that abdominal guarding is masking an acutely inflamed gallbladder, the right subcostal area should be palpated while the patient inhales deeply. Inspiration will be arrested abruptly by pain **(Murphy's sign),** or the gallbladder fundus may be felt as it strikes the examining fingers during descent of the diaphragm.

Deeper masses may be adherent to the posterior or lateral abdominal wall and are often partially walled off by overlying omentum and small bowel. As a result, their borders are ill-defined, and only dull pain may be elicited by palpation. Examples include pancreatic phlegmon and ruptured aortic aneurysm.

Even if a mass cannot be directly felt, its presence may be inferred by other maneuvers. A large psoas abscess arising from a perinephric abscess or perforated Crohn's enteritis may cause pain when the hip is passively extended or actively flexed against resistance **(iliopsoas sign).** Similarly, internal and external rotation of the flexed thigh may exert painful pressure **(obturator sign)** on a loop of the small bowel entrapped within the obturator canal (obturator hernia). **Punch tenderness** over the lower costal ribs indicates an inflammatory condition affecting the diaphragm, liver, or spleen or its adjacent structures. While this may suggest a hepatic, splenic, or subphrenic abscess, it is also common in acute cholecystitis, acute hepatitis, or splenic infarct. **Costovertebral angle tenderness** is common in acute pyelonephritis. Since they are not invariably present, these special signs are helpful only in conjunction with a compatible history and related physical findings.

(f) Inguinal and femoral rings; male genitalia: The inguinal and femoral rings in both sexes and the genitalia in male patients should be examined next.

(g) Rectal examination: A rectal examination must always be performed in patients with an acute abdomen. Diffuse tenderness is nonspecific, but right-sided rectal tenderness accompanied by lower abdominal rebound tenderness is indicative of peritoneal irritation due to pelvic appendicitis or abscess. Other useful findings include a rectal tumor, blood-stained stool, or occult blood (detected by guaiac testing).

(h) Pelvic examination: The pelvic examination deserves emphasis. An acute abdomen is incorrectly diagnosed more often in women than in men, particularly in younger age groups. A properly performed pelvic examination is invaluable in differentiating among acute pelvic inflammatory diseases that do not require operation and acute appendicitis, twisted ovarian cyst, or tubo-ovarian abscess (see Chapter 42).

INVESTIGATIVE STUDIES

The history and physical examination by themselves provide the diagnosis in two-thirds of cases of an acute abdomen. Supplementary laboratory and radiologic examinations are indispensable for diagnosis of many surgical conditions, for exclusion of medical causes ordinarily not treated by operation, and for assistance in preoperative preparation. Even in the absence of a specific diagnosis, there may already be enough information on which to base a rational decision about management. Additional studies are worthwhile only if they are likely to significantly alter or improve therapeutic decisions. A more liberal use of diagnostic studies is justified in elderly or seriously ill patients, in whom the history and physical findings may be less reliable and an early diagnosis vital to ensure a successful outcome.

The availability and reliability of certain studies vary in different hospitals. The invasiveness, risks, and cost-effectiveness of a test should be weighed when the physician selects diagnostic studies. Test results must always be interpreted within the clinical context of each case. As a rule, basic studies should be obtained in all but the most desperately ill patients. Other less vital tests may be requested later as indicated (Table 21–5).

Laboratory Investigations

A. Blood Studies: Hemoglobin, hematocrit, and **white blood cell and differential counts** taken on admission are highly informative. Only a rising or marked leukocytosis ($> 13,000/\mu L$), especially in the presence of a shift to the left on the blood smear, is indicative of serious infection. Moderate leukocytosis, commonly encountered in medical as well as surgical inflammatory conditions, is nonspecific and may even be absent in elderly or debilitated patients with infections. A low white blood cell count ($< 8000/\mu L$) is a feature of viral infections such as mesenteric adenitis or gastroenteritis and nonspecific abdominal pain.

A specimen of clotted blood for cross-matching should be sent whenever urgent surgery is anticipated. An additional tube of clotted blood may be reserved in case of such need.

Serum electrolytes, urea, and **creatinine** are important, especially if hypovolemia is expected (ie, due to shock, copious vomiting or diarrhea, tense abdominal distention, or delay of several days after onset of symptoms). **Arterial blood gas determinations** should be obtained in patients with hypotension, generalized peritonitis, pancreatitis, possible ischemic bowel, and septicemia. Unsuspected metabolic acidosis may be the first clue to serious disease.

A raised **serum amylase** level corroborates a clinical diagnosis of acute pancreatitis. Moderately elevated values must be interpreted with caution, since

Table 21–5. General principles of timing of diagnostic studies in acute abdomen.

	Immediate	Same Day[1]	Next Day[1]
Blood	Hematocrit, white blood cell count, urea, creatinine, cross-matching,[1] arterial gases.[1]	Clotting studies, amylase, liver function tests.	Specific tests.
Urine	Microscopy, dipstick testing, culture.[1]		Specific tests.
Stool	Occult blood.	Warm smear, culture.	
Radiography and ultrasound	Chest, abdomen.	Ultrasonography or CT scan, angiography, water-soluble upper gastrointestinal series, HIDA scan (see Chapter 26).	Repeat abdominal films; barium enema or small bowel follow-through, intravenous urogram, and PTC (see Chapter 26); liver-spleen, gallium, and technetium scans.
Endoscopy		Proctosigmoidoscopy, upper endoscopy.	ERCP (see Chapter 26), colonoscopy, peritoneoscopy.
Other		Paracentesis, culdocentesis.	

[1]When indicated.

abnormal levels frequently accompany strangulated or ischemic bowel, twisted ovarian cyst, or perforated ulcer. Moreover, a normal or even low amylase value may be seen in hemorrhagic pancreatitis or pseudocyst. Cloudy (lactescent) serum in a patient with abdominal pain suggests pancreatitis even though the serum amylase is normal.

In patients with suspected hepatobiliary disease, **liver function tests** (serum bilirubin, alkaline phosphatase, AST, ALT, albumin, and globulin) are useful to differentiate medical from surgical hepatic disorders and to gauge the severity of underlying parenchymal disease.

Clotting studies (platelet counts; prothrombin time and partial thromboplastin time) and a **peripheral blood smear** should be requested if the history hints at a possible hematologic abnormality (cirrhosis, petechiae, etc). The erythrocyte sedimentation rate, often nonspecifically raised in the acute abdomen, is of dubious diagnostic value; a normal value does not exclude serious surgical illness.

Antibody titers for amebic or viral disease and other special blood tests may pinpoint a specific disease, but therapeutic decisions often cannot await their results.

B. Urine Tests: So easily performed yet frequently overlooked, urinalysis may unexpectedly reveal useful information. Dark urine or a raised specific gravity reflects mild dehydration in patients with normal renal function. Hyperbilirubinemia may give rise to tea-colored urine that froths when shaken. Microscopic hematuria or pyuria can confirm ureteral colic or urinary tract infection and obviate a needless operation. Initial antibiotic treatment should be adjusted after culture and sensitivity reports are available. **Dipstick testing** (for albumin, bilirubin, glucose, and ketones) may reveal a medical cause of an acute abdomen.

C. Stool Tests: Gastrointestinal bleeding is not a common feature of the acute abdomen. Nonetheless, testing for **occult fecal blood** should be routinely performed in all patients. A positive test points to a mucosal lesion that may be responsible for large bowel obstruction or chronic anemia, or it may reflect an unsuspected carcinoma.

Warm stool smears for bacteria, ova, and animal parasites may demonstrate amebic trophozoites in patients with bloody or mucous diarrhea. Stool samples for culture should be taken in patients with suspected gastroenteritis, dysentery, or cholera.

Imaging Studies

A. Plain Chest X-Ray Studies: An erect chest x-ray is essential in all cases of an acute abdomen. Not only is it vital for preoperative assessment, but it may also demonstrate supradiaphragmatic conditions that simulate an acute abdomen (eg, basal pneumonia or ruptured esophagus). An elevated hemidiaphragm or pleural effusion may direct attention to subphrenic inflammatory lesions.

B. Plain Abdominal X-Ray Studies: Plain supine films of the abdomen should be obtained only selectively. In general, erect (or lateral decubitus) views contribute little additional information except in suspected intestinal obstruction. Even though radiologic abnormalities are present in up to 40% of patients, these are diagnostic only half the time. Plain films are indicated in patients who have appreciable abdominal tenderness or distention or who are suspected of having intestinal obstruction or ischemia, perforated viscus, renal or ureteral calculi, or acute cholecystitis. They are seldom of value in patients suspected clinically to have appendicitis or urinary tract infection. They should not be requested in pregnant patients, unstable individuals in whom clear-cut physical signs mandating laparotomy already exist, or patients with only mild, resolving nonspecific pain. Maximal information is obtained by an experienced radiologist apprised of the clinical situation. However, the surgeon who is familiar with the clinical details should review all x-rays.

One should observe the gas pattern of the hollow viscera; free or abnormal air patterns under the diaphragm, within the biliary radicles, or outside the bowel wall; the outline of solid organs and the peritoneal fat lines; and radiopaque densities.

An abnormal bowel gas pattern suggests paralytic ileus, mechanical bowel obstruction, or pseudoobstruction. A diffuse gas pattern with air outlining the rectal ampulla suggests paralytic ileus, especially if bowel sounds are absent. Gaseous distention is the rule in bowel obstruction. Air-fluid levels are usually seen in distal small bowel obstruction and a distended cecum with small bowel dilation in large bowel obstruction. Along with the clinical findings, the distinctive radiologic appearances of colonic dilation in toxic megacolon or volvulus establish the diagnosis (see Figure 31–15). Adynamic ileus associated with long-standing acute appendicitis or with an atypical appendix location often produces a pattern that suggests localized right lower quadrant ileus. This radiologic picture in a patient without previous abdominal surgery should influence the diagnostic decision toward appendicitis or other ileocecal disease (tumor, inflammatory disorders). "Thumbprint" impressions on the colonic wall are noted in about half of patients with ischemic colitis. A displaced gastric or colonic air shadow may be the only sign of subcapsular splenic hematoma.

Free gas under the hemidiaphragm may be missed unless specifically looked for. Its presence in approximately 80% of perforated ulcers corroborates the clinical diagnosis. Massive pneumoperitoneum is seen in free colonic perforations.

Biliary tree air designates a biliary-enteric communication, such as a choledochoduodenal fistula or gallstone ileus. Air delineating the portal venous system characterizes pylephlebitis. Air between loops of small bowel may arise from a small localized perforation.

Obliteration of the psoas muscle margins or enlargement of the kidney shadows indicates retroperitoneal disease.

Radiopaque densities of characteristic appearance and location may confirm a clinical suspicion of biliary, renal staghorn, or ureteral calculi; appendicitis; or aortic aneurysm. Whereas pelvic phleboliths are readily distinguishable, a migrant gallstone may be mistaken for a calcified mesenteric lymph node if the accompanying small bowel distention or biliary tree air is overlooked in gallstone ileus.

C. Angiography: Angiographic studies are indicated if intra-abdominal intestinal ischemia or ongoing hemorrhage is suspected. They should precede any gastrointestinal contrast study that might obscure film interpretation. Selective visceral angiography is a reliable method of diagnosing mesenteric infarction. Emergency angiography may disclose a ruptured liver adenoma or carcinoma or an aneurysm of the splenic artery or other visceral artery. In patients with massive lower gastrointestinal bleeding, angiography may identify the bleeding site, may suggest the likely diagnosis (eg, vascular ectasia, polyarteritis nodosa), and may even be therapeutic if embolization can be performed. Angiography is of little value in ruptured aortic aneurysm or if frank peritoneal findings (peritonitis) are present. It is contraindicated in unstable patients with severe shock or sepsis and seldom warranted if other findings or tests already dictate the need for laparotomy or laparoscopy.

D. Contrast X-Ray Studies: Gastrointestinal contrast studies should not be requested routinely or be regarded as screening studies. They are helpful only if a specific condition being considered can be verified or treated by a contrast x-ray examination. For suspected perforations of the esophagus or gastroduodenal area without pneumoperitoneum, a water-soluble contrast medium (eg, meglumine diatrizoate [Gastrografin]) is preferred. If there is no clinical evidence of bowel perforation, barium enema may identify the level of a large bowel obstruction or reduce a sigmoid volvulus or intussusception. Only if there is no likelihood of large bowel obstruction should a barium bowel follow-through study be used to study a partial small bowel obstruction or to look for an intramural duodenal (or jejunal) hematoma that is best managed conservatively.

An emergency intravenous urogram is seldom necessary to evaluate nontraumatic causes of hematuria. It should be performed electively after microscopic examination of a stained and centrifuged urine specimen and cystoscopic examination. Ultrasonography and HIDA scans have largely replaced intravenous cholangiography in the evaluation of jaundiced patients and those suspected of having acute cholecystitis.

E. Ultrasonography and CT Scan: Ultrasonography is useful in evaluating upper abdominal pain that does not resemble ulcer pain or bowel obstruction and in investigating abdominal masses. Ultrasonography has a diagnostic sensitivity of about 80% for acute appendicitis and is most useful in pregnant patients and those presenting with features suggestive of atypical appendicitis or pelvic inflammatory disease. CT scanning may be necessary if excessive bowel gas precludes satisfactory ultrasound examination. It is particularly helpful in pancreatic and retropancreatic lesions and any severe localized infections (eg, acute diverticulitis). A CT scan may detect the presence of intramural bowel or venous (mesenteric or portal) gas that is highly indicative of bowel infarction.

Thus far, motion artifacts have limited the application of MRI in the acute abdomen.

F. Radionuclide Scans: Liver-spleen scans, HIDA scans, and gallium scans are useful for localizing intra-abdominal abscesses. Radionuclide blood pool or Tc sulfur colloid scans may identify sources of intestinal bleeding. Technetium pertechnetate scans may reveal ectopic gastric mucosa in Meckel's diverticulum.

Endoscopy

Proctosigmoidoscopy is indicated in any patient with suspected large bowel obstruction, grossly bloody stools, or a rectal mass. Minimal air should be used for bowel insufflation. Besides reducing sigmoid volvulus, **colonoscopy** may also locate the source of bleeding in cases of lower gastrointestinal hemorrhage that has subsided. **Gastroduodenoscopy** and **ERCP** are usually done electively to evaluate less urgent inflammatory conditions (eg, gastritis, peptic disease) in patients without alarming abdominal signs.

Paracentesis

The finding of free blood or turbid, infected ascites on abdominal paracentesis is invaluable in patients with free peritoneal fluid. Aspiration of blood, bile, or bowel contents is a strong indication for urgent laparatomy. On the other hand, infected ascitic fluid may establish a diagnosis in spontaneous bacterial peritonitis, tuberculous peritonitis, or chylous ascites (see Chapter 22), which rarely require surgery. **Culdocentesis** may be useful for suspected ruptured corpus luteum cyst.

Peritoneal cytology (obtained by direct aspiration through a fine catheter) or diagnostic peritoneal lavage may disclose an acute intra-abdominal inflammatory problem. More importantly, in equivocal cases, it may indicate a nonsurgical condition.

Laparoscopy

Laparoscopy has an established role prior to laparotomy in women in whom the diagnosis of appendicitis is uncertain. A ruptured graafian follicle, pelvic inflammatory disease, or other tubo-ovarian conditions can be readily diagnosed, thereby averting an unnecessary laparotomy. Where appendicitis is confirmed, laparoscopic appendectomy may be performed. Laparoscopy is also a useful diagnostic tool in managing obtunded, elderly, or critically ill patients who may have subdued manifestations of an acute abdomen.

DIFFERENTIAL DIAGNOSIS

The **age** and **sex** of the patient help in the differential diagnosis: Mesenteric adenitis is apt to mimic acute appendicitis in the young; gynecologic disorders complicate the evaluation of lower abdominal pain in women of childbearing age; and malignant and vascular diseases are more common in the elderly. Causes of an acute abdomen reflect the disease patterns of the indigenous population, and an awareness of common causes within the physician's locale will improve diagnostic accuracy.

The differential diagnosis of specific acute surgical conditions is dealt with elsewhere in this book. The clinical picture in early cases is often unclear. The following observations should be borne in mind:

(1) **Any patient** with acute abdominal pain persisting for over 6 hours should be regarded as having a surgical problem requiring in-hospital evaluation. Well-localized pain and tenderness usually indicate a surgical condition. Patients with generalized abdominal pain due to surgical disorders (eg, diffuse peritonitis) often have associated systemic toxicity; this is uncommon when pain is due to an undiagnosed medical problem.

(2) **Acute cholecystitis, appendicitis, bowel obstruction, cancer,** and **acute vascular conditions** are the most common causes of the surgical acute abdomen in older patients. In children, appendicitis accounts for one-third of all cases and nonspecific abdominal pain for nearly all the remainder.

(3) **Acute appendicitis** and **intestinal obstruction** are the most frequent final diagnoses in cases erroneously believed at first to be nonsurgical. Appendicitis should always remain a foremost concern if sepsis or an inflammatory lesion is suspected. It is the commonest cause of bizarre peritoneal findings that produce ileus or intestinal obstruction. Half of children with appendicitis present with a marked facial flush (due to high serotonin levels). The presence of the gas stoppage sign or x-ray findings of right lower quadrant ileus should raise the possibility of retrocecal or retroileal appendicitis.

Pelvic appendicitis, with mild abdominal pain, vomiting, and frequent loose stools, simulates gastroenteritis. The initial abdominal signs may be mild and the rectal and pelvic examinations unremarkable. A low white blood cell count or lymphocytosis favors gastroenteritis.

Atypical presentations of appendicitis are encountered during pregnancy. Maternal illness and fetal death in such cases are caused mainly by complications following delayed diagnosis. Appendectomy is well tolerated during pregnancy.

(4) **Salpingitis, dysmenorrhea, ovarian lesions,** and **urinary tract infections** complicate the evaluation of the acute abdomen in young women. Many diagnostic errors can be avoided by taking a careful menstrual history and performing a proper pelvic examination and urinalysis. Ultrasound study and pregnancy tests are helpful in appropriate cases. Compared with patients with appendicitis, patients with acute salpingitis tend to present with a longer history of pain, often related to the menstrual cycle, and to have higher fever and a markedly elevated white blood cell count.

(5) **Unusual types or atypical manifestations of intestinal obstruction,** especially early cases, are easily missed. Emesis, abdominal distention, and air-fluid levels on x-ray may be negligible in Richter's hernia, proximal or closed-loop small bowel obstructions, and early cecal volvulus.

Intestinal obstruction in an elderly woman who has not had a previous operation strongly suggests an incarcerated femoral hernia or, rarely, an obturator hernia or gallstone ileus. There may be no pain in the area of the hernia, and the palpable bulge may not be tender. Carefully examine the inguinofemoral region; repeat the rectal and pelvic examinations; and check for an obturator sign. Transient mild upper abdominal pain followed several days later by signs of intestinal obstruction is typical of gallstone ileus. Look for a radiopaque stone and air outlining the biliary tree on the plain abdominal x-ray.

(6) Elderly or cardiac patients with severe unrelenting diffuse abdominal pain but without commensurate peritoneal signs or abnormalities on plain abdominal films may have **intestinal ischemia.** Arterial blood pH should be measured and visceral angiography performed early.

(7) **Medical causes of the acute abdomen** should be excluded before exploratory laparotomy is considered (Table 21–6). Upper abdominal pain may be encountered in myocardial infarction, acute pulmonary conditions (pneumothorax, basal pneumonia, pleurisy, empyema, infarction), and acute hepatitis. Generalized or migratory abdominal discomfort may be felt in acute rheumatic fever, polyarteritis nodosa and other types of diffuse vasculitis, acute intermittent porphyria, and acute pleurodynia. Sharp flank pain, often accompanied by rectus spasm and cutaneous hyperesthesia, may be caused by osteoarthritis with thoracic or spinal nerve compression. Likewise, acute bursitis and hip joint disorders may produce pain ra-

Table 21–6. Medical causes of acute abdomen for which surgery is not indicated.

Endocrine and metabolic disorders	**Infections and inflammatory disorders**
Uremia	Tabes dorsalis
Diabetic crisis	Herpes zoster
Addisonian crisis	Acute rheumatic fever
Acute intermittent porphyria	Henoch-Schönlein purpura
Acute hyperlipoproteinemia	Systemic lupus erythematosus
Hereditary Mediterranean fever	Polyarteritis nodosa
Hematologic disorders	**Referred pain**
Sickle cell crisis	Thoracic region
Acute leukemia	Myocardial infarction
Other dyscrasias	Acute pericarditis
Toxins and drugs	Pneumonia
Lead and other heavy metal poisoning	Pleurisy
Narcotic withdrawal	Pulmonary embolus
Black widow spider poisoning	Pneumothorax
	Empyema
	Hip and back

diating into the lower quadrants. Exquisite tingling or pinpricking sensations along a flank dermatome are characteristic of preeruptive herpes zoster.

Medical conditions usually can be distinguished from surgical ones by a careful assessment of the history and physical examination. The family history may furnish the first clue. The history is usually atypical in some aspects, and thoughtful scrutiny will disclose details such as unusual or exaggerated symptoms—or concomitant extra-abdominal complaints—that point to the true cause. Despite the apparent severity of pain, localized abdominal tenderness with involuntary guarding is seldom present. Fever and associated systemic signs may be disproportionate to the degree of pain. Laboratory and x-ray studies will verify the diagnosis and avoid an operation.

(8) Beware of **acute cholecystitis, acute appendicitis,** and **perforated peptic ulcer** in patients already hospitalized for an illness affecting another organ system. Their presentation is often atypical, leading to delayed diagnosis and complications.

(9) **Exploration** is most often **mistakenly undertaken** for salpingitis, mesenteric adenitis, gastroenteritis, pyelonephritis, and acute viral hepatitis.

(10) **Nonspecific abdominal pain,** representing one-third of all cases, is the most common cause of the acute abdomen. Generally mild, short-lived, and seldom associated with other serious symptoms, it resolves without specific treatment. Most cases represent undiagnosed viral and bacterial infections, worm infestation, abdominal wall pain, irritable bowel syndrome, gynecologic problems, or psychosomatic pain.

INDICATIONS FOR LAPAROTOMY

The need for operation is apparent when the diagnosis is certain, but surgery sometimes must be undertaken before a precise diagnosis is reached. Table 21–7 lists some indications for urgent laparotomy. Among patients with acute abdominal pain, those over age 65 more often require operation (33%) than do younger patients (15%).

A liberal policy of exploration is advisable in patients with inconclusive but persistent right lower quadrant tenderness. Pain in the left upper quadrant infrequently requires urgent laparotomy, and its cause can usually await elective confirmatory studies.

PREOPERATIVE MANAGEMENT

After initial assessment, narcotic **analgesics** for pain relief should not be withheld. In moderate doses, analgesics neither obscure useful physical findings nor mask their subsequent development. Indeed, abdominal masses may become obvious once rectus spasm is relieved. Pain that persists in spite of adequate doses of narcotics suggests a serious condition often requiring operative correction.

Resuscitation of acutely ill patients is outlined in Chapter 2. Medications should be restricted to only essential requirements. Particular care should be given to use of cardiac drugs and corticosteroids and to control of diabetes. **Antibiotics** are indicated for some infectious conditions or as prophylaxis during the perioperative period (see Chapter 8).

Table 21–7. Indications for urgent operation in patients with acute abdomen.

Physical findings
Involuntary guarding or rigidity, especially if spreading
Increasing or severe localized tenderness
Tense or progressive distention
Tender abdominal or rectal mass with high fever or hypotension
Rectal bleeding with shock or acidosis
Equivocal abdominal findings along with—
   Septicemia (high fever, marked or rising leukocytosis, mental changes, or increasing glucose intolerance in a diabetic patient)
   Bleeding (unexplained shock or acidosis, falling hematocrit)
   Suspected ischemia (acidosis, fever, tachycardia)
   Deterioration on conservative treatment
Radiologic findings
Pneumoperitoneum
Gross or progressive bowel distention
Free extravasation of contrast material
Space-occupying lesion on scan, with fever
Mesenteric occlusion on angiography
Endoscopic findings
Perforated or uncontrollably bleeding lesion
Paracentesis findings
Blood, bile, pus, bowel contents, or urine

A **nasogastric tube** should be inserted in patients likely to undergo surgery and for those with hematemesis or copious vomiting, suspected bowel obstruction, or severe paralytic ileus. This precaution may prevent aspiration in patients suffering from drug overdose or alcohol intoxication, patients who are comatose or debilitated, or elderly patients with impaired cough reflexes. However, since the tube interferes with coughing and is uncomfortable, it should be removed once it is safe to do so.

Constipation rarely produces a genuine acute abdomen. Enemas, laxatives, and cathartics should never be administered until the possibility of bowel obstruction has been excluded.

Informed consent for surgery may be difficult to obtain when the diagnosis is uncertain. It is prudent to discuss with the patient and family the possibility of multiple staged operations; temporary or permanent stomal openings; impotence or sterility; and postoperative intubation for mechanical ventilation.

REFERENCES

Adams Computer aided diagnosis of acute abdominal pain. A multicentre study. Br Med J 1986;293:800.

Austin H: Acute right upper quadrant abdominal pain: Ultrasound approach. J Clin Ultrasound 1983;11:187.

Bender JS: Approach to the acute abdomen. Med Clin North Am 1989;73:1413.

Berci G et al: Emergency laparoscopy. Am J Surg 1991;161:332.

Brewer RJ et al: An analysis of 1,000 consecutive cases in a university hospital emergency room. Am J Surg 1976;131:219.

Campbell JPM, Gunn AA: Plain abdominal radiographs and abdominal pain. Br J Surg 1988;75:554.

de Dombal FT: *Diagnosis of Acute Abdominal Pain,* 2nd ed. Churchill Livingstone, 1991.

Dickson JAS et al: Acute abdominal pain in children. Scand J Gastroenterol 1988;144(Suppl):43.

Dixon JM et al: Rectal examination in patients with pain in the right lower quadrant of the abdomen. Br Med J 1991;302:386.

Gallegos NC, Hobsley M: Abdominal wall pain: An alternative diagnosis. Br J Surg 1990;77:1167.

Gray DWR, Collin J: Non-specific abdominal pain as a cause of acute admission to hospital. Br J Surg 1987;74:239.

Merten DF: The acute abdomen in childhood. Curr Probl Diagn Radiol 1986;15:333.

Mirvis SE et al: Plain film evaluation of patients with abdominal pain: Are three radiographs necessary? AJR 1986;147:501.

Paterson Brown S et al: Laparoscopy as an adjunct to decision making in the acute abdomen. Br J Surg 1986;73:1022.

Paterson-Brown S, Vipond MN: Modern aids to clinical decision-making in the acute abdomen. Br J Surg 1990;77:13.

Ridge JA, Way LW: Abdominal pain and acute abdomen. In: *Gastrointestinal Disease,* 5th ed. Sleisenger MH, Fordtran JS (editors). Saunders, 1993.

Sawyers JL, Williams LF (editors): The acute abdomen. Surg Clin North Am 1988;68:233.

Shaff MI et al: Computed tomography and magnetic resonance imaging of the acute abdomen. Surg Clin North Am 1988;68:233.

Silen W: *Cope's Early Diagnosis of the Acute Abdomen,* 18th ed. Oxford Univ Press, 1991.

Steinheber FV: Medical conditions mimicking the acute surgical abdomen. Med Clin North Am 1973;57:1559.

Telfer S et al: Acute abdominal pain in patients over 50 years of age. Scand J Gastroenterol 1988;144(Suppl):47.

Peritoneal Cavity

22

John H. Boey, MD

THE PERITONEUM & ITS FUNCTIONS

The peritoneal cavity is lined by the **parietal peritoneum,** a mesothelial lining. This lining is called the **visceral peritoneum** where it is reflected onto the enclosed abdominal organs. The relationship to intraperitoneal structures defines discrete compartments within which abscesses may form (see Intraabdominal Abscesses). The peritoneal surface area is a semipermeable membrane with an area comparable to that of the cutaneous body surface. Nearly 1 m^2 of the total 1.7-m^2 area participates in fluid exchange with the extracellular fluid space at rates of 500 mL or more per hour. Normally, there is less than 50 mL of free peritoneal fluid, a transudate with the following characteristics: specific gravity below 1.016; protein concentration less than 3 g/dL; white blood cell count less than 3000/μL; complement-mediated antibacterial activity; and lack of fibrinogen-related clot formation. The circulation of peritoneal fluid is directed toward lymphatics in the undersurface of the diaphragm. There, particulate matter—including bacteria up to 20 μm in size—is cleared via stomas in the diaphragmatic mesothelium and lymphatics and discharged mainly into the right thoracic duct.

The peritoneal cavity is normally sterile. Small numbers of bacteria can be efficiently disposed of, but peritonitis ensues if the defense mechanisms are overwhelmed by massive or continued contamination. In response to tissue damage, mast cells in the delicate mesothelial lining discharge histamine and other vasoactive substances that enhance vascular permeability. The resulting fibrinogen-rich plasma exudate supplies complement and opsonic proteins that promote bacterial destruction. Tissue thromboplastin released by injured mesothelial cells converts fibrinogen into fibrin, which may in turn lead to collagen deposition and formation of fibrous adhesions. In health, this reaction is limited by a plasminogen activator in the cell lining, but the plasminogen activator is inactivated by injury or infection. Fibrin clots segregate bacterial deposits, which are the source of endotoxins that contribute to sepsis, but segregation

may also inadvertently shield bacteria from bacteria-clearing mechanisms.

The **omentum** is a well-vascularized pliable, mobile double fold of peritoneum and fat that participates actively in the control of peritoneal inflammation and infection. Its composition is well suited to sealing off a leaking viscus (eg, perforated ulcer) or area of infection (eg, resulting from a ruptured appendix) and for carrying a collateral blood supply to ischemic viscera. Its bacteria scavenger functions include absorption of small particles and delivery of phagocytes that destroy unopsonized bacteria.

DISEASES & DISORDERS OF THE PERITONEUM

ACUTE SECONDARY BACTERIAL PERITONITIS

Pathophysiology

Peritonitis is an inflammatory or suppurative response of the peritoneal lining to direct irritation. Peritonitis can occur after perforating, inflammatory, infectious, or ischemic injuries of the gastrointestinal or genitourinary system. Common examples are listed in Table 22–1. **Secondary peritonitis** results from bacterial contamination originating from within viscera or from external sources (eg, penetrating injury). It most often follows disruption of a hollow viscus. Extravasated bile and urine, although only mildly irritating when sterile, are markedly toxic if infected and provoke a vigorous peritoneal reaction. Gastric juice from a perforated duodenal ulcer remains mostly sterile for several hours, during which time it produces a chemical peritonitis with large fluid losses; but if left untreated, it evolves within 6–12 hours into bacterial peritonitis. Intraperitoneal fluid dilutes opsonic proteins and impairs phagocytosis. Furthermore, when hemoglobin is present in the peritoneal cavity, *Escherichia coli* growing within the cavity can elaborate leukotoxins that reduce bactericidal activity. Limited, localized infection can be

Table 22–1. Common causes of peritonitis.

Severity	Cause	Mortality Rate
Mild	Appendicitis Perforated gastroduodenal ulcers Acute salpingitis	<10%
Moderate	Diverticulitis (localized perforations) Nonvascular small bowel perforation Gangrenous cholecystitis Multiple trauma	<20%
Severe	Large bowel perforations Ischemic small bowel injuries Acute necrotizing pancreatitis Postoperative complications	20–80%

eradicated by host defenses, but continued contamination invariably leads to generalized peritonitis and eventually to septicemia with multiple organ failure (see Chapter 8).

Factors that influence the severity of peritonitis include the type of bacterial contamination, the nature of the initial injury, and the host's nutritional and immune status. The grade of peritonitis varies with the cause. Clean (eg, proximal gut perforations) or well-localized (eg, ruptured appendix) contaminations progress to fulminant peritonitis relatively slowly (eg, 12–24 hours). In contrast, bacteria associated with distal gut or infected biliary tract perforations quickly overwhelm host peritoneal defenses. This degree of toxicity is also characteristic of postoperative peritonitis due to anastomotic leakage or contamination. Conditions that ordinarily cause mild peritonitis may produce life-threatening sepsis in a compromised host.

Causative organisms. Systemic sepsis due to peritonitis occurs in varying degrees depending on the virulence of the pathogens, the bacterial load, and the duration of bacterial proliferation and synergistic interaction. Except for spontaneous bacterial peritonitis, peritonitis is almost invariably polymicrobial; cultures usually contain more than one aerobic and more than two anaerobic species. The microbial picture reflects the bacterial flora of the involved organ. As long as gastric acid secretion and gastric emptying are normal, perforations of the proximal bowel (stomach or duodenum) are generally sterile or associated with relatively small numbers of gram-positive organisms. Perforations or ischemic injuries of the distal small bowel (eg, strangulated hernia) lead to infection with aerobic bacteria in about 30% of cases and anaerobic organisms in about 10% of cases. Fecal spillage, with a bacterial load of 10^{12} or more organisms per gram, is extremely toxic. Positive cultures with gram-negative and anaerobic bacteria are characteristic of infections originating from the appendix, colon, and rectum. The predominant aerobic pathogens include the gram-negative bacteria *E coli,* streptococci, *Proteus,* and the *Enterobacter-*

Klebsiella groups. Besides *Bacteroides fragilis,* anaerobic cocci and clostridia are the prevalent anaerobic organisms. Synergism between fecal anaerobic and aerobic bacteria increases the severity of infections.

Clinical Findings

By estimating the severity of peritonitis from clinical and laboratory findings, the need for specific organ-supportive care and surgery can be determined.

See Chapter 21 for details of radiologic and other investigations.

A. Symptoms and Signs: The clinical manifestations of peritonitis reflect the severity and duration of infection and the age and general health of the patient. Physical findings can be divided into (1) abdominal signs arising from the initial injury and (2) manifestations of systemic infection. Acute peritonitis frequently presents as acute abdomen. **Local findings** include abdominal pain, tenderness, guarding or rigidity, distention, free peritoneal air, and diminished bowel sounds—signs that reflect parietal peritoneal irritation and resulting ileus. **Systemic findings** include fever, chills or rigors, tachycardia, sweating, tachypnea, restlessness, dehydration, oliguria, disorientation, and, ultimately, refractory shock. Shock is due to the combined effects of hypovolemia and septicemia with multiple organ dysfunction. *Recurrent unexplained shock is highly predictive of serious intraperitoneal sepsis.*

The findings in abdominal sepsis are modified by the patient's age and general health. Physical signs of peritonitis are subtle or difficult to interpret in either very young or very old patients or in those who are chronically debilitated, immunosuppressed, receiving corticosteroids, or recently postoperative. Diagnostic peritoneal lavage may be employed in equivocal cases in senile or confused patients. There are virtually no false-positive and only minimal false-negative errors. Delayed recognition is a major cause of the high mortality rate of peritonitis.

B. Laboratory Findings: Laboratory studies gauge the severity of peritonitis and guide therapy. Blood studies should include a complete blood cell count, cross-matching, arterial blood gases, a blood clotting profile, and liver and renal function tests. Samples for culture of blood, urine, sputum, and peritoneal fluid should be taken before antibiotics are started. A positive blood culture is usually present in toxic patients.

Differential Diagnosis

Specific kinds of infective (eg, gonococcal, amebic, candidal) and noninfective peritonitis may be seen. In the elderly, systemic diseases (eg, pneumonia, uremia) may produce intestinal ileus so striking that it resembles bowel obstruction or peritonitis.

Familial Mediterranean fever (periodic peritonitis, familial paroxysmal polyserositis) is a rare genetically transmitted cause of acute peritonitis that primarily affects individuals of southern and eastern Mediterranean genetic background. Its cause is unknown, but enzymatic defects in catecholamine metabolism and a deficiency of C5a inhibitor in synovial fluid have been postulated. Recurring bouts of abdominal pain with direct and rebound tenderness occur along with pleuritic or joint pains. Fever and leukocytosis accompany the attacks. Renal amyloidosis is a late and serious complication.

Colchicine (1–1.5 mg daily)—effective in preventing but not treating acute attacks—can be used as a diagnostic test. Intravenous metaraminol infusion (10 mg) is a safe and specific provocative test that precipitates abdominal pain within 2 days in afflicted patients.

Laparotomy is often performed during the initial episodes. The peritoneal surfaces may be inflamed and there may be free fluid, but smears and cultures of peritoneal fluid are negative. Even though it may appear normal, the appendix should be removed to exclude appendicitis from the differential diagnosis in subsequent attacks. Late illness results from amyloidosis and renal failure, complications that also appear to be preventable by long-term colchicine therapy.

Treatment

Fluid and electrolyte replacement, operative control of sepsis, and systemic antibiotics are the mainstays of treatment of peritonitis.

A. Preoperative Care:

1. Intravenous fluids–The massive transfer of fluid into the peritoneal cavity must be replaced by an appropriate amount of intravenous fluid. If systemic toxicity is evident or if the patient is old or in fragile health, a central venous pressure (or pulmonary artery wedge pressure) line and bladder catheter should be inserted; a fluid balance chart should be kept; and serial body weight measurements should be taken to monitor fluid requirements. Several liters of balanced salt or lactated Ringer's solution may be required to correct hypovolemia. Intravenous infusions must be given rapidly enough to restore blood pressure and urine output promptly to satisfactory levels. Potassium supplements are withheld until tissue and renal perfusion are adequate. Blood is reserved for anemic patients or those with concomitant bleeding.

2. Care for advanced septicemia–Cardiovascular agents and mechanical ventilation in an intensive care unit are essential in patients with advanced septicemia. An arterial line for continuous blood pressure recording and blood sampling is helpful. Cardiac monitoring with a Swan-Ganz catheter is essential if inotropic drugs are used. (See Chapters 8, 9, and 12 for details of fluid resuscitation and the management of septic shock.)

3. Antibiotics–Loading doses of intravenous antibiotics directed against the anticipated bacterial pathogens should be given after fluid samples have been obtained for culture. Initial regimens include cephalosporins or imipenem-cilastatin for gram-negative coliforms, ampicillin for enterococci, and metronidazole or clindamycin for anaerobic organisms. The empirically chosen antibiotic regimen should be modified after results of culture and sensitivity studies are available. Because renal impairment is often a feature of peritonitis, serum levels of potentially nephrotoxic agents (especially aminoglycosides) should be checked regularly. Antibiotics should be continued until the patient has remained afebrile with a normal WBC and a differential count of less than 3% bands.

4. Other measures–Other therapeutic measures are of secondary importance or of equivocal value. Pharmacologic doses of methylprednisolone have not been shown to be of value in controlled trials and would rarely be appropriate in light of their detrimental effects on the immune system. The experimental use of fibronectin and immune-stimulating drugs (eg, glucan, muramyl dipeptide) or polyvalent immunoglobulins to counter sepsis-related immunosuppression may soon find clinical application.

B. Operative Management:

1. Control of sepsis–The objectives of surgery for peritonitis are to remove all infected material, correct the underlying cause, and prevent late complications. Except in early, localized peritonitis, a midline incision offers the best surgical exposure. Materials for aerobic and anaerobic cultures of fluid and infected tissue are obtained immediately after the abdomen is opened. Occult pockets of infection are located by thorough exploration, and contaminated or necrotic material is removed. Routine radical debridement of all peritoneal and serosal surfaces does not increase survival rates. The primary disease is then treated. This may require resection (eg, ruptured appendix or gallbladder), repair (eg, perforated ulcer), or drainage (eg, acute pancreatitis). Attempts to reanastomose resected bowel in the presence of extensive sepsis or intestinal ischemia often lead to leakage. Temporary stomas are safer, and these can be taken down several weeks later after the patient has recovered from the acute illness.

2. Peritoneal lavage–In diffuse peritonitis, lavage with copious amounts (> 3 L) of warm isotonic crystalloid solution removes gross particulate matter as well as blood and fibrin clots and dilutes residual bacteria. Fears that this maneuver might spread infection to uncontaminated areas have proved to be unfounded. The addition of antiseptics or antibiotics to the irrigating solution is generally useless (eg, noxythiolin) or even harmful because of induced adhesions (eg, tetracycline, povidone-iodine). Antibiotics given parenterally will reach bactericidal levels in peritoneal fluid and may afford no additional benefit when given by lavage. Furthermore, lavage with aminoglycosides can produce respiratory depression and complicate anesthesia because of the neuromuscular blocking action of this group of drugs. After lavage is completed, all fluid in the peritoneal cavity must be aspirated because it may hamper local defense mechanisms by diluting opsonins and removing surfaces upon which phagocytes destroy bacteria.

Continuous peritoneal lavage for up to 3 days postoperatively with a balanced crystalloid or antibiotic-containing solution is recommended by some groups. The solution is infused hourly through soft sump drains placed in the right suprahepatic and left paracolic gutters, and the effluent is collected via sump drains in the pelvic cul-de-sac. This method requires careful postoperative monitoring of the fluid and electrolyte status and attention to the irrigating system. Heparin may be added to reduce intraperitoneal fibrin clot formation. Postoperative lavage is unnecessary in perforated appendicitis and should be considered only in severe peritonitis associated with systemic sepsis.

3. Peritoneal drainage–Drainage of the free peritoneal cavity is ineffective and often undesirable. As foreign bodies, drains are quickly isolated from the rest of the peritoneal cavity, but they still provide a channel for exogenous contamination. Prophylactic drainage in diffuse peritonitis does not prevent abscess formation and may even predispose to abscesses or fistulas. Drainage is useful chiefly for residual focal infection or when continued contamination is present or likely to occur (eg, fistula). Drains are indicated for localized inflammatory masses that cannot be resected or for cavities that cannot be obliterated. Soft sump drains with continuous suction through multiple side perforations are effective for large volumes of fluid. Smaller volumes of fluid are best handled with closed drainage systems (eg, Jackson-Pratt drains). Large cavities with thick walls may be drained better by several large Penrose drains placed in a dependent position.

To achieve more effective peritoneal drainage in severe peritonitis, some surgeons have left the entire abdominal wound open to widely expose the peritoneal cavity. Besides requiring intensive nursing and medical support to cope with massive protein and fluid losses (averaging 9 L the first day), there are serious complications such as spontaneous fistulization, wound sepsis, and large incisional hernias.

An alternative method is to reexplore the abdomen every 1–3 days until all loculations have been adequately drained. The wound may be closed temporarily with a sheet of polypropylene (Marlex) mesh that contains a nylon zipper or Velcro to avoid a tight abdominal closure and to facilitate repeated opening and closing. Exploration may even be performed in the intensive care unit without general anesthesia. Available data suggest that this method should be restricted to selected patients with long-standing (more than 48 hours) extensive intraperitoneal sepsis associated with multiple organ failure (high sepsis

scores). The mortality rate still is about 30% in these critically septic patients.

4. Management of abdominal distention–Abdominal distention caused by ileus frequently accompanies peritonitis, and decompression of the intestine is often useful to facilitate abdominal closure and minimize postoperative respiratory problems. This is best accomplished by nasal passage of a long intestinal tube (eg, Baker or Dennis tube) to avoid an enterotomy and to act as a sutureless intestinal stent. A **gastrostomy** may be advantageous if prolonged nasogastric decompression is expected, especially in elderly patients or those with chronic respiratory disease. A feeding **jejunostomy** is indicated whenever prolonged nutritional support is anticipated.

C. Postoperative Care: Fluid, nutritional, and other supportive measures are continued postoperatively. Antibiotics are given for 10–14 days, depending on the severity of peritonitis. A favorable clinical response is evidenced by well-sustained perfusion with good urine output, reduction in fever and leukocytosis, resolution of ileus, and a returning sense of well-being. The rate of recovery varies with the duration and degree of peritonitis.

Postoperative **complications** can be divided into local and systemic problems. Residual abscesses and intraperitoneal sepsis, deep wound infections, anastomotic breakdown, and fistula formation require reexploration or percutaneous drainage. Progressive or uncontrolled sepsis leads to multiple organ failure affecting the respiratory, renal, hepatic, clotting, and immune systems. Supportive measures, including mechanical ventilation, transfusions, total parenteral nutrition, and hemodialysis, are ineffectual unless primary septic foci are eliminated by combined surgical and antibiotic therapy.

Prognosis

The overall mortality rate of generalized peritonitis is about 40% (Table 22–1). Factors contributing to a high mortality rate include the type of primary disease and its duration, associated multiple organ failure before treatment, and the age and general health of the patient. Mortality rates are consistently below 10% in patients with perforated ulcers or appendicitis; in young patients; in those having less extensive bacterial contamination; and in those diagnosed and operated upon early. Patients with distal small bowel or colonic perforations or postoperative sepsis tend to be older, to have concurrent medical illnesses and greater bacterial contamination, and to have a greater propensity to renal and respiratory failure; their mortality rates are about 50%.

Barakat MH et al: Familial Mediterranean fever (recurrent hereditary polyserositis) in Arabs: A study of 175 patients and review of the literature. Quart J Med (New Series) 1986;233:837. Bohnen J et al: Prognosis in generalized peritonitis. Arch Surg 1983;118:285.

Bohnen JM et al: APACHE II score and abdominal sepsis. A prospective study. Arch Surg 1988;123:225.

Christou NV: Systemic and peritoneal host defense in peritonitis. World J Surg 1990;14:184.

Cuesta MA et al: Sequential abdominal reexploration with the zipper technique. World J Surg 1991;15:74.

Dobrin PB et al: The value of continuous 72-hour peritoneal lavage for peritonitis. Am J Surg 1989;157:368.

Farthmann EH, Schoffel U: Principles and limitations of operative management of intraabdominal infections. World J Surg 1990;12:210.

Hau T: Bacteria, toxins, and the peritoneum. World J Surg 1990;12: 167.

Hoffman J et al: Peritoneal lavage in the diagnosis of acute peritonitis. Am J Surg 1988;155:359.

Kinney EV, Polk HC Jr.: Open treatment of peritonitis: An argument against. Adv Surg 1988;21:19.

Korepanov VI: Open abdomen technique in the treatment of peritonitis. Br J Surg 1989;76:471.

Kumar GV et al: Postoperative peritoneal lavage in generalised peritonitis. A prospective analysis. Int Surg 1989;74:20.

Leiboff AR, Soroff HS: The treatment of generalized peritonitis by closed postoperative peritoneal lavage. Arch Surg 1987;122.1005.

Maddaus MA et al: The biology of peritonitis and implications for treatment. Surg Clin North Am 1988;68:431.

Mustard RA et al: Pneumonia complicating abdominal sepsis: An independent risk factor for mortality. Arch Surg 1991;126:170.

O'Brien PE et al: Management of diffuse peritonitis by prolonged postoperative peritoneal lavage. Aust N Z J Surg 1987;57:181.

Poenaru D et al: Clinical outcome of seriously ill surgical patients with intra-abdominal infection depends on both physiologic (APACHE II score) and immunologic (DTH score) alterations. Ann Surg 1991;213:130.

Polk HC, Fry DE: Radical peritoneal debridement for established peritonitis. Ann Surg 1980;192:350.

Roger PN, Wright IH: Postoperative intra-abdominal sepsis. Br J Surg 1987;74:973. Schein M et al: Aggressive treatment of severe diffuse peritonitis. a prospective study. Br J Surg 1988,75.173.

Solomon JS et al: Results of a multicenter trial comparing imipenem/cilastatin to tobramycin/clindamycin for intra-abdominal infection. Ann Surg 1990;212:58:1.

Walsh GL et al: The open abdomen. The Marlex mesh and zipper technique. a method of managing intraperitoneal infection. Surg Clin North Am 1988;68.25.

Wittmann DH et al: Etappenlavage: Advanced diffuse peritonitis managed by planned multiple laparotomies utilizing zippers, slide fastener, and Velcro analogue for temporary abdominal closure. World J Surg 1990; 12:218.

Zemer D et al: Colchicine in the prevention and treatment of the amyloidosis of familial Mediterranean fever. N Engl J Med 1986;314:1001.

INTRA-ABDOMINAL ABSCESSES

1. INTRAPERITONEAL ABSCESSES

Pathophysiology

An intra-abdominal abscess is a collection of infected fluid within the abdominal cavity. Currently, gastrointestinal perforations, operative complications, penetrating trauma, and genitourinary infections are the most common causes. An abscess forms by one of two modes: It may develop (1) adjacent to a diseased viscus (eg, with perforated appendix or diverticulitis) or (2) as a result of external contamination (eg, postoperative subphrenic abscesses). In one-third of cases, the abscess occurs as a sequela of generalized peritonitis. Interloop and pelvic abscesses form if extravasated fluid gravitating into a dependent or localized area becomes secondarily infected (Figure 22–1).

Bacteria-laden fibrin and blood clots and neutrophils contribute to the formation of an abscess. The pathogenic organisms are similar to those responsible for peritonitis, but anaerobic organisms occupy an important role. Lowering of the redox potential by *E coli* is conducive to *Bacteroides* proliferation.

Sites of Abscesses

The areas in which abscesses commonly occur are defined by the configuration of the peritoneal cavity with its dependent lateral and pelvic basins (Figure 22–1), together with the natural divisions created by the transverse mesocolon and the small bowel mesentery. The supracolic compartment, located above the transverse mesocolon, broadly defines the subphrenic spaces (Figure 22–2A). Within this area, the subdiaphragmatic (suprahepatic) and subhepatic areas of the subphrenic space may be distinguished. **The subdiaphragmatic space** on each side occupies the con cavity between the hemidiaphragms and the domes of the hepatic lobes. The inferior limits of its posterior recess are the attachments of the coronary and triangular ligaments on the dorsal—not superior—aspect of the diaphragm. Anteriorly, the lower limits are defined on the right by the transverse colon and on the left by the anterior stomach surface, omentum, transverse colon, spleen, and phrenicocolic ligament. Although each subdiaphragmatic space is continuous over the convex liver surface, inflammatory adhesions may delimit an abscess in an anterior or posterior position (Figure 22–2B). The falciform ligament separates the right and left subdiaphragmatic divisions.

The **right subhepatic division** (Figure 22–2B) of the subphrenic space is located between the undersurfaces of the liver and gallbladder superiorly and the right kidney and mesocolon inferiorly. The anterior bulge of the kidney partitions this space into an ante-

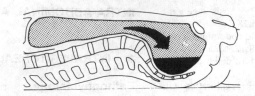

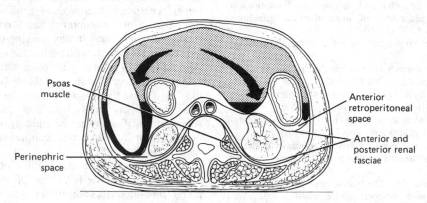

Figure 22–1. Lateral (top) and cross-sectional (bottom) views of the abdomen, showing fluid gravitating to the dependent areas of the peritoneal cavity. The retroperitoneal compartments are also outlined.

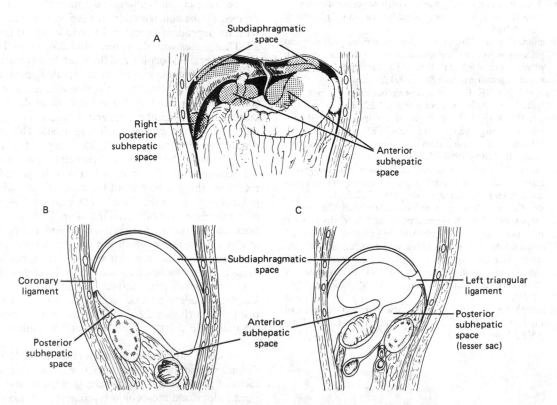

Figure 22–2. Subphrenic spaces. **A:** Anterior view. **B:** Right lateral view. **C:** Left lateral view.

rior (gallbladder fossa) and posterior (Morison's pouch) section.

The **left subhepatic space** also has an anterior and posterior part (Figure 22–2C). The smaller anterior subhepatic space lies between the undersurface of the left lobe and the anterior surface of the stomach. Left subdiaphragmatic collections often extend into this anterior subhepatic area. The posterior subhepatic space is the lesser sac, which is situated behind the lesser omentum and stomach and lies anterior to the pancreas, duodenum, transverse mesocolon, and left kidney. It extends posteriorly to the attachment of the left triangular ligament to the hemidiaphragm. The lesser sac communicates with both the right subhepatic and right paracolic spaces through the narrow foramen of Winslow.

The **infracolic compartment,** below the transverse mesocolon, includes the pericolic and pelvic areas (Figure 22–3). The diagonally aligned root of the small bowel mesentery divides the midabdominal area between the fixed right and left colons into right and left infracolic spaces. Each lateral paracolic gutter and lower quadrant area communicates freely with the pelvic cavity. However, while right paracolic collections may track upward into the subhepatic and subdiaphragmatic spaces, the phrenicocolic ligament hinders fluid migration along the left paracolic gutter into the left subdiaphragmatic area.

The most common abscess sites are in the lower quadrants, followed by the pelvic, subhepatic, and subdiaphragmatic spaces (Table 22–2).

Clinical Findings

A. Symptoms and Signs: An intraperitoneal abscess should be suspected in any patient with a predisposing condition. Fever, tachycardia, and pain may be mild or absent, especially in patients receiving antibiotics. A deep-seated or posteriorly situated abscess may exist in seemingly well individuals whose only symptom is persistent fever. Not infrequently, prolonged ileus, sluggish recovery in a patient who has had recent abdominal surgery or peritoneal sepsis, rising leukocytosis, or nonspecific radiologic abnormality provides the initial clue. A mass is seldom felt except in patients with lower quadrant or pelvic lesions. In patients with subphrenic abscesses, irritation of contiguous structures may produce lower chest pain, dyspnea, referred shoulder pain or hiccup, or basilar atelectasis or effusion; in patients with pelvic abscesses, it may produce diarrhea or urinary urgency. The diagnosis is more difficult in postoperative, chronically ill, or diabetic patients and in those receiving immunosuppressive drugs, a group particularly susceptible to septic complications.

Sequential multiple organ failure—principally respiratory, renal, or hepatic failure—or stress gastrointestinal bleeding with disseminated intravascular

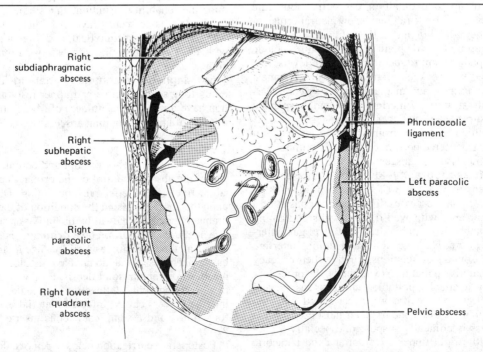

Figure 22–3. The infracolic peritoneal compartment and common abscess sites. Note how paracolic fluid on the right side can migrate up into the subphrenic spaces, whereas collections on the left side are prevented from doing so by the phrenicocolic ligament.

Table 22–2. Common sites and causes of intraperitoneal abscesses.

Site	Cause
Right lower quadrant	Appendicitis, perforated ulcer, regional enteritis
Left lower quadrant	Colorectal perforation (diverticulitis, carcinoma, inflammatory bowel diseases)
Pelvis	Appendicitis, colorectal perforation, gynecologic sepsis, postoperative complications
Subphrenic region	Postoperative complications following gastric or hepatobiliary surgery or splenectomy, perforated ulcer, acute cholecystitis, appendicitis, pancreatitis (lesser sac)
Interloop	Postoperative bowel perforation

coagulopathy is highly suggestive of intra-abdominal infection.

B. Laboratory Findings: Blood studies may suggest infection. A raised leukocyte count, abnormal liver or renal function test results, and abnormal arterial blood gases are nonspecific signs of infection. Persistently positive blood cultures point strongly to an intra-abdominal focus. A cervical smear demonstrating gonococcal infection is of specific value in diagnosing tubo-ovarian abscess.

C. Imaging Studies:

1. X-ray studies–Plain x-rays may suggest an abscess in up to one-half of cases. In subphrenic abscesses, the chest x-ray may show pleural effusion, a raised hemidiaphragm, basilar infiltrates, or atelectasis. Abnormalities on plain abdominal films include an ileus pattern, soft tissue mass, air-fluid levels, free or mottled gas pockets, effacement of properitoneal or psoas outlines, and displacement of viscera. Barium contrast studies interfere with and have been largely superseded by other imaging techniques. A water-soluble upper gastrointestinal series may reveal an unsuspected perforated viscus or outline perigastric and lesser sac abscesses.

2. Ultrasonography–Real-time ultrasonography is sensitive (about 80% of cases) in diagnosing intra-abdominal abscesses. The findings consist of a sonolucent area with well-defined walls containing fluid or debris of variable density. Bowel gas, intervening viscera, skin incisions, and stomas interfere with ultrasound examinations, limiting their efficacy in postoperative patients. Nevertheless, the procedure is readily available, portable, and inexpensive, and the findings are specific when correlated with the clinical picture. Ultrasonography is most useful when an abscess is clinically suspected, especially for lesions in the right upper quadrant and the paracolic and pelvic areas.

3. CT scan–CT scan of the abdomen, the best diagnostic study, is highly sensitive (over 95% of cases) and specific. Neither gas shadows nor exposed wounds interfere with CT scanning in postoperative patients, and the procedure is reliable even in areas poorly seen on ultrasonography. Abscesses appear as cystic collections with density measurements of between 0 and 15 attenuation units (Figure 22–4). Resolution is increased by contrast media (eg, sodium diatrizoate) injected intravenously or instilled into hollow viscera adjacent to the abscess. One drawback of CT scan is that diagnosis may be difficult in areas with multiple thick-walled bowel loops or if a pleural effusion overlies a subphrenic abscess, so that occasionally a very large abscess is missed. CT- or ultrasonography-guided needle aspiration can distinguish between sterile and infected collections in uncertain cases.

4. Radionuclide scan–Radionuclide scanning has a secondary but complementary role. Combined liver-lung scans to delineate subphrenic pockets have been replaced by ultrasonography or CT scanning. If peritoneal sepsis is clinically questionable or if the site of an abscess is uncertain, scanning with gallium-67 citrate or indium-111-labeled autologous leukocytes may sometimes disclose an abscess or another unexpected extra-abdominal site of infection. These radionuclide studies are sensitive (over 80% of cases), but many false-positive errors occur as a result of nonpyogenic inflammatory conditions, bowel accumulation of labeled leukocytes, or surgical drains and other foreign bodies in postoperative patients. Leukopenia in debilitated patients can undermine the reliability of indium-111 studies. Unfortunately, leukocyte scans may not be helpful in cases where CT scans are equivocal, and this fact coupled with the time-consuming process has limited their clinical usefulness.

5. Magnetic resonance imaging–The currently long scanning time and upper respiratory motion have limited the usefulness of MRI in the investigation of upper abdominal abscesses.

Treatment

Treatment consists of prompt and complete drainage of the abscess, control of the primary cause, and adjunctive use of effective antibiotics. Depending upon the abscess site and the condition of the patient, drainage may be achieved by operative or nonoperative methods. **Percutaneous drainage** is the preferred method for single, well-localized, superficial bacterial abscesses that do not have fistulous communications or contain solid debris. Following CT scan or ultrasonographic delineation, a needle is guided into the abscess cavity; infected material is aspirated for culture; and a sump catheter is inserted (Figure 22–4).

Postoperative irrigation helps to remove debris and ensure catheter patency. This technique is not appropriate for multiple or deep (especially pancreatic) abscesses or for patients with ongoing contamination,

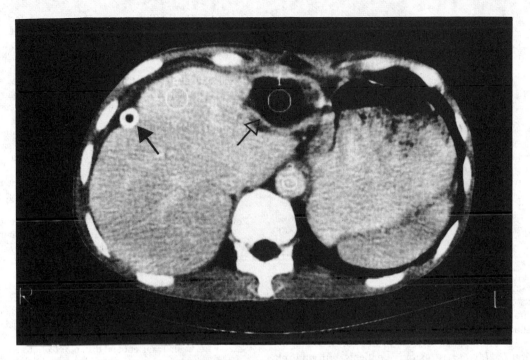

Figure 22–4. CT scan of a right subphrenic abscess. The subdiaphragmatic abscess has been drained by a percutaneous catheter (solid arrowhead), but an anterior subhepatic collection (hollow arrowhead) is still present.

fungal infections, or thick purulent or necrotic material. Percutaneous drainage can be performed in about 75% of cases. The success rate exceeds 80% in simple abscesses but is only 25% in more complex ones; it is heavily influenced by the training and experience of the radiologist performing the drainage. Complications include septicemia, fistula formation, bleeding, and peritoneal contamination.

Open drainage is reserved for abscesses for which percutaneous drainage is inappropriate or unsuccessful. The direct extraserous route has the advantage of establishing dependent drainage without contaminating the rest of the peritoneal cavity. Only light general anesthesia or even local anesthesia is necessary, and surgical trauma is minimized. Right anterior subphrenic abscesses can be drained by a subcostal incision (Clairmont incision, Figure 22–5). Posterior subdiaphragmatic and subhepatic lesions can be decompressed posteriorly through the bed of the resected twelfth rib (Nather-Ochsner incision, Figure 22–5) or by a lateral extraserous method (DeCosse incision). Most lower quadrant and flank abscesses can be drained through a lateral extraperitoneal approach. Pelvic abscesses can often be detected on pelvic or rectal examination as a fluctuant mass distorting the contour of the vagina or rectum. If needle aspiration directly through the vaginal or rectal wall returns pus, the abscess is best drained by making an incision in that area (Figure 22–6). In all cases, digital

or direct exploration must ensure that all loculations are broken down. Penrose and sump drains are used to allow continued drainage postoperatively until the infection has resolved. Serial sonograms or imaging studies help document obliteration of the abscess cavity.

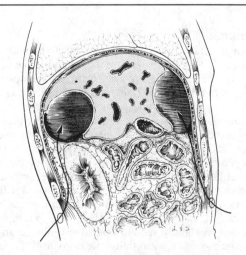

Figure 22–5. Extraperitoneal approaches to the right subphrenic spaces. An abscess in the anterior subhepatic space usually requires transperitoneal drainage. Posterior abscesses may also be drained laterally.

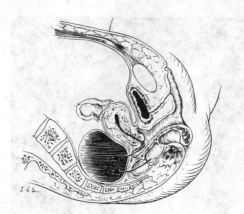

Figure 22–6. A pelvic abscess may be drained through the rectum or vagina.

Transperitoneal exploration is indicated if the abscess cannot be localized preoperatively, if there are several or deep-lying lesions, if an enterocutaneous fistula or bowel obstruction exists, or if previous drainage attempts have been unsuccessful. This is especially likely in postoperative patients with multiple abscesses and persistent peritoneal soiling. The need to achieve complete drainage fully justifies the greater stress of laparotomy and the small possibility that infection might be spread to other uninvolved areas.

Satisfactory drainage is usually evident by improving clinical findings within 3 days of treatment. Failure to improve indicates inadequate drainage, another source of sepsis, or organ dysfunction. Additional localizing studies and repeated percutaneous or operative drainage should be undertaken urgently (ie, within 24–48 hours, depending on the seriousness of the case).

Prognosis

The mortality rate of serious intra-abdominal abscesses is about 30%. Deaths are related to the severity of the underlying cause, delay in diagnosis, multiple organ failure, and incomplete drainage. Right lower quadrant and pelvic abscesses are usually caused by perforated ulcers and appendicitis in younger individuals. They are readily diagnosed and treated, and the mortality rate is less than 5%. Diagnosis is often delayed in older patients; this increases the likelihood of multiple organ failure. Decompensation of two major organ systems is associated with a mortality rate of over 50%. Shock is an especially ominous sign. Subphrenic, deep, and multiple abscesses frequently require operative drainage and are associated with a mortality rate of over 40%. An untreated residual abscess is nearly always fatal.

Deveney CW et al: Improved treatment of intraabdominal abscess. Arch Surg 1988;123:1126.

Gerzof SC, Oates ME: Imaging techniques for infections in the surgical patient. Surg Clin North Am 1988;68:89.

Haaga JR: Imaging intraabdominal abscesses and nonoperative drainage procedures. World J Surg 1990;14:204.

Hau T et al: Pathophysiology, diagnosis, and treatment of abdominal abscesses. Curr Probl Surg 1984;21:1.

Hinsdale JG, Jaffe BM: Re-operation for intra-abdominal sepsis: Indications and results in modern critical care setting. Ann Surg 1984;199:31.

Hoogewoud H-M et al: The role of computerized tomography in fever, septicemia and multiple system organ failure after laparotomy. Surg Gynecol Obstet 1986; 162:539.

Lang EK et al: Abdominal abscess drainage under radiologic guidance: Causes of failure. Radiology 1986; 159:329.

Levison MA et al: Correlation of APACHE II score, drainage technique and outcome in postoperative intra-abdominal abscesses. Surg Gynecol Obstet 1991;172:89.

Mughal MM et al: "Laparostomy": A technique for the management of intractable intraabdominal sepsis. Br J Surg 1986;73:253.

Pruett TL, Simmons R: Status of percutaneous catheter drainage of abscesses. Surg Clin North Am 1988;68:89.

Riberio MB et al: Intra-abdominal abscess in regional enteritis. Ann Surg 1991;213:23.

Sawyer RG et al: Transient and distant infections alter later intraperitoneal abscess formation. Arch Surg 1991; 126:164.

Stone HH et al: Extraperitoneal versus transperitoneal drainage of the intra-abdominal abscess. Surg Gynecol Obstet 1984;159:549.

van der Sluis RF et al: The value of traditional methods of diagnosing subphrenic abscess. Infect Surg 1986;5:337.

2. RETROPERITONEAL & RETROFASCIAL ABSCESSES

Pathophysiology

The large retroperitoneal space, extending from the diaphragm to the pelvis, is divided into anterior and posterior compartments (Figure 22–1). The **anterior portion** includes structures between the posterior peritoneum and the perinephric fascia (pancreas; parts of the duodenum and the ascending and descending colon). The **posterior portion** contains the adrenals, kidneys, and perinephric spaces. The compartment posterior to the transversalis fascia is involved in retrofascial abscesses.

Abscesses occur less commonly in the retroperitoneum than in the peritoneal cavity. Retroperitoneal abscesses arise chiefly from injuries or infections in adjacent structures: gastrointestinal tract abscesses due to appendicitis, pancreatitis, penetrating posterior ulcers, regional enteritis, diverticulitis, or trauma; genitourinary tract abscesses due to pyelonephritis; and spinal column abscesses due to osteomyelitis or disk space infections.

Psoas abscesses may be primary or secondary. Primary psoas abscesses, which occur without associated disease of other organs, are caused by hematogenous spread of *Staphylococcus aureus* from an occult source and are predominantly seen in children and young adults. They are more common in underdeveloped countries. Secondary psoas abscesses result from spread of infection from adjacent organs, principally from the intestine, and are therefore most often polymicrobial. The most common cause is Crohn's disease.

The pyogenic bacteria *(E coli, Bacteroides, Proteus, Klebsiella)* have replaced *Mycobacterium tuberculosis* as the major causative organism. Surprisingly, only a single causative organism is involved in over one-half of cases. A positive blood culture—especially with *Bacteroides*—is an ominous finding.

Clinical Findings

Although they may be symptomless, retroperitoneal abscesses tend to develop in patients with obvious acute illnesses. Fever and abdominal or flank pain are prominent features, sometimes accompanied by anorexia, weight loss, and nausea and vomiting. The clinical findings in patients with psoas abscess consist of hip pain, flexion of the hip and pain on extension, and a positive iliopsoas sign. Abdominal, thigh, and back pain may also occur. The diagnosis is apt to be overlooked when pain in the hip aggravated by walking is the major complaint. The differential diagnosis includes retroperitoneal tumors and hematomas. Radionuclide scanning, bowel contrast studies, and urograms are the common preliminary investigations, but CT scanning most accurately delineates these lesions. Gas bubbles are diagnostic of an abscess. Abscesses are confined to specific compartments, whereas malignant lesions, by contrast, frequently violate peritoneal and fascial barriers and can invade bone.

Treatment

Failure to institute prompt and adequate drainage in addition to systemic antibiotics leads to a fatal outcome. Apart from multiloculated pancreatic abscesses, many retroperitoneal abscesses are amenable to percutaneous CT scan-guided needle aspiration and catheter drainage. Drainage by catheter, however, has a lower success rate for retroperitoneal than intraperitoneal abscesses for the following reasons: (1) Retroperitoneal abscesses often dissect along planes, giving a stellate instead of globular shape; (2) they often contain necrotic debris that will not pass through catheters; and (3) they often invade adjacent muscle (eg, psoas abscess). Operation is indicated if there is no clinical improvement after 2 days of percutaneous drainage. An extraperitoneal approach via the flank is preferred for upper retroperitoneal and perirenal abscesses—and one via the perineum presacrally between the anus and the coccyx for pelvic lesions. Transperitoneal exploration may be unavoidable for deep anterior retroperitoneal abscesses. Resection of necrotic or diseased organs, debridement

of the affected compartment, and thorough drainage should be accomplished. In general, retroperitoneal abscesses are difficult to drain completely, and residual or recurrent abscesses are common (especially with regional enteritis). Psoas abscesses may invade the spine or ipsilateral hip to cause osteomyelitis or may track across the midline to cause a contralateral psoas abscess.

The surgical mortality rate is about 25%. Failure of the fever to subside within 3 days indicates inadequate drainage and persistent sepsis that will prove fatal if not corrected promptly.

Altemeier WA, Alexander JW: Retroperitoneal abscess. Arch Surg 1961;83:512.

Bresee J et al: Psoas abscess in children. Pediatr Infect Dis J 1990;9:201.

Crepps JT et al: Management and outcome of retroperitoneal abscesses. Ann Surg 1987;205:276.

Gordon DII et al: Percutaneous management of retroperitoneal abscesses. Urology 1987;30:299.

Ricci MA et al: Pyogenic psoas abscess: Worldwide variations in etiology. World J Surg 1986;10:834.

Rubenstein WA, Whalen JP: Extraperitoneal spaces. AJR Am J Roentgenol 1986;147:1162.

PRIMARY PERITONITIS

Primary ("spontaneous") peritonitis occurring in the absence of gastrointestinal perforation is caused mainly by hematogenous spread but occasionally by transluminal or direct bacterial invasion of the peritoneal cavity. It occurs mostly in patients with cirrhosis or the nephrotic syndrome, with systemic lupus erythematosus, or after splenectomy during childhood. Recurrence is common in cirrhosis and often proves fatal.

Clinical Findings

The clinical presentation simulates secondary bacterial peritonitis, with abrupt onset of fever, abdominal pain, distention, and rebound tenderness. However, one-fourth of patients have minimal or no peritoneal symptoms. Most have clinical and biochemical manifestations of advanced cirrhosis or nephrosis. Leukocytosis, hypoalbuminemia, and a prolonged prothrombin time are characteristic findings. The diagnosis hinges upon examination of the ascitic fluid, which reveals a white blood cell count greater than $500/\mu L$ and more than 25% polymorphonuclear leukocytes. A blood-ascitic fluid albumin gradient greater than 1.1 g/dL, a raised serum lactic acid level (> 33 mg/dL), or a reduced ascitic fluid pH (< 7.31) supports the diagnosis. Bacteria are seen on gram-stained smears in only 25% of cases. Culture of ascitic fluid inoculated immediately into blood culture media at the bedside usually reveals a single enteric organism, most commonly *E coli, Klebsiella,* or streptococci.

Treatment

Systemic antibiotics (cefotaxime or a combination of an aminoglycoside and ampicillin) and supportive treatment should be started as soon as the diagnosis is established. The mortality rate is about 60% but is attributable to peritonitis in only half of cases. Progressive hepatic encephalopathy and renal failure are ominous signs.

Albillos A et al: Ascitic fluid polymorphonuclear cell count and serum to ascites albumin gradient in the diagnosis of bacterial peritonitis. Gastroenterology 1990;98:134.

Hallak A: Spontaneous bacterial peritonitis. Am J Gastroenterol 1989;84:345.

Tito L et al: Recurrence of spontaneous bacterial peritonitis in cirrhosis: frequency and predictive factors. Hepatology 1988;8:27.

Wilcox CM, Dismukes WE: Spontaneous bacterial peritonitis: A review of pathogenesis, diagnosis and treatment. Medicine 1987;66:447.

TUBERCULOUS PERITONITIS

Pathophysiology

Tuberculosis peritonitis is encountered in 0.5% of new cases of tuberculosis. It presents as a primary infection without active pulmonary, intestinal, renal, or uterine tube involvement. Its cause is reactivation of a dormant peritoneal focus derived from hematogenous dissemination from a distant nidus or breakdown of mesenteric lymph nodes. Some cases occur as a systemic manifestation of extra-abdominal infection. Multiple small, hard, raised, whitish tubercles studding the peritoneum, omentum, and mesentery are the distinctive finding. A cecal tuberculoma, matted lymph nodes, or omental involvement may form a palpable mass.

The disease affects young persons, particularly women, and is more prevalent in countries where tuberculosis is still endemic. AIDS patients are especially susceptible to development of extrapulmonary tuberculosis.

Clinical Findings

Chronic symptoms (lasting more than a week) include abdominal pain and distention, fever, night sweats, weight loss, and altered bowel habits. Ascites is present in about half of cases, especially if the disease is of long standing, and may be the primary manifestation. A mass may be felt in a third of cases. The differential diagnosis includes Crohn's disease, carcinoma, hepatic cirrhosis, and intestinal lymphoma. One-fourth of patients have acute symptoms suggestive of acute bowel obstruction or peritonitis that mimics appendicitis, cholecystitis, or a perforated ulcer.

Detection of an extra-abdominal site of tuberculosis, evident in half of cases, is the single most useful diagnostic clue. Pleural effusion is present in up to 50% of patients. Paracentesis, laparoscopy, or peritoneal biopsy is applicable only in patients with ascites. The peritoneal fluid is characterized by a protein concentration above 3 g/dL with less than 1.1 g/dL serum-ascitic fluid albumin difference and lymphocyte predominance among white blood cells. Definitive diagnosis is possible in 80% of cases by culture and direct smear. A PPD skin test is useful only when positive (about 80% of cases). Hematologic and biochemical studies are seldom helpful, and leukocytosis is uncommon. The sedimentation rate is elevated in many cases. The presence of high-density ascites or soft tissue masses on CT scan supports the diagnosis and may obviate operation.

Treatment

In chronic cases, nonoperative therapy is preferable if the diagnosis can be established. Most patients presenting with acute symptoms are diagnosed only by laparotomy. In the absence of intestinal obstruction or perforation, only a biopsy of a peritoneal or omental nodule should be taken. Obstruction due to constriction by a tuberculous lesion usually develops in the distal ileum and cecum, although multiple skip areas along the small bowel may exist. Localized short segments of diseased bowel are best treated by resection with primary anastomosis. Multiple strictured areas may be managed either by side-to-side bypass or a stricturoplasty of partially narrowed segments.

Combination antituberculosis chemotherapy should be started once the diagnosis is confirmed or considered likely. A favorable response is the rule, but isoniazid and rifampin must be continued for 18 months postoperatively.

Akhan O et al: Tuberculous peritonitis: Ultrasonic diagnosis. JCU J Clin Ultrasound 1990;18:711.

Akinoglu A et al: Tuberculous enteritis and peritonitis. Can J Surg 1988;31:55.

Haddad FS et al: Abdominal tuberculosis. Dis Colon Rectum 1987;30:724.

Jakubowski A et al: Clinical features of abdominal tuberculosis. J Infect Dis 1988;158:687.

Khoury GA et al: Tuberculosis of the peritoneal cavity. Br J Surg 1978;65:808.

Rosengart TK, Coppa GF: Abdominal mycobacterial infections in immunocompromised patients. Am J Surg 1990;159:125.

GRANULOMATOUS PERITONITIS

Pathophysiology

Talc (magnesium silicate), cornstarch glove lubricants, gauze fluffs, and cellulose fibers from disposable surgical fabrics may elicit a vigorous granulomatous (probably a delayed hypersensitivity) response in some patients 2–6 weeks after laparotomy. The condition became much less common after surgeons became aware of its cause and made a practice of wiping surgical gloves clean before handling abdominal viscera.

Clinical Findings

Besides abdominal pain, which is often out of proportion to the low-grade fever, there may be nausea and vomiting, ileus, and other systemic complaints. Abdominal tenderness is usually diffuse but mild. Free abdominal fluid, if detectable, should be tapped and inspected for the diagnostic Maltese cross pattern of starch particles.

Treatment

Reoperation achieves little and should be avoided if the diagnosis can be made. Most patients undergo reexploration because they present an erroneous impression of postoperative bowel obstruction or peritoneal sepsis. The diffuse hard, white granulomatous masses studding the peritoneum and omentum are easily mistaken for cancer or tuberculosis unless a biopsy specimen is taken to demonstrate foreign body granulomas.

If granulomatous peritonitis is suspected, the response to treatment with corticosteroids or other anti-inflammatory agents is often so dramatic as to be diagnostic in itself. After clinical improvement, intravenous methylprednisolone can be replaced by oral prednisone for 2–3 weeks. The disease is self-limited and does not predispose to late intestinal obstruction.

Sheikh KMA: Granulomatous reactions to surgical glove powders. Infect Surg 1985;4:733.

Tinker MA et al: Cellulose granulomas and their relationship to intestinal obstruction. Am J Surg 1977;133:134.

Tolbert TW, Brown JL: Surface powders on surgical gloves. Arch Surg 1980;115:729.

FEVER OF UNKNOWN ORIGIN

Fever of unknown origin is fever of 38.5 °C (100.6 °F) or higher lasting longer than 3 weeks, the cause of which remains unknown even after more than 1 week of in-hospital investigations. Malignant neoplasms, occult infections, and connective tissue disorders each account for about one-third of eventual diagnoses. Abdominal (especially liver) and pelvic abscesses account for one-third of infectious cases.

Clinical Findings

A. Symptoms and Signs: Systemic symptoms include malaise, chills, night sweats, weight loss, and vague abdominal or musculoskeletal discomfort. Specific signs are frequently absent but include hepatosplenomegaly, lymphadenopathy, and joint or skin abnormalities.

B. Laboratory Findings: An ESR greater than 100 mm/h along with thrombocytopenia strongly suggest tuberculosis, cancer, or connective tissue disease. The alkaline phosphatase is often raised in cases associated with hepatobiliary disease, lymphoma, and renal carcinoma.

The presence of hepatomegaly is an indication for liver biopsy. Bone marrow examination should be performed in most patients. Peritoneoscopy with biopsy under local anesthesia is worthwhile if superficial lesions are identified on scanning studies.

C. Imaging Studies: Basic x-rays include contrast studies of the alimentary and urinary tracts and liver-spleen scans. Ultrasonography, CT scans, and MRI scans can often uncover septic or inflammatory foci and malignant tumors that were previously undetected without laparotomy. Radionuclide scans, with gallium-67 preferred over indium-111-labeled leukocytes, have a low sensitivity (50–60%) but are more useful in the postoperative setting. These tests are associated with more false-negative errors in the presence of diffuse processes such as vasculitis or noncaseating granulomatous diseases.

D. Laparotomy: Exploratory laparotomy or laparoscopy is advisable if all investigations prove inconclusive, because it will disclose the cause in over two-thirds of cases, and the morbidity rate is low. Laparotomy is of more value if the fever is of long standing and objective findings of intra-abdominal disease are present. Because some patients have a protracted acute viral or hypersensitivity condition, a period of observation may be considered in those without obvious intra-abdominal disease. However, a therapeutic trial of aspirin, corticosteroids, or antibiotics without a firm diagnosis is seldom helpful and potentially hazardous.

At laparotomy, multiple biopsies and cultures of the liver, spleen, mesenteric and retroperitoneal lymph nodes, omental and mesenteric fat, muscle, and iliac crest should be taken. Lymphoproliferative neoplasms and obscure adenocarcinomas (biliary tree, pancreas, kidney) are the most common types of malignant disease associated with fever of unknown cause, and tuberculosis and hepatobiliary infection are the most common types of infectious disease. Among patients in whom exploration does not reveal a cause, fever resolves spontaneously in some cases or the cause becomes evident subsequently, most often in an extra-abdominal site.

Brusch JL et al: Fever of unknown origin. Med Clin North Am 1988;72:1247. Coon WW: Diagnostic celiotomy for fever of undetermined origin. Surg Gynecol Obstet 1983;157:467.

Greenall MJ et al: Laparotomy in the investigation of patients with pyrexia of unknown origin. Br J Surg 1983;70:356.

MacSweeney JE et al: Indium-labelled leucocyte scanning in pyrexia of unknown origin. Clin Radiol 1990;42:414.

Smith JW: Fever of undetermined origin: Not what it used to be. Am J Med Sci 1986;292:56.

ASCITES*

1. CHYLOUS ASCITES

The accumulation of free chyle in the peritoneal cavity is a rare form of ascites. Most patients are adults—many of them elderly women—with occult cancer, often a lymphoma or adenocarcinoma (of the pancreas or stomach), causing lymphatic obstruction. Chylous ascites resulting from external trauma or operative mishap (portosystemic decompression, abdominal aneurysmectomy and retroperitoneal lymphadenectomy procedures) has a more favorable prognosis. About 15% of cases occur in young children (usually < 1 year old) with congenital lymphatic anomalies.

Clinical Findings

The typical presentation is of abdominal distention and pain along with vague constitutional symptoms. Physical findings—besides ascites—include concomitant pleural effusion and peripheral edema. The combination of fever, night sweats, and lymphadenopathy should arouse suspicion of a lymphoma. The discovery of milky ascitic fluid on paracentesis suggests the correct diagnosis. Only a rough correlation exists between the gross appearance of the fluid and its triglyceride content (200 mg/dL, with a mean level of 1500 mg/dL). The fluid leukocyte count (mostly lymphocytes) averages $1000/\mu L$. Hypoalbuminemia, lymphocytopenia, and anemia are frequently present.

Conventional radiologic investigations, particularly CT scan of the abdomen, may be helpful. Lymph node biopsy, where applicable, and laparotomy have the highest diagnostic value.

Treatment

Treatment of spontaneous chylous ascites is largely supportive rather than operative. Symptomatic relief can be obtained by intermittent abdominal and pleural tapping. Repeated punctures seldom arrest the chylous leakage and are not without hazard. Dietary measures should begin with a low-fat diet supplemented by medium-chain triglycerides, the latter being transported via the portal rather than the lymphatic circulation. Two-thirds of pediatric cases resolve spontaneously on expectant management within a month or so as collaterals develop. If dietary measures fail, oral findings should be halted and total parenteral nutrition instituted. In adults, the most hopeful situation is if an underlying cancer (which is rarely amenable to curative resection) producing the chylous ascites regresses with chemotherapy or irradiation. Spontaneous improvement is the rule in posttraumatic cases.

*Cirrhotic ascites is discussed in Chapter 25.

Except for resectable congenital chylous cysts, surgery has little to offer. In refractory traumatic cases, intraoperative lymphangiography or perioperative injection of lipophilic dyes at times identifies a leaking site that can be plicated. At operation, the root of the small bowel mesentery around the superior mesenteric vessels should be carefully examined, as a discrete tear is more common at this site. Peritoneovenous shunting has been successful in some postoperative cases. Other surgical endeavors such as bowel resection and retroperitoneal dissection are uniformly futile.

Ablan CJ et al: Postoperative chylous ascites: Diagnosis and treatment. A series report and literature review. Arch Surg 1990;125:270.

Ohri SK et al: The management of postoperative chylous ascites: A case report and literature review. J Clin Gasteroenterol 1990;12:693.

2. MALIGNANT ASCITES

Ascites due to advanced cancer is a distressing complication that often necessitates in-hospital care. Peritoneal implants stimulate production of ascitic fluid while impeding its resorption by diaphragmatic lymphatics. Malignant ascites also occurs in the absence of free peritoneal tumor cells if there is advanced venous or lymphatic obstruction. A positive cytologic diagnosis is obtained in 60–90% of cases and supported by a high LDH (> 500 IU/L) or CEA content. DNA aneuploidy on flow cytometry analysis is confirmatory in cytology-negative cases.

Since this is often a preterminal condition, conservative management is preferred, with diuretics (especially spironolactone), paracentesis if warranted by the symptoms, and chemotherapy.

Peritoneovenous shunting (preferably with the Denver shunt) should be considered in symptomatic patients who have ascites refractory to conservative methods and an expected survival time of at least 2 months. Shunting is not effective for viscous or loculated ascites, heavily bloodstained ascites, or ascites with an unusually high cell count. The procedure is most suitable in patients with breast, gastric, or ovarian adenocarcinoma or cytology-negative ascites. Complications include shunt obstruction, disseminated intravascular coagulation, fluid overload, and sepsis. Surprisingly, dissemination of the tumor is rare. About half of the patients derive substantial benefits but few survive beyond 6 months.

Edney JA et al: Peritoneovenous shunts palliate malignant ascites. Am J Surg 1989;158:598.

Garrison RN et al: Malignant ascites: Clinical and experimental observations. Ann Surg 1986;203:644.

Greenway B, Johnson PJ, Williams R: Control of malignant ascites with spironolactone. Br J Surg 1982;69:441.

LeVeen HH et al: Coagulopathy post peritoneovenous shunt. Ann Surg 1987;205:305.

Smith DA et al: Peritoneovenous shunt (PVS) for malignant ascites. An analysis of outcome. Am Surg 1989;55:445.

Sonnenfeld T, Tyden G: Peritoneovenous shunts for malignant ascites. Acta Chir Scand 1986;152:117.

Souter RG, Tarin D, Kettlewell MG: Peritoneovenous shunts in the management of malignant ascites. Br J Surg 1983;70:478.

INTERNAL HERNIAS

Internal hernias occur in a large fossa, fovea, or foramen. The four major categories of internal hernias, all extremely rare, are paraduodenal hernias, hernias into the foramen of Winslow, mesenteric hernias, and omental hernias.

Clinical Findings

Internal hernias may produce chronic digestive complaints, including pain and acute or chronic intestinal obstruction. Most patients have chronic symptoms for years before the diagnosis is made. Plain films of the abdomen show a cluster of air-filled loops of bowel. The trapped bowel can be even better demonstrated on a small bowel series, provided that total obstruction is not present.

Treatment

One should attempt either to reduce the hernia without opening the sac or to open the anterior wall of the sac and divide any adhesions present. Great care should be taken not to injure major arteries or veins that may run in the margin of the sac orifice. The dilated bowel should be decompressed. Herniated bowel should be reduced by pressure from within and traction from without and the hernial defect then closed or the wall of the hernia area resected. Strangulated bowel requiring resection is encountered in about one-quarter of patients with mesenteric hernias and carries a 30% mortality risk.

Berardi RS: Paraduodenal hernias. Surg Gynecol Obstet 1981;152:99.

Brigham RA, d'Avis JC: Paraduodenal hernia. In: *Hernia,* 3rd ed. Nyhus LM, Condon RE (editors). Lippincott, 1989.

Janin Y et al: Mesenteric hernia. In: *Hernia,* 3rd ed. Nyhus LM, Condon RE (editors). Lippincott, 1989.

Turley K: Right paraduodenal hernia: A source of chronic abdominal pain in the adult. Arch Surg 1979;114:1072.

PERITONEAL ADHESIONS

Tissue ischemia, mechanical or thermal trauma, infection, and foreign body reaction predispose to adhesion formation. The peritoneal injury underlying these noxious stimuli evokes a serosanguineous inflammatory reaction that leads to fibrin deposition. Ordinarily, local plasminogen activators initiate lysis of the fibrin strands within 3 days of their formation. Metamorphosis of mesodermal cells regenerates a single layer of new mesothelium as early as 5 days after injury. Inadequate fibrinolysis due to reduced mesothelial plasminogen activator activity allows fibroblastic proliferation to produce fibrous adhesions. Adhesions are now the most prevalent cause of acute and recurrent small bowel obstruction (see Chapter 30) and a persistent bane of abdominal and especially pelvic surgery. However, adhesions may also provide useful vascular bridges that promote tissue healing, such as in ischemic areas of a bowel anastomosis.

Adhesions develop in two-thirds of patients after laparotomy, especially after extensive procedures, pelvic operations, or multiple abdominal operations. Spontaneous adhesions, presumably related to subclinical inflammation, are also found in one-quarter of patients on postmortem examination. Postoperative adhesions are most heavily distributed near the operative site. The omentum, small bowel, colon, and rectum (in descending order of frequency) are involved most often. Short obese female patients seem to have a greater tendency to form adhesions.

Prevention & Treatment

A. Operative Treatment: Precise operative technique with avoidance of serosal trauma will reduce but not eliminate adhesion formation. Ischemic tissue trauma caused by crushing, cautery, and mass ligation should be minimized. Reperitonealization of the pelvic floor under tension has been shown to promote rather than hinder adhesion formation. Indeed, well-vascularized peritoneal edges will resurface adjacent denuded areas with epithelium within 2 weeks. The use of an omental flap or synthetic absorbable or nonabsorbable material (eg, Goretex) appears useful after extensive pelvic dissections. Abdominal packs, moist or dry, should be used sparingly, because they produce abrasive serosal tears. Blood and foreign bodies alone induce only a slight peritoneal reaction, but this becomes extensive when there are accompanying serosal injuries. Precise hemostasis is vital, because unclotted blood in the peritoneal cavity acts as an additional source of fibrin, and platelets themselves stimulate serosal inflammation. Starch glove powder, lint gauze fluffs, and cellulose fibers from disposable drapes provoke a rigorous foreign body reaction, and care should be taken to prevent such contamination. The differences between similar types of nonreactive suture material are less critical than the manner in which they are employed: A large number of coarse sutures creates more adhesions than well-placed finer sutures. Laparoscopic procedures tend to produce fewer adhesions than laparotomy.

B. Prevention: Prophylactic measures to minimize adhesions aim to lessen the intensity of the inflammatory response, reduce coagulability, and prevent prolonged contact between apposing surfaces. These should be considered in radical pelvic operations and when reoperating for recurrent adhesive obstruction. Dexamethasone combined with promethazine has deleterious side effects that may outweigh its alleged usefulness. Nonsteroidal anti-inflammatory drugs, such as colchicine and ibuprofen, have been used with inconsistent results. Prostacyclin, found in high concentrations in the peritoneum, inhibits platelet aggregation and may eventually have therapeutic applications. Intraperitoneal irrigation with the glucose polymer dextran 70 (Hyskon) reduced adhesion formation in some studies. Its action is based upon hydroflotation and siliconizing effects that separate raw serosal surfaces. It is not suitable in potentially septic conditions because it reduces peritoneal lymphocyte and macrophage activity. A prospective trial failed to show any advantage of steroids, promethazine, heparin, or Hyskon over peritoneal irrigation with lactated Ringer's solution in preventing adhesion formation after primary pelvic surgery. Encouraging experimental reports may lead to the clinical application of recombinant tissue plasminogen activator, calcium-channel blockers (eg, verapamil), and prokinetic agents (eg, cisapride).

Adhesion Study Group: Reduction of postoperative pelvic adhesions with intraperitoneal 32% dextran 70: A prospective, randomized clinical trial. Fertil Steril 1983; 40:612.

Breland U, Bengmark S: Peritoneum and adhesion formation. In: The Peritoneum and Peritoneal Access. Bengmark S (editor). Wright, 1989.

Fayez JA et al: Prevention of pelvic adhesion formation by different modalities of treatment. Am J Obstet Gynecol 1987;157:1184.

Sparnon AL, Spitz L: Pharmacological manipulation of postoperative intestinal adhesions. Aust N Z J Surg 1989;59:725.

Steinleitner A et al: Reduction of primary postoperative adhesion formation under calcium channel blockade in the rabbit. J Surg Res 1990;48:42.

Thompson JN et al: Reduced human peritoneal plasminogen activating activity: Possible mechanism of adhesion formation. Br J Surg 1989;76:382.

TUMORS OF THE PERITONEUM & RETROPERITONEUM

Most tumors affecting the peritoneum are secondary implants from primary intraperitoneal cancers. Some unusual peritoneal and retroperitoneal lesions present with abdominal masses or ascites that may be confused with carcinomatosis or chronic inflammatory peritonitis.

Peritoneal Mesothelioma

These rare primary neoplasms are derived from the mesodermal lining of the peritoneum. The malignant variety develops most commonly in men, with a long latent period (averaging 40 years) after prolonged asbestos exposure. Pleural malignant mesotheliomas outnumber peritoneal ones by a ratio of 3:1. Patients present typically with weight loss, crampy abdominal pain, a large mass or distention due to ascites, and a history of asbestos contact. Fewer than half of these patients have asbestosis demonstrated on plain chest films. In contrast to peritoneal carcinomatosis, mesotheliomas are associated with less ascites than the degree of abdominal distention would suggest, and cytologic studies of ascitic fluid are rarely positive. CT scan of the lower thorax and abdomen will demonstrate ascites, peritoneal and mesenteric thickening, pleural plaques, and soft tissue masses involving the omentum and peritoneum. Multiple fine-needle aspiration biopsies guided by ultrasonography, CT scan, or laparoscopy can establish the diagnosis. Electron microscopy is confirmatory in equivocal cases.

Patients usually undergo laparotomy either for diagnosis or because of bowel obstruction. Localized masses should be resected to avoid subsequent obstruction. Metastases to the liver and lung occur late. Long-term survivors (beyond 1 year) have been reported with combined treatment by surgical debulking, intraperitoneal cisplatin-doxorubicin, and whole-abdomen irradiation. One should differentiate malignant mesotheliomas from cystic mesotheliomas and well-differentiated papillary mesotheliomas in women, which are less malignant and carry an excellent prognosis even though they tend to recur locally.

Asensio JA et al: Primary malignant peritoneal mesothelioma: A report of seven cases and a review of the literature. Arch Surg 1990;125:1477.

Daya D, McCaughey WTE: Well-differentiated papillary mesothelioma: A clinicopathologic study of 22 cases. Cancer 1990;65:292.

Katsube Y et al: Cystic mesothelioma of the peritoneum: A report of five cases and review of the literature. Cancer 1982;50:1615.

Lederman GS et al: Long-term survival in peritoneal mesothelioma: The role of radiotherapy and combined modality treatment. Cancer 1987;59:1882.

Plaus WJ: Peritoneal mesothelioma. Arch Surg 1988; 123:763.

Pseudomyxoma Peritonei

This unusual disease is caused by a mucinous cystadenocarcinoma of the ovary or appendix that secretes large amounts of mucus-containing epithelial cells. It should be distinguished from benign appendiceal mucocele, which may also have local mucinous deposits but carries a favorable outlook. Patients seldom complain until advanced stages of disease, at which time they have abdominal distention and pain and, in many instances, intermittent or chronic partial small bowel obstruction. Weight loss and other features of cancer are uncommon. The neoplastic cells spread freely on serosal surfaces, but they rarely metastasize elsewhere or invade visceral structures. Ultrasonography and CT scans show a distinctive peritoneal scalloping of the liver margin, calcified plaques, ascites, and low-density masses.

Preoperative mucolysis with intraperitoneal 5% dextrose has been successful occasionally. At laparotomy, the surgeon should remove as much of the primary lesion and gelatinous material as possible. The omentum also should be resected and existing or impending bowel obstruction relieved. This often necessitates right hemicolectomy. If there is no apparent primary tumor, the appendix and, in women, both ovaries should be removed.

Postoperative chemotherapy is reasonably effective, particularly for ovarian carcinomas. Reexploration should be undertaken either as a planned second-look laparotomy or to debulk residual tumor responsible for recurrent obstruction or debilitating mucous ascites. Prolonged survival has been achieved by radical surgical debulking of tumor combined with intraperitoneal fluorouracil and intravenous mitomycin C. Intraperitoneal cisplatin and other chemotherapeutic agents have been used with only minimal benefit. Radiotherapy to the abdomen with a pelvic boost should be given in cases unresponsive to chemotherapy. Two-thirds of patients eventually succumb to local or regional disease. The survival rate is about 50% at 5 years and 20% at 10 years.

Lee HH: Pseudomyxoma peritonei: radiologic features. J Clin Gastroenterol 1986;8:312.

Mann WJ Jr et al: The management of pseudomyxoma peritonei. Cancer 1990;66:1636.

Sugarbaker PH et al: Malignant pseudomyxoma peritonei of colonic origin: Natural history and presentation of a curative approach to treatment. Dis Colon Rectum 1987; 30:772.

Cysts of the Mesentery & Retroperitoneum

These rare developmental lesions are usually ectopic pockets of lymphatic tissue or, more rarely, mucinous ovarian cystadenomas. Patients present with an asymptomatic abdominal mass, chronic pain, or acute abdomen. The mass is often large, smooth, round, compressible, and more mobile transversely than longitudinally. CT or ultrasonographic scans along with contrast studies of the gastrointestinal and urinary tracts reveal the cystic nature and location of the mass. The differential diagnosis includes pancreatic pseudocysts, enteric duplication (in children), inflammatory cysts, and retroperitoneal tumors. Laparotomy reveals the cyst, which contains serous fluid if it is in the mesocolon; chylous fluid if it is in the small bowel mesentery; or blood-stained fluid. Most lesions are benign, and enucleation suffices. Segmental resection may be necessary for cysts that impinge upon the bowel wall or its blood supply. Recurrences are more frequent with retroperitoneal cysts, because they may not be amenable to complete excision, and marsupialization may be required instead.

Kurtz RJ et al: Mesenteric and retroperitoneal cysts. Ann Surg 1986;203:109.

Rod PR et al: Mesenteric and retroperitoneal cysts: Histologic classification with imaging correlation. Radiology 1987;164:327.

Takiff H et al: Mesenteric cysts and intra-abdominal cystic lymphangiomas. Arch Surg 1985;120:1266.

Vane VW, Phillips AK: Retroperitoneal, mesenteric, and omental cysts. Arch Surg 1984;119:838.

Retroperitoneal Tumors

Retroperitoneal tumors include lymphomas as well as sarcomatous derivatives composed of mesodermal tissue (eg, liposarcoma, leiomyosarcoma, fibrosarcoma), nervous tissue (eg, schwannoma, neuroblastoma), and embryonic remnant (eg, malignant teratoma, chordoma). In addition to nonspecific abdominal pain, weight loss, and fever, a palpable mass is present in most cases. Contrast-enhanced CT and MRI imaging are the best diagnostic studies. Intravenous urography, angiography, venacavography, and myelography are performed as needed. Although transperitoneal fine-needle biopsy under ultrasound guidance can establish the correct diagnosis preoperatively, an open biopsy is preferred whenever a retroperitoneal sarcoma is suspected.

Complete surgical resection with en bloc removal of affected contiguous structures provides the best chance of cure. Vascular spread to the lungs, bones and liver occurs in more than half of patients. Local recurrence occurs in up to 90% of cases even after complete resections and is the primary cause of death. Postoperative irradiation and doxorubicin-based chemotherapy have been utilized with only slight benefit. Nevertheless, cytoreductive surgery is beneficial, and even local recurrences should be subjected to repeat resections. Tumor grade is the single most important prognostic factor. The overall 5-year survival rate of about 30% has been increased to over 50% with systematic radical resection.

Bevilacque RG et al: Prognostic factors in primary retroperitoneal soft-tissue sarcomas. Arch Surg 1991;126:328.

Jaques DP et al: Management of primary and recurrent soft-tissue sarcoma of the retroperitoneum. Ann Surg 1990; 212:51.

Kinsella TJ et al: Preliminary results of a randomized study of adjuvant radiation therapy in resectable adult retroperitoneal soft tissue sarcomas. J Clin Oncol 1988;6:18.

Sondak VK et al: Soft tissue sarcomas of the extremity and retroperitoneum: advances in management. Adv Surg 1991;24:333.

Storm FK, Mahvi DM: Diagnosis and management of retroperitoneal soft-tissue sarcoma. Ann Surg 1991;214:2.

Mesenteric Lipodystrophy (Mesenteric Panniculitis)

There are fewer than 200 reported cases of mesenteric lipodystrophy, in which chronic fat degeneration and fibrosis affecting the root of the mesentery produce diffuse mesenteric thickening or masses. Its cause is unknown, but it may be a localized form of Weber-Christian disease.

The patient, often an elderly man, has recurrent abdominal pain, weight loss, or symptoms of partial intestinal obstruction. A hard irregular abdominal mass, usually in the left upper quadrant, is felt in over half of patients. CT or ultrasound examination and barium follow-up studies can outline the lesion. CT scanning shows the characteristic features of nonhomogeneous masses of fat and soft tissue density. MRI may suggest the fibrous nature of the lesion and delineates vascular involvement. The diagnosis is usually made only by biopsy at laparotomy, but resection is neither feasible nor indicated. An occasional patient will require a side-to-side intestinal bypass to relieve obstruction.

The process subsides spontaneously in most cases. A more serious variant (**retractile mesenteritis**) associated with obstruction of the mesenteric lymphatics and veins often proves fatal. Corticosteroids, cyclophosphamide, and azathioprine should be reserved for such cases and for patients with clinical deterioration. Lymphoma occurs in 15% of cases on follow-up.

Bush RW et al: Sclerosing mesenteritis: response to cyclophosphamide. Arch Intern Med 1986;146:503.

Durst AL et al: Mesenteric panniculitis: A review of the literature and presentation of cases. Surgery 1977;81:203.

Kronthal AJ et al: MRI imaging in sclerosing mesenteritis. AJR Am J Roentgenol 1991;156:517.

Wexner SE, Attiyeh FF: Mesenteric panniculitis to the sigmoid colon. Dis Colon Rectum 1987;30:812.

RETROPERITONEAL FIBROSIS

This uncommon entity is characterized by extensive fibrotic encasement of retroperitoneal tissues. Over two-thirds of cases are idiopathic and the rest secondary to drugs (eg, methysergide, beta-adrenergic blocking agents), retroperitoneal hemorrhage, perianeurysmal inflammation, irradiation, urinary extravasation, or cancer. The fibrosis represents an allergic reaction to insoluble lipid (ceroid) that has leaked from atheromatous plaques, especially those within the aorta. The urinary tract may be involved with a diagnostic triad of hydronephrosis and hydroureter (usually bilateral), medial deviation of the ureters, and extrinsic ureteric compression near the L4–5 level. Desmoplastic involvement of the small and large bowel may give rise to obstructive symptoms. Most patients are men over age 50 who present with renal failure or obstructive uropathy. Pain in the low back or flank is common. Pyuria is present in most patients. The diagnosis is suggested by a CT scan that shows the fibrotic process and any coexisting aneurysmal changes in the aorta. MRI may distinguish fibrosis from lymphoma or metastatic carcinoma. Withdrawal of suspect drugs is usually followed by gradual improvement.

Severe urinary obstruction should be decompressed by ureteric stents or nephrostomy. Prednisone (30–60 mg daily) and immunosuppression have been tried but with inconclusive benefits. These agents should be started early postoperatively before marked fibrosis develops. If surgery becomes necessary, a thick rubbery or fibrotic plaque containing chronic inflammatory cells is found at exploration. Multiple biopsy specimens should be taken to exclude cancer. Ureterolysis should be attempted, and there may be some advantage to wrapping omentum around the freed ureters to reduce the risk of subsequent entrapment. The outlook is good as long as there is no underlying cancer.

Brooks AP et al: Magnetic resonance imaging in idiopathic retroperitoneal fibrosis: Measurement of T1 relaxation time. Br J Radiol 1990;63:842.

Bullock N: Idiopathic retroperitoneal fibrosis. Br Med J 1988;297:240.

Carini M et al: Surgical treatment of retroperitoneal fibrosis with omentoplasty. Surgery 1982;91:137.

Cerfolio RJ et al: Idiopathic retroperitoneal fibrosis: Is there a role for postoperative steroids? Curr Surg 1990;47:423.

Higgins PH et al: Non-operative management of retroperitoneal fibrosis. Br J Surg 1988;75:573. McDougal WS et al: Treatment of idiopathic retroperitoneal fibrosis by immunosuppression. J Urol 1991;145:112.

Mitchinson MJ: Retroperitoneal fibrosis revisited. Arch Pathol Lab Med 1986;110:784.

DISORDERS INVOLVING THE OMENTUM

Infection

The omentum plays an important role in protecting against spreading peritonitis. In chronic infections such as tuberculosis, it may become infected and appear as a rolled-up thickened, inflamed mass. Nonspecific inflammation of the omentum, often a sequela of previous torsion, causes vague abdominal pain.

Torsion & Infarction

Primary (spontaneous) torsion of the omentum may develop if a free portion is fixed by an adhesion or trapped within a hernia. Rotation around the pedicle occludes the blood supply and leads to ischemic necrosis. Infarction may also be secondary to abdominal trauma or vascular conditions such as polyarteritis nodosa. Paraesophageal omental herniation may predispose to a hiatal hernia and may mimic a mediastinal lipoma.

Clinically, torsion presents as acute abdominal pain with nausea and vomiting. Tenderness is confined to the involved area, usually on the right side but away from McBurney's point. A mobile, tender mass is noted in one-third of cases. These features may suggest acute appendicitis or cholecystitis but are not typical of those diseases. The clinical findings usually mandate surgical exploration, which reveals serosanguineous fluid, a normal appendix, and the hemorrhagic necrotic segment of omentum. Resection of the affected portion is curative.

Adams JT: Primary torsion of the omentum. Am J Surg 1973;126:102.
Crofoot DD: Spontaneous segmental infarction of the greater omentum. Am J Surg 1980;139:262.

Tumors & Cysts of the Omentum

The omentum is frequently involved secondarily by intra-abdominal malignant tumors, especially gastrointestinal and ovarian adenocarcinomas. Primary cysts or vascular anomalies, usually incidentally discovered at laparotomy, are readily resected.

Lee MJ et al: CT and MRI findings in paraoesophageal omental herniation. Clin Radiol 1990;42:207.
Molander ML et al: Omental and mesenteric cysts in children. Acta Paediatr Scand 1982;71:227.

Stomach & Duodenum

Lawrence W. Way, MD

I. STOMACH

The stomach receives food from the esophagus and has four functions: (1) It acts as a reservoir that permits eating reasonably large quantities of food at intervals of several hours. (2) Food contained in the stomach is mixed, triturated, and delivered into the duodenum in amounts regulated by its chemical nature and texture. (3) The first stages of protein and carbohydrate digestion are carried out in the stomach. (4) A few substances are absorbed across the gastric mucosa.

ANATOMY
(Figures 23–1, 23–2, 23–3)

The **cardia** is located at the gastroesophageal junction. The **fundus** is the portion of the stomach that lies cephalad to the gastroesophageal junction. The **corpus** is the capacious central part; division of the corpus from the pyloric antrum is marked approximately by the angular incisure, a crease on the lesser curvature just proximal to the "crow's-foot" terminations of the nerves of Latarjet (Figure 23–3). The **pylorus** is the boundary between the stomach and the duodenum.

The **cardiac gland area** is the small segment located at the gastroesophageal junction. Histologically, it contains principally mucus-secreting cells, though a few parietal cells are sometimes present. The **oxyntic gland area** is the portion containing parietal (oxyntic) cells and chief cells (Figure 23–2). The boundary between this region and the adjacent pyloric gland area is reasonably sharp, since the zone of transition spans a segment of only 1–1.5 cm. The **pyloric gland** area constitutes the distal 30% of the stomach and contains the G cells that manufacture gastrin. Mucous cells are common in the oxyntic and pyloric gland areas.

As in the rest of the gastrointestinal tract, the muscular wall of the stomach is composed of an outer longitudinal and an inner circular layer. An additional incomplete inner layer of obliquely situated fibers is most prominent near the lesser curvature but is of less substance than the other two layers.

Blood Supply

The blood supply of the stomach and duodenum is illustrated in Figure 23–3. The left gastric artery supplies the lesser curvature and connects with the right gastric artery, a branch of the common hepatic artery. In 60% of persons, a posterior gastric artery arises off the middle third of the splenic artery and terminates in branches on the posterior surface of the body and the fundus. The greater curvature is supplied by the right gastroepiploic artery (a branch of the gastroduodenal artery) and the left gastroepiploic artery (a branch of the splenic artery). The mid portion of the greater curvature corresponds to a point at which the gastric branches of this vascular arcade change direction. The fundus of the stomach along the greater curvature is supplied by the vasa brevia, branches of the splenic and left gastroepiploic arteries.

The blood supply to the duodenum is from the superior and inferior pancreaticoduodenal arteries, which are branches of the gastroduodenal artery and the superior mesenteric artery, respectively. The stomach contains a rich submucosal vascular plexus. Venous blood from the stomach drains into the coronary, gastroepiploic, and splenic veins before entering the portal vein. The lymphatic drainage of the stomach, which largely parallels the arteries, partially determines the direction of spread of gastric neoplasms.

Nerve Supply

The parasympathetic nerves to the stomach are shown in Figure 23–3. As a rule, two major vagal trunks pass through the esophageal hiatus in close approximation to the esophageal muscle. The nerves are originally located to the right and left of the esophagus and stomach during embryonic development. When the foregut rotates, the lesser curvature turns to the right and the greater curvature to the left, and corresponding shifts in location of the vagal trunks follow. Hence, the right vagus supplies the posterior and the left the anterior gastric surface. About 90% of the vagal fibers are sensory afferent; the remaining 10% are efferent.

In the region of the gastroesophageal junction,

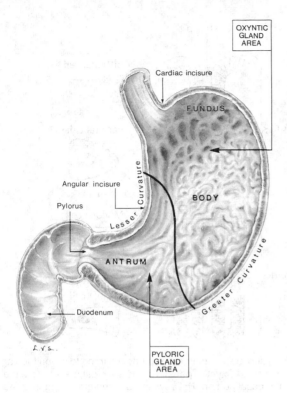

Figure 23–1. Names of the parts of the stomach. The line drawn from the lesser to the greater curvature depicts the approximate boundary between the oxyntic gland area and the pyloric gland area. No prominent landmark exists to distinguish between antrum and body (corpus). The fundus is the portion craniad to the esophagogastric junction.

each trunk bifurcates. The anterior trunk sends to the liver a division that travels in the lesser omentum. The bifurcation of the posterior trunk gives rise to fibers that enter the celiac plexus and supply the parasympathetic innervation to the remainder of the gastrointestinal tract as far as the mid transverse colon. Both trunks, after giving rise to their extragastric divisions, send some fibers directly onto the surface of the stomach and others along the lesser curvature (anterior and posterior nerves of Latarjet) to supply the distal part of the organ. As shown in Figure 23–3, a variable number of vagal fibers ascend with the left gastric artery after having passed through the celiac plexus.

The preganglionic motor fibers of the vagal trunks synapse with ganglion cells in Auerbach's plexus (plexus myentericus) between the longitudinal and circular muscle layers. Postganglionic cholinergic fibers are distributed to the cells of the smooth muscle layers and the mucosa.

The adrenergic innervation to the stomach consists of postganglionic fibers that pass along the arterial vessels from the celiac plexus.

PHYSIOLOGY

Motility

Storage, mixing, trituration, and regulated emptying are accomplished by the muscular apparatus of the stomach. Peristaltic waves originate in the body and pass toward the pylorus. The thickness of the smooth muscle increases in the antrum and corresponds to the stronger contractions that can be measured in the distal stomach. The pylorus behaves as a sphincter, though it normally allows a little to-and-fro movement of chyme across the junction.

An electrical pacemaker situated in the fundal musculature near the greater curvature gives rise to regular (3/min) electrical impulses (pacesetter potential, basic electrical rhythm) that pass toward the pylorus in the outer longitudinal layer. Every impulse is not always followed by a peristaltic muscular contraction, but the impulses determine the maximal peristaltic rate. The frequency of peristalsis is governed by a variety of stimuli mentioned below. Each contraction follows sequential depolarization of the underlying circular muscle resulting from arrival of the pacesetter potential.

Peristaltic contractions are more forceful in the antrum than the body and travel faster as they progress distally. Gastric chyme is forced into the funnel-shaped antral chamber by peristalsis; the volume of contents delivered into the duodenum by each peristaltic wave depends on the strength of the advancing wave and the extent to which the pylorus closes. Most of the gastric contents that are pushed into the antral funnel are propelled backward as the pylorus closes and pressure within the antral lumen rises. Five to 15 mL enter the duodenum with each gastric peristaltic wave.

The volume of the empty gastric lumen is only 50 mL. By a process called receptive relaxation, the stomach can accommodate about 1000 mL before intraluminal pressure begins to rise. Receptive relaxation is an active process mediated by vagal reflexes and abolished by vagotomy. Peristalsis is initiated by the stimulus of distention after eating. Various other factors have positive or negative influences on the rate and strength of contractions and the rate of gastric emptying. Vagal reflexes from the stomach have a facilitating influence on peristalsis. The texture and volume of the meal both play a role in the regulation of emptying; small particles are emptied more rapidly than large ones, which the organ attempts to reduce in size (trituration). The osmolality of gastric chyme and its chemical makeup are monitored by duodenal receptors. If osmolality is greater than 200 mosm/L, a long vagal reflex (the enterogastric reflex) is activated, delaying emptying. Gastrin causes delay in emptying. Gastrin is the only circulating gastrointestinal hormone to have a physiologic effect on emptying.

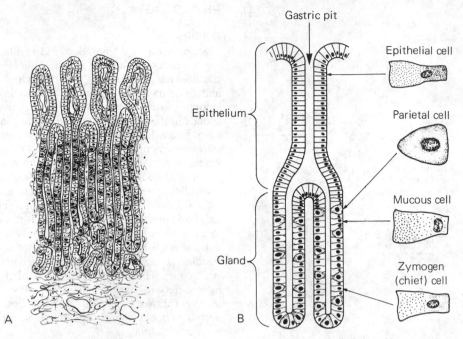

Figure 23–2. Histologic features of the mucosa in the oxyntic gland area. Each gastric pit drains three to seven tubular gastric glands. **A:** The neck of the gland contains many mucous cells. Oxyntic (parietal) cells are most numerous in the mid portion of the glands; peptic (chief) cells predominate in the basal portion. **B:** Drawing from photomicrograph of the gastric mucosa.

Gastric Juice

The output of gastric juice in a fasting subject varies between 500 and 1500 mL/d. After each meal, about 1000 mL are secreted by the stomach.

The components of gastric juice are as follows:

A. Mucus: Mucus is a heterogeneous mixture of glycoproteins manufactured in the mucous cells of the oxyntic and pyloric gland areas. Mucus provides a weak barrier to the diffusion of H^+ and probably protects the mucosa. It also acts as a lubricant and impedes diffusion of pepsin.

B. Pepsinogen: Pepsinogens are synthesized in the chief cells of the oxyntic gland area (and to a lesser extent in the pyloric area) and are stored as visible granules. Cholinergic stimuli, either vagal or intramural, are the most potent pepsigogues, though gastrin and secretin are also effective. The precursor zymogen is activated when pH falls below 5.00, a process that entails severance of a polypeptide fragment from the larger molecule. Pepsin cleaves peptide bonds, especially those containing phenylalanine, tyrosine, or leucine. Its optimal pH is about 2.00. Pepsin activity is abolished at pH greater than 5.00, and the molecule is irreversibly denatured at pH greater than 8.00.

C. Intrinsic Factor: Intrinsic factor, a mucoprotein secreted by the parietal cells, binds with vitamin B_{12} of dietary origin and greatly enhances absorption of the vitamin. Absorption occurs by an active process in the terminal ileum.

Intrinsic factor secretion is enhanced by stimuli that evoke H^+ output from parietal cells. Pernicious anemia is characterized by atrophy of the parietal cell mucosa, deficiency in intrinsic factor, and anemia. Subclinical deficiencies in vitamin B_{12} have been described after operations that reduce gastric acid secretion, and abnormal Schilling tests in these patients can be corrected by the administration of intrinsic factor. Total gastrectomy creates a dependence on parenteral administration of vitamin B_{12}.

D. Blood Group Substances: Seventy-five percent of people secrete blood group antigens into gastric juice. The trait is genetically determined and is associated with a lower incidence of duodenal ulcer than in nonsecretors.

E. Electrolytes: The unique characteristic of gastric secretion is its high concentration of hydrochloric acid, a product of the parietal cells. As the concentration of H^+ rises during secretion, that of Na^+ drops in a reciprocal fashion. K^+ remains relatively constant at 5–10 meq/L. Chloride concentration remains near 150 meq/L, and gastric juice maintains its isotonicity at varying secretory rates.

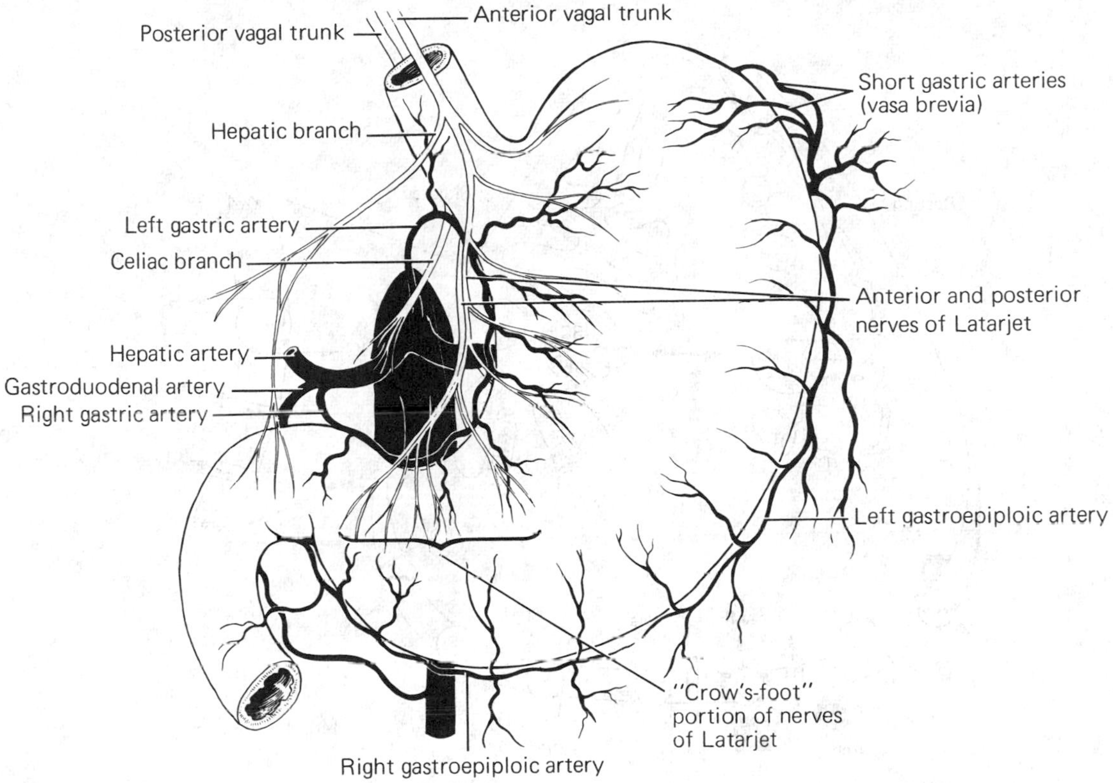

Figure 23–3. Blood supply and parasympathetic innervation of the stomach and duodenum.

The Parietal Cell & Acid Secretion

Many of the key events in acid secretion by gastric parietal cells are illustrated in Figure 23–4. The onset of secretion is accompanied by striking morphologic changes in the apical membranes. Resting parietal cells are characterized by an infolding of the apical membrane, called the secretory canaliculus, which is lined by short microvilli. Multiple membrane-bound tubulovesicles and mitochondria are present in the cytoplasm. With stimulation, the secretory canaliculus expands, the microvilli become long and narrow and filled with microfilaments, and the cytoplasmic tubulovesicles disappear. The proton pump mechanism for acid secretion is located in the tubulovesicles in the resting state and in the secretory canaliculus in the stimulated state.

The basal lateral membrane contains the receptors for secretory stimulants and transfers HCO_3^- out of the cell to balance the H^+ output at the apical membrane. Active uptake of Cl^- and K^+ conduction also occur at the basal lateral membrane. Separate membrane-bound receptors exist for histamine (H_2 receptor), gastrin, and acetylcholine. The intracellular second messengers are thought to be cAMP for histamine and Ca^{2+} for gastrin and acetylcholine.

Acid secretion at the apical membrane is accomplished by a membrane-bound H^+/K^+-ATPase (the proton pump); H^+ is secreted into the lumen in exchange for K^+.

Mucosal Resistance in the Stomach & Duodenum

The healthy mucosa of the stomach and duodenum is provided with mechanisms that allow it to withstand the potentially injurious effects of high concentrations of luminal acid. Disruption of these mechanisms may contribute to acute or chronic ulceration.

The surface of the gastric mucosa is coated with mucus and secretes HCO_3^- in addition to H^+. Protected by the blanket of mucus, the surface pH is much higher than the luminal pH. HCO_3^- secretion is stimulated by cAMP, prostaglandins, cholinomimetics, glucagon, CCK, and by as yet unidentified paracrine hormones. Inhibitors of HCO_3^- secretion include nonsteroidal anti-inflammatory agents, alpha-adrenergic agonists, bile acids, ethanol, and acetazolamide. Increases in luminal H^+ result in increased HCO_3^- secretion, probably mediated by tissue prostaglandins.

Gastric mucus is a gel composed of high-molecular-weight glycoproteins and 95% water. Since it forms an unstirred layer, it helps the underlying mucosa to maintain a higher pH than that of gastric juice,

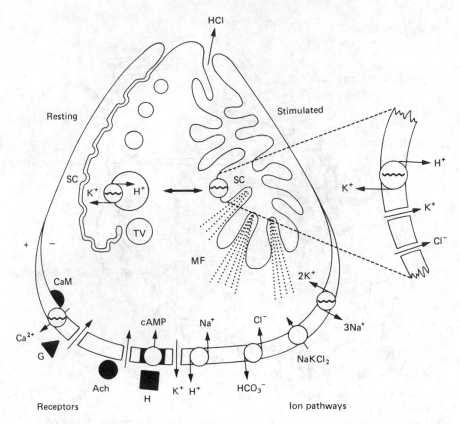

Figure 23–4. Diagram of a parietal cell, showing the receptor systems and ion pathways in the basal lateral membrane and the apical membrane transition from a resting to a stimulated state. Ach, acetylcholine; CaM, calmodulin; G, gastrin; H, histamine; MF, microfilaments; SC, secretory canaliculus; TV, tubulovesicles. (Redrawn and reproduced, with permission, from Malinowska DH, Sachs G: Cellular mechanisms of acid secretion. Clin Gastroenterol 1984;13:309.)

and it also acts as a barrier to the diffusion of pepsin. At the surface of the layer of mucus, peptic digestion continuously degrades mucus, while below it is continuously being replenished by mucous cells. Gastric acid is thought to enter the lumen through thin spots in the mucus overlying the gastric glands. Secretion of mucus is stimulated by luminal acid and perhaps by cholinergic stimuli. The layer of mucus is damaged by exposure to nonsteroidal anti-inflammatory agents and is enhanced by topical prostaglandin E_2.

Mucosal defects produced by mechanical or chemical trauma are rapidly repaired by adjacent normal cells that spread to cover the defect, a process that can be enhanced experimentally by adding HCO_3^- to the nutrient side of the mucosa. This important phenomenon has not yet been thoroughly studied.

The duodenal mucosa possesses defenses similar to those in the stomach: the ability to secrete HCO_3^- and mucus and rapid repair of mucosal injuries.

Regulation of Acid Secretion

The regulation of acid secretion can best be described by considering separately those factors that

enhance gastric acid production and those that depress it. The interaction of these forces is what determines the levels of secretion observed during fasting and after meals.

A. Stimulation of Acid Secretion: Acid production is usually described as the result of three phases that are excited simultaneously after a meal. The separation into phases is of value principally for descriptive purposes.

1. Cephalic phase–Stimuli that act upon the brain lead to increased vagal efferent activity and acid secretion. The sight, smell, taste, or even thought of appetizing food may elicit this response. The effect is entirely vagally mediated and is abolished by vagotomy. The vagal stimuli have a direct effect on the parietal cells to increase acid output.

2. Gastric phase–Food in the stomach (principally protein hydrolysates and hydrophobic amino acids) stimulates gastrin release from the antrum. Gastric distention has a similar but less intense effect.

The presence of food in the stomach excites long vagal reflexes, impulses that pass to the central nervous system via vagal afferents and return to stimulate the parietal cells.

A third aspect of the gastric phase involves the sensitizing effect of distention of the parietal cell area to gastrin that is probably mediated through local intramural cholinergic reflexes.

3. Intestinal phase–The role of the intestinal phase in the stimulation of gastric secretion has been incompletely investigated. Various experiments have shown that the presence of food in the small bowel releases a humoral factor, named entero-oxyntin, that evokes acid secretion from the stomach.

B. Inhibition of Acid Secretion: Without systems to limit secretion, unchecked acid production could become a serious clinical problem. Examples can be found (eg, Billroth II gastrectomy with retained antrum) where acid production rose after surgical procedures that interfered with these inhibitory mechanisms.

1. Antral inhibition–pH below 2.50 in the antrum inhibits the release of gastrin regardless of the stimulus. When the pH reaches 1.20, gastrin release is almost completely blocked. If the normal relationship of parietal cell mucosa to antral mucosa is changed so that acid does not flow past the site of gastrin production, serum gastrin may increase to high levels, with marked acid stimulation. Somatostatin in gastric antral cells serves a physiologic role as an inhibitor of gastrin release (a paracrine function).

2. Intestinal inhibition–The intestine participates in controlling acid secretion by liberating hormones that inhibit both the release of gastrin and its effects on the parietal cells. Secretin blocks acid secretion under experimental conditions but not as a physiologic action. Fat in the intestine is the most potent method of inhibition, affecting gastrin release and acid secretion. Neither somatostatin nor GIP, both released by food in the intestine, seems able to account for the inhibition, and the term enterogastrone is used to denote the still unidentified hormone presumably responsible.

Integration of Gastric Physiologic Function

Ingested food is mixed with salivary amylase before it reaches the stomach. The mechanisms stimulating gastric secretion are activated. Serum gastrin levels increase from a mean fasting concentration of about 50 pg/mL to 200 pg/mL, the peak occurring about 30 minutes after the meal. Food in the lumen of the stomach is exposed to high concentrations of acid and pepsin at the mucosal surface. Food settles in layers determined by sequence of arrival, but fat tends to float to the top. The greatest mixing occurs in the antrum. Antral contents therefore become more uniformly acidic than those in the body of the organ, where the central portion of the meal tends to remain

alkaline for a considerable time, allowing continued activity of the amylase.

Peptic digestion of protein in the stomach is only about 5–10% complete. Carbohydrate digestion may reach 30–40%. A lipase originating from the tongue initiates the first stages of lipolysis in the stomach.

The gastric contents are delivered to the duodenum at a rate determined by the volume and texture of the meal, its osmolality and acidity, and its content of fat. A meal of lean meat, potatoes, and vegetables leaves the stomach within 3 hours. A meal with a very high fat content may remain in the stomach for 6–12 hours.

Debas HT, Mulvihill SJ: Neuroendocrine design of the gut. Am J Surg 1991;161:243.
Thompson JC: Humoral control of gut function. Am J Surg 1991;161:6.
Walsh JH: Gastrin: A normal and pathologic regulator of gastric function. West J Med 1991;154:33.

PEPTIC ULCER

Peptic ulcers result from the corrosive action of acid gastric juice on a vulnerable epithelium. Depending on circumstances, they may occur in the esophagus, the duodenum, the stomach itself, the jejunum after surgical construction of a gastrojejunostomy, or the ileum in relation to ectopic gastric mucosa in Meckel's diverticulum. When the term peptic ulcer was first used, it was thought that the most important factor was the peptic activity in gastric juice. Since then, evidence has implicated acid as the chief injurious agent; in fact, it is axiomatic that if gastric juice contains no acid, a (benign) peptic ulcer cannot be present. Appreciation of the role of acid has led to the emphasis on therapy with antacids and H_2 blocking agents for the medical therapy of ulcers and to operations that reduce acid secretion as the major surgical approach. In the case of duodenal and gastric ulcers, *Helicobacter pylori* must colonize and weaken the mucosa before acid is able to do the damage, and therapy directed against this organism has a more definitive effect on the disease.

It has been estimated that about 2% of the adult population in the USA suffers from active peptic ulcer disease, and about 10% of the population will have the disease during their lifetime. Men are affected three times as often as women. Duodenal ulcers are ten times more common than gastric ulcers in young patients, but in the older age groups the frequency is about equal. Probably as a result of a declining prevalence of *H pylori* infection, the incidence has declined to less than half what it was 20 years ago.

In general terms, the ulcerative process can lead to four types of disability: (1) **Pain** is the most common. (2) **Bleeding** may occur as a result of erosion of submucosal or extraintestinal vessels as the ulcer becomes deeper. (3) Penetration of the ulcer through all layers of the affected gut results in **perforation** if other viscera do not seal the ulcer. (4) **Obstruction** may result from inflammatory swelling and scarring and is most likely to occur with ulcers located at the pylorus or gastroesophageal junction, where the lumen is narrowest.

The clinical features and prognosis of duodenal ulcer and gastric ulcer are sufficiently different to be dealt with separately here.

DUODENAL ULCER

Essentials of Diagnosis

- Epigastric pain relieved by food or antacids.
- Epigastric tenderness.
- Normal or increased gastric acid secretion.
- Signs of ulcer disease on upper gastrointestinal x-rays or endoscopy.
- Evidence of *Helicobacter pylori* infection.

General Considerations

Duodenal ulcers may occur in any age group but are most common in the young and middle-aged (20–45 years). They appear in men more often than women. About 95% of duodenal ulcers are situated within 2 cm of the pylorus, in the duodenal bulb.

Considerable evidence implicates *H pylori* as the principal cause of duodenal ulcer disease. This microaerophilic gram-negative curved bacillus can be found colonizing patches of gastric metaplasia within the duodenum in 90% of patients with this disease. The bacilli remain on the surface of the mucosa rather than invading it. They are thought to render the duodenum more vulnerable to the injurious effects of acid and pepsin by releasing urease or other toxins.

The epidemiology of peptic ulcer disease reflects the prevalence of *H pylori* infection in different populations. In areas of the world where peptic ulcer is uncommon (eg, rural Africa), human infection is rare. Duodenal ulcer disease has emerged as a major clinical entity in Western society only since the latter part of the 19th century. The incidence reached a peak about 30 years ago and then declined to reach a lower plateau a few years ago. These changes are thought to be explained by variations in *H pylori* infection resulting from public health factors. Within countries like the USA, the distribution of *H pylori* is explainable by a fecal-oral theory of transmission. The prevalence of infection is higher among lower socioeconomic groups. Interestingly, only a minority of infected persons develop ulcers. *H pylori* also has an important role in the etiology of gastric ulcer, gastric cancer, and gastritis. The 10% of duodenal ulcers that are not associated with *Helicobacter* infection are caused by nonsteroidal anti-inflammatory drugs and other agents.

Gastric acid secretion is characteristically higher than normal in patients with duodenal ulcer compared with normal subjects, but only one-sixth of the duodenal ulcer population have secretory levels that exceed the normal range (ie, acid secretion in normal subjects and those with duodenal ulcer overlap considerably), so the disease cannot be explained simply as a manifestation of increased acid production. Whether acid secretion increases in response to *Helicobacter* infection is doubted. One possibility is that the patches of metaplastic gastric epithelium in the duodenum on which *Helicobacter* take up residence result from the action of acid. Then the colonized patches undergo ulceration.

Chronic liver disease, chronic lung disease, and chronic pancreatitis have all been implicated as increasing the possibility of duodenal ulceration.

Clinical Findings

A. Symptoms and Signs: Pain, the presenting symptom in most patients, is usually located in the epigastrium and is variably described as aching, burning, or gnawing. Radiologic survey studies indicate, however, that some patients with active duodenal ulcer have no gastrointestinal complaints.

The daily cycle of the pain is often characteristic. The patient usually has no pain in the morning until an hour or more after breakfast. The pain is relieved by the noon meal, only to recur in the later afternoon. Pain may appear again in the evening, and in about half of cases it arouses the patient during the night. Food, milk, or antacid preparations give temporary relief.

When the ulcer penetrates the head of the pancreas posteriorly, back pain is noted; concomitantly, the cyclic pattern of pain may change to a more steady discomfort, with less relief from food and antacids.

Varying degrees of nausea and vomiting are common. Vomiting may be a major feature even in the absence of obstruction.

The abdominal examination may reveal localized epigastric tenderness to the right of the midline, but in many instances no tenderness can be elicited.

B. Endoscopy: Gastroduodenoscopy is useful in evaluating patients with an uncertain diagnosis, those with bleeding from the upper intestine, and those who have obstruction of the gastroduodenal segment and for assessing response to therapy.

C. Diagnostic Tests:

1. Gastric analysis–A gastric analysis may be indicated in certain cases. The standard gastric analysis consists of the following: (1) Measurement of acid production by the unstimulated stomach under basal fasting conditions; the result is expressed as H^+ secretion in meq/h and is termed the **basal acid output (BAO).** (2) Measurement of acid production during stimulation by histamine or pentagastrin given in a dose maximal for this effect. The result is expressed as H⁺ secretion in meq/h and is termed the **maximal acid output (MAO).**

Interpretation of the results is outlined in Table 23–1.

2. Serum gastrin–Depending on the laboratory, normal basal gastrin levels average 50–100 pg/mL, and levels over 200 pg/mL can almost always be considered high.

Gastrin concentrations may rise in hyposecretory and hypersecretory states. In the former conditions (eg, atrophic gastritis, pernicious anemia), the cause is higher antral pH with loss of antral inhibition for gastrin release. More important clinically is elevated gastrin levels with concomitant hypersecretion, where the high gastrin level is responsible for the increased acid and resulting peptic ulceration. The best-defined clinical condition in this category is Zollinger-Ellison syndrome (gastrinoma)

A fasting serum gastrin determination should be obtained in patients with peptic ulcer disease that is unusually severe or refractory to therapy.

D. Radiographic Studies: On an upper gastrointestinal series, the changes induced by duodenal ulcer consist of duodenal deformities and an ulcer niche. Inflammatory swelling and scarring may lead to distortion of the duodenal bulb, eccentricity of the pyloric channel, or pseudodiverticulum formation. The ulcer itself may be seen either in profile or, more commonly, en face.

Differential Diagnosis

The most common diseases simulating peptic ulcer are (1) chronic cholecystitis, in which cholecystograms show either nonfunctioning of the gallbladder or stones in a functioning gallbladder; (2) acute pancreatitis, in which the serum amylase is elevated; (3) chronic pancreatitis, in which ERCP shows an abnormal pancreatic duct; (4) functional indigestion, in which x-rays are normal; and (5) reflux esophagitis.

Complications

The common complications of duodenal ulcer are hemorrhage, perforation, and duodenal obstruction. Each of these is discussed in a separate section. Less common complications are pancreatitis and biliary obstruction.

Table 23–1. Mean values for acid output during gastric analysis for normals and patients with duodenal ulcer. The upper limits of normal are: Basal (BAO), 5 meq/h; maximal (MAO), 30 meq/h.

		Mean Acid Output (meq/h)	
	Sex	**Normal**	**Duodenal Ulcer**
Basal	Male	2.5	5.5
	Female	1.5	3
Maximal (pentagastrin)	Male	30	40
	Female	20	30

Prevention

Prevention of ulcer disease entails avoidance of *H pylori* infection.

Treatment

Acute duodenal ulcer can be controlled by suppressing acid secretion in most patients, but the long-term course of the disease (ie, frequency of relapses and of complications) is unaffected unless *H pylori* infection is eradicated. Surgical therapy is recommended principally for the treatment of complications: bleeding, perforation, or obstruction.

A. Medical Treatment: The goals of medical therapy are (1) to heal the ulcer and (2) to cure the disease. Treatment in the first category is aimed at decreasing acid secretion or neutralizing acid. The principal drugs consist of H_2 receptor antagonists (eg, cimetidine, ranitidine) and proton pump blockers (eg, omeprazole). One of the H_2 receptor antagonists is usually the first choice, and when given in therapeutic doses, it will bring about healing of the ulcer in 80% of patients within 6 weeks. Omeprazole is reserved for patients whose ulcers are refractory to H_2 antagonists or for those with Zollinger-Ellison syndrome. Antacids may be used alternatively as primary therapy or on an as-needed basis to treat ulcer pain. Antacids are just as effective as H_2 receptor antagonists but slightly more difficult to administer.

After the ulcer has healed, discontinuation of therapy results in an 80% recurrence rate within 1 year, which may be avoided by chronic nighttime administration of a single dose of H receptor antagonists. A better approach is to treat the *H pylori* infection along with the ulcer, since eradication of *H pylori* eliminates recurrent ulceration unless the infection recurs—an uncommon event. At present, the optimal daily regimen consists of the following combination of drugs: (1) an H_2 receptor antagonist (eg, cimetidine, 1.2 g); (2) a bismuth compound (PeptoBismol, 8 tablets; DeNol); (3) tetracycline, 2 g; and (4) metronidazole, 750 mg. The H_2 receptor antagonist is given until the ulcer has healed or for 16 weeks; the last three drugs are given for 3 weeks.

B. Surgical Treatment: If medical treatment has been optimal, a persistent ulcer may be judged intractable, and surgical treatment is indicated. This is now uncommon.

The surgical procedures that can cure peptic ulcer are aimed at reduction of gastric acid secretion. Excision of the ulcer itself is not sufficient for either duodenal or gastric ulcer; recurrence is nearly inevitable with such procedures.

The surgical methods of treating duodenal ulcer are vagotomy (several varieties) and antrectomy plus vagotomy. All of these procedures can be performed laparoscopically. With rare exceptions, one of the vagotomy operations is sufficient (Figure 23–5).

1. Vagotomy—Truncal vagotomy consists of resection of a 1- or 2-cm segment of each vagal trunk as

Antrectomy and vagotomy
(Billroth I)

Subtotal gastrectomy
(Billroth II)

Total gastrectomy

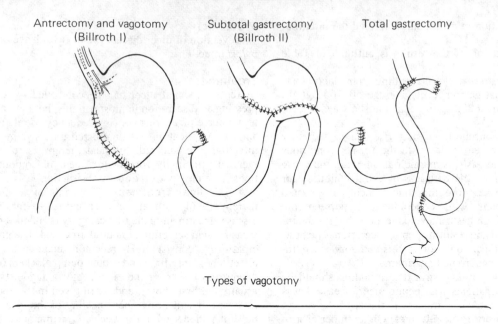

Types of vagotomy

Truncal

Selective

Parietal cell

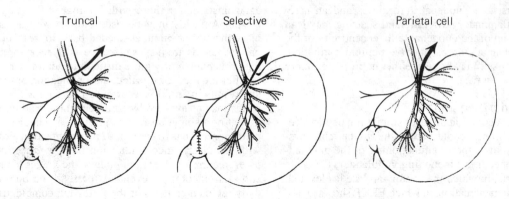

Figure 23–5. Various types of operations currently popular for treating duodenal ulcer disease. Total gastrectomy is reserved for Zollinger-Ellison syndrome. The choice among the other procedures should be individualized according to principles discussed in the text.

it enters the abdomen on the distal esophagus. The resulting vagal denervation of the gastric musculature produces delayed emptying of the stomach in many patients unless a drainage procedure is performed. The method of drainage most often selected is **pyloroplasty (Heineke-Mikulicz procedure;** Figure 23–6); **gastrojejunostomy** is used less often. Neither procedure gives a superior functional result, and pyloroplasty is less time-consuming.

Vagal denervation of just the parietal cell area of the stomach is called **parietal cell vagotomy** or **proximal gastric vagotomy.** The technique spares the main nerves of Latarjet (Figures 23–3 and 23–5) but divides all vagal branches that terminate on the proximal two-thirds of the stomach. Since antral innervation is preserved, gastric emptying is relatively normal, and a drainage procedure is unnecessary.

Nevertheless, parietal cell vagotomy plus pyloroplasty gives better results (ie, fewer recurrent ulcers) than parietal cell vagotomy alone. Parietal cell vagotomy appears to have about the same effectiveness as truncal or selective vagotomy for curing the ulcer disease, but dumping and diarrhea are much less frequent. It is probably the procedure of choice for intractable and perforated duodenal ulcers and is relatively less useful for obstructing and bleeding ulcers.

The vagotomy procedures have the advantages of technical simplicity and preservation of the entire gastric reservoir capacity. The principal disadvantage is recurrent ulceration in about 10% of patients. The recurrence rate after parietal cell vagotomy is about twice as high in patients with prepyloric ulcer, and

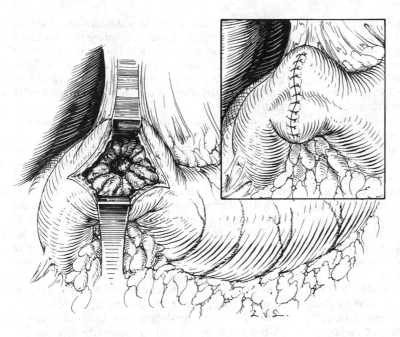

Figure 23–6. Heineke-Mikulicz pyloroplasty. A longitudinal incision has been made across the pylorus, revealing an active ulcer in the duodenal bulb. The insert shows the transverse closure of the incision that widens the gastric outlet. The accompanying vagotomy is not shown.

most surgeons use a different operation for an ulcer in this location.

2. Antrectomy and vagotomy–This operation entails a distal gastrectomy of 50% of the stomach, with the line of gastric transection carried high on the lesser curvature to conform with the boundary of the gastrin-producing mucosa.

The terms antrectomy and hemigastrectomy are loosely synonymous. The proximal remnant may be reanastomosed to the duodenum (**Billroth I resection**) or to the side of the proximal jejunum (**Billroth II resection**). The Billroth I technique is most popular, but there is no conclusive evidence that the results are superior. When creating a Billroth II (gastrojejunostomy) reconstruction, the surgeon may bring the jejunal loop up to the gastric remnant either anterior to the transverse colon or posteriorly through a hole in the transverse mesocolon. Since either method is satisfactory, an antecolic anastomosis is elected in most cases because it is simpler. Truncal vagotomy is performed as described in the preceding section; antrectomy by itself will not prevent a high recurrence rate. In most instances, the surgeon will be able to remove the ulcerated portion of duodenum in the course of resection.

Vagotomy and antrectomy is associated with a low incidence of marginal ulceration (2%) and a generally good overall outcome, but the risk of complications is higher than after vagotomy without resection.

3. Subtotal gastrectomy–This operation consists of resection of two-thirds to three-fourths of the distal stomach. After subtotal gastrectomy for duodenal ulcer, a Billroth II reconstruction is preferable. Subtotal gastrectomy is largely of historical interest.

Complications of Surgery for Peptic Ulcer

A. Early Complications: Duodenal stump leakage, gastric retention, and hemorrhage may develop in the immediate postoperative period.

B. Late Complications:

1. Recurrent ulcer (marginal ulcer, stomal ulcer, anastomotic ulcer)–Recurrent ulcers form in about 10% of duodenal ulcer patients treated by vagotomy and pyloroplasty or parietal cell vagotomy; and in 2–3% after vagotomy and antrectomy or subtotal gastrectomy. Recurrent ulcers nearly always develop immediately adjacent to the anastomosis on the intestinal side.

The usual complaint is upper abdominal pain, which is often aggravated by eating and improved by antacids. In some patients, the pain is felt more to the left in the epigastrium, and left axillary or shoulder pain is occasionally reported. About a third of patients with stomal ulcer will experience major gastrointestinal hemorrhage. Free perforation is less common (5%).

Diagnosis and treatment are essentially the same as for the original ulcer.

2. Gastrojejunocolic and gastrocolic fistula–A deeply eroding ulcer may occasionally produce a fistula between the stomach and colon. Most examples have resulted from recurrent peptic ulcer after an operation that included a gastrojejunal anastomosis.

Severe diarrhea and weight loss are the presenting symptoms in over 90% of cases. Abdominal pain typical of recurrent peptic ulcer often precedes the onset of the diarrhea. Bowel movements number 8–12 or more a day; they are watery and often contain particles of undigested food.

The degree of malnutrition ranges from mild to very severe. Laboratory studies reveal low serum proteins and manifestations of fluid and electrolyte depletion. Appropriate tests may reflect deficiencies in both water-soluble and fat-soluble vitamins.

An upper gastrointestinal series reveals the marginal ulcer in only 50% of patients and the fistula in only 15%. Barium enema unfailingly demonstrates the fistulous tract.

Initial treatment should replenish fluid and electrolyte deficits. The involved colon and ulcerated gastrojejunal segment should be excised and colonic continuity reestablished. Vagotomy, partial gastrectomy, or both are required to treat the ulcer diathesis and prevent another recurrent ulcer. Results are excellent in benign disease. In general, the outlook for patients with a malignant fistula is poor.

3. Dumping syndrome–Symptoms of the dumping syndrome are noted to some extent by most patients who have an operation that impairs the ability of the stomach to regulate its rate of emptying. Within several months, however, dumping is a clinical problem in only 1–2% of patients. Symptoms fall into two categories: cardiovascular and gastrointestinal. Shortly after eating, the patient may experience palpitations, sweating, weakness, dyspnea, flushing, nausea, abdominal cramps, belching, vomiting, diarrhea, and, rarely, syncope. The degree of severity varies widely, and not all symptoms are reported by all patients. In severe cases, the patient must lie down for 30–40 minutes until the discomfort passes.

Diet therapy to reduce jejunal osmolality is successful in all but a few cases. The diet should be low in carbohydrate and high in fat and protein content. Sugars and carbohydrates are least well tolerated; some patients are especially sensitive to milk. Meals should be taken dry, with fluids restricted to between meals. This dietary regimen ordinarily suffices, but anticholinergic drugs may be of help in some patients; others have reported improvement with supplemental pectin in the diet, and the use of somatostatin analogues offers some promise.

4. Alkaline gastritis–Reflux of duodenal juices into the stomach is an invariable and usually innocuous situation after operations that interfere with pyloric function, but in some patients, it may cause marked gastritis. The principal symptom is postprandial pain, and the diagnosis rests on endoscopic and biopsy demonstration of an edematous inflamed gastric mucosa. Since a minor degree of gastritis is found in most patients after Billroth II gastrectomy, the endoscopic findings are to some degree nonspecific. Persistent severe pain is an indication for surgical reconstruction. Roux-en-Y gastrojejunostomy with a 40-cm efferent jejunal limb is the treatment of choice.

5. Anemia–Iron deficiency anemia develops in about 30% of patients within 5 years after partial gas-

trectomy. It is caused by failure to absorb food iron bound in an organic molecule. Before this diagnosis is accepted, the patient should be checked for blood loss, marginal ulcer, or an unsuspected tumor. Inorganic iron—ferrous sulfate or ferrous gluconate—is indicated for treatment and is absorbed normally after gastrectomy.

Vitamin B_{12} deficiency and megaloblastic anemia appear in a few cases after gastrectomy.

6. Postvagotomy diarrhea–About 5–10% of patients who have had truncal vagotomy require treatment with antidiarrheal agents at some time, and perhaps 1% are seriously troubled by this complication. The diarrhea may be episodic, in which case the onset is unpredictable after symptom-free intervals of weeks to months. An attack may consist of only one or two watery movements or, in severe cases, may last for a few days. Other patients may continually produce 3–5 loose stools per day.

Most cases of postvagotomy diarrhea can be treated satisfactorily with constipating agents.

7. Chronic gastroparesis–Chronic delayed gastric emptying is seen occasionally after gastric surgery. Prokinetic agents (eg, metoclopramide) are often helpful, but some cases are refractory to any therapy except a completion gastrectomy and Roux-en-Y esophagojejunostomy (ie, total gastrectomy).

Allison MC et al: Gastrointestinal damage associated with the use of nonsteroidal antiinflammatory drugs. N Engl J Med 1992;327:749.

Beardshall K et al: Suppression of *Helicobacter pylori* reduces gastrin releasing peptide stimulated gastrin release in duodenal ulcer patients. Gut 1992;33:601.

Cuschieri A: Laparoscopic vagotomy. Surg Clin North Am 1992;72:357.

Donahue PE et al: Experimental basis and clinical application of extended highly selective vagotomy for duodenal ulcer. Surg Gynecol Obstet 1993;176:39.

Eagon JC, Miedema BW, Kelly KA: Postgastrectomy syndromes. Surg Clin North Am 1992;72:445.

Emas S, Eriksson B: Twelve-year follow-up of a prospective, randomized trial of selective vagotomy with pyloroplasty and selective proximal vagotomy with and without pyloroplasty for the treatment of duodenal, pyloric, and prepyloric ulcers. Am J Surg 1992;164:4.

Emas S, Grupcev G, Eriksson B: Six-year results of a prospective, randomized trial of selective proximal vagotomy with and without pyloroplasty in the treatment of duodenal, pyloric, and prepyloric ulcers. Ann Surg 1993;217:6.

Eysselein VE et al: Regulation of gastric acid secretion by gastrin in duodenal ulcer patients and healthy subjects. Gastroenterology 1992;102:1142.

Folkman J et al: Duodenal ulcer: Discovery of a new mechanism and development of angiogenic therapy that accelerates healing. Ann Surg 1991;214:414.

Geer RJ et al: Efficacy of octreotide acetate in treatment of severe postgastrectomy dumping syndrome. Ann Surg 1990;212:678.

Gompertz RH et al: Duodenal ulcer: A model of impaired mucosal defence. Gut 1992;33:1044.

Graham DY et al: Effect of treatment of *Helicobacter pylori* infection on the long-term recurrence of gastric or duodenal ulcer: A randomized, controlled study. Ann Intern Med 1992;116:705.

Hentschel E et al: Effect of ranitidine and amoxicillin plus metronidazole on the eradication of *Helicobacter pylori* and the recurrence of duodenal ulcer. N Engl J Med 1993;328:308.

Lee A: *H pylori*-initiated ulcerogenesis: Look to the host. Lancet 1993;341:280.

McCallum RW, Polepalle SC, Schirmer B: Completion gastrectomy for refractory gastroparesis following surgery for peptic ulcer disease. Dig Dis Sci 1991;36:1556.

McCarthy DM: Sucralfate. N Engl J Med 1991;325:1017.

Maton PN: Omeprazole. N Engl J Med 1991;324:965.

Megraud F; Lamouliatte H: *Helicobacter pylori* and duodenal ulcer: Evidence suggesting causation. Dig Dis Sci 1992;37:769.

Mertz HR, Walsh JH: Peptic ulcer pathophysiology. Med Clin North Am 1991;75:799.

Miedema BW, Kelly KA: The Roux operation for postgastrectomy syndromes. Am J Surg 1991;161:256.

Moss SF et al: Effect of *Helicobacter pylori* on gastric somatostatin in duodenal ulcer disease. Lancet 1992; 340:930.

Saita H et al: Link between *Helicobacter pylori*-associated gastritis and duodenal ulcer. Dig Dis Sci 1993;38:117.

Stabile BE: Current surgical management of duodenal ulcers. Surg Clin North Am 1992;72:335.

Valen B et al: Proximal gastric vagotomy for peptic ulcer disease: Follow-up of 483 patients for 3 to 14 years. Surgery 1991;110:824.

Valenzuela JE et al: U.S. experience with omeprazole in duodenal ulcer: Multicenter double-blind comparative study with ranitidine. The Omeprazole DU Comparative Study Group. Dig Dis Sci 1991;36:761.

Walt RP: Misoprostol for the treatment of peptic ulcer and antiinflammatory-drug-induced gastroduodenal ulceration. N Engl J Med 1992;327:1575.

ZOLLINGER-ELLISON SYNDROME (Gastrinoma)

Essentials of Diagnosis

- Peptic ulcer disease (often severe) in 95%.
- Gastric hypersecretion.
- Elevated serum gastrin.
- Non-B islet cell tumor of the pancreas or duodenum.

General Considerations

Zollinger-Ellison syndrome is manifested by gastric acid hypersecretion caused by a gastrin-producing tumor (gastrinoma). Although the normal pancreas does not contain appreciable amounts of gastrin, most gastrinomas occur in the pancreas; others are found submucosally in the duodenum and rarely in the antrum or ovary. The gastrin-producing lesions (called **apudomas** from the theory of their histogenesis) in the pancreas are non-B islet cell carcinomas (60%), solitary adenomas (25%), and hyperplasia or microadenomas (10%); the remaining cases (5%) are due to solitary submucosal gastrinomas in the first or second portion of the duodenum. About one-third of patients have the multiple endocrine neoplasia type I syndrome (MEN I), which is characterized by a family history of endocrinopathy and the presence of tumors in other glands, especially the parathyroids and pituitary. Patients with MEN I usually have multiple benign gastrinomas. Those without MEN I usually have solitary gastrinomas that are often malignant. The tumors may be as small as 2–3 mm and are often difficult to find. In about one-third of cases, the tumor cannot be located at laparotomy.

The diagnosis of cancer can be made only with findings of metastases or blood vessel invasion, because the histologic pattern is similar for benign and malignant tumors. In most patients with malignant gastrinomas, the illness caused by hypergastrinemia (ie, severe peptic ulcer disease) is a greater threat to health than the illness caused by malignant growth and spread.

Clinical Findings

A. Symptoms and Signs: Symptoms associated with gastrinoma are principally a result of acid hypersecretion—usually from peptic ulcer disease. Some patients with gastrinoma have severe diarrhea from the large amounts of acid entering the duodenum, which can destroy pancreatic lipase and produce steatorrhea, damage the small bowel mucosa, and overload the intestine with gastric and pancreatic secretions. About 5% of patients present with diarrhea only.

Ulcer symptoms are often refractory to large doses of antacids or standard doses of H_2 blocking agents. Hemorrhage, perforation, and obstruction are common complications. Marginal ulcers appear after surgical procedures that would cure the ordinary ulcer diathesis.

B. Laboratory Findings: Hypergastrinemia in the presence of acid hypersecretion is almost pathognomonic for gastrinoma. Gastrin levels are normally inversely proportionate to gastric acid output; therefore, diseases that result in increased gastric pH may cause a rise in serum gastric concentration (eg, pernicious anemia, atrophic gastritis, gastric ulcer, postvagotomy state). Serum gastrin levels should be measured in any patient with suspected gastrinoma or ulcer disease severe enough to warrant consideration of surgical treatment. H_2 receptor blocking agents, omeprazole, or antacids may increase serum gastrin concentrations and should be avoided for several days before gastrin measurements are made. It is often helpful to measure gastric acid secretion to rule out H^+ hyposecretion as a cause of hypergastrinemia.

The normal gastrin value is less than 200 pg/mL. Patients with gastrinoma usually have levels exceeding 500 pg/mL and sometimes 10,000 pg/mL or higher. Very high gastrin levels (eg, > 5000 pg/mL) or the presence of alpha chains of hCG in the serum usually indicates cancer. Patients with borderline gastrin values (eg, 200–500 pg/mL) and acid secretion in the range associated with ordinary duodenal ulcer disease should have a secretin provocative test. Following intravenous administration of secretin (2 units/kg as a bolus), a rise in the gastrin level of ≥150 pg/mL within 15 minutes is diagnostic.

Marked basal acid hypersecretion (> 15 meq H^+ per hour) occurs in most Zollinger-Ellison patients who have an intact stomach. In a patient who has previously undergone gastrectomy, a basal acid output of 5 meq/h or more is highly suggestive. Since the parietal cells are already under near maximal stimulation from hypergastrinemia, there is little increase in acid secretion following an injection of pentagastrin, and the ratio of basal to maximal acid output (BAO/MAO) characteristically exceeds 0.6.

Hypergastrinemia and gastric acid hypersecretion may be seen in gastric outlet obstruction, retained antrum after a Billroth II gastrojejunostomy, and in antral gastrin cell hyperactivity (hyperplasia). These conditions may be differentiated from gastrinoma by use of the secretin test. Because associated hyperparathyroidism is so common, serum calcium concentrations should be measured in all patients with gastrinoma.

Serum levels of neuron-specific enolase, β-hCG, and chromogranin-A are often elevated in patients with functioning apudomas. Although they are probably of no physiologic importance, the high levels of these peptides may be useful in diagnosing apudomas and following the results of therapy.

C. Imaging Studies: An upper gastrointestinal series usually shows ulceration in the duodenal bulb, though ulcers sometimes appear in the distal duodenum or proximal jejunum. The presence of ulcers in these distal ("ectopic") locations is nearly diagnostic of gastrinoma. The stomach contains prominent rugal folds, and secretions are present in the lumen despite overnight fasting. The duodenum may be dilated and exhibit hyperactive peristalsis. Edema may be detected in the small bowel mucosa. The barium flocculates in the intestine, and transit time is accelerated. A CT or MR scan will often demonstrate the pancreatic tumors. Misleading results are common with angiography. Transhepatic portal vein blood sampling to find hot spots of gastrin production has largely failed to help in localizing the tumor preoperatively.

Treatment

A. Medical Treatment: Initial treatment should consist of H_2 blocking agents (eg, cimetidine, 300–600 mg, four times daily; ranitidine, 300–450 mg, four times daily). The dose should be adjusted to keep gastric H^+ output below 5 meq in the hour preceding the next dose. Although the response to H_2 blocking agents is usually excellent at first. With time, the dose must be increased in order to maintain the same level of control, and control eventually becomes unsatisfactory even at high doses. Omeprazole, a proton pump blocker, is indicated sooner or later in nearly all patients.

A combination of streptozocin, fluorouracil, and doxorubicin is the most effective chemotherapeutic regimen for advanced cancer.

B. Surgical Treatment: Although resection is the ideal treatment for gastrinoma, this is only possible in the 30% of patients who have solitary lesions or multiple lesions that can be removed. All of the gastrin-producing tissue cannot be resected when there are multiple metastases, diffuse microadenomatosis of the pancreas (as in MEN I), or when the tumor cannot be located. Surgical cure may still be possible, however, when there are just a few localized metastases in peripancreatic lymph nodes or the liver.

Every patient with sporadic Zollinger-Ellison syndrome should be considered a candidate for tumor resection. The preoperative workup should include a CT or MR scan of the pancreas and, if that does not show the tumor, selective angiography. Regardless of other findings, exploratory laparotomy is then recommended in the absence of evidence of unresectable metastatic disease. If the tumor is found in the pancreas, it is enucleated if possible. Operative ultrasound may help in the examination of the pancreas. Most lesions will be found either in the head of the pancreas or in the duodenum. If enucleation cannot be performed, a distal pancreatectomy is indicated. A Whipple procedure should usually be avoided. The mucosal surface of the duodenum must be carefully palpated through a duodenotomy in every patient, since the duodenal lesions may be so tiny that they cannot be felt from the outside.

Prognosis

Since H_2 blocking agents become less effective with time, omeprazole is eventually required in medically treated patients. If all visible tumor has been resected and serum gastrin levels return to normal postoperatively, recurrence is rare. Because it is usually multifocal, the disease can rarely be cured surgically in patients with MEN I. A few malignant gastrinomas cause death from growth of metastases.

Berg CL, Wolfe MM: Zollinger-Ellison syndrome. Med Clin North Am 1991;75:903.

Cherner JA, Sawyers JL: Benefit of resection of metastatic gastrinoma in multiple endocrine neoplasia type I. Gastroenterology 1992;102:1049.

Delcore R, Friesen SR: Role of pancreatoduodenectomy in the management of primary duodenal wall gastrinomas in patients with Zollinger-Ellison syndrome. Surgery 1992;112:1016.

Donow C et al: Surgical pathology of gastrinoma: Site, size, multicentricity, association with multiple endocrine neoplasia type 1, and malignancy. Cancer 1991;68:1329.

Doppman JL: Pancreatic endocrine tumors: The search goes on. N Engl J Med 1992;326:1770.

Grama D et al: Pancreatic tumors in multiple endocrine neoplasia type 1: Clinical presentation and surgical treatment. World J Surg 1992;16:611.

Howard TJ et al: Biologic behavior of sporadic gastrinoma located to the right and left of the superior mesenteric artery. Am J Surg 1993;165:101.

Imamura M et al: Clinicopathological characteristics of duodenal microgastrinomas. World J Surg 1992;16:703.

MacGillivray DC et al: The significance of gastrinomas found in peripancreatic lymph nodes. Surgery 1991;109:558.

Mozell EJ et al: Long-term efficacy of octreotide in the treatment of Zollinger-Ellison syndrome. Arch Surg 1992;127:1019.

Norton JA et al: Intraoperative ultrasonographic localization of islet cell tumors. A prospective comparison to palpation. Ann Surg 1988;207:160.

Norton JA, Jensen RT: Unresolved surgical issues in the management of patients with Zollinger-Ellison syndrome. World J Surg 1991;15:151.

Pisegna JR et al: Effects of curative gastrinoma resection on gastric secretory function and antisecretory drug requirement in the Zollinger-Ellison syndrome. Gastroenterology 1992;102:767.

Sawicki MP et al: The dichotomous distribution of gastrinomas. Arch Surg 1990;125:1584.

Thom AK et al: Location, incidence, and malignant potential of duodenal gastrinomas. Surgery 1991;110:1086.

Thom AK et al: Prospective study of the use of intraarterial secretin injection and portal venous sampling to localize duodenal gastrinomas. Surgery 1992;112:1002.

Tompson NW, Vinik AI, Eckhauser FE: Microgastrinomas of the duodenum. A cause of failed operations for the Zollinger-Ellison syndrome. Ann Surg 1989;209:396.

Van Heerden JA et al: Management of the Zollinger-Ellison syndrome in patients with multiple endocrine neoplasia type I. Surgery 1986;100:971.

Vinayek R et al: Pharmacokinetics of oral and intravenous omeprazole in patients with the Zollinger-Ellison syndrome. Gastroenterology 1991;101:138.

Wilson SD: Zollinger-Ellison syndrome in children: A 25-year follow-up. Surgery 1991;110:696.

GASTRIC ULCER

Essentials of Diagnosis

- Epigastric pain.
- Ulcer demonstrated by x-ray.
- Acid present on gastric analysis.

General Considerations

The peak incidence of gastric ulcer is in patients aged 40–60 years, or about 10 years older than the average for those with duodenal ulcer. Ninety-five percent of gastric ulcers are located on the lesser curvature, and 60% of these are within 6 cm of the pylorus. The symptoms and complications of gastric ulcer closely resemble those of duodenal ulcer.

Gastric ulcers may be separated into three types with different causes and different treatments. **Type I ulcers,** the most common variety, are found in patients who on the average are 10 years older than patients with duodenal ulcers and who have no clinical or radiographic evidence of previous duodenal ulcer disease; gastric acid output is normal or low. The ulcers are usually located within 2 cm of the boundary between parietal cell and pyloric mucosa, but always in the latter. As noted above, 95% are on the lesser curvature, usually near the incisura angularis.

Antral gastritis is universally present, being most severe near the pylorus and gradually diminishing. This is associated in most cases with the presence of *H pylori* beneath the mucus layer, on the luminal surface of epithelial cells, and gastric ulcer disease is probably the result of infection with this organism.

Type II ulcers are located close to the pylorus (prepyloric ulcers) and occur in association with (most often following) duodenal ulcers. The risk of cancer is very low in these gastric ulcers. Acid secretion measured by gastric analysis is in the range associated with duodenal ulcer.

Type III ulcers occur in the antrum as a result of chronic use of nonsteroidal anti-inflammatory agents.

One must always consider whether the ulcer seen on x-ray or by endoscopy represents an ulcerated malignant tumor rather than a simple benign ulcer. Efforts must be expended during the *initial* stage of the workup to establish this distinction. Despite the generally discouraging results of surgery for gastric adenocarcinoma, those whose tumors are difficult to distinguish from benign ulcer have a 50–75% chance of cure after gastrectomy.

Clinical Findings

A. Symptoms and Signs: The principal symptom is epigastric pain relieved by food or antacids, as in duodenal ulcer. Epigastric tenderness is a variable finding. Compared with duodenal ulcer, the pain in gastric ulcer tends to appear earlier after eating, often within 30 minutes. Vomiting, anorexia, and aggravation of pain by eating are also more common with gastric ulcer.

Achlorhydria is defined as no acid (pH > 6.00) after pentagastrin stimulation. Achlorhydria is incompatible with the diagnosis of benign peptic ulcer and suggests a malignant gastric ulcer. About 5% of malignant gastric ulcers will be associated with this finding.

B. Gastroscopy and Biopsy: Gastroscopy should be performed as part of the initial workup to attempt to find malignant lesions. The rolled-up margins of the ulcer that produce the meniscus sign on x-ray can often be distinguished from the flat edges characteristic of a benign ulcer. Multiple (preferably six) biopsy specimens and brush biopsy should be obtained from the edge of the lesion. False-positives are rare; false-negatives occur in 5–10% of malignant ulcers.

C. Imaging Studies: Upper gastrointestinal

x-rays will show an ulcer, usually on the lesser curvature in the pyloric area. In the absence of a tumor mass, the following suggest that the ulcer is malignant: (1) the deepest penetration of the ulcer is not beyond the expected border of the gastric wall; (2) the meniscus sign is present, ie, a prominent rim of radiolucency surrounding the ulcer, caused by heaped-up edges of tumor; and (3) cancer is more common (10%) in ulcers greater than 2 cm in diameter. Coexistence of duodenal deformity or ulcer favors a diagnosis of benign ulcer in the stomach.

Differential Diagnosis

The characteristic symptoms of gastric ulcer are often clouded by numerous nonspecific complaints. Uncomplicated hiatal hernia, atrophic gastritis, chronic cholecystitis, irritable colon syndrome, and undifferentiated functional problems are distinguishable from peptic ulcer only after appropriate radiologic studies and sometimes not even then.

Gastroscopy and biopsy of the ulcer should be performed to rule out malignant gastric ulcer.

Complications

Bleeding, obstruction, and perforation are the principal complications of gastric ulcer. They are discussed separately elsewhere in this chapter.

Treatment

A. Medical Treatment: Medical management of gastric ulcer is the same as for duodenal ulcer. The patient should be questioned regarding the use of ulcerogenic agents, which should be eliminated as far as possible.

Repeat endoscopy should be obtained to document the rate of healing. After 4–16 weeks (depending on the initial size of the lesion and other factors), healing usually has reached a plateau. In order to cure the disease and avoid recurrent ulcers, *H pylori* must be eradicated. The success of therapy in this regard can be checked by serologic testing for *H pylori* antibodies.

B. Surgical Treatment: Before the significance of *H pylori* in the etiology of gastric ulcer was appreciated, the most effective surgical treatment was distal hemigastrectomy (including the ulcer); somewhat less effective but still useful in high-risk patients was vagotomy and pyloroplasty. Parietal cell vagotomy for prepyloric ulcers was followed by a high (eg, 30%) recurrence rate, but parietal cell vagotomy plus pyloroplasty worked well.

Intractability to medical therapy has now become a rare indication for surgery in gastric ulcer disease, since H_2 receptor antagonists or omeprazole can bring the condition under control, and treatment of *H pylori* infection can almost eliminate the problem of recurrence. Consequently, surgery will be needed principally for complications of the disease: bleeding, perforation, or obstruction.

Chua CL, Jeyaraj PR, Low CH: Relative risks of complications in giant and nongiant gastric ulcers. Am J Surg 1992;164:94.

Emas S, Eriksson B: Twelve-year follow-up of a prospective, randomized trial of selective vagotomy with pyloroplasty and selective proximal vagotomy with and without pyloroplasty for the treatment of duodenal, pyloric, and prepyloric ulcers. Am J Surg 1992;164:4.

Emas S, Grupcev G, Eriksson B: Six-year results of a prospective, randomized trial of selective proximal vagotomy with and without pyloroplasty in the treatment of duodenal, pyloric, and prepyloric ulcers. Ann Surg 1993;217:6.

Emas S, Hammarberg C: Prospective, randomized trial of selective proximal vagotomy with ulcer excision and partial gastrectomy with gastroduodenostomy in the treatment of corporeal gastric ulcer. Am J Surg 1983;146:631.

Graham DY et al: Effect of treatment of *Helicobacter pylori* infection on the long-term recurrence of gastric or duodenal ulcer: A randomized, controlled study. Ann Intern Med 1992;116:705.

Greenall MJ, Lehnert T: Vagotomy or gastrectomy for elective treatment of benign gastric ulceration? Dig Dis Sci 1985;30:353.

Jensen HE, Hoffmann J, Jorgensen PW: High gastric ulcer. World J Surg;1987;11:325.

Leung KM et al: *Helicobacter pylori*-related gastritis and gastric ulcer: A continuum of progressive epithelial degeneration. Am J Clin Pathol 1992;98:569.

Walan A et al: Effect of omeprazole and ranitidine on ulcer healing and relapse rates in patients with benign gastric ulcer. N Engl J Med 1989;320:69.

Walt RP: Misoprostol for the treatment of peptic ulcer and antiinflammatory-drug-induced gastroduodenal ulceration. N Engl J Med 1992;327:1575.

UPPER GASTROINTESTINAL HEMORRHAGE

Upper gastrointestinal hemorrhage may be mild or severe but should always be considered an ominous manifestation that deserves thorough evaluation. Bleeding is the most common serious complication of peptic ulcer, portal hypertension, and gastritis, and these conditions taken together account for most episodes of upper gastrointestinal bleeding in the average hospital population.

The major factors that determine the diagnostic and therapeutic approach are the amount and rate of bleeding. Estimates of both should be made promptly and monitored and revised continuously until the episode has been resolved. It is important to know at the outset that bleeding stops spontaneously in 75% of cases; the remainder includes those who will require surgery, experience complications, or die.

Hematemesis or melena is present except when the rate of blood loss is minimal. **Hematemesis** of either bright-red or dark blood indicates that the source is proximal to the ligament of Treitz. It is more common from bleeding that originates in the stomach or esophagus. In general, hematemesis denotes a more rapidly bleeding lesion, and a high percentage of patients who vomit blood require surgery. Coffee-ground vomitus is due to vomiting of blood that has been in the stomach long enough for gastric acid to convert hemoglobin to methemoglobin.

Most patients with **melena** (passage of black or tarry stools) are bleeding from the upper gastrointestinal tract, but melena can be produced by blood entering the bowel at any point from mouth to cecum. The conversion of red blood to dark depends more on the time it resides in the intestine than on the site of origin. The black color of melenic stools is probably caused by hematin, the product of oxidation of heme by intestinal and bacterial enzymes. Melena can be produced by as little as 50–100 mL of blood in the stomach. When 1 L of blood was instilled into the upper intestine of experimental subjects, melena persisted for 3–5 days, which shows that the rate of change in character of the stool is a poor guide to the time bleeding stops after an episode of hemorrhage.

Hematochezia is defined as the passage of bright-red blood from the rectum. Bright-red rectal blood can be produced by bleeding from the colon, rectum, or anus. However, if intestinal transit is rapid during brisk bleeding in the upper intestine, bright-red blood may be passed unchanged in the stool.

Tests for Occult Blood

Normal subjects lose about 2.5 mL of blood per day in their stools, presumably from minor mechanical abrasions of the intestinal epithelium. Between 50 and 100 mL of blood per day will produce melena. Tests for occult blood in the stool should be able to detect amounts between 10 and 50 mL/d. False-positive results may be due to dietary hemoglobin, myoglobin, or peroxidases of plant origin. Iron ingestion does not give positive reactions. The various tests using guaiac, benzidine, phenolphthalein, or orthotoluidine have similar specificities. The sensitivity of the guaiac slide test (Hemoccult) is in the desired range, and this is the best test available at present.

Initial Management

In an apparently healthy patient, melena of a week or more suggests that the bleeding is slow. In this type of patient, admission to the hospital should be followed by a deliberate but nonemergency workup. However, patients who present with hematemesis or melena of less than 12 hours' duration should be handled as if exsanguination were imminent. The approach entails a simultaneous series of diagnostic and therapeutic steps with the following initial goals: (1) Assess the status of the circulatory system and replace blood loss as necessary. (2) Determine the amount and rate of bleeding. (3) Slow or stop the bleeding by ice-water lavage. (4) Discover the lesion responsible for the episode. The last step may lead to

more specific treatment appropriate to the underlying condition.

The patient should be admitted to the hospital and a history and physical examination performed. Experienced clinicians are able to make a correct diagnosis of the cause of bleeding from clinical findings in only 60% of patients. Peptic ulcer, acute gastritis, esophageal varices, esophagitis, and Mallory-Weiss tear account for over 90% of cases (see Table 23–2). Questions concerning the symptoms and predisposing factors should be asked. The patient should be questioned about salicylate intake and any history of a bleeding tendency.

Of the diseases commonly responsible for acute upper gastrointestinal bleeding, only portal hypertension is associated with diagnostic clues on physical examination. However, gastrointestinal bleeding should not be automatically attributed to esophageal varices in a patient with jaundice, ascites, splenomegaly, spider angiomas, or hepatomegaly; over half of cirrhotic patients who present with acute hemorrhage are bleeding from gastritis or peptic ulcer.

Blood should be drawn for cross-matching, hematocrit, hemoglobin, creatinine, and tests of liver function. An intravenous infusion should be started and, in the massive bleeder, a large-bore nasogastric tube inserted. In cases of melena, the gastric aspirate should be examined to verify the gastroduodenal source of the hemorrhage, but about 25% of patients with bleeding duodenal ulcers have gastric aspirates that test negatively for blood. The tube must be larger than the standard nasogastric tube (16F) so the stomach can be lavaged free of liquid blood and clots. After its contents have been removed, the stomach should be irrigated with copious amounts of ice water or saline solution until blood no longer returns. If the patient was bleeding at the time the nasogastric tube was inserted, iced saline irrigation usually stops it. The large tube can then be exchanged for a standard nasogastric tube attached to continuous suction so further blood loss can be measured.

It is common to give H_2 receptor antagonists or omeprazole, though controlled trials have shown no benefit. If bleeding continues or if tachycardia or hypotension is present, the patient should be monitored and treated as for hemorrhagic shock.

In acute rapid hemorrhage, the hematocrit may be normal or only slightly low. A very low hematocrit without obvious signs of shock indicates more gradual blood loss.

All of the above tests and procedures can be performed within 1 or 2 hours after admission. By this time, in most instances, bleeding is under control, blood volume has been restored to normal, and the patient is being adequately monitored so that recurrent bleeding can be detected promptly. When this stage is reached, additional diagnostic tests should be performed.

Diagnosis of Cause of Bleeding
(Table 23–2)

Once the patient is stabilized, endoscopy should be the first study. In general, endoscopy should be performed within 24 hours after admission, and under these circumstances the source of bleeding can be demonstrated in about 80% of cases. Longer delays will give a lower diagnostic yield. Two lesions are seen in about 15% of patients. An upper gastrointestinal series should be performed if endoscopy is equivocal or unavailable. Although the diagnostic information provided by endoscopy does not appear to have resulted in decreased blood loss or improved outcome, endoscopic therapy, in the form of sclerosis of varices or injection of a bleeding ulcer, may do so. Having the diagnosis will also help in planning subsequent treatment, including the surgical approach if surgery becomes necessary.

Rarely, selective angiography will have diagnostic or therapeutic usefulness. For diagnosis, it is most helpful when other studies fail to demonstrate the cause of bleeding. Infusion through the angiographic catheter of vasoconstrictors (eg, vasopressin) and embolization of the bleeding vessel with Gelfoam may be able to halt the bleeding in special cases.

Later Management

Although a precise diagnosis of the cause of the bleeding may be valuable in later management, the patient must not be allowed to slip out of clinical control during the search for definitive diagnostic information. *The decision for emergency surgery depends more on the rate and duration of bleeding than on its specific cause.*

The need for transfusion should be determined on a continuing basis, and blood volume must be maintained. Blood pressure, pulse, central venous pressure, hematocrit, hourly urinary volume, and amount of blood obtained from the gastric tube or from the rectum all enter into this assessment. Many studies have shown the tendency to underestimate blood loss and inadequately transfuse massively bleeding patients who truly need aggressive therapy. Continued slow bleeding is best monitored by serial determinations of the hematocrit.

The following criteria define patients with a very low risk of serious bleeding: age less than 75 years, no unstable comorbid illness, no ascites evident on physical examination, normal prothrombin time, and, within 1 hour after admission, a systolic blood pressure above 100 mm Hg and nasogastric aspirate free of fresh blood. Patients with all six of these findings may be spared emergency endoscopy and discharged from the hospital early to undergo outpatient workup.

Several factors are associated with a worse prognosis with continued medical management of the bleeding episode. These are not absolute indications for laparotomy, but they should alert the clinician that emergency surgery may be required.

High rates of bleeding or amounts of blood loss predict high failure rates with medical treatment. Hematemesis is usually associated with more rapid bleeding and a greater blood volume deficit than melena. The presence of hypotension on admission to the hospital or the need for more than four units of blood to achieve circulatory stability implies a worse prognosis; if bleeding continues and subsequent transfusion requirements exceed 1 unit every 8 hours, continued medical management is usually unwise. The level of serum fibrin degradation products, indicating endogenous fibrinolysis, correlates with the severity of hemorrhage and the death rate. This may be a useful prognostic test, and the results could be used as a guide for the administration of fibrinolytic inhibitors in therapy. Evidence for or against this view is not yet available.

Total transfusion requirements also correlate with death rates. Death is uncommon when fewer than seven units of blood have been used, and the death rate rises progressively thereafter.

In general, bleeding from a gastric ulcer is more dangerous than bleeding from gastritis or duodenal ulcer, and patients with gastric ulcer should always be considered for early surgery. Regardless of the cause, if bleeding recurs after it has once stopped, the chances of success without operation are low. Most patients who rebleed in the hospital should have surgery.

Patients over age 60 tolerate continued blood loss less well than younger patients, and their bleeding should be stopped before secondary cardiovascular, pulmonary, or renal complications arise.

In 85% of patients, bleeding stops within a few hours of admission. About 25% of patients rebleed once bleeding has stopped. Rebleeding episodes are concentrated within the first 2 days of hospitalization, and if the patient has had no further bleeding for a period of 5 days, the chance of rebleeding is only 2%. Rebleeding is most common in patients with varices, peptic ulcer, anemia, or shock. About 10% of patients require surgery to control bleeding, and most

Table 23–2. Causes of massive upper gastrointestinal hemorrhage. Note that cancer is rarely the cause.

	Relative Incidence	
Common causes		
Peptic ulcer		45%
Duodenal ulcer	25%	
Gastric ulcer	20%	
Esophageal varices		20%
Gastritis		20%
Mallory-Weiss syndrome		10%
Uncommon causes		5%
Gastric carcinoma		
Esophagitis		
Pancreatitis		
Hemobilia		
Duodenal diverticulum		

of these patients have bleeding ulcers or, less commonly, esophageal varices. The death rate is 30% among patients who rebleed and 3% among those who do not. The mortality rate is also high in the elderly and in patients who are already hospitalized at the onset of bleeding. Analyses of large series of patients suggest that a number of those who died would not have done so if operations had been performed earlier and more often.

al-Mohana JM et al: Association of fibrinolytic tests with outcome of acute upper-gastrointestinal-tract bleeding. Lancet 1993;341:518.

Bordley DR et al: Early clinical signs identify low-risk patients with acute upper gastrointestinal hemorrhage. JAMA 1985;253:3282.

Branicki FJ et al: Emergency surgical treatment for nonvariceal bleeding of the upper part of the gastrointestinal tract. Surg Gynecol Obstet 1991;172:113.

Clason AE, Macleod DAD, Elton RA: Clinical factors in the prediction of further haemorrhage or mortality in acute upper gastrointestinal haemorrhage. Br J Surg 1986;73:985.

Cook DJ et al: Endoscopic therapy for acute nonvariceal upper gastrointestinal hemorrhage: A meta-analysis. Gastroenterology 1992;102:139.

Daneshmend TK et al: Omeprazole versus placebo for acute upper gastrointestinal bleeding: Randomised double blind controlled trial. Br Med J 1992;304:143.

Henry DA: Fibrinolysis and upper gastrointestinal bleeding. Lancet 1993;341:527.

Laine L et al: Prospective evaluation of immediate versus delayed refeeding and prognostic value of endoscopy in patients with upper gastrointestinal hemorrhage. Gastroenterology 1992;102:314.

Laine L: Upper gastrointestinal tract hemorrhage. West J Med 1991;155:274.

Laporte JR et al: Upper gastrointestinal bleeding in relation to previous use of analgesics and non-steroidal anti-inflammatory drugs. Catalan Countries Study on Upper Gastrointestinal Bleeding. Lancet 1991;337:85.

Morgan AG, Clamp SE: OMGE international upper gastrointestinal bleeding survey, 1978–1986. Scand J Gastroenterol 1988;23(Suppl 144):51.

Morris AJ, Wasson LA, MacKenzie JF: Small bowel enteroscopy in undiagnosed gastrointestinal blood loss. Gut 1992;33:887.

Sugawa C et al: Upper GI bleeding in an urban hospital: Etiology, recurrence, and prognosis. Ann Surg 1990;212:521.

HEMORRHAGE FROM PEPTIC ULCER

Approximately 20% of patients with peptic ulcer will experience a bleeding episode, and this complication is responsible for about 40% of the deaths from peptic ulcer. Peptic ulcer is the most common cause of massive upper gastrointestinal hemorrhage, accounting for over half of all cases. Chronic gastric and duodenal ulcers have about the same tendency to bleed, but the former produce more severe episodes. Bleeding ulcers are more common in persons with blood group O, though the reason for this association is not known.

Bleeding ulcers in the duodenum are usually located on the posterior surface of the duodenal bulb. As the ulcer penetrates, the gastroduodenal artery is exposed and may become eroded. Since no major blood vessels lie on the anterior surface of the duodenal bulb, ulcerations at this point are not as prone to bleed. Patients with concomitant bleeding and perforation usually have two ulcers, a bleeding posterior ulcer and a perforated anterior one. Postbulbar ulcers (those in the second portion of the duodenum) bleed frequently, though ulcers are much less common in this site than near the pylorus.

In some patients, the bleeding is sudden and massive, manifested by hematemesis and shock. In others, chronic anemia and weakness due to slow blood loss are the only findings. The diagnosis is unreliable when based on clinical findings, so endoscopy should be performed early (ie, within 24 hours) in most cases.

In the preceding section, the management of acute upper gastrointestinal hemorrhage, the selection of diagnostic tests, and the factors suggesting the need for operation were discussed. Most patients (75%) with bleeding peptic ulcer can be successfully managed by medical means alone. Initial therapeutic efforts usually halt the bleeding. H_2 Cimetidine decreases the risk of rebleeding, but blockers and omeprazole decrease the risk of rebleeding but have no effect on active bleeding.

After 12–24 hours have passed and the bleeding has clearly stopped, a patient who feels hungry should be fed. Twice-daily hematocrit readings should be ordered as a check on slow continued blood loss. Stools should be tested daily for the presence of blood; they will usually remain guaiac-positive for several days after bleeding stops.

Rebleeding in the hospital has been attended by a death rate of about 30%. A policy of early surgery for those who rebled would improve this figure. Patients who are over age 60, present with hematemesis, are actively bleeding at the time of endoscopy, or whose admission hemoglobin is below 8 g/dL have a higher risk of rebleeding. About three times as many patients with gastric ulcer (30%) rebled compared with those with duodenal ulcer. Most instances of rebleeding occur within 2 days from the time the first episode has stopped. In one study, only 3% of patients who stopped bleeding for this long bled again.

Endoscopic Therapy

Treatments administered through the endoscope may stop active bleeding or prevent rebleeding. Effective methods include injection into the ulcer of epinephrine, epinephrine plus 1% polidocanol (a sclerosing agent), or ethanol; or cautery using the heater probe, monopolar electrocautery, or the YAG laser. At least two modalities should be available to the endoscopist in the event one is unsuitable for a specific case or fails to work. Except for the laser, all are inexpensive. The indications for treatment are (1) active bleeding at the time of endoscopy and (2) the presence of a visible vessel in the base of the ulcer. Endoscopic therapy decreases transfusion requirements (by about half) and the rate of rebleeding (by about three-quarters) compared with sham-treated controls. When treatment fails the first time, it may often be repeated with a good chance of success. It is important, however, not to allow the patient to deteriorate during nonoperative attempts at halting the bleeding.

Emergency Surgery

About 10% of patients bleeding from a peptic ulcer require emergency surgery. Selection of those most likely to survive with surgical compared with medical treatment rests on the rate of blood loss and the other factors associated with a poor prognosis.

The overall death rate is significantly less after vagotomy and pyloroplasty than after gastrectomy for bleeding ulcer, and rebleeding occurs with about equal frequency after either procedure.

During laparotomy, the first step is to make a pyloroplasty incision if the endoscopic diagnosis is a bleeding duodenal ulcer. If a duodenal ulcer is found, the bleeding vessel should be suture-ligated and the duodenum and antrum inspected for additional ulcers. The pyloroplasty incision should then be closed and a truncal vagotomy performed. If the posterior wall of the duodenal bulb has been destroyed by a giant duodenal ulcer, a gastrectomy and Billroth II gastrojejunostomy may be preferable, since this somewhat uncommon ulcer is especially prone to bleed again if left in continuity with the stomach. Gastric ulcers can be handled by either gastrectomy or vagotomy and pyloroplasty. A thorough search should always be made for second ulcers or other causes of bleeding.

Prognosis

The death rate for an acute massive hemorrhage is about 15%. Careful study of the causes of death suggests that this figure could be improved by (1) more precise blood replacement–since undertransfusion is the cause of some complications and deaths; and (2) earlier surgery in selected patients who fall into serious-risk categories–since the tendency has been to perform surgery on too few patients too late in the illness. Patients who stop bleeding should be treated as outlined in the section on duodenal ulcer.

Branicki FJ et al: Emergency surgical treatment for nonvariceal bleeding of the upper part of the gastrointestinal tract. Surg Gynecol Obstet 1991;172:113.

Chung SCS et al: Injection or heat probe for bleeding ulcer. Gastroenterology 1991;100:33.

Cook DJ et al: Endoscopic therapy for acute nonvariceal upper gastrointestinal hemorrhage: A meta-analysis. Gastroenterology 1992;102:139.

Daneshmend TK et al: Omeprazole versus placebo for acute upper gastrointestinal bleeding: Randomised double blind controlled trial. Br Med J 1992;304:143.

Faulkner G et al: Aspirin and bleeding peptic ulcers in the elderly. Br Med J 1988;297:1311.

Garrigues-Gil V et al: Do the stigmata of recent haemorrhage have additional prognostic value in patients with bleeding duodenal ulcer? Scand J Gastroenterol 1988;23(Suppl 144):59.

Laine L et al: Prospective evaluation of immediate versus delayed refeeding and prognostic value of endoscopy in patients with upper gastrointestinal hemorrhage. Gastroenterology 1992;102:314.

Laine L: Multipolar electrocoagulation versus injection therapy in the treatment of bleeding peptic ulcers: A prospective, randomized trial. Gastroenterology 1990; 99:1303.

Matthewson K et al: Which peptic ulcer patients bleed? Gut 1988;29:70.

Miedema BW et al: Proximal gastric vagotomy in the emergency treatment of bleeding duodenal ulcer. Am J Surg 1991;161:64.

Richter JM et al: Practice patterns and costs of hospitalization for upper gastrointestinal hemorrhage. J Clin Gastroenterol 1991;13:268.

Sugawa C, Joseph AL: Endoscopic interventional management of bleeding duodenal and gastric ulcers. Surg Clin North Am 1992;72:317.

MALLORY-WEISS SYNDROME

Mallory-Weiss syndrome is responsible for about 10% of cases of acute upper gastrointestinal hemorrhage. The lesion consists of a 1- to 4-cm longitudinal tear in the gastric mucosa near the esophagogastric junction; it usually follows a bout of forceful retching. The disruption extends through the mucosa and submucosa but not usually into the muscularis mucosae. About 75% of these lesions are confined to the stomach; 20% straddle the esophagogastric junction; and 5% are entirely within the distal esophagus. Two-thirds of patients have a hiatal hernia.

The majority of patients are alcoholics, but the tear may appear after severe retching for any reason. Several cases have been reported following closed chest cardiac compression.

Clinical Findings

Typically, the patient first vomits food and gastric contents. This is followed by forceful retching and then bloody vomitus. Rapid increases in gastric pressure, sometimes aggravated by hiatal hernia, cause the tear. Actual rupture of the distal esophagus can also be produced by vomiting (Boerhaave's syndrome), but the difference seems to depend on vomiting of food in rupture and nonproductive retching in gastric mucosal tear.

Esophagogastroscopy is the most practical means of making the diagnosis.

Treatment & Prognosis

Initially, the patient is handled according to the general measures prescribed for upper gastrointestinal hemorrhage. In about 90% of patients, the bleeding stops spontaneously after ice-water lavage of the stomach. Patients who are still bleeding vigorously by the time endoscopy is performed are likely to require surgery. The bleeding can sometimes be controlled by endoscopic therapy (eg, electrocautery). If bleeding persists, surgical repair of the tear will be required.

If the diagnosis has been made before laparotomy, the surgeon should make a long, high gastrotomy after the abdomen is opened. The tear may be difficult to expose adequately. The search must be thorough, since in about 25% of patients there are two tears. A running polyglycolic acid (not catgut) suture should be used to oversew the lesion. Postoperative recurrence is rare.

Hastings PR, Peters KW, Cohn I: Mallory-Weiss syndrome: Review of 69 cases. Am J Surg 1981;142:560.

Michel L, Serrano A, Malt RA: Mallory-Weiss syndrome: Evolution of diagnostic and therapeutic patterns over two decades. Ann J Surg 1980;192:716.

Paquet KJ, Mercado-Diaz M, Kalk JF: Frequency, significance and therapy of the Mallory-Weiss syndrome in patients with portal hypertension. Hepatology 1990;11:879.

Sugawa C, Benishek D, Walt AJ: Mallory-Weiss syndrome: A study of 224 patients. Am J Surg 1983;145:30.

PYLORIC OBSTRUCTION DUE TO PEPTIC ULCER

The cycles of inflammation and repair in peptic ulcer disease may cause obstruction of the gastroduodenal junction as a result of edema, muscular spasm, and scarring. To the extent that the first two factors are involved, the obstruction may be reversible with medical treatment. Obstruction is usually due to duodenal ulcer and is less common than either bleeding or perforation. The few gastric ulcers that obstruct are close to the pylorus. Obstruction due to peptic ulcer must be differentiated from that caused by a malignant tumor of the antrum or of the pancreas. Malignancy is becoming the more common cause, and it may be difficult to identify.

Clinical Findings

A. Symptoms and Signs: Most patients with obstruction have a long history of symptomatic peptic ulcer, and as many as 30% have been treated for perforation or obstruction in the past. The patient often notes gradually increasing ulcer pains over weeks or months, with the eventual development of anorexia, vomiting, and failure to gain relief from antacids. The vomitus often contains food ingested several hours previously, and absence of bile staining reflects the site of blockage. Weight loss may be marked if the patient has delayed seeking medical care.

Dehydration and malnutrition may be obvious on physical examination but are not always present. A succussion splash can often be elicited from the retained gastric contents. Peristalsis of the distended stomach may be visible on gross inspection of the abdomen, but this sign is relatively rare. Most patients have upper abdominal tenderness. Tetany may appear with advanced alkalosis.

B. Laboratory Findings: Anemia is found in about 25% of patients. Prolonged vomiting leads to a unique form of metabolic alkalosis with dehydration. Measurement of serum electrolytes shows hypochloremia, hypokalemia, hyponatremia, and increased bicarbonate. Vomiting depletes the patient of Na^+, K^+, and Cl^-; the latter is lost in excess of Na^+ and K^+ as HCl. Gastric HCl loss causes extracellular HCO_3^- to rise, and renal excretion of HCO_3^- increases in an attempt to maintain pH. Large amounts of Na^+ are excreted in the urine with the HCO_3^-. Increasing Na^+ deficit evokes aldosterone secretion, which in turn brings about renal Na^+ conservation at the expense of more renal loss of K^+ and H^+. GFR may drop and produce a prerenal azotemia. The eventual result of the process is a marked deficit of Na^+, Cl^-, K^+, and H_2O. Treatment involves replacement of water and NaCl until a satisfactory urine flow has been established. KCl replacement should then be started. Details of management are found in Chapter 9.

C. Saline Load Test: This is a simple means of assessing the degree of pyloric obstruction and is useful in following the patient's progress during the first few days of nasogastric suction.

Through the nasogastric tube, 700 mL of normal saline (at room temperature) is infused over 3–5 minutes, and the tube is clamped. Thirty minutes later, the stomach is aspirated and the residual volume of saline recorded. Recovery of more than 350 mL indicates obstruction. It must be recognized that the results of a saline load test do not predict how well the stomach will handle solid food. Solid emptying can be measured with technetium Tc 99m-labeled chicken liver.

D. Imaging Studies: Plain abdominal x-rays may show a large gastric fluid level. An upper gastrointestinal series should not be performed until the stomach has been emptied, because dilution of the barium in the retained secretions makes a worthwhile study impossible.

E. Endoscopy: Gastroscopy is usually indicated to rule out the presence of an obstructing neoplasm.

Treatment

A. Medical Treatment: A large (32F) Ewald tube should be passed and the stomach emptied of its contents and lavaged until clean. After the stomach has been completely decompressed, a smaller tube should be inserted and placed on suction for several days to allow pyloric edema and spasm to subside and to permit the gastric musculature to regain its tone. A saline load test may be performed at this point to provide a baseline for later comparison. If chronic obstruction has produced severe malnutrition, total parenteral nutrition should be instituted.

After decompression of the stomach for 48–72 hours, the saline load test should be repeated. If this indicates sufficient improvement, the tube should be withdrawn and a liquid diet may be started. Gradual resumption of solid foods is permitted as tolerated.

B. Surgical Treatment: If 5–7 days of gastric aspiration do not result in relief of the obstruction, the patient should be treated surgically. Persistence of nonoperative effort beyond this point in the absence of progress rarely achieves the result hoped for. Failure of the obstruction to resolve completely (eg, if the patient can take only liquids) and recurrent obstruction of any degree are indications for surgery.

Surgical treatment may consist of a truncal or parietal cell vagotomy and drainage procedure (Figure 23–5). Truncal vagotomy and gastrojejunostomy is the easiest to perform laparoscopically.

Prognosis

About two-thirds of patients with acute obstruction fail to improve sufficiently on medical therapy and require operation to relieve the blockage. Patients who respond to medical treatment should be treated as outlined in the section on duodenal ulcer.

Donahue PE et al: Proximal gastric vagotomy with drainage for obstructing duodenal ulcer. Surgery 1988;104:757.

Ellis H: Pyloric stenosis complicating duodenal ulceration. World J Surg 1987;11:315.

Hom S et al: Postoperative gastric atony after vagotomy for obstructing peptic ulcer. Am J Surg 1989;157:282.

Jaffin BW, Kaye MD: The prognosis of gastric outlet obstruction. Ann Surg 1985;201:176.

PERFORATED PEPTIC ULCER

Perforation complicates peptic ulcer about half as often as hemorrhage. Most perforated ulcers are located anteriorly, though occasionally gastric ulcers perforate into the lesser sac. The 15% death rate correlates with increased age, female sex, and gastric perforations. The diagnosis is overlooked in about 5% of patients, most of whom do not survive.

Anterior ulcers tend to perforate instead of bleed because of the absence of protective viscera and major blood vessels on this surface. In less than 10% of cases, acute bleeding from a posterior "kissing" ulcer complicates the anterior perforation, an association that carries a high death rate. Immediately after perforation, the peritoneal cavity is flooded with gastroduodenal secretions that elicit a chemical peritonitis. Early cultures show either no growth or a light growth of streptococci or enteric bacilli. Gradually, over 12–24 hours, the process evolves into bacterial peritonitis. Severity of illness and occurrence of death are directly related to the interval between perforation and surgical closure.

In an unknown percentage of cases, the perforation becomes sealed by adherence to the undersurface of the liver. In such patients, the process may be self-limited, but a subphrenic abscess will develop in many.

Clinical Findings

A. Symptoms and Signs: The perforation usually elicits a sudden, severe upper abdominal pain whose onset can be recalled precisely. The patient may or may not have had preceding chronic symptoms of peptic ulcer disease. Perforation rarely is heralded by nausea or vomiting, and it typically occurs several hours after the last meal. Shoulder pain, if present, reflects diaphragmatic irritation. Back pain is uncommon.

The initial reaction consists of a chemical peritonitis caused by gastric acid or bile and pancreatic enzymes. The peritoneal reaction dilutes these irritants with a thin exudate, and as a result the patient's symptoms may temporarily improve before bacterial peritonitis occurs. The physician who sees the patient for the first time during this symptomatic lull must not be misled into interpreting it as representing bona fide improvement.

The patient appears severely distressed, lying quietly with the knees drawn up and breathing shallowly to minimize abdominal motion. Fever is absent at the start. The abdominal muscles are rigid owing to severe involuntary spasm. Epigastric tenderness may not be as marked as expected because the board-like rigidity protects the abdominal viscera from the palpating hand. Escaped air from the stomach may enter the space between the liver and abdominal wall, and upon percussion the normal dullness over the liver will be tympanitic. Peristaltic sounds are reduced or absent. If delay in treatment allows continued escape of air into the peritoneal cavity, abdominal distention and diffuse tympany may result.

The above description applies to the typical case of perforation with classic findings. In as many as one-third of patients, the presentation is not as dramatic, diagnosis is less obvious, and serious delays in treatment may result from failure to consider this condition and to obtain the appropriate abdominal x-rays. Many of these atypical perforations occur in patients already hospitalized for some unrelated illness, and the significance of the new symptom of abdominal pain is not appreciated. The only way to improve this record is to routinely obtain abdominal films on patients with abdominal pain of recent onset.

Lesser degrees of shock with minimal abdominal findings occur if the leak is small or rapidly sealed. A small duodenal perforation may slowly leak fluid that runs down the lateral peritoneal gutter, producing pain and muscular rigidity in the right lower quadrant and thus raising a problem of confusion with acute appendicitis.

Perforations may be sealed by omentum or by the liver, with the later development of a subhepatic or subdiaphragmatic abscess.

B. Laboratory Findings: A mild leukocytosis in the range of 12,000/µL is common in the early stages. After 12–24 hours, this may rise to 20,000/µL or more if treatment has been inadequate. The mild rise in the serum amylase value that occurs in many patients is probably caused by absorption of the enzyme from duodenal secretions within the peritoneal cavity. Direct measurement of fluid obtained by paracentesis may show very high levels of amylase.

C. Imaging Studies: Plain x-rays of the abdomen reveal free subdiaphragmatic air in 85% of patients. Films should be taken with the patient both supine and upright. A film in the left lateral decubitus position may be a more practical way to demonstrate free air in the uncomfortable patient. If the findings are questionable, 400 mL of air can be insufflated into the stomach through a nasogastric tube and the films repeated. Free air in the abdomen in a patient with sudden upper abdominal pain should clinch the diagnosis.

If no free air is demonstrated and the clinical picture suggests perforated ulcer, an emergency upper gastrointestinal series should be performed. If the perforation has not sealed, the diagnosis is established by noting escape of the contrast material from the lumen. Barium is more reliable than water-soluble contrast media, and, contrary to previous views, does not appear to aggravate infection or to be difficult to remove.

Differential Diagnosis

The differential diagnosis includes acute pancreatitis and acute cholecystitis. The former does not have as explosive an onset as perforated ulcer and is usually accompanied by a high serum amylase level. Acute cholecystitis with perforated gallbladder could mimic perforated ulcer closely but free air would not be present with ruptured gallbladder. Intestinal obstruction has a more gradual onset and is characterized by less sever pain that is crampy and accompanied by vomiting.

The simultaneous onset of pain and free air in the abdomen in the absence of trauma usually means perforated peptic ulcer. Free perforation of colonic diverticulitis and acute appendicitis are other rare causes.

Treatment

The diagnosis is often suspected before the patient is sent for confirmatory x-rays. Whenever a perforated ulcer is considered, the first step should be to pass a nasogastric tube and empty the stomach to reduce further contamination of the peritoneal cavity. Blood should be drawn for laboratory studies, and intravenous antibiotics (eg, cefazolin, cefoxitin) should be started. If the patient's overall condition is precarious owing to delay in treatment, fluid resuscitation should precede diagnostic measures. X-rays should be obtained as soon as the clinical status will permit.

The simplest surgical treatment, laparoscopy (or laparotomy) and suture closure of the perforation solves the immediate problem. The closure most often consists of securely plugging the hole with omentum (Graham-Steele closure) sutured into place rather than bringing together the two edges with sutures. All fluid should be aspirated from the peritoneal cavity, but drainage is not indicated. Reperforation is rare in the immediate postoperative period.

About three-fourths of patients whose perforation is the culmination of a history of chronic symptoms continue to have clinically severe ulcer disease after simple closure. This has gradually led to a more aggressive treatment policy involving a definitive ulcer operation for most patients with acute perforation, eg, parietal cell vagotomy plus closure of the perforation or truncal vagotomy and pyloroplasty. Now that ulcer disease can be cured by eradicating *H pylori,* the value of anything more than simple closure will have to be reexamined.

Concomitant hemorrhage and perforation are most often due to two ulcers, an anterior perforated one and a posterior one that is bleeding. Perforated ulcers that also obstruct obviously cannot be treated by suture closure of the perforation alone. Vagotomy plus gastroenterostomy or pyloroplasty should be performed. Perforated anastomotic ulcers require a vagotomy or gastrectomy, since in the long run, closure alone is nearly always inadequate.

Nonoperative treatment of perforated ulcer consists of continuous gastric suction and the administration of antibiotics in high doses. Although this has been shown to be effective therapy, with a low death rate, it is occasionally accompanied by a peritoneal and subphrenic abscess, and side effects are greater than with laparoscopic closure.

Prognosis

About 15% of patients with perforated ulcer die, and about a third of these are undiagnosed before surgery. The death rate of perforated ulcer seen early is low. Delay in treatment, advanced age, and associated systemic diseases account for most deaths.

Berne TV, Donovan AJ: Nonoperative treatment of perforated duodenal ulcer. Arch Surg 1989;124:830.
Boey J et al: Proximal gastric vagotomy. The preferred op-

eration for perforations in acute duodenal ulcer. Ann Surg 1988;208:169.

George RL; Smith IF: Long-term results after omental patch repair in patients with perforated duodenal ulcers: A 5- to 10-year follow-up study. Can J Surg 1991;34:447.

Macintyre IM, Millar A: Impact of H$_2$-receptor antagonists on the outcome of treatment of perforated duodenal ulcer. J R Coll Surg Edinb 1990;35:348.

Rabinovici R, Manny J: Perforated duodenal ulcer in the elderly. Eur J Surg 1991;157:121.

Shinagawa N et al: A bacteriological study of perforated duodenal ulcers. Jpn J Surg 1991;21:1.

Svanes C et al: A multifactorial analysis of factors related to lethality after treatment of perforated gastroduodenal ulcer. Ann Surg 1989;209:418.

Tanphiphat C et al: Surgical treatment of perforated duodenal ulcer: A prospective trial between simple closure and definitive surgery. Br J Surg 1985;72:370.

STRESS GASTRODUODENITIS, STRESS ULCER & ACUTE HEMORRHAGIC GASTRITIS

The term stress ulcer has been used to refer to a heterogeneous group of acute gastric or duodenal ulcers that develop following physiologically stressful illnesses. There are four major etiologic factors associated with such lesions: (1) shock, (2) sepsis, (3) burns, and (4) central nervous system tumors or trauma.

Etiology

A. Stress Ulcer: Acute ulcers following major surgery, mechanical ventilation, shock, sepsis, and burns (Curling's ulcers) have enough common features to suggest they evolve by a similar pathogenetic mechanism

Hemorrhage is the major clinical problem, though perforation occurs in about 10% of cases. Despite the predilection of stress ulcers to develop in the parietal cell mucosa, in about 30% of patients the duodenum is affected, and sometimes both stomach and duodenum are involved. Morphologically, the ulcers are shallow, discrete lesions with congestion and edema but little inflammatory reaction at their margins. Gastroduodenal endoscopy performed early in traumatized or burned patients has shown acute gastric erosions in the majority of patients within 72 hours after the injury (Figures 23–7 and 23–8). Such studies illustrate how frequently the disease process remains subclinical; clinically apparent ulcers develop in about 20% of susceptible patients. Clinically evident bleeding is usually seen 3–5 days after the injury, and massive bleeding generally does not appear until 4–5 days later.

Decreased mucosal resistance is the first step, which may involve the effects of ischemia (with production of toxic superoxide and hydroxyl radicals) and circulating toxins, followed by decreased muco-

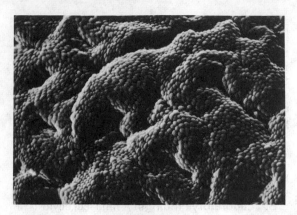

Figure 23–7. Scanning electron photomicrograph of the surface epithelium of a normal subject showing individual cells and numerous gastric pits. (Reduced from × 350.) (Courtesy of Jeanne M. Riddle.)

sal renewal, decreased production of endogenous prostanoids, and thinning of the surface mucus layer. Decreased gastric mucosal blood flow also plays a role by decreasing the supply of blood buffers available to neutralize hydrogen ions that are diffusing into the weakened mucosa. Experimental evidence has implicated platelet-activating factor, released by endotoxin, as a possible mediator of gut ulceration in sepsis. The mucosa is thus rendered more vulnerable to acid-pepsin ulceration and lysosomal enzymes. Acid hypersecretion may be involved to some extent, since burn patients who manifest serious bleeding have higher gastric acid output than patients with a more benign course. Disruption of the gastric mucosal barrier to back diffusion of acid has been found in less than half of patients and is now thought to be a manifestation of the disease rather than a cause.

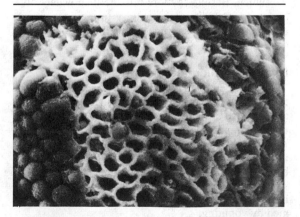

Figure 23–8. Scanning electron photomicrograph of the surface epithelium of a patient with acute gastric mucosal erosions, showing a patch of cellular defoliation. Lesions such as this may account for back diffusion of H$^+$. (Reduced from × 1145.) (Courtesy of Jeanne M. Riddle.)

B. Cushing's Ulcers: Acute ulcers associated with central nervous system tumors or injuries differ from stress ulcers because they are associated with elevated levels of serum gastrin and increased gastric acid secretion. Morphologically, they are similar to ordinary gastroduodenal peptic ulcers. Cushing's ulcers are more prone to perforate than other kinds of stress ulcers.

C. Acute Hemorrhagic Gastritis: This disorder may share some causative factors with the above conditions, but the natural history is different and the response to treatment considerably better. Most of these patients can be controlled medically. When surgery is required for alcoholic gastritis, a high proportion of patients are cured by pyloroplasty and vagotomy.

Clinical Findings

Hemorrhage is nearly always the first manifestation. Pain rarely occurs. Physical examination is not contributory except to reveal gross or occult fecal blood or signs of shock.

Prevention

H_2 receptor antagonists given prophylactically to critically ill patients decrease the incidence of stress erosions and overt bleeding. The drug may be given orally (eg, ranitidine, 150 mg through a nasogastric tube every 12 hours) or intravenously (eg, cimetidine, 50–100 mg/h). Sucralfate is also effective. Patients receiving total parenteral nutrition appear to be protected by this therapy and experience no increased benefit from H_2 antagonists. A concern that decreasing gastric acidity with H_2 blocking agents would increase the rate and severity of nosocomial pneumonia (from gastric bacterial overgrowth) has not been justified by experience.

Treatment

Initial management should consist of gastric lavage with chilled solutions and measures to combat sepsis if present. H_2 receptor blockers are of no value in the actively bleeding patient, but they probably decrease the rate of rebleeding once bleeding has stopped.

Some success has been reported with the selective infusion of vasoconstricting agents (eg, vasopressin) into the left gastric artery through a percutaneously placed catheter. In the sickest patients, if facilities and trained personnel are available, this technique should probably be attempted before operation is considered.

Perform laparotomy if the nonoperative regimen fails to halt the bleeding. Surgical treatment should consist of vagotomy and pyloroplasty, with suture of the bleeding points, or vagotomy and subtotal gastrectomy. There is a trend toward the first of these options, particularly in the sickest patients. When it occurs, rebleeding is nearly always from an ulcer left behind at the initial procedure. Rarely, total gastrectomy has had to be used because of the extent of ulceration and severity of bleeding or because of rebleeding after a lesser operation.

Cook DJ et al: Stress ulcer prophylaxis in the critically ill: A meta-analysis. Am J Med 1991;91:519.

Fabian TC et al: Pneumonia and stress ulceration in severely injured patients: A prospective evaluation of the effects of stress ulcer prophylaxis. Arch Surg 1993;128:185.

Kitler ME et al: Preventing postoperative acute bleeding of the upper part of the gastrointestinal tract. Surg Gynecol Obstet 1990;171:366.

Lamothe PH et al: Comparative efficacy of cimetidine, famotidine, ranitidine, and Mylanta in postoperative stress ulcers: Gastric pH control and ulcer prevention in patients undergoing coronary artery bypass graft surgery. Gastroenterology 1991;100:1515.

Martin LF et al: Continuous intravenous cimetidine decreases stress-related upper gastrointestinal hemorrhage without promoting pneumonia. Crit Care Med 1993;21:19.

Martin LF et al: Stress ulcers and organ failure in intubated patients in surgical intensive care units. Ann Surg 1992;215:332.

Miller TA, Tornwall MS, Moody FG: Stress erosive gastritis. Curr Probl Surg 1991 Jul 28(7):453.

Pemberton LB et al: Oral ranitidine as prophylaxis for gastric stress ulcers in intensive care unit patients: Serum concentrations and cost comparisons. Crit Care Med 1993;21:339.

Rosen HR, Vlahakes GJ, Rattner DW: Fulminant peptic ulcer disease in cardiac surgical patients: Pathogenesis, prevention, and management. Crit Care Med 1992;20:354.

Ruiz-Santana S et al: Stress-induced gastroduodenal lesions and total parenteral nutrition in critically ill patients: Frequency, complications, and the value of prophylactic treatment. A prospective, randomized study. Crit Care Med 1991;19:887.

Schuster DP: Stress ulcer prophylaxis: In whom? With what? Crit Care Med 1993;21:4.

GASTRIC CARCINOMA

There are about 20,000 new cases of carcinoma of the stomach in the USA annually. The incidence has dropped to one-third of what it was 30 years ago. This may reflect changes in the prevalence of *H pylori* infection, which has a role in the etiology of this disease. *H pylori* is known to be a cause of chronic atrophic gastritis, which in turn is a recognized precursor of gastric adenocarcinoma. Epidemiologic studies have linked gastric *H pylori* infection with a 3.6- to 18-fold (all patients versus women) increase in the risk of developing carcinoma of the body or antrum (not the cardia), and the risk is proportionate to serum levels of *H pylori* antibodies.

The present incidence in American males is ten new cases per 100,000 population per year. The highest rate, 63 per 100,000 males, is seen in Costa Rica; in eastern and central European countries, it is about 35 per 100,000 per year. Epidemiologic studies suggest that the incidence of gastric carcinoma is related to low dietary intake of vegetables and fruits and high intake of starches. Carcinoma of the stomach is rare under age 40, from which point the risk gradually climbs. The mean age at discovery is 63. It is about twice as common in men as in women.

Gastric epithelial cancers are nearly always adenocarcinomas. Squamous cell tumors of the proximal stomach involve the stomach secondarily from the esophagus. Five morphologic subdivisions correlate loosely with the natural history and outcome.

(1) Ulcerating carcinoma (25%): This consists of a deep, penetrating ulcer-tumor that extends through all layers of the stomach. It may involve adjacent organs in the process. The edges are shallow by contrast with overhanging edges noted in benign ulcers.

(2) Polypoid carcinomas (25%): These are large, bulky intraluminal growths that tend to metastasize late.

(3) Superficial spreading carcinoma (15%): Also known as early gastric cancer, superficial spreading carcinoma is confined to the mucosa and submucosa. Metastases are present in only 30% of cases. Even when metastases are present, the prognosis after gastrectomy is much better than for the more deeply invading lesions of advanced gastric cancer. In Japan, screening programs have been so successful that early gastric cancer now constitutes 30% of surgical cases, and survival rates have improved accordingly.

(4) Linitis plastica (10%): This variety of spreading tumor involves all layers with a marked desmoplastic reaction in which it may be difficult to identify the malignant cells. The stomach loses its pliability. Cure is rare because of early spread.

(5) Advanced carcinoma (35%): This largest category contains the big tumors that are found partly within and partly outside the stomach. They may originally have qualified for inclusion in the preceding groups but have outgrown that early stage.

Gastric adenocarcinomas can also be classified by degree of differentiation of their cells. In general, rate and extent of spread correlate with lack of differentiation. Some tumors are found histologically to excite an inflammatory cell reaction at their borders, and this feature indicates a relatively good prognosis. Tumors whose cells form glandular structures (intestinal type) have a somewhat better prognosis than tumors whose cells do not (diffuse type); the diffuse type is often associated with a substantial stromal component. The intestinal type of tumor accounts for a much larger proportion of cases in countries such as Japan and Finland where gastric cancer is especially common. The gradual decline in incidence in these areas is due principally to decreased occurrence of the intestinal type of tumor. Signet ring carcinomas, which contain more than 50% signet ring cells, have become increasingly more common and now constitute one-third of all cases. They behave as the diffuse type of cancer and occur more frequently in women, in younger patients, and in the distal part of the stomach. Previous *H pylori* infection is not associated with the development of any specific histologic type of gastric cancer.

Extension occurs by intramural spread, direct extraluminal growth, and lymphatic metastases. Pathologic staging, which correlates closely with survival, is illustrated in Figure 23–9. Three-fourths of patients have metastases when first seen. Within the stomach, proximal spread exceeds distal spread. The pylorus acts as a partial barrier, but tumor is found in 25% of cases in the first few centimeters of the bulb.

Early gastric cancer, defined as a primary lesion confined to the mucosa and submucosa with or without lymph node metastases, is associated with an excellent prognosis (5-year survival rate of 90%) after resection. In Japan, mass screening programs detect about 30% of patients with this lesion, whereas in the USA, only 10% of patients have early gastric cancer.

Forty percent of tumors are in the antrum, predominantly on the lesser curvature; 30% arise in the body and fundus, 25% at the cardia, and 5% involve the entire organ. Frequency of location has gradually changed, so that proximal lesions are more common now than 10–20 years ago. Benign ulcers develop at the greater curvature and cardia less commonly than malignant ones. Ulcers at these points are particularly suspect for neoplasm.

Clinical Findings

A. Symptoms and Signs: The earliest symptom is usually vague postprandial abdominal heaviness that the patient does not identify as a pain. Sometimes the discomfort is no different from other vague dyspeptic symptoms that have been intermittently present for years, but the frequency and persistence are new.

Anorexia develops early and may be most pronounced for meat. Weight loss, the most common symptom, averages about 6 kg. True postprandial pain suggesting a benign gastric ulcer is relatively uncommon, but if it is present one may be misled if subsequent x-rays show an ulcer. Vomiting may be present and becomes a major feature if pyloric obstruction occurs. It may have a coffee-ground appearance owing to bleeding by the tumor. Dysphagia may be the presenting symptom of lesions at the cardia.

An epigastric mass can be felt on examination in about one-fourth of cases. Hepatomegaly is present in 10% of cases. The stool will be positive for occult blood in half of patients, and melena is seen in a few. Otherwise, abnormal physical findings are confined to signs of distant spread of the tumor. Metastases to

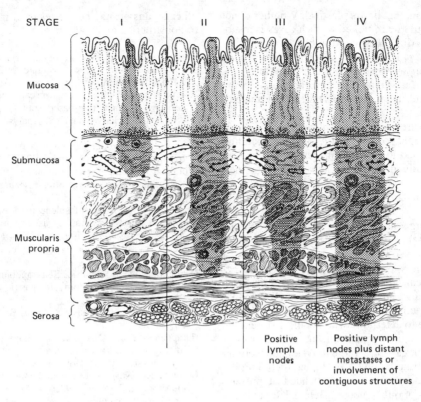

STAGE   I   II   III   IV

Mucosa

Submucosa

Muscularis propria

Serosa

Positive lymph nodes

Positive lymph nodes plus distant metastases or involvement of contiguous structures

Figure 23–9. Staging system for gastric carcinoma. The darkly shadowed areas represent cancers with different depths of mucosal penetration.

the neck along the thoracic duct may produce a Virchow node. Rectal examination may reveal a Blumer shelf, a solid peritoneal deposit anterior to the rectum. Enlarged ovaries (Krukenberg tumors) may be caused by intraperitoneal metastases. Further dissemination may involve the liver, lungs, brain, or bone.

B. Laboratory Findings: Anemia is present in 40% of patients. Carcinoembryonic antigen (CEA) levels are elevated in 65%, usually indicating extensive spread of the tumor.

C. Imaging Studies: An upper gastrointestinal series is diagnostic for many tumors, but the overall false-negative rate is about 20%. Major diagnostic problems are posed by ulcerating tumors, a few of which may not be distinguishable radiologically from benign peptic ulcers. The differential features are listed in the section on gastric ulcer, but x-rays alone will not establish a diagnosis of benign ulcer. All patients with a newly discovered gastric ulcer should undergo gastroscopy and gastric biopsy.

D. Gastroscopy and Biopsy: Large gastric carcinomas can usually be identified as such by their gross appearance at endoscopy. All gastric lesions, whether polypoid or ulcerating, should be examined by taking multiple biopsy and brush cytology specimens during endoscopy. False results are seen occa-

sionally as a result of sampling error, and a minimum of six biopsies is necessary for greatest accuracy.

Treatment

Surgical resection is the only curative treatment. About 85% of patients are operable, and in 50% the lesions are amenable to resection; of the resectable lesions, half are potentially curable (ie, no signs of spread beyond the limits of resection).

The surgical objective should be to remove the tumor, an adjacent uninvolved margin of stomach and duodenum, the regional lymph nodes, and, if necessary, portions of involved adjacent organs. The proximal margin should be a minimum of 6 cm from the gross tumor. If the tumor is located in the antrum, a curative resection would entail distal gastrectomy with en bloc removal of the omentum, a 3- to 4-cm cuff of duodenum and the subpyloric lymph nodes, and, in some instances, excision of the left gastric artery and nearby lymph nodes. Reconstruction after gastrectomy may be by either a Billroth I or II procedure, but the latter is preferable because postoperative growth of residual tumor near the pylorus may obstruct a gastroduodenal anastomosis early.

Total gastrectomy with splenectomy is required for tumors of the proximal half of the stomach and for extensive tumors (eg, linitis plastica). Whether or not the spleen should be removed in such cases is a subject of debate. Alimentary continuity is most often reestablished by a Roux-en-Y esophagojejunostomy. Construction of an intestinal pouch as a substitute food reservoir (eg, Hunt-Lawrence pouch) is of no nutritional value, and it increases the risks of immediate complications.

Esophagogastrectomy plus splenectomy with intrathoracic esophagogastrostomy is the operation usually performed for tumors of the cardia. The procedure is usually done through two separate incisions: first, a laparotomy for the gastric part, and then a right posterolateral thoracotomy for the anastomosis.

Japanese surgeons have devised a more detailed staging system than the one used in most other countries and have also recommended more aggressive lymphadenectomy as a matter of routine in the resection of gastric cancers. The results of resections as reported from Japan are better than those obtained by the standard operations described above, so attempts are being made to determine whether the difference is due to the more radical operations. Most Western surgeons are skeptical, and radical lymphadenectomy (eg, clearing all nodal levels up to and including the para-aortic nodes) is not recommended at present. For an analysis of this issue, see Behrns KE et al: Extended lymph node dissection for gastric cancer. Surg Clin North Am 1992;72:433.

The propensity for proximal submucosal spread must be appreciated at surgery. It is often advisable to perform a frozen section at the proximal margin before constructing the anastomosis. If tumor is found, the gastrectomy should be extended.

Palliative resection is usually indicated if the stomach is still movable and life expectancy is estimated to be more than 1–2 months. Palliative gastrectomy is usually performed to remove an antral lesion and prevent obstruction, but in selected cases, total gastrectomy is appropriate palliative treatment if the operation can be done safely and the amount of extragastric tumor is minimal. Whenever technically feasible, palliative gastrectomy is preferable to palliative gastrojejunostomy.

Adjuvant chemotherapy after curative surgery has not been of value with the regimens tested to date. For advanced disease, doxorubicin or fluorouracil alone, each of which results in a 20% response rate, is as good as a combination of chemotherapeutic agents.

Prognosis

In the USA, the overall 5-year survival rate is about 12%. The 5-year survival rate for patients with early gastric cancer is about 90%. The 5-year survival rates in relation to the extent of spread are stage I, 70%; stage II, 30%; stage III, 10%; and stage IV, 0%.

Death from tumor may follow dissemination to other organs or may be the result of progressive gastric obstruction and malnutrition.

Akoh JA, Macintyre IM: Improving survival in gastric cancer: Review of 5-year survival rates in English language publications from 1970. Br J Surg 1992;79:293.

Arveux P et al: Prognosis of gastric carcinoma after curative surgery: A population-based study using multivariate crude and relative survival analysis. Dig Dis Sci 1992;37:757.

Behrns KE et al: Extended lymph node dissection for gastric cancer. Surg Clin N Amer 1992;72:433.

Blomjous JG et al: Adenocarcinoma of the gastric cardia. Recurrence and survival after resection. Cancer 1992; 70:569.

Brady MS et al: Effect of splenectomy on morbidity and survival following curative gastrectomy for carcinoma. Arch Surg 1991;126:359.

Correa P: Is gastric carcinoma an infectious disease? N Engl J Med 1991;325:1170.

Dent DM, Madden MV, Price SK: Randomized comparison of R1 and R2 gastrectomy for gastric carcinoma. Br J Surg 1988;75:110.

Farley DR et al: Early gastric cancer. Br J Surg 1992;79: 539.

Haraguchi M et al: DNA ploidy is a major prognostic factor in advanced gastric carcinoma: Univariate and multivariate analysis. Surgery 1991;110:814.

Hermann RE: Newer concepts in the treatment of cancer of the stomach. Surgery, 1993;113:361.

Jaehne J et al: Lymphadenectomy in gastric carcinoma: A prospective and prognostic study. Arch Surg 1992; 127:290.

Kim JP et al: Results of surgery on 6589 gastric cancer patients and immunochemosurgery as the best treatment of advanced gastric cancer. Ann Surg 1992;216:269.

Korenaga D et al: DNA ploidy is closely linked to tumor invasion, lymph node metastasis, and prognosis in clinical gastric cancer. Cancer 1988;62:309.

Korenaga D et al: Results of resection of gastric cancer extending to adjacent organs. Br J Surg 1988;75:12.

Korenaga D et al: Trends in survival rates in Japanese patients with advanced carcinoma of the stomach. Surg Gynecol Obstet 1992;174:387.

Lauren P: Histogenesis of intestinal and diffuse types of gastric carcinoma. Scand J Gastroenterol 1991;26(Suppl 180):160.

Lawrence M, Shiu MH: Early gastric cancer. Ann Surg 1991,213:327.

Maehara Y et al: Predictors of lymph node metastasis in early gastric cancer. Br J Surg 1992;79:245.

Maehara Y et al: Prophylactic lymph node dissection in patients with advanced gastric cancer promotes increased survival time. Cancer 1992;70:392.

Monson JR et al: Total gastrectomy for advanced cancer. A worthwhile palliative procedure. Cancer 1991;68:1863.

Moreaux J, Msika S: Carcinoma of the gastric cardia: Surgical management and long-term survival. World J Surg 1988;12:229.

Nakamura K et al: Pathology and prognosis of gastric carcinoma: Findings in 10,000 patients who underwent primary gastrectomy. Cancer 1992;70:1030.

Nomura A et al: *Helicobacter pylori* infection and gastric

carcinoma among Japanese Americans in Hawaii. N Engl J Med 1991;325:1132.

Parsonnet J et al: *Helicobacter pylori* infection and the risk of gastric carcinoma. N Engl J Med 1991;325:1127.

Podolsky I et al: Gastric adenocarcinoma masquerading endoscopically as benign gastric ulcer. A five-year experience. Dig Dis Sci 1988;33:1057.

Sindelar WF et al: Randomized trial of intraoperative radiotherapy in carcinoma of the stomach. Am J Surg 1993;165:178.

Smith JW et al: Morbidity of radical lymphadenectomy in the curative resection of gastric carcinoma. Arch Surg 1991;126:1469.

Smith JW, Brennan MF: Surgical treatment of gastric cancer: Proximal, mid, and distal stomach. Surg Clin North Am 1992;72:381.

Sue-Ling HM et al: Early gastric cancer: 46 cases treated in one surgical department. Gut 1992;33:1318.

Wang LS et al: Lymph node metastasis in patients with adenocarcinoma of gastric cardia. Cancer 1993;71:1948.

Wright PA; Williams GT: Molecular biology and gastric carcinoma. Gut 1993;34:145.

GASTRIC POLYPS

Gastric polyps are single or multiple benign tumors that occur predominantly in the elderly. Those located in the distal stomach are more apt to cause symptoms. Whenever gastric polyps are discovered, gastric cancer must be ruled out.

Gastric polyps can be classified histologically as hyperplastic, adenomatous, or inflammatory. Other polypoid lesions, such as leiomyomas and carcinoid tumors, are discussed elsewhere. Hyperplastic polyps, which constitute 80% of cases, consist of an overgrowth of normal epithelium; they are not true neoplasms and have no relationship to gastric cancer. About 30% of adenomatous polyps contain a focus of adenocarcinoma, and adenocarcinoma can be found elsewhere in the stomach in 20% of patients with a benign adenomatous polyp. The incidence of cancer in an adenomatous polyp rises with increasing size. Lesions with a stalk and those less than 2 cm in diameter are usually not malignant. About 10% of benign adenomatous polyps undergo malignant change during prolonged follow-up.

Anemia may develop from chronic blood loss or deficient iron absorption. Over 90% of patients are achlorhydric after maximal stimulation. Vitamin B_{12} absorption is deficient in 25%, although megaloblastic anemia is present in only a few. Exfoliative cytologic examination of specimens obtained by endoscopy and brush biopsy should be performed in all patients.

Excision with a snare through the endoscope can be performed safely for most polyps. Otherwise, laparotomy is indicated for polyps greater than 1 cm in diameter or when cancer is suspected. Single polyps may be excised through a gastrotomy and a frozen section performed. If the polyp is found to be carcinoma, an appropriate type of gastrectomy is indicated. Partial gastrectomy should be performed for multiple polyps in the distal stomach. If 10–20 polyps are distributed throughout the stomach, the antrum should be removed and the fundic polyps excised. Total gastrectomy may be required for symptomatic diffuse multiple polyposis.

These patients should be followed because they have an increased risk of late development of pernicious anemia or gastric cancer. Recurrent polyps are uncommon.

Chua CL: Gastric polyps: the case for polypectomy and endoscopic surveillance. J R Coll Surg Edinb 1990;35:163.

Church JM et al: Gastroduodenal polyps in patients with familial adenomatous polyposis. Dis Colon Rectum 1992;35:1170.

Cristallini EG, Ascani S, Bolis GB: Association between histologic type of polyp and carcinoma in the stomach. Gastrointest Endosc 1992;38:481.

Dekker W: Clinical relevance of gastric and duodenal polyps. Scand J Gastroenterol 1990;178(Suppl):7.

Rugge M et al: Gastric epithelial dysplasia: a prospective multicenter follow-up study from the Interdisciplinary Group on Gastric Epithelial Dysplasia. Hum Pathol 1991;22:1002.

GASTRIC LYMPHOMA & PSEUDOLYMPHOMA

Lymphoma is the second most common primary cancer of the stomach but constitutes only 2% of the total number, 95% being adenocarcinomas. Almost all are non-Hodgkin's lymphomas and are generally classified as B cell mucosa-associated lymphoid tissue (MALT) lymphomas. They are further subclassified as low-grade or high-grade based on nuclear pattern. About 20% of patients manifest a second primary cancer in another organ.

The principal symptoms are epigastric pain and weight loss, similar to those of carcinoma. Characteristically, the tumor has attained bulky proportions by the time it is discovered; by comparison with adenocarcinoma of the stomach, the symptoms from a gastric lymphoma are usually mild in relation to the size of the lesion. A palpable epigastric mass is present in 50% of patients. Barium x-ray studies will demonstrate the lesion, although it usually is mistaken for adenocarcinoma or, in 10% of cases, for benign gastric ulcer. Gastroscopy with biopsy and brush cytology provides the correct diagnosis preoperatively in about 75% of cases. If a pathologic diagnosis has not been made, the surgeon may incorrectly judge the lesion to be inoperable carcinoma because of its large size. Preoperative staging should include a CT scan and bone marrow biopsy.

Treatment of low-grade gastric lymphoma consists of long-term chemotherapy with cyclophosphamide. Surgical resection followed by total abdominal radiotherapy may be the treatment of choice for high-grade lymphomas, but the subject is debated. Intraoperative staging should consist of needle biopsies of both lobes of the liver and biopsies of celiac and para-aortic lymph nodes. Splenectomy should be performed only if the spleen is directly invaded. Extension into the duodenum or esophagus should not lead to resection of these organs but to postoperative adjunctive therapy. The 5-year disease-free survival rate is 50%. Survival correlates with stage of disease, extent of penetration of the gastric wall, and histologic grade of the tumor. Most recurrences appear within 2 years of surgery. Because two-thirds of recurrences are outside the abdomen, patients at high risk of recurrence should receive postoperative chemotherapy also.

Gastric pseudolymphoma consists of a mass of lymphoid tissue in the gastric wall, often associated with an overlying mucosal ulcer. It is thought to represent a response to chronic inflammation. The lesion is not malignant, though the presentation, which includes pain, weight loss, and a mass on barium studies, cannot be distinguished from that of a malignant lesion.

Treatment of gastric pseudolymphoma consists of resection. The distinction from lymphoma is made on histologic examination of the specimen, which shows mature germinal centers in pseudolymphoma. No additional therapy is indicated postoperatively.

Blazquez M et al: Low grade B cell mucosa associated lymphoid tissue lymphoma of the stomach: clinical and endoscopic features, treatment, and outcome. Gut 1992;33:1621.

Castrillo JM et al: Gastric B-cell mucosa associated lymphoid tissue lymphoma: A clinicopathological study in 56 patients. Gut 1992;33:1307.

Cogliatti SB et al: Primary B-cell gastric lymphoma: A clinicopathological study of 145 patients. Gastroenterology 1991;101:1159.

Frazee RC, Roberts J: Gastric lymphoma treatment: Medical versus surgical. Surg Clin North Am 1992;72:423.

Shutze WP, Halpern NB: Gastric lymphoma. Surg Gynecol Obstet 1991;172:33.

Sweeney JF et al: Gastric pseudolymphoma: Not necessarily a benign lesion. Dig Dis Sci 1992;37:939.

GASTRIC LEIOMYOMAS & LEIOMYOSARCOMAS

Leiomyomas are common submucosal growths that are usually asymptomatic but may cause intestinal bleeding. Leiomyosarcomas may grow to a large size and most often present with bleeding. Radiologically, the tumor usually contains a central ulceration caused by necrosis from outgrowth of its blood supply. In most cases the tumor arises from the proximal stomach. It may grow into the gastric lumen, remain entirely on the serosal surface, or even become pedunculated within the abdominal cavity. Spread is by direct invasion or blood-borne metastases. CT scans provide useful information on the amount of extragastric extension. Leiomyomas should be removed by enucleation or wedge resection. After the more radical resections required for leiomyosarcomas, the 5-year survival rate is 20%. If technically possible, complete resection of metastases (eg, peritoneal, hepatic) in addition to the primary may improve the outcome. The results are affected by tumor size, DNA ploidy pattern, and tumor grade. Lesions that exhibit ten or more mitoses in a high-powered field rarely can be cured. The tumor is resistant to radiotherapy.

Eng-Hen Ng, Pollock RE, Romsdahl MM: Prognostic implications of patterns of failure for gastrointestinal leiomyosarcomas. Cancer 1992;69:1334.

Graham SM, Ballantyne GH, Modlin IM: Gastric epithelioid leiomyomatous tumors. Surg Gynecol Obstet 1987;164:391.

Megibow AJ et al: CT evaluation of gastrointestinal leiomyomas and leiomyosarcomas. AJR 1985;144:727.

Tsushima K et al: Leiomyosarcomas and benign smooth muscle tumors of the stomach: Nuclear DNA patterns studied by flow cytometry. Mayo Clin Proc 1987;62:275.

MÉNÉTRIER'S DISEASE

Ménétrier's disease, a form of hypertrophic gastritis, consists of giant hypertrophy of the gastric rugae; high, normal, or low acid secretion; and excessive loss of protein from the thickened mucosa into the gut, with resulting hypoproteinemia. The etiology may involve altered expression of TGFα. Clinical manifestations include edema, diarrhea, anorexia, weight loss, and skin rash. Chronic blood loss may also be a problem. Indigestion may respond to antacids, but this treatment does not improve the gastric pathologic process or secondary hypoproteinemia. The hypertrophic rugae present as enormous filling defects on upper gastrointestinal series and are frequently misinterpreted as carcinoma. The protein leak from the gastric mucosa may respond to atropine (and other anticholinergic drugs), hexamethonium bromide, or H_2 blocking agents or omeprazole. Rarely, total gastrectomy is indicated for severe intractable hypoproteinemia, anemia, or inability to exclude cancer. Medical management is best for most patients, though the gastric abnormalities and hypoproteinemia may persist. Some cases gradually evolve into atrophic gastritis. In children the disease characteristically is self-limited and benign. There is an increased risk of adenocarcinoma of the stomach in adults with Ménétrier's disease.

Bradburn DM et al: Medical therapy of Ménétrier's disease with omeprazole. Digestion 1992;52:204.

Dempsey PJ et al: Possible role of transforming growth factor alpha in the pathogenesis of Ménétrier's disease: Supportive evidence form humans and transgenic mice. Gastroenterology 1992;103:1950.

Komorowski RA, Caya JG: Hyperplastic gastropathy: Clinicopathologic correlation. Am J Surg Pathol 1991;15:577.

Mosnier JF et al: Hypertrophic gastropathy with gastric adenocarcinoma: Ménétrier's disease and lymphocytic gastritis? Gut 1991;32:1565.

Sundt TM, III, Compton CC, Malt RA: Ménétrier's disease: A trivalent gastropathy. Ann Surg 1988;208:694.

PROLAPSE OF THE GASTRIC MUCOSA

This uncommon lesion occasionally accompanies small prepyloric gastric ulcers. Episodes of vomiting and abdominal pain simulate peptic ulcer disease. X-ray shows prolapse of antral folds into the duodenum. One must be alert to the presence of gastric or duodenal ulcer as the underlying cause.

Antrectomy with a Billroth I anastomosis is occasionally required. Generally, conservative treatment suffices.

Shepherd HA et al: Recurrent retching with gastric mucosal prolapse. Dig Dis Sci 1984;29:121.

GASTRIC VOLVULUS

The stomach may rotate about its longitudinal axis (organo-axial volvulus) or a line drawn from the mid lesser to the mid greater curvature (mesenterioaxial volvulus). The former is more common and is often associated with a paraesophageal hiatal hernia. In other patients, eventration of the left diaphragm allows the colon to rise and twist the stomach by pulling on the gastrocolic ligament.

Acute gastric volvulus produces severe abdominal pain accompanied by a diagnostic triad (Brochardt's triad): (1) vomiting followed by retching and then inability to vomit, (2) epigastric distention, and (3) inability to pass a nasogastric tube. The situation calls for immediate laparotomy to prevent death from acute gastric necrosis and shock. An emergency upper gastrointestinal series will show a block at the point of the volvulus. The death rate is high.

Chronic volvulus is more common than acute. It may be asymptomatic or may cause crampy intermittent pain. Cases associated with paraesophageal hiatal hernia should be treated by repair of the hernia and anterior gastropexy. When cases are due to eventration of the diaphragm, the gastrocolic ligament should be divided the entire length of the greater curvature. The colon rises to fill the space caused by the eventration, and the stomach will resume its normal position, to be fastened by a gastropexy.

Carter R, Brewer LA III, Hinshaw DB: Acute gastric volvulus: Study of 25 cases. Am J Surg 1980;140:99.

Patel NM: Chronic gastric volvulus: Report of a case and review of literature. Am J Gastroenterol 1985;80:170.

GASTRIC DIVERTICULA

Gastric diverticula are uncommon and usually asymptomatic. Most are pulsion diverticula consisting of mucosa and submucosa only, located on the lesser curvature within a few centimeters of the esophagogastric junction. Those in the prepyloric region generally possess all layers and are more likely to be symptomatic. A few patients have symptoms from hemorrhage of inflammation within a gastric diverticulum, but for the most part these lesions are incidental findings on upper gastrointestinal series. Radiologically, they can be confused with a gastric ulcer.

Hughes W, Pierce WS: Surgical implications of gastric diverticula. Surg Gynecol Obstet 1970;131:99.

BEZOAR

Bezoars are concretions formed in the stomach. Trichobezoars are composed of hair and are usually found in young girls who pick at their hair and swallow it. Phytobezoars consist of agglomerated vegetable fibers. Pressure by the mass can create a gastric ulcer that is prone to bleed or perforate.

The postgastrectomy state predisposes to bezoar formation because pepsin and acid secretion are reduced and the triturating function of the antrum is gone. Orange segments or other fruits that contain a large amount of cellulose have been implicated in most cases. Improper mastication of food is a contributing factor that can sometimes be obviated by providing the patient with properly fitted dentures. The fruit may remain in the stomach or pass into the small intestine and cause obstruction. Some surgeons routinely warn postgastrectomy patients to avoid citrus fruits.

Large semisolid bezoars of *Candida albicans* have also been found in postgastrectomy patients. Some can be fragmented with the gastroscope. The patient should also be treated with oral nystatin.

Patients with symptomatic gastric bezoars may complain of abdominal pain. Ulceration and bleeding are associated with a death rate of 20%.

Nearly all gastric bezoars can be broken up and dispersed by endoscopy. Neglected lesions with complications (ie, bleeding or perforation) require gastrectomy.

Calabuig R et al: Gastric emptying and bezoars. Am J Surg 1989;157:287.

Chisholm EM et al: Phytobezoar: an uncommon cause of small bowel obstruction. Ann R Coll Surg Engl 1992;74:342.

Cifuentes Tebar J et al: Gastric surgery and bezoars. Dig Dis Sci 1992;37:1694.

Afridi SA, Fichtenbaum CJ, Taubin H: Review of duodenal diverticula. Am J Gastroenterol 1991;86:935.

Duarte B, Nagy KK, Cintron J: Perforated duodenal diverticulum. Br J Surg 1992;79:877.

Karoll MP et al: Diagnosis and management of intraluminal duodenal diverticulum. Dig Dis Sci 1983;28:411.

Trondsen E, Rosseland AR, Bakka AO: Surgical management of duodenal diverticula. Acta Chir Scand 1990;156:383.

II. DUODENUM*

DUODENAL DIVERTICULA

Diverticula of the duodenum are found in 20% of autopsies and 5–10% of upper gastrointestinal series. Symptoms are uncommon, and only 1% of those found by x-ray warrant surgery.

Duodenal pulsion diverticula are acquired outpouchings of the mucosa and submucosa, 90% of which are on the medial aspect of the duodenum. They are rare before age 40. Most are solitary and within 2.5 cm of the ampulla of Vater. There is a high incidence of gallstone disease of the gallbladder in patients with juxtapapillary diverticula. Diverticula are not seen in the first portion of the duodenum, where diverticular configurations are due to scarring by peptic ulceration or cholecystitis.

A few patients have chronic postprandial abdominal pain or dyspepsia caused by a duodenal diverticulum. Treatment is with antacids and anticholinergics.

Serious complications are hemorrhage or perforation from inflammation, pancreatitis, and biliary obstruction. Bile acid-bilirubinate enteroliths are occasionally formed by bile stasis in a diverticulum. Enteroliths can precipitate diverticular inflammation or biliary obstruction and, rarely, have caused bowel obstruction after entering the intestinal lumen.

Surgical treatment is required for complications and, rarely, for persistent symptoms. Excision and a two-layer closure are usually possible after mobilization of the duodenum and dissection of the diverticulum from the pancreas. Removal of the diverticulum and closure of the defect are superior to simple drainage in the case of perforation. If biliary obstruction appears in a patient whose bile duct empties into a diverticulum, excision might be more hazardous than a side-to-side choledochoduodenostomy.

The rare wind sock type of intraluminal diverticulum usually presents with vague epigastric pain and postprandial fullness, though intestinal bleeding or pancreatitis is occasionally seen. The diagnosis can be made by barium x-ray studies. The diverticulum can be excised through a nearby duodenotomy. In some cases, the narrow diverticular outlet can be enlarged endoscopically.

DUODENAL TUMORS

Tumors of the duodenum are rare. Carcinoma of the ampulla of Vater is discussed in Chapter 27.

1. MALIGNANT DUODENAL TUMORS

Most malignant duodenal tumors are adenocarcinomas, leiomyosarcomas, or lymphomas. They appear in the descending duodenum more often than elsewhere. Pain, obstruction, bleeding, obstructive jaundice, and an abdominal mass are the modes of presentation. Duodenal carcinomas, particularly those in the third and fourth portions of the duodenum, are often missed on barium x-ray studies. Endoscopy and biopsy will usually be diagnostic if the examiner is suspicious enough and can reach the lesion.

If possible, adenocarcinomas and leiomyosarcomas should be resected. Pancreaticoduodenectomy is usually necessary if the tumor is localized. Unresectable lesions should be treated by radiotherapy. Biopsy and radiotherapy are recommended for lymphoma.

After curative resections, the 5-year survival rate is 30%. The overall 5-year survival rate is 18%.

2. BENIGN DUODENAL TUMORS

Brunner's gland adenomas are small submucosal nodules that have a predilection for the posterior duodenal wall at the junction of the first and second portions. Sessile and pedunculated variants are seen. Symptoms are due to bleeding or obstruction. Leiomyomas may also be found in the duodenum and ordinarily are asymptomatic.

Carcinoid tumors of the duodenum are often endocrinologically active, producing gastrin, somatostatin, or serotonin. Simple excision is the treatment of choice.

Heterotopic gastric mucosa, presenting as multiple small mucosal nodules, is an occasional endoscopic finding of no clinical significance.

Villous adenomas of the duodenum may give rise to intestinal bleeding or may obstruct the papilla of Vater and cause jaundice. As in the colon, the risk of

---

*Duodenal ulcer is discussed on p 466.

malignant change is high—about 50%. Small pedunculated villous adenomas may be snared during endoscopy, but sessile tumors must be locally excised via laparotomy. Tumors that contain malignant tissue should be treated by a Whipple procedure.

Beckwith PS, van Heerden JA, Dozois RR: Prognosis of symptomatic duodenal adenomas in familial adenomatous polyposis. Arch Surg 1991;126:825.

Bjork KJ et al: Duodenal villous tumors. Arch Surg 1990;125:961.

Burke AP et al: Carcinoid tumors of the duodenum: A clinicopathologic study of 99 cases. Arch Pathol Lab Med 1990;114:700.

Burke AP et al: Somatostatin-producing duodenal carcinoids in patients with von Recklinghausen's neurofibromatosis: A predilection for black patients. Cancer 1990;65:1591.

Kazerooni EA, Quint LE, Francis IR: Duodenal neoplasms: Predictive value of CT for determining malignancy and tumor resectability. AJR Am J Roentgenol 1992;159:303.

Lowell JA et al: Primary adenocarcinoma of third and fourth portions of duodenum: Favorable prognosis after resection. Arch Surg 1992;127:557.

Michelassi F et al: Experience with 647 consecutive tumors of the duodenum, ampulla, head of the pancreas, and distal common bile duct. Ann Surg 1989;210:544.

Remmele W et al: Three other types of duodenal polyps: Mucosal cysts, focal foveolar hyperplasia, and hyperplastic polyp originating from islands of gastric mucosa. Dig Dis Sci 1989;34:1468.

SUPERIOR MESENTERIC ARTERY OBSTRUCTION OF THE DUODENUM

Rarely, obstruction of the third portion of the duodenum is produced by compression between the superior mesenteric vessels and the aorta. It most commonly appears after rapid weight loss following injury, including burns. Patients in body casts are particularly susceptible.

The superior mesenteric artery normally leaves the aorta at an angle of 50–60 degrees, and the distance between the two vessels where the duodenum passes between them is 10–20 mm. These measurements in patients with superior mesenteric artery syndrome average 18 degrees and 2.5 mm. Acute loss of mesenteric fat is thought to permit the artery to drop posteriorly, trapping the bowel like a scissors.

Skepticism exists regarding the frequency of this condition in adults who have not experienced acute loss of weight. Most often the patient in question is a thin, nervous woman whose complaints of dyspepsia and occasional emesis are more properly explained on a functional basis. When a clear-cut example is encountered, it may actually represent a form of intestinal malrotation with duodenal bands.

The patient complains of epigastric bloating and crampy pain relieved by vomiting. The symptoms may remit in the prone position. Anorexia and postprandial pain lead to additional malnutrition and weight loss.

Upper gastrointestinal x-rays demonstrate a widened duodenum proximal to a sharp obstruction at the point where the artery crosses the third portion of the duodenum. When the patient moves to the knee-chest position, the passage of barium is suddenly unimpeded. Further verification can be provided if angiography shows an angle of 25 degrees or less between the superior mesenteric artery and the aorta. However, this procedure is not recommended for routine evaluation of obvious cases.

Many patients whose superior mesenteric artery makes a prominent impression on the duodenum are asymptomatic, and in ambulatory patients one should hesitate to attribute vague chronic complaints to this finding.

Involvement of the duodenum by scleroderma leads to duodenal dilatation and hypomotility and an x-ray and clinical picture highly suggestive of superior mesenteric artery syndrome. In the latter, increased duodenal peristalsis should be demonstrable proximal to the arterial blockage, whereas diminished peristalsis characterizes scleroderma. Patients with duodenal scleroderma usually have dysphagia from concomitant esophageal involvement.

Malrotation with duodenal obstruction by congenital bands can mimic this syndrome.

Postural therapy may suffice. The patient should be placed prone when symptomatic or in anticipation of postprandial difficulties. Ambulatory patients should be instructed to assume the knee-chest position, which allows the viscera and the artery to rotate forward off the duodenum.

Chronic obstruction may require section of the suspensory ligament and mobilization of the duodenum, or a duodenojejunostomy to bypass the obstruction. Patients with various forms of malrotation should be treated by mobilizing the duodenojejunal flexure, which releases the duodenum from entrapment by congenital bands.

Hines JR et al: Superior mesenteric artery syndrome: Diagnostic criteria and therapeutic approaches. Am J Surg 1984;148:630.

Hutchinson DT, Bassett GS: Superior mesenteric artery syndrome in pediatric orthopedic patients. Clin Orthop 1990 Jan;(250):250.

Ylinen P, Kinnunen J, Hockerstedt K: Superior mesenteric artery syndrome: A follow-up study of 16 operated patients. J Clin Gastroenterol 1989;11:386.

REGIONAL ENTERITIS
OF THE STOMACH & DUODENUM

The proximal intestine and stomach are rarely involved in regional enteritis, though this disease has now been reported in every part of the gastrointestinal tract from the lips to the anus. Most patients with Crohn's disease in the stomach or duodenum have ileal involvement as well.

Pain can in many instances be relieved by antacids. Intermittent vomiting from duodenal stenosis or pyloric obstruction is frequent. The x-ray finding of a cobblestone mucosa or stenosis would be suggestive when associated with typical changes in the ileum. The endoscopic appearance is fairly characteristic, and biopsy with the peroral suction device usually gives an adequate specimen for histologic confirmation of the diagnosis.

Medical treatment is nonspecific and consists principally of corticosteroids during exacerbations. Surgery may be indicated for disabling pain or obstruction. If the disease is localized to the stomach, a partial gastrectomy can be performed. Duodenal involvement most often requires a gastrojejunostomy to bypass the obstruction. Vagotomy should also be performed to prevent development of a marginal ulcer. Recurrent Crohn's disease involving the anastomosis is an occasional late complication, but it can usually be managed successfully by reoperation.

Internal fistulas involving the stomach or duodenum usually represent extensions from primary disease in the ileum or colon. Surgical treatment consists of resection of the diseased ileum or colon and closure of the fistulous opening in the upper gut.

Jacobson IM et al: Gastric and duodenal fistulas in Crohn's disease. Gastroenterology 1985;89:1347.

Ross TM, Fazio VW, Farmer RG: Long-term results of surgical treatment for Crohn's disease of the duodenum. Ann Surg 1983;197:399.

Shepherd AFI et al: The surgical treatment of gastroduodenal Crohn's disease. Ann R Coll Surg Engl 1985;67:382.

Liver

24

Lawrence W. Way, MD

Liver transplantation is discussed in Chapter 48. The physiology of bilirubin metabolism and the diagnostic approach to the jaundiced patient are covered in Chapter 26.

SURGICAL ANATOMY

Segments

The liver develops as an embryologic outpouching from the duodenum by a process described in Chapter 26. The liver is one of the largest organs in the body, representing 2% of the total body weight. In classic descriptions, the liver was characterized as having four lobes: right, left, caudate, and quadrate. However, these traditional lobes do not describe the true segmental anatomy of the liver, which is depicted in Figure 24–1. The main lobar fissure can be thought of as represented by an oblique plane passing posteriorly from the gallbladder bed to the vena cava, dividing the anatomic right and left lobes. This primary division is to the right of the falciform ligament. The right lobe is subdivided into anterior and posterior segments by the right segmental fissure. The left lobe is subdivided into medial and lateral segments by the left segmental fissure, marked by the position of the falciform ligament.

The relationship of the liver to the other abdominal organs is shown in Figure 24–2.

Venous Blood Supply (Figure 24–3)

Both the portal and hepatic venous systems lack valves. The portal vein terminates in the porta hepatis by dividing into right and left lobar branches. The right lobar branch immediately follows the course of the segmental ducts and arteries. The left lobar branch has two portions: the transverse part and the umbilical part. The former is a short segment coursing through the porta hepatis. The latter descends into the umbilical fossa and supplies the medial and lateral segments of the left lobe.

The hepatic veins represent the final common pathway for the central veins of the lobules of the liver. There are three major hepatic veins: left, right, and middle. The middle hepatic vein lies in the major lobar fissure and drains blood from the medial segment of the left lobe and the inferior portion of the anterior segment of the right lobe. The left hepatic vein drains the lateral segment of the left lobe, and the right hepatic vein drains the posterior segment and much of the anterior segment of the right lobe. Several small accessory veins enter the inferior vena cava directly from the posterior segment of the right lobe and must be carefully ligated during a right hemihepatectomy. The middle hepatic vein usually joins the left hepatic vein before they meet the inferior vena cava.

Arterial Blood Supply

The common hepatic artery arises from the celiac axis, ascends in the hepatoduodenal ligament, and gives rise to the right gastric and gastroduodenal arteries before dividing into right and left branches in the hilum. The hepatic artery supplies approximately 25% of the 1500 mL of blood that enters the liver each minute; the remaining 75% is supplied by the portal vein. In 10% of individuals, the common hepatic artery has an anomalous origin. In the most common variants, the common hepatic or the right hepatic artery arises from the superior mesenteric artery. The left hepatic originates from the left gastric artery in 15% of subjects. The common hepatic artery divides to follow the segmental ducts. Once they enter the liver and divide, the various segmental branches are termed end-arteries, since they do not communicate with each other via collaterals.

Biliary Drainage

Segmental bile ducts drain each segment. The right anterior and right posterior segmental ducts unite to form the right hepatic duct, and the left lateral and left medial segmental ducts form the left hepatic duct. These lobar ducts join outside the parenchyma to form the common hepatic duct. Anatomic variations are common. In over 25% of specimens, the duct from the right posterior segment joins the left hepatic duct independently. Variations are far less common on the left side.

Lymphatics

Superficial lymphatics arise from superficial por-

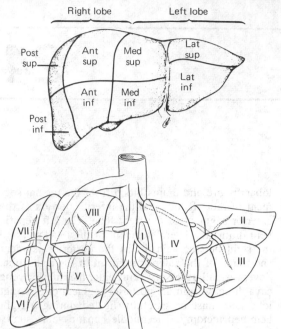

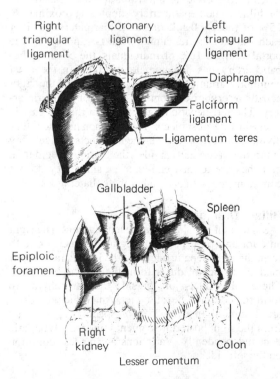

Figure 24–1. Segmental anatomy of the liver with the two most popular versions of segmental terminology. The major lobar fissure, separating the right and left lobes, passes from the inferior vena cava through the gallbladder bed.

Figure 24–2. Relationships of the liver to adjacent abdominal organs.

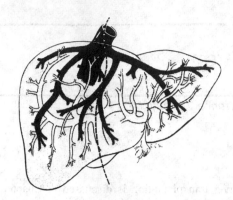

Figure 24–3. Anatomy of the veins of the liver. The major lobar fissure is represented by the dashed line. Branches of the hepatic artery and biliary ducts follow those of the portal vein. The darker vessels represent the hepatic veins and vena cava; the lighter system represents the portal vein and its branches.

tions of the lobules and pass beneath the capsule to enter the posterior mediastinum via the diaphragm and the suspensory ligaments of the liver. Some enter the porta hepatis and others enter the coronary chain. Other lymphatics arise deep in the liver lobules and pass either with the hepatic veins along the vena cava or with the portal veins into the porta hepatis.

HEPATIC RESECTION

The indications for resection of portions of the liver include primary and secondary malignant tumors, benign tumors, traumatic ruptures, cysts, and abscesses. Removal of as much as 80–85% of the normal liver is consistent with survival. Liver function may be decreased for several weeks after extensive resection, but the extraordinary regenerative capacity of the liver rapidly provides new functioning hepatocytes. Within 24 hours after partial hepatectomy, cell replication becomes active and continues until the original weight of the organ is restored. Considerable regeneration occurs within 10 days, and the process is essentially complete by 4–5 weeks. Excised lobes are not re-formed as such. Rather, the growth consists of formation of new lobules and expansion of residual lobules. The stimuli for hepatic regeneration are thought to include the following: hepatocyte growth factor, TGFα, heparin binding growth factor, hepatopoietin B, and disinhibition by TGFβ_1 (ie, decreased levels of this inhibitor of hepatic growth).

Preoperative Evaluation

Since liver function is compromised after major hepatic resection, the decision to perform such operations must take into account the preoperative functional status. Cirrhosis is a relative contraindication for partial hepatectomy because the limited reserve of the residual cirrhotic liver is usually insufficient to meet essential metabolic demands and the cirrhotic liver has little capacity for regeneration. These factors prohibit resection of some primary hepatic tumors that develop in cirrhotics.

Extent of Hepatic Resection

Based upon the labor anatomy, hepatic resections are classified as segmental or nonsegmental. Wedge resections and resectional debridement of devitalized tissue are examples of the latter. Major lobar resections must be planned in accordance with the segmental vascular anatomy (Figure 24–3). The terminology and extent of the common types of resections are depicted in Figure 24–4. The operation entails removal of a lobe or segment with its afferent and efferent vessels while avoiding injury to vessels and bile ducts supplying the residual tissue. An extended right hepatectomy—the most extensive—removes all but 15–20% of the hepatic mass.

Most elective hepatic lobectomies can be performed through an abdominal incision, though some surgeons prefer a thoracoabdominal approach for right lobectomies. The key to technical success is hemostasis.

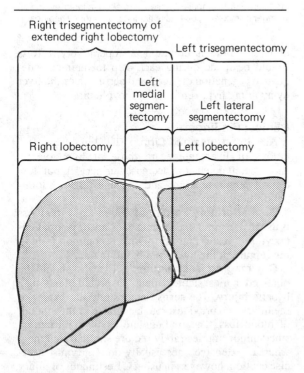

Figure 24–4. Terminology of various segmental resections of the liver. Lobectomy is sometimes referred to as hemihepatectomy.

Postoperative Course

If 50% or more of the liver has been removed, the patient will require close monitoring for the first week or two after operation. Patients without cirrhosis usually exhibit few metabolic changes postoperatively and are often ready for discharge on the seventh or eighth day after surgery. In the presence of cirrhosis or septic complications, postoperative liver function may be impaired.

The blood glucose level may fall immediately after surgery if it is not maintained by parenteral infusions. The glucose concentration should be measured twice daily for the first 2 days and 5% or 10% glucose administered intravenously to avoid hypoglycemia. The serum albumin concentration may drop. If the prothrombin level falls, vitamin K should be given. Low concentrations of fibrinogen and factor IX usually improve spontaneously and require no treatment.

Occasionally, the serum bilirubin will rise several days after resection, but it usually returns to normal within 1–2 weeks. The alkaline phosphatase usually remains normal. AST and serum LDH rise for several days and then return to normal levels.

Complications

Postoperative fever may be due to pulmonary complications or perihepatic abscess formation, but in many cases no cause can be identified, and convalescence in the latter patients may be otherwise unmarred. Abscesses formed in the space created by the resection can usually be drained by percutaneous catheters.

Because partial hepatectomy is attended by a relatively high incidence of stress ulcers, prophylactic H_2 receptor antagonists should be given routinely after operation. Liver failure may result if the residual tissue is diseased or has been compromised by prolonged ischemia during the operation. Ascites, varices, and coma are the manifestations.

Prognosis

The death rate of elective hepatectomy is now less than 5% and is largely related to postoperative liver failure, infection, or associated conditions.

Elias D et al: Prolonged intermittent clamping of the portal triad during hepatectomy. Br J Surg 1991;78:42.

Iwatsuki S, Sheahan DG, Starzl TE: The changing face of hepatic resection. Curr Probl Surg 1989;26:287.

Jamieson GG et al: Major liver resection without a blood transfusion: Is it a realistic objective? Surgery 1992; 112:32.

Launois B, Jamieson GG: The importance of Glisson's capsule and its sheaths in the intrahepatic approach to resection of the liver. Surg Gynecol Obstet 1992;174:7.

Launois B, Jamieson GG: The posterior intrahepatic approach for hepatectomy or removal of segments of the liver. Surg Gynecol Obstet 199;174:155.

Lerut J et al: Resection of the caudate lobe of the liver. Surg Gynecol Obstet 1990;171:160.

Matsumata T et al: Modified technique of Pringle's maneuver in resection of the liver. Surg Gynecol Obstet 1991;172:245.

Mentha G et al: Elective hepatic resection in the elderly. Br J Surg 1992;79:557.

Paul AM et al: Hepatic failure and coma after liver resection is reversed by manipulation of gut contents: The role of endotoxin. Surgery 1991;110:169.

Selden AC, Hodgson HJF: Growth factors and the liver. Gut 1991;32:601.

Suc Bet al: "Natural history" of hepatectomy. Br J Surg 1992;79:39.

Sukru E et al: Liver resection under total vascular isolation. Ann Surg 1993;217:15.

Taniguchi H et al: Vascular inflow exclusion and hepatic resection. Br J Surg 1992;79:672.

DISEASES & DISORDERS OF THE LIVER

HEPATIC TRAUMA
(Table 24–1)

Based on the mechanism of injury, liver trauma is classified as penetrating or blunt. Penetrating wounds, constituting more than half of cases, are due to bullets, knives, etc. In civilian practice, most of these tend to be clean wounds—dangerous because of abdominal bleeding but not producing much devitalization of liver substance. In contrast, high-velocity missiles, in addition to piercing the liver, shatter the parenchyma for a variable distance from the track of the missile.

Blunt trauma can be inflicted by a direct blow to the upper abdomen or lower right rib cage or can follow sudden deceleration, as occurs with a fall from a great height. Most often a consequence of automobile accidents, direct blunt trauma tends to produce explosive bursting wounds or linear lacerations of the hepatic surface, often with considerable parenchymal destruction. The stellate, bursting type of injury tends to affect the posterior superior segment of the right lobe because of its relatively vulnerable location, convex surface, fixed position, and concentration of hepatic mass. Damage to the left lobe is much less common than damage to the right. Injuries that involve shearing forces can tear the hepatic veins where they enter the liver substance, producing an exsanguinating retrohepatic injury in an area difficult to surgically expose and repair. The staging system described in Table 24–1 is used to categorize liver injuries and provide a common language in order to allow comparisons of results of treatment between institutions.

The principal surgical goals are to stop bleeding and debride devitalized liver. Because some degree

Table 24–1. Liver Injury Scale.[1]

Grade	Type	Description
I	Hematoma	Subcapsular, nonexpanding, <10% surface area.
	Laceration	Capsular tear, nonbleeding; <1 cm deep in parenchyma.
II	Hematoma	Subcapsular, nonexpanding, 10–50% surface area; intraparenchymal, nonexpanding, <2 cm in diameter.
	Laceration	Capsular tear, active bleeding; 1–3 cm deep into the parenchyma, <10 cm long.
III	Hematoma	Subcapsular, >50% surface area or expanding; ruptured subcapsular hematoma with active bleeding; intraparenchymal hematoma >2 cm or expanding.
	Laceration	>3 cm deep into the parenchyma.
IV	Hematoma	Ruptured intraparenchymal hematoma with active bleeding.
	Laceration	Parenchymal disruption involving >50% of hepatic lobe.
V	Laceration	Parenchymal disruption involving >50% of hepatic lobe.
	Vascular	Juxtahepatic venous injuries; ie, retrohepatic vena cava or major hepatic veins.
VI	Vascular	Hepatic avulsion.

[1]Increase by one grade when there are two or more injuries to the liver. Grading applied based on best available evidence, whether from x-rays, operative findings, or autopsy findings.

of liver failure is common postoperatively, efforts should be made during each step to maintain adequate oxygenation of blood and perfusion of the liver by avoiding hypoxemia and hypovolemia.

Clinical Findings

A. Symptoms and Signs: The clinical manifestations of liver injury are those of hypovolemic shock, ie, hypotension, decreased urinary output, low central venous pressure, and, in some cases, abdominal distention.

B. Laboratory Findings: The rate of blood loss is usually so rapid that anemia does not develop. Leukocytosis greater than 15,000/μL is common following rupture of the liver from blunt trauma.

C. Imaging Techniques: CT scans should be obtained in most stable patients suspected of having a hepatic injury. The scans demonstrate the extent of the injury and provide a rough estimate of the amount of blood loss. The findings are useful for triaging, since minor injuries rarely require surgical treatment whereas extensive ones usually do. One must exercise caution, however, in using CT estimates of injury grade, since they correlate poorly (ie, they both understage and overstage) with what is found at surgery.

Sonography has not been helpful. Angiography is diagnostic in hemobilia.

Treatment

Patients with stable minor injuries may be managed expectantly unless symptoms or signs of bleeding appear. The CT findings in patients who may be considered for nonoperative management include contained subcapsular or intrahepatic hematoma, unilobar fracture, absence of devitalized liver, minimal intraperitoneal blood, and absence of injuries to other intra-abdominal organs. Serial CT scans should be obtained to verify the assumption that the lesion is stable rather than expanding.

Most patients have CT or clinical evidence of active bleeding or a major injury, however, and require prompt exploration.

Most lacerations have stopped bleeding by the time operation is performed. In the absence of active hemorrhage, these wounds should be drained but not sutured. Active bleeding should be managed by clipping or direct suture of identifiable vessels, not by mass ligatures. Subcapsular hematomas often overlie an active bleeding site or parenchyma in need of debridement and should be explored even though the injury appears to be tamponaded and of limited severity. Blunt injuries associated with substantial amounts of parenchymal destruction may be particularly difficult to manage. Rarely, a very severe pulverizing injury requires formal lobectomy.

Temporary occlusion of the hepatic artery and portal vein with a vascular clamp (Pringle's maneuver) for periods of 15–20 minutes may permit more accurate ligation of bleeding vessels in the wound. If this is unsuccessful, the bleeding area should be packed; the packing is removed under general anesthesia 2–3 days later. Absorbable gauze mesh (eg, polyglycolic acid) can sometimes be wrapped around an injured lobe and sutured in a way that maintains pressure and tamponades the bleeding. In a few cases, control of arterial hemorrhage requires ligation of the hepatic artery or one of the accessible lobar branches in the hilum.

The most difficult problems involve lacerations of the major hepatic veins behind the liver. Temporary clamping of the inflow vessels may or may not slow blood loss enough to allow inspection and suturing of the bleeding point. For persistent bleeding, the abdominal incision should be extended into a median sternotomy to improve exposure. An ancillary technique, which is used only rarely, is to place a tube through the atrial appendage into the inferior vena cava past the origin of the hepatic veins. Appropriately placed ligatures around the cava permit total isolation of the liver circulation without interrupting venous return from the lower extremities to the heart. Lobectomy, usually of the right lobe, may be required to manage these retrohepatic injuries.

Nevertheless, the great majority of patients who come to surgery require only drainage of the hepatic wound. Suture ligation of bleeding hepatic vessels and debridement of devitalized tissue are indicated in about 30% and 10% of cases, respectively. The other procedures are indicated even less often.

Penetrating injuries that involve the hepatic flexure of the colon as well as the liver are apt to result in subhepatic sepsis if managed by primary colonic anastomosis. After the liver is repaired and the injured colon is resected, a temporary ileostomy and mucous fistula may avoid this complication.

Postoperative Complications

With present techniques, hemorrhage at laparotomy is rarely uncontrollable except with retrohepatic venous injuries. Patients who rebleed from the liver wound after initial suture ligation should be treated by reexploration and lobectomy. Angiography and CT scanning may provide useful diagnostic information preoperatively in such patients.

Subhepatic sepsis develops in about 20% of cases; it is more frequent if lobectomy has been done.

Hemobilia may be responsible for gastrointestinal bleeding in the postoperative period and can be diagnosed by selective angiography. Treatment consists of embolization through the arteriography catheter.

Bleeding from stress ulcers is common after hepatic trauma, so patients with liver injuries should be given H_2 receptor antagonists after operation.

Prognosis

The death rate of 10–15% following hepatic trauma depends largely on the type of injury and the extent of associated injury to other organs. About one-third of patients admitted in shock cannot be saved. Only 1% of penetrating civilian wounds are lethal, whereas a 20% death rate attends blunt trauma. The death rate in blunt hepatic injury is 10% when only the liver is injured. If three major organs are damaged, the death rate is close to 70%. Bleeding causes more than half of deaths.

Buechter KJ, Zeppa R, Gomez G: The use of segmental anatomy for an operative classification of liver injuries. Ann Surg 1990;211:669.

Bynoe RP et al: Complications of nonoperative management of blunt hepatic injuries. J Trauma 1992;32:308.

Durham RM et al: Management of blunt hepatic injuries. Am J Surg 1992;164:477.

Fabian TC et al: Factors affecting morbidity following hepatic trauma: A prospective analysis of 482 injuries. Ann Surg 1991;213:540.

Feliciano DV: Continuing evolution in the approach to severe liver trauma. Ann Surg 1992;216:521.

Harris LM, Booth FV, Hassett JM Jr: Liver lacerations A marker of severe but sometimes subtle intra-abdominal injuries in adults. J Trauma 1991;31:894.

Jacobson LE, Kirton OC, Gomez GA: The use of an absorbable mesh wrap in the management of major liver injuries. Surgery 1992;111:455.

Knudson MM et al: Nonoperative management of blunt liver injuries in adults: The need for continued surveillance. J Trauma 1990;30:1494.

Pachter HL et al: Significant trends in the treatment of hepatic trauma: Experience with 411 injuries. Ann Surg 1992;215:492.

Reed RL 2d et al: Continuing evolution in the approach to severe liver trauma. Ann Surg 1992;216:524.

Ringe B et al: Management of severe hepatic trauma by two-stage total hepatectomy and subsequent liver transplantation. Surgery 1991;109:792.

Sharp KW, Locicero RJ: Abdominal packing for surgically uncontrollable hemorrhage. Ann Surg 1992;215:467.

Sherlock DJ, Bismuth H: Secondary surgery for liver trauma. Br J Surg 1991;78:1313.

SPONTANEOUS HEPATIC RUPTURE

Spontaneous rupture of the liver is not common. Most cases of ruptured normal liver are due to pre-eclampsia-eclampsia, and most cases of ruptured diseased liver are due to hepatic tumors. Hepatic rupture should be suspected in any pregnant or postpartum patient (especially if hypertensive) who complains of acute discomfort in the upper abdomen. Spontaneous rupture has also been reported in association with hepatic hemangioma, gallstone obstruction, typhoid fever, malaria, tuberculosis. syphilis, polyarteritis nodosa, and diabetes mellitus. The diagnosis can be made by ultrasound or CT scanning. Rupture of the liver in the newborn is related to birth trauma in larger infants after difficult deliveries. The common course is intrahepatic hemorrhage expanding to capsular rupture.

Treatment consists of emergency surgery as for traumatic rupture (see above).

Smith LG Jr et al: Spontaneous rupture of liver during pregnancy: Current therapy. Obstet Gynecol 1991;77:171.

Wilkinson ML: Diagnosis and management of liver disease in pregnancy. Adv Intern Med 1990;35:289.

PRIMARY LIVER CANCER

Primary hepatic cancer is uncommon in the USA. However, the incidence is high and is increasing in parts of Asia and Africa. In some regions, hepatoma is the single most frequent abdominal tumor. The etiologic factors in these high-risk areas are environmental or cultural, since persons of similar racial background in the USA are at only slightly greater risk than Caucasians. About 9000 cases—distributed equally between men and women—occur in the USA each year. Most arise in persons over age 50, but a few are found in children, mainly under 2 years of age.

Chronic hepatitis B and C virus (HBV and HCV) infection is the principal etiologic factor worldwide. Patients chronically seropositive for HBsAg constitute a high-risk group for development of hepatoma, which in some cases may be detected early by screening for serum alpha-fetoprotein levels. Hepatitis B virus DNA has been detected integrated into the genome of host hepatocytes and hepatoma cells, but whether it has any direct oncogenic effect is unknown. Cirrhosis from almost any cause (eg, alcoholism, hemochromatosis, α_1-antitrypsin deficiency, or primary biliary cirrhosis) is associated with an increased risk of hepatocellular carcinoma. Widespread infection with liver flukes *(Clonorchis sinensis)* is at least partly responsible for the higher incidence of these tumors in Asia. Certain fungus metabolites called aflatoxins have been shown experimentally to be capable of producing liver tumors. These substances are present in staple foods (eg, ground nuts and grain) in some parts of Africa where hepatomas are common.

Three main cellular types of primary liver cancer are recognized: hepatocellular carcinoma (hepatoma), cholangiocellular carcinoma (cholangiocarcinoma), and a mixed form (hepatocholangioma). In children, the hepatocellular tumor is sometimes termed a hepatoblastoma because of its cellular similarly to fetal liver and the occasional presence of hematopoiesis.

Hepatomas constitute about 80% of primary hepatic cancers. Their gross morphology allows separation into three classes: a **massive** form, characterized by a single predominant mass clearly demarcated from the surrounding liver, occasionally with small satellite nodules; a **nodular** form, composed of multiple nodules, often distributed throughout the liver; and a **diffuse** variety, characterized by infiltration of tumor throughout the remaining parenchyma. About 50% of resectable tumors are surrounded by a fibrous capsule, a structure that develops as a result of compression and collagenization of adjacent liver stroma. Encapsulated tumors exhibit a lower incidence of direct liver invasion, tumor microsatellites, and venous permeation compared with nonencapsulated ones, and the finding is a favorable sign. An uncommon variety of the massive type, **fibrolamellar hepatoma,** contains numerous fibrous septa and may resemble focal nodular hyperplasia. Fibrolamellar hepatoma occurs in a younger age group (average 25 years) and is not associated with cirrhosis or hepatitis B virus infection.

In 70% of patients, tumor has spread outside the liver when hepatoma is first diagnosed. Metastases are almost invariably present with the nodular or diffuse forms, but 40% of the massive type are confined to the liver. The hilar and celiac lymph nodes are most commonly involved. Metastases to lung and the peritoneal surface also occur frequently. The portal or hepatic veins are often invaded by tumor, and venous occlusion may occur in either case.

Microscopically, there is usually little stroma between the malignant cells, and the tumor has a soft consistency. The tumor may be highly vascularized, a feature that sometimes produces massive intraperitoneal hemorrhage following spontaneous rupture. Hepatocellular function occurs in some, as indicated by the presence of bile pigment between or in the tumor cells.

Cholangiocarcinomas make up about 15% of primary liver cancers. They are usually well-differentiated adenocarcinomas that spread invasively in the liver substance. Extrahepatic metastases are the rule by the time the tumor is detected.

The mixed tumors resemble hepatomas in their pathologic and clinical behavior.

Angiosarcoma of the liver, a rare fatal tumor, has been seen in workers intensively exposed to vinyl chloride for prolonged periods in polymerization plants.

Clinical Findings

A. Symptoms and Signs: The diagnosis is often difficult. Early cases present with right upper quadrant pain, which may be associated with referred pain in the right shoulder. Weight loss is usually present, and jaundice is evident in about one-third of cases.

Hepatomegaly or a mass is palpable in many patients. An arterial bruit or a friction rub may be audible over the liver. Intermittent fever may be a presenting feature. Ascites or gastrointestinal bleeding from varices indicates advanced disease, and ascites fluid with blood in it should always suggest hepatoma.

The patterns of presentation are as follows: (1) pain with or without hepatomegaly; (2) sudden deterioration of the condition of a cirrhotic patient owing to the appearance of hepatic failure, bleeding varices, or ascites; (3) sudden, massive intraperitoneal hemorrhage; (4) acute illness with fever and abdominal pain; (5) distant metastases; and (6) no clinical findings.

B. Laboratory Findings: The serum bilirubin is elevated in one-third of patients. In another 25%, serum alkaline phosphatase is increased but the serum bilirubin is normal. Since many of these patients have cirrhosis, the significance of these alterations is often difficult to assess. About 75% of patients are positive for HBsAg or hepatitis C.

C. Liver Scan: CT scans, ultrasound scans, and MRI scans demonstrate the principal lesion in 80% of patients. MRI scans are the best way to show extension into the hepatic veins. CT portography is superior to ordinary contrast-enhanced CT scans.

D. Angiography: Hepatomas are usually supplied by the hepatic artery, and 80% are more vascular than adjacent parenchyma. In some cases, the center of the tumor has become necrotic, and only the peripheral areas are hypervascular. Cholangiocarcinomas usually appear less vascular than adjacent

tissue. Hemangiomas can be recognized by a characteristic picture of patchy vascular pooling.

The venous phase of a superior mesenteric arterial injection may show invasion or occlusion of the portal vein by tumor.

Angiography may be equivocal in small tumors, which may be demonstrated with greater certainty by a selective injection of iodized oil (Lipiodol) followed 1–2 weeks later by CT scans. Normal liver clears the contrast medium, but hepatomas cannot do so and remain opacified.

E. Special Tests: Alpha-fetoprotein (AFP), an α_1-globulin normally present only in the fetal circulation, is present in high concentrations in the serum of about 80% of patients with primary hepatomas and a few others with testicular tumors. It is also elevated to a lesser degree in chronic active hepatitis and acute viral and alcoholic hepatitis, where it seems to reflect the extent of liver regeneration.

Combined ultrasound scanning and AFP measurement is the screening protocol currently used to detect early cases of liver cancer in high-risk areas in Asia.

Changes in AFP levels in patients with hepatoma correlate with growth activity of the tumor and can be used postoperatively as an index of the success of hepatic resection.

F. Liver Biopsy: The diagnosis can be established by percutaneous core biopsy or aspiration biopsy in most patients if the biopsy site is selected according to the scan. Percutaneous biopsy is risky, however (rate of fatal hemorrhage is 0.4%), because these tumors are so vascular.

G. Screening: Attempts have been made to detect hepatocellular carcinomas early at a surgically more favorable stage by screening patients with chronic liver disease with periodic hepatic ultrasound examinations. These programs appear to have been worthwhile in Asia, with about two-thirds of detected lesions being under 2 cm in diameter, a majority of which are resectable. A similar effort in Italy, however, was disappointing. The explanation may be that the disease simply follows a more aggressive course in Europe than in Asia.

H. Tumor Markers: Alpha-fetoprotein (AFP), a glycoprotein normally present only in the fetal circulation, is present in high concentrations in the serum of many patients with primary hepatomas and testicular tumors. Increased levels may also be seen rarely as a product of tumors elsewhere in the body, such as the lung, stomach, pancreas, and biliary tree.

The upper limit of normal in the serum is 20 ng/mL; values above 200 ng/mL are suggestive of hepatoma. Levels in the intermediate range may occur with other kinds of liver disease, such as cirrhosis and chronic hepatitis, where they represent a manifestation of liver cell proliferation. As imaging methods have improved, the diagnosis of liver cancer is being made earlier and the frequency of AFP levels above 200 ng/mL in newly diagnosed cases has declined to about 25%. In general, whether or not AFP levels are abnormal is related to the size of the tumor, whereas the absolute level, which may exceed 10,000 ng/mL, is related to lack of differentiation histologically. Consequently, the prognosis is worse when AFP levels are high.

Differential Diagnosis

The clinical picture is usually nonspecific. Because of weight loss and weakness, liver cancer is most often confused with other abdominal carcinomas. Once hepatomegaly and a filling defect in the liver are found, it must be determined whether the liver harbors a primary neoplasm or a metastasis. Arteriography, biopsy, and serum AFP levels establish the diagnosis in most cases. However, it may be difficult to distinguish hepatic cancer from benign tumors or cysts or, if the patient is febrile, from liver abscess.

When complications develop suddenly in a cirrhotic patient, the possibility of hepatoma must always be considered. Portacaval shunts have been performed for recent variceal hemorrhage in cirrhotic patients without the physician suspecting that a hepatoma was responsible for the portal hypertension.

In rare instances, primary hepatocellular cancer is associated with metabolic or endocrine abnormalities such as erythrocytosis, hypercalcemia, hypoglycemic attacks, Cushing's syndrome, or virilization.

Complications

Sudden intra-abdominal hemorrhage may occur from spontaneous bleeding. Obstruction of the portal vein may produce portal hypertension, and obstruction of the hepatic veins may produce the Budd-Chiari syndrome. Liver failure is a common cause of death.

Treatment

A. Partial Hepatectomy: Resection of the tumor offers the only possibility of cure. The operation should usually begin with a diagnostic laparoscopy, for this may reveal previously undetected spread of tumor within the liver or abdominal cavity that militates against resection. The criteria of resectability are that (1) the tumor must be confined to the liver (ie, distant metastases or extension into the hepatic or portal veins must be absent) and (2) the lesion must be entirely encompassed by local excision, lobectomy, or extended lobectomy. Small lesions, particularly in cirrhotics, may be removed by local excision. About 25% of patients with primary liver cancer meet these requirements.

If visible tumor is left behind or if the margins of resection are less than 0.5 cm, progressive disease is the rule. After what is thought to be a complete resection, the outlook is worse with any of the following: (1) age over 50 years, (2) coexistent hepatocellular

disease (ie, cirrhosis), (3) vascular invasion, (4) portal vein thrombosis, (5) tumor located deep in the liver, (6) intracapsular infiltration of tumor cells, (7) bilobar involvement, and (8) more than one deposit of tumor. In general, however, cirrhosis constitutes the major obstacle. Any but the most limited resection is apt to trigger acute liver failure in cirrhotic patients, but in addition to this immediate concern, there is a late risk of death from bleeding esophageal varices or liver failure, and a high rate (> 75%) of new tumors developing in the residual liver. This is why liver transplantation has been tried for this group.

Overall, the rate of tumor recurrence is about 50% (though it is higher, as mentioned above, in patients with cirrhosis). The 5-year survival rate for patients with cirrhosis is close to zero, but for those without cirrhosis, it is about 40%. The results are still better (5-year survival about 60%) for fibrolamellar carcinomas.

After surgery, the patient should be followed by imaging studies and AFP measurements, and a localized recurrence should be considered for repeat resection or palliative therapy if technically feasible.

B. Liver Transplantation: Liver transplantation is of theoretic advantage because it should overcome the following problems: (1) lesions that are unresectable because of size or multifocal distribution (2) the inability of a cirrhotic liver to tolerate any but the most limited resection and (3) the likelihood in many cases that an undetectable second tumor is located remote from the index lesion. The results of liver transplantation have been good for fibrolamellar carcinoma and hemangioblastoma: 5-year survival rates for each are about 50%. There have been no survivors among those with hemangiosarcoma.

In patients with clinically apparent hepatomas complicating cirrhosis, 5-year survival is about 35%, good enough to encourage further efforts. The results are almost twice as good for patients with just one locus of tumor. Therefore, although the logistical problems and expense are enormous, transplantation is presently the best treatment for hepatoma in a cirrhotic liver.

The immunosuppressive therapy required to support the transplant is thought to impair the host's defenses against the tumor: Calculated tumor doubling time for lesions in transplanted patients was 37 days compared with 274 days in patients treated by hepatic resection (no immunosuppression).

C. Ethanol Injection: Using ultrasound guidance, 95% ethanol (5–20 mL) is injected through a 22-gauge needle into the neoplasm, which results in complete necrosis of the lesion in 75% of patients and partial (90%) necrosis in 20%. The patient is followed and re-treatment given for residual or new primary tumors. In one multi-institutional series from Italy, survival 1, 2, and 3 years after treatment for patients with solitary tumors was 90%, 80%, and 63%, respectively.

D. Arterial Chemoembolization: This approach takes advantage of the fact that primary liver cancers obtain their blood supply almost exclusively from the hepatic artery, whereas the rest of the liver is supplied more by the portal vein than by the artery. The strategy is to combine selective hepatic arterial injection of cancer chemotherapeutic agents with embolization, the latter to produce ischemia and slow the washout of the drugs. Patients with Child class C cirrhosis or thrombosis of the portal vein are not suitable candidates.

A variety of techniques have been used. Embolization is usually performed with Gelfoam, which dissolves after a few weeks, allowing repeated treatment. Doxorubicin, mitomycin, and cisplatin in various combinations are the drugs most often given. Lipiodol, which lodges in the tumor, has occasionally been used as a carrier for the drugs. A reduction in tumor size of 50% or more is seen in about 25% of patients. The best 3-year survival rates are around 50%. Histologic studies of tumors resected shortly after treatment reveal viable neoplastic cells in the tumor capsule, which receives blood from the portal vein as well as the hepatic artery.

Prognosis

Most patients with unresectable lesions succumb within a year after diagnosis. Patients generally die from the effects of the expanding hepatic neoplasm rather than from metastases.

Arii S et al: Predictive factors for intrahepatic recurrence of hepatocellular carcinoma after partial hepatectomy. Cancer 1992;69:913.

Belghiti J et al: Intrahepatic recurrence after resection of hepatocellular carcinoma complicating cirrhosis. Ann Surg 1991;214:114.

Belghiti J: Resection of hepatocellular carcinoma complicating cirrhosis. Br J Surg 1991;78:257.

Bismuth H et al: Primary treatment of hepatocellular carcinoma by arterial chemoembolization. Am J Surg 1992;163:387.

Colombo M et al: Hepatocellular carcinoma in Italian patients with cirrhosis. N Engl J Med 1991;325:675.

Ikeda K et al: Effect of repeated transcatheter arterial embolization on the survival time in patients with hepatocellular carcinoma. Cancer 1991;68:2150.

Ikeda K et al: Risk factors for tumor recurrence and prognosis after curative resection of hepatocellular carcinoma. Cancer 1993;71:19.

Iwatsuki S et al: Hepatic resection versus transplantation for hepatocellular carcinoma. Ann Surg 1991;214:221.

Jwo S-C et al: Risk factors linked to tumor recurrence of human hepatocellular carcinoma after hepatic resection. Hepatology 1992;16:1367.

Lai ECS et al: Hepatectomy for large hepatocellular carcinoma: The optimal resection margin. World J Surg 1991;15:141.

Lai ECS et al: Hepatic resection for small hepatocellular carcinoma: The Queen Mary Hospital experience. World J Surg 1991;15:654.

Livraghi T et al: Percutaneous ethanol injection in the treatment of hepatocellular carcinoma in cirrhosis: A study on 207 patients. Cancer 1992;69:925.

Matsuda Y et al: Rationale of surgical management for recurrent hepatocellular carcinoma. Ann Surg 1993;217:28.

Merine D, Takayasu K, Wakao F: Detection of hepatocellular carcinoma: Comparison of CT during arterial portography with CT after intraarterial injection of iodized oil. Radiology 1990;175:707.

Okuda K: Hepatocellular carcinoma: Recent progress. Hepatology 1992;15:948.

Paquet K-J et al: Limited hepatic resection for selected cirrhotic patients with hepatocellular or cholangiocellular carcinoma: A prospective study. Br J Surg 1991;78:459.

Penn I: Hepatic transplantation for primary and metastatic cancers of the liver. Surgery 1991;110:726.

Ringe B et al: Surgical treatment of hepatocellular carcinoma: Experience with liver resection and transplantation in 198 patients. World J Surg 1991;15:270.

Shiina S et al: Percutaneous ethanol injection therapy for hepatocellular carcinoma: A histopathologic study. Cancer 1991;68:1524.

Shirabe K et al: Factors linked to early recurrence of small hepatocellular carcinoma after hepatectomy: Univariate and multivariate analyses. Hepatology 1991;14:802.

Simonetti RG et al: Hepatocellular carcinoma: A worldwide problem and the major risk factors. Dig Dis Sci 1991;36:962.

Sitzmann JV, Abrams R: Improved survival for hepatocellular cancer with combination surgery and multimodality treatment. Ann Surg 1993;217:149.

Suenaga M et al: Hepatic resection for hepatocellular carcinoma. World J Surg 1992;16:97.

Taketa K: α-Fetoprotein: Reevaluation in hepatology. Hepatology 1990;12:1420.

Tanaka S et al: Effectiveness of periodic checkup by ultrasonography for the early diagnosis of hepatocellular carcinoma. Cancer 1990;66:2210.

Venook AP et al: Chemoembolization for hepatocellular carcinoma. J Clin Oncol 1990;8:1108.

Wernecke K et al: Detection of hepatic masses in patients with carcinoma: Comparative sensitivities of sonography, CT, and MR imaging. AJR Am J Roentgenol 1991;157:731.

Yu Y-Q et al: Experience with liver resection after hepatic arterial chemoembolization for hepatocellular carcinoma. Cancer 1993;71:62.

METASTATIC NEOPLASMS OF THE LIVER

Metastatic cancer is 20 times more common than primary tumors in the liver. Cancers of the breast, lung, pancreas, stomach, large intestine, kidney, ovary, and uterus account for about 75% of cases. Spread to the liver may be via the systemic circulation, portal vein, or, less often, the lymphatics. The cirrhotic liver, which often gives rise to primary hepatic tumors, is less susceptible than normal liver to implantation of metastases.

Over 90% of patients with hepatic metastases have

tumor implants in other organs. The lung is most commonly involved and contains tumor in 30% of cases. About 20% of patients with hepatic metastases have gross tumor deposits demonstrable on hepatic section that cannot be seen or felt from the surface of the liver during laparotomy.

Clinical Findings

A. Symptoms and Signs: Weight loss, fatigue, and anorexia are the presenting general complaints. Right upper abdominal pain, ascites, and jaundice are the usual symptoms. Fever without demonstrable infection is present in 15% of cases and bears only a loose relationship to leukocytosis.

In 60% of cases, physical examination reveals hepatomegaly or a palpable metastatic tumor in the upper abdomen. Either may be tender. Portal hypertension may be manifested by abdominal venous collaterals or splenomegaly. A friction rub is sometimes heard over the liver.

B. Laboratory Findings: Laboratory investigation reveals a hematocrit between 30% and 36%. The serum bilirubin is elevated in almost half of patients, and half of these have values over 4 mg/dL. The alkaline phosphatase is also usually increased.

The diagnosis can be established in most cases by percutaneous liver biopsy or fine-needle aspiration for malignant cells, especially if scans are used to direct the site of the biopsy.

C. Imaging Studies: The detection of liver metastases usually relies on CT or ultrasound scans. MRI provides useful additional information, however, and it may be superior to CT scans. CT portography is superior to ordinary contrast-enhanced CT. Where available, MRI and CT portography should both be performed if the patient is being considered for resection of hepatic metastases or insertion of a hepatic artery infusion pump. During surgery the liver should be further examined by ultrasound to check for lesions that might have been missed by preoperative studies.

Treatment

Little effective treatment is available for the average patient with diffuse metastases throughout the liver or with combined hepatic and extrahepatic disease.

A. Hepatic Resection: Partial hepatectomy—either wedge resection or lobectomy—is indicated for the 5% of patients with liver metastases from colorectal cancer whose disease is resectable. If all gross tumor can be removed, about 25% of patients are cured. The only absolute requirements are that no extrahepatic disease be present and that resection be technically feasible. The following indicate a worse prognosis after resection: (1) original tumor stage Dukes C compared with Dukes B; (2) four or more liver lesions; (3) over 25% of the mass of the liver replaced by tumor; (4) less than 1 year since resection

of the colon primary; and (5) 1 cm or less margin of resection. Variables that do not influence the outcome include (1) lobectomy versus wedge resection; (2) histologic pattern of the tumor; (3) bilateral rather than unilateral disease; (4) site of the primary tumor within the large intestine; and (5) the sex of the patient. The mortality rate for resection of hepatic metastases is about 2% in hospitals where this operation is performed frequently.

When the disease returns following a resection that removed all detectable tumor, the median time to recurrence is 9 months. The initial recurrence in about half of these patients is confined to the liver. Another resection may be performed if the criteria listed above are once again met, which amounts to perhaps 30% of cases. The chances of permanently eradicating the disease by a second resection is about 15%.

Other tumors that occasionally produce disease localized to one lobe of the liver and amenable to curative resection include pancreatic islet cell carcinomas, renal cell carcinomas, and carcinoids. Debulking liver resections may provide palliation of the carcinoid syndrome even when it is impossible to remove all the tumor. Partial hepatectomy is also sometimes worthwhile to extirpate a tumor invading directly from a contiguous organ. Hepatic resection of apparently solitary metastases from cancers of the breast, pancreas, stomach, female pelvic organs, and lung has been fruitless.

B. Chemotherapy: In as many as 30% of cases, the liver is the only evident site of metastases from colorectal cancer. If the lesion cannot be resected, local chemotherapy of these lesions can be given by placing a catheter in the hepatic artery connected to an implantable infusion pump (Infusaid pump), which allows the delivery of much higher concentrations of drug to the tumor than is possible with systemic administration. This regimen is not used for metastases from other kinds of tumors. The pump is primed with floxuridine, which is delivered by continuous infusion (0.3 mg/kg/d) for 14-day periods alternating with 14-day rests. The discovery of extrahepatic lesions at laparotomy for pump placement is considered an absolute contraindication to proceeding with this approach. Treatment is continued until toxicity or relapse occurs, or rarely until the response is complete. Toxicity consists mainly of gastroduodenal erosions (caused by unintentional perfusion of these areas), chemical hepatitis, or chemical sclerosing cholangitis. Extrahepatic lesions that appear during therapy are treated by concomitant systemic chemotherapy. Survival is related principally to the initial amount of liver involvement by tumor, objective response to treatment (which is seen in about 50% of patients), and extent of weight loss. Median survival of patients with less than 30% of liver replaced by tumor is 24 months, compared with 10 months if the extent of replacement exceeds 30%. There is a general feeling that hepatic artery infusion therapy improves survival, but the objective evidence is inconclusive. Cure is not a realistic objective.

Systemic chemotherapy (eg, with fluorouracil) does not improve survival, though it is often prescribed.

C. Miscellaneous: Hepatic artery ligation or angiographic embolization of the tumor has been of benefit in a few patients with hepatic metastases from various tumors.

Prognosis

Survival varies with the extent of disease, ranging from 3 months for patients with extensive hepatic replacement by multiple lesions to 2–3 years for patients with small solitary lesions. Survival is slightly longer in patients with metastases from colonic cancer than in patients with metastases from pancreatic or gastric tumors.

Bozzetti F et al: Repeated hepatic resection for recurrent metastases from colorectal cancer. Br J Surg 1992; 79:146.

Cady B et al: Technical and biological factors in disease-free survival after hepatic resection for colorectal cancer metastases. Arch Surg 1992;127:561.

Doci R et al: One hundred patients with hepatic metastases from colorectal cancer treated by resection: Analysis of prognostic determinants. Br J Surg 1991;78:797.

Hohenberger P et al: Tumor recurrence and options for further treatment after resection of liver metastases in patients with colorectal cancer. J Surg Oncol 1990;44:245.

Kemeny N et al: A pilot study of hepatic artery floxuridine combined with systemic 5-fluorouracil and leucovorin: A potential adjuvant program after resection of colorectal hepatic metastases. Cancer 1993;71:1964.

Nakamura S et al: Results of extensive surgery for liver metastases in colorectal carcinoma. Br J Surg 1992;79:35.

Scheele J, Stangl R, Altendorf-Hofmann A: Hepatic metastases from colorectal carcinoma: Impact of surgical resection on the natural history. Br J Surg 1990;77:1241.

Soyer P et al: Preoperative assessment of resectability of hepatic metastases from colonic carcinoma: CT portography vs sonography and dynamic CT. AJR Am J Roentgenol 1992;159:741.

Soyer P et al: Surgical treatment of hepatic metastases: Impact of intraoperative sonography. AJR Am J Roentgenol 1993;160:511.

Sterchi JM et al: Chemoinfusion of the hepatic artery for metastases to the liver. Surg Gynecol Obstet 1989; 168:291.

Stone MD et al: Surgical therapy for recurrent liver metastases from colorectal cancer. Arch Surg 1990;125:718.

Uetsuji S et al: Absence of colorectal cancer metastasis to the cirrhotic liver. Am J Surg 1992;164:176.

Wolf RF et al: Results of resection and proposed guidelines for patient selection in instances of non-colorectal hepatic metastases. Surg Gynecol Obstet 1991;173:454.

BENIGN TUMORS & CYSTS OF THE LIVER*

Hemangiomas

Hemangioma is the most common benign hepatic tumor, and—except for the skin and mucous membranes—the liver is the most common location for hemangiomas. Women are affected more often than men in a ratio of 6:1. Histologically, hepatic hemangiomas are of the cavernous type. Most are small solitary subcapsular growths that are found incidentally during laparotomy or at autopsy. Those greater than 4 cm in diameter may cause abdominal pain or a palpable mass. Rare patients have presented with hemorrhagic shock resulting from spontaneous rupture. Large congenital hemangiomas of the liver may be associated with others in the skin. Occasionally, a hemangioma may behave as an arteriovenous fistula and produce cardiac hypertrophy and congestive heart failure.

Large-bore needle biopsy is hazardous, but aspiration biopsy with a fine needle is safe. Nevertheless, biopsy is rarely indicated, since the diagnosis can be made with certainty in most cases by scintigraphy, contrast-enhanced CT scans, MRI, or angiography. CT scans show a vascular lesion with delayed clearing of the contrast medium. Similar features are seen with technetium-labeled red blood cell scintigrams. Arteriograms demonstrate puddling of contrast medium within the tumor that clears slowly.

Symptomatic hemangiomas should be excised by lobectomy or enucleation. Even large lesions can be safely removed with modest blood loss if they are confined to one lobe. Radiotherapy or embolization via a catheter in the hepatic artery may be tried in patients who are poor candidates for surgery. It has been suggested that exogenous estrogens may contribute to the occasional recurrence of giant hemangiomas, so they should probably be proscribed.

The natural history of asymptomatic hemangiomas, whether large or small, is benign. If discovered as an incidental finding during laparotomy, a hemangioma should not be biopsied or removed, because of potential difficulties with hemostasis.

Baer HU et al: Enucleation of giant hemangiomas of the liver: Technical and pathologic aspects of a neglected procedure. Ann Surg 1992;216:673.

Belli L et al: Surgical treatment of symptomatic giant hemangiomas of the liver. Surg Gynecol Obstet 1992;174:474.

Gandolfi L et al: Natural history of hepatic haemangiomas: Clinical and ultrasound study. Gut 1991;32:677.

Lise M et al: Giant cavernous hemangiomas: Diagnosis and surgical strategies. World J Surg 1992;16:516.

Nelson RC, Chezmar JL: Diagnostic approach to hepatic hemangiomas. Radiology 1990;176:11.

---

*Echinococcal cysts are discussed in Chapter 8.

Pateron D et al: Giant hemangioma of the liver with pain, fever, and abnormal liver tests: Report of two cases. Dig Dis Sci 1991;36:524.

Cysts

Hepatic cysts are usually solitary unilocular lesions that produce no symptoms. The occasional large cyst may present as an upper abdominal mass or discomfort. Polycystic liver disease is associated in about half of cases with polycystic renal disease. The possibility of echinococcosis (see Chapter 8) should always be considered in patients with just one or two cysts.

Most solitary cysts have a serous lining. Solitary cysts lined with cuboidal epithelium are classified as cystadenomas and should be resected, since they are premalignant. Multilocular (septated) cysts (if not echinococcal) are usually neoplastic. There are few indications for aspirating hepatic cysts, because simple cysts reaccumulate fluid quickly; neoplastic cysts must be excised; and parasitic cysts might be ruptured and the parasite thus allowed to spread. On the other hand, it may be possible to eliminate a small cyst by aspiration of the contents followed by an injection into the lumen of 20–100 mL of absolute alcohol.

Large symptomatic cysts are difficult to eradicate with alcohol injections, and serious superinfection of the cyst cavity may occur. The simplest method of treatment consists of laparoscopic excision of the superficial portion (about 20–40%) of the cyst wall. A tongue of omentum is fixed so it lies in the residual cyst cavity as an ancillary measure to prevent the edges from coapting. The operation is curative in nearly all patients.

Multiple cysts do not usually require treatment, but large polycystic livers that cause discomfort or are associated with obstructive jaundice can be managed by surgically unroofing the cysts on the surface of the liver and creating windows between superficial cysts and adjacent deep cysts. The opened cysts are allowed to drain into the abdominal cavity. Postoperatively, the liver shrinks to about half its previous size. In some cases, the liver returns to its original size quickly; in others, it remains smaller.

Gabow PA et al: Risk factors for the development of hepatic cysts in autosomal dominant polycystic kidney disease. Hepatology 1990;11:1033.

Kairaluoma MI et al: Percutaneous aspiration and alcohol sclerotherapy for symptomatic hepatic cysts: An alternative to surgical intervention. Ann Surg 1989;210:208.

Lai EC, Wong J: Symptomatic nonparasitic cysts of the liver. World J Surg 1990;14:452.

Newman KD et al: Treatment of highly symptomatic polycystic liver disease: Preliminary experience with a combined hepatic resection-fenestration procedure. Ann Surg 1990;212:30.

Sanchez H et al: Surgical management of nonparasitic cystic liver disease. Am J Surg 1991;161:113.

Starzl TE et al: Liver transplantation for polycystic liver disease. Arch Surg 1990;125:575.

Telenti A et al: Hepatic cyst infection in autosomal dominant polycystic kidney disease. Mayo Clin Proc 1990;65:933.

Hepatic Adenoma

Hepatic adenomas occur almost exclusively in women and are increasing in frequency, apparently because of the widespread use of oral contraceptives. Mestranol-containing compounds have been associated with a disproportionate number of cases, but mestranol has been in use longer than the other agents.

The tumors are soft, yellow-tan, well-circumscribed masses that measure 2–15 cm in diameter. Most of those that cause symptoms are in the 8- to 15-cm range. Two-thirds of hepatic adenomas are solitary; the remainder are multiple. A few are pedunculated. Transition from benign hepatic adenoma to hepatocellular carcinoma may occur, with liver cell dysplasia as an intermediate step. Histologically, hepatic adenomas consist of an encapsulated homogeneous mass of normal-appearing hepatocytes without bile ducts or central veins. Hemorrhage may be present.

About half of patients are asymptomatic. Most of those with symptoms present with right upper quadrant pain or acute intra-abdominal hemorrhage and shock. These complications are due to spontaneous hemorrhage into the substance of the tumor, which may rupture into the peritoneal cavity. There is a strong association of acute bleeding episodes with menstruation. Patients with symptoms usually have a palpable mass in the liver.

Liver function tests and AFP levels are usually normal. Hepatic CT and ultrasound scans show a focal defect. On hepatic angiography, the lesions range from avascular to hypervascular and cannot usually be distinguished from malignant hepatoma. Aspiration biopsy is safe, but core needle biopsy is risky because of the danger of bleeding.

Symptomatic hepatic adenomas should be resected; in acutely bleeding patients, this may be lifesaving. Some may be removed by wedge resection, but deep-seated or large lesions usually require partial hepatectomy. Hepatic adenomas may regress when oral contraceptive agents are discontinued, and expectant management is appropriate for asymptomatic or mildly symptomatic lesions smaller than about 6 cm. The tumor should be followed by periodic ultrasound or CT scan and resection recommended if it enlarges. The possibility that the tumor may be a hepatoma must always be kept in mind, because there is no completely reliable means of making the differentiation. In fact, even at laparotomy it may be difficult to distinguish between hepatoma and hepatic adenoma by gross inspection or frozen section examination. Large hepatic adenomas should be removed without a period of expectant management, because they are more likely to bleed or be malignant.

Most patients recover without sequelae after surgical removal; recurrence is rare. Oral contraceptives should be proscribed permanently in all cases. Radiotherapy and chemotherapy are of no value.

See references at end of next section.

Focal Nodular Hyperplasia

Focal nodular hyperplasia is a benign lesion with no malignant potential. It is found in women twice as often as in men. The average age is about 40 years, but the tumor can occur at any age. The use of oral contraceptive agents may stimulate the development or growth of this tumor.

Grossly, the tumor is a well-circumscribed, firm, tan, usually subcapsular mass measuring 2–3 cm in diameter. In patients with symptoms, the lesions average 4–7 cm in diameter and occasionally are multiple. Eighty percent are solitary. The appearance on cut section is pathognomonic, consisting of a central stellate scar with radiating fibrous septa that compartmentalize the lesion into lobules. Histologically, there are nodular aggregations of normal-appearing hepatocytes without central veins or portal triads. Bile duct proliferation is present in the nodules.

Most patients with focal nodular hyperplasia are asymptomatic. The few with symptoms present with a right upper quadrant mass, discomfort, or both. Unlike hepatic adenomas, these lesions rarely grow or bleed, and the natural history of asymptomatic lesions is benign. A few patients with diffuse focal nodular hyperplasia develop portal hypertension.

Hepatic function tests and AFP levels are usually normal. Hepatic scintiscans usually do not show a filling defect; CT scans demonstrate the tumor and usually the central stellate scar. The arteriographic pattern is one of hypervascularity.

Patients taking oral contraceptives should have these drugs withdrawn. Symptomatic lesions should be removed; asymptomatic ones (the majority) should be left undisturbed. Focal nodular hyperplasia can be reliably identified on examination of frozen sections.

Brady MS, Coit DG: Focal nodular hyperplasia of the liver. Surg Gynecol Obstet 1990;171:377.

Iwatsuki S; Todo S; Starzl TE: Excisional therapy for benign hepatic lesions. Surg Gynecol Obstet 1990;171:240.

Muguti G et al: Hepatic focal nodular hyperplasia: A benign incidentaloma or a marker of serious hepatic disease? HPB Surg 1992;5:171.

Nichols FC 3d, van Heerden JA, Weiland LH: Benign liver tumors. Surg Clin North Am 1989;69:297.

Ros PR, Li KC: Benign liver tumors. Curr Probl Diagn Radiol 1989;18:125.

Shortell CK, Schwartz SI: Hepatic adenoma and focal nodular hyperplasia. Surg Gynecol Obstet 1991;173:426.

Tao LC: Oral contraceptive-associated liver cell adenoma and hepatocellular carcinoma: Cytomorphology and mechanism of malignant transformation. Cancer 1991;68:342.

HEPATIC ABSCESS

Hepatic abscesses may be bacterial, parasitic, or fungal in origin. In the USA, pyogenic abscesses are the most common and amebic abscesses (see Chapter 8) the next most common. Unless otherwise specified, these remarks refer to bacterial abscesses.

Cases are about evenly divided between those with a single abscess and those with many abscesses. About 90% of right lobe abscesses are solitary, while only 10% of left lobe abscesses are solitary.

In most cases, the development of a hepatic abscess follows a suppurative process elsewhere in the body. Many abscesses are due to direct spread from biliary infections such as empyema of the gallbladder or protracted cholangitis. Abdominal infections such as appendicitis or diverticulitis may spread through the portal vein to involve the liver with abscess formation. About 40% of patients have an underlying malignancy. Other cases develop after generalized sepsis from bacterial endocarditis, renal infection, or pneumonitis. In 25% of cases, no antecedent infection can be documented ("cryptogenic" abscesses). Rare causes include secondary bacterial infection of an amebic abscess, hydatid cyst, or congenital hepatic cyst.

In most cases, the organism is of enteric origin. *Escherichia coli, Klebsiella pneumoniae, Bacteroides,* enterococci (eg, *Streptococcus faecalis*), anaerobic streptococci (eg, *Peptostreptococcus*), and microaerophilic streptococci are most common. Staphylococci, hemolytic streptococci, or other gram-positive organisms are usually found if the primary infection is bacterial endocarditis or pneumonitis.

Clinical Findings

A. Symptoms and Signs: When liver abscess develops in the course of another intra-abdominal infection such as diverticulitis, it is accompanied by increasing toxicity, higher fever, jaundice, and a generally deteriorating clinical picture. Right upper quadrant pain and chills may appear.

In other cases, the diagnosis is much less obvious, since the illness develops insidiously in a previously healthy person. In these, the first symptoms are usually malaise and fatigue, followed after several weeks by fever. Epigastric or right upper quadrant pain is present in about half of cases. The pain may be aggravated by motion or may be referred to the right shoulder.

The course of fever is often erratic, and spikes to 40–41 °C (104–105.8 °F) are common. Chills are present in about 25% of cases. The liver is usually enlarged and may be tender to palpation. If tenderness is severe, the condition may be confused with cholecystitis.

Jaundice is unusual in solitary abscesses unless the patient's condition is seriously worsening. It is often present in patients with multiple abscesses and primary disease in the biliary tree and in general is a bad prognostic sign.

B. Laboratory Findings: Leukocytosis is present in most cases and is usually over 15,000/µL. A small group of patients—including some of the most seriously ill—fail to develop leukocytosis. Anemia is present in most. The average hematocrit is 33%.

Serum bilirubin is usually normal except in patients with multiple abscesses or biliary obstruction or when hepatic failure has supervened. Alkaline phosphatase is often elevated even in the presence of a normal bilirubin.

C. Imaging Studies: X-ray changes present in the right lung in about one-third of cases consist of basilar atelectasis or pleural effusion. The right diaphragm may be elevated and less mobile than the left.

Plain films of the abdomen are usually normal or show only hepatomegaly. In a few patients, an air-fluid level in the region of the liver reveals the presence and location of the abscess. Distortion of the contour of the stomach on upper gastrointestinal series may be seen with large abscesses involving the left lobe.

Ultrasound and CT scans are the most useful diagnostic tests, providing accurate information regarding the presence, size, number, and location of abscesses within the liver. CT scans have the added advantage of being able to demonstrate abscesses or neoplasms elsewhere in the abdomen. The radioisotope liver scintiscan is able to demonstrate most liver abscesses but given no information about the rest of the abdomen.

Differential Diagnosis

In many cases, early findings may be so vague that hepatic abscess is not even considered. The multiple other causes of malaise, weight loss, and anemia would enter into the differential diagnosis. With spiking fevers, one must consider all the causes of fever of unknown origin. Failure to entertain the idea of hepatic abscess and to obtain the necessary scans leads to most errors in diagnosis.

Once imaging tests have demonstrated the abscess, the responsible organisms must be identified. Amebiasis should be considered in every case of solitary abscess. Compared with amebic abscesses, pyogenic liver abscesses are seen more often in patients older than 50 years and are associated with jaundice, pruritus, sepsis, a palpable mass, and elevated bilirubin and alkaline phosphatase levels. Patients with amebic abscesses more often have been to an endemic area and have abdominal pain and tenderness, diarrhea, hepatomegaly, and positive serologic tests for amebiasis.

Complications

Intrahepatic spread of infection may create multiple additional abscesses and is responsible for some failures after treatment of an apparently solitary abscess. As the untreated abscess expands, rupture may occur into the pleural or peritoneal cavity, usually with catastrophic results. Septicemia and septic shock are common terminal complications of diffuse hepatic infection. Hepatic failure may develop in addition to uncontrolled sepsis, or it may predominate over signs of infection.

Hemobilia may follow bleeding from the vascular wall into the abscess cavity. In this case, hepatic artery embolization or ligation may be required to control bleeding.

Treatment

Antibiotics should be started promptly. Initial coverage, before culture results are available, should be adequate for *E coli, K pneumoniae, Bacteroides,* enterococcus, and anaerobic streptococci and consequently would usually include an aminoglycoside, clindamycin or metronidazole, and ampicillin. The regimen may be modified later according to the results of cultures.

About 80% of patients with liver abscesses are adequately treated by suction catheters inserted percutaneously under ultrasound or CT guidance. Whether the patient has a single abscess or multiple abscesses, this is usually the most appropriate initial therapy. The catheters can be removed in 1–2 weeks after output becomes nonpurulent and scant.

In about 40% of patients, the catheters do not drain well following initial placement and must be repositioned. The principal advantage of percutaneous drainage is lower morbidity (not lower mortality). It is easier to provide thorough drainage surgically, so when difficulties are encountered with percutaneous drainage, laparotomy should be performed promptly. Surgical therapy may also be called for in patients whose underlying disease requires an operation.

In many cases, multiple abscesses cannot be drained satisfactorily. Rarely, multiple abscesses are confined to a single lobe and can be cured by lobectomy. Biliary obstruction or other causes of sepsis must also be corrected.

Prognosis

The overall mortality rate of 15% is more closely related to the underlying disease than to any other factor. The mortality rate is about 40% in patients with malignant disease. Pleural effusion, leukocytosis over 20,000/µL, hypoalbuminemia, and polymicrobial infection correlate with a poor outcome. In the USA, whether the abscess is solitary or multiple no longer has a major influence on survival, but where benign biliary disease remains a major cause of this disease, multiple hepatic abscesses are associated with a worse prognosis. Death is rare in patients with a cryptogenic liver abscess.

Branum GD et al: Hepatic abscess: Changes in etiology, diagnosis, and management. Ann Surg 1990;212:655.

Cohen JL et al: Liver abscess: The need for complete gastrointestinal evaluation. Arch Surg 1989;124:561.

Do H et al: Percutaneous drainage of hepatic abscesses: Comparison of results in abscesses with and without intrahepatic biliary communication. AJR Am J Roentgenol 1991;157:1209.

Frey CF et al: Liver abscesses. Surg Clin North Am 1989;69:259.

Matthews JB et al: Hepatic abscess after biliary tract procedures. Surg Gynecol Obstet 1990;170:469.

Stain SC et al: Pyogenic liver abscess: Modern treatment. Arch Surg 1991;126:991.

25

Portal Hypertension

Lawrence W. Way, MD

In the USA, portal hypertension is mainly caused by cirrhosis of the liver; worldwide, schistosomiasis is a more common cause. The high portal pressure stimulates expansion of rudimentary venous collaterals between the portal and systemic venous systems. The most significant is the venous plexus at the gastroesophageal junction, which drains into the azygos veins. Under the stimulus to transport greater volumes, these collaterals can develop into large fragile submucosal varices susceptible to rupture and massive hemorrhage. This is the major complication of portal hypertension and the usual reason the surgeon becomes involved in the care of these patients. The other common clinical sequelae include ascites, hepatic encephalopathy, and secondary hypersplenism. If the surgeon can construct a large-diameter anastomosis (shunt) between the portal and systemic venous circulations, the elevated portal pressure drops and the risk of variceal hemorrhage is eliminated. However, decisions about the care of these patients are rarely simple, since portacaval shunts tend to impair hepatic function and lower the threshold for encephalopathy. Potential candidates for operation must be carefully evaluated to ensure optimal surgical results.

ANATOMY OF THE PORTAL CIRCULATION

The portal vein is formed by the confluence of the splenic and superior mesenteric veins at the level of the second lumbar vertebra behind the head of the pancreas (Figure 25–1). It runs for 8–9 cm to the hilum of the liver, where it divides into lobar branches. The left gastric vein usually enters the portal vein on its anteromedial aspect just cephalad to the margin of the pancreas, in which case it usually must be ligated during the surgical construction of a portacaval shunt; in 25% of cases, the left gastric vein joins the splenic vein. Other small venous tributaries from the pancreas and duodenum are less constant but must be anticipated during surgical mobilization of the portal vein.

The inferior mesenteric vein generally drains into the splenic vein several centimeters to the left of the junction with the superior mesenteric vein; not uncommonly, it empties directly into the superior mesenteric vein.

In the hepatoduodenal ligament, the portal vein lies dorsal and slightly medial to the common bile duct. A large lymph node is often encountered lateral to the vein and must be dissected off before a shunt can be performed.

PHYSIOLOGY

Total hepatic blood flow (about 1500 mL/min; 30 mL/min per kg body weight) constitutes 25% of the cardiac output, though the liver accounts for only 2.5% of body weight. About 30% of the hepatic volume is blood (12% of total blood volume). Two-thirds of the flow enters through the portal vein and one-third through the hepatic artery. Pressure in the portal vein is normally 10–15 cm H_2O (7–11 mm Hg). The liver derives half of its oxygen from hepatic arterial blood and half from portal venous blood.

Portal venous and hepatic arterial blood becomes pooled after entering the periphery of the hepatic sinusoid (Figure 25–2). Hepatic arterial flow increases or decreases reciprocally with changes in portal flow. The regulatory mechanism for hepatic arterial flow involves an adenosine washout phenomenon: adenosine is released into the space of Mall surrounding the hepatic arterial resistance vessels. High concentrations of adenosine dilate the vessels, which increases flow and washes out the adenosine. Blood flow within the liver is uniform, as demonstrated by an even distribution of microspheres injected into the hepatic artery or portal vein.

Sudden occlusion of the portal vein results in an immediate 60% rise in hepatic arterial flow. In a matter of weeks, total flow gradually returns toward normal. On the other hand, sudden reductions in hepatic arterial supply are not immediately met by significant increases in portal vein flow. In both normal subjects and cirrhotics, total hepatic flow and portal pressure drop following hepatic arterial occlusion. Arterial collaterals develop over the ensuing months, and arterial perfusion is ultimately restored.

ETIOLOGY

The causes of portal hypertension are listed in Table 25–1. In all but a few instances, the basic lesion

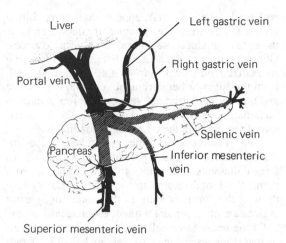

Figure 25–1. Anatomic relationships of portal vein and branches.

Table 25–1. Causes of portal hypertension.

I. Increased resistance to flow
  A. Prehepatic (portal vein obstruction)
    1. Congenital atresia or stenosis
    2. Thrombosis of portal vein
    3. Thrombosis of splenic vein
    4. Extrinsic compression (eg, tumors)
  B. Hepatic
    1. Cirrhosis
      a. Portal cirrhosis (nutritional, alcoholic, Laennec's)
      b. Postnecrotic cirrhosis
      c. Biliary cirrhosis
      d. Others (Wilson's disease, hemochromatosis)
    2. Acute alcoholic liver disease
    3. Congenital hepatic fibrosis
    4. Idiopathic portal hypertension (hepatoportal sclerosis)
    5. Schistosomiasis
  C. Posthepatic
    1. Budd-Chiari syndrome
    2. Constrictive pericarditis
II. Increased portal blood flow
  A. Arterial-portal venous fistula
  B. Increased splenic flow
    1. Banti's syndrome
    2. Splenomegaly (eg, tropical splenomegaly, myeloid metaplasia)

is increased resistance to portal flow. Those associated with increased resistance can be subclassified according to the site of the block as prehepatic, hepatic, and posthepatic. Cirrhosis accounts for about 85% of cases of portal hypertension in the USA, and the most common form is that due to alcoholism. Postnecrotic cirrhosis is next in frequency, followed by biliary cirrhosis. The other intrahepatic causes of portal hypertension are relatively rare in this country, although in some parts of the world hepatic schistosomiasis constitutes the largest single group. Idiopathic portal hypertension occurs with greater frequency in southern Asia.

Next to cirrhosis, extrahepatic portal venous occlusion is the most common cause of portal hypertension in the USA. These patients are generally younger than the cirrhotics, and many are children. Posthepatic obstruction due to Budd-Chiari syndrome or constrictive pericarditis is rare.

PATHOPHYSIOLOGY

Since pressure in the portal venous system is determined by the relationship $P = F \times R$, portal hypertension could result either from increased volume of portal blood flow or increased resistance to flow. In practice, however, all but a few cases are caused by increased resistance, though the site of the resistance varies in different diseases. A pathophysiologic classification of the causes of portal hypertension is given in Table 25–1.

Portal venous pressure normally ranges from 7 to 10 mm Hg. In portal hypertension, portal pressure exceeds 10 mm Hg, averaging around 20 mm Hg and occasionally rising as high as 50–60 mm Hg.

In alcoholic liver disease, the abnormal resistance is predominantly at the postsinusoidal position, as shown by the results of wedged hepatic vein pressure studies.* The causes of increased resistance in this disease are thought to be (1) distortion of the hepatic veins by regenerative nodules and (2) fibrosis of the hepatic veins and perisinusoidal areas.

Even in the absence of cirrhosis, acute alcoholism can raise portal pressure by producing centrilobular

---

*A catheter wedged in a tributary of the hepatic vein permits estimation of the pressure in the afferent veins to the sinusoid. The gradient between the wedged pressure and that in the hepatic vein reflects resistance at any point between the wedged position and the periphery of the sinusoid. The current view holds that the site of principal resistance in normal persons is in reasonably large hepatic veins. In cirrhosis, it is probably in the sinusoids as well as the hepatic veins.

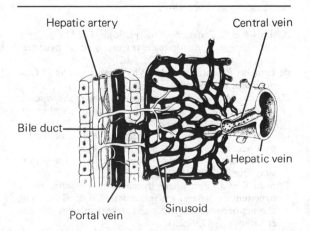

Figure 25–2. Vascular anatomy of the liver lobule.

swelling and fibrosis. Sinusoidal resistance to flow is also increased by engorgement of adjacent hepatocytes with fat and resultant distortion and narrowing of the vascular pathway. Cases have been documented where the elevated portal pressure dropped with resolution of the pathologic changes.

Schistosomiasis alone produces a presinusoidal block as a consequence of deposition of parasite ova in small portal venules. However, many patients with schistosomiasis who have bleeding varies or other complications of liver disease also harbor chronic hepatitis B infection, which produces concomitant cirrhosis.

Fluctuations in the level of portal hypertension also occur in conjunction with changes in blood volume, and patients with ascites are especially sensitive. Administration of colloid solutions to a patient with a normal or expanded blood volume could theoretically aggravate the clinical manifestations of portal hypertension.

Budd-Chiari syndrome (see p 522) is produced by restriction to flow through the hepatic veins or the inferior vena cava above the liver. The resulting sinusoidal hypertension produces prominent ascites and hepatomegaly.

Banti's syndrome was defined as liver disease secondary to primary splenic disease and was incorrectly considered to explain the average case of portal hypertension now known to result from cirrhosis and other kinds of hepatic disease.

The average portal flow in cirrhotic patients with complications of portal hypertension is about 30% of normal, ranging from 0 to 700 mL/min. Hepatic arterial flow is usually reduced by a similar proportion. The range of portal flow rates in different patients may vary greatly; in a few, blood in the portal vein moves only sluggishly, and in rare instances the direction of flow may even be reversed so that the portal vein functions as an outflow tract from the liver. These states of low flow predispose to spontaneous thrombosis of the portal vein, a complication of cirrhosis that usually renders the portal vein unsuitable for a shunt.

The obstacle to flow through the liver stimulates expansion of collateral channels between the portal and systemic venous systems. As the pathologic process develops, portal pressure increases until a level of about 40 cm H_2O (30 mm Hg) is reached. At this point, increasing hepatic resistance, even to the point of occlusion of the portal vein, diverts a greater fraction of portal flow through the collaterals without significant increments in portal pressure.

The type of collateral that develops depends partly on the cause of the portal hypertension. In extrahepatic portal vein thrombosis (without liver disease), collaterals (hepatopetal) in the diaphragm, in the hepatocolic and hepatogastric ligaments, etc, transport blood into the liver around the occluded vein. In both cirrhosis and portal vein thrombosis,

collaterals (hepatofugal) appear that carry blood around the liver into the systemic circulation, and it is these that produce esophageal and gastric varices. Other common spontaneous collaterals are through a recanalized umbilical vein to the abdominal wall, from the superior hemorrhoidal vein into the middle and inferior hemorrhoidal veins, and through numerous small veins (of Retzius) connecting the retroperitoneal viscera with the posterior abdominal wall.

Isolated thrombosis of the splenic vein causes localized splenic venous hypertension and gives rise to large collaterals from spleen to gastric fundus. From there, the blood returns to the main portal system through the coronary vein. In this condition, gastric varices are often present without esophageal varices.

Of the many large collaterals that form as a result of portal hypertension, spontaneous bleeding is rare except from those at the gastroesophageal junction; the reason for this bleeding is only vaguely understood. Compared with adjacent areas of the esophagus and stomach, this segment is especially rich in submucosal veins, which expand disproportionately in patients with portal hypertension. The cause of variceal bleeding is most probably rupture of one of these veins due to sudden increases in hydrostatic pressure. Esophagitis is not present.

Increased flow may contribute to portal hypertension in patients with traumatic arterial-portal venous fistulas and perhaps in some cases of giant splenomegaly, as in myeloid metaplasia or tropical splenomegaly. When an arteriovenous fistula occurs, portal hypertension and its clinical manifestations usually do not appear for several months, because sinusoidal capacity is so great that the immediate rise in portal pressure is only moderate. With time, however, sinusoidal sclerosis develops, resistance increases, and portal pressure gradually reaches high levels and stimulates variceal formation. Even in cirrhosis, the increased splenic blood flow accompanying "congestive" splenomegaly may occasionally be great enough so that splenic artery ligation or splenectomy decreases portal pressure.

Albillos A et al: Sequence of morphological and hemodynamic changes of gastric microvessels in portal hypertension. Gastroenterology 1992;102:2066.

de Franchis R, Primignani M: Why do varices bleed? Gastroenterol Clin North Am 1992;21:85.

Hashizume M et al: Three-dimensional view of the vascular structure of the lower esophagus in clinical portal hypertension. Hepatology 1988;8:1482.

Lautt WW, Greenway CV: Conceptual review of the hepatic vascular bed. Hepatology 1987;7:952.

MacMathuna P et al: Pathophysiology of portal hypertension. Dig Dis 1992;10(Suppl 1):3.

Ohnishi K et al: Portal hemodynamics in idiopathic portal hypertension (Banti's syndrome): Comparison with chronic persistent hepatitis and normal subjects. Gastroenterology 1987;92:751.

Rector WG Jr et al: Hepatofugal portal flow in cirrhosis:

observations on hepatic hemodynamics and the nature of the arterioportal communications. Hepatology 1988;8:16.

Rikkers LF: New concepts of pathophysiology and treatment of portal hypertension. Surgery 1990;107:481.

Vianna A et al: Normal venous circulation of the gastroesophageal junction. A route to understanding varices. Gastroenterology 1987;93:876.

Villeneuve JP, Huet PM: Microcirculatory abnormalities in liver diseases. Hepatology 1987;7:186.

Watanabe K et al: Portal hemodynamics in patients with gastric varices: A study in 230 patients with esophageal and/or gastric varices using portal vein catheterization. Gastroenterology 1988;95:434.

Whittle BJR, Moncada S: Nitric oxide: The elusive mediator of the hyperdynamic circulation of cirrhosis? Hepatology 1992;16:1089.

CIRRHOSIS OF THE LIVER

The death rate from cirrhosis of the liver exceeds 23,000 per year in the USA. The incidence of the disease is increasing, and at present it is the third most common cause of death in men in the fifth decade of life.

The alcoholic satisfies caloric needs from dietary alcohol to the exclusion of other important nutrients such as protein, vitamins, and minerals. Alcohol exerts direct toxic effects on the liver that are magnified in the presence of protein deficiency, but it is not known why only 15% of alcoholics develop cirrhosis. Alcohol induces a specific cytochrome P450 in the liver (ie, P450IIE1) that participates in the metabolism of alcohol. Acetaldehyde production is increased, which has a host of deleterious effects—antibody formation, decreased DNA repair, enzyme inactivation, and alterations in microtubules, mitochondria, and plasma membranes. Acetaldehyde also promotes glutathione depletion, toxicity mediated by free radicals, lipid peroxidation, and hepatic collagen synthesis. Hepatic steatosis and alcoholic hepatitis are stages of alcoholic liver injury that precede cirrhosis. Alcoholic hyalin, a glycoprotein, accumulates in centrilobular hepatocytes of patients with alcoholic hepatitis. There is some evidence that immunologic responses to alcoholic hyalin may be important in the pathogenesis of cirrhosis.

Collagen deposition in cirrhosis results from primary increased fibroblastic activity as well as from repair following hepatocellular necrosis. The ultimate result is a liver containing regenerative nodules and connective tissue septa linking portal fields with central canals.

The natural history of cirrhosis is not fully known. Once the diagnosis has been established, about 30% or more of patients are dead within a year. In newly diagnosed cirrhotics, the chances of dying within the subsequent 2–3 years are influenced by the status of liver function (as reflected by the Child-Pugh classi-

fication), the presence of large varices, and the absolute height of the portal pressure. A group of cirrhotics with varices followed by the Boston Interhospital Liver Group experienced a 1-year death rate of 66%. Cirrhotics without varices may benefit substantially by returning to a nutritious diet and abstaining from alcohol. Bleeding occurs in about 40% of all patients with cirrhosis, and the initial episode of variceal hemorrhage is fatal to 50–80%. At least two-thirds of those who survive their initial hemorrhage will bleed again, and the risk of dying from the second is about the same as from the first episode. It is principally for such patients that portacaval shunts are recommended.

Callea F et al: Cirrhosis of the liver: A regenerative process. Dig Dis Sci 1991;36:1287.

Gluud C et al: Prognostic indicators in alcoholic cirrhotic men. Hepatology 1988;8:222.

Lieber CS: Biochemical and molecular basis of alcohol-induced injury to liver and other tissues. N Engl J Med 1988;319:1639.

Stark ME, Szurszewski JH: Role of nitric oxide in gastrointestinal and hepatic function and disease. Gastroenterology 1992;103:1928.

ACUTELY BLEEDING VARICES

About half of patients with massive bleeding from varices die as a result of the acute event. This high death rate reflects not only the amount and rate of hemorrhage but also the frequent presence of severely compromised liver function and other systemic disease that may or may not be related to alcoholism. Malnutrition, pulmonary aspiration and infection, and coronary artery disease are frequent coexistent factors. The alcoholic patient often does not cooperate during therapy, and if delirium tremens ensues, even physical control of the patient may present a major challenge.

Clinical Findings
A. Symptoms and Signs: The initial management of the patient with massive gastrointestinal hemorrhage is discussed in Chapter 23. It must be emphasized that bleeding from varices cannot be accurately diagnosed on clinical grounds alone even though the history or the appearance of the patient may strongly suggest the presence of cirrhosis or portal hypertension. Most patients with bleeding varices have alcoholic cirrhosis, and the diagnosis may seem obvious in a patient with hepatomegaly, jaundice, and vascular spiders who admits to a recent alcoholic binge. Splenomegaly, the most constant physical finding, is present in 80% of patients with portal hypertension regardless of the cause. Ascites is frequently present. Massive ascites and hepatosplenomegaly in a nonalcoholic would suggest the rare

Budd-Chiari syndrome. If cirrhosis or varices have been documented on previous examinations, hematemesis later may point toward bleeding varices.

B. Laboratory Findings: Most alcoholics with acute upper gastrointestinal bleeding have compromised liver function. The bilirubin is usually elevated, and the serum albumin is often below 3 g/dL. The leukocyte count may be elevated. Anemia may be a reflection of chronic alcoholic liver disease or hypersplenism as well as acute hemorrhage. The development of a hepatoma by a cirrhotic sometimes is first manifested by bleeding varices; CT scan and determination of serum alpha-fetoprotein will make the diagnosis. The prothrombin time and partial thromboplastin time may be abnormal.

C. Special Examinations:

1. Esophagogastroscopy–Emergency esophagogastroscopy is the most useful procedure for diagnosing bleeding varices and should be scheduled as soon as the patient's general condition is stabilized by blood transfusion and other supportive measures. Varices appear as three or four large, tortuous submucosal bluish vessels running longitudinally in the distal esophagus. The bleeding site may be identified, but sometimes the lumen fills with blood so rapidly that the lesion is obscured.

2. Upper gastrointestinal series–A barium swallow outlines the varices in about 90% of affected patients, but barium studies are neither as sensitive nor as specific as endoscopy.

Treatment of Acute Bleeding

The general goal of treatment is to control the bleeding as quickly and reliably as possible using methods with the fewest possible side effects. The methods currently in use for acute variceal bleeding are listed in Table 25–2.

The patient's condition is stabilized to the extent possible by following the general guidelines for treating upper gastrointestinal bleeding described in Chapter 23. Other therapy should include measures to treat or prevent encephalopathy, parenteral vitamin K to correct a prolonged prothrombin time, and electro-

lytes (especially potassium) as required to restore electrolyte balance.

Acute endoscopic sclerotherapy is the first treatment recommended by most experts. Vasopressin or propranolol may or may not be included in the initial resuscitative regimen. Balloon tamponade is no longer used as a routine—as it once was—but is reserved for special situations when simpler methods fail.

These measures are successful in stopping the bleeding in about 90% of cases, but the early rebleeding rate is about 30%. When bleeding continues and if the patient is a good operative risk, emergency shunt is the preferred treatment.

Death rates rise rapidly in patients receiving more than ten units of blood, and in general, patients still bleeding after six units—or those whose bleeding is still unchecked 24 hours after admission—should be considered for operation. Whether or not the bleeding is brought under control, the mortality rate among patients who present with acutely bleeding varices is high (about 35%) as a result of liver failure and other complications.

A. Specific Measures:

1. Acute endoscopic sclerotherapy or ligation–Via fiberoptic endoscopy, 1–3 mL of sclerosant solution is injected into the lumen of each varix, causing it to become thrombosed. Variations in the kind of endoscope, different sclerosant solutions, whether or not the varices are physically compressed, etc, appear to have little influence on the outcome. Endoscopy is usually repeated within 48 hours and then once or twice again at weekly intervals, at which time any residual varices are injected.

Sclerotherapy controls acute bleeding in 80–95% of patients, and rebleeding during the same hospitalization is about half (25% versus 50%) the rebleeding rate of patients treated with a combination of vasopressin and balloon tamponade. Even though controlled trials show improvement in the control of bleeding, the evidence is conflicting on whether this results in increased patient survival.

A somewhat similar effect can be achieved by endoscopic rubber band ligation of the varices. The varix is lifted with a suction tip, and a small rubber band is slipped around the base. The varix necroses to leave a superficial ulcer. A controlled trial has reported rubber band ligation to be more effective in controlling bleeding (eg, fewer episodes of rebleeding; lower mortality rate) than sclerotherapy.

2. Vasopressin and terlipressin (triglycyl lysine vasopressin)–Vasopressin and terlipressin lower portal blood flow and portal pressure by a direct constricting action on splanchnic arterioles. Acute bleeding is controlled in about 80% of patients—when used in conjunction with balloon tamponade, in about 95% of patients. Cardiac output, oxygen delivery to the tissues, hepatic blood flow, and renal blood flow are also decreased—effects that oc-

---

Table 25–2. Measures to control acute bleeding from esophageal varices.

A. **Noninterventional**
  1. Vasopressin, terlipressin
  2. Somatostatin
  3. Balloon tamponade
B. **Interventional, nonsurgical**
  4. Endoscopic sclerotherapy
  5. Transphepatic embolization and sclerotherapy
C. **Surgical**
  6. Emergency portasystemic shunts
  7. Esophageal transection and reanastomosis
  8. Esophagogastric devascularization
  9. Suture ligation of varices

casionally produce complications such as myocardial infarction, cardiac arrhythmias, and intestinal necrosis. These unwanted side effects may sometimes be prevented without interfering with the decrease in portal pressure by simultaneous administration of nitroglycerin or isoproterenol.

Although the results are somewhat contradictory, controlled trials generally indicate that vasopressin plus nitroglycerin is superior to vasopressin alone and that vasopressin alone is superior to placebo in controlling active variceal bleeding. Survival is not increased, however. Vasopressin is given as a peripheral intravenous infusion (at about 0.4 units/min), which is safer than bolus injections. The nitroglycerin can be given intravenously or sublingually. Terlipressin, a synthetic vasopressin analogue, undergoes gradual conversion to vasopressin in the body and is safe to give by intravenous bolus injection (2 mg intravenously every 6 hours). It may cause fewer cardiac side effects than vasopressin.

3. Octreotide acetate–Somatostatin and the synthetic longer-lasting analogue octreotide have the same effect on the splanchnic circulation as vasopressin but without significant side effects. These drugs are as effective as vasopressin in controlling acute variceal bleeding and are now the first choice for the pharmacologic control of acutely bleeding varices. Octreotide is given as an initial bolus of 100 μg followed by a continuous infusion of 25 μ/h for 24 hours.

4. Balloon tamponade–(Figure 25–3.) Tubes designed for tamponade have two balloons that can be inflated in the lumen of the gut to compress bleed-

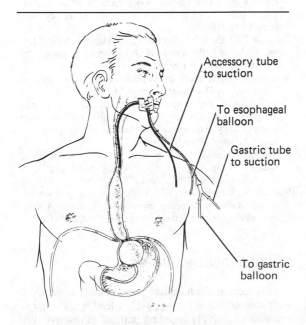

Figure 25–3. Sengstaken-Blakemore (SB) tube with both gastric and esophageal balloons inflated.

ing varices. There are three or four lumens in the tube: two are for filling the balloons and the third permits aspiration of gastric contents. A fourth lumen in the Minnesota tube is used to aspirate the esophagus orad to the esophageal balloon. The main effect is due to traction applied to the tube, which forces the gastric balloon to compress the collateral veins at the cardia of the stomach. Inflating the esophageal balloon probably contributes little, since barium x-rays suggest that it does not actually compress the varices.

The most common serious complication is aspiration of pharyngeal secretions and pneumonitis.

Another serious hazard is the occasional instance of esophageal rupture caused by inflation of the esophageal balloon. To avoid this risk, the instructions packaged with the tube must be followed carefully.

About 75% of actively bleeding patients can be controlled by balloon tamponade. When bleeding has stopped, the balloons are left inflated for another 24 hours. They are then decompressed, leaving the tube in place. If bleeding does not recur, the tube should be withdrawn.

5. Transjugular intrahepatic portasystemic shunt (TIPS)–This is a minimally invasive way of creating a shunt between the portal vein and the hepatic vein through the liver. A catheter is introduced through the jugular vein and, under radiologic control, positioned in the hepatic vein. From this point, the portal vein is accessed through the liver, the tract is dilated, and the channel is kept open by inserting an expandable metal stent, which is left in place. This technique is of great value in controlling portal hypertension and variceal bleeding and can be used to stop acute bleeding or to prevent rebleeding in a patient who has recovered from an acute episode. The shunts remain open in most patients for up to a year, at which point intimal overgrowth and thrombosis occlude a gradually increasing number.

TIPS has its greatest usefulness as a bridge to transplantation. With current materials, it should probably not be regarded as definitive therapy, though the shunt will usually remain patent for many months. Thus, patients with advanced liver disease are the principal candidates for TIPS, whereas those with less severe disease should be considered for propranolol therapy or a standard shunt operation.

6. Surgery–The operative procedures to control active bleeding are emergency portasystemic shunt and variceal ligation or esophageal transection.

a. Emergency portacaval shunt–An emergency portasystemic shunt has a 95% rate of success in stopping variceal bleeding. The death rate of the operation is related to the status of the patient's liver function (eg, Child-Pugh classification) (Table 25–3) as well as the rate and amount of bleeding and its effects on cardiac, renal, and pulmonary function. Some patients with advanced liver disease—especially those with severe encephalopathy and ascites—are so unlikely to survive that surgery is unwar-

Table 25–3. Child-Pugh classification of functional status in liver disease.

	Class: Risk:	A Low	B Moderate	C High
Ascites		Absent	Slight to moderate	Tense
Encephalopathy		None	Grades I–II	Grades III–IV
Serum albumin (g/dL)		>3.5	3.0–3.5	<3.0
Serum bilirubin (mg/dL)		<2.0	2.0–3.0	>3.0
Prothrombin time (seconds above control)		<4.0	4.0–6.0	>6.0

ranted for them despite continued bleeding. On the other hand, patients with good liver function usually recover after an emergency shunt. The only relevant controlled trial showed that the death rate in acutely bleeding Child's C patients was insignificantly lower after endoscopic sclerotherapy (44%) than after emergency portacaval shunt (50%).

For active bleeding, an end-to-side portacaval shunt or H-mesocaval shunt is most commonly performed.

The distal splenorenal (Warren) shunt is usually too time-consuming for use in emergency operations. The central splenorenal shunt is more complicated than an end-to-side portacaval shunt and has no specific advantages. A side-to-side portacaval shunt might be preferable in an acutely bleeding patient with severe ascites, and it or a variant (eg, H-mesocaval shunt) would be required for someone with Budd-Chiari syndrome.

Hepatic failure is the cause of death in about two-thirds of those who succumb after an emergency portacaval shunt. Renal failure, which is often accompanied by ascites, is another potentially lethal problem. Metabolic alkalosis and delirium tremens are common postoperatively in alcoholics. Antacids should be given for 1–2 weeks after surgery to prevent stress ulceration.

b. Esophageal transection–Varices may be obliterated by firing the end-to-end stapler in the distal esophagus after tucking a full-thickness ring of tissue into the cartridge with a circumferential tie. This procedure has gained popularity in the past decade, and in many surgical units it is the first choice for therapy when nonsurgical methods fail. If transection is performed, it must be done as soon as it is recognized that a second attempt at sclerotherapy or band ligation has failed. As a last-ditch effort—after many units of blood have been transfused—death from liver failure is all but certain. The results (eg, survival) are better in patients with nonalcoholic cirrhosis. Stapled transection has replaced the older technique of direct suture ligation of the varices.

Transection must be viewed as an emergency measure to stop persistent bleeding—not as definitive treatment—because varices recur months later in many patients.

Burroughs AK: Medical management of bleeding esophageal varices. Dig Dis 1992;10(Suppl 1):30.

Cello JP et al: Endoscopic sclerotherapy versus portacaval shunt in patients with severe cirrhosis and acute variceal hemorrhage. N Engl J Med 1987;316:11.

Dudley FJ: Somatostatin and portal hypertensive bleeding: a safe therapeutic alternative? Gastroenterology 1992;103:1973.

Gostout CJ et al: Acute gastrointestinal bleeding. Experience of a specialized management team. Journal of Clinical Gastroenterology 1992;14:260.

Hwang SJ et al: A randomized controlled trial comparing octreotide and vasopressin in the control of acute esophageal variceal bleeding. J Hepatol 1992;16:320.

Jenkins SA, Shields R: Non-surgical management of the acute variceal bleed. Br J Surg 1992;79:859.

Kochman ML, Elta GH, Laine L: Bleeding esophageal varices: Inject or band? Gastroenterology 1992;103:1979.

Lee H et al: Intensive care treatment of patients with bleeding esophageal varices: Results, predictors of mortality, and predictors of the adult respiratory distress syndrome. Crit Care Med 1992;20:1555.

Le Moine O et al: Factors related to early mortality in cirrhotic patients bleeding from varices and treated by urgent sclerotherapy. Gut 1992;33:1381.

Lewis JJ, Basson MD, Modlin IM: Surgical therapy of acute esophageal variceal hemorrhage. Dig Dis 1992;10(Suppl 1):46.

Matloff DS: Treatment of acute variceal bleeding. Gastroenterol Clin North Am 1992;21:103.

Orloff MJ et al: Is portal-systemic shunt worthwhile in Child's class C cirrhosis? Long-term results of emergency shunt in 94 patients with bleeding varices. Ann Surg 1992;216:256.

Pasquale MD, Cerra FB: Sengstaken-Blakemore tube placement: Use of balloon tamponade to control bleeding varices. Crit Care Clin 1992;8:743.

Scarpignato C: Clinical pharmacology of active variceal bleeding. Dig Dis 1992;10(Suppl 1):16.

Shields R et al: A prospective randomised controlled trial comparing the efficacy of somatostatin with injection sclerotherapy in the control of bleeding oesophageal varices. J Hepatol 1992;16:128.

Stiegmann GV et al: Endoscopic sclerotherapy as compared with endoscopic ligation for bleeding esophageal varices. N Engl J Med 1992;326:1527.

Walker S, Kreichgauer HP, Bode JC: Terlipressin vs. somatostatin in bleeding esophageal varices: A controlled, double-blind study. Hepatology 1992;15:1023.

NONBLEEDING VARICES

This section discusses the management of patients with varices that are not actively bleeding. The management of actively bleeding patients is discussed in the preceding section and in Chapter 24.

Patients with varices that have never bled have a

30% chance of bleeding; and of those who bleed, 50% die. For patients who do not bleed during the first year after diagnosis of varices, the risk of bleeding subsequently decreases by half and continues to drop thereafter. Patients who have bled once from esophageal varices have a 70% chance of bleeding again, and about two-thirds of repeat bleeding episodes are fatal.

Evaluation

A. Severity of Hepatic Disease and Operative Risk: The immediate death rate of an elective shunt procedure can be predicted from the patient's hepatic function as reflected by the Child-Pugh classification (Table 25–3). In addition to operative death rate, the figures also correlate with the death rate in the first postshunt year. Thereafter, survival curves of the different risk classes become reasonably parallel.

The severity of histopathologic changes in liver biopsies correlates with the immediate surgical death rate, the most ominous findings being hepatocellular necrosis, polymorphonuclear leukocyte infiltration, and the presence of Mallory bodies. The extent of histologic change also correlates with the more easily obtained data in the Child-Pugh classification (ie, severe changes occur in class C patients), so results of biopsies have no independent predictive value.

B. Portal Flow and Pressure Measurements: Measurements of pressure and flow in the splanchnic vasculature have been used for diagnosis and as a guide to therapy and prognosis in portal hypertension. Portal pressure can be measured directly at surgery or preoperatively by any of the following techniques: (1) Wedged hepatic venous pressure (WHVP), which accurately reflects free portal pressure when portal hypertension is caused by a postsinusoidal (or sinusoidal) resistance, as in cirrhosis. The measurement obtained with the catheter in the wedged position should be corrected by subtracting the free hepatic venous pressure (FHVP). This is the most commonly used technique. (2) Direct measurement of splenic pulp pressure by a percutaneously placed needle. (3) Percutaneous transhepatic catheterization of the intrahepatic branches of the portal vein. This is the method of choice in patients thought to have presinusoidal block or Budd-Chiari syndrome. (4) Catheterization of the umbilical vein through a small incision, the catheter being threaded into the portal system. With each of these methods, one may also obtain anatomic information by performing angiography through the catheter.

It is not customary in the average case to measure portal pressure preoperatively, however, since the information obtained does not influence management of the average case.

Duplex ultrasonography is an accurate noninvasive means of assessing the amount and direction of flow in the portal vein. Preoperatively, duplex ultrasonography is useful to determine patency of the por-

tal vein and direction of flow. Because of spontaneous thrombosis, about 10% of patients with cirrhosis have a portal vein unsuitable for a portacaval shunt. If flow in the portal vein is reversed (hepatofugal), a selective shunt is not recommended, because it compromises the ability of portal tributaries to serve as an outflow tract for liver blood. Duplex ultrasonography can also be used to follow changes in portal perfusion after shunt operations.

C. Portal Angiography: The portal venous anatomy is often studied preoperatively by angiographic techniques. The objectives are to determine the patency, location, and size of the veins tentatively chosen for a shunt, to demonstrate the presence of varices, and to estimate the degree of prograde portal flow. Some of this information can now be obtained less invasively by duplex ultrasonography. When a splenorenal shunt is contemplated, the left renal vein should be opacified, either by injection of the renal artery or renal vein.

Treatment

The treatment options consist of expectant management, endoscopic sclerotherapy, propranolol, portasystemic shunts, devascularization of the esophagogastric junction, and miscellaneous rarely used operations. The treatment of patients with varices that have never bled is usually referred to as "prophylactic" therapy (eg, "prophylactic" sclerotherapy or "prophylactic" propranolol). By convention, procedures performed on patients who have bled previously are referred to as "therapeutic" (eg, "therapeutic" shunts).

A. Prophylactic Therapy: Prophylactic therapy could theoretically be of value since the mortality rate of variceal bleeding is high (50%), the risk of bleeding in patients with varices is relatively high (30%), and varices can often be diagnosed before the initial episode of bleeding. In patients who have never bled before, the following have been shown to be related to the risk of bleeding: Child-Pugh classification, the size of the varices, and the presence of red wale markings (longitudinal dilated venules resembling whip marks) on the varices. This information can be used to identify and consider for prophylactic propranolol those patients who have a 65% chance of bleeding within a year.

B. Therapy of Patients Who Have Bled Previously: As noted earlier, patients who recover from an episode of variceal bleeding have about a 70% chance of bleeding again. Much effort is being expended in attempts to ascertain the best treatment regimen for these patients. The methods of greatest interest include endoscopic sclerotherapy, propranolol, and various kinds of portasystemic shunts.

1. Endoscopic sclerotherapy–The technique of endoscopic sclerotherapy was described earlier in this chapter. Chronic sclerotherapy has been disappointing as a method for preventing future bleeding, and most have come to think of it principally as a way to stop acute bleeding when bleeding recurs.

2. Propranolol–Propranolol, a β-adrenergic blocking agent, decreases cardiac output and splanchnic blood flow and consequently portal blood pressure. Chronic propranolol therapy, 20–160 mg twice daily (a dose that reduces resting pulse rate by 25%), decreases by about 40% the frequency of rebleeding from esophageal or gastric varices, deaths from rebleeding, and overall mortality. The benefits are greater in Child's A and B than in Child's C cirrhotics. The addition of chronic sclerotherapy to the propranolol regimen does not improve the outcome. Abstinence from alcohol may not be critical to success, as was initially thought.

C. Surgery: The objective of the surgical procedures used to treat portal hypertension is either to obliterate the varices or to reduce blood flow and pressure within the varices (Table 25–4). A more recent option is liver transplantation.

1. Liver transplantation–Any relatively young patient with cirrhosis who has survived an episode of variceal hemorrhage should be considered a candidate for liver transplantation, since any other form of

Table 25–4. Surgical procedures for esophageal varices.

A. Direct variceal obliteration
 1. Variceal suture ligation
  a. Transthoracic
  b. Transabdominal
 2. Esophageal transection and reanastomosis
  a. Suture technique
  b. Staple technique
 3. Variceal sclerosis
  a. Esophagoscopic
  b. Transhepatic
 4. Variceal resection
  a. Esophagogastrectomy
  b. Subtotal esophagectomy
B. Reduction of variceal blood flow and pressure
 1. Portasystemic shunts
  a. End-to-side
  b. Side-to-side
   1. Side-to-side portacaval
   2. Mesocaval
   3. Central splenorenal
   4. Renosplenic
 2. Selective shunts
  a. Distal splenorenal (Warren)
  b. Left gastric vena caval (Inokuchi)
 3. Reduction of portal blood flow
  a. Splenectomy
  b. Splenic artery ligation
 4. Reduction of proximal gastric blood flow
  a. Esophagogastric devascularization
  b. Gastric transection and reanastomosis (Tanner)
 5. Stimulation of additional portasystemic venous collaterals
  a. Omentopexy
  b. Splenic transposition
C. Measures to preserve hepatic blood flow after portacaval shunt
 1. Arterialization of portal vein stump

therapy carries a much higher (about 80%) mortality rate within the subsequent year or two as a result of repeated bleeding or complications of hepatic failure. Obviously, continued alcoholism will serve as an absolute contraindication to transplantation in most patients. The good transplantation candidates, however, should not be subjected to portasystemic shunts or other procedures if it appears that they will come to transplantation in the near future. In general, Child's class A patients are candidates for portal decompression; Child's class C patients are candidates for a transplant. A transjugular intrahepatic shunt (see previous section) is an excellent way to control bleeding while the patient is being prepared for a transplant.

2. Portasystemic shunts–Portasystemic shunts can be grouped into those that shunt the entire portal system (total shunts) and those that selectively shunt blood from the gastrosplenic region while preserving the pressure-flow relationships in the rest of the portal bed (selective shunts). All of the shunt operations commonly used today reduce the incidence of rebleeding to less than 10%, compared with about 75% in unshunted patients. Unfortunately, the price of this achievement is an operative mortality rate of 5–20% (depending on the Child-Pugh classification [Table 25–3]), decreased liver function, and an increase in encephalopathy (at least with total shunts). Therefore, since shunts have these drawbacks in addition to the ability to prevent bleeding, experimental trials are needed to pinpoint their place within an overall treatment strategy.

In one well-designed trial, patients who had bled previously were randomized to chronic sclerotherapy or a distal splenorenal shunt (Warren shunt). Patients randomized to chronic sclerotherapy who had recurrent episodes of bleeding during treatment (ie, treatment failures, which amounted to 30% of the sclerotherapy group) were then treated surgically (ie, shunted). The results showed that 2-year survival was better among those originally randomized to sclerotherapy (90%) than among those originally assigned to the shunt group (60%). This trial supports a general treatment plan consisting initially of sclerotherapy and reserving portasystemic shunts for the patients in whom sclerotherapy fails to control bleeding adequately.

The choice of what kind of shunt to use has been the subject of much debate and several randomized trials. The principal question in recent years has been whether encephalopathy and survival are better with a selective shunt (eg, a distal splenorenal shunt) than with a total shunt (eg, a mesocaval or an end-to-side portacaval shunt). The results are conflicting, but in general they support the contention that there is about half as much severe encephalopathy following selective shunts. None of the trials have shown any particular shunt to be associated with longer survival than other shunts.

 a. Types of portasystemic shunts–Figure

25–4 depicts the various shunts in use at this time. Although they differ technically, physiologically there are only three different types: end-to-side, side-to-side, and selective.

(1) Total shunts–The end-to-side shunt completely disconnects the liver from the portal system. The portal vein is transected near its bifurcation in the liver hilum and anastomosed to the side of the inferior vena cava. The hepatic stump of the vein is oversewn. Postoperatively, the wedged hepatic venous pressure (sinusoidal pressure) drops slightly, reflecting the inability of the hepatic artery to compensate fully for the loss of portal inflow. The side-to-side portacaval, mesocaval, mesorenal, and central splenorenal shunts are all physiologically similar, since the shunt preserves continuity between the hepatic limb of the portal vein, the portal system, and the anastomosis. Flow through the hepatic limb of the standard side-to-side shunt is nearly always away from the liver and toward the anastomosis. The extent to which hepatofugal flow is produced by the other types of "side-to-side" shunts listed above is not known.

The end-to-side portacaval shunt gives immediate and permanent protection from variceal bleeding and is somewhat easier to perform than a side-to-side portacaval or central splenorenal shunt. Encephalopathy may be slightly more common after side-to-side than end-to-side portacaval shunts. Side-to-side shunts are required in patients with Budd-Chiari syndrome or refractory ascites (when the latter is treated by a portasystemic shunt).

The mesocaval shunt interposes a segment of prosthetic graft or internal jugular vein between the inferior vena cava and the superior mesenteric vein where the latter passes in front of the uncinate process of the pancreas. The mesocaval shunt is particularly useful in the presence of severe scarring in the right upper quadrant or portal vein thrombosis, and in some cases it may be technically easier than a conventional side-to-side portacaval shunt if a side-to-side type of shunt is necessary. In most cases, portal flow to the liver is lost after this shunt. Evidence has been presented, however, that by limiting the diameter of the prosthetic graft to 8 mm (compared with 12- to 20-mm grafts), prograde flow is preserved in the portal vein, which decreases the incidence of postoperative encephalopathy while still preventing variceal hemorrhage.

(2) Selective shunts–Selective shunts lower pressure in the gastroesophageal venous plexus while preserving blood flow through the liver via the portal vein.

The distal splenorenal (Warren) shunt involves anastomosing the distal (splenic) end of the transected splenic vein to the side of the left renal vein, plus ligation of the major collaterals between the remaining portal and isolated gastrosplenic venous system. The latter step involves division of the gastric vein, the right gastroepiploic vein, and the vessels in the splenocolic ligament. The operation is more difficult and time-consuming than conventional shunts and except for the experienced operator is probably too complex for emergency portal decompression. If mobilization of the splenic vein is hazardous, the renal vein may be transected and its caval end joined to the side of the undisturbed splenic vein. The segment of splenic vein between the anastomosis and the portal vein is then ligated. Surprisingly, this seems to have little permanent effect on renal function as long as the remaining tributaries are preserved on the oversewn renal vein stump.

In contrast to total shunts, the Warren shunt does not improve ascites and should not be performed in patients whose ascites has been difficult to control. Preoperative angiography should be performed to determine if the splenic vein and left renal vein are large enough and close enough together for performance of

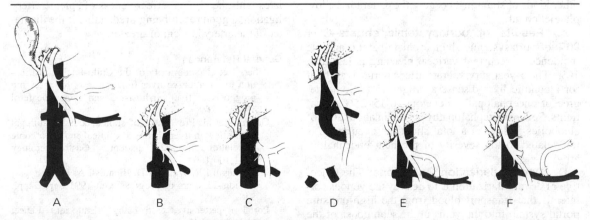

Figure 25–4. Types of portacaval anastomoses: **A:** Normal. **B:** Side-to-side. **C:** End-to-side. **D:** Mesocaval. **E:** Central splenorenal. **F:** Distal splenorenal (Warren). The H-mesocaval shunt is not illustrated.

this shunt. Recent pancreatitis may preclude safe dissection of the splenic vein from the undersurface of the pancreas.

Another type of selective shunt (Inokuchi shunt) consists of joining the left gastric vein to the inferior vena cava by a short segment of autogenous saphenous vein. The procedure has not become popular, perhaps because of its technical complexity.

Selective shunts tend to become less selective over several years as new collaterals develop between the high- and low-pressure regions of the portal system. This is accompanied by a gradual decrease in portal pressure (measured by WHVP) and evolution of the procedure into a version of side-to-side total shunt. The enlargement postoperatively of small venous tributaries entering the distal splenic vein from the pancreas suggests that this is the path by which nonselectivity develops. It is possible that this can be avoided by mobilizing the splenic vein all the way to the hilum (dividing these small vessels) before performing the splenorenal anastomosis.

b. Choice of shunt–Our current approach to shunt selection is as follows: The distal splenorenal shunt is the first choice for elective portal decompression. If ascites is present or the anatomy is unfavorable, an end-to-side portacaval shunt is preferred. Side-to-side shunts would be done for patients with severe ascites or Budd-Chiari syndrome. We reserve the H-mesocaval and central splenorenal shunts for special anatomic situations in which the above operations are unsuitable. An end-to-side shunt or H-mesocaval shunt is performed for emergency decompression.

Portacaval and distal splenorenal shunts are often followed by a rise in platelet count in patients with secondary hypersplenism. Even though the response is unpredictable, however, hypersplenism rarely produces clinical manifestations, so it does not have to be taken into account in making a choice of shunt. A central splenorenal shunt, in which splenectomy is performed, should not be considered preferable to other kinds of shunt just because the patient has a low platelet count.

c. Results of portasystemic shunts–Over 90% of portasystemic shunts remain patent, and the incidence of recurrent variceal bleeding is less than 10%. The 5-year survival rate after a portacaval shunt for alcoholic liver disease averages 45%. Some degree of encephalopathy develops in 15–25% of patients. Severe encephalopathy is seen in about 20% of alcoholics following a total shunt; its occurrence is not related to the severity of preshunt encephalopathy.

D. Devascularization Operations: The objective of devascularization is to destroy the venous collaterals that transport blood from the high-pressure portal system into the veins in the submucosa of the esophagus.

The Sugiura procedure is done in two stages. In the first stage, performed through a thoracotomy, the dilated venous collaterals between esophagus and adjacent structures are divided, and the esophagus at the level of the diaphragm is transected and reanastomosed. The second stage, a laparotomy, is performed immediately after the thoracotomy if the patient is actively bleeding, but for elective cases it is deferred 4–6 weeks. The upper two-thirds of the stomach is devascularized, selective vagotomy and pyloroplasty are performed, and the spleen is removed. It is possible in some cases to perform the entire operation through the left chest. An analogous operation has been described that consists of splenectomy, gastroesophageal devascularization, and resection of a 5-cm segment of the gastroesophageal junction. Continuity of the gut is restored by an end-to-side esophagogastrostomy, and pyloroplasty is performed.

In the reports from Japan, where these operations originated, there was a 5% operative death rate, a 2–4% rate of variceal rebleeding, and an 80% 5-year survival rate. The new operations of this type performed in alcoholic patients in North America have had poor results, owing to a high rate (40%) of late rebleeding.

E. Miscellaneous Operations: Attempts have also been made to decrease portal pressure by decreasing splanchnic inflow through splenectomy or splenic artery ligation. Diseases characterized by marked splenomegaly may rarely be associated with portal hypertension as a consequence of increased splenic blood flow, which has been known to reach levels as high as 1000 mL/min. Splenic blood flow may occasionally be increased enough in patients with cirrhosis to contribute significantly to the portal hypertension. However, splenectomy or splenic artery ligation in cirrhosis most often gives only a transient decrease in portal pressure, and over half of patients having these operations bleed again. Some workers have suggested that the absolute size of the splenic artery (a crude index of splenic flow) correlates with the clinical effectiveness of splenic artery ligation, a good result being predictable if the diameter of the artery is 1 cm or greater.

General References

Albers I et al: Superiority of the Child-Pugh classification to quantitative liver function tests for assessing prognosis of liver cirrhosis. Scand J Gastroenterol 1989;24:269.

Gaiani S et al: Prevalence of spontaneous hepatofugal portal flow in liver cirrhosis: Clinical and endoscopic correlation in 228 patients. Gastroenterology 1991;100:160.

MacDougall BR, Westaby D, Blendis LA: Portal hypertension–25 years of progress. Gut 1991 Sep; Suppl: S18.

Portal hypertensive gastropathy. (Editorial.) Lancet 1991;338:1045.

Ready JB et al: Assessment of the risk of bleeding from

esophageal varices by continuous monitoring of portal pressure. Gastroenterology 1991;100(5 Part 1):1403.

Rice S et al: Portal venous system after portosystemic shunts or endoscopic sclerotherapy: Evaluation with Doppler sonography. AJR Am J Roentgenol 1991; 156:85.

Sarin SK et al: Prevalence, classification and natural history of gastric varices: A long-term follow-up study in 568 portal hypertension patients. Hepatology 1992;16:1343.

Sclerotherapy

Heaton ND, Howard ER: Complications and limitations of injection sclerotherapy in portal hypertension. Gut 1993;34:7.

Ink O et al: Does elective sclerotherapy improve the efficacy of long-term propranolol for prevention of recurrent bleeding in patients with severe cirrhosis? A prospective multicenter, randomized trial. Hepatology 1992;16:912.

Kochhar R, Goenka MK, Mehta SK: Esophageal strictures following endoscopic variceal sclerotherapy: Antecedents, clinical profile, and management. Dig Dis Sci 1992;37:347.

Parikh SS, Desai HG: What is the aim of esophageal variceal sclerotherapy—prevention of rebleeding or complete obliteration of veins? J Clin Gastroenterol 1992;15:186.

Propranolol

Hayes PC et al: Meta-analysis of value of propranolol in prevention of variceal haemorrhage. Lancet 1990; 336:153.

Perez-Ayuso RM et al: Propranolol in prevention of recurrent bleeding from severe portal hypertensive gastropathy in cirrhosis. Lancet 1991;337:1431.

Transjugular Intrahepatic Portal-Systemic Shunts (TIPS)

Bleeding oesophageal varices: IST, EVL, or TIPS? (Editorial.) Lancet 1992;340:515.

Conn HO: Transjugular intrahepatic portal-systemic shunts: The state of the art. Hepatology 1993;17:148.

Haskal ZJ et al: Role of parallel transjugular intrahepatic portosystemic shunts in patients with persistent portal hypertension. Radiology 1992;185:813.

Shunts

Adam R, Diamond T, Bismuth H: Partial portacaval shunt: Renaissance of an old concept. Surgery 1992; 111:610.

Bismuth H et al: Options for elective treatment of portal hypertension in cirrhotic patients in the transplantation era. Am J Surg 1990;160:105.

Galloway JR, Henderson JM: Management of variceal bleeding in patients with extrahepatic portal vein thrombosis. Am J Surg 1990;160:122.

Gongliang J, Rikkers LF: Cause and management of upper gastrointestinal bleeding after distal splenorenal shunt. Surgery 1992;112:719.

Henderson JM: The distal splenorenal shunt. Surg Clin North Am 1990;70:405.

Henderson JM et al: Selective shunt in the management

of variceal bleeding in the era of liver transplantation. Ann Surg 1992;216:248.

Johansen K: Prospective comparison of partial versus total portal decompression for bleeding esophageal varices. Surg Gynecol Obstet 1992;175:528.

Levine BA, Sirinek KR: The portacaval shunt. Surg Clin N Amer 1990;70:361.

Lillemoe KD, Cameron JL: The interposition mesocaval shunt. Surg Clin North Am 1990;70:379.

Millikan WJ Jr et al: Surgical rescue for failures of cirrhotic sclerotherapy. Am J Surg 1990;160:117.

Myburgh JA: Selective shunts: The Johannesburg experience. Am J Surg 1990;160:67.

Orozco H et al: Selective splenocaval shunt for bleeding portal hypertension: Fifteen-year evaluation period. Surgery 1993;113:260.

Orozco H et al: Elective treatment of bleeding varices with the Sugiura operation over 10 years. Am J Surg 1992;163:585.

Rikkers LF: New concepts of pathophysiology and treatment of portal hypertension. Surgery 1990;107:481.

Rypins EB, Sarfeh IJ: Small-diameter portacaval H-graft for variceal hemorrhage. Surg Clin North Am 1990;70:395.

Spina GP et al: Distal spleno-renal shunt versus endoscopic sclerotherapy in the prevention of variceal rebleeding: A meta-analysis of 4 randomized clinical trials. J Hepatol 1992;16:338.

EXTRAHEPATIC PORTAL VENOUS OCCLUSION

Idiopathic portal vein thrombosis (in the absence of liver disease) accounts for most cases of portal hypertension in childhood and for a few cases in adults. Neonatal septicemia, omphalitis, umbilical vein catheterization for exchange transfusion, and dehydration have all been incriminated as possible causes, but collectively they can be implicated in less than half of cases. The causes of portal vein thrombosis in adults include hepatic tumors, cirrhosis, trauma, pancreatitis, pancreatic pseudocyst, myelofibrosis, thrombotic states (eg, protein C deficiency), and sepsis.

Although clinical manifestations may be delayed until adulthood, 80% of patients present between 1 and 6 years of age with variceal bleeding. About 70% of hemorrhages are preceded by a recent upper respiratory tract infection. Some of these children first come to medical attention because of splenomegaly and pancytopenia. Failure to recognize the underlying problem has occasionally led to splenectomy, with the result that portal decompression using the splenic vein is precluded. Ascites is uncommon except transiently after bleeding. Liver function is either normal or only slightly impaired, which probably accounts for the low incidence of overt encephalopathy. There is an increased frequency of neuropsychiatric problems, which may be a subtle form of encephalopathy.

Because the patient's general condition and liver

function are good, the death rate for sudden massive bleeding is about 20%, much below the rate in other types of portal hypertension. The diagnosis can be confirmed radiologically by percutaneous mesenteric angiography. Wedged hepatic venous pressure is normal.

Bleeding episodes in children under age 8 are usually self-limited and often do not require endoscopic sclerotherapy, administration of vasopressin, or Sengstaken tube tamponade. In general, however, the bleeding episodes are self-limited and uncommonly fatal, so emergency operations are rarely necessary.

The thrombosed portal vein is unsuitable for a shunt. A cavomesenteric shunt is best for young children, whose vessels are small. In older individuals, treatment should be started with sclerotherapy; if that fails to control the bleeding, a distal splenorenal shunt is preferred. Splenectomy alone has no permanent effect and sacrifices the splenic vein, which might be needed later for a shunt. Because shunts in small children have a high rate of spontaneous thrombosis, variceal bleeding is preferably managed without a shunt until the child is 8–10 years of age and the vessels are larger. Nevertheless, using silk sutures and precise technique, some surgeons have obtained a high rate of anastomotic patency even in the very young. Patients with encephalopathy and hepatic dysfunction many years after a total shunt may be improved if they are converted to a selective shunt.

Splenectomy alone is never indicated in this disease, either for hypersplenism or in an attempt to reduce portal pressure, because the rebleeding rate is 90% and fatal postsplenectomy sepsis is not uncommon. If it is not possible to construct an adequate shunt, expectant management is the best regimen. Repeated severe hemorrhages should be treated by transendoscopic sclerosis. Esophagogastrectomy with colon interposition is a last resort.

Galloway JR, Henderson JM: Management of variceal bleeding in patients with extrahepatic portal vein thrombosis. Am J Surg 1990;160:122.

Orozco H et al: The Sugiura procedure for patients with hemorrhagic portal hypertension secondary to extrahepatic portal vein thrombosis. Surg Gynecol Obstet 1991;173:45.

Sahni P, Parde GK, Nundy S: Extrahepatic portal vein obstruction. Br J Surg 1990;77:1201.

Szczepanik AB, Rudowski WJ: Extrahepatic portal hypertension: Long-term results of surgical treatment. Ann R Coll Surg Engl 1989;71:222.

Valla D et al: Etiology of portal vein thrombosis in adults: A prospective evaluation of primary myeloproliferative disorders. Gastroenterology 1988;94:1063.

Warren WD et al: Management of variceal bleeding in patients with noncirrhotic portal vein thrombosis. Ann Surg 1988;207:623.

SPLENIC VEIN THROMBOSIS

Isolated thrombosis of the splenic vein is a rare cause of variceal bleeding that can be cured by splenectomy. The splenic venous blood, blocked from its normal route, flows through the short gastric vessels to the gastric fundus and then into the left gastric vein, continuing toward the liver. As the blood traverses the stomach, large gastric varices are produced that may rupture and bleed. Characteristically, the collateral pattern does not involve the esophagus, so esophageal varices are uncommon.

The principal causes of this syndrome are pancreatitis, pancreatic pseudocyst, neoplasm, and trauma. Splenomegaly is present in two-thirds of patients. Diagnosis can be made by selective splenic arteriography that opacifies the venous phase. Splenectomy is curative. Many cases of splenic vein thrombosis are unaccompanied by bleeding varices, and in such cases, no therapy is required.

Little AG, Moossa AR: Gastrointestinal hemorrhage from left-sided portal hypertension: An unappreciated complication of pancreatitis. Am J Surg 1981;141:153.

Madsen MS, Petersen TH, Sommer H: Segmental portal hypertension. Ann Surg 1986;204:72.

BUDD-CHIARI SYNDROME

Budd-Chiari syndrome is a rare disorder resulting from obstruction of hepatic venous outflow. Most cases are caused by spontaneous thrombosis of the hepatic veins, often associated with polycythemia vera or the use of birth control pills. Some patients present with idiopathic membranous stenosis of the inferior vena cava located between the hepatic veins and right atrium, which is usually associated with thrombosis of one or both hepatic veins. Most patients with this lesion are HBsAg-positive, and many have malignancies (eg, hepatocellular carcinoma). It was originally thought that these lesions were congenital, but they are now known to consist of stenosis resulting from thrombosis and scar formation.

The posthepatic (postsinusoidal) obstruction raises sinusoidal pressure, which is transmitted upstream to cause portal hypertension. Because the parenchyma is relatively free of fibrosis, filtration across the sinusoids and hepatic lymph formation increase greatly, producing marked ascites.

Symptoms usually begin with a mild prodrome consisting of vague right upper quadrant abdominal pain, postprandial bloating, and anorexia. After weeks or months, a more florid picture develops consisting of gross ascites, hepatomegaly, and hepatic failure. At this stage the AST is usually markedly increased, the serum bilirubin is slightly elevated, and the alkaline phosphatase is inconsistently abnormal.

Except in patients with membranous obstruction of

the vena cava, liver scan usually demonstrates absent function through most of the liver except for a small central area representing the caudate lobe, whose venous outflow is spared (it goes directly to the vena cava through multiple small tributaries). CT scans show pooling of intravenous contrast media in the periphery of the liver; patent hepatic veins cannot be seen on ultrasound scans. An enlarged azygos vein may be seen on chest x-rays of patients with caval obstruction. Liver biopsy reveals grossly dilated central veins and sinusoids, pericentral necrosis, and replacement of hepatocytes by red blood cells. Centrilobular fibrosis develops late. The clinical diagnosis should be confirmed by venography, which shows the hepatic veins to be obstructed, usually with a beak-like deformity at their orifice. The inferior vena cava should be opacified to verify that it is patent—a requirement for a successful portacaval shunt. The x-rays may show compression of the intrahepatic cava by the congested liver.

A side-to-side portacaval or mesocaval shunt should be constructed when the obstruction is confined to the hepatic veins. Focal membranous obstruction of the suprahepatic cava may be treated by excision of the lesion with or without the addition of a patch angioplasty. Some cases may be managed nonsurgically by percutaneous transluminal balloon dilation of the stenosis.

Occlusion of the inferior vena cava by thrombosis or compression from the liver requires a mesoatrial shunt using a prosthetic vascular graft. Because the incidence of graft thrombosis is relatively high, it may be advisable to perform a second-stage side-to-side portacaval shunt a few months after mesoatrial shunt decompression of the liver in patients with hepatic vein thrombosis whose vena cava was originally blocked by a congested liver. Development of hepatocellular carcinoma is common in patients with membranous obstruction of the vena cava. The postoperative results are excellent in patients without malignant neoplasms.

Liver transplantation is indicated in patients with advanced hepatic decompensation either from cirrhosis or as part of the acute syndrome. The results are excellent, and the risk of later hepatocellular carcinoma is eliminated.

Bismuth H, Sherlock DJ: Portasystemic shunting versus liver transplantation for the Budd-Chiari syndrome. Ann Surg 1991;214:581.

Henderson JM: Portal hypertension and shunt surgery. Adv Surg 1993;26:233.

Hobbs KE: Budd-Chiari syndrome. Lancet 1992;339:115.

Kage M et al: Histopathology of membranous obstruction of the inferior vena cava in the Budd-Chiari syndrome. Gastroenterology 1992;102:2081.

Klein AS et al: Current management of the Budd-Chiari syndrome. Ann Surg 1990;212:144.

Langnas AN et al: Surgical management of the Budd-Chiari

syndrome: No place for a procrustean bed. Hepatology 1992;16:1303.

Lim JH, Park JH, Auh YH: Membranous obstruction of the inferior vena cava: Comparison of findings at sonography, CT, and venography. AJR Am J Roentgenol 1992;159:515.

Lopez RR Jr et al: Expandable venous stents for treatment of the Budd-Chiari syndrome. Gastroenterology 1991;100(5 Part 1):1435.

Orloff MJ, Daily PO, Girard B: Treatment of Budd-Chiari syndrome due to inferior vena cava occlusion by combined portal and vena caval decompression. Am J Surg 1992;163:137.

Orloff MJ, Orloff MS, Daily PO: Long-term results of treatment of Budd-Chiari syndrome with portal decompression. Arch Surg 1992;127:1182.

Shaked A et al: Portosystemic shunt versus orthotopic liver transplantation for the Budd-Chiari syndrome. Surg Gynecol Obstet 1992;174:453.

Soyer P et al: Mesoinnominate shunt for the treatment of Budd-Chiari syndrome: Evaluation with multimodality imaging. Eur J Radiol 1993;16:131.

ASCITES

Ascites in hepatic disease results from (1) increased formation of hepatic lymph (from sinusoidal hypertension), (2) increased formation of splanchnic lymph, (3) hypoalbuminemia, and (4) salt and water retention by the kidneys. Before therapy is started, paracentesis should be performed and the following examinations made on a sample of ascitic fluid: (1) Culture and leukocyte count: Spontaneous bacterial peritonitis is common and may be clinically silent. A white count above 250/μL is highly suggestive of infection. (2) LDH levels: A ratio of LDH in ascites to serum that exceeds 0.6 suggests the presence of cancer or infection. (3) Serum amylase: A high level indicates pancreatic disease. (4) Albumin: The ratio of serum to ascites albumin concentrations is above 1.1 in liver disease and below 1.1 in malignant ascites.

Medical Treatment

In general, the intensity of medical therapy required to control ascites can be predicted from the pretreatment 24-hour urine Na^+ output as follows: A Na^+ output above 5 meq/24 h will require strong diuretics; 5–25 meq/24 h, mild diuretics; and above 25 meq/24 h, no diuretics. Initial treatment is usually with spironolactone, 200 mg/d. The objective is to stimulate a weight loss of 0.5–0.75 kg/d, except in patients with peripheral edema who can mobilize fluid faster. If spironolactone alone is insufficient, another drug such as furosemide should be added. A loop diuretic (eg, furosemide, ethacrynic acid) should be given only in combination with a distally acting diuretic (eg, spironolactone, triamterene). Alternatively, massive ascites may be treated by one or more large (eg, 5-L) paracenteses accompanied by an intravenous infusion of albumin. If albumin is not given, the incidence of renal and electrolyte complications is high. Salt or water restriction is no longer recommended except in the most refractory cases.

Surgical Treatment

A. Portacaval Shunt: A history of ascites that has been easy to control need not influence the choice of shunt operation intended to treat variceal bleeding. When ascites has been severe, however, a side-to-side shunt (eg, side-to-side portacaval, H-mesocaval, central splenorenal) may be considered, because it reduces sinusoidal as well as splanchnic venous pressure. A side-to-side portacaval shunt is indicated rarely just to treat ascites—eg, in patients in whom several LeVeen shunts have thrombosed—although the incidence of severe postoperative encephalopathy is high under these circumstances.

B. Peritoneal-Jugular Shunt (LeVeen Shunt): Refractory ascites can be treated with a LeVeen shunt—a subcutaneous Silastic catheter that transports ascitic fluid from the peritoneal cavity to the jugular vein. A small unidirectional valve sensitive to a pressure gradient of 3–5 cm H_2O prevents backflow of blood. A modification called the Denver shunt contains a small chamber that can be used as a pump to clear the line by external pressure. In practice, Denver shunts become blocked more often than LeVeen shunts.

In patients with ascites due to cirrhosis, use of a LeVeen shunt should be confined to those who fail to respond to high doses of diuretics (eg, 400 mg of spironolactone and 400 mg of furosemide daily) or who repeatedly develop encephalopathy or azotemia during diuretic therapy.

Peritoneovenous shunts may also be used for ascites associated with cancer. The best results occur in patients whose ascitic fluid contains no malignant cells. A LeVeen shunt is of benefit in Budd-Chiari syndrome but is ineffective for chylous ascites. Because the incidence of complications and early shunt thrombosis is high, a LeVeen shunt is relatively contraindicated if the ascitic fluid is grossly bloody, contains many malignant cells, or has a high protein concentration (> 4.5 g/dL). The incidence of tumor embolization is low (5%).

The ascitic fluid should be cultured a few days before the shunt is inserted. Antibiotics are given pre- and postoperatively. The operation is best performed under general anesthesia but can be done with local anesthesia.

Postoperatively, the patient is outfitted with an abdominal binder and instructed to perform respiratory exercises against mild pressure to increase abdominal pressure and flow through the shunt. Dietary salt should not be restricted. A functioning LeVeen shunt is unable by itself to eliminate ascites, but it renders the patient much more responsive to diuretics. Therefore, furosemide should be administered postoperatively.

An average of 10 kg of weight is lost during the first 10 days after the operation, and eventually the abdomen assumes a normal configuration. Nutrition and serum albumin levels often improve postoperatively. Urinary sodium excretion increases promptly, and renal function may improve in patients with the hepatorenal syndrome. Serious complications and deaths are most common in patients with advanced hepatorenal syndrome or a serum bilirubin level greater than 4 mg/dL. Although some patients eventually bleed from varices following insertion of a LeVeen shunt, the risk of bleeding is not increased by the shunt, which actually decreases portal pressure. Thus, a previous episode of variceal bleeding is not a contraindication for this procedure. Disseminated intravascular coagulation (DIC), manifested by increased fibrin split products, decreased platelet count, etc, occurs in more than half of cases but presents a clinical problem in only a few. The frequency and severity of DIC may be minimized by emptying most of the ascitic fluid from the abdomen during operation and partially replacing it with Ringer's lactate solution. Lethal septicemia may occur if the ascitic fluid is infected at the time the shunt is inserted.

In about 10% of cases, the valve becomes thrombosed and must be replaced.

Hydrothorax, usually on the right side, may develop in patients with cirrhosis and ascites. The fluid reaches the chest through a pinhole opening in the membranous portion of the diaphragm, a pathway that can be demonstrated by aspirating the thoracic fluid, injecting technetium Tc 99m colloid into the ascites fluid, and observing rapid accumulation of the label in the chest. Treatment consists of a peritoneovenous shunt and injection of a sclerosing agent into the pleural cavity after it has been tapped dry. If a leak persists, it may be closed surgically by thoracotomy.

Gines P et al: Paracentesis with intravenous infusion of albumin as compared with peritoneovenous shunting in cirrhosis with refractory ascites. N Engl J Med 1991;325:829.

Gough IR, Balderson GA: Malignant ascites: A comparison of peritoneovenous shunting and nonoperative management. Cancer 1993;71:2377.

Herrera JL: Current medical management of cirrhotic ascites. Am J Med Sci 1991;302:31.

Hillaire S et al: Peritoneovenous shunting of intractable ascites in patients with cirrhosis: Improving results and predictive factors of failure. Surgery 1993;113:373.

Lee CM et al: Serum-ascites albumin concentration gradient and ascites fibronectin in the diagnosis of malignant ascites. Cancer 1992;70:2057.

Longmire-Cook SJ: Pathophysiologic factors and management of ascites. Surg Gynecol Obstet 1993;176:191.

Runyon BA et al: The serum-ascites albumin gradient is superior to the exudate-transudate concept in the differential diagnosis of ascites. Ann Intern Med 1992;117:215.

Wilkinson SP, Moore KP, Arroyo V: Pathogenesis of ascites and hepatorenal syndrome. Gut 1991 Sep;Suppl:S12.

HEPATIC ENCEPHALOPATHY

Central nervous system symptoms may be seen in patients with chronic liver disease and are especially prone to develop after portacaval shunt. Portal-systemic encephalopathy, ammonia intoxication, hepatic coma, and meat intoxication are terms used to refer to this condition. The manifestations range from lethargy to coma—from minor personality changes to psychosis—from asterixis to paraplegia. Hypothermia and hyperventilation may precede coma.

Pathogenesis

Hepatic encephalopathy is a reversible metabolic neuropathy that results from the effects of toxins absorbed from the gut on the brain. Increased exposure of the brain to these toxins is the result of decreased detoxification by the liver due to diminished function and spontaneous or surgically created shunts of portal venous blood around the liver and increased permeability of the blood-brain barrier. The toxins form from the action of colonic bacteria on protein within the gut. Potential aggravating factors include gastrointestinal hemorrhage, constipation, azotemia, hypokalemic alkalosis, infection, excessive dietary protein, and sedatives (Table 25–5). Four main theories concerning mediation of this syndrome currently attract the most attention.

A. Amino Acid Neurotransmitters: Gamma-aminobutyric acid (GABA), the principal inhibitory neurotransmitter in the brain, produces a state similar to hepatic encephalopathy when given experimentally. It is synthesized in the brain and by bacteria within the colon, is degraded by the liver, and is found in increased levels in the serum of patients with hepatic encephalopathy. The passage of GABA across the blood-brain barrier is increased in hepatic encephalopathy. Experiments also indicate the presence of increased numbers of GABA receptors in encephalopathy and increased GABA ergic tone, perhaps due to a benzodiazepine receptor agonist ligand on the receptor complex (GABA/benzodiazepine receptor). This has raised the possibility of treating encephalopathy with benzodiazepine antagonists, and the drug flumazenil has shown promise in preliminary trials.

B. Ammonia: Ammonia is produced in the colon by bacteria and is absorbed and transported in portal venous blood to the liver, where it is extracted and converted to glutamine. Ammonia concentrations are elevated in the arterial blood and cerebrospinal fluid of patients with encephalopathy, and experimental administration of ammonia produces central nervous system symptoms.

C. False Neurotransmitters: According to this theory, cerebral neurons become depleted of normal neurotransmitters (norepinephrine and dopamine), which are partially replaced by false neurotransmitters (octopamine and phenylethanolamine). The result is inhibition of neural function. Serum levels of branched-chain amino acids (leucine, isoleucine, valine) are decreased and levels of aromatic amino acids (tryptophan, phenylalanine, tyrosine) are elevated in patients with encephalopathy. Because these two classes of amino acids compete for transport across the blood-brain barrier, the aromatic amino acids have increased access to the central nervous system, where they serve as precursors for false neurotransmitters. Trials of therapy with supplements of branched-chain amino acids have given conflicting results.

D. Synergistic Neurotoxins: This theory postulates that ammonia, mercaptans, and fatty acids, none of which accumulate in brain in amounts capable of producing encephalopathy, have synergistic effects that produce the full-blown syndrome.

Prevention

Encephalopathy is a major side effect of portacaval shunt and is to some extent predictable. Elderly patients are considerably more susceptible. Alcoholics fare better than those with postnecrotic or cryptogenic cirrhosis, apparently owing to the invariable progression of liver dysfunction in the latter. Good liver function partially protects the patients from encephalopathy. If the liver has adapted to complete or nearly complete diversion of portal blood before operation, a surgical shunt is less apt to depress liver function further. For example, patients with thrombosis of the portal vein (complete diversion and normal liver function) rarely experience encephalopathy after portal-systemic shunt. Encephalopathy is less common after a distal splenorenal (Warren) shunt than after other kinds of shunts.

Increased intestinal protein whether of dietary origin or from intestinal bleeding aggravates encephalopathy by providing more substrate for intestinal bacteria. Constipation allows more time for bacterial action on colonic contents. Azotemia results in higher concentration of blood urea, which diffuses into the intestine, is converted to ammonia, and is

Table 25–5. Factors contributing to encephalopathy.

A.	**Increased systemic toxin levels**
1.	Extent of portal-systemic venous shunt
2.	Depressed liver function
3.	Intestinal protein load
4.	Intestinal flora
5.	Azotemia
6.	Constipation
B.	**Increased sensitivity of central nervous system**
1.	Age of patient
2.	Hypokalemia
3.	Alkalosis
4.	Diuretics
5.	Sedatives, narcotics, tranquilizers
6.	Infection
7.	Hypoxia, hypoglycemia, myxedema

then reabsorbed. Hypokalemia and metabolic alkalosis aggravate encephalopathy by shifting ammonia from extracellular to intracellular sites where the toxic action occurs.

Laboratory Findings

Arterial ammonia levels are usually high. The presence of high levels of glutamine in the cerebrospinal fluid may help distinguish hepatic encephalopathy from other causes of coma. Electroencephalography is more sensitive than clinical evaluation in detecting minor involvement. The changes are nonspecific and consist of slower mean frequencies. Studies performed at different times can be compared to assess the effects of therapy.

Treatment

Acute encephalopathy is treated by controlling precipitating factors, halting all dietary protein intake, cleansing the bowel with purgatives and enemas, and administering antibiotics (neomycin or ampicillin) or lactulose. Neomycin may be given orally or by gastric tube (2–4 daily) or rectally as an enema (1% solution 1–2 times daily). At least 1600 kcal of carbohydrate should be provided daily, along with therapeutic amounts of vitamins. Blood volume must be maintained to avoid prerenal azotemia. After the patient responds to initial therapy, dietary protein may be started at 20 g/d and increased by increments of 10–20 g every 2–5 days as tolerated.

Chronic encephalopathy is treated by restriction of dietary protein, avoidance of constipation, and elimination of sedatives, diuretics, and tranquilizers. To avoid protein depletion, protein intake must not be chronically reduced below 50 g/d. Vegetable protein in the diet is tolerated better than is animal protein. Lactulose, a disaccharide unaffected by intestinal enzymes, is the drug of choice for long-term control. When given orally (20–30 g three or four times daily), it reaches the colon, where it stimulates bacterial anabolism (which increases ammonia uptake) and inhibits bacterial enzymes (which decreases the generation of nitrogenous toxins). Its effect is independent of colonic pH. A related compound, lactitol (β-galactoside sorbitol), is also effective and appears to work faster. As a powder, it is easier to use than liquid lactulose. Intermittent courses of oral neomycin or metronidazole may be given if lactitol therapy and preventive measures are inadequate.

Butterworth RF: Pathogenesis and treatment of portal-systemic encephalopathy: An update. Dig Dis Sci 1992;37:321.

Kreis R et al: Metabolic disorders of the brain in chronic hepatic encephalopathy detected with H-1 MR spectroscopy. Radiology 1992;182:19.

Mullen KD: Benzodiazepine compounds and hepatic encephalopathy. N Engl J Med 1991;325:509.

Record CO: Neurochemistry of hepatic encephalopathy. Gut 1991;32:1261.

Biliary Tract

26

Lawrence W. Way, MD

EMBRYOLOGY & ANATOMY

The anlage of the biliary ducts and liver consists of a diverticulum that appears on the ventral aspect of the foregut in 3 mm embryos. The cranial portion becomes the liver; a caudal bud forms the ventral pancreas; and an intermediate bud develops into the gallbladder. Originally hollow, the hepatic diverticulum becomes a solid mass of cells that later recanalizes to form the ducts. The smallest ducts—the bile canaliculi—are first seen as a basal network between the primitive hepatocytes that eventually expands throughout the liver (Figure 26–1). Numerous microvilli increase the canalicular surface area. Bile secreted here passes through the interlobular ductules (canals of Hering) and the lobar ducts and then into the hepatic duct in the hilum. In most cases, the common hepatic duct is formed by the union of a single right and left duct, but in 25% of individuals, the anterior and posterior divisions of the right duct join the left duct separately. The origin of the common hepatic duct is close to the liver but always outside its substance. It runs about 4 cm before joining the cystic duct to form the common bile duct. The common duct begins in the hepatoduodenal ligament, passes behind the first portion of the duodenum, and runs in a groove on the posterior surface of the pancreas before entering the duodenum. Its terminal 1 cm is intimately adherent to the duodenal wall. The total length of the common duct is about 9 cm.

In 80–90% of individuals, the main pancreatic duct joins the common duct to form a common channel about 1 cm long. The intraduodenal segment of the duct is called the hepatopancreatic ampulla, or ampulla of Vater.

The gallbladder is a pear-shaped organ adherent to the undersurface of the liver in a groove separating the right and left lobes. The fundus projects 1–2 cm below the hepatic edge and can often be felt when the cystic or common duct is obstructed. It rarely has a complete peritoneal covering, but when this variation does occur, it predisposes to infarction by torsion. The gallbladder holds about 50 mL of bile when fully distended. The neck of the gallbladder tapers into the narrow cystic duct, which connects with the common duct. The lumen of the cystic duct contains a thin mucosal septum, the spiral valve of Heister, that offers mild resistance to bile flow. In 75% of persons, the cystic duct enters the common duct at an angle. In the remainder, it runs parallel to the hepatic duct or winds around it before joining the common duct (Figure 26–2).

In the hepatoduodenal ligament, the hepatic artery is to the left of the common duct and the portal vein is posterior and medial. The right hepatic artery usually passes behind the hepatic duct and then gives off the cystic artery before entering the right lobe of the liver, but variations are common.

The mucosal epithelium of the bile ducts varies from cuboidal in the ductules to columnar in the main ducts. The gallbladder mucosa is thrown into prominent ridges when the organ is collapsed, and these flatten during distention. The tall columnar cells of the gallbladder mucosa are covered by microvilli on their luminal surface. Wide channels, which play an important role in water and electrolyte absorption, separate the individual cells.

The walls of the bile ducts contain only small amounts of smooth muscle, but the termination of the common duct is enveloped by a complex sphincteric muscle. The gallbladder musculature is composed of interdigitated bundles of longitudinal and spirally arranged fibers.

The biliary tree receives parasympathetic and sympathetic innervation. The former contains motor fibers to the gallbladder and secretory fibers to the ductal epithelium. The afferent fibers in the sympathetic nerves mediate the pain of biliary colic.

PHYSIOLOGY

Bile Flow

Bile is produced at a rate of 500–1500 mL/d by the hepatocytes and the cells of the ducts. Active secretion of bile salts into the biliary canaliculus is responsible for most of the volume of bile and its fluctuations. Na^+ and water follow passively to establish isosmolality and electrical neutrality. Lecithin and cholesterol enter the canaliculus at rates that correlate with variations in bile salt output. Bilirubin and a number of other organic anions—estrogens, sulfobromophthalein, etc—are actively secreted by the

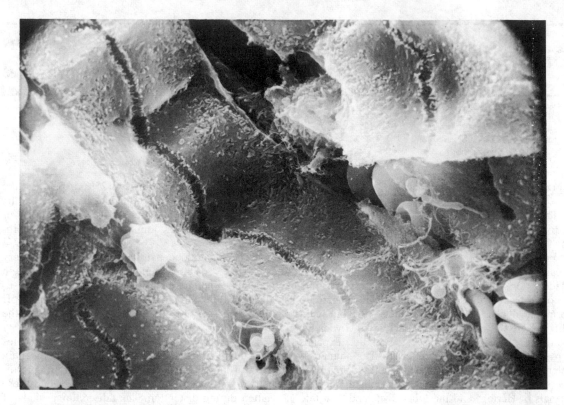

Figure 26–1. Scanning electron photomicrograph of a hepatic plate with adjacent sinusoids and sinusoidal microvilli and a bile canaliculus running in the center of the liver cells. Although their boundaries are indistinct, about four hepatocytes constitute the section of the plate in the middle of the photograph. Occasional red cells are present within the sinusoids. (Reduced from × 2000.) (Courtesy of Dr James Boyer.)

hepatocyte by a different transport system from that which handles bile salts.

The columnar cells of the ducts add a fluid rich in HCO_3^- to that produced in the canaliculus. This involves active secretion of Na^+ and HCO_3^- by a cellular pump stimulated by secretin, VIP, and cholecystokinin. K^+ and water are distributed passively across the ducts (Figure 26–3).

Between meals, bile is stored in the gallbladder, where it is concentrated at rates of up to 20% per hour. Na^+ and either HCO_3^- or Cl^- are actively transported from its lumen during absorption. The changes in composition brought about by concentration are shown in Figure 26–4.

Three factors regulate bile flow: hepatic secretion, gallbladder contraction, and choledochal sphincteric resistance. In the fasting state, pressure in the common bile duct is 5–10 cm H_2O, and bile produced in the liver is diverted into the gallbladder. After a meal, the gallbladder contracts, the sphincter relaxes, and bile is forced into the duodenum in squirts as ductal pressure intermittently exceeds sphincteric resistance. During contraction, pressure within the gallbladder reaches 25 cm H_2O and that in the common bile duct 15–20 cm H_2O.

Cholecystokinin (CCK) is the major physiologic stimulus for postprandial gallbladder contraction and relaxation of the sphincter, but vagal impulses facilitate its action. CCK is released into the bloodstream from the mucosa of the small bowel by fat or lipolytic products in the lumen. Amino acids and small polypeptides are weaker stimuli, and carbohydrates are ineffective. Bile flow during a meal is augmented by turnover of bile salts in the enterohepatic circulation and stimulation of ductal secretion by secretin, VIP, and CCK. Motilin stimulates episodic partial gallbladder emptying in the interdigestive phase.

Bile Salts & the Enterohepatic Circulation (Figures 26–4 and 26–5)

Bile salts, lecithin, and cholesterol comprise about 90% of the solids in bile, the remainder consisting of bilirubin, fatty acids, and inorganic salts. Gallbladder bile contains about 10% solids and has a bile salt concentration between 200 and 300 mmol/L.

Bile salts are steroid molecules formed from cholesterol by hepatocytes. The rate of synthesis is under feedback control and can be increased a maximum of about 20-fold. Two **primary** bile salts—cholate and chenodeoxycholate—are produced by the liver. Be-

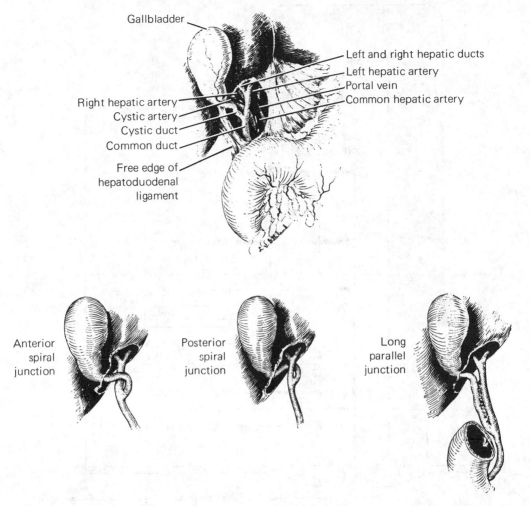

Figure 26–2. Anatomy of the gallbladder and variations in anatomy of the cystic duct.

fore excretion into bile, they are conjugated with either glycine or taurine, which enhances water solubility. Intestinal bacteria alter these compounds to produce the **secondary** bile salts, deoxycholate and lithocholate. The former is reabsorbed and enters bile, but lithocholate is insoluble and is excreted in the stool. Bile is composed of 40% cholate, 40% chenodeoxycholate, and 20% deoxycholate, conjugated with glycine or taurine in a ratio of 3:1.

The functions of bile salts are (1) to induce the flow of bile, (2) to transport lipids, and (3) to bind calcium ions in bile. The importance of the last of these is unknown. Bile acid molecules are amphipathic—ie, they have hydrophilic and hydrophobic poles. In bile, they form multimolecular aggregates called micelles in which the hydrophilic poles become aligned to face the aqueous medium. Water-insoluble lipids, such as cholesterol, can be dissolved within the hydrophobic centers of bile salt micelles. Molecules of lecithin, a water-insoluble but

polar lipid, aggregate into hydrated bilayers that form vesicles in bile, and they also become incorporated into bile acid micelles to form mixed micelles. Mixed micelles have an increased lipid-carrying capacity compared with pure bile acid micelles. Cholesterol in bile is transported within the phospholipid vesicles and the bile salt micelles.

Bile salts remain in the intestinal lumen throughout the jejunum, where they participate in fat digestion and absorption. Upon reaching the distal small bowel, they are reabsorbed by an active transport system located in the terminal 200 cm of ileum. Over 95% of bile salts arriving from the jejunum are transferred by this process into portal vein blood; the remainder enter the colon, where they are converted to secondary bile salts. The entire bile salt pool of 2.5–4 g circulates twice through the enterohepatic circulation during each meal, and six to eight cycles are made each day. The normal daily loss of bile salts in

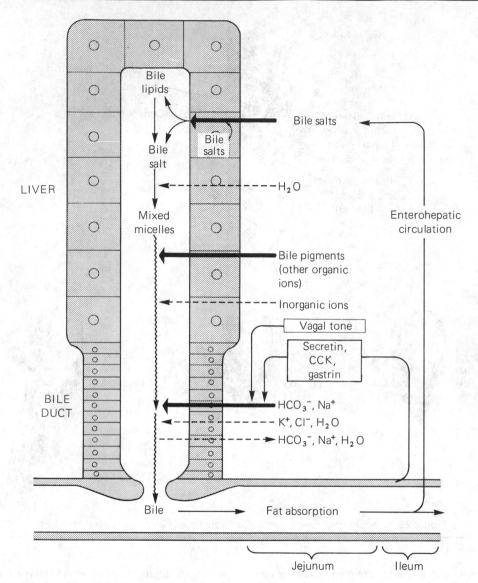

Figure 26–3. Bile formation. Solid lines into the ductular lumen indicate active transport; dotted lines represent passive diffusion.

the stool amounts to 10–20% of the pool and is restored by hepatic synthesis.

Arias IM et al: The biology of the bile canaliculus. Hepatology 1993;17:318.

Buanes T et al: Secretin empties bile duct cell cytoplasm of vesicles when it initiates ductular HCO_3^- secretion in the pig. Gastroenterology 1988;95:417.

Burwen SJ, Schmucker DL, Jones AL: Subcellular and molecular mechanisms of bile secretion. Int Rev Cytol 1992;135:269.

Cohen DE, Carey MC: Physical chemistry of biliary lipids during bile formation. Hepatology 1990;12(3 Part 2):143S.

Coleman R, Rahman K: Lipid flow in bile formation. Biochim Biophys Acta 1992;23;1125:113.

Goff JS: The human sphincter of Oddi. Arch Intern Med 1988;148:2673.

Hofmann AF: Bile acid secretion, bile flow and biliary lipid secretion in humans. Hepatology 1990;12(3 Part 2):17S.

Marzio L et al: Gallbladder contraction and its relationship to interdigestive duodenal motor activity in normal human subjects. Dig Dis Sci 1988;33:540.

Motta PM: The three-dimensional microanatomy of the liver. Arch Histol Jpn 1984;47:1.

Nathanson MH, Boyer JL: Mechanisms and regulation of bile secretion. Hepatology 1991;14:551.

Renner EL, Reichen J: The role of bile salt uptake in canalicular bile formation. Transport systems and acinar heterogeneity. J Hepatol 1991;13:140.

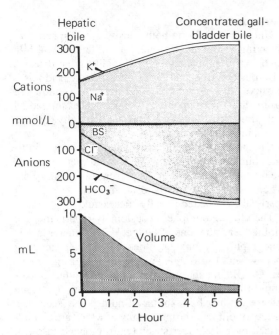

Figure 26–4. Changes in gallbladder bile composition with time. (Courtesy of J Dietschy.)

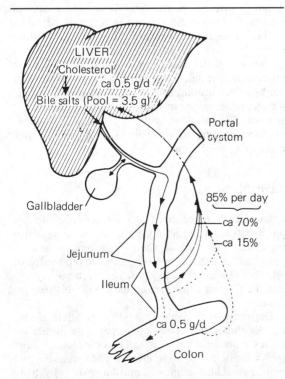

Figure 26–5. Enterohepatic circulation of bile salts. (Courtesy of M Tyor.)

Bilirubin

About 250–300 mg of bilirubin is excreted each day in the bile, 75% of it from breakdown of red cells in the reticuloendothelial system and 25% from turnover of hepatic heme and hemoproteins. First, heme is liberated from hemoglobin, and the iron and globin are removed for reuse by the organism. Biliverdin, the first pigment formed from heme, is reduced to unconjugated bilirubin, the indirect-reacting bilirubin of the van den Bergh test. Unconjugated bilirubin is insoluble in water and is transported in plasma bound to albumin.

Unconjugated bilirubin is extracted from blood by hepatocytes, where it is conjugated with glucuronic acid to form bilirubin diglucuronide, the water-soluble direct bilirubin. Conjugation is catalyzed by glucuronyl transferase, an enzyme on the endoplasmic reticulum. Bilirubin is transported within the hepatocyte by cytosolic binding proteins, which rapidly deliver the molecule to the canalicular membrane for active secretion into bile. Within bile, conjugated bilirubin is largely transported in association with mixed lipid micelles.

After entering the intestine, bilirubin is reduced by intestinal bacteria to several compounds known as urobilinogens, which are subsequently oxidized and converted to pigmented urobilins. The term urobilinogen is often used to refer to both urobilins and urobilinogens.

DIAGNOSTIC EXAMINATION OF THE BILIARY TREE

Plain Abdominal Film

The posteroanterior supine view of the abdomen will show gallstones in the 10–15% of cases where they are radiopaque. The bile itself sometimes contains sufficient calcium (milk of calcium bile) to be seen. An enlarged gallbladder can occasionally be identified as a soft tissue mass in the right upper quadrant indenting an air-filled hepatic flexure.

In several types of biliary disease, the diagnosis may be suggested by air seen in the bile ducts on a plain film. This usually signifies the presence of a biliary-intestinal fistula (from disease or surgery) but also occurs rarely in severe cholangitis, emphysematous cholecystitis, and biliary ascariasis.

Oral Cholecystography

Tyropanoate sodium (Bilopaque) or iopanoic acid (Telepaque) is taken orally the night before the examination, along with a light meal. The drug is absorbed, bound to albumin in portal blood, extracted by hepatocytes, and secreted in bile. Opacification occurs only with concentration in the gallbladder and on the average is optimal 10 hours after tyropanoate ingestion. Posteroanterior and oblique supine views and an upright or lateral decubitus film are obtained.

Oral cholecystograms are unsatisfactory if the contrast agent is inefficiently absorbed from the intestine or poorly excreted by the liver. Absorption is often impaired in acute abdominal illnesses with ileus, vomiting, or diarrhea. If the bilirubin level is over 3 mg/dL, hepatic excretion will probably be inadequate. False-negative results are obtained in 5% of tests. A normal gallbladder may not opacify for several weeks after severe trauma or a major illness.

Nonopacification occurs in 20% of patients after the usual single-dose regimen. When a second dose is given and x-rays repeated the following day, opacification is obtained in 25% of these patients. Persistent nonopacification is a highly reliable (> 95% true positive) indication of gallbladder disease. Instead of performing a double-dose oral cholecystogram as the next step when a single dose fails to opacify, it is simpler to obtain an ultrasound scan.

Percutaneous Transhepatic Cholangiography (THC, PTC)

Percutaneous transhepatic cholangiography is performed by passing a fine needle through the right lower rib cage and the hepatic parenchyma and into the lumen of a bile duct. Water-soluble contrast material is injected, and x-ray films are taken.

The technical success is related to the degree of dilatation of the intrahepatic bile ducts. THC is especially valuable in demonstrating the biliary anatomy in patients with benign biliary strictures, malignant lesions of the proximal bile duct, or when ERCP (see below) has been unsuccessful. Failure of the contrast medium to enter a duct does not prove that obstruction is absent. THC should not be done in patients with cholangitis until the infection has been controlled with antibiotics. Virtually all patients should be premedicated with antibiotics regardless of whether they have cholangitis—septic shock has been produced by sudden inoculation of organisms from bile into the systemic circulation. Otherwise, the contraindications are the same as for percutaneous liver biopsy.

Endoscopic Retrograde Cholangiopancreatography (ERCP)

ERCP involves cannulating the sphincter of Oddi under direct vision through a side-viewing duodenoscope. It requires special training involving more than familiarity with the use of fiberoptic endoscopes. Usually it is possible to opacify the pancreatic as well as the bile ducts. This method of cholangiography is especially applicable to patients with an abnormal clotting mechanism who would not be candidates for transhepatic puncture of the ducts. It is usually the preferred method of examining the biliary tree in patients with presumed choledocholithiasis or obstructing lesions in the periampullary region.

Ultrasound

Ultrasonography is both sensitive and specific in detecting gallbladder stones and dilatation of bile ducts. In the investigation of gallbladder disease, false-positive diagnoses for stones are rare, and false-negative reports owing to small stones or a contracted gallbladder occur in only 5% of patients examined by real time ultrasound. Ultrasound usually misses stones in the common duct.

Dilatation of bile ducts in a jaundiced patient indicates bile duct obstruction, but it is fairly common for the ducts to be normal in the presence of obstruction. When ultrasound shows dilated ducts, THC will nearly always be technically successful.

The ultrasonographer occasionally reports that the gallbladder contains "sludge." This material is sonographically opaque, does not cast an acoustic shadow, and forms a dependent layer in the gallbladder. On clinical analysis, it is a fine precipitate of calcium bilirubinate. Sludge may accompany gallstone disease or may be a solitary finding. It is seen in a variety of clinical settings, many of which are characterized by gallbladder stasis (eg, prolonged fasting). By itself, sludge is not an indication for cholecystectomy.

Radionuclide Scan (HIDA Scan)

Technetium 99m-labeled derivatives of iminodiacetic acid (IDA) are excreted in high concentration in bile and produce excellent gamma camera images. Following intravenous injection of the radionuclide, imaging of the bile ducts and gallbladder normally appears within 15–30 minutes and of the intestine within 60 minutes. In patients with acute right upper quadrant pain and tenderness, a good image of the bile duct accompanied by no image of the gallbladder indicates cystic duct obstruction and strongly supports a diagnosis of acute cholecystitis. The test is easy to perform and is currently the best method of confirming this diagnosis.

JAUNDICE

Jaundice is categorized as prehepatic, hepatic, or posthepatic, depending upon the site of the underlying disease. Hemolysis, the most common cause of prehepatic jaundice, involves increased production of bilirubin. Less common causes of prehepatic jaundice are Gilbert's disease and the Crigler-Najjar syndrome.

Hepatic parenchymal jaundice is subdivided into hepatocellular and cholestatic types. The former includes acute viral hepatitis and chronic alcoholic cirrhosis. Some cases of intrahepatic cholestasis may be indistinguishable clinically and biochemically from cholestasis due to bile duct obstruction. Primary biliary cirrhosis, toxic drug jaundice, cholestatic jaundice of pregnancy, and postoperative cholestatic jaundice are the most common forms.

Extrahepatic jaundice most often results from biliary obstruction by a malignant tumor, choledocholithiasis, or biliary stricture. Pancreatic pseudocyst, chronic pancreatitis, sclerosing cholangitis, metastatic cancer, and duodenal diverticulitis are less common causes.

The cause of jaundice can be ascertained in the majority of patients from clinical and laboratory findings alone. In the remainder, THC or ERCP and ultrasound or CT scans will be necessary. The indications for these tests are discussed in later sections.

History

The age, sex, and parity of the patient and possible deleterious habits should be noted. Most cases of infectious hepatitis occur in patients under age 30. A history of drug addiction may suggest serum hepatitis transmitted by shared hypodermic equipment. Chronic alcoholism can usually be documented in patients with cirrhosis, and acute jaundice in alcoholics usually follows a recent binge. Obstructing gallstones or tumors are more common in older people.

Patients with jaundice due to choledocholithiasis may have associated biliary colic, fever, and chills and may report previous similar attacks. The pain in malignant obstruction is deep-seated and dull and may be affected by changes in position. Pain in the region of the liver is frequently experienced in the early stages of viral hepatitis and acute alcoholic liver injury. The patient with extrahepatic obstruction may report that stools have become lighter in color and the urine dark.

Cholestatic diseases are often accompanied by pruritus–a source of severe discomfort in some cases. Pruritus may precede jaundice, but usually it appears at about the same time. The itching is most severe on the extremities and is aggravated by warm, humid weather. The cause remains obscure; itching does not correlate with bile salt levels in the skin, as was once believed. Cholestyramine, an anion exchange resin, usually provides relief by binding bile salts in the intestinal lumen and preventing their reabsorption.

Physical Examination

Hepatomegaly is common in both hepatic and posthepatic jaundice. In some cases, palpation of the liver may suggest cirrhosis or metastatic cancer, but impressions of this kind are unreliable. Secondary stigmas of cirrhosis usually accompany acute alcoholic jaundice; liver palms, spider angiomas, ascites, collateral veins on the abdominal walls, and splenomegaly suggest cirrhosis. A nontender, palpable gallbladder in a jaundiced patient suggests malignant obstruction of the common duct (Courvoisier's law), but absence of a palpable gallbladder is of little significance in ruling out cancer.

Laboratory Tests

In hemolytic disease, the increased bilirubin is principally in the unconjugated indirect fraction. Since unconjugated bilirubin is insoluble in water, the jaundice in hemolysis is acholuric. The total bilirubin in hemolysis rarely exceeds 4–5 mg/dL, because the rate of excretion increases as the bilirubin concentration rises, and a plateau is quickly reached. Greater values suggest concomitant hepatic parenchymal disease.

Jaundice due to hepatic parenchymal disease is characterized by elevations of both conjugated and unconjugated serum bilirubin. An increase in the conjugated fraction always signifies disease within the hepatobiliary system. The direct bilirubin predominates in about half of cases of hepatic parenchymal disease.

Both intrahepatic cholestasis and extrahepatic obstruction raise the direct bilirubin fraction, though the indirect fraction also increases somewhat. Since direct bilirubin is water-soluble, bilirubinuria develops. With complete extrahepatic obstruction, the total bilirubin rises to a plateau of 25–30 mg/dL, at which point loss in the urine equals the additional daily production. Higher values suggest concomitant hemolysis or decreased renal function. Obstruction of a single hepatic duct does not usually cause jaundice.

In extrahepatic obstruction caused by neoplasms, the serum bilirubin usually exceeds 10 mg/dL, and the average concentration is about 18 mg/dL. Obstructive jaundice due to common duct stones often produces transient bilirubin increases in the range of 2–4 mg/dL, and the level rarely exceeds 15 mg/dL. Serum bilirubin values in patients with alcoholic cirrhosis and acute viral hepatitis vary widely in relation to the severity of the parenchymal damage.

In extrahepatic obstruction, modest rises of AST levels are common, but levels as high as 1000 units are seen (though rarely) in patients with common duct stones and cholangitis. In the latter patients, the high values last for only a few days and are associated with increases in LDH concentrations. In general, AST levels above 1000 units suggest viral hepatitis.

Serum alkaline phosphatase comes from three sites: liver, bone, and intestine. In normal subjects, liver and bone contribute about equally, and the intestinal contribution is small. Hepatic alkaline phosphatase is a product of the epithelial cells of the cholangioles, and increased alkaline phosphatase levels associated with liver disease are the result of increased enzyme production. Alkaline phosphatase levels go up with intrahepatic cholestasis, cholangitis, or extrahepatic obstruction. Since the elevation is from overproduction, it may occur with focal hepatic lesions in the absence of jaundice. For example, a solitary hepatic metastasis or pyogenic abscess in one lobe or a tumor obstructing only one hepatic duct may fail to obstruct enough hepatic parenchyma to cause jaundice but usually is associated with increased alkaline phosphatase. In cholangitis with incomplete extrahepatic obstruction, serum bilirubin levels may be normal or mildly elevated, but serum alkaline phosphatase may be very high.

Bone disease may complicate the interpretation of abnormal alkaline phosphatase levels (Figure 26–6). If one suspects that the increased serum enzyme may be from bone, serum calcium, phosphorus, and 5′-nucleotidase or leucine aminopeptidase levels should be determined. These last two enzymes are also produced by cholangioles and are elevated in cholestasis, but their serum concentrations remain unchanged with bone disease.

Changes in serum protein levels may reflect hepatic parenchymal dysfunction. In cirrhosis, the serum albumin falls and the globulins increase. Serum globulins reach high values in some patients with primary biliary cirrhosis. Biliary obstruction generally produces no changes unless secondary biliary cirrhosis has developed.

Diagnosis

The principal diagnostic objective is to distinguish surgical (obstructive) from nonsurgical jaundice. The history, physical examination, and basic laboratory data allow an accurate diagnosis to be made in most cases without invasive tests (eg, liver biopsy, cholangiograms).

Since most jaundiced patients are not critically ill when first seen, diagnosis and therapy may be conducted in a stepwise fashion, with each test selected according to the information available at that point. Only severe or worsening cholangitis requires urgent intervention. If the jaundice is mild and recent, it often passes within 24–48 hours, at which time an oral cholecystogram or ultrasound scan can be ordered to verify gallstone disease.

In patients with persistent jaundice, the first test will usually be an ultrasound scan, which may show dilated intrahepatic bile ducts (indicating ductal obstruction) or gallbladder stones. The lesion may be further delineated by ERCP or THC. ERCP is preferable when the lower end of the duct is thought to be obstructed (eg, suspected carcinoma of the pancreas or other periampullary tumors). THC is usually preferred for proximal lesions (eg, biliary stricture, neoplasm of the bifurcation of the hepatic ducts), because it gives better opacification of the ducts proximal to the obstruction and therefore provides more information that can be used in planning surgery. If the clinical presentation suggests neoplastic obstruction, a CT scan could be selected in preference to an ultrasound scan, because CT gives better definition of mass lesions while also demonstrating the presence and general location of bile duct obstruction.

If ultrasound or CT scans suggest biliary obstruction, a decision must be made about whether cholangiograms are indicated. In general, patients with gallstone disease do not require preoperative cholangiograms, whereas cholangiograms would be routine in patients with neoplastic obstruction, benign biliary stricture, or rare or unknown causes of obstructive jaundice.

PATHOGENESIS OF GALLSTONES (Figure 26–7)

More than 20 million people in the USA have gallstones in their gallbladders; about 300,000 operations are performed annually for this disease, and at least 6000 deaths result from its complications or treatment. The incidence of gallstones rises with age, so that between 50 and 65 years of age about 20% of women and 5% of men are affected.

The gallstones in 75% of patients are composed predominantly (70–95%) of cholesterol and are called cholesterol stones. The remaining 25% are pigment stones. Regardless of composition, all gallstones give rise to similar clinical sequelae.

Cholesterol Gallstones

Cholesterol gallstones result from secretion by the liver of bile supersaturated with cholesterol. Influenced by various factors present in bile, the cholesterol precipitates from solution and the newly formed crystals grow to macroscopic stones. Except when the common bile duct is dilated or partially obstructed, the stones in this disease form almost exclusively within the gallbladder. Those found in the

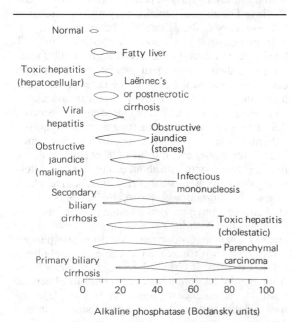

Figure 26–6. Range of alkaline phosphatase values in various hepatobiliary disorders.

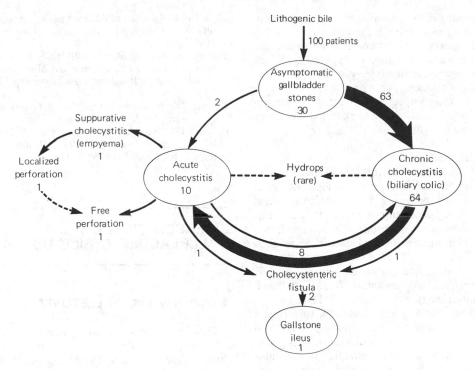

Figure 26–7. The natural history of gallbladder stones. The numbers approximate the percentage of patients in each category. Note that most patients with acute cholecystitis have previously had biliary colic.

ducts usually reach that location after passing through the cystic duct.

The incidence of cholesterol gallstone disease is highest in American Indians, lower in Caucasians, and lowest in blacks, with a twofold gradient from one group to the next. More than 75% of American Indian women over age 40 are affected. Before puberty, the disease is rare but of equal frequency in both sexes. Thereafter, women are more commonly affected than men until after menopause, when the discrepancy lessens. Hormonal effects are also reflected in the increased incidence of gallstones with multiparity and the increased cholesterol saturation of bile and greater incidence of gallstones following ingestion of oral contraceptives. Obesity is the other major risk factor. The relative risk rises proportionately to the extent of overweight due to a progressively increasing output of cholesterol in bile.

As noted previously, cholesterol is insoluble and in bile must be transported within bile salt micelles and phospholipid (lecithin) vesicles. When the amount of cholesterol in bile exceeds the cholesterol holding capacity, cholesterol crystals begin to precipitate from the phospholipid vesicles.

The secretion of bile salt and cholesterol into bile is linked. Bile salt elutes cholesterol from the hepatocyte membrane during passage into the bile canaliculus. At higher bile salt output levels, the amount of cholesterol relative to bile salt entering bile decreases. This means that during low bile flow (eg, during fasting), bile holding capacity for cholesterol is more saturated than during high bile flow. In fact, almost half of persons in Western cultures have bile supersaturated with cholesterol in the morning after an overnight fast. The bile salt pool in patients with cholesterol gallstone disease is about half the size of that of normal subjects, but this is a result of the gallstone disease (eg, gallstones displace bile in the gallbladder) and not a cause.

The occurrence of cholesterol gallstone disease requires cholesterol supersaturation of bile, but that in itself is not sufficient. Cholesterol in supersaturated bile from individuals without gallstone disease precipitates spontaneously at a much slower rate than does the cholesterol in similar bile from patients with gallstones. Furthermore, among individuals with supersaturated bile, only those with gallstone disease demonstrate cholesterol crystal formation in vivo. These observations are the result of specific bile proteins that either stabilize or destabilize cholesterol-laden phospholipid vesicles. For gallstone formation, the pronucleating factors (eg, immunoglobulin, mucus glycoprotein, fibronectin, orosomucoid) appear to be more important than the antinucleating factors (eg, glycoprotein, apolipoprotein, cytokeratin). Variations in these proteins may be the critical factor determining which of the many individuals with saturated bile develop gallstones.

The fact that gallstones form almost exclusively in the gallbladder even though the composition of hepatic bile is abnormal underscores the important role of the gallbladder in gallstone pathogenesis. This includes concentrating the bile, providing nidi (eg, small grains of pigment) for crystallization of cholesterol, supplying mucoprotein to paste the stones together, and serving as an area of stasis to allow stone formation and growth.

Pigment Stones

Pigment stones account for 25% of gallstones in the USA and 60% of those in Japan. Pigment stones are black to dark brown, 2–5 mm in diameter, and amorphous. They are composed of a mixture of calcium bilirubinate, complex bilirubin polymers, bile acids, and other unidentified substances. About 50% are radiopaque, and in the USA they constitute two-thirds of all radiopaque gallstones. The incidence is similar in men and women and in blacks and whites. Pigment stones are rare in American Indians.

Predisposing factors are cirrhosis, bile stasis (eg, a strictured or markedly dilated common duct), and chronic hemolysis. Some patients with pigment stones have increased concentrations of unconjugated bilirubin in their bile. Scanning electron microscopy demonstrates that about 90% of pigment stones are composed of dense mixtures of bacteria and bacterial glycocalix along with pigment solids. This suggests that bacteria have a primary role in pigment gallstone formation, and it also helps to explain why patients with pigment gallstone disease have sepsis more often than do those with cholesterol gallstone disease. It seems likely that bacterial β-glucuronidase is responsible for deconjugating the soluble bilirubin-diglucuronide to insoluble unconjugated bilirubin, which subsequently becomes agglomerated by glycocalix into macroscopic stones.

Abei M et al: Isolation and characterization of a cholesterol crystallization promoter from human bile. Gastroenterology 1993;104:539.

Cetta F: The role of bacteria in pigment gallstone disease. Ann Surg 1991;213:315.

Diehl AK: Epidemiology and natural history of gallstone disease. Gastroenterol Clin North Am 1991;20:1.

Donovan JM, Carey MC: Physical-chemical basis of gallstone formation. Gastroenterol Clin North Am 1991;20:47.

Johnston DE, Kaplan MM: Pathogenesis and treatment of gallstones. N Engl J Med 1993;328:412.

Jungst D et al: Cholesterol nucleation time in gallbladder bile of patients with solitary or multiple cholesterol gallstones. Hepatology 1992;15:804.

Knyrim K, Vakil N: Bile composition, microspheroliths, antinucleating activity, and gallstone calcification. Gastroenterology 1992;103:552.

Miquel JF et al: Isolation and partial characterization of cholesterol pronucleating hydrophobic glycoproteins associated to native biliary vesicles. FEBS Lett 1993;318:45.

Ohya T et al: Isolation of a human biliary glycoprotein inhibitor of cholesterol crystallization. Gastroenterology 1993;104:527.

Shaffer EA: Abnormalities in gallbladder function in cholesterol gallstone disease: Bile and blood, mucosa and muscle—the list lengthens. Gastroenterology 1992;102:1808.

Trotman BW: Pigment gallstone disease. Gastroenterol Clin North Am 1991;20:111.

Upadhya GA, Harvey PR, Strasberg SM: Effect of human biliary immunoglobulins on the nucleation of cholesterol. J Biol Chem 1993;268:5193.

DISEASES OF THE GALLBLADDER & BILE DUCTS

ASYMPTOMATIC GALLSTONES

Data on the prevalence of gallstones in the USA indicate that only about 30% of people with cholelithiasis come to surgery. Symptoms of gallstone disease generally do not change in severity. Each year, about 2% of patients with asymptomatic gallstones develop symptoms, usually biliary colic rather than one of the complications of gallstone disease. Patients with chronic colic tend to have symptoms of the same level of severity and frequency. The present practice of operating only on symptomatic patients, leaving the millions without symptoms alone, seems appropriate. A question is often raised about what to advise the asymptomatic patient found to have gallstones during the course of unrelated studies. The presence of either of the following portends a more serious course and should probably serve as a reason for prophylactic cholecystectomy: (1) large stones (> 2 cm in diameter), because they produce acute cholecystitis more often than small stones; and (2) a calcified gallbladder, because it so often is associated with carcinoma. However, most asymptomatic patients have no special features. If coexistent cardiopulmonary or other problems increase the risk of surgery, operation should not be considered. For the average asymptomatic patient, it is not reasonable to make a strong recommendation for cholecystectomy. The tendency, however, is to operate on younger patients and temporize in the elderly.

Diehl AK: Epidemiology and natural history of gallstone disease. Gastroenterol Clin North Am 1991;20:1.

McSherry CK et al: The natural history of diagnosed gallstone disease in symptomatic and asymptomatic patients. Ann Surg 1985;202:59.

Ransohoff DF et al: Prophylactic cholecystectomy or expectant management for silent gallstones: A decision analysis to assess survival. Ann Intern Med 1983;99:199.

Strasberg SM, Clavien P-A: Cholecystolithiasis: Litho-therapy for the 1990's. Hepatology 1992;16:820.

GALLSTONES & CHRONIC CHOLECYSTITIS (Biliary Colic)

Essentials of Diagnosis
- Episodic abdominal pain.
- Dyspepsia.
- Gallstones on cholecystography or ultrasound scan.

General Considerations

Chronic cholecystitis is the most common form of symptomatic gallbladder disease and is associated with gallstones in nearly every case. In general, the term cholecystitis is applied whenever gallstones are present regardless of the histologic appearance of the gallbladder. Repeated minor episodes of obstruction of the cystic duct cause intermittent biliary colic and contribute to inflammation and subsequent scar formation. Gallbladders from symptomatic patients with gallstones who have never had an attack of acute cholecystitis are of two types: (1) In some, the mucosa may be slightly flattened, but the wall is thin and unscarred and, except for the stones, appears normal. (2) Others exhibit obvious signs of chronic inflammation, with thickening, cellular infiltration, loss of elasticity, and fibrosis. The clinical history in these two groups cannot always be distinguished, and inflammatory changes may also be found in patients with asymptomatic gallstones.

Clinical Findings

A. Symptoms and Signs: Biliary colic, the most characteristic symptom, is caused by transient gallstone obstruction of the cystic duct. The pain usually begins abruptly and subsides gradually, lasting for a few minutes to several hours. The pain of biliary colic is usually steady—not intermittent, like that of intestinal colic. In some patients, attacks occur postprandially; in others, there is no relationship to meals. The frequency of attacks is quite variable, ranging from nearly continuous trouble to episodes many years apart. Nausea and vomiting may accompany the pain.

Biliary colic is usually felt in the right upper quadrant, but epigastric and left abdominal pain are common, and some patients experience precordial pain. The pain may radiate around the costal margin into the back or may be referred to the region of the scapula. Pain on top of the shoulder is unusual and suggests direct diaphragmatic irritation. In a severe attack, the patient usually curls up in bed, changing position frequently in order to be more comfortable.

During an attack, there may be tenderness in the right upper quadrant, and, rarely, the gallbladder is palpable.

Fatty food intolerance, dyspepsia, indigestion, heartburn, flatulence, nausea, and eructations are other symptoms associated with gallstone disease. Because they are also frequent in the general population, their presence in any given patient may only be incidental to the gallstones.

B. Laboratory Findings: An ultrasound scan of the gallbladder should usually be the first test. Gallstones can be demonstrated in about 95% of cases, and a positive reading for gallstones is almost never in error. An oral cholecystogram should be obtained if the ultrasound study is equivocal, if the patient is a candidate for lithotripsy or ursodiol therapy, or if symptoms are highly suggestive and an ultrasound study has been read as normal.

About 2% of patients with gallstone disease have normal ultrasound studies and oral cholecystograms. Therefore, if the clinical suspicion of gallbladder disease is high and these two tests are negative, the patient should be studied by ERCP (to opacify the gallbladder in the search for stones) or duodenal intubation and examination of duodenal bile for cholesterol crystals or bilirubinate granules.

Differential Diagnosis

Gallbladder colic may be strongly suggested by the history, but the clinical impression should always be verified by an ultrasound study. Biliary colic may simulate the pain of duodenal ulcer, hiatal hernia, pancreatitis, and myocardial infarction.

An ECG and a chest x-ray should be obtained to investigate cardiopulmonary disease. It has been suggested that biliary colic may sometimes aggravate cardiac disease, but angina pectoris or an abnormal ECG should rarely be indications for cholecystectomy.

Right-sided radicular pain in the T6–T10 dermatomes may be confused with biliary colic. Osteoarthritic spurs, vertebral lesions, or tumors may be shown on x-rays of the spine or may be suggested by hyperesthesia of the abdominal skin.

An upper gastrointestinal series may be indicated to search for esophageal spasm, hiatal hernia, peptic ulcer, or gastric tumors. In some patients, the irritable colon syndrome may be mistaken for gallbladder discomfort. Carcinoma of the cecum or ascending colon may be overlooked on the assumption that postprandial pain in these conditions is due to gallstones.

Complications

Chronic cholecystitis predisposes to acute cholecystitis, common duct stones, and adenocarcinoma of the gallbladder. The longer the stones have been present, the higher the incidence of all of these complications. Complications are infrequent, however, and the presence of gallstones is not reason enough for prophylactic cholecystectomy in a person with asymptomatic or mildly symptomatic disease.

Treatment

A. Medical Treatment: Avoidance of offending foods may be helpful.

1. Dissolution—Cholesterol gallstones in the gallbladder can be dissolved in some cases by chronic treatment with ursodiol, which reduces the cholesterol saturation of bile by inhibiting cholesterol secretion. The resulting undersaturated bile slowly dissolves the solid cholesterol in the gallstones.

Unfortunately, bile salt therapy has marginal efficacy. The gallstones must be small (eg, < 5 mm) and devoid of calcium (ie, nonopaque on CT scans), and the gallbladder must opacify on oral cholecystography (an indication of unobstructed flow of bile between bile duct and gallbladder). About 15% of patients with gallstones are candidates for treatment. Dissolution is achieved within 2 years in about 50% of highly selected patients. Stones recur, however, in 50% of cases within 5 years. In general, dissolution therapy—alone or in conjunction with lithotripsy—is used only rarely.

2. Lithotripsy and dissolution—Extracorporeal shock wave lithotripsy (ESWL) involves focusing shock waves, which pass through tissue and fluids, upon the gallstones. The stones are fragmented by explosion of small air bubbles within interstices of the solid material.

Both cholesterol and pigment stones can be fragmented by ESWL, but only cholesterol stones can be eliminated after fragmentation. The objective of treatment is to reduce the stones to fragments less than 5 mm in diameter, at which point they are amenable to dissolution therapy. Total stone load is the principal factor limiting the success of fragmentation, which is ineffective if there are more than three stones. The ideal patient is one who has a solitary cholesterol stone no larger than 2 cm in diameter.

Lithotripsy by itself is of little therapeutic value, because the fragments remain in the gallbladder unless they can be dissolved. Consequently, candidates for lithotripsy must satisfy the same criteria as patients who are being considered for ursodiol therapy without lithotripsy, except the stones can be larger. Thus, the stones must be composed of cholesterol and be free of calcium, and the gallbladder must opacify on oral cholecystography. Complete elimination of gallbladder stones is attained within 9 months in about 25% of appropriately selected patients. Because of the many drawbacks of this form of treatment, it has not been approved by the FDA in the United States.

B. Surgical Treatment: Cholecystectomy is indicated in most patients with symptoms. The procedure can be scheduled at the patient's convenience, within weeks or months after diagnosis. Active concurrent disease that increases the risk of surgery should be treated before operation. In some chronically ill patients, surgery should be deferred indefinitely.

Cholecystectomy is most often performed laparoscopically, but when the laparoscopic approach is contraindicated (eg, too many adhesions) or unsuccessful, it may be performed through a laparotomy. The difference consists of 4 fewer days in the hospital and several fewer weeks off work when done laparoscopically. Regardless of how it is done, operative cholangiography is usually included to look for common duct stones. If stones are found, common duct exploration is performed (see under choledocholithiasis).

Prognosis

Serious complications and deaths related to the operation itself are rare. The operative death rate is about 0.1% in patients under age 50 and about 0.5% in patients over age 50. Most deaths occur in patients recognized preoperatively to have increased risks. The operation relieves symptoms in 95% of cases.

Aranha GV, Kruss D. Greenlee HB: Therapeutic options for biliary tract disease in advanced cirrhosis. Am J Surg 1988;155:374.

Bailey RW et al: Laparoscopic cholecystectomy. Ann Surg 1991;214:531.

Diehl AK, Beral V: Cholecystectomy and changing mortality from gallbladder cancer. Lancet 1981;2:187.

Dixon NP, Faddis DM, Silberman H: Aggressive management of cholecystitis during pregnancy. Am J Med 1987;154:292.

Gallstones and laparoscopic cholecystectomy. (NIH Consensus conference.) JAMA 1993;269:1018.

Gilliland TM, Traverso LW: Modern standards for comparison of cholecystectomy with alternative treatments for symptomatic cholelithiasis with emphasis on long-term relief of symptoms. Surg Gynecol Obstet 1990;170:39.

Gleeson D et al: Final outcome of ursodeoxycholic acid treatment in 126 patients with radiolucent gallstones. Q J Med 1990;279:711.

Johnston DE, Kaplan MM: Pathogenesis and treatment of gallstones. N Engl J Med 1993;328:412.

Jorgensen T: Abdominal symptoms and gallstone disease: An epidemiological investigation. Hepatology 1989; 9:856.

Konsten J et al: Long-term followup after open cholecystectomy. Br J Surg 1993;80:100.

Meyers WC et al: A prospective analysis of 1518 laparoscopic cholecystectomies. N Engl J Med 1991;324:1073.

Miles RH et al: Laparoscopy: The preferred method of cholecystectomy in the morbidly obese. Surgery 1992;112:818.

Minoli G et al: Circadian periodicity and other clinical features of biliary pain. J Clin Gastroenterol 1991;13:546.

Morgenstern L, Wong L, Berci G: Twelve hundred open cholecystectomies before the laparoscopic era. Arch Surg 1992;127:400.

O'Leary DP, Johnson AG: Future directions for conservative treatment of gallbladder calculi. Br J Surg 1993; 80:143.

Schoenfield LJ et al: The effect of ursodiol on the efficacy and safety of extracorporeal shock-wave lithotripsy of gallstones. The Dornier National Biliary Lithotripsy Study. N Engl J Med 1990;323:1239.

Strasberg SM, Clavien P-A: Cholecystolithiasis: Lithotherapy for the 1990's. Hepatology 1992;16:820.

Wetter LA, Way LW: Surgical therapy for gallstone disease. Gastroenterol Clin North Am 1991;20:157.

ACUTE CHOLECYSTITIS

Essentials of Diagnosis

- Acute right upper quadrant pain and tenderness.
- Fever and leukocytosis.
- Palpable gallbladder in one-third of cases.
- Nonopacified gallbladder on radionuclide excretion scan.
- Sonographic Murphy's sign.

General Considerations

In 80% of cases, acute cholecystitis results from obstruction of the cystic duct by a gallstone impacted in Hartmann's pouch. The gallbladder becomes inflamed and distended, creating abdominal pain and tenderness. The natural history of acute cholecystitis varies, depending on whether the obstruction becomes relieved, the extent of secondary bacterial invasion, the age of the patient, and the presence of other aggravating factors such as diabetes mellitus. Most attacks resolve spontaneously without surgery or other specific therapy, but some progress to abscess formation or free perforation with generalized peritonitis.

The pathologic changes in the gallbladder evolve in a typical pattern. Subserosal edema and hemorrhage and patchy mucosal necrosis are the first changes. Later, PMNs appear. The final stage involves development of fibrosis. Gangrene and perforation may occur as early as 3 days after onset, but most perforations occur during the second week. In cases that resolve spontaneously, acute inflammation has largely cleared by 4 weeks, but some residual evidence of inflammation may last for several months. About 90% of gallbladders removed during an acute attack show chronic scarring, although many of these patients deny having had any previous symptoms.

The cause of acute cholecystitis is still partially conjectural. Obstruction of the cystic duct is present in most cases, but in experimental animals, cystic duct obstruction does not result in acute cholecystitis unless the gallbladder is filled with concentrated bile or bile saturated with cholesterol. There is also evidence that trauma from gallstones releases phospholipase from the mucosal cells of the gallbladder. This is followed by conversion of lecithin in bile to lysolecithin, which is a toxic compound that may cause more inflammation. Bacteria appear to have a minor role in the early stages of acute cholecystitis,

even though most complications of the disease involve suppuration.

About 20% of cases of acute cholecystitis occur in the absence of cholelithiasis (acalculous cholecystitis). Some of these are due to cystic duct obstruction by another process such as a malignant tumor. Rarely, acute acalculous cholecystitis results from cystic artery occlusion or primary bacterial infection by *E coli,* clostridia, or, occasionally, *Salmonella typhi.* Most cases occur in patients hospitalized with some other illness; acute acalculous cholecystitis is particularly common in trauma victims (civilian or military) and in patients receiving total parenteral nutrition. Small-vessel occlusion occurs early, and unless treatment is given promptly, the disease progresses rapidly to gangrenous cholecystitis and septic complications, at which point the death rate is high.

Clinical Findings

A. Symptoms and Signs: The first symptom is abdominal pain in the right upper quadrant, sometimes associated with referred pain in the region of the right scapula. In 75% of cases, the patient will have had previous attacks of biliary colic, at first indistinguishable from the present illness. However, in acute cholecystitis, the pain persists and becomes associated with abdominal tenderness. Nausea and vomiting are present in about half of patients, but the vomiting is rarely severe. Mild icterus occurs in 10% of cases. The temperature usually ranges from 38 to 38.5 °C (100.4–101.3 °F). High fever and chills are uncommon and should suggest the possibility of complications or an incorrect diagnosis.

Right upper quadrant tenderness is present, and in about a third of patients the gallbladder is palpable (often in a position lateral to its normal one). Voluntary guarding during examination may prevent detection of an enlarged gallbladder. In others, the gallbladder is not enlarged because scarring of the wall restricts distention. If instructed to breathe deeply during palpation in the right subcostal region, the patient experiences accentuated tenderness and sudden inspiratory arrest (Murphy's sign).

B. Laboratory Findings: The leukocyte count is usually elevated to 12,000–15,000/μL. Normal counts are common, but if the count goes much above 15,000, one should suspect complications. A mild elevation of the serum bilirubin (in the range of 2–4 mg/dL) is common, presumably owing to secondary inflammation of the common duct by the contiguous gallbladder. Bilirubin values above this range would most likely indicate the associated presence of common duct stones. A mild increase in alkaline phosphatase may accompany the attack. Occasionally, the serum amylase concentration transiently reaches 1000 units/dL or more.

C. Imaging Studies: A plain x-ray of the abdomen may occasionally show an enlarged gallbladder shadow. In 15% of patients, the gallstones contain enough calcium to be seen on the plain film.

Ultrasound scans show gallstones, sludge, and thickening of the gallbladder wall, and the ultrasonographer can determine even better than the clinician whether the point of maximum tenderness is over the gallbladder (ultrasonographic Murphy's sign). This last finding is often absent, however, when the gallbladder is gangrenous. Usually, ultrasound is the only test needed to make the diagnosis of acute cholecystitis.

If additional diagnostic information is desirable (eg, if ultrasound is equivocal or negative), a radionuclide excretion scan (eg, HIDA scan) should be performed. This test cannot demonstrate gallstones, but if the gallbladder is imaged, acute cholecystitis is ruled out except in rare cases of acalculous cholecystitis (the test is positive in most cases of acute acalculous cholecystitis). Imaging of the duct but not the gallbladder supports the diagnosis of acute cholecystitis. A few false positives are seen in advanced gallstone disease without acute inflammation and in acute biliary pancreatitis.

Differential Diagnosis

The differential diagnosis includes other common causes of acute upper abdominal pain and tenderness. An acute peptic ulcer with or without perforation might be suggested by a history of epigastric pain relieved by food or antacids. Most cases of perforated ulcer demonstrate free air under the diaphragm on x-ray. An emergency upper gastrointestinal series may help.

Acute pancreatitis can be confused with acute cholecystitis, especially if cholecystitis is accompanied by an elevated amylase level. Furthermore, HIDA scans fail to outline the gallbladder in most cases of acute biliary pancreatitis. Sometimes the two diseases coexist, but pancreatitis should not be accepted as a second diagnosis without specific findings.

Acute appendicitis in patients with a high cecum may closely simulate acute cholecystitis.

Severe right upper quadrant pain with high fever and local tenderness may develop in acute gonococcal perihepatitis (Fitz-Hugh-Curtis syndrome). Clues to the proper diagnosis may be found in tenderness in the adnexa, vaginal discharge that shows gonococci on a Gram-stained smear, and a disparity between the patient's high fever and her general lack of toxicity.

Complications

The major complications of acute cholecystitis are empyema, gangrene, and perforation.

A. Empyema: In empyema (suppurative cholecystitis), the gallbladder contains frank pus, and the patient becomes more toxic, with high spiking fever (39–40 °C [102.2–104 °F]), chills, and leukocytosis greater than 15,000/μL. Parenteral antibiotics should

be given, and percutaneous cholecystostomy or cholecystectomy should be performed.

B. Perforation: Perforation may take any of three forms: (1) localized perforation with pericholecystic abscess; (2) free perforation with generalized peritonitis; and (3) perforation into an adjacent hollow viscus, with the formation of a fistula. Perforation may occur as early as 3 days after the onset of acute cholecystitis or not until late in the second week. The total incidence of perforation is about 10%.

1. Pericholecystic abscess—Pericholecystic abscess, the most common form of perforation, should be suspected when the signs and symptoms progress, especially when accompanied by the appearance of a palpable mass. The patient often becomes toxic, with fever to 39 °C (102.2 °F) and a leukocyte count above 15,000/μL, but sometimes there is no correlation between the clinical signs and the development of local abscess. Cholecystectomy and drainage of the abscess can be performed safely in many of these patients, but if the patient's condition is unstable, percutaneous cholecystostomy is preferable.

2. Free perforation—Free perforation occurs in only 1–2% of patients, most often early in the disease when gangrene develops before adhesions wall off the gallbladder. The diagnosis is made preoperatively in less than half of cases. In some patients with localized pain, sudden spread of pain and tenderness to other parts of the abdomen suggests the diagnosis. Whenever it is suspected, free perforation must be treated by emergency laparotomy. Abdominal paracentesis may be misleading and has proved to be of little diagnostic usefulness. Cholecystectomy should be performed if the patient's condition will permit; otherwise, cholecystostomy is done. The death rate depends partly on whether the cystic duct remains obstructed or the stone becomes dislodged after perforation. The former leads to a purulent peritonitis that is lethal in 20% of cases. In the latter, a true bile peritonitis ensues and over 50% of patients die. The earlier operation is performed, the better the prognosis.

3. Cholecystenteric fistula—If the acutely inflamed gallbladder becomes adherent to adjacent stomach, duodenum, or colon and necrosis develops at the site of one of these adhesions, perforation may occur into the lumen of the gut. The resulting decompression often allows the acute disease to resolve. If the gallbladder stones discharge through the fistula and if they are large enough, they may obstruct the small intestine (gallstone ileus; see below). Rarely, patients vomit gallstones that have entered the stomach through a cholecystogastric fistula. In most patients, the acute attack subsides and the cholecystenteric fistula is clinically unsuspected.

Cholecystenteric fistulas do not usually cause symptoms unless the gallbladder is still partially obstructed by stones or scarring. Neither oral nor intravenous cholangiograms will opacify the gallbladder or the fistula, but the latter may be shown on upper gastrointestinal series, where it must be differentiated from a fistula due to perforated peptic ulcer. Malabsorption and steatorrhea have been reported in isolated cases of cholecystocolonic fistulas. Steatorrhea in this situation could be due either to absence of bile in the proximal bowel following diversion into the colon or, more rarely, to excess bacteria in the upper intestine.

Symptomatic cholecystenteric fistulas should be treated by cholecystectomy and closure of the fistula. The majority are discovered incidentally during cholecystectomy for symptomatic gallbladder disease.

Treatment

Intravenous fluids should be given to correct dehydration and electrolyte imbalance, and a nasogastric tube should be inserted. For acute cholecystitis of average severity, parenteral cefazolin (2–4 g daily) should be given. Parenteral penicillin (20 million units daily), clindamycin, and an aminoglycoside should be given for severe disease. Single-drug therapy using imipenem appears to be a good alternative.

There are two schools of thought about the treatment of acute cholecystitis. Since the disease resolves spontaneously in about 60% of cases, one approach is to manage the patient expectantly, with a plan to perform elective cholecystectomy after recovery, reserving surgery during the acute attack for those with severe or worsening disease. (This approach is untenable in acute acalculous cholecystitis.)

The preferred plan is to perform cholecystectomy in all patients unless there are specific contraindications to operation (eg, serious concomitant disease). Four controlled trials have supported this approach with the following data: (1) the incidence of technical complications is no greater with early surgery; (2) early surgery reduces the total duration of illness by approximately 30 days, length of hospitalization by 5–7 days, and direct medical costs by several thousand dollars; and (3) the death rate is slightly lower with early surgery because of earlier treatment for some patients whose condition would have worsened during expectant management. Since these trials were completed, the average case appears to have become more severe, and the arguments against expectant management are now even more compelling.

The following are the major factors that affect the decision (Figure 26–8): (1) whether the diagnosis is established; (2) the general health of the patient as modified by coexistent disease or the present illness; and (3) signs of local complications of acute cholecystitis. The diagnosis should be clear-cut and the patient optimally prepared; if perforation or empyema is suspected, emergency surgery is indicated.

In about 30% of cases, the diagnosis of acute cholecystitis is established but the general condition of the patient is unsatisfactory. If possible, surgery should be postponed in these cases until the ancillary disease is controlled. Expectant management cannot

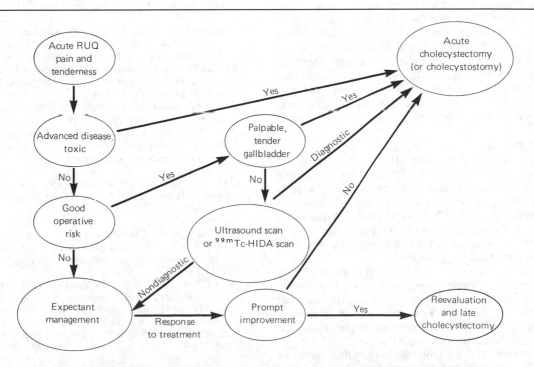

Figure 26–8. Scheme for the management of acute cholecystitis.

be rigidly adhered to, however, if the manifestations of cholecystitis worsen.

About 10% of patients require emergency treatment. These are generally clinical situations in which the disease appears to have become complicated or is about to. High fever (39 °C [102.2 °F]), marked leukocytosis (> 15,000/µL), or chills suggest suppurative progression. Acalculous acute cholecystitis should automatically be placed in this category. When the patient's general condition is poor, percutaneous catheter cholecystostomy is the preferable treatment. Patients in better overall health should be treated by cholecystectomy.

The sudden appearance of generalized abdominal pain may indicate free perforation. Appearance of a mass while the patient is under observation may be a sign of local perforation and abscess formation. Changes of this sort are indications for emergency surgery.

Cholecystectomy is the preferable operation in acute cholecystitis, and it can be performed laparoscopically in about 50% of patients. Operative cholangiography should be performed in most cases, and the common bile duct explored if appropriate indications are present (see section on choledocholithiasis). Patients with severe acute cholecystitis who are in poor condition for emergency cholecystectomy should be treated by percutaneous cholecystostomy. Percutaneous cholecystostomy may also be the preferred therapy for acute acalculous cholecystitis. A catheter inserted under ultrasound or CT guidance is allowed to drain the gallbladder of its bile or pus. The resulting decompression controls the acute disease, including any local infection, but the gallstones cannot be removed. Therefore, cholecystectomy should be performed after the patient recovers in order to avoid recurrent attacks. Cholecystectomy is definitive therapy in the patient with acalculous cholecystitis. At one time, cholecystostomy was performed surgically, but most hospitals now have radiologists skilled in the simpler percutaneous method.

Prognosis

The overall death rate of acute cholecystitis is about 5%. Nearly all of the deaths are in patients over age 60 or those with diabetes mellitus. In the older age group, secondary cardiovascular or pulmonary complications contribute substantially to the death rate. Uncontrolled sepsis with peritonitis and intrahepatic abscesses are the most important local conditions responsible for death.

Common duct stones are present in about 15% of patients with acute cholecystitis, and some of the more seriously ill patients have simultaneous cholangitis from biliary obstruction. Acute pancreatitis may also complicate acute cholecystitis, and the combination carries a greater risk.

Patients who develop the suppurative forms of gallbladder disease such as empyema or perforation are less likely to recover. Earlier admission to the hospital and early cholecystectomy reduce the chances of these complications.

Acute Cholecystitis: General

Babb RR: Acute acalculous cholecystitis: A review. J Clin Gastroenterol 1992;15:238.

Edlund G, Ljungdahl M: Acute cholecystitis in the elderly. Am J Surg 1990;159:414.

Gouma DJ, Obertop H: Acute calculous cholecystitis: What is new in diagnosis and therapy? HPB Surg 1992;6:69.

Hidalgo LA et al: The influence of age on early surgical treatment of acute cholecystitis. Surg Gynecol Obstet 1989;169:393.

Imhof M et al: Acute acalculous cholecystitis complicating trauma: A prospective sonographic study. World J Surg 1992;16:1160.

Jivegard L, Thornell E, Svanvik J: Pathophysiology of acute obstructive cholecystitis: Implications for nonoperative management. Br J Surg 1987;74:1084.

Kaminski DL et al: The role of prostanoids in the production of acute acalculous cholecystitis by platelet-activating factor. Ann Surg 1990;212:455.

Kaufman M et al: Cholecystostomy as a definitive operation. Surg Gynecol Obstet 1990;170:533.

Lee MJ et al: Treatment of critically ill patients with sepsis of unknown cause: Value of percutaneous cholecystostomy. AJR Am J Roentgenol 1991;156:1163.

Myers S, Bartula L, Kalley-Taylor B: The role of prostaglandin I_2 and biliary lipids during evolving cholecystitis in the rabbit. Gastroenterology 1993;104:248.

Reiss R et al: Changing trends in surgery for acute cholecystitis. World J Surg 1990;14:567.

Reiss R, Deutsch AA: State of the art in the diagnosis and management of acute cholecystitis. Dig Dis 1993;11:55.

vanSonnenberg E et al: Percutaneous gallbladder puncture and cholecystostomy: Results, complications, and caveats for safety. Radiology 1992;183:167.

Vauthey JN et al: Indications and limitations of percutaneous cholecystostomy for acute cholecystitis. Surg Gynecol Obstet 1993;176:49.

Warren BL: Small vessel occlusion in acute acalculous cholecystitis. Surgery 1992;111:163.

Yellin AE et al: Intramuscular imipenem as adjuvant therapy for acute cholecystitis and perforated or gangrenous appendicitis. Chemotherapy 1991;37(Suppl 2):37.

Zucker KA, Bailey RW, Flowers J: Laparoscopic management of acute and chronic cholecystitis. Surg Clin North Am 1992;72:1045.

Acute Cholecystitis: Complications

Ackerman NB et al: Consequences of intraperitoneal bile: Bile ascites versus bile peritonitis. Am J Surg 1985;149:244.

Ong CI, Wong TH, Rauff A: Acute gall bladder perforation: A dilemma in early diagnosis. Gut 1991;32:956.

Siskind BN et al: Gallbladder perforation. An imaging analysis. J Clin Gastroenterol 1987;9:670.

Stull JR, Thomford NR: Biliary intestinal fistula. Am J Surg 1970;120:27.

Thornton JR et al: Empyema of the gallbladder: Reappraisal of a neglected disease. Gut 1983;24:1183.

EMPHYSEMATOUS CHOLECYSTITIS

Emphysematous cholecystitis is a rare condition in which bubbles of gas from anaerobic infection appear in the lumen of the gallbladder, its wall, the pericholecystic space, and, on occasion, the bile ducts. Clostridia species are the most commonly implicated organisms, but other gas-forming anaerobes such as *E coli* or anaerobic streptococci may be found. Three times as many men as women are affected, and 20% of patients have diabetes mellitus. In contrast to the usual form of acute cholecystitis, the disease probably is a bacterial infection from the earliest moment. In many cases, the gallbladder contains no stones.

The disease begins with sudden and rapidly progressive right upper quadrant pain. Fever and leukocytosis reach high levels quickly, and the patient is considerably more toxic than is usually the case in acute cholecystitis. On examination, a mass can usually be found in the right upper quadrant.

Plain films of the abdomen show tissue emphysema outlining the gallbladder and, in some cases, an air-fluid level in the lumen. The clinical and x-ray pictures are characteristic enough so that the diagnosis is usually obvious. If the changes on plain films are equivocal, a CT scan may bring them out.

The patient should be treated with high doses of antibiotics effective against clostridia and the other species mentioned above. Emergency surgical treatment should follow the initial resuscitative measures. Cholecystectomy can be safely performed in most cases, but the most critically ill might fare better with cholecystostomy. The types of complications are the same as in other forms of acute cholecystitis, but illness is more severe and death rates are higher.

Andreu J et al: Computed tomography as the method of choice in the diagnosis of emphysematous cholecystitis. Gastrointest Radiol 1987;12:315.

May RE, Strong R: Acute emphysematous cholecystitis. Br J Surg 1971;58:453.

Rosoff L, Meyers H: Acute emphysematous cholecystitis. Am J Surg 1966;111:410.

GALLSTONE ILEUS

Gallstone ileus is mechanical intestinal obstruction caused by a large gallstone lodged in the lumen. It is seen most often in women, and the average age is about 70.

Clinical Findings

A. Symptoms: The patient usually presents with obvious small bowel obstruction, either partial or complete. The obstructing gallstone enters the intestine through a cholecystenteric fistula located in the duodenum, colon, or, rarely, the stomach or jejunum. The gallbladder may contain one or several stones, but stones that cause gallstone ileus are almost always 2.5 cm or more in diameter. The lumen in the proximal bowel will allow most of these large calculi to pass caudally until the ileum is reached. Obstruction of the large intestine may follow passage of a gallstone through a fistula at the hepatic flexure or may occur even after the stone has traversed the entire small bowel.

B. Signs: In most patients, the findings on physical examination are typical of distal small bowel obstruction. Obstruction of the duodenum or jejunum may give a perplexing clinical picture because of the lack of distention. Right upper quadrant tenderness and a mass may be present in some cases, but the distended abdomen may be difficult to examine accurately.

C. Imaging Studies: In addition to dilated small intestine, plain films of the abdomen may show a radiopaque gallstone, and unless one is alert to the possibility of gallstone ileus, the ectopic stone can be a puzzling finding. In about 40% of cases, careful examination of the film will reveal gas in the biliary tree, a manifestation of the cholecystenteric fistula. When the clinical picture is unclear, an upper gastrointestinal series should be obtained, which will demonstrate the cholecystoduodenal fistula and verify intestinal obstruction.

Treatment

The proper treatment is emergency laparotomy and removal of the obstructing stone through a small enterotomy. The proximal intestine must be carefully inspected for the presence of a second calculus that might cause a postoperative recurrence. The gallbladder should be left undisturbed at the original operation.

Once the patient has recovered, an elective cholecystectomy should be scheduled if the patient complains of chronic gallbladder symptoms. On this basis, interval cholecystectomy will be required in about 30% of patients. The fistula itself is rarely the source of trouble and closes spontaneously in most patients.

Prognosis

The death rate of gallstone ileus remains about 20%, largely because of the poor general condition of elderly patients at the time of laparotomy. In many cases, the patient has developed cardiac or pulmonary complications during a preoperative delay when the diagnosis was unclear.

Deitz DM et al: Improving the outcome in gallstone ileus. Am J Surg 1986;151:572.

Kurtz RJ et al: Patterns of treatment of gallstone ileus over a 45-year period. Am J Gastroenterol 1985;80:95.

Schutte H et al: Gallstone ileus. Hepatogastroenterology 1992;39:562.

Way LW: Gallstone ileus. In: *Surgery of the Gallbladder and Bile Ducts.* Way LW, Pellegrini CA (editors). Saunders, 1987.

CHOLANGITIS
(Bacterial Cholangitis)

Bacterial infection of the biliary ducts always signifies biliary obstruction, since in the absence of obstruction even heavy bacterial contamination of the ducts fails to produce symptoms or pathologic changes. The block to flow may be partial or, less commonly, complete. The principal causes are choledocholithiasis, biliary stricture, and neoplasm. Less common causes are chronic pancreatitis, ampullary stenosis, pancreatic pseudocyst, duodenal diverticulum, congenital cyst, and parasitic invasion. Iatrogenic cholangitis may complicate transhepatic or T tube cholangiography. Not all obstructing lesions are followed by cholangitis, however. For example, biliary infection develops in only 15% of patients with neoplastic obstruction. The likelihood of cholangitis is greatest when the obstruction occurs after the duct has acquired a resident bacterial population.

With obstruction, ductal pressure rises, and bacteria proliferate and escape into the systemic circulation via the hepatic sinusoids. Experimentally, the incidence of positive blood cultures with ductal infection is directly proportionate to the absolute height of the pressure in the duct.

The symptoms of cholangitis (sometimes referred to as Charcot's triad) are biliary colic, jaundice, and chills and fever, though a complete triad is present in only 70% of cases. Laboratory findings include leukocytosis and elevated serum bilirubin and alkaline phosphatase levels. The predominant organisms in bile (in approximately decreasing frequency) are *E coli, Klebsiella, Pseudomonas,* enterococci, and *Proteus. Bacteroides fragilis* and other anaerobes (eg, *Clostridium perfringens*) can be detected in about 25% of cases, and their presence correlates with multiple previous biliary operations (often including a biliary enteric anastomosis), severe symptoms, and a high incidence of postoperative suppurative complications. Anaerobes are nearly always seen in the company of aerobes. Two species of bacteria can be cultured in about 50% of cases. Bacteremia probably occurs in most cases, and blood cultures obtained at the appropriate time contain the same organisms as the bile. Early in an attack, an ultrasound scan will often give useful diagnostic information. Further workup (THC, ERCP, etc) can proceed later after the acute manifestations are brought under control.

Cholangiography is dangerous during active cholangitis.

The term **suppurative cholangitis** has been used for the most severe form of this disease, when manifestations of sepsis overshadow those of hepatobiliary disease. The diagnostic pentad of suppurative cholangitis consists of abdominal pain, jaundice, fever and chills, mental confusion or lethargy, and shock. The diagnosis is often missed because the signs of biliary disease are overlooked.

Most cases of cholangitis can be controlled with intravenous antibiotics. A cephalosporin antibiotic (eg, cefazolin, cefoxitin) is the drug of choice in the average mild to moderately severe case. If disease is severe or progressively worsens, an aminoglycoside plus clindamycin should be added to the regimen.

For patients with severe cholangitis or unremitting cholangitis despite antibiotic therapy, the bile duct must be promptly decompressed. Most cases of severe acute cholangitis are associated with choledocholithiasis, where the best treatment consists of emergency endoscopic sphincterotomy. In the uncommon case where this is unsuccessful, laparotomy is indicated in order to decompress the bile duct. Cholangitis accompanying neoplastic obstruction may be managed by insertion of a transhepatic drainage catheter into the bile duct. A cholangiogram should not be obtained because the procedure could worsen sepsis.

Urgent intervention (eg, endoscopic sphincterotomy, percutaneous transhepatic drainage, or operative decompression) is required in about 10% of patients with acute cholangitis. The remaining 90% are eventually treated by elective surgery or endoscopic sphincterotomy following antibiotic therapy and a thorough diagnostic evaluation.

Csendes A et al: Risk factors and classification of acute suppurative cholangitis. Br J Surg 1992;79:655.

Gigot JF et al: Acute cholangitis: Multivariate analysis of risk factors. Ann Surg 1989;209:435.

Lai EC et al: Endoscopic biliary drainage for severe acute cholangitis. N Engl J Med 1992;326:1582.

Lipsett PA, Pitt HA: Acute cholangitis. Surg Clin North Am 1990;70:1297.

Magun A. Acute cholangitis: Endoscopic drainage or emergency surgery? Gastroenterology 1990;99:1530.

Nahrwold DL: Acute cholangitis. Surgery 1992;112:487.

Raper SE et al: Anatomic correlates of bacterial cholangiovenous reflux. Surgery 1989;105:352.

CHOLEDOCHOLITHIASIS

Essentials of Diagnosis
- Biliary pain.
- Jaundice.
- Episodic cholangitis.
- Gallstones in gallbladder or previous cholecystectomy.

General Considerations

Approximately 15% of patients with stones in the gallbladder are found to harbor calculi within the bile ducts. Common duct stones are usually accompanied by others in the gallbladder, but in 5% of cases, the gallbladder is empty. The number of duct stones may vary from one to more than 100.

There are two possible origins for common duct stones. The evidence suggests that most cholesterol stones develop within the gallbladder and reach the duct after traversing the cystic duct. These are called secondary stones. Pigment stones may have a similar pedigree or, more often, develop de novo within the common duct. These are called primary common duct stones. About 60% of common duct stones are cholesterol stones and 40% are pigment stones. The latter are, on the average, associated with more severe clinical manifestations.

Patients may have one or more of the following principal clinical findings, all of which are caused by obstruction to the flow of bile or pancreatic juice: biliary colic, cholangitis, jaundice, and pancreatitis (Figure 26–9). It seems likely, however, that as many as 50% of patients with choledocholithiasis remain asymptomatic.

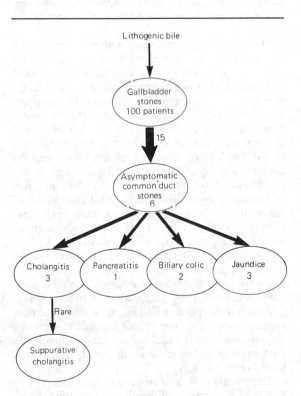

Figure 26–9. The natural history of common duct stones. Of every 100 patients with gallbladder stones, 15 will have common duct stones, which will produce the spectrum of syndromes illustrated. Note that the individual syndromes overlap, indicating that they may appear together in various combinations.

The common duct may dilate to 2–3 cm proximal to an obstructing lesion, and truly huge ducts develop in patients with biliary tumors. In choledocholithiasis or biliary stricture, the inflammatory reaction restricts dilation, so the dilatation is less marked. Dilation of the ductal system within the liver can also be limited by cirrhosis.

Biliary colic is the result of rapid rises in biliary pressure whether the block is in the common duct or neck of the gallbladder. Gradual occlusion of the duct—as in cancer—rarely produces the same kind of pain as gallstone disease.

Clinical Findings

A. Symptoms: Choledocholithiasis may be asymptomatic or may produce sudden toxic cholangitis, leading to a rapid demise. The seriousness of the disease parallels the degree of obstruction, the length of time it has been present, and the extent of secondary bacterial infection (see Cholangitis, above). Biliary colic, jaundice, or pancreatitis may be isolated findings or may occur in any combination along with signs of infection (cholangitis).

Biliary colic from common duct obstruction cannot be distinguished from that caused by stones in the gallbladder. The pain is felt in the right subcostal region, epigastrium, or even the substernal area. Referred pain to the region of the right scapula is common.

Choledocholithiasis should be strongly suspected if intermittent chills, fever, or jaundice accompanies biliary colic. Some patients notice transient darkening of their urine during an attack even though jaundice is not evident.

Pruritus is usually the result of persistent long-standing obstruction. The itching is more intense in warm weather when the patient perspires and is usually worse on the extremities than on the trunk. It is much more common with neoplastic obstruction than with gallstone obstruction.

B. Signs: The patient may be icteric and toxic, with high fever and chills, or may appear to be perfectly healthy. A palpable gallbladder is unusual in patients with obstructive jaundice from common duct stone because the obstruction is transient and partial, and scarring of the gallbladder renders it inelastic and nondistensible. Tenderness may be present in the right upper quadrant but is not often as marked as in acute cholecystitis, perforated peptic ulcer, or acute pancreatitis. Tender hepatic enlargement may occur.

C. Laboratory Findings: In cholangitis, leukocytosis of 15,000/μL is usual, and values above 20,000/μL are common. A rise in serum bilirubin often appears within 24 hours after the onset of symptoms. The absolute level usually remains under 10 mg/dL, and most are in the range of 2–4 mg/dL. The direct fraction exceeds the indirect, but the latter becomes elevated in most cases. Bilirubin levels do not ordinarily reach the high values seen in malignant tumors because the obstruction is usually incomplete and transient. In fact, fluctuating jaundice is so characteristic of choledocholithiasis that it fairly reliably differentiates between benign and malignant obstruction.

The serum alkaline phosphatase level usually rises and may be the only chemical abnormality in patients without jaundice. When the obstruction is relieved, the alkaline phosphatase and bilirubin levels should return to normal within 1–2 weeks, with the exception that the former may remain elevated longer if the obstruction was prolonged.

Mild increases in AST and ALT are often seen with extrahepatic obstruction of the ducts; rarely, AST levels transiently reach 1000 units.

D. Imaging Studies: Radiopaque gallstones may be seen on plain abdominal films or CT scans. Ultrasound scans will usually show gallbladder stones and, depending on the degree of obstruction, dilatation of the bile duct. Ultrasound and CT scans are insensitive in the search for stones in the common duct. ERCP is indicated if the patient has had a previous cholecystectomy. If cholecystectomy has not been performed, cholangiography should be part of operative management. Preoperative ERCP would rarely be indicated in a patient scheduled for cholecystectomy.

Bilirubin values above 10 mg/dL are so uncommon in choledocholithiasis that when this finding is present, cholangiography should be performed to rule out the possibility of neoplastic obstruction.

Differential Diagnosis

The workup should consider the same possibilities in differential diagnosis as for cholecystitis.

Serum amylase levels above 500 units/dL can result from acute pancreatitis, acute cholecystitis, or choledocholithiasis. Other manifestations of pancreatic disease should be documented before an unqualified diagnosis of pancreatitis is accepted.

Alcoholic cirrhosis or acute alcoholic hepatitis may present with jaundice, right upper quadrant tenderness, and leukocytosis. The differentiation from cholangitis may be impossible from clinical data. A history of a recent binge suggests acute liver disease. A percutaneous liver biopsy may be specific.

Intrahepatic cholestasis from drugs, pregnancy, chronic active hepatitis, or primary biliary cirrhosis may be difficult to distinguish from extrahepatic obstruction. ERCP would be appropriate to make the distinction, particularly if other studies (eg, ultrasound scan) failed to provide evidence of gallstone disease. If jaundice has persisted for 4–6 weeks, a mechanical cause is probable. Since most patients improve during this interval, persistent jaundice should never be assumed to be the result of parenchymal disease unless a normal cholangiogram rules out obstruction of the major ducts.

Intermittent jaundice and cholangitis after chole-cystectomy are compatible with biliary stricture, and the distinction require ERCP.

Biliary tumors usually produce intense jaundice without biliary colic or fever, and once it begins, the jaundice rarely remits.

Complications

Long-standing ductal infection can produce intrahepatic abscesses. Hepatic failure or secondary biliary cirrhosis may develop in unrelieved obstruction of long duration. Since the obstruction is usually incomplete and intermittent, cirrhosis develops only after several years in untreated disease. Acute pancreatitis, a fairly common complication of calculous biliary disease, is discussed in Chapter 27. Rarely, a stone in the common duct may erode through the ampulla, resulting in gallstone ileus. Hemorrhage (hemobilia) is also a rare complication.

Treatment

Patients with acute cholangitis should be treated with systemic antibiotics and other measures as described in the preceding section; this usually controls the attack within 24–48 hours. If the patient's condition worsens or if marked improvement is not observed within 2–4 days, endoscopic sphincterotomy or surgery and common bile duct exploration should be performed.

The typical patient presents with mild cholangitis and evidence on ultrasound scans of gallbladder stones. Laparoscopic cholecystectomy is indicated and, depending on the experience of the surgeon, laparoscopic exploration of the common duct if an operative cholangiogram demonstrates the expected common duct stones. Laparoscopic common duct exploration is usually accomplished through the cystic duct (which may have to be dilated), but when the common duct is enlarged (> 1.5 cm), it may be accomplished through a choledochotomy incision, just as in open surgery. Eventually, nearly all cases of common duct stones should be manageable by laparoscopic techniques, but at this stage many surgeons are still acquiring the requisite laparoscopic skills. If the surgeon thinks the common duct stones cannot be removed laparoscopically, it is probably best to remove the gallbladder laparoscopically and the common duct stones by endoscopic sphincterotomy. Opinion on this point is divided, however, and some surgeons would recommend that the cholecystectomy be performed open and accompanied by common bile duct exploration, which was the standard approach until a few years ago.

There is also a lack of consensus regarding the importance of operative cholangiography during cholecystectomy when there are no clues suggesting stones in the duct. In such cases the chances of finding a stone are only 3–5%, and some consider the effort unwarranted. On the other hand, operative cholangiograms also provide confirmation of the biliary anatomy, which contributes to avoidance of bile duct injuries, and the natural history of the few overlooked stones is worrisome. Therefore, we side with those who perform operative cholangiography liberally in such cases.

When the common duct is explored through the cystic duct and gallstones are removed, the cystic duct must be ligated, but a drainage catheter is not usually left within the common duct. When the common duct is explored through a choledochotomy (either during a laparoscopic or open operation), a T tube is usually left in the duct, and cholangiograms are taken a week or so postoperatively. Any residual stones discovered on these postoperative x-rays can be extracted 4–6 weeks later through the T tube tract.

Patients with common duct stones who have had a previous cholecystectomy are best treated by **endoscopic sphincterotomy.** Using a side-viewing duodenoscope, the ampulla is cannulated, and a 1-cm incision is made in the sphincter with an electrocautery wire. The opening created in the sphincter permits stones to pass from the duct into the duodenum. Endoscopic sphincterotomy is unlikely to be successful in patients with large stones (eg, > 2 cm), and it is contraindicated in the presence of stenosis of the bile duct proximal to the sphincter. Endoscopic removal of large impacted stones may be facilitated by preliminary lithotripsy (ESWL). Laparotomy and common duct exploration are required in a few cases.

Stones in the intrahepatic branches of the bile duct can usually be removed without difficulty during common duct exploration. In some cases, however one or more of the intrahepatic ducts have become packed with stones, and the associated chronic inflammation has produced stenosis of the duct near its junction with the common hepatic duct. It is often impossible in these cases to clear the duct of stones, and if the disease involves only one lobe (usually the left lobe), hepatic lobectomy is indicated.

Bernhoft RA et al: Composition and morphologic and clinical features of common duct stones. Am J Surg 1984;148:77.

Bland KI et al: Extracorporeal shock-wave lithotripsy of bile duct calculi. Ann Surg 1989;209:743.

Choi TJ: Intrahepatic stones. Br J Surg 1989;76:213.

Csendes A et al: Risk factors and classification of acute suppurative cholangitis. Br J Surg 1992;79:655.

Hauer-Jensen M et al: Prospective randomized study of routine intraoperative cholangiography during open cholecystectomy: Long-term follow-up and multivariate analysis of predictors of choledocholithiasis. Surgery 1993;113:318.

Hunter JG, Soper NJ: Laparoscopic management of bile duct stones. Surg Clin North Am 1992;72:1077.

Lai EC et al: Endoscopic biliary drainage for severe acute cholangitis. N Engl J Med 1992;326:1582.

Lillemoe KD et al: Selective cholangiography: Current role in laparoscopic cholecystectomy. Ann Surg 1992;215:669.

Neoptolemos JP et al: Study of common bile duct explora-

tion and endoscopic sphincterotomy in a consecutive series of 438 patients. Br J Surg 1987;74:916.

Neoptolemos JP, Carr-Locke DL, Fossard DP: Prospective randomised study of preoperative endoscopic sphincterotomy versus surgery alone for common bile duct stones. Br Med J 1987;294:470.

Neoptolemos JP, Shaw DE, Carr-Locke DL: A multivariate analysis of preoperative risk factors in patients with common bile duct stones: Implications for treatment. Ann Surg 1989;209:157.

Ponsky JL: Alternative methods in the management of bile duct stones. Surg Clin North Am 1992;72:1099.

Ramirez P et al: Long term results of surgical sphincterotomy in the treatment of choledocholithiasis. Surg Gynecol Obstet 1993;176:246.

Schwab G et al: Treatment of calculi of the common bile duct. Surg Gynecol Obstet 1992;175:115.

Smith AL et al: Gallstone disease: The clinical manifestations of infectious stones. Arch Surg 1989;124:629.

Stiegmann GV et al: Precholecystectomy endoscopic cholangiography and stone removal is not superior to cholecystectomy, cholangiography, and common duct exploration. Am J Surg 1992;163:227.

Wilson MS, Tweedle DE, Martin DF: Common bile duct diameter and complications of endoscopic sphincterotomy. Br J Surg 1992;79:1346.

POSTCHOLECYSTECTOMY SYNDROME

This term has been used to signify the heterogeneous group of disorders affecting patients who continue to complain of symptoms after cholecystectomy. It is not really a syndrome, and the term is confusing.

The usual reason for incomplete relief after cholecystectomy is that the preoperative diagnosis of chronic cholecystitis was incorrect. The only symptom entirely characteristic of chronic cholecystitis is biliary colic. When a calculous gallbladder is removed in the hope that the patient will gain relief from dyspepsia, fatty food intolerance, belching, etc, the operation may leave the symptoms unchanged.

The presenting symptom may be dyspepsia or pain. An organic cause for the symptoms is more likely to be discovered in patients with severe episodic pain than in those with other complaints. Abnormal liver function studies, jaundice, and cholangitis are other manifestations that indicate residual biliary disease. Patients with suspicious findings should be studied by ERCP or THC. Choledocholithiasis, biliary stricture, and chronic pancreatitis are the most common causes of symptoms. Evidence is accumulating to implicate sphincter of Oddi dysmotility as a cause of pain in some patients. The diagnosis may be possible by biliary manometry, but experience is still too meager to justify acceptance of this entity without question. Relief of pain may follow endoscopic sphincterotomy. Stenosis of the hepatobiliary ampulla, a long cystic duct remnant, and neuromas have been blamed for continued symptoms, but well-verified cases are uncommon.

Geenen JE et al: The efficacy of endoscopic sphincterotomy after cholecystectomy in patients with sphincter-of-Oddi dysfunction. New Engl J Med 1989;320:82.

Lasson A: The postcholecystectomy syndrome: Diagnostic and therapeutic strategy. Scand J Gastroenterol 1987; 897.

Ros E, Zambon D: Postcholecystectomy symptoms. A prospective study of gall stone patients before and two years after surgery. Gut 1987;28:1500.

CARCINOMA OF THE GALLBLADDER

Carcinoma of the gallbladder is an uncommon neoplasm that occurs in elderly patients. It is associated with gallstones in 70% of cases, and the risk of malignant degeneration correlates with the length of time gallstones have been present. The tumor is twice as common in women as in men, as one would expect from the association with gallstones.

Most primary tumors of the gallbladder are adenocarcinomas that appear histologically to be scirrhous (60%), papillary (25%), or mucoid (15%). Dissemination of the tumor occurs early by direct invasion of the liver and hilar structures and by metastases to the common duct lymph nodes, liver, and lungs. In an occasional case, where carcinoma is an incidental finding after cholecystectomy for gallstone disease, the tumor is confined to the gallbladder as a carcinoma in situ or an early invasive lesion. Most invasive carcinomas, however, have spread by the time of surgery, and spread is virtually certain if the tumor has progressed to the point where it causes symptoms.

Clinical Findings

A. Symptoms and Signs: The most common presenting complaint is of right upper quadrant pain similar to previous episodes of biliary colic but more persistent. Obstruction of the cystic duct by tumor sometimes initiates an attack of acute cholecystitis. Other cases present with obstructive jaundice and, occasionally, cholangitis due to secondary involvement of the common duct.

Examination usually reveals a mass in the region of the gallbladder, which may not be recognized as a neoplasm if the patient has acute cholecystitis. If cholangitis is the principal symptom, a palpable gallbladder would be an unusual finding with choledocholithiasis alone and should suggest gallbladder carcinoma.

B. Imaging Studies: Oral cholecystograms almost never opacify except in patients with small incidental cancers. CT and ultrasound scans may demonstrate the extent of disease, but more often they show only gallstones.

The correct diagnosis is made preoperatively in only 10% of cases.

Complications

Obstruction of the common duct may produce multiple intrahepatic abscesses. Abscesses in or next to the tumor-laden gallbladder are frequent.

Prevention

The incidence of gallbladder cancer has decreased in recent years as the frequency of cholecystectomy has increased. It has been estimated that one case of gallbladder cancer is prevented for every 100 cholecystectomies performed for gallstone disease.

Treatment

If a localized carcinoma of the gallbladder is recognized at laparotomy, cholecystectomy should be performed along with en bloc wedge resection of an adjacent 3–5 cm of normal liver and dissection of the lymph nodes in the hepatoduodenal ligament. If a small invasive carcinoma overlooked during cholecystectomy for gallstone disease is later discovered by the pathologist, reoperation is indicated to perform a wedge resection of the liver bed plus regional lymphadenectomy. Some surgeons also recommend that the common duct be included routinely (ie, even in the absence of gross invasion) in the lymph node dissection for any lesion that involves the full thickness of the gallbladder wall. In the few cases where cancer has not penetrated the muscularis mucosae, cholecystectomy alone should suffice. More extensive hepatectomies (eg, right lobectomy) are not worthwhile. Lesions that invade the bile duct and produce jaundice should be resected if possible. When not, a stent should be inserted endoscopically or percutaneously. There is little that surgery can offer in cases with hepatic metastases or more distant spread.

Prognosis

Radiotherapy and chemotherapy are not effective palliative measures. About 85% of patients are dead within a year after diagnosis.

The 10% of patients who presently survive more than 5 years consist of those whose carcinoma was an incidental finding during cholecystectomy for symptomatic gallstone disease and those in whom an aggressive resection has removed all gross tumor.

Aldridge MC, Bismuth H: Gallbladder cancer: The polyp-cancer sequence. Br J Surg 1990;77:363.

Chijiiwa K, Sumiyoshi K, Nakayama F: Impact of recent advances in hepatobiliary imaging techniques on the preoperative diagnosis of carcinoma of the gallbladder. World J Surg 1991;15:322.

Henson DE, Albores-Saavedra J, Corle D: Carcinoma of the

gallbladder: Histologic types, stage of disease, grade, and survival rates. Cancer 1992;70:1493.

Matsumoto Y et al: Surgical treatment of primary carcinoma of the gallbladder based on the histologic analysis of 48 surgical specimens. Am J Surg 1992;163:239.

Mimura H et al: Block resection of the hepatoduodenal ligament for carcinoma of the bile duct and gallbladder: Surgical technique and a report of 11 cases. Hepatogastroenterology 1991;38:561.

Nakamura S et al: Aggressive surgery for carcinoma of the gallbladder. Surgery 1989;106:467.

Ootani T et al: Relationship between gallbladder carcinoma and the segmental type of adenomyomatosis of the gallbladder. Cancer 1992;69:2647.

Ouchi K et al: Do recent advances in diagnosis and operative management improve the outcome of gallbladder carcinoma? Surgery 1993;113:324.

Paraskevopoulos JA, Dennison AR, Johnson AG: Primary carcinoma of the gallbladder. HPB Surg 1991;4:277.

Shirai Y et al: Inapparent carcinoma of the gallbladder: An appraisal of a radical second operation after simple cholecystectomy. Ann Surg 1992;215:326.

Shirai Y et al: Radical surgery for gallbladder carcinoma. Long-term results. Ann Surg 1992;216:565.

Sumiyoshi K et al: Pathology of carcinoma of the gallbladder. World J Surg 1991;15:315.

Yamaguchi K, Tsuneyoshi M: Subclinical gallbladder carcinoma. Am J Surg 1992;163:382.

MALIGNANT TUMORS OF THE BILE DUCT

Essentials of Diagnosis

- Intense cholestatic jaundice and pruritus.
- Anorexia and dull right upper quadrant pain.
- Dilated intrahepatic bile ducts on ultrasound or CT scan.
- Focal stricture on transhepatic or retrograde endoscopic cholangiogram.

General Considerations

Primary bile duct tumors are not more common in patients with cholelithiasis, and men and women are affected with equal frequency. Tumors appear at an average age of 60 years but may appear at any time between 20 and 80 years of age. More young people have been seen with this disease in recent years. Ulcerative colitis is a common associated condition, and in occasional cases bile duct cancer develops in a patient with ulcerative colitis who has been known to have sclerosing cholangitis for several years. Chronic parasitic infestation of the bile ducts in the Orient may be responsible for the greater incidence of bile duct tumors in that area.

Most malignant biliary tumors are adenocarcinomas located in the hepatic or common bile duct. The histologic pattern varies from typical adenocarcinoma to tumors composed principally of fibrous stroma and few cells. The acellular tumors may be mistaken for benign strictures or sclerosing cholangitis if adequate biopsies are not obtained. About 10% are bulky papillary tumors, which tend to be less invasive and less apt to metastasize.

At presentation, metastases are uncommon, but the tumor has often grown into the portal vein or hepatic artery.

Clinical Findings

A. Symptoms and Signs: The illness presents with gradual onset of jaundice or pruritus. Chills, fever, and biliary colic are usually absent, and except for a deep discomfort in the right upper quadrant the patient feels well. Bilirubinuria is present from the start, and light-colored stools are usual. Anorexia and weight loss develop insidiously with time.

Icterus is the most obvious physical finding. If the tumor is located in the common duct, the gallbladder may distend and become palpable in the right upper quadrant. The tumor itself is never palpable. Patients with tumors of the hepatic duct do not develop palpable gallbladders. Hepatomegaly is common. If obstruction is unrelieved, the liver may eventually become cirrhotic, and splenomegaly, ascites, or bleeding varices become secondary manifestations.

B. Laboratory Findings: Since the duct is often completely obstructed, the serum bilirubin is usually over 15 mg/dL. Serum alkaline phosphatase is also increased. Fever and leukocytosis are not common, since the bile is sterile in most cases. The stool may contain occult blood, but this is more common with tumors of the pancreas or hepatopancreatic ampulla than those of the bile ducts.

C. Imaging Studies: Ultrasound or CT scans usually detect dilated intrahepatic bile ducts. THC or ERCP clearly depicts the lesion, and both are indicated in most cases. THC is of greater value, since it better demonstrates the ductal anatomy on the hepatic side of the lesion. With tumors involving the bifurcation of the common hepatic duct (Klatskin tumors), it is important to determine the proximal extent of the lesion (ie, whether the first branches of the lobar ducts are also involved). ERCP is of value with proximal tumors because if it shows concomitant obstruction of the cystic duct, the diagnosis will most often prove to be gallbladder cancer invading the common duct (not a primary common duct neoplasm). The typical pattern with distal bile duct cancers consists of stenosis of the bile duct with sparing of the pancreatic duct. Adjacent stenoses of both ducts (the double-duct sign) indicate primary cancer of the pancreas.

Occasionally, bile samples obtained at the time of THC will show malignant cells on cytologic study, but this is not a particularly useful test since the diagnosis of cancer must be presumed from the cholangiographic findings and a negative cytologic study is unreliable. Angiography may suggest invasion of the portal vein or encasement of the hepatic artery. False positives may occur, however.

Differential Diagnosis

The differential diagnosis must consider other causes of extrahepatic and intrahepatic cholestatic jaundice. Choledocholithiasis is characterized by episodes of partial obstruction, pain, and cholangitis, which contrast with the unremitting jaundice of malignant obstruction. Bilirubin concentrations rarely surpass 15 mg/dL and are usually below 10 mg/dL in gallstone obstruction, whereas bilirubin levels almost always exceed 10 mg/dL and are usually above 15 mg/dL in neoplastic obstruction. A rapid rise of the bilirubin level to above 15 mg/dL in a patient with sclerosing cholangitis should suggest superimposed neoplasm. Dilatation of the gallbladder may occur with tumors of the distal common duct but is rare with calculous obstruction.

The combination of an enlarged gallbladder with obstructive jaundice is usually recognized as being due to tumor. If the gallbladder cannot be felt, primary biliary cirrhosis, drug-induced jaundice, chronic active hepatitis, metastatic hepatic cancer, and common duct stone must be ruled out. In general, any patient with cholestatic jaundice of more than 2 weeks' duration whose diagnosis is uncertain should be studied by THC or ERCP. The finding of focal bile duct stenosis in the absence of previous biliary surgery is almost pathognomonic of neoplasm.

Treatment

Patients without evidence of metastases or other signs of advanced cancer (eg, ascites) are candidates for laparotomy. The 30% of patients who do not qualify may be treated by insertion of a tube stent into the bile duct transhepatically under radiologic control or from the duodenum under endoscopic control. The tube is positioned so that holes above and below the tumor reestablish flow of bile into the duodenum. If both lobar ducts are blocked by a tumor at the bifurcation of the common hepatic duct, it is usually necessary to place a transhepatic tube into only one lobar duct. If the lesion blocks the takeoff of the segmental ducts, stents are rarely beneficial.

Laparotomy is indicated in most cases, however, with the objective of removing the tumor. Preoperative decompression of the bile duct with a percutaneous catheter to relieve jaundice does not lower the incidence of postoperative complications. At operation, which may be immediately preceded by diagnostic laparoscopy, the extent of the tumor should be determined by external examination of the bile duct and the adjacent portal vein and hepatic artery.

Tumors of the distal common duct should be treated by radical pancreaticoduodenectomy (Whipple procedure) (Figure 27–5) if it appears that all tumor would be removed. Secondary involvement of the portal vein is the usual reason for unresectability of tumors in this location. Mid common duct or low hepatic duct tumors should also be removed if possible. If the tumor cannot be excised, bile flow should be reestablished into the intestine by a cholecystojejunostomy or Roux-en-Y choledochojejunostomy. The choice is based on technical considerations.

Tumors at the hilum of the liver should be resected if possible and a Roux-en-Y hepaticojejunostomy performed. The anastomosis is usually between hilum and bowel rather than between individual bile ducts and bowel. A curative operation nearly always requires resection of either the right or the left lobe of the liver and, in all cases, the caudate lobe. Extension into the lobar and segmental ducts and secondary involvement of the hepatic artery and portal vein are the most common reasons for inability to resect the tumor. Subtotal resections offer little in the way of palliation.

Postoperative radiotherapy is commonly recommended.

Prognosis

The average patient with adenocarcinoma of the bile duct survives less than a year. The overall 5-year survival rate is 15%. Following a thorough radical operation, 5-year survival is about 40%. Biliary cirrhosis, intrahepatic infection, and general debility with terminal pneumonitis are the usual causes of death. Palliative resections and stents may improve the length and quality of survival in this disease even though surgical cure is uncommon. Limited experience with liver transplantation for this disease has been discouraging: tumor has recurred postoperatively in most patients.

Baer HU et al: Improvements in survival by aggressive resections of hilar cholangiocarcinoma. Ann Surg 1993;217:20.

Flickinger JC et al: Radiation therapy for primary carcinoma of the extrahepatic biliary system: An analysis of 63 cases. Cancer 1991;68:289.

Grove MK et al: Role of radiation after operative palliation in cancer of the proximal bile ducts. Am J Surg 1991;161:454.

Henson DE, Albores-Saavedra J, Corle D: Carcinoma of the extrahepatic bile ducts: Histologic types, stage of disease, grade, and survival rates. Cancer 1992;70:1498.

Koyama K et al: Experience in twenty patients with carcinoma of hilar bile duct treated by resection, targeting chemotherapy and intracavitary irradiation. Surg Gynecol Obstet 1993;176:239.

Reding R et al: Surgical management of 552 carcinomas of the extrahepatic bile ducts (gallbladder and periampullary tumors excluded): Results of the French Surgical Association Survey. Ann Surg 1991;213:236.

Rosen CB et al: Cholangiocarcinoma complicating primary sclerosing cholangitis. Ann Surg 1991;213:21.

Saunders KD et al: The natural history of carcinoma of the bile duct in patients less than forty-five years of age. Surg Gynecol Obstet 1992;174:1.

Tashiro S et al: Prolongation of survival for carcinoma at the hepatic duct confluence. Surgery 1993;113:270.

Tsuzuki T et al: Carcinoma of the main hepatic duct junction: Indications, operative morbidity and mortality, and long-term survival. Surgery 1990;108:495.

Verbeek PC et al: Benign fibrosing disease at the hepatic confluence mimicking Klatskin tumors. Surgery 1992;112:866.

Wetter LA et al: Differential diagnosis of sclerosing cholangiocarcinomas of the common hepatic duct (Klatskin tumors). Am J Surg 1991;161:57.

Yeo CJ, Pitt HA, Cameron JL: Cholangiocarcinoma. Surg Clin North Am 1990;70:1429.

BENIGN TUMORS & PSEUDOTUMORS OF THE GALLBLADDER

Various unrelated lesions appear on the cholecystogram as projections from the gallbladder wall. The differentiation from gallstones is based upon observing whether a shift in position of the projections follows changes in posture of the patient, since stones are not fixed. Cancer should be suspected in any polypoid lesion that exceeds 1 cm in diameter.

Polyps

Most of these are not true neoplasms but cholesterol polyps, a local form of cholesterosis. Histologically, they consist of a cluster of lipid-filled macrophages in the submucosa. They easily become detached from the wall when the gallbladder is handled at surgery. It is not known whether cholesterol polyps are important in the genesis of gallstones. Some patients experience gallbladder pain, but whether this is related to the presence of the polyps per se or is a manifestation of functional gallbladder disease has not been established.

Inflammatory polyps have also been reported, but they are quite rare.

Adenomyomatosis

On cholecystography, this entity presents as a slight intraluminal convexity that is often marked by central umbilication. It is usually found in the fundus but may occur elsewhere. It is unclear whether adenomyomatosis is an acquired degenerative lesion or a developmental abnormality (ie, hamartoma). The following synonyms for this lesion appear in the literature: adenomatous hyperplasia, cholecystitis glandularis proliferans, and diverticulosis of the gallbladder. Although the condition is probably asymptomatic in many cases, adenomyomatosis can cause abdominal pain. Cholecystectomy should be performed in such patients.

Adenomas

These appear as pedunculated adenomatous polyps, true neoplasms that may be papillary or nonpapillary histologically. In a few cases they have been found in association with carcinoma in situ of the gallbladder.

Albores-Saavedra J, Vardaman CJ, Vuitch F: Non-neoplastic polypoid lesions and adenomas of the gallbladder. Pathol Annu 1993;28(Part 1):145.

Aldridge MC, Bismuth H: Gallbladder cancer: the polyp-cancer sequence. Br J Surg 1990;77:363.

Farinon AM et al: "Adenomatous polyps of the gallbladder" adenomas of the gallbladder. HPB Surg 1991;3:251.

Ishikawa O et al: The difference in malignancy between pedunculated and sessile polypoid lesions of the gallbladder. Am J Gastroenterol 1989;84:1386.

Jorgensen T, Jensen KH: Polyps in the gallbladder: A prevalence study. Scand J Gastroenterol 1990;25:281.

Yang HL, Sun YG, Wang Z: Polypoid lesions of the gallbladder: Diagnosis and indications for surgery. Br J Surg 1992;79:227.

BENIGN TUMORS OF THE BILE DUCTS

Benign papillomas and adenomas may arise from the ductal epithelium. Only 90 cases have been reported to date. The neoplastic propensity of the ductal epithelium is widespread, so the tumors are often multiple, and recurrence is common after excision. The affected duct must be radically excised for permanent cure to result.

Bruhans R, Myers RT: Benign neoplasms of the extrahepatic biliary ducts. Am Surg 1971;37:161.

Gouma DJ et al: Intrahepatic biliary papillomatosis. Br J Surg 1984;71:72.

Mercadier M et al: Papillomatosis of the intrahepatic bile ducts. World J Surg 1984;8:30.

BILE DUCT INJURIES & STRICTURES

Essentials of Diagnosis

- Episodic cholangitis.
- Previous biliary surgery.
- Transhepatic cholangiogram often diagnostic.

General Considerations

Benign biliary injuries and strictures are caused by surgical trauma in about 95% of cases. The remainder result from external abdominal trauma or, rarely, from erosion of the duct by a gallstone. Prevention of injury to the duct depends on a combination of technical skill, experience, and a thorough knowledge of the normal anatomy and its variations in the hilum of the liver. The number of bile duct injuries has risen sharply in the past few years along with the shift from open to laparoscopic cholecystectomy.

The most common lesion consists of excision of a segment of the common duct as a result of mistaking it for the cystic duct. Partial transection, occlusion with metal clips, injury to the right hepatic duct, and leakage from the cystic duct are other examples. A full discussion of how these injuries occur and how they can be prevented is beyond the scope of this text.

A clean incision of the duct without additional damage is best managed by opening the abdomen and suturing the incision with fine absorbable suture material.

Clinical Findings

A. Symptoms: Manifestations of injury to the duct may or may not be evident in the postoperative period. Following laparoscopic surgery, bile ascites, manifested by abdominal distention, bloating, and pain plus mild jaundice, is the usual presentation, since the duct is usually open to the abdomen. The symptoms are relatively mild and may for a time be thought to represent only ileus until a worsening picture requires further investigation.

Injuries following open cholecystectomy more often present with intermittent cholangitis or jaundice as a consequence of a biliary stricture. The first clear-cut symptoms may not be evident for weeks or months after surgery.

B. Signs: Findings are not distinctive. Bile ascites produces abdominal distention and ileus and, rarely, true bile peritonitis with toxicity. The right upper quadrant may be tender but usually is not. Jaundice is usually present during an attack of cholangitis.

C. Laboratory Findings: The serum alkaline phosphatase concentration is elevated in cases of stricture. The serum bilirubin fluctuates in relation to symptoms but usually remains well below 10 mg/dL.

Blood cultures are usually positive during acute cholangitis.

D. Imaging Studies: Bile ascites can be suspected on ultrasound or CT scan. Fluid should be aspirated, and if it is bile, the diagnosis is clear. THC and ERCP are necessary to depict the anatomy. After laparoscopic cholecystectomy, the most common pattern is a blocked (by a metal clip) lower duct and an upper duct draining freely into the abdomen. With a stricture, the findings most often consist of focal narrowing of the common hepatic duct within 2 cm of the bifurcation and mild to moderate dilatation of the intrahepatic ducts.

Differential Diagnosis

Choledocholithiasis is the condition that most often must be differentiated from biliary stricture because the clinical and laboratory findings can be identical. A history of trauma to the duct would point toward stricture as the more likely diagnosis. The final distinction must often await radiologic or surgical findings. THC or ERCP should be definitive.

Other causes of cholestatic jaundice may have to be ruled out in some cases.

Complications

Complications develop quickly if the leak is not controlled. Bile peritonitis and abscesses may form. With stricture, persistent cholangitis may progress to multiple intrahepatic abscesses and a septic death.

Treatment

Bile duct injuries should be surgically repaired in all but a few patients who are likely to improve with a nonoperative approach. Excision of the damaged duct and Roux-en-Y hepaticojejunostomy is indicated for most acute and chronic injuries. The entire biliary tree must be outlined by cholangiograms preoperatively. The key to success is the thoroughness of the dissection and the ability ultimately to suture healthy duct to healthy bowel. This, in turn, depends on the experience of the surgeon with this particular operation.

When a definitive repair is technically impossible, the stricture may be dilated with a transhepatic balloon-tipped catheter. This is particularly applicable to patients with portal hypertension, whose hepatic hilum contains numerous venous collaterals that make operation hazardous.

Prognosis

The death rate from biliary injuries is about 5%, and severe illness is frequent. If the stricture is not repaired, episodic cholangitis and secondary liver disease are inevitable.

Surgical correction of the stricture should be successful in about 90% of cases. Experience at centers with a special interest in this problem indicates that good results can be obtained even if several previous attempts did not relieve the obstruction. There is essentially no place for liver transplantation in this disease.

Berci G: Biliary ductal anatomy and anomalies: The role of intraoperative cholangiography during laparoscopic cholecystectomy. Surg Clin North Am 1992;72:1069.

Csendes A et al: Indications and results of hepaticojejunostomy in benign strictures of the biliary tract. Hepatogastroenterology 1992;39:333.

Davidoff AM et al: Mechanisms of major biliary injury during laparoscopic cholecystectomy. Ann Surg 1992; 215:196.

Deziel DJ et al: Complications of laparoscopic cholecystectomy: A national survey of 4,292 hospitals and an analysis of 77,604 cases. Am J Surg 1993;165:9.

Hunter JG: Avoidance of bile duct injury during laparoscopic cholecystectomy. Am J Surg 1991;162:71.

Lillemoe KD, Pitt HA, Cameron JL: Current management of benign bile duct strictures. Adv Surg 1992;25:119.

Miller TA: Biliary stricture: Is dilatation an acceptable alternative to operation? Gastroenterology 1990;98:1089.

Moossa AR, Mayer AD, Stabile B: Iatrogenic injury to the bile duct: Who, how, where? Arch Surg 1990;125:1028.

Pellegrini CA et al: Recurrent biliary stricture: Patterns of recurrence and outcome of surgical therapy. Am J Surg 1984;147:175.

Terblanche J et al: High or low hepaticojejunostomy for bile duct strictures? Surgery 1990;108:828.

Way LW: Bile duct injury during laparoscopic cholecystectomy. Ann Surg 1992;215:195.

Way LW: Biliary strictures. In: Surgery of the Gallbladder and Bile Ducts. Way LW, Pellegrini CA (editors). Saunders, 1987.

UNCOMMON CAUSES OF BILE DUCT OBSTRUCTION

Congenital Choledochal Cysts

About 30% of congenital choledochal cysts produce their first symptoms in adults, usually presenting with jaundice, cholangitis, and a right upper quadrant mass. Diagnosis can be made by THC or ERCP. The optimal surgical procedure is excision of the cyst and construction of a Roux-en-Y hepaticojejunostomy. If this is not technically possible or if the patient's condition will not permit a prolonged operation, the cyst should be emptied of precipitated biliary sludge and a cystenteric anastomosis constructed. Congenital cysts of the biliary tree have a high incidence of malignant degeneration, which is another argument for excision rather than drainage.

Chijiiwa K, Koga A: Surgical management and long-term follow-up of patients with choledochal cysts. Am J Surg 1993;165:238.

Gertler JP, Cahow CE: Choledochal cysts in the adult. J Clin Gastroenterol 1988;10:315.

Martin RF et al: Symptomatic choledochoceles in adults: Endoscopic retrograde cholangiopancreatography recognition and management. Arch Surg 1992;127:536.

O'Neill JA Jr: Choledochal cyst. Curr Probl Surg 1992;29:361.

Savader SJ et al: Choledochal cysts: classification and cholangiographic appearance. AJR Am J Roentgenol 1991; 156:327.

Shemesh E et al: The role of endoscopic retrograde cholangiopancreatography in the diagnosis and treatment of adult choledochal cyst. Surg Gynecol Obstet 1988;167:423.

Caroli's Disease

Caroli's disease, another form of congenital cystic disease, consists of saccular intrahepatic dilatation of the ducts. In some cases, the biliary abnormality is an isolated finding, but more often it is associated with congenital hepatic fibrosis and medullary sponge kidney. The latter patients often present in childhood or as young adults with complications of portal hypertension. Others have cholangitis and obstructive jaundice as initial manifestations. There is no definitive surgical solution to the problem except in rare cases with isolated involvement of one hepatic lobe, where lobectomy is curative. Intermittent antibiotic therapy for cholangitis is the usual regimen.

Desmet VJ: Congenital diseases of intrahepatic bile ducts:

Variations on the theme "ductal plate malformation." Hepatology 1992;16:1069.

Hopper KD: The role of computed tomography in the evaluation of Caroli's disease. Clin Imaging 1989;13:68.

Summerfield JA et al: Hepatobiliary fibropolycystic diseases: A clinical and histological review of 51 patients. J Hepatol 1986;2:141.

Tandon RK et al: Caroli's syndrome: A heterogeneous entity. Am J Gastroenterol 1990;85:170.

Hemobilia

Hemobilia presents with the triad of biliary colic, obstructive jaundice, and occult or gross intestinal bleeding. Most cases in Western cultures follow several weeks after hepatic trauma with bleeding from an intrahepatic branch of the hepatic artery into a duct. It is seen with less frequency now, because the general principles of management of hepatic trauma are better understood. In the Orient, hemobilia usually follows ductal parasitism (*Ascaris lumbricoides*) or Oriental cholangiohepatitis. Other causes are hepatic neoplasms, rupture of a hepatic artery aneurysm, hepatic abscess, and choledocholithiasis. The diagnosis may be suspected from a technetium 99m-labeled red blood cell scan, but an arteriogram is usually required for diagnosis and planning of therapy. Sometimes the bleeding can be stopped by embolizing the lesion with stainless steel coils, Gelfoam, or autologous blood clot infused through a catheter selectively positioned in the hepatic artery. If this is unsuccessful, either direct ligation of the bleeding point in the liver or proximal ligation of an upstream branch of the hepatic artery in the hilum is required.

Czerniak A et al: Hemobilia: A disease in evolution. Arch Surg 1988;123:718.

Jackson DE Jr et al: Hemobilia associated with hepatic artery aneurysms: Scintigraphic detection with technetium-99-m-labeled red blood cells. J Nucl Med 1986; 27:491.

Lygidakis NJ, Okazaki M, Damtsios G: Iatrogenic hemobillia: How to approach it. Hepatogastroenterology 1991;38:454.

Merrell SW, Schneider PD: Hemobilia: Evolution of current diagnosis and treatment. West J Med 1991;155:621.

Sandblom P: Why should every physician know about hemobilia? West J Med 1991;155:660.

Savader SJ et al: Hemobilia after percutaneous transhepatic biliary drainage: Treatment with transcatheter embolotherapy. J Vasc Intervent Radiol 1992;3:345.

Pancreatitis

Pancreatitis can cause obstruction of the intrapancreatic portion of the bile duct by inflammatory swelling, encasement with scar, or compression by a pseudocyst. The patient may present with painless jaundice or cholangitis. Occasionally, a distended gallbladder can be felt on abdominal examination. Differentiation from choledocholithiasis and secondary acute pancreatitis depends on biliary x-rays or surgical exploration if the jaundice persists. Jaundice due to inflammation alone rarely lasts more than 2 weeks; persistent jaundice following an attack of acute pancreatitis suggests the development of a pseudocyst, underlying chronic pancreatitis with obstruction by fibrosis, or even an obstructing neoplasm.

Biliary obstruction from chronic pancreatitis may have few or no clinical manifestations. Jaundice is usually present, but the average peak bilirubin level is only 4–5 mg/dL. Some patients with functionally significant stenosis have persistently elevated alkaline phosphatase levels as the only abnormality; when surgical decompression of the bile duct is not performed, these patients often develop secondary biliary cirrhosis within a year or so. Diagnosis of stricture is made by ERCP, which shows a long stenosis of the intrapancreatic portion of the duct, proximal dilatation, and either a gradual or abrupt tapering of the lumen at the pancreatic border, occasionally accompanied by ductal angulation. If cholangiograms show stenosis and if alkaline phosphatase or bilirubin levels remain more than twice normal for longer than 2 months, the stenosis is functionally significant and unlikely to resolve and requires surgical correction. Choledochoduodenostomy is done in most cases. Cholecystoduodenostomy is unreliable because the cystic duct is often too narrow to provide continued biliary decompression.

Patients with obstructive jaundice and pseudocyst usually respond to surgical drainage of the pseudocyst. However, occasionally they do not respond, because chronic scarring—not the cyst—is the cause of obstruction. Procedures to drain both the bile duct and the pseudocyst are indicated if operative cholangiograms demonstrate persistent bile duct obstruction after the cyst has been decompressed.

Bradley EL: Parapancreatic biliary and intestinal obstruction in chronic obstructive pancreatitis. Is prophylactic bypass necessary? Am J Surg 1986;151:256.

Petrozza JA, Dutta SK: The variable appearance of distal common bile duct stenosis in chronic pancreatitis. J Clin Gastroenterol 1985;7:447.

Skellenger ME et al: Cholestasis due to compression of the common bile duct by pancreatic pseudocysts. Am J Surg 1983;145:343.

Stahl TJ et al: Partial biliary obstruction caused by chronic pancreatitis. Ann Surg 1988;207:26.

Sugerman HJ et al: Selective drainage for pancreatic, biliary, and duodenal obstruction secondary to chronic fibrosing pancreatitis. Ann Surg 1986;203:558.

Ampullary Dysfunction & Stenosis

Stenosis of the hepatopancreatic ampulla (ampullary stenosis) has been implicated as a cause of pain and other manifestations of ampullary obstruction and is often considered as a cause of postcholecystectomy complaints. Some cases are idiopathic, whereas others may be the result of trauma from gallstones. If the patient has secondary manifestations of biliary obstruction (eg, jaundice, increased alkaline phosphatase concentration, cholangitis) in the absence of gallstones or some other obstructing lesion, and cholangiography shows dilatation of the common duct, ampullary stenosis is a plausible explanation. However, the diagnosis is more often proposed as a reason for upper abdominal pain without these more objective findings. Ampullary dysfunction is postulated in these cases.

Sphincter of Oddi dysfunction may be the cause of biliary-like pain and is often considered in patients who remain uncomfortable after cholecystectomy. The pathogenesis of the symptoms is thought to be similar to that of esophageal dysmotility and the irritable bowel syndrome, The patients typically experience severe, intermittent upper abdominal pain that lasts for 1–3 hours, sometimes following a meal.

Residual gallstone and pancreatic disease must first be ruled out. Ampullary dysfunction can then be diagnosed by sphincter of Oddi manometry. Patients are placed in one of three groups depending on the presence of three objective manifestations of biliary obstruction: abnormal liver function tests, prolonged (> 45 minutes) common bile duct emptying of contrast media after ERCP; and a common duct greater than 12 mm in diameter. Patients in group I have all three findings; patients in group II have one or two findings; and patients in group III have none of the findings. Group I patients are thought to have enough evidence of disease that sphincterotomy should be performed without manometry. Group I patients have abnormal motility so rarely that they should not be considered further for sphincterotomy. Thus, motility studies are most often of value in determining which of the group II patients will improve after sphincterotomy.

The abnormalities sought on the motility studies include an elevated (> 40 mm Hg) basal sphincter pressure and a paradoxic rise in sphincter pressure in response to CCK. The former is most reliable. About 50% of group II patients have elevated sphincter pressures, and these are the ones who benefit from sphincterotomy.

A scintigraphic test may be just as accurate. The patient is given a bolus of CCK followed by ^{99m}Tc-DISIDA. Gamma camera images of the liver and bile duct are obtained for 60 minutes. A scoring system (score: 0–12) is based on the rate of passage of the imaging agent past various relevant points (eg, appearance and clearance through the liver, bile duct, and bowel). The normal range is 0–5; abnormal is 6–12.

Sphincter of Oddi dysfunction is an uncommon explanation for abdominal pain, and it is appropriate to remain skeptical unless the objective findings of biliary obstruction are clear-cut. In well-selected cases, however, endoscopic sphincterotomy is truly beneficial.

Dodds WJ: Biliary tract motility and its relationship to clinical disorders. AJR Am J Roentgenol 1990;155:247.

Elta GH et al: Delayed biliary drainage is common in asymptomatic post-cholecystectomy volunteers. Gastrointest Endosc 1992;38:435.

Elta GH: Sphincter of Oddi manometry in patients with possible sphincter of Oddi dysfunction. Gastroenterology 1991;101:1747.

Funch-Jensen P, Thommesen P, Jensen SL: Sphincter of Oddi motility and its disorders. Dig Dis 1991;9:229.

Geenen JE et al: The efficacy of endoscopic sphincterotomy after cholecystectomy in patients with sphincter-of-Oddi dysfunction. N Engl J Med 1989;320:82.

Gilbert DA et al: Status evaluation: sphincter of Oddi manometry. American Society for Gastrointestinal Endoscopy. Technology Assessment Committee. Gastrointest Endosc 1992;38:757.

Meshkinpour H, Mollot M: Sphincter of Oddi dysfunction and unexplained abdominal pain: Clinical and manometric study. Dig Dis Sci 1992;37:257.

Moody FG et al: Stenosis of the sphincter of Oddi. Surg Clin North Am 1990;70:1341.

Raddawi HM et al: Pressure measurements from biliary and pancreatic segments of sphincter of Oddi: Comparison between patients with functional abdominal pain, biliary, or pancreatic disease. Dig Dis Sci 1991;36:71.

Sherman S et al: Frequency of abnormal sphincter of Oddi manometry compared with the clinical suspicion of sphincter of Oddi dysfunction. Am J Gastroenterol 1991;86:586.

Sostre S, Kalloo AN, Spiegler EJ: A noninvasive test of sphincter of Oddi dysfunction in postcholecystectomy patients: The scintigraphic score. J Nucl Med 1992;33:1216.

Thune A et al: Reproducibility of endoscopic sphincter of Oddi manometry. Dig Dis Sci 1991;36:1401.

Toouli J: Clinical relevance of sphincter of Oddi dysfunction. Br J Surg 1990;77:723.

Duodenal Diverticula

Duodenal diverticula usually arise on the medial aspect of the duodenum within 2 cm of the orifice of the bile duct, and in some individuals the duct empties directly into a diverticulum. Even in the latter circumstance, duodenal diverticula are usually innocuous. Occasionally, distortion of the duct entrance or obstruction by enterolith formation in the diverticulum produces symptoms. Either choledochoduodenostomy or Roux-en-Y choledochojejunostomy is usually a safer method of reestablishing biliary drainage than attempts to excise the diverticulum and reimplant the duct.

McSherry CK, Glenn F: Biliary tract obstruction and duodenal diverticula. Surg Gynecol Obstet 1970;130:829.

Ascariasis

When the worms invade the duct from the duodenum, ascariasis can produce symptoms of ductal obstruction. Air may sometimes be seen within the ducts on plain films. Antibiotics should be used until cholangitis is controlled, and anthelmintic therapy (mebendazole, albendazole, or pyrantel pamoate) should then be given. The acute symptoms usually subside with antibiotics, but if they do not, endoscopic sphincterotomy should be performed and attempts made to extricate the worms. If this is unsuccessful and the patient remains acutely ill, the duct should be emptied surgically.

Khuroo MS, Zargar SA, Mahajan R: Hepatobiliary and pancreatic ascariasis in India. Lancet 1990;335:1503.

Wani NA, Chrungoo RK: Biliary ascariasis: Surgical aspects. World J Surg 1992;16:976.

Recurrent Pyogenic Cholangitis (Oriental Cholangiohepatitis)

Oriental cholangiohepatitis is a type of chronic recurrent cholangitis prevalent in coastal areas from Japan to Southeast Asia. In Hong Kong it is the third most common indication for emergency laparotomy and the most frequent type of biliary disease. The disease is currently thought to result from chronic portal bacteremia, with portal phlebitis antedating the biliary disease. *E coli* causes secondary infection of the bile ducts, which initiates pigment stone formation within the ducts.

Biliary obstruction from the stones gives rise to recurrent cholangitis, which, unlike gallstone disease in Western countries, may be unaccompanied by gallbladder stones. The gallbladder is usually distended during an attack and may contain pus.

Chronic recurrent infection often leads to biliary strictures and hepatic abscess formation. The strictures are usually located in the intrahepatic bile ducts, and for some unknown reason the left lobe of the liver is more severely involved. Intrahepatic gallstones are common, and their surgical removal may be difficult or impossible. Acute abdominal pain, chills, and high fever are usually present, and jaundice develops in about half of cases. Right upper quadrant tenderness is usually marked, and in about 80% of cases the gallbladder is palpable. ERCP or THC is the best way to study the biliary tree and can help in determining the need for surgery and the type of procedure.

Systemic antibiotics should be given for acute cholangitis. Surgical treatment consists of cholecystectomy, common duct exploration, and removal of stones. Sphincteroplasty should also be performed to allow any residual or recurrent stones to escape from the duct. A Roux-en-Y choledochojejunostomy is indicated for patients with strictures, markedly dilated ducts (eg, > 3 cm), or recurrent disease after a previous sphincteroplasty. The results of surgery are good in 80% of patients. Chronic intrahepatic stones and infection, which often involve only one lobe, may require hepatic lobectomy.

Although many patients are cured, prolonged illness from repeated infection is almost unavoidable once strictures have appeared or the intrahepatic ducts have become packed with stones.

Chan FL et al: Evaluation of recurrent pyogenic cholangitis with CT: Analysis of 50 patients. Radiology 1989;170(1 Part 1):165.

Fan ST, Choi TK, Wong J: Recurrent pyogenic cholangitis: Current management. World J Surg 1991;15:248.

Khuroo MS et al: Oddi's sphincter motor activity in patients with recurrent pyogenic cholangitis. Hepatology 1993; 17:53.

Kusano S et al: Oriental cholangiohepatitis: Correlation between portal vein occlusion and hepatic atrophy. AJR Am J Roentgenol 1992;158:1011.

Lim JH et al: Oriental cholangiohepatitis: Sonographic findings in 48 cases. AJR Am J Roentgenol 1990;155:511.

Lim JH: Oriental cholangiohepatitis: Pathologic, clinical, and radiologic features. AJR Am J Roentgenol 1991; 157:1.

Sclerosing Cholangitis

Sclerosing cholangitis is a rare chronic disease of unknown cause characterized by nonbacterial inflammatory narrowing of the bile ducts. About 60% of cases occur in patients with ulcerative colitis, and sclerosing cholangitis develops in about 5% of patients with that disorder. Other less commonly associated conditions are thyroiditis, retroperitoneal fibrosis, and mediastinal fibrosis. The disease chiefly affects men 20–50 years of age. In most cases, the entire biliary tree is affected by the inflammatory process, which causes irregular partial obliteration of the lumen of the ducts. The narrowing may be confined, however, to the intrahepatic or extrahepatic ducts, though it is almost never so short as to resemble a posttraumatic or focal malignant stricture. The woody-hard duct walls contain increased collagen and lymphoid elements and are thickened at the expense of the lumen.

The clinical onset usually consists of the gradual appearance of mild jaundice and pruritus. Symptoms of bacterial cholangitis (eg, fever and chills) are uncommon in the absence of previous biliary surgery. Laboratory findings are typical of cholestasis. The total serum bilirubin averages about 4 mg/dL and rarely exceeds 10 mg/dL. ERCP is usually diagnostic, demonstrating ductal stenoses and irregularity, which often gives a beaded appearance. Liver biopsy may show pericholangitis and bile stasis, but the changes are nonspecific.

The complications of sclerosing cholangitis include gallstone disease and adenocarcinoma of the bile duct. The latter is most common in patients with ulcerative colitis. Furthermore, patients with ulcerative colitis and sclerosing cholangitis appear to be at greater risk for colonic mucosal dysplasia and colon cancer than those with ulcerative colitis not associated with sclerosing cholangitis.

Ursodiol (ursodeoxycholic acid), 10 mg/kg/d, improves liver function tests and symptoms. Cholestyramine will give relief from pruritus. Percutaneous transhepatic balloon dilatation can be of value to treat dominant strictures. In cases where the disease is largely confined to the distal extrahepatic duct and the proximal ducts are dilated, a Roux-en-Y hepaticojejunostomy may be indicated. For patients with severe intrahepatic involvement, hepatic transplantation should be considered.

The natural history of sclerosing cholangitis is one of chronicity and unpredictable severity. Some patients seem to obtain nearly complete remission after treatment, but this is not common. Bacterial cholangitis may develop after operation if adequate drainage has not been established. In these cases, antibiotics will be required at intervals. Most patients experience the gradual evolution of secondary biliary cirrhosis after many years of mild to moderate jaundice and pruritus. Liver transplantation is indicated when the disease becomes advanced. The results are good.

Beuers U et al: Ursodeoxycholic acid for treatment of primary sclerosing cholangitis: A placebo-controlled trial. Hepatology 1992;16:707.

Cameron JL: Primary sclerosing cholangitis: Palliative surgery or transplantation? HPB Surg 1992;5:275.

Chapman RW: Aetiology and natural history of primary sclerosing cholangitis A decade of progress? Gut 1991;32:1433.

Hanauer S: Primary sclerosing cholangitis and ulcerative colitis: Potential cofactors in the dysplasia sequence. Gastroenterology 1992;102:2161.

Harrison RF, Hubscher SG: The spectrum of bile duct lesions in end-stage primary sclerosing cholangitis. Histopathology 1991;19:321.

Farrant JM et al: Natural history and prognostic variables in primary sclerosing cholangitis. Gastroenterology 1991;100:1710.

Ismail T et al: Primary sclerosing cholangitis: Surgical options, prognostic variables and outcome. Br J Surg 1991;78:564.

Jansen PL, Sanders JB: Primary sclerosing cholangitis: An unresolved enigma. Scand J Gastroenterol 1992; 194(Suppl):76.

Martin M: Primary sclerosing cholangitis. Annu Rev Med 1993;44:221.

Martin FM, Braasch JW: Primary sclerosing cholangitis. Curr Probl Surg 1992;29:133.

Olsson R et al: Prevalence of primary sclerosing cholangitis in patients with ulcerative colitis. Gastroenterology 1991;100(5 Part 1):1319.

Rasmussen HH et al: Primary sclerosing cholangitis in patients with ulcerative colitis. Scand J Gastroenterol 1992;27:732.

Wiesner RH et al: Selection and timing of liver transplantation in primary biliary cirrhosis and primary sclerosing cholangitis. Hepatology 1992;16:1290.

Pancreas

27

Howard A. Reber, MD, & Lawrence W. Way, MD

EMBRYOLOGY

The pancreas arises in the fourth week of fetal life from the caudal part of the foregut as dorsal and ventral pancreatic buds. Both anlagen rotate to the right and fuse near the point of origin of the ventral pancreas. Later, as the duodenum rotates, the pancreas shifts to the left. In the adult, only the caudal portion of the head and the uncinate process are derived from the ventral pancreas. The cranial part of the head and all of the body and tail are derived from the dorsal pancreas. Most of the dorsal pancreatic duct joins with the duct of the ventral pancreas to form the main pancreatic duct **(duct of Wirsung);** a small part persists as the accessory duct **(duct of Santorini).** In 5–10% of people, the ventral and dorsal pancreatic ducts do not fuse, and most regions of the pancreas drain through the duct of Santorini and the orifice of the minor papilla. In this case, only the small ventral pancreas drains with the common bile duct through the papilla of Vater.

ANATOMY

The pancreas is a thin elliptic organ that lies within the retroperitoneum in the upper abdomen (Figures 27–1 and 27–2). In the adult, it is 12–15 cm long and weighs 70–100 g. The gland can be divided into three portions—head, body, and tail. The head of the pancreas is intimately adherent to the medial portion of the duodenum and lies in front of the inferior vena cava and superior mesenteric vessels. A small tongue of tissue called the uncinate process lies behind the superior mesenteric vessels as they emerge from the retroperitoneum. Anteriorly, the stomach and the first portion of the duodenum lie partly in front of the pancreas. The common bile duct passes through a posterior groove in the head of the pancreas adjacent to the duodenum. The body of the pancreas is in contact posteriorly with the aorta, the left crus of the diaphragm, the left adrenal gland, and the left kidney. The tail of the pancreas lies in the hilum of the spleen. The main pancreatic duct (the duct of Wirsung) courses along the gland from the tail to the head and joins the common bile duct just before entering the duodenum at the ampulla of Vater. The accessory pancreatic duct (the duct of Santorini) enters the duodenum 2–2.5 cm proximal to the ampulla of Vater (Figure 27–1).

The blood supply of the pancreas is derived from branches of the celiac and superior mesenteric arteries (Figure 27–2). The superior pancreaticoduodenal artery arises from the gastroduodenal artery, runs parallel to the duodenum, and eventually meets the inferior pancreaticoduodenal artery, a branch of the superior mesenteric artery, to form an arcade. The splenic artery provides tributaries that supply the body and tail of the pancreas. The main branches are termed the dorsal pancreatic, pancreatica magna, and caudal pancreatic arteries. The venous supply of the gland parallels the arterial supply. Lymphatic drainage is into the peripancreatic nodes located along the veins.

The innervation of the pancreas is derived from the vagal and splanchnic nerves. The efferent fibers pass through the celiac plexus from the celiac branch of the right vagal nerve to terminate in ganglia located in the interlobular septa of the pancreas. Postganglionic fibers from these synapses innervate the acini, the islets, and the ducts. The visceral afferent fibers from the pancreas also travel in the vagal and splanchnic nerves, but those that mediate pain are confined to the latter. Sympathetic fibers to the pancreas pass from the splanchnic nerves through the celiac plexus and innervate the pancreatic vasculature.

PHYSIOLOGY

Exocrine Function

The external secretion of the pancreas consists of a clear, alkaline (pH 7.0–8.3) solution of 1–2 L/d containing digestive enzymes. Secretion is stimulated by the hormones secretin and cholecystokinin (CCK) and by parasympathetic vagal discharge. Secretin and cholecystokinin are synthesized, stored, and released from duodenal mucosal cells in response to specific stimuli. Acid in the lumen of the duodenum causes the release of secretin, and luminal digestion products of fat and protein cause the release of cholecystokinin.

The water and electrolyte secretion is formed by the centroacinar and intercalated duct cells principally in response to secretin stimulation. The secre-

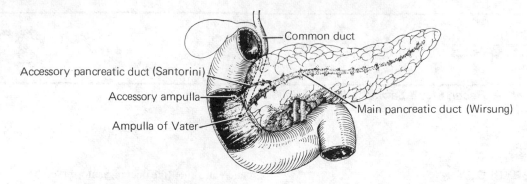

Figure 27–1. Anatomic configuration of pancreatic ductal system. (Courtesy of W Silen.)

tion is modified by exchange processes and active secretion in the ductal collecting system. The cations sodium and potassium are present in the same concentrations as in plasma. The anions bicarbonate and chloride vary in concentration according to the rate of secretion: with increasing rate of secretion, the bicarbonate concentration increases and chloride concentration falls, so that the sum of the two is the same throughout the secretory range. Pancreatic juice helps neutralize gastric acid in the duodenum and adjusts luminal pH to the level that gives optimal activity of pancreatic enzymes.

Pancreatic enzymes are synthesized, stored (as zymogen granules), and released by the acinar cells of the gland, principally in response to cholecystokinin and vagal stimulation. Pancreatic enzymes are proteolytic, lipolytic, and amylolytic. Lipase and amylase are stored and secreted in active forms. The proteolytic enzymes are secreted as inactive precursors and are activated by the duodenal enzyme enterokinase. Other enzymes secreted by the pancreas include ribonucleases and phospholipase A. Phospholipase A is secreted as an inactive proenzyme activated in the duodenum by trypsin. It catalyzes the conversion of biliary lecithin to lysolecithin.

Turnover of protein in the pancreas exceeds that of any other organ in the body. Intravenously injected amino acids are incorporated into enzyme protein and may appear in the pancreatic juice within 1 hour. Three mechanisms prevent autodigestion of the pancreas by its proteolytic enzymes: (1) The enzymes are stored in acinar cells as zymogen granules, where they are separated from other cell proteins. (2) The enzymes are secreted in an inactive form. (3) Inhibitors of proteolytic enzymes are present in pancreatic juice and pancreatic tissue.

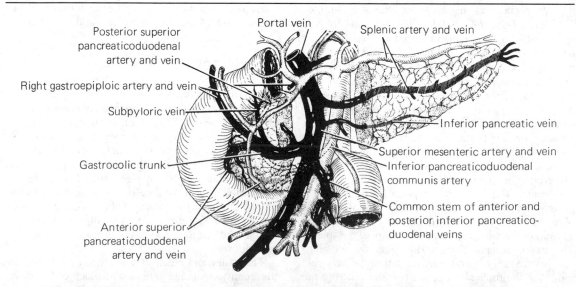

Figure 27–2. Arterial supply and venous drainage of the pancreas. (Courtesy of W Silen.)

Endocrine Function

The function of the endocrine pancreas is to facilitate storage of foodstuffs by release of insulin after a meal and to provide a mechanism for their mobilization by release of glucagon during periods of fasting. Insulin and glucagon, as well as pancreatic polypeptide and somatostatin, are produced by the islets of Langerhans.

Insulin, a polypeptide (MW 5734) consisting of 51 amino acid residues, is formed in the beta cells of the pancreas via the precursor proinsulin. Insulin secretion is stimulated by rising or high serum concentrations of metabolic substrates such as glucose, amino acids, and perhaps short-chain fatty acids. The major normal stimulus for insulin release appears to be glucose. The release and synthesis of insulin are stimulated by activation of specific glucoreceptors located on the surface membrane of the beta cell. Insulin release is also stimulated by glucagon, secretin, cholecystokinin, vasoactive intestinal polypeptide (VIP), and gastrin, all of which sensitize the receptors on the beta cell to glucose. Epinephrine, tolbutamide, and chlorpropamide release insulin by acting on the adenylyl cyclase system.

Glucagon, a polypeptide (MW 3485) consisting of 29 amino acid residues, is formed in the α cells of the pancreas. The release of glucagon is stimulated by a low blood glucose concentration, amino acids, catecholamines, sympathetic nervous discharge, and cholecystokinin. It is suppressed by hyperglycemia and insulin.

The principal functions of insulin are to stimulate anabolic reactions involving carbohydrates, fats, proteins, and nucleic acids. Insulin decreases glycogenolysis, lipolysis, proteolysis, gluconeogenesis, ureagenesis, and ketogenesis. Glucagon stimulates glycogenolysis from the liver and proteolysis and lipolysis in adipose tissue as well as in the liver. With the increase in lipolysis, there is an increase in ketogenesis and gluconeogenesis. Glucagon increases cAMP in the liver, heart, skeletal muscle, and adipose tissue. The short-term regulation of gluconeogenesis depends on the balance between insulin and glucagon. Studies on insulin and glucagon suggest that the hormones exert their effects via receptors on the cell membrane. Before entering the systemic circulation, blood draining from the islets of Langerhans perfuses the pancreatic acini, and this exposure to high levels of hormones is thought to influence acinar function.

ANNULAR PANCREAS

Annular pancreas is a rare congenital condition in which a ring of pancreatic tissue from the head of the pancreas surrounds the descending duodenum. The abnormality usually presents in infancy as duodenal obstruction with postprandial vomiting. There is bile in the vomitus if the constriction is distal to the entrance of the common bile duct. X-rays show a dilated stomach and proximal duodenum (double bubble sign) and little or no air in the rest of the small bowel.

After correction of fluid and electrolyte imbalance, the obstructed segment should be bypassed by a duodenojejunostomy or other similar procedure. No attempt should be made to resect the obstructing pancreas, because a pancreatic fistula or acute pancreatitis often develops postoperatively.

Occasionally, annular pancreas will present in adult life with similar symptoms.

PANCREATITIS

Pancreatitis is a common nonbacterial inflammatory disease caused by activation, interstitial liberation, and autodigestion of the pancreas by its own enzymes. The process may or may not be accompanied by permanent morphologic and functional changes in the gland. Much is known about the causes of pancreatitis, but despite the accumulation of much experimental data, understanding of the pathogenesis of this disorder is still incomplete.

In **acute pancreatitis,** there is sudden upper abdominal pain, nausea and vomiting, and elevated serum amylase. **Chronic pancreatitis** is characterized by chronic pain, pancreatic calcification on x-ray, and exocrine (steatorrhea) or endocrine (diabetes mellitus) insufficiency. Attacks of acute pancreatitis often occur in patients with chronic pancreatitis. **Acute relapsing pancreatitis** is defined as multiple attacks of pancreatitis without permanent pancreatic scarring, a picture most often associated with biliary pancreatitis. The unsatisfactory term **chronic relapsing pancreatitis,** denoting recurrent acute attacks superimposed on chronic pancreatitis, will not be used in this chapter. Alcoholic pancreatitis often behaves in this way. The term **subacute pancreatitis** has also been used by some to denote the minor acute attacks that typically appear late in alcoholic pancreatitis.

Etiology

Most cases of pancreatitis are caused by gallstone disease or alcoholism; a few result from hypercalcemia, trauma, hyperlipidemia, and genetic predisposition; and the remainder are idiopathic. Important differences exist in the manifestations and natural history of the disease as produced by these various factors.

A. Biliary Pancreatitis: About 40% of cases of pancreatitis are associated with gallstone disease, which, if untreated, usually gives rise to additional acute attacks. For unknown reasons, even repeated attacks of acute biliary pancreatitis seldom produce chronic pancreatitis. Eradication of the biliary disease nearly always prevents recurrent pancreatitis.

The etiologic mechanism most likely consists of transient obstruction of the ampulla of Vater and pancreatic duct by a gallstone. Choledocholithiasis is found in only 25% of cases, but because over 90% of patients excrete a gallstone in feces passed within 10 days after an acute attack, it is assumed that most attacks are caused by a gallstone or biliary sludge traversing the common duct and ampulla of Vater. Other possible steps in pathogenesis initiated by passage of the gallstone are discussed below.

B. Alcoholic Pancreatitis: In the USA, alcoholism accounts for about 40% of cases of pancreatitis. Characteristically, the patients have been heavy users of hard liquor or wine; the condition is relatively infrequent in countries where beer is the most popular alcoholic beverage. Most commonly, 6 years or more of alcoholic excess precede the initial attack of pancreatitis, and even with the first clinical manifestations, signs of chronic pancreatitis can be detected if the gland is examined microscopically. Thus, alcoholic pancreatitis is often considered to be synonymous with chronic pancreatitis no matter what the clinical findings.

Acetaldehyde, an ethanol metabolite, has been implicated as a mediator, since it can generate toxic oxygen metabolites under the influence of xanthine oxidase. In experimental studies, alcohol decreases incorporation of phosphate into parenchymal phospholipids, decreases zymogen synthesis, and produces ultrastructural changes in acinar cells. Acute administration of alcohol stimulates pancreatic secretion and induces spasm in the sphincter of Oddi. This has been compared to experiments that produce acute pancreatitis by combining partial ductal obstruction and secretory stimulation. If the patient can be persuaded to stop drinking, acute attacks may be prevented, but parenchymal damage continues to occur owing to persistent ductal obstruction and fibrosis.

C. Hypercalcemia: Hyperparathyroidism and other disorders accompanied by hypercalcemia are occasionally complicated by acute pancreatitis. With time, chronic pancreatitis and ductal calculi appear. It is thought that the increased calcium concentrations in pancreatic juice that result from hypercalcemia may prematurely activate proteases. They may also facilitate precipitation of calculi in the ducts.

D. Hyperlipidemia: In some patients—especially alcoholics—hyperlipidemia appears transiently during an acute attack of pancreatitis; in others with primary hyperlipidemia (especially those associated with elevated chylomicrons and very low density lipoproteins), pancreatitis seems to be a direct consequence of the metabolic abnormality. Hyperlipidemia during an acute attack of pancreatitis is usually associated with normal serum amylase levels, because the lipid interferes with the chemical determination for amylase; urinary output of amylase may still be high. One should inspect the serum of every patient with acute abdominal pain, because if it is lactescent, pancreatitis will almost always be the correct diagnosis. If a primary lipid abnormality is present, dietary control reduces the chances of additional attacks of pancreatitis as well as other complications.

E. Familial Pancreatitis: In this condition, attacks of abdominal pain usually begin in childhood. The genetic defect appears to be transmitted as a non-X-linked dominant with variable penetrance. Some affected families also have aminoaciduria, but this is not a universal finding. Diabetes mellitus and steatorrhea are uncommon. Chronic calcific pancreatitis develops eventually in most patients, and many patients become candidates for operation for chronic pain. Pancreatic carcinoma is more frequent in patients with familial pancreatitis.

F. Protein Deficiency: In certain populations where dietary protein intake is markedly deficient, the incidence of chronic pancreatitis is high. The reason for this association is obscure, especially in view of the observation that pancreatitis afflicts alcoholics with higher dietary protein and fat intake than those who consume less protein and fat.

G. Postoperative (Iatrogenic) Pancreatitis: Most cases of postoperative pancreatitis follow common bile duct exploration, especially if sphincterotomy was performed. Two practices, now largely abandoned, were often responsible: (1) use of a common duct T tube with a long arm passing through the sphincter of Oddi, and (2) dilation of the sphincter to 5–7 mm during common duct exploration. Operations on the pancreas, including pancreatic biopsy, are another cause. A few cases follow gastric surgery or even operations remote from the pancreas. Pancreatitis is particularly common after cardiac surgery with cardiopulmonary bypass, where the risk factors are preoperative renal failure, valve surgery, postoperative hypotension, and (particularly) the perioperative administration of calcium chloride (> 800 mg calcium chloride per square meter of body surface area). Pancreatitis may also complicate endoscopic retrograde pancreatography or endoscopic sphincterotomy.

Rarely, pancreatitis follows Billroth II gastrectomy, owing to acute obstruction of the afferent loop and reflux of duodenal secretions under high pressure into the pancreatic ducts. The condition has been recreated experimentally in dogs (Pfeffer loop preparation).

H. Drug-Induced Pancreatitis: Drugs are probably responsible for more cases of acute pancreatitis than is generally suspected. The most commonly incriminated drugs are corticosteroids, estrogen-containing contraceptives, azathioprine, thiazide diuretics, and tetracyclines. Pancreatitis associated with use of estrogens is usually the result of drug-induced hypertriglyceridemia. The mechanisms involved in the case of other drugs are unknown.

I. Obstructive Pancreatitis: Chronic partial

obstruction of the pancreatic duct may be congenital or may follow healing after injury or inflammation. Over time, the parenchyma drained by the obstructed duct is replaced by fibrous tissue, and chronic pancreatitis develops. Sometimes there are episodes of acute pancreatitis as well.

Pancreas divisum may predispose to a kind of obstructive pancreatitis. If this anomaly is present and further narrowing of the opening of the minor papilla occurs (eg, by an inflammatory process), the orifice may be inadequate to handle the flow of pancreatic juice. The diagnosis of pancreas divisum may be made by ERCP. If a patient with the anomaly is found to have documented episodes of acute pancreatitis and no other cause is found, it is reasonable to assume that the anomaly is the cause.

Surgical sphincteroplasty of the minor papilla or the insertion of a stent has been proposed as treatment, but results have been suboptimal. This may be due to the presence of irreversible parenchymal changes and the persistence of chronic inflammation. In patients with obvious changes of chronic pancreatitis, surgical treatment should consist of pancreatic resection or drainage (see p 573).

J. Idiopathic Pancreatitis and Miscellaneous Causes: In about 15% of patients, representing the third largest group after biliary and alcoholic pancreatitis, there is no identifiable cause of the condition. If investigated in greater than usual detail (eg, duodenal drainage examination for cholesterol crystals), many of these patients will be found to have gallstones or biliary sludge undetectable by ultrasound scans.

Viral infections and scorpion stings may cause pancreatitis.

Pathogenesis

The concept that pancreatitis is due to enzymatic digestion of the gland is supported by the finding of proteolytic enzymes in ascitic fluid and increased amounts of phospholipase A and lysolecithins in pancreatic tissue from patients with acute pancreatitis. Experimentally, pancreatitis can be created readily if activated enzymes are injected into the pancreatic ducts under pressure. Trypsin has not been found in excessive amounts in pancreatic tissue from affected humans, possibly because of inactivation by trypsin inhibitors. Nevertheless, although the available evidence is inconclusive, the autodigestion theory is almost universally accepted. Other proposed factors are vascular insufficiency, lymphatic congestion, and activation of the kallikrein-kinin system.

For many years, trypsin and other proteases were held to be the principal injurious agents, but recent evidence has emphasized phospholipase A, lipase, and elastase as perhaps of greater importance. Trypsin ordinarily does not attack living cells, and even when trypsin is forced into the interstitial spaces, the resulting pancreatitis does not include coagulation necrosis, which is so prominent in human pancreatitis.

Phospholipase A, in the presence of small amounts of bile salts, attacks free phopholipids (eg, lecithin) and those bound in cellular membranes to produce extremely potent lyso- compounds. Lysolecithin, which would result from the action of phospholipase A on biliary lecithin, or phospholipase A itself, plus bile salts, is capable of producing severe necrotizing pancreatitis. Trypsin is important in this scheme, because small amounts are needed to activate phospholipase A from its inactive precursor.

Elastase, which is both elastolytic and proteolytic, is secreted in an inactive form. Because it can digest the walls of blood vessels, elastase has been thought to be important in the pathogenesis of hemorrhagic pancreatitis.

If autodigestion is the final common pathway in pancreatitis, earlier steps must account for the presence of active enzymes and their reaction products in the ducts and their escape into the interstitium. The following are the most popular theories that attempt to link the known etiologic factors with autodigestion:

A. Obstruction-Secretion: In animals, ligation of the pancreatic duct generally produces mild edema of the pancreas that resolves within a week. Thereafter, atrophy of the secretory apparatus occurs. On the other hand, partial or intermittent ductal obstruction, which more closely mimics what seems to happen in humans, can produce frank pancreatitis if the gland is simultaneously stimulated to secrete. The major shortcoming of these experiments has been the difficulty encountered in attempting to cause severe pancreatitis in this way. However, since the human pancreas manufactures ten times as much phospholipase A as does the dog or rat pancreas, the consequences of obstruction in humans conceivably could be more serious.

B. Common Channel Theory: Opie, having observed pancreatitis in a patient with a gallstone impacted in the ampulla of Vater, speculated that reflux of bile into the pancreatic ducts might have initiated the process. Flow between the biliary and pancreatic ducts requires a common channel connecting these two systems with the duodenum. Although these ducts converge in 90% of humans, only 10% have a common channel long enough to permit biliary-pancreatic reflux if the ampulla contained a gallstone. Experimentally, pancreatitis produced by pancreatic duct obstruction alone is similar in severity to pancreatitis following obstruction of a common channel, so biliary reflux is discounted as an etiologic factor in this disease.

C. Duodenal Reflux: The above theories do not explain activation of pancreatic enzymes, a process that normally takes place through the action of enterokinase in the duodenum. In experimental animals, if the segment of duodenum into which the pancreatic duct empties is surgically converted to a closed loop, reflux of duodenal juice initiates severe pancreatitis (Pfeffer loop). Pancreatitis associated with acute afferent loop obstruction after Billroth II gastrectomy is probably the result of similar factors. Other than in this specific example, there is no direct evidence for duodenal reflux in the pathogenesis of pancreatitis in humans.

D. Back Diffusion Across the Pancreatic Duct: Just as the gastric mucosa must serve as a barrier to maintain high concentrations of acid, so must the epithelium of the pancreatic duct prevent diffusion of luminal enzymes into the pancreatic parenchyma. Experiments in cats have shown that the barrier function of the pancreatic duct is vulnerable to several injurious agents, including alcohol and bile acids. Furthermore, the effects of alcohol can occur even after oral ingestion, because alcohol is secreted in the pancreatic juice. Injury to the barrier renders the duct permeable to molecules as large as MW 20,000, and enzymes from the lumen may be able to enter the gland and produce pancreatitis.

The studies by Steer and his coworkers have shown that a very early event in several forms of experimental pancreatitis, including that due to pancreatic duct obstruction, consists of zymogen activation within acinar cells by lysosomal hydrolases (eg, cathepsin B). This may represent the long-sought unifying explanation. Other factors must be postulated, however, to account for the variations in severity of the disease. In biliary pancreatitis, transient obstruction of the ampulla of Vater by a gallstone is most likely the first event. Alcoholic pancreatitis probably has several causes, including partial ductal obstruction, secretory stimulation, acute effects on the ductal barrier, and toxic actions of alcohol on parenchymal cells.

E. Systemic Manifestations: Severe acute pancreatitis may be complicated by multiple organ failure, principally respiratory insufficiency (adult respiratory distress syndrome [ARDS]), myocardial depression, renal insufficiency, and gastric stress ulceration. The pathogenesis of these complications is similar in many respects to that of multiple organ failure in sepsis, and in fact, sepsis due to pancreatic abscess formation is a contributing factor in some of the most severe cases of acute pancreatitis. During acute pancreatitis, pancreatic proteases, bacterial endotoxins, and other active agents are liberated into the systemic circulation. The concentrations of serum factors able to complex with the proteases (eg, α_2-macroglobulin) decrease in proportion to the severity of the illness, and complexed α_2-macroglobulin, which normally is cleared rapidly by macrophages, accumulates. These circulating complexes, which retain proteolytic activity, are thought to contribute to systemic toxicity. The endotoxin probably originates from bacteria that translocate through an abnormally permeable intestinal mucosa. Within the

circulation, the proteases and the endotoxin activate the complement system (especially C5) and kinins. Complement activation leads to granulocyte aggregation and accumulation of aggregates in the pulmonary capillaries. The granulocytes release neutrophil elastase, superoxide anion, hydrogen peroxide, and hydroxide radicals, which in concert with bradykinin exert local toxic effects on the pulmonary epithelium that result in increased permeability. Arachidonate metabolites (eg, PGE_2, PGI_2, leukotriene B_4) may also be involved in some way. Analogous events are thought to occur in other organs.

Dubick M et al: Digestive enzymes and protease inhibitors in plasma from patients with acute pancreatitis. Pancreas 1987;2:187.

Fernandez-del Castillo C: Risk factors for pancreatic cellular injury after cardiopulmonary bypass. N Engl J Med 1991;325:382

Guice KS et al: Pancreatitis-induced acute lung injury: An ARDS model. Ann Surg 1988;208:71.

Harvey MH, Cates MC, Reber HA: Possible mechanisms of acute pancreatitis induced by ethanol. Am J Surg 1988;155:49.

Lankisch PG, Ihse I: Bile-induced acute experimental pancreatitis. Scand J Gastroenterol 1987;22:257.

Larvin M et al: Impaired mononuclear phagocyte function in patients with severe acute pancreatitis: Evidence from studies of plasma clearance of trypsin and monocyte phagocytosis. Digest Dis Sci 1993;38:18

Lee SP, Nicholls JF, Park HZ: Biliary sludge as a cause of acute pancreatitis. N Engl J Med 1992;326:589

Lerch MM et al: Pancreatic duct obstruction triggers acute necrotizing pancreatitis in the opossum. Gastroenterology 1993;104:853.

Medich DS et al: Pathogenesis of pancreatic sepsis. Am J Surg 1993;165:46.

Miller AR, Nagorney DM, Sarr MG: The surgical spectrum of hereditary pancreatitis in adults. Ann Surg 1992; 215:39.

Nordback IH et al: The role of acetaldehyde in the pathogenesis of acute alcoholic pancreatitis. Ann Surg 1991;214:671.

Ros E et al: Occult microlithiasis in "idiopathic" acute pancreatitis: Prevention of relapses by cholecystectomy or ursodeoxycholic acid therapy. Gastroenterology 1991; 101:1701.

Sarr MG, Bulkley GB, Cameron JL: The role of leukocytes in the production of oxygen-derived free radicals in acute experimental pancreatitis. Surgery 1987;101:292.

Searles GE, Ooi TC: Underrecognition of chylomicronemia as a cause of acute pancreatitis. Can Med Assoc J 1992;147:1806.

Steer ML: How and where does acute pancreatitis begin? Arch Surg 1992;127:1350.

Terry TR, Grant DAW, Hermon-Taylor J: Intraductal enterokinase is lethal in rats with experimental bile-salt pancreatitis. Br J Surg 1987;74:40.

Wedgwood KR, et al: Effects of oral agents on pancreatic duct permeability. Dig Dis Sci. 1986;31:1081.

1. ACUTE PANCREATITIS

Essentials of Diagnosis
- Abrupt onset of epigastric pain, frequently with back pain.
- Nausea and vomiting.
- Elevated serum or urinary amylase.
- Cholelithiasis or alcoholism (many patients).

General Considerations

While edematous and hemorrhagic pancreatitis are manifestations of the same pathologic processes and the general principles of treatment are the same, hemorrhagic pancreatitis has more complications and a higher death rate. In edematous pancreatitis, the glandular tissue and surrounding retroperitoneal structures are engorged with interstitial fluid, and the pancreas is infiltrated with inflammatory cells that surround small foci of parenchymal necrosis. Hemorrhagic pancreatitis is characterized by bleeding into the parenchyma and surrounding retroperitoneal structures and extensive pancreatic necrosis. In both forms, the peritoneal surfaces may be studded with small calcifications representing areas of fat necrosis.

Clinical Findings

A. Symptoms and Signs: The acute attack frequently begins following a large meal and consists of severe epigastric pain that radiates through to the back. The pain is unrelenting and usually associated with vomiting and retching. In severe cases, the patient may collapse from shock.

Depending on the severity of the disease, there may be profound dehydration, tachycardia, and postural hypotension. Myocardial function is depressed in severe pancreatitis, presumably because of circulating factors that affect cardiac performance. Examination of the abdomen reveals decreased or absent bowel sounds and tenderness that may be generalized but more often is localized to the epigastrium. Temperature is usually normal or slightly elevated in uncomplicated pancreatitis. Clinical evidence of pleural effusion may be present, especially on the left. If an abdominal mass is found, it probably represents a swollen pancreas (phlegmon) or, later in the illness, a pseudocyst or abscess. In 1–2% of patients, bluish discoloration is present in the flank **(Grey Turner's sign)** or periumbilical area **(Cullen's sign),** indicating hemorrhagic pancreatitis with dissection of blood retroperitoneally into these areas.

B. Laboratory Findings: The hematocrit may be elevated as a consequence of dehydration or low as a result of abdominal blood loss in hemorrhagic pancreatitis. There is usually a moderate leukocytosis, but total white blood cell counts over 12,000/µL are unusual in the absence of suppurative complications. Liver function studies are usually normal, but there may be a mild elevation of the serum bilirubin concentration (usually < 2 mg/dL).

The serum amylase concentration rises to more than 2½ times normal within 6 hours after the onset of an acute episode and generally remains elevated for several days. Values in excess of 1000 IU/dL occur early in the attack in 95% of patients with biliary pancreatitis and 85% of patients with acute alcoholic pancreatitis. Those with the most severe disease are more apt to have amylase levels below 1000 IU/dL.

Elevated serum lipase is detectable early and for several days after the acute attack. Since the lipase level tends to be higher in alcoholic pancreatitis and the amylase level higher in gallstone pancreatitis, the lipase/amylase ratio has been suggested as a means to help distinguishing the two.

Elevated amylase levels may occur in other acute abdominal conditions, such as gangrenous cholecystitis, small bowel obstruction, mesenteric infarction, and perforated ulcer, though levels rarely exceed 500 IU/dL. Episodes of acute pancreatitis may occur without rises in serum amylase; this is the rule if hyperlipidemia is present. Furthermore, high levels may return to normal before blood is drawn.

The methods most commonly used for measuring amylase in the serum detect pancreatic amylase, salivary amylase, and macroamylase. However, hyperamylasemia is sometimes present in patients with abdominal pain when the elevated amylase levels consist entirely of salivary amylase or macroamylase and the pancreas is not inflamed.

Urine amylase excretion is also increased and is of diagnostic value. Excretion of more than 5000 IU/24 h is abnormal. The urinary clearance of amylase increases during acute pancreatitis owing to a decrease in tubular reabsorption of amylase (normally 75% of filtered amylase). This was once thought to be specific, and the amylase-to-creatinine clearance ratio was used as a diagnostic test for acute pancreatitis. However, the increased amylase clearance results from overload of the tubular reabsorptive pathway with various urine proteins and is a nonspecific effect of tissue damage seen in many acute illnesses or following trauma.

In severe pancreatitis, the serum calcium concentration may fall as a result of calcium being complexed with fatty acids (liberated from retroperitoneal fat by lipase) and impaired reabsorption from bone owing to the action of calcitonin (liberated by high levels of glucagon). Relative hypoparathyroidism and hypoalbuminemia have also been implicated.

C. Imaging Studies: In about two-thirds of cases, a plain abdominal film is abnormal. The most frequent finding is isolated dilatation of a segment of gut **(sentinel loop)** consisting of jejunum, transverse colon, or duodenum adjacent to the pancreas. Gas distending the right colon that abruptly stops in the mid or left transverse colon **(colon cutoff sign)** is due to colonic spasm adjacent to the pancreatic inflammation. Both of these findings are relatively nonspecific. Glandular calcification may be evident, signifying chronic pancreatitis. An upper gastrointestinal series may show a widened duodenal loop, swollen ampulla of Vater, and, occasionally, evidence of gastric irritability. Chest films may reveal pleural effusion on the left side.

A CT scan of the pancreas using intravenous contrast media should be obtained in any patient with acute pancreatitis whose illness is not resolving after 48–72 hours. The radiologic findings may be consistent with any of the following: relatively normal appearing pancreas, pancreatic **phlegmon,** pancreatic phlegmon with extension of the inflammatory process to adjacent extrapancreatic spaces, pancreatic **necrosis**, or pancreatic pseudocyst or **abscess** formation.

Occasionally, radiopaque gallstones will be apparent on plain x-rays. Ultrasound study may demonstrate gallstones early in the attack and may be used as a baseline for sequential examinations of the pancreas.

Several weeks after the pancreatitis has subsided, ERCP may be of value in patients with a tentative diagnosis of idiopathic pancreatitis (ie, those who have no history of alcoholism and no evidence of gallstones on ultrasound and oral cholecystogram). This examination demonstrates gallstones or changes of chronic pancreatitis in about 40% of such patients.

Differential Diagnosis

To some extent, acute pancreatitis is a diagnosis of exclusion, for other acute upper abdominal conditions such as acute cholecystitis, penetrating or perforated duodenal ulcer, high small bowel obstruction, acute appendicitis, and mesenteric infarction must always be seriously considered. In most cases, the distinction is possible on the basis of the clinical picture, laboratory findings, and CT scans. The critical point is that the diseases with which acute pancreatitis is most likely to be confused are often lethal if not treated surgically. Therefore, diagnostic laparotomy is indicated if they cannot be ruled out on clinical grounds.

Chronic hyperamylasemia occurs rarely without any relation to pancreatic disease. Some cases are associated with renal failure, chronic sialadenitis, salivary tumors, ovarian tumors, or liver disease, but often there is no explanation. Analysis of serum amylase isoenzymes is the only way to determine whether the amylase originates from salivary glands or pancreas. **Macroamylasemia** is a chronic hyperamylasemia in which normal amylase (usually salivary) is bound to a large serum glycoprotein or immunoglobulin molecule and is therefore not excreted into urine. The diagnosis rests on the combination of hyperamylasemia and low urinary amylase. Macroamylasemia has been found in patients with other diseases such as malabsorption, alcoholism, and cancer. Many patients have abdominal pain, but the relationship of the pain and the macroamylasemia is uncertain.

Complications

The principal complications of acute pancreatitis are abscess and pseudocyst formation. These are discussed in separate sections. Gastrointestinal bleeding may occur from adjacent inflamed stomach or duodenum, ruptured pseudocyst, or peptic ulcer. Intraperitoneal bleeding may occur spontaneously from the celiac or splenic artery or from the spleen following acute splenic vein thrombosis. Involvement of the transverse colon or duodenum by the inflammatory process may result in partial obstruction, hemorrhage, necrosis, or fistula formation.

Early identification of patients at greatest risk of complications allows them to be managed more aggressively, which appears to decrease the mortality rate. The criteria of severity that have been found to be reliable are based either on the systemic manifestations of the disease as reflected in the clinical and laboratory findings or on the local changes in the pancreas as reflected by the findings on CT scan. Ranson used the former approach to develop the staging criteria listed in Table 27–1. Just the single finding of fluid sequestration (ie, fluid administered minus urine output) exceeding 2 L/d for more than 2 days is a reasonably accurate dividing line between severe (life-threatening) and mild-to-moderate disease. The local changes in the pancreas as shown on CT scans may be even more revealing. The presence of any of the following indicates a high risk of local infection in the pancreatic bed: involvement of extrapancreatic spaces in the inflammatory process, pancreatic necrosis (areas in the pancreas that do not enhance with intravenous contrast media), and early signs of abscess formation (eg, gas bubbles in the tissue).

Treatment

A. Medical Treatment: The goals of medical

Table 27–1. Ranson's criteria of severity of acute pancreatitis.[1]

Criteria present initially
Age >55 years
White blood cell count >16,000/μL
Blood glucose >200 mg/dL
Serum LDH >350 IU/L
AST (SGOT) >250 IU/dL

Criteria developing during first 24 hours
Hematocrit fall >10%
BUN rise >8 mg/dL
Serum Ca^{2+} <8 mg/dL
Arterial Po_2 <60 mm Hg
Base deficit >4 meq/L
Estimated fluid sequestration >600 mL

[1]Morbidity and mortality rates correlate with the number of criteria present. Mortality rates correlate as follows: 0–2 criteria present = 2%; 3 or 4 = 15%; 5 or 6 = 40%; 7 or 8 = 100%.

therapy are reduction of pancreatic secretory stimuli and correction of fluid and electrolyte derangements.

1. Gastric suction–Oral intake is withheld, and a nasogastric tube is inserted to aspirate gastric secretions, although the latter has no specific therapeutic effect. Oral feeding should be resumed only after the patient appears much improved, appetite has returned, and serum amylase levels have dropped to normal. Premature resumption of eating may result in exacerbation of disease.

2. Fluid replacement–Patients with acute pancreatitis sequester fluid in the retroperitoneum, and large volumes of intravenous fluids are necessary to maintain circulating blood volume and renal function. Patients with severe pancreatitis should receive albumin to combat the capillary leak that contributes to the pathophysiology. In severe hemorrhagic pancreatitis, blood transfusions may also be required. The adequacy of fluid replacement is the single most important aspect of medical therapy. In fact, undertreatment with fluids may actually contribute to the progression of pancreatitis. Fluid replacement may be judged most accurately by monitoring the volume and specific gravity of urine.

3. Antibiotics–Antibiotics are not useful in the average case of acute pancreatitis and should be reserved for treatment of specific suppurative complications. Prophylactic broad-spectrum antibiotics are often used in patients with severe pancreatitis, since the likelihood of infection is high in this group.

4. Calcium and magnesium–In severe attacks of acute pancreatitis, hypocalcemia may require parenteral calcium replacement in amounts determined by serial calcium measurements. Recognition of hypocalcemia is important because it may produce cardiac dysrhythmias. Hypomagnesemia is also common, especially in alcoholics, and magnesium should also be replaced as indicated by serum levels.

5. Oxygen–Hypoxemia severe enough to require therapy develops in about 30% of patients with acute pancreatitis. It is often insidious, without clinical or x-ray signs, and out of proportion to the severity of the pancreatitis. The most pronounced examples accompany severe pancreatitis, often in association with hypocalcemia. The basic lesion, a form of adult respiratory distress syndrome, is poorly understood. The pathogenesis is discussed on p 563. Pulmonary changes include decreased vital capacity and an oxygen diffusion defect.

Hypoxemia must be suspected in every patient, and arterial blood gases should be measured every 12 hours for the first few hospital days. Supplemental oxygen therapy is indicated for Pao_2 levels below 70 mm Hg. An occasional patient requires endotracheal intubation and mechanical ventilation. Diuretics may be useful in decreasing lung water and improving arterial oxygen saturation.

6. Peritoneal lavage–Peritoneal lavage has been employed in severe refractory cases to remove toxins in the peritoneal fluid that would otherwise have been absorbed into the systemic circulation. Some patients appear to improve in response to this therapy although controlled trials have not substantiated its efficacy. Severe pancreatitis that fails to show clinical improvement after 24–48 hours of standard inpatient treatment is the usual indication for peritoneal lavage. The technique involves infusing and withdrawing 1–2 L of lactated Ringer's solution through a peritoneal dialysis catheter every hour for 1–3 days. If a response occurs, it is usually seen within 8 hours. If the patient improves following lavage, laparotomy can be avoided. If improvement does not occur, laparotomy is often required.

7. Nutrition–Total parenteral nutrition avoids pancreatic stimulation and should be used for nutritional support in any severely ill patient who will be unable to eat for more than 1 week. Elemental diets ingested orally or given by tube into the small intestine do not avoid secretory stimulation. Neither form of nutrition directly affects recovery of the pancreas.

8. Other drugs–Octreotide, H_2 receptor blockers, anticholinergic drugs, glucagon, and aprotinin have shown no beneficial effects in controlled trials.

B. Endoscopic Sphincterotomy: Biliary pancreatitis is caused by a gallstone becoming lodged in the ampulla of Vater. In most cases, the stone passes into the intestine but occasionally it becomes impacted in the ampulla, which results in more severe disease. Less than 10% of cases of biliary pancreatitis are severe (ie, three or more three Ranson criteria), but in severe cases, endoscopic sphincterotomy performed within 72 hours of the onset of the disease has been shown to decrease the incidence of concomitant biliary sepsis and lower the mortality rate from the pancreatitis.

C. Surgical Treatment: Surgery is generally contraindicated in uncomplicated acute pancreatitis. However, when the diagnosis is uncertain in a patient with severe abdominal pain, diagnostic laparotomy is not thought to aggravate pancreatitis.

When laparotomy has been performed for diagnosis and mild to moderate pancreatitis is found, cholecystectomy and operative cholangiography should be performed if gallstones are present, but the pancreas should be left undisturbed. For *severe* edematous pancreatitis, the gastrocolic omentum should be divided and the pancreas inspected. Although some surgeons place drains and irrigating catheters in the region of the pancreas, we prefer to keep foreign bodies out of this area.

The diagnosis of biliary pancreatitis can usually be suspected on the basis of ultrasound studies of the gallbladder early in the acute attack. Cholecystectomy should be performed on these patients during hospitalization for the acute attack soon after the attack resolves. A longer delay (even a few weeks) is associated with a high incidence (80%) of recurrent pancreatitis. Since life-threatening attacks are uncommon in gallstone pancreatitis, operation (common duct exploration; sphincteroplasty) or endoscopic therapy (sphincterotomy) early in an attack is rarely justified. However, when the attack is especially severe, elective cholecystectomy should be deferred up to several months to allow complete recovery from pancreatitis.

It is currently thought that debridement of dead peripancreatic tissue, which is often (40% of cases) colonized by bacteria, lowers the mortality rate of acute severe necrotizing pancreatitis. Historical controls place the mortality rate at 50–80% in the absence of operative treatment and 10–40% among patients subjected to necrosectomy. The diagnosis of necrotizing pancreatitis is suspected from the clinical findings; patients treated surgically have three or more Ranson criteria and average about 4½ criteria. Contrast-enhanced CT scans obtained early in the course of the disease are studied for the presence of nonenhancing areas, which indicate lack of vascular perfusion and reflect the presence of necrotic peripancreatic fat or pancreatic parenchyma. Percutaneous needle aspiration of these areas is used to detect the presence of bacterial colonization. A distinction is made between these cases of "infected necrotizing pancreatitis" and "pancreatic abscess," which may appear later in the course of the disease. Patients with infected necrotizing pancreatitis and severe clinical findings benefit most from surgical therapy, but laparotomy may be undertaken just because of a deteriorating condition in patients with necrotizing pancreatitis in the absence of bacterial colonization. At surgery, all peripancreatic spaces are opened and any necrotic tissue is removed by gentle blunt dissection. A T-tube is inserted if there is bile duct obstruction, and cholecystectomy is performed for gallstone disease. Two large drains are placed within the debrided spaces and are used postoperatively for sterile lavage. About 8 L of fluid are infused through this system daily for an average of 2 weeks. Other than CT evidence of necrotic tissue with or without infection, there are presently no other criteria in general use that call for pancreatic surgery in patients with severe pancreatitis.

Surgery for complications of acute pancreatitis, such as abscess, pseudocyst, and pancreatic ascites, is discussed below.

Prognosis

The death rate associated with acute pancreatitis is about 10%, and nearly all deaths occur in a first attack and among patients with three or more Ranson criteria of severity. Respiratory insufficiency and hypocalcemia indicate a poor prognosis. The death rate associated with severe necrotizing pancreatitis is 50% or more, but surgical therapy lowers the figure to about 20%. Persistent fever or hyperamylasemia 3 weeks or longer after an attack of pancreatitis usually indicates the presence of a pancreatic abscess or pseudocyst.

General

Aldridge MC et al: Colonic complications of severe acute pancreatitis. Br J Surg 1988;76:362.

Aldridge MC: Diagnosis of pancreatic necrosis. Br J Surg 1988;75:99.

Beger HG: Surgical management of necrotizing pancreatitis. Surg Clin North Am 1989;69:529.

Bouillot JL, Alexandre JH, Vuong NP: Colonic involvement in acute necrotizing pancreatitis: Results of surgical treatment. World J Surg 1989;13:84.

Bradley EL 3d, Allen K: A prospective longitudinal study of observation versus surgical intervention in the management of necrotizing pancreatitis. Am J Surg 1991;161:19.

Clavien PA et al: Value of contrast-enhanced computerized tomography in the early diagnosis and prognosis of acute pancreatitis: A prospective study of 202 patients. Am J Surg 1988;155:457.

Dominguez-Munoz JE et al: Clinical usefulness of polymorphonuclear elastase in predicting the severity of acute pancreatitis: results of a multicentre study. Br J Surg 1991;78:1230.

Fan ST et al: Pancreatic phlegmon: What is it? Am J Surg 1989;157:544.

Gjorup I et al: A double-blinded multicenter trial of somatostatin in the treatment of acute pancreatitis. Surg Gynecol Obstet 1992;175:397.

Gumaste VV et al: Lipase/amylase ratio: A new index that distinguishes acute episodes of alcoholic from nonalcoholic acute pancreatitis. Gastroenterology 1991;101:1361.

Howard JM, Wagner SM: Pancreatography after recovery from massive pancreatic necrosis. Ann Surg 1989;209:31.

Howard JM: Delayed debridement and external drainage of massive pancreatic or peripancreatic necrosis. Surg Gynecol Obstet 1989;168:25.

Larvin M, McMahon M: Apache-II score for assessment and monitoring of acute pancreatitis. Lancet 1989;2:201.

Lesse T, Shaw D: Comparison of three Glasgow multifactor prognostic scoring systems in acute pancreatitis. Br J Surg 1988;75:460.

London NJM et al: Contrast-enhanced abdominal computed tomography scanning and prediction of severity of acute pancreatitis: A prospective study. Br J Surg 1989;76:258.

Mayer AD et al: Controlled clinical trial of peritoneal lavage for the treatment of severe acute pancreatitis. N Engl J Med 1985;312:399.

Neoptolemos JP, London NJ, Carr-Locke DL: Assessment of main pancreatic duct integrity by endoscopic retrograde pancreatography in patients with acute pancreatitis. Br J Surg 1993;80:94.

Pisters PW, Ranson JH: Nutritional support for acute pancreatitis. Surg Gynecol Obstet 1992;175:275.

Rutledge PL, Warshaw AL: Persistent acute pancreatitis: A variant treated by pancreatoduodenectomy. Arch Surg 1988;123:597.

Sarr MG et al: Acute necrotizing pancreatitis: management by planned, staged pancreatic necrosectomy/debridement and delayed primary wound closure over drains. Br J Surg 1991;78:576.

Teerenhovi O, Nordback I, Isolauri J: Influence of pancreatic resection on systemic complications in acute necrotizing pancreatitis. Br J Surg 1988;75:793.

Thompson JS et al: Postoperative pancreatitis. Surg Gynecol Obstet 1988;167:377.

Wilson C, Imrie CW, Carter DC: Fatal acute pancreatitis. Gut 1988;29:782.

Winslet M et al: Relation of diagnostic serum amylase levels to aetiology and severity of acute pancreatitis. Gut 1992;33:982.

Gallstone Pancreatitis

Fan ST et al: Early treatment of acute biliary pancreatitis by endoscopic papillotomy. N Engl J Med 1993;328:228.

Kelly TR, Wagner DS: Gallstone pancreatitis; A prospective randomized trial of the timing of surgery. Surgery 1988;104:600.

Kelly TR: Gallstone pancreatitis: Local predisposing factors. Ann Surg 1984;200:479.

Moreau JA et al: Gallstone pancreatitis and the effect of cholecystectomy: A population-based cohort study. Mayo Clin Proc 1988;63:466.

Neoptolemos JP et al: Controlled trial of urgent endoscopic retrograde cholangiopancreatography and endoscopic sphincterotomy versus conservative treatment for acute pancreatitis due to gallstones. Lancet 1988;2:979.

Neoptolemos JP et al: ERCP findings and the role of endoscopic sphincterotomy in acute gallstone pancreatitis. Br J Surg 1988;75:954.

Ros E et al: Occult microlithiasis in "idiopathic" acute pancreatitis: Prevention of relapses by cholecystectomy or ursodeoxycholic acid therapy. Gastroenterology 1991;101:1701.

Scholmerich J et al: Detection of biliary origin of acute pancreatitis. Dig Dis Sci 1989;34:830.

Williamson RC: Endoscopic sphincterotomy in the early treatment of acute pancreatitis. N Engl J Med 1993;328:279.

2. PANCREATIC PSEUDOCYST

Essentials of Diagnosis

- Epigastric mass and pain.
- Mild fever and leukocytosis.
- Persistent serum amylase elevation.
- Pancreatic cyst demonstrated by ultrasound or CT scan.

General Considerations

Pancreatic pseudocysts are encapsulated collections of fluid with high enzyme concentrations that arise from the pancreas. They are usually located either within or adjacent to the pancreas in the lesser sac, but pancreatic pseudocysts have also been found in the neck, mediastinum, and pelvis. The walls of a pseudocyst are formed by inflammatory fibrosis of the peritoneal, mesenteric, and serosal membranes, which limits spread of the pancreatic juice as the lesion develops. The term pseudocyst denotes absence of an epithelial lining, whereas true cysts are lined by epithelium.

Two different processes are involved in the pathogenesis of pancreatic pseudocysts. Many occur as complications of severe acute pancreatitis, where extravasation of pancreatic juice and glandular necrosis form a sterile pocket of fluid that is not reabsorbed as inflammation subsides. Superinfection of such collections leads to pancreatic abscess instead of pseudocyst. In other patients, usually alcoholics or trauma victims, pseudocysts appear without preceding acute pancreatitis. The mechanism in these cases consists of ductal obstruction and formation of a retention cyst that loses its epithelial lining as it grows beyond the confines of the gland. In posttraumatic pseudocyst, symptoms usually do not appear until several weeks after the injury. Some are iatrogenic, eg, occurring during splenectomy; others follow an external blow to the abdomen.

Pseudocysts develop in about 2% of cases of acute pancreatitis. The cysts are single in 85% of cases and multiple in the remainder.

Clinical Findings

A. Symptoms and Signs: A pseudocyst should be suspected when a patient with acute pancreatitis fails to recover after a week of treatment or when, after improving for a time, symptoms return. Since it is now fairly routine to obtain a CT scan early in an attack of severe acute pancreatitis, the early stages of pseudocyst formation are often demonstrated radiographically before specific clinical findings appear. The first clinical manifestation is usually a palpable tender mass in the epigastrium, consisting of a swollen pancreas and contiguous viscera (a phlegmon). With time, the mass may subside, but if it persists it most likely represents a pseudocyst.

In other cases, the pseudocyst develops insidiously without an obvious attack of acute pancreatitis.

Regardless of the type of prodromal phase, pain is the most common finding. Fever, weight loss, tenderness, and a palpable mass are present in about half of patients. A few have jaundice, a manifestation of obstruction of the intrapancreatic segment of the bile duct.

B. Laboratory Findings: An elevated serum amylase and leukocytosis are present in about half of patients. When present, elevated bilirubin levels reflect biliary obstruction. Of those patients with acute pancreatitis whose serum amylase remains elevated for as long as 3 weeks, about half will have a pseudocyst.

C. Imaging Studies: CT scan (Figure 27–3) is the diagnostic study of choice. The size and shape of the cyst and its relationship to other viscera can be seen. Acute pseudocysts are often irregular in shape; chronic pseudocysts are most often circular or nearly

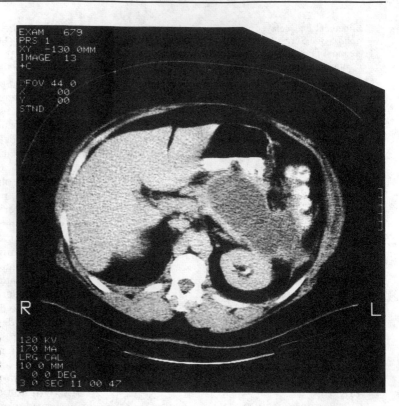

Figure 27–3. CT scan of a large unilocular pseudocyst impinging on the posterior wall of the stomach (which contains contrast media). A cyst in this location is usually best drained into the stomach.

so. An enlarged pancreatic duct may be demonstrated in patients with chronic pancreatitis. A dilated common bile duct would suggest biliary obstruction, either from the cyst or from underlying chronic pancreatitis.

The gallbladder should be studied by ultrasound to look for gallstones, especially in patients with acute pancreatitis. Although ultrasound can also demonstrate pseudocysts, the amount of important detail obtained is less than that from CT scans, and consequently the role of ultrasound is mainly to follow changes in size of an acute pseudocyst already imaged by CT scans, so the amount of x-ray exposure can be kept to a minimum.

ERCP should be performed if there are thought to be significant abnormalities of the bile or pancreatic duct as suggested by CT scans or the results of liver function tests. Either duct may be dilated and in need of surgical drainage in conjunction with drainage of the pseudocyst. ERCP usually opacifies the pseudocyst as well, but the information is not usually of major value in planning treatment, so ERCP is not obtained routinely.

An upper gastrointestinal series will often reveal a mass in the lesser sac that distorts the stomach or duodenum, but this is not particularly useful information. The principal indication for an upper gastrointestinal series is to search for a site of gastric or duodenal obstruction in patients who are vomiting.

With wide use of sensitive imaging studies in the diagnosis of pancreatic disease, small asymptomatic pseudocysts are often demonstrated. The natural history of these subclinical lesions is benign, and there is no indication for prophylactic surgical treatment.

Differential Diagnosis

Pancreatic pseudocysts must be distinguished from pancreatic abscess and acute pancreatic phlegmon. Patients with an abscess exhibit signs of infection.

Rarely, patients with pseudocyst present with weight loss, jaundice, and a nontender palpable gallbladder and are first thought to have pancreatic carcinoma. CT scans show that the lesion is fluid-filled, which suggests the correct diagnosis.

Neoplastic cysts—either cystadenoma or cystadenocarcinoma—account for about 5% of all cases of cystic pancreatic masses and may be indistinguishable preoperatively from pseudocyst. The correct diagnosis can be made from the gross appearance supplemented by a biopsy obtained at operation.

Complications

A. Infection: Infection is a rare complication resulting in high fever, chills, and leukocytosis. Drainage is required as soon as the diagnosis is suspected. Some lesions can be drained externally via a catheter placed percutaneously using ultrasound guidance. Internal drainage of infected pseudocysts adherent to the stomach can be achieved surgically by cystogastrostomy; otherwise, drainage should be external, because the suture line of a Roux-en-Y cystojejunostomy may not heal.

B. Rupture: Sudden perforation into the free peritoneal cavity produces severe chemical peritonitis, with board-like abdominal rigidity and severe pain. Rapid enlargement of the pseudocyst is sometimes noted before it ruptures. The treatment is emergency surgery with irrigation of the peritoneal cavity and a drainage procedure for the pseudocyst. The wall of a ruptured pseudocyst is usually too flimsy to hold sutures securely, so most ruptured cysts must be drained externally. Rupture of a pseudocyst occurs in less than 5% of cases, but even with prompt treatment it may be fatal.

C. Hemorrhage: Bleeding may occur into the cyst cavity or an adjacent viscus into which the cyst has eroded. Intracystic bleeding may present as an enlarging abdominal mass with anemia resulting from blood loss. If the cyst has eroded into the stomach, there may be hematemesis, melena, and blood in the nasogastric aspirate. The rapidity of the blood loss often produces hemorrhagic shock, which may preclude arteriography. If time permits, however, emergency arteriography should be performed to delineate the site of bleeding, which is usually a false aneurysm of an artery in the cyst wall, and to embolize it if possible. If embolization successfully occludes the bleeding vessel, several weeks should elapse to ensure that bleeding will not recur, and at that point the pseudocyst should be drained surgically in the same fashion as a nonbleeding pseudocyst. If the bleeding cannot be stopped by embolization, emergency surgery should be performed. Usually all that can be done is to open the cyst and suture ligate the bleeding vessel in the cyst wall, followed by external or internal drainage of the cyst. Sometimes it is possible to excise the cyst, which is desirable because doing so more certainly avoids the risk of recurrent hemorrhage.

Treatment

The principal indications for treating pancreatic pseudocysts are to improve symptoms and to prevent complications. Recent data indicate that the natural history of these lesions is more benign than previously thought—that in the absence of symptoms or radiographic evidence of enlargement (and irrespective of cyst size), expectant management is not unreasonable, and that a few untreated cysts resolve spontaneously even after being stable for months. Expectant management is especially important in the first 6–12 weeks of existence of cysts that have arisen during an attack of acute pancreatitis. The chances of spontaneous resolution are about 40%; catheter drainage at this stage is meddlesome; and internal drainage of the cyst by surgery may be difficult or even impossible. Thereafter, for cysts greater than 5

cm, treatment is usually recommended over expectant management (in the absence of contraindications, such as serious concomitant disease), because most cysts can be promptly eliminated by percutaneous catheter drainage or surgical drainage into the stomach or intestine. This obviates the need for prolonged follow-up with repeated ultrasound or CT scans and avoids the risks, albeit low, of complications. Patients who present with a symptomatic pseudocyst and no history of recent acute pancreatitis may be treated without the 6- to 12-week delay, because their cyst wall is tough (mature) enough to hold sutures and allow an anastomosis with the gut. Jaundice in a patient with a pseudocyst is usually caused by pressure from the cyst on the bile duct. Draining the pseudocyst usually relieves the obstruction, but an operative cholangiogram should be obtained just to make sure.

A. Excision: Excision is the most definitive treatment but is usually confined to chronic pseudocysts in the tail of the gland. This approach is recommended especially for cysts that follow trauma, where the head and body of the gland are normal. Most cysts should be drained either externally or internally into the gut.

B. External Drainage: External drainage is best for critically ill patients or when the cyst wall has not matured sufficiently for anastomosis to other organs. A large tube is sewn into the cyst lumen, and its end is brought out through the abdominal wall. External drainage is complicated in a third of patients by a pancreatic fistula that sometimes requires surgical drainage but on the average closes spontaneously in several months. The incidence of recurrent pseudocyst is about four times greater after external drainage than after drainage into the gut.

C. Internal Drainage: The preferred method of treatment is internal drainage, where the cyst is anastomosed to a Roux-en-Y limb of jejunum (cystojejunostomy), to the posterior wall of the stomach (cystogastrostomy), or to the duodenum (cystoduodenostomy). The interior of the cyst should be inspected for evidence of a tumor and biopsy performed as appropriate. Cystogastrostomy is preferable for cysts behind and densely adherent to the stomach. This may well be done laparoscopically in the future. To accomplish free, dependent drainage, Roux-en-Y cystojejunostomy provides better drainage of cysts in various other locations. Cystoduodenostomy is indicated for cysts deep within the head of the gland and adjacent to the medial wall of the duodenum—lesions that would be difficult to drain by any other technique. The procedure consists of making a lateral duodenotomy, opening into the cyst through the medial wall of the duodenum, and then closing the lateral duodenotomy. Following internal drainage, the cyst cavity becomes obliterated within a few weeks. Even after cystogastrostomy, an unrestricted diet can be allowed within a week after surgery, and x-rays taken at this time usually show only a small residual cyst cavity.

D. Nonsurgical Drainage: External drainage can be established by a percutaneous catheter placed into the cyst under radiographic or ultrasound control. This is the preferred method for infected pseudocysts. In some centers, it is also used for the majority of uncomplicated pseudocysts as the primary mode of therapy. About two-thirds of cysts so treated are permanently eradicated. It may also be useful to shrink a truly huge pseudocyst (eg, one that occupies half of the abdominal cavity), because it is technically difficult to obtain adequate internal drainage of these lesions into the gut. Occasionally, a sterile cyst may become infected when a narrow catheter is inserted into it. This is more likely when the cyst lumen contains debris that is not drained effectively by this technique. Chronic external pancreatic fistula is a potential complication of this method.

Two other drainage techniques have been tried: (1) Passing a catheter percutaneously through the anterior abdominal wall, the anterior wall of the stomach, and through the posterior stomach into the cyst. After several weeks, the catheter is removed, and a chronic tract remains from cyst to gastric lumen. 2) Using a fiberoptic gastroscope to make a small incision through the back wall of the stomach into the cyst. Because of questions about efficacy and safety, neither method is really being used.

Prognosis

The recurrence rate for pancreatic pseudocyst is about 10%, and recurrence is more frequent after treatment by external drainage. Serious postoperative hemorrhage from the cyst occurs rarely—most often after cystogastrostomy. In most cases, however, surgical treatment of pseudocysts is uncomplicated and definitively solves the immediate problem. Many patients later experience chronic pain as a manifestation of underlying chronic pancreatitis.

Adams DB, Anderson MC: Percutaneous catheter drainage compared with internal drainage in the management of pancreatic pseudocyst. Ann Surg 1992;215:571.

Ahearne PM et al: An endoscopic retrograde cholangiopancreatography (ERCP)-based algorithm for the management of pancreatic pseudocysts. Am J Surg 1992;163:111.

Bourliere M, Sarles H: Pancreatic cysts and pseudocysts associated with acute and chronic pancreatitis. Dig Dis Sci 1989;34:343.

Bradley EL: Complications of chronic pancreatitis. Surg Clin North Am 1989;69:431.

Criado E et al: Long term results of percutaneous catheter drainage of pancreatic pseudocysts. Surg Gynecol Obstet 1992;175:293.

D'Egidio A, Schein M: Percutaneous drainage of pancreatic pseudocysts: A prospective study. World J Surg 1992;16:141.

el Hamel A et al: Bleeding pseudocysts and pseudo-aneurysms in chronic pancreatitis. Br J Surg 1991;78:1059.

Farrar T: Direct cystogastrostomy for pancreatic pseudocysts. Surg Gynecol Obstet 1988;166:477.

Himal HS, Cusimano RJ: Pancreatic pseudocysts: The role of percutaneous catheter drainage. Can J Surg 1992;35:403.

Imrie CW, Buist LJ, Shearer MG: Importance of cause in the outcome of pancreatic pseudocysts. Am J Surg 1988;156:159.

Johnson LB, Rattner DW, Warshaw AL: The effect of size of giant pancreatic pseudocysts on the outcome of internal drainage procedures. Surg Gynecol Obstet 1991;173:171.

Kloppel G, Maillet B: Pseudocysts in chronic pancreatitis: A morphological analysis of 57 resection specimens and 9 autopsy pancreata. Pancreas 1991;6:266.

Lee YT: Cystadenocarcinoma versus pseudocyst of the pancreas: A difficult differential diagnosis. Curr Surg 1989;46:202.

Lewandrowski KB et al: Cyst fluid analysis in the differential diagnosis of pancreatic cysts: A comparison of pseudocysts, serous cystadenomas, mucinous cystic neoplasms, and mucinous cystadenocarcinoma. Ann Surg 1993;217:41.

Lewis G et al: Traumatic pancreatic pseudocysts. Br J Surg 1993;80:89.

London NJ et al: Serial computed tomography scanning in acute pancreatitis: A prospective study. Gut 1989;30:397.

Mainwaring R et al: Differentiating pancreatic pseudocyst and pancreatic necrosis using computerized tomography. Ann Surg 1989;209:562.

Munn JS et al: Simultaneous treatment of chronic pancreatitis and pancreatic pseudocyst. Arch Surg 1987;122:662.

Newell KA et al: Are cystgastrostomy and cystjejunostomy equivalent operations for pancreatic pseudocysts? Surgery 1990;108:635.

Pitkaranta P et al: Diagnostic evaluation and aggressive surgical approach in bleeding pseudoaneurysms associated with pancreatic pseudocysts. Scand J Gastroenterol 1991;26:58.

Vitas GJ, Sarr MG: Selected management of pancreatic pseudocysts: Operative versus expectant management. Surgery 1992;111:123.

Yeo CJ et al: The natural history of pancreatic pseudocysts documented by computed tomography. Surg Gynecol Obstet 1990;170:411.

3. PANCREATIC ABSCESS

Pancreatic abscess, which complicates about 5% of cases of acute pancreatitis, is invariably fatal if it is not treated surgically. It tends to develop in severe cases accompanied by hypovolemic shock and pancreatic necrosis and is an especially frequent complication of postoperative pancreatitis. Abscess formation follows secondary bacterial contamination of necrotic pancreatic debris and hemorrhagic exudate. The organisms may spread to the pancreas hematogenously as well as directly through the wall of the transverse colon. It is unknown whether prophylactic antibiotics given early in the course of severe acute pancreatitis decrease the incidence of abscess.

Clinical Findings

An abscess should be suspected when a patient with severe acute pancreatitis fails to improve and develops rising fever or when symptoms return after a period of recovery. In most cases, there is improvement for a while before signs of infection appear 2–4 weeks after the attack began. Epigastric pain and tenderness and a palpable tender mass are clues to diagnosis. In many cases, the findings are not especially striking—ie, the temperature is only modestly elevated and the patient does not appear septic. Vomiting or jaundice may be present, but in some cases fever and leukocytosis are the only findings. The serum amylase may be elevated but usually is normal. Characteristically, the serum albumin is below 2.5 g/dL and the alkaline phosphatase is elevated. Pleural fluid and diaphragmatic paralysis may be evident on chest x-rays. An upper gastrointestinal series may show deformity of the stomach or duodenum by a mass, but it usually does not, and the changes are nonspecific in any case. Diagnostic CT scans will usually indicate the presence of a fluid collection in the area of the pancreas. Gas in the collection on plain films or CT scans is virtually diagnostic. Percutaneous CT scan-guided aspiration may be used to aid in diagnosis and obtain a specimen for Gram stain and culture.

In general, the diagnosis is difficult, treatment is often instituted late, illness is severe, and death rates are high.

Treatment

The collection of pus must be drained. Percutaneous catheter drainage may be helpful as a first step in order to decrease toxicity or to obtain a specimen for culture. In some cases, catheter drainage will prove to be definitive, but most often the infected retroperitoneal space is honeycombed and contains necrotic debris that cannot pass through the catheter, so surgical debridement is necessary. It is best to consider catheter drainage as a preparatory step for surgery rather than a curative treatment, for that is the usual relationship. Otherwise, there may be a tendency to delay surgery for too long as futile efforts are repeatedly made to manipulate the catheters into better positions. In fact, the two measures—surgical debridement and catheter drainage—are complementary.

Preoperatively, the patient should be given broad-spectrum antibiotics, since the organisms are usually a mixed flora, most often *Escherichia coli, Bacteroides, Staphylococcus, Klebsiella, Proteus, Candida albicans,* etc. Necrotic debris should be removed and external drainage instituted.

Postoperative hemorrhage (immediate or delayed) from the abscess cavity occurs occasionally.

Prognosis

The death rate is about 20%, a consequence of the severity of the condition, incomplete surgical drainage, and the inability in some cases to make the diagnosis.

Adams DB, Harvey TS, Anderson MC: Percutaneous catheter drainage of infected pancreatic and peripancreatic fluid collections. Arch Surg 1990;125:1554.

Bradley EL 3d, Olson RA: Current management of pancreatic abscess. Adv Surg 1991;24:361.

Fedorak IJ et al: Secondary pancreatic infections: Are they distinct clinical entities? Surgery 1992;112:824.

Fink A et al: Indolent presentation of pancreatic abscess. Arch Surg 1988;123:1067.

Lang EK, Paolini RM, Pottmeyer A: The efficacy of palliative and definitive percutaneous versus surgical drainage of pancreatic abscesses and pseudocysts: A prospective study of 85 patients. South Med J 1991;84:55.

Ranson JHC et al: Computed tomography and the prediction of pancreatic abscess in acute pancreatitis. Ann Surg 1985;201:656.

Rotman N et al: Failure of percutaneous drainage of pancreatic abscesses complicating severe acute pancreatitis. Surg Gynecol Obstet 1992;174:141.

Stricker PD, Hunt DR: Surgical aspects of pancreatic abscess. Br J Surg 1986;73:644.

Vernacchia FS et al: Pancreatic abscess: Predictive value of early abdominal CT. Radiology 1987;162:435.

4. PANCREATIC ASCITES & PANCREATIC PLEURAL EFFUSION

Pancreatic ascites consists of accumulated pancreatic fluid in the abdomen without peritonitis or severe pain. Since many of these patients are alcoholic, they are often thought at first to have cirrhotic ascites. The syndrome is most often due to chronic leakage of a pseudocyst, but a few cases are due to disruption of a pancreatic duct. The principal causative factors are alcoholic pancreatitis in adults and traumatic pancreatitis in children. Marked recent weight loss is a major clinical manifestation, and unresponsiveness of the ascites to diuretics is an additional diagnostic clue. The ascitic fluid, which ranges in appearance from straw-colored to blood-tinged, contains elevated protein (> 2.9 g/dL) and amylase levels. Once this condition is suspected, definitive diagnosis is based on chemical analysis of the ascitic fluid and endoscopic retrograde pancreatography. The latter procedure frequently demonstrates the point of fluid leak and allows a rational surgical approach if operation is required.

Initial therapy should consist of a period of intravenous hyperalimentation and somatostatin. This often cures the problem. If considerable improvement has not occurred within 2–3 weeks, surgery should be performed. A preoperative ERCP is essential to demonstrate the site of the leak. If it is not entirely obvious from the films taken during ERCP, a CT scan should be performed immediately afterward, while contrast media is still in the pancreatic duct. The greater sensitivity of the CT scan will be enough to reveal the tiny trickle from the pancreatic duct into the abdomen. The operation involves suturing a Roux-en-Y limb of jejunum to the site of the leak on the surface of the pancreas or a pancreatic pseudocyst. With appropriate therapy, the outlook is excellent. The death rate is low in patients treated before debilitation becomes severe.

Chronic pleural effusions of pancreatic origin represent a variant in which the pancreatic fistula drains into the chest. The diagnosis is made by measuring high concentrations of amylase (usually > 3000 IU/dL) in the fluid. A CT scan of the pancreas and retrograde pancreatogram should be obtained. Medical therapy consists of draining the fluid with a chest tube, somatostatin, and total parenteral nutrition. If after several weeks the fistula persists or if it recurs after the tube has been removed, the source of the leak on the pancreas should either be drained into a Roux-en-Y limb of jejunum or excised as part of a distal pancreatectomy.

Adler J, Barkin JS: Management of pseudocysts, inflammatory masses, and pancreatic ascites. Gastroenterol Clin North Am 1990;19:863.

Gislason H, Gronbech JE, Soreide O: Pancreatic ascites: Treatment by continuous somatostatin infusion. Am J Gastroenterol 1991;86:519.

Lipsett PA, Cameron JL: Internal pancreatic fistula. Am J Surg 1992;163:216.

Martin FM et al: Management of pancreatic fistulas. Arch Surg 1989;124:571.

Pottmeyer EW, Frey CF, Massuno S: Pancreaticopleural fistulas. Arch Surg 1987;122:648.

Rockey DC, Cello JP: Pancreaticopleural fistula: Report of 7 patients and review of the literature. Medicine 1990; 69:332.

5. CHRONIC PANCREATITIS

Essentials of Diagnosis

- Persistent or recurrent abdominal pain.
- Pancreatic calcification on x-ray in 50%.
- Pancreatic insufficiency in 30%; malabsorption and diabetes mellitus.
- Most often due to alcoholism.

General Considerations

Chronic alcoholism causes most cases of chronic pancreatitis, but a few are due to gallstones, hypercalcemia, hyperlipidemia, duct obstruction from any cause, or inherited predisposition (familial pancreatitis). Direct trauma to the gland, either from an external blow or from surgical injury, can produce chronic pancreatitis if a ductal stricture develops during the healing process. In such cases, disease is often localized to the segment of gland drained by the obstructed duct. Although gallstone disease may cause repeated attacks of acute pancreatitis, this uncommonly leads to chronic pancreatitis.

There is evidence that pancreatic juice normally contains a specific protein responsible for maintaining calcium carbonate in solution. Levels of this protein are decreased in patients with chronic pancreatitis, a situation that allows calcium carbonate to precipitate and form calculi. Pressure within the duct is increased in patients with chronic pancreatitis (about 40 cm H_2O) compared with normal subjects (about 15 cm H_2O). This is a result of increased viscosity of pancreatic juice, partial obstruction by calculi, and impaired distensibility of the gland because of diffuse fibrosis (eg, a compartment syndrome). Sphincteric pressure remains in the normal range. The increased pressure causes dilation of the duct in the patient whose pancreas has not yet become fixed by scarring. It may also impair nutrient blood flow, causing further functional damage. Pathologic changes in the gland include destruction of parenchyma, fibrosis, dedifferentiation of acini, calculi, and ductal dilatation.

Clinical Findings

A. Symptoms and Signs: Chronic pancreatitis may be asymptomatic, or it may produce abdominal pain, malabsorption, diabetes mellitus, or (usually) all three manifestations. The pain is typically felt deep in the upper abdomen and radiating through to the back, and it waxes and wanes from day to day. Early in the course of the disease, the pain may be episodic, lasting for days to weeks and then vanishing for several months before returning again. Attacks of acute pancreatitis may occur, superimposed on the pattern of chronic pain. Many patients become addicted to the narcotics prescribed for pain.

B. Laboratory Findings: Abnormal laboratory findings may result from (1) pancreatic inflammation, (2) pancreatic exocrine insufficiency, (3) diabetes mellitus, (4) bile duct obstruction, or (5) other complications such as pseudocyst formation or splenic vein thrombosis.

1. Amylase–In acute exacerbations, serum and urinary amylase levels may be elevated, but most often they are not, perhaps because pancreatic fibrosis has destroyed so much of the enzyme-forming capacity of the parenchyma.

2. Tests of exocrine pancreatic function– The secretin and cholecystokinin stimulation tests are the most sensitive tests to detect exocrine malfunction but are difficult to perform. Other practical tests are discussed on p 575.

3. Diabetes mellitus–About 75% of patients with calcific pancreatitis and 30% of those with noncalcific pancreatitis have insulin-dependent diabetes. Most of the rest have either abnormal glucose tolerance curves or abnormally low serum insulin levels after a test meal. The margin of reserve is such that partial pancreatectomy is quite likely to convert a patient who does not require insulin into one who does require it postoperatively.

4. Biliary obstruction–Elevated bilirubin or alkaline phosphatase levels may result from fibrotic entrapment of the lower end of the bile duct. The differential diagnosis of biliary obstruction in these patients must consider acute pancreatic inflammation, pseudocyst, or pancreatic neoplasm.

5. Miscellaneous–Splenic vein thrombosis may produce secondary hypersplenism or gastric varices.

C. Imaging Studies: Endoscopic retrograde pancreatography is helpful in establishing the diagnosis of chronic pancreatitis, in ruling out pancreatic pseudocyst and neoplasm, and in preoperative planning for patients thought to be candidates for surgery. The typical findings are ductal stones and irregularity, with dilatation and stenoses and, occasionally, ductal occlusion. The discovery of small unsuspected pseudocysts is common. Retrograde cholangiography should be performed simultaneously to determine whether the common bile duct is narrowed by the pancreatitis, to determine whether biliary calculi are present, and to aid the surgeon in avoiding injury to the bile duct during operation.

Complications

The principal complications of chronic pancreatitis are pancreatic pseudocyst, biliary obstruction, duodenal obstruction, malnutrition, and diabetes mellitus. Adenocarcinoma of the pancreas occurs with greater frequency in patients with familial chronic pancreatitis than in the general population.

Treatment

A. Medical Treatment: The treatment of malabsorption and steatorrhea is discussed on p 575. Controlled trials have shown that administering pancreatic enzymes has little effect on the pain.

Patients with chronic pancreatitis should be urged to discontinue the use of alcohol. Abstention from alcohol will reduce chronic or episodic pain in more than half of cases even though damage to the pancreas is irreversible. Psychiatric treatment may be beneficial. Diabetes in these patients usually requires insulin.

B. Surgical Treatment: (Figure 27–4.) Surgical therapy is principally of value to relieve chronic intractable pain. It is essential that every effort be made to eliminate alcohol abuse. The best surgical candidates are those whose pain persists after alcohol has been abandoned.

Surgical treatment in most cases involves a procedure that facilitates drainage of the pancreatic duct or resects diseased pancreas—or that serves both purposes. The choice of operation can usually be made preoperatively based on the findings of a retrograde pancreatogram and CT scans. Coincidental bile duct

obstruction is common and should be treated by simultaneous choledochoduodenostomy.

1. Drainage procedures–A dilated ductal system reflects obstruction, and when dilatation is present, procedures to improve ductal drainage usually relieve pain. Calcific alcoholic pancreatitis most often falls into this category.

The usual finding is an irregular, widely dilated duct (1–2 cm in diameter) with points of stenosis ("chain of lakes" appearance) and ductal calculi. For such patients, a longitudinal pancreaticojejunostomy **(Puestow procedure)** is appropriate (Figure 27–4). The duct is opened anteriorly from the tail into the head of the gland and anastomosed side-to-side to a Roux-en-Y segment of proximal jejunum. Pain improves postoperatively in about 80% of patients, but improvement of pancreatic insufficiency is uncommon. This procedure, however, has a low rate of success when the pancreatic duct is narrow (ie, < 8 mm).

Sphincteroplasty and distal (caudal) pancreaticojejunostomy **(Du Val procedure)** are other drainage techniques that were used more often in the past. The latter is only of historical interest, but surgical sphincteroplasty plus extraction of pancreatic ductal calculi has been used with some success in recent years. Attempts are currently being made to accomplish something similar by subjecting pancreatic cal-

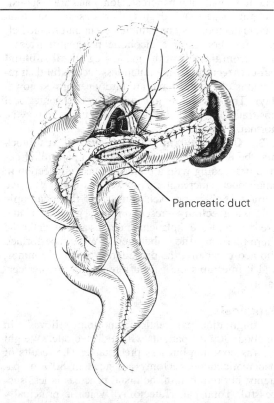

Figure 27–4. Longitudinal pancreaticojejunostomy (Puestow) for chronic pancreatitis.

culi to external shock wave lithotripsy, followed by endoscopic sphincterotomy and stone extraction. Another experimental method involves decompression of the duct by an endoscopically placed stent. Questions of safety and efficacy have tempered the early enthusiasm for these procedures.

2. Pancreatectomy–In the absence of a dilated duct, pancreatectomy is the best procedure, and the extent of resection can often be determined from a CT scan and pancreatogram. In patients with small ducts, the most severe disease is usually located in the head of the gland, and **pancreaticoduodenectomy** (Whipple procedure) is the operation of choice. A variant of this procedure involves resection of the head of the gland while preserving the duodenum. A Roux-en-Y limb of jejunum is anastomosed to both cut surfaces of the pancreas. If the duct is also dilated in the body and tail, resection of the head can also be combined with longitudinal pancreaticojejunostomy in that part of the gland. Pain relief is satisfactory in about 80% of patients treated by these operations. **Total pancreatectomy** is indicated when a previous pancreaticoduodenectomy or distal pancreatectomy has failed to give satisfactory pain relief. The reported results are contradictory; pain relief has been excellent in reports from the UK but less than excellent in reports from the USA. Difficulties in controlling diabetes mellitus occur in 30–40% of patients who have had total pancreatectomy and are responsible for occasional deaths. For this reason, total pancreatectomy is contraindicated in unreformed alcoholics. For chronic alcoholic pancreatitis, resections from the left of the gland—eg, **distal subtotal pancreatectomy,**—are much less successful than resections of the head and are rarely performed nowadays. The most common indication is chronic focal posttraumatic pancreatitis, in which the head may be normal.

3. Celiac plexus block–Celiac plexus block may be used in an attempts to obtain pain relief before proceeding with a major pancreatic resection in small duct pancreatitis. A newer and more effective variant of this approach consists of **thoracoscopic splanchnicectomy**—resection of segments of the greater and lesser splanchnic nerves as they enter the thorax from the abdomen. When performed thoracoscopically, the procedure is relatively minor, and it interrupts the pain afferents with greater certainty.

Prognosis

Longitudinal pancreaticojejunostomy relieves pain in about 80% of patients with a dilated duct. Weight gain is common but less predictable. The results of pancreaticoduodenectomy are good in 80% of patients, but removal of the distal pancreas is less successful. Total pancreatectomy, which is principally reserved for failures of other operations, gives satisfying relief in 30–90% of patients depending on the

series. The reasons for these widely differing results are not known. Celiac plexus block is of lasting benefit to no more than 30% of patients. In some patients, pain subsides with advancing pancreatic insufficiency.

Except in advanced cases with continuous pain, alcoholics who can be persuaded to stop drinking often experience relief from pain and recurrent attacks of pancreatitis. In familial pancreatitis, the progress of the disease is inexorable, and many of these patients require surgery. The results of longitudinal pancreaticojejunostomy are excellent in familial pancreatitis. Narcotic addiction, diabetes, and malnutrition are serious problems in many patients.

Ammann RW et al: Evolution and regression of pancreatic calcification in chronic pancreatitis. Gastroenterology 1988;95:1018.

Beger HG et al: Duodenum-preserving resection of the head of the pancreas in severe chronic pancreatitis: Early and late results. Ann Surg 1989;209:273.

Bradley E: Long-term results of pancreatojejunostomy in patients with chronic pancreatitis. Am J Surg 1987;153:207.

Bradley EL III: Complications of chronic pancreatitis. Surg Clin North Am 1989;69:481.

Cooper MJ et al: Total pancreatectomy for chronic pancreatitis. Br J Surg 1987;74:912.

Drake DH, Fry WJ: Ductal drainage for chronic pancreatitis. Surgery 1989;105:131.

Frey CF et al: Pancreatic resection for chronic pancreatitis. Surg Clin North Am 1989;69:499.

Frey CF, Suzuki M, Isaji S: Treatment of chronic pancreatitis complicated by obstruction of the common bile duct or duodenum. World J Surg 1990;14:59.

Gulliver DJ et al: Stent placement for benign pancreatic diseases: Correlation between ERCP findings and clinical response. AJR Am J Roentgenol 1992;159:751.

Ihse I, Borch K, Larsson J: Chronic pancreatitis: Results of operations for relief of pain. World J Surg 1990;14:33.

Jalleh RP, Aslam M, Williamson RC: Pancreatic tissue and ductal pressures in chronic pancreatitis. Br J Surg 1991;78:1235.

Mossner J et al: Treatment of pain with pancreatic extracts in chronic pancreatitis: Results of a prospective placebo-controlled multicenter trial. Digestion 1992;53:54.

Nealon WH, Townsend CM Jr, Thompson JC: Operative drainage of the pancreatic duct delays functional impairment in patients with chronic pancreatitis. Ann Surg 1988;208:321.

Nealon WH, Townsend CM Jr, Thompson JC: The time course of beta cell dysfunction in chronic ethanol-induced pancreatitis: A prospective analysis. Surgery 1988;104:1074.

Sarles H, Bernard JP, Gullo L: Pathogenesis of chronic pancreatitis. Gut 1990;31:629.

Stone WM et al: Chronic pancreatitis: Results of Whipple's resection and total pancreatectomy. Arch Surg 1988;123:815.

Walsh TN et al: Minimal change chronic pancreatitis. Gut 1992;33:1566.

Warshaw AL, Jin G, Ottinger LW: Recognition and clinical

implications of mesenteric and portal vein obstruction in chronic pancreatitis. Arch Surg 1987;122:410.

Williamson RCN, Cooper MJ: Resection in chronic pancreatitis. Br J Surg 1987;74:807.

Wilson JS, Korsten MA, Pirola RC: Alcohol-induced pancreatic injury (Part I): Unexplained features and ductular theories of pathogenesis. Int J Pancreatol 1989;4:109.

PANCREATIC INSUFFICIENCY (Steatorrhea; Malabsorption)

Pancreatic exocrine insufficiency may follow pancreatectomy or pancreatic disease, especially chronic pancreatitis. Many patients with varying degrees of pancreatic insufficiency have no symptoms and require no treatment, whereas others may benefit greatly from a rational medical regimen.

Malabsorption and steatorrhea do not appear until more than 90% of pancreatic exocrine function is lost; with 2–10% of normal function, steatorrhea is mild to moderate; with less than 2% of normal function, steatorrhea is severe. On a diet containing 100 g of fat per day, normal subjects excrete 5–7 g/d, and the efficiency of assimilation is similar over a wide range of fat intake. Total pancreatectomy causes about 70% fat malabsorption. If the pancreatic remnant is normal, subtotal resections may have little effect on absorption.

Pancreatic insufficiency affects fat absorption more than that of protein or carbohydrate, because protein digestion is aided by gastric pepsin and carbohydrate digestion by salivary and intestinal amylase. Malabsorption of vitamins is rarely a significant problem. Water-soluble B vitamins are absorbed throughout the small intestine, and fat-soluble vitamins, although dependent on micellar solubilization by bile salts, do not require pancreatic enzymes for absorption. Vitamin B_{12} malabsorption has been detected in some patients with pancreatic insufficiency, but it is rarely a clinical problem, and vitamin B_{12} replacement is unnecessary.

Thus, the principal problem in otherwise uncomplicated pancreatic insufficiency is fat malabsorption and accompanying caloric malnutrition.

Tests of Pancreatic Exocrine Function
A. Secretin or Cholecystokinin Test: Pancreatic juice is obtained by peroral duodenal intubation, and the response to an intravenous injection of secretin or cholecystokinin is measured. The results vary, depending on the dose and preparation of hormone used. Both tests (using purified hormones or the synthetic octapeptide of cholecystokinin) seem to be reliable. Pancreatic fluid should normally have a bicarbonate concentration greater than 80 meq/L and bicarbonate output above 15 meq/30 min.

B. Pancreolauryl Test: Fluorescein dilaurate is given orally with breakfast, and urinary fluorescein excretion is measured. Release and absorption of fluorescein depend on the action of pancreatic esterase. The test is relatively specific, but considerable exocrine insufficiency is required for a positive result. It is currently the most widely used test of exocrine function because it is inexpensive and easy to do.

C. PABA Excretion (Bentiromide) Test: The patient ingests 1 g of the synthetic peptide bentiromide (Bz-Ty-PABA), and urinary excretion of aromatic amines (PABA) is measured. Cleavage of the peptide to liberate PABA depends on intraluminal chymotrypsin activity. Patients with chronic pancreatitis excrete about 50% of the normal amount of PABA.

D. Fecal Fat Balance Test: The patient ingests a diet containing 75–100 g fat each day for 5 days. The amounts of dietary fat should be measured and should be the same each day. Excretion of less than 7% of ingested fat is normal. Clinically significant steatorrhea is present when fat malabsorption exceeds about 25%. Total pancreatectomy results in about 70% fat malabsorption.

Examination of a stool specimen for fat globules (obviously much simpler than the fat balance test) is specific and relatively sensitive for fat malabsorption.

Treatment
The diet should aim for 3000–6000 kcal/d, emphasizing carbohydrate (400 g or more) and protein (100–150 g). Patients with steatorrhea may or may not have diarrhea, and dietary restriction of fat is important mainly to control diarrhea. Patients with diarrhea may be restricted to 50 g of fat and the amount increased until diarrhea appears. Permissible fat intake averages 100 g/d distributed equally among four meals.

Pancreatic enzyme replacement may be accomplished with pancreatic extracts (eg, Cotazym, Ilozyme, Pancrease, Viokase) containing 30,000–50,000 units of lipase distributed throughout each of four daily meals. Lesser amounts are much less effective; an hourly dosage regimen probably has no advantages.

If enzymes alone do not improve the malabsorption enough, the problem is probably due to destruction of lipase by gastric acid. This can be largely alleviated by adding an H2 receptor blocking agent to the enzyme regimen. A preparation of enzymes as enteric-coated microspheres (Pancrease) is less vulnerable to low pH and may be more effective in refractory cases.

Medium-chain triglycerides (MCT), which can be obtained as a powder or an oil, may be used as a caloric supplement. This product is more rapidly hydrolyzed and the fatty acids more readily absorbed than are long-chain triglycerides, which make up 98% of the fat in a normal diet. Unfortunately, MCT oil is relatively unpalatable and is frequently associated with nausea and vomiting, bloating, and diarrhea, which limit patient acceptance.

Choosing and using a pancreatic enzyme supplement. Drug Ther Bull 1992;30:37.

Doty JE, Fink AS, Meyer JH: Alterations in digestive function caused by pancreatic disease. Surg Clin North Am 1989;69:44.

Li Y, Chiverton SG, Hunt RH: Exocrine pancreatic function tests. J Clin Gastroenterol 1989;11:376.

Marotta F et al: Pancreatic enzyme replacement therapy. Importance of gastric acid secretion, H2-antagonists, and enteric coating. Dig Dis Sci 1989;34:456.

Roberts IM et al: Utility of fecal fat concentrations as screening test in pancreatic insufficiency. Dig Dis Sci 1986;31:1021.

Romano TJ, Dobbins JW: Evaluation of the patient with suspected malabsorption. Gastroenterol Clin North Am 1989;18:467.

ADENOCARCINOMA OF THE PANCREAS

Until recently, the incidence of carcinoma of the pancreas was increasing in the USA at an annual rate of 15%, but now it seems to have reached a plateau. About 28,000 new cases of pancreatic cancer occur each year. After tumors of the lung and colon, pancreatic carcinoma is the third leading cause of death due to cancer in men between ages 35 and 54. Factors associated with an increased risk of pancreatic cancer are cigarette smoking, dietary consumption of meat (especially fried meat) and fat, previous gastrectomy (> 20 years earlier), and race (in the USA but not Africa, blacks are more susceptible than whites). Factors for which the data are inconsistent include coffee drinking, alcohol intake, occupation, and diabetes mellitus. High intake of fruits and vegetables has been shown to exert a protective effect. Over 90% of pancreatic adenocarcinomas exhibit a mutation of the Ki-*ras* oncogene on codon 12.

The peak incidence is in the fifth and sixth decades. In two-thirds of cases, the tumor is located in the head of the gland; the remainder occur in the body or tail. Ductal adenocarcinoma, mainly of a poorly differentiated cell pattern, accounts for 80% of the cancers; the remainder are islet cell tumors and cystadenocarcinomas, tumors that are discussed later in this chapter. Pancreatic adenocarcinoma is characterized by early local extension to contiguous structures and metastases to regional lymph nodes and the liver. Pulmonary, peritoneal, and distant nodal metastases occur later.

Clinical Findings

A. Symptoms and Signs:

1. Carcinoma of the head of the pancreas– About 75% of patients with carcinoma of the head of the pancreas present with weight loss, obstructive jaundice, and deep-seated abdominal pain. Back pain occurs in 25% of patients and is associated with a worse prognosis. In general, smaller tumors confined to the pancreas are associated with less pain. Weight loss averages about 20 lb (44 kg). Hepatomegaly is present in half of patients but does not necessarily indicate spread to the liver. A palpable mass, which is found in 20%, nearly always signifies surgical incurability. Jaundice is unrelenting in most patients but fluctuates in about 10%. Cholangitis occurs in only 10% of patients with bile duct obstruction. A palpable nontender gallbladder in a jaundiced patient suggests neoplastic obstruction of the common duct **(Courvoisier's law),** most often due to pancreatic cancer; this finding is present in about half of cases. Jaundice is often accompanied by pruritus, especially of the hands and feet.

2. Carcinoma of the body and tail of the pancreas–Since carcinomas of the body and tail of the pancreas are remote from the bile duct, less than 10% of patients are jaundiced. The presenting complaints are weight loss and pain, which sometimes occurs in excruciating paroxysms. In the few patients with jaundice or hepatomegaly, metastatic involvement has usually occurred. Migratory thrombophlebitis develops in 10% of cases. Once considered relatively specific as a clue to pancreatic cancer, this complication is now known to affect patients with other types of malignant disease.

The diagnosis of pancreatic carcinoma may be extremely difficult. The typical patient who presents with abdominal pain, weight loss, and obstructive jaundice rarely presents a problem, but those with just weight loss, vague abdominal pain, and nondiagnostic x-rays are occasionally labeled psychoneurotics until the existence of cancer becomes obvious. If back pain predominates, orthopedic or neurosurgical causes may be sought at first. One characteristic feature is the tendency for the patient to seek relief of pain by assuming a sitting position with the spine flexed. Recumbency, on the other hand, aggravates the discomfort and sometimes makes sleeping in bed impossible. Sudden onset of diabetes mellitus is an early manifestation in 25% of patients.

B. Laboratory Findings: Elevated alkaline phosphatase and bilirubin levels reflect either common duct obstruction or hepatic metastases. The bilirubin level with neoplastic obstruction averages 18 mg/dL, much higher than that generally seen with benign disease of the bile ducts. Only rarely are serum aminotransferase levels markedly elevated. Repeated examination of stool specimens for occult blood gives a positive reaction in many cases.

Serum levels of the tumor marker CA 19-9 are elevated in most patients with pancreatic cancer, but the sensitivity in resectable (< 4cm) lesions is probably too low (50%) to serve as a screening tool. Elevated levels also occur with other gastrointestinal cancers. The greatest usefulness of CA 19-9 measurements may be in following the results of treatments. After complete resection of a tumor, elevated levels drop to normal, but they rise again with recurrence.

C. Imaging Studies: Nearly all patients should have a CT scan.

1. CT scan–CT scans show a pancreatic mass in 95% of cases, usually with a central zone of diminished attenuation, and in over 90% of patients with a mass there are signs of extension beyond the boundaries of the pancreas. The upstream pancreatic duct is noted to be dilated in 70% of patients, and the bile duct is dilated in 60% (principally in those with jaundice). The presence of both bile duct and pancreatic duct dilatation is strong evidence for pancreatic cancer even in the absence of a mass. Findings suggesting unresectability include local tumor extension (eg, behind the pancreas; into the liver hilum), contiguous organ invasion (eg, duodenum, stomach), distant metastases, involvement of the superior mesenteric or portal vessels, or ascites. In general, size of the mass is only loosely related to resectability. CT scans using modern dynamic scanning techniques are as accurate as angiography in assessing vascular involvement.

2. ERCP–In patients with a typical clinical history and a pancreatic mass on CT, ERCP is unnecessary. In the absence of a mass, an ERCP is indicated. It is the most sensitive test (95%) for detecting pancreatic cancer, though specificity in differentiating between cancer and pancreatitis is low. Consequently, a pancreatogram should be obtained early in cases where the existence of a pancreatic lesion is suspected but unproved. The findings consist of stenosis or obstruction of the pancreatic duct. Adjacent lesions of the bile duct and pancreatic duct ("double-duct sign") are highly suggestive of neoplastic disease, especially if the biliary involvement is focal. Although ERCP is useful to distinguish between the various kinds of periampullary tumors, that information rarely alters management.

3. Upper gastrointestinal series–An upper gastrointestinal series is not sensitive in detecting pancreatic cancer, but it provides information about patency of the duodenum that may be useful in deciding whether a gastrojejunostomy will have to be performed. The classic findings consist of widening of the duodenal sweep, narrowing of the lumen, and the "reversed-3 sign," named for the duodenal configuration.

4. Other studies–Angiography has not proved reliable in detecting or staging pancreatic neoplasms, and ultrasound is a poor second to CT scans for imaging.

D. Aspiration Biopsy: Percutaneous aspiration biopsy of pancreatic mass lesions is positive in 85% of malignant tumors. The procedure is relatively safe, but there is a risk of spreading a localized (resectable) tumor, so it is contraindicated in patients who are candidates for surgery. Aspiration biopsy in them should be performed, if desired, during laparotomy. Percutaneous aspiration biopsy is principally of value to verify a presumptive diagnosis of adenocarcinoma of the pancreas in patients with radiographic evidence of unresectability. In these cases, cytologic proof is important, for treatment decisions should not be made solely on the basis of the indirect evidence provided by CT scans, etc. There is too great a risk of misdiagnosing something unusual, such as a retroperitoneal lymphoma or sarcoma, and administering inappropriate treatment.

Differential Diagnosis

The other periampullary neoplasms—carcinoma of the ampulla of Vater, distal common bile duct, or duodenum—may also present with pain, weight loss, obstructive jaundice, and a palpable gallbladder. Preoperative cholangiography and gastrointestinal x-rays may suggest the correct diagnosis, but laparotomy is sometimes required.

Complications

Obstruction of the splenic vein by tumor may cause splenomegaly and segmental portal hypertension with bleeding gastric or esophageal varices.

Treatment

Pancreatic resection for pancreatic cancer is appropriate only if all gross tumor can be removed with a standard resection. The lesion is considered resectable if the following areas are free of tumor: (1) the hepatic artery near the origin of the gastroduodenal artery; (2) the superior mesenteric artery where it courses under the body of the pancreas; and (3) the liver and regional lymph nodes. Since the pancreas is so close to the portal vein and the superior mesenteric vessels, these structures may be involved early. About 20% of cancers of the head of the pancreas can be resected, but because of local and distant spread, this is rarely possible for lesions of the body and tail.

A histologic diagnosis can usually be made at operation by aspiration biopsy. With small lesions of the head of the gland, it may be difficult to obtain a specimen for histologic diagnosis because much of the palpable mass may consist of inflamed pancreatic tissue. Occasionally, histologic diagnosis is impossible, and clinical decisions must rest on indirect evidence.

For curable lesions of the head, pancreaticoduodenectomy **(Whipple operation)** is required (Figure 27–5). This involves resection of the common bile duct, the gallbladder, the duodenum, and the pancreas to the mid body. There is an increasing tendency to preserve the antrum and pylorus. Involvement of a short (< 1.5 cm) segment of the portal vein is not a contraindication to a curative resection. This is managed by a partial or circumferential resection of the affected area.

When the procedure is performed by surgeons who do it frequently, the operative mortality rate is less than 5%. When it is performed by less experienced

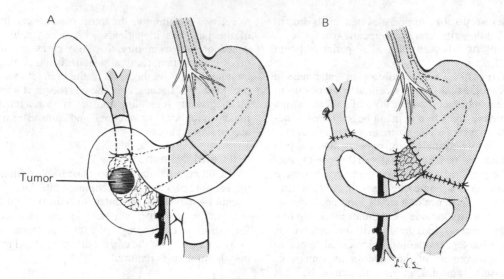

Figure 27–5. Pancreaticoduodenectomy (Whipple procedure). **A:** Preoperative anatomic relationships showing a tumor in the head of the pancreas. **B:** Postoperative reconstruction showing pancreatic, biliary, and gastric anastomoses. A cholecystectomy and bilateral truncal vagotomy are also part of the procedure. In many cases, the distal stomach and pylorus can be preserved, and vagotomy is then unnecessary.

surgeons, the mortality rate is 20–30%. Postoperative deaths are due to complications such as pancreatic and biliary fistulas, hemorrhage, and infection.

In an attempt to increase the cure rate, total pancreatectomy has been given a trial on the theory that many pancreatic cancers are multicentric. However, total pancreatectomy produces a brittle type of diabetes mellitus that compromises the quality of life, and cure rates were not higher.

For unresectable lesions, cholecystojejunostomy or choledochojejunostomy provides relief of jaundice and pruritus. A cholangiogram should be obtained to verify patency between the cystic and common bile ducts unless it is grossly obvious. Percutaneous or endoscopically placed biliary stents may also provide effective palliation and are preferable to surgical biliary decompression if the lesion is known to be unresectable. Gastrojejunostomy is required if the tumor blocks the duodenum. If laparotomy has been performed, gastrojejunostomy should be considered regardless of the presence of duodenal obstruction, because with time this often develops before other life-threatening complications.

An operative strategy gaining in popularity is to perform laparoscopy as the first step in patients scheduled for a possible Whipple procedure. If metastases are seen that militate against a curative resection, laparoscopic gastrojejunostomy or cholecystojejunostomy (or both) can be performed. If not, one should proceed with the laparotomy. About 15% of patients thought to have localized disease from preoperative studies will be found to be unresectable at laparoscopy.

Radiotherapy should be combined with chemotherapy (fluorouracil) for palliation. Radiotherapy alone has been shown to be of no benefit.

Prognosis

The mean survival following palliative therapy is 7 months. Following a Whipple procedure, survival averages about 18 months. Factors associated with tumor recurrence and shorter survival include lymph node involvement, tumor size over 2.5 cm, blood vessel invasion, and amount of blood transfused. If tumor cells extend to the margins of the resected specimen, long-term survival is rare. If the margins are clear, about 20% of patients live more than 5 years. Overall 5-year survival is about 10%, but only 60% of these patients are actually free of tumor.

Cameron JL et al: Factors influencing survival after pancreaticoduodenectomy for pancreatic cancer. Am J Surg 1991;161:120.

Carey LC: Pancreaticoduodenectomy. Am J Surg 1992;164:153.

Dalton RR et al: Carcinoma of the body and tail of the pancreas: Is curative resection justified? Surgery 1992;111:489.

de Rooij, Rogatko A, Brennan MF: Evaluation of palliative surgical procedures in unresectable pancreatic cancer. Br J Surg 1991;78:1053.

Fontham ETH, Correa P: Epidemiology of pancreatic cancer. Surg Clin North Am 1989;69:551.

Freeny PC et al: Pancreatic ductal adenocarcinoma: Diagnosis and staging with dynamic CT. Radiology 1988;166:125.

Geer RJ, Brennan MF: Prognostic indicators for survival

after resection of pancreatic adenocarcinoma. Am J Surg 1993;165:68.

Haddock G, Carter DC: Aetiology of pancreatic cancer. Br J Surg 1990;77:1159.

Ishikawa O et al: Preoperative indications for extended pancreatectomy for locally advanced pancreas cancer involving the portal vein. Ann Surg 1992;215:231.

Kalser MH, Ellenberg SS: Pancreatic cancer: Adjuvant combined radiation and chemotherapy following curative resection. Arch Surg 1985;120:899.

Klinkenbijl JH et al: The advantages of pylorus-preserving pancreatoduodenectomy in malignant disease of the pancreas and periampullary region. Ann Surg 1992;216:142.

Launois B et al: Total pancreatectomy for ductal adenocarcinoma of the pancreas with special reference to resection of the portal vein and multicentric cancer. World J Surg 1993;17:122.

Lillemoe KD et al: Current status of surgical palliation of periampullary carcinoma. Surg Gynecol Obstet 1993; 176:1.

McAfee MK, van Heerden JA, Adson MA: Is proximal pancreatoduodenectomy with pyloric preservation superior to total pancreatectomy? Surgery 1989;105:347.

Miedema BW et al: Complications following pancreaticoduodenectomy. Arch Surg 1992;127:945.

Motojima K et al: Distinguishing pancreatic carcinoma from other periampullary carcinomas by analysis of mutations in the Kirsten-ras oncogene. Ann Surg 1991; 214:657.

Nix GAJJ, et al: ERCP diagnosis of tumors in the region of the head of the pancreas: Analysis of criteria and computer-aided diagnosis. Dig Dis Sci 1988;33:577.

Nordback I et al: Carcinoma of the body and tail of the pancreas. Am J Surg 1992;164:26.

Parsons L Jr, Palmer CH: How accurate is fine-needle biopsy in malignant neoplasia of the pancreas? Arch Surg 1989;124:681.

Pellegrini CA et al: An analysis of the reduced morbidity and mortality rates after pancreaticoduodenectomy. Arch Surg 1989;124:778.

Rosa JA et al: New-onset diabetes mellitus as a harbinger of pancreatic carcinoma. J Clin Gastroenterol 1989;11:211.

Satake K et al: Surgical curability and prognosis for standard versus extended resection for T1 carcinoma of the pancreas. Surg Gynecol Obstet 1992;175:259.

Shimi S, Banting S, Cuschieri A: Laparoscopy in the management of pancreatic cancer: Endoscopic cholecystojejunostomy for advanced disease. Br J Surg 1992; 79:317.

Sperti C et al: CA 19-9 as a prognostic index after resection for pancreatic cancer. J Surg Oncol 1993;52:137.

Tashiro S et al: Surgical indication and significance of portal vein resection in biliary and pancreatic cancer. Surgery 1991;109:481.

Tian F et al: Prognostic value of serum CA 19-9 levels in pancreatic adenocarcinoma. Ann Surg 1992;215:350.

van der Schelling GP et al: Is there a place for gastroenterostomy in patients with advanced cancer of the head of the pancreas? World J Surg 1993;17:128.

van Heerden JA et al: Total pancreatectomy for ductal adenocarcinoma of the pancreas: An update. World J Surg 1988;12:658.

Warshaw AL, Fernandez-del Castillo C: Pancreatic carcinoma. N Engl J Med 1992;326:455.

Warshaw AL: Implications of peritoneal cytology for staging of early pancreatic cancer. Am J Surg 1991;161:26.

Watanapa P, Williamson RC: Surgical palliation for pancreatic cancer: Developments during the past two decades. Br J Surg 1992;79:8.

Willett CG et al: Resection margins in carcinoma of the head of the pancreas: Implications for radiation therapy. Ann Surg 1993;217:144.

CYSTIC NEOPLASMS

Cystic neoplasms of the pancreas usually present with abdominal pain, a mass, or jaundice and are diagnosed from the findings on CT scans.

Cystadenomas can be classified as serous or mucinous. Serous cystadenomas, which are usually microcystic adenomas, are well-circumscribed lesions consisting of multiple small cysts ranging in size from microscopic to about 2 cm. The cut surface has the appearance of a sponge. The multicystic nature of the lesion is usually—but not always—evident on CT scans, which may also show a few calcifications. The epithelium, which is flat to cuboidal, has no malignant potential. Treatment usually entails excision, but in the rare case where this is too hazardous, the lesion may be left in place with the knowledge that complications are rare. An occasional serous cystadenoma will consist of one or more large cysts (ie, macrocystic).

Mucinous cystadenomas (macrocystic adenomas), which are much more common in women than in men, are unilocular or, more often, multilocular lesions that have a smooth lining with papillary projections. The septate appearance on CT scans is characteristic. The cystic spaces measure 2–20 cm in diameter and contain mucus. The lining consists of tall columnar and goblet cells, which are often arranged in a papillary pattern. In time, most mucinous cystadenomas will evolve into cystadenocarcinomas, so total excision is the required treatment.

Cystadenocarcinomas invariably present as a focus of malignancy within an existing mucinous cystadenoma. The tumors are often quite large (eg, 10–20 cm) at the time of diagnosis. Metastases occur in about 25% of cases. Complete excision results in a 5-year survival rate of 70%.

An uncommon lesion, referred to as solid-and-papillary or papillary-cystic neoplasm of the pancreas, occurs almost exclusively in young women (under age 25 years). The tumor is usually large. It may be locally invasive, but metastases are uncommon, and cure is to be expected after resection.

Delcore R et al: Characteristics of cystic neoplasms of the pancreas and results of aggressive surgical treatment. Am J Surg 1992;164:437.

Itoh S et al: Mucin-producing pancreatic tumor: CT findings and histopathologic correlation. Radiology 1992; 183:81.

Lewandrowski KB et al: Cyst fluid analysis in the differential diagnosis of pancreatic cysts: A comparison of pseudocysts, serous cystadenomas, mucinous cystic neoplasms, and mucinous cystadenocarcinoma. Ann Surg 1993;217:41.

Lewandrowski K, Warshaw A, Compton C: Macrocystic serous cystadenoma of the pancreas: A morphologic variant differing from microcystic adenoma. Hum Pathol 1992;23:871.

Nishihara K et al: Papillary cystic tumors of the pancreas: Assessment of their malignant potential. Cancer 1993;71:82.

Pettinato G et al: Papillary cystic tumor of the pancreas: A clinicopathologic study of 20 cases with cytologic, immunohistochemical, ultrastructural, and flow cytometric observations, and a review of the literature. Am J Clin Pathol 1992;98:478.

Pyke CM, et al: The spectrum of serous cystadenoma of the pancreas: Clinical, pathologic, and surgical aspects. Ann Surg 1992;215:132.

Rickaert F et al: Intraductal mucin-hypersecreting neoplasms of the pancreas. Gastroenterology 1991;101:512.

Sclafani LM et al: The malignant nature of papillary and cystic neoplasm of the pancreas. Cancer 1991;68:153.

Talamini MA et al: Spectrum of cystic tumors of the pancreas. Am J Surg 1992;163:117.

Yamada M et al: Mucin-producing tumor of the pancreas. Cancer 1991;68:159.

Zinner MJ, Shurbaji MS, Cameron JL: Solid and papillary epithelial neoplasms of the pancreas. Surgery 1990;108:475.

ADENOMA & ADENOCARCINOMA OF THE AMPULLA OF VATER

Adenoma and adenocarcinoma of the ampulla of Vater account for about 10% of neoplasms that obstruct the distal bile duct. One-third are adenomas and two-thirds adenocarcinomas. Since a remnant of benign adenoma can be found in a majority of adenocarcinomas, it is suspected that malignant change in an adenoma gives rise to most carcinomas. The presenting symptom is most often jaundice or occasionally gastrointestinal bleeding. Weight loss and pain are more common with carcinoma than with adenoma, but the differences are not great enough to allow a distinction to be made on this basis alone.

CT and ultrasound scans reveal dilatation of the biliary tree and pancreatic duct. Gallstones are an incidental finding in 20% of patients, and when common duct stones are present, they may incorrectly be held responsible for the biliary obstruction. The most important diagnostic study is ERCP. In 75% of cases, tumor is visible on duodenoscopy as an exophytic papillary lesion, an ulcerated tumor, or an infiltrating mass. An adequate biopsy usually can be obtained of these lesions. In 25% of cases, there is no intraduodenal growth, and endoscopic sphincterotomy is necessary to display the tumor. It is best to wait 10–14 days to biopsy these tumors because of transient artifacts that result from the sphincterotomy. ERCP also demonstrates dilatation of the biliary and pancreatic ducts. It has become common to perform a sphincterotomy whenever possible, not only to facilitate performance of a biopsy but also to decompress the biliary tree and allow jaundice to subside in anticipation of subsequent surgical therapy. The value of this step has not been established.

Although some adenomas have been successfully treated by snare excision or, preferably, by neodymium:YAG laser destruction, local resection or pancreaticoduodenectomy is preferable because of the significant chance that an invasive carcinoma will be undertreated at a time that it is curable. These nonsurgical methods should be reserved for patients who are poor candidates for resection.

Treatment of adenocarcinoma consists of pancreaticoduodenectomy as for pancreatic carcinoma. The operative mortality rate is less than 5%, and the 5-year survival rate is about 50%. The presence of metastases in resectable peripancreatic lymph nodes is not a contraindication to pancreaticoduodenectomy, for the 5-year survival rate under these circumstances is still a respectable 25%. Local excision is an alternative for noninfiltrating papillary adenocarcinomas in patients who are too poor a risk for pancreaticoduodenectomy, but this operation is not as successful as pancreaticoduodenectomy. Endoscopic sphincterotomy alone or with retrograde stent placement (the combination is usually required) is indicated when there is definite evidence (eg, hepatic metastases) that the tumor is incurable. Survival averages less than a year with this approach, however.

Dawson PJ, Connolly MM: Influence of site of origin and mucin production on survival in ampullary carcinoma. Ann Surg 1989;210:173.

Farouk M et al: Indications for and the technique of local resection of tumors of the papilla of Vater. Arch Surg 1991;126:650.

Gray G, Browder W: Villous tumors of the ampulla of Vater. South Med J 1989;82:917.

Kimura W, Ohtsubo K: Incidence, sites of origin, and immunohistochemical and histochemical characteristics of atypical epithelium and minute carcinoma of the papilla of Vater. Cancer 1988;61:1394.

Monson JRT et al: Radical resection for carcinoma of the ampulla of Vater. Arch Surg 1991;126:353.

Ponchon T et al: Contribution of endoscopy to diagnosis and treatment of tumors of the ampulla of Vater. Cancer 1989;64:161.

Yamaguchi K, Enjoji M: Carcinoma of the ampulla of Vater: A clinicopathologic study and pathologic staging of 109 cases of carcinoma and five cases of adenoma. Cancer 1987;59:506.

PANCREATIC ISLET CELL TUMORS

Islet cell tumors may be functioning (ie, hormone-producing) or nonfunctioning, malignant or nonmalignant. More than half are functioning; less than half are malignant. Insulinoma, the most common functioning islet cell neoplasm, arises from beta cells and produces insulin and symptoms of hypoglycemia. Tumors of the δ or α_1 cells produce gastrin and the Zollinger-Ellison syndrome. Alpha$_2$ cell neoplasms may produce excess glucagon and hyperglycemia. Non-beta islet cell tumors may secrete serotonin, ACTH, MSH, and kinins (and evoke the carcinoid syndrome). Some produce pancreatic cholera, a severe diarrheal illness.

1. NONFUNCTIONING ISLET CELL TUMORS

Most of these lesions are malignant tumors of the head of the gland, which present with abdominal and back pain, weight loss, and, in many cases, a palpable abdominal mass. Jaundice is seen occasionally. The patients do not have MEN-I syndrome. CT scans reveal a pancreatic mass, and angiography typically shows it to be hypervascular. The histologic pattern on biopsy specimens is diagnostic of islet cell tumor, but whether or not the lesion is malignant rests on evidence of invasiveness or metastases, not the appearance of the cells. Immunohistochemical staining of the tissue is positive for chromogranin and neuron-specific enolase (markers of APUD tumors). Metastases are present at the time of diagnosis in 80% of patients. Resection of all gross tumor (eg, by a Whipple procedure), the preferred treatment, is possible in less than half of patients because of local extension or distant metastases. A combination of streptozocin and doxorubicin is the most effective chemotherapeutic regimen. The 5-year disease-free survival rate is about 15%.

Legaspi A, Brennan MF: Management of islet cell carcinoma. Surgery 1988;104:1018.

Moertel CG, et al: Streptozocin-doxorubicin, streptozocin-fluorouracil or chlorozotocin in the treatment of advanced islet-cell carcinoma. N Engl J Med 1992; 326:519.

Thompson GB et al: Islet cell carcinomas of the pancreas: A twenty-year experience. Surgery 1988;104:1011.

Venkatesh S et al: Islet cell carcinoma of the pancreas. Cancer 1990;65:354.

2. INSULINOMA

Insulinomas have been reported in all age groups. About 75% are solitary and benign. About 10% are malignant, and metastases are usually evident at the time of diagnosis. The remaining 15% are manifestations of multifocal pancreatic disease—either adenomatosis, nesidioblastosis, or islet cell hyperplasia.

The symptoms (related to cerebral glucose deprivation) are bizarre behavior, memory lapse, or unconsciousness. Patients may be mistakenly treated for psychiatric illness. There may be profuse sympathetic discharge, with palpitations, sweating, and tremulousness. Hypoglycemic episodes are usually precipitated by fasting and are relieved by food, so weight gain is common. The classic diagnostic criteria (**Whipple's triad**) are present in most cases: (1) hypoglycemic symptoms produced by fasting, (2) blood glucose below 50 mg/dL during symptomatic episodes, and (3) relief of symptoms by intravenous administration of glucose.

The most useful diagnostic test and the only one indicated in all but a few patients is demonstration of fasting hypoglycemia in the presence of inappropriately high levels of insulin. The patient is fasted, and blood samples are obtained every 6 hours for glucose and insulin measurements. The fast is continued until hypoglycemia or symptoms appear or for a maximum of 72 hours. If hypoglycemia has not developed after 70 hours, the patient should be exercised for the final 2 hours. Although insulin levels are not always elevated in patients with insulinoma, they will be high relative to the blood glucose concentration. A ratio of plasma insulin to glucose greater than 0.3 is diagnostic. Ratios should be calculated before and during the fast. Proinsulin, which constitutes more than 25% of total insulin (the upper limit of normal) in about 85% of patients with insulinomas, should also be measured. Proinsulin levels greater than 40% suggest a malignant islet cell tumor.

Drugs that release insulin (tolbutamide, glucagon, leucine, arginine, calcium) were used in the past as provocative tests. The tolbutamide test is safe in patients whose fasting glucose exceeds 50 mg/dL, and it is still occasionally used.

Localization of the tumor is important but may be difficult. In about 10% of cases, the tumor is so small or located so deeply that it is difficult or impossible to find at laparotomy. High-resolution CT and MR scans are successful in demonstrating about 40% of tumors. Endoscopic (gastroscopic) ultrasound examination of the pancreas may be able to show a much higher percentage, but data are still sparse. Angiography gives a yield of about 50%. Transhepatic portal venous sampling has proved to be the most accurate preoperative localizing method, demonstrating the position in the pancreas of about 95% of lesions. This test, which is time consuming and somewhat invasive, involves entering the portal vein with a catheter passed percutaneously through the liver and testing blood at various sites within the portal, superior mesenteric, and splenic veins for insulin levels. The point where insulin concentrations rise sharply indicates the site of the tumor. This procedure may be considered when arteriography is negative and in patients with MEN-I, who may have multiple tumors only one of which is secreting insulin. Probably the most important simple way to search for small insulinomas is by using operative ultrasound.

Differential Diagnosis

Fasting hypoglycemia may be a manifestation of some nonpancreatic, non-islet cell tumors. Clinically, the condition is identical to that resulting from insulinoma, but the cause is rarely secretion of insulin by the tumors, as serum insulin levels are normal. Most non-islet cell tumors associated with hypoglycemia are large and readily detected on physical examination. The majority are of mesenchymal origin (eg, hemangiopericytoma, fibrosarcoma, leiomyosarcoma) and are located in the abdomen or thorax, but hepatoma, adrenocortical carcinoma, and a variety of other lesions may also produce hypoglycemia. The principal means by which these tumors produce hypoglycemia are the following: (1) secretion by the tumor of insulin-like growth factor II (IGF-II), an insulin-like peptide that normally mediates the effects of growth hormone; and (2) inhibition of glycogenolysis or gluconeogenesis. Rapid utilization of glucose by the tumor, replacement of liver tissue by metastases, and secretion of insulin are other postulated mechanisms that are probably uncommon.

Surreptitious self-administration of insulin is seen occasionally, most often in an individual with access to insulin on the job. If insulin injections have been given for as long as 2 months, insulin antibodies will be detectable in the patient's serum. Circulating C peptide levels are normal in these patients but elevated in most patients with insulinoma. Sulfonylurea ingestion can be detected by measuring the drug in plasma.

Treatment

Surgery should be done promptly, because with repeated hypoglycemic attacks, permanent cerebral damage occurs and the patient becomes progressively more obese. Moreover, the tumor may be malignant. Medical treatment is reserved for surgically incurable lesions.

A. Medical Treatment: Diazoxide is administered to suppress insulin release. For incurable islet cell carcinomas, streptozocin is the best chemotherapeutic agent. Sixty percent of patients live up to 2 additional years. Toxicity is considerable; streptozocin is not recommended as a routine adjunct to surgical therapy.

B. Surgical Treatment: At surgery, the entire pancreas must be palpated carefully, because the tumors are usually small and difficult to find. The gland should also be examined intraoperatively with ultrasound, which may be able to locate a tumor that cannot be felt, or to demonstrate signs of invasion (ie, irregular borders) that indicate malignancy—something that cannot be detected by palpation. When the tumor is found, it may be enucleated if it is superficial or resected as part of a partial pancreatectomy if it is

deep-seated or invasive. Insulinomas in the head of the gland can nearly always be enucleated.

In the past, the tumor could not be detected in about 5% of cases by these methods. The traditional recommendation was to resect the distal half of the pancreas and have the pathologist slice the specimen into thin sections and look for the tumor. If the tumor was found, the operation was concluded; if it was not found, additional pancreas would be resected until an 80% distal pancreatectomy had been performed. Since the tumors are evenly distributed, this strategy is 80% successful in removing the tumor. Intraoperative monitoring of blood glucose is often done as a means of determining if the tumor has been excised, but it is unreliable. With the use of preoperative measurement of insulin levels in splenic and portal vein blood and operative ultrasound scanning, however, no more than 1–2% of insulinomas remain occult, and blind distal pancreatectomy is rarely even considered.

Patients with insulinoma associated with MEN-1 usually have multiple (average of three) lesions. Because persistence of the disease is much more likely in this condition following the standard surgical approach, the operation recommended here is distal pancreatectomy plus enucleation of any lesions found in the head of the gland.

For islet cell hyperplasia, nesidioblastosis, or multiple benign adenomas, distal subtotal pancreatectomy usually decreases insulin levels enough that medical management is simplified. For islet cell carcinomas, resection of both primary and metastatic lesions is warranted if technically feasible.

Patients with sporadic insulinomas lead a normal life after the tumor has been removed. The outcome is less predictable in patients with MEN-1, who usually have several insulin-producing tumors.

Axelrod L, Ron D: Insulin-like growth factor II and the riddle of tumor-induced hypoglycemia. N Engl J Med 1988;319:1477.

Demeure MJ et al: Insulinomas associated with multiple endocrine neoplasia type I: The need for a different surgical approach. Surgery 1991;110:998.

Doherty GM et al: Results of a prospective strategy to diagnose, localize, and resect insulinomas. Surgery 1991; 110:989.

Fedorak IJ et al: Localization of islet cell tumors of the pancreas: A review of current techniques. Surgery 1993;113:242.

Grama D et al: Pancreatic tumors in multiple endocrine neoplasia type 1: Clinical presentation and surgical treatment. World J Surg 1992;16:611.

Grunberger G et al: Factitious hypoglycemia due to surreptitious administration of insulin: Diagnosis, treatment, and long-term follow-up. Ann Intern Med 1988;108:252.

Marks V: Recognition and differential diagnosis of spontaneous hypoglycaemia. Clin Endocrinol 1992;37:309.

Norton JA et al: Localization and surgical treatment of occult insulinomas. Ann Surg 1990;212:615.

Pasieka JL et al: Surgical approach to insulinomas: Assessing the need for preoperative localization. Ann Surg 1992;127:442.

Rosch T et al: Localization of pancreatic endocrine tumors by endoscopic ultrasonography. N Engl J Med 1992; 326:1721.

Service FJ et al: Functioning insulinoma: Incidence, recurrence, and long-term survival of patients. Mayo Clin Proc 1991;66:711.

Service FJ: Hypoglycemias. West J Med 1991;154:442.

van Heerden JA et al: Occult functioning insulinomas: which localizing studies are indicated? Surgery 1992; 112:1010.

Vinik AI et al: Transhepatic portal vein catheterization for localization of insulinomas: A ten-year experience. Surgery 1991;109:1.

3. PANCREATIC CHOLERA (WDHA Syndrome: Watery Diarrhea, Hypokalemia, & Achlorhydria)

Most cases of pancreatic cholera are caused by a non-beta islet cell tumor of the pancreas that secretes VIP (vasoactive intestinal polypeptide) and peptide histidine isoleucine. The syndrome is characterized by profuse watery diarrhea, massive fecal loss of potassium, low serum potassium, and extreme weakness. Gastric acid secretion is usually low or absent even after stimulation with betazole or pentagastrin. Stool volume averages about 5 L/d during acute episodes and contains over 300 meq of potassium (20 times normal). Severe metabolic acidosis frequently results from loss of bicarbonate in the stool. Many patients are hypercalcemic, possibly from secretion by the tumor of a parathyroid hormone-like substance. Abnormal glucose tolerance may result from hypokalemia and altered sensitivity to insulin. Patients who complain of severe diarrhea must be studied carefully for other causes before the diagnosis of WDHA syndrome is entertained seriously. Chronic laxative abuse is a frequent explanation.

Preoperative angiography should be used in an attempt to localize the tumor. Approximately 80% of the tumors are solitary, located in the body or tail, and can be removed easily. About half of the lesions are malignant, and three-fourths of those have metastasized by the time of exploration. Even if all of the tumor cannot be removed, resection of most of it alleviates symptoms in about 40% of patients even though the average survival is only 1 year. If the neoplasm cannot be identified grossly at operation, distal pancreatectomy should be performed. Streptozocin has produced remissions in several cases, but nephrotoxicity may limit its effectiveness. Selective arterial administration is preferred when renal function is impaired. Treatment with long-acting somatostatin analogs decreases VIP levels, controls diarrhea, and may even reduce tumor size. The effect persists indefinitely in most patients, but in a few it is transient. Calcitonin has also been useful in some patients.

4. GLUCAGONOMA

Glucagonoma syndrome is characterized by migratory necrolytic dermatitis (usually involving the legs and perineum), weight loss, stomatitis, hypoaminoacidemia, anemia, and mild to moderate diabetes mellitus. Scotomas and changes in visual acuity have been reported in some cases. The age range is 20–70 years, and the condition is more common in women. The diagnosis may be suspected from the distinctive skin lesion; in fact, the presence of a prominent rash in a patient with diabetes mellitus should be enough to raise suspicions. Glucagonoma should also be suspected in any patient with new onset of diabetes after age 60. Confirmation of the diagnosis depends on measuring elevated serum glucagon levels. CT scans demonstrate the tumor and sites of spread. Angiography is not essential but reveals a hypervascular lesion.

Glucagonomas arise from α_2 cells in the pancreatic islets. Most are large at the time of diagnosis. About 25% are benign and confined to the pancreas. The remainder have metastasized by the time of diagnosis, most often to the liver, lymph nodes, adrenal gland, or vertebrae. A few cases have been the result of islet cell hyperplasia.

Severe malnutrition should be corrected preoperatively with a period of total parenteral nutrition. Surgical removal of the primary lesion and resectable secondaries is indicated if technically feasible. If the tumor is confined to the pancreas, cure is possible. Even if it is not possible to remove all the tumor deposits, considerable palliation may result from subtotal removal, so surgery is indicated in almost every case. Low-dose heparin therapy should be administered pre- and postoperatively because of a high risk of deep venous thrombosis and pulmonary embolism. Streptozocin and dacarbazine are the most effective chemotherapeutic agents for unresectable lesions. Somatostatin therapy normalizes serum glucagon and amino acid levels, clears the rash, and promotes weight gain. The clinical course generally parallels changes in serum levels of glucagon in response to therapy.

Boden G: Glucagonomas and insulinomas. Gastroenterol Clin North Am 1989;18:831,

Edney JA et al: Glucagonoma syndrome is an underdiagnosed clinical entity. Am J Surg 1990;160:625.

Holmes A et al: Reversal of a neurologic paraneoplastic syndrome with octreotide (Sandostatin) in a patient with glucagonoma. Am J Med 1991;91:434.

Howard TJ et al: Anatomic distribution of pancreatic endocrine tumors. Am J Surg 1990;159:258.

Mozell E et al: Functional endocrine tumors of the pancreas: Clinical presentation, diagnosis, and treatment. Curr Probl Surg 1990(Jun);27:301.

Shepherd ME et al: Treatment of necrolytic migratory erythema in glucagonoma syndrome. J Am Acad Dermatol 1991;25(5 Part 2):925.

5. SOMATOSTATINOMA

Somatostatinomas are characterized by diabetes mellitus (usually mild), diarrhea and malabsorption, and dilatation of the gallbladder (usually with cholelithiasis). Serum calcitonin and IgM concentrations may be elevated. The syndrome results from secretion of somatostatin by an islet cell tumor of the pancreas, half of which are malignant and accompanied by hepatic metastases. The lesion is usually large and readily demonstrated by CT scan. The diagnosis may be made by recognizing the clinical syndrome and measuring increased concentrations of somatostatin in the serum. Often, however, the somatostatin syndrome is unsuspected until histologic evidence of metastatic islet cell carcinoma has been obtained. When the disease is localized, resection is able to cure about 50% of cases. Enucleation is inappropriate for these tumors. Chemotherapy with streptozocin, dacarbazine, doxorubicin, etc, is the best treatment for unresectable tumors. Small somatostatin-rich tumors of the duodenum or ampulla of Vater have also been reported, but none of these lesions have been associated with high serum levels of somatostatin or the clinical syndrome.

Vinik AI, Moattari AR: Treatment of endocrine tumors of the pancreas. Endocrinol Metab Clin North Am 1989;18:483.

REFERENCES

Howard JM, Jordan GL, Reber HA (editors): *Surgical Diseases of the Pancreas.* Lea & Febiger, 1987.

Reber HA (guest editor): The pancreas. Surg Clin North Am 1989;69:447.

Spleen

28

David C. Hohn, MD

ANATOMY

The spleen is a dark purplish, highly vascular, coffee bean-shaped organ situated in the left upper quadrant of the abdomen at the level of the eighth to eleventh ribs between the fundus of the stomach, the diaphragm, the splenic flexure of the colon, and the left kidney (Figure 28–1). The adult spleen weighs 100–150 g, measures about 12 × 7 × 4 cm, and usually cannot be palpated. It is attached to adjacent viscera and the abdominal wall by peritoneal folds or "ligaments." The gastrosplenic ligament carries the short gastric vessels. The other ligaments are avascular except in patients with portal hypertension or myelofibrosis.

The splenic capsule consists of peritoneum overlying a 1- to 2-mm fibroelastic layer that contains a few smooth muscle cells. The fibroelastic layer sends into the pulp numerous fibrous bands (trabeculae) that form the framework of the spleen. In dogs and cats, but not humans, the spleen stores blood that is autotransfused when the organ contracts in response to circulating catecholamines.

The splenic artery enters the hilum of the spleen, branches into the trabecular arteries, and then branches into the central arteries that course through the surrounding white pulp and send terminal branches to the peripheral marginal zone and the more distant red pulp. The white pulp consists of lymphatic tissue and lymphoid follicles containing predominantly lymphocytes, plasma cells, and macrophages distributed throughout a reticular network. The vascular spaces of the marginal zone between the red and white pulp contain mostly plasma and are a preferential location for sequestration of foreign material and abnormal cells. The red pulp is made up of cords of reticular cells and sinuses forming a honeycombed vascular space.

PHYSIOLOGY

Although the human spleen has reticuloendothelial, immunologic, and storage functions, normal life is possible without a spleen.

Although the spleen contains only 1% of the total red cell mass, each red cell averages 1000 passes through the spleen each day. Normal blood cells pass rapidly through the spleen, while abnormal and senescent cells are retarded and entrapped. As they travel through the hypoxic, acidotic, glucose-deprived splenic channels, red cells are "conditioned," becoming more susceptible to subsequent trapping and destruction. In the presence of splenomegaly and other disease states, the flow patterns of the spleen become more circuitous, so that even normal cells may be trapped.

The adult spleen produces monocytes, lymphocytes, and plasma cells. Production of other blood elements occurs in patients with myeloid metaplasia and in the fetal spleen.

Lymphocytes, the predominant cells of the spleen, produce antibodies (immunoglobulins). The spleen is particularly well suited to antibody formation, since plasma is skimmed by the trabecular arteries and delivered to the lymphoid follicles, bringing soluble antigens into direct contact with immunologically competent cells. Cells and particulate matter, including particulate antigens (eg, bacteria), travel through the sluggish sinuses and cords and make direct contact with the macrophages that line these vascular channels. Although phagocytosis and synthesis of immunoglobulins also occur in other organs, the spleen appears to have a central role in the development of new antibodies (especially IgM) after initial exposure to foreign antigens. This is especially important in infancy and explains the special susceptibility to infection that follows splenectomy in children under 2 years of age. Even in adults, splenectomy leads to a slight but definite reduction in immune function.

Normally, about 30% of the total platelet pool is sequestered in the spleen, but as much as 80% can be sequestered in patients with splenomegaly. Sequestration and increased splenic destruction of platelets account for the thrombocytopenia that often accompanies splenomegaly.

HYPERSPLENISM

In the past, the term hypersplenism has been used to denote the syndrome characterized by splenic enlargement, deficiency of one or more blood cell lines, normal or hyperplastic cellularity of deficient cell

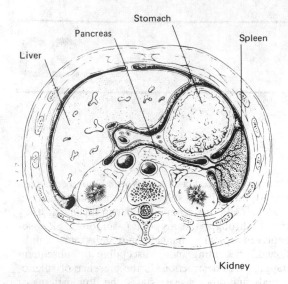

Figure 28–1. Normal anatomic relations of the spleen.

lines in the marrow, and increased turnover of affected cells. If the defect was not corrected by splenectomy, the diagnosis was considered incorrect.

It is now recognized that some disorders in which there is spleen-dependent destruction of blood elements do not manifest all features of hypersplenism. For example, splenomegaly is rarely a feature of immune thrombocytopenic purpura, and splenectomy is not always curative. In disorders with known pathogenesis, the recent trend has been to classify them as separate disease entities rather than as hypersplenic conditions.

The defects in hypersplenism are exaggerations of normal splenic functions, such as removal and destruction of aged or defective cells, sequestration of normal cells, and production of immunoglobulins. The principal cause of cytopenias in hypersplenism is increased sequestration and destruction of blood cells in the spleen. Etiologic factors include (1) splenic enlargement, (2) intrinsic defects in blood cells, or (3) autoimmune destruction of blood cells. The hyperplastic spleen is not selective in its hyperfunction. For example, even though the splenomegaly may have been induced by sequestration of abnormal red cells (eg, hemolytic anemia), platelets and leukocytes may also be destroyed more rapidly than normal.

Primary hypersplenism is a diagnosis of exclusion reached after a careful search (including pathologic examination of the spleen) for conditions that can produce secondary hypersplenism. True primary hypersplenism is exceedingly rare; most cases diagnosed as primary hypersplenism involve intrinsic defects in the blood cells or the presence of unrecognized blood cell antibodies. What appears to be primary hypersplenism may be an early manifesta-

tion of lymphoma or leukemia, since these cancers develop in some patients after splenectomy.

Secondary hypersplenism occurs in association with splenomegaly of known cause. It is most often due to congestive splenomegaly caused by portal hypertension (cirrhosis or portal or splenic vein obstruction) or by neoplastic diseases involving the spleen (eg, lymphoma, myeloid metaplasia, leukemia) (Table 28–1).

About 60% of patients with cirrhosis develop splenomegaly and 15% develop hypersplenism. The hypersplenism of cirrhosis is seldom of clinical significance; the anemia and thrombocytopenia are usually mild and rarely are indications for splenectomy.

If portal decompression is indicated for bleeding esophageal varices, any procedure that lowers the portal pressure tends to improve the thrombocytopenia and anemia and reduce the size of the spleen. It is rare for hypersplenism to develop after a successful portal-systemic shunt. In the rare case of portal hypertension caused by massive splenomegaly and huge splenic blood flow, splenectomy alone will cure the hypersplenism and portal hypertension.

Several inflammatory diseases cause secondary hypersplenism. Sarcoidosis is complicated by splenomegaly in 25% of patients and secondary hypersplenism in about 5%. Patients with chronic rheumatoid arthritis may develop splenomegaly and neutropenia, an association known as **Felty's syndrome.**

Hairy-cell leukemia (leukemic reticuloendotheliosis) is a B lymphocyte cancer that usually presents with hypersplenism and palpable splenomegaly. Infection due to leukopenia is common. Alpha interferon is now the preferred treatment for most patients. The response rate is about 80%. Splenectomy is indicated as initial therapy for patients with massive splenomegaly, cytopenia, and a low number of hairy cells in the marrow. Adenosine deaminase inhibitors (oxycoformycin, chlorodeoxyadenosine) remain experimental but show promise.

In occasional patients with chronic leukemia or lymphoma, the spleen may be the predominant site of residual disease, or hypersplenism may preclude fur-

Table 28–1. Disorders associated with secondary hypersplenism.

Congestive splenomegaly (cirrhosis, portal or splenic vein obstruction)
Neoplasm (leukemia, lymphoma, metastatic carcinoma)
Inflammatory disease (sarcoid, lupus erythematosus, Felty's syndrome)
Acute infections with splenomegaly
Chronic infection (tuberculosis, brucellosis, malaria)
Storage diseases (Gaucher's disease, Letterer-Siwe disease, amyloidosis)
Chronic hemolytic diseases (spherocytosis, thalassemia, glucose 6-phosphate dehydrogenase deficiency, elliptocytosis)
Myeloproliferative disorders (myelofibrosis with myeloid metaplasia)

ther chemotherapy. Splenectomy may benefit such patients.

Clinical Findings

A. Symptoms and Signs: The clinical findings depend largely on the underlying disorder. Manifestations of hypersplenism usually develop gradually, and the diagnosis often follows a routine physical or laboratory examination. Some patients experience left upper quadrant fullness or discomfort, which can be severe. Others have hematemesis due to gastroesophageal varices.

Purpura, bruising, and diffuse mucous membrane bleeding are unusual symptoms despite the presence of thrombocytopenia. Recurrent infections and chronic leg ulcers are sometimes seen in patients with Felty's syndrome and severe leukopenia.

B. Laboratory Findings: Patients with primary hypersplenism usually exhibit pancytopenia of moderate degree and generalized marrow hyperplasia. Severe deficiency of one or more cell lines may imply (1) bleeding, (2) marrow aplasia, or (3) an underlying disorder causing secondary hypersplenism (hemolytic anemia, Felty's syndrome, etc). Abnormalities of red cell morphology are seen with thalassemia, clliptocytosis, and myclofibrosis.

C. Evaluation of Splenic Size: Before it becomes palpable, an enlarged spleen may cause dullness to percussion above the left costal margin. Splenomegaly is manifested on supine x-rays of the abdomen by medial displacement of the stomach and downward displacement of the transverse colon and splenic flexure. Technetium-99m sulfur colloid imaging and CT scans are useful for differentiating the spleen from other abdominal masses and for demonstrating splenic enlargement or intrasplenic lesions.

D. Evaluation of Splenic Function: Reduced red cell or platelet survival can be measured by labeling the patient's cells with ^{51}Cr or the platelets with indium-111 and measuring the rate of disappearance of radioactivity from the blood. The spleen's role in producing the anemia or thrombocytopenia can be determined by measuring the ratio of radioactivity that accumulates in the liver and spleen during destruction of the tagged cells; a spleen/liver ratio greater than 2:1 indicates significant splenic pooling and suggests that splenectomy would be beneficial.

Differential Diagnosis

Leukemia and lymphoma are diagnosed by marrow aspiration, lymph node biopsy, and examination of the peripheral blood (white count and differential). In hereditary spherocytosis there are spherocytes, osmotic fragility is increased, and platelets and white cells are normal. The hemoglobinopathies with splenomegaly are differentiated on the basis of hemoglobin electrophoresis or the demonstration of an unstable hemoglobin. Thalassemia major becomes apparent in early childhood, and the blood smear

morphology is characteristic. In myelofibrosis, the bone marrow shows proliferation of fibroblasts and replacement of normal elements. In idiopathic thrombocytopenic purpura, the spleen is normal or only slightly enlarged. In aplastic anemia, the spleen is not enlarged and the marrow is fatty.

Treatment & Prognosis

The course, response to treatment, and prognosis of the hypersplenic syndromes differ widely depending on the underlying disease and its response to treatment. For example, hypersplenism in malaria responds to antimalarial therapy. In some diseases, especially those involving immune reactions, corticosteroids are effective.

The indications for splenectomy are given in Table 28–2. Splenectomy should be performed for primary hypersplenism. In secondary hypersplenism, the severity and prognosis of the primary disease and the risk of surgery must be considered. Splenectomy may decrease transfusion requirements, decrease the incidence and number of infections, prevent hemorrhage, and reduce pain. Because many patients with hypersplenism are poor surgical risks, splenic embolization, a form of nonsurgical splenectomy, has been developed. Substances such as absolute alcohol, polyvinyl alcohol foam, polystyrene, or silicone are

Table 28–2. Indications for splenectomy.

Splenectomy always indicated
    Primary splenic tumor (rare)
    Hereditary spherocytosis (congenital hemolytic anemia)
Splenectomy usually indicated
    Primary hypersplenism
    Chronic immune thrombocytopenic purpura
    Splenic vein thrombosis causing esophageal varices
    Splenic abscess (rare)
Splenectomy sometimes indicated
    Splenic injury
    Autoimmune hemolytic disease
    Elliptocytosis with hemolysis
    Nonspherocytic congenital hemolytic anemias (eg, pyruvate kinase deficiency)
    Hemoglobin H disease
    Hodgkin's disease (for staging)
    Thrombotic thrombocytopenic purpura
    Myelofibrosis
Splenectomy rarely indicated
    Chronic leukemia
    Splenic lymphoma
    Macroglobulinemia
    Thalassemia major
    Splenic artery aneurysm
    Sickle cell anemia
    Congestive splenomegaly and hypersplenism due to portal hypertension
Splenectomy not indicated
    Asymptomatic hypersplenism
    Splenomegaly with infection
    Splenomegaly associated with elevated IgM
    Hereditary hemolytic anemia of moderate degree
    Acute leukemia
    Agranulocytosis

injected into the splenic artery to decrease splenic mass and function. Partial embolization has also been performed in an effort to ablate enough splenic tissue to improve the hematologic status while still preserving immune function. Transarterial placement of metal coils has also been used to occlude the splenic artery preoperatively in an effort to reduce hemorrhage at surgery. Splenic abscesses, pain due to tissue infarction, and even death from pancreatitis have been reported with these procedures. The optimal technique for occlusion and the clinical indications for splenic embolization are still to be defined.

Splenectomy may not be necessary when hypersplenism is mild. Operation is also contraindicated in the following diseases where it has been shown to have no therapeutic benefit: acute leukemia, agranulocytosis, paroxysmal nocturnal hemoglobinuria, and Wiskott-Aldrich syndrome. In sickle cell anemia, splenectomy is rarely necessary, because autosplenectomy has usually occurred by age 10.

Some of the best results have followed splenectomy for Felty's syndrome, myeloid metaplasia, chronic malaria, and tuberculosis of the spleen. Less satisfactory results have been achieved in thalassemia major, sickle cell anemia, and the secondary hypersplenism of lymphoma and the leukemias. Splenectomy may rarely be required in patients with leukemia and lymphoma when severe cytopenias limit further treatment or bone marrow transplantation or when the spleen is thought to be the major site of residual disease. Hypersplenism develops in 5–10% of uremic patients undergoing long-term hemodialysis. Therapeutic splenectomy is being performed with increasing frequency in such patients.

The course of congestive splenomegaly due to portal hypertension depends upon the degree of venous obstruction and liver damage. The hypersplenism is rarely a major problem and is almost always overshadowed by variceal bleeding or liver dysfunction.

Black LM et al: Hazards of splenic embolization. Clin Pediatr 1987;26:292.

Brandt CT et al: Splenic embolization in children: Long-term efficacy. J Pediatr Surg 1989;24:642.

Coon WW: Splenectomy for thrombocytopenia due to secondary hypersplenism. Arch Surg 1988;123:369.

Damasio EE et al: Splenectomy after initial therapy with alpha-IFN in patients with hairy-cell leukemia (HCL): A multi-center study by the Italian Cooperative Group for HCL. Eur J Haematol 1990;45(Suppl 52):29.

Danforth DN, Fraker DL: Splenectomy for the massively enlarged spleen. Am Surg 1991;56:108.

Dawson AA, Jones PF, King DJ: Splenectomy in the management of haematological disease. Br J Surg 1987;74:353.

Delpero JR et al: Splenectomy for hypersplenism in chronic lymphocytic leukaemia and malignant non-Hodgkin's lymphoma. Br J Surg 1990;77:443.

Dodds WJ et al: Radiologic imaging of splenic anomalies. Am J Roentgenol 1990;155:805.

Fleshner PR et al: A 27-year experience with splenectomy for Gaucher's disease. Am J Surg 1991;161:69.

Grant IR et al: Elective splenectomy in hematologic disorders. Ann R Coll Surg Engl 1988;70:29.

Lill MCC, Golde DW: Treatment of hairy-cell leukemia. Blood Rev 1990;4:238.

Shah R et al: Partial splenic embolization. Am Surg 1990;56:774.

Sills RH: Splenic function: Physiology and splenic hypofunction. CRC Crit Rev Oncol Hematol 1987;7:1.

Vasquez EJ et al: Partial splenic embolization in hypersplenism. Acta Paediatr Scand 1988;77:593.

Wilhelm MC et al: Splenectomy in hematologic disorders. The ever-changing indications. Ann Surg 1988;207:581.

DISORDERS POTENTIALLY AMENABLE TO SPLENECTOMY

1. HEREDITARY SPHEROCYTOSIS

Essentials of Diagnosis

- Malaise, abdominal discomfort.
- Jaundice, anemia, splenomegaly.
- Spherocytosis, increased osmotic fragility of red cells, negative Coombs test.

General Considerations

Hereditary spherocytosis (congenital hemolytic jaundice, familial hemolytic anemia), the commonest congenital hemolytic anemia, is transmitted as an autosomal dominant trait; it appears to be caused by deficiency of ankyrin, a protein required for assembly of the structural protein spectrin into the red cell membrane. The abnormality produces small, dense, round red cells with increased osmotic fragility and a rigid nondeformable shape. The lack of deformability delays the cells as they pass through the normal gaps and channels in the splenic pulp, resulting in glucose and ATP deprivation, damage to the red cell membranes, and, finally, membrane fragmentation and cell disruption. Significant cell destruction occurs only in the presence of the spleen. Hemolysis is largely relieved by splenectomy.

The condition is seen in all races but is more frequent in whites than in blacks. When discovered early in infancy, it may resemble hemolytic disease of the newborn due to ABO incompatibility. In occasional instances the diagnosis is not made until later in adult life, but it is usually discovered in the first 3 decades.

Clinical Findings

A. Symptoms and Signs: The principal manifestations are splenomegaly, mild to moderate anemia, and jaundice. The patient may complain of easy fatigability. The spleen is almost always enlarged and may cause fullness and discomfort in the left upper quadrant. However, most patients are diagnosed during a family survey at a time when they are asymptomatic.

Periodic exacerbations of hemolysis can occur. The rare hypoplastic crises, which often follow acute viral illnesses, may be associated with profound anemia, headache, nausea, abdominal pain, pancytopenia, and hypoactive marrow.

B. Laboratory Findings: The red cell count and hemoglobin are moderately reduced. Some of the asymptomatic patients detected by family surveys have normal red cell counts when first seen. The red cells are usually normocytic, but microcytosis may occur. Macrocytosis may present during periods of marked reticulocytosis. Spherocytes in varying numbers, sizes, and shapes are seen on a Wright-stained smear. The reticulocyte count is increased to 5–20%.

The indirect serum bilirubin and stool urobilinogen are usually elevated, and serum haptoglobin is usually decreased to absent. The Coombs test is negative. Osmotic fragility is increased; hemolysis of 5–10% of cells may be observed at saline concentrations of 0.6%. Occasionally, the osmotic fragility is normal but the incubated fragility test (defibrinated blood incubated at 37 °C for 24 hours) will show increased hemolysis. Autohemolysis of defibrinated blood incubated under sterile conditions for 48 hours is usually greatly increased (10–20%, compared to a normal value of < 5%). The addition of 10% glucose before incubation will decrease the abnormal osmotic fragility and autohemolysis. Infusion of the patient's own blood labeled with ^{51}Cr shows a greatly shortened red cell life span and sequestration in the spleen. Normal red cells labeled with ^{51}Cr have a normal life span when transfused into a spherocytotic patient, indicating that splenic function is normal.

Differential Diagnosis

At present there is no pathognomonic test for hereditary spherocytosis. Spherocytes in large numbers may occur in autoimmune hemolytic anemias, in which osmotic fragility and autohemolysis may be increased but are usually not improved by incubation with glucose. The positive Coombs test, negative family history, and sharply reduced survival of normal donor red cells are diagnostic of autoimmune hemolysis. Spherocytes are also seen in hemoglobin C disease, in some alcoholics, and in some severe burns.

Complications

Pigment gallstones occur in about 85% of adults with spherocytosis but are uncommon under age 10. On the other hand, gallstones in a child should suggest congenital spherocytosis.

Chronic leg ulcers unrelated to varicosities are a rare complication but, when present, will heal only after the spleen is removed.

Treatment

Splenectomy is the sole treatment for hereditary spherocytosis and is indicated even when the anemia is fully compensated and the patient is asymptomatic. The longer the hemolytic process persists, the greater the potential risk of complications such as hypoplastic crises and cholelithiasis. At operation, the gallbladder should be inspected for stones and accessory spleens should be sought. When there is associated cholelithiasis, cholecystectomy should be performed along with the splenectomy. Unless the clinical manifestations are severe, splenectomy should be delayed in children until age 6 to avoid the risk of increased infection due to loss of reticuloendothelial function.

Prognosis

Splenectomy cures the anemia and jaundice in all patients. The membrane abnormality, spherocytosis, and increased osmotic fragility persist, but red cell life span becomes almost normal. An overlooked accessory spleen is an occasional cause of failure of splenectomy. The presence of Howell-Jolly bodies in red cells makes the presence of accessory spleens unlikely.

Boyd AS: Hereditary spherocytosis. Am Fam Phys (Feb) 1989;39:167.

Costa FF et al: Linkage of dominant hereditary spherocytosis to the gene for the erythrocyte membrane-skeleton protein ankyrin. N Eng J Med 1990;323:1046.

Hanspal M et al: Molecular basis of spectrin and ankyrin deficiencies in severe hereditary spherocytosis: evidence implicating a primary defect of ankyrin. Blood 1991; 77:165.

2. HEREDITARY ELLIPTOCYTOSIS

This familial disorder, also known as ovalocytosis, is usually of little clinical significance. Normally, up to 15% oval or elliptic red blood cells can be seen on a peripheral blood smear. In elliptocytosis, at least 25% and up to 90% of circulating erythrocytes are elliptic. As with hereditary spherocytosis, a structural defect in the red cell membrane is responsible for the abnormal shape and the increased splenic destruction.

Most affected individuals are asymptomatic; about 10% have clinical manifestations consisting of moderate anemia, slight jaundice, and a palpable spleen.

Symptomatic patients should have splenectomy, and cholecystectomy if gallstones are present. The red cell defect persists after splenectomy, but the hemolysis and anemia are cured.

Chabanel A et al: Viscoelastic properties of red cell membrane in hereditary elliptocytosis. Blood 1989;73:592.

Liu SC et al: Alteration of the erythrocyte membrane skeletal ultrastructure in hereditary spherocytosis, hereditary elliptocytosis, and pyropoikilocytosis. Blood 1990;76: 198.

3. HEREDITARY NONSPHEROCYTIC HEMOLYTIC ANEMIA

This is a heterogeneous group of rare hemolytic anemias caused by inherited intrinsic red cell defects. Included in the group are pyruvate kinase deficiency and glucose 6-phosphate dehydrogenase (G6PD) deficiency. They are usually manifested in early childhood with anemia, jaundice, reticulocytosis, erythroid hyperplasia of the marrow, and normal osmotic fragility. As with other hemolytic anemias, there may be associated cholelithiasis.

Multiple blood transfusions are often required. Splenectomy, while not curative, may ameliorate some of these conditions, especially pyruvate kinase deficiency. In G6PD deficiency, splenectomy is not beneficial.

Valentine WN et al: Hemolytic anemias and erythrocyte enzymopathies. Ann Intern Med 1985;103:245.

4. THALASSEMIA MAJOR (Mediterranean Anemia; Cooley's Anemia)

In this autosomal dominant disorder, a structural defect in one of the globin chains of the hemoglobin molecule produces abnormal red cells (eg, target cells). Heterozygotes usually have mild anemia (thalassemia minor); however, starting early in infancy, homozygotes have severe chronic anemia accompanied by jaundice, hepatosplenomegaly (often massive), retarded body growth, and enlargement of the head. The peripheral blood smear reveals target cells, nucleated red cells, and a hypochromic microcytic anemia. Gallstones are present in about 25% of patients. A characteristic feature is the persistence of fetal hemoglobin (Hb F).

Although iron chelation is the usual treatment, splenectomy is helpful in some patients by reducing hemolysis and transfusion requirements and by removing an enlarged, uncomfortable spleen.

Cohen A, Gayer R, Mizanin J: Long-term effect of splenectomy on transfusion requirements in thalassemia major. Am J Hematol 1989;30:254.

Maurer HS et al: A prospective evaluation of iron chelation therapy in children with severe beta-thalassemia: A six-year study. Am J Dis Child 1988;142:287.

5. ACQUIRED HEMOLYTIC ANEMIA

Essentials of Diagnosis
- Fatigue, pallor, jaundice.
- Splenomegaly.
- Persistent anemia and reticulocytosis.

General Considerations

Acquired hemolytic anemias were previously classified as either idiopathic (40–50%) or secondary to drug use or an underlying disease (Table 28–3). The **autoimmune hemolytic anemias** have also been classified according to the optimal temperature at which autoantibodies react with the red cell surface (warm or cold antibodies). This classification is particularly useful, since patients with cold antibodies will not benefit from splenectomy but those with warm antibodies may.

Although hemolysis without demonstrable antibody (Coombs test-negative) may occur in uremia, cirrhosis of the liver, cancer, and certain infections, in most cases the red cell membranes are coated with either immunoglobulin or complement (Coombs test-positive). Studies using specific antisera have shown that red cells in warm-antibody hemolytic anemia are coated with IgG, complement (usually C3), or both. Specific IgG receptors are present on macrophages in the spleen and in the reticuloendothelial system, and these cells appear to be responsible for hemolysis. In cold-antibody hemolytic anemia, IgM is bound to a specific antigen on the red cell and mediates fixation of complement (C3b). Erythrocytes in this disorder are removed by hepatic macrophages, and splenectomy is not effective.

About 20% of cases of secondary immune hemolytic anemia are due to drug use, and hemolysis is usually mediated by warm antibodies. Penicillin, quinidine, hydralazine, and methyldopa have been most commonly implicated in this syndrome.

Clinical Findings

A. Symptoms and Signs: Autoimmune hemolytic anemia may be encountered at any age but is most common after age 50; it occurs twice as often in women. The onset is usually acute, consisting of anemia, mild jaundice, and sometimes fever. The spleen is palpably enlarged in over 50% of patients, and pigment gallstones are present in about 25%. Rarely, a sudden severe onset produces hemoglobinuria, renal tubular necrosis, and a 40–50% death rate.

Table 28–3. Disorders associated with immune hemolysis.

Immune drug reaction (penicillin, quinidine, hydralazine, methyldopa, cimetidine)
Collagen vascular disease (lupus erythematosus, rheumatoid arthritis)
Tumors (lymphoma, myeloma, leukemia, dermoid cysts, ovarian teratoma)
Infection (*Mycoplasma*, malaria, syphilis, viremia)

B. Laboratory Findings: Hemolytic anemia is diagnosed by demonstrating a normocytic normochromic anemia, reticulocytosis (over 10%), erythroid hyperplasia of the marrow, and elevation of serum indirect bilirubin. Stool urobilinogen may be greatly increased, but there is no bile in the urine. Serum haptoglobin is usually low or absent. The direct Coombs test is positive because the red cells are coated with immunoglobulins or complement (or both).

Treatment

Associated diseases must be carefully sought and appropriately treated. Corticosteroids produce a remission in about 75% of patients, but only 25% of remissions are permanent. Transfusion should be avoided if possible, since cross-matching may be extremely difficult, requiring washed red cells and saline-active antisera.

Splenectomy is indicated for patients with warm-antibody hemolysis who fail to respond to 4–6 weeks of high-dose corticosteroid therapy, for patients who relapse after an initial response when steroids are withdrawn, and for patients in whom steroid therapy is contraindicated (eg, those with active pulmonary tuberculosis). Patients who require chronic high-dose steroid therapy should also be considered for splenectomy, since the risks of long-term steroid administration are substantial.

Splenectomy is effective because it removes the principal site of red cell destruction. Occasionally, splenectomy discloses the presence of an underlying disorder such as lymphoma. Enthusiasm for routine preoperative use of ^{51}Cr red cell splenic sequestration studies has waned, because predictions of outcome after splenectomy have not been reliable. About half of patients who fail to respond to splenectomy will respond to azathioprine (Imuran) or cyclophosphamide (Cytoxan). Plasmapheresis has recently been employed as salvage therapy in patients with refractory hemolytic anemia.

Prognosis

Relapses may occur after splenectomy but are less frequent if the initial response was good. The ultimate prognosis in the secondary cases depends upon the underlying disorder.

Nydegger UE, Kazatchkine MD, Miescher PA: Immunopathologic and clinical features of hemolytic anemia due to cold agglutinins. Semin Hematol 1991;28:66.

Petz LD: Transfusing the patient with autoimmune hemolytic anemia. Clin Lab Med 1982;2:193.

6. IMMUNE THROMBOCYTOPENIC PURPURA
(Idiopathic Thrombocytopenic Purpura, ITP)

Essentials of Diagnosis

- Petechiae, ecchymoses, epistaxis, easy bruising.
- No splenomegaly.
- Decreased platelet count, prolonged bleeding time, poor clot retraction, normal coagulation time.

General Considerations

Immune thrombocytopenic purpura is a hemorrhagic syndrome with diverse causes and is characterized by marked reduction in the number of circulating platelets, abundant megakaryocytes in the bone marrow, and a shortened platelet life span. It may be idiopathic or secondary to a lymphoproliferative disorder, drugs or toxins, bacterial or viral infection (especially in children), systemic lupus erythematosus, or other conditions. An increased incidence of immune thrombocytopenic purpura has also been identified in homosexual males and appears to be associated with the acquired immunodeficiency syndrome (AIDS). Although responses to corticosteroids and to splenectomy in these patients are comparable to the responses observed in other patients with immune thrombocytopenic purpura, splenectomy should be reserved for those with signs of blood loss, since surgical complications are high and survival may be short. These patients may also have associated opportunistic infections, making corticosteroid treatment more hazardous.

The pathogenesis of both primary and secondary disorders involves a circulating antiplatelet autoantibody that binds to platelets, making them more vulnerable to destruction. The precise role of the spleen in the pathogenesis is unclear; it appears that the spleen may be both a source of antiplatelet antibody and a site of increased platelet destruction. Splenomegaly, present in only 2% of cases, is usually a manifestation of another underlying disease such as lymphoma or lupus erythematosus.

Clinical Findings

A. Symptoms and Signs: The onset may be acute, with ecchymoses or showers of petechiae, and may be accompanied by bleeding gums, vaginal bleeding, gastrointestinal bleeding, and hematuria. Central nervous system bleeding occurs in 3% of patients. The acute form is most common in children, usually occurring before 8 years of age, and often begins 1–3 weeks after a viral upper respiratory illness.

The chronic form, which may start at any age, is more common in women. It characteristically has an insidious onset, often with a long history of easy bruisability and menorrhagia. Showers of petechiae may occur, especially over pressure areas. Cyclic remissions and exacerbations may continue for several years.

B. Laboratory Findings: The platelet count is moderately to severely decreased (always below 100,000/μL), and platelets may be absent from the peripheral blood smear. Although white and red cell counts are usually normal, iron deficiency anemia may be present as a result of bleeding. The bone marrow shows increased numbers of large megakaryocytes without platelet budding.

The bleeding time is prolonged, capillary fragility (Rumpel-Leede test) greatly increased, and clot retraction poor. Partial thromboplastin time, prothrombin time, and coagulation time are normal.

It is now recognized that splenic sequestration studies using ^{51}Cr-tagged platelets correlate poorly with response to splenectomy and are of little value.

Differential Diagnosis

Other causes of nonimmunologic thrombocytopenia must be ruled out, such as leukemia, aplastic anemia, and macroglobulinemia. Thrombocytopenia and purpura may be caused by ineffective thrombocytopoiesis (eg, pernicious anemia, preleukemic states) or by nonimmune platelet destruction (eg, septicemia, disseminated intravascular coagulation, or other causes of hypersplenism).

The diagnosis of immune thrombocytopenic purpura is usually made by exclusion. Through use of anti-IgG monoclonal antibodies, a Coombs test for platelets is being developed that may allow more precise differential diagnosis and treatment selection.

Treatment

Treatment of immune thrombocytopenic purpura depends on the age of the patient, the severity of the disease, the duration of the thrombocytopenia, and the clinical variant. Secondary immune thrombocytopenias are best managed by treating the underlying primary disorder (eg, if it is drug-induced, the drug should be stopped).

Patients with mild or no symptoms need no specific therapy but should avoid contact sports, elective surgery, and all unessential medications. Corticosteroids are indicated in patients with moderate to severe purpura of short duration. Steroids increase the platelet count in 75% of cases, which will avert the danger of severe hemorrhage. Usually, 60 mg of prednisone (or equivalent) is required daily; this is continued until the platelet count returns to normal and then is gradually tapered after 4–6 weeks. Corticosteroids produce sustained remissions in about 20% of adults.

Splenectomy is the most effective form of therapy and is indicated for patients who do not respond to corticosteroids, for those who relapse after an initial remission on steroids, and for those whose disease has lasted for more than 1 year. Corticosteroid therapy is not necessary in the immediate preoperative period unless bleeding is severe or the patient was receiving steroids before the operation. Intracranial bleeding is an indication for emergency splenectomy.

Splenectomy produces a sustained remission in about 80% of patients. As with corticosteroids, success rates are better with acute than chronic immune thrombocytopenic purpura. The platelet count usually rises promptly following splenectomy (eg, it may double in 24 hours) and reaches a peak after 1–2 weeks. If the platelet count remains elevated after 2 months, the patient can be considered cured. Occasionally, the platelet count reaches 1–2 million/μL. Although this is generally considered to be harmless and not an indication for anticoagulation, some recommend the administration of anti-platelet-aggregating agents (eg, aspirin). When corticosteroids and splenectomy have failed, immunosuppressive drugs (azathioprine, vincristine) will achieve a remission in 25% of cases. Gamma globulin given intravenously in large doses may also cause transient increases in the platelet count, but this treatment is expensive, and clinical indications for its use are unclear. Administration of danazol has also been reported to increase platelet counts in some patients with immune thrombocytopenic purpura. Patients without adequate marrow megakaryocytes are extremely unlikely to respond to splenectomy.

Prognosis

Acute immune thrombocytopenic purpura in children under age 16 has an excellent prognosis; approximately 80% of patients have a complete and permanent spontaneous remission. This occurs rarely in adults. Splenectomy is successful in about 80% of patients, but more often in idiopathic cases than in those secondary to another disorder.

Akwari OE et al: Splenectomy for primary and recurrent immune thrombocytopenic purpura (ITP). Current criteria for patient selection and results. Ann Surg 1987;206:529.

Berchtold P, McMillan R: Therapy of chronic idiopathic thrombocytopenic purpura in adults. Blood 1989;74:2309.

Burrows RF, Kelton JG: Low fetal risks in pregnancies associated with idiopathic thrombocytopenic purpura. Am J Obstet Gynecol 1990;163:1147.

Bussel JB: The use of intravenous γ-globulin in idiopathic thrombocytopenic purpura. Clin Immunol Immunopathol 1989;53:S147.

Edelmann DZ et al: Danazol in non-splenectomized patients with refractory idiopathic thrombocytopenic purpura. Postgrad Med J 1990;66:827.

Gibson J et al: Management of splenectomy failures in chronic thrombocytopenic purpura: Role of accessory splenectomy. Aust NZ J Med 1986;16:695.

McMillian R et al: Platelet-associated and plasma anti-glycoprotein autoantibodies in chronic ITP. Blood 1987;70:1040.

Schneider PA et al: Immunodeficiency-associated thrombocytopenic purpura (IDTP): Response to splenectomy. Arch Surg 1987;122:1175.

Siegel RS et al: Platelet survival and turnover: Important factors in predicting response to splenectomy in immune thrombocytopenic purpura. Am J Hematol 1989;30:206.

7. THROMBOTIC THROMBOCYTOPENIC PURPURA (TTP)

Thrombotic thrombocytopenic purpura is a rare disease with a pentad of clinical features: (1) fever, (2) thrombocytopenic purpura, (3) hemolytic anemia, (4) neurologic manifestations, and (5) renal failure. The cause is unknown, but autoimmunity to endothelial cells has been implicated and its occurrence in patients with the AIDS complex has been reported. It is most common between ages 10 and 40 years.

The thrombocytopenia is probably due to a shortened platelet life span. The microangiopathic hemolytic anemia is produced by passage of red cells over damaged small blood vessels containing fibrin strands. Rigid red cells are trapped and fragmented in the spleen, whereas those that escape the spleen may be more vulnerable to damage and destruction in the abnormal microvasculature. The anemia is often severe, and it may be aggravated by hemorrhage secondary to thrombocytopenia.

Fluctuating neurologic manifestations are frequent, and intracerebral hemorrhage is a common cause of death. Renal dysfunction is manifested by proteinuria, gross or microscopic hematuria, and elevated blood urea nitrogen and serum creatinine. Acute renal failure is common. Microinfarctions in the pancreas and gastrointestinal tract commonly cause abdominal pain. Hepatomegaly and splenomegaly occur in 35% of cases.

Histologic examination of biopsy specimens confirms the diagnosis. Subintimal deposits of PAS-positive material are seen at arteriolocapillary junctions, along with hyaline thrombi, vessel wall thickening, and aneurysmal dilatations. The lesions are widespread and may be seen in muscle, skin, bone marrow, kidney, and lymph nodes.

Treatment & Prognosis

Until recently, there was no effective therapy for this disorder, and mortality rates as high as 95% were reported. Most patients died of renal failure or cerebral bleeding. Plasmapheresis with plasma exchange has recently emerged as an effective form of treatment which is superior to simple plasma infusion. The plasma supernatant after cryoprecipitation may be more effective than whole plasma. When combined with other therapies, including corticosteroids, dextran, splenectomy, and antiplatelet drugs, prolonged remission can be achieved in most patients.

Bell WR et al: Improved survival in thrombotic thrombocytopenic purpura-hemolytic uremic syndrome. N Eng J Med 1991;325:398.

Byrnes JJ et al: Effectiveness of the cryosupernatant fraction of plasma in the treatment of refractory thrombotic thrombocytopenic purpura. Am J Hematol 1990;34:169.

Rock GA et al: Comparison of plasma exchange with plasma infusion in the treatment of thrombotic thrombocytopenic purpura. N Eng J Med 1991;325:393.

Schneider PA et al: The role of splenectomy in the multimodality treatment of thrombotic thrombocytopenic purpura. Ann Surg 1985;202:318.

8. IDIOPATHIC MYELOFIBROSIS (Agnogenic Myeloid Metaplasia)

Myelofibrosis is a myeloproliferative disorder of unknown cause that is closely related to polycythemia vera and myelogenous leukemia. It is characterized by moderate to massive splenomegaly, leukoerythroblastic blood reaction, and hypocellularity and fibrosis of the bone marrow. The spleen is typically huge, hard, and irregular.

The bone marrow is usually almost completely replaced by fibrous tissue, although in some cases it is hyperplastic and fibrosis is minimal. Extramedullary hematopoiesis develops mainly in the spleen, liver, and long bones. Symptoms are attributable to anemia (weakness, fatigue, dyspnea) and to splenomegaly (abdominal fullness and pain, which may be severe). Pain over the spleen from splenic infarcts is common. Spontaneous bleeding, secondary infection, bone pain, and a hypermetabolic state are frequent. Portal hypertension develops in some cases as a result of fibrosis of the liver, greatly increased splenic blood flow, or both.

Hepatomegaly is present in 75% of cases and splenomegaly in all cases. Striking changes are seen in the peripheral blood. Red cells vary greatly in size and shape, and many are distorted and fragmented. The white count is usually high (20,000–50,000/μL). The platelet count may be elevated, but values less than 100,000/μL are seen in 30% of cases. Secondary hypersplenism is common and may lead to thrombocytopenia and hemolytic anemia. It was once incorrectly thought that the spleen performed a crucial function of extramedullary hematopoiesis in this disease and that splenectomy could be lethal. In fact, many patients with myeloid metaplasia feel better if the massive spleen is removed, and their hypersplenism is often corrected.

About 30% of patients are asymptomatic at the time of initial diagnosis and require no therapy. When anemia and splenomegaly produce symptoms, transfusions, androgenic steroids, antimetabolites, and radiation therapy are indicated. Splenectomy is indicated in the following situations: (1) major hemolysis unresponsive to medical management, (2) severe symptoms of massive splenomegaly, (3) life-threatening thrombocytopenia, and (4) portal hypertension with variceal hemorrhage. This is one of the rare occasions when portal hypertension may be cured by splenectomy.

Splenectomy in myeloid metaplasia is associated with a 13% death rate and frequent complications. For unknown reasons, women have fewer complications and live longer following splenectomy than men. The high operative death rate of splenectomy in the past was at least partly related to excessive delay in performing the operation.

Brenner B, Tavori S, Tatarsky I: Influence of splenectomy on hemostasis in agnogenic myeloid metaplasia. Haemostasis 1987;17:141.

Brenner B et al: Splenectomy in agnogenic myeloid metaplasia and postpolycythemic myeloid metaplasia. A study of 34 cases. Arch Intern Med 1988;148:2501.

Coon WW: Splenectomy for thrombocytopenia due to secondary hypersplenism. Arch Surg 1988;123:369.

SPLENECTOMY FOR STAGING HODGKIN'S DISEASE

The staging system used for classification of Hodgkin's disease is shown in Table 28–4. Exploratory laparotomy with splenectomy has been widely performed in early-stage Hodgkin's disease, so that therapy can be planned according to the extent of disease. Following laparotomy, staging will be revised upward in about 25% and downward in about 10% of patients. Lymphangiography accurately predicts nodal involvement in about 80% of cases; CT scans are less accurate. These studies should be used to guide biopsy of suspicious nodes at laparotomy. Patients with obvious stage IV disease or systemic symptoms require chemotherapy and will not benefit from laparotomy. Patients with stage IA or IIA disease to be treated with radiotherapy and those with associated hypersplenism are candidates for staging laparotomy. Those with stage IIIA disease are the subject of controversy, as chemotherapy is usually required in this group, and the utility of splenectomy is

unclear. Some authorities initially treat all stage III patients with chemotherapy and utilize surgical staging for planning abdominal radiation fields only in those with clinically or radiographically apparent residual disease.

Some authorities believe that staging laparotomy is no longer needed regardless of stage, arguing that patients with limited disease in whom local radiation fails may be effectively managed by salvage chemotherapy and that laparotomy findings would not really alter the outcome. Others advocate more extended radiation or combined chemotherapy and radiation in early-stage patients, obviating the need for laparotomy. Recently, an association has been recognized between splenectomy and secondary acute myeloid leukemias in patients receiving combination chemotherapy. Although many centers still base treatment in early-stage Hodgkin's disease on the results of staging laparotomy, the indications for laparotomy are being restricted. Laparotomy for restaging may occasionally be required, especially when results of radiologic studies are equivocal or when a change in histologic type is suspected. Patients with non-Hodgkin's lymphoma do not require staging laparotomy.

Staging laparotomy involves splenectomy, liver biopsy, and thorough abdominal exploration with generous biopsy of portal-celiac, iliofemoral, and periaortic lymph nodes and any others that appear abnormal on lymphangiogram or by gross inspection. Extensive retroperitoneal dissection is unnecessary. Metallic clips placed next to involved nodes at the time of surgery will aid the radiation therapist. In addition to the diagnostic information obtained, removal of the spleen improves tolerance to chemotherapy in patients with hypersplenism. Radiation injury to the left kidney and lung is avoided, because the spleen need not be irradiated. Although it has been suggested that partial splenectomy may provide adequate diagnostic information and prevent postsplenectomy sepsis, splenic involvement is frequently focal rather than diffuse and is often inapparent at surgery.

Table 28–4. Staging of Hodgkin's disease.

Stage*	Definition
0	No detectable disease following excisional biopsy
I	Single abnormal lymph node
II	Two or more discrete abnormal nodes, limited to one side of diaphragm
III	Disease on both sides of diaphragm but limited to the lymph nodes, spleen, or Waldeyer's ring
IV	Involvement of bone, bone marrow, lung parenchyma, pleura, liver, skin, gastrointestinal tract, central nervous system, kidney, or sites other than lymph nodes, spleen, or Waldeyer's ring

*All stages are subclassified to describe the absence (A) or presence (B) of systemic symptoms.

Aragon-de-la-Cruz G et al: Individual risk of abdominal disease in patients with stages I and II supradiaphragmatic Hodgkin's disease: A rule index based on 341 laparotomized patients. Cancer 1989;63:1799.

Edwards MJ, Balch CM: Surgical aspects of lymphoma. Adv Surg 1989;22:225.

Leibenhaut MH et al: Prognostic indicators of laparotomy findings in clinical stage I–II supradiaphragmatic Hodgkin's disease. J Clin Oncol 1989;7:81.

Rosenberg SA: Exploratory laparotomy and splenectomy for Hodgkin's disease: A commentary. J Clin Oncol 1988;6:574.

Skillings JR et al: A prospective study of magnetic resonance imaging in lymphoma staging. Cancer 1991;67:1838.

Taylor MA, Kaplan HS, Nelsen TS: Staging laparotomy

with splenectomy for Hodgkin's disease: The Stanford experience. World J Surg 1985;9:449.

Tubiana M et al: Toward comprehensive management tailored to prognostic factors of patients with clinical stages I and II Hodgkin's disease. Blood 1989;73:47.

ANEURYSM OF THE SPLENIC ARTERY

Splenic artery aneurysm is uncommon even though this is the second most frequent abdominal artery to undergo aneurysmal change. It occurs twice as often in women as in men. The patients can be divided into two groups: (1) elderly people whose aneurysms are manifestations of atherosclerosis and (2) young women with apparently congenital aneurysms, which have a predilection for rupture during pregnancy, perhaps related to hormonal and hemodynamic changes of pregnancy. Portal hypertension and splenomegaly may be associated with some cases, and inflammatory processes involving the vessel wall (eg, pancreatitis) occasionally lead to aneurysm. Portal hypertension may result from splenic vein thrombosis caused by compression from the aneurysm. These lesions are usually asymptomatic and are noted on abdominal x-rays as an eggshell rim of calcification in the left upper quadrant. Sometimes they are responsible for pain, nausea, and vomiting. The presence of symptoms suggests impending rupture, and splenectomy with ligation of the splenic artery is indicated.

When a calcified atherosclerotic aneurysm is discovered in a patient over age 60, surgical excision is not indicated in the absence of symptoms or splenic enlargement. In younger patients, aneurysmectomy and splenectomy are advisable to prevent rupture. Sudden intra-abdominal hemorrhage during pregnancy suggests rupture of the splenic artery and calls for prompt laparotomy. The aneurysm is usually found within several centimeters of the hilum of the spleen. Control of bleeding followed by excision of the aneurysm and splenectomy is the treatment of choice. A nonsurgical approach has been successful in thrombosing splenic artery aneurysms by packing them with foreign material introduced through a catheter.

Lambert CJ, Williamson JW: Splenic artery aneurysm: A rare cause of upper gastrointestinal bleeding. Am Surg 1990;56:543.

Reidy JF, Rowe PH, Ellis FG: Splenic artery aneurysm embolization: The preferred technique to surgery. Clin Radiol 1990;41:281.

CYSTS & TUMORS OF THE SPLEEN

Parasitic cysts are almost always echinococcal (see Chapter 8). They may be asymptomatic, but usually the patient notices splenomegaly. Calcification of the cyst wall may be seen on x-ray. Eosinophilia may be found, and serologic tests may confirm the diagnosis. The treatment of choice is splenectomy.

Other cysts are dermoid, epidermoid, endothelial, and pseudocysts. The latter are thought to be late results of infarction or trauma. Splenectomy may be indicated to exclude tumor; however, partial splenectomy or observation has been advocated.

The rare primary tumors of the spleen include lymphoma, sarcoma, hemangioma, and hamartoma. Hamartomas may be confused grossly with splenic lymphoma at laparotomy. These lesions are usually asymptomatic until splenomegaly causes abdominal discomfort or a palpable mass. The benign vascular tumors of the spleen (angiomas) can produce hypersplenism. Spontaneous rupture with massive hemorrhage can occur. Splenectomy is indicated if the tumor appears to be limited to the spleen.

The spleen is a common site for metastases in advanced cancers, especially of the lung and breast. Splenic metastases are common autopsy findings but are rarely clinically significant.

Brown MF et al: Partial splenectomy: The preferred alternative for the treatment of splenic cysts. J Pediatr Surg 1989;24:694.

Hahn PF et al: MR imaging of focal splenic tumors. Am J Roentgenol 1988;150:823.

Moir C et al: Splenic cysts: Aspiration, sclerosis, or resection. J Pediatr Surg 1989;24:646.

Sagar PM, McMahon MJ: Partial splenectomy for splenic cysts. Br J Surg 1988;75:488.

ABSCESS OF THE SPLEEN

Splenic abscesses are uncommon but are important because the death rate is so high. They may be caused by hematogenous seeding of the spleen with bacteria from remote sepsis, by direct spread of infection from adjacent structures, or by splenic trauma resulting in a secondarily infected splenic hematoma. In 80% of cases, one or more abscesses exist in organs other than the spleen, and the splenic abscess develops as a terminal manifestation of uncontrolled sepsis in other organs. In some patients, unexplained sepsis, progressive splenic enlargement, and abdominal pain are the presenting manifestations. The spleen may not be palpable, because of left upper quadrant tenderness and guarding. Splenic abscess is a complication of intravenous drug abuse. The finding of gas in the spleen on plain abdominal x-ray is pathognomonic of splenic abscess. Ultrasound and CT scans also reveal splenic abscess.

Most splenic abscesses remain localized, periodically seeding the bloodstream with bacteria, but spontaneous rupture and peritonitis may occur. Splenectomy is essential for cure if sepsis is localized to the spleen. Percutaneous drainage of large, solitary juxtacapsular abscesses may occasionally be feasible.

Faught WE, Gilbertson JJ, Nelson EW: Splenic abscess: Presentation, treatment options, and results. Am J Surg 1989;158:612.

Gadacz TR: Splenic abscess. World J Surg 1985;9:410.

Nelken N et al: Changing clinical spectrum of splenic abscess: A multicenter study and review of the literature. Am J Surg 1987;154:27.

ACCESSORY & ECTOPIC SPLEEN

Ectopic spleen (wandering spleen) is an unusual condition in which a long splenic pedicle allows the spleen to move about the abdomen. The mass can be identified as spleen by radionuclide scan. It often resides in the lower abdomen or pelvis, where even a normal-sized spleen can be felt as a mass. The condition is 13 times more common in women than in men. Acute torsion of the pedicle occurs occasionally, necessitating emergency splenectomy. Elective removal of pelvic spleens is indicated.

Accessory spleens are found in about 10% of routine postmortem autopsies, usually near the hilum of the spleen and the tail of the pancreas. Ordinarily of no significance, they may play a role in the recurrence of certain hematologic disorders for which splenectomy was performed; removal of accessory spleens may lead to remission of disease in these patients. Patients who fail to respond to the initial splenectomy should undergo scanning with technetium 99m-labeled heated red cells or indium 111-labeled platelets. Intraoperative use of a sterile isotopic detector may be helpful in locating accessory spleens.

Gibson J et al: Management of splenectomy failures in chronic immune thrombocytopenic purpura: Role of accessory splenectomy. Aust NZ J Med 1986;16:695.

Guze BH, Hawkins R: The utility of SPECT liver-spleen imaging in the evaluation of a possible accessory spleen. Clin Nucl Med 1988;13:496.

RUPTURE OF THE SPLEEN

Essentials of Diagnosis

- Trauma to the abdomen or flank; often a fractured rib on the left.
- Abdominal pain and tenderness.
- Pain in the left shoulder or left side of the neck.
- Tachycardia.
- Anemia or hypotension.

General Considerations

Disruption of the parenchyma, capsule, or blood supply of the spleen is termed rupture. It is the most common indication for splenectomy and the most common major injury from blunt abdominal trauma.

The spleen may be ruptured by penetrating, nonpenetrating, or operative thoracic or abdominal trauma, or it may rupture spontaneously. Even trivial trauma has been reported to cause splenic rupture. The spleen is highly vascular but friable and bleeds profusely when injured.

Most penetrating abdominal injuries are obvious, and surgical exploration is routine; if a splenic rupture is present, it will be readily discovered. Penetrating thoracic injuries must penetrate the lung, pleura, and diaphragm before reaching the spleen.

Automobile accidents are the most common cause of blunt trauma to the spleen. With blunt injury, the spleen may be fractured through the parenchyma and capsule, avulsed from its pedicle, or disrupted beneath an intact capsule to produce a subcapsular or contained hematoma. Approximately 5% of blunt injuries to the spleen result in **delayed rupture,** which begins as a subcapsular hematoma that grows and becomes clinically manifest days to weeks later. Delayed splenic rupture is believed to evolve as follows: There is a minor rupture of the splenic pulp, but the lesion is either intraparenchymal or contained within peritoneal folds. As the red cells disintegrate, the hematoma liquefies, and increased osmolality of its contents attracts additional fluid. This leads to expansion of the cavity, secondary hemorrhage, and eventually rupture. It frequently produces sudden shock from profuse bleeding. Approximately 75% of delayed ruptures occur within 2 weeks of the initial injury, but in rare instances, months or years may pass before secondary bleeding occurs. Some patients present with anemia and left upper quadrant mass suggesting a retroperitoneal tumor.

Operative trauma to the spleen, which accounts for about 20% of splenectomies, is most common during upper abdominal operations on adjacent viscera (stomach, esophageal hiatus, vagus nerves, splenic flexure of the colon, etc). The usual mechanisms of injury are avulsion of the splenic capsule by traction on the peritoneal attachments and direct injury by a misplaced retractor.

The spleen may also rupture spontaneously (no antecedent trauma). Spontaneous rupture of a normal spleen is rare; it most frequently occurs in malaria, mononucleosis, lymphoma, leukemia, typhoid fever, and other conditions accompanied by an enlarged, diseased spleen. Spontaneous rupture of the spleen is a rare complication of pregnancy and of oral anticoagulant therapy.

Clinical Findings

A. Symptoms and Signs: The clinical spectrum varies from severe hypovolemic shock to minimal or no symptoms. Most patients fall between these extremes. There is usually a history of a blow to the upper abdomen, particularly to the left flank, but the trauma may have seemed so trivial as to be overlooked by the patient. This is especially true in children. Most patients complain of generalized abdominal pain that is most severe in the left upper quadrant. About one-third of patients have pain confined to the left upper quadrant. Referred pain is often felt in the left shoulder or cervical region (Kehr's sign). This is a reliable indication of diaphragmatic irritation and can often be elicited by placing the patient in the Trendelenburg position or by palpation in the left upper quadrant. Mild nausea and vomiting may sometimes occur.

The abdominal findings are those of low-grade peritoneal irritation (ie, tenderness, mild spasm, and distention). The area of splenic dullness may be increased to percussion, or a mass may be palpable in the left upper quadrant. With marked bleeding, the abdomen may distend rapidly and the characteristic signs of acute blood loss (ie, tachycardia, hypotension, and shock) will appear. An important early diagnostic clue is tenderness over the ninth and tenth ribs on the left. A fractured rib in that area should arouse a strong suspicion of the possibility of a ruptured spleen. It occurs in about 20% of cases.

Deaths from splenic rupture may be attributed to delay in diagnosis and concomitant injuries. The diagnosis may be difficult even when suspected. Associated injuries are often present and may mask the physical signs. Abdominal pain and tenderness are usually present, but the peritoneal reaction to bleeding varies greatly, and some patients will have minimal findings even when intraperitoneal bleeding is massive. In doubtful cases, paracentesis is indicated to look for free intra-abdominal blood.

B. Laboratory Findings: With acute rupture, the initial hematocrit is usually normal, but serial determinations will show a fall. The leukocyte count is often increased to 15,000–20,000/μL with a shift to the left.

C. Imaging Studies: Plain films of the abdomen may show fractured ribs or an enlarged spleen. The gastric air bubble may be displaced medially and the transverse colon inferiorly. A serrated appearance of the greater curvature of the stomach due to dissection of blood into the gastrosplenic ligament is a useful radiographic sign but is uncommon.

Contrast-enhanced CT scanning is the preferred method of diagnosis in patients who do not require urgent laparotomy. It may also be used to monitor splenic healing. Grading systems are not accurate enough to allow selection of patients for nonoperative management. Selective splenic arteriograms are helpful in doubtful cases and are particularly useful in evaluating for delayed rupture.

Treatment & Prognosis

Laparotomy is indicated in about 75% of patients and nonoperative management in about 25%. Selection of patients for nonoperative management should be based on the following criteria: (1) The mode of injury is blunt rather than penetrating trauma; (2) other injuries do not require operation (ie, the injury severity score is low); (3) the patient is hemodynamically stable, and signs of blood loss and peritonitis

do not progress during observation; and (4) total transfusion requirements do not exceed two units. Changes in the lesion in the spleen can be detected by comparing follow-up CT scans with studies obtained shortly after the injury.

Of the 75% of patients who come to laparotomy, only one-third (25% of all splenic injuries) require splenectomy. The remainder (50% of all splenic injuries) can be managed by techniques that preserve the spleen. Small capsular tears can usually be successfully treated by application of a hemostatic agent such as microcrystalline collagen. Larger injuries that do not involve the hilar vessels can often be repaired by debridement of devitalized tissue, ligation of individual vessels, and approximation of the remaining cut surfaces **(splenorrhaphy).** Partial removal of the spleen can also be successful in some cases. The death rate of isolated splenic rupture is 10%; with other serious concomitant injuries, the death rate approaches 25%.

Chung SW, Nagy AG: Preservation of the spleen using human fibrin seal. Can J Surg 1988;31:195.

Lally KP et al: Evolution in the management of splenic injury in children. Surg Gynecol Obstet 1990;170:245.

Lange DA et al: The use of absorbable mesh in splenic trauma. J Trauma 1988;28:269.

Pickhardt B et al: Operative splenic salvage in adults. J Trauma 1989;29:1386.

Pitcher ME, Cade RJ, Mackay JR: Splenectomy for trauma: Morbidity, mortality and associated abdominal injuries. Aust NZ J Surg 1989;59:461.

Safran D, Bloom GP: Spontaneous splenic rupture following infectious mononucleosis. Am Surg 1990;56:601.

Sivit CJ, Peclet MH, Taylor GA: Life-threatening intraperitoneal bleeding: Demonstration with CT. Radiology 1989;171:430.

Umlas SL, Cronan JJ: Splenic trauma: can CT grading systems enable prediction of successful nonsurgical treatment? Radiology 1991;178:481.

Villalba MR et al: Nonoperative management of the adult ruptured spleen. Arch Surg 1990;125:836.

SPLENOSIS

In splenosis, multiple small implants of splenic tissue grow in scattered areas on the peritoneal surfaces throughout the abdomen. They arise from dissemination and autotransplantation of splenic fragments following traumatic rupture of the spleen. Although splenic implants or intentional autotransplants are capable of cell culling, their immunologic function appears to be insignificant. Aggressive attempts at surgical excision are not warranted. Splenosis is usually an incidental finding discovered much later during laparotomy for an unrelated problem. However, the implants stimulate formation of adhesions and may be a cause of intestinal obstruction. They must be distinguished from peritoneal nodules of metastatic carcinoma and from accessory spleens. Histologically, they differ from accessory spleens by the absence of elastic or smooth muscle fibers in the delicate capsule.

Holdsworth RJ: Regeneration of the spleen and splenic autotransplantation. Br J Surg 1991;78:270.

Maillard JC et al: Intraperitoneal splenosis: Diagnosis by ultrasound and computed tomography. Gastrointest Radiol 1989;14:179.

SPLENECTOMY

Preoperative preparation of patients undergoing elective splenectomy should correct coagulation abnormalities and deficits in red cell mass, treat infections, and control immune reactions. Because platelets are removed so rapidly from the circulation, they usually are not given for thrombocytopenia until after the splenic artery has been ligated. Antibodies in the patient's serum may complicate cross-matching of blood. Many patients with autoimmune disorders require corticosteroid coverage in the perioperative period. For emergency splenectomy, hypovolemia should be corrected by whole blood transfusions.

Details of surgical technique are not within the scope of this text, but it should be noted that there are two methods of splenectomy (Figure 28–2). In one, which is of value chiefly in traumatic rupture of the spleen, the organ is immediately mobilized and the splenic artery is secured from behind as it enters the hilum. In the other, which is of vital importance in the removal of massively enlarged spleens, the organ is left in situ. The gastrocolic ligament is opened, and the splenic artery is ligated as it courses along the upper edge of the pancreas. This permits blood to leave the spleen through the splenic vein while all other attachments (ie, the short gastric vessels and colic attachments) are divided before the spleen is delivered. This method permits the removal of massively enlarged vascular spleens with practically no loss of blood.

Cooper MJ, Williamson RC: Splenectomy: Indications, hazards and alternatives. Br J Surg 1984;71:173.

Danforth DN, Fraker DL: Splenectomy for the massively enlarged spleen. Am Surg 1991;56:108.

Graham RA, Hohn DC: The spleen: Splenectomy for hematologic disorders. In: *Current Surgical Therapy–3*. Cameron JL (editor). BC Decker, 1989.

Johansson T et al: Splenectomy for haematological diseases. Acta Chir Scand 1990;156:8.

Shaw JH, Clark M: Splenectomy for massive splenomegaly. Br J Surg 1989;76:395.

1. HEMATOLOGIC EFFECTS OF SPLENECTOMY

Absence of the spleen in a normal adult usually has few clinical consequences. Red cell count and indices do not change, but red cells with cytoplasmic inclusions may appear, eg, Heinz bodies, Howell-Jolly bodies, and siderocytes. Granulocytosis occurs immediately after splenectomy but is replaced in several weeks by lymphocytosis and monocytosis. Platelets are usually increased, occasionally markedly so, and may stay at levels of 400,000–500,000/μL for over a year. Even more striking thrombocytosis (eg, 2–3 million/μL) may develop after splenectomy for hemolytic anemia. A platelet count of over a million is

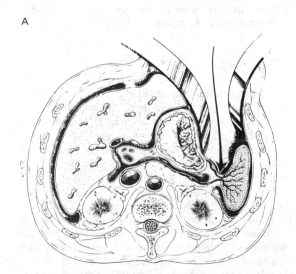

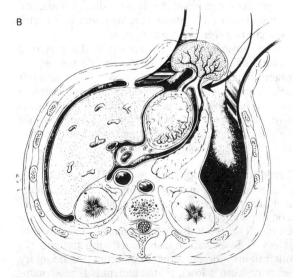

Figure 28–2. *A:* Anterior approach to splenic artery. *B:* Mobilization of spleen with posterior exposure of splenic artery.

not an indication for anticoagulants, but antiplatelet agents such as aspirin may help prevent thrombosis.

2. POSTSPLENECTOMY SEPSIS & OTHER POSTSPLENECTOMY PROBLEMS

Complications related to splenectomy per se are relatively few, with atelectasis, pancreatitis, and postoperative hemorrhage being the most common. If splenectomy is done for thrombocytopenia, secondary bleeding may occur even though the platelet count usually rises promptly. Platelet transfusions should be given if primary hemostasis is abnormal (ie, oozing occurs) and the platelet count remains low. Thromboembolic complications may be more common following splenectomy, but this complication does not correlate with the degree of thrombocytosis.

Individuals are more susceptible to fulminant bacteremia after splenectomy. This is a result of the following changes that occur after splenectomy: (1) decreased clearance of bacteria from the blood, (2) decreased levels of IgM, and (3) decreased opsonic activity. The risk is greatest in young children, especially in the first 2 years after surgery (80% of cases) and when the disorder for which splenectomy was required was a disease of the reticuloendothelial system. In general, the younger the patient undergoing splenectomy and the more severe the underlying condition, the greater the risk for developing overwhelming postsplenectomy infection. There is a low but significant risk of infection even in otherwise normal adults following splenectomy. Most of these infections occur after the first year, and nearly half occur more than 5 years after splenectomy. Lethal sepsis is very rare in adults. There is a distinct clinical syndrome: mild, nonspecific symptoms are followed by high fever and shock from sepsis, which may rapidly lead to death. *Streptococcus pneumoniae, Haemophilus influenzae,* and meningococci are the most common pathogens. Disseminated intravascular coagulation is a common complication. Awareness of this fatal complication has led to efforts to avoid splenectomy or to perform partial splenectomy or splenic repair for ruptured spleens (analogous to surgical management of liver trauma) to maintain adequate splenic function. Splenic autotransplantation may also achieve partial restoration of splenic function after splenectomy.

The risk of fatal sepsis is less after splenectomy for trauma than for hematologic disorders. Prophylactic vaccination against pneumococcal sepsis should be used in all surgically or functionally asplenic patients. Since splenic function may be important in the immune response to vaccine, early administration of polyvalent pneumococcal vaccine (Pneumovax) is advisable. The vaccine provides protection in adults and older children for 4–5 years, after which revaccination is advisable. Since the vaccine is only effective against about 80% of organisms, some authorities have recommended a 2-year course of prophylactic penicillin following splenectomy. Others have advocated use of ampicillin to provide coverage for *H influenzae* as well as pneumococci. Antibiotic prophylaxis is essential in children under 2 years of age. In general, splenectomy should be deferred until age 6 unless the hematologic problem is especially severe.

Chattopadhyay B: Splenectomy, pneumococcal vaccination and antibiotic prophylaxis. Br J Hosp Med 1989;41:172.

Cooper MJ, Williamson RCN: Splenectomy: Indications, hazards and alternatives. Br J Surg 1984;71:173.

Cullingford GL et al: Severe late postsplenectomy infection. Br J Surg 1991;78:716.

Pimpl W et al: Incidence of septic and thromboembolic-related deaths after splenectomy in adults. Br J Surg 1989;76:517.

Powell RW et al: The efficacy of postsplenectomy sepsis prophylactic measures: The role of penicillin. J Trauma 1988;28:1285.

Rao GN: Predictive factors in local sepsis after splenectomy for trauma in adults. J R Coll Surg Edinb 1988;33:68.

Shaw JHF, Print CG: Postsplenectomy sepsis. Br J Surg 1989;76:1074.

Siber GR et al: Antibody responses to pretreatment immunization and post-treatment boosting with bacterial polysaccharide vaccines in patients with Hodgkin's disease. Ann Intern Med 1986;104:467.

Traub A et al: Splenic reticuloendothelial function after splenectomy, spleen repair, and spleen autotransplantation. N Engl J Med 1987;317:1559.

REFERENCES

Cooper MJ, Williamson RCN: Splenectomy: Indications, hazards and alternatives. Br J Surg 1984;71:173.

Danforth DN, Fraker DL: Splenectomy for the massively enlarged spleen. Am Surg 1991;56:108.

Enriquez P: *The Pathology of the Spleen: A Functional Approach.* American Society of Clinical Pathologists, 1976.

Graham RA, Hohn DC: The spleen: Splenectomy for hematologic disorders. In: *Current Surgical Therapy–3.* Cameron JL (editor). BC Decker, 1989.

Sandusky WR, Hess CE: Splenectomy in hematologic disorders. The ever-changing indications. Ann Surg 1988;207:581.

Vevon PA, Ellison EC, Carey LC: Splenectomy for hematologic disease. Adv Surg 1989;22:105.

29

Appendix

Lawrence W. Way, MD

ANATOMY & PHYSIOLOGY

In infants, the appendix is a conical diverticulum at the apex of the cecum, but with differential growth and distention of the cecum, the appendix ultimately arises on the left and dorsally approximately 2.5 cm below the ileocecal valve. The taeniae of the colon converge at the base of the appendix, an arrangement that helps in locating this structure at operation. The appendix is fixed retrocecally in 16% of adults and is freely mobile in the remainder.

The appendix in youth is characterized by a large concentration of lymphoid follicles that appear 2 weeks after birth and number about 200 or more at age 15. Thereafter, progressive atrophy of lymphoid tissue proceeds concomitantly with fibrosis of the wall and partial or total obliteration of the lumen.

If the appendix has a physiologic function, it is probably related to the presence of lymphoid follicles. Reports of a statistical relationship between appendectomy and subsequent carcinoma of the colon and other neoplasms in humans are not supported by controlled studies.

ACUTE APPENDICITIS

Essentials of Diagnosis

- Abdominal pain.
- Anorexia, nausea and vomiting.
- Localized abdominal tenderness.
- Low-grade fever.
- Leukocytosis.

General Considerations

Approximately 7% of individuals in Western countries develop appendicitis at some time during their lives, and about 200,000 appendectomies for acute appendicitis are performed annually in the USA. Acute appendicitis is uncommon in parts of Africa and Asia, perhaps because of the high-residue diets ingested by inhabitants of these areas.

In about two-thirds of acutely inflamed appendices, obstruction of the proximal lumen by fibrous bands, lymphoid hyperplasia, fecaliths, parasites (eg, pinworms), etc, can be demonstrated. Luminal obstruction is not found in the remaining one-third. A

fecalith or calculus is found in the lumen of about 10% of acutely inflamed appendices. Since they are seen in only 2% of incidentally removed (uninflamed) appendices, fecaliths and calculi appear to be causative factors in appendicitis. Fecaliths are five times as common as calculi. The appendicitis is complicated by perforation or abscess formation in half of patients with an appendiceal calculus and in 20% of those with an appendiceal fecalith, while the overall incidence of these complications is about 12%.

As appendicitis progresses, the blood supply is impaired by bacterial infection in the wall and distention of the lumen by pus; gangrene and perforation occur at about 24 hours, though the timing is highly variable. Gangrene implies microscopic perforation and bacterial peritonitis (which may be localized by adhesions from nearby viscera).

Clinical Findings

Acute appendicitis has protean manifestations. It may simulate almost any other acute abdominal illness and in turn may be mimicked by a variety of conditions. Progression of symptoms and signs is the rule—in contrast to the fluctuating course of some other diseases.

A. Symptoms and Signs: Typically, the illness begins with vague midabdominal discomfort followed by nausea, anorexia, and indigestion. The pain is persistent and continuous but not severe, with occasional mild cramps. There may be an episode of vomiting, and within several hours the pain shifts to the right lower quadrant, becoming localized and causing discomfort on moving, walking, or coughing. The patient may feel constipated.

Examination at this point shows localized tenderness to one-finger palpation and possibly slight muscular rigidity. Rebound tenderness is referred to the same area. Peristalsis is normal or slightly reduced. Rectal and pelvic examinations are likely to be negative. The temperature is only slightly elevated (eg, 37.8 °C [100 °F]) in the absence of perforation.

Although it was long held that inflammation of a retrocecal appendix produces an atypical syndrome, this is now known to be incorrect; the findings are the same as for ordinary (antececal) appendicitis.

Rarely, the cecum may lie on the left side of the abdomen, and appendicitis may be mistaken for sigmoid diverticulitis. An inflamed appendix in the right upper quadrant may mimic acute cholecystitis or perforated ulcer. Even when the cecum is normally situated, a long appendix may reach to other parts of the abdomen, and acute appendicitis in these circumstances may be very confusing indeed.

A couple of general points are worth remembering: (1) People with early (nonperforated) appendicitis often do not appear ill and may even apologize for taking your time. Finding localized tenderness over McBurney's point is the cornerstone of diagnosis. (2) A rule that will help considerably with atypical cases is never to place appendicitis lower than second in the differential diagnosis of acute abdominal pain in a previously healthy person.

B. Laboratory Findings: The average leukocyte count is 15,000/μL, and 90% of patients have counts over 10,000/μL. In three-fourths of patients, the differential white count shows more than 75% neutrophils. It must be emphasized, however, that one patient in ten with acute appendicitis has a leukocyte count indistinguishable from normal, and many have normal differential cell counts. Appendicitis in patients infected with HIV produces the same syndrome as in other people, but the white blood cell count is usually normal.

The urine is usually normal, but a few leukocytes and erythrocytes and occasionally even gross hematuria may be noted, particularly in retrocecal or pelvic appendicitis.

C. Imaging Studies: Localized air-fluid levels, localized ileus, or increased soft tissue density in the right lower quadrant is present in 50% of patients with early acute appendicitis. Less common findings are a calculus, an altered right psoas shadow, or an abnormal right flank stripe. The finding on plain films of a calculus in the right lower quadrant coupled with pain in this area strong supports a diagnosis of appendicitis. Although perforated peptic ulcer is by far the most common cause of free intraperitoneal air, free air is also a rare manifestation of perforated appendicitis. In general, however, the findings on plain films are nonspecific and rarely of help in diagnosis. A suggestion that barium enema may contribute to the diagnosis has not been supported by experience.

Ultrasound or CT examination of the appendix may be helpful in patients with atypical symptoms, such as children and elderly persons, in whom the diagnosis is often delayed. The findings consist of a dilated appendiceal lumen and a thickened wall. The sensitivity of ultrasound has been reported to be 100% in diagnosing obstructive appendicitis and 30% in diagnosing catarrhal appendicitis. When appendicitis is accompanied by a right lower quadrant mass, an ultrasound or CT scan should be obtained to differentiate between a periappendiceal phlegmon and an abscess.

D. Appendicitis During Pregnancy: Appendi-

citis is the most common nonobstetric surgical disease of the abdomen during pregnancy. Pregnant women develop appendicitis with the same frequency as do nonpregnant women of the same age, and the cases are equally distributed through the three trimesters of pregnancy. Diagnosis may be difficult, because as the uterus enlarges, the appendix is progressively shoved farther out of the pelvis toward the right upper quadrant. Pain, anorexia, fever, leukocytosis, and abdominal tenderness are usually present. The main problem is to recognize the possibility of appendicitis and perform appendectomy promptly. Delay in operation runs a higher than usual risk of perforation and diffuse peritonitis, because omentum is less available to wall off the infection. The mother is in greater jeopardy of serious abdominal infection, and the fetus is more vulnerable to premature labor with complications. Early appendectomy has decreased the maternal death rate to under 0.5% and the fetal death rate to under 10%.

Differential Diagnosis

The diagnosis of acute appendicitis is particularly difficult in the very young and in the elderly. These are the groups where diagnosis is most often delayed and perforation most common. Infants manifest only lethargy, irritability, and anorexia in the early stages, but vomiting, fever, and pain are apparent as the disease progresses. Classic symptoms may not be elicited in aged patients, and the diagnosis is often not considered by the examining physician. The course of appendicitis is more virulent in the elderly, and suppurative complications occur earlier.

The highest incidence of false-positive diagnosis (30–40%) is in women between ages 20 and 40 and is attributable to pelvic inflammatory disease and other gynecologic conditions. Compared with appendicitis, pelvic inflammatory disease is more often associated with bilateral lower quadrant tenderness, left adnexal tenderness, onset of illness within 5 days of the last menstrual period, and a history that does not include nausea and vomiting. Cervical motion tenderness is common in both diseases.

Complications

The complications of acute appendicitis include perforation, peritonitis, abscess, and pylephlebitis.

A. Perforation: Perforation is accompanied by more severe pain and higher fever (average, 38.3 °C [100 °F]) than in appendicitis. It is unusual for the acutely inflamed appendix to perforate within the first 12 hours. The appendicitis has progressed to perforation by the time of appendectomy in about 50% of patients under age 10 or over age 50. Nearly all deaths occur in the latter group.

The acute consequences of perforation vary from generalized peritonitis to formation of a tiny abscess that may not appreciably alter the symptoms and signs of appendicitis. Perforation in young women increases the subsequent risk of tubal infertility about fourfold.

B. Peritonitis: Localized peritonitis results from microscopic perforation of a gangrenous appendix, while spreading or generalized peritonitis usually implies gross perforation into the free peritoneal cavity. Increasing tenderness and rigidity, abdominal distention, and adynamic ileus are obvious in patients with peritonitis. High fever and severe toxicity mark progression of this catastrophic illness in untreated patients. Peritonitis is discussed in Chapter 22.

C. Appendiceal Abscess (Appendiceal Mass): Localized perforation occurs when the periappendiceal infection becomes walled off by omentum and adjacent viscera. The clinical presentation consists of the usual findings in appendicitis plus a right lower quadrant mass. An ultrasound or CT scan should be performed; if an abscess is found, it is best treated by percutaneous ultrasound-guided aspiration. Opinion differs about how very small abscesses and phlegmons should be handled. Some surgeons prefer a regimen consisting of antibiotics and expectant management followed by elective appendectomy 6 weeks later. The purpose is to avoid spreading the localized infection, which usually resolves in response to the antibiotics. Other surgeons recommend immediate appendectomy, which considerably shortens the duration of the illness. The trend is in favor of the latter approach, since it is more expeditious and appears to be just as safe.

When the surgeon encounters an unsuspected abscess during appendectomy, it is usually best to proceed and remove the appendix. If the abscess is large and further dissection would be hazardous, drainage alone is appropriate.

Appendicitis recurs in only 10% of patients whose initial treatment consisted of antibiotics or antibiotics plus drainage of an abscess. Therefore, when the presence of ancillary conditions increases the risks of surgery, interval appendectomy may be postponed unless symptoms recur.

D. Pylephlebitis: Pylephlebitis is suppurative thrombophlebitis of the portal venous system. Chills, high fever, low-grade jaundice, and, later, hepatic abscesses are the hallmarks of this grave condition. The appearance of shaking chills in a patient with acute appendicitis demands vigorous antibiotic therapy to prevent the development of pylephlebitis.

CT scanning is the best means of detecting thrombosis and gas in the portal vein. In addition to antibiotics, prompt surgery is indicated to treat appendicitis or other primary sources of infection (eg, diverticulitis).

Prevention

Appendectomy is commonly performed as an incidental procedure during laparotomy for other conditions. Experience has shown that this is a safe and reasonable practice as long as the following criteria are satisfied: (1) The main operation is elective and the patient is stable. (2) The main operation entails no special risk factors for infection, such as insertion of a prosthetic vascular graft. (3) The appendectomy would not require extending the abdominal incision or a time-consuming dissection through adhesions from a previous abdominal operation. (4) The patient has given preoperative consent. (5) The patient is under age 50—even the low risks of incidental appendectomy outweigh benefits of attempts to prevent appendicitis in older patients.

Treatment

With few exceptions, the treatment of appendicitis is surgical. The technique of open appendectomy is illustrated in Figure 29–1. Performing appendectomy by laparoscopic methods has the following advantages compared with open appendectomy: (1) the diagnosis can be made with certainty before treatment is rendered (eg, patients found to have gynecologic disorders can be treated appropriately); (2) the postoperative hospital stay averages 1 day less than after open appendectomy; (3) the operation is technically easier in obese patients when done laparoscopically; (4) postoperative complications (eg, ileus, wound infection) are less common; and (5) recuperation and return to normal activity is faster. The direct costs are slightly higher, but this is offset by the economic dividends of the speedier recovery. The use of prophylactic antibiotics decreases the incidence of septic complications in both perforated and nonperforated appendicitis. The treatment of appendiceal mass is discussed above.

Prognosis

Although a death rate of zero is theoretically attainable in acute appendicitis, deaths still occur, some of which are avoidable. The death rate in simple acute appendicitis is approximately 0.1% and has not changed significantly since 1930. Progress in pre- and postoperative care—particularly the emphasis on fluid replacement before operation—has reduced the death rate from perforation to about 5%. Nonetheless, postoperative infections still occur in 30% of cases of gangrenous or perforated appendix. Although most of these patients survive, many near fatalities require prolonged hospitalization. The substantial increase in tubal infertility that follows perforation in young women is also avoidable by early appendectomy.

Further reduction of illness and death rates due to appendicitis rests with prevention of perforation. The greatest need for improvement lies in the diagnosis of appendicitis in young children and the elderly; in both of these groups, the incidence of perforation reaches 75% or higher. Delay by patient or parent may be unavoidable, but failure on the part of physicians to recognize the disease is disturbing. In one series of children with appendiceal perforation, 40%

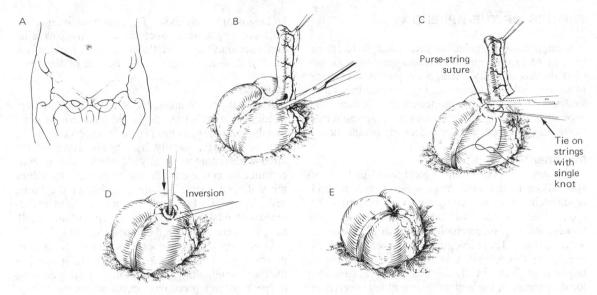

Figure 29–1. Technique of appendectomy. **A:** Incision. **B:** After delivery of the tip of the cecum, the mesoappendix is divided. **C:** The base is clamped and ligated with a simple throw of the knot. The next step—inversion of the stump—is optional. **D:** A clamp is placed to hold the knot during inversion with a purse-string suture of fine silk. **E:** The loosely tied inner knot on the stump assures that there is no closed space for the development of a stump abscess.

had been seen by a physician who failed to make the correct diagnosis before perforation.

In order to minimize the incidence of perforation, it is necessary to remove a certain number of normal appendices in patients with acute illnesses suggesting appendicitis. In early cases when the diagnosis is in doubt, repeated careful reappraisal of the progress of symptoms and signs will permit avoidance of unnecessary operations without increasing the risk of perforation. The incidence of normal appendices removed varies from 10% to 15%.

Allen JR, Helling TS, Langenfeld M: Intraabdominal surgery during pregnancy. Am J Surg 1989;158:567.

Attwood SEA et al: A prospective randomized trial of laparoscopic versus open appendectomy. Surgery 1992; 112:497.

Bennion RS et al: The bacteriology of gangrenous and perforated appendicitis. Ann Surg 1990;211:165.

Binderow SR, Shaked AA: Acute appendicitis in patients with AIDS/HIV infection. Am J Surg 1991;162:9.

Brown JJ: Acute appendicitis: the radiologist's role. Radiology 1991;180:13.

Fisher KS, Ross DS: Guidelines for therapeutic decision in incidental appendectomy. Surg Gynecol Obstet 1990; 171:95.

Gamal R, Moore TC: Appendicitis in children aged 13 years and younger. Am J Surg 1990;159:589.

Graff L, Radford MJ, Werne C: Probability of appendicitis before and after observation. Ann Emerg Med 1991; 20:503.

Meller JL et al: One-drug versus two-drug antibiotic therapy in pediatric perforated appendicitis: A prospective randomized study. Surgery 1991;110:764.

Nitecki S et al: Appendiceal calculi and fecaliths as indications for appendectomy. Surg Gynecol Obstet 1990; 171:185.

Scott-Conner C et al: Laparoscopic appendectomy. Ann Surg 1992;215:660.

Seidman JD et al: Recurrent abdominal pain due to chronic appendiceal disease. S Med J 1991;84:913.

Shen GK et al: Does the retrocecal position of the vermiform appendix alter the clinical course of acute appendicitis? Arch Surg 1991;126:569.

Tamir IL, Bongard FS, Klein SR: Acute appendicitis in the pregnant patient. Am J Surg 1990;160:571.

CHRONIC APPENDICITIS

Chronic abdominal pain is a common problem, and when the complaints are confined to the right lower quadrant, the question of chronic appendicitis is usually raised. Occasionally it is clear that the patient has had recurrent acute appendicitis with pain between attacks that have occurred at intervals of several months or more. However, the patient with chronic intermittent pain is more of a problem, since the symptoms are unlikely to be caused by chronic appendicitis. If there is an organic cause, it most often will be some other condition such as Crohn's disease or renal disease. Barium x-rays are sometimes helpful, particularly in children. In many patients, the diagnosis is not obvious. Appendectomy relieves symptoms occasionally, but laparotomy for chronic abdominal pain is generally unproductive in the absence of objective findings (eg, localized tenderness, palpable mass, leukocytosis).

TUMORS OF THE APPENDIX

Benign tumors, including carcinoids, were found in 4.6% of 71,000 human appendix specimens examined microscopically. Benign neoplasms may arise from any cellular element and are usually incidental findings. Occasionally, a neoplasm obstructs the appendiceal lumen and produces acute appendicitis. No treatment other than appendectomy is indicated.

Malignant Tumors

Primary malignant tumors were found in 1.4% of appendices in the same large series. Carcinoid and argentaffin tumors comprise the majority of appendiceal cancers, and the appendix is the commonest location of carcinoid tumors of the gastrointestinal tract. The biologic behavior of carcinoids arising in the appendix is usually benign; tumors larger than 2 cm in diameter are rare, and though local invasion of the appendiceal wall is observed in 25% of cases, only 3% metastasize to lymph nodes and only isolated reports of hepatic metastases and the carcinoid syndrome have appeared. Appendectomy is adequate therapy unless the lymph nodes are obviously involved, the tumor is greater than 2 cm in diameter, or the mesoappendix or the base of the cecum is invaded. Right hemicolectomy is the treatment of choice for these more advanced lesions.

Adenocarcinoma of the colonic type can arise in the appendix and spread rapidly to regional lymph nodes or implant on ovaries or other peritoneal surfaces. Ten percent of patients have widespread metastases when first seen. Adenocarcinoma is virtually never diagnosed preoperatively; about half of cases present as acute appendicitis, and 15% have formed appendiceal abscesses. Right hemicolectomy should be performed if disease is localized to the appendix and regional lymph nodes. The 5-year survival rate is 60% after right hemicolectomy and only 20% after appendectomy alone, but the latter group includes patients with distant metastases at the time of diagnosis.

Mucocele

Mucocele of the appendix is a cystic, dilated appendix filled with mucin. Simple mucocele is not a neoplasm and results from chronic obstruction of the proximal lumen, usually by fibrous tissue. If the appendiceal contents distally are sterile, mucous cells continue to secrete until distention of the lumen thins the wall and interferes with nutrition of the lining cells; histologically, simple mucocele is lined by flattened cuboidal epithelium or no epithelium at all. Simple mucocele is cured by appendectomy.

Less commonly, mucocele is caused by a neoplasm—cystadenoma, or adenocarcinoma grade 1 in the older terminology. This lesion may arise de novo or (perhaps) in a preceding simple mucocele. In cystadenoma, the lumen is filled with mucin but the wall is lined by columnar epithelium with papillary projections. Tumor does not infiltrate the appendiceal wall and does not metastasize, although it may recur locally after appendectomy. Cystadenoma is believed to undergo malignant change in some instances. Appendectomy is adequate treatment.

Bowman GA, Rosenthal D: Carcinoid tumors of the appendix. Am J Surg 1983;146:700.

Conte CC et al: Adenocarcinoma of the appendix. Surg Gynecol Obstet 1988;166:451.

Harris GJ et al: Adenocarcinoma of the vermiform appendix. J Surg Oncol 1990;44:218.

Lenriot JP, Huguier M: Adenocarcinoma of the appendix. Am J Surg 1988;155:470.

Small Intestine

30

Theodore R. Schrock, MD

The small intestine is the portion of the alimentary tract extending from the pylorus to the cecum. The structure, function, and diseases of the duodenum are discussed in Chapter 23; the jejunum and ileum are described in this chapter.

ANATOMY

Gross Anatomy

The small intestine in an adult is 5–6 m long from the ligament of Treitz to the ileocecal valve. The upper two-fifths of the small intestine distal to the duodenum are termed the **jejunum** and the lower three-fifths the **ileum.** There is no sharp demarcation between the jejunum and the ileum; however, as the intestine proceeds distally, the lumen narrows, the mesenteric vascular arcades become more complex, and the circular mucosal folds become shorter and fewer (Figure 30–1). In general, the jejunum resides in the left side of the peritoneal cavity, and the ileum occupies the pelvis and right lower quadrant.

The small bowel is attached to the posterior abdominal wall by the mesentery, a reflection from the posterior parietal peritoneum. This peritoneal fold arises along a line originating just to the left of the midline and passing obliquely to the right lower quadrant. Although the mesentery joins the intestine along one side, the peritoneal layer of the mesentery envelops the bowel and is called the visceral peritoneum, or serosa.

The mesentery contains fat, blood vessels, lymphatics, lymph nodes, and nerves. The arterial blood supply to the jejunum and ileum derives from the superior mesenteric artery. Branches within the mesentery anastomose to form arcades (Figure 30–1), and small straight arteries travel from these arcades to enter the mesenteric border of the gut. The antimesenteric border of the intestinal wall is less richly supplied with arterial blood than the mesenteric side, so when blood flow is impaired, the antimesenteric border becomes ischemic first. Venous blood from the small intestine drains into the superior mesenteric vein and then enters the liver through the portal vein.

Submucosal lymphoid aggregates (Peyer's patches) are much more numerous in the ileum than in the jejunum. Lymphatic channels within the mesentery drain through regional lymph nodes and terminate in the cisterna chyli.

Parasympathetic nerves from the right vagus and sympathetic fibers from the greater and lesser splanchnic nerves reach the small intestine through the mesentery. Both types of autonomic nerves contain efferent and afferent fibers, but intestinal pain appears to be mediated by the sympathetic afferents only.

Microscopic Anatomy

The wall of the small intestine consists of four layers: mucosa, submucosa, muscularis, and serosa.

A. Mucosa: The absorptive surface of the mucosa is multiplied by circular mucosal folds termed plicae circulares (valvulae conniventes) that project into the lumen; they are taller and more numerous in the proximal jejunum than in the distal ileum (Figure 30–1). On the surface of the plicae circulares are delicate villi less than 1 mm in height, each containing a central lacteal, a small artery and vein, and fibers from the muscularis mucosae that lend contractility to the villus. Villi are in turn covered by columnar epithelial cells that have a brush border consisting of microvilli 1 μm in height (Figure 30–2). The presence of villi multiplies the absorptive surface about eight times, and microvilli increase it another 14–24 times; the total absorptive area of the small intestine is 200–500 m².

The major cell types in the epithelium of the small intestine are absorptive enterocytes, mucous cells, Paneth cells, endocrine cells, and M cells. Absorptive enterocytes are responsible for absorption; they arise from continually proliferating undifferentiated cells in the crypts of Lieberkühn (Figure 30–3) and migrate to the tips of villi over a 3- to 7-day period. The life span of enterocytes in humans is 5–6 days.

Mucous cells originate in crypts and migrate to the tips of villi also; mature mucous cells are termed goblet cells. Paneth cells are found only in the crypts; their function is unknown but may be secretory. Endocrine cells have abundant cytoplasmic granules that contain 5-hydroxtryptamine and various peptides. Enterochromaffin cells are the most numerous; N cells (containing neurotensin), L cells (glucagon), and other cells containing motilin and cholecystokinin are also present. M cells are thin membra-

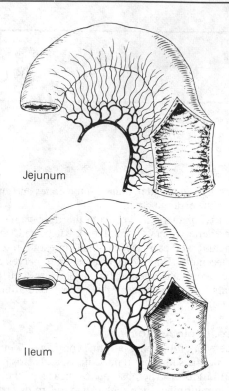

Jejunum

Ileum

Figure 30–1. Blood supply and luminal surface of the small bowel. The arterial arcades of the small intestine increase in number from one or two in the proximal jejunum to four or five in the distal ileum, a finding that helps to distinguish proximal from distal bowel at operation. Plicae circulares are more prominent in the jejunum.

nous cells that cover Peyer's patches. They have the ability to sample luminal antigens such as proteins and microorganisms. Mast cells in the lamina propria are closely applied to nerve fibers, thus providing an anatomic basis for communication between these two structures in disease processes such as inflammation.

B. Other Layers: The submucosa is a fibroelastic layer containing blood vessels and nerves. Submucosa is the strongest component of bowel wall and must be included in intestinal sutures. The muscularis consists of an inner circular layer and an outer longitudinal coat of smooth muscle. The serosa is the outermost covering of the intestine.

Allan LE, Trier JS: Structure and permeability differ in subepithelial villus and Peyer's patch follicle capillaries. Gastroenterology 1991;100:1172.

Furness JB, Bornstein JC, Smith TK: The normal structure of gastrointestinal innervation. J Gastroenterol Hepatol 1990;(Suppl 1):1.

PHYSIOLOGY

The principal function of the small intestine is absorption.

Motility

Smooth muscles of the small intestine undergo spontaneous oscillations of membrane potential; these cyclic changes are termed pacesetter potentials or electrical control activity. Each segment of intestine has a characteristic frequency of pacesetter potentials; it is highest proximally, and it decreases progressively from duodenum to ileum. In intact intestine, higher frequency pacesetter potentials can drive adjacent distal intestine so that both segments have the same frequency (said to be phase-locked). In humans, the duodenum determines the frequency of pacesetter potentials for the entire small intestine.

As pacesetter potentials spread distally, they bring the onset of action potentials and muscular contractions into phase. One type of muscular contraction causes segmentation, which mixes chyme with digestive juices, repeatedly exposes the mixture to the absorptive surface, and moves chyme slowly in an aboral direction. Another type of muscular contraction is peristaltic. Normal peristalsis is a short, weak propulsive movement that travels at about 1 cm/s for a distance of 10–15 cm before subsiding. Mean transit time for a solid meal is 4 hours from mouth to colon.

The enteric nervous system is a dominant regulator of all aspects of motility of the small intestine. The two major types of nerve plexuses in the enteric nervous system are the myenteric plexus, mainly responsible for control of peristaltic activity and the submucosal plexus, which regulates secretion and absorption. The enteric nervous system contains four types of neurons: motor, secretory, sensory, and interneurons (which provide communication between neurons in the intestinal wall). Neurotransmitters found in the enteric nervous system include cholinergic, adrenergic, serotonergic, and peptidergic substances. Among the numerous peptides secreted by neurons in the enteric nervous system are cholecystokinin, vasoactive intestinal peptide (VIP), somatostatin, neurotensin, enkephalin, galanin, and substance P. In general, intestinal action potentials and muscular contractions are stimulated by substance P and galanin, and motility is inhibited by VIP, somatostatin, neurotensin, and enkephalin.

Peristalsis is initiated by stretch of the intestinal wall by a food bolus, and a dual reflex is set in motion. The circular smooth muscle orad to the bolus contracts; this reflex is mediated by enteric neurons with acetylcholine and substance P as neurotransmitters. Simultaneous relaxation of the intestinal circular muscle below is mediated by enteric neurons using VIP as the neurotransmitter. Relaxation of gut sphincters, including the ileocecal valve, is mediated

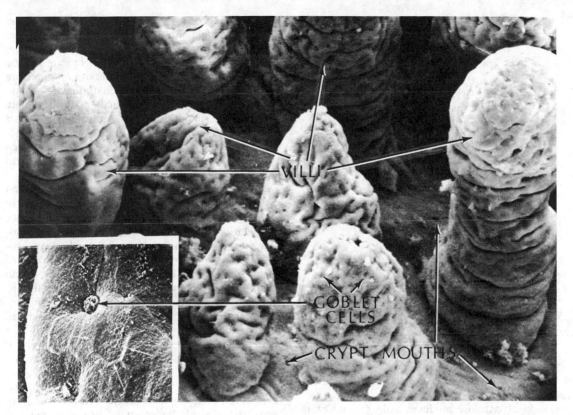

Figure 30–2. Scanning electron microscopic photo of small intestinal villi from the human terminal ileum. (Reduced from × 320.) **Inset:** Detail of a villous surface showing a mucous (goblet) cell surrounded by polygonal columnar cells. (Reduced from × 2100.) Epithelial cell borders are visible (white arrows). The pebbled columnar cell surface represents closely packed microvilli seen end-on. (Courtesy of Robert L. Owen, MD, and Albert L. Jones, MD.)

by VIP, and contraction of sphincters is effected by cholinergic or adrenergic neurons (or both).

The interdigestive migrating myoelectric complex (MMC), which originates every 1½–2 hours in the stomach and duodenum of fasting mammals, is under control of the enteric nervous system; motilin may be the responsible hormone. It is an aborally progressive front of action potentials and muscular contractions. As the MMC reaches the colon, another burst of potentials and contractions begins proximally. The MMC serves to clean up remnants of the preceding meal and propel them into the colon; the complex is abolished by ingestion of food and by major abdominal operations.

Numerous peptides have been found to act in the brain to alter gastrointestinal motility. Hypothalamic hormones (eg, corticotropin-releasing factor and thyrotropin-releasing hormone), calcitonin, and nearly all of the enteric nervous system neurotransmitters have central nervous system actions that affect motility, at least in animals. Exogenous opioids, including codeine and loperamide, exert antidiarrheal action by inhibition or disruption of the pattern of circular muscle contraction; some of these effects may be mediated in the central nervous system. The vagus plays an important role in many of these phenomena.

Paralytic (adynamic) ileus is routine after abdominal operations, and it also accompanies inflammatory conditions in the abdomen, intestinal ischemia, ureteral colic, pelvic fractures, and back injuries. Abdominal surgery abolishes gastrointestinal motility for a period of time that varies with the type of operation; the MMC returns within 3 hours after cholecystectomy, but it may take up to 6 days following colon resection. The small intestine recovers in 12–24 hours, and the colon may not regain normal motility until the sixth postoperative day. The clinical manifestations of postoperative ileus do not correlate well with the myoelectric parameters, however, and the pathophysiology of ileus remains incompletely understood. Recent data suggest that corticotropin-releasing factor is an important mediator of postoperative ileus.

Orocecal transit time is an important indicator of small bowel function. Transit may be accelerated in patients with diarrhea and delayed in constipation; a variety of disease states are responsible. Orocecal transit time can be measured by the lactulose breath

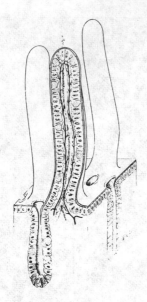

Figure 30–3. Schematic representation of villi and crypts of Lieberkühn.

hydrogen test. An ingested solution of lactulose reaches the cecum in about 90 minutes; colonic fermentation of lactulose produces hydrogen, which is detected in the breath. Gamma scintigraphy is another method of estimating small bowel transit time.

Digestion, Secretion, & Absorption

With a few exceptions (eg, iron, calcium), the normal small intestine absorbs indiscriminately without regard to body composition. Absorption of fat, carbohydrate, and protein is just as complete in the obese patient as in the slender individual. The enteric nervous system regulates secretion and absorption in the small intestine; VIP is one mediator, and neuropeptide Y may be another.

A. Water and Electrolytes: Ingested fluid and salivary, gastric, biliary, pancreatic, and intestinal secretions present a total of 5–9 L of water to the absorptive surface of the small intestine each day, and 1–2 L are discharged from the ileum into the colon. Water is absorbed throughout the intestine, but the major site of absorption after a meal is in the upper tract.

The net flow of water and electrolytes across the intestinal mucosa is equal to the difference between absorption and secretion. The villi are mainly absorbing structures, and secretion of water and electrolytes is localized to the crypts. Much of the transfer of water and small solutes occurs via paracellular "shunt" pathways. The intercellular tight junctions between cells are actually rather loose, and it is through these "pores" that water moves passively in response to osmotic and hydrostatic pressures in the

lumen and in the interstitial fluid. The pores are larger in the jejunum (0.7–0.9 nm) than in the ileum (0.3–0.4 nm). Hypertonic solutions in the duodenum and upper jejunum are rapidly brought into osmotic equilibrium with blood, and as the osmotic pressure of luminal contents is increased further by breakdown of large molecules into smaller ones, still more water enters the lumen. Net absorption of water accompanies active transport of ions and small molecules such as glucose and amino acids. If the lumen contains nonabsorbable solute, water is retained to maintain isotonicity.

Three mechanisms are responsible for sodium and chloride absorption in the small intestine: (1) active electrogenic transport of sodium, which establishes an electrical gradient for passive absorption of chloride, mostly through the paracellular pathway; (2) sodium absorption directly coupled to the absorption of water-soluble organic solutes such as hexoses, amino acids, and triglycerides, with passive absorption of chloride; and (3) neutral sodium chloride cotransport, in which a carrier at the mucosal membrane mediates the one-for-one entry of both ions into the cell. The ileum has low permeability to chloride, so that active absorption processes are needed for chloride in that part of the gut.

Potassium diffuses passively along electrical and concentration gradients. Calcium diffuses passively and also is actively transported, a process stimulated by vitamin D. Calcium absorption is most efficient in the duodenum, but because intestinal contents are in the jejunum and ileum longer, most calcium is absorbed in these areas. Magnesium is absorbed by all segments of the intestine, but relatively poorly. Iron is absorbed in the duodenum and jejunum, primarily as the ferrous ion.

Bicarbonate is absorbed by secretion of hydrogen ions in exchange for sodium ions; one bicarbonate ion is released into the interstitial fluid for every hydrogen ion secreted, and CO_2 is generated in the intestinal lumen. Phosphate is absorbed in all portions of the small bowel.

Epithelial transport of water and electrolytes is under partial control of the enteric nervous system. Intramural nervous reflexes elicited by luminal stimuli increase fluid secretion from the crypts. The afferent part of these reflexes is not well understood, but acetylcholine and perhaps substance P and VIP are secretory neurotransmitters on the efferent side. Absorption and secretion are influenced by other polypeptides such as somatostatin, corticosteroids, prostaglandins, cAMP, various drugs, and bacterial toxins.

B. Carbohydrate: The polysaccharides starch and glycogen and the disaccharides sucrose and lactose comprise about half the calories ingested by humans. Digestion of starch is begun by salivary amylase and is completed by pancreatic amylase in the duodenum and upper jejunum. The products of hydrolysis are further hydrolyzed by contact with enzymes contained in the brush border of intestinal epithelial cells. The monosaccharides glucose, galactose, and fructose are actively transported against a concentration gradient by a carrier-mediated mechanism that is dependent on and coupled to the absorption of sodium. Monosaccharides are delivered directly into portal blood from the intestinal mucosa.

Although the entire small intestine has the capacity for carbohydrate digestion and absorption, under normal circumstances most absorption of monosaccharides occurs in the duodenum and proximal jejunum. About 10% of dietary starch passes unabsorbed into the colon.

Fiber is insoluble matrix substance of plant cells and is mostly indigestible by human enzymes. It is composed of the carbohydrates cellulose and hemicellulose and the noncarbohydrate lignin. Dietary fiber increases the osmotic load to the distal small intestine and colon and therefore increases stool mass.

C. Protein: Protein is denatured and partially digested in the stomach, but these steps are not essential. Pancreatic enzymes digest protein to form free amino acids and oligopeptides; oligopeptides are attacked by carboxypeptidases and aminopeptidases in the brush border, liberating amino acids, dipeptides, and tripeptides. Amino acids are absorbed by means of an active, carrier-mediated transport mechanism. Dipeptides and tripeptides are actively absorbed into columnar cells, where they are hydrolyzed completely to constituent amino acids. More than 80% of protein absorption occurs in the proximal 100 cm of jejunum. Absorption of ingested protein is virtually complete, and the protein excreted in feces is derived from bacteria, desquamated cells, and mucoproteins.

Important changes occur in the intestine during critical illness, eg, following trauma or abdominal surgery. The intestinal epithelial barrier to absorption of bacteria and endotoxins may be compromised, permitting translocation of bacteria into the circulation. Furthermore, glutamine extraction from the circulation by the small intestine is impaired in septic patients. Glutamine is the preferred fuel for oxidative metabolism by the enterocyte, and diminished uptake of this mucosal nutrient may be significant. In stressed states, glutamine deficiency is associated with mucosal atrophy.

D. Fat: Dietary fat is largely in the form of triglycerides, which are water-insoluble oil droplets until attacked by pancreatic lipase. Colipase, a protein in pancreatic juice, helps lipase adhere to the surface of these oil droplets as the triglycerides are partially hydrolyzed to fatty acids and 2-monoglycerides. These products of digestion are also water-insoluble, and their efficient absorption depends on the presence of bile acids. When the concentration of bile acids exceeds a certain level (the critical micellar concentration), they spontaneously aggregate to form micelles. Bile acids in micelles are arranged with the fat-soluble portion of the molecule toward the center of the aggregate and the water-soluble portion at the periphery; hydrophobic molecules such as fatty acids, monoglycerides, cholesterol, and fat-soluble vitamins are carried in the centers of the micelles.

Micelles release monoglycerides and fatty acids to enter the mucosal cells, where triglycerides are resynthesized, aggregated with phospholipid and cholesterol, and delivered to the lymph as chylomicrons. Medium-chain triglyceride is a synthetic substance that is hydrolyzed to water-soluble fatty acids which do not require bile acids for absorption. Also, these fatty acids are not reesterified to triglycerides in the mucosal cells; they pass directly into portal blood.

Normally, most of the ingested fat is digested and absorbed in the duodenum and proximal jejunum. Conjugated bile acids are actively absorbed in the distal ileum and returned via portal blood to the liver, where they again are secreted into the bile. Disease or resection of the terminal ileum disrupts this enterohepatic circulation, and increased amounts of bile acids enter the colon, where they induce net secretion of water and electrolytes and cause diarrhea (cholerheic diarrhea). Malabsorbed fatty acids contribute to diarrhea by an effect similar to that of castor oil.

E. Vitamins: Vitamin B_{12} (cyanocobalamin) is a water-soluble cobalt compound that requires a special mechanism for absorption, because of its large molecular weight. Dietary vitamin B_{12} complexes with intrinsic factor, a mucoprotein secreted by the gastric parietal cells. The complex dissociates at the surface of cells in the distal ileum, and vitamin B_{12} enters the cells, perhaps by receptor-mediated endocytosis. Folic acid, thiamin, and ascorbic acid are also absorbed by active transport. Other water-soluble vitamins diffuse passively across the mucosa.

Fat-soluble vitamins—notably vitamins A, D, E, and K—are dissolved in mixed micelles and absorbed like other lipids. Since they are totally nonpolar lipids, the absence of bile seriously impairs their absorption.

Debas HT, Mulvihill SJ: Neuroendocrine design of the gut. Am J Surg 1991;161:243.

Edmiston DE Jr., Condon RE: Bacterial translocation. Surg Gynecol Obstet 1991;173:73.

Field M, Rao MC, Chang EB: Intestinal electrolyte transport and diarrheal disease. N Engl J Med 1989;321:800.

Field FJ, Kam NTP, Mathur SN: Regulation of cholesterol metabolism in the intestine. Gastroenterology 1990;99:539.

Gilmore IT: Orocaecal transit time in health and disease. Gut 1990;31:250.

Holmes R, Lobley RW: Intestinal brush border revisited. Gut 1989;30:1667.

Madsen JL, Dahl K: Human migrating myoelectric complex in relation to gastrointestinal transit of a meal. Gut 1990;31:1003.

Rouillon J-M, Azpiroz F, Malagelada J-R: Sensorial and intestinointestinal reflex pathways in the human jejunum. Gastroenterology 1991;101:1606.

Salloum RM, Copeland EM, Souba WW: Brush border transport of glutamine and other substrates during sepsis and endotoxemia. Ann Surg 1991;213:401.

Schippers E et al: Return of interdigestive motor complex after abdominal surgery. End of postoperative ileus? Dig Dis Sci 1991;36:621.

Taché Y, Garrick T, Raybould H: Central nervous system action of peptides to influence gastrointestinal motor function. Gastroenterology 1990;98:517.

BLIND LOOP SYNDROME

The normal concentration of bacteria in the small intestine is about 10^5/mL. Mechanisms that limit bacterial populations include the continual flow of luminal contents, resulting from peristalsis; the interdigestive migrating myoelectric complex, which sweeps away remnants of food; gastric acidity; local effects of immunoglobulins; and the prevention of reflux of colonic contents by the ileocecal valve. Disturbance of any of these mechanisms can lead to bacterial overgrowth and the blind loop (contaminated small bowel, intestinal bacterial overgrowth) syndrome. Strictures, diverticula, fistulas, or blind (poorly emptying) segments of intestine are anatomic lesions that cause stagnation and permit bacterial proliferation. In many patients, stasis of intestinal contents is the result of a functional abnormality of motility (eg, scleroderma). Bacterial overgrowth is observed in patients with immunodeficiency syndromes.

Steatorrhea, diarrhea, megaloblastic anemia, and malnutrition are the hallmarks of the blind loop syndrome. Steatorrhea is the consequence of bacterial deconjugation and dehydroxylation of bile salts in the proximal small bowel. Deconjugated bile salts have a higher critical micellar concentration, and micelle formation is inadequate to solubilize ingested fat in preparation for absorption. The presence of partially digested triglycerides in the distal ileum inhibits jejunal motility ("ileal brake" reflex); nevertheless, the unabsorbed fatty acids enter the colon, where they increase net secretion of water and electrolytes, and diarrhea results. Hypocalcemia occurs because calcium is bound to unabsorbed fatty acids in the intestinal lumen. Macrocytic anemia is due to malabsorption of vitamin B_{12}, largely because of binding of the vitamin by anaerobic bacteria. Malabsorption of carbohydrate and protein is due partly to bacterial catabolism and partly to impaired absorption of these nutrients because of direct damage to the small intestinal mucosa. All of these mechanisms contribute to malnutrition in blind loop syndrome.

Quantitative culture of upper intestinal aspirates is valuable if properly performed; bacterial counts of more than 10^5 per milliliter are generally abnormal. Laboratory studies reveal impaired absorption of orally administered vitamin B_{12} (Schilling test), D-xylose, and ^{14}C triolein. Fecal fat measurement is an obsolete procedure. A large variety of breath tests have been studied, but most have proved to be unreliable. The ^{14}C-D-xylose breath test is the best of these methods available at present. Anaerobic bacteria in the small bowel metabolize xylose, releasing $^{14}CO_2$, which is detected in the breath.

Surgical treatment of the underlying neoplasm, fistula, blind loop, diverticula, or other lesion is carried out whenever possible. A majority of patients do not have a problem that is amenable to surgical correction, however, and treatment consists of broad-spectrum antibiotics and drugs to control diarrhea. It may be necessary to use different antibiotics in sequence, guided by culture results and response to therapy. Damage to enterocytes appears to be reversible with treatment. Octreotide (somatostatin analogue) reduced bacterial overgrowth and improved abdominal symptoms in patients with scleroderma according to a recent report.

Corazza GR et al: The diagnosis of small bowel bacterial overgrowth. Reliability of jejunal culture and inadequacy of breath hydrogen testing. Gastroenterology 1990;98:302.

Corazziari E et al: Perendoscopic manometry of the distal ileum and ileocecal junction in humans. Gastroenterology 1991;101:1314.

Kirsch M: Bacterial overgrowth. Am J Gastroenterol 1990;85:231.

Peled Y et al: D-Xylose absorption test: Urine or blood? Dig Dis Sci 1991;36:188.

Pignata C et al: Jejunal bacterial overgrowth and intestinal permeability in children with immunodeficiency syndromes. Gut 1990;31:879.

Soudah HC, Hasler WL, Owyang C: Effect of octreotide on intestinal motility and bacterial overgrowth in scleroderma. N Engl J Med 1991;325:1461.

Stewart BA et al: The blind loop syndrome in children. J Pediatr Surg 1990;25:905.

SHORT BOWEL SYNDROME

Essentials of Diagnosis

- Extensive small bowel resection.
- Diarrhea.
- Steatorrhea.
- Malnutrition.

General Considerations

The absorptive capacity of the small intestine is normally far in excess of need. The short bowel syndrome may develop after extensive resection of the small intestine for trauma, mesenteric thrombosis, regional enteritis, radiation enteropathy, strangulated small bowel obstruction, or neoplasm. Necrotizing enterocolitis and congenital atresia are the most common pediatric causes.

The ability of a patient to maintain nutrition after massive small bowel resection depends on the extent and site of resection, the presence of the ileocecal valve and the colon, the absorptive function of the intestinal remnant, adaptation of remaining bowel, and the nature of the underlying disease process and its complications. When 3 m or less of the small intestine remain, serious nutritional abnormalities develop. With 2 m or less remaining, function is clinically impaired in most patients, and many patients with 1 m or less of normal bowel require parenteral nutrition at home indefinitely. Some patients with a very short small bowel are net absorbers, and others are net secretors—ie, they put out more intestinal fluid than they take orally.

If the jejunum is resected, the ileum is able to take over most of its absorptive function. Because transport of bile salts, vitamin B$_{12}$, and cholesterol is localized to the ileum, resection of this region is poorly tolerated (Figure 30–4). Bile salt malabsorption causes diarrhea, and steatorrhea occurs if 100 cm or more of distal ileum is resected. Abdominal gamma counting after oral administration of 23-selena-25-homocholyltaurine (^{75}SeHCAT) is a test of bile acid absorption in the distal ileum. Steatorrhea and diarrhea are more pronounced if the ileocecal valve is removed, because this sphincter retards transit into the colon, and it also helps prevent reflux of bacteria from the colon. Blind loop syndrome due to bacterial overgrowth in the shortened small bowel (see above) compounds the problems. Patients who have colectomy in addition to extensive small bowel resection are among the most difficult to manage.

Calcium oxalate urinary tract calculi form in 7–10% of patients who have extensive ileal resection (or disease) and an intact colon. This condition, called **enteric hyperoxaluria,** results from excessive absorption of oxalate from the colon. Two synergistic mechanisms are responsible: (1) Unabsorbed fatty acids combine with calcium, preventing the formation of insoluble calcium oxalate and allowing oxalate to remain available for absorption. (2) Unabsorbed fatty acids and bile acids increase the permeability of the colon to oxalate.

D-Lactic acidosis may result from colonic fermentation of unabsorbed carbohydrate; symptoms of confusion, loss of memory, slurred speech, unsteady gait, and inappropriate behavior resemble those associated with alcoholic intoxication. Treatment includes correction of the acidosis with bicarbonate infusion, thiamine replacement, and antibiotics to reduce colonic flora.

Some patients develop gastric hypersecretion after extensive small bowel resection. It is more marked after proximal resection, and it improves with time. The outpouring of gastric juice may damage the mucosa of the upper intestine, inactivate lipase and trypsin by lowering intraluminal pH, and present an excessive solute load to the intestinal remnant. The increased acid production results from loss of inhibitory hormones normally secreted by the small intestine. Elevated basal and postprandial serum gastrin levels have been detected in some cases.

Clinical Course

During the immediate postoperative period, more than 2 L of daily fluid and electrolyte losses from diarrhea are characteristic. The diarrhea is less severe after a few weeks, and eventually a reasonably normal existence is possible in most cases. The progression of a patient from strict dependence on intravenous feeding to nutritional maintenance by oral intake is possible because of intestinal **adaptation,** a compensatory increase of absorptive capacity in the intestinal remnant. The mucosa becomes hyperplastic, the villi lengthen and the crypts become deeper, the wall thickens, and the intestine elongates and dilates. The intensity of these responses is proportionate to the amount of intestine removed, the segment remaining (greater after proximal than after distal small bowel resection), and the presence of a luminal stream. Nutritional support is essential, and although

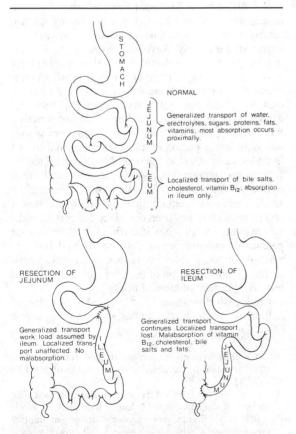

Figure 30–4. The consequences of complete resection of jejunum or ileum are predictable in part from the loss of regionally localized transport processes.

nutrition must be provided intravenously at first, food in the lumen of the intestine is required for full adaptation. Short-chain fatty acids and triglycerides are important trophic nutrients. Glutamine is the principal fuel utilized by the small intestine, and gut glutamine extraction is increased in the first week after massive small bowel resection in animals, but it is not clear whether glutamine needs to be provided specifically to aid in adaptation. Systemic circulating factors are no doubt important; enteroglucagon is strongly implicated, and epidermal growth factor (urogastrone) may also play a role. Somatostatin (octreotide) may impair postresectional hyperplasia.

Treatment

A. General Measures: Treatment of severe short bowel syndrome may be divided into three stages:

1. Stage 1 (intravenous feeding)–During this stage, which lasts 1–3 months, patients should receive nothing by mouth. Careful intravenous fluid and electrolyte therapy and parenteral nutrition must be given. Other important measures include reduction of gastric secretion with intravenous H_2 blockers, control of diarrhea (eg, with loperamide), and protection of perianal skin from irritation. Somatostatin has limited value in reduction of fecal output.

2. Stage 2 (intravenous and oral feeding)– Oral feedings should not be initiated until diarrhea subsides to less than 2.5 L/d. Intravenous nutrition should continue while oral intake begins. Oral rehydration solutions that are used for diarrheal diseases in developing countries are applicable to short bowel syndrome as well. An oral solution of sodium and potassium salts and glucose (or a starch) takes advantage of the phenomenon of cotransport whereby sodium ions are absorbed with the hexose molecules across the intestinal epithelium. Other liquid diets are best tolerated if they are isotonic. Liquid polymeric diets are the next step, and then a more liberal selection of food is allowed. A diet with normal fat content is more palatable and just as effective as a low-fat diet.

Milk may aggravate diarrhea, because total intestinal lactase activity is severely reduced after extensive resection; cheese is tolerated because lactose has been digested in this product. There may be some advantage in making breakfast the largest meal of the day, because as a result of gallbladder filling during the overnight fast, morning may be the time when the greatest amount of bile salts are present in the proximal intestine.

3. Stage 3 (complete oral feeding)–After about 6 months, complete dependence on oral intake may be expected in patients with 1–2 m of remaining small bowel, but full adaptation may require up to 2 years. Maintenance of body weight at levels 20% or more below normal, acceptable bowel habits, and return to productive life are reasonable expectations in many patients. Chronic parenteral nutrition at home is required if oral intake is not tolerated.

Patients with extensive ileal resection require parenteral vitamin B_{12} (1000 µg intramuscularly every 2–3 months) for life. Hyperoxaluria often can be prevented by a diet low in fat and oxalate; supplementary oral calcium or citrate may be helpful. An organic hydrocolloid charged with calcium that has the ability to bind oxalate and reduce urinary oxalate excretion is under study. Oral cholestyramine to minimize diarrhea is usually rejected by patients; loperamide (Imodium) is well tolerated. Pancreatic enzyme supplements may reduce diarrhea also. Deficiencies in magnesium, vitamins D, A, and K, and water-soluble vitamins should be prevented. Osteomalacia is common, and x-rays are falsely negative in many cases; the diagnosis can only be made by bone biopsy. Blind loop syndrome may require treatment. H_2 receptor antagonists reduce acid secretion and improve absorption in the early stages but probably are not needed long-term. The incidence of cholelithiasis is increased in patients with short bowel syndrome, and symptoms should be investigated. Interestingly, the stones may be composed of pigment rather than cholesterol.

B. Adjunctive Surgical Procedures: Surgical procedures to slow intestinal transit, reduce gastric acidity, or increase the absorptive surface are not recommended routinely. Reversed segments, recirculating loops, and construction of valve mechanisms have been tried in the hope of slowing transit and improving absorption. None of these methods have a clearly established role. By enhancing bacterial growth, damaging additional bowel, and obstructing the intestine, they are likely to make matters worse. An implantable pacing unit to slow intestinal transit is under study. Gastric hyperacidity is controlled by H_2 receptor antagonists, and operation is rarely necessary for this problem. A method of lengthening the small intestine by longitudinal division of the bowel and its mesentery has been described for certain pediatric situations. In vivo growth of neomucosa on patches of colonic serosa that are sutured into the wall of the small intestine is promising but experimental. Transplantation of the small intestine has not reached the stage of clinical utility.

Cholecystectomy should be avoided, if possible, to help conserve the bile salt pool and limit the degree of fat malabsorption.

Albert V et al: Systemic factors are trophic in bypassed rat small intestine in the absence of luminal contents. Gut 1990;31:311.

Avery ME, Snyder JD: Oral therapy for acute diarrhea: The underused simple solution. N Engl J Med 1990;323:891.

Bass BL et al: Somatostatin analogue treatment inhibits post-resectional adaptation of the small bowel in rats. Am J Surg 1991;161:107.

Hudson M, Pocknee R, Mowat NA: D-Lactic acidosis in

short bowel syndrome: An examination of possible mechanisms. Q J Med 1990;74:157.

Klimberg VS et al: Intestinal glutamine metabolism after massive small bowel resection. Am J Surg 190;159:27.

Lindsjo M et al: Treatment of enteric hyperoxaluria with calcium-containing organic marine hydrocolloid. Lancet 1989;2:701.

Messing B et al: Intestinal absorption of free oral hyperalimentation in the very short bowel syndrome. Gastroenterology 1991;100:1502.

Miedema BW et al: Absorption and motility of the bypassed human ileum. Dis Colon Rectum 1990;33:829.

Miura S et al: Long-term outcome of massive small bowel resection. Am J Gastroenterol 1991;86:454.

Nightingale JMD et al: Jejunal efflux in short bowel syndrome. Lancet 1990;336:765.

Pigot F et al: Severe short bowel syndrome with a surgically reversed small bowel segment. Dig Dis Sci 1990;35:137.

Pokorny WJ, Fowler CL: Isoperistaltic intestinal lengthening for short bowel syndrome. Surg Gynecol Obstet 1991;172:39.

Weber TR, Tracy TJ, Connors RH: Short-bowel syndrome in children: Quality of life in an era of improved survival. Arch Surg 1991;126:841.

INTESTINAL BYPASS FOR HYPERCHOLESTEROLEMIA

Bypass of the distal third of the small intestine is performed in rare individuals with hypercholesterolemia uncontrollable by medical means. The enterohepatic circulation of bile salts is interrupted, and conversion of cholesterol to bile salts is increased. Plasma cholesterol levels fall about 25%. The LDL cholesterol drops about 40%, and the HDL cholesterol rises an average of 8%. These effects are maintained for 20 years or more. A recent controlled trial found that partial ileal bypass produced sustained improvement in blood lipid patterns of hypercholesterolemic patients who had a myocardial infarction and reduced their subsequent morbidity from coronary heart disease. There is variable disappearance of xanthelasmas (subcutaneous lipid deposits) and tendon xanthomas. Diarrhea is not usually severe. Weight loss averages about 10%.

Partial ileal bypass is performed most often for patients with heterozygous familial hypercholesterolemia. Homozygous familial hypercholesterolemia is more serious than the heterozygous form, and the results of intestinal bypass are not as good. Intestinal bypass is contraindicated in familial hypertriglyceridemia.

Buchwald H et al: Partial ileal bypass for hypercholesterolemia: 20- to 26-year follow-up of the first 57 consecutive cases. Ann Surg 1990;212:318.

Buchwald H et al: Effect of partial ileal bypass surgery on mortality and morbidity from coronary heart disease in patients with hypercholesterolemia. Report of the program on the surgical control of the hyperlipidemias (POSCH). N Engl J Med 1990;323:946.

Campos CT et al: Lipid results of partial ileal bypass in patients with heterozygous, type II-A hyperlipoproteinemia. Surgery 1990;108:601.

Field FJ, Kam NTP, Mathur SN: Regulation of cholesterol metabolism in the intestine. Gastroenterology 1990;99: 539.

OBSTRUCTION OF THE SMALL INTESTINE

Essentials of Diagnosis

Complete proximal obstruction:
- Vomiting.
- Abdominal discomfort.
- Abnormal oral contrast x-rays.

Complete mid or distal obstruction:
- Colicky abdominal pain.
- Vomiting.
- Abdominal distention.
- Constipation-obstipation.
- Peristaltic rushes.
- Dilated small bowel on x-ray.

General Considerations

Obstruction is the most common surgical disorder of the small intestine.

Mechanical obstruction implies a physical barrier that impedes aboral progress of intestinal contents; it may be complete or partial. **Simple obstruction** occludes the lumen only; **strangulation obstruction** impairs the blood supply also and leads to necrosis of the intestinal wall. Most simple obstructions occur at only one point. Closed loop obstruction, in which the lumen is occluded in at least two places (eg, in a volvulus), is commonly associated with strangulation. Ileus is a term whose definition includes mechanical obstruction, but in the USA it usually refers to **paralytic ileus** (adynamic ileus), a disorder in which there is neurogenic failure of peristalsis to propel intestinal contents but no mechanical obstruction.

A. Etiology: (Table 30–1)

1. Adhesions–Adhesions are by far the most common cause of mechanical small bowel obstruction. Congenital bands are seen in children, but adhesions acquired from abdominal operations or inflammation are much more frequent in adults. Surgical glove dusting powders evoke an inflammatory response and contribute to adhesion formation.

Table 30–1. Causes of obstruction of the small intestine in adults.

Causes	Relative Incidence (%)	
Adhesions	60	
External hernia	10	
Neoplasms	20	
Intrinsic		3
Extrinsic		17
Miscellaneous	10	

2. Hernia–Incarceration of an external hernia is the second most common cause of intestinal obstruction, though it is less frequent since prophylactic repair of hernias became common. Inguinal, femoral, or umbilical hernias may have been present for years, or the patient may be unaware of the defect before the onset of obstructive symptoms. An incarcerated hernia may be overlooked by the examining surgeon, particularly if the patient is obese or if the hernia is of the femoral type, and a careful search for external hernias must be made during evaluation of every patient with acute abdominal illness. Internal hernias into the obturator foramen, foramen epiploicum (Winslow), or other anatomic defects are rare, but internal herniation is one of several mechanisms by which acquired adhesions produce obstruction. Surgical defects—lateral to an ileostomy, for example—also provide sites for internal herniation of small bowel loops.

3. Neoplasms–Intrinsic small bowel neoplasms can progressively occlude the lumen or serve as a leading point in intussusception. Symptoms may be intermittent, onset of obstruction is slow, and signs of chronic anemia are present. Neoplasms extrinsic to small bowel may entrap loops, and strategically situated lesions of the colon—particularly those near the ileocecal valve—may present as small bowel obstruction.

4. Intussusception–Invagination of one loop of intestine into another is rarely encountered in adults and is usually caused by a polyp or other intraluminal lesion. Intussusception is more often seen in children; an organic lesion is not required, and the syndrome of colicky pain, passage of blood per rectum, and a palpable mass (the intussuscepted segment) is characteristic.

5. Volvulus–Volvulus results from rotation of bowel loops about a fixed point, often the consequence of congenital anomalies or acquired adhesions. Onset of obstruction is abrupt, and strangulation develops rapidly. Malrotation of the intestine is a cause of volvulus in infants and rarely in adults.

6. Foreign bodies–Bezoars and ingested foreign bodies may pass into the intestine and block the lumen.

7. Gallstone ileus–Passage of a large gallstone into the intestine through a cholecystenteric fistula may produce obstruction of the small bowel. Gallstone ileus is discussed in Chapter 26.

8. Inflammatory bowel disease–Inflammatory bowel disease often causes obstruction when the lumen is narrowed by inflammation or fibrosis of the wall.

9. Stricture–Stricture due to ischemia or radiation injury or surgical trauma can result in mechanical obstruction.

10. Cystic fibrosis–Cystic fibrosis causes chronic partial obstruction of the distal ileum and

right colon in adolescents and adults. It is equivalent to meconium ileus in newborns.

11. Hematoma–Hematoma may develop spontaneously in the intestinal wall in a patient taking anticoagulants.

B. Pathophysiology: The small bowel proximal to a point of obstruction distends with gas and fluid. Swallowed air is the major source of gaseous distention, at least in the early stages, because nitrogen is not well absorbed by mucosa. When bacterial fermentation occurs later on, other gases are produced; the partial pressure of nitrogen within the lumen is lowered, and a gradient for diffusion of nitrogen from blood to lumen is established.

Enormous quantities of fluid from the extracellular space are lost into the gut and from the serosa into the peritoneal cavity. Fluid fills the lumen proximal to the obstruction, because the bidirectional flux of salt and water is disrupted and net secretion is enhanced. Mediator substances (eg, endotoxin, prostaglandins) released from proliferating bacteria in the static luminal contents are responsible. Somatostatin effectively inhibits secretion in animal models of intestinal obstruction, but it has no defined role in humans. Reflexly induced vomiting accentuates the fluid and electrolyte deficit. Hypovolemia leads to multi-organ system failure and is the cause of death in patients with nonstrangulating obstruction.

Audible peristaltic rushes are manifestations of attempts by the small bowel to propel its contents past the obstruction. The vomitus becomes feculent—particularly with distal obstruction—as the illness progresses. Bacterial translocation from lumen to mesenteric nodes and the bloodstream occurs even in simple obstruction. Abdominal distention elevates the diaphragm and impairs respiration, so that pulmonary complications are frequent.

Strangulation is a threat early in the course of closed loop obstruction but must be feared in any complete mechanical obstruction. Incarcerated inguinal hernia and volvulus are examples of obstructing mechanisms that occlude the vascular supply as well as the intestinal lumen. Strangulation rarely if ever results just from progressive distention. Venous drainage is more apt to be interrupted than arterial inflow when the mesentery is trapped. Gangrenous intestine bleeds into the lumen and into the peritoneal cavity, and eventually it perforates. The luminal contents of strangulated intestine are a toxic mixture of bacteria, bacterial products, necrotic tissue, and blood. Some of this fluid may enter the circulation by way of intestinal lymphatics or by absorption from the peritoneal cavity; septic shock is the result.

Clinical Findings
A. Simple Obstruction:
1. Symptoms and signs–(Figure 30–5.) Proximal (high) small bowel obstruction usually presents as profuse vomiting that seldom becomes feculent

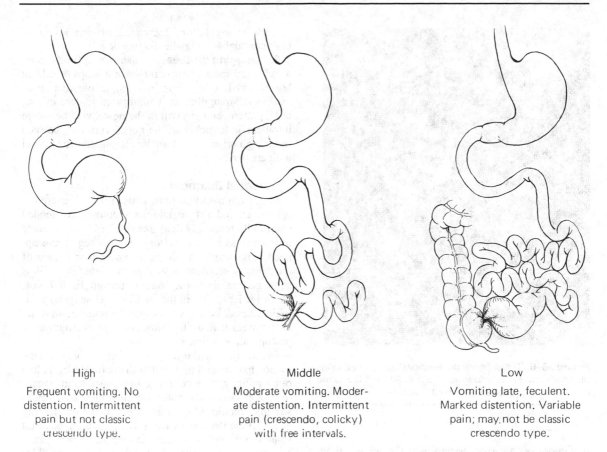

High	Middle	Low
Frequent vomiting. No distention. Intermittent pain but not classic crescendo type.	Moderate vomiting. Moderate distention. Intermittent pain (crescendo, colicky) with free intervals.	Vomiting late, feculent. Marked distention. Variable pain; may not be classic crescendo type.

Figure 30–5. Small bowel obstruction. Variable manifestations of obstruction depend upon the level of blockage of the small bowel.

even in prolonged obstruction. Abdominal pain is variable and often is described as upper abdominal discomfort rather than cramping pain.

Obstruction of the mid or distal small intestine causes cramping periumbilical or poorly localized abdominal pain. Each episode of cramps has a crescendo-decrescendo pattern, lasts for a few seconds to a few minutes, and recurs every few minutes. Between cramps, the patient may be entirely free of pain. Vomiting follows the onset of pain after an interval that varies with the level of obstruction; it may not occur until several hours later. The more distal the obstruction, the more likely it is that vomitus will become feculent. Gas and feces present in the colon may be expelled after the onset of pain, but obstipation always occurs eventually in complete obstruction.

Vital signs may be normal in the early stages, but dehydration is noted with continued loss of fluid and electrolytes. Temperature is normal or mildly elevated. Abdominal distention is minimal to absent in proximal obstruction but is pronounced in more distal obstruction. Peristalsis in dilated loops of small bowel may be visible beneath the abdominal wall in thin patients. Mild tenderness may be elicited. Peristaltic rushes, gurgles, and high-pitched tinkles are audible in coordination with attacks of cramping pain in distal obstruction. Computer analysis of bowel sounds has been suggested to avoid the subjectivity of auscultation. Incarcerated hernias should be sought. Rectal examination is usually normal.

2. Laboratory findings–In the early stages, laboratory findings may be normal; with progression of disease, there are hemoconcentration, leukocytosis, and electrolyte abnormalities that depend on the level of obstruction and the severity of dehydration. Serum amylase is often elevated.

3. Imaging studies–Supine and upright plain abdominal films reveal a ladder-like pattern of dilated small bowel loops with air-fluid levels (Figure 30–6). These features may be minimal or absent in early obstruction, proximal obstruction, or closed loop obstruction or in some cases when fluid-filled loops contain little gas. The colon is often devoid of gas unless the patient has been given an enema, has undergone sigmoidoscopy, or has only a partial obstruction. Opaque gallstones and air in the biliary tree should be looked for. Administration of contrast

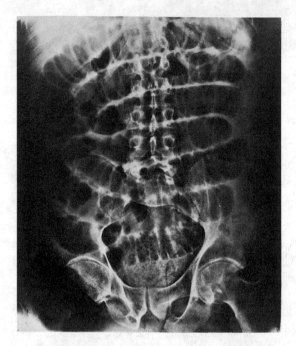

Figure 30–6. Small bowel obstruction. Note dilated loops of small bowel in a ladder-like pattern. Air-fluid levels are not obvious, because the patient is supine.

media orally confirms the presence of mechanical obstruction and its completeness. Enteroclysis gives more detail about the level and cause of obstruction, and it may diagnose closed loop obstruction. CT scan is useful in patients with a history of abdominal malignancy and in some other situations.

B. Strangulation Obstruction: Although certain clinical features should make the surgeon suspicious of strangulation, no historical, physical, or laboratory findings entirely exclude the possibility of strangulation in complete small bowel obstruction. At least one-third of strangulation obstructions are unsuspected before operation, which underscores the need for early operation whenever obstruction is complete. Newer tools may have an impact on this problem in the future. Computer-assisted prediction of strangulation has shown promise, and enteroclysis may detect closed-loop obstruction before strangulation can occur.

1. Symptoms and signs–Shock that appears early in the course of obstruction suggests a strangulated closed loop. When strangulation supervenes in simple obstruction, high fever may develop, previously cramping abdominal pain may become a severe continuous ache, vomitus may contain gross or occult blood, and abdominal tenderness and rigidity may appear.

2. Laboratory findings–Marked leukocytosis not accounted for by hemoconcentration alone should suggest strangulation. Increased plasma levels of malondialdehyde may be diagnostic

3. Imaging studies–Intraperitoneal fluid is seen as widened spaces between adjacent loops of dilated bowel and is often found in simple obstruction as well as in strangulation. Thumbprinting, loss of mucosal pattern, and gas within the bowel wall or within intrahepatic branches of the portal vein may be seen in strangulation. Air-fluid levels outside the bowel indicate perforation.

Differential Diagnosis

Pain from paralytic ileus is usually not severe but is constant and diffuse, and the abdomen is distended and mildly tender. If ileus has resulted from an acute intraperitoneal inflammatory process (eg, acute appendicitis), there should be symptoms and signs of the primary problem as well as the ileus. Plain films show gas mainly in the colon in uncomplicated postoperative ileus; gas in the small bowel suggests peritonitis. Small bowel x-rays may be required in order to distinguish ileus from mechanical obstruction in postoperative patients.

Obstruction of the large intestine is characterized by obstipation and abdominal distention; pain is less often colicky, and vomiting is an inconstant symptom. X-rays usually make the diagnosis by demonstrating colonic dilation proximal to the obstructing lesion. If the ileocecal valve is incompetent, the distal small bowel will be dilated, and a barium enema may be needed to determine the level of obstruction. This subject is covered in detail in Chapter 31.

Acute gastroenteritis, acute appendicitis, and acute pancreatitis can mimic simple intestinal obstruction. Strangulation obstruction may be confused with acute hemorrhagic pancreatitis or mesenteric vascular occlusion.

Intestinal pseudo-obstruction is a diverse group of disorders in which there are symptoms and signs of intestinal obstruction without evidence for an obstructing lesion. Acute pseudo-obstruction of the colon carries the risk of cecal perforation and is discussed in Chapter 31. Chronic or recurrent pseudo-obstruction affecting the small bowel with or without colonic involvement is often idiopathic. In other cases, pseudo-obstruction is associated with scleroderma, myxedema, lupus erythematosus, amyloidosis, drug abuse (eg, phenothiazine ingestion), radiation injury, or progressive systemic sclerosis. Several variations of familial visceral *myopathy* have been identified with seemingly distinct patterns of intestinal pseudo-obstruction. Patients with familial visceral *neuropathy* have degeneration of axons and neurons of the myenteric plexus of the gastrointestinal tract, and pseudo-obstruction results.

Patients with chronic pseudo-obstruction have recurrent attacks of vomiting, cramping abdominal pain, and abdominal distention. In some patients the esophagus, stomach, small bowel, colon, and urinary bladder all have abnormal motility, but in others one or more of these organs may be spared. Treatment is directed at the underlying disease if there is one. Metoclopramide should be tried, but management of idiopathic pseudo-obstruction is largely supportive.

Treatment

Partial small bowel obstruction can be treated expectantly as long as there is continued passage of stool and flatus. Plain abdominal x-rays show gas in the colon, and small bowel contrast x-rays prove the diagnosis. Decompression with a nasogastric or long intestinal tube is successful in 90% of such patients. Operation is required if obstruction persists for several days even though it is incomplete.

Complete obstruction of the small intestine is treated by operation after a period of careful preparation. The compelling reason for operation is that strangulation cannot be excluded with certainty, and strangulation is associated with high rates of complications and death. The surgeon must avoid being lulled into a false sense of security by the improvement in symptoms and signs that almost invariably occurs after resuscitation.

There are exceptions to the general rule that operation must be performed promptly: Incomplete obstruction, postoperative obstruction, a history of numerous previous operations for obstruction, radiation therapy, inflammatory bowel disease, and abdominal carcinomatosis are situations demanding mature judgment, and judicious nonoperative management may be in the patient's best interests. A long intestinal tube (eg, Miller-Abbott tube) may be passed in these cases to decompress the intestine.

A. Preparation: Proper timing of the operation is determined by the requirements of individual patients. The risk of strangulation must be weighed against the severity of fluid and electrolyte abnormalities and the need for evaluation and treatment of associated systemic diseases.

1. Nasogastric suction–A nasogastric tube should be inserted immediately upon admission to the emergency ward in order to relieve vomiting, avoid aspiration, and reduce the contribution of further swallowed air to the abdominal distention. A few surgeons routinely attempt to pass a long intestinal tube. Endoscopy may be of use when manipulating a tube through the pylorus.

2. Fluid and electrolyte resuscitation–Depending upon the level and duration of obstruction, fluid and electrolyte deficits are mild to severe. Hemoconcentration induced by long-standing obstruction cannot be corrected by dextrose solutions alone. Fluid losses are isotonic, and resuscitation should begin with infusion of isotonic saline solution. Losses of gastrointestinal fluid also entail acid-base deficits, and since there is no neuroendocrine mechanism for correcting these deficits, the surgeon must do so. Serum electrolyte concentrations and arterial

blood gas determinations are guides to electrolyte therapy; potassium is best withheld until urine output is satisfactory, but patients should not undergo operation until hypokalemia has been treated. The volume of fluid required and its exact electrolyte composition must be calculated for each patient, and careful monitoring of clinical signs and associated systemic diseases is imperative. Some patients—notably those with strangulation obstruction—require plasma or blood. Antibiotics should be given if strangulation is even remotely suspected.

B. Operation: Operation may commence when the patient has been rehydrated and vital organs are functioning satisfactorily. Occasionally, the toxic effects of strangulation may force operation at an earlier time.

A standard groin incision is used for patients with incarcerated inguinal or femoral hernias, but other types of obstruction require an abdominal incision. Wide exposure is essential, and the position of the incision is partly dictated by the location of scars from previous operations.

Details of the operative procedure vary according to the cause of obstruction. Adhesive bands causing obstruction should be lysed; an obstructing tumor should be resected; and an obstructing foreign body should be removed through an enterotomy. Gangrenous intestine must be resected, but it may be difficult to determine whether obstructed bowel is viable or not. The loop should be wrapped in a warm saline-soaked pack and inspected for color, mesenteric pulsation, and peristalsis several minutes later. Intraoperative use of Doppler ultrasound has been suggested as a method of determining viability of obstructed intestine, but it is not reliable. The qualitative fluorescein test may be helpful; 1000 mg of fluorescein is injected into a peripheral vein over a 30- to 60-second period, and the bowel is then inspected under ultraviolet (Wood's) light. If the loop appears nonviable, resection with end-to-end anastomosis is the safest course.

Extirpation of the obstructing lesion is not possible in some patients with carcinoma or radiation injury. Anastomosis of proximal small bowel to small or large intestine distal to the obstruction (bypass) may be the best procedure in these patients. Rarely, adhesions are so dense that the intestine cannot be freed and bypass cannot be accomplished. Prolonged decompression through a gastrostomy tube or Baker tube and provision of nutrition via the parenteral route may allow spontaneous resolution over a period of a few weeks.

Decompression of massively dilated small bowel loops facilitates closure of the abdomen and may shorten the time for recovery of bowel function postoperatively. Decompression is accomplished by threading down a long tube passed orally or by needle aspiration through the bowel wall.

Attempts to prevent uncontrolled adhesion formation by suturing loops of bowel so that they are fixed in a suitable relation to one another (Nobel plication procedures) are unsuccessful. However, another procedure in which a long tube is inserted through a gastrostomy or jejunostomy for 10 days to provide intraluminal stenting has some proponents. Attempts to prevent adhesions by placement of various substances in the peritoneal cavity have met limited success; a 5% solution of polyethylene glycol 4000 has shown promise.

Prognosis

Nonstrangulating obstruction has a death rate of about 2%; most of these deaths occur in the elderly. Strangulation obstruction has a mortality rate of approximately 8% if operation is performed within 36 hours of the onset of symptoms and 25% if operation is delayed beyond 36 hours. Recurrent obstruction after lysis of adhesions is uncommon.

Camilleri M, Carbone LD, Schuffler MD: Familial enteric neuropathy with pseudoobstruction. Dig Dis Sci 1991; 36:1168.

Czyrko C et al: Blunt abdominal trauma resulting in intestinal obstruction: When to operate? J Trauma 1990; 30:1567.

Deitch EA et al: Obstructed intestine as a reservoir for systemic infection. Am J Surg 1990;159:394.

Ellis CN et al: Small bowel obstruction after colon resection for benign and malignant diseases. Dis Colon Rectum 1991;34:367.

Ellis H: The hazards of surgical glove dusting powders. Surg Gynecol Obstet 1990;171:521.

Gallegos NC et al: Risk of strangulation in groin hernias. Br J Surg 1991;78:1171.

Livingston EH, Passaro EPJ: Postoperative ileus. Dig Dis Sci 1990;35:121.

Maglinte DDT, Nolan DJ, Herlinger H: Preoperative diagnosis by enteroclysis of unsuspected closed loop obstruction in medically managed patients. J Clin Gastroenterol 1991;13:308.

Megibow AJ et al: Bowel obstruction: Evaluation with CT. Radiology 1991;180:313.

Neville R et al: Vascular responsiveness in obstructed gut. Dis Colon Rectum 1991;34:229.

O'Sullivan D et al: Peritoneal adhesion formation after lysis: Inhibition by polyethylene glycol 4000. Br J Surg 1991;78:427.

Shrake PD et al: Radiographic evaluation of suspected small bowel obstruction. Am J Gastroenterol 1991; 86:175.

Snyder CL et al: Nonoperative management of small-bowel obstruction with endoscopic long intestinal tube placement. Am Surgeon 1990;56:587.

Welch JP: *Bowel Obstruction. Differential Diagnosis and Clinical Management.* Saunders, 1990.

Yoshino H et al: Clinical application of spectral analysis of bowel sounds in intestinal obstruction. Dis Colon Rectum 1990;33:753.

ACQUIRED INTESTINAL DIVERTICULA*

Congenital diverticula of the jejunum are rare, but acquired diverticula are found in the jejunum (or ileum) in 1.3% of radiographic studies or autopsy series when specifically sought. Jejunal diverticula are wide-mouthed sacs measuring 1–25 cm in diameter. Most contain all layers of the intestinal wall (true diverticula), but some consist of mucosa and submucosa herniated through thickened muscularis (false diverticula). Diverticula in the small bowel are often multiple; they diminish in frequency from the ligament of Treitz to the ileocecal valve and are associated with diverticulosis of the duodenum or colon in 30% of cases. Most symptomatic patients are over age 60.

Jejunal diverticulosis is a heterogeneous disorder associated with abnormalities of smooth muscle or the myenteric plexus. Intestinal pseudo-obstruction is a common associated problem, also reflecting the presence of an underlying motility disorder such as familial visceral myopathy or progressive systemic sclerosis.

Symptoms may be due to pseudo-obstruction or to inflammation of the diverticula. Acute intestinal bleeding and diverticulitis leading to perforation may occur. Blind loop syndrome is caused by bacterial overgrowth in the stagnant bowel with pseudo-obstruction or in large diverticula.

Barium x-rays may outline the diverticula (Figure 30–7) and reveal the underlying motility disorder. The primary cause should be sought.

Operation is required for perforation or bleeding. Symptoms of the underlying motility disorder are not improved by resection of the segment containing diverticula.

Garrett JP, Nolan DJ: Diverticula of the terminal ileum. Clin Radiol 1989;40:178.

Palder SB, Frey CB: Jejunal diverticulosis. Arch Surg 1988;123:889.

Wilcox RD, Shatney CH: Surgical significance of acquired ileal diverticulosis. Am Surgeon 1990;56:222.

CROHN'S DISEASE*
(Regional Enteritis)

Essentials of Diagnosis
- Diarrhea.
- Abdominal pain and palpable mass.
- Low-grade fever, lassitude, weight loss.
- Anemia.
- Radiographic findings of thickened, stenotic bowel with ulceration and internal fistulas.

---

*Meckel's diverticulum and other congenital diverticula of the small intestine are discussed in Chapter 46.

*Crohn's disease of the colon is discussed in Chapter 31.

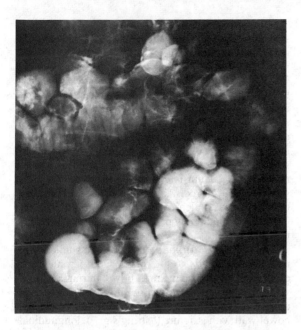

Figure 30–7. Jejunal diverticula.

General Considerations

Crohn's disease is a chronic progressive granulomatous inflammatory disorder of the gastrointestinal tract. From two to nine cases per 100,000 population are detected annually in Europe and the USA. The prevalence ranges broadly from 20 to 90 per 100,000 population. There is geographic variation (more common in urban dwellers and Northern residents of the USA), and there is a relatively high incidence among Ashkenazi Jews. The peak incidence occurs between the second and fourth decades. Cigarette smoking and a high intake of sugar are independent risk factors for Crohn's disease.

A. Etiology: The cause of Crohn's disease is unknown. Theories holding that Crohn's disease is caused by bovine milk products or is the result of psychophysiologic abnormalities have been discarded. The favored hypothesis is that Crohn's disease results from the interaction of genetic and environmental factors. A genetic influence is suggested by a family history of inflammatory bowel disease in 15–20% of patients. Offspring of couples, both of whom have inflammatory bowel disease, have a high risk (36%) of developing the illness. Transmissible agents, including small viruses, cell wall-deficient *Pseudomonas*-like bacteria, mycobacteria, chlamydiae, and *Yersinia,* have been isolated from tissues of patients with Crohn's disease. Data thus far lack reproducibility and specificity, but this type of environmental influence is a likely candidate for an important role in the causation of Crohn's disease. Numerous immunologic abnormalities have been reported, but the importance of these changes remains conjectural.

B. Pathology: Crohn's disease may affect any part of the gastrointestinal tract from the lips to the anus and may even spill over into the larynx or extend beyond the gut to the skin. "Metastatic" skin lesions have been described. The distal ileum is the most frequent site of involvement, eventually becoming diseased in about three-fourths of patients. The small bowel alone is involved in 15–30%, both the distal ileum and the colon in 40–60%, and the large bowel alone in 25–30%. Duodenal Crohn's disease is found in 0.5–7% of patients. Discontinuous areas of disease with segments of normal bowel between ("skip lesions") occur in 15% of patients. Subtle histologic changes can be seen in "normal," grossly uninvolved intestine of patients with Crohn's disease, suggesting that the mucosa of the entire bowel may be abnormal in this disorder.

The earliest Crohn's lesion is a focal accumulation of inflammatory cells adjacent to an epithelial crypt. Candidate mediators of inflammation include plasma activating factor, leukotrienes, complement, kinins, enterotoxin, interleukins, tumor necrosis factor, and neurotransmitters of the enteric nervous system. In a process similar to that seen in ischemia, reactive molecules such as oxygen radicals are generated; they propagate the inflammatory response and contribute to tissue damage. Erosions, crypt abscesses, and granulomas result.

Granulomas are seen in the bowel wall in 50–70% and in mesenteric lymph nodes in 25% of patients. The number of granulomas is related to the duration of the history and the site of involvement. It has been speculated that granuloma formation reflects efforts to localize or eliminate the causative agent of Crohn's disease. Mucosal lesions appear grossly as tiny (pinpoint) hemorrhagic spots or shallow ulcers with white bases and elevated margins (aphthous ulcers). Punched out ulcers are seen with progression of the disease. The next stage is development of fissures—knife-like clefts beginning in mucosa and extending deeply into the wall. These fissures and the serpiginous or linear ulcers surrounding islands of intact mucosa overlying edematous submucosa give a cobblestone appearance to the luminal surface. Crohn's disease ultimately becomes a transmural inflammatory process with thickening of the bowel wall, and it often progresses to stricture formation. The bowel and its mesentery are foreshortened in advanced cases, and on gross inspection mesenteric fat seems to have advanced over the surface of the bowel toward the antimesenteric border.

Clinical Findings

A. Symptoms and Signs: Crohn's disease has many modes of presentation:

1. Diarrhea—Continuous or episodic diarrhea is noted in about 90% of patients. Stools are liquid or semisolid and characteristically contain no blood if small bowel alone is diseased. One-third of patients with colonic involvement pass blood, and a few present with bloody diarrhea resembling that seen in ulcerative colitis.

2. Recurrent abdominal pain–Mild colic initiated by meals, centered in the lower abdomen, and relieved by defecation is common. These symptoms are due to chronic partial obstruction of the small bowel, colon, or both. Some patients progress to complete obstruction, and they have severe cramping, vomiting, and abdominal distention.

3. Abdominal symptoms and constitutional effects–Episodic attacks of abdominal pain and diarrhea accompanied by lassitude, malaise, weight loss, fever, and anemia are a common syndrome. A mass is often palpable in the right lower quadrant in these patients. Occasionally, fever of unknown origin is the only clinical finding.

4. Anorectal lesions–Chronic anal fissures, large ulcers, complex anal fistulas, or pararectal abscesses are seen in 15–25% of patients with Crohn's disease confined to small bowel and in 50–75% of those with colonic involvement. These problems may appear many years before the intestinal disease. Histologic features of Crohn's disease, including granulomas, are often found in biopsies of anorectal lesions even when the only other identifiable disease is located much higher in the gastrointestinal tract.

5. Anemia–Iron deficiency anemia or macrocytic anemia due to vitamin B_{12} or folate deficiency may occur in the absence of abdominal symptoms.

6. Malnutrition–Protein-losing enteropathy, steatorrhea, chronic obstruction, and diminished dietary intake from chronic illness contribute to malnutrition and weight loss. Mineral and vitamin deficiencies (especially vitamin D deficiency) are common. Deficiencies of water-soluble and fat-soluble vitamins are common in patients with Crohn's disease of the small intestine, but clinical symptoms of vitamin deficiency are rare. Zinc deficiency has been recognized. Children afflicted with extensive Crohn's disease fail to grow and may have severely retarded sexual maturation. Reversal of growth arrest by parenteral feeding emphasizes the importance of malnutrition as a cause of growth failure in Crohn's disease. Somatomedin C levels may be a reliable marker of nutritional adequacy.

7. Acute onset–Acute abdominal pain and right lower quadrant tenderness mimicking acute appendicitis may be found at operation to be due to acute inflammation of the distal ileum. Only 15% of such cases evolve into chronic Crohn's disease, suggesting that most patients with acute ileitis have an infectious process unrelated to Crohn's disease. This condition is discussed further in the section on acute enteritis and mesenteric lymphadenitis.

8. Systemic complications–Any of the systemic complications described below may prompt the patient to seek medical advice.

B. Laboratory Findings: Tests results are nonspecific and vary greatly according to the site of intestinal involvement, the severity of disease, and the presence of complications such as abscess or fistula. The sedimentation rate may not be elevated in patients with disease of the small intestine. Hypoalbuminemia, anemia, and steatorrhea are common. Abnormal D-xylose absorption suggests extensive disease or fistula formation, since carbohydrate is normally absorbed in the jejunum. Breath tests, as described in the section on blind loop syndrome, are abnormal if the ileum is diseased or if bacterial overgrowth has occurred. Abnormal fecal α_1-antitrypsin (α_1-antiprotease) clearance and concentration reflect inflammation and may predict recurrence after resection.

C. Imaging Studies: Radiographic studies contribute substantially to the diagnosis of Crohn's disease. The appearance of small bowel during a barium study is a composite of proliferative and destructive changes. The principal findings include thickened bowel wall with stricture ("string sign"), longitudinal ulceration that is shallow at first but becomes deep and undermining, deep transverse fissures resembling spicules, and cobblestone formation (Figure 30–8). Deformity of the cecum, fistulas, abscesses, and skip lesions are additional findings of importance. Enteroclysis provides excellent detail. CT scan, ultrasound, and MRI have diagnostic value in some cases.

^{111}In-tagged granulocytes accumulate in Crohn's lesions over 2–3 hours and can be detected by scintiscan. Autologous ^{99m}Tc-labeled phagocyte scanning assesses disease activity. Gamma scanning after oral administration of ^{75}SeHCAT is a nonspecific test for the presence of diseased or dysfunctional distal ileum. Sucralfate complexed to ^{99m}Tc helps localize

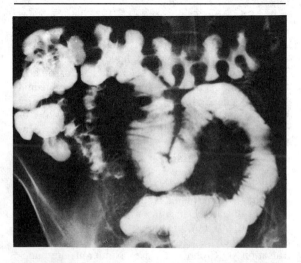

Figure 30–8. Barium x-ray showing spicules, edema, and ulcers in Crohn's disease.

Crohn's disease. Other isotope tests include ^{51}Cr-EDTA for intestinal permeability and ^{99m}Tc-porphyrins for assessing intestinal inflammation.

D. Endoscopy: Upper gastrointestinal endoscopy diagnoses esophageal, gastric, and duodenal lesions. Colonoscopy reveals typical changes of Crohn's disease in the colon if it is involved or in the ileum if it can be examined. Ileoscopy after colectomy is accurate for the diagnosis of Crohn's disease in the ileum.

Differential Diagnosis

A. Ulcerative Colitis: Crohn's disease of the colon may be difficult to distinguish from ulcerative colitis. This topic is covered in detail in Chapter 31.

B. Appendicitis: Acute ileitis may be the presenting manifestation, and differentiation from appendicitis may be impossible without operation.

C. Tuberculosis: Tuberculosis may affect any part of the gastrointestinal tract but is uncommon distal to the cecum. Small bowel tuberculosis is discussed elsewhere in this chapter.

D. Lymphoma: Radiographic findings help differentiate lymphoma from Crohn's disease, but histologic examination of the tissue is occasionally required before the diagnosis is certain. Rectal or colonic biopsies that show granulomas or colitis may support the diagnosis of Crohn's disease.

E. Other Diseases: Carcinoma, amebiasis, ischemia, eosinophilic gastroenteritis, and other inflammatory conditions may simulate Crohn's disease. Enteropathy from nonsteroidal anti-inflammatory agents has recently been added to this list.

Complications

A. Intestinal: Some intestinal complications, such as obstruction, abscess, fistula, and anorectal lesions, are so common that they are regarded as part of the characteristic clinical picture. Free perforation and massive hemorrhage are uncommon. The risk of cholelithiasis is increased. Oral manifestations of Crohn's disease may cause disabling pain. Carcinoma may occur in segments of small or large bowel that are involved with Crohn's disease, especially in segments excluded from the fecal stream by surgical bypass procedures.

B. Systemic: Systemic complications such as hepatobiliary disease, uveitis, arthritis, ankylosing spondylitis, aphthous ulcers, erythema nodosum, amyloidosis, thromboembolism, and vascular disorders are found both in Crohn's disease and in ulcerative colitis. These manifestations are described more fully in Chapter 31. "Metastatic" (distant cutaneous) Crohn's disease is a cutaneous ulcer with a granulomatous reaction at a site separated from gut by normal skin. Urinary complications include cystitis, calculi, and ureteral obstruction.

Treatment

The initial treatment of Crohn's disease is nonoperative. Physical rest, relief of emotional stress, and a confiding patient-doctor relationship have favorable effects. A low-residue, milk-free, high-protein diet may provide adequate nutrition. Malnourished patients benefit from elemental or polymeric diets if standard food is not tolerated, and total or supplementary parenteral nutrition is an important adjunct. As nutrition improves, infection is more successfully treated, and complications such as fistulas may be reversed. Chronic intermittent elemental diet improves growth failure in prepubertal children. Most clinicians prefer enteral feeding over the parenteral route when conditions permit, though comparative studies are inconclusive on this issue. Preoperative total parenteral nutrition prolongs the hospital stay and should be restricted to patients with severe active disease. Chronic parenteral nutrition at home allows some patients with extensive disease to postpone operation, but it does not reduce the necessity of operation over the long term.

Enteral nutrition alone is insufficient therapy for active Crohn's disease compared with pharmacologic treatment. The standard drugs for Crohn's disease are steroids, sulfasalazine, immunosuppressives, and antibiotics. Prednisone, prednisolone, and methylprednisolone are the most common corticosteroids for this purpose. Studies suggest that steroids are most effective for Crohn's disease of the small intestine, but they are applied to Crohn's colitis as well. Prednisone (0.25–0.75 mg/d) and sulfasalazine (1 g/15 kg/d) are each superior to placebo in the control of acute disease over the short term. These two agents often are given in combination. The utility of prednisone is limited by side effects, and the use of sulfasalazine is complicated by adverse reactions. The active principle of sulfasalazine is 5-aminosalicylic acid; oral forms (mesalamine in the USA and mesalazine in Europe) are now available. Other aminosalicylate preparations are in development. Azathioprine and mercaptopurine are the immunosuppressive drugs with the longest records. They are effective in Crohn's colitis and less so in ileitis; they spare steroids (allow reduction of steroid doses), help close fistulas, maintain remissions, and heal perianal disease. The disadvantage of azathioprine and mercaptopurine is their slow action, often requiring 4 months or more before effects are seen. Cyclosporine is another immunosuppressive agent that is used in inflammatory bowel disease; 59% of patients with active chronic Crohn's disease benefited from cyclosporine in a controlled trial, and the drug worked quickly—within days or weeks. Various broad-spectrum antibiotics have been tried, but only metronidazole is used regularly. Metronidazole is effective for Crohn's colitis, particularly perianal disease.

The indication for operation in Crohn's disease of the small bowel is obstruction in about half of cases;

perforation, internal fistula, external fistula, abscess, perianal disease, and growth failure in children are other reasons for operation. Over the long term, about 70% of patients with Crohn's disease undergo definitive surgery. Conservative resection of diseased bowel with end-to-end anastomosis is the preferred surgical procedure. If an inflammatory mass adheres to vital structures, however, it may be necessary to bypass rather than resect the involved segment. Extensive involvement of small bowel, either diffusely or by skip lesions, is unfavorable for curative resection. Resection is usually limited to the area responsible for the complications that prompted operation. If multiple symptomatic strictures are encountered, they can be treated by "strictureplasty," a procedure in which the bowel is incised through the stricture and the wall is sutured in such a way that the lumen is widened. Strictureplasty can be accomplished with staples as well.

Prognosis

Crohn's disease is a chronic condition. It may progress to involve additional portions of bowel or may seem to spread no farther. Surgical procedures are palliative, not curative, but operations contribute greatly to rehabilitation of patients with refractory disease. The recurrence rate after resection of ileal or ileocolic disease increases with time; symptomatic recurrence rates range from 25% to 50% at 5 years, from 35% to 80% at 10 years, and from 45% to 85% at 15 years. The marked variability is due to differences in patient populations, type of surgical procedures, and criteria for recurrence. Extensive confluent ulcers seen endoscopically in the ileum at the anastomosis within 1 year after ileocolectomy strongly predict symptomatic recurrence. Strictureplasty is surprisingly effective for obstructive lesions, and there are few postoperative complications. Reoperation is needed in about 10% of patients within a year after strictureplasty, and in one-third of patients by 10 years, but the strictureplasty sites show no evidence of inflammation and are not the source of symptoms.

Surgery should be used to manage complications in coordination with medical therapy. This team approach enables 80–85% of patients who require surgery to lead normal lives. The long-term risk of death is twice normal in patients with Crohn's disease. There is little evidence that pregnancy affects the course of Crohn's disease or that inactive Crohn's disease alters the course of pregnancy.

Andrews HA et al: Strategy for management of distal ileal Crohn's disease. Br J Surg 1991;78:679.

Bello C, Goldstein F, Thornton JJ: Alternate-day prednisone treatment and treatment maintenance in Crohn's disease. Am J Gastroenterol 1991;86:460.

Bennett RA, Rubin PH, Present DH: Frequency of inflammatory bowel disease in offspring of couples both presenting with inflammatory bowel disease. Gastroenterology 1991;100:1638.

Brynskov J et al: A placebo-controlled, double-blind, randomized trial of cyclosporine therapy in active chronic Crohn's disease. N Engl J Med 1989;321:845.

Cravo M et al: Nutritional support in Crohn's disease: Which route? Am J Gastroenterol 1991;86:317.

Drossman DA et al: Health status and health care use in persons with inflammatory bowel disease: A national sample. Dig Dis Sci 1991;36:1746.

Ekbom A et al: The epidemiology of inflammatory bowel disease: A large, population-based study in Sweden. Gastroenterology 1991;100:350.

Galandiuk S et al: A century of home parenteral nutrition for Crohn's disease. Am J Surg 1990;159:540.

Gitnick G (editor): *Inflammatory Bowel Disease. Diagnosis and Treatment.* Igaku-Shoin, 1991.

Jayanthi V et al: Current concepts of the etiopathogenesis of inflammatory bowel disease. Am J Gastroenterol 1991; 86:1566.

Lochs H et al: Comparison of enteral nutrition and drug treatment in active Crohn's disease: Results of the European Cooperative Crohn's Disease Study IV. Gastroenterology 1991;101:881.

Michelassi F et al: Primary and recurrent Crohn's disease. Experience with 1379 patients. Ann Surg 1991;214:230.

Modigliani R et al: Clinical, biological, and endoscopic picture of attacks of Crohn's disease: Evolution on prednisolone. Gastroenterology 1990;98:811.

Nelson RL et al: Indium 111-labeled granulocyte scan in the diagnosis and management of acute inflammatory bowel disease. Dis Colon Rectum 1990;33:451.

O'Brien CJ et al: Elemental diet in steroid-dependent and steroid-refractory Crohn's disease. Am J Gastroenterol 1991;86:1614.

O'Brien JJ, Bayless TM, Bayless JA: Use of azathioprine or 6-mercaptopurine in the treatment of Crohn's disease. Gastroenterology 1991;101:39.

Olaison G, Sjödahl R, Tagesson C: Glucocorticoid treatment in ileal Crohn's disease: Relief of symptoms but not of endoscopically viewed inflammation. Gut 1990; 31:325.

Plauth M, Henss H, Meyle J: Oral manifestations of Crohn's disease. An analysis of 79 cases. J Clin Gastroenterol 1991;13:29.

Podolsky DK: Inflammatory bowel disease. N Engl J Med 1991;325:928.

Pritchard TJ et al: Strictureplasty of the small bowel in patients with Crohn's disease: An effective surgical option. Arch Surg 1990;125:715.

Ribeiro MB et al: Adenocarcinoma of the small intestine in Crohn's disease. Surg Gynecol Obstet 1991;173:343.

Ribeiro MB et al: Intra-abdominal abscess in regional enteritis. Ann Surg 1991;213:32.

Rigaud D et al: Controlled trial comparing two types of enteral nutrition in treatment of active Crohn's disease: elemental v polymeric diet. Gut 1991;32:1492.

Rutgeerts P et al: Predictability of the postoperative course of Crohn's disease. Gastroenterology 1990;99:956.

Sachar DB: Inflammatory bowel disease: Back to the future. Am J Gastroenterol 1990;85:373.

Sedgwick DM et al: Population-based study of surgery in juvenile onset Crohn's disease. Br J Surg 1991;78:171.

Sonnenberg A, McCarty DJ, Jacobsen SJ: Geographic variation of inflammatory bowel disease within the United States. Gastroenterology 1991;100:143.

Stowe SP et al: An epidemiologic study of inflammatory bowel disease in Rochester, New York: Hospital incidence. Gastroenterology 1990;98:104.

Tonelli F, Ficari F: Pathological features of Crohn's disease determining perforation. J Clin Gastroenterol 1991;13:226.

Williams JG et al: Recurrence of Crohn's disease after resection. Br J Surg 1991;78:10.

OTHER INFLAMMATORY & ULCERATIVE DISEASES OF THE SMALL INTESTINE

Acute Enteritis & Mesenteric Lymphadenitis

Acute inflammation of the small intestine (enteritis) often also affects the stomach (**gastroenteritis**) or the colon (**enterocolitis**). Involvement of regional lymph nodes is termed **mesenteric adenitis.** These usually self-limiting illnesses may be caused by viruses, bacteria, parasites, toxins, or unknown agents.

Gastrointestinal infections are frequent in AIDS patients. Enteric pathogens recoverable from these patients include *Cryptosporidium,* cytomegalovirus, *Entamoeba histolytica, Giardia lamblia, Mycobacterium avium-intracellulare, Salmonella typhimurium, Shigella,* and *Campylobacter jejuni.* The most common pathogen associated with diarrhea in one study was *Cryptosporidium.* Stool examination identifies the infection in 60% of cases, and endoscopy with biopsies adds to diagnostic accuracy. Intestinal perforation is a rare but devastating complication in these patients.

Blacklow NR, Greenberg HB: Viral gastroenteritis. N Engl J Med 1991;325:252.

Conlon CP, Peto TEA: Infectious diarrhoea. Int J Colorect Dis 1990;5:236.

Fry RD: Infectious enteritis: A collective review. Dis Colon Rectum 1990;33:520.

Guerrant RL, Bobak DA: Bacterial and protozoal gastroenteritis. N Engl J Med 1991;325:327.

Yersinia Enteritis

Much attention has focused on *Yersinia enterocolitica;* this pathogen may cause acute gastroenteritis, terminal ileitis, enterocolitis, colitis, mesenteric lymphadenitis, hepatic and splenic abscesses, and autoimmune processes such as erythema nodosum and polyarthritis. *Y enterocolitica* has also been implicated in other disease (especially in women), including carditis, glomerulonephritis, Graves' disease, and Hashimoto's thyroiditis.

Acute gastroenteritis with fever, diarrhea, and sometimes vomiting is the most common clinical syndrome, especially in children. Acute mesenteric lymphadenitis and acute terminal ileitis are more frequent in adolescents and adults. These infections may cause enough abdominal pain and tenderness that ap-

pendicitis seems a likely diagnosis. If operation is performed, large inflamed lymph nodes are found in the mesentery of the distal ileum, and the bowel itself may be grossly inflamed. In these circumstances, appendectomy is usually performed. Organisms can be cultured from stool, and antibody titers may rise and then fall in some patients. *Y enterocolitica* may respond to trimethoprim-sulfamethoxazole or doxycycline, and complicated *Y enterocolitica* infections should be treated. Fatal septicemia has been reported. No patient with *Y enterocolitica* enteritis has progressed to classic Crohn's disease.

Lee LA et al: *Yersinia enterocolitica* O:3 infections in infants and children, associated with the household preparation of chitterlings. N Engl J Med 1990;322:984.

Matsumoto T et al: Endoscopic findings in *Yersinia enterocolitica* enterocolitis. Gastrointest Endosc 1990;36:583.

Tripoli LC et al: Disseminated *Yersinia enterocolitica.* Case report and review of the literature. J Clin Gastroenterol 1990;12:85.

Campylobacter Enteritis

Campylobacter jejuni is a gram-negative rod that is now recognized as an important cause of human illness in all parts of the world. *C jejuni* infection is more common than infection by either *Salmonella* or *Shigella.* Raw milk, untreated drinking water, and undercooked poultry are recognized vehicles of transmission. Clinical features vary from mild abdominal pain, fever, emesis, and diarrhea indistinguishable from viral gastroenteritis to severe chronic or relapsing bloody diarrhea that resembles ulcerative or granulomatous colitis. *C jejuni* produces an enterotoxin that may play a role in causing diarrhea.

Darkfield or phase-contrast microscopy of stool samples may reveal the characteristic darting motility of *C jejuni* and allow for a presumptive diagnosis. Stool and occasionally blood cultures are positive. Colonoscopy may reveal colonic lesions, and x-rays show inflammation of the small bowel or colon.

Although *C jejuni* infection is self-limited in most patients and symptoms subside within a week, relapses occur in 20% of untreated patients. The appropriate antibiotic is erythromycin, ciprofloxacin, or doxycycline, depending on the results of in vitro sensitivity studies. Disease can be spread by symptomatic patients; once diarrhea subsides, transmission is unlikely.

Echeverria P et al: Case-control study of endemic diarrheal disease in Thai children. J Infect Dis 1989;159:543.

Popovic UT: *Campylobacter jejuni* and *Campylobacter coli* diarrhoea in rural and urban populations in Yugoslavia. Epidemiol Infect 1989;102:59.

Tuberculosis

Primary tuberculous infection of the intestine, caused by ingestion of the bovine strain of *Mycobac-*

terium tuberculosis, is rare in the USA. Secondary infection is due to swallowing the human tubercle bacillus. About 1% of patients with pulmonary tuberculosis have intestinal involvement. Recent immigration from endemic areas has increased the incidence. Tuberculosis is prevalent in individuals infected with HIV.

The distal ileum is the most common site of disease. The bacillus localizes in the mucosal glands and spreads to Peyer's patches, where inflammation, sloughing of tissue, and local attempts at walling off give rise to symptoms. The pathologic reaction is hypertrophic or ulcerative. Hypertrophic tuberculous enteritis results in stenosis, and the symptoms and signs are those of obstruction. The ulcerative form causes abdominal pain, alternating constipation and diarrhea, and, occasionally, progressive inanition. Free perforation, fistula formation, or hemorrhage may occur in severe untreated disease.

The diagnosis of intestinal tuberculosis can be difficult, but medical treatment should not be based on clinical suspicion alone, since carcinoma and Crohn's disease cause similar symptoms and signs. Less than half of patients in a recent study had an abnormality on chest x-ray, and none had a positive sputum. Biopsy by colonoscopy, laparoscopy, or even laparotomy is needed to demonstrate the organism.

Antituberculosis chemotherapy is the mainstay of management. Surgery is required if the diagnosis is uncertain, if disease is resistant to chemotherapy, or if complications develop. Some surgeons recommend early operation because medical treatment results in healing by fibrosis with resultant obstruction. Resection is the preferred surgical procedure, and bypass is done only if abscesses or fistulas are present. The prognosis is good if the patient is operated on in the early stages of the illness

Guth AA, Kim U: The reappearance of abdominal tuberculosis. Surg Gynecol Obstet 1991;172:432.

Harries AD: Tuberculosis and human immunodeficiency virus infection in developing countries. Lancet 1990; 335:387.

Rieder HL et al: Tuberculosis in the United States. JAMA 1989;262:385.

Typhoid

Salmonella typhi may cause ulcers in the distal ileum or cecum. Bleeding or perforation presents a formidable surgical challenge. Early operation offers the best hope for survival.

Santillana M: Surgical complications of typhoid fever: Enteric perforation. World J Surg 1991;15:170.

Enteropathy From Nonsteroidal Anti-inflammatory Drugs

Nonsteroidal anti-inflammatory drugs increase intestinal permeability within hours after ingestion, exposing the mucosa to macromolecules and toxins in the lumen. Bacterial invasion may contribute to inflammation. Perhaps 70% of patients of any age and either sex who have taken these agents for 6 months or longer develop enteropathy, with subclinical intestinal inflammation and occult blood loss. Fewer than 1% of patients develop mucosal ulceration or transmural inflammation with submucosal fibrosis and circumferential diaphragm-like strictures. These patients may have obstruction, perforation, or anemia. The differential diagnosis includes Crohn's disease, ischemia, tuberculosis, and lymphoma.

The drug should be withdrawn. Strictures require resection.

Banerjee AK: Enteropathy induced by non-steroidal anti-inflammatory drugs. Br Med J 1989;298:1539.

Morris AJ et al: Enteroscopic diagnosis of small bowel ulceration in patients receiving non-steroidal anti-inflammatory drugs. Lancet 1991;337:520.

Radiation Enteropathy

Aggressive radiation therapy for abdominal or pelvic cancer is almost always associated with some gastrointestinal injury, because proliferating intestinal epithelial cells are extremely radiosensitive. Degeneration of cells and edema of bowel wall may produce abdominal pain, nausea and vomiting, and sometimes bloody diarrhea during therapy or a few months later. Symptoms are usually minor and transient for most patients with modern irradiation techniques.

Injury to blood vessels in the bowel wall is far more serious than the early mucosal lesion. Endothelial proliferation and fibrosis in the media may gradually obliterate the vessel lumen over months or years, producing chronic intestinal ischemia. Carcinoma arising in irradiated small intestine is a rare late complication.

The incidence of significant bowel injury is dose-related and varies from 5% after 4500 cGy to 30% after 6000 cGy. Fixation of small bowel loops in the radiation field by adhesions from previous operations greatly increases the risk of intestinal complications. Absorbable polyglycolic acid mesh can be used to keep the small bowel out of the pelvis when radiation therapy is planned following pelvic surgery. Oral glutamine protects the small bowel mucosa from some of the morbidity of irradiation in preliminary animal studies.

Symptoms necessitating operation appear as early as 1 month or as late as 30 years after completion of therapy. Operation is required for obstruction due to stricture or entrapment in pelvic fibrosis, perforation with abscess or fistula formation, or hemorrhage from ulcerated mucosa. Symptoms should not be attributed to cancer until residual cancer is proved to be present.

The objective of operation is relief of symptoms. If resection of the involved segment is not possible, bypass is performed. It is imperative that normal bowel be used for anastomoses, because suture lines in irradiated bowel are likely to disrupt. The bowel is friable despite its thickness, and care must be taken in freeing adhesions. If the distal colon and rectum are involved, diverting colostomy is the safest course. Radiation proctitis is discussed in Chapter 32.

The operative death rate is 10–15%, and the prognosis thereafter depends on the extent of involvement and the presence of untreatable fistulas, short bowel syndrome, and cancer. Only 30–45% of patients with significant intestinal complications of radiation therapy are alive 5 years after operation.

Dasmahapatra KS, Swaminathan AP: The use of a biodegradable mesh to prevent radiation-associated small-bowel injury. Arch Surg 1991;126:366.

Fernández-Bañares F et al: Acute effects of abdominopelvic irradiation on the orocecal transit time: Its relation to clinical symptoms, and bile salt and lactose malabsorption. Am J Gastroenterol 1991;86:1771.

Klimberg VS et al: Oral glutamine accelerates healing of the small intestine and improves outcome after whole abdominal radiation. Arch Surg 1990;125:1040.

Sher ME, Bauer J: Radiation-induced enteropathy. Am J Gastroenterol 1990;85:121.

SMALL INTESTINE FISTULAS

Essentials of Diagnosis

- Fever and sepsis.
- Abdominal pain.
- Localized abdominal tenderness.
- External drainage of small bowel contents.
- Dehydration and malnutrition.

General Considerations

External fistulas of the small bowel may form spontaneously as a result of disease, but about 95% are complications of surgical procedures (anastomotic dehiscence or injury to bowel during dissection). Fistulas are particularly prone to develop when the surgeon encounters extensive adhesions, inflamed intestine, or radiation enteropathy.

Fistulas can be classified according to anatomic site, characteristics of the tract (simple or complex), and volume of output (high or low). A high-output fistula produces more than 500 mL/24 h. Other descriptive terms are also used, eg, end fistula, which encompasses the entire diameter of the bowel, and lateral fistula, which arises from one side only.

Clinical Findings

A. Symptoms and Signs: Postoperative fistula formation is heralded by fever and abdominal pain until bowel contents discharge through the abdominal incision. Spontaneous fistulas from neoplasms or inflammatory disease usually develop in a more indolent manner. Most fistulas are associated with one or more abscesses, which often drain incompletely with fistulization, so that persistent sepsis is a common feature. Intestinal fluid escaping through the fistula may severely excoriate the skin and abdominal wall tissues. Fluid and electrolyte losses may be severe, especially if the fistula is large, if it is located in the upper tract, or if there is partial or complete intestinal obstruction distal to the fistula. Persistent sepsis and difficulty in nourishing the patient contribute to rapid weight loss.

B. Laboratory Findings: Routine laboratory tests reflect the severity of deficits in red cell mass, plasma volume, and electrolytes. Leukocytosis due to sepsis and hemoconcentration is common. Disease of other organs such as liver and kidneys may be detected.

C. Imaging Studies: Abscesses and intestinal obstruction may be evident on plain abdominal films. Contrast medium administered orally, per rectum, or through the fistula (fistulogram) delineates the abnormal anatomy, including intrinsic bowel disease, and demonstrates the location and number of fistulas, the length and course of fistula tracts, associated abscess cavities, and the presence of distal obstruction. Radiologists can manipulate catheters into tracts and provide detailed diagnostic information; this procedure may also be therapeutic (see below). Chest films, CT scans, ultrasound, endoscopy, and other special studies may be indicated in certain individuals.

Complications

Fluid and electrolyte losses, malnutrition, and sepsis contribute to multiple organ failure and death unless effective therapy is instituted promptly.

Treatment

A systematic approach combining diagnostic, supportive, and operative procedures is essential in the management of patients with fistulas (Table 30–2). In few other conditions is the proper timing of operative intervention more critical.

Table 30–2. Treatment of fistulas.

First:
Restore blood volume and begin correction of fluids and electrolyte imbalance.
Drain accessible abscesses.
Control fistula and measure losses.
Begin nutritional support.
Second:
Delineate anatomy of fistulas by radiographic studies.
Third:
Maintain caloric intake of 2000–3000 kcal or more per day, depending on status of nutrition and energy expenditure.
Drain abscesses as they appear.
Fourth:
Operate if fistula fails to close.

A. Fluid and Electrolyte Resuscitation: Many fistula patients are profoundly depleted of intravascular and interstitial volume, and replacement of this fluid with isotonic saline solution takes first priority. Central venous pressure, urine output, and skin turgor are guides to the progress of volume resuscitation. Blood is sent to the laboratory for measurement of serum electrolyte concentrations and arterial blood gases. Results of these studies assist in correcting electrolyte deficits and deranged acid-base balance. Fluid should be collected from fistula output, nasogastric suction, and urine for measurement of volume and electrolyte composition. Body weight is recorded daily. Fluid and electrolyte resuscitation can usually be accomplished within the first day or two. Subsequent maintenance of homeostasis depends on accurately measuring losses and replacing them.

B. Control of Fistula: Fistula drainage fluid must be collected to avoid excoriation of skin and abdominal wall tissues and to record volume losses. An ostomy appliance may fit around the fistula or a catheter inserted by a radiologist under x-ray guidance may work best. Skilled and experienced nursing care is indispensable.

C. Control of Sepsis: Abscesses should be drained as soon as they are diagnosed. The source of sepsis is often obscure, and a continuous diligent search for abscesses must be made by repeated physical examination and imaging studies until the infection is located and treated. Blind therapy with broad-spectrum antibiotics is not a substitute for drainage of abscesses. In many cases, an incompletely drained abscess can be managed by an interventional radiologist, who passes a catheter through a fistula tract into the associated abscess cavity. Drainage is accomplished, and the fistula may close as the sump tube is gradually withdrawn over a period of weeks.

D. Delineation of Fistula: Radiographic contrast studies (see above) should be obtained as soon as feasible.

E. Nutrition: Adequate nutrition and control of sepsis make the difference between survival and death for these patients. A useful general rule is to avoid all oral intake at the outset. Nasogastric suction may be necessary temporarily. As soon as intravascular fluid and electrolytes are restored, parenteral nutrition should be instituted via a central intravenous catheter.

For many patients, total parenteral nutrition is the principal exogenous source of calories and nitrogen until the fistula heals or is closed surgically. For patients with low-output or distal fistulas, the enteral route for nutrition is preferred, and elemental or polymeric diets can be delivered into the distal gut in some patients with proximal fistulas.

F. Other Measures: H_2 receptor antagonists are useful adjuncts in patients with proximal fistulas. By reducing gastric acid secretion, fistula output is decreased and fluid and electrolyte management is sim-

plified. Somatostatin decreases fistula output and accelerates fistula closure. The short half-life of this agent, its inhibitory effects on pancreatic insulin secretion, and rebound recurrences after fistula closure leave the value of somatostatin unclear. New somatostatin analogues may prove more useful in the future.

G. Operation: About 30% of fistulas close spontaneously; Crohn's disease, irradiated bowel, cancer, foreign body, distal obstruction, extensive disruption of intestinal continuity, and a short (< 2 cm) fistula tract are associated with failure of fistulas to heal. An experimental approach is instillation of fibrin glue into the tract directly or through an endoscope inserted into the fistula; despite promising reports, this method has not been proved safe and effective, and it is not applicable to most fistulas that come to operation. If they are going to heal spontaneously, fistulas usually close within a month after eradication of infection and institution of adequate nutritional support, and persistence much beyond a month indicates the need for surgical closure in most cases. The operation should be postponed, however, until one can predict that intra-abdominal inflammation has resolved—typically 3 months after the last operation. The fistulous segment should be resected, associated obstruction relieved, and continuity reestablished by end-to-end anastomosis. Bypass without resection rarely is indicated.

Prognosis

The plan of management outlined above results in survival rates of 80–95% in patients with external fistulas. Uncontrolled sepsis is the chief cause of death.

Altomare DF et al: Prediction of mortality by logistic regression analysis in patients with postoperative enterocutaneous fistulae. Br J Surg 1990;77:450.

Buechter KJ et al: Enterocutaneous fistulas following laparotomy for trauma. Am Surg 1991;57:354.

Lange V et al: Fistuloscopy—an adjuvant technique for sealing gastrointestinal fistulae. Surg Endosc 1990;4:212.

Rinsema W et al: Primary conservative management of external small-bowel fistulas: Changing composition of fistula series? Acta Chir Scand 1990;156:457.

Schein M, Decker GAG: Gastrointestinal fistulas associated with large abdominal wall defects: Experience with 43 patients. Br J Surg 1990;77:97.

ACUTE VASCULAR LESIONS OF THE SMALL INTESTINE & MESENTERY

Lesions producing acute or chronic ischemia or hemorrhage may result from intrinsic vascular disease, systemic illness, pharmacologic agents, and surgical procedures. Chronic occlusion may be amenable to vascular reconstruction and is discussed in Chapter 35. Acute mesenteric ischemia is discussed here.

1. ACUTE MESENTERIC VASCULAR OCCLUSION

Essentials of Diagnosis
- Severe, diffuse abdominal pain.
- Gross or occult intestinal bleeding.
- Minimal physical findings.
- Radiographic findings (sometimes).
- Operative findings.

General Considerations

Sudden occlusion of major small bowel arteries or veins is catastrophic. It is predominantly a disease of the elderly and is highly lethal. Mesenteric **arterial emboli** account for 30% of cases; they most commonly originate from mural thrombus in an infarcted left ventricle or clot in a fibrillating left atrium in patients with mitral stenosis. **Thrombosis of a mesenteric artery** (25% of cases) is the end result of atherosclerotic stenosis, and these patients often give a history of intestinal angina before the acute thrombosis occurs. Other causes of acute arterial occlusions, such as dissecting aortic aneurysm or fusiform aortic aneurysm, are rare. Occlusions of smaller mesenteric arteries often are associated with connective tissue or other systemic disorders. Cocaine ingestion is another cause. These miscellaneous problems are responsible for about 20% of patients with acute mesenteric ischemia.

Thrombosis of mesenteric veins is associated with portal hypertension, abdominal sepsis, hypercoagulable states, or trauma, or there may be no apparent underlying disease. Mesenteric venous or arterial thrombosis can occur in women taking oral contraceptives. Some venous occlusions develop peripherally and progress insidiously, causing segmental infarction that resembles strangulation obstruction. Others have acute, severe, rapidly progressive ischemia.

The consequences of major vascular occlusion depend on the vessel involved, the level of occlusion, the status of other visceral vessels, the development of collaterals, the establishment of reperfusion, and other factors. Tissue injury is caused by events related to the ischemia itself (ischemic injury) and by return of blood flow, either spontaneous or as a result of treatment (reperfusion injury). Complete interruption of oxygen supply to the intestine produces necrosis first at the tips of villi. Mucosal slough begins within 3 hours after onset of ischemia, and ulceration and bleeding soon become extensive. Full-thickness infarction of bowel wall occurs as early as 6 hours after onset in total ischemia; in partial ischemia, it may take several days for this stage to be reached. Hemorrhage into the lumen, accumulation of bloody abdominal fluid, perforation, and death from sepsis are the end results of infarction. Sepsis and multiorgan system failure may develop even in the absence of full-thickness necrosis or perforation; bacteria proliferate in the necrotic segment; the mucosal barrier is disrupted; and bacteria and their toxic products translocate into the circulation. A variety of plasma substances including tumor necrosis factor and platelet-activating factor arise at the site of intestinal injury, enter the circulation, and damage target organs such as the lung.

There is increasing recognition of the importance of reperfusion injury in the outcome of intestinal ischemia. Return of arterial blood flow from spontaneous events, lysis of clot by anticoagulants, or arterial reconstruction converts the enzyme xanthine dehydrogenase to xanthine oxidase, resulting in the release of superoxide and hydrogen peroxide. These oxygen radicals destabilize cell membranes, disrupt the mucosal barrier, and flood the systemic circulation with mediators of damage to other organs. Most of the data come from experimental animals, but there is little doubt that reperfusion injury is an important and potentially lethal phenomenon in patients. In some animal studies, pretreatment with superoxide dismutase or dimethyl sulfoxide (both scavengers of oxygen radicals) seems to be protective. Allopurinol, an inhibitor of xanthine oxidase, also is effective in the laboratory. Drug prophylaxis against ischemic and reperfusion injury has not reached the stage of clinical utility.

Clinical Findings

A. Symptoms and Signs: The most constant symptom is severe, poorly localized abdominal pain that is often unresponsive to narcotics. Nausea and vomiting, diarrhea, and constipation are variable in occurrence.

In the early stages there is a striking paucity of abdominal findings; in fact, pain out of proportion to the objective findings is a hallmark of mesenteric vascular occlusion. Ischemia can also occur with much less severe pain, and serious illness may be recognized only when secondary toxicity develops. Later in the course, abdominal distention and tenderness occur. Shock and generalized peritonitis eventually develop, but by that time the opportunity for salvage has been lost. In some instances—particularly with a high venous occlusion—shock is an early finding. Stool or gastric contents contain blood in 75–95% of patients later in the course. Paracentesis does not help to establish the diagnosis in the reversible stages.

B. Laboratory Findings: Striking leukocytosis is present. Serum amylase is elevated in about half of patients, and creatine kinase (BB isoenzyme) correlates with intestinal infarction. Significant base deficits may be observed. Increased inorganic phosphate levels in serum and peritoneal fluid are a sign of irreversible ischemia. Hemoconcentration and the effects of hemorrhage into the lumen or mesentery are reflected in laboratory tests in the late stages. Antithrombin III deficiency and other abnormalities of coagulation should be sought.

C. Imaging Studies: Plain abdominal films allow a presumptive diagnosis of vascular occlusion to be made in about 20% of patients. Absence of intestinal gas, diffuse distention with air-fluid levels, and distention of small bowel and colon up to the splenic flexure are nonspecific but suggestive. Blunt plicae, thickened bowel wall, and small bowel loops that remain unchanged over several hours are seen occasionally. Specific findings of intestinal necrosis, including intramural gas and gas in the portal venous system, occur late. Barium studies may reveal "thumbprinting" and disordered motility (either slow or rapid). CT gives useful information in 50% of patients, though a specific diagnosis is possible in only 25% of cases. MRI may be useful. Mesenteric arteriography may be helpful but is logistically cumbersome in acutely ill patients and is not sensitive enough to rule out the diagnosis.

D. Special Studies: Use of xenon Xe 133 has been promising for early diagnosis of intestinal ischemia. This inert gas is dissolved in saline and injected into the peritoneal cavity; it is then absorbed by passive diffusion into the gut. Normally perfused tissue rapidly clears the gas, but ischemic bowel retains labeled xenon, which is detected by external camera imaging. Indium In 111-labeled leukocyte scans are useful for detection of infarcted bowel in some cases.

Differential Diagnosis

Acute pancreatitis and strangulation obstruction of the intestine may be difficult to distinguish from mesenteric vascular occlusion. A very high serum amylase early in the disease or a swollen pancreas on CT scan suggests pancreatitis. Differentiation from strangulation obstruction is less important, since both conditions require operation. Angiography may be definitive. Even surgeons with a special interest in this condition are unable to make an early diagnosis in more than half of cases.

Treatment

Survival depends upon diagnosis and operative treatment within 12 hours after onset of symptoms. Although acute occlusion of major arteries or veins requires operation, pre- and postoperative intra-arterial infusion of papaverine (30–60 mg/h) has been recommended if the angiogram demonstrates embolic occlusion of the superior mesenteric artery.

Acute venous thrombosis is diagnosed by the edematous mesentery and extrusion of clots when mesenteric veins are cut. Resection of all of the involved gut and its mesentery is the treatment of choice; direct mesenteric venous surgery (thrombectomy) is seldom successful. Administration of heparin postoperatively is recommended. Antithrombin III deficiency and other causes of hypercoagulability should be treated.

In arterial occlusion, there is segmental or diffuse ischemia or infarction of small bowel and colon in the distribution of the occluded vessel. Arterial pulsations are absent or reduced, and mesenteric edema is not so striking as in venous occlusion. Many methods of helping the surgeon judge viability have been suggested, but most have not proved their worth. The Doppler ultrasonic flowmeter is of little help, but the laser Doppler system is promising. The qualitative fluorescein test is not as sensitive as once believed. Quantitative fluorescence, as measured by a perfusion fluorometer, is under investigation. Oxygen electrodes that can be used intraoperatively, an electronic contractility meter, and other innovative techniques have been proposed.

Necrotic bowel should be resected unless the extent of damage is so great that satisfactory life could not be expected. With the availability of home parenteral nutrition, more patients are salvageable now than before. It is not clear how to integrate the new information about reperfusion injury into management of patients with reversibly ischemic bowel. Perhaps it is better to just resect the affected intestine, particularly in the elderly, even though vascular reconstruction may be technically possible by embolectomy, thromboendarterectomy, or arterial bypass. Vascular reconstruction was attempted in 10% or less of patients before reperfusion injury became recognized, and it is likely that even fewer patients will be treated by a direct approach to the vessels in the future.

Massive volume support and antibiotics are mandatory, and anticoagulants or drugs that inhibit platelet aggregation are given by some surgeons. A second-look operation is performed 12–24 hours later if marginally viable bowel was left in.

Percutaneous transluminal angioplasty has been used to treat acute mesenteric ischemia, but its role is yet to be defined, and abdominal operation remains the standard treatment.

Prognosis

Acute mesenteric vascular occlusion is often lethal, because diagnosis and treatment are delayed, infarction is extensive, and arterial reconstruction is difficult. The overall mortality rate of arterial occlusion is about 45%, although a recent report of deaths occurring in only 24% is encouraging. If infarction is so extensive that over half of the small bowel must be resected, the death rate is 45–85%. Reconstruction of acutely thrombosed visceral arteries is often not feasible, and patency rates are poor. In a few patients, the acute ischemic episode goes unrecognized, and the process resolves spontaneously with stricture formation. The prognosis is excellent in this situation. Acute venous thrombosis has a death rate of 30%, and if long-term anticoagulants are not used, approximately 25% of patients have another episode of thrombosis. Administration of coumarin anticoagulants for at least 3 months is recommended to minimize the possibility of recurrence.

2. NONOCCLUSIVE INTESTINAL ISCHEMIA

In about one-fourth of patients with intestinal ischemia, vascular occlusion does not involve a major artery or vein (although arterial stenosis is usually present). In the presence of some other acute disease such as a cardiac dysrhythmia or sepsis, splanchnic vasoconstriction occurs, and the intestine becomes ischemic because of low perfusion pressure and flow. Arterial blood is shunted away from the villi in these circumstances, and the ischemic villi are destroyed if the condition persists.

The diagnosis is suspected when a potentially susceptible patient develops acute abdominal pain. The clinical picture is similar to that of arterial thrombosis, but the onset is less often sudden. Arteriography documents the absence of major vascular occlusion but is not otherwise diagnostic in most cases.

Direct infusion of vasodilator agents into the superior mesenteric artery may reverse splanchnic vasoconstriction in selected cases. Papaverine is the drug of choice, but other drugs are under investigation. Operation is usually required to exclude other diseases that simulate intestinal ischemia and to resect infarcted bowel.

Patchy or diffuse ischemia varies in extent and severity. Ischemia is most pronounced on the antimesenteric border, and the mucosa may be extensively involved before abnormalities are visible on the serosal surface. There are often ischemic areas in other organs such as liver and spleen. Vascular reconstruction is ineffective, and surgical procedures are limited to resection of infarcted bowel. Decisions about when to perform a primary anastomosis or second look operation are individualized. The death rate was about 90% until recently, mainly because the underlying disease often could not be corrected. Intraarterial vasodilator therapy has lowered this figure.

Brewster DC et al: Intestinal ischemia complicating abdominal aortic surgery. Surgery 1991;109:447.

Caty MG et al: Evidence for tumor necrosis factor-induced pulmonary microvascular injury after intestinal ischemia-reperfusion injury. Ann Surg 1990;212:694.

Fried MW et al: Creatine kinase isoenzymes in the diagnosis of intestinal infarction. Dig Dis Sci 1991;36:1589.

Grieshop RJ et al: Acute mesenteric venous thrombosis revisited in a time of diagnostic clarity. Am Surg 1991; 57:573.

Landreneau RJ, Fry WJ: The right colon as a target organ of nonocclusive mesenteric ischemia: Case report and review of the literature. Arch Surg 1990;125:591.

Levy PJ, Krausz MM, Manny J: The role of second-look procedure in improving survival time for patients with mesenteric venous thrombosis. Surg Gynecol Obstet 1990;170:287.

Levy PJ, Krausz MM, Manny J: Acute mesenteric ischemia: Improved results—a retrospective analysis of ninety-two patients. Surgery 1990;107:372.

Marston A: Acute intestinal ischaemia. Resection rather than revascularisation. Br Med J 1990;301:1174.

Park PO et al: The sequence of development of intestinal tissue injury after strangulation ischemia and reperfusion. Surgery 1990;107:574.

Smerud MJ, Johnson CD, Stephens DH: Diagnosis of bowel infarction: A comparison of plain films and CT scans in 23 cases. Am J Roentgenol 1990;154:99.

Wilkerson DK et al: Magnetic resonance imaging of acute occlusive intestinal ischemia. J Vasc Surg 1990;11:567.

3. OTHER VASCULAR LESIONS

Vasculitis

Vascular lesions associated with systemic disorders such as polyarteritis nodosa and systemic lupus erythematosus may cause patchy infarction of the small intestine. Similar lesions have been seen in patients with a history of amphetamine abuse. The presenting manifestation is usually perforation with peritonitis or intraluminal bleeding. The prognosis depends on the underlying pathologic process and the severity of peritoneal contamination. These patients are often on corticosteroid therapy and do not tolerate infection well. Survival is rare.

Ljungström K-G, Strandberg O, Sandstedt B: Infarction of the small bowel caused by giant cell arteritis: Case report. Acta Chir Scand 1989;155:361.

Mesenteric Apoplexy

Mesenteric apoplexy is a rare disorder caused by spontaneous rupture of mesenteric arteries. The more general category of **abdominal apoplexy** includes spontaneous hemorrhage into the peritoneal cavity from tumors (particularly hepatomas), the spleen, or other organs. Arteriosclerotic lesions are the cause of arterial rupture in older individuals; the superior mesenteric, right colic, and branches of the celiac artery are the usual sites. Sudden hemorrhage from congenital aneurysms occurs in younger patients; the splenic artery is most commonly involved and is particularly prone to rupture during pregnancy (see Chapter 42). The typical picture is sudden onset of diffuse abdominal pain followed by hypotension. Operation is imperative.

Greene DR et al: The diagnosis and management of splenic artery aneurysms. J Royal Soc Med 1988;81:387.

Bleeding Lesions

Arteriovenous malformations and other bleeding lesions in the small intestine are discussed under

Acute Lower Gastrointestinal Hemorrhage in Chapter 31.

GAS CYSTS
(Pneumatosis Cystoides Intestinalis)

Pneumatosis cystoides intestinalis is a rare condition characterized by gas-filled cysts in the wall of the gut and sometimes in the mesentery. When the process is limited to the large intestine, the term **pneumatosis coli** is used. Cysts vary in size from microscopic to several centimeters in diameter.

Pneumatosis may be primary or secondary. About 15% of cases are primary and idiopathic; the cysts are submucosal and usually are limited to the left colon. Secondary pneumatosis comprises 85% of cases. Cysts are subserosal and may be located anywhere in the gastrointestinal tract or its mesentery. Conditions that underlie secondary pneumatosis intestinalis or pneumatosis coli include inflammatory bowel disease, infectious gastroenteritis or colitis, steroid therapy, connective tissue disorders, intestinal obstruction, diverticulitis, chronic obstructive pulmonary disease, acute leukemia, lymphoma, AIDS, and organ transplantation.

The mechanism of cyst formation may not be the same in all patients. In some, anaerobic bacterial fermentation of carbohydrates leads to excess production of hydrogen gas, which enters the intestinal wall by diffusion. Patients with impaired pulmonary function are less able to excrete excessive hydrogen gas through the lungs, and they are more prone to develop pneumatosis. Cysts are maintained because additional hydrogen is generated with each meal, thus replacing gas that may have diffused into the bloodstream since the previous meal. High breath hydrogen levels have been reported in pneumatosis patients even during fasting.

Symptoms are absent or nonspecific. In secondary pneumatosis, symptoms are due to the underlying disease. In the primary form, abdominal discomfort, distention, and altered bowel habits may be present. Rarely, perforation of a cyst, hemorrhage, obstruction, or malabsorption may bring benign pneumatosis to medical attention. **Fulminant pneumatosis** is associated with acute bacterial infection and necrosis of the bowel wall. Such patients are toxic and may have underlying impaired immunologic defenses. Gas may also be seen within the intestinal wall late in intestinal infarction.

Treatment of secondary pneumatosis intestinalis is directed toward the underlying disease. Resolution of cysts can be accomplished in either primary or secondary pneumatosis by having patients breathe oxygen by mask for several days interrupted only at mealtime. Response to hyperbaric oxygen is more rapid. Recurrence of cysts after oxygen treatment reflects continued production of hydrogen, and in these patients it is necessary to reduce the amount of gas being generated. The amount of substrate can be controlled by dietary manipulation, and the fecal flora can be suppressed by antibacterial agents such as ampicillin or metronidazole. Surgical resection of bowel involved with benign primary pneumatosis is rarely required, but underlying disease may need operative treatment in the secondary form of this condition. Fulminant pneumatosis is treated surgically, but the mortality rate is high.

Andorsky RI: Pneumatosis cystoides intestinalis after organ transplantation. Am J Gastroenterol 1990;85:189.

Knechtle SJ, Davidoff AM, Rice RP: Pneumatosis intestinalis. Surgical management and clinical outcome. Ann Surg 1990;212:160.

Rogy MA et al: Pneumatosis cystoides intestinalis (PCI). Int J Colorect Dis 1990;5:120.

TUMORS OF THE SMALL INTESTINE

Neoplasms of the jejunum and ileum comprise 1–5% of all tumors of the gastrointestinal tract. The terminal ileum is the favored site, followed by proximal jejunum. Approximately 85% of patients are over age 40. There is a high correlation of small bowel tumors with primary neoplasms elsewhere.

Only 10% of small bowel tumors are symptomatic. Benign lesions are ten times as common as malignant ones. Lymphoma is now the most common primary malignant tumor of the small intestine. At least 75% of symptomatic neoplasms are malignant. Bleeding and obstruction, sometimes due to intussusception, are the most frequent symptoms.

1. BENIGN TUMORS

Polyps

Adenomatous or villous polyps of the type seen in the colon are rare in the small bowel; they are usually solitary and cause symptoms by intussusception or bleeding.

Polypoid **hamartomas** may be solitary in patients who are free of associated anomalies. Hamartomas are multiple in 50% of cases, and 10% of these have **Peutz-Jeghers syndrome,** a familial disorder characterized by diffuse gastrointestinal polyposis and mucocutaneous pigmentation. The malignant potential of these polyps is very small. Operation is indicated only for symptoms (eg, obstruction, bleeding), at which time all polyps greater than about 1 cm should be removed. A combined surgical and endoscopic approach is the best strategy.

Familial adenomatous polyposis (familial polyposis coli, Gardner's syndrome; see Chapter 31) is characterized by multiple intestinal and colonic polyps, osteomas, and subcutaneous cysts or fibromas.

The polyps are true neoplasms, and malignant degeneration of colonic polyps is common; there is a predilection for periampullary duodenal cancer as well.

Juvenile (retention) polyps may bleed or obstruct. They are more common in the colon than the small bowel and usually autoamputate before adolescence. Some pathologists regard these lesions as hamartomas.

Other Tumors

Leiomyomas, lipomas, neurofibromas, and fibromas may cause symptoms that require operation. Endometriosis can implant on the small bowel. Hemangiomas are discussed in the section on Acute Lower Gastrointestinal Hemorrhage in Chapter 31.

Cappell MS, Friedman D, Mikhail N: Endometriosis of the terminal ileum simulating the clinical, roentgenographic, and surgical findings in Crohn's disease. Am J Gastroenterol 1991;86:1057.

Morgan BK et al: Benign smooth muscle tumors of the gastrointestinal tract: A 24-year experience. Ann Surg 1990; 211:63.

Panos RG, Opelka RG, Nogueras JJ: Peutz-Jeghers syndrome: A call for intraoperative enteroscopy. Am Surg 1990;56:331.

Spigelman AD, Thomson JPS, Phillips RKS: Towards decreasing the relaparotomy rate in the Peutz-Jeghers syndrome: The role of perioperative small bowel endoscopy. Br J Surg 1990;77:301.

2. MALIGNANT TUMORS

Primary

Adenocarcinoma is often asymptomatic or causes only minimal symptoms for prolonged periods. It usually arises in the proximal jejunum, except in Crohn's disease, in which bypassed distal ileum is at greatest risk. Metastases are present in 80% of cases at the time of operation. Segmental resection of bowel and adjacent mesentery is done when possible, but metastases near the superior mesenteric artery may make the procedure difficult. Five-year survival is 25% in patients undergoing intestinal resection.

Primary small intestinal lymphomas of the Western type arise focally. These lymphomas develop in the proximal jejunum in patients with celiac disease, and in another group of patients the lymphomas arise de novo in the distal ileum. In the Middle East, primary small bowel lymphoma is the most common form of extranodal lymphomatous disease. **Immunoproliferative small intestinal disease** is a geographic variant in that part of the world; it is characterized by diffuse infiltration of the small intestine by abnormal lymphoid cells. The infiltrate is probably benign in the initial phase of alpha-chain disease, but the other cases are malignant. AIDS-associated non-Hodgkin's lymphomas of B cell origin can in-

volve the small intestine; the prognosis in these patients is very poor.

Western-type lymphomas develop as a nodular, polypoid, or ulcerating mass. Lesions are multiple in 20% of patients. Obstruction, bleeding, and perforation bring the lesion to attention. Abdominal operation is often required to establish a histologic diagnosis by conservative resection of the intestinal lesion. Operation is followed by whole abdominal radiation, with or without chemotherapy, in some patients. The overall 5-year survival rate is about 40%.

Leiomyosarcoma in small bowel tends to ulcerate centrally and bleed. Other types of primary malignant neoplasm are rare.

Metastatic

Small bowel metastases are found in 50% of patients dying of malignant melanoma. Carcinomas of the cervix, kidney, breast, lung, etc, may also spread to bowel. Obstruction or hemorrhage may require operation if life expectancy is reasonably good. Significant palliation may be achieved, particularly in patients with solitary metastatic lesions.

Auger MJ, Allan NC: Primary ileocecal lymphoma: A study of 22 patients. Cancer 1990;65:358.

Branum GD, Seigler HF: Role of surgical intervention in the management of intestinal metastases from malignant melanoma. Am J Surg 1991;162:428.

Caputy GG et al: Metastatic melanoma of the gastrointestinal tract: Results of surgical management. Arch Surg 1991;126:1353.

Desa LAJ et al: Primary jejunoileal tumors: A review of 45 cases. World J Surg 1991;15:81.

Dougherty MJ et al: Sarcomas of the gastrointestinal tract. Separation into favorable and unfavorable prognostic groups by mitotic count. Ann Surg 1991;214:569.

Ihde JK, Coit DG: Melanoma metastatic to stomach, small bowel, or colon. Am J Surg 1991;162:208.

Iida M et al: Double-contrast radiographic features in primary small intestinal lymphoma of the "Western" type: Correlation with pathological findings. Clin Radiol 1991; 44:322.

Kimura H et al: Prognostic factors in primary gastrointestinal leiomyosarcoma: A retrospective study. World J Surg 1991;15:771.

Koretz MJ, Graham R: Primary adenocarcinoma of the jejunum. Am Surg 1989;55:539.

Talamonti MS et al: Gastrointestinal lymphoma. A case for primary surgical resection. Arch Surg 1990;125:972.

3. CARCINOID TUMORS & CARCINOID SYNDROME

Carcinoid tumors are apudomas that arise from enterochromaffin cells throughout the gut. Carcinoids may be associated with multiple endocrine neoplasia (MEN) type 1 and type 2. Rare familial clustering not associated with MEN has been reported. Neoplasms of other organs—most commonly the colon, lung, stomach, or breast—are present in 15% of patients. Carcinoids occur in patients 25–45 years of age.

The origin of carcinoid tumors of the gastrointestinal tract is foregut, 5%; midgut, 88%; and hindgut, 6%. Most carcinoids associated with MEN are of foregut origin. Midgut carcinoids produce serotonin and substance P; neurotensin, gastrin, somatostatin, motilin, secretin, and pancreatic polypeptide are also common. Foregut and hindgut carcinoids do not produce serotonin, but they often contain gastrin, somatostatin, pancreatic polypeptide, and glucagon.

The appendix is the most common site of carcinoid tumors, and the small intestine is the second most common location; about ten times as many originate in the ileum as in the jejunum. Multiple tumors are present in 40% of cases. Grossly, carcinoids are firm, yellowish submucosal nodules. Special stains may demonstrate argentaffin or argyrophil reactions in microscopic sections.

Carcinoid of the small bowel should be regarded as "a malignant neoplasm in slow motion." At the time of surgical diagnosis, 40% of tumors have invaded the muscularis and 45% have metastasized to lymph nodes or liver. Of primary tumors less than 1 cm in diameter, fewer than 2% metastasize, but 80% of those larger than 2 cm have spread at the time of operation. Huge metastatic deposits emanating from a minute primary are sometimes encountered.

Clinical Findings

A. Symptoms and Signs: Small tumors are usually asymptomatic. Overall, 30% of small bowel carcinoids cause symptoms of obstruction, pain, bleeding, or the carcinoid syndrome. Obstruction due to sclerosis and kinking of the bowel may be related to elaboration of vasoactive materials by metastases in the mesentery. Intestinal ischemia has been reported.

About 10% of patients with small bowel carcinoids present with **carcinoid syndrome,** and others develop it later. The syndrome consists of cutaneous flushing, diarrhea, bronchoconstriction, and right-sided cardiac valvular disease due to collagen deposition. Biologically active substances secreted by carcinoids are usually inactivated in the liver, but hepatic metastases or primary ovarian or bronchial carcinoids release these compounds directly into the systemic circulation, where they produce symptoms. Serotonin production in large quantities occurs in almost all cases of carcinoid syndrome; it is responsible for much of the diarrhea. A host of other active materials may participate, including substance P, neurotensin, histamine, catecholamines, pancreatic polypeptide, chorionic gonadotropin, gastrin, glucagon, prostaglandins, ACTH, and calcitonin.

B. Laboratory Findings: Some carcinoid tumors are detected by radiographic methods. Elevated urinary levels of 5-hydroxyindoleacetic acid (5-HIAA) are the diagnostic hallmark of carcinoid syndrome. An injection of pentagastrin can be used as a provocative test: Symptoms appear, and serum levels of serotonin and substance P increase.

Treatment

All accessible carcinoid tumor in small bowel, mesentery, and the peritoneal cavity should be removed. If metastases are present in the mesentery but all gross disease can be removed, a second-look operation is often recommended 6 months later.

If intestinal obstruction is the principal serious manifestation of incurable abdominal disease, it should be treated aggressively because tumor growth is so slow. Extensive enterectomy followed by chronic total parenteral nutrition may even be justified in some cases.

Localized hepatic metastases should be resected. Unresectable hepatic metastases can sometimes be palliated by hepatic artery embolization or hepatic artery infusion chemotherapy. Doxorubicin gives a 20% response rate. A combination of fluorouracil, doxorubicin, cyclophosphamide, and streptozocin gives a response rate of 30%. Suppression of tumor growth in animals is achieved by interferon, octreotide, and difluoromethylornithine in combination.

Carcinoid syndrome can be treated by various pharmacologic agents designed to block the effects of active substances. Among the agents sometimes used are phenothiazines, corticosteroids, and histamine H_1 and H_2 receptor antagonists. Cyproheptadine, an antihistamine that blocks serotonin 1, serotonin 2, and histamine H_1 receptors, is useful for the control of diarrhea. Octreotide inhibits release of gastrointestinal hormones; in carcinoid syndrome, it relieves flushing, wheezing, and severe diarrhea refractory to other measures. Interferon has a mixed record of tumor suppression and reduction of symptoms of carcinoid syndrome.

Prognosis

Carcinoid tumors grow slowly over months and years. The overall 5-year survival rate after resection of small bowel carcinoid is 70%; 40% of patients with inoperable metastases and 20% of those with hepatic metastases survive 5 years or longer. Median survival from the time of histologic diagnosis is 14 years, and from onset of the carcinoid syndrome it is 8 years.

Eller R, Frazee R, Roberts J: Gastrointestinal carcinoid tumors. Am Surg 1991;57:434.

Evers BM et al: Expression of neurotensin messenger RNA in a human carcinoid tumor. Ann Surg 1991;214:448.

Evers BM et al: Novel therapy for the treatment of human carcinoid. Ann Surg 1991;213:411.

MacGillivray DD et al: Carcinoid tumors: The relationship between clinical presentation and the extent of disease. Surgery 1991;110:68.

Makridis C et al: Surgical treatment of mid-gut carcinoid tumors. World J Surg 1990;14:377.

Moertel CG, Kvols LK, Rubin J: A study of cyproheptadine in the treatment of metastatic carcinoid tumor and the malignant carcinoid syndrome. Cancer 1991;67:33.

Vinik A, Moattari AR: Use of somatostatin analog in management of carcinoid syndrome. Dig Dis Sci 1989;34:14.

Vlalimaki M et al: Is the treatment of metastatic carcinoid tumor with interferon not as successful as suggested? Cancer 1991;67:547.

Large Intestine

Theodore R. Schrock, MD

ANATOMY

The colon extends from the end of the ileum to the rectum. The cecum, ascending colon, hepatic flexure, and proximal transverse colon comprise the **right colon.** The distal transverse colon, splenic flexure, descending colon, sigmoid colon, and rectosigmoid comprise the **left colon** (Figure 31–1). The ascending and descending portions are fixed in the retroperitoneal space, and the transverse colon and sigmoid colon are suspended in the peritoneal cavity by their mesocolons. The caliber of the lumen is greatest at the cecum and diminishes distally. The wall of the colon has four layers: mucosa, submucosa, muscularis, and serosa (Figure 31–2). The muscularis propria consists of an inner circular layer and an outer longitudinal layer. The longitudinal muscle completely encircles the colon in a very thin layer, and at three points around the circumference it is gathered into thick bands called taeniae. Sacculations (haustra) are the result of shortening of the colon by the taeniae and contractions of the circular muscle. The haustra are not fixed anatomic structures and may be observed to move longitudinally. There are fatty appendages (the appendices epiploicae) on the serosal surface. The wall of the colon is so thin that it becomes markedly distended when obstructed.

The rectum is 12–15 cm in length. The taeniae coli spread out at the rectosigmoid junction and are not apparent distal to that area. The upper rectum is invested by peritoneum anteriorly and laterally, but posteriorly it is retroperitoneal up to the rectosigmoid. The anterior peritoneal reflection dips low into the pelvis to approximately 7 cm above the anal verge—a fact to be noted when rectal lesions are biopsied or fulgurated; perforation into the peritoneal cavity can occur at a much lower level anteriorly than posteriorly. The anterior peritoneal reflection lies behind the bladder in males and behind the uterus (the rectouterine pouch of Douglas) in females. Tumor masses or abscesses in this location are readily palpated on digital rectal or pelvic examination. The rectum is normally capacious and distensible. When its capacity to distend is lost or impaired by surgery or disease, fecal urgency and frequency are noted.

The rectal valves of Houston are prominent spirally arranged mucosal folds within the rectum. Less than half of people have the so-called normal three valves, two on the left and one on the right. The valves are at variable distances from the anal verge in different individuals. Normally, the valves appear thin with sharp edges, but they become thickened and blunted when inflamed. A rectal valve may hide a small lesion from endoscopic view, and during rigid sigmoidoscopy the valve must be "ironed out" so its superior surface can be examined. The most difficult level to pass with the sigmoidoscope is the rectosigmoid junction, because of angulation and local muscular contraction. The presence of a rectosigmoid sphincter was postulated long ago and has received support from physiologic studies.

In males, the prostate gland, the seminal vesicles, and the seminal ducts lie anterior to the rectum. The prostate usually is easily felt, but the seminal vesicles are not palpable unless distended, because the firm, unyielding rectovesical fascia of Denonvilliers intervenes. In females, the rectovaginal septum and uterus lie anterior and the uterine adnexa anterolateral to the rectum. The structures are easily palpated with one finger in the vagina and one in the rectum.

Blood Supply & Lymphatic Drainage

The arterial supply of the right colon, from the ileocecal junction to approximately the mid transverse colon, is from the superior mesenteric artery through its ileocolic, right colic, and middle colic branches.

The inferior mesenteric artery arises from the abdominal aorta and gives off the left colic and sigmoid branches before it becomes the superior hemorrhoidal artery. The vasa recta are the terminal arterial branches to the colon and run directly to the mesocolic wall or through the bowel wall to the antimesocolic border.

The colic arteries bifurcate and form arcades about 2.5 cm from the mesocolic border of the bowel, forming a pathway of communicating vessels called the marginal artery of Drummond. The marginal artery thus forms an anastomosis between the superior mesenteric and inferior mesenteric arteries. The configuration of the blood supply, however, varies greatly; the typical pattern is present in only 15% of individuals.

The middle hemorrhoidal artery arises on each side

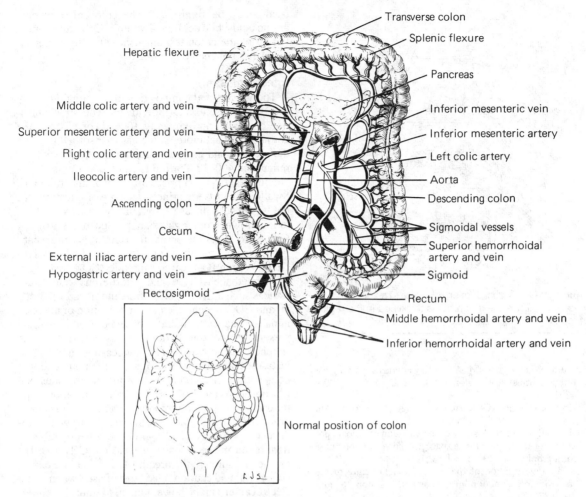

Normal position of colon

Figure 31–1. The large intestine: anatomic divisions and blood supply. The veins are shown in black. The insert shows the usual configuration of the colon.

from the anterior division of the internal iliac artery or from the internal pudendal artery and runs inward in the lateral ligaments of the rectum. The inferior hemorrhoidal arteries derive from the internal pudendal arteries and pass through Alcock's canal. The anastomoses between the superior hemorrhoidal vessels and branches of the internal iliac arteries provide collateral circulation; this is important after surgical interruption or atherosclerotic occlusion of the vascular supply of the left colon.

The veins accompany the corresponding arteries and drain into the liver through the portal vein or into the systemic circulation by way of the hypogastric veins. Continuous lymphatic plexuses in the submucous and subserous layers of the bowel wall drain into the lymphatic channels and lymph nodes that accompany the blood vessels.

Nerve Supply

The sympathetic nerves originating in T10–12 travel in the thoracic splanchnic nerves to the celiac plexus and then to the preaortic and superior mesenteric plexuses, from which postganglionic fibers are distributed along the superior mesenteric artery and its branches to the right colon. The left colon is supplied by sympathetic fibers that arise in L1–3, synapse in the paravertebral ganglia, and accompany the inferior mesenteric artery to the colon. The parasympathetic nerves to the right colon come from the right vagus and travel with the sympathetic nerves. The parasympathetic supply to the left colon derives from S2–4. These fibers emerge from the spinal cord as the nervi erigentes, which form the pelvic plexus and send branches to the transverse, descending, and pelvic portions of the colon.

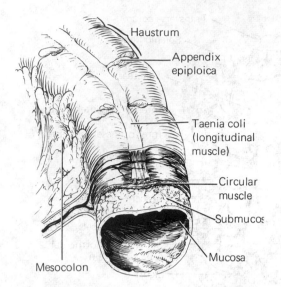

Figure 31–2. Cross section of colon. The longitudinal muscle encircles the colon but is thickened in the region of the taeniae coli.

Koizumi M, Horiguchi M: Accessory arteries supplying the human transverse colon. Acta Anat (Basel) 1990; 137:246.

Levin DS, Haggitt RC: Normal histology of the colon. Am J Surg Pathol 1989;13:966.

Prassopoulos P et al: A study of the variation of colonic positioning in the pararenal space as shown by computed tomography. Eur J Radiol 1990;10:44.

Stoss F: Investigation of the muscular architecture of the rectosigmoid junction in humans. Dis Colon Rectum 1990;33:378.

PHYSIOLOGY

The primary functions of the colon are absorption, secretion, motility, and intraluminal digestion. These interrelated phenomena process ileal effluent and convert it into semisolid feces that are stored until defecation is convenient. Regional variations in function are significant. The proximal colon absorbs electrolytes and water more efficiently than do the descending colon and rectum, and motility and intraluminal digestion differ by region also.

Loss of colonic function through disease or surgery results in a continuous discharge of food wastes and increases daily intestinal losses of water and electrolytes, chiefly sodium chloride.

The small intestine digests and absorbs most nutrients from ingested foods. The role of the colon in human nutrition is not well defined. Metabolism of carbohydrate to absorbable volatile fatty acids is probably important. Ureolysis—conversion of circulating urea to ammonia, which is reabsorbed and re-used—may be significant. The colon also absorbs amino acids, bile acids, and vitamin K, but the contribution of the colon to homeostasis by these mechanisms has not been quantitated.

Intestinal Gas

The volume and composition of intestinal gas vary greatly among normal individuals. The small intestine contains approximately 100 mL of gas and the colon somewhat more. Some gas is absorbed through the mucosa and excreted through the lungs, and the remaining 400–1200 mL/d is emitted as flatus.

Nitrogen (N_2) comprises 30–90% of intestinal gas. Swallowed air is the principal source of intestinal N_2, but N_2 also can diffuse across the mucosa from blood to lumen when other gases are produced in sufficient volume to lower the partial pressure of N_2 and establish a gradient for diffusion. Other intestinal gases include oxygen (O_2), carbon dioxide (CO_2), hydrogen (H_2), methane (CH_4), and odoriferous trace substances such as hydrogen sulfide, indole, and skatole. H_2 and CO_2 are generated by fermentation of ingested nonabsorbed carbohydrate, especially carbohydrate present in polysaccharides (eg, fiber) and some starches. Lactose in milk provides the substrate in lactase-deficient persons. Mucus is the main endogenous source of carbohydrate in the colon; intestinal glycoproteins are 80% carbohydrate. Only about one-third of the population produces CH_4, which is also a product of colonic bacteria that use hydrogen to reduce CO_2. Stools of CH_4-producers nearly always float, even in the absence of fecal fat. CH_4, like H_2, can be measured in the breath. H_2 and CH_4 are explosive gases, and caution must be exercised when using electrocautery in the bowel lumen. Mannitol, a carbohydrate alcohol that is not absorbed by the small bowel, has been used to cleanse the bowel for colonoscopy. Since colonic bacteria ferment mannitol to produce hydrogen, this agent should not be used.

Patients with "excessive gas" may complain of abdominal pain and distention, increased flatus, and watery stools. Some of these patients have irritable bowel syndrome. "Increased" flatus may reflect extreme sensitivity of the rectum to small volumes, resulting in frequent passage of gas. Alternatively, gas may be produced in excessive quantities in symptomatic patients. Almost invariably, hydrogen is the culprit. Measurement of breath hydrogen is a potentially useful test for malabsorption states. Treatment of overproduction at present is directed toward elimination of lactose, legumes, and wheat from the diet.

Motility

Motor activity of the colon occurs in three patterns, and there is marked regional variation between the right and left colon. A pacemaker in the transverse colon has been postulated, perhaps pacing the proximal colon retrograde to facilitate storage and absorption while pacing the distal colon in the aborad direction to favor propulsion. **Retrograde peristalsis (antiperistalsis),** annular contractions moving orad, dominates in the right colon. This kind of activity churns the contents and tends to confine them to the cecum and ascending colon. As ileal effluent continually enters the cecum, some of the column of liquid stool in the right colon is displaced and flows into the transverse colon. **Segmentation** is the most common type of motor activity in the transverse and descending colon. Annular contractions divide the lumen into uniform segments, propelling feces over short distances in both directions. Segmental contractions form, relax, and re-form in different locations, seemingly at random. **Mass movement** is a strong ring contraction moving abroad over long distances in the transverse and descending colon. It occurs infrequently, perhaps only a few times daily, most commonly after meals.

The enteric nervous system (ENS) coordinates and programs motility (see Chapter 30). Eating produces a group of alterations in colonic myoelectrical and motor activity collectively termed the gastrocolic response. As a result, more fluid is emptied from the ileum into the colon, mass movements are increased, and the urge to defecate is perceived. The magnitude of the gastrocolic response depends on the caloric content of the meal. Dietary fat is the principal stimulus. Gut hormones also participate in the regulation of these events.

Physical activities such as changes in posture, walking, and lifting are physiologically important stimuli to the movement of colonic contents. Colonic motility is also affected by emotional states. Transit through the colon is speeded by a diet containing large amounts of fiber from vegetables or bran. Fiber is defined as insoluble plant cell matrix and consists of cellulose, hemicellulose, and lignin. Dietary fiber slows transit through the jejunum.

Normal colonic movements are slow, complex, and extremely variable, making it difficult to define altered motility in disease states. The fecal stream itself does not move along in anything resembling orderly laminar flow. Some of the material entering the cecum flows past feces remaining from earlier periods. Portions of the stream enter the periphery of haustra, where they may fail to progress for 24 hours or more. In most persons with normal bowel function, residue from a meal reaches the cecum after 4 hours and the rectosigmoid by 24 hours. The transverse colon is the primary site for fecal storage. Mixing of bowel content in the colon results in passage of residue from a single meal in movements for up to 3–4 days afterward.

The urge to defecate is perceived when small amounts of feces enter the rectum and stimulate stretch receptors in the rectal wall or the levator muscles. The sensation may be temporarily suppressed by voluntarily contracting the sphincter and pelvic diaphragm. Eventually, increased rectal filling may make the urge to defecate impossible to deny. When defecation is performed, it is aided by assumption of a position with the thighs flexed, so that intra-abdominal pressure can be increased by abdominal wall contraction. The internal and external anal sphincters relax, and the rectal or rectosigmoid contents are extruded by contraction of the colon and by increasing abdominal pressure via a Valsalva maneuver. The pelvic floor relaxes and the rectum loses its curves as the feces are discharged from the anus. Afterward, the sphincters resume their tone and the rectum remains empty until shortly before the next movement, when arrival of more feces from the sigmoid evokes the urge to defecate once again.

Absorption

The colon participates in maintaining the body economy by absorption of water and electrolytes, but the absorptive function of the colon is not essential to life. Although amino acids, fatty acids, and some vitamins can be absorbed slowly from the large bowel, only a small amount of these nutrients reaches the colon normally. Perhaps 10–20% of ingested starch, however, passes unabsorbed into the colon, where bacterial fermentation converts starch to short-chain volatile fatty acids (eg, acetate). Absorption of fatty acids contributes importantly to assimilation of calories. Dietary celluloses and hemicelluloses are degraded by colonic bacteria.

Approximately 1000–2000 mL of ileal effluent containing 90% water enters the cecum each day. This material is desiccated during transit through the colon, so that only 100–200 mL of water is excreted in the feces. Table 31–1 gives average values for the electrolyte and water composition of ileal effluent and feces; the differences provide a rough estimate of colonic absorption and secretion. Data are listed also for the estimated maximal absorptive capacity, which is greater in the right colon than in the left. This capacity depends on the rate at which fluid enters the cecum. Normally, formed feces are composed of 70% water and 30% solids. Almost half of these solids are bacteria; the remainder is food waste and desquamated epithelium.

Sodium is absorbed by an active transport mechanism that is enhanced by mineralocorticoids, glucocorticoids, and volatile fatty acids produced by bacteria. Volatile fatty acids may be essential mucosal nutrients for normal colonic absorption of electrolytes and water. There are segmental differences in the mode of absorption of sodium and water. Normally, sodium absorption is so efficient that a person can remain in balance on as little as 5 meq in the daily diet, but colectomy increases the minimum daily requirements to 80–100 meq to offset losses from the ileostomy. Potassium enters feces by passive diffusion and by secretion in mucus. Excessive mucus production may occur in colitis or with certain tumors such as villous adenomas and may lead to substantial

Table 31–1. Mean values for electrolyte and water balance in the normal colon. A plus (+) sign indicates absorption from the colonic lumen; a minus (–) sign indicates secretion into the lumen.

	Ileal Effluent		Fecal Fluid		Net Colonic Absorption (per 24 h)	
	Concentration (meq/L)	Quantity (per 24 h)	Concentration (meq/L)	Quantity (per 24 h)	Normal	Maximal Capacity
Na^+	120	180 meq	30	2 meq	+178 meq	+400 meq
K^+	6	10 meq	67	5 meq	+5 meq	–45 meq
Cl^-	67	100 meq	20	1.5 meq	+98 meq	+500 meq
HCO_3^-	40	60 meq	50	4 meq	+56 meq	
H_2O		1500 mL		100 mL	+1400 mL	+5000 mL

potassium losses in the stool. Chloride is absorbed in exchange for bicarbonate.

Bowel Habits

The frequency of defecation is influenced by social and dietary customs. The average interval between bowel movements among the population of Western countries is a little over 24 hours but may vary in normal subjects from 8–12 hours to 2–3 days. Dietary fiber content and physical activity influence stool frequency to a great extent. Many bedridden patients have infrequent, hard stools. Self-reported constipation in the general population of the USA has a prevalence of about 10% in men and 20% in women; diarrhea is reported by 5% of men and women. These complaints are more frequent with aging.

A change in bowel habits demands investigation for organic disease. Diarrhea may be debilitating and even fatal, because it is associated with loss of large amounts of water and electrolytes. Diarrhea is usually said to be present if stools contain more than 300 mL of fluid daily. Osmotic diarrhea results when excess water-soluble molecules remain in the bowel lumen, causing osmotic retention of water; this is one mechanism by which saline laxatives act. Colonic diseases that produce diarrhea usually cause excessive fluid secretion more than impaired absorption. Bile salts, hydroxy fatty acids, and castor oil (ricinoleic acid) are a few of the many substances that stimulate secretion of fluid by the colon by increasing mucosal cAMP. Increased secretion by the small bowel may also cause diarrhea. Loss of absorptive surface (eg, after intestinal resection) and exudative diseases are other reasons for feces to contain excess fluid. Disordered intestinal motility is not primarily responsible for increased fecal excretion of water. The physician should be alert to surreptitious laxative abuse among patients who complain of diarrhea.

Constipation means infrequent stools (less than two per week), excessive straining, or incomplete evacuation. Recent onset of this complaint in an adult should prompt a search for obstructing lesions.

Severe idiopathic constipation refractory to usual remedies is more common in women; it often begins in adolescence and worsens during the 20s or 30s, or

it may be precipitated by childbirth or hysterectomy. A heterogeneous group of disorders is responsible. Slow colonic transit (colonic inertia) is one mechanism of constipation, and failure of the pelvic floor to relax during defecation (obstructed defecation) is a separate category. A classification of disorders in which constipation and obstructed defecation are symptoms is given in Table 31–2. Conditions giving rise to obstructed defecation are part of a larger group of abnormalities termed "disorders of the pelvic floor."

A thorough history and physical examination may elucidate the origin of the symptoms, eg, depression, psychotropic or other drugs, or anatomic abnormalities. Further investigation of chronic idiopathic constipation requires assessment of colonic transit and study of pelvic floor function. Colonic transit is evaluated by obtaining serial plain abdominal x-rays after ingestion of tiny radiopaque markers or by scintigraphy after ingestion of radiolabeled solid pellets. Tests of pelvic floor function include defecography, anorectal manometry, electromyography, and nerve conduction studies.

Severe slow-transit constipation does not respond to dietary fiber; an irritant laxative (eg, Senokot, Dulcolax) may be necessary. Cisapride, a prokinetic agent, may be superior. Selected patients qualify for a

Table 31–2. Classification of constipation and obstructed defecation.[1]

Constipation
  Normal colon
    Normal transit
    Slow transit
  Megacolon/megarectum
    Congenital
    Acquired
Obstructed defecation
    Solitary rectal ulcer syndrome
    Descending perineum syndrome
    Rectal intussusception
    Complete rectal prolapse
    Anismus (inappropriate sphincter contraction)

[1]Modified from Bartolo DCG: Pelvic floor disorders: Incontinence, constipation, and obstructed defecation. Perspect Colon Rectal Surg 1988;1:1.

surgical procedure (colectomy and ileorectal anastomosis). Obstructed defecation related to rectal prolapse responds to operation to repair the prolapse. Rectal intussusception should be repaired also, but relief of symptoms is less predictable. Surgical treatment of the other conditions is unsatisfactory at present.

Bazzocchi G et al: Effect of eating on colonic motility and transit in patients with functional diarrhea. Simultaneous scintigraphic and manometric evaluations. Gastroenterology 1991;101:1298.

Bazzocchi G et al: Postprandial colonic transit and motor activity in chronic constipation. Gastroenterology 1990; 98:686.

Beaugerie L et al: Digestion and absorption in the human intestine of three sugar alcohols. Gastroenterology 1990;99:717.

Bertomeu A et al: Chronic diarrhea with normal stool and colonic examinations: Organic or functional? J Clin Gastroenterol 1991;13:531.

Brown SR, Cann PA, Read NW: Effect of coffee on distal colon function. Gut 1990;31:450.

Garcia D et al: Colonic motility: Electric and manometric description of mass movement. Dis Colon Rectum 1991; 34:577.

Grimble G: Fibre, fermentation, flora, and flatus. Gut 1989;30:6.

Heaton KW: Dietary fibre. Br Med J 1990;300:1479.

Klauser AG et al: Behavioral modification of colonic function: Can constipation be learned? Dig Dis Sci 1990; 35:1271.

Koch TR et al: Inhibitory neuropeptides and intrinsic inhibitory innervation of descending human colon. Dig Dis Sci 1991;36:712.

Pemberton JH, Rath DM, Ilstrup DM: Evaluation and surgical treatment of severe chronic constipation. Ann Surg 1991;214:403.

Royall D, Wolever TMS, Jeejeebhoy KN: Clinical significance of colonic fermentation. Am J Gastroenterol 1990;85:1307

Sandle GI et al: Cellular basis for defective electrolyte: Transport in inflamed human colon. Gastroenterology 1990;99:97.

Sarna SK: Physiology and pathophysiology of colonic motor activity. (Two parts.) Dig Dis Sci 1991;36:827, 998.

Schoetz DJ Jr: Postcolectomy syndromes. World J Surg 1991;15:605.

Smith AN et al: Disordered colorectal motility in intractable constipation following hysterectomy. Br J Surg 1990; 77:1361.

Staiano A et al: Effect of cisapride on chronic idiopathic constipation in children. Dig Dis Sci 1991;36:733.

Steadman CJ et al: Variation of muscle tone in the human colon. Gastroenterology 1991;101:373.

Stivland T et al: Scintigraphic measurement of regional gut transit in idiopathic constipation. Gastroenterology 1991; 101:107.

Van Tilburg AJP et al: Na$^+$-dependent bile acid transport in the ileum: The balance between diarrhea and constipation. Gastroenterology 1990;98:25.

Walsh RM, Aranha GV, Freeark RJ: Mortality and quality of life after a total abdominal colectomy. Arch Surg 1990;125:1564.

Ziegenhagen DJ et al: Adding more fluid to wheat bran has no significant effects on intestinal functions of healthy subjects. J Clin Gastroenterol 1991;13:525.

MICROBIOLOGY

The colon of the fetus is sterile, and the bacterial flora is established soon after birth. The type of organisms present in the colon depends in part on dietary and environmental factors. It is estimated that stool contains up to 400 different species of autochthonous (native) bacteria.

Over 99% of the normal fecal flora is anaerobic. *Bacteroides fragilis* is most prevalent, and counts average 10^{10}/g of wet feces. *Lactobacillus bifidus,* clostridia, and cocci of various types are other common anaerobes. Aerobic fecal bacteria are mainly coliforms and enterococci. *Escherichia coli* is the predominant coliform and is present in counts of 10^7/g of feces; other aerobic coliforms include *Klebsiella, Proteus,* and *Enterobacter. Streptococcus faecalis* is the principal enterococcus. *Methanobrevibacter smithii* is the predominant methane-producing organism in humans.

The fecal flora participates in numerous physiologic processes. Bacteria degrade bile pigments to give the stool its brown color, and the characteristic fecal odor is due to the amines indole and skatole produced by bacterial action. Fecal organisms deconjugate bile salts (only free bile salts are found in feces) and alter the steroid nucleus. Bacteria influence colonic motility and absorption, generate intestinal gases, supply vitamin K to the host, and may be important in the defense against infection. Nutrition of colonic mucosal cells may be partially derived from fuels (eg, fatty acids) produced by bacteria. Intestinal bacteria participate in the pathophysiology of a variety of disease processes. Bacterial translocation from the small and large bowel in critically ill or traumatized patients is believed to contribute to multiple organ system failure. There is evidence that bacteria play a role in the pathogenesis of carcinoma of the large bowel.

Benno Y, Mitsuoka T, Kanazawa K: Human faecal flora in health and colon cancer. Acta Chir Scand Suppl 1991; 562:15.

Dunn DL: Autochthonous microflora of the gastrointestinal tract. Perspect Colon Rectal Surg 1990;2:105.

Latella G, Caprilli R: Metabolism of large bowel mucosa in health and disease. Int J Colorect Dis 1991;6:127.

Strocchi A et al: Competition for hydrogen by human faecal bacteria: Evidence for the predominance of methane producing bacteria. Gut 1991;32:1498.

ROENTGENOLOGIC EXAMINATION

Plain films of the abdomen depict the distribution of gas in the intestines, calcifications, tumor masses, and the size and position of the liver, spleen, and kidneys. In the presence of acute intra-abdominal disease, erect, lateral, and oblique projections and lateral decubitus views are helpful.

The lumen of the colon can be seen radiographically by instilling a suspension of barium sulfate through the anus (barium enema) (Figure 31–3). Adequate preparation of the bowel is imperative before barium enema examination so that the colon will be as free as possible of fecal material and gas. Although many rectal lesions can be demonstrated by barium enema, x-rays are not as accurate here as with lesions above the rectosigmoid. Proctosigmoidoscopy is the best method for inspecting the rectum. Postevacuation films reveal the mucosal pattern and small lesions.

Double contrast (air contrast) barium enema (sometimes called a pneumocolon examination) is more sensitive than the single column technique for detection of small intraluminal lesions such as polyps. A higher-density, more viscous barium is used. After the mucosa is first coated with barium, carbon dioxide or air is insufflated to distend the colon and provide a second contrast medium.

Arteriography is used to detect bleeding sites and is discussed in the section on massive hemorrhage.

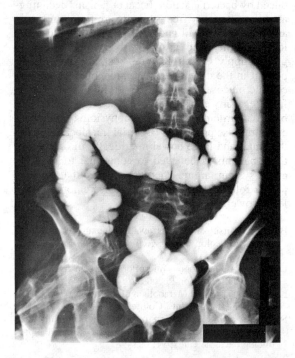

Figure 31–3. Roentgenogram of normal colon. The colon has been rendered radiopaque by a barium enema (single-column technique).

CT scan and sonography (external, endorectal, and endovaginal) help diagnose masses (neoplasms and abscesses). MRI is proving reliable for staging of cancers. Single-photon emission CT (SPECT), positron emission tomography (PET), and other potentially useful radiographic techniques are in development.

Feczko PJ: Increased frequency of reactions to contrast materials during gastrointestinal studies. Radiology 1990; 174:367.

Gelfand DW, Chen MYM, Ott DJ: Preparing the colon for the barium enema examination. Radiology 1991; 178:609.

Levine MS et al: Diagnosis of pneumoperitoneum on supine abdominal radiographs. AJR Am J Roentgenol 1991; 56:731.

Limberg B: Diagnosis of large bowel tumours by colonic sonography. Lancet 1990;335:144.

Markus JB et al: Double-contrast barium enema studies: Effect of multiple reading on perception error. Radiology 1990;175:155.

Marshall JB et al: Air-contrast barium enema studies after flexible proctosigmoidoscopy: Randomized controlled clinical trial. Radiology 1990;176:549.

Taylor PN, Beckly DE: Use of air in double contrast barium enema: Is it still acceptable? Clin Radiol 1991;44:183.

Wheatley MJ, Eckhauser FE: Portal venous barium intravasation complicating barium enema examination. Surgery 1991;109:788.

FIBEROPTIC COLONOSCOPY & SIGMOIDOSCOPY

The flexible colonoscope permits examination of the entire colon in most individuals, and biopsies or cytologic material can be obtained under direct vision. Video technology is replacing fiberoptic viewing systems.

Diagnostic colonoscopy is indicated in patients with the following: (1) abnormal or equivocal barium enema; (2) unexplained rectal bleeding; (3) abnormal sigmoidoscopy (eg, polyps); (4) inflammatory bowel disease; or (5) previous colon cancer or polyp. Therapeutic uses of colonoscopy include (1) excision of polyps; (2) control of bleeding; (3) removal of foreign body; (4) detorsion of volvulus; (5) decompression of pseudo-obstruction; (6) dilation of strictures; and (7) laser destruction of neoplasms. Relative contraindications to colonoscopy are fulminant colitis and suspected colonic perforation. Complications (mainly perforation and bleeding) occur in 0.35–0.8% of diagnostic colonoscopy procedures. Success may be limited by such technical difficulties as diverticular disease, strictures, sharp flexures, redundant colon, or previous pelvic surgery. Colonoscopy is performed intraoperatively on occasion.

Flexible sigmoidoscopy uses an instrument 30–65 cm long. The diagnostic yield is two to six times greater than with the rigid sigmoidoscope because two to three times more colon can be seen. Flexible sigmoidoscopy is especially suitable for screening asymptomatic patients for neoplasms; the presence of gross or occult blood may be an indication for total colonoscopy. Flexible sigmoidoscopy has few complications when performed expertly, but the technique must be learned under supervision. Flexible sigmoidoscopes have replaced the rigid variety for most but not all purposes.

Fennerty MB et al: Physiologic changes during colonoscopy. Gastrointest Endosc 1990;36:22.

Hall C et al: Colon perforation during colonoscopy: Surgical versus conservative management. Br J Surg 1991; 78:542.

Morrissey JF, Reichelderfer M: Gastrointestinal endoscopy. (Two parts.) N Engl J Med 1991;325:1142, 1214.

Perry RE et al: Office colonoscopy: A safe procedure in selected patients. Dis Colon Rectum 1989;32:1031.

Rösch T et al: Colonic endoscopic ultrasonography: First results of a new technique. Gastrointest Endosc 1990; 36:382.

Schapiro M, Lehman GA (editors): *Flexible Colonoscopy. Techniques and Utilization.* Williams & Wilkins, 1990.

Soon JCC et al: Perforation of the large bowel during colonoscopy in Singapore. Am Surg 1990;56:285.

Waye JD, Bashkoff E: Total colonoscopy: is it always possible? Gastrointest Endosc 1991;37:152.

Webb WA: Colonoscoping the "difficult" colon. Am Surg 1991;57:178.

Wolff WI: Colonoscopy: History and development. Am J Gastroenterol 1989;84:1017.

DISEASES OF THE COLON & RECTUM

OBSTRUCTION OF THE LARGE INTESTINE

Essentials of Diagnosis

- Constipation or obstipation.
- Abdominal distention and sometimes tenderness.
- Abdominal pain.
- Nausea and vomiting (late).
- Characteristic x-ray findings.

General Considerations

Approximately 15% of intestinal obstructions in adults occur in the large bowel. The obstruction may be in any portion of the colon but most commonly is in the sigmoid. Complete colonic obstruction is most often due to carcinoma; volvulus, diverticular disease, inflammatory disorders, benign tumors, fecal impaction, and miscellaneous rare problems account for the remainder (Table 31–3). Adhesive bands sel-

Table 31–3. Causes of colonic obstruction in adults.

Cause	Relative Incidence (%)*
Carcinoma of colon	65
Diverticulitis	20
Volvulus	5
Miscellaneous	10

*Obstruction due to diverticulitis is usually incomplete; volvulus is second to carcinoma as a cause of complete obstruction.

dom obstruct the colon, and intussusception is uncommon in adults.

Obstruction by a lesion at the ileocecal valve produces the symptoms and signs of small bowel obstruction. The pathophysiology of more distal colonic obstruction depends on the competence of the ileocecal valve (Figure 31–4). In 10–20% of patients, the ileocecal valve is incompetent, and colonic pressure

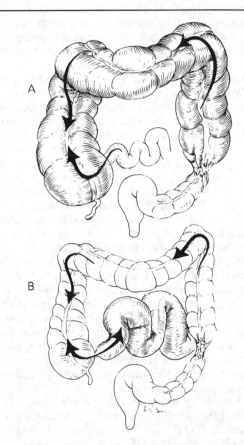

Figure 31–4. The role of the ileocecal valve in obstruction of the colon. The obstruction is in the upper sigmoid. *A:* The ileocecal valve is competent, creating a closed loop between the obstruction and the valve. Tension in the closed loop is increased further by emptying of gas and fluid from the ileum into the colon. *B:* The ileocecal valve is incompetent. Reflux into the ileum is permitted. The colon is relieved of some of its distention, and the small bowel has become distended.

is relieved by reflux into the ileum. If the colon is not decompressed through the ileocecal valve, a "closed loop" is formed between the valve and the obstructing point. The colon distends progressively, because the ileum continues to empty gas and fluid into the obstructed segment. If luminal pressure becomes very high, circulation is impaired and gangrene and perforation can result. The wall of the right colon is thinner than that of the left colon and its luminal caliber is larger, so the cecum is at greatest risk of perforation in these circumstances (law of Laplace). In general, if the cecum acutely reaches a diameter of 10–12 cm, the risk of perforation is great.

Clinical Findings

A. Symptoms and Signs: Simple mechanical obstruction of the colon may develop insidiously. Deep, visceral, cramping pain from obstruction of the colon is usually referred to the hypogastrium. Lesions of the fixed portions of the colon (cecum, hepatic flexure, splenic flexure) may cause pain that is felt immediately anteriorly. Pain originating from the sigmoid is often located to the left in the lower abdomen. Severe, continuous abdominal pain suggests intestinal ischemia or peritonitis. Borborygmus may be loud and coincident with cramps. Constipation or obstipation is a universal feature of complete obstruction, although the colon distal to the obstruction may empty after the initial symptoms begin. Vomiting is a late finding and may not occur at all if the ileocecal valve prevents reflux. If reflux decompresses the cecal contents into the small intestine, the symptoms of small bowel as well as large bowel obstruction appear. Feculent vomiting is a late manifestation.

Physical examination discloses abdominal distention and tympany, and peristaltic waves may be seen if the abdominal wall is thin. High-pitched, metallic tinkles associated with rushes and gurgles may be heard on auscultation. Localized tenderness or a tender, palpable mass may indicate a strangulated closed loop. Signs of localized or generalized peritonitis suggest gangrene or rupture of the bowel wall. Fresh blood may be found in the rectum in intussusception and in carcinoma of the rectum or colon. Sigmoidoscopy may disclose a neoplasm. Colonoscopy may be diagnostic and perhaps therapeutic in some patients with strictures or neoplasms.

B. Imaging Studies: The distended colon frequently creates a "picture frame" outline of the abdominal cavity. The colon can be distinguished from the small intestine by its haustral markings, which do not cross the entire lumen of the distended colon. Barium enema will confirm the diagnosis of colonic obstruction and identify its exact location. Water-soluble contrast medium should be used if strangulation or perforation is suspected. Once the obstruction is seen, the procedure should be discontinued. Barium must not be given orally in the presence of suspected colonic obstruction.

Differential Diagnosis

A. Small Versus Large Bowel Obstruction: Large bowel obstruction is frequently slow in onset, causes less pain, and may not cause vomiting in spite of considerable distention. Elderly patients with no history of abdominal surgery or prior attacks of obstruction frequently have carcinoma of the large bowel. Plain abdominal x-rays are essential to make the differential diagnosis, and barium contrast studies are often helpful.

B. Paralytic Ileus: The distinguishing features of paralytic ileus are signs of peritonitis or a history of trauma to the back or pelvis. The abdomen is silent, and abdominal cramping is not present. There may be tenderness. Plain films show a dilated colon. Contrast enema may be required to exclude an obstruction.

C. Pseudo-obstruction: Acute pseudo-obstruction of the colon (**Ogilvie's syndrome**) is massive colonic distention in the absence of a mechanically obstructing lesion. It is a severe form of ileus and arises in bedridden patients who have serious extraintestinal illness (renal, cardiac, respiratory) or trauma (eg, vertebral fracture). Aerophagia and impairment of colonic motility by drugs are contributory factors. Abdominal distention without pain or tenderness is the earliest manifestation, but later symptoms mimic those of true obstruction. Plain x-rays of the abdomen show marked gaseous distention of the colon. Although the entire colon may contain gas, the distention is typically localized to the right colon, with a cutoff at the hepatic or splenic flexure. Contrast enema proves the absence of obstruction, but instillation of radiopaque material should cease as soon as the dilated colon is reached.

The risk of cecal perforation is high in this condition, and decompression of the colon should be attempted. Enemas may help evacuate gas from the colon in mild cases. In more severe distention, fiberoptic colonoscopy is the treatment of choice, provided there are no clinical or x-ray signs of perforation. Colonoscopic decompression is successful initially in 90% of patients, and the complication rate is low. Recurrence is frequent (20% or more); techniques are available for colonoscopic placement of a tube in the proximal colon to maintain decompression. Cecostomy is reserved for patients in whom colonoscopy fails. Endoscopic percutaneous cecostomy, similar to the technique for gastrostomy, is a new method of longer-term decompression. Laparoscopic cecostomy is performed by a few specialists. Open surgical cecostomy is an established procedure that is widely available.

Complications

Cecal perforation, described above, is a potentially lethal complication. Partially obstructive lesions of the colon may be complicated by acute colitis in the bowel proximal to the obstruction; it is probably a form of ischemic colitis secondary to impaired mucosal blood flow in the distended segment.

Treatment

The primary goal of treatment is decompression of the obstructed segment to prevent perforation; an operation is almost always required. Removal of the obstructing lesion is a secondary goal, but a single operation to accomplish both objectives is preferred whenever possible.

Colonoscopic balloon dilation of obstructing benign strictures or neoplasms is applicable sometimes. Laser photocoagulation of an obstructing cancer, especially in the rectum, may enlarge the lumen to permit an elective operation later under better circumstances, and occasionally a patient with advanced cancer may avoid operation entirely. Permanent diverting colostomy may be the only possible choice in a debilitated patient with unresectable obstructing rectal cancer.

Obstructing lesions of the right colon are resected in one stage, with ileotransverse colostomy if the patient's condition is good. If the patient's condition is precarious or if the colon has perforated, the bowel is resected but no anastomosis is done; an ileostomy is established, and anastomosis is performed at a second operation. Nonresectable lesions may be bypassed. Cecostomy is seldom used for obstruction in this area.

Obstructing lesions of the left colon are best treated by resection in patients who seem likely to tolerate this procedure. It is advantageous to immediately remove the lesion (often a malignant tumor) rather than delay for days or weeks after a preliminary decompressive maneuver. There are four choices of operation. Anastomosis may be postponed and a temporary end colostomy created (2-stage procedure; Figure 31–12). Alternatively, intraoperative colonic lavage can be carried out by inserting a tube into the ileum or appendix and then into the cecum; a large-bore tube is placed into the colon proximal to the obstruction to allow effluent to drain out of the sterile field. This procedure may cleanse the colon well enough so that primary anastomosis can be performed safely. Primary anastomosis with the aid of an intraluminal bypass tube (Coloshield) to prevent anastomotic leakage is another option; the early results are encouraging. Total abdominal colectomy with ileorectal anastomosis in one stage is another acceptable option because it avoids the risks of anastomosing unprepared obstructed colon.

Cecostomy (Figure 31–5) is the operation of choice in patients whose surgical risk is prohibitive. It gives adequate decompression if the distal colon is not packed with feces and complete diversion of the fecal stream is not necessary. Cecostomy has the advantage that it does not interfere with subsequent extensive resection of the left colon. **Transverse colostomy** can provide complete fecal diversion, but a

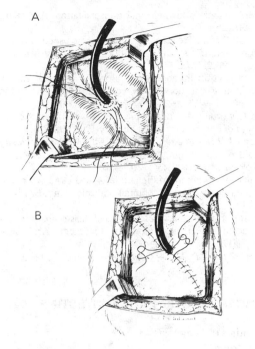

Figure 31–5. Cecostomy. **A:** Through a small incision overlying the cecum, a tube has been inserted through the wall of the cecum into its lumen and secured with a purse-string suture. **B:** Peritoneal closure. The cecum is fixed to the peritoneum. **Note:** A useful modification is to suture the peritoneum to the cecum circumferentially around the proposed cecostomy before the bowel is opened; this maneuver excludes the cecum from the peritoneal cavity and avoids the risk of fecal contamination of the abdomen.

serious disadvantage is the need for a total of three operations if this approach is followed: (1) colostomy, (2) resection of the obstructing lesion, and (3) closure of colostomy.

Prognosis

The prognosis depends upon the age and general condition of the patient, the extent of vascular impairment of the bowel, the presence or absence of perforation, the cause of obstruction, and the promptness of surgical management. The overall mortality rate is about 20%. Cecal perforation carries a 40% mortality rate. Obstructing cancer of the colon has a worse prognosis than nonobstructing cancer because it is more likely to be locally extensive or metastatic to nodes or distant sites.

Ericksen AS et al: Use of gastrointestinal contrast studies in obstruction of the small and large bowel. Dis Colon Rectum 1990;33:56.

Garcia-Valdecasas JC et al: Obstructing colorectal carcinomas: Prospective study. Dis Colon Rectum 1991;34:759.

Koneru B et al: Nonobstructing colonic dilatation and colon

perforations following renal transplantation. Arch Surg 1990;125:610.

MacColl C et al: Treatment of acute colonic pseudoobstruction (Ogilvie's syndrome) with cisapride. Gastroenterology 1990;98:773.

Murray JJ et al: Intraoperative colonic lavage and primary anastomosis in nonelective colon resection. Dis Colon Rectum 1991;34:527.

Oz MC, Forde KA: Endoscopic alternatives in the management of colonic strictures. Surgery 1990;108:513.

Sariego J, Matsumoto T, Kerstein MD: Colonoscopically guided tube decompression in Ogilvie's syndrome. Dis Colon Rectum 1991;34:720.

Stephenson BM et al: Malignant left-sided large bowel obstruction managed by subtotal/total colectomy. Br J Surg 1990;77:1098.

Tan SG et al: Primary resection and anastomosis in obstructed descending colon due to cancer. Arch Surg 1991;126:748.

Welch JP (editor): Bowel Obstruction. Saunders, 1990.

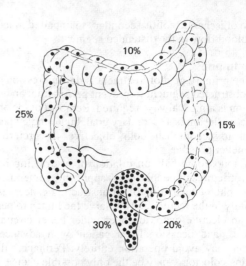

Figure 31–6. Distribution of cancer of the colon and rectum.

CANCER OF THE LARGE INTESTINE

Essentials of Diagnosis

Right colon:
- Unexplained weakness or anemia.
- Occult blood in feces.
- Dyspeptic symptoms.
- Persistent right abdominal discomfort.
- Palpable abdominal mass.
- Characteristic x-ray findings.
- Characteristic colonoscopic findings.

Left colon:
- Change in bowel habits.
- Gross blood in stool.
- Obstructive symptoms.
- Characteristic x-ray findings.
- Characteristic colonoscopic or sigmoidoscopic findings.

Rectum:
- Rectal bleeding.
- Alteration in bowel habits.
- Sensation of incomplete evacuation.
- Intrarectal palpable tumor.
- Sigmoidoscopic findings.

General Considerations

In Western countries, cancer of the colon and rectum ranks second after cancer of the lung in incidence and death rates. An estimated 150,000 new cases of colorectal cancer are diagnosed and 60,000 people die of this disease in the USA each year. The incidence increases with age, from 0.39 per 1000 persons per year at age 50 to 4.5 per 1000 persons per year at age 80. Carcinoma of the colon, particularly the right colon, is more common in women, and carcinoma of the rectum is more common in men. The distribution of cancers of the colon and rectum is shown in Figure 31–6; these percentages reflect an increased inci-

dence of cancer in the sigmoid and in the right colon and a decreased incidence in the rectum over the past 30 years. Multiple synchronous colonic cancers—ie, two or more carcinomas occurring simultaneously—are found in 5% of patients. Metachronous cancer is a new primary lesion in a patient who has had a previous resection for cancer. The cumulative risk of metachronous colorectal cancer is as high as 30% after 4 decades of follow-up. Ninety-five percent of malignant tumors of the colon and rectum are adenocarcinomas.

Genetic predisposition to cancer of the large bowel is well recognized in persons with familial adenomatous polyposis. In addition, at least two varieties of autosomal dominant hereditary nonpolyposis colorectal cancer (HNPCC) have been identified: (1) cancer family syndrome (CFS; Lynch syndrome II), with early onset (age 20–30), proximal dominance, and other associated extracolonic adenocarcinomas, especially endometrial carcinoma; and (2) hereditary site-specific colon cancer (HSSCC; Lynch syndrome I), which shows the same characteristics except for extracolonic cancers. An estimated 6% of patients with cancer of the colon and rectum have HNPCC. In the absence of these syndromes, first-degree relatives of patients with colorectal cancer have a two- to threefold increased risk of large bowel cancer.

Ulcerative colitis, Crohn's colitis, schistosomal colitis, exposure to radiation, colorectal polyps, and the presence of a ureterocolostomy are conditions that predispose to cancer of the large bowel. Association between Barrett's esophagus and colonic cancer has been reported. Data on the risk of large bowel cancer after cholecystectomy are conflicting; some studies find a greater likelihood of right-sided colonic cancer in women after cholecystectomy, but the effect is small, and it may reflect sharing of common etiologic factors rather than a consequence of cholecystectomy. Association of human papillomavirus (HPV) types 16 and 18 and colorectal adenocarcinoma has been reported. Mean plasma levels of gastrin are higher in patients with colorectal cancer than in controls; the significance is unknown.

A high incidence of colorectal cancer occurs in populations that are economically prosperous. This observation has focused attention on environmental factors, particularly diet, in the etiology of this tumor. Increased intake of fat, increased caloric intake, decreased dietary calcium, and decreased intake of fermentable fiber are among the possible dietary influences. Dietary fat enhances cholesterol and bile acid synthesis by the liver, and the amounts of these sterols in the colon increase. Anaerobic colonic bacteria convert these compounds to secondary bile acids, which are promoters of carcinogenesis. Fermentable dietary fiber contains plant lignans which are converted to a group of human lignans by bacterial action in the colon. Lignans may be protective against cancer by as yet unclear mechanisms. Ingested calcium affects colonic epithelial cell proliferation topically and by absorption into the blood stream. If these concepts are correct, the risk of colorectal cancer can be minimized by reducing dietary fat and calories and increasing the intake of calcium and fermentable fiber. It is of note that populations with a high incidence of colon cancer tend to have low serum cholesterol levels, and average serum cholesterol levels are higher in groups with less cancer of the colon. Dietary balance seems to be the best advice.

Carcinogenesis in the large bowel and elsewhere is a long multistep process. Heredity may make cells susceptible to cancer by the presence of oncogenes; expression of these genes results in an abnormal product or abnormal quantities of a product. Another class of cancer genes (tumor suppressor genes) inhibit tumor growth, and oncogenesis occurs when these genes are lost. In familial adenomatous polyposis, a segment of the long arm of chromosome 5 is lost, and deletions of genes from chromosomes 17 and 18 are linked to benign and malignant colorectal tumors. Mutational activation of oncogenes (eg, *ras* gene) or loss of tumor suppressor genes is initiated by carcinogenic agents. Promoters, such as bile acids, may stimulate growth of a benign neoplasm, and perhaps still other promoters cause malignant change to occur. There is evidence that female hormones are promoters, perhaps by influencing the availability of secondary bile acids in the colon. Another series of changes, termed progression, make cancer cells more aggressive in their behavior. This sequence is the basis for an enormous amount of current research in colorectal cancer. It was recently reported that regular use of aspirin may reduce the risk of death from colon cancer, perhaps by inhibition of prostaglandin synthesis or some other mechanism.

Cancer of the colon and rectum spreads in the following ways:

A. Direct Extension: Carcinoma grows circumferentially and may completely encircle the bowel before it is diagnosed; this is especially true in the left colon, which has a smaller caliber than the right. It takes about 1 year for a tumor to encircle three-fourths of the circumference of the bowel. Longitudinal submucosal extension occurs with invasion of the intramural lymphatic network, but it rarely goes beyond 2 cm from the edge of the tumor unless there is concomitant spread to lymph nodes. As the lesion extends radially, it penetrates the outer layers of the bowel wall, and it may extend by contiguity into neighboring structures: the liver, the greater curvature of the stomach, the duodenum, the small bowel, the pancreas, the spleen, the bladder, the vagina, the kidneys and ureters, and the abdominal wall. Cancer of the rectum may invade the vaginal wall, bladder, prostate, or sacrum, and it may extend along the levators. Subacute perforation with inflammatory attachment of bowel to an adjacent viscus may be indistinguishable from actual invasion on gross examination.

B. Hematogenous Metastasis: The tumor may invade colonic veins and be carried via portal venous blood to the liver to establish hepatic metastases. Tumor embolization also occurs through lumbar and vertebral veins to the lungs and elsewhere. Rectal cancer spreads through tributaries of the hypogastric veins. Metastases to ovaries are mostly hematogenous; they are found in 4% of women with colorectal cancer. Venous invasion occurs in 15–50% of cases even though it does not always cause distant metastases. An attempt is made to avoid producing hematogenous metastases during operation by minimizing manipulation of the tumor.

C. Regional Lymph Node Metastasis: This is the most common form of tumor spread (Figure 31–7). Longitudinal spread via extramural lymphatics is an important mechanism. Rectal cancer metastasizes radially along lymphatics to the pelvic side walls, where obturator nodes can become involved. The lymphatic drainage of the tumor must be removed in curative operations, and some nodal involvement will be found in over half of the specimens. Regional nodes are not necessarily involved in a progressive or orderly fashion: Positive nodes may be found at some distance from the primary site with normal nodes intervening. The size of the lesion bears little relationship to the degree of nodal involvement. The more anaplastic the lesion, the more likely that lymph node metastasis will occur.

D. Transperitoneal Metastasis: "Seeding" may occur when the tumor has extended through the serosa and tumor cells enter the peritoneal cavity, producing local implants or generalized abdominal carcinomatosis. Large metastatic deposits in the pel-

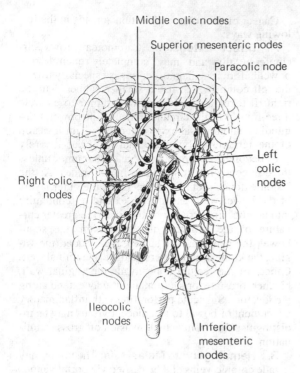

Figure 31–7. Lymphatic drainage of the colon. The lymph nodes (black) are distributed along the blood vessels to the bowel.

vic cul-de-sac are palpable as a hard shelf (Blumer's shelf).

E. Intraluminal Metastasis: Malignant cells shed from the surface of the tumor can be swept along in the fecal current. Implantation more distally on intact mucosa occurs rarely, if ever, but viable exfoliated cells presumably can be trapped in an anastomotic suture or staple line during operation. Most "anastomotic recurrences," however, are believed to arise from malignant cells outside the bowel wall (eg, in lymphatics in the mesocolon) that invade the intestine secondarily.

Clinical Findings

A. Symptoms and Signs: Adenocarcinoma of the colon and rectum has a median doubling time (the time required for the tumor to double in volume) of 130 days, suggesting that at least 5 years—and often 10–15 years—of silent growth are required before a cancer reaches symptom-producing size. During this asymptomatic phase, diagnosis depends on routine examination.

The value of routine screening of asymptomatic populations who lack high-risk factors for development of large bowel cancer is still an open question, because no study to date has proved conclusively that screening confers a survival advantage. There is indirect evidence that screening detects cancers at an ear-

lier stage, and for that reason improved survival is expected, but it has not been established to the satisfaction of many critics that the great effort and cost of screening large populations of asymptomatic people can be justified. Even the detection and removal of polyps, believed by most authorities to be a form of cancer prevention, does not make the case for screening convincingly. Opinion is divided on the best course of action at this time. For a physician who takes care of patients and is not responsible for public health policy, it is prudent to follow the recommendations of the American Cancer Society: annual digital rectal examination beginning at age 40, guaiac slide testing for fecal occult blood annually after age 50, and flexible sigmoidoscopy every 3–5 years beginning at age 50.

Screening of patients in high-risk groups is less controversial, and questions remain about the choice and timing of various tests. Children with possible familial adenomatous polyposis should have sigmoidoscopy at puberty. Annual colonoscopy beginning at age 25 is the recommendation for members of families with Lynch syndrome. Colonoscopy every year is probably the best advice for patients with ulcerative colitis for longer than 10 years. The best method of screening for people with a history of colorectal cancer in a first-degree relative is unclear, but there is increasing preference for colonoscopy rather than sigmoidoscopy with or without fecal occult blood testing. Dissatisfaction with the poor specificity of guaiac slide tests has led to development of alternative methods, including a quantitative assay specific for heme and an immunologic method using an antibody to hemoglobin. If fecal occult blood is detected, total colonoscopy is the single best study. If colonoscopy to the cecum in a well-prepared patient is unrevealing, further diagnostic evaluation of the lower or upper gastrointestinal tract is probably unnecessary. The yield of upper tract neoplasms is nil in asymptomatic patients.

Symptoms in patients with large bowel cancer depend upon the anatomic location of the lesion, its type and extent, and upon complications, including perforation, obstruction, and hemorrhage. Marked systemic manifestations such as cachexia are indications of advanced disease. The average delay between the onset of symptoms and definitive therapy is 7–9 months; both patients and physicians are responsible.

The **right colon** has a large caliber and a thin and distensible wall, and the fecal content is fluid. Because of these anatomic features, carcinoma of the right colon may attain a large size before it is diagnosed. Patients often see a physician for complaints of fatigability and weakness due to severe anemia. Unexplained microcytic hypochromic anemia should always raise the question of carcinoma of the ascending colon. Gross blood may not be visible in the stool, but occult blood may be detected. Patients may complain of vague right abdominal discomfort, which is often postprandial and may be mistakenly attributed to gallbladder or gastroduodenal disease. Alterations in bowel habits are not characteristic of carcinoma of the right colon, and obstruction is uncommon. In about 10% of cases, the first evidence of the disease is discovery of a mass by the patient or the physician.

The **left colon** has a smaller lumen than the right, and the feces are semisolid. Tumors of the left colon can gradually occlude the lumen, causing changes in bowel habits with alternating constipation and increased frequency of defecation (not true watery diarrhea). Partial or complete obstruction may be the initial picture. Bleeding is common but is rarely massive. The stool may be streaked or mixed with bright red or dark blood, and mucus is often passed together with small blood clots.

In **cancer of the rectum,** the most common symptom is the passage of red blood with bowel movements (hematochezia). Bleeding is usually persistent; it may be slight or (rarely) copious. Blood may or may not be mixed with stool or mucus. Predictions of an anal source of bleeding based on color and pattern are unreliable. *Whenever rectal bleeding occurs in a middle-aged or older individual, even in the presence of hemorrhoids, coexisting cancer must be ruled out.* There may be tenesmus (painful incomplete evacuation).

Physical examination is important to determine the extent of the local disease, to reveal distant metastases, and to detect diseases of other organ systems that may influence treatment. The supraclavicular areas should be carefully palpated for metastatic nodes. Examination of the abdomen may disclose a mass, enlargement of the liver, ascites, or engorgement of the abdominal wall veins if there is portal obstruction. If a mass is palpated, its location and extent of fixation are important.

Distal rectal cancers can be felt as a flat, hard, oval or encircling tumor with rolled edges and a central depression. Its extent, the size of the lumen at the site of the tumor, and the degree of fixation should be noted. Blood may be found on the examining finger. Vaginal and rectovaginal examination will yield additional information on the extent of the tumor. Retrorectal nodes may be palpable.

B. Laboratory Findings: Urinalysis, leukocyte count, and hemoglobin determination should be done. Serum proteins, calcium, bilirubin, alkaline phosphatase, and creatinine should be measured.

Carcinoembryonic antigen (CEA) is a glycoprotein found in the cell membranes of many tissues, including cancerous tissue in the colon and rectum. Some of the antigen enters the circulation and is detected by radioimmunoassay of serum; CEA is also detectable in various other body fluids, secretions, urine, and feces.

Elevated serum CEA is not specifically associated with colorectal cancer; abnormally high levels of CEA are also found in sera of patients with other gastrointestinal cancers, nonalimentary cancers, and various benign diseases. CEA levels are high in 70% of patients with cancer of the large intestine, but less than half of patients with localized disease are CEA-positive. CEA does not, therefore, serve as a useful screening procedure, nor is it an accurate diagnostic test for colorectal cancer in a curable stage.

Preoperative CEA levels correlate with the postoperative recurrence rate, and failure of serum CEA to fall to normal levels after resection implies a poor prognosis. CEA is helpful in detecting recurrence after curative surgical resection; if high CEA levels return to normal after operation and then rise progressively during the follow-up period, recurrence of cancer is likely. CEA is just one of many putative chemical markers for the presence of colorectal cancer. Screening for *ras*-oncogene products in urine or serum may become a practical test for colorectal cancer in the future.

Radioactively labeled monoclonal antibodies directed against tumor-associated antigens can be injected intravenously. In such patients, gamma scintiscanning (radioimmunoscintigraphy) detects tumor deposits preoperatively. A hand-held gamma detecting probe can be used intraoperatively to search for radioactively labeled tumor deposits that otherwise would escape detection. This procedure, termed radioimmunoguided surgery, is still investigative.

C. Imaging Studies: Chest films should be obtained routinely. Barium enema examination is the most important radiographic means of diagnosing cancer of the colon, although cancers are increasingly being diagnosed by colonoscopy, and contrast x-rays are unnecessary in those cases. Carcinoma of the left colon appears as a fixed filling defect, usually 2–6 cm long, with an annular ("apple core") configuration (Figure 31–8). Lesions of the right colon may appear as a constriction or an intraluminal mass. The bowel wall is inflexible at the site of the lesion, and the mucosal pattern is destroyed. It is important to remember that this is the typical picture of locally advanced carcinoma. Earlier stages of the disease produce less characteristic filling defects that should be investigated with the colonoscope. Artifacts (stool, spasm) can resemble carcinoma. Barium should not be administered by mouth if there is evidence of carcinoma of the colon, especially on the left side, since it may precipitate acute large bowel obstruction. X-rays are unreliable in detecting cancer of the rectum. Such growths are more accurately diagnosed by palpation and sigmoidoscopy.

CT scans are not essential in patients with cancer of the colon, but they are helpful in assessing extramural extension in patients with rectal cancer. MRI is probably even more accurate for this purpose. Detection of liver metastases by CT scan and other methods is discussed in Chapter 24. Endorectal ultrasonography provides very accurate information about

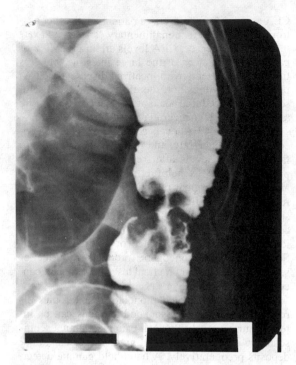

Figure 31–8. Barium enema roentgenogram of an encircling carcinoma of the descending colon presenting an "apple core" appearance. Note the loss of mucosal pattern, the "hooks" at the margins of the lesion owing to undermining by the growth, the relatively short (6 cm) length of the lesion, and its abrupt ends.

the depth of penetration of rectal cancer into or through the bowel wall. It also reveals the presence of enlarged pararectal lymph nodes but cannot at present distinguish between cancerous and reactive nodes.

D. Special Examinations:

1. Proctosigmoidoscopy–From 50% to 65% of colorectal cancers are within the reach of a 60-cm flexible sigmoidoscope. Only 30–40% are accessible with a 30-cm flexible sigmoidoscope, and still fewer (perhaps 20%) can be seen with a rigid sigmoidoscope. The typical cancer is raised, red, centrally ulcerated, and bleeding slightly. Mobility of the lesion can be determined by manipulation with the tip of the instrument. The size of the lumen should be noted, and the sigmoidoscope should be passed beyond the lesion to inspect the proximal bowel if possible. The tumor should be biopsied.

2. Colonoscopy–Endoscopic examination of the entire colon should be performed in every patient with suspected or known cancer of the colon or rectum if the intention is curative treatment. Preoperative colonoscopy is preferred, unless obstructing cancer or other circumstances do not allow it. Increasingly today, a patient with rectal bleeding will undergo prompt total colonoscopy; a cancer is found and biopsied; synchronous lesions are excluded (or treated); and operation is planned without the need for barium enema x-rays. If barium studies are done first, colonoscopy is still necessary to prove that the defect is neoplastic and, more importantly, to detect synchronous polyps or cancers. Data vary, but barium enema x-rays miss about 20% of neoplastic lesions greater than 5 mm in diameter that are seen on colonoscopy. Colonoscopy can miss lesions too—hidden around folds or in flexures—and the cecum is not reached in every patient. Barium enema still has a role if colonoscopy is incomplete or if the findings do not explain the symptoms.

Differential Diagnosis

An initial erroneous diagnosis is made in as many as 25% of patients with cancer of the colon and rectum after gastrointestinal symptoms appear. Symptoms may be attributed mistakenly to disease of the upper gastrointestinal tract, particularly gallstones or peptic ulcer. Chronic anemia may be attributed to a primary hematologic disorder if a specimen of stool is not examined for occult blood. Acute pain in the right side of the abdomen owing to carcinoma can simulate appendicitis.

Most errors are made when the clinical findings are ascribed to benign disease, and patients may even be operated upon for benign anorectal conditions in the presence of undetected cancer. Cancer must be searched for in every patient with recent onset of significant rectal bleeding, even if there are obvious hemorrhoids.

Carcinoma may be difficult to distinguish from diverticular disease; colonoscopy is useful in these cases. Other colonic diseases, including ulcerative colitis, Crohn's colitis, ischemic colitis, and amebiasis, usually can be diagnosed by sigmoidoscopy, colonoscopy, and barium enema. Symptoms should be attributed to irritable bowel syndrome only after neoplasm has been ruled out.

Treatment

A. Cancer of the Colon: Treatment consists of wide surgical resection of the lesion and its regional lymphatic drainage after preparation of the bowel. The primary tumor is resected, even if distant metastases have occurred, since prevention of obstruction or bleeding may offer palliation for long periods.

The abdomen is explored to determine resectability of the tumor and to search for multiple primary carcinomas of the colon, distant metastases, and associated abdominal disease. Care is taken not to contribute to spread of the tumor by unnecessary palpation. The bowel is occluded tightly with an encircling tape on either side of the lesion to contain exfoliated cancer cells within the segment to be resected. The cancer-bearing portion of colon is then mobilized and removed. Most surgeons irrigate the two open ends of bowel with saline solution, povidone-iodine, 1:500 bichloride of mercury, or other fluids before anastomosis in the hope that tumor cells in the lumen will be washed away or destroyed. The extent of resection of the colon and mesocolon for cancers in various locations and the methods for restoration of continuity are shown in Figure 31–9.

B. Cancer of the Rectum: For cancer of the rectum, the choice of operation depends on the height of the lesion above the anal verge, the configuration (whether polypoid or infiltrative), the gross extent of the tumor, the degree of differentiation, and the patient's size, habitus, and general condition. Preoperative staging by digital rectal examination followed by CT, MRI, endorectal ultrasound, or some combi-

nation of these tests helps tailor the treatment to the patient. Preservation of the anal sphincter and avoidance of colostomy are desirable if possible.

The principal procedures for rectal tumors are as follows:

1. Abdominoperineal resection of the rectum–The distal sigmoid, rectosigmoid, rectum, and anus are removed through combined abdominal and perineal incisions. A permanent end sigmoid colostomy is required. The procedure is not performed in the presence of peritoneal seeding or fixation to the bony pelvis.

2. Low anterior resection of the rectum–This operation, performed through an abdominal incision, is the curative procedure of choice provided a margin

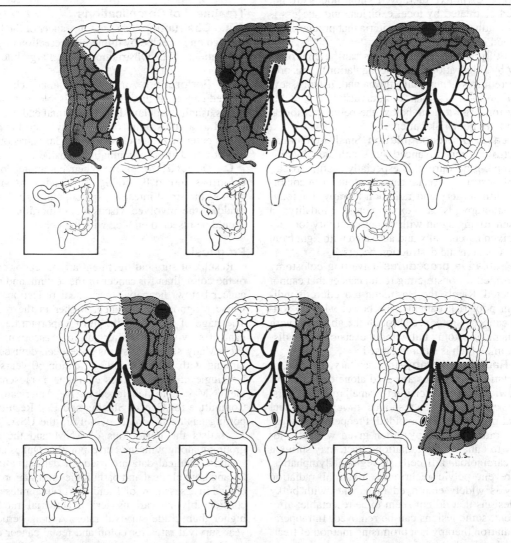

Figure 31–9. Extent of surgical resection for cancer of the colon at various sites. The cancer is represented by a black disk. Anastomosis of the bowel remaining after resection is shown in the small insets. The extent of resection is determined by the distribution of the regional lymph nodes along the blood supply. The lymph nodes may contain metastatic cancer.

of at least 2 cm of normal bowel, as estimated at operation, can be resected below the lesion. At least 10 cm of bowel proximal to the growth should also be removed along with the lymph node-bearing tissue. It is important to excise 5 cm of mesorectum distal to the tumor to minimize the chance of local recurrence from cancer in lymph nodes. The descending or sigmoid colon is anastomosed to the rectum. This type of resection is likely to fail in patients with extensive carcinoma and local spread. The end-to-end stapling device facilitates very low anastomosis, sometimes even as low as the anal canal (colon-anal anastomosis).

3. Local excision–In carefully selected patients with small, well-differentiated mobile polypoid lesions, a disk of rectum containing the tumor can be excised as definitive therapy. Lymph nodes are not sampled or treated by local excision, and success is based on adherence to strict criteria that predict a low likelihood of nodal spread.

4. Fulguration–Some tumors can be controlled locally by fulguration (electrocoagulation). This procedure requires general anesthesia and, usually, several fulguration sessions at intervals. It is suitable mostly for large lesions below the pelvic peritoneal reflection in poor-risk patients.

5. Laser photocoagulation–Small tumors can be destroyed and advanced ones palliated by this endoscopic procedure. It is especially useful in treatment of obstructing rectal cancers alone or in combination with surgery and radiation therapy. Photodynamic therapy is an experimental modality; a photosensitizing agent with some selectivity for cancer is given parenterally and activated with light from a laser. Local tissue destruction occurs.

6. Palliative procedures–Diverting colostomy is performed for obstructing rectal cancer that cannot be resected. Rarely the Hartmann procedure is indicated in poor-risk patients; the bowel with its contained cancer is removed through the abdomen with permanent colostomy but without excision of the distal rectum, which is sutured closed.

7. Radiation therapy–Intracavitary, external, or implantation techniques are used alone or in combination with surgical excision for small rectal cancers. In some cases, the lesion responds so well that radical surgical procedures are avoided. Preoperative megavoltage radiation therapy, often given with chemotherapy to enhance the radiation effect, may shrink a rectal carcinoma, kill cells in regional lymphatics, and prevent pelvic recurrence. External radiation therapy is widely employed in patients with bulky fixed lesions that do not seem to be resectable; after treatment, some lesions can be removed. Intraoperative radiation therapy is a promising method of treatment of local pelvic recurrences.

C. Adjuvant Therapy: Chemotherapy and radiation therapy have been studied extensively as adjuvants to curative resection of cancer of the large intestine. A recent NIH Consensus Development Conference reviewed available data and clarified many of the issues in the controversy surrounding this subject. It is apparent that strategies should be different for cancer of the colon and cancer of the rectum. Patients with stage I lesions in either site do not benefit from adjuvant therapy. Stage II and stage III rectal cancer patients have improved local control and survival with combined postoperative chemotherapy and radiation therapy. Patients with stage II colon cancer should enter clinical trials; no particular adjuvant regimen can be recommended outside of a trial. Stage III colon cancer patients also should enroll in clinical trials, but if that is not possible, a combination of oral levamisole and intravenous fluorouracil is acceptable.

Treatment of Complications

A. Obstruction: Obstructing cancer of the left or right colon is treated by immediate resection in good-risk patients. (See Obstruction of the Large Intestine, above.)

B. Perforation: An aggressive approach to perforated cancer of the colon is advisable, but anastomosis usually is delayed. The proximal end is exteriorized as a colostomy (or ileostomy), and the distal end is exteriorized or closed. Secondary anastomosis is performed after inflammation subsides.

C. Direct Extension: When carcinoma of the colon has spread by contiguity to adjacent viscera such as the small intestine, spleen, uterus, or urinary bladder, the involved viscus—or a portion of it—should be resected en bloc with the colon.

Prognosis

Results of surgical treatment are better for cancer of the colon than for cancer of the rectum, and rectal cancer below the pelvic peritoneal reflection has a worse prognosis than cancer higher in the rectum. The stage of disease is the most important determinant of survival rates after surgical resection, however. Many staging systems have been devised, beginning with the Dukes classification 60 years ago. No single method satisfies everyone at present, but the TNM system developed by the American Joint Committee for Cancer Staging and End Results Reporting has been adopted widely in the USA. Table 31–4 lists the definitions of TNM and the stage grouping along with the corresponding Dukes classification. Clinical data are used for determination of M, and both clinical and pathologic information is included in assessment of T and N. Survival rates differ considerably in various series; actuarial rates are higher than crude survival rates. Average crude 5-year survival rates for colon and rectal cancer using the Dukes system are as follows: stage A, 80%; stage B, 60%; stage C, 30%; stage D, 5%.

Approximately 10% of lesions are not resectable at the time of operation, and an additional 20% of pa-

Table 31–4. TNM classification of cancer of the colon and rectum.[1]

PRIMARY TUMOR (T)

TX	Primary tumor cannot be assessed
T0	No evidence of primary tumor
Tis	Carcinoma in situ
T1	Tumor invades submucosa
T2	Tumor invades muscularis propria
T3	Tumor invades through the muscularis propria into the subserosa, or into nonperitonealized pericolic or perirectal tissues
T4	Tumor perforates the visceral peritoneum, or directly invades other organs or structures

REGIONAL LYMPH NODES (N)

NX	Regional lymph nodes cannot be assessed
N0	No regional lymph node metastasis
N1	Metastasis in one to three pericolic or perirectal lymph nodes
N2	Metastasis in four or more pericolic or perirectal lymph nodes
N3	Metastasis in any lymph node along the course of a named vascular trunk

DISTANT METASTASIS (M)

MX	Presence of distant metastasis cannot be assessed
M0	No distant metastasis
M1	Distant metastasis

STAGE GROUPING

				Dukes
Stage 0	Tis	N0	M0	
Stage I	T1	N0	M0	A
	T2	N0	M0	A
Stage II	T3	N0	M0	B
	T4	N0	M0	B
Stage III	Any T	N1	M0	C
	Any T	N2, N3	M0	C
Stage IV	Any T	Any N	M1	

[1]From Beahrs OH et al (editors): *Manual for Staging of Cancer*, 3rd ed. Lippincott, 1988.

tients have liver or other distant metastases. Hence, operation for cure can be performed on only about 70% of patients. The operative mortality rate is 2–6%. The survival rate of patients undergoing curative resection is about 55%; the overall survival rate (all stages) is about 35%.

The prognosis is adversely affected by complications such as obstruction or perforation. The histologic features—including the degree of differentiation of the tumor, colloid content, intravascular tumor cells, or malignant cells in the perineural space—also have a bearing on prognosis. Tumor DNA content determined by flow cytometry may be an important prognostic factor; aneuploid tumors are more aggressive than diploid cancers. Suggestions that colorectal

cancer has a worse prognosis in patients younger than age 40 compared with older people have not been substantiated by recent studies. Perioperative blood transfusions may adversely affect long-term survival of patients with colorectal cancer, but data are conflicting. Patients should be followed after curative resection of cancer of the large bowel. The goals are detection of recurrent, metastatic, or metachronous lesions. The program varies with the location of the original tumor, the operation performed, and the stage of the disease. Serum CEA levels should be determined every 1–2 months in patients with stage II or stage III lesions. Fecal occult blood is tested every 12 months. Colonoscopy is performed 1 year after operation; if no neoplasms are seen in a thorough examination, it is probably safe to wait 2–3 years before doing colonoscopy again. Better data on the timing of these studies will be forthcoming from studies now in progress. Barium contrast x-rays are not used routinely in most follow-up programs. CT scans are recommended in patients with rectal cancer.

If recurrent or metastatic cancer is discovered, the patient is evaluated for potential surgical resection of the lesions; this may be feasible in cases of hepatic or pulmonary metastases, and it may be possible to remove some local (eg, pelvic) recurrences in combination with intraoperative radiation therapy. If recurrent cancer is suggested on the basis of rising serum CEA levels and if the responsible lesion cannot be located, a second-look laparotomy may be undertaken. The impact of this approach on survival is uncertain, but apparently resectable cancer is found in 30–60% of patients.

Ahnen DJ: Genetics of colon cancer. West J Med 1991; 154;700.

Arbeit JM: The molecular conspiracy in the mucosa: A review of the molecular biology of colorectal carcinogenesis. Perspect Colon Rectal Surg 1991;4:85.

Beahrs OH et al (editors): *Manual for Staging of Cancer*, 3rd ed. Lippincott, 1988.

Beart RW (editor): Progress symposium: Carcinoma of the large bowel. World J Surg 1991;15:561.

Bülow S, Svendsen LB, Mellemgaard A: Metachronous colorectal carcinoma. Br J Surg 1990;77:502.

Chu DZJ et al: Prognostic significance of carcinoembryonic antigen in colorectal carcinoma. Arch Surg 1991;126: 314.

Dawson PM et al: The value of radioimmunoguided surgery in first and second look laparotomy for colorectal cancer. Dis Colon Rectum 1991;34:217.

Doerr RJ et al: Radiolabeled antibody imaging in the management of colorectal cancer: Results of a multicenter clinical study. Ann Surg 1991;214:118.

Eisenberg SB, Kraybill WG, Lopez MJ: Long-term results of surgical resection of locally advanced colorectal carcinoma. Surgery 1990;108:779.

Eisner MS, Lewis, JH: Diagnostic yield of a positive fecal occult blood test found on digital rectal examination. Arch Intern Med 1991;151:2180.

Enker WE: Flow cytometric determination of tumor cell

DNA content and proliferative index as prognostic variables in colorectal cancer. Perspect Colon Rectal Surg 1990;3:1.

Fantini GA, DeCosse JJ: Surveillance strategies after resection of carcinoma of the colon. Surg Gynecol Obstet 1990;171,267.

Isbister WH, Fraser J: Large-bowel cancer in the young: A national survival study. Dis Colon Rectum 1990;33:366.

Itoh H, Houlston RS, Slack J: Risk of cancer death in first-degree relatives of patients with hereditary non-polyposis cancer syndrome (Lynch type II): A study of 130 kindreds in the United Kingdom. Br J Surg 1990; 77:1367.

Jass JR: Subsite distribution and incidence of colorectal cancer in New Zealand, 1974–1983. Dis Colon Rectum 1991;34:56.

Juhl G et al: Six-year results of annual colonoscopy after resection of colorectal cancer. World J Surg 1990; 14:255.

Kirgan D et al: Association of human papillomavirus and colon neoplasms. Arch Surg 1990;125:862.

Korn JE: Colon cancer epidemiology: Fat, fiber, and fertility. Perspect Colon Rectal Surg 1990;3:297.

Kune GA et al: Survival in patients with large-bowel cancer. A population-based investigation from the Melbourne Colorectal Cancer Study. Dis Colon Rectum 1990;33:938.

Lanspa SJ et al: The colonoscopist and the Lynch syndromes. Gastrointest Endosc 1990;36:156.

Lieberman DA, Smith FW: Screening for colon malignancy with colonoscopy. Am J Gastroenterol 1991;86:946.

Martin EW Jr, Carey LC: Second-look surgery for colorectal cancer: The second time around. Ann Surg 1991; 214:321.

Moertel CG et al: Levamisole and fluorouracil for adjuvant therapy of resected colon carcinoma. N Engl J Med 1990;322:352.

Morris JB et al: A critical analysis of the largest reported mass fecal occult blood screening program in the United States. Am J Surg 1991;161:101.

NIH Consensus Conference: Adjuvant therapy for patients with colon and rectal cancer. JAMA 1990;264:1444.

Narisawa T et al: Clinical observation on the association of gallstones and colorectal cancer. Cancer 1991;67:1696.

Ransohoff DF, Lang CA: Screening for colorectal cancer. N Engl J Med 1991;325:37.

Rex DK et al: Screening colonoscopy in asymptomatic average-risk persons with negative fecal occult blood tests. Gastroenterology 1991;100:64.

Rigas B: Editorial. Oncogenes and suppressor genes: Their involvement in colon cancer. J Clin Gastroenterol 1990; 12:494.

Runkel NS et al: Outcome after emergency surgery for cancer of the large intestine. Br J Surg 1991;78:183.

Schubert W: Dukes' classification: American chaos versus British order. Can J Surg 1990;33:8.

Slater G, Aufses AH Jr, Szporn A: Synchronous carcinoma of the colon and rectum. Surg Gynecol Obstet 1990;171: 283.

Stephenson BM et al: Frequency of familial colorectal cancer. Br J Surg 1991;78:1162.

Thoeni RF: Colorectal cancer: Cross-sectional imaging for staging of primary tumor and detection of local recurrence. AJR Am J Roentgenol 1991;156:909.

Thun MJ et al: Aspirin use and reduced risk of fatal colon cancer. N Engl J Med 1991;325:1593.

Unger SW et al: Endoscopic Nd-YAG laser treatment of colorectal neoplasms: A four-year longitudinal study. Am Surg 1990;56:153.

Vukasin AP et al: Increasing incidence of cecal and sigmoid carcinoma. Data from the Connecticut Tumor Registry. Cancer 1990;66:2442.

Willett WC et al: Relation of meat, fat, and fiber intake to the risk of colon cancer in a prospective study among women. N Engl J Med 1990;323:1664.

Winawer SJ et al: Declining serum cholesterol levels prior to diagnosis of colon cancer. A time-trend, case-control study. JAMA 1990;263:2083.

Woolfson K: Tumor markers in cancer of the colon and rectum. Dis Colon Rectum 1991;34:506.

POLYPS OF THE COLON & RECTUM

Essentials of Diagnosis

- Passage of blood per rectum.
- Possible family history.
- Sigmoidoscopic, colonoscopic, or radiologic discovery of polyps.

General Considerations

Colorectal polyps are masses of tissue that project into the lumen. They comprise a heterogeneous group of sessile or pedunculated, benign or malignant, mucosal, submucosal, or muscular lesions. "Polyp" is a morphologic term, and no histologic diagnosis is implied. The most common epithelial polyps of the colon and rectum are listed in Table 31–5. Most adenomas are tubular, tubulovillous, or villous. Hyperplastic polyps are diminutive lesions most often found in the left colon. Hamartomas are uncommon. Polyposis, discussed later in this section, is a term reserved for the presence of many polyps in the large bowel.

Estimates of the incidence of colonic and rectal polyps in the general population range from 9% to 60%; the higher figure includes small polyps found at

Table 31–5. Polyps of the large intestine.

Type	Histologic Diagnosis
Neoplastic	Adenoma
	Tubular adenoma (adenomatous polyp)
	Tubulovillous adenoma (villoglandular adenoma)
	Villous adenoma (villous papilloma)
	Carcinoma
Hamartomas	Juvenile polyp
	Peutz-Jeghers polyp
Inflammatory	Inflammatory polyp (pseudopolyp)
	Benign lymphoid polyp
Unclassified	Hyperplastic polyp
Miscellaneous	Lipoma, leiomyoma, carcinoid

autopsy. Adenomatous polyps are found in about 25% of asymptomatic adults who undergo screening colonoscopy. The prevalence of adenomatous polyps is 30% at age 50 years, 40% at age 60, 50% at age 70, and 55% at age 80. The mean age of patients with adenoma is 55 years, about 5–10 years younger than the mean age of patients with colorectal cancer. About 50% of polyps occur in the sigmoid or rectum. About 50% of patients with adenoma have more than one lesion, and 15% have more than two lesions. An increased incidence of adenomatous polyps in breast cancer patients has been reported.

Inflammatory polyps have no malignant potential, and cancer developing in association with hamartomas is rare. Hyperplastic polyps are not neoplastic and therefore do not become malignant. It has been suggested that hyperplastic polyps in the left colon are markers for neoplastic polyps elsewhere in the colon, but the weight of evidence is against this concept at present.

Adenomas are a premalignant lesion, and most authorities believe that the majority of adenocarcinomas of the large bowel evolve from adenomas (adenoma to carcinoma sequence). Both adenomas and cancer increase in incidence with age, and the distribution of adenomas and cancer in the bowel is similar. Approximately 25% of patients who have five or more adenomatous polyps have a synchronous colon cancer at the initial colonoscopy. About one-third of colonic and rectal specimens resected for cancer also harbor adenomas; if a surgical specimen contains two or more synchronous carcinomas, the incidence of associated adenomas is 75%. All gradations of malignancy—from total absence, to dysplasia, to a microscopic cytologic cancer, to invasive cancer, to a gross cancer with remnants of benign tumor at one margin—may be seen in colonic neoplasms; on the other hand, cancers that are smaller than 0.5 cm in diameter and contain no benign adenoma are extremely rare. Additional support for the malignant potential of adenomas is as follows: (1) Patients with familial adenomatous polyposis die of cancer at a young age unless the colon is removed. (2) Chemical carcinogens produce adenomas and cancers indiscriminately in the colons of experimental animals. (3) Routine removal of adenomas from the rectum reduces the incidence of subsequent rectal cancer.

The malignant potential of an adenoma depends on size, growth pattern, and the degree of epithelial atypia. Cancer is found in 1% of adenomas under 1 cm in diameter, 10% of adenomas 1–2 cm in size, and 45% of adenomas larger than 2 cm. So-called flat adenomas, small flat or depressed tubular adenomas that tend to occur in the right colon, may be an exception to these guidelines; they may become malignant when still only a few millimeters in diameter. The three histologic patterns of adenoma are variations of one neoplastic process; about 5% of tubular adenomas, 22% of tubulovillous adenomas, and 40% of villous adenomas become malignant. The potential for cancerous transformation rises with increasing degrees of epithelial dysplasia. Sessile lesions are more apt to be malignant than pedunculated ones. It probably takes at least 5 years, and more often 10–15 years, for an adenoma to become malignant.

Clinical Findings

A. Symptoms and Signs: Many polyps are asymptomatic; the larger the lesion, the more likely it is to cause symptoms. Rectal bleeding is by far the most frequent complaint. Blood is bright red or dark red depending on the location of the polyp, and bleeding is usually intermittent. Profuse hemorrhage from polyps is rare.

Alterations in bowel habits are more common in the presence of frank carcinoma, but large benign tumors may produce tenesmus, constipation, or increased frequency of bowel movements. Some polyps, notably large villous adenomas, may secrete copious amounts of mucus that are evacuated per rectum. Polypoid tumors may induce peristaltic cramps or varying degrees of intussusception, but most often obstructive symptoms are due to associated diverticular disease or irritable bowel syndrome and persist after polypectomy. Occasionally, a polyp on a very long pedicle will prolapse through the anus; this is most apt to occur with juvenile polyps.

General physical examination yields little information about the colonic polyps themselves, although other manifestations of diseases such as Peutz-Jeghers syndrome may be found. A polyp may be palpable by digital rectal examination, and proctosigmoidoscopy may disclose polyps in the rectum or sigmoid. Blood-tinged mucus strongly suggests the presence of a neoplasm situated farther proximally. Since polyps are often multiple and may occur synchronously with cancer, further investigation of the colon is mandatory even if a lesion is found by sigmoidoscopy.

B. Imaging Studies (Barium Enema): A polyp appears as a rounded filling defect with smooth, sharply defined margins. Double-contrast (pneumocolon) examination is recommended. Thorough cleansing of the colon and examination by a skilled radiologist are essential if small polyps are to be demonstrated; even so, polyps smaller than 0.5 cm in diameter often cannot be detected on x-ray.

C. Colonoscopy: This is the most reliable way to diagnose colonic polyps, and polypectomy can be done at the same time. The entire colon should be examined by colonoscopy in every patient with known polyps or symptoms suggestive of their presence.

Differential Diagnosis

Artifacts seen on barium enema x-ray examination may be confused with polyps. These include bits of feces, air bubbles, diverticula, indenting appendices epiploicae, calcified lymph nodes, and others. Colonoscopy is essential in doubtful situations.

Polyps of various histologic types can be differentiated only by microscopic examination of the entire lesion, although clues may be gained from clinical and radiographic features.

Treatment

Polyps of the colon and rectum are treated because they produce symptoms, because they may be malignant when first discovered, or because they may become malignant later. In a study of untreated colonic polyps, the cumulative risk of eventual cancer at the polyp site was 2.5% at 5 years, 8% at 10 years, and 24% at 20 years.

Small polyps can be removed with an electrocautery snare passed through a rigid or flexible sigmoidoscope, but since total colonoscopy is recommended in all patients who have a polyp, it is best to wait and do the polypectomy in a well-prepared colon during that procedure.

Large, sessile, soft, velvety lesions in the rectum are usually villous adenomas; these tumors have a high malignant potential and must be excised completely. With the patient anesthetized, this can be accomplished through the anus in most instances. Only if histologic sections show invasive cancer at the margins of excision is further therapy necessary. Management of villous tumors by endoscopic Nd:YAG laser photocoagulation may be useful for extensive carpet-like tumors. Excision has the advantage of permitting histologic examination of the specimen.

Pedunculated polyps and small sessile lesions in the sigmoid and above should be removed with a hot biopsy forceps or an electrocautery snare passed through the colonoscope. Colonoscopic polypectomy is usually successful, but technical obstacles occasionally seem insurmountable. Only experts should attempt colonoscopic removal of large sessile lesions, because the risk of perforation, bleeding, and incomplete excision is greater if there is no pedicle. Colonoscopic polypectomy is safer than laparotomy; the combined incidence of perforation and hemorrhage is 2%, and deaths are rare. Colonoscopy is less expensive and incurs much less disability than laparotomy.

Laparotomy should be considered if colonoscopy is unsuccessful, if the lesion is large and sessile, or if there are many polyps. Operation for large sessile tumors usually consists of resection of the segment of colon containing the lesion. If numerous polyps are present in different anatomic parts of the colon, total abdominal colectomy with ileorectal anastomosis may be the best course in good-risk patients. The presence of other factors such as family history may strongly influence a decision in favor of extensive resection.

From 2% to 4% of colonoscopically excised pol-

yps contain invasive adenocarcinoma, and a decision must be made whether to resect the segment of colon or simply follow the patient. Carcinoma-in-situ is a cytologic abnormality equivalent to severe dysplasia and does not require further treatment. (Some authorities recommend abandoning the term carcinoma-in-situ because it gives a misleading impression.) Only when malignant cells penetrate the muscularis mucosae is there any potential for metastasis (because there are no lymphatics in the lamina propria of the large intestine), and only these lesions should be labeled as cancers. The incidence of metastasis is low, and resection of the colon is not required if the following criteria are met: (1) Gross margin is clear at endoscopy; (2) microscopic margin is clear; (3) cancer is well-differentiated; (4) there is no lymphatic or venous invasion; and (5) cancer does not invade the stalk. Other malignant polyps of the colon should be managed by resection of involved bowel. Since rectal cancers are sometimes treated definitively by local excision, it may not be necessary to do a radical resection if the malignant polyp arose in the distal rectum.

Familial adenomatous polyposis (adenomatous polyposis coli) is a rare but important disease because colorectal cancer develops before age 40 in nearly all untreated patients. The trait is autosomal dominant, and it is not X-linked. The FAP (APC) gene has been localized to the long arm of chromosome 5. More than a hundred (occasionally fewer) polyps of varying size and configuration are present in the colon and rectum. An increasing list of benign and malignant extracolonic manifestations are associated with familial adenomatous polyposis (Table 31–6). **Gardner's syndrome** (polyposis, desmoid tumors, osteomas of mandible or skull, and sebaceous cysts) and **Turcot's syndrome** (polyposis and a medulloblastoma or glioma) are examples of familial adenomatous polyposis with variations in expression of the ex-

Table 31–6. Extracolonic manifestations of familial adenomatous polyposis.[1]

Benign	Malignant
Endocrine adenoma	Duodenal carcinoma
Osteoma	Bile duct carcinoma
Epidermoid cyst	Pancreatic carcinoma
Hypertrophic retinal pigmentation	Desmoid tumor
Gastric fundic gland polyp	Carcinoma of the stomach
Duodenal adenoma	Adrenal carcinoma
Small bowel adenoma	Medulloblastoma
	Glioblastoma
	Thyroid carcinoma
	Small bowel carcinoma
	Carcinoid tumor of the ileum
	Osteogenic sarcoma
	Hepatoblastoma

[1]Reproduced, with permission, from Jagelman DG: The expanding spectrum of familial adenomatous polyposis. Perspect Colon Rectal Surg 1988;1:30.

tracolonic manifestations; there is no genetic distribution among the syndromes. Congenital hypertrophy of retinal pigment epithelium is present as early as 3 months of age in affected members of two-thirds of families with familial adenomatous polyposis; this abnormality (always bilateral, more than four lesions on each side) predicts familial adenomatous polyposis with 97% sensitivity. Polyps begin to appear at puberty. If a family lacks the retinal pigment abnormality, flexible sigmoidoscopy will need to be done from puberty until age 40 or 50 to be certain the family members do not have polyposis. Once polyposis is diagnosed, colectomy should be done. Upper gastrointestinal endoscopy is advised to look for gastroduodenal lesions.

Although total proctocolectomy eliminates the risk of cancer, it leaves the patient with a permanent ileostomy. Abdominal colectomy ("subtotal colectomy") with ileorectal anastomosis is favored by many surgeons because an ileostomy is not required; rectal polyps regress in some patients after this procedure, and, it is hoped, cancer can be prevented by sigmoidoscopic destruction of polyps every 3 months. The long-term success rate varies in different reports, and the incidence of cancer in the remaining rectum may be very low or quite high (50% after 20 years). Sulindac has been reported to induce regression of rectal polyps after ileorectal anastomosis. Total colectomy, mucosal proctectomy, and ileoanal anastomosis eliminates the neoplasm-prone mucosa completely while preserving good rectal function. This procedure (see Ulcerative Colitis, below) is preferred for patients with carpets of adenomas in the rectum. Prophylactic colectomy does not alter the extracolonic manifestations. Desmoid tumor is a locally invasive nonmetastasizing fibrous tumor that occurs in the mesentery or abdominal wall of some patients after the colectomy. Results of attempts to excise desmoids are poor, with 80% recurrence. Sulindac, tamoxifen, prednisolone, and progesterone have been reported to halt the growth of desmoids, but chemotherapeutic agents and radiation therapy are disappointing. Desmoids grow slowly and capriciously, but they prove fatal in 10% of patients with familial adenomatous polyposis. Upper gastrointestinal cancer occurs in up to 10% of these patients, and medulloblastoma is also a significant risk.

Hereditary flat adenoma syndrome has been described recently. It is separable from familial adenomatous polyposis, and it is either a variant of hereditary nonpolyposis colorectal cancer or a distinct entity. Three syndromes of juvenile polyposis have been defined: (1) **juvenile polyposis coli,** (2) **generalized juvenile gastrointestinal polyposis,** and (3) the **Cronkhite-Canada syndrome** (juvenile polyposis and ectodermal lesions). The first two are inherited with an autosomal dominant pattern. Although juvenile polyps are hamartomas with a low malignant potential, the risk of gastrointestinal cancer is increased in familial juvenile polyposis patients and their relatives. Furthermore, hamartomas can coexist with adenomas, and one must not assume that a polyp is a hamartoma without proof. Colonoscopic excision is performed for large or symptomatic (bleeding, intussusception) lesions. Some juvenile polyps autoamputate. Colectomy is required in some patients with familial forms of juvenile polyposis.

Peutz-Jeghers syndrome is an uncommon autosomal dominant disease in which multiple hamartomatous polyps appear in the stomach, small bowel, and colon. Affected individuals have melanotic pigmentation of the skin and mucous membranes, especially about the lips and gums. The malignant potential of the hamartomas is small, and generally polyps are removed only if symptomatic. Carcinoma develops at an increased rate in other tissues, eg, stomach, duodenum, pancreas, small intestine, and breast.

Prognosis

Villous adenomas recur (presumably because of incomplete excision) in about 15% of cases after local removal. Tubular adenomas seldom recur, but new ones may develop, and a patient who has had any type of adenoma is at greater risk of developing adenocarcinoma than the general population. In one study, the cumulative risk of developing further adenomas was linear over time, reaching about 50% by 15 years after removal of one or more colorectal adenomas; the cumulative incidence of cancer in the same population rose to 7% at 15 years. Multiple adenomas signal a greater risk of further neoplasms than single polyps, and more men than women seem to develop new polyps or cancers. Based on these and other observations, if the colon is cleared by total colonoscopy at the time of excision of the index polyps, it is probably wise to repeat the colonoscopy 1 year later. Thereafter, colonoscopy every 3 years is probably sufficient. Opinion is divided on details of this surveillance program, but it seems clear that colonoscopic follow-up is essential, probably for the patient's remaining years of life. Barium enema x-rays are no longer routinely used for surveillance in these patients.

Adachi M et al: Clinicopathologic features of the flat adenoma. Dis Colon Rectum 1991;34:981.

Arvanitis ML et al: Mortality in patients with familial adenomatous polyposis. Dis Colon Rectum 1990;33:639.

Blue MG et al: Hyperplastic polyps seen at sigmoidoscopy are markers for additional adenomas seen at colonoscopy. Gastroenterology 1991;100:564.

Demers RY et al: Pathologist agreement in the interpretation of colorectal polyps. Am J Gastroenterol 1990; 85:417.

DiSario JA et al: Prevalence and malignant potential of colorectal polyps in asymptomatic, average-risk men. Am J Gastroenterol 1991;86:941.

Heyen F et al: Predictive value of congenital hypertrophy of the retinal pigment epithelium as a clinical marker for familial adenomatous polyposis. Dis Colon Rectum 1990; 33:1003.

Hixson LJ et al: Prospective blinded trial of the colonoscopic miss-rate of large colorectal polyps. Gastrointest Endosc 1991;37:125.

Kinzler KW et al: Identification of FAP locus genes from chromosome 5q21. Science 1991;253:661.

Kronborg O (editor): Symposium: Colorectal polyps. World J Surg 1991;15:1.

Labayle D et al: Sulindac causes regression of rectal polyps in familial adenomatous polyposis. Gastroenterology 1991;101:635.

Lynch HT et al: Phenotypic variation in colorectal adenoma/cancer expression in two families. Hereditary flat adenoma syndrome. Cancer 1990;66:909.

Madden MV et al: Comparison of morbidity and function after colectomy with ileorectal anastomosis or restorative proctocolectomy for familial adenomatous polyposis. Br J Surg 1991;78:789.

Mathus-Vliegen EMH, Tytgat GNJ: The potential and limitations of laser photoablation of colorectal adenomas. Gastrointest Endosc 1991;37:9.

Molecular secrets of colorectal cancer. Lancet 1991; 338:1363.

Nishisho I et al: Mutations of chromosome 5q21 genes in FAP and colorectal cancer patients. Science 1991;253: 665.

O'Brien MJ et al: The National Polyp Study: Patient and polyp characteristics associated with high-grade dysplasia in colorectal adenomas. Gastroenterology 1990; 98:371.

Sakamoto GD, MacKeigan JM, Senagore AJ: Transanal excision of large, rectal villous adenomas. Dis Colon Rectum 1991;34:880.

Schuman BM, Simsek H, Lyons RC: The association of multiple colonic adenomatous polyps with cancer of the colon. Am J Gastroenterol 1990;85:846.

Skinner MA et al: Subtotal colectomy for familial polyposis: A clinical series and review of the literature. Arch Surg 1990;125:621.

Tierney RP, Ballantyne GH, Modlin IM: The adenoma to carcinoma sequence. Surg Gynecol Obstet 1990;171:81.

Vasen HFA et al: The value of screening and central registration of families with familial adenomatous polyposis: A study of 82 families in the Netherlands. Dis Colon Rectum 1990;33:227.

Williams CB, Bedenne L: Management of colorectal polyps: Is all the effort worthwhile? J Gastroenterol Hepatol 1990;1(Suppl):144.

Wolff WL et al: Cancerous colonic polyps: "Hands on" or "hands off?" Am Surg 1990;56:148.

Woolfson IK et al: Usefulness of performing colonoscopy one year after endoscopic polypectomy. Dis Colon Rectum 1990;33:389.

OTHER TUMORS OF THE COLON & RECTUM

Carcinoids of the large bowel are uncommon, and most of them occur in the rectum. Lesions less than 2 cm in diameter usually are asymptomatic, behave benignly, and can be managed by local excision. Larger tumors arising in the colon (mainly the right side) or rectum cause local symptoms, often metastasize, and require standard cancer operations. Carcinoid syndrome appears in less than 5% of patients with metastatic carcinoid of the large bowel.

Lymphomas are the most common of the noncarcinomatous malignant tumors of the large bowel. Diffuse lymphomatous polyposis is a rare gastrointestinal manifestation. Non-Hodgkin's lymphoma and Kaposi's sarcoma are two AIDS-related cancers that affect the colon and rectum. Lymphoma is often aggressive, but Kaposi's sarcoma may cause few colonic or systemic symptoms.

Lipomas may be difficult to distinguish radiographically from mucosal neoplasms, but colonoscopy most often permits accurate diagnosis. Lipomas are usually asymptomatic but can cause obstruction. Removal is recommended if they cause symptoms.

Leiomyomas are much less common in the colon than in the stomach or small intestine. Colonic tumors are less apt to cause significant hemorrhage than those of the upper bowel. Some leiomyomas become malignant.

Endometriomas are masses of endometrial tissue that implant on the surface of the rectum, sigmoid colon, appendix, cecum, or distal ileum and may invade locally into the muscularis or submucosa. The ectopic tissue responds to cyclic hormonal stimulation, causing inflammation and fibrosis. Intestinal symptoms of endometriosis include altered bowel habits and occasionally rectal bleeding during menstruation. Tender nodularities are palpable in the pelvis in 90% of cases. Sigmoidoscopy, fiberoptic colonoscopy, and barium enema x-rays may make the diagnosis. Operation is performed only if symptoms are not controlled by endocrine therapy or if cancer cannot be excluded. Operation in severe cases usually requires hysterectomy and oophorectomy; intestinal lesions are excised or the diseased segment is resected.

Other benign colorectal tumors include neurofibromas associated with Recklinghausen's disease, teratomas, enterocystomas (duplication of rectum), lymphangiomas, and cavernous hemangiomas. Adenosquamous carcinoma, primary squamous cell carcinoma, sarcomas, and primary melanoma of the colon or rectum are extremely rare malignant tumors.

Collin GR, Russell JC: Endometriosis of the colon: Its diagnosis and management. Am Surg 1990;56:275.

Federspiel BH et al: Rectal and colonic carcinoids: A clinicopathologic study of 84 cases. Cancer 1990;65:135.

Järvinen HJ: Other gastrointestinal polyps. World J Surg 1991;15:50.

Meijer S et al: Primary colorectal sarcoma: A retrospective review and prognostic factor study of 50 consecutive patients. Arch Surg 1990;125:1163.

Pfeil SA et al: Colonic lipomas: Outcome of endoscopic removal. Gastrointest Endosc 1990;36:435.

Rogy MA et al: Submucous large-bowel lipomas: Presentation and management. An 18-year study. Eur J Surg 1991;157:51.

Urschel JD, Berendt RC, Anselmo JE: Surgical treatment of colonic ganglioneuromatosis in neurofibromatosis. Can J Surg 1991;34:271.

DIVERTICULAR DISEASE OF THE COLON

Diverticula are more common in the colon than in any other portion of the gastrointestinal tract. Colonic diverticula are acquired and are classified as false because they consist of mucosa and submucosa that have herniated through the muscular coats. True diverticula containing all layers of the bowel wall are rare in the colon. Colonic diverticula are pulsion (rather than traction) diverticula, because they are pushed out by intraluminal pressure. They vary from a few millimeters to several centimeters in diameter; the necks may be narrow or wide; and some contain inspissated fecal matter. Approximately 95% of patients with diverticula have involvement of the sigmoid colon. The descending, transverse, and ascending portions of the colon are involved in decreasing order of frequency. The presence of a solitary diverticulum of the cecum and the occurrence of multiple diverticula limited to the right colon are distinct entities often seen in Asian people but seldom encountered in other populations. Giant colonic diverticulum is a very rare lesion of huge dimensions, usually arising from the sigmoid colon.

In Western countries, perhaps 50% of individuals develop diverticula—10% by age 40 years and 65% by age 80 years. Diverticular disease is more common in Western nations than in Japan or in developing countries of the tropics. The prevalence of diverticulosis is 20% in Singapore; 70% of the cases are right-sided. Cultural factors, especially diet, play an important etiologic role. Chief among the dietary influences is the fiber content of ingested food.

The pathogenesis of diverticula requires defects in the colonic wall and increased pressure in the lumen relative to the serosal surface. Small openings in the circular muscle layer for penetration of nutrient blood vessels are the sites of diverticula formation in many individuals (Figure 31–10). Diverticulosis of the colon comprises a spectrum with two extremes: (1) diverticulosis associated with hypermotility, and (2) simple massed diverticulosis. In the first type, colonic musculature is shortened and thickened (myochosis coli); colonic pressures are high in response to meals or pharmacologic stimuli; patients may have pain and altered bowel habits; and diverticula are limited to the sigmoid, at least initially. It is hypothesized that myochosis reflects work hypertrophy from a lifetime of fiber-deficient diet and the consequent scybalous stools. High intraluminal pressures are possible because the colon forms closed compart-

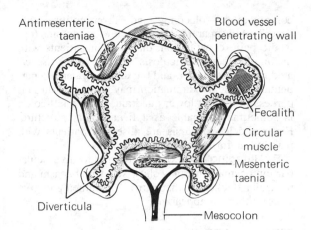

Figure 31–10. Cross section of the colon depicting the sites where diverticula form. Note that the antimesocolic portion is spared. The longitudinal layer of muscle completely encircles the bowel and is not limited to the taeniae as depicted here.

ments when opposite walls of the thickened bowel actually touch and occlude the lumen. The propensity for diverticula to develop in the sigmoid is explained by the law of Laplace, which states that pressure within a tube is inversely proportionate to the radius. It had been speculated that the irritable bowel syndrome is a prediverticular state, but patterns of colonic motility are different in diverticular disease and irritable bowel syndrome. Moreover, it is clear that irritable bowel syndrome can affect the esophagus and small bowel in addition to the colon, so an etiologic link to colonic diverticula now seems unlikely. The two conditions can coexist, however, and irritable bowel syndrome may be the reason for symptoms.

Patients with simple massed diverticulosis have grossly normal colonic musculature, normal pressures, often no symptoms, and diverticula throughout the colon. Presumably, the primary abnormality is weakness of the colonic wall from aging or illness. It is of interest that Ehlers-Danlos syndrome and Marfan's syndrome, both of which involve abnormal connective tissue, are associated with colonic diverticulosis.

1. DIVERTICULOSIS

Diverticulosis is the presence of multiple false diverticula.

Clinical Findings

A. Symptoms and Signs: Diverticulosis probably remains asymptomatic in about 80% of people and is detected incidentally on barium enema x-rays or endoscopy if it is discovered at all. Symptoms attributable to the diverticula themselves are actually complications—bleeding and diverticulitis—each described in separate sections below. Symptoms (episodic pain, constipation, diarrhea) in patients with uncomplicated diverticulosis are due to the associated motility disorder, and the diverticula are coincidental. Physical examination may disclose mild tenderness in the left lower quadrant, and the left colon is sometimes palpable as a firm tubular structure. Fever and leukocytosis are absent in patients with pain but no inflammation.

B. Imaging Studies: In addition to diverticula, barium enema films may show segmental spasm and muscular thickening that narrow the lumen and give it a saw-toothed appearance.

Differential Diagnosis

Pain from the colonic muscular abnormality in the absence of inflammation can be difficult to differentiate from diverticulitis. The presence or absence of systemic signs of inflammation is the chief differential point, but the natural history of the acute episode may be the only way to make the distinction. Diverticulosis must be differentiated from other causes of rectal bleeding, especially carcinoma. Colonoscopy is essential in patients with bleeding.

Complications

Diverticulitis and massive hemorrhage are discussed below.

Treatment

A. Medical Treatment: Asymptomatic persons with diverticulosis may be given a high-fiber diet, although it is not certain that complications of diverticulosis can be avoided by dietary changes once the diverticula have formed. Symptomatic patients also can be treated with a high-fiber diet; constipation is improved, but abdominal pain is not. Unprocessed bran is the least expensive source of fiber; patients should take 10–25 g daily with cereal, soup, salad, or other food. More palatable sources of wheat fiber include whole-grain bread and breakfast cereals. Commercial bulk agents (eg, psyllium seed products) are also available at greater cost. One problem in prescribing bulk agents is that different types of fiber may have dissimilar effects on the colon. Anticholinergic agents, sedatives, tranquilizers, antidepressants, and antibiotics have no value. The analgesic of choice is pentazocine, 0.5 mg/kg body weight given intramuscularly. Education, reassurance, and a warm personal relationship between physician and patient are important to successful management.

B. Surgical Treatment: Operation is necessary for massive hemorrhage or to rule out carcinoma in some patients, but colonoscopy usually resolves the question of cancer. Colon resection for uncomplicated diverticular disease or irritable bowel syndrome is rarely necessary or advisable.

Prognosis

The natural history of diverticulosis has not been defined. Ten to 20% of patients with diverticulosis develop diverticulitis or hemorrhage when followed for many years. These patients are selected, however, and the incidence of complications in the population at large may be much lower. About 75% of complications of diverticular disease develop in patients with no prior colonic symptoms. Some evidence suggests that diverticulitis is more common with the hypermotility type of diverticulosis, and bleeding is the more frequent complication in simple massed diverticulosis. Irritable bowel syndrome is a chronic relapsing disorder that affects patients over long periods of their lives. There is hope that better understanding of the pathophysiologic mechanisms will soon lead to more rational therapy.
See references at end of next section.

2. DIVERTICULITIS

Essentials of Diagnosis

- Acute abdominal pain.
- Left lower quadrant tenderness and mass.
- Fever and leukocytosis.
- Characteristic radiologic signs.

General Considerations

Acute colonic diverticulitis is the result of perforation due to intraluminal pressure, or it begins as infection in a diverticulum. Corticosteroids or nonsteroidal anti-inflammatory drug use may contribute to this complication. With either mechanism, only one diverticulum is involved at a time, usually in the sigmoid colon. Infection limited to a tiny diverticulum may not cause symptoms, but when infection extends through the wall of the colon into peridiverticular tissue **(peridiverticulitis),** it becomes clinically significant. Peridiverticulitis implies that the diverticulum has perforated, but the process evolves slowly rather than suddenly, as may occur when intraluminal pressure causes perforation.

Microperforation of a diverticulum leads to localized inflammation in the colonic wall or paracolic tissues. Macroperforation results in more extensive bacterial contamination and more serious infection such as an abscess or generalized peritonitis. An abscess may be confined by adjacent structures or may enlarge and spread; it may resorb with antibiotic treatment or drain spontaneously into the lumen of the bowel or into an adjacent viscus to form a fistula; it may require surgical drainage; it may rupture into the peritoneal cavity and produce generalized purulent peritonitis; or it may become chronic. The other mechanism for development of generalized peritonitis is rupture of a diverticulum into the free peritoneal cavity, which contaminates the abdomen with feces. Intraluminal pressure is responsible. Fortunately, this form of diverticulitis is uncommon. Chronic colonic obstruction can result from fibrosis in response to repeated episodes of microperforation. Also, small bowel may adhere acutely to an inflamed area and cause small bowel obstruction. Cecal diverticulitis resembles appendicitis clinically.

It was once believed that nearly all perforated diverticula maintain a connection with the bowel lumen (**communicating diverticulitis**). It is now known that in many cases, the original perforation seals quickly and the paracolic infection is isolated from the colonic lumen (**noncommunicating diverticulitis**). This concept has implications for surgical treatment.

Clinical Findings

A. Symptoms and Signs: The acute attack consists of localized abdominal pain that is mild to severe, aching, and either steady or cramping; it resembles acute appendicitis except that it is situated in the left lower quadrant. Occasionally, pain is suprapubic, in the right lower quadrant, or throughout the lower abdomen. Constipation or increased frequency of defecation (or both in the same patient) is common, and passage of flatus may give some relief of pain. Inflammation adjacent to the bladder may produce dysuria. Nausea and vomiting depend on the location and severity of the inflammation. Physical findings characteristically include low-grade fever, mild abdominal distention, left lower quadrant tenderness, and a left lower quadrant or pelvic mass. Occult or, less commonly, gross blood is present in stools; massive hemorrhage is rare in the presence of peridiverticular inflammation. Leukocytosis is mild to moderate.

The clinical picture described above is typical, but acute diverticulitis has other modes of presentation. Free perforation of a diverticulum produces generalized peritonitis rather than localized inflammation. An acute attack of diverticulitis may go unnoticed until a complication develops, and the complication may be the reason for the patient to seek help. The course of diverticulitis may be so insidious, particularly in advanced age groups, that vague abdominal pain associated with an abscess in the groin or a colovesical fistula is the initial presentation. In some cases, pain and inflammatory signs are not marked, but a palpable mass and signs of large bowel obstruction are present, so that carcinoma of the left colon seems the more likely diagnosis. In one series of women with proved diverticulitis, 38% were initially misdiagnosed as having a gynecologic pelvic mass, because gastrointestinal symptoms and signs were mild or absent.

B. Imaging Studies: Plain abdominal films may show free abdominal air if a diverticulum has perforated into the general peritoneal cavity. If inflammation is localized, there is a picture of ileus, partial colonic obstruction, small bowel obstruction, or left lower quadrant mass.

CT scan is replacing water-soluble contrast enema as the initial imaging study. CT can be obtained early in the patient's course, with intravenous and usually oral contrast to enhance the image. Effacement of pericolic fat is seen in diverticulitis, and complications such as abscess or fistula may be evident. The finding of an abscess that is accessible for percutaneous drainage provides a major therapeutic advantage over contrast enemas. CT findings of perforated diverticulitis are not specific; colonoscopy and sometimes contrast enema must be obtained subsequently. Ultrasound and MRI are helpful in some cases.

Barium enema is contraindicated during the initial stages of an acute attack of diverticulitis lest barium leak into the peritoneal cavity, but water-soluble contrast media used under low pressure is safe. Barium enema can be performed a week or more after the attack began if the patient has recovered promptly. Radiographic signs include the following: (1) an abscess cavity or sinus tract outside the colonic wall communicating with the lumen; (2) an intramural abscess producing indentation of the barium column; (3) extrinsic compression by a paracolic mass; (4) intramural sinuses; and (5) fistulas. (See Figure 31–11.)

C. Special Examinations: The rigid sigmoidoscope usually cannot be passed beyond the rectosigmoid junction, because of acute angulation and fixation at that level with a decrease in size of the lumen. Erythema, edema, and spasm may be noted. A

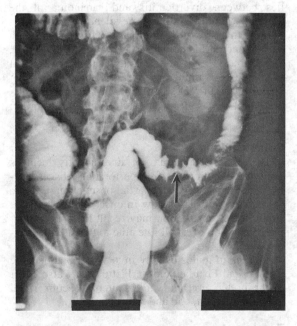

Figure 31–11. Barium enema roentgenogram showing upper sigmoid colon involved with diverticulitis. Note the long segment of narrowing, the spasm, and the deformity (arrow) produced by an intramural abscess.

purulent discharge can sometimes be seen coming from above. Flexible sigmoidoscopy or colonoscopy should be avoided during an acute attack but is very helpful in evaluating strictures and other persistent abnormalities later. Small-bore upper tract instruments may be needed to examine narrow segments. Cystoscopy may reveal bullous edema of the bladder wall.

Differential Diagnosis

Free perforation of a diverticulum with generalized peritonitis often cannot be differentiated from the other causes of perforation, including foreign bodies and stercoraceous perforation. Acute diverticulitis with localized perforation may simulate appendicitis, perforated colonic carcinoma, strangulation obstruction, mesenteric vascular insufficiency, Crohn's disease, and many other conditions. One source of confusion is that diverticulitis can be precipitated by Crohn's disease, but the length of the paracolic fistulous tract is a differential point: a short tract (< 4 cm) is due to diverticulitis, and a long tract (> 8 cm) reflects either diverticulitis alone or Crohn's disease in association with diverticulitis. Differentiation from appendicitis is especially difficult when a redundant sigmoid colon lies in the right lower quadrant. A history of colonic symptoms on prior occasions, palpation of a mass, ultrasonography, CT, or water-soluble contrast enema may be helpful in differentiating these conditions. Sigmoidoscopy may detect carcinoma, vascular insufficiency, or inflammatory disease of the colon. A difficult differential diagnosis lies between diverticulitis and carcinoma of the colon, particularly in the more silent forms of diverticulitis that present with a mass or fistula. Although barium enema and colonoscopy may clarify the issue, the diagnosis may not be known until the surgical specimen is examined by the pathologist. Persistent bleeding should not be attributed to diverticular disease until cancer has been excluded as a possibility; this nearly always requires colonoscopy.

Complications

The clinical spectrum of diverticulitis includes such complications as free perforation, abscess formation, fistulization, and partial obstruction. Colonic obstruction is usually slow in onset and incomplete; small bowel obstruction may result from the attachment of a loop of small intestine to the inflamed sigmoid.

Fistulas in males usually involve the bladder (see Colovesical Fistula, below). Fistulas may also occur to the ureter, urethra, vagina, uterus, cecum, small bowel, perineum, and abdominal wall.

Treatment

A. Expectant Treatment: Patients with acute diverticulitis may need to be hospitalized. Details of management vary with the severity of the attack; generally, nothing is given by mouth, nasogastric suction is instituted, intravenous fluids are given, and systemic broad-spectrum antibiotics are administered. Oral nonabsorbable antibacterial drugs are of little value. Pentazocine is the preferred analgesic; morphine increases colonic pressure, and meperidine has less of this side effect. As acute manifestations subside, oral feeding is resumed gradually, and bulk-forming agents such as unprocessed bran are prescribed if there is no stricture.

Barium enema x-rays are obtained a week or so after the attack began. Colonoscopy is mandatory in the presence of rectal bleeding or if x-rays show a possible neoplasm (stricture, mass, equivocal findings). It is recommended in patients with abdominal pain or change in bowel habits attributed to diverticular disease, even if barium x-rays reveal only diverticula. Colonoscopy will disclose a colonic neoplasm in about 30% of such patients.

B. Surgical Treatment: Cecal diverticulitis is usually treated by right colectomy. Immediate operation for sigmoid diverticulitis is required if spreading or generalized peritonitis is present upon entry into the hospital or if peritonitis develops during the hospital stay. Abdominal pain, mass, fever, or leukocytosis that fails to improve after 3–4 days of medical therapy also indicates that intervention is necessary. Obstruction and fistula seldom become indications for urgent operation during acute diverticulitis; both of these clinical problems are discussed separately in this chapter.

Percutaneous catheter drainage of well-localized paracolic abscesses can be performed by interventional radiologists. This technique is especially useful because it converts a potential emergency operation to an elective one when the patient is in better condition. Colonic resection will be needed eventually in most of these patients.

At laparotomy for severe acute diverticulitis, peritoneal fluid varies from turbid to purulent to grossly fecal. The sigmoid colon is involved in an inflammatory mass comprised of large bowel, mesocolon, omentum, and sometimes small bowel. Except in cases of free perforation with generalized fecal peritonitis, the diseased diverticulum may not be visible. An abscess cavity may be hidden beneath colon or omentum and discovered when the bowel is mobilized; abscesses are commonly found lateral or medial to the colon, in the mesocolon, or in the pelvis. Microperforation of a diverticulum is not associated with a grossly apparent abscess. The extent of colonic inflammation, the amount of peritonitis, the patient's general condition, and the surgeon's experience and preferences determine the type of operation to be performed.

1. Primary resection with anastomosis–Resection of the diseased colon and performance of colonic anastomosis at the same time have the advantage of solving the entire problem in one operation. It is not possible to anastomose the colon safely if the bowel is edematous or if there is gross infection in the surgical field, because the risk of anastomotic leakage is great. Intraoperative lavage of the colon and the intracolonic bypass tube are advocated in this situation as in colonic obstruction.

2. Primary resection without anastomosis (2-stage procedure)–The diseased bowel is removed, the proximal end of the colon is brought out as a temporary colostomy, and the distal colonic stump is closed (Hartmann procedure, Figure 31–12) or exteriorized as a mucous fistula. Intestinal continuity is restored in a second operation after the inflammation subsides. Increasingly, percutaneous drainage of abscesses avoids the need for staged procedures.

3. Three-stage procedure–The three-stage procedure consists of a first operation during which a transverse colostomy is created and the paracolic abscess is drained; a second operation during which the left colon is resected; and, still later, a third operation during which the colostomy is taken down. The three-stage approach is seldom used today.

Definitive resection for sigmoid diverticulitis should include the rectosigmoid distally to the point where the taeniae become confluent; anastomosis is performed to the proximal rectum, which is always free of diverticula. The distal descending colon is removed, but it is unnecessary to resect additional bowel proximally; even if it is involved with diverticula, they do not become symptomatic in the absence of the sigmoid high-pressure zone.

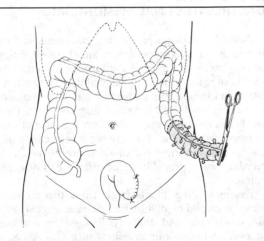

Figure 31–12. Primary resection for diverticulitis of the colon. The affected segment (shaded) has been divided at its distal end. If primary anastomosis is to be done, the proximal margin (dotted line) is transected, and the bowel is anastomosed end-to-end. If a two-stage procedure will be used, a colostomy is formed at the proximal margin, and the distal stump is oversewn (Hartmann procedure, as shown), or exteriorized as a mucous fistula. The second state consists of colostomy takedown and anastomosis.

Prognosis

Approximately 25% of patients hospitalized with acute diverticulitis require surgical treatment. The operative mortality rate is about 5% in recent reports, compared with 25% a few years ago. Some of this improvement is attributable to the greater use of primary resection following percutaneous drainage of abscess.

Diverticulitis recurs in about one-third of medically treated cases. Most of these recurrences develop within the first 5 years. It is unknown whether recurrent attacks of diverticulitis can be prevented by increasing dietary fiber, although this measure is generally recommended. Indications for elective colon resection are recurrent diverticulitis, persistent diverticulitis (pain, tenderness, mass, dysuria), age under 50 years, and inability to rule out carcinoma. The mortality rate of elective left colectomy is 2–4%. Recurrent diverticulitis after resection is very unusual (about 3–7%).

Campbell K, Steele RJC: Non-steroidal anti-inflammatory drugs and complicated diverticular disease: A case-control study. Br J Surg 1991;78:190.

Chia JG et al: Trends of diverticular disease of the large bowel in a newly developed country. Dis Colon Rectum 1991;34:498.

Cho KC et al: Sigmoid diverticulitis: Diagnostic role of CT: Comparison with barium enema studies. Radiology 1990;176:111.

Cook IJ et al: Effect of dietary fiber on symptoms and rectosigmoid motility in patients with irritable bowel syndrome. A controlled, crossover study. Gastroenterology 1990;98:66.

Cortesini C, Pantalone D: Usefulness of colonic motility study in identifying patients at risk for complicated diverticular disease. Dis Colon Rectum 1991;34:339.

Hold M, Denck H, Bull P: Surgical management of perforating diverticular disease in Austria. Int J Colorect Dis 1990;5:195.

Moreaux J, Vons C: Elective resection for diverticular disease of the sigmoid colon. Br J Surg 1990;77:1036.

Peoples JB et al: Reassessment of primary resection of the perforated segment for severe colonic diverticulitis. Am J Surg 1990;159:291.

Schmit PJ, Bennion RS, Thompson JE Jr: Cecal diverticulitis: A continuing diagnostic dilemma. World J Surg 1991;15:367.

Shrier D, Skucas J, Weiss S: Diverticulitis: An evaluation by computed tomography and contrast enema. Am J Gastroenterol 1991;86:1466.

Stillman AE, Painter R, Hollister DW: Ehlers-Danlos syndrome type IV: Diagnosis and therapy of associated bowel perforation. Am J Gastroenterol 1991;86:360.

Talley NJ et al: Epidemiology of colonic symptoms and the irritable bowel syndrome. Gastroenterology 1991;101:927.

Tyau ES et al: Acute diverticulitis. A complicated problem in the immunocompromised patient. Arch Surg 1991;126:855.

vanSonnenberg E et al: Percutaneous abscess drainage: Current concepts. 1991;181:617.

Watters DAK, Smith AN: Strength of the colon wall in diverticular disease. Br J Surg 1990;77:257.

Wilson SR, Toi A: The value of sonography in the diagnosis of acute diverticulitis of the colon. AJR Am J Roentgenol 1990;154:1199.

COLOVESICAL FISTULA

Colovesical fistula is the most common type of fistulous communication between the urinary bladder and the gastrointestinal tract. There is a 3:1 ratio of men to women with this condition, presumably because the uterus and adnexa are situated between the colon and the bladder in women.

Diverticulitis is the most common cause of colovesical fistula. This complication occurs in 2–4% of cases of diverticulitis, although an even higher incidence is reported from specialized referral centers. Carcinoma of the colon, cancer of other organs such as the bladder, Crohn's disease, radiation bowel injury, external trauma, foreign bodies, and iatrogenic injuries are other causes or underlying conditions.

A colovesical fistula may cause surprisingly little disturbance to the patient, and some patients remain completely asymptomatic. The appearance of a fistula from diverticulitis or colonic cancer is seldom accompanied by dramatic or sudden abdominal symptoms; more typically, refractory urinary tract infection is the presenting complaint. Fecaluria and pneumaturia may have been obvious to the patient, or it may be recollected only in response to direct questioning. The episode of diverticulitis may have gone entirely unnoticed.

Physical examination may disclose a pelvic mass or no abnormalities. Leukocytosis is absent in most cases, and routine blood chemistries are normal. Urinalysis may reveal fecaluria or infected urine. Rigid sigmoidoscopy is usually unrevealing; flexible sigmoidoscopy or colonoscopy may disclose colonic cancer or inflammation at the fistula site. Cystoscopy shows bullous edema, but the fistula is usually not visible. Barium enema, CT scan, sonography, and cystography may demonstrate the fistula, but small communications escape detection. In some cases, the fistula is not demonstrable because it has closed, at least temporarily. If doubt exists about the presence of a fistula, a dye marker such as methylene blue can be instilled into the rectum or bladder.

Colovesical fistulas usually require surgical treatment if they persist, but there is no need for emergency or urgent operation. Patients may recover well from spontaneous drainage of a paracolic abscess through a fistula into the bladder, and operation can be delayed to be sure it is necessary and by then the conditions will be more favorable. Inability to rule out cancer may prompt earlier operation. If a fistula closes spontaneously, as it may do in up to 50% of patients with diverticulitis, requirements for resection depend on the nature of the underlying colonic disease. Some patients tolerate a colovesical fistula so well that operation is deferred indefinitely.

At operation, patients with diverticulitis or colonic carcinoma have mild to moderate inflammatory reaction around the sigmoid colon, which has dropped into the pelvis and adhered to the bladder; severe active diverticulitis with abscess or peritonitis is exceptional. If the fistula has been caused by cancer of the colon, the adherent bladder should not be separated from the colon lest tumor cells be spilled into the pelvis; a disk of bladder wall should be excised in continuity with the colon, the bladder closed primarily, and catheter drainage of the bladder provided for 7–10 days. Fortunately, most colovesical fistulas enter the bladder away from the trigone. Diverticulitis is managed by bluntly dissecting the colon from the bladder, resecting the colon, and performing a primary anastomosis.

Many of these fistulous tracts are tiny, and if the opening into the bladder is not apparent, the bladder should be distended with fluid containing methylene blue. The opening into the bladder need not be sutured unless it is very large. It is seldom necessary to delay performance of the colonic anastomosis.

Grissom R, Snyder TE: Colovaginal fistula secondary to diverticular disease. Dis Colon Rectum 1991;34:1043.

Kirsh GM et al: Diagnosis and management of vesicoenteric fistulas. Surg Gynecol Obstet 1991;173:91.

ACUTE LOWER GASTROINTESTINAL HEMORRHAGE

Acute hemorrhage per rectum can originate from lesions in the gastroduodenum, small bowel, colon, or anorectum. A source in the lower gastrointestinal tract is suggested by the passage of dark to bright red blood, but the color of evacuated blood is a function of the length of time it remained in the intestinal tract, and bright red blood may come from a duodenal ulcer or hemorrhoids as well as any point in between. If a patient passing bright red blood is not in shock, the bleeding site is probably in the distal small bowel or colon.

Exsanguinating hemorrhage from the colon in adults is caused by diverticular disease, angiodysplasia, solitary ulcer, ulcerative colitis, ischemic colitis, or a variety of uncommon lesions such as coagulation disorders, radiation injury, chemotherapeutic toxicity, and others. Bleeding occurs in the right colon about as often as in the left colon, probably because angiodysplasias are more prominent on the right side, but right-sided diverticula can also bleed. Bleeding lesions in the small intestine are rare and include hereditary hemorrhagic telangiectasia (Rendu-Osler-Weber syndrome).

Chronic rectal bleeding, typically seen in patients

with cancer, polyps, hemorrhoids, fissures, and other conditions, does not require urgent evaluation. Anorectal examination, colonoscopy, and x-rays if indicated can be performed electively. Acute severe hemorrhage, however, is a potentially life-threatening problem, and prompt evaluation and treatment are critical. Some patients bleed rapidly, but the bleeding stops spontaneously after only a small amount of blood is lost, and these patients are never in danger. Usually, however, one cannot be sure that bleeding will not recur, so this type of bleeding must be taken seriously too, which means that aggressive evaluation is needed.

A plan of management of acute lower gastrointestinal hemorrhage is outlined in Figure 31–13. Many decisions depend on the rate of bleeding, which is difficult to include in an algorithm. Bleeding stops spontaneously in 90% of patients before transfusion requirements exceed two units.

The patient with severe rectal bleeding is resuscitated with intravenous fluids and transfusions while the diagnostic procedures are begun. Clotting param-

eters should be measured and deficits corrected, and associated medical conditions should be identified and treated as soon as possible. Digital rectal examination, anoscopy, and sigmoidoscopy should be performed with no attempt to prepare the bowel. If a bleeding lesion is found in the anorectum, it should be treated. Examples include hemorrhoids, polypoid neoplasm, and ulcerative proctitis.

A nasogastric tube should be inserted and the aspirate inspected for bile, gross blood, and occult blood. Blood in the stomach is an indication of bleeding from a site proximal to the ligament of Treitz—ie, upper gastrointestinal bleeding—and esophagogastroduodenoscopy (EGD) is performed. Occasionally, a patient bleeds from the duodenum, but blood does not reflux back into the stomach; bile in the nasogastric aspirate would seem to eliminate this possibility, but in the absence of blood or bile, EGD should be done.

If EGD is negative and bleeding has presumably stopped or continues at a slow rate, the colon can be prepared with polyethylene glycol-sodium sulfate so-

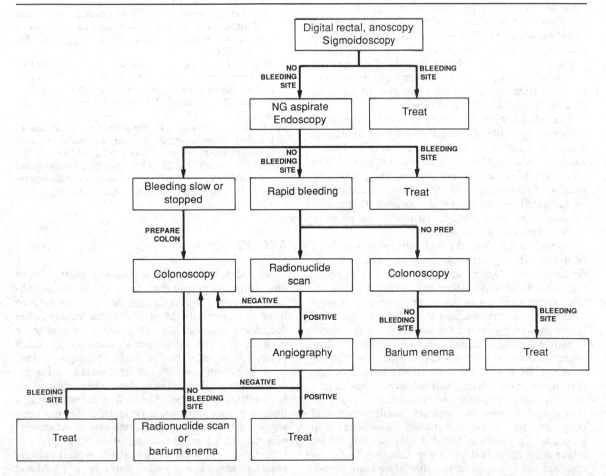

Figure 31–13. Plan for diagnosis and treatment of acute lower gastrointestinal hemorrhage. (NG = nasogastric.)

lution, and colonoscopy is performed within a few hours. The bleeding site is identified in 25–94% of cases, depending in part on skill, experience, and, very importantly, the criteria for inclusion of a patient in this category of bleeding. Some bleeding lesions can be treated colonoscopically with a bipolar probe, heater probe, or laser. Colonoscopy with negative results probably means that bleeding has stopped. Barium enema discloses abnormalities such as diverticula but does not reveal which lesions have been bleeding.

The optimal method of evaluating patients who are bleeding rapidly is controversial, and the decision may hinge on available resources. Radionuclide "bleeding" scan after injection of ^{99m}Tc-sulfur colloid or ^{99m}Tc-labeled red blood cells may show whether bleeding persists. The results using ^{99m}Tc-labeled red blood cells are superior to those with ^{99m}Tc-sulfur colloid, but localization of bleeding is not reliable by either method, and enthusiasm for bleeding scans generally has waned recently. Angiography is seldom successful in demonstrating an active bleeding site if the bleeding scan is negative, so colonoscopy should be undertaken. Active bleeding shown on radionuclide scan should be followed by angiography.

Selective mesenteric angiography identifies the bleeding site in 14–70% of patients; here, too, enthusiasm of the angiographer is important. If the bleeding site is seen, intra-arterial infusion of vasopressin controls bleeding, at least transiently, in 35–90% of patients. Bleeding recurs after cessation of vasoconstrictor therapy in 50% of instances.

The other option for rapid bleeding is emergency colonoscopy without preliminary bowel cleansing. Blood is a cathartic, and the colon may be free of stool. Even so, colonoscopy in this situation is difficult. Experts are able to see the bleeding point in up to 50% of patients, and in 70% of cases bleeding can be localized to one region. Endoscopic therapeutic measures can be applied in up to 40% of patients, with success in one-half of them.

Operation is indicated for bleeding that persists or recurs despite angiographic and endoscopic therapeutic maneuvers. Operation is advisable also in good-risk patients who have stopped bleeding if the bleeding source is known and cannot be managed in some other way (eg, colonoscopic coagulation). Operation is limited to segmental colonic resection if the bleeding site has been localized conclusively. More extensive resection is usually warranted in patients who are bleeding from the right colon and have multiple diverticula in the left colon. If the surgeon has no preoperative localizing data and intraoperative examination is unrevealing, the stomach, small bowel, and colon can be endoscoped during the procedure to search for the source of blood. If all localizing efforts fail and the colon is the likely bleeding site, total abdominal colectomy (usually with primary anastomo-

sis) may be the only recourse. Fortunately, extensive "blind" colectomy is seldom required today.

The mortality rate from lower gastrointestinal hemorrhage is about 10–15%.

Bender JS, Wiencek RG, Bouwman DL: Morbidity and mortality following total abdominal colectomy for massive lower gastrointestinal bleeding. Am Surg 1991; 57:536.

Bentley DE, Richardson JD: The role of tagged red blood cell imaging in the localization of gastrointestinal bleeding. Arch Surg 1991;126:821.

Church JM: Analysis of the colonoscopic findings in patients with rectal bleeding according to the pattern of their presenting symptoms. Dis Colon Rectum 1991; 34:391.

Dent OF et al: Rectal bleeding. Patient delay in presentation. Dis Colon Rectum 1990;33:851.

Desa LA et al: Role of intraoperative enteroscopy in obscure gastrointestinal bleeding of small bowel origin. Br J Surg 1991;78:192.

Foutch PG, Sawyer R, Sanowski RA: Push-enteroscopy for diagnosis of patients with gastrointestinal bleeding of obscure origin. Gastrointest Endosc 1990;36:337.

Lewis BS et al: Small bowel enteroscopy and intraoperative enteroscopy for obscure gastrointestinal bleeding. Am J Gastroenterol 1991;86:171.

Naveau S et al: Long-term results of treatment of vascular malformations of the gastrointestinal tract by Neodymium YAG laser photocoagulation. Dig Dis Sci 1990;35:821.

Rex DK et al: Flexible sigmoidoscopy plus air contrast barium enema versus colonoscopy for suspected lower gastrointestinal bleeding. Gastroenterology 1990;98:855.

Richardson JD: : Vascular lesions of the intestines. Am J Surg 1991;161:284.

van Cutsem E, Rutgeerts P, Vantrappen G: Treatment of bleeding gastrointestinal vascular malformations with oestrogen-progesterone. Lancet 1990:335:953.

Voeller GR, Bunch G, Britt LG: Use of technetium-labeled red blood cell scintigraphy in the detection and management of gastrointestinal hemorrhage. Surgery 1991; 110:799.

ANGIODYSPLASIA

Angiodysplasia is an acquired condition most often affecting people over age 60. It is a focal submucosal vascular ectasia that has a propensity to bleed spontaneously. Most lesions are located in the cecum and proximal ascending colon, but in younger persons, they are occasionally found in the small bowel, principally the jejunum. Multiple lesions occur in 25% of cases. Aortic stenosis is found in patients with angiodysplasias, but whether they are truly related is still being argued. Von Willebrand's disease is present in some patients, and it has been suggested that the two conditions may be reflections of a generalized tissue disorder. Bleeding is typically intermittent and is rarely massive; a typical episode requires transfusion of two to four units of blood and is not associated with hypotension. Angiodysplasia may also present clinically as melena or as iron deficiency anemia and guaiac-positive stools.

The diagnosis is made in some cases by colonoscopy, and colonoscopic therapy is often successful. Incidental angiomas should be ignored. The lesions are characterized angiographically by (1) an early-filling vein (ie, within 4–5 seconds after injection), (2) a vascular tuft, and (3) a delayed-emptying vein. It is generally thought that two of the three features should be seen for the diagnosis to be secure. Active bleeding (ie, extravasation) is rarely demonstrated by angiography. As many as 25% of persons over age 60 with no history of gastrointestinal bleeding have angiodysplasias of the cecum, so the finding of a lesion is not proof that it has caused bleeding.

The natural history of angiodysplasia is not as yet well delineated, and in elderly, poor-risk patients who have bled only once or twice, expectant management may be preferable to surgery if colonoscopic therapeutic methods are unsuccessful. Operation should consist of a right hemicolectomy if the right colon was shown to be the bleeding site. It may be wise to resect the entire colon, with ileorectal anastomosis, in good-risk patients who also have extensive left-sided diverticulosis. In one series, 23% of patients who underwent operation for presumably bleeding colonic angiodysplasias were eventually found to have a small bowel lesion also.

Belli A-M, Hemingway AP: Malignant "angiodysplasia." Clin Radiol 1991;44:31.

Cottone C et al: Use of BICAP in a case of colon angiodysplasia. Surg Endosc 1991;5:99.

Helmrich GA, Stallworth JR, Brown JJ: Angiodysplasia: Characterization, diagnosis, and advances in treatment. South Med J 1990;83:1450.

Navab F et al: Angiodysplasia in patients with renal insufficiency. Am J Gastroenterol 1989;84:1297.

Richter JM et al: Angiodysplasia. Natural history and efficacy of therapeutic interventions. Dig Dis Sci 1989; 34:1542.

Vu H, Adams CZ Jr, Hoover EL: Jejunal angiodysplasia presenting as acute lower gastrointestinal bleeding. Am Surg 1990;56:302.

VOLVULUS

Essentials of Diagnosis

- Colicky abdominal pain, usually with persistence of pain between spasms.
- Abdominal distention.
- Vomiting sometimes.
- Usually older age groups.
- Characteristic x-ray findings.

General Considerations

Rotation of a segment of the intestine on an axis formed by its mesentery may result in partial or complete obstruction of the lumen and may be followed

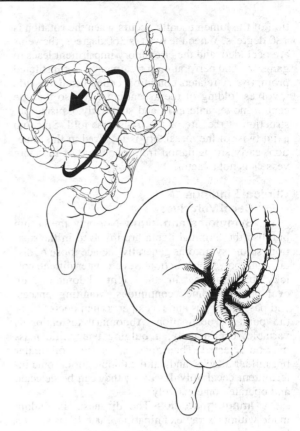

Figure 31–14. Volvulus of the sigmoid colon. The twist is counterclockwise in most cases of sigmoid volvulus.

by circulatory impairment of the bowel (Figure 31–14). Volvulus of the colon involves the cecum (30%), sigmoid (65%), transverse colon (3%), or splenic flexure (2%). Volvulus of the colon accounts for 5–10% of cases of large bowel obstruction in the USA and is the second most common cause of complete colonic obstruction. In certain developing countries where the population consumes a high-residue diet, volvulus is the most frequent cause of large bowel obstruction. Volvulus—sigmoid more often than cecal—accounts for 25% of intestinal obstructions during pregnancy; it occurs most often in the last trimester, probably because the enlarging uterus displaces the colon.

Elongation of the sigmoid and rectosigmoid is a predisposing factor in sigmoid volvulus; 50% of patients are over age 70, and many patients are mentally ill or bedridden persons who do not evacuate stool with regularity. Chagas' disease of the colon is an important cause of sigmoid volvulus in South America. Formation of cecal volvulus requires a cecum that is hypermobile owing to incomplete embryologic fixation of the ascending colon. The bowel twists about the mesentery, forming a closed loop obstruction as the entry and exit points of the twist engage; obstruction of the lumen usually occurs when the rotation is 180 degrees. When the twist is 360 degrees, the veins are occluded, and the circulatory impairment leads to gangrene and perforation if treatment is not instituted promptly. A related condition called **cecal bascule** involves folding of the ascending colon so that the cecum moves anteriorly and superiorly, causing obstruction at the site of the transverse fold. Since no axial twist of the mesentery is involved in this situation, early strangulation from occlusion of the main vessels is not a factor.

Clinical Findings

A. Cecal Volvulus:

1. Symptoms and signs—Not only the cecum but also the terminal ileum are involved in the rotation, so the symptoms generally include those of distal small bowel obstruction. Severe, intermittent, colicky pain begins in the right abdomen. Pain eventually becomes continuous, vomiting ensues, and passage of gas and feces per rectum decreases to the point of obstipation. Abdominal distention is variable; occasionally, a bulging tympanitic mass may be detected. There may be a history of similar but milder attacks, and valid examples of chronic intermittent cecal volvulus exist; they can be detected and operated on electively.

2. Imaging studies—The diagnosis is seldom made without x-ray examination. Plain films show a hugely dilated ovoid cecum that may change position but favors the epigastrium or left upper quadrant. In the early stages, there is a single fluid level that may be mistaken for gastric dilation, but large amounts of gas or fluid cannot be aspirated from the stomach, and the x-ray picture is not changed by this maneuver. Later, the radiologic findings of small bowel obstruction are superimposed on the cecal volvulus. The success rate of diagnosis based on plain abdominal films is extremely variable, ranging from 5% to 90%. Barium enema may be pathognomonic.

B. Sigmoid Volvulus:

1. Symptoms and signs—In volvulus of the sigmoid, there are intermittent cramp-like pains, increasing in severity as obstipation becomes complete. Abdominal distention may be marked. There may be a history of transient attacks in which spontaneous reduction of the volvulus has occurred.

2. Imaging studies—On a plain film of the abdomen, a single, greatly distended loop of bowel that has lost its haustral markings is usually seen rising up out of the pelvis, frequently as high as the diaphragm. The distended loop may assume a "coffee bean" shape. In cecal volvulus, the concavity of the "coffee bean" points toward the right lower abdominal quadrant, and in sigmoid volvulus it points toward the left lower quadrant. On barium enema, a "bird's beak" or "ace of spades" deformity with spiral narrowing of the upper end of the lower segment is pathognomonic (Figure 31–15). Between attacks, barium enema may

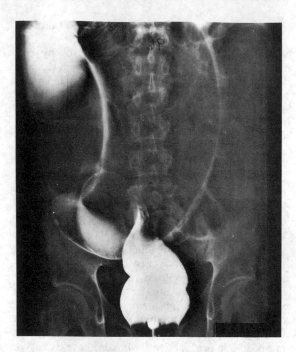

Figure 31–15. Volvulus of the sigmoid colon. Barium enema taken with the patient in the supine position. Note the massively dilated sigmoid colon. The distinct vertical crease, which represents juxtaposition of adjacent walls of the dilated loop, points toward the site of torsion. The barium column resembles a "bird's beak" or "ace of spades" because of the way in which the lumen tapers toward the volvulus.

reveal sigmoid megacolon. The entire colon may be termed a megacolon in some cases.

Differential Diagnosis

Cecal volvulus must be differentiated from colonic pseudo-obstruction and from other causes of small bowel and colonic obstruction. Sigmoid volvulus mimics other types of large bowel obstruction. Alertness to the possibility and correct interpretation of x-rays are the essentials of diagnosis.

Complications

Early diagnosis and treatment are imperative because perforation may occur if circulation to the bowel is impaired. Delay may be due to incorrect diagnosis or to futile attempts at proximal decompression by gastric intubation.

Treatment

In **cecal volvulus,** operation usually is advisable as soon as the patient can be prepared by replacing fluid and electrolyte deficits. Colonoscopic detorsion and decompression may be attempted instead in selected patients who have serious associated disease that would make operation hazardous. At laparotomy, the loop is untwisted and carefully inspected. If the bowel is viable, cecopexy (suture fixation of the bowel to the parietal peritoneum) gives good immediate results, but the long-term success rate is controversial; recurrent volvulus developed in 29% of patients after cecopexy in one review. Tube cecostomy both decompresses the cecum and fixes it, and this procedure is favored by some surgeons. Resection and anastomosis is preferred by others even if the bowel is viable, arguing that long-term results are better than with lesser procedures. Gangrenous colon or small bowel is found in about 20% of cases and requires right hemicolectomy; immediate anastomosis is performed in good-risk patients; otherwise, a temporary ileostomy is constructed, and continuity is restored later.

In many patients with **sigmoid volvulus,** the distended sigmoid can be decompressed by gentle insertion of a flexible colonoscope or sigmoidoscope. Decompression by passage of a tube through a rigid sigmoidoscope works well too, and some authorities argue that it should be tried first. Endoscopic decompression is contraindicated if there is evidence of strangulation or perforation. Percutaneous decompression of sigmoid volvulus has been reported, but it cannot be recommended for general use. If decompression is successful, good-risk young patients should be scheduled for elective resection as soon as the colon can be prepared, because the recurrence rate after decompression alone is 50%. No operation is indicated after endoscopic decompression of the first episode of sigmoid volvulus in elderly patients or those with severe disease of other organ systems. Emergency operation is performed if strangulation or perforation is suspected or if attempts to decompress the bowel per rectum are unsuccessful. Gangrenous bowel is found in about one-third of such patients and is treated by resection without anastomosis. If the sigmoid is viable, most surgeons proceed with resection, deferring anastomosis to a later time if the bowel is unprepared. If the entire colon is a megacolon, total abdominal colectomy should be considered. Recurrent volvulus in nonoperated patients is managed by transrectal decompression followed by a definitive surgical procedure in all patients but those with very severe associated disease.

Prognosis

The mortality rate after emergency operation in patients with cecal volvulus is 12%; if the bowel is gangrenous, 35% of patients die after resection. Recurrence after cecopexy or resection is very unusual.

Sigmoid volvulus is fatal in about 50% of patients with perforation; mortality rates are much lower with gangrene alone, and only 5% of patients die after operation if the bowel is viable. Elective resection after endoscopic decompression has a low mortality rate, and recurrent volvulus is rare.

Geer DA et al: Colonic volvulus: The Army Medical Center experience 1983–1987. Am Surg 1991;57:295.

Gibney EJ: Volvulus of the sigmoid colon. Surg Gynecol Obstet 1991;173:243.

Jacobs DM, Bubrick MP: Volvulus of the large intestine. Perspect Colon Rectal Surg 1990;3:34.

Peoples JB, McCafferty JC, Scher KS: Operative therapy for sigmoid volvulus: Identification of risk factors affecting outcome. Dis Colon Rectum 1990;33:643.

Rabinovici R et al: Cecal volvulus. Dis Colon Rectum 1990;33:765.

Theuer C, Cheadle WG: Volvulus of the colon. Am Surg 1991;57:145.

COLITIS

Colitis is a nonspecific term. Patients have diarrhea, abdominal pain, systemic symptoms, and abnormal endoscopic, radiographic, and laboratory tests. The task of the clinician is to differentiate among the various causes of colitis discussed below.

1. IDIOPATHIC MUCOSAL ULCERATIVE COLITIS

Essentials of Diagnosis

- Diarrhea, usually bloody.
- Abdominal cramps.
- Fever, weight loss, anemia.
- Absence of specific fecal pathogens.
- Endoscopic and radiographic abnormalities.

General Considerations

The age at onset of ulcerative colitis has a bimodal distribution, with the first peak between ages 15 and 30 years and a second, lower peak in the sixth to eighth decade. Females are affected slightly more often than males. The annual incidence varies from 5 to 12 per 100,000 population, and the prevalence is 50–150 per 100,000 population. The disease is found worldwide but is more common in Western countries. In 15–40% of patients, there is a family history of ulcerative colitis or Crohn's disease. In the USA, Jews are more commonly affected than non-Jews, but in Israel the prevalence among new immigrants is low.

The cause of ulcerative colitis is not known. The current hypothesis is that external agents, host responses, and genetic immunologic influences interact in the pathogenesis of inflammatory bowel disease. According to this concept, ulcerative colitis and Crohn's disease are different manifestations of a single disease process. The host becomes sensitized to the antigens of the inciting external agent or agents (eg, microbial, viral, or dietary). Once immunologic priming of the gut is established—perhaps during the period of microbial colonization in infancy—any insult that increases mucosal permeability to these antigens can precipitate an inflammatory reaction in the bowel wall. The types of antigens and many other factors determine the nature of the inflammatory process (eg, Crohn's disease or ulcerative colitis). Eicosanoids, metabolites of arachidonic acid, and platelet-activating factor are just two of many putative mediators of inflammation in colitis. A negative association between cigarette smoking and ulcerative colitis has been reported, but the significance is unclear.

Ulcerative colitis is a diffuse inflammatory disease confined to the mucosa initially. Abscesses form in the crypts of Lieberkühn, penetrate the superficial submucosa, and by spreading horizontally cause the overlying mucosa to slough. Vascular congestion and hemorrhage are prominent. The margins of the ulcers are raised as mucosal tags that project into the lumen (pseudopolyps or inflammatory polyps). Except in the most severe forms, the muscular layers are spared; the serosal surface usually shows only dilated congested blood vessels. In fulminant disease, when the full thickness is involved, the colon may dilate or perforate. The colon is shortened, but the mesocolon remains thin—in contrast to Crohn's disease.

Ulcerative colitis involves the rectum in most, but not all, patients. If confined to the rectum, as it is in one-half of cases, it is termed ulcerative proctitis. Inflammation may spread proximally to affect the left colon, and in about one-third of patients the entire colon becomes involved (pancolitis). A few centimeters of distal ileum are ulcerated in 10% of patients with pancolitis (backwash ileitis). The diseased areas are contiguous, ie, segmental disease or skip lesions are rare.

Clinical Findings

A. Symptoms and Signs: The cardinal symptoms are rectal bleeding and diarrhea: frequent discharges of watery stool mixed with blood, pus and mucus accompanied by tenesmus, rectal urgency, and even anal incontinence. Nearly two-thirds of patients have cramping abdominal pain and variable degrees of fever, vomiting, weight loss, and dehydration. The onset may be insidious or acute and fulminating, and the clinical findings differ accordingly. Mild disease may be manifested only by loose or frequent stools, and, paradoxically, a few patients complain of constipation. In isolated instances, the only symptoms may be from systemic complications such as arthropathy or pyoderma. Dairy products may aggravate diarrhea.

If the disease is mild, physical examination may be normal, but in severe disease the abdomen is tender, especially in the left lower quadrant, and the colon may be distended. The anus is often fissured, tender, and spastic, and the rectal mucosa feels gritty. The gloved examining finger may be covered with blood, mucus, or pus.

Sigmoidoscopy is essential. An enema should not be given before the examination. The rectal mucosa is granular, dull, hyperemic, and friable, so that the touch of a cotton swab causes oozing of blood. The submucosal vascular pattern is lost because of edema. Gross ulcers are not visible in the rectum in ulcerative colitis because of the superficial nature of these lesions. In more advanced disease, the mucosa is purplish-red, velvety, and extremely friable. Blood mixed with mucopus is evident in the lumen. The disease is uniform in the affected bowel, and patches of normal mucosa are not seen. If the mucosa is not grossly diseased, biopsy may be helpful to confirm the diagnosis. In the recovery phase, mucosal hyperemia and edema subside and inflammatory polyps may be seen. The healing mucosa is typically dull and granular and has a neovascular pattern of telangiectatic vessels that differs from the normal pink mucosa.

B. Laboratory Findings: Anemia, leukocytosis, and elevated sedimentation rate are usually present. Severe disease leads to hypoalbuminemia; depletion of water, electrolytes, and vitamins; and laboratory evidence of steatorrhea. Reduced plasma antithrombin III levels may contribute to thromboembolic complications. Smears of the stool should be examined for parasites, bacteria, and leukocytes, and stool should be sent for cultures.

C. Imaging Studies: Barium enema examination should not be preceded by catharsis in acute cases and should not be performed at all in severely ill patients, because it may precipitate acute colonic dilation. Plain films of the abdomen should be obtained serially during fulminant attacks in order to detect colonic dilation (megacolon) if it occurs.

Barium x-rays in acute ulcerative colitis show mucosal irregularity that varies from fine serrations to rough, ragged, undermined ulcers. As the disease progresses, haustrations are gradually effaced, and the colon narrows and shortens because of muscular rigidity (Figure 31–16). Pseudopolyposis signifies severe ulceration. Widening of the space between the sacrum and rectum is due either to periproctitis or to shortening of the bowel. The presence of a stricture should always arouse suspicion of cancer, although most strictures are benign.

The indium 111-labeled leukocyte scan is useful if the presence of inflammation in the colon is in question.

D. Colonoscopic Findings: Colonoscopy should be performed if sigmoidoscopic and radiographic findings are not diagnostic, and in fact endoscopy substitutes for barium enema in most situations. Usually the instrument need be inserted only into the sigmoid in order to make the initial diagnosis. Because of the danger of perforation, colonoscopy should be performed with great care if the disease is active, and it should not be done in the presence of colonic dilation. In chronic disease, colonoscopy with biopsies is valuable in surveillance for cancer. Strictures and other x-ray abnormalities can be investigated by colonoscopy also.

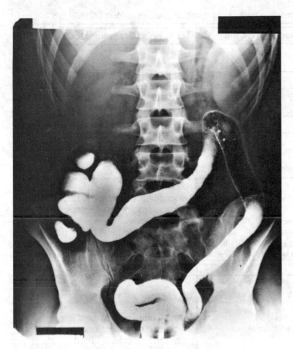

Figure 31–16. Ulcerative colitis. Barium enema roentgenogram of colon. Note shortening of colon, loss of haustral markings ("lead pipe" appearance), and fine serrations at the edges of the bowel wall that represent multiple small ulcers.

Differential Diagnosis

Malignant neoplasms of the colon (including lymphomas) and diverticular disease must be considered in the differential diagnosis. Salmonellosis and other bacillary dysenteries are diagnosed by repeated stool cultures. Shigellosis may be suspected on the basis of a positive methylene blue stain for fecal leukocytes. *Campylobacter jejuni* is a common cause of bloody diarrhea; the organisms can be cultured from the stool, and serum antibody titers rise during the illness. Hemorrhagic colitis—a syndrome of bloody diarrhea and abdominal cramps but no fever—is associated with infection by *Escherichia coli* O157:H7. *Legionella* infections can mimic ulcerative colitis. Gonococcal proctitis is detected by culture of rectal swabs. Herpes simplex virus is the most common cause of nongonococcal proctitis in homosexual men. *Chlamydia trachomatis* infections are also common in this group; the mucosa is markedly inflamed and resembles Crohn's disease; the organism can be cultured. It is most important in every case to rule out amebiasis (see Chapter 8) by microscopic examination of stool, rectal swabs, or rectal biopsies; serologic tests confirm that clinical infection has occurred. Corticosteroids must never be given to a patient with presumed idiopathic ulcerative colitis until amebiasis has been excluded.

Rare cases of histoplasmosis, tuberculosis, cytomegalovirus disease, schistosomiasis, amyloidosis, or Behçet's disease may be very difficult to diagnose. AIDS-related gastrointestinal infections are increasingly common. Colitis caused by antibiotics is discussed separately below; the history is important in this type of disease. Ischemic colitis has a segmental pattern of involvement quite unlike the usual distribution of ulcerative colitis. Functional diarrhea can mimic colitis, but organic disease must be excluded before it can be concluded that the diarrhea is functional. Malacoplakia is a rare chronic granulomatous disease that can cause colonic strictures and resemble colitis. Collagenous colitis has been reported; persistent watery diarrhea is the main symptom, mostly in middle-aged women, and sigmoidoscopy and colonoscopy are grossly normal. Biopsy specimens, however, show a thickened band of collagen just beneath the surface. The cause is obscure and treatment is difficult, but most patients are not seriously troubled by this condition.

Diversion colitis is inflammation of a previously normal segment of colon or rectum following construction of a temporary colostomy, eg, in a two-stage approach to diverticulitis. Deficiency of mucosal nutrients may be responsible, and inflammation may resolve with topical application of short-chain fatty acids. Restoration of intestinal continuity also solves the problem.

The most difficult differential diagnosis is between mucosal ulcerative colitis and Crohn's colitis (Table 31–7). None of the features is specific for one or the other disease, and often the differentiation can be made only after all the data have been assembled. About 10% of cases cannot be classified (indeterminate colitis).

Complications

The following **extracolonic manifestations** may occur in association with ulcerative colitis. There is an inexact relationship between the severity of the colitis and these complications: (1) lesions of the skin and mucous membranes, eg, erythema nodosum, erythema multiforme, pyoderma gangrenosum, pustular dermatitis, and aphthous stomatitis; (2) uveitis; (3) bone and joint lesions, eg, arthralgia, arthritis, and ankylosing spondylitis; (4) hepatobiliary and possibly pancreatic lesions, eg, fatty infiltration, pericholangitis, cirrhosis, sclerosing cholangitis, bile duct carcinoma, gallstones, and pancreatic insufficiency; (5) anemia, usually due to iron deficiency; (6) malnutrition and growth retardation; and (7) pericarditis. Sclerosing cholangitis may require liver transplantation.

Anorectal complications occur in 15–20% of patients with ulcerative colitis, a smaller percentage than in Crohn's colitis. Anal fissures are most common (about 12% of patients), and anorectal abscesses and fistulas are seen in 5% of patients.

Table 31–7. Comparison of various features of ulcerative colitis with those of granulomatous colitis.

	Ulcerative (Mucosal) Colitis	Crohn's (Granulomatous) Colitis
Signs and symptoms		
Diarrhea	Marked.	Present; less severe.
Gross bleeding	Characteristic.	Infrequent.
Perianal lesions	Infrequent, mild.	Frequent, complex; may precede diagnosis of intestinal disease.
Toxic dilatation	Yes (3–10%).	Yes (2–5%).
Perforation	Free.	Localized.
Systemic manifestations (arthritis, uveitis, pyoderma, hepatitis)	Common.	Common.
X-ray studies	Confluent, diffuse. Tiny serrations, coarse mucosa, mucosal tags. Concentric involvement. Internal fistulas very rare. Colon only except in backwash ileitis; may be limited to left side.	Skip areas. Longitudinal ulcers, transverse ridges, "cobblestone" appearance. Eccentric involvement. Internal fistulas common. Any portion of intestinal tract may be involved; may be limited to ileum and right colon.
Morphology		
Gross	Confluent involvement. Rectum usually involved. Mesocolon not involved; nodes enlarged. Widespread ragged superficial ulceration. Inflammatory polyps (pseudopolyps) common. No thickening of bowel wall.	Segmental involvement with or without skip areas. Rectum often not involved. Thickened mesocolon; pronounced lymph node enlargement. Large longitudinal ulcers or transverse fissures. Inflammatory polyps not prominent. Thickened bowel wall.
Microscopic	Inflammatory reaction usually limited to mucosa and submucosa; only in severe disease are muscle coats involved; no fibrosis. Granulomas rare.	Chronic inflammation of all layers of bowel wall; damage to muscle layers usual; submucosal fibrosis. Granulomas frequent.
Natural history	Exacerbations, remissions; may be explosive, lethal.	Indolent, recurrent.
Treatment		
Response to medical treatment	Good response in 85% of cases.	Difficult to evaluate; less well controlled over long term.
Type of surgical treatment and response	Colectomy with ileoanal anastomosis; proctocolectomy with conventional or continent ileostomy. No recurrence.	Segmental colectomy; total colectomy with ileorectal anastomosis; proctocolectomy if rectum severely diseased. Recurrence common.

Perforation of the colon, which occurs in about 3–5% of hospitalized patients, is responsible for more deaths than any other complication of ulcerative colitis. The risk of perforation is highest in the initial attack of the disease and correlates well with its extent and severity. It occurs most commonly in the sigmoid or splenic flexure and may result in a localized abscess or generalized fecal peritonitis. Any severely diseased colon may perforate, but patients with toxic dilation (megacolon) are especially vulnerable. Systemic therapy (corticosteroids and antibiotics) may mask the development of this complication.

Acute colonic dilation (toxic megacolon) occurs in approximately 3–10% of patients and in about 9% of patients coming to emergency operation. The pa-

tients are severely ill (toxic) and usually exhibit one or more of the following contributory factors: inflammation involving the muscular coats, hypokalemia, opiates, anticholinergics, and barium enema examinations. Toxic megacolon is diagnosed by plain abdominal x-rays or barium enemas, which show a thickened bowel wall and dilated lumen (greater than 6 cm in the transverse colon); often, the luminal air outlines irregular nodular pseudopolyps (Figure 31–17). Toxic dilation also occurs in Crohn's disease and in other types of colitis such as amebiasis and salmonellosis.

Massive hemorrhage is an uncommon but life-threatening complication.

Strictures develop in 10% of patients with ulcera-

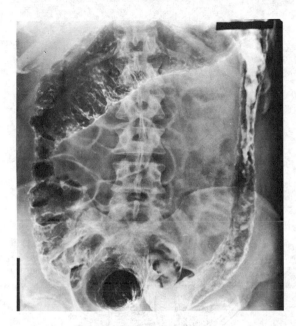

Figure 31–17. Barium enema showing acute colonic dilation in ulcerative colitis. Note dilation of the transverse colon, the multiple irregular densities in the lumen that represent pseudopolyps, and the loss of haustral markings.

tive colitis. They are more common in chronic disease, although they also appear in acute cases. Benign strictures are caused by thickening of the muscular coats, fibrosis, clusters of inflammatory polyps, or a combination of these processes. Carcinoma is of greatest concern.

Carcinoma of the colon or rectum begins to appear 5–8 years after onset of ulcerative colitis. By 10 years after onset, about 5% of patients have developed colorectal cancer; the cumulative incidence is 20–25% after 20 years and 30–40% by 30 years. Most of the factors previously thought to identify patients at greatest risk of cancer are unreliable (eg, age at onset, severity of first attack, and degree of activity of disease). The extent of colitis has limited usefulness as a predictor; although cancer develops earlier in the course of disease in pancolitis, left-sided colitis eventually gives rise to carcinoma at about the same rate. Cancers in colitis tend to be multicentric, less well differentiated, and perhaps more often right-sided. Some of them are difficult to recognize grossly by endoscopy or x-ray because they are small and flat. Vigilant surveillance is required; the most sensitive screening technique is annual or biennial colonoscopy with multiple mucosal biopsies to search for epithelial dysplasia. If high-grade dysplasia persists on serial biopsies, the chances of finding cancer in the colon are 30–50%, and colectomy should be performed promptly.

Treatment

A. Conservative Measures: The goals of conservative therapy are to terminate the acute attack as rapidly as possible and to prevent relapse. Management depends on the severity of the attack and the age group; children and the elderly present special problems.

1. Mild attack–Mild or insidious disease limited to the rectum and sigmoid usually can be checked with outpatient management. Reduced physical activity, even bed rest, is advisable. Diet should be free of bovine milk products and any other food that exacerbates diarrhea in the individual patient. Sulfasalazine, 2–8 g/d orally, is effective in controlling acute attacks. The active moiety of sulfasalazine is 5-aminosalicylic acid (5-ASA), which is also effective topically in a retention enema. Oral forms of 5-ASA (eg, mesalamine or olsalazine) are as effective as sulfasalazine and do not have as many adverse effects. Topical corticosteroids are indicated in many cases and may be administered as an enema (100 mg hydrocortisone in 60 mL of saline) or hydrocortisone acetate rectal foam. If these measures fail to relieve symptoms promptly, therapy should be intensified.

2. Severe attack–Severe or fulminating ulcerative colitis requires hospitalization. Nasogastric suction is required in patients with colonic dilation or those at risk of developing this complication. Although "bowel rest" has no special benefit, many ill patients are incapable of maintaining nutrition by oral intake, and total parenteral nutrition should be started early in these patients.

Corticosteroids are given intravenously initially as hydrocortisone (100–300 mg/d) or prednisolone (20–80 mg/d). Alternatively, corticotropin (ACTH) may be administered as an intravenous drip (20–40 units/8 h). Corticosteroids are given orally when oral feeding is resumed, and doses are tapered gradually over a period of 1–3 months. Topical corticosteroids may be instituted when the diarrhea abates. Sulfasalazine should be given orally if the patient is allowed to eat, but the most severely ill patients require intravenous broad-spectrum antibiotics. Hypokalemia is common and should be corrected. Caution should be exercised in administering anticholinergics and opiates, because they may precipitate acute dilation of the colon.

3. Maintenance–Controlled trials have shown that chronic administration of sulfasalazine (2 g/d orally) reduces relapse rates. A nightly enema of 5-ASA maintains remission in left-sided colitis. A suppository form also seems effective. Oral corticosteroids in doses small enough to avoid side effects are ineffective in preventing relapse. Topical corticosteroids may be useful maintenance therapy in patients with proctitis or proctosigmoiditis. Immunosuppressive therapy (mercaptopurine, azathioprine) is used by some physicians to treat ulcerative colitis in patients who cannot tolerate discontinuation of corticosteroid therapy. Cyclosporine is effective for patients who do not respond to steroids. The efficacy of metronidazole in ulcerative colitis remains unclear.

B. Surgical Treatment:

1. Indications–

a. Acute disease–Emergency operation is indicated for proved or suspected perforation of the colon. Urgent operation is performed for an acute problem (toxic megacolon, hemorrhage, or fulminating colitis) that is treated medically at first and then surgically if the response is inadequate. There are no firm guidelines for when to switch from medical to surgical therapy in these cases. If toxic megacolon does not respond to treatment within a few hours (*not* a few days), operation is necessary to avoid perforation. Fulminating disease without megacolon should improve in 4–5 days or less; otherwise, operation may be advisable.

b. Chronic disease–Intractable disease is difficult to define. Frequent exacerbations, chronic continuous symptoms, malnutrition, weakness, inability to work, incapacity to enjoy a full social and sexual life—all are elements of intractable disease. Exacerbation of disease when corticosteroids are tapered—and thus inability to discontinue these drugs over months or even years—is a compelling indication for colectomy. Children with chronic colitis may have impaired growth and development. Prevention or treatment of carcinoma is an important indication for operation. Severe extracolonic manifestations such as arthritis, pyoderma gangrenosum, or hepatobiliary disease may respond to colectomy. Some of these problems (eg, ankylosing spondylitis) do not improve after the diseased colon is removed.

2. Surgical procedures– Total colectomy with ileoanal anastomosis (restorative proctocolectomy, ileal pouch-anal anastomosis) is the elective operation of choice in most patients. Obesity and advanced age are limiting factors. In this procedure, the entire colon and rectum are excised, and the ileum (made into a reservoir or pouch) is brought into the pelvis and anastomosed to the anal canal just above the dentate line (Figure 31–18). Rectal mucosectomy was once routine, but many surgeons now do not strip the mucosa at all; instead, the full thickness of rectum is excised to eliminate disease while preserving good rectal function. A temporary ileostomy is used by most surgeons to protect the ileoanal anastomosis for 2–3 months. A successful outcome is expected in 95% of patients. Pouchitis (inflammation of the reservoir, presumably from bacterial overgrowth) is a complication.

Proctocolectomy with permanent conventional ileostomy or continent ileostomy is chosen in patients who may not be candidates for the ileoanal procedure. In an emergency operation, the rectum is preserved to minimize operative complications in an ill patient and to make it possible to do an ileoanal pro-

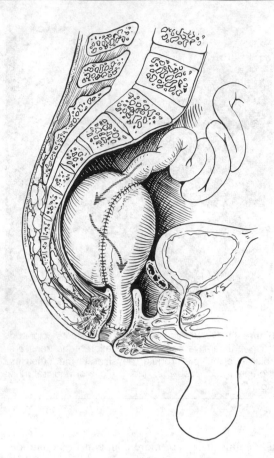

Figure 31–18. Lateral view of the pelvis after colectomy and ileoanal anastomosis in a male. The S pouch, shown here, is one of several types of reservoirs; the J pouch and the W pouch have come to be favored by most surgeons in recent years. The pouch is anastomosed to the anal canal just above the dentate line. The distal anorectal stump as depicted is longer than is usually the practice today.

cedure later. The operation therefore usually consists of total abdominal colectomy (subtotal colectomy) and ileostomy with a distal mucous fistula or Hartmann procedure. Ileorectal anastomosis (ileoproctostomy, ileorectostomy) is seldom used for ulcerative colitis today.

Prognosis

The mortality rate of ulcerative colitis has dropped sharply in the last decade or two, and older figures no longer apply. First attacks are seldom fatal when treated by specialists. In one large series, emergency colectomy was required in 25% of patients with severe first attacks; 60% responded rapidly to medical therapy; and 15% improved slowly on medications alone. Overall, the colitis-related mortality rate during the year after onset is about 1%. Colorectal cancer arising in association with ulcerative colitis has a prognosis similar to cancer in the absence of colitis if equivalent stages are compared, but colitis-associated cancer is more often diagnosed at a later stage.

The long-term prognosis of ulcerative proctitis is good; about 10% of patients will develop colonic disease by 10 years, and the mortality rate is very low. If colitis involves the left colon, the prognosis is worse, and in patients with pancolitis, the likelihood of operation during the first year is about 25% and the mortality rate is 5% over 10 years.

Emergency colectomy has a mortality rate of 6%; most of these deaths are due to perforation, a complication that has a fatal outcome in 40% of cases. The operative mortality rate is less than 1% for elective colectomy. In an estimated 90% of survivors, colectomy with ileostomy is consistent with normal life, but a few patients experience problems such as small bowel obstruction and ileostomy dysfunction. Altered sexual function after proctectomy occurs in about 12% of men overall, limited mostly to those over age 50. True impotence is found in 3% of men. Sexual dysfunction in women relates to change of body image, the presence of an ileostomy, and pelvic fibrosis. Most patients believe that ileoanal anastomosis gives a better quality of life than does an ileostomy.

Adler DJ, Korelitz BI: The therapeutic efficacy of 6- mercaptopurine in refractory ulcerative colitis. Am J Gastroenterol 1990;85:717.

Alemayehu G, Järnerot G: Colonoscopy during an attack of severe ulcerative colitis is a safe procedure and of great value in clinical decision making. Am J Gastroenterol 1991;86:187.

Asztély M et al: Radiological study of changes in the pelvis in women following proctocolectomy. Int J Colorect Dis 1991;6:103.

Biddle WL, Miner PB Jr: Long-term use of mesalamine enemas to induce remission in ulcerative colitis. Gastroenterology 1990;99:113.

Christie PM, Hill GL: Effect of intravenous nutrition on nutrition and function in acute attacks of inflammatory bowel disease. Gastroenterology 1990;99:730.

de Silva HJ et al: Clinical and functional outcome after restorative proctocolectomy. Br J Surg 1991;78:1039.

Ekbom A et al: Ulcerative colitis and colorectal cancer. A population-based study. N Engl J Med 1990;323:1228.

Ekbom A et al: Ulcerative proctitis in Central Sweden 1965–1983: A population-based epidemiological study. Dig Dis Sci 1991;36:97.

Ferguson CM, Siegel RJ: A prospective evaluation of diversion colitis. Am Surg 1991;57:46.

Gitnick G (editor): *Inflammatory Bowel Disease. Diagnosis and Treatment.* Igaku-Shoin, 1991.

Guillemot F et al: Treatment of diversion colitis by short-chain fatty acids: A prospective and double-blind study. Dis Colon Rectum 1991;34:861.

Jenkins D, Goodall A, Scott BB: Ulcerative colitis: One disease or two? (Quantitative histological differences between distal and extensive disease.) Gut 1990;31:426.

Köhler LW et al: Quality of life after proctocolectomy: A comparison of Brooke ileostomy, Kock pouch, and ileal pouch-anal anastomosis. Gastroenterology 1991;101:679.

LaRosa D et al: Maintenance oral sulfasalazine prolongs remission in ulcerative proctitis and proctosigmoiditis. Am J Gastroenterol 1991;86:1456.

Leijonmarck CE, Persson PG, Hellers G: Factors affecting colectomy rate in ulcerative colitis: An epidemiologic study. Gut 1990;31:329. Lennard-Jones JE et al: Precancer and cancer in extensive ulcerative colitis: Findings among 401 patients over 22 years. Gut 1990;31:800.

Lichtiger S, Present DH: Preliminary report: Cyclosporin in treatment of severe active ulcerative colitis. Lancet 1990;336:16.

Löfberg R et al: Colonoscopic surveillance in long-standing total ulcerative colitis: A 15-year follow-up study. Gastroenterology 1990;99:1021.

Madden MV, Farthing MJG, Nicholls RJ: Inflammation in ileal reservoirs: "pouchitis." Gut 1990;31:247.

McLeod RS et al: Quality of life of patients with ulcerative colitis preoperatively and postoperatively. Gastroenterology 1991;101:1307.

Monsén U et al: Extracolonic diagnoses in ulcerative colitis: An epidemiological study. Am J Gastroenterol 1990;85:711.

Niv Y, Abukasis G: Prevalence of ulcerative colitis in the Israeli Kibbutz population. J Clin Gastroenterol 1991;13:98.

Nugent FW, Haggitt RC, Gilpin PA: Cancer surveillance in ulcerative colitis. Gastroenterology 1991;100:1241.

Olsson R et al: Prevalence of primary sclerosing cholangitis in patients with ulcerative colitis. Gastroenterology 1991;100:1319.

Orholm M et al: Familial occurrence of inflammatory bowel disease. N Engl J Med 1991;324:84.

Prantera C et al: The plain abdominal film accurately estimates extent of active ulcerative colitis. J Clin Gastroenterol 1991;13:231.

Podolsky DK: Inflammatory bowel disease. (Two parts.) N Engl J Med 1991;325:928, 1008.

Riddell RH (editor): *Dysplasis and Cancer in Colitis.* Elsevier, 1991.

Riley SA et al: Why do patients with ulcerative colitis relapse? Gut 1990;31:179.

Samuelsson S-M et al: Risk factors for extensive ulcerative colitis and ulcerative proctitis: A population based case-control study. Gut 1991;32:1526.

Sedgwick DM et al: Population-based study of surgery in juvenile onset ulcerative colitis. Br J Surg 1991;78:176.

Stampfl DA, Friedman LS: Collagenous colitis: Pathophysiologic considerations. Dig Dis Sci 1991;36:705.

Steinhart AH et al: Azathioprine therapy in chronic ulcerative colitis. J Clin Gastroenterol 1990;12:271.

Telander RL et al: Long-term follow-up of the ileoanal anastomosis in children and young adults. Surgery 1990;108:717.

Walsh RM, Aranha GV, Freeark RJ: Mortality and quality of life after total abdominal colectomy. Arch Surg 1990;125:1564.

Wells AD et al: Natural history of indeterminate colitis. Br J Surg 1991;78:179.

Wexner SD, James K, Jagelman DG: The double-stapled ileal reservoir and ileoanal anastomosis: A prospective review of sphincter function and clinical outcome. Dis Colon Rectum 1991;34:487.

Zinberg J, Molinas S, Das KM: Double-blind placebo-controlled study of olsalazine in the treatment of ulcerative colitis. Am J Gastroenterol 1990;85:562.

2. CROHN'S COLITIS (Granulomatous Colitis)

The general features of Crohn's disease (regional enteritis, granulomatous colitis, transmural colitis) are described in Chapter 30. Approximately 50% of patients with Crohn's disease have both small and large bowel involvement, 25% have colonic disease alone, and another 3% have anorectal involvement only. Diarrhea, cramping abdominal pain, constitutional effects, and extraintestinal manifestations are approximately the same in colonic and enteric disease. Internal fistulas and abscesses and intestinal obstruction are usually complications of small bowel disease. Anorectal complications (anal fistula, fissure, abscess, and rectal stricture) and hemorrhage are more common when the large bowel is affected, and toxic dilation is limited to patients with inflammation of the colon.

Typical anal lesions of Crohn's disease are large undermined indolent ulcers. The perianal skin has a violaceous hue, and if fistulas are present, they tend to be multiple and complex. Proctosigmoidoscopy discloses a normal rectum in 50% of patients with Crohn's colitis. Diseased mucosa is patchily involved, with irregular ulcerations separated by edematous or even normal-appearing mucosa. Biopsy may confirm the diagnosis. Radiographic features include sparing of the rectum, right colonic and ileal involvement, skip areas, transverse fissures, longitudinal ulcers, strictures, and fistulas. Features differentiating Crohn's from ulcerative colitis are summarized in Table 31–7. Ischemic colitis is another disease that may be confused with Crohn's colitis, and the differential diagnosis is discussed below. *Chlamydia trachomatis* infection is diagnosed by culture of the organism. Malacoplakia is a rare chronic granulomatous disease that can cause colonic strictures, and Behçet's disease is another rare condition that can mimic inflammatory bowel disease. Tuberculosis and amebiasis must be considered too.

Frank blood in the stools is observed in about one-third of patients with granulomatous colitis, but massive hemorrhage is unusual. Acute colonic dilation (toxic megacolon) occurs in 5%; it responds to nonoperative treatment more often than it does in ulcerative colitis.

Actuarial methods suggest that the risk of colonic cancer in granulomatous colitis patients is 4–20 times that of the general population, and it appears that segments of intestine excluded from the fecal stream (eg, an isolated rectal stump or bypassed ileum) are especially vulnerable. Carcinoma can also arise in anorectal or rectovaginal fistulas. The small bowel is at risk for development of cancer in patients with regional enteritis with or without colitis. Epithelial dysplasia is associated with cancer in Crohn's disease as well as in ulcerative colitis, but this indicator is not helpful for the areas at greatest risk (eg, bypassed segments of small bowel or colon) because they cannot be examined endoscopically. Surveillance colonoscopy may be worthwhile in colonic Crohn's disease, though it has not been routine in the past.

Medical management of Crohn's disease of the small bowel is described in Chapter 30. Steroids are effective for acute attacks, but they are not advisable for maintenance therapy because of limited benefit and frequent complications. Sulfasalazine (4 g daily) is effective in the treatment of Crohn's colitis. Oral 5-ASA preparations are beneficial also, and both 5-ASA enemas and 5-ASA suppositories are helpful for Crohn's disease of the rectum and sigmoid. These agents are steroid-sparing, ie, they allow the dosage of steroids to be reduced. Metronidazole, 10–20 mg/kg/d orally in three to five doses, is used for treatment of anal complications of Crohn's disease. Abscesses and fistulas improve with less pain and drainage, but full permanent healing is unusual, and the disease worsens when the drug is discontinued. Immunosuppressants (azathioprine, mercaptopurine) are steroid-sparing drugs that seem to control Crohn's colitis well enough that surgery is delayed or avoided. Cyclosporine is effective in refractory cases.

Surgical treatment is indicated for intractability, abscess or fistula, obstruction, fulminant disease, anorectal disease, hemorrhage, or cancer. Segmental colectomy with primary anastomosis is useful for limited disease. Total colectomy with ileorectal anastomosis is done more frequently in Crohn's than in ulcerative colitis. Proctocolectomy with ileostomy is needed if rectal disease is severe and the colon needs resection also. Internal bypass of severe disease is seldom used today. Diverting ileostomy improves the clinical status of patients, but few patients obtain lasting benefit. Colostomy may relieve pain in patients with anorectal disease. Perianal complications can be treated directly (eg, by fistulotomy) in carefully selected patients whose Crohn's disease is inactive.

There is a high rate of recurrence at intestinal anastomoses (50–75% at 15 years). Recurrence is less common following proctocolectomy and ileostomy (about 15% at 15 years, but there is a wide disparity—3–46%—among different reports on this controversial topic).

Surgical procedures—like medical therapy—should be regarded as palliative, not curative, in patients with Crohn's disease. Although recurrence rates are high and chronic disease is common, a productive life is usually possible with the aid of combined medical and surgical management. The mortality rate is about 15% over 30 years. Urolithiasis is a common sequela of resection for Crohn's disease.

Brynskov J et al: A placebo-controlled, double-blind, randomized trial of cyclosporine therapy in active chronic Crohn's disease. N Engl J Med 1989;321:845.

Deutsch AA et al: Results of the pelvic-pouch procedure in patients with Crohn's disease. Dis Colon Rectum 1991; 34:475.

Ekbom A et al: The epidemiology of inflammatory bowel disease: A large, population-based study in Sweden. Gastroenterology 1991;100:350.

Fasoli R et al: Response to faecal challenge in defunctioned colonic Crohn's disease: prediction of long-term course. Br J Surg 1990;77:616.

Harling H et al: Fate of the rectum after colectomy and ileostomy for Crohn's colitis. Dis Colon Rectum 1991;34:931.

Levitt MD et al: Pyoderma gangrenosum in inflammatory bowel disease. Br J Surg 1991;78:676.

Okada M et al: Minute lesions of the rectum and sigmoid colon in patients with Crohn's disease. Gastrointest Endosc 1991;37:319.

Rubio CA et al: Crohn's disease and adenocarcinoma of the intestinal tract: Report of four cases. Dis Colon Rectum 1991;34:174.

Sachar DB: Inflammatory bowel disease: Back to the future. Am J Gastroenterol 1990;85:373.

Savoca PE, Ballantyne GH, Cahow CE: Gastrointestinal malignancies in Crohn's disease: A 20-year experience. Dis Colon Rectum 1990;33:7.

Sitzmann JV, Converse RL Jr, Bayless TM: Favorable response to parenteral nutrition and medical therapy in Crohn's colitis: A report of 38 patients comparing severe Crohn's and ulcerative colitis. Gastroenterology 1990;99:1647.

Stowe SP et al: An epidemiologic study of inflammatory bowel disease in Rochester, New York: Hospital incidence. Gastroenterology 1990;98:104.

Van Outryve MJ et al: Value of transrectal ultrasonography in Crohn's disease. Gastroenterology 1991;101:1171.

Williams JG, Hughes LE: Abdominoperineal resection for severe perianal Crohn's disease. Dis Colon Rectum 1990;33:402.

Yamazaki Y et al: Malignant colorectal strictures in Crohn's disease. Am J Gastroenterol 1991;86:882.

3. ANTIBIOTIC-ASSOCIATED COLITIS

A spectrum of adverse colonic responses may develop in hospitalized patients during or after antibiotic therapy. There may be diarrhea without gross mucosal abnormality (antibiotic-associated diarrhea), gross inflammation of the mucosa, or whitish-green or yellow plaques on the inflamed mucosa (pseudomembranous colitis). It is not clear whether one or several pathologic processes are responsible. Patients may progress from mild to more severe disease. The differential diagnosis among these variations is based on endoscopic findings and the clinical picture.

Clostridium difficile is a resident of the gut in 3% of people in the general population and about 10% of patients admitted to hospital. It is the major known cause of nosocomial antibiotic-associated diarrhea and colitis. Certain antibiotics allow the organism to proliferate, and then it is transmitted among patients and hospital personnel. Epidemics of *C difficile* infection have been noted on surgical wards.

C. difficile may colonize the upper gastrointestinal tract as well as the colon, but the symptomatic infection appears at present to be colonic alone. The organism elaborates at least four toxins, including toxin A (an enterotoxin) and toxin B (a cytotoxin). Together these substances—and perhaps others—produce the symptoms and signs. Clindamycin causes watery diarrhea in 15–30% of patients and true pseudomembranous colitis in 1–10%. Lincomycin, ampicillin, cephalosporins, and penicillin are also common inciting antibiotics. Many others have been implicated, including metronidazole. Parenteral aminoglycosides seem to be an exception. Colitis may develop as early as 2 days after beginning antibiotics or as late as 3 weeks after they are discontinued.

Symptoms and signs include diarrhea (usually watery, occasionally bloody), abdominal cramps, vomiting, fever, and leukocytosis. Sigmoidoscopy in pseudomembranous colitis shows elevated plaques or a confluent pseudomembrane, and the mucosa is erythematous and edematous. Biopsies reveal acute inflammation; the pseudomembrane is made up of leukocytes, necrotic epithelial cells, and fibrin. The rectum is spared in about one-fourth of cases, and colonoscopy may be necessary to detect the presence of pseudomembranous colitis. Culture of *C difficile* and detection of *C difficile* cytotoxin in the stool are necessary to prove that this organism is responsible for the colitis. Barium enema, CT, or ultrasound may assist with the diagnosis.

Management consists first of discontinuing the inciting antibiotic agent. In most patients, the colitis resolves in 1–2 weeks after the offending agent is withdrawn, but severe symptoms or persistent diarrhea calls for additional treatment. Oral cholestyramine (4 g every 6 hours for 5 days) is sufficient in mild cases; it acts by binding clostridial toxin. Vancomycin (125–500 mg orally four times daily for 7–10 days) is expensive but effective, although the relapse rate is 15–20% after vancomycin is discontinued. Metronidazole, 1.5–2 g/d orally for 7–14 days, is also effective and much less expensive. Paradoxically, metronidazole can also cause antibiotic-associated colitis. Bacitracin is an effective drug and, like vancomycin, is not absorbed from the gastrointestinal tract. Antidiarrheal drugs may prolong symptoms and should be avoided. Oral administration of *Saccharomyces boulardii,* a nonpathogenic yeast, has been successful in treatment of recurrent *C difficile* colitis in an experimental setting.

The outcome of pseudomembranous colitis and the other forms of antibiotic-associated colonic disease is usually excellent if the disease is recognized and treated. Untreated pseudomembranous colitis, however, may lead to severe dehydration and electrolyte imbalance, toxic megacolon, or colonic perforation. Operation is required for perforation or toxic dilation. Chronic relapsing *C difficile* diarrhea has been treated by rectal instillation of mixed colonic bacteria (bacteriotherapy).

Bergstein JM et al: Pseudomembranous colitis: How useful is endoscopy? Surg Endosc 1990;4:217.

Fishman EK et al: Pseudomembranous colitis: CT evaluation of 26 cases. Radiology 1991;180:57.

Gerding DN et al: *Clostridium difficile* diarrhea and colonization after treatment with abdominal infection regimens containing clindamycin or metronidazole. Am J Surg 1990;159:212.

Johnson S et al: Nosocomial *Clostridium difficile* colonisation and disease. Lancet 1990;336:97.

Johnson S et al: Prospective, controlled study of vinyl glove use to interrupt *Clostridium difficile* nosocomial transmission. Am J Med 1990;88:137.

Kimmey M et al: Prevention of further recurrences of *Clostridium difficile* colitis with *Saccharomyces boulardii.* Dig Dis Sci 1990;35:897.

Kofsky P et al: *Clostridium difficile*: A common and costly colitis. Dis Colon Rectum 1991;34:244.

Triadafilopoulos G, Hallstone AE: Acute abdomen as the first presentation of pseudomembranous colitis. Gastroenterology 1991;101:685.

Yee J et al: *Clostridium difficile* disease in a Department of Surgery. Arch Surg 1991;126:241.

4. ISCHEMIC COLITIS

Ischemic colitis is caused by mesenteric vascular occlusion or nonocclusive mechanisms (Chapter 30). A common precipitating event is abdominal aortic reconstruction with interruption of a vital blood supply such as the inferior mesenteric artery. An entity that resembles ischemic colitis sometimes develops proximal to obstructing colonic carcinoma. Isolated ischemia of the right colon is seen in patients with chronic heart disease, especially aortic stenosis. Ischemic colitis most often afflicts the elderly (average age 60 years), but it also occurs in younger adults in association with diabetes mellitus, systemic lupus erythematosus, or sickle cell crisis. Pancreatitis can occlude mesocolic vessels.

Ischemic colitis is categorized as reversible or irreversible. Reversible ischemia heals with nonoperative treatment, sometimes with stricture formation. Over half of the patients have a reversible injury. The severe form is fulminant from onset or may pursue an indolent course without resolution for weeks. Both of the severe forms require operation.

Patients with ischemic colitis have an abrupt onset of abdominal pain, diarrhea (commonly bloody), and systemic symptoms. The abdomen may be tender diffusely, in a localized area (eg, left lower quadrant), or not at all. Blood is seen coming from above at sigmoidoscopy; if the rectum itself is ischemic—an unusual occurrence—the mucosa is edematous, hemorrhagic, friable, and sometimes ulcerated. A grayish membrane may be present, resembling pseudomembranous colitis. The same abnormalities are seen in the ischemic segment examined with the flexible sigmoidoscope or colonoscope. Serum alkaline phosphatase is elevated in some cases. Plain abdominal x-rays are nonspecific. Barium enema x-rays show "thumbprints" or pseudotumors, typically limited to a 6- to 20-cm segment; 75% or more have involvement of the left colon. CT scan shows a thickened colonic wall, and it also helps exclude other conditions. Mesenteric arteriography may show major arterial occlusion or no abnormalities and is not recommended as a rule.

Differentiating ischemic colitis from carcinoma, ulcerative colitis, and diverticulitis should not be difficult, but Crohn's disease presents a greater diagnostic problem. Rectal bleeding—especially gross hemorrhage—is less common in Crohn's disease, and the rapid onset of ischemic colitis is also different from Crohn's disease. Radiographic findings and, in some cases, the colonoscopic appearance may be helpful, but often the natural history of the acute attack is the only way to make the distinction. Acute mesenteric ischemia may be difficult to exclude (see Chapter 30), but the more benign presentations of reversible ischemic colonic injury are not seen with ischemia of the small intestine. *C difficile* is cultured from stool in pseudomembranous colitis.

Therapy for reversible ischemic colitis consists of intravenous fluids, antibiotics, and observation to be certain the problem is in fact reversible. Irreversible disease, whether fulminant from the beginning, becoming more severe over several days, or just failing to resolve after treatment, should be treated by operation. The diseased colon is resected; anastomosis is usually deferred if the colon is unprepared. Because patients with severe ischemia often have multiple other medical problems, the overall mortality rate is 50%.

Boley SJ: Colonic ischemia: 25 years later. Am J Gastroenterol 1990;85:931.

Brewster DC et al: Intestinal ischemia complicating abdominal aortic surgery. Surgery 1991;109:447.

Kaleya RN, Boley SJ: Colonic ischemia. Perspect Colon Rectal Surg 1990;3:62.

Parish KL, Chapman WC, Williams LF Jr: Ischemic colitis: An ever-changing spectrum? Am Surg 1991;57:118.

5. NEUTROPENIC COLITIS

Neutropenic colitis (neutropenic typhlitis, ileocecal syndrome, necrotizing enteropathy, agranulocytic colitis) occurs as colonic necrosis in neutropenic patients. Although the cecum and right colon are most often affected, all parts of the large bowel can be involved. Acute leukemia, aplastic anemia, and cyclic neutropenia are the underlying diseases in which this lesion occurs. Colonic perforation during treatment with interleukin-2 is probably related. The pathogenesis is not well understood, but responsible factors probably include mucosal ischemia, necrosis of intramural leukemic infiltrates, shock, hemorrhage into the bowel wall, chemotherapy, and corticosteroid therapy. The mucosa ulcerates, permitting bacterial invasion into the bowel wall, thrombosis of intramural vessels, necrosis, and perforation.

As many as 25% of patients with acute myeloblastic leukemia may develop typhlitis, and during induction chemotherapy the incidence may be much higher. Fever, watery or bloody diarrhea, abdominal discomfort and distention, and nausea are noted first. Pain and tenderness may then become localized to the right lower quadrant, and systemic toxicity increases. Careful examination and x-ray studies are required. Nasogastric suction, parenteral nutrition, and antibiotic therapy are instituted. Operation (resection of the involved colon) is performed for persistent unresponsive sepsis, perforation, obstruction, severe bleeding, or abscess formation. Neutropenic colitis can recur after medical therapy.

Katz JA et al: Typhlitis: An 18-year experience and post-mortem review. Cancer 1990;65:1041.

Musher DR et al: Neutropenic typhlitis simulating carcinoma of the cecum. Gastrointest Endosc 1989;35:449.

Wade DS et al: Abdominal pain in neutropenic patients. Arch Surg 1990;125:1119.

INTESTINAL STOMAS
(Ileostomy & Colostomy)

An intestinal stoma is an opening of the bowel onto the surface of the abdomen. It may be temporary or permanent. Esophagostomy, gastrostomy, jejunostomy, and cecostomy are usually temporary, but ileostomy, colostomy, and some urinary tract stomas are often permanent. Although "stoma" is the preferred medical term, "ostomy" is used by lay organizations devoted to the rehabilitation of these patients.

Few surgical alterations of anatomy are surrounded by as much misunderstanding as intestinal stomas, and few pronouncements by surgeons are as horrifying to patients as the indication that a stoma will be necessary. For these and other reasons, a paramedical profession, **enterostomy therapy,** has developed. The enterostomal therapist (ET) is usually a registered nurse who has taken specialized training and is certified in the field. The enterostomal therapist provides the following services: (1) preoperative education and counseling of patient and family; (2) immediate postoperative care of the stoma; (3) training in the use of equipment and supervision of self-care; (4) fitting of a permanent appliance; (5) advice on day-to-day living with a stoma; (6) management of skin problems and odor control; (7) recognition of surgical stoma problems; (8) long-term emotional, moral, and physical support; and (9) information about the United Ostomy Association, an organization with chapters in many localities.

ILEOSTOMY

Permanent ileostomy is performed most commonly after proctocolectomy for ulcerative colitis; patients with Crohn's disease, familial polyposis, and other conditions may also require ileostomy. A temporary (loop) ileostomy often is used to divert the fecal stream for several weeks when ileoanal anastomosis is performed. An ileostomy discharges small quantities of liquid material continuously; it does not require irrigation; and an appliance must be worn at all times.

The optimal position of the stoma is in the right lower quadrant (Figure 31–19). The ileum is brought through the rectus abdominis muscle, everted upon itself, and the mucosa is sutured to the skin (surgically matured). An appliance is placed immediately; it consists of a plastic bag attached to a square sheet of protective material containing a central opening for the stoma. A reusable appliance can be fitted after a few weeks, but modern disposable appliances are so satisfactory that most patients never do change to the other type. Appliances lie flat against the abdomen, adhere firmly to the skin, are inconspicuous and odor-proof, and need be changed only every 3–5 days in most cases. They are drained at intervals during the day through an opening in the bottom of the pouch.

A **continent ileostomy** (reservoir ileostomy, Kock pouch) is designed to avoid the continual discharge of ileal effluent that necessitates construction of a protruding stoma and the wearing of an appliance at all times. A reservoir is constructed out of the distal ileum, and the outlet from the reservoir is arranged as a valve so that fluid cannot escape onto the abdominal wall. The reservoir is emptied several times a day by inserting a catheter into the stoma. Continent ileostomy is successful in 70–90% of patients. Problems with the valve, fistulas, and "pouchitis" (mucosal inflammation in the reservoir, presumably due to bacterial stasis) are causes of failure. Crohn's disease is a contraindication, because of the risk of recurrence necessitating excision of the reservoir.

Physiologic changes after ileostomy are due to the loss of the water- and salt-absorbing capacity of the colon. If the small bowel is free of disease and extensive resection has not been done, an ileostomy puts out 1–2 L of fluid per day initially (Table 31–1). The volume of effluent diminishes to between 500 and

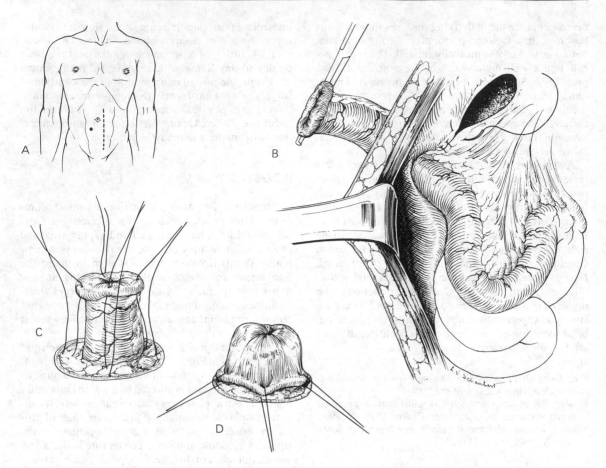

Figure 31–19. Ileostomy after colectomy. **A:** A paramedian incision for colectomy is indicated by the dotted line and the site of the ileostomy by the black dot. (A midline incision is favored by many surgeons.) **B:** The ileum has been brought through the abdominal wall. **C and D:** The ileostomy stoma has been everted and its margins sutured to the edges of the wound.

800 mL/d after a month or two. This loss of fluid is obligatory and is not reduced by manipulations of diet. Obligatory sodium losses are about 50 meq/d greater than in patients with an intact colon, and potassium losses are also increased. Healthy ileostomy patients have low total exchangeable sodium and potassium but normal serum electrolyte concentrations. The depletion, therefore, is primarily intracellular. The patient with an ileostomy is susceptible to acute or subacute salt and water depletion manifested by fatigue, anorexia, irritability, headache, drowsiness, muscle cramps, and thirst. Gastroenteritis or diarrhea from any cause and exposure to hot weather or vigorous exercise are situations that require caution; salt and water intake must be increased in these circumstances. Ileostomy patients must never be in a position where salt and water are unavailable, eg, on long hikes in the desert. Low-salt diets and diuretics may induce salt depletion or dehydration also. Patients should be counseled to salt food liberally, but salt tablets will not be required in usual circumstances.

Patients with unusually high ileostomy outputs may need supplemental potassium in the form of bananas or orange juice. Water intake in response to thirst may not be adequate to maintain hydration, and patients should consume enough water to keep the urine pale or to maintain a urine output of at least 1 L/d.

Patients must be informed about these physiologic alterations and measures to compensate for them. Otherwise, instructions are simple, and patients should live normally. A low-residue diet should be advised at least initially. Certain foods (eg, fish, eggs) may cause excessive odor or gas. Ordinary physical activity, employment, and social activities are encouraged. Bathing, swimming, sexual intercourse, and pregnancy and delivery are unrestricted.

Complications are reported in about 40% of patients with conventional ileostomy; about 15% require operative correction, usually minor. Complications include the following:

(1) Intestinal obstruction: Obstruction may be

due to adhesive bands, volvulus, or paraileostomy herniation of bowel.

(2) Stenosis: Circumferential scar formation at the skin or subcutaneous level is usually at fault. Stenosis may cause profuse watery discharge from the ileostomy. Treatment requires a minor local procedure to release the scar.

(3) Retraction: The stoma should protrude 2–3 cm above the skin level to avoid leakage beneath the ileostomy pouch. A flush or retracted stoma functions poorly and should be revised.

(4) Prolapse: This is uncommon if the mesentery has been sutured to the parietal peritoneum.

(5) Paraileostomy abscess and fistula: Perforation of the ileum by sutures, pressure necrosis from an ill-fitted appliance, or recurrent disease may cause abscess and fistula.

(6) Skin irritation: This is the single most common complication of ileostomy and is due to leakage of ileal effluent onto the peristomal skin; it is usually minor but can be very severe if neglected. Treatment is directed toward the cause of leakage, usually an ill-fitted pouch. Protection of the skin by a barrier material (eg, karaya [*Sterculia*] gum, or a variety of synthetic products will resolve the problem. Enterostomal therapists manage these problems expertly.

(7) Offensive odors: Odor-proof appliances, commercial deodorants placed in the appliance, and attention to diet usually control the problem.

(8) Diarrhea: Excessive output should be reported to the physician promptly, and supplemental water, salt, and potassium should be given. Codeine, diphenoxylate with atropine (Lomotil), or loperamide (Imodium) may slow the output. Recurrent intestinal disease, bowel obstruction, or ileostomy stenosis should be looked for.

(9) Urinary tract calculi: Uric acid and calcium stones occur in about 5–10% of patients after ileostomy and are probably the result of chronic dehydration due to inadequate fluid intake. Ileostomy is associated with lower urinary pH and volume and higher urinary concentration of calcium, oxalate, and uric acid than an intact gastrointestinal tract.

(10) Gallstones: Cholesterol gallstones are three times more common in ileostomy patients than in the general population. Altered bile acid absorption preoperatively may be responsible.

(11) Ileitis: Patients who develop inflammation of the ileum just proximal to the ileostomy usually have recurrence of their original inflammatory bowel disease. Stenosis of the stoma is another cause.

(12) Varices: Varices develop around the stoma in patients with portal hypertension. Bleeding can be troublesome.

In long-term follow-up of ileostomy patients, most return to their previous occupation, and they consider their health to be good or excellent. Continent ileostomy is preferable to conventional ileostomy in the view of some patients who have had both types of stoma.

Sexual consequences of proctocolectomy should be discussed before and after operation. Some degree of sexual impairment occurs in 10–15% of men after removal of the rectum for inflammatory bowel disease. Up to three-fourths of women report dyspareunia or reduced orgasmic sensation in the first few months after proctectomy and ileostomy. Infertility is more frequent among women after excision of the rectum, and cesarean delivery is necessary more often; both problems are related to pelvic fibrosis and not the ileostomy.

COLOSTOMY

Colostomies are made for the following purposes: (1) to decompress an obstructed colon; (2) to divert the fecal stream in preparation for resection of an inflammatory, obstructive, or perforated lesion or following traumatic injury; (3) to serve as the point of evacuation of stool when the distal colon or rectum is removed; and (4) to protect a distal anastomosis following resection. The colostomy may be temporary, in which event it is subsequently closed, or it may be permanent. Colostomies can be constructed by making an opening in a loop of colon (**loop colostomy**) or by dividing the colon and bringing out one end (**end [terminal] colostomy**). A colostomy is double-barreled if a loop or both ends of a colon are exteriorized, and it is single-barreled if only one end is brought out.

The most common permanent colostomy is a **sigmoid (iliac) colostomy** made at the time of abdominoperineal resection for cancer of the rectum (Figure 31–20). Such a colostomy is compatible with a normal life except for the route of fecal evacuation. A sigmoid colostomy expels stool approximately once a day, but the frequency varies among individuals just as bowel habits vary in the general population. An appliance is not required, although many patients find that wearing a light pouch is reassuring. Some patients achieve a regular pattern of evacuation on their own; others require irrigation daily or every other day. Irrigation is performed by inserting a catheter into the stoma and instilling water, 500 mL at a time, by gravity flow from a reservoir held at shoulder height. A plastic olive-shaped tip on the catheter fits snugly into the stoma and greatly reduces the risk of perforation. Diet is individualized; generally, patients are able to eat the same foods they enjoyed preoperatively. Fresh fruits, fruit juices, and other foods may cause diarrhea. A properly functioning colostomy need not be dilated.

Transverse colostomy should not be constructed as a permanent stoma if it can be avoided. Unlike sigmoid colostomy, transverse colostomy is "wet"—ie,

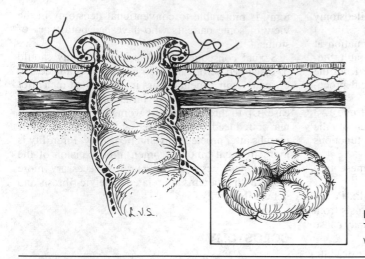

Figure 31–20. Single-barreled end colostomy. The margins of the stoma are fixed to the skin with sutures.

it discharges semiliquid waste frequently—and usually requires an appliance. These stomas are bulky, foul-smelling, and extremely difficult to manage. They are prone to leak under the appliance, and prolapse is common. The needs of most patients who require a permanent stoma are better served by an ileostomy than by a transverse colostomy.

The overall complication rate of colostomies is 20%, and 15% of these require operative correction. Chronic paracolostomy hernia is a frequent complication; it develops because the abdominal wall aperture enlarges with time, allowing colon, omentum, or small bowel to herniate adjacent to the colostomy. Hernia—and prolapse—are more apt to occur in obese patients. Stenosis is largely avoided by maturing the colostomy at the operating table as with ileostomy. Necrosis and retraction are due to technical errors in constructing the stoma. Paracolostomy abscess occurs occasionally regardless of precautions. Perforation is avoided by the plastic catheter tip and by maintaining the irrigation reservoir at no greater than shoulder height. Less serious complications include diarrhea, fecal impaction, and skin irritation.

Clague MB, Heald RJ: Achievement of stomal continence in one-third of colostomies by use of a new disposable plug. Surg Gynecol Obstet 1990;170:390.

Dini D et al: Irrigation for colostomized cancer patients: A rational approach. Int J Colorect Dis 1991;6:9.

Foulis W, Mayberry JF: Elderly ileostomists and their social problems. J Clin Gastroenterol 1990;12:276.

Fucini C, Wolff BG, Dozois RR: Bleeding from peristomal varices: Perspectives on prevention and treatment. Dis Colon Rectum 1991;34:1073.

Hayashi AH, Lau HYC, Gillis DA: Topical sucralfate: Effective therapy for the management of resistant peristomal and perineal excoriation. J Pediatr Surg 1991;26:1279.

Öjerskog B et al: Long-term follow-up of patients with continent ileostomies. Dis Colon Rectum 1990;33:184.

Roberts PL et al: Bleeding stomal varices. The role of local treatment. Dis Colon Rectum 1990;33:547.

Sjödahl R et al: Complications, surgical revision and quality of life with conventional and continent ileostomy. Acta Chir Scand 1990;156:403.

Williams JG et al: Paraileostomy hernia: A clinical and radiological study. Br J Surg 1990;77:1355.

Winslet MC et al: Assessment of the defunctioning efficiency of the loop ileostomy. Dis Colon Rectum 1991;34:699.

PREOPERATIVE PREPARATION OF THE COLON

Complications of colonic surgery such as wound infection and anastomotic dehiscence are partially related to the high bacterial content of the large bowel. It is advisable to eliminate the fecal mass and reduce the numbers of bacteria as much as possible prior to operation. Measures taken to achieve this purpose are known as the "bowel prep."

The fecal mass is reduced by allowing the patient only clear liquids orally for 1 day before operation. Chemically defined diets also leave a small fecal residue; because of their nutritional advantages, they are useful in patients whose colons are especially difficult to cleanse and who require prolonged periods of preparation (eg, children with Hirschsprung's disease). These liquid diets have little or no effect on fecal flora, however.

Mechanical cleansing is employed except in patients with obstructing lesions or, perhaps, severe inflammatory bowel disease. There has been a strong trend toward whole-gut lavage, which involves ingestion (or instillation through a nasogastric tube) of large quantities of fluid; the absorptive capacity of the small bowel is overwhelmed, and the colon is cleared of fecal matter. A solution containing polyethylene glycol (PEG) minimizes the risk of fluid overload and excessive dehydration. Most patients prefer this to preparation with laxatives and enemas. The original PEG solutions contained sodium sulfate as the predominant intraluminal anion. Recently, the sulfate has been deleted from some of these products in an attempt to avoid the unpleasant salty taste that some patients found disagreeable.

Direct attack on the bacteria of the large bowel may be undertaken with systemic antibiotics (see Chapter 8) or oral nonabsorbable antibiotics. Oral antibiotics remain controversial despite many years of study. An important reason for disparate opinions is the difficulty of performing prospective trials in which all the variables are strictly controlled. The numbers of fecal bacteria can be reduced by giving oral neomycin and erythromycin base (1 g each at 1:00 PM, 2:00 PM, and 11:00 PM the day before operation). Metronidazole (Flagyl) has also been shown to be effective, but an aminoglycoside should probably be added to cover against aerobic bacteria. The dose of metronidazole is 200–750 mg orally three times daily for 2 days preoperatively. Significant levels of these agents are found in the serum, and it is possible that the systemic effect is as important as the benefit from reduction of flora intraluminally. Tinidazole, a nitroimidazole similar to metronidazole, is under trial in several centers.

It is agreed that some form of antibiotic prophylaxis is essential. At present, surgeons have a choice among various systemic antibiotics or one of several oral antibiotic regimens in addition to mechanical cleansing. It is unclear whether a combination of oral and systemic antibiotics compares favorably with either alone. Pseudomembranous colitis is a complication of antibiotic preparation.

Beck DE, Fazio VW: Current preoperative bowel cleansing methods. Results of a survey. Dis Colon Rectum 1990; 33:12.

Beck DE, DiPalma JA: A new oral lavage solution vs cathartics and enema method for preoperative colonic cleansing. Arch Surg 1991;126:552.

DiPalma JA, Marshall JB: Comparison of a new sulfate-free polyethylene glycol electrolyte lavage solution versus a standard solution for colonoscopy cleansing. Gastrointest Endosc 1990;36:285.

Fordtran JS, Santa Ana CA, Cleveland MB: A low-sodium solution for gastrointestinal lavage. Gastroenterology 1990;98:11.

Froehlich F et al: Palatability of a new solution compared with standard polyethylene glycol solution for gastrointestinal lavage. Gastrointest Endosc 1991;37:325.

Sakanoue Y et al: The efficacy of whole gut irrigation with polyethylene glycol electrolyte solution in elective colorectal surgery for cancer. Acta Chir Scand 1990; 156:463.

Schoetz DJ Jr et al: Addition of parenteral cefoxitin to regimen of oral antibiotics for elective colorectal operations: A randomized prospective study. Ann Surg 1990; 212:209.

Smith MB et al: Suppression of the human mucosal-related colonic microflora with prophylactic parenteral and/or oral antibiotics. World J Surg 1990;14:636.

Solla JA, Rothenberger DA: Preoperative bowel preparation. A survey of colon and rectal surgeons. Dis Colon Rectum 1990;33:154.

Stellato TA et al: Antibiotics in elective colon surgery: A randomized trial of oral, systemic, and oral/systemic antibiotics for prophylaxis. Am Surg 1990;56:251.

LAPAROSCOPIC COLECTOMY

The first reports of laparoscopic or laparoscopically assisted colon resections have now appeared. Building on experience with diagnostic laparoscopy and laparoscopic cholecystectomy, surgeons are tackling more difficult procedures with this technique, including colectomy. Most reports to date involve laparoscopic mobilization of the colon with an extracorporeal anastomosis through a small incision. Intracorporeal anastomosis is possible in the rectum, and new instruments are appearing now that will make it possible to anastomose the bowel entirely through the laparoscopic approach. This field is in its infancy, and many questions remain about its indications, contraindications, and outcome compared with standard open colectomy.

Jacobs M, Verdeja JC, Goldstein HS: Minimally invasive colon resection (laparoscopic colectomy). Surg Lap Endosc 1991;1:144.

Schlinkert RT: Laparoscopic-assisted right hemicolectomy. Dis Colon Rectum 1991;34:1030.

Wexner SD et al: Laparoscopic total abdominal colectomy: A prospective trial. Dis Colon Rectum 1992;35:651.

REFERENCES

Corman MW: *Colon and Rectal Surgery,* 2nd ed. Lippincott, 1989.

Fazzio VW (editor): *Current Therapy in Colorectal Surgery.* BC Decker, 1989.

Gordon PH, Nivatvongs S: *Principles and Practice of Surgery for the Colon, Rectum, and Anus.* Quality Medical Publishing, 1992.

Norris HT (editor): *Contemporary Issues in Surgical Pathology: Pathology of the Colon, Small Intestine, and Anus,* 2nd ed. Churchill Livingstone, 1991.

Shackelford RT, Zuidema GD (editors): *Surgery of the Alimentary Tract.* Vol 4: *Colon and Anorectum,* 3rd ed. Saunders, 1989.

Sleisenger M, Fordtran J: *Gastrointestinal Disease,* 5th ed. Saunders, 1993.

Anorectum

32

Thomas R. Russell, MD

SURGICAL ANATOMY & PHYSIOLOGY

The anal canal is derived from the proctodeum, an invagination of the ectoderm. The rectum is of entodermal origin. Because of the difference in their origins, the arterial and nerve supply and the venous and lymphatic drainage differ in the two structures, as do their linings also. Thus, the rectum is lined with glandular mucosa and the anal canal with anoderm, a continuation of the external stratified epithelium. It is incorrect to speak of anal "mucosa." The marginal zone between the rectum and the anal canal contains transitional cells. The anal canal and adjacent external skin are generously supplied with somatic sensory nerves and are highly susceptible to painful stimuli; the rectal mucosa has an autonomic nerve supply and is relatively insensitive to pain. Pain is not an early symptom in patients with rectal neoplasm.

Venous drainage above the anorectal juncture is through the portal system; drainage of the anal canal is through the caval system. This distribution is important in understanding the modes of spread of malignant disease and infection and the formation of hemorrhoids. The lymphatic return from the rectum is along the superior hemorrhoidal vascular pedicle to the inferior mesenteric and aortic nodes, but the lymphatics from the anal canal pass through Alcock's canal to the internal iliac nodes and ventrally to the inguinal nodes.

The **anal canal** is about 3 cm long (Figure 32–1). It points toward the umbilicus and forms a distinct angle with the rectum in its resting state. During defecation, the angle straightens out. At the superior boundary of the anal canal is the **anorectal juncture** (mucocutaneous juncture, pectinate line, or dentate line). At this level are found anal crypts and the openings of the anal glands. Infections may lead to anorectal abscess and fistula formation. The intersphincteric groove can be palpated in the canal and denotes the separation of the internal sphincter from the external sphincter.

The **anorectal sphincteric ring** encircles the anal canal. Posteriorly and laterally, it is composed of the fusion of the internal sphincter, the longitudinal muscle, the central portion of the levators (puborectalis), and components of the external sphincter. Anteriorly, it is more vulnerable to trauma because the pubo-rectalis muscle passes directly anteriorly and takes no part in the formation of the ring. The internal sphincter is composed of smooth involuntary muscle; the remaining muscles are striated voluntary ones.

Supporting Structures

The puborectalis forms a muscular sling around the rectum to give it support. The rectum is further supported by the **fascia of Waldeyer,** a heavy avascular layer of the parietal pelvic fascia; the **lateral ligaments,** through which pass the middle hemorrhoidal vessels; and the posterior **mesorectum.** The ligaments and mesorectum fix the rectum to the anterior surface of the sacrum (see Rectal Prolapse).

Arteries

The **superior hemorrhoidal artery** is a direct continuation of the inferior mesenteric artery. It divides into two main branches: left and right. The right branch again bifurcates. These three terminal divisions probably account for the characteristic location of internal hemorrhoids, ie, two in each of the right quadrants and one in the left lateral quadrant. The **middle hemorrhoidal artery** arises on each side from the anterior division of the internal iliac artery or from the internal pudendal artery and runs inward in the lateral ligaments of the rectum. The **inferior hemorrhoidal arteries** are branches of the internal pudendal arteries and pass through Alcock's canal. The anastomoses between the superior and inferior vascular arcades provide collateral circulation that is of importance after surgical interruption or atherosclerotic occlusion of the vascular supply of the left colon.

Veins

The **superior hemorrhoidal veins** originate in the internal hemorrhoidal venous plexus and pass cephalad to the inferior mesenteric veins and thence to the portal venous system. They have no valves. Rectal cancer may be disseminated by venous embolism to the liver, and septic emboli may cause pylephlebitis. The **inferior hemorrhoidal veins** drain into the internal pudendal veins and to the internal iliac and caval system. Enlargement of the hemorrhoidal veins may produce symptomatic hemorrhoids.

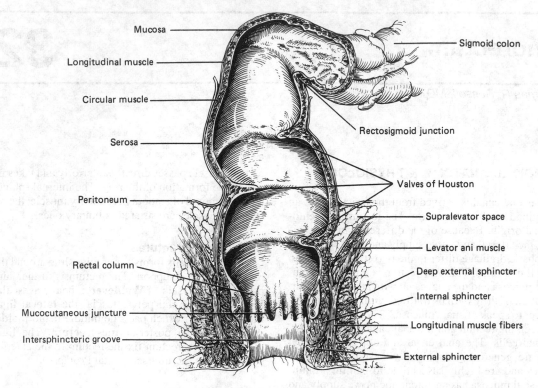

Figure 32–1. Anatomy of the anorectal canal.

Lymphatics

The lymphatics of the anal canal form a fine plexus draining into larger collecting vessels leading to the inguinal lymph nodes, whose efferents lead to the external iliac or common iliac lymph nodes. Infections and cancer in the region of the anus may result in inguinal lymphadenopathy. The lymphatics of the rectum above the level of the anorectal juncture accompany the veins of the superior hemorrhoidal vascular pedicle and thence to the inferior mesenteric and aortic lymph nodes. Posterior to the rectum lie the nodes of Gerota. Radical operations for eradication of cancer of the rectum and anus are based upon lymphatic anatomy.

Nerves

The nerve supply of the rectum is derived from the sympathetic and parasympathetic systems. The sympathetic fibers are derived from the inferior mesenteric plexus and the hypogastric (presacral) nerve, which arises by three roots from the second, third, and fourth lumbar sympathetic ganglia. Sympathetic control from this plexus extends to the genital structures and smooth muscle controlling emission and ejaculation. The parasympathetic supply (nervi erigentes) is derived from the second, third, and fourth sacral nerves. Fibers extend to the erectile tissue of the penis and clitoris and control erection by the

shunting of blood to these tissues. Thus, injuries to these nerves during radical operations on the rectum may cause bladder and sexual dysfunction.

Cherry D, Rothenberger D: Pelvic floor physiology. Surg Clin North Am 1988;68:1217.

Ger R: Surgical anatomy of the pelvis. Surg Clin North Am 1988;68:1201.

Levi AC, Borghi F, Garavaglia M: Development of the anal canal muscles. Dis Colon Rectum 1991;34:262.

Shafik A: A concept of the anatomy of the anal sphincter mechanism and the physiology of defecation. Dis Colon Rectum 1987;30:970.

Shafik A: A concept of the anatomy of the anal sphincter mechanism and the physiology of defecation. Dis Colon Rectum 1987;30:970.

Siddharth P, Ravo B: Colorectal neurovasculature and anal sphincter. Surg Clin North Am 1988;68:1185.

PROCTOLOGIC EXAMINATION

Most disorders affecting the anorectum can be diagnosed by history and physical examination, including perianal inspection and palpation, digital rectal examination, anoscopic examination, and proctosigmoidoscopic examination.

With the patient in either the lateral Sims or the inverted knee-chest position, the perianal region is inspected and palpated. The buttocks are then gently retracted in order to inspect the lower portion of the anal canal. These initial steps allow for the diagnosis of many common painful anorectal disorders such as anal fissure, perianal abscess, and thrombosed external hemorrhoids without inserting a finger or instrument into the rectum.

Digital rectal examination need not be painful. In addition to palpating for masses or induration of the anal canal and lower rectal segment, other structures such as the prostate, cervix, coccyx, and the pubococcygeus muscle may be felt. Sphincter tone, stenosis of the anal canal, and the presence of blood on the examining finger should be noted.

Anoscopic examination evaluates the anal canal and lowest portion of the rectum. A tubular or slotted anoscope should be used with good lighting to see what has already been felt.

Proctosigmoidoscopy may be done with a rigid lighted instrument, generally 25 cm long. Proctoscopy (inspection of the rectum for a distance of 14–18 cm from the anus) can be accomplished in nearly all patients without discomfort. Advancing from the rectum to the distal sigmoid colon (sigmoidoscopy) is often uncomfortable and may not be possible. Perforation or injury of the proximal rectum or distal sigmoid colon is exceedingly rare if the lumen of the bowel is in direct vision while the scope is being advanced. All patients should have a stool specimen examined for occult blood.

A flexible fiberoptic sigmoidoscope (60 cm) is a more complete way of examining the rectum and entire sigmoid colon. Since a greater length of bowel is examined, the diagnostic yield exceeds that of rigid proctosigmoidoscopy. This screening examination procedure is safe, and patient acceptance is favorable.

Church JM: Analysis of the colonoscopic findings in patients with rectal bleeding according to the pattern of their presenting symptoms. Dis Colon Rectum 1991; 34.391.

Forde KA, Waye JD: Is there a need to perform full colonoscopy in a middle-aged person with episodic bright red blood per rectum and internal hemorrhoids? Am J Gastroenterol 1989;84:1227.

Rosen L: Physical examination of the anorectum: A systematic technique. Dis Colon Rectum 1990;33:439.

Wilking N et al: A comparison of the 25-cm rigid proctosigmoidoscope with the 65-cm flexible endoscope in the screening of patients for colorectal carcinoma. Cancer 1986;57:669.

Wilking N et al: A comparison of the 25-cm rigid proctosigmoidoscope with the 65-cm flexible endoscope in the screening of patients for colorectal carcinoma. Cancer 1986;57:669.

DISEASES OF THE ANORECTUM

HEMORRHOIDS (Piles)

Essentials of Diagnosis

- Rectal bleeding, protrusion, discomfort.
- Mucoid discharge from rectum.
- Possible secondary anemia.
- Characteristic findings on external anal inspection and anoscopic examination.

General Considerations

Hemorrhoids (meaning flowing blood) represent a normal anatomic state and occur in all adults. Only when hemorrhoids become enlarged and symptomatic is treatment indicated.

Hemorrhoids are classified as internal or external. **Internal hemorrhoids** are a plexus of superior hemorrhoidal veins above the mucocutaneous junction which are covered by mucosa. They represent a vascular cushion in the loose areolar submucosal tissues of the lower rectum. As shown in Figure 32–2, they occur in three primary positions: right anterior, right posterior, and left lateral. Smaller hemorrhoids occur between the primary locations.

External hemorrhoids (inferior hemorrhoidal plexus) occur below the mucocutaneous junction in the tissues beneath the anal epithelium of the anal canal and the skin of the perianal region. The two plexuses of internal and external hemorrhoids anastomose freely and comprise the venous return of the lower rectum and anus. Internal hemorrhoids drain to the superior hemorrhoidal veins and thence to the portal vein. External hemorrhoids drain into the systemic circulation.

Hemorrhoids become symptomatic for many reasons. The most common cause is straining in the

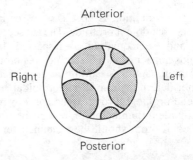

Figure 32–2. The usual arrangement of primary and secondary internal hemorrhoids. The anal canal as seen with the patient in the lithotomy position.

squatting position at the time of bowel movement, which increases venous pressure and distends the veins. This may create redundancy and enlargement of the vascular cushions, allowing for eventual bleeding or protrusion. Other important causative factors of symptomatic hemorrhoids include chronic constipation, pregnancy, obesity, the low-fiber diet of Western society, etc.

Clinical Findings

A. Symptoms and Signs: Patients will frequently complain of "hemorrhoids" regardless of their specific rectal or anal symptoms. It is important to remember that severe pain is not associated with internal hemorrhoids and occurs only with external hemorrhoid thrombosis.

Bleeding is usually the first symptom of internal hemorrhoids. It is bright red, unmixed with the stool, and may vary in quantity from streaks on the toilet tissue to amounts sufficient to be noticed in the water. Occasionally, recurrent hemorrhoidal bleeding may result in marked anemia. As the hemorrhoids gradually enlarge, they may protrude (prolapse). At first this occurs only with defecation and is followed by spontaneous reduction. At a later stage, it may be necessary for the patient to manually replace the internal hemorrhoids after defecation. Finally, the hemorrhoids may progress to the point where they are permanently prolapsed and incapable of being reduced. Mucoid discharge and soiled underclothing are most marked when the hemorrhoids are permanently prolapsed. The perianal skin may become irritated as a result of constant leakage of mucus. Discomfort and pain occur only when there is extensive thrombosis with edema and inflammation.

B. Examination: External hemorrhoids may be seen on inspection, particularly if they are thrombosed. If internal hemorrhoids are prolapsed, the redundant covering of mucin-secreting epithelium will be observed in one or several quadrants. Prolapse can be produced when the physician asks the patient to strain while the buttocks are gently spread.

On digital examination of the rectum, internal hemorrhoids usually cannot be felt, and they should not be tender.

Anoscopic evaluation is necessary to see internal hemorrhoids that do not protrude. The anoscope is introduced, and each quadrant is inspected. Internal hemorrhoids appear as vascular structures protruding into the lumen. Gentle straining by the patient may allow better determination of hemorrhoidal size and the degree of prolapse. Proctosigmoidoscopy must be done to exclude inflammatory or malignant disease at a higher level. Stool should be examined for occult blood.

Differential Diagnosis

Rectal bleeding, the most common manifestation of internal hemorrhoids, also occurs with carcinoma of the colon and rectum, diverticular disease, adenomatous polyps, ulcerative colitis, and other less common diseases of the colon and rectum. Sigmoidoscopic examination must be performed. Barium enema x-ray studies and colonoscopy should be ordered selectively, depending on symptoms and findings.

Rectal prolapse (procidentia) must be differentiated from mucosal prolapse owing to internal hemorrhoids. In rectal prolapse, a circle of protruding bowel appears which is greater anteriorly and which involves the full thickness of bowel wall with concentric mucosal folds. The double full thickness of the wall can be perceived on bidigital palpation. Hemorrhoids and procidentia may coexist.

Perianal condylomas and anorectal tumors are so characteristic in their appearance that differentiation should not be difficult. Thrombosed external hemorrhoids are described below. External skin tags are the result of prior thrombosis of external hemorrhoids and also should be easy to identify. The presence of a midline sentinel tag may signify an adjacent fissure.

Complications

Rarely, prolapsed internal hemorrhoids become irreducible because of congestion, edema, and thrombosis. This may progress to circumferential thrombosis of internal and external hemorrhoids, an exquisitely painful condition that may result in infarction of the overlying mucosa and skin. Septic emboli occur rarely via the portal system and may produce liver abscesses. Iron deficiency anemia may occur.

Hemorrhoids may serve as a portasystemic shunt in portal hypertension, and bleeding in this situation can be profuse.

Treatment

The treatment of symptomatic internal hemorrhoids must be individualized. Hemorrhoids are normal, and therefore the goal of treatment is not to obliterate hemorrhoidal plexuses but rather to render the patient asymptomatic. For this reason, hemorrhoidectomy is done less often today, and other modalities of treatment are more frequently used.

Treatment is based on the presenting findings according to the following classification: **First-degree** internal hemorrhoids cause painless, bright red rectal bleeding at the time of defecation. At this early stage, there is no prolapse, and anoscopic examination reveals enlarged hemorrhoids projecting into the lumen. **Second-degree** hemorrhoids protrude through the anal canal on gentle straining but spontaneously reduce. **Third-degree** hemorrhoids protrude with straining and must be reduced manually after defecation. Fixed protrusion defines fourth-degree hemorrhoids.

A. Medical Treatment: Most patients with early hemorrhoids (first- and second-degree) can be managed by simple local measures and dietary advice. The diet should be high in fiber (vegetables, fruits), and increased water intake must be stressed. Unrefined bran added to food or other commercially available hydrophilic agents can be used to augment dietary bulk. These measures aid defecation and obviate the need to strain.

Suppositories and rectal ointments have no known therapeutic value except for their anesthetic and astringent effects.

For prolapsed edematous internal hemorrhoids, gentle reduction followed by bed rest and local astringent compresses (witch hazel) decreases swelling. Warm sitz baths may also offer symptomatic relief. Patients with underlying inflammatory bowel disease (particularly Crohn's disease) should be treated medically when hemorrhoids become symptomatic.

B. Injection Treatment: Injection treatment, a form of sclerotherapy, consists of injecting an irritating chemical solution (eg, 5% phenol in vegetable oil) submucosally into the loose areolar tissue above the internal hemorrhoid. One to 2 mL injected into symptomatic quadrants causes inflammation and eventually fibrosis and scarring. Injection is performed with a long hemorrhoidal needle through an anoscope, and the injection must be above the mucocutaneous junction. There is minimal pain if the injection is in the correct location. Complications are rare but include sloughing of the mucosa, infection, acute prostatitis, and sensitivity reactions to the injected material.

Injection therapy combined with dietary counseling is effective treatment for bleeding and early prolapse of internal hemorrhoids (first- and second-degree hemorrhoids).

C. Rubber Band Ligation: For enlarged or prolapsing hemorrhoids, band ligation is excellent treatment. With the aid of an anoscope, the redundant mucosa above the hemorrhoid is grasped with forceps and advanced through the barrel of a special ligator. The rubber band is then placed snugly around the mucosa and hemorrhoidal plexus. Ischemic necrosis occurs over several days, with eventual slough, fibrosis, and fixation of the tissues. One hemorrhoidal complex at a time is treated, with repeat ligations done at 2- and 4-week intervals as needed.

The major complication of this technique is pain severe enough to require removal of the band. To avoid this, the band must be placed high and well above the mucocutaneous juncture, where few sensory fibers exist. Persistent pain may herald serious infection, and prompt evaluation must follow. Bleeding may occur at the time the hemorrhoid sloughs (generally in 7–10 days), and the patient should be warned of this possibility.

D. Cryosurgery: Hemorrhoids can be necrosed by freezing with a cryoprobe, using CO_2 or N_2O. The technique has not gained wide acceptance because of uncontrolled slough of mucosa and associated foul-smelling discharge from the anus. Wound healing may be delayed.

E. Hemorrhoidectomy: Surgical excision is reserved for patients with chronic symptoms and third-degree or fourth-degree prolapse; surgical candidates often have chronic bleeding and anemia and have failed to respond to simpler therapeutic measures. Patients with acute painful thrombosed fourth-degree hemorrhoids are most expeditiously treated by hemorrhoidectomy.

Important principles of hemorrhoidectomy include excision of redundant tissue only and conservative excision of normal anoderm and skin. The underlying sphincter should not be disrupted, and mucosal flaps should be developed to excise venous channels beneath the mucosa and anoderm. This may be accomplished using standard techniques or more recently the CO_2 or Nd:YAG laser.

F. Other Operative Procedures: Anal dilation may be performed under anesthesia to disrupt bands of the anal canal. It is believed by proponents of this technique that these submucosal bands produce partial anal outlet obstruction (spasm) that is important in hemorrhoidal formation. Anal dilation has not gained wide acceptance in the USA.

Infrared photocoagulation, bipolar diathermy, and the galvanic generator and probe are newer office-based treatments. Each is relatively painless, but all create tissue injury with resultant fibrosis and fixation. Long-term efficacy is unknown.

Prognosis

With appropriate treatment, all patients with symptomatic hemorrhoids should become asymptomatic. A conservative approach should be used initially in nearly all cases, with hemorrhoidectomy reserved for treatment failures and selected severe cases. The results of hemorrhoidectomy, however, are excellent. Following treatment, straining must be minimized to prevent recurrence of symptoms. Caution and conservatism are emphasized in the treatment of any patient with Crohn's disease.

Cocchiara JL: Hemorrhoids: A practical approach to an aggravating problem. Postgrad Med 1991;89:149.

Dennison AR, Wherry DC, Morris DL: Hemorrhoids: Nonoperative management. Surg Clin North Am 1988;68:1401.

Dennison A, Whiston RJ: A randomized comparison of infrared photocoagulation with bipolar diathermy for the outpatient treatment of hemorrhoids. Dis Colon Rectum 1990;33:32.

Dennison AR et al: The management of hemorrhoids. Am J Gastroenterol 1989;84:475.

Deutsch AA et al: Anal pressure measurements in the study of hemorrhoid etiology and their relation to treatment. Dis Colon Rectum 1987;30:855.

Ferguson EF Jr: Alternatives in the treatment of hemorrhoidal disease. South Med J 1988;81:606.

Gibbons CP, Bannister JJ, Read NW: Role of constipation

and anal hypertonia in the pathogenesis of haemorrhoids. Br J Surg 1988;75:656.

Johanson JF, Sonnenberg A: Temporal changes in the occurrence of hemorrhoids in the United States and England. Dis Colon Rectum 1991;34:585.

Khubchandani I: Operative hemorrhoidectomy. Surg Clin North Am 1988;68:1411.

Smith LE: Hemorrhoids: A review of current techniques and management. Gastroenterol Clin North Am 1987; 16:79.

Wang JY, Chang-Chien CR: The role of lasers in hemorrhoidectomy. Dis Colon Rectum 1991;34:78.

THROMBOSED EXTERNAL HEMORRHOID

This common lesion is not a true hemorrhoid but rather a thrombosis of the subcutaneous external hemorrhoidal veins of the anal canal. It is more appropriately termed a perianal hematoma. It is characterized by a painful, tense, bluish elevation beneath the skin or anoderm, varying in size from a few millimeters to several centimeters. It may be multilobular, and there may be several such lesions. Although rupture may occur through the vein wall, it is usually incomplete, so that a thin layer of adventitia remains over the clot. Thrombosis of an external hemorrhoid generally follows a sudden increase in venous pressure (eg, after heavy lifting, coughing, sneezing, straining at stool, or parturition). It most often affects otherwise healthy young persons and is not related necessarily to internal hemorrhoidal disease.

Pain is greatest at the onset and gradually subsides in 2–3 days as the acute edema resolves. Spontaneous rupture may occur with disgorgement of the thrombus, followed by bleeding. Spontaneous resolution will occur without treatment.

Symptoms may be alleviated by warm sitz baths, applications of petrolatum to minimize friction in walking, and mild sedation. Bed rest is important to minimize swelling and additional thrombosis.

If the patient is examined within the first 48 hours, the course may be hastened and immediate relief obtained either by evacuation of the thrombus or by complete excision ("external hemorrhoidectomy") under local anesthesia. When the thrombus is evacuated, an ellipse of skin should be removed to prevent agglutination of the skin edges and re-formation of the underlying clot. After the clot has begun to organize, it cannot be evacuated, and in this situation conservative measures should be employed. No attempt should be made to reduce a thrombosed external hemorrhoid, since it belongs in an external position.

It is important to differentiate this lesion from a prolapsed internal hemorrhoid. The pathologic features and methods of treatment are entirely different.

Grosz CR: A surgical treatment of thrombosed external hemorrhoids. Dis Colon Rectum 1990;33:249.

ANAL FISSURE
(Fissure-in-Ano, Anal Ulcer)

Essentials of Diagnosis

- Rectal pain related to defecation.
- Bleeding.
- Constipation.
- Spasm of sphincters.
- Anal tenderness.
- Ulceration of anal canal.
- Stenosis.
- Hypertrophic anal papilla.
- Sentinel pile.

General Considerations

Fissures represent denuded epithelium of the anal canal overlying the internal sphincter. They are painful because of their location below the mucocutaneous juncture. Anal ulcers are usually single and occur in the posterior midline or, less commonly, in the anterior midline. They may occur first in the lower portion of the anal canal or may involve its entire length. Ulcers tend to occur in the posterior midline position because of the acute angulation between the anal canal and the rectum.

Infection of the adjacent crypt results in chronic inflammation. Edema of the anal papilla adjacent to the crypt occurs with enlargement and fibrosis of the papilla, so that it may become a firm, whitish, polypoid structure. It is then called a **hypertrophic papilla.** Hypertrophic papillae are not neoplastic but are often confused with adenomatous polyps. External to the anal ulcer, the adjacent skin likewise is involved in chronic inflammatory changes and interference with its lymphatic drainage. A fibrotic nubbin of skin may form at the anal verge. This is termed a **sentinel pile** because it stands as a sentinel just below the ulcer. Thus, the fissure triad has been formed: (1) the ulcer itself, (2) the hypertrophic papilla, and (3) the sentinel pile (Figure 32–3).

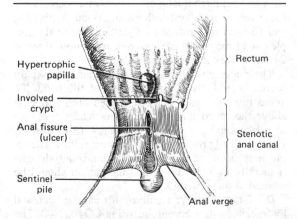

Figure 32–3. Diagram of the anorectum showing the fissure or ulcer triad.

Two of the most important factors in the genesis of fissures are irritant diarrheal stools and tightening of the anal canal secondary to nervous tension. Manometric studies have shown increased basal sphincter pressures. Other factors may be habitual use of cathartics, chronic diarrhea, avulsion of an anal valve, childbirth trauma, laceration by a sharp foreign body, or iatrogenic trauma such as the passage of a large speculum or prostatic massage. Often a cause cannot be definitely identified.

Fissures of the perianal skin may be associated with pruritus ani and may be the cause of a localized perianal dermatitis.

Clinical Findings

A. Symptoms and Signs: The classic history of a painful bowel movement associated with bright red bleeding is often given. The pain may be severe and is described as tearing, burning, or cutting. It occurs during passage of stool, then usually subsides somewhat and becomes more severe when secondary sphincteric spasm occurs. Fissures are characterized by their chronicity, with periods of exacerbation and remission, often over a number of years. Bleeding is bright red, not mixed with the stool, usually noted on the toilet tissue, and small in amount. Constipation develops as a result of fear of defecation, which is so frequently postponed that regular bowel habits become disrupted. A cycle develops that must be interrupted to promote healing.

The sentinel pile can be observed externally. Gentle eversion of the anus will often reveal the inferior portion of the ulcer. Application of a topical anesthetic should precede a very gentle digital examination to ascertain the site of the ulcer, the degree of induration and stenosis, etc. There is often marked spasm of the sphincters.

B. Special Examinations: A small-caliber anoscope can be introduced with pressure on the side of the anal canal opposite the lesion. The hypertrophic papilla, ulcer, and associated lesions can then be seen. Sigmoidoscopic examination should be deferred (but not omitted) until it can be done painlessly.

Differential Diagnosis

Other anal ulcerations that must be differentiated from fissure include the primary lesion of syphilis, anal carcinoma, tuberculous ulceration, and ulceration associated with blood dyscrasias, Crohn's disease, and AIDS. Each of these lesions has its own characteristics, but any lesion not in the midline or displaying the typical findings outlined above should be investigated by means of further diagnostic tests. Anal fissure often occurs concomitantly with internal hemorrhoids and may be overlooked. Internal hemorrhoids are not painful; when pain occurs, fissure must be suspected. The persistence of pain following

hemorrhoidectomy is frequently due to a missed fissure.

Treatment

A. Medical Treatment: Softening the stools is the mainstay of medical treatment. This is done with changes in diet and use of hydrophilic bulk agents. Water intake should be increased. Topical agents such as ichthammol 10% or 1% hydrocortisone applied in the anal canal with a "pile pipe" may be helpful. Warm sitz baths after a painful bowel movement may offer symptomatic relief and help reduce spasm. Suppositories are of no value.

B. Surgical Treatment: Surgical treatment (lateral internal sphincterotomy) should be considered if the fissure remains refractory after 1 month of supervised conservative therapy. Intolerable pain may hasten the decision for surgery.

The fissure or ulcer is left alone except for excising the external skin tag (sentinel pile) to promote drainage. The internal sphincter is identified in a lateral position at the intersphincteric groove, and its lower portion is transected. Sphincterotomy allows the fissure to heal promptly with few complications and can be performed on an outpatient basis.

Forceful anal dilation under general anesthesia has also been used; the procedure essentially causes divulsion of the sphincter.

Prognosis

Anal ulcers tend to become chronic, with alternate periods of healing and exacerbation. They do not become malignant. Surgical treatment is highly successful in selected patients.

Brown AC, Sumfest JM, Rozwadowski JV: Histopathology of the internal anal sphincter in chronic anal fissure. Dis Colon Rectum 1989;32:680.

Carr ND, Mercey D, Slack WW: Non-condylomatous, perianal disease in homosexual men. Br J Surg 1989;76:1064.

Case JB: Chronic anal fissure. A new method of treatment by anoplasty. Dis Colon Rectum 1991;34:198.

Khubchandani IT, Reed JF: Sequelae of internal sphincterotomy for chronic fissure in ano. Br J Surg 1989;76:431.

Lewis TH et al: Long-term results of open and closed sphincterotomy for anal fissure. Dis Colon Rectum 1988;31:368.

Lin JK: Anal manometric studies in hemorrhoids and anal fissures. Dis Colon Rectum 1989;32:839.

Marks CG: Anal lesions in Crohn's disease. Ann R Coll Surg Engl 1990;72:158.

McNamara MJ, Percy JP, Fielding IR: A manometric study of anal fissure treated by subcutaneous lateral internal sphincterotomy. Ann Surg 1990;211:235.

Notaras MJ: Anal fissure and stenosis. Surg Clin North Am 1988;68:1427.

Smith LE: Anal fissures. Neth J Med 1990;37:S33.

ANORECTAL ABSCESS

Essentials of Diagnosis
- Persistent throbbing rectal pain.
- External evidence of abscess, such as palpable induration and tenderness, may or may not be present.
- Systemic evidence of infection.

General Considerations
Anorectal abscess results from the invasion of the pararectal spaces by pathogenic microorganisms. A mixed infection usually occurs, with *Escherichia coli, Proteus vulgaris,* streptococci, staphylococci, and *Bacteroides* predominating. Anaerobes are often present. The abscess may appear small but often contains a large amount of foul-smelling pus.

The incidence is much higher in men. The most common cause is infection extending from an anal crypt into one of the pararectal spaces. The internal sphincter is an important barrier and influences the intermuscular spread of infection. Less commonly, abscesses superficial to the corrugator muscle may result from infection of hair follicles or sebaceous and sweat glands of the skin; abrasions due to scratching; infection of a perianal hematoma; as a complication of deep anal fissure; infection of a prolapsed internal hemorrhoid; or following sclerosing injection of hemorrhoids. Deeper abscesses usually arise in the crypts but may also result from trauma, foreign bodies, etc. Underlying disorders such as Crohn's disease are associated with abscesses.

Abscesses are classified according to the anatomic space they occupy (Figure 32–4): (1) Perianal abscess lies immediately beneath the skin of the anus and the lowermost part of the anal canal. (2) Ischiorectal abscess occupies the ischiorectal fossa; this type is uncommon, although the term is often improperly used to describe most anorectal abscesses. (3) Retrorectal (deep postanal) abscess is situated in the retrorectal space. (4) Submucous abscess is situated in the submucosa immediately above the anal canal. (5) Marginal abscess is located in the anal canal beneath the anoderm. (6) Pelvirectal (supralevator) abscess lies above the levator ani muscle and below the peritoneum. (7) Intermuscular abscess lies between the layers of the sphincter muscles. A lateral abscess may extend through the triangle just posterior to the anal canal and pass around to the opposite side to form a horseshoe abscess. Abscesses may extend from the supralevator space down through the levator into the ischiorectal fossa to form an hourglass abscess.

After they are drained, most abscesses result in fistulas.

Clinical Findings
Superficial abscesses are the most painful, with pain related to sitting and walking but not necessarily

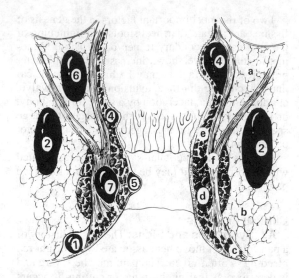

Figure 32–4. Composite diagram of acute anorectal abscesses and spaces. (a) Pelvirectal (supralevator) space. (b) Ischiorectal space. (c) Perianal (subcutaneous) space. (d) Marginal (mucocutaneous) space. (e) Submucous space. (f) Intermuscular space. Numbers designate abscesses as enumerated in text above. (Retrorectal abscess is not shown.)

to bowel movement. Inspection discloses the characteristic evidence of external swelling, with redness, induration, and tenderness. Deeper abscesses may cause systemic sepsis, but localized pain may not be severe. External inspection shows no swelling. Digital rectal examination reveals the tender swelling, and on bidigital examination with the index finger in the rectum and the thumb external, the abscess may be readily felt. High pelvirectal abscesses may cause minimal or no rectal symptoms and may be associated with lower abdominal pain and fever of undetermined origin. Diagnosis may be difficult.

Complications
Unless the abscess is evacuated promptly by surgery or ruptures spontaneously, it will extend into other adjacent anatomic spaces. Rarely, an anaerobic infection will spread extensively without respect for anatomic planes of cleavage.

Treatment
The treatment of pararectal abscesses is prompt incision and adequate drainage. In healthy individuals with superficial abscesses, this may be accomplished on an outpatient basis with local anesthesia. In patients who are immunologically compromised (due to diabetes, leukemia, etc) or are otherwise poor risks, drainage should be performed in the operating room with adequate anesthesia. Despite a lack of palpable fluctuance, suppuration will almost always have oc-

curred when the diagnosis is first made. One should not wait for the abscess to point externally. Antibiotics are of limited value, may only serve to mask the infection temporarily, and may result in the overgrowth of resistant organisms. Warm sitz baths and analgesics are palliative.

Before operation, the patient should be advised that after the abscess is drained there may be a persistent fistula. If, under anesthesia, the primary origin of the fistula can be found, and if the tract connecting it to the abscess can be incised without dividing a significant portion of the sphincteric ring, the abscess can be drained and fistulotomy performed at the same time. A second operation for fistula will then be avoided. If the fistulous tract is deep, the abscess should simply be drained and fistulectomy delayed until infection clears. The wound should not be packed, since this may result in a broad scar that may interfere with the ability of the sphincters to close the anal canal, resulting in leakage or partial incontinence.

The wound should be inspected at frequent intervals to make certain that it heals from the base, so bridging of the wound and recurrent abscess formation will not occur.

Prognosis

Abscesses that rupture spontaneously or are drained without removal of the fistulous connection will frequently recur until the underlying cause is removed.

Fry RD et al: Techniques and results in the management of anal and perianal Crohn's disease. Surg Gynecol Obstet 1989;168:42.

Law PJ et al: Anal endosonography in the evaluation of perianal sepsis and fistula in ano. Br J Surg 1989;76:752.

Milsom JW, Graffner H: Intrarectal ultrasonography in rectal cancer staging and in the evaluation of pelvic disease: Clinical uses of intrarectal ultrasound. Ann Surg 1990; 212:602.

Piazza DJ, Radhakrishnan J: Perianal abscess and fistula-in-ano in children. Dis Colon Rectum 1990;33:1014.

Pritchard TJ et al: Perirectal abscess in Crohn's disease: Drainage and outcome. Dis Colon Rectum 1990;33:933.

Schouten WR, van Vroonhoven TJ: Treatment of anorectal abscess with or without primary fistulectomy: Results of a prospective randomized trial. Dis Colon Rectum 1991;34:60.

Ustynoski K et al: Horseshoe abscess fistula: Seton treatment. Dis Colon Rectum 1990;33:602.

ANORECTAL FISTULAS

Essentials of Diagnosis

- Chronic purulent discharge from a para-anal opening.
- Tract that may be palpated or probed leading to rectum.

General Considerations

By definition, a fistula must have at least two openings connected by a hollow tract—as opposed to a sinus, which is a tract with but one opening. Most anorectal fistulas originate in the anal crypts at the anorectal juncture. The crypt becomes injured or infected (cryptitis), the infection extends along one of several well-defined planes, and an abscess occurs. When the abscess is opened or when it ruptures, a fistula is formed. The fistula may be subcutaneous, submucosal, intramuscular, or submuscular. It may be anterior or posterior, single, complex, or horseshoe.

Fistulas are usually due to pyogenic infection or, less commonly, to granulomatous disease of the intestine or to tuberculosis. Those that do not originate in the crypts may result from diverticulitis, neoplasm, or trauma. Cryptogenic fistulas that have their secondary (external) opening posterior to an imaginary line passing transversely through the center of the anal orifice usually have their primary (internal) opening in a crypt in the posterior midline. When the secondary (external) opening is anterior to the transverse line, the primary (internal) opening is usually in a crypt immediately opposite the secondary opening (Salmon-Goodsall rule; Figure 32–5).

Clinical Findings

A. Symptoms and Signs: The chief complaint is intermittent or constant drainage or discharge. There is usually a history of a recurrent abscess that ruptured spontaneously or was surgically drained. There may be a pink or red elevation exuding pus, or it may have healed. In Crohn's disease or tuberculosis, the margins may be violaceous and the discharge watery. On palpation, a cord-like tract can be felt, and

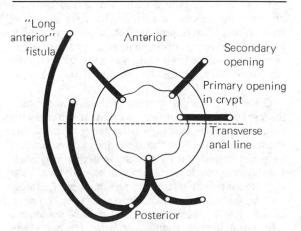

Figure 32–5. Salmon-Goodsall rule. The usual relation of the primary and secondary openings of fistulas. When there is an anterior and also a posterior opening of the same fistula, the rule of the posterior opening applies; the "long anterior" fistula is an exception to the rule.

its course, both in relation to the sphincter and to its primary orifice, can be determined. A probe can be inserted into the tract to determine its depth and course. This maneuver should not be done if it is too painful, in which case it can be completed under anesthesia at the time of operation. Bidigital examination is helpful.

Anorectal fistulas in infants are congenital, may cause abscesses, are more common in boys, and are anterior, straight, and superficial. The treatment is the same as in adults. Rectovaginal fistulas are commonly related to anterior anorectal infection or injury at the time of childbirth. Other causes include radiation injury, neoplasm, or inflammatory bowel disease. The most common complaint is the passage of flatus or feces per vaginam. Vaginal and anoscopic examination will generally reveal the fistulous tract.

B. Special Examinations: Digital rectal examination will frequently reveal a defect at the site of the scarred internal opening. Using this information in conjunction with Salmon-Goodsall's rule, one attempts to confirm the location using a curved crypt hook. Through an anoscope, one probes at the crypt level. Proctoscopy is an essential examination before any operative procedure. If there is evidence of proctitis or symptoms that could be due to inflammatory bowel disease, contrast x-ray studies should be obtained of the colon and small bowel. For the complex elusive fistula, fistulography may prove useful in selected cases.

Differential Diagnosis

Hidradenitis suppurativa is a disease of the apocrine sweat glands characterized by the formation of multiple, deep perianal sinuses. Other sites of predilection are the axillas and the inguinal and pubic areas. There may be scrotal or labial involvement.

Pilonidal sinus with a tract leading into the perianal area may resemble a fistula. The direction of the tract on palpation or probing, the presence of another opening in the sacrococcygeal area, and the possible presence of tufts of hair in the sinus may establish the diagnosis, although the differentiation may be difficult.

Granulomatous disease (regional enteritis, Crohn's disease) of the small or large bowel is associated with anorectal fistulas in a high percentage of cases. The fistula may be the first manifestation of proximal disease and precedes it by months or even years. Such fistulas are indolent in appearance and have pale granulations and characteristic microscopic findings.

Tuberculous fistulas are now rare. They too have an indolent appearance and are usually associated with pulmonary, glandular, or osseous tuberculosis elsewhere in the body.

Infected comedones, infected sebaceous cysts, chronic folliculitis, and bartholinitis are other dermal sources of draining sinuses. The history, the location of the sinus in relation to the anus or vulva, and the absence of an anorectal source are helpful in the diagnosis. Examination under anesthesia may be necessary.

Rectorectal dermoid cysts are more common in females and form chronic perianal sinuses.

Coloperineal fistulas may occur in diverticulitis of the sigmoid colon. Whenever a probe can be passed deeply into a perianal fistula and sigmoidal diverticular disease coexists, the intracolonic origin of the fistula should be suspected and checked by fistulography.

Sinuses from trauma and foreign bodies may occur. The foreign body may gain entrance from the outside by penetration or from within the canal from the ingestion of a sharp piece of bone, etc. An unabsorbed suture remaining from perineorrhaphy or episiotomy or a piece of drainage tubing may act as a foreign body.

Urethroperineal fistulas are often traumatic in origin, resulting from urethral instrumentation or direct external trauma. Rectourethral fistulas may be congenital or may follow urethral instrumentation or prostatectomy. The chief complaint is pneumaturia or fecaluria. Small, recent fistulas may close spontaneously, or urinary diversion by cystostomy and repair may be required.

Less common causes of perianal sinuses and fistulas are tubo-ovarian abscess, actinomycosis, osteomyelitis, and carcinoma. In these instances the history, physical findings, x-ray examination, and laboratory studies will provide the differential diagnosis.

Complications

Without treatment, chronically infected fistulas may be the source of systemic infection. Although carcinoma develops rarely in a chronic untreated anorectal fistula, many such cases have been reported, and effective removal of the fistula is a prophylactic measure against such an eventuality.

Treatment

Small acute fistulas may heal spontaneously, but in most cases the only effective treatment is fistulotomy (commonly termed fistulectomy). The following principles must be observed: (1) The primary opening must be found and excised. (2) The fistulous tract or tracts must be identified completely. (3) The tract must be unroofed throughout its entire length so that the fistulous tunnel is converted into an open wound. (4) The wound must be constructed so as to make certain that the cavity will heal from within outward. Fistulotomy should never be performed in the presence of chronic diarrhea, active ulcerative colitis, or active granulomatous enterocolitis. Delayed wound healing may present a severe problem as well as fecal incontinence if the sphincter is cut.

A staged operation is indicated when the fistula passes deep to the entire anorectal ring, so that all the muscles must be divided in order to extirpate the tract. If the deeper portions of the sphincteric ring and the levator ani muscles are left intact, incontinence will not occur.

Frequent follow-up examination of the wound after fistulotomy is of great importance to make certain that bridging and re-formation of the fistula do not occur.

Prognosis

The prognosis after surgery is excellent. Fistulas persist for the following reasons: (1) The primary opening of the fistula is not removed; (2) collateral tracts are missed; (3) the operation is inadequate for fear of creating incontinence; (4) there is a mistaken diagnosis; and (5) postoperative care is inadequate.

Goebell H: Perianal complications in Crohn's disease. Neth J Med 1990;37:S47.

Morrison JG et al: Surgical management of anorectal fistula in Crohn's disease. Dis Colon Rectum 1989;32:492.

Ross S: Fistula in ano. Surg Clin North Am 1988;68:1417.

Schouten WR, van Vroonhoven TJ: Treatment of anorectal abscess with or without primary fistulectomy: Results of a prospective randomized trial. Dis Colon Rectum 1991;34:60.

Ustynoski K, Rosen L, Riether R: Horseshoe abscess fistula: Seton treatment. Dis Colon Rectum 1990;33:602.

Williams JG et al: Fistula-in-ano in Crohn's disease: Results of aggressive surgical treatment. Dis Colon Rectum 1991;34:378.

Wise WE et al: Surgical treatment of low rectovaginal fistulas. Dis Colon Rectum 1991;34:271.

PILONIDAL DISEASE

Essentials of Diagnosis

- Acute abscess or chronic draining sinus in the sacrococcygeal area.
- Pain, tenderness, induration.

General Considerations

Pilonidal disease presents either as a draining sinus or as an acute abscess in the sacrococcygeal area. There is an underlying cyst with associated granulation tissue, fibrosis, and, frequently, tufts of hair.

Controversy continues about whether pilonidal cysts are congenital or acquired. Some still believe they are remnants of the medullary canal or represent faulty development of the sacrococcygeal raphe, leading to dermal inclusions. The cause in most cases, however, is probably infection, irritation, and trapping of hair in the deep tissues of the sacrococcygeal area (ie, they are acquired). Pilonidal disease more commonly affects men than women and particularly those with abundant hair in the gluteal fold of the buttocks. The disease often presents initially at puberty, when hair growth and activity of the sebaceous glands increases. The midline postanal dimple,

commonly noted in infants, rarely is a precursor of pilonidal disease.

Clinical Findings

The lesion is usually asymptomatic until it becomes acutely infected. The symptoms and findings of acute suppuration are similar to those of acute abscesses in other locations. The inflammatory process may subside or progress until relief is obtained by spontaneous rupture or surgical drainage. After drainage has occurred, the purulent discharge may cease completely or, more commonly, may recur intermittently with drainage from one or more sinus openings. On examination, one or several midline or eccentric cutaneous openings in the skin of the sacral region are found. Hairs can often be seen projecting from the openings. A probe may be passed into the sinuses for several millimeters to many centimeters.

Differential Diagnosis

The diagnosis is usually readily apparent. Other conditions that should be considered are a perianal abscess arising from the posterior midline crypt, hidradenitis suppurativa, and simple carbuncle or furuncle.

Complications

Untreated pilonidal infection may result in the formation of multiple, sometimes long draining sinuses. Rarely, malignant degeneration has occurred.

Treatment

The acute abscess should be treated by incision and drainage, which can often be done in the office or emergency room using local anesthesia. With gentle probing, it may be possible to extract tufts of hair that act as a foreign body to perpetuate the infection.

There are a variety of surgical treatments for chronic disease with persistent drainage or recurrent abscess formation and pain. It is important to be conservative and excise only diseased tissue, leaving normal skin, fat, etc. Wide excisions that were often done in the past are generally not indicated, because the wound heals slowly and causes unnecessarily prolonged disability in an otherwise healthy, productive individual. Surgical options currently range from simple pilonidal cystotomy to excision of the sinus tract and cyst with either primary closure or healing by secondary intention. Whatever technique is used, careful follow-up is essential. The patient should be instructed to keep the area clean and dry, to avoid direct trauma, and to shave the skin or apply a depilatory regularly to prevent further entrapment of hair. Weekly outpatient visits are important until the physician is confident that the process has resolved and the prophylactic regimen is being followed faithfully.

Prognosis

Recurrence may follow any therapy, but the chance of recurrence is least if the wound is left open and postoperative care is diligent. The patient should be able to return to normal activity promptly in most cases.

Allen-Mersh TG: Pilonidal sinus: Finding the right track for treatment. Br J Surg 1990;77:123.

Bascom JU: Repeat pilonidal operations. Am J Surg 1987; 154:118.

Jensen SL, Harling H: Prognosis after simple incision and drainage for a first-episode acute pilonidal abscess. Br J Surg 1988;75:60.

Solla JA, Rothenberger DA: Chronic pilonidal disease: An assessment of 150 cases. Dis Colon Rectum 1990;33: 758.

PRURITUS ANI

The perianal skin has a "maximum readiness to itch." Pruritus ani is due to a wide variety of causes and is not in itself a specific clinical entity or disease.

Etiology

Note: Contrary to popular belief, hemorrhoids are not a cause of pruritus ani.

A. Dermatologic: Psoriasis, seborrheic dermatitis, atopic eczema, lichen planus, etc.

B. Contact Dermatitis: Resulting from the use of local anesthetics (all "-caine" preparations must be suspected), topical antihistamines, various ointments, suppositories, douches, aromatic and other chemical substances used in soap.

C. Fungal: Dermatophytosis, candidiasis, etc.

D. Bacterial: Secondary infection due to scratching.

E. Parasitic: Pinworms *(Enterobius vermicularis)* and, less commonly, scabies or pediculosis.

F. After Oral Antibiotic Therapy: Especially tetracyclines.

G. Systemic Diseases: Diabetes (usually candidiasis), liver disease, etc.

H. Proctologic Disorders: Skin tags, cryptitis, draining fistulas or sinuses, ectropion, sphincter dysfunction, and stool leakage.

I. Neoplasms: Intradermal carcinoma (Bowen's disease), extramammary Paget's disease, etc.

J. Hygiene: Poor hygiene with residual irritating feces or overmeticulous hygiene with excessive use of soap and rubbing.

K. Warmth and Hyperhidrosis: Due to a tight girdle, jockey shorts, warm bedclothing, obesity, climate.

L. Dietary: Excessive consumption of alcohol, coffee, milk, and certain fruit juices.

M. Psychogenic: The importance of the anxiety-itch-anxiety cycle varies from trivial to overwhelming. The significance of this area as an erotic zone in its relation to pruritus ani is not firmly established.

N. Idiopathic.

Clinical Findings

A. Symptoms and Signs: Itching of the anogenital area may be related to sleeping, defecation, warmth, emotional stress, activity, or ingestion of certain foods. It may vary from intermittent and mild to constant and severe. The clinical manifestations are consistent with the underlying cause. Skin changes may be minimal. Characteristic changes may be masked by excoriation caused by scratching and secondary infection. There may be erythema, fissuring, maceration, lichenification, thickening and fibrosis of the skin, changes suggestive of fungal infection, the presence of pinworms (seen with the endoscope), and lesions elsewhere on the body.

The etiologic diagnosis is based upon a careful history and physical examination and laboratory tests. Characteristic lesions must be searched for elsewhere on the body. The use of oral or topical medication and the patient's hygienic habits should be determined.

B. Laboratory Findings: Direct microscopic examination or culture of tissue scrapings may reveal yeasts, other fungi, or parasites. The Scotch Tape test may be used to disclose pinworm ova. In the case of persistent pruritus that does not respond to treatment, a biopsy must be taken to detect unusual but important malignant or premalignant lesions.

Complications

Complications include local secondary infection, dermatitis medicamentosa, and signs associated with loss of sleep and persistent severe discomfort.

Prevention

The use of any kind of soap directly applied to the perianal area during bath or shower is interdicted. Self-medication with anesthetic or antihistamine ointments must be avoided. Scratching leads to secondary infection and should be discouraged, as should vigorous rubbing with harsh toilet paper. Clothing should be loose. Women should avoid elastic girdles or body stockings that press the buttocks together. Bedclothing should be light. Systemic causes should be treated. Dietary practices that prevent frequent loose bowel movements and perianal staining should be followed.

Treatment

The underlying cause should be specifically treated. In addition, all patients should be instructed to stop using soap in the perianal region. Soap is alkaline, whereas the perianal skin is slightly acid. The area should be thoroughly cleansed after each bowel movement, using a soft, moistened tissue paper or cloth. A water-soluble corticosteroid cream with an acid pH may be applied three or four times daily. Dietary changes may also be necessary.

X-ray treatment and surgical procedures or injections designed to cure or create local anesthesia are rarely if ever indicated. Dermatologic and psychiatric consultation may be useful in chronic or refractory cases.

Eusebio EB: New treatment of intractable pruritus ani. Dis Colon Rectum 1991;34:289.

Eusebio EB, Graham J, Mody N: Treatment of intractable pruritus ani. Dis Colon Rectum 1990;33:770.

Hanno R, Murphy P: Pruritus ani: Classification and management. Dermatol Clin 1987;5:811.

Silverman SH, et al: The fecal microflora in pruritus ani. Dis Colon Rectum 1989;32:466.

Stolz E, Vuzevski VD, van der Stek J: General perianal skin problems. Neth J Med 1990;37:S43.

RECTAL PROLAPSE

Essentials of Diagnosis

- Protrusion of the rectum through the anus.
- Partial or complete fecal incontinence.
- Rectal bleeding and discharge.

General Considerations

Rectal prolapse (procidentia) is an unusual condition in which the full thickness of the rectum descends through the anus. It must be differentiated from mucosal prolapse (hemorrhoidal), which is common. Postulated causes range from colonic intussusception to a sliding type of hernia involving the rectum. The basic defect is a deficit in one or more of the supporting structures of the rectum, which, combined with increased intra-abdominal pressure, may result in rectal prolapse.

The normal rectal support consists of a mesentery posteriorly, peritoneal folds, fascial attachments, the rectal curvature, and the levator muscle. In the resting state, the puborectalis portion of the levator establishes an acute angle between the lower rectum and anus by pulling anteriorly. This is an especially important supporting element because it closes the opening in the pelvic floor.

When seen in infants and children, rectal prolapse is usually congenital and related to lack of skeletal support and fixation. In adults it is acquired and may be related to injury of the levator muscle (puborectalis), muscular degeneration in elderly or psychotic patients, paralysis of the cauda equina, increased pressure with attenuated tissues, etc.

Clinical Findings

A. Symptoms and Signs: The most obvious manifestation is a protruding mass from the anus. Initially, the prolapse is small, occurs with straining, and reduces spontaneously. Further progression leads to continuous prolapse, which must be manually replaced. In the prolapsed position, the mucosa becomes irritated, bleeds readily, and secretes mucus. This leads to local discomfort and problems with hygiene. With enlargement of the descensus, the anal sphincter dilates and becomes weakened and atonic, leading to incontinence of feces and flatus.

When these patients are examined, it is essential that the prolapse be demonstrated. It is often necessary to have the patient stand or squat and strain to fully demonstrate the prolapse. Concentric mucosal folds characterize this condition. The extent of the weakness of the pelvic musculature and sphincteric ring should be evaluated by observing muscular tone and ability to contract around the examining finger.

On endoscopic examination, the mucosa is often engorged and thickened in the area of prolapse.

B. Special Examinations: Colonoscopy or barium enema x-ray examination of the colon must be done to exclude other disease processes. A neurologic examination is necessary to rule out a primary neurologic disorder. The anal rectal sphincter should be evaluated.

Differential Diagnosis

Many patients with an initial diagnosis of rectal prolapse really have mucosal hemorrhoidal prolapse. In the latter condition, the prolapse is relatively small and often involves just one quadrant, although it may involve several or may be circumferential. The mucosal folds are arranged in a radial fashion, and a sulcus separates the various quadrants. Prolapsing internal hemorrhoids are recognizable by their varicose appearance and separation by a sulcus into discrete masses. Other prolapsing lesions include polyps, tumors, and hypertrophic anal papillae.

Complications

The prolapsing mucosa frequently shows signs of superficial friability, ulceration, and edema. Irreducibility is uncommon. Gangrene or rupture of the anterior rectal wall with extrusion of small bowel is a rare serious complication.

Treatment

A. Medical Treatment: In infants and children, conservative treatment is most satisfactory, since most frequently the prolapse is mucosal.

Stool softeners can be used to prevent straining, and submucosal sclerotherapy may be indicated to create scarring and fixation.

B. Surgical Treatment: Many surgical procedures have been described for complete rectal prolapse which attempt to correct an anatomic defect that has allowed the prolapse. The appropriate one depends in large part on the general condition of the patient. For the elderly, poor-risk, or demented patient, no corrective procedure may be elected. The simplest surgical approach is to use a circumferential loop of synthetic mesh, which is placed in the peri-anal space to constrict the anus at the sphincteric ring and prevent prolapse. Complications of this procedure include fecal impaction, infection, and erosion of the foreign body into the rectum.

For better risk patients, a more definitive transabdominal procedure may be used. The rectum is mobilized by entering the presacral space posteriorly. Gentle traction is then used, and the mobilized rectum is anchored to the sacrum. A Teflon mesh graft is sutured to the upper rectum and then anchored to the presacral fascia (Ripstein procedure). Similarly, Ivalon sponge is popular in England to fix the rectum to the hollow of the sacrum, thus preventing prolapse. In addition, adhesions and fibrosis occur in the tissue planes entered to anchor the rectum. This reinforces the posterior fixation of the rectum and helps to prevent prolapse. Following these procedures, obstruction can occur if the mesh graft is placed too snugly around the bowel or if the bowel undergoes torsion above the point of fixation. Infection in the mesh or sponge and recurrence of the prolapse may occur.

Excisional therapy of the redundant prolapsed rectum is another approach to be considered in the appropriate good-risk patient. This can be done transabdominally by resecting the rectum and performing a low anterior anastomosis between the colon and lower rectum. Rectopexy may also be performed following resection.

Another technique in appropriate patients is via a perineal approach. This can be performed in the lithotomy or preferably the prone jackknife position. The prolapse after mobilization can be excised. This may consist of excision of full-thickness rectum and colon (Altmeier procedure) or just the mucosa with appropriate fixation of the underlying muscle (Delorme procedure). These operations remove the prolapse and are less invasive than the transabdominal approaches.

Other procedures, such as the puborectalis sling operation, have been designed in an attempt to stabilize the rectum and provide additional pelvic support. A Teflon graft is used, and the normal anorectal angle is restored by suturing the sling to the pubic bone. Multiple other operative procedures have been described in the past.

There is continued uncertainty about the exact physiologic defects that allow procidentia of the rectum. Thus, the ideal operation, which can be applied to all, does not exist.

Prognosis

If patients are incontinent before prolapse repair, there will usually be some incontinence postoperatively. The success rate of definitive repairs is about 85%. Recurrences have been reported after all of the commonly used procedures.

Allen-Mersh TG, Turner MJ, Mann CV: Effect of abdominal Ivalon rectopexy on bowel habit and rectal wall. Dis Colon Rectum 1990;33:550.

Berman IR, Harris MS, Robeler MB: Delorme's transrectal excision for internal rectal prolapse: Patient selection, technique and three year follow-up. Dis Colon Rectum 1990;33:573.

Corman ML: Rectal prolapse: Surgical techniques. Surg Clin North Am 1988;68:1255.

Dietzen CD, Pemberton JH: Perineal approaches for the treatment of complete rectal prolapse. Neth J Surg 1989;41:140.

Hiltunen KM et al: Clinical and manometric evaluation of anal sphincter function in patients with rectal prolapse. Am J Surg 1986;151:489.

Monson JR et al: Delorme's operation: The first choice in complete rectal prolapse. Ann R Coll Surg Engl 1986;68:143.

Prasad ML et al: Perineal proctectomy, posterior rectopexy, and postanal levator repair for the treatment of rectal prolapse. Dis Colon Rectum 1986;29:547.

Solla JA, Rothenberger DA, Goldberg SM: Colonic resection in the treatment of rectal prolapse. Neth J Surg 1989;41:132.

Wassef R et al: Rectal prolapse. Curr Probl Surg (June) 1986;23:397.

Williams J et al: Incontinence and rectal prolapse: A prospective manometric study. Dis Colon Rectum 1991;34:209

Yoshioka K, Heyen F, Keighley MRB: Functional results after posterior abdominal rectopexy for rectal prolapse. Dis Colon Rectum 1989;33:835.

SOLITARY RECTAL ULCER

Solitary rectal ulcer is an unusual lesion seen frequently in association with complete rectal prolapse. Symptoms vary but generally consist of the passage of mucus and blood per rectum.

The ulcer is typical in appearance and is generally solitary, occurring on the anterior wall of the rectum and generally 5–10 cm from the anal verge. A rim of hyperemia surrounds the ulcer, with associated fibrosis and necrosis at the base of the lesion. This benign ulcer must be differentiated from carcinoma of the rectum, ulcerative proctitis, Crohn's disease, and other inflammatory conditions.

Patients with solitary rectal ulcer often have a history of bowel irregularity and increased consciousness of bowel function. It has been suggested that the ulcer represents ischemic necrosis of the anterior rectal wall caused by repeated straining with increased intra-abdominal pressure and trauma from internal mucosal prolapse.

Surgical treatment is not indicated. General measures to aid defecation may be of benefit, as well as reassurance to the patient of the benign nature of the lesion.

Mackle EJ, Parks TG: Solitary rectal ulcer syndrome: Aetiology, investigation and management. Dig Dis 1990; 8:294.

Sun WM et al: A common pathophysiology for full thickness rectal prolapse, anterior mucosal prolapse and solitary rectal ulcer. Br J Surg 1989;76:290.

Womack NR et al: Anorectal function in the solitary rectal ulcer syndrome. Dis Colon Rectum 1987;30:319.

Zargar SA, Khuroo MS, Mahajan R: Sucralfate retention enemas in solitary rectal ulcer. Dis Colon Rectum 1991;34:455.

FECAL INCONTINENCE

Essentials of Diagnosis

- Loss of voluntary control of passage of feces from anus.
- Fecal soiling of clothing.

General Considerations

The complex voluntary control of passage of flatus and stool depends on sensory fibers in and around the rectum that discern the need for evacuation. The process involves muscles under voluntary (external sphincter) and involuntary (levator and internal sphincter) control. Therefore, any disease process that interferes with sensation of the rectum or affects function of the anorectal musculature may produce incontinence.

Clinical Findings

In neurogenic incontinence, there is atony of the pelvic musculature with laxity of the anal canal, insensibility to tactile stimulation, inability to contract the anal musculature voluntarily, and absence of anal reflexes. In traumatic or postoperative incontinence, the circumference of the anorectal ring has been disrupted, and the defect can be seen and felt. A clue to the site of the defect is the loss of corrugation, or wrinkling, of the perianal skin because the underlying subcutaneous corrugator cutis ani muscle is absent. Functional ability of the sphincteric muscular ring can be determined by anal-rectal manometry. Extensive inflammatory or malignant disease can give a readily diagnosed rigidity of the rectal outlet.

Prevention

During surgical operations on the anorectum, forceful dilation and inadvertent division of the sphincters must be avoided. In operations for fistula, enough of the anorectal ring must remain to allow control. Postoperative packing must be avoided as well as excision of the sphincter. Obstetric injuries to the sphincters must be immediately recognized and repaired.

Treatment

A. Medical Measures: For mild incontinence, nonsurgical measures (ie, a low-residue diet and anti-cholinergic drugs) may suffice. Daily enemas with a device to allow for retention of the irrigating fluid may be useful. Daily exercises of the sphincter muscles may be of long-term benefit. Patients with neurogenic incontinence may be trained to initiate defecation by digital stimulation of the anal canal.

B. Surgical Treatment: A damaged sphincter may be repaired at the time of injury (following obstetric tears), or electively much later after an injury in patients with established incapacitating incontinence.

Preoperatively, a complete mechanical and antibiotic preparation of the bowel is carried out. Elective surgery is deferred until all local infection has resolved. The tissues should be noninfected and pliable so wound healing can occur primarily.

The divided ends of the muscle are reapproximated. Muscle bundles, which are often encased in scar tissue, are found and mobilized so they can be approximated without tension. Other operations are used when muscle cannot be found. These include fascia lata sling, transplantation of the gracilis muscle from the medial side of the thigh, or encircling of the anus with mesh. In some cases, it may be wise to perform a temporary colostomy at the time of repair or even a permanent one if previous repairs have been unsuccessful.

Prognosis

Prevention of surgical injury to the anorectal sphincter is paramount. Minor incontinence can be controlled with conservative measures. In selected patients, surgical repair will improve voluntary control.

Bielefeldt K, Enck P, Wienbeck M: Diagnosis and treatment of fecal incontinence. Dig Dis 1990;8:179.

Miller R et al: Prospective study of conservative and operative treatment for faecal incontinence. Br J Surg 1988; 75:101.

Pearl R et al: Bilateral gluteus maximus transposition for anal incontinence. Dis Colon Rectum 1991;34:478

Pinho M et al: Assessment of noninvasive intra-anal electromyography to evaluate sphincter function. Dis Colon Rectum 1991;34:69.

Pinho M, Keighley MR: Result of surgery in idiopathic faecal incontinence. Ann Med 1990;22:425.

Wexner SD, Marchetti F, Jagelman DG: The role of sphincteroplasty for fecal incontinence reevaluated: A prospective physiologic and functional review. Dis Colon Rectum 1991;34:22.

Wong WD, Rothenberger DA: Surgical approaches to anal incontinence. Ciba Found Symp 1990;151:246.

Yoshioka K, Keighley MR: Sphincter repair for fecal incontinence. Dis Colon Rectum 1989;32:39.

IDIOPATHIC ANAL PAIN

After exclusion of organic causes, some patients present with anal pain without a specific cause. Levator syndrome is one variant consisting of episodic pain, fullness, and pressure in the rectum and sacrococcygeal area, often aggravated by sitting. Some patients describe a sensation of an intrarectal object. A variant of the syndrome is sharp rectal pain awaking the individual at night (proctalgia fugax). The term coccygodynia was often used in the past for this condition, but few patients actually have coccygeal pain.

Clinical Findings

Many patients have sought previous consultation for their discomfort, but the diagnosis has been missed. There is often an association between stress and symptoms.

A complete examination fails to reveal other painful lesions of the anorectum. Rectal examination reveals a tender levator muscle which, when digitally pressed, reproduces the patient's discomfort. The levator muscle (puborectalis, pubococcygeus) can be felt as it passes from the tip of the coccyx posteriorly to the symphysis pubica anteriorly. Additionally, the coccyx should be palpated and articulated to exclude coccygodynia. Further testing may include manometric studies to investigate sphincter tone and spasm. In addition, defecography may reveal abnormalities of the pelvic muscles.

Differential Diagnosis

Thrombosed external hemorrhoids, anal fissure, and deep perianal abscess must be excluded. Generally, the chronic intermittent symptoms of rectal pain and specific levator tenderness establish the diagnosis.

Treatment & Prognosis

Reassurance about the cause of pain helps. In addition, periodic massage of the painful spastic muscle or electrogalvanic stimulation combined with warm baths and muscle relaxants may be useful. Biofeedback training is also effective.

Levator syndrome may be chronic, with exacerbations often related to stress.

Grimaud JC et al: Manometric and radiologic investigations and biofeedback treatment of chronic idiopathic anal pain. Dis Colon Rectum 1991;34:690.

West L, Abell TL, Cutts T: Anorectal manometry and EMG in the diagnosis of the levator ani syndrome. Gastroenterology 1990;98:A401.

INFECTION & TRAUMA

A history of anal sexual exposure should be sought when any of the conditions in this section are being considered.

Infection

A. Gonococcal Proctitis: Rectal gonorrhea may be present with irritation, itching, drainage, and pain. Examination should include a smear and culture of the discharge. Anoscopy may reveal pus and blood in the rectal ampulla, with edematous and friable mucosa. Treatment consists of penicillin or tetracycline followed by repeated cultures.

B. Syphilis: Perianal or anal ulcers from syphilis are common. The chancre is indurated but generally nontender. Diagnosis is based on darkfield examination and serologic testing. Penicillin is the best treatment. Follow-up as well as treatment of contacts is important.

C. Condylomata Acuminata (Venereal Warts): Venereal warts are caused by a virus. They may occur on the perianal skin, anal canal, and lower rectum, and are often difficult to eradicate. Examination reveals typical cauliflower-like excrescences that may be isolated, scattered, or coalesced. Symptoms include irritation, odor, or bleeding. Before treatment is started, serologic testing and cultures may be indicated. A biopsy should be obtained from unusual-appearing perianal warts before treatment to exclude cancer.

All methods of treatment are painful, and recurrences are frequent. Sexual contact should be stopped while treatment is in progress.

Most patients can be treated in the clinic, but a few severe refractory cases may require treatment in the hospital under anesthesia. Podophyllum resin, 25% in compound tincture of benzoin, should be applied to the warts every 2–3 weeks. Podophyllum resin causes local discomfort and should be washed off after 4–6 hours. Other treatment options include excision, electrocoagulation, and cryosurgical destruction. Immunotherapy using a vaccine obtained from the patient's excised tissue has been attempted in refractory cases.

Carcinoma has been rarely associated with perianal condyloma. An unusual variant, **giant condyloma** (Buschke-Löwenstein tumor), may appear histologically benign but is locally invasive and malignant. Awareness of signs, clinical evaluation, and biopsy are necessary for diagnosis of this rare malignant form.

D. Other Infections: Amebiasis, shigellosis, giardiasis, hepatitis B, infections due to *Chlamydia,* lymphogranuloma venereum, and herpes simplex may be transmitted through sexual contact and may have manifestations in the rectum or anus.

E. AIDS: A number of infections or cancers related to HIV infection and associated immunosuppression may present as anorectal problems. Among them are Kaposi's sarcoma, lymphoma, and squamous carcinoma. Among the causes of ulceration and infection are cytomegalovirus (CMV) infection, herpes simplex virus infection, cryptosporidiosis, isosporiasis, and *Mycobacterium avium-intracellulare* infection, as well as many others. Appropriate biopsies and cultures usually yield the diagnosis. A significant number of patients who are immunosuppressed will present with anorectal infections or malignancy. Physicians must be aware of this in order to correctly diagnose and council.

Trauma & Foreign Bodies

Insertion of foreign bodies into the rectum as part of sexual activity may cause tears, avulsion of the sphincter, excessive bleeding, or perforation of the rectum or intra-abdominal colon. Perirectal or deep abscesses may form following a tear or perforation. Foreign bodies usually can be removed either without anesthesia or with local anesthesia of the anal canal and sphincter. On occasion, general or spinal anesthesia is needed for transrectal extraction; rarely, laparotomy is necessary.

Andrews H et al: Prevalence of sexually transmitted disease among male patients presenting with proctitis. Gut 1988;29:332.

Hyder JW, Mackeigan JM: Anorectal and colonic disease and the immunocompromised host. Dis Colon Rectum 1988;31:971.

Miles AJ et al: Surgical management of anorectal disease in HIV-positive homosexuals. Br J Surg 1990;77:869.

Safavi A, Gottesman L, Dailey TH: Anorectal surgery in the HIV+ patient: Update. Dis Colon Rectum 1991;34:299.

Wexner SD: Sexually transmitted diseases of the colon, rectum, and anus. The challenge of the nineties. Dis Colon Rectum 1990;33:1048.

ANAL STENOSIS

Stenosis of the anal canal leads to increasing difficulty and straining at defecation, with small, painful bowel movements. Frequently there is a history of prior anorectal surgery—primarily hemorrhoidectomy. The narrowing may be at the skin level or higher in the anal canal if an excessive amount of skin or anoderm has been excised. Chronic laxative abuse and spasm due to anal fissure are also common causes of anal stenosis. Other less frequent causes include lymphogranuloma venereum, ulcerative colitis, Crohn's disease, anorectal cancer, irradiation, and congenital abnormalities.

Treatment must be based on the cause. Any suspicious lesion should be biopsied. Mild stenosis may be treated with gentle digital dilation and increased bulk residue in the diet. For severe stenosis, excision of scar, sphincterotomy, and anoplasty may be performed if there is no active coexisting disease (Crohn's disease, etc).

Caplin DA, Kodner IJ: Repair of anal stricture and mucosal ectropion by simple flap procedures. Dis Colon Rectum 1986;29:92

Milsom JW, Mazier WP: Classification and management of postsurgical anal stenosis. Surg Gynecol Obstet 1986;163:60.

Pearl RK et al: Island flap anoplasty for the treatment of anal stricture and mucosal ectropion. Dis Colon Rectum 1990;33:581.

FECAL IMPACTION

Hard desiccated stool impacted in the rectum and unable to pass through the anal canal is common in debilitated or hospitalized patients. A common symptom is diarrhea, because only liquid stool can pass around the impaction. Some patients complain of severe pain in the rectum owing to spasm of the rectal and anal musculature in response to pressure from the impaction.

Fecal impaction can be prevented in hospitalized patients by stool softeners, laxatives, or enemas. Once an impaction is recognized, it must be digitally dislodged. If this is too painful, a local block of the anal sphincter will achieve relaxation and anesthesia. Oil retention enema or 5 mL of 1% docusate sodium in 30 mL of mineral oil taken as an enema may be helpful. Cathartics by mouth will also be useful.

After the impaction is relieved, sigmoidoscopy should be performed to ensure that an inflammatory or neoplastic process does not exist.

Berman IR, Manning DH, Harris MS: Streamlining the management of defecation disorders. Dis Colon Rectum 1990;33:778.

Vanheuverzwym R et al: Chronic idiopathic constipation with outlet obstruction. Hepatogastroenterology 1990; 37:585.

RADIATION PROCTITIS

Exposure to radium, ^{60}Co, and x-ray during treatment of malignant lesions of the pelvis, especially cancer of the cervix, uterus, bladder, and prostate, may cause reaction in the adjacent bowel. With the advent of high-voltage x-ray and ^{60}Co irradiation, skin effects no longer limit the deep dose, as was the case with 200- to 400-kV x-ray therapy. The rectal mucosa is much more sensitive to irradiation than normal vaginal mucosa.

There may be no demonstrable external abnormalities or skin changes at the site of the x-ray exposure. On rectal examination, the anal canal may be tender and spastic. The rectal mucosa may feel indurated, and an ulcer may be felt.

In the first few weeks after exposure, proctosigmoidoscopy shows a red, edematous mucosa that bleeds easily with slight trauma. It later becomes indurated and then flat, pale, and atrophic, and it develops persistent telangiectasis. When ulcers occur, they are gray, well-defined, and oval or circular. A barium enema may demonstrate mucosal abnormalities, fistulas, or a stricture. The rectosigmoid may be involved, resulting in a stenosing ulcerative lesion closely resembling cancer. Stenosis may not develop for months or years after treatment.

Small increments of radiation therapy to multiple fields, megavoltage, and cobalt teletherapy reduce the incidence of injury to the rectum and sigmoid colon. Direct exposure of bladder, bowel, and ureters must be avoided wherever possible. Special shield applicators for radium insertion and positioning of the patient for external beam therapy should be used.

Symptoms related to radiation proctitis include bleeding, frequent loose irritating movements, spasms, and incontinence. Treatment depends on the severity of symptoms and the amount of time elapsed since irradiation. Symptoms occurring soon after irradiation is started may be transient and require no treatment. Rectal instillation of hydrocortisone in enema or as a suppository may be effective for more severe symptoms. Patients with severe bleeding, pain, stenosis, or fistulas to the bladder or vagina may require a proximal diverting colostomy with mucous fistula in nonirradiated bowel or, in selected cases, resection of the involved segment. The injury to the bowel may progress over a period of years, with the development of fibrosis and obliterative arterial changes.

Buchi K: Radiation proctitis: Therapy and prognosis. JAMA 1991;265:1180.

Galland RB, Spencer MS: Surgical management of radiation enteritis. Surgery 1986;99:133.

Gazet JC: Parks' coloanal pull-through anastomosis for severe, complicated radiation proctitis. Dis Colon Rectum 1985;28:110.

Jao SW, Beart RW Jr, Gunderson LL: Surgical treatment of radiation injuries of the colon and rectum. Am J Surg 1986;151:272.

Kimose H-H et al: Late radiation injury of the colon and rectum: Surgical management and outcome. Dis Colon Rectum 1989;32:684.

MALIGNANT TUMORS OF THE ANAL CANAL & PERINEUM

Several relatively uncommon tumors arise from the epithelial surface distal to the mucocutaneous juncture. Symptoms are nonspecific and include bleeding, drainage, pain, mass, pruritus, etc. The examining physician must be aware of these lesions and differentiate them from benign conditions such as hemorrhoids, leukoplakia, lymphogranuloma venereum, venereal warts, chronic fissure, and chronic skin changes. The diagnosis can often be established only by biopsy.

Epidermoid Carcinoma of the Anorectum (Squamous Cell Carcinoma)

This is the most common tumor of the anal canal and perineum, accounting for 75% of malignant growths in this area. It is uncommon (3–5%) compared with adenocarcinoma of the rectum. Transitional cell, cloacogenic, basiloid, basosquamous, or mucoepidermoid tumors are considered variants of epidermoid carcinoma. There is a probable viral link and association with sexual transmission.

When diagnosed early, the lesion may be small, mobile, and verrucous. Large lesions are ulcerated and indurated and produce a palpable mass. There may be skin satellitosis and palpable inguinal lymph nodes. The rectum and sphincter may be invaded, giving a false appearance of a primary rectal cancer. Leukoplakia, lymphogranuloma venereum, chronic fistulas, and irradiated anal skin are predisposing causes.

Anal carcinoma may spread along the lymphatics of the rectum to the perirectal and mesenteric lymph nodes as well as to the inguinal lymph nodes. Carcinoma arising external to the anus metastasizes to the inguinal nodes either across the perineum to the superficial inguinal lymph nodes or along the middle hemorrhoidal lymphatics to the hypogastric and obturator nodes and from there to the external iliac and inguinal lymph nodes.

Treatment depends upon the stage of the tumor, its location, and the depth of invasion. The lesion must be inspected carefully and often, using general anesthesia if the examination causes undue pain. CT scan and ultrasound may assist in determining local penetration and spread. Superficial mobile and small lesions arising below the mucocutaneous juncture may be treated by local excision. Larger tumors that invade the sphincter or rectum must be approached differently. External radiation with simultaneous chemotherapy (fluorouracil and mitomycin or fluorouracil and cisplatin) is preferred as primary therapy (Table 32–1). The tumor is controlled in about 80% of patients treated in this way. Radical surgery (eg, abdominoperineal resection) is reserved for treatment failures or recurrent disease.

Malignant Melanoma

Malignant melanoma arising in the anorectum has an extremely poor prognosis. Often undetected for long periods, the lesion frequently presents as a dark mass protruding from the anus or as an ulcer. Over half of such lesions are pigmented. Lymph node involvement and distant metastasis occur early. Surgical treatment ranges from local excision to abdominal perineal resection and pelvic lymph node dissection. Radical surgery, however, has not been shown to increase survival and is rarely indicated. Systemic or perfusion chemotherapy and immunologic agents with autologous vaccine are under study. No specific treatment has proved superior.

Table 32–1. Treatment of anal carcinoma

T Stage	N Stage	Radiation Therapy	Adjuvant Chemotherapy[1]
T0	N0	None (local excision)	None
T1<1 cm	N0	None (local excision)	None
T1>1 cm	N0	Local[2]	None
T2	N0	Local	Yes
T3	N0	Regional[3]	Yes
T4	N0	Regional	Yes
All	N1–3	Regional	Yes

[1]Combination cisplatin and fluorouracil.
[2]Local irradiation: 5400–5800 cGy given to tumor site by external irradiation using a three-field technique (two lateral and one sacral field).
[3]Regional irradiation: 5400–5800 cGy given to tumor site and regional nodes by external irradiation using a two-field technique (two anteroposterior-posteroanterior opposed fields).

Bowen's Disease

Bowen's disease (intraepidermal squamous cell carcinoma) may present in the perianal area as it does on the face, hands, and trunk. Patients are seen frequently for pruritus and a dull, red, spreading, irregular plaque-like eczematoid lesion. Biopsy reveals carcinoma in situ, with hyperkeratosis and a characteristic intraepidermoid, haloed giant cell. Treatment consists of local excision with adequate margins or topical use of fluorouracil.

Extramammary Paget's Disease

Extramammary Paget's disease of the anus (intraepithelial adenocarcinoma) is a rare condition appearing as a pale gray, plaque-like lesion with surrounding induration and sometimes an underlying mass. In contrast with Paget's disease of the nipple, there may not be an underlying tumor. Diagnosis depends on biopsy and histologic findings of large intraepithelial cells. If there is a deep tumor, it is an infiltrating, usually colloid carcinoma arising from a perianal gland or other skin appendage. Treatment consists of local excision if tumor is absent, to more radical excisional therapy, chemotherapy, and radiation therapy for cancer.

Basal Cell Carcinoma

Basal cell carcinoma is an uncommon ulcerating tumor presenting at the anal verge and is similar to the more frequent "rodent ulcer" seen on exposed skin surfaces. Local excision is the treatment of choice, since this tumor does not metastasize.

Malignant Tumors: Kaposi's Sarcoma

An uncommon malignancy in the anorectal area, it has been recently recognized in immunosuppressed patients following transplantation or in those with AIDS. It presents as small brown-red nodules. Biopsy will confirm the diagnosis. Kaposi's sarcoma is radiosensitive, with chemotherapy reserved for systemic disease.

Beart RW Jr: Colon, rectum, and anus. Cancer 1990;65:684.
Cho CC et al: Squamous-cell carcinoma of the anal canal: Management with combined chemo-radiation therapy. Dis Colon Rectum 1991;34:675.
Gordon PH: Current status: Perianal and anal canal neoplasms. Dis Colon Rectum 1990;33:799.
Leichman LP, Cummings BJ: Anal carcinoma. Curr Probl Cancer 1990;14:117.
Lopez MJ et al: Carcinoma of the anal region. Curr Probl Surg 1989;26:525.
Nigro ND, Vaitkeviceus VK; Herskovic AM: Preservation of function in the treatment of cancer of the anus. Important Adv Oncol 1989;:161.
Nigro N: The force of change in the management of squamous-cell cancer of the anal canal: Harry E. Bacon Oration. Dis Colon Rectum 1991;34:482.
Scherrer A et al: CT of malignant anal canal tumors. Radiographics 1990;10:433.
Shutze WP, Gleysteen JJ: Perianal Paget's disease. Classification and review of management: Report of two cases. Dis Colon Rectum 1990;33:502.
Tanum G et al: Chemotherapy and radiation therapy for anal carcinoma: Survival and late morbidity. Cancer 1991;67:2462.
Ward MWN et al: The surgical treatment of anorectal malignant melanoma. Br J Surg 1986;73:68.

REFERENCES

Corman ML: *Colon and Rectal Surgery,* 2nd ed. Lippincott, 1984.
Goligher JC: *Surgery of the Anus, Rectum and Colon,* 5th ed. Bailliere Tindall, 1983.

Gordon PH, Nivatvongs S: *Principles and Practice of Surgery for the Colon, Rectum, and Anus.* Quality Medical Publishing, 1991.

33

Hernias & Other Lesions of the Abdominal Wall*

Karen E. Deveney, MD

HERNIAS

An external hernia is an abnormal protrusion of intra-abdominal tissue through a fascial defect in the abdominal wall. About 75% of hernias occur in the groin (indirect inguinal, direct inguinal, femoral). Incisional and ventral hernias comprise about 10%; umbilical, 3%; and others, about 3%. Generally, a hernial mass is composed of covering tissues (skin, subcutaneous tissues, etc), a peritoneal sac, and any contained viscera. Particularly if the neck of the sac is narrow where it emerges from the abdomen, bowel protruding into the hernia may become obstructed or strangulated. If the hernia is not repaired early, the defect may enlarge, and operative repair may become more complicated. The definitive treatment of hernia is early operative repair.

A **reducible hernia** is one in which the contents of the sac return to the abdomen spontaneously or with manual pressure when the patient is recumbent.

An **irreducible (incarcerated) hernia** is one whose contents cannot be returned to the abdomen, usually because they are trapped by a narrow neck. The term incarceration does not imply obstruction, inflammation, or ischemia of the herniated organs, though incarceration is necessary for obstruction or strangulation to occur.

Though the lumen of a segment of bowel within the hernia sac may become **obstructed,** there may initially be no interference with blood supply. Compromise to the blood supply of the contents of the sac (eg, omentum or intestine) results in a **strangulated hernia,** in which gangrene of the sac and its contents has occurred. The incidence of strangulation is higher in femoral than in inguinal hernias, but strangulation may occur in other hernias as well.

An uncommon and dangerous type of hernia, a **Richter hernia,** occurs when only a part of the cir-cumference of the bowel becomes incarcerated or strangulated in the fascial defect. A strangulated Richter hernia may spontaneously reduce and the gangrenous piece of intestine be overlooked at operation. The bowel may subsequently perforate, with resultant peritonitis.

HERNIAS OF THE GROIN

Anatomy

All hernias of the abdominal wall consist of a peritoneal sac that protrudes through a weakness or defect in the muscular layers of the abdomen. The defect may be congenital or acquired.

Just outside the peritoneum is the **transversalis fascia,** an aponeurosis whose weakness or defect is the major source of groin hernias. Next are found the **transversus abdominis, internal oblique,** and **external oblique muscles,** which are fleshy laterally and aponeurotic medially. Their aponeuroses form investing layers of the strong **rectus abdominis muscles** above the semilunar line. Below this line, the aponeurosis lies entirely in front of the muscle. Between the two vertical rectus muscles, the aponeuroses meet again to form the **linea alba,** which is well defined only above the umbilicus. The subcutaneous fat contains Scarpa's fascia—a misnomer, since it is only a condensation of connective tissue with no substantial strength.

In the groin, an **indirect inguinal hernia** results when obliteration of the processus vaginalis, the peritoneal extension accompanying the testis in its descent into the scrotum, fails to occur. The resultant hernia sac passes through the **internal inguinal ring,** a defect in the transversalis fascia halfway between the anterior iliac spine and the pubic tubercle. The sac is located anteromedially within the spermatic cord and may extend partway along the **inguinal canal** or accompany the cord out through the subcutaneous (external) inguinal ring, a defect medially in the external oblique muscle just above the pubic tubercle. A hernia that passes fully into the scrotum is known as a **complete hernia.** The sac and the spermatic cord

---

*See Chapter 46 for further discussion of hernias in the pediatric age group and Chapter 22 for a discussion of internal hernias.

are invested by the **cremaster muscle,** an extension of fibers of the internal oblique muscle.

Other anatomic structures of the groin that are important in understanding the formation of hernias and types of hernia repairs include the **conjoined tendon,** or falx inguinalis, a fusion of the medial aponeurotic transversus abdominis and internal oblique muscles that passes along the inferolateral edge of the rectus abdominis muscle and attaches to the pubic tubercle. Between the pubic tubercle and anterior iliac spine passes the **inguinal (Poupart) ligament,** formed by the lowermost border of the external oblique aponeurosis as it rolls on itself and thickens into a cord.

The lower end of the inguinal ligament is reflected dorsally and laterally from the pubic tubercle back along the iliopectineal line of the pubis as the **lacunar (Gimbernat) ligament.** The lacunar ligament is about 1.25 cm long and triangular in shape. The sharp, crescentic lateral border of this ligament is the unyielding noose for the strangulation of a femoral hernia.

Cooper's ligament is a strong, fibrous band that extends laterally for about 2.5 cm along the iliopectineal line on the superior aspect of the superior pubic ramus, starting at the lateral base of the lacunar ligament.

Hesselbach's triangle is bounded by the inguinal ligament, the inferior epigastric vessels, and the lateral border of the rectus muscle. A weakness or defect in the transversalis fascia, which forms the floor of this triangle, results in a **direct inguinal hernia.** In most direct hernias, the transversalis fascia is diffusely attenuated, though a discrete defect in the fascia may occasionally occur. This **funicular** type of direct inguinal hernia is more likely to become incarcerated, since it has distinct borders.

A **femoral hernia** passes beneath the inguinal ligament into the upper thigh. The predisposing anatomic feature for femoral hernias is a small empty space between the lacunar ligament medially and the femoral vein laterally—the **femoral canal.** Because its borders are distinct and unyielding, a femoral hernia has the highest risk of incarceration and strangulation.

Causes

Nearly all inguinal hernias in infants, children, and young adults are **indirect inguinal hernias.** Although these "congenital" hernias most often present during the first year of life, the first clinical evidence of hernia may not appear until middle or old age, when increased intra-abdominal pressure and dilatation of the internal inguinal ring allow abdominal contents to enter the previously empty peritoneal diverticulum. An untreated indirect hernia will inevitably dilate the internal ring and displace or attenuate the inguinal floor. The peritoneum may protrude on either side of the inferior epigastric vessels to give a combined direct and indirect hernia, called a **pantaloon hernia.**

In contrast, **direct inguinal hernias** are acquired as the result of a developed weakness of the transversalis fascia in Hesselbach's area. There is some evidence that direct inguinal hernias may be related to hereditary or acquired defects in collagen synthesis or turnover. **Femoral hernias** involve an acquired protrusion of a peritoneal sac through the femoral ring. In women, the ring may become dilated by the physical and biochemical changes during pregnancy.

Any condition that chronically increases intra-abdominal pressure may contribute to the appearance and progression of a hernia. Marked obesity, abdominal strain from heavy exercise or lifting, cough, constipation with straining at stool, and prostatism with straining on micturition are often implicated. Cirrhosis with ascites, pregnancy, chronic ambulatory peritoneal dialysis, and chronically enlarged pelvic organs or pelvic tumors may also contribute. Loss of tissue turgor in Hesselbach's area, associated with a weakening of the transversalis fascia, occurs with advancing age and in chronic debilitating disease.

That colonic cancer may predispose in some way to inguinal herniation was initially suggested a half century ago, and the concept and has gained renewed credibility from several recent studies. While there is no clear mechanism whereby colon cancer could cause hernia, the prevalence of colonic neoplasia and the insensitivity of tests for occult blood in the stool argue in favor of routine flexible sigmoidoscopy in all patients over age 50.

Skandalakis JE et al: Surgical anatomy of the inguinal area. World J Surg 1989;13:490.

Wheeler WE et al: Flexible sigmoidoscopy screening for asymptomatic colorectal disease in patients with and without inguinal hernia. South Med J 1991;84:876.

1. INDIRECT & DIRECT INGUINAL HERNIAS

Clinical Findings

A. Symptoms: Most hernias produce no symptoms until the patient notices a lump or swelling in the groin, though some patients may describe a sudden pain and bulge that occurred while lifting or straining. Frequently, hernias are detected in the course of routine physical examinations such as pre-employment examinations. Some patients complain of a dragging sensation and, particularly with indirect inguinal hernias, radiation of pain into the scrotum. As a hernia enlarges, it is likely to produce a sense of discomfort or aching pain, and the patient must lie down to reduce the hernia.

In general, direct hernias produce fewer symptoms than indirect inguinal hernias and are less likely to become incarcerated or strangulated.

B. Signs: Examination of the groin reveals a mass that may or may not be reducible. The patient should be examined both supine and standing and also with coughing and straining, since small hernias may be difficult to demonstrate. The external ring can be identified by invaginating the scrotum and palpating with the index finger just above and lateral to the pubic tubercle (Figure 33–1). If the external ring is very small, the examiner's finger may not enter the inguinal canal, and it may be difficult to be sure that a pulsation felt on coughing is truly a hernia. At the other extreme, a widely patent external ring does not by itself constitute hernia. Tissue must be felt protruding into the inguinal canal during coughing in order for a hernia to be diagnosed.

Differentiating between direct and indirect inguinal hernia on examination is difficult and is of little importance since most groin hernias should be repaired regardless of type. Nevertheless, each type of inguinal hernia has specific features more common to it. A hernia that descends into the scrotum is almost certainly indirect. On inspection with the patient erect and straining, a direct hernia more commonly appears as a symmetric, circular swelling at the external ring; the swelling disappears when the patient lies down. An indirect hernia appears as an elliptic swelling that may not reduce easily.

On palpation, the posterior wall of the inguinal canal is firm and resistant in an indirect hernia but relaxed or absent in a direct hernia. If the patient is asked to cough or strain while the examining finger is directed laterally and upward into the inguinal canal, a direct hernia protrudes against the side of the finger, whereas an indirect hernia is felt at the tip of the finger.

Compression over the internal ring when the patient strains may also help to differentiate between in-direct and direct hernias. A direct hernia bulges forward through Hesselbach's triangle, but the opposite hand can maintain reduction of an indirect hernia at the internal ring.

These distinctions are obscured as a hernia enlarges and distorts the anatomic relationships of the inguinal rings and canal. In most patients the type of inguinal hernia cannot be established accurately before surgery.

Differential Diagnosis

Groin pain of musculoskeletal or obscure origin may be difficult to distinguish from hernia. Herniography, in which x-rays are obtained after intraperitoneal injection of contrast medium, may aid in the diagnosis in cases of groin pain when no hernia can be felt even after multiple maneuvers to increase intra-abdominal pressure.

Herniation of properitoneal fat through the inguinal ring into the spermatic cord ("lipoma of the cord") is commonly misinterpreted as a hernia sac. Its true nature may only be confirmed at operation. Occasionally, a femoral hernia that has extended above the inguinal ligament after passing through the fossa ovalis femoris may be confused with an inguinal hernia. If the examining finger is placed on the pubic tubercle, the neck of the sac of a femoral hernia lies lateral and below, while that of an inguinal hernia lies above.

Inguinal hernia must be differentiated from hydrocele of the spermatic cord, lymphadenopathy or abscesses of the groin, varicocele, and residual hematoma following trauma or spontaneous hemorrhage in patients taking anticoagulants. An undescended testis in the inguinal canal must also be considered when the testis cannot be felt in the scrotum.

The presence of an impulse in the mass with coughing, bowel sounds in the mass, and failure to transilluminate are features which indicate that an irreducible mass in the groin is a hernia.

Treatment

Inguinal hernias should always be repaired unless there are specific contraindications. The same advice applies to patients of all ages; the complications of incarceration, obstruction, and strangulation are greater threats than are the risks of operation.

Elderly patients tolerate elective repair of a groin hernia very well, especially when other medical problems are optimally controlled and local anesthetic is used. Emergency operation carries a much greater risk for the elderly than carefully planned elective operation.

If the patient has significant prostatic hyperplasia, it is prudent to solve this problem first, since the risks of urinary retention and urinary tract infection are high following hernia repair in patients with significant prostatic obstruction.

Although most direct hernias do not carry as high a

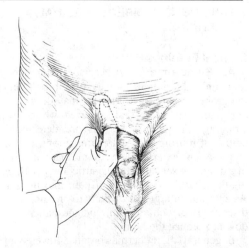

Figure 33–1. Insertion of finger through upper scrotum into external inguinal ring.

risk of incarceration as indirect hernias, the difficulty in reliably differentiating them from indirect hernias makes the repair of all inguinal hernias advisable. Funicular hernias, which are particularly likely to incarcerate, should always be repaired.

Because of the possibility of strangulation, an incarcerated, painful, or tender hernia usually requires an emergency operation. In patients with serious concomitant disease, nonoperative reduction of the incarcerated hernia may first be attempted. The patient is placed with hips elevated and given analgesics and sedation sufficient to promote muscle relaxation. Repair of the hernia may be deferred if the hernia mass reduces with gentle manipulation and if there is no clinical evidence of strangulated bowel. Though strangulation is usually clinically evident, gangrenous tissue can occasionally be reduced into the abdomen by manual or spontaneous reduction. It is therefore safest to repair the reduced hernia at the earliest opportunity.

At surgery, one must decide whether to explore the abdomen to make certain that the intestine is viable. If the patient has leukocytosis or clinical signs of peritonitis or if the hernia sac contains dark or bloody fluid, the abdomen should be explored.

A. Principles of Operative Treatment of Inguinal Hernia:

1. Successful repair requires that any correctable aggravating factors be identified and treated (chronic cough, prostatic obstruction, colonic tumor, ascites, etc) and that the defect be reconstructed with the best available tissues that can be approximated without tension.

2. An indirect hernia sac should be anatomically isolated, dissected to its origin from the peritoneum, and ligated (Figure 33–2). In infants and young adults in whom the inguinal anatomy is normal, repair can usually be limited to high ligation, removal of the sac, and reduction of the internal ring to an appropriate size. For most adult hernias, the inguinal floor should also be reconstructed. The internal ring should be reduced to a size just adequate to allow egress of the cord structures. In women, the internal ring can be totally closed to prevent recurrence through that site. To construct a solid inguinal floor in men with recurrent hernias, it may rarely be necessary to divide the cord and completely close the internal ring. The testicle may be removed or left in the scrotum.

3. In direct inguinal hernia (Figure 33–3), the inguinal canal may be so wide and its floor so weak that the repair appears to be under tension. In such cases, a vertical relaxing incision in the anterior rectus abdominis sheath will allow the repair to rest without tension.

4. Even though a direct hernia is found, the cord should always be carefully searched for a possible indirect hernia as well.

5. In patients with large hernias, bilateral repair should not usually be performed as one procedure,

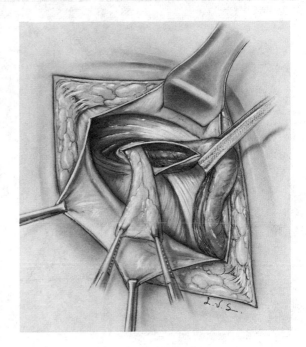

Figure 33–2. Indirect inguinal hernia. Inguinal canal opened, showing spermatic cord retracted medially and indirect hernia peritoneal sac dissected free to above the level of the internal inguinal ring.

since greater tension in the repairs increases the recurrence rate and surgical complications. In children and adults with small hernias, bilateral hernia repair is recommended because it spares the patient a second anesthetic.

6. Recurrent hernia within a few months or a year of operation usually indicates an inadequate repair, such as overlooking an indirect sac or failing to repair the fascial defect securely. Any repair completed under tension is subject to early recurrence. Recurrences two or more years after repair are more likely to be caused by progressive weakening of the patient's fascia. Repeated recurrence after careful repair by an experienced surgeon suggests a defect in collagen synthesis. Because the fascial defect is often small, firm, and unyielding, recurrent hernias are much more likely to develop incarceration or strangulation than unoperated inguinal hernias, and they should nearly always be repaired again.

If recurrence is due to an overlooked indirect sac, the posterior wall is often solid and removal of the sac may be all that is required. Occasionally, a recurrence is discovered to consist of a small, sharply circumscribed defect in the previous hernioplasty, in which case closure of the defect suffices. More diffuse weakness of the posterior inguinal wall or repeated recurrences occasionally require more elaborate repair using fascia lata from the thigh or polypropylene (Marlex) mesh.

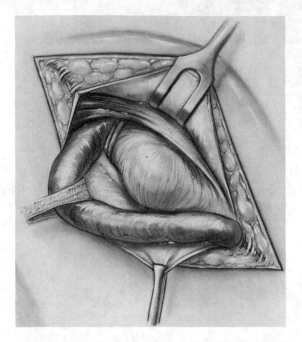

Figure 33–3. Direct inguinal hernia. Inguinal canal opened and spermatic cord retracted inferiorly and laterally to reveal the hernia bulging through the floor of Hesselbach's triangle.

B. Types of Operations for Inguinal Hernia: Different operative techniques are designed to deal with variations in the size and location of a hernia and the extent of associated tissue weakness.

Simple high ligation of the sac through an inguinal incision is the key to the repair of indirect hernias in infants and children. Combined with a tightening of the internal ring, it is called the **Marcy repair.**

Repair of inguinal hernias in adults can be accomplished successfully through an inguinal, properitoneal, or abdominal approach, though inguinal repairs are most widely used today. Though a given repair may be championed by a particular surgeon or group, there is no comparative study demonstrating the superiority of any one type; in fact, it seems likely that all the methods in common use give equivalent results. Details of technique and the experience and skill of the surgeon are more likely to account for differences in results.

Though most methods of repairing indirect inguinal hernias in adults emphasize high ligation of the sac, as in children, elimination of the sac by reducing it may suffice. The factor common to all successful methods of inguinal hernia repairs in adults is repair of the inguinal floor.

The **Bassini repair,** the most widely used method, approximates the conjoined tendon to Poupart's ligament and leaves the spermatic cord in its normal anatomic position under the external oblique aponeuro-

sis. The **Halsted repair** places the external oblique beneath the cord but otherwise resembles the Bassini repair. **Cooper's ligament (Lotheissen-McVay) repair** brings conjoined tendon farther posteriorly and inferiorly to Cooper's ligament. Unlike the Bassini and Halsted methods, McVay's repair is effective for femoral hernia but always requires a relaxing incision to relieve tension. Though the **Shouldice repair** has a low reported recurrence rate, it is not widely used, perhaps because of the more extensive dissection required and a belief that the skill of the surgeons may be as important as the method itself. In the Shouldice repair, the transversalis fascia is first divided and then imbricated to Poupart's ligament. Finally, the conjoined tendon and internal oblique muscle are also approximated in layers to the inguinal ligament.

The **properitoneal approach** exposes the groin from between the transversalis fascia and peritoneum via a lower abdominal incision to effect closure of the fascial defect. Because it requires more initial dissection and is associated with higher morbidity and recurrence rates in less experienced hands, it is not widely favored.

A desire to decrease the recurrence rate of hernias has prompted an increased use of prosthetic materials in repair of both recurrent and first-time hernias. Methods include "plugs" of mesh inserted into the internal ring and sheets of mesh to reinforce the repair. However, whether mesh has a useful role in routine hernia repair has not yet been established.

Within the past 2 years, serious investigation has begun into methods of repairing inguinal hernias laparoscopically. The method currently thought to have the greatest promise involves the use of staples to secure a patch of mesh over the internal ring. While the initial experience is encouraging, the efficacy—in particular, the long-term results—and the comparative morbidity of laparoscopic hernia repair are as yet unknown. Until these issues are settled, such operations should probably be restricted to prospective clinical trials.

C. Nonsurgical Management (Use of a Truss): The surgeon is occasionally called upon to prescribe a truss when a patient refuses operative repair or when there are absolute contraindications to operation. A truss should be fitted to provide adequate external compression over the defect in the abdominal wall. It should be taken off at night and put on in the morning before the patient arises. The use of a truss does not preclude later repair of a hernia, although it may cause fibrosis of the anatomic structures, so that subsequent repair may be difficult.

Pre- & Postoperative Course

The preoperative evaluation should be completed before hospitalization. The patient usually enters the hospital on the morning of operation. The anesthetic may be general, spinal, or local. Local anesthetic is effective for most patients, and the incidence of urinary retention and pulmonary complications is lowest with local anesthesia. Recurrent hernias are more easily repaired with the patient under spinal or general anesthesia, since local anesthetic does not readily diffuse through scar tissue. In the past, the patient was routinely kept in the hospital for a few days after operation, but "come-and-go" hernia repair has been shown to be safe and effective, particularly for younger and healthier patients, and is now common. A sedentary worker may return to work within a few days; heavy manual labor has traditionally not been performed for up to 4–6 weeks after hernia repair, though recent studies document no increase in recurrence when full activity is resumed as early as 3 weeks after surgery.

Prognosis

In addition to chronic cough, prostatism, and constipation, poor tissue quality and poor operative technique may contribute to recurrence of inguinal hernia. Because tissue is often more attenuated in direct hernias, recurrence rates are higher than for indirect hernias. Placing the repair under tension and using absorbable suture are technical errors that lead to recurrence. Failure to find an indirect hernia, to dissect the sac high enough, or to adequately close the internal ring may lead to recurrence of indirect hernia. Postoperative wound infection is associated with increased recurrence. The recurrence rate is considerably increased in patients receiving chronic peritoneal dialysis—in one report, the rate was as high as 27%.

Recurrence rates after indirect hernia repair in adults are reported at best to be 0.6–3%, though the incidence is more probably 5–10%. Inadequate sac reduction or internal ring closure and failure to identify a femoral or direct hernia contribute to recurrence, as does inadequate repair of the inguinal canal. A wide range of figures is quoted for recurrence after repair of direct hernias, from less than 1% to as high as 28%. The point of recurrence is most often just lateral to the pubic tubercle, implicating excessive tension on the repair and adding evidence to favor the routine use of a relaxing incision in the rectus sheath in the repair of direct hernias.

Barbier J, Carretier M, Richer JP: Cooper ligament repair: An update. World J Surg 1989;13:499.

Curtsinger LJ III et al: Orchiectomy during herniorrhaphy: What should we tell the patient? Am J Surg 1987; 154:636.

Greenburg AG: Revisiting the recurrent groin hernia. Am J Surg 1987;154:35.

Gullmo A: Herniography. World J Surg 1989;13:560.

Heydorn WH et al: A five-year U.S. Army experience with 36,250 abdominal hernia repairs. Am Surg 1990;56:596.

Johnson J et al: Radionuclide imaging in the diagnosis of hernias related to peritoneal dialysis. Arch Surg 1987; 122:952.

Lichtenstein IL: Herniorrhaphy: A personal experience with 6,321 cases. Am J Surg 1987;153:553.

Lichtenstein IL et al: The tension-free hernioplasty. Am J Surg 1989;157:188.

Rutledge RH: Cooper's ligament repair: A 25-year experience with a single technique for all groin hernias in adults. Surgery 1988;103:1.

Stoppa RE: The treatment of complicated groin and incisional hernias. World J Surg 1989;13:545.

Young DV: Comparison of local, spinal, and general anesthesia for inguinal herniorrhaphy. Am J Surg 1987; 153:560.

2. SLIDING INGUINAL HERNIA (Figures 33–4 and 33–5)

A sliding inguinal hernia is a type of indirect inguinal hernia in which the wall of a viscus forms a portion of the wall of the hernia sac. On the right side the cecum is most commonly involved, and on the left side the sigmoid colon. The development of a sliding hernia is related to the variable degree of posterior fixation of the large bowel or other sliding components (eg, bladder, ovary) and their proximity to the internal inguinal ring.

Clinical Findings

Though sliding hernias have no special signs that

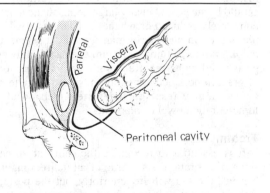

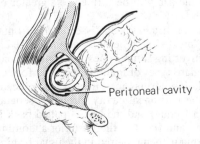

Figure 33–4. Right-sided sliding hernia. ***Top:*** Note cecum and ascending colon sliding on fascia of posterior abdominal wall. ***Bottom:*** Hernia has entered internal inguinal ring. Note that one-fourth of the hernia is not related to the peritoneal sac.

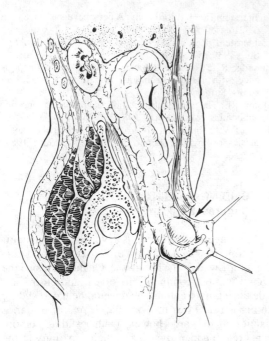

Figure 33–5. Right-sided sliding hernia seen in sagittal section. (After Linden in Thorek.) At arrow, the wall of the cecum forms a portion of the hernia sac.

distinguish them from other inguinal hernias, they should be suspected in any large hernia that cannot be completely reduced or whenever a large scrotal hernia is seen in an elderly man. Finding a segment of colon in the scrotum on barium enema strongly suggests a sliding hernia. Recognition of this variation is of great importance at operation, since failure to recognize it may result in inadvertent incision of the lumen of the bowel or bladder.

Treatment

It is essential to recognize the entity at an early stage of operation. As is true of all indirect inguinal hernias, the sac will lie anteriorly, but the posterior wall of the sac will be formed to a greater or lesser degree by colon.

After the cord has been dissected free from the hernia sac, most sliding hernias can be reduced by a series of inverting sutures (Bevan technique) and one of the standard types of inguinal repair performed. Very large sliding hernias may have to be reduced by entering the peritoneal cavity through a separate incision (La Roque) and the bowel pulled back into the abdomen and fixed to the posterior abdominal wall. The hernia is then repaired in the usual fashion.

Prognosis

Sliding hernias have a higher recurrence rate than uncomplicated indirect hernias.

The surgical complications most often encountered

following sliding hernia repair are encroachment on the circulation to the large bowel, with bowel necrosis, and actual strangulation of a portion of the large bowel when attempting a high ligation of the hernia sac.

Mackie JA Jr, Berkowitz HD: Sliding inguinal hernia. In: *Hernia,* 3rd ed. Nyhus LM, Condon RE (editors). Lippincott, 1989.

3. FEMORAL HERNIA

A femoral hernia descends through the femoral canal beneath the inguinal ligament. Because of its narrow neck, it is prone to incarceration and strangulation. Femoral hernia is much more common in women than in men, but in both sexes femoral hernia is less common than inguinal hernia. Femoral hernias comprise about one-third of groin hernias in women and about 2% of groin hernias in men.

Clinical Findings

A. Symptoms: Femoral hernias are notoriously asymptomatic until incarceration or strangulation occurs. Even with obstruction or strangulation, the patient may feel discomfort more in the abdomen than in the femoral area. Thus, colicky abdominal pain and signs of intestinal obstruction frequently are the presenting manifestations of a strangulated femoral hernia, without discomfort, pain, or tenderness in the femoral region.

B. Signs: A femoral hernia may present in a variety of ways. If it is small and uncomplicated, it usually appears as a small bulge in the upper medial thigh just below the level of the inguinal ligament. Because it may be deflected anteriorly through the fossa ovalis femoris to present as a visible or palpable mass at or above the inguinal ligament, it can be confused with an inguinal hernia.

Differential Diagnosis

Femoral hernia must be distinguished from inguinal hernia, a saphenous varix, and femoral adenopathy. A saphenous varix transmits a distinct thrill when a patient coughs, and it appears and disappears instantly when the patient stands or lies down—in contrast to femoral hernias, which are either irreducible or reduce gradually on pressure.

Treatment

A. Principles: The principles of femoral hernia repair are as follows: (1) complete excision of the hernia sac, (2) the use of nonabsorbable sutures, (3) repair of the defect in the transversalis fascia that is responsible for the hernia, and (4) use of Cooper's ligament for the repair, since it gives a firm support for sutures and forms the natural line for closure of the defect.

B. Types of Repair for Femoral Hernia: A femoral hernia can be repaired through an inguinal, thigh, properitoneal, or abdominal approach, though the inguinal approach is most commonly used. No matter what the approach, the hernia is often difficult to reduce. Reduction may be facilitated by carefully incising the iliopubic tract, Gimbernat's ligament, or even the inguinal ligament. Occasionally, a counterincision in the thigh is required to free attachments below the inguinal ligament.

Irrespective of the approach used, successful femoral hernia repair must close the femoral canal. The Lotheissen-McVay repair, also used for inguinal hernia, is most commonly employed.

If the hernia sac and mass reduce when the patient is given opiates or anesthesia and if bloody fluid appears in the hernia sac when it is exposed and opened, one must strongly suspect the possibility of nonviable bowel in the peritoneal cavity. In such cases, it is mandatory to open and explore the abdomen, usually through a separate midline incision.

Prognosis

Recurrence rates usually approximate the middle range for direct inguinal hernia, ie, about 5–10%.

Bendavid R: A femoral "umbrella" for femoral hernia repair. Surg Gynecol Obstet 1987;165:153.
Glassow F: Femoral hernia: Review of 2,105 repairs in a 17 year period. Am J Surg 1985;150:353.

OTHER TYPES OF HERNIAS

1. UMBILICAL HERNIAS IN ADULTS

Umbilical hernia in adults occurs long after closure of the umbilical ring and is due to a gradual yielding of the cicatricial tissue closing the ring. It is more common in women than in men.

Predisposing factors include (1) multiple pregnancies with prolonged labor, (2) ascites, (3) obesity, and (4) large intra-abdominal tumors.

Clinical Findings

In adults, umbilical hernia does not usually obliterate spontaneously, as in children, but instead increases steadily in size. The hernia sac may have multiple loculations. Umbilical hernias usually contain omentum, but small and large bowel may be present. Emergency repair is often necessary, because the neck of the hernia is usually quite narrow compared to the size of the herniated mass and strangulation is common.

Umbilical hernias with tight rings are often associated with sharp pain on coughing or straining. Very large umbilical hernias more commonly produce a dragging or aching sensation.

Treatment

Umbilical hernia in an adult should be repaired expeditiously to avoid incarceration and strangulation. The umbilical dimple should be preserved if possible and the fascia approximated with nonabsorbable suture. A transverse closure of the aponeurotic defect results in the strongest repair. Large umbilical hernia defects that cannot be closed without undue tension may be closed with an inlay of Marlex mesh.

The presence of cirrhosis and ascites should not discourage repair of an umbilical hernia, since incarceration, strangulation, and rupture are particularly dangerous in patients with these disorders. If significant ascites exists, however, it should first be controlled medically or by peritoneovenous shunt if necessary, since morbidity and recurrence are higher after hernia repair in patients with ascites. Preoperative correction of fluid and electrolyte imbalance and improvement of nutrition will improve the outcome in these patients.

Prognosis

Factors that may lead to high rates of complication and death after surgical repair include large size of the hernia, old age or debility of the patient, and the presence of related intra-abdominal disease. In healthy individuals, surgical repair of the umbilical defects gives good results with a low rate of recurrence.

Kirkpatrick S et al: Umbilical hernia rupture in cirrhotics with ascites. Dig Dis Sci 1988;33:762.

2. EPIGASTRIC HERNIA
(Figure 33–6)

An epigastric hernia protrudes through the linea alba above the level of the umbilicus. The hernia may develop through one of the foramens of egress of the small paramidline nerves and vessels or through an area of congenital weakness in the linea alba.

About 3–5% of the population have epigastric hernias. They are more common in men than in women and most common between the ages of 20 and 50. About 20% of epigastric hernias are multiple, and about 80% occur just off the midline.

Clinical Findings
A. Symptoms: Most epigastric hernias are painless and are found on routine abdominal examination. If symptomatic, their presentation ranges from mild epigastric pain and tenderness to deep, burning epigastric pain with radiation to the back or the lower abdominal quadrants. The pain may be accompanied

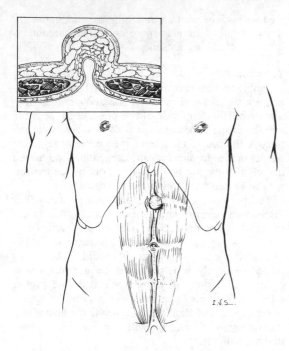

Figure 33–6. Epigastric hernia. Note closeness to midline and presence in upper abdomen. The herniation is through the linea alba.

by abdominal bloating, nausea, or vomiting. The symptoms often occur after a large meal and on occasion may be relieved by reclining, probably because the supine position causes the herniated mass to drop away from the anterior abdominal wall. The smaller masses most frequently contain only properitoneal fat and are especially prone to incarceration and strangulation. These smaller hernias are often tender. Larger hernias seldom strangulate and may contain, in addition to properitoneal fat, a portion of the nearby omentum and, occasionally, a loop of small or large bowel.

B. Signs: If a mass is palpable, the diagnosis can often be confirmed by any maneuver that will increase intra abdominal pressure and thereby cause the mass to bulge anteriorly. The diagnosis is difficult to make when the patient is obese, since a mass is hard to palpate; ultrasound or computed tomography may be needed in the very obese patient.

Differential Diagnosis

Differential diagnosis includes peptic ulcer, gallbladder disease, hiatal hernia, pancreatitis, and upper small bowel obstruction. On occasion, it may be impossible to distinguish the hernial mass from a subcutaneous lipoma, fibroma, or neurofibroma.

Treatment

Most epigastric hernias should be repaired, since small ones are likely to become incarcerated and large ones are often symptomatic and unsightly. The defect can usually be closed primarily. Herniated fat contents are usually dissected free and removed. Intraperitoneal herniating structures are reduced, but no attempt is made to close the peritoneal sac.

Prognosis

The recurrence rate is 10–20%, a higher incidence than with the routine inguinal or femoral hernia repair. This high recurrence rate may be partly due to failure to recognize and repair multiple small defects.

3. INCISIONAL HERNIA (Ventral Hernia)

About 10% of abdominal operations result in incisional hernias. The incidence of this iatrogenic type of hernia is not diminishing in spite of an awareness of the many causative factors.

Etiology

The factors most often responsible for incisional hernia are listed below. When more than one factor coexists in the same patient, the likelihood of postoperative wound failure is greatly increased.

(1) Poor surgical technique. Inadequate fascial bites, tension on the fascial edges, or too tight a closure are most often responsible for incisional failure.

(2) Postoperative wound infection.

(3) Age. Wound healing is usually slower and less solid in older patients.

(4) General debility. Cirrhosis, carcinoma, and chronic wasting diseases are factors that affect wound healing adversely. Any condition that compromises nutrition increases the likelihood of incision breakdown.

(5) Obesity. Fat patients frequently have increased intra-abdominal pressure. The presence of fat in the abdominal wound masks tissue layers and increases the incidence of seromas and hematomas in wounds.

(6) Postoperative pulmonary complications that stress the repair as a result of vigorous coughing. Smokers and patients with chronic pulmonary disease are therefore at increased risk of fascial disruption.

(7) Placement of drains or stomas in the primary operative wound.

Treatment

Incisional hernia should be treated by early repair. In addition to its unsightliness and the pain it causes, it may cause bowel obstruction. If the patient is unwilling to undergo surgery or is a poor surgical risk, symptoms may be controlled by an elastic corset.

Defects too large to close easily may be left without surgical repair if they are asymptomatic, since they are unlikely to incarcerate.

A. Small Hernias: Small incisional hernias usually require only a direct fascia-to-fascia repair for satisfactory closure. Interrupted or continuous closure may be used, but the sutures should be nonabsorbable. Sutures tied too tightly or tension on the repair will predispose to recurrence.

B. Large Hernias: Although no specific diameter distinguishes a small from a large hernia, a hernia can be considered large when the fascial edges cannot be approximated without tension. In repair of large hernias, spinal or epidural anesthesia gives superior relaxation, though general anesthesia with the addition of muscle relaxants is also excellent.

In performing the repair, excess and scarred skin and subcutaneous tissues over the hernia are removed. The hernia sac is then carefully dissected free from the underlying muscles and fascial tissues. If there are no adherent intraperitoneal structures, the sac may be inverted and the repair done over the inverted sac. If there is incarceration or adhesion of intraperitoneal contents, the abdominal contents should be dissected free from the sac and dropped back into the abdomen. The fascial edges of the defect should be cleaned so that the closure will be to solid tissues rather that to scar.

Primary closure of a large defect is not advisable, since tension on the closure increases the risk of hernia recurrence. Increasingly, repair of large or recurrent defects is performed using nonabsorbable mesh. Although a variety of techniques exist for placement of the mesh, an inlay or sandwich technique achieves a lower recurrence rate than an edge-to-edge or onlay placement. If a large dead space persists, a closed drainage system should be employed. The patient's own tissue should be used only if the wound can be closed without tension.

Prognosis

The recurrence rate for first-time incisional hernia repairs varies directly with the size of the fascial defect. Small hernias have a recurrence rate of 2–5%; medium-sized hernias recur in 5–15% of cases; and large hernias, too often closed under tension, have a recurrence rate as high as 25%. Repair of recurrent incisional hernias is even less likely to succeed, with a recurrence rate as high as 50%.

Houck JP et al: Repair of incisional hernia. Surg Gynecol Obstet 1989;169:397.

Krukowski ZH et al: Polydioxanone or polypropylene for closure of midline abdominal incisions: A prospective comparative clinical trial. Br J Surg, 1987;74:828.

Molloy RG et al: Massive incisional hernia: Abdominal wall replacement with Marlex mesh. Br J Surg 1991; 78:242.

Read RC et al: Recent trends in the management of incisional herniation. Arch Surg 1989;124:485.

Wantz GE: Incisional hernioplasty with Mersilene. Surg Gynecol Obstet 1991;172:129.

Wissing J et al: Fascia closure after midline laparotomy: Results of a randomized trial. Br J Surg, 1987;74:738.

4. VARIOUS RARE HERNIATIONS THROUGH THE ABDOMINAL WALL

Littre's Hernia

A Littre hernia is a hernia that contains a Meckel diverticulum in the hernia sac. Although Littre first described the condition in relation to a femoral hernia, the relative distribution of Littre's hernias is as follows: inguinal, 50%; femoral, 20%; umbilical, 20%; and miscellaneous, 10%. Littre's hernias of the groin are more common in men and on the right side. The clinical findings are similar to those of Richter's hernia; when strangulation is present, pain, fever, and manifestations of small bowel obstruction occur late.

Treatment consists of repair of the hernia plus, if possible, excision of the diverticulum. If acute Meckel's diverticulitis is present, the acute inflammatory mass may have to be treated through a separate abdominal incision.

Trupo FJ et al: Meckel's diverticulum in femoral hernia: A Littre's hernia. South Med J 1987;80:655.

Spigelian Hernia

Spigelian hernia is an acquired ventral hernia through the linea semilunaris, the line where the sheaths of the lateral abdominal muscles fuse to form the lateral rectus sheath. Spigelian hernias are nearly always found above the level of the inferior epigastric vessels. They most commonly occur where the semicircular line (fold of Douglas) crosses the linea semilunaris.

The presenting symptom is pain that is usually localized to the hernia site and may be aggravated by any maneuver that increases intra-abdominal pressure. With time, the pain may become more dull, constant, and diffuse, making diagnosis more difficult.

If a mass can be demonstrated, the diagnosis presents little difficulty. The diagnosis is most easily made with the patient standing and straining; a bulge then presents in the lower abdominal area and disappears with a gurgling sound on pressure. Following reduction of the mass, the hernia orifice can usually be palpated.

Diagnosis is often made more difficult because the hernial defect may lie beneath an intact external oblique layer and therefore not be palpable. The hernia often dissects within the layers of the abdominal wall and may not present a distinct mass, or the mass may be located at a distance from the linea semilunaris. Patients with spigelian hernias should have a tender point over the hernia orifice, though tenderness alone is not sufficient to make the diagnosis. Both ultrasound and CT scan may help to confirm the diagnosis.

Spigelian hernias have a high incidence of incarceration and should be repaired. These hernias are quite easily cured by primary aponeurotic closure.

Spangen L: Spigelian hernia. World J Surg 1989;13:573.

Lumbar or Dorsal Hernia (Figure 33–7)

Lumbar or dorsal hernias are hernias through the posterior abdominal wall at some level in the lumbar region. The most common sites (95%) are the superior (Grynfeltt's) and inferior (Petit's) lumbar triangles. A "lump in the flank" is the common complaint, associated with a dull, heavy, pulling feeling. With the patient erect, the presence of a reducible, often tympanitic mass in the flank usually makes the diagnosis. Incarceration and strangulation occur in about 10% of cases. Hernias in the inferior lumbar triangle are most often small and occur in young, athletic women. They present as tender masses producing backache and usually contain fat. Lumbar hernia must be differentiated from abscesses, hematomas, soft tissue tumors, renal tumors, and muscle strain.

Acquired hernias may be traumatic or nontraumatic. Severe direct trauma, penetrating wounds, abscesses, and poor healing of flank incisions are the usual causes. Congenital hernias occur in infants and are usually isolated unilateral congenital defects.

Lumbar hernias increase in size and should be repaired when found. Repair is by mobilization of the nearby fascia and obliteration of the hernia defect by precise fascia-to-fascia closure. The recurrence rate is very low.

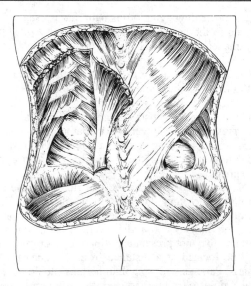

Figure 33–7. Anatomic relationships of lumbar or dorsal hernia. (Adapted from Netter.) On the left, lumbar or dorsal hernia into space of Grynfeltt. On the right, hernia into Petit's triangle (inferior lumbar space).

Faro SH et al: Traumatic lumbar hernia: CT diagnosis. AJR Am J Roentgenol 1990;154:757.
Thor K: Lumbar hernia. Acta Chir Scand 1985;151:389.

Obturator Hernia

Herniation through the obturator canal is more frequent in elderly women and is difficult to diagnose preoperatively. The mortality rate (13–40%) of these hernias makes them the most lethal of all abdominal hernias. These hernias most commonly present as small bowel obstruction with cramping abdominal pain and vomiting. The hernia is rarely palpable in the groin, though a mass may be felt on pelvic or rectal examination. The most specific finding is a positive Howship-Romberg sign, in which pain extends down the medial aspect of the thigh with abduction, extension, or internal rotation of the knee. Since this sign is present in fewer than half of cases, diagnosis should be suspected in any elderly debilitated woman without previous abdominal operations who presents with a small bowel obstruction. Though diagnosis can be confirmed by CT scan, operation should not be unduly delayed if complete bowel obstruction is present.

The abdominal approach gives the best exposure; these hernias should not be repaired from the thigh approach. The Cheatle-Henry approach (retropubic) may also be used. Simple repair is most often possible, though bladder wall has been used when the defect cannot be approximated primarily.

Bjork KJ et al: Obturator hernia. Surg Gynecol Obstet 1988;167:217.
Young A et al: Strangulated obturator hernia: Can mortality be reduced? South Med J 1988;81:1117.

Perineal Hernia

A perineal hernia protrudes through the muscles and fascia of the perineal floor. It may be primary but is usually acquired following perineal prostatectomy, abdominoperineal resection of the rectum, or pelvic exenteration.

These hernias present as easily reducible perineal bulges and usually are asymptomatic, but may present with pain, dysuria, bowel obstruction, or perineal skin breakdown.

Repair is usually done by an abdominal approach, with an adequate fascial and muscular perineal repair. Occasionally polypropylene (Marlex) mesh or flaps using the gracilis or gluteus may be necessary, when the available tissues are too attenuated for adequate primary repair.

Beck DE et al: Postoperative perineal hernia. Dis Colon Rectum 1987;30:21.
Brotschi E, Noe JM, Silen W: Perineal hernias after proctectomy: A new approach to repair. Am J Surg 1985; 149:301.

Interparietal Hernia

Interparietal hernias, in which the sac insinuates itself between the layers of the abdominal wall, are usually of an indirect inguinal type but, rarely, may be direct or ventral hernias. Although interparietal hernias are rare, it is essential to recognize them, because strangulation is common and the mass is easily mistaken for a tumor or abscess. The lesion usually can be suspected on the basis of the physical examination provided it is kept in mind. In most cases, extensive studies for intra-abdominal tumors have preceded diagnosis. A lateral film of the abdomen will usually show bowel within the layers of the abdominal wall in cases with intestinal incarceration or strangulation, and an ultrasound or CT scan may be diagnostic.

As soon as the diagnosis is established, operation should be performed, usually through the standard inguinal approach.

Sciatic Hernia

Sciatic hernia is the rarest of abdominal hernias and consists of an outpouching of intra-abdominal contents through the greater sciatic foramen. The diagnosis is made after incarceration or strangulation of the bowel occurs. The repair is usually made through the abdominal approach. The hernia sac and contents are reduced, and the weak area is closed by making a fascial flap from the superficial fascia of the piriformis muscle.

TRAUMATIC HERNIA

Abdominal wall hernias occur rarely as a direct consequence of direct blunt abdominal injury. The patient presents with abdominal pain. On examination, ecchymosis of the abdominal wall and a bulge are usually present. The existence of a hernia may not be obvious, however, and the patient may require CT scan to confirm it. Because of the high incidence of associated intra-abdominal injuries, laparotomy is usually required. The defect should be repaired primarily if possible.

Otero C et al: Injury to the abdominal wall musculature: The full spectrum of traumatic hernia. South Med J 1988; 81:517.
Wood RJ et al: Traumatic abdominal hernia: A case report and review of the literature. Am Surg 1988;54:648.

OTHER LESIONS OF THE ABDOMINAL WALL

CONGENITAL DEFECTS

Congenital defects of the abdominal wall other than hernias or lesions of the urachus and umbilicus are rare. The important ones involving the urachus and umbilicus are discussed in Chapter 47.

TRAUMA

Hematoma of the Rectus Sheath

This is a rare but important entity that may follow mild trauma to the abdominal wall or may occur secondary to disorders of coagulation, blood dyscrasia, or degenerative vascular diseases.

Abdominal pain, usually in the right lower abdomen, is a presenting sign. It may be sudden and severe in onset or slowly progressive. The key to diagnosis is the physical examination. Careful palpation will reveal an exquisitely tender mass within the abdominal wall. If the patient tenses the rectus muscles by raising the head or body, the swelling becomes more tender and distinct on palpation, in contrast to an intra-abdominal mass or tenderness that disappears when the rectus muscles are contracted (Fothergill's sign). In addition, there may be detectable discoloration or ecchymosis. If the physical signs are not diagnostic, ultrasound or CT scan can demonstrate the hematoma in the abdominal wall.

Usually, the condition can be treated without operation. The acute pain and discomfort should disappear within 2 or 3 days, although a residual mass may persist for several weeks. If pain is severe, an acceptable alternative is evacuation of the clot and control of the bleeding.

Gocke JE, MacCarty RL, Foulk WT: Rectus sheath hematoma: Diagnosis by computed tomography scanning. Mayo Clin Proc 1981;56:757.
Zainea GG et al: Rectus sheath hematomas: Their pathogenesis, diagnosis, and management. Am Surg 1988;54:630.

PAIN IN THE ABDOMINAL WALL

A number of conditions are characterized by pain in the abdominal wall without a demonstrable organic lesion. Pain from a diaphragmatic, supradiaphragmatic, or spinal cord lesion may be referred to the abdomen. Herpes zoster (shingles) may present as abdominal pain, in which case it will follow a dermatomal distribution.

Scars may be sensitive or painful, particularly in the first 6 months after surgery.

Entrapment of a nerve by a nonabsorbable suture may cause persistent incisional pain, sometimes quite severe. Hyperesthesia of the skin over the involved dermatome may provide a clue to the cause.

In all cases of epigastric pain in the abdominal wall, careful search should be made for a small epigastric hernia, as noted earlier.

ABDOMINAL WALL TUMORS

Tumors of the abdominal wall are quite common, but most are benign, eg, lipomas, hemangiomas, and fibromas. Musculoaponeurotic fibromatoses (desmoid tumors), which often occur in abdominal wall scars or after parturition in women, are discussed in more detail in Chapter 48. Most malignant tumors of the abdominal wall are metastatic. Metastases may appear by direct invasion from intra-abdominal lesions or by vascular dissemination. The sudden appearance of a sensitive nodule anywhere in the abdominal wall that is clearly not a hernia should arouse suspicion of an occult cancer, the lung and pancreas being the more likely primary sites.

REFERENCES

Nyhus LM, Condon RE (editors): *Hernia,* 3rd ed. Lippincott, 1989.

Skandalakis JE et al: *Surgical Anatomy and Technique.* McGraw-Hill, 1989.

Adrenals

34

Quan-Yang Duh, MD, Thomas K. Hunt, MD, Edward G. Biglieri, MD, & J. Blake Tyrrell, MD

Operations on the adrenal glands are performed for primary hyperaldosteronism, pheochromocytoma, hyperadrenocorticism (Cushing's disease or Cushing's syndrome), and, less commonly, other adrenocortical tumors. These conditions are usually characterized by hypersecretion of one or more of the adrenal hormones.

Anatomy & Surgical Principles

The normal combined weight of the adrenals is 7–12 g. The right gland lies posterior and lateral to the vena cava and superior to the kidney (Figure 34–1). The left gland lies medial to the superior pole of the kidney, just lateral to the aorta and immediately posterior to the superior border of the pancreas. An important surgical feature is the remarkable constancy of the adrenal veins. The right adrenal vein, 2–5 mm long and several millimeters wide, connects the anterior aspect of the adrenal gland with the posterolateral aspect of the vena cava. The left adrenal vein is several centimeters long and travels inferiorly from the lower pole of the gland, joining the left renal vein after receiving the inferior phrenic vein. The adrenal arteries are small, multiple, and inconstant. They usually come from the inferior phrenic artery, the aorta, and the renal artery.

With the exception of rare nonsecreting cancers, indications for adrenal surgery result from hypersecretory states. Diagnosis and treatment begin with confirmation of a hypersecretory state (ie, measurement of excess cortisol, aldosterone, or catecholamines in blood or urine). In order to determine whether the problem originates in the adrenal, levels of the stimulator of the hormone in question (ie, ACTH or renin) must be measured. If stimulator levels are low or normal but hormone secretion is excessive, autonomous secretion is proved. The next step, except in pheochromocytoma, is to determine the degree of autonomy, a process that usually distinguishes hyperplasias (which respond to most but not all controlling mechanisms) from adenomas and adenomas from cancers. In general, cancers are under little if any feedback control. If the primary problem is not in the adrenal, as in Cushing's disease, treatment must be directed elsewhere when possible.

Adrenal masses are usually detected (and localized) by CT scan or MRI. Functioning tumors of the adrenal can be localized by adrenal scintigraphy, [131]I-6 beta-iodomethylnorcholesterol (NP-59) for cortical tumors and ^{131}I-metaiodobenzylguanidine (MIBG) for medullary tumors. Functioning adrenal or pituitary tumors can also be localized by demonstrating a gradient of hormone levels between their venous drainage and a peripheral vein.

The major principles of adrenal surgery are as follows:

(1) The surgeon must be certain of the diagnosis before undertaking the operation and must not hesitate to undertake an exhaustive search for the tumor. Sometimes the surgeon must be prepared to take definitive action based on the preoperative diagnosis even if no visible lesion is found.

(2) Since the gross pathologic changes are often subtle, the surgeon must work with complete hemostasis and must be able to recognize even minor variations from normal.

(3) The patient must be carefully prepared in order to withstand the metabolic problems caused by the disease and the operation.

(4) The surgeon and consultants must be able to detect and treat any metabolic crisis that occurs during operation or afterward.

Surgical Approaches

The anterior or transperitoneal approach through a long vertical midline incision or a bilateral subcostal incision facilitates bilateral exploration and is used for patients with potentially bilateral diseases of the adrenals, such as pheochromocytomas. It permits wide exposure of the abdominal organs and the retroperitoneum. Unfortunately, this incision causes significant pain, ileus, and atelectasis. The patients—especially those with Cushing's syndrome—are exposed to the risks of poor wound healing, such as evisceration (Table 34–1).

The posterior approach, performed through incisions on each side of the spine with the patient lying prone, is better tolerated postoperatively but gives only limited exposure. In this retroperitoneal operation, poor healing does not have the potential of evisceration, and return of intestinal function is rapid. The posterior approach can be made through incisions varying from transpleural to those through the bed of the 11th or 12th rib. The 12th rib incision is

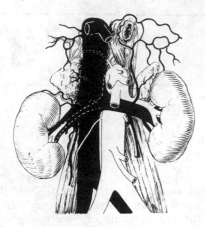

Figure 34–1. Anatomy of the adrenals, showing venous return.

best tolerated by the patient and is best for lesions smaller than 4–5 cm. Because of the limited exposure, the posterior approach is used only when the location of the lesion is identified in advance by radiographic, scintigraphic, or angiographic studies. A lateral approach through the bed of the 11th rib, exposing the adrenals retroperitoneally, is useful for known large unilateral tumors or for bilateral disease in obese or very poor risk patients. Adrenalectomy can also be performed by a laparoscopic approach, and this will probably become the preferred method as experience accumulates.

Table 34–1. Estimated frequency of manifestations of hyperadrenocorticism.

	Percentage
Obesity	90
Hypertension	80
Evidence of diabetes with normal fasting blood glucose	80
Centripetal distribution of fat	80
Weakness	80
Muscle atrophy in upper and lower extremities	70
Hirsutism	70
Menstrual disturbance or impotence	70
Purple striae	70
Plethoric facies	60
Atrophic skin, connective tissues, or bone (osteoporosis)	50
Easy bruisability	50
Acne or skin pigmentation	50
Mental changes	50
Edema	50
Headache	40
Poor wound healing	40
Leukocytosis with lymphopenia	Frequent

DISEASES OF THE ADRENALS

PRIMARY HYPERALDOSTERONISM

Essentials of Diagnosis

- Hypertension, polyuria. polydipsia, muscle weakness, tetany.
- Hypokalemia, alkalosis.
- Elevated autonomous urine and plasma aldosterone and low plasma renin.
- Small adrenal lesions demonstrable by CT scan.
- Adrenal vein sampling showing unilateral elevation of aldosterone level.

General Considerations

Aldosterone, the most potent mineralocorticoid secreted by the adrenal cortex, regulates the body's electrolyte composition, fluid volume, and blood pressure. Excess aldosterone increases total body sodium, decreases potassium, increases extracellular fluid volume (without edema), and increases blood pressure. Aldosterone secretion is regulated by the renin-angiotensin system in a feedback fashion and is also stimulated transiently by ACTH.

Hyperaldosteronism may occur in several forms: (1) primary hyperaldosteronism, caused by adrenal adenoma or adrenal hyperplasia; (2) secondary hyperaldosteronism, usually in hypertensive nonedematous patients with renal vascular disease; and (3) hyperaldosteronism in nonhypertensive edematous patients taking diuretics. Operation is useful only in primary hyperaldosteronism—and then only in patients with adrenal adenomas. Hypertension in patients with hyperplasia rarely responds even to total adrenalectomy.

Primary hyperaldosteronism is diagnosed by a triad of hypertension, hypokalemia, and low plasma renin activity. Adrenal adenoma is the cause in about 70% of patients, bilateral hyperplasia in 30%, and adrenal cancer rarely. The syndrome was first described in 1955 by Jerome Conn. Aldosterone-secreting adrenal adenoma can be (though rarely) part of the multiple endocrine neoplasia syndrome (MEN) I, and familial Conn's syndrome has been described.

Almost all adenomas are unilateral, and most are 1-2 cm in diameter. They have a characteristic chrome yellow color when sectioned. On light microscopic examination, most adenomas appear to arise from the zona fasciculata of the adrenal cortex, but on electron microscopy the cells are more like granulosa cells. Hyperplasia is characterized by diffuse micronodularity in the cortex. Hyperplasia is also often seen in glands with adenomas.

Clinical Findings

Hypertension and hypokalemia usually lead to investigation of hyperaldosteronism. Because the hypertension is less severe and not episodic, the diagnosis of hyperaldosteronism in hypertensive patients tends to be delayed, usually for years after the onset of symptoms.

A. Symptoms and Signs: The usual clinical symptoms are muscle weakness, cramps, polydipsia, polyuria, nocturia, and headache. Carpopedal spasm and paresthesias sometimes occur from hypokalemic alkalosis. Rhabdomyolysis may occur with severe hypokalemia. Hypertension is moderate. The patient may have signs of chronic hypertension but rarely has retinopathy. Although extracellular fluid volume is increased, edema is not seen until renal failure occurs.

B. Laboratory Findings: Aldosterone facilitates the exchange of sodium for potassium and hydrogen ions in the distal nephron. Therefore, when aldosterone secretion is chronically elevated, serum potassium and hydrogen ion concentrations fall (hypokalemia and alkalosis), total body sodium rises, and hypertension results. Hypokalemia in response to salt loading is characteristic of primary hyperaldosteronism. Patients who are not taking diuretics or potassium are given 1 g of sodium chloride with each meal for 4 days. If hypokalemia occurs, primary hyperaldosteronism is likely, and urinary or plasma aldosterone and plasma renin activity should be measured.

In primary hyperaldosteronism, the plasma renin level is low; in secondary hyperaldosteronism, the plasma renin level is high. In primary hyperaldosteronism due to adrenal hyperplasia, plasma renin levels are suppressed but to a lesser degree than those seen in patients with adrenal adenoma. In order for the following tests to be meaningful, patients should not be taking diuretics and should not be on salt restriction; both cause secondary hyperaldosteronism by elevating the plasma renin concentration.

Aldosterone-secreting adenomas (aldosteronoma) and hyperplasia (idiopathic hyperplasia) can be distinguished by their response to various stimuli; adenomas are more autonomous, whereas hyperplasia tends to retain normal control. Aldosteronomas secrete aldosterone autonomously and are independent of the control of the renin-angiotensin system. The secretion of aldosteronoma is thus not decreased by the suppression of plasma renin activity, by fludrocortisone, desoxycorticosterone acetate (DOCA), or by plasma volume expansion (saline infusion); and is not increased by the stimulation of plasma renin activity, ie, by standing after overnight recumbency.

Diurnal variations in aldosterone secretion are retained in adenomas, but responses to postural changes are not; this is the basis for the postural stimulation test to distinguish adenoma from hyperplasia. Normal subjects follow the normal diurnal pattern if they remain supine for 24 hours; aldosterone levels decrease between 8 AM and 10 AM. If they stand during this time, plasma renin rises because of pooling of blood by gravity, and the aldosterone level will increase. Patients with adenomas, on the other hand, are not responsive to postural stimulation and will have a paradoxic decrease in plasma aldosterone when standing. The postural stimulation test has a 35% false-negative rate (increase in plasma aldosterone in patients with adenoma) and a 15% false-positive rate (paradoxic decrease in plasma aldosterone in patients with hyperplasia).

The response to saline infusion after overnight recumbency also differs between adenoma and hyperplasia; the plasma renin level decreases in patients with hyperplasia, and the aldosterone/cortisol ratio increases in patients with adenoma.

Differential Diagnosis

Hypertensive patients may have secondary hyperaldosteronism caused by malignant hypertension, renovascular hypertension, or the use of diuretics or birth control pills. Estrogens (particularly birth control pills) must be withdrawn for at least 2 months before renin or aldosterone is measured to avoid a mistaken diagnosis of primary hyperaldosteronism. Plasma renin activity also increases with stress, pregnancy, diabetes, and alcohol intoxication.

Complications

Uncontrolled hypertension can lead to renal failure, stroke, and myocardial infarction. Severe hypokalemia can cause weakness and paralysis. Patients who are taking digitalis are at high risk for developing dysrhythmia from hypokalemia.

Treatment

A. Medical Treatment: Unilateral adrenalectomy is curative for aldosteronoma and should be performed electively unless the patient has contraindications to operation and general anesthesia. Spironolactone and amiloride are specific antihypertensive medications for patients with primary hyperaldosteronism. High doses of spironolactone, however, may cause impotence, gynecomastia, and postural hypotension. Short-term treatment using less than 150 mg/d of spironolactone or 40 mg/d of amiloride is well tolerated. Ironically, patients with adenomas, who would benefit most from adrenalectomy, are also more responsive to medical treatment; whereas patients with bilateral hyperplasia, who would be less likely to benefit from the operation, are more likely to escape from medical treatment. Refractory hypokalemia or weakness make operation more urgent.

B. Surgical Treatment:

1. Selection of patients for operation–Patients with aldosterone-secreting adenomas respond well to unilateral adrenalectomy, whereas those with bilateral hyperplasia tend to have persistent disease after operation. Biochemical studies should be performed to distinguish patients with adenomas from those with hyperplasia. CT and MRI may aid the diagnosis of adenoma by disclosing a unilateral adrenal tumor and a normal contralateral gland. Carcinomas causing hyperaldosteronism are very rare and tend to have very high or erratic plasma aldosterone levels. A good initial response to spironolactone predicts a good result from operation.

2. Localization of tumor–CT and MRI scans will localize adenomas as small as 0.5 cm in diameter in over 80% of patients with aldosteronoma. Dexamethasone suppression NP-59 scintigraphy frequently will show uptake by the tumor with contralateral suppression. NP-59 scan is more accurate when the adenoma is larger and secreting more aldosterone and is less helpful in smaller adenomas. Adrenal venous sampling for aldosterone is indicated when other studies are nondiagnostic or equivocal. Venous sampling should be performed with concurrent measurement of cortisol as controls and with stimulation by ACTH. Measuring the aldosterone/cortisol ratio corrects for the inexact position of the catheter in the adrenal vein.

3. Preoperative preparation–Spironolactone, a competitive aldosterone antagonist, or amiloride, a potassium-sparing diuretic, or both, will normalize blood pressure and reverse hypokalemia and can be continued to the day of operation. Because extracellular fluid and plasma volume are reduced by the medications, the patient may require more saline infusion in the immediate postoperative period. A sodium-restricted diet with potassium supplementation has almost the same effect as the drugs and may be sufficient for patients with milder disease. Other antihypertensive medications may be required if hypertension is severe. Hypokalemia increases the risk of general anesthesia and should be corrected before operation.

4. Surgical procedures–A unilateral posterior approach or the lateral approach is suitable for most patients because the adenoma is usually small and its location known from preoperative localization studies. Bilateral adenomas and aldosterone-secreting carcinomas are extremely rare. If abdominal exploration is required or if the side of the adenoma is not known, an anterior approach is preferable.

Adrenals containing adenomas are often also hyperplastic. Knowing this sometimes facilitates discovery of adenomas. We prefer to excise the entire adrenal together with the adenoma, because enucleation of the adenoma is frequently more difficult and confers no advantage.

Because patients with bilateral hyperplasia frequently can be diagnosed by biochemical and imaging studies and because operation rarely cures the hyperaldosteronism associated with hyperplasia, very few of these patients will come to operation. If an operation is undertaken, however, bilateral total adrenalectomy or right total and left subtotal adrenalectomy should be performed. Subtotal adrenalectomy should leave about 30% of the left gland, which is easier to resect than the right if reoperation is required.

5. Postoperative care–The patient undergoing unilateral adrenalectomy for hyperaldosteronism does not require administration of corticosteroids pre- or postoperatively. Blood losses are minimal. Large volumes of intravenous saline are not usually necessary unless spironolactone has been used up to the day of operation. It is rarely necessary to give potassium if the serum potassium level was normal before the operation.

A few patients may have transient aldosterone deficiency because the normal adrenal gland has been suppressed by the hyperfunctioning adenoma. The signs of hypoaldosteronism are continuing weight loss, postural hypotension, and hyperkalemia occurring 1 week after operation. Fludrocortisone, 0.1 mg/d orally, is given until the remaining adrenal gland has regained its ability to secrete aldosterone, usually within a month after operation.

Prognosis

Hyperaldosteronism usually follows a prolonged and subtly changing course. Untreated hypertension causes stroke, myocardial infarction, and renal failure.

When adenomas are removed, the blood pressure becomes normal in 70% of cases. The other 30% will require modest antihypertensive therapy. When hyperplasia is the cause, hypertension requiring medications usually persists. The patient with a solitary adenoma within a normal gland achieves better improvement of blood pressure than one with an adenoma within a multinodular gland.

Beckers A et al: Aldosterone-secreting adrenal adenoma as part of multiple endocrine neoplasia type 1 (MEN 1): Loss of heterozygosity for polymorphic chromosome 11 deoxyribonucleic acid markers, including the MEN 1 locus. J Clin Endocrinol Metab 1992;75:564.

Doppman JL et al: Distinction between hyperaldosteronism due to bilateral hyperplasia and unilateral aldosteronoma: Reliability of CT. Radiology 1992;184:677.

Dunnick NR et al: CT in the diagnosis of primary aldosteronism: Sensitivity in 29 patients. AJR Am J Roentgenol 1993;160:321.

Gordon RD et al: Primary aldosteronism: hypertension with a genetic basis. Lancet 1992;340:159.

Ito Yet al: Clinical significance of associated nodular lesions of the adrenal in patients with aldosteronoma. World J Surg 1990;14:330.

Merrell RC: Aldosterone-producing tumors (Conn's syndrome). Semin Surg Oncol 1990;6:66.

Nomura K et al: Iodomethylnorcholesterol uptake in an aldosteronoma shown by dexamethasone-suppression scintigraphy: Relationship to adenoma size and functional activity. J Clin Endocrinol Metab 1990;71:825.

Schwarz RJ, Schmidt N: Efficient management of adrenal tumors. Am J Surg 1991;161:576.

PHEOCHROMOCYTOMA

Essentials of Diagnosis

- Episodic headache, severe sweating, palpitation and visual blurring.
- Hypertension, often paroxysmal but frequently sustained; cardiac enlargement.
- Postural tachycardia and hypotension.
- Elevated urinary catecholamines or their metabolites, hypermetabolism, hyperglycemia.

General Considerations

Pheochromocytomas are tumors of the adrenal medulla and related chromaffin tissues elsewhere in the body that secrete dopamine, epinephrine, or norepinephrine, resulting in sustained or episodic hypertension and other symptoms of excess catecholamine.

Pheochromocytoma is found in 0.1% of autopsies and 0.5% of patients with hypertension and accounts for 5% of adrenal tumors incidentally discovered by CT scanning. Most pheochromocytomas occur sporadically without other diseases, but they may occur also in patients with various syndromes such as MEN IIa (medullary thyroid carcinoma, pheochromocytoma, and hyperparathyroidism), MEN IIb (medullary thyroid carcinoma, pheochromocytoma, mucosal neuromas, marfanoid habitus, and ganglioneuromatosis), Recklinghausen's neurofibromatosis, Griffith's syndrome (pheochromocytoma, neurofibroma, and duodenal somatostatinoma) and Lindau's syndrome (cerebellar, medullary, and spinal cord hemangioblastoma, pheochromocytoma, and retinal angioma).

On pathologic examination, pheochromocytoma appears gray and frequently has areas of necrosis. The usual size is about 100 g, though much larger tumors also occur. Cells are pleomorphic, showing prominent nucleoli and frequent mitoses, and the veins and capsules may be invaded even in clinically benign tumors. Malignancy can only be diagnosed in the presence of metastases or invasion into surrounding tissues.

Clinical Findings

A. Symptoms and Signs: The clinical findings of pheochromocytoma are variable, and mild cases may not be apparent. Classically, the patient has episodic hypertension associated with the triad of palpitation, headache, and sweating. Patients may also complain of nervousness, anxiety, weight loss, and constipation. The physical examination may be unremarkable except during an attack, when pallor, flushing, and excess sweating may be observed. Tachycardia, postural hypotension, and hypertensive retinopathy are other signs.

Half of patients with pheochromocytoma have *sustained* hypertension with or without other manifestations of excessive catecholamine secretion, and the diagnosis may be missed. In some cases severe hypertension occurs only while the patient is under stress, such as general anesthesia or trauma. Patients with diastolic hypertension and postural hypotension, who are not receiving antihypertensive medications, may have pheochromocytoma. Epinephrine raises blood glucose and norepinephrine decreases insulin secretion, and patients therefore may have hyperglycemia.

About 10% of pheochromocytomas are malignant, 10% familial, 10% bilateral, 10% extra-adrenal, and 10% multiple. In children, hypertension is less prominent, and about 50% have multiple or extra-adrenal tumors. Malignant tumors are more common in children and in extra-adrenal pheochromocytomas. Pheochromocytomas occur in 50% of patients with MEN II; they tend to be bilateral and multiple but are rarely extra-adrenal or malignant. Screening of MEN II patients and family members by urine vanillylmandelic acid and metanephrine measurements can diagnose pheochromocytomas before they become clinically apparent.

B. Laboratory Findings: Twenty-four-hour urine collection for determination of metanephrine and 3-methoxy-4-hydroxymandelic acid (vanillylmandelic acid, VMA) is useful for screening. Very few patients with pheochromocytomas will have normal urinary metanephrine and VMA. Urinary catecholamine levels may be useful in equivocal cases. Plasma epinephrine and norepinephrine should only be measured under standard, controlled conditions, since these levels may be falsely low if the tumor secretes episodically and falsely elevated if the patient is under stress.

The levels of catecholamines and their metabolites do not correlate with the size of tumor. Provocative tests—using glucagon, histamine, or tyramine—are inaccurate and potentially dangerous. They are almost never indicated in these patients. Suppression tests are used only if essential for diagnosis. Successful treatment of hypertensive crisis by phentolamine can be both diagnostic and therapeutic. Clonidine does not decrease plasma catecholamine levels in patients with pheochromocytoma, as it may in normal anxious individuals (Figure 34–2).

Most tumors secrete both norepinephrine and epinephrine. Extra-adrenal pheochromocytomas are not in an environment with a high enough cortisol level to induce phenylethanolamine-N-methyltransferase (PNMT), the methylating enzyme that converts norepinephrine to epinephrine. Hence, they may secrete only norepinephrine (Figure 34–3). When epinephrine levels are elevated, the tumor is almost always in or near the adrenal area.

Supportive laboratory findings are hyperglycemia and polycythemia. Many pheochromocytomas also

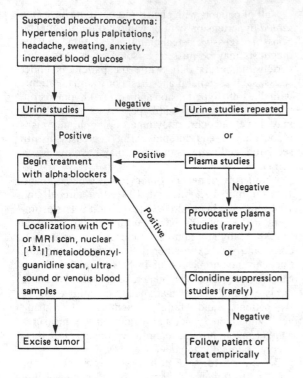

Figure 34–2. Scheme for evaluation of patient with suspected pheochromocytoma.

sampling for catecholamines may rarely be helpful to localize extra-adrenal pheochromocytomas.

Differential Diagnosis

The differential diagnosis includes all causes of hypertension. Hyperthyroidism and pheochromocytoma have many features in common (weight loss, tremor, and tachycardia). The diagnosis of pheochromocytoma is easier if episodic hypertension is present. Diastolic hypertension distinguishes patients with pheochromocytoma from those with hyperthyroidism, who usually have wide pulse pressures and only systolic hypertension. Acute anxiety attacks mimic the symptoms and may precipitate hypertensive episodes, but anxiety alone rarely produces severe hypertension. Carcinoid syndrome causing episodes of flushing may also be mistaken for pheochromocytoma. The urinary 5-HIAA level is usually elevated, and CT scan usually shows liver metastases in patients with carcinoid syndrome. Labile essential hypertension is not associated with elevated catecholamine levels.

Pheochromocytoma in pregnancy, if not recognized, will kill half of the fetuses and nearly half of the mothers. Hypertension in pregnancy is usually ascribed to preeclampsia-eclampsia. The diagnosis of pheochromocytomas requires the same biochemical studies; radiation (CT) and radioisotopes (MIBG) are usually not used. Alpha- and beta-adrenergic blockers appear to be well tolerated. Timing of the operation is individualized. If recognized early, the tumor is best removed early in the second trimester. Otherwise, cesarean section followed by tumor resection can be performed when the fetus reaches term.

Some patients with pheochromocytoma may develop crisis, with multisystem failure, mimicking severe sepsis. If the disease is not recognized, death is the usual result. Emergent operation is indicated in these cases.

Complications

Pheochromocytoma causes complications because of hypertension, dysrhythmia, and hypovolemia. The sequelae of hypertension are stroke, renal failure, myocardial infarction, and congestive heart failure. Sudden death can be caused by ventricular dysrhyth-

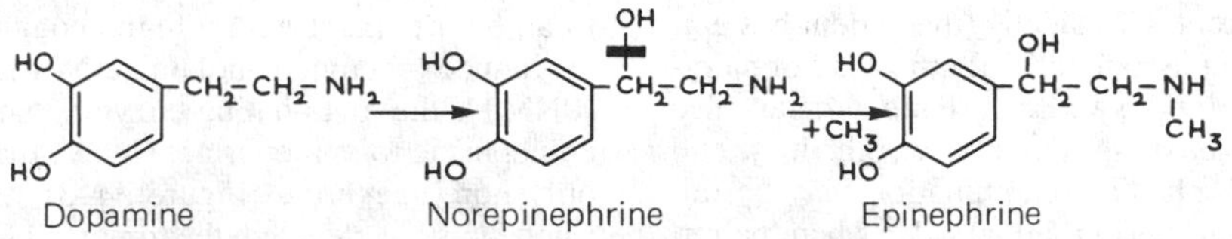

secrete vasoactive peptides—VIP, somatostatin, etc—which may add to the symptomatology. Secretion of multiple vasoactive peptides suggests malignancy.

C. Localization of Tumor: Because pheochromocytomas are usually large, they may be apparent on plain films of the abdomen. CT is the most sensitive test for localization of adrenal pheochromocytoma. MRI of pheochromocytoma shows a characteristic bright lesion on T2-weighted imaging. Nuclear scanning with MIBG is more sensitive than CT scanning for localizing extra-adrenal pheochromocytomas. Arteriography and fine-needle biopsy can precipitate a hypertensive crisis, do not contribute to the diagnosis, and are not indicated. Venous

Figure 34–3. Sequence of catecholamine synthesis from dopamine. The more primitive extra-adrenal pheochromocytomas lack the methylating enzyme necessary to convert norepinephrine to epinephrine. Thus, when norepinephrine levels are high and epinephrine levels are normal or low, extra-adrenal tumor becomes a good diagnostic possibility.

mia. Alpha-adrenergic stimulation by the catecholamines causes vasoconstriction and a low total blood volume. These patients are therefore unable to compensate for a sudden loss of blood volume (bleeding) or catecholamines (tumor removal) and are at risk for cardiovascular collapse. Preoperative alpha-adrenergic blockade and blood volume expansion can prevent these complications.

Congestive heart failure is a significant risk postoperatively, especially in patients with long-standing disease, and some have developed cardiomyopathy.

Treatment

A. Medical Treatment: *Treatment with alpha-adrenergic blocking agents should be started as soon as the biochemical diagnosis is established.* The aims of preoperative therapy are (1) to restore the blood volume, which has been depleted by excessive catecholamines; (2) to relieve the patient of the danger of a severe attack, with its potential complications; and (3) to allow the patient to recover from myocardiopathy. Close control of hypertension is necessary in order to keep blood volume normal. Even 15 minutes of hypertension due to release of catecholamines can significantly reduce blood volume.

Phenoxybenzamine, an α_1-adrenergic antagonist, has a long duration of action and is the preferred treatment. It should be started at a dosage of 10 mg every 8 hours, and the dosage should be increased—as postural hypotension allows—until signs of excess catecholamine stimulation have disappeared and blood volume is clinically normal. Doses as high as 150 mg/d may be necessary.

Metyrosine, 250-500 mg once a day, inhibits tyrosine hydroxylase and reduces catecholamine synthesis and can be used as preoperative therapy. Prazosin and verapamil have also been used successfully.

Beta-adrenergic blocking agents are often useful to treat dysrhythmias and tachycardia but should only be given after the alpha blockade has been achieved. Otherwise, a hypertensive crisis may be precipitated because of the unopposed alpha-adrenergic effect of the catecholamines. Sedatives and tranquilizers are also useful in treating the anxiety that often accompanies pheochromocytoma. Opiates should be avoided because they may stimulate histamine release and precipitate a pheochromocytoma crisis.

B. Surgical Treatment: The definitive treatment of pheochromocytoma is excision. The transabdominal approach is traditionally used in order to explore both adrenals and other areas in the abdomen for extra-adrenal pheochromocytomas. A transabdominal approach is indicated in children and in patients with MEN, since they are more likely to have bilateral tumors and extra-adrenal pheochromocytomas. Otherwise, if the tumor has been localized by CT, MRI, or MIBG and is less than 5 cm in diameter, it can be removed by the posterior or lateral approach.

Lines in a peripheral artery and the pulmonary artery are useful for intraoperative monitoring. Phentolamine or nitroprusside should be immediately available to treat sudden hypertension and propranolol to treat the cardiac dysrhythmias that often occur when the tumor is manipulated. The surrounding tissues should be dissected away from the tumor and the tumor itself not manipulated to reduce hypertension during the operation. The adrenal veins draining the tumor should be divided early in the operation to avoid a sudden influx of catecholamine during tumor removal.

The major surgical problems arise in excising large malignant tumors and in detecting multiple and ectopic tumors. Extra-adrenal pheochromocytomas are usually found along the abdominal aorta and in the organ of Zuckerkandl (para-aortic at the level of the inferior mesenteric artery). However, tumors have been found in widely scattered sites such as the vagina, the mediastinum, the neck, and even the skull and pericardium.

Many patients undergoing resection of pheochromocytoma have dysrhythmias and wide variations in blood pressure and heart rate. Catecholamine levels rise to as high as 150,000 µg/L (normal, 300 µg/L) during manipulation of the tumor. Blood pressure will almost always fall when all functioning tissue has been removed. If the patient has been properly prepared with alpha-blockers, the changes in blood pressure will not be severe. Otherwise, intravenous infusion of large amounts of saline and catecholamine may be necessary to maintain blood pressure after the tumor is removed.

After operation, the patient may develop hypoglycemia from a rebound in the secretion of insulin. Congestive heart failure is also common because of myocardiopathy.

Prognosis

The outlook for patients with untreated pheochromocytoma is grim, whereas the operative mortality rate is less than 5% with preoperative alpha-adrenergic blockade and blood volume expansion. Mild to moderate essential hypertension often persists. Second tumors in the remaining adrenal can occur years after excision of the primary pheochromocytoma; long-term follow-up is thus mandatory. Metastatic or recurrent malignant pheochromocytoma should be resected if possible to reduce the catecholamine load. Treatment with high-dose MIBG may be helpful in these patients.

Campeau RJ et al: Pheochromocytoma: Diagnosis by scintigraphy using iodine 131 metaiodobenzylguanidine. South Med J 1991;84:1221.

Caty MG et al: Current diagnosis and treatment of pheochromocytoma in children: Experience with 22 consecutive tumors in 14 patients. Arch Surg 1990;125:978.

Daly PA, Landsberg L: Phaeochromocytoma: Diagnosis

and management. Baillieres Clin Endocrinol Metab 1992;6:143.

Grossman E et al: Glucagon and clonidine testing in the diagnosis of pheochromocytoma. Hypertension 1991;17:733.

Hanson MW et al: Iodine 131-labeled metaiodobenzylguanidine scintigraphy and biochemical analyses in suspected pheochromocytoma. Arch Intern Med 1991;151:1397.

Herrera MF et al: Pheochromocytoma producing multiple vasoactive peptides. Arch Surg 1992;127:105.

Hsiao RJ et al: Chromogranin A storage and secretion: Sensitivity and specificity for the diagnosis of pheochromocytoma. Medicine 1991;70:33.

Ito Y et al: The role of epinephrine, norepinephrine, and dopamine in blood pressure disturbances in patients with pheochromocytoma. World J Surg 1992;16:759.

Krempf M et al: Treatment of malignant pheochromocytoma with [131I] metaiodobenzylguanidine: A French multicenter study. J Nucl Biol Med 1991;35:284.

Perry RR et al: Surgical management of pheochromocytoma with the use of metyrosine. Ann Surg 1990;212:621.

Revillon Y et al: Pheochromocytoma in children: 15 cases. J Ped Surg 1992;27:910.

Sheps SG et al: Recent developments in the diagnosis and treatment of pheochromocytoma. Mayo Clinic Proc 1990;65:88.

Stein PP, Black HR: A simplified diagnostic approach to pheochromocytoma: A review of the literature and report of one institution's experience. Medicine 1991;70:46.

van Heerden JA et al: Long-term evaluation following resection of apparently benign pheochromocytoma(s)/paraganglioma(s). World J Surg 1990;14:325.

HYPERADRENOCORTICISM (Cushing's Disease & Cushing's Syndrome)

Essentials of Diagnosis

- Buffalo hump, truncal obesity, easy bruisability, psychosis, hirsutism. purple striae, acne, impotence or amenorrhea, and moon facies.
- Osteoporosis, hypertension, glycosuria.
- Elevated autonomous cortisol secretion, low serum potassium and chloride, low total eosinophils, and lymphopenia.
- CT scan may reveal a tumor or hyperplasia of the adrenals.

General Considerations

Cushing's syndrome is due to an excess of cortisol and corticosterone. It may be caused by bilateral adrenal hyperplasia due to increased stimulation by excess ACTH (corticotropin) or by adrenocortical tumors that are independent of ACTH stimulation. Excess ACTH may be produced by pituitary overactivity (increased corticotropin-releasing hormone, CRH), pituitary adenomas (Cushing's disease), or extrapituitary ACTH-producing tumors (ectopic ACTH syndrome). Cushing's syndrome not dependent on ACTH may be caused by primary adrenal diseases such as adrenocortical adenoma, nodular hyperplasia, or carcinoma.

The natural history of Cushing's syndrome depends on the underlying disease and varies from a mild, indolent disease to rapid progression and death.

Clinical Findings

A. Symptoms and Signs: (Table 34–1). The classic description of Cushing's syndrome includes truncal obesity, hirsutism, moon facies, acne, buffalo hump, purple striae, hypertension, and diabetes, but other signs and symptoms are common. Weakness and depression are striking features. Weakness and other features are also seen after prolonged and excessive administration of adrenocortical steroids or ACTH. Pituitary tumors and tumors producing ectopic ACTH usually secrete melanotropins (MSH) as well as ACTH. Chronic MSH stimulation increased skin pigmentation.

In children, Cushing's syndrome is most commonly caused by adrenal cancers, but adenomas and nodular hyperplasia have been described. Cushing's syndrome in children also causes growth retardation or arrest.

B. Pathologic Examination: The pathologic features of the adrenal gland depend on the underlying disease. Normal adrenal glands weigh 7–12 g combined. The usual hyperplastic adrenal glands in patients with Cushing's syndrome weigh below 25 g combined, but they can be as large as 70 g.

Adrenal adenomas in Cushing's syndrome range in weight from a few grams to over 100 g and are larger than aldosterone-producing adenomas. The typical cells usually resemble those of the zona fasciculata. Variable degrees of anaplasia are seen, and differentiation of benign from malignant tumors is often difficult. These adrenal adenomas occur in women and are very rare in men. Adrenal cancers are frequently very large, undifferentiated, invade the surrounding tissue, and metastasize via the blood vessels.

Adrenal hyperplasia in patients with ACTH-dependent Cushing's syndrome is usually macronodular hyperplasia, whereas ACTH-independent primary adrenal hyperplasia is usually micronodular hyperplasia. Pigmented micronodular hyperplasia is associated with the syndrome of Carney's complex that also includes cardiac myxoma and lentigines. Massive enlargement of the adrenal glands with macronodular hyperplasia is a distinct form of macronodular hyperplasia that is ACTH-independent; it is treated by adrenalectomy.

Rare ectopic adrenal tissue can also be the source of excessive cortisol secretion. It has been found in various locations, most commonly near the abdominal aorta.

Cushing's disease is most commonly caused by basophilic pituitary adenomas.

Ectopic ACTH syndrome is usually caused by

small-cell lung cancers and carcinoid tumors, but tumors of the pancreas, thymus, thyroid, prostate, esophagus, colon, and ovaries may also secrete ACTH.

C. Laboratory Findings: Since no one test is specific, a combination of tests must be used.

Normal subjects have a circadian rhythmic of ACTH secretion that is paralleled by cortisol secretion. Levels are highest in the morning and decline during the day to their lowest in the evening. Normal variation is responsible for the inexactness of many of the tests, which can be improved by taking circadian rhythms into account.

In Cushing's disease, the circadian rhythm is abolished, and total secretion of cortisol is increased. In mild cases, the plasma cortisol and ACTH levels may be within the normal range during much of the day but abnormally high in the evening.

When Cushing's syndrome is suspected, the first objective is to establish the diagnosis; the second is to establish the cause. An algorithm for the diagnosis is presented in Figure 34–4. When hyperadrenocorticism is suspected, an **overnight dexamethasone suppression test** is the best first diagnostic step. Unstressed normal subjects produce about 30 mg of

cortisol a day. Dexamethasone, 1 mg orally (equivalent to about 30 mg of cortisol), will suppress ACTH secretion and stop cortisol production. This low dose dexamethasone, however, will not suppress excessive cortisol production from autonomous adrenocortical tumors or adrenals that are being stimulated by excess ACTH. Since dexamethasone does not crossreact in the assay for plasma cortisol, suppression of endogenous circulating cortisol is easily demonstrated. The test is done as follows: At 11 PM, the patient is given 1 mg of dexamethasone by mouth. A fasting plasma cortisol is measured the following morning. Normally, the morning plasma cortisol level will be suppressed to less than 5 µg/dL. In patients with Cushing's syndrome, the levels will not be suppressed below 12 µg/dL.

In patients receiving estrogen therapy, such as birth control pills, the plasma cortisol levels are elevated because of increased cortisol-binding globulin. In these patients, a basal fasting plasma sample (drawn before the dexamethasone suppression) is required to evaluate suppression. The response is normal if the plasma cortisol level is suppressed more than 50% below basal levels by the dexamethasone.

Absence of suppression by the dexamethasone in-

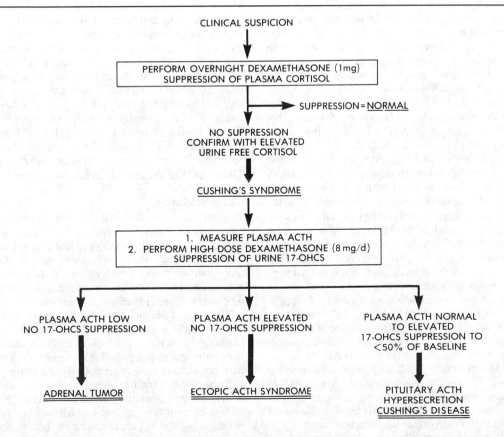

Figure 34–4. Cushing's syndrome: diagnosis and differential diagnosis. (17-OHCS, 17-hydroxycorticosteroids.)

dicates fixed production of ACTH or cortisol, ie, Cushing's syndrome. Partial suppression may occur in patients with thyrotoxicosis or acromegaly, in patients receiving other corticosteroids, and in patients who are chronically ill or under chronic physical stress. These conditions are almost always clinically obvious.

The results of the dexamethasone test should be confirmed with a measurement of 24-hour urinary excretion of free cortisol. It directly measures the physiologically active form of circulating cortisol, integrates the daily variations of cortisol production, and is very sensitive for the diagnosis of Cushing's syndrome. Free urinary cortisol excretion exceeds 120 μg/24 h in patients with Cushing's syndrome. The excessive cortisol production also increases the urinary excretion of 17-hydroxycorticosteroids and 17-ketogenic steroids.

If the plasma cortisol level is not suppressed by the overnight dexamethasone suppression test and the urinary free cortisol is elevated, the patient has Cushing's syndrome. The next step is to determine the cause. Plasma ACTH measurement by radioimmunoassay is the most direct method. A very high ACTH level is diagnostic of hyperadrenocorticism due to pituitary adenoma or ectopic ACTH secretion. Very low ACTH levels are diagnostic of hyperadrenocorticism due to a primary adrenal cause such as adenoma, nodular hyperplasia, or carcinoma.

To distinguish among the causes of ACTH-dependent hyperadrenocorticism, the high-dose dexamethasone suppression test is useful. This supraphysiologic dose of dexamethasone usually suppresses pituitary adenomas but does not suppress ectopic sources of ACTH. The test is done as follows: 8 mg of dexamethasone is given over 24 hours. This is then followed by a 24-hour urine collection to determine urinary cortisol or urinary 17-hydroxycorticosteroids. In patients with pituitary adenoma, the urinary excretion of steroids is suppressed to less than 50% of baseline, whereas patients with ectopic ACTH syndrome do not respond. Since primary adrenal diseases (adenoma, nodular hyperplasia, or carcinoma) are independent of ACTH, they will not be suppressed by the high-dose dexamethasone.

In summary, patients with elevated urinary free cortisol, in whom the plasma cortisol level is not suppressed by low-dose dexamethasone of the overnight suppression test, have Cushing's *syndrome.* Inappropriately normal or elevated plasma ACTH and suppression of urinary 17-hydroxycorticosteroids by high dose dexamethasone indicate Cushing's *disease,* a pituitary adenoma. Elevated plasma ACTH and no suppression of urinary 17-hydroxycorticosteroids by high-dose dexamethasone indicates ectopic ACTH syndrome. Low plasma ACTH and no suppression of urinary 17-hydroxycorticosteroids by high-dose dexamethasone indicate primary adrenal diseases.

The high-dose dexamethasone suppression test can accurately distinguished between pituitary adenoma and ectopic ACTH syndrome in 80% of cases. Many occult ACTH-secreting tumors can be suppressed by high-dose dexamethasone, however, making the differential diagnosis difficult.

Inferior petrosal sinus sampling to measure the ACTH gradient is the most sensitive and specific study to determine the presence of an ACTH-secreting pituitary adenoma. The test requires simultaneous bilateral venous sampling from the inferior petrosal sinuses. The inferior petrosal sinus connects the cavernous sinus with the ipsilateral internal jugular vein and drains the pituitary. A central to peripheral ACTH ratio of 2 or greater is diagnostic of pituitary adenoma. Corticotropin-releasing hormone (CRH), 100 μg intravenously as a bolus injection, can increase the diagnostic sensitivity to almost 100%; a peak central to peripheral ACTH ratio of 3 or greater is diagnostic of pituitary adenoma. The lack of a central to peripheral ACTH gradient is diagnostic of an ectopic ACTH secreting tumor. Although inferior petrosal sinus sampling is very accurate, the risk of brain stem injury from the catheter is 0.2–0.5%.

For Cushing's syndrome caused by primary adrenal diseases, carcinoma becomes more likely if the tumor is large and if 17-ketogenic steroid, 11-deoxycortisol, or aldosterone levels are elevated. Pregnenolone is often elevated in adrenal cancers.

D. Imaging Studies: CT scan and MRI are sensitive enough to detect most pituitary and adrenal adenomas and adrenal hyperplasia. Small pituitary adenomas, however, may not be apparent on CT or MRI. NP-59 scanning is useful in localizing the adrenal tumors and determining their functioning status; adenomas and hyperplasia take up NP-59; carcinomas only rarely do. Angiography is rarely helpful to find an ectopic source of cortisol or ACTH. Occult tumors that secrete ACTH ectopically are almost always in the chest—bronchial carcinoids or thymic carcinoids. Thin-cut CT of the chest is indicated in these cases.

Complications

Severe or terminal complications are most often those associated with hypertension (renal failure, strokes, myocardial infarction), diabetes (hyperglycemia, insulin reactions, infections), or severe debilitating muscle wasting and weakness. Cancer of the adrenals and pituitary tumors also cause characteristic complications. Psychosis is common.

The truncal obesity (which only rarely surpasses 90 kg) and muscle weakness in patients with Cushing's syndrome predispose them to postoperative pulmonary complications. Atrophic skin and easy bruisability also cause poor wound healing.

Nelson's syndrome, due to progression of an ACTH-secreting pituitary adenoma, occurs in about 20% of cases following bilateral adrenalectomy. The patient develops hyperpigmentation, headaches, exophthalmos, and hypopituitarism. Blindness may result from optic nerve compression.

Treatment

Cushing's syndrome can be treated by excision or irradiation of the pituitary adenoma, by excision of the adrenals, or by decreasing the synthesis of adrenal hormones using medications.

A. Medical Treatment: Temporary control of Cushing's disease is possible with metyrapone, ketoconazole, or aminoglutethimide, which inhibit steroid biosynthesis. Eventual escape from medical control is the rule in ACTH-dependent Cushing's syndrome, but medical treatment can be used before the definitive operation. Medical treatment is also often effective for prolonged periods in patients with adrenocortical adenomas. It may be the only treatment when the operative risk is prohibitive.

Mitotane is a DDT derivative that is toxic to the adrenal cortex. It has been used with modest success in treatment of adrenal hypersecretory states, especially adrenocortical carcinoma. Unfortunately, serious side effects are common at effective doses.

B. Pituitary Ablation or Excision of Adenoma: Patients with Cushing's disease are usually treated by transsphenoidal microsurgical excision of the pituitary adenomas. Relief of symptoms is rapid, and the prognosis for adequate residual pituitary-adrenal function is good. Total or subtotal hypophysectomy may be performed in older patients if a discrete tumor is not found. Pituitary procedures fail in about 15–25% of patients. This is due to failure to find the adenoma; to pituitary hyperplasia caused by suprasellar disease; or to recurrence of adenoma. Patients who fail pituitary operation may respond to pituitary irradiation. In some patients, total adrenalectomy will be necessary.

Primary irradiation treatment of pituitary adenomas is effective; however, it may take a year or longer before significant effects are achieved—too long for patients with rapidly progressive disease. Recurrences after radiotherapy are common.

C. Adrenalectomy: Patients with severe Cushing's syndrome are at high risk for postoperative complications, such as wound infection, hemorrhage, peptic ulceration, and pulmonary embolism. Adrenalectomy, however, is usually successful in reversing the devastating effect of hypercortisolism.

Unilateral adrenalectomy is indicated for adrenal adenomas or carcinomas that secrete cortisol. The contralateral adrenal gland and the hypothalamic-pituitary-adrenal axis will usually recover from the suppression 1–2 years after the operation.

Total bilateral adrenalectomy is indicated for selected patients with Cushing's disease or ectopic ACTH syndrome in whom the ACTH secreting tumor can not be found or resected. It is also indicated for patients with bilateral primary adrenal disease, such as pigmented micronodular hyperplasia or massive macronodular hyperplasia.

Bilateral adrenalectomy can be accomplished by the transabdominal, bilateral flank, bilateral posterior, or a laparoscopic approach. The transabdominal approach provides wide access to both adrenals and other abdominal and retroperitoneal organs. The posterior approach is associated with the least operative morbidity but with limited operative access. Early experience in the laparoscopic approach showed that it may provide good access with low morbidity.

Subtotal resection is not recommended in patients with Cushing's syndrome, because it usually leaves inadequate adrenocortical reserve initially, and the disease recurs in 40% with continuing ACTH stimulation. Total bilateral adrenalectomy with adrenal gland autotransplantation—in the groin with microvascular anastomosis or as small sections implanted in the muscle—offers little advantage over pharmacologic replacement.

D. Postoperative Maintenance Therapy: After total adrenalectomy, lifelong corticosteroid maintenance therapy becomes necessary. The following schedule is commonly used: No cortisol is given until the adrenals are removed during surgery. On the first day, give 100 mg of cortisol phosphate or hemisuccinate intramuscularly or intravenously every 8 hours. On the second day, give 50–75 mg every 8 hours. Thereafter, the dose should be tapered as tolerated. The same tapering process is used after excision of unilateral adenoma, because the remaining adrenal may not function normally for months.

As the hydrocortisone dose is reduced below 50 mg/d, it is often necessary to add fludrocortisone (a mineralocorticoid), 0.1 mg daily orally, to avoid excessive urinary electrolyte losses. The usual maintenance doses are about 20–30 mg of hydrocortisone and 0.1 mg of fludrocortisone daily. More than half the dose is given in the morning.

Patients who have had a total bilateral adrenalectomy and are on maintenance therapy can develop addisonian crisis when under stress, such as general anesthesia or infection. Adrenal insufficiency causes fever, hyperkalemia, abdominal pain, and hypertension and should be promptly recognized and treated with saline infusion and cortisol.

Prognosis

The prognosis of Cushing's syndrome due to benign causes of short duration is good after resection; hypertension, diabetes, depression, fatigue, and obesity improve in 80–90% of patients. Patients with long-standing disease tend to have persistent symptoms. Occult ACTH-secreting tumor may become apparent and require resection. These patients should be followed with serial chest CT scan even after adrenalectomy. Cushing's disease can recur after excision of pituitary adenoma. Malignant ectopic ACTH-secreting tumors tend to recur after resection.

Residual adrenal or adenoma tissue is present in about 10% of patients after total adrenalectomy, Cushing's syndrome can recur if the residual adrenal tissue continues to be stimulated by ACTH.

Cheung PS, Thompson NW: Carney's complex of primary pigmented nodular adrenocortical disease and pigmentous and myxomatous lesions. Surg Gynecol Obstet 1989;168:413.

Doherty GM et al: Time to recovery of the hypothalamic-pituitary-adrenal axis after curative resection of adrenal tumors in patients with Cushing's syndrome. Surgery 1990;108:1085.

Findlay JC et al: Familial adrenocorticotropin-independent Cushing's syndrome with bilateral macronodular adrenal hyperplasia. J Clin Endocrinol Metab 1993;76:189.

Gagner M et al: Laparoscopic adrenalectomy in Cushing's syndrome and pheochromocytoma. N Engl J Med 1992; 327:1033.

Kemink L et al: Residual adrenocortical function after bilateral adrenalectomy for pituitary-dependent Cushing's syndrome. J Clin Endocrinol Metab 1992;75:1211.

Leinung MC et al: Diagnosis of corticotropin-producing bronchial carcinoid tumors causing Cushing's syndrome. Mayo Clinic Proc 1990;65:1314.

Oldfield EH et al: Petrosal sinus sampling with and without corticotropin-releasing hormone for the differential diagnosis of Cushing's syndrome. N Engl J Med 1991; 325:897.

Pasieka JL et al: Adrenal scintigraphy of well-differentiated (functioning) adrenocortical carcinomas: Potential surgical pitfalls. Surgery 1992;112:884.

Sarkar R et al: The role of adrenalectomy in Cushing's syndrome. Surgery 1990;108:1079.

Tahir AH, Sheeler LR: Recurrent Cushing's disease after transsphenoidal surgery. Arch Intern Med 1992;152:977.

Tindall GT et al: Cushing's disease: Results of transsphenoidal microsurgery with emphasis on surgical failures. J Neurosurg 1990;72:363.

Xu YM et al: The value of adrenal autotransplantation with attached blood vessels for the treatment of Cushing's disease: A preliminary report. J Urol 1992;147:1209.

Zeiger MA et al: Primary bilateral adrenocortical causes of Cushing's syndrome. Surgery 1991;110:1106.

VIRILIZING ADRENAL TUMORS

Congenital adrenal hyperplasia is the most common cause of virilization. Other causes are exogenous administration of androgen, ovarian tumors, testicular tumors, ovarian dysfunction, Cushing's syndrome, and adrenal cortical carcinoma.

Congenital virilizing adrenal hyperplasia is usually caused by deficiency of an enzyme that is required in the synthesis of cortisol and mineralocorticoids. The manifestations of congenital adrenal hyperplasia are due to deficiency of the final product and accumulation of the precursors.

The three major patterns of congenital virilizing adrenal hyperplasia are simple virilism, virilism with renal sodium loss and virilism with hypertension. A defect in 21-hydroxylase leads to deficient synthesis of 21-hydroxycorticosteroids and accumulation of 17-hydroxyprogesterone. The blocked hydrocortisone synthesis leads to a feedback increase of ACTH, which in turn leads to increased production of androgens. Overproduction of the androgens, especially testosterone, leads to virilization.

A partial defect in 21-hydroxylase allows some escape in the production of mineralocorticoid; it causes simple virilism. A severe defect of 21-hydroxylase impairs aldosterone synthesis; it causes virilism with sodium loss. Virilism with hypertension is caused by incomplete 11-hydroxylation that leads to an increase in deoxycorticosterone.

Congenital adrenal hyperplasia is treated by administration of hydrocortisone, the end product of the blocked synthetic pathway. ACTH is suppressed and the androgen level is lowered.

Virilization can also be caused by adrenal tumors that oversecrete androgens. These patients are older, usually have no salt wasting, do not have elevated ACTH, and are not responsive to treatment with hydrocortisone. These adrenal tumors are frequently large and palpable.

To distinguish congenital virilizing adrenal hyperplasia and virilizing adrenal carcinoma, ACTH stimulation and dexamethasone suppression tests can be used. Virilizing adrenal carcinomas are not responsive to ACTH stimulation or dexamethasone suppression. CT and MRI are also useful in showing unilateral adrenal mass or bilateral hyperplasia.

Treatment of virilizing adrenal carcinoma consists of excision.

Dorr HG, Sippell WG: Prenatal dexamethasone treatment in pregnancies at risk for congenital adrenal hyperplasia due to 21-hydroxylase deficiency: Effect on midgestational amniotic fluid steroid levels. J Clin Endocrinol Metab 1993;76:117.

Migeon CJ, Donohoue PA: Congenital adrenal hyperplasia caused by 21-hydroxylase deficiency: Its molecular basis and its remaining therapeutic problems. Endocrinol Metab Clin North Am 1991; 20:277.

Morales L et al: Adrenocortical tumors in childhood: A report of four cases. J Pediatr Surg 1989;24:276.

Strumberg D et al: Molecular detection of genetic defects in congenital adrenal hyperplasia due to 21-hydroxylase deficiency: A study of 27 families. Eur J Pediatr 1992; 151:821.

FEMINIZING ADRENAL TUMORS

Feminization is most commonly caused by adrenocortical carcinoma. The diagnosis is based on a finding of increased urinary or plasma estrogens. Ovarian tumors, testicular feminization, and administration of exogenous estrogen should be ruled out.

Definitive treatment is by excision of the carcinoma. The prognosis is guarded.

Saadi HF et al: Feminizing adrenocortical tumor: steroid hormone response to ketoconazole. J Clin Endocrinol Metab 1990; 70:540.

ADRENOCORTICAL CARCINOMA

Adrenal cortical carcinomas are rare tumors. Fifty to 70 percent of patients have symptoms related to hypersecretion of hormones, most commonly Cushing's syndrome. Virilizing, feminizing, and purely aldosterone-secreting carcinomas account for 15% of cases. An additional 10% of cases of adrenal carcinoma will be found to secrete hormones only by biochemical studies. A palpable abdominal mass is a common finding. The mean diameter of adrenal carcinoma is 12 cm (range, 3–30 cm). Adrenocortical carcinoma invades the surrounding tissues, and about half of the patients have metastases (lung, liver, and elsewhere) at the time of diagnosis.

Treatment is by radical resection. Resection is possible in 80% of cases. Curative resection improves survival. Median survival is 15 months, and 5-year actuarial survival is 30–40% after resection. Patients over age 40 with metastases have a poor prognosis.

Mitotane controls hormone secretion and is useful for palliation. Chemotherapy using mitotane or doxorubicin induces tumor regression in about 20% of cases but does not improve survival rates. If the tumor recurs, repeat resection is indicated because some patients can have prolonged survival.

Decker RA et al: Eastern Cooperative Oncology Group study 1879: Mitotane and Adriamycin in patients with advanced adrenocortical carcinoma. Surgery 1991; 110:1006.

Icard P et al: Adrenocortical carcinoma in surgically treated patients: A retrospective study on 156 cases by the French Association of Endocrine Surgery. Surgery 1992; 112:972.

Icard P et al: Survival rates and prognostic factors in adrenocortical carcinoma. World J Surg 1992;16:753.

Jensen JC et al: Recurrent or metastatic disease in select patients with adrenocortical carcinoma: Aggressive resection vs chemotherapy. Arch Surg 1991;126:457.

Loriaux DL: The treatment of Cushing's syndrome and adrenal cancer. Endocrinol Metab Clin North Am 1991;20:767.

Luton JP et al: Clinical features of adrenocortical carcinoma, prognostic factors, and the effect of mitotane therapy. N Engl J Med 1990;322:1195.

Soreide JA et al: Adrenal cortical carcinoma in Norway, 1970–1984. World J Surg 1992;16:663.

INCIDENTALOMAS

Adrenal tumors are usually diagnosed by clinical symptoms of excess hormone secretion. The increased use of ultrasonography, CT, and MRI for various diseases in the abdomen have led to some incidentally discovered adrenal tumors called incidentalomas. Most of the incidentalomas are small, nonfunctioning adrenal cortical adenomas; some are functioning adenomas or pheochromocytomas with subclinical secretion of hormones; and a few are adrenocortical carcinomas.

Incidentalomas are found in 1–2% of CT scans; this is consistent with autopsy findings. There may be a familial predisposition. Patients who are heterozygous for congenital adrenal hyperplasia have a high incidence of adrenal masses (about 40%). Simple adrenal cysts, myelolipomas, and adrenal hemorrhages can be identified by the CT characteristics alone. Adrenal cysts can be large but are rarely malignant. Myelolipomas are benign tumors that may rarely cause Cushing's syndrome.

The major issue in managing a patient with an incidentaloma is to determine whether the tumor is hormonally active and whether it is a cancer; either would be an indication for resection. Since most incidentalomas are nonfunctioning adenomas, the workup of these patients should be selective to avoid unnecessary expense and procedures.

The workup of incidentaloma should include a complete history and physical examination to search for signs and symptoms of Cushing's syndrome, hyperaldosteronism, pheochromocytoma, and virilizing or feminizing adrenocortical carcinoma. Further laboratory studies may be indicated depending on the clinical presentation.

The management of incidentaloma depends on the functional status and the size of the tumor. All functioning tumors should be excised. Large nonfunctioning tumors also should be excised because of the risk of cancer. Small nonfunctioning tumors are almost always benign adenomas; they can be followed with serial CT scans to look for changes in size.

All patients—even those who do not have hypertension—should have a 24-hour urine collection for VMA and metanephrine to search for pheochromocytoma; the risk of unrecognized pheochromocytoma is high, and the hypertension may be episodic. Most pheochromocytomas are over 2 cm in diameter and characteristically bright on T2-weighted MRI.

All patients should also have a 24-hour urine collection for cortisol and an overnight dexamethasone suppression test. Autonomous cortisol production ("subclinical Cushing's syndrome") may be present in up to 10% of incidentalomas.

Patients who are hypertensive and hypokalemic should also have plasma aldosterone renin activity measurements to diagnose primary hyperaldosteronism.

If the above studies show that the tumor does not secrete hormone, the size of the tumor and the patient's overall medical condition will determine the appropriate treatment. Nonfunctioning adrenal tumors larger than 5 cm in diameter should usually be removed because of the high risk for cancer (as high as one-third). Nonfunctioning adrenal tumors smaller than 3 cm are unlikely to be cancers and can be safely followed. The patient's overall medical condition and the CT scan findings (irregular borders and heterogeneity, making cancers more likely) will usually determine whether a tumor 3–5 cm in size should be resected.

In patients who have a known cancer outside of the adrenals, such as lung cancer, an adrenal mass larger than 3 cm is very likely a metastasis. Unilateral adrenal masses smaller than 3 cm are likely to be benign adenomas. This is the only situation when the result of fine-needle aspiration biopsy may influence management. No adrenal tumor should be biopsied until one is certain that it is not a pheochromocytoma, in which case biopsy may induce severe hypertension and kill the patient. Resection of a solitary adrenal metastasis from a primary lung cancer can result in long-term survival and should be considered when there is no other metastasis.

Herrera MF et al: Incidentally discovered adrenal tumors: An institutional perspective. Surgery 1991;110:1014.

Khafagi FA et al: Clinical significance of the large adrenal mass. Br J Surg 1991 78:828.

Reincke M et al: Preclinical Cushing's syndrome in adrenal "incidentalomas": Comparison with adrenal Cushing's syndrome. J Clin Endocrinol Metab 1992;75:826.

Ross NS, Aron DC: Hormonal evaluation of the patient with an incidentally discovered adrenal mass. N Engl J Med 1990;323:1401.

REFERENCES

Biglieri EG (editor): Endocrine hypertension. In: *Comprehensive Endocrinology 1990*. Raven Press, 1990.

Gross MD, Shapiro B: Scintigraphic studies in adrenal hypertension. Semin Nucl Med 1989;19:122.

James VHT (editor): The adrenal gland. In: *Comprehensive Endocrinology 1992*. Raven Press, 1992.

Lack EE (editor): Pathology of the adrenal glands. In: *Contemporary Issues in Surgical Pathology*, vol 14. Churchill Livingstone, 1990.

Pommier RF, Brennan MF: Management of adrenal neoplasms. Curr Probl Surg 1991 Oct;28(10):661.

Schwartz RW et al: Diagnosis and treatment of primary adrenal tumors. Curr Opin Oncol 1991;3:121.

Arteries

35

William C. Krupski, MD, & David J. Effeney, MB, BS, FRACS

ATHEROSCLEROSIS

Atherosclerosis is the major degenerative disease of human arteries. The lesions of atherosclerosis are characterized by intimal proliferation of smooth muscle cells, with accumulation of large amounts of connective tissue matrix and lipids. The "response to injury" hypothesis proposes that atherosclerosis results from continuous repair in response to continuous injury of the arterial intima. According to this hypothesis, the endothelial lining of arteries can be damaged by factors such as hyperlipidemia, shear stress, hypertension, and hormone dysfunction. Growth factors released from platelets and arterial wall macrophages influence this process. While this theory is widely accepted, there is no in vivo evidence of spontaneous endothelial injury or disruption with or without platelet adherence.

Atheromas most commonly occur adjacent to arterial bifurcations, at the origins of major arterial branches, and at sites where an artery passes beneath or through a fascial sling. For example, the superficial femoral artery is often most severely diseased where the vessel passes through the adductor hiatus. Although atherosclerosis is a diffuse disease, patterns of distribution vary widely. Young patients with accelerated atherosclerosis most commonly have aortoiliac arterial stenoses, while elderly diabetics have disease involving the superficial femoral and tibioperoneal arteries. Lesions are usually symmetrically distributed on both sides of the body. Variations in symmetry may result from a local complication, such as hemorrhage or dissection within a plaque.

Hypertension, hypercholesterolemia, and cigarette smoking are the major risk factors for atherosclerosis. Diabetes mellitus, hypertriglyceridemia, obesity, sedentary and stressful life-style, and positive family history are more variably associated. Hyperhomocysteinemia is an independent risk factor for arterial occlusive disease. The progress of atherosclerosis may be slowed or even reversed by controlling these risk factors.

Clinical manifestations of atherosclerosis include arterial insufficiency, aneurysm formation, and embolism. Usually, manifestations of only one of these conditions are present, but they may coexist.

Arterial insufficiency, or circulatory hypoperfusion, may result from atherosclerotic plaques that have become large enough to narrow the arterial lumen. In medium-sized and large arteries, a 50% reduction in arterial diameter on arteriogram correlates roughly with 75% stenosis of a cross-sectional area and enough resistance to decrease flow and downstream pressure.

The hemodynamic circuit consists of the diseased major artery, a parallel system of collateral vessels, and the peripheral runoff bed. Collateral vessels are smaller, more circuitous, and more numerous than the major arteries they replace and always have a higher resistance than the original unobstructed artery. The stimuli for collateral development are the presence of an abnormal pressure gradient across the collateral system and increased velocity of flow through intramuscular channels that connect stem distributing branches with reentry vessels. This explains the improvement in collateral circulation that results from a regular exercise program in patients with ischemia of the lower extremities.

When the stenosis approaches total occlusion, the sharply reduced blood flow eventually leads to thrombosis. The clot propagates in the stagnant column of blood both proximally and distally to the first major tributary. Persistent flow at these sites halts the propagation of clot. The end result is a totally occluded segment bypassed by a collateral system (Figure 35–1). Clinical manifestations of ischemia are related to the effectiveness of the collateral system. The development of additional arterial stenoses further reduces blood flow; severe chronic ischemia is nearly always due to multiple sites of occlusion of the major vessels proximal to the affected tissues.

Atherosclerotic aneurysms occur because the arterial wall is unable to withstand the tensile stress imposed by the distending pressure of the pulsatile column of blood. Alterations in the architecture, composition, nutrition, or metabolism of the arterial wall may be the primary cause of this mechanical failure. Why atherosclerosis results in occlusive disease in some patients and aneurysmal disease in others is unknown. It may be that atheromatous change

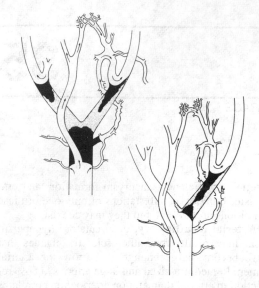

Figure 35–1. Development of collateral channels in response to occlusion of the right common iliac artery and the aortic bifurcation.

is due to intimal injury, whereas aneurysmal change occurs because of medial injury. Elastic fibers of the media become fatigued, fracture, and disintegrate, and collagen-to-elastin ratios are higher in aneurysms. A hereditary deficiency of the pyridinoline cross-linkage in collagen has been found in some patients with aneurysms. Abnormal copper metabolism and positive family histories have also been found in patients with aneurysms. Finally, there is an association of abdominal aortic aneurysms and specific genes on the long arm of chromosome 16.

Emboli may arise from the lining of aneurysms or from debris in necrotic atherosclerotic plaques. They are composed of aggregated platelets, thrombi, cholesterol crystals, lipids, or other plaque constituents. Symptoms produced by an embolus depend on its size; the affected organ and its arterial anatomy; the available collateral vessels; and the composition of the embolus, which largely determines its rate of dissolution.

Criqui MH et al: Peripheral arterial disease in large vessels is epidemiologically distinct from small vessel disease. Am J Epidemiol 1989;29:1110.

Krupski WC: The peripheral vascular consequences of smoking. Ann Vasc Surg 1991;5:291.

Malinow MR et al: Prevalence of hyperhomocysteinemia in patients with peripheral arterial occlusive disease. Circulation 1989;79:1180.

Powell JT et al: Genetic variation on chromosome 16 is associated with abdominal aortic aneurysm. Clin Sci 1990; 78:13.

Ross R: The pathogenesis of atherosclerosis: An update. N Engl J Med 1986;314:488.

Tilson MD: Status of research on abdominal aortic aneurysm disease. J Vasc Surg 1989;9:367.

PERIPHERAL ARTERIAL INSUFFICIENCY

Essentials of Diagnosis

- Intermittent claudication; rest pain.
- Impotence.
- Decreased pulses, hardening of arteries.
- Bruit.
- Pallor of foot on elevation, rubor on dependency.
- Necrosis and atrophy.

General Considerations

Peripheral arterial insufficiency is predominantly a disease of the lower extremities. In the arms, arterial lesions are confined mostly to the subclavian and axillary arteries. Stenoses of the radial and ulnar arteries occur primarily in patients with long-standing diabetes mellitus. Because collateral pathways are so abundant, upper extremity atherosclerosis rarely produces symptoms. In the lower extremities, obstructive lesions are distributed widely (Figure 35–2), and symptoms are related to the location and number of obstructions. Involvement of the femoropopliteal system is more common than aortoiliac disease. Tandem lesions are often present, increasing the degree of ischemia.

Clinical Findings

A. Symptoms:

1. Intermittent claudication–Intermittent claudication is pain or fatigue in muscles of the lower extremity caused by walking and relieved by rest. The

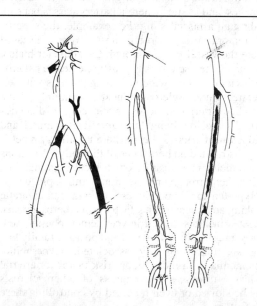

Figure 35–2. Common sites of stenosis and occlusion of the visceral and peripheral arterial systems.

pain is a deep-seated ache gradually progressing to a degree that forces the patient to stop walking. Patients occasionally describe "cramping" or "tiredness" in the muscle and report that it is completely relieved after 2–5 minutes of inactivity. It is distinguished from other pains in the extremities in that some exertion is always required before it appears, it does not occur at rest, and it is relieved by cessation of walking. Relief of symptoms is not dependent upon sitting or other positional change. The distance a patient can walk varies with the rate of walking, the level of incline, the degree of arterial obstruction, and the development of collateral circulation. The average patient with obstruction of a single arterial segment can walk 90–180 meters on a level terrain at a moderate pace before pain appears. The presence of additional lesions may reduce the walking tolerance to a few meters.

Claudication most commonly occurs in the calf muscles, regardless of which arterial segment is involved. Occlusions proximal to the origin of the profunda femoris can extend the pain to involve the thigh. Gluteal pain is added by lesions in or proximal to the hypogastric arteries; impotence often accompanies these symptoms. The LeRiche syndrome occurs in men as a result of aortoiliac disease and includes claudication of the hip, thigh, and buttock muscles, atrophy of the leg muscles, impotence, and diminished or absent femoral pulses. Occasionally, patients describe transient numbness of the extremity accompanying the pain and fatigue of claudication.

The two conditions that most often mimic claudication are osteoarthritis of the hip or knee and neurospinal compression due to osteophytic narrowing of the lumbar neurospinal canal (spinal stenosis). Osteoarthritis can be differentiated because pain occurs mostly in joints, the amount of exercise required to elicit symptoms varies, symptoms are characteristically worse in the morning, rest does not relieve symptoms promptly, and the severity of symptoms changes from day to day (and may be related to changes in the weather). Neurospinal compression symptoms are produced by increasing lumbar lordosis; therefore, standing as well as walking causes symptoms, which are not relieved until the patient straightens the lumbar spine by sitting or lying down.

2. Rest pain–Ischemic rest pain—a grave symptom caused by ischemic neuritis and tissue necrosis—indicates far-advanced arterial insufficiency that usually terminates in gangrene and amputation of the extremity if arterial reconstruction cannot be performed. It is *not* pain in a muscle group but rather a severe burning pain usually confined to the foot distal to the metatarsals. It may be localized to the vicinity of an ischemic ulcer or pregangrenous toe. It is aggravated by elevation of the extremity or by bringing the leg to the horizontal position. Thus, it appears at bed rest and may prevent sleep. When rest pain first ap-

pears, the patient typically rubs the painful foot and walks about. Pain is relieved somewhat when the patient is standing erect, as gravity aids the delivery of arterial blood. The patient with continuous rest pain hangs the leg over the side of the bed to obtain relief or sleeps sitting in a chair. Because of constant dependency, the leg and foot of a patient with severe rest pain may be swollen, causing some confusion in diagnosis. Extreme pain may require narcotics for relief. Rest pain indicates an advanced stage of ischemia; it is classically preceded by claudication but may occur de novo in patients whose walking is limited by other illness (eg, angina pectoris). The differentiation of ischemic rest pain from neuropathy in patients with long-standing diabetes mellitus may be difficult. Characteristically, patients with ischemic rest pain experience some relief by placing their limbs in a dependent position, whereas patients with neuropathy do not.

3. Impotence–Inability to attain or maintain an erection may be produced by lesions that obstruct blood flow through both hypogastric arteries and is commonly found in association with obstruction of the terminal aorta. Vasculogenic impotence is less common than impotence due to most other causes (see Chapter 41).

4. Sensation–Although the patient may report numbness in the extremity, sensory abnormalities are generally absent on examination. If decreased sensation is found in the foot, peripheral neuropathy should be suspected.

B. Signs: Physical examination is of paramount importance in assessing the presence and severity of vascular disease. The physical findings of peripheral atherosclerosis are related to changes in the peripheral arteries and to tissue ischemia.

1. Arterial palpation–Hardening and rubbery firmness of the arterial wall are palpable in vessels near the surface of the extremity. Decreased amplitude of the pulse denotes proximal stenosis. It is unusual for collateral flow to be sufficient to produce a pulse distal to an occluded artery.

Grading of Pulses

4+	Normal
3+	Slightly reduced
2+	Markedly reduced
1+	Barely palpable
0	Pulse absent

2. Bruits–A bruit is the sound produced by dissipation of energy as blood flows through a stenotic arterial segment. The sound is caused partly by blood turbulence and partly by arterial wall vibrations. It is heard loudest during systole and, with greater stenosis, may extend into diastole. The bruit is transmitted distally along the course of the artery. Thus, when a bruit is heard through a stethoscope placed over a peripheral artery, stenosis is present *at* or *proximal* to that level. The pitch of the bruit rises as the stenosis becomes more marked, until a critical stenosis is reached or the vessel becomes occluded, when the bruit may disappear.

3. Pallor–Pallor of the foot on elevation of the extremity indicates advanced ischemia. Lesser degrees of elevation are necessary to produce pallor in patients with advanced lesions. The ischemia produced by elevation results in maximum cutaneous vasodilatation. When the extremity is returned to a dependent position, blood returning to the dilated vascular bed produces an intense red color in the foot, called *reactive hyperemia*. The rate of return of skin color when the extremity is returned to a dependent position is proportionate to the efficiency of the collateral circulation.

4. Rubor–In advanced atherosclerotic disease, the skin of the foot displays a characteristic ruborous cyanosis on dependency. Because of reduced inflow, the blood in the capillary network of the foot is relatively stagnant, and oxygen extraction is high. Hemoglobin becomes deoxygenated, and the capillary blood becomes the color of that found in the venous side of the circulation. The concurrent vasodilatation due to ischemia causes blood to suffuse the cutaneous plexus, imparting a purple color to the skin. The purple discoloration due to chronic congestion from venous insufficiency does not clear on elevation.

5. Response to exercise–Exercise in a normal individual increases the pulse rate without producing arterial bruits or changes in pulse amplitude. In an individual who complains of claudication but who has minimal findings at rest, exercise will sometimes produce an audible bruit and a decrease in pulse strength and distal arterial pressure, unmasking an otherwise inapparent stenosis.

6. Temperature–With chronic ischemia, the temperature of the skin of the foot decreases. A fall in skin temperature can best be detected by palpation with the back of the examiner's hand against the dorsum of the patient's foot.

7. Ulceration–Ischemic ulcers are usually very painful and accompanied by rest pain in the foot. They occur in toes or at a site where trauma from a shoe or bedding causes additional ischemia or infection. The margin of the ulcer is sharply demarcated or punched–out, and the base is devoid of healthy granulation tissue. The surrounding skin is pale and mottled, and signs of chronic ischemia are invariably present. Scraping or debriding the ulcer results in little bleeding.

8. Necrosis–Tissue necrosis first becomes apparent in the most distal portions of the extremity, often at an ulcer site. Necrosis halts proximally at a line where the blood supply is sufficient to maintain viability and results in dry gangrene. If the part is infected (wet gangrene), necrosis may extend into tissues that would normally remain viable.

9. Atrophy–Moderate to severe degrees of chronic ischemia produce gradual muscle atrophy and loss of strength in the ischemic zone. A frequently associated complaint is reduction of joint mobility in the forefeet, as atrophy of the muscles of the feet produces increasing prominence of the interosseous spaces. Subsequent changes in foot structure and gait increase the possibility of developing foot ulceration.

10. Integumentary changes–Chronic ischemia commonly produces loss of hair over the dorsum of the toes and foot and may be associated with thickening of the toenails due to slowed keratin turnover. With more advanced ischemia, there is atrophy of the skin and subcutaneous tissue, so that the foot becomes shiny, scaly, and skeletonized. Hence, a simple glance at a foot can identify the presence or absence of serious arterial insufficiency.

C. Noninvasive Vascular Tests: Noninvasive vascular testing may aid in the management of patients with symptoms of peripheral vascular disease. In a patient with severe ischemia, rest pain, or tissue loss, in whom arteriography is clearly indicated, noninvasive tests are not essential but are useful for comparison purposes. Noninvasive assessment is helpful in a patient with claudication and decreased pulses below the femoral artery, because testing can reveal the severity of hypoperfusion and the sites of hemodynamically significant stenoses or occlusions.

A peripheral vascular testing laboratory should be equipped with a Doppler velocity detector, blood pressure cuffs of different sizes, a sphygmomanometer, and a motorized treadmill set at about 1.5 miles per hour with an incline of 12%. A device to measure the partial pressure of oxygen in tissues (transcutaneous [TC] Po_2) is also useful. With these instruments, blood pressure can be measured at rest and during exercise in the arm, ankle, calf, and thigh, and the rate of recovery of an ischemic area after exercise can be determined. The TC Po_2 in potentially ischemic locations correlates with wound healing.

A quick screening test consists of measurement of resting systolic blood pressure at the brachial artery and the posterior tibial or dorsalis pedis artery. The **ankle-brachial index (ABI)** is determined by dividing the pressure obtained at the ankle by the brachial arterial pressure. Normally, the ABI is 1.0 or greater; a value below 1.0 indicates occlusive disease proximal to the point of measurement. ABIs correlate roughly with the degree of ischemia; eg, rest pain usually appears when the ratio is 0.3 or lower. An important limitation of the indirect measurement of extremity pressure is in patients with extreme stiffening and calcification of the vessel wall. Since such a vessel cannot be compressed, an elevated pressure is recorded even though the intraluminal pressure may be low. Extreme wall stiffness should be suspected whenever the ABI is above 1.2 or when the value is out of proportion to the patient's clinical status. Patients with diabetes mellitus most commonly exhibit this phenomenon.

D. Imaging Studies: Calcification in the walls of atherosclerotic arteries is often visible on standard x-ray films and may occur without narrowing of the arterial lumen; for this reason, it is not an index of the functional status of the artery.

Arteriography supplements the physical findings by defining precisely (1) the site and degree of arterial obstruction, (2) the status of the proximal and distal arterial tree, and (3) the status of the collateral pathways.

Investigation of occlusive disease in the lower extremities can be accomplished by injection of contrast media directly into the abdominal aorta by the translumbar route or through a catheter threaded into the aorta from a peripheral artery, the Seldinger technique. A series of films of the opacified arteries of the abdomen and lower extremities is then taken.

Digital subtraction angiography (DSA) electronically digitizes x-ray signals and enhances the images using computer subtraction techniques. Although the images produced by DSA have contrast, the spatial resolution is less than with conventional arteriography. DSA was first used as a means of producing intravenous angiography. It has been used along with arterial injections to decrease the amount of contrast media and to better delineate small vessels in the foot.

Complications of angiography are related to technique and contrast media. Technical complications include puncture site hematoma, arteriovenous fistula, false aneurysm, retroperitoneal hematoma, subintimal dissection, and distal embolization of blood clot or atheromatous plaque. Contrast agents may precipitate allergic reactions ranging from mild rash to severe anaphylaxis. Because of their high osmolality, standard chemicals cause heat, vasodilatation, and pain upon injection. Use of nonionic agents lessens symptoms. Both standard and nonionic agents cause a transient decrease in renal blood flow and increased vascular resistance; in a small proportion of patients, angiography induces acute renal insufficiency. Patients with renal failure, proteinuria, diabetes, and dehydration are at increased risk for contrast-induced renal failure. Adequate hydration of patients before and after angiography reduces the incidence of this complication.

Magnetic resonance imaging can image arteries without using contrast agents. The basic principle of MRI is that the vector of the proton spin becomes aligned with the brief application of a magnetic field. The MRI signal is generated as the protons return to a nonexcited or random alignment. MRI is potentially able to define the components of atherosclerotic plaque, which vary in water and lipid composition, and to differentiate plaque from thrombus.

Treatment & Prognosis

The objectives of treatment are relief of symptoms and prevention of limb loss. In the lower extremity, the goal is to maintain bipedal gait. In the upper extremity, symptoms are rarely severe enough to require arterial operation, although revascularization is occasionally required for severe symptoms precipitated by exercise of the arm. Viability of fingers or of the hand is rarely jeopardized by arterial disease, unless repeated emboli occur.

The operative risk must be assessed for each patient. Evaluation of the cardiac and respiratory systems is particularly relevant, because most patients with peripheral vascular disease also have ischemic heart disease or chronic obstructive pulmonary disease due to prolonged tobacco use. At least 50% of patients with peripheral vascular disease have concomitant coronary artery obstructions. If the patient is apt to remain incapacitated by angina or dyspnea, there is little to be gained by operation for mild or moderate claudication. The death rates for various operations may not be an accurate gauge of risk for every patient, because rates are higher for patients with associated ischemic cardiac disease and pulmonary disease, which can vary greatly in severity among patients.

In general, patients with peripheral vascular disease have shortened life expectancies. Nondiabetic patients with ischemic disease of the lower extremity have a 5-year survival rate of 70%. The survival rate is 60% in patients with associated ischemic heart disease or cerebrovascular insufficiency. Most deaths are due to myocardial infarction. If the patient also has diabetes mellitus, death and amputation rates are almost four times as high.

A. Medical Treatment: Medical treatment consists of (1) reducing risk factors, (2) improving collateral circulation, and (3) avoiding foot trauma.

1. Reduction of risk factors–Cigarette smoking has a substantial influence on the progression of atherosclerosis, and all patients should be urged to stop smoking. Hypertension should be controlled. Hyperlipidemia should be treated by weight reduction, decreased consumption of cholesterol and saturated fats, and moderation in the use of alcohol both to reduce calories and to lower serum triglyceride levels. When diet therapy fails to control hyperlipidemia, a bile acid-binding resin such as cholestyramine or colestipol will cause low-density lipoprotein (LDL) (the most injurious circulating lipoprotein) to fall to levels 25% below those achieved by diet alone. Niacin or nicotinic acid can further lower LDL levels by limiting the mobilization of free fatty acids from adipose tissue; this reduces hepatic synthesis of very low density lipoprotein. The most effective drugs to treat hypercholesterolemia inhibit hydroxymethylglutaryl coenzyme A (HMG-CoA) reductase. One such agent, lovastatin, can lower LDL cholesterol by more than 60% when combined with other drugs.

2. Improvement of collateral circulation–Since walking stimulates the development of collateral circulation, patients with arterial insufficiency should be encouraged to walk to tolerance regularly. Exercise also decreases LDL levels slightly while raising high-density lipoprotein (HDL) levels (which has a protective effect). The increased flow with exercise also serves to limit flow stasis and decrease the time available for atherogenic stimuli to interact with vessel walls. The lowered resting heart rate induced by exercise therapy decreases coronary atherosclerosis. Not all reports support the antiatherogenic effects of exercise, however.

Drugs used to preserve or improve blood flow include anticoagulants, antiplatelet agents, vasodilators, and hemorrheologic agents. The ten% major complication rate associated with warfarin therapy probably outweighs its benefits. Aspirin, the most commonly used antiplatelet agent, is beneficial in cerebrovascular disease but has no proved role in treating atherosclerosis elsewhere in the body. Vasodilators are of no value in treating limb ischemia. Pentoxifylline, a drug that increases red blood cell flexibility, may increase blood flow and oxygen tension in ischemic muscles and walking distance in patients with claudication. In general, however, the modest improvement in walking distance produced by pentoxifylline does not warrant the cost and inconvenience of therapy.

3. Avoidance of foot trauma–The feet should be inspected and washed daily and kept dry. Clean cotton socks should be worn beneath dress socks, and shoes must fit properly. Mechanical and thermal trauma to the feet should be avoided. Toenails should be trimmed carefully, and corns and calluses should be attended to promptly. Because even minor foot infections may produce complications that will result in amputation (especially in patients with diabetes mellitus), foot infections or injuries should be treated immediately. Educating the patient to understand peripheral vascular insufficiency and the importance of foot care is a central aspect of treatment.

B. Surgical Treatment: Arterial reconstruction is performed both for limb salvage and for incapacitating claudication. For patients with more advanced disease (eg, rest pain, impending gangrene), operation is mandatory. The choice of operative procedure depends upon the location and distribution of arterial lesions and the presence of associated heart, pulmonary, or other disease.

Direct revascularization operations are applicable for patients with obstructive lesions located anywhere from the abdominal aorta to the arteries of the calf, providing there is demonstrable patency of the arteries distal to the segment to be revascularized.

1. Aortoiliofemoral reconstruction–The operation performed for atherosclerotic narrowing of the aortoiliac and common femoral arteries usually involves placement of a bypass graft of knitted Dacron. An inverted Y-shaped prosthesis is interposed between the infrarenal abdominal aorta and the femoral arteries. On occasion, the lesion is confined to the aorta and common iliac arteries, and endarterectomy is preferable (Figure 35–3). The goal of operation is restoration of blood flow to the common femoral artery or, when occlusive disease of the superficial femoral artery is present, to the profunda femoris artery.

The clinical results of aortoiliofemoral reconstruction are excellent. The operative death rate is 5%; early patency rate, 95%; and late patency rate (5–10 years postoperatively), about 80%. Complications associated with aortoiliac reconstruction include infection, aortointestinal fistula formation, false aneurysm formation at the site of anastomosis, occlusion of a limb of the graft, bowel infarction, peripheral embolization with limb loss, renal failure, and impotence.

Although the risks of aortoiliac reconstruction are acceptably low in the average patient, simpler procedures may be preferable in high-risk patients. If the clinically important lesions are confined to one side, a femorofemoral or iliofemoral bypass graft can be used. A long graft from the axillary to the femoral artery (ie, axillofemoral graft) is used for treating patients with infected abdominal aortic Dacron grafts or aortoenteric fistulas. These "extra-anatomic" methods of arterial reconstruction, however, are much more prone to late occlusion than are direct reconstructions.

2. Femoropopliteal reconstruction–When disease affects both the aortoiliac and femoropopliteal segments of the artery, aortofemoral bypass (with profundaplasty if indicated) is generally adequate. When disease is confined to the femoropopliteal segment, femoropopliteal bypass is used. The principal indication for these operations is limb salvage. In patients with claudication alone, the indications for femoropopliteal bypass are more difficult to define

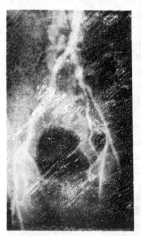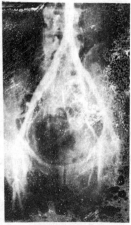

Figure 35–3. Left: Aortogram showing atherosclerotic occlusive disease of the infrarenal aorta and iliac arteries. **Right:** Postoperative aortogram showing wide patency after aortoiliac endarterectomy.

but must include substantial disability resulting from the claudication symptoms.

A femoropopliteal bypass graft is performed to provide pulsatile blood flow to the popliteal artery (Figure 35–4). The best graft for this purpose is autologous saphenous vein. The saphenous vein may be left in situ or removed and reversed for use as an arterial conduit. In the former instance, the vein is left in its normal position, special instruments are used to render the valves incompetent, and the venous tributaries are ligated. Expanded polytetrafluoroethylene (PTFE) may also be used as a conduit, particularly when bypassing to the supragenicular popliteal artery. Below the knee PTFE conduits produce much lower patency rates than saphenous veins. Operative death rates are low (2%), and 5-year patency rates range from 60% to 80%. Limb salvage rates are higher than graft patency rates. Patients undergoing femoropopliteal bypass for limb salvage have a survival rate of only about 50% within 5 years. Myocardial infarctions and strokes cause most deaths.

When profundaplasty alone is performed for limb salvage, the goal is improvement of flow to the profunda femoris artery and thereby through collaterals to the popliteal or tibial arteries. The operative death rate is only 1%, but the 5-year survival rate is 50%. Limb salvage in patients undergoing profundaplasty is 80% when the popliteal artery is patent and 40–50% when the popliteal artery is occluded. Profundaplasty is rarely helpful for treating claudication.

3. Distal arterial reconstruction– Reconstruction of distal arteries (ie, bypass to the tibial, peroneal, or pedal vessels) is performed only for limb salvage. Autogenous saphenous vein is the best graft material, and either in situ or reversed technique may be used. If the greater saphenous vein is unavailable, a composite graft of lesser saphenous or arm veins is the next best choice. The operative death rate is about 5%, and the graft failure rate during the first 30 days is 15–35%. Five years after operation, about half of the grafts at risk are still functioning. The survival rate of patients undergoing distal arterial reconstruction is lower than for those undergoing operation for femoropopliteal disease.

Successful revascularization results in lower costs ($28,000) than primary amputation ($40,500) or failed reconstruction ($56,800). Obviously, improvements in patient selection and in vascular reconstructive techniques reduce the high cost of caring for such patients.

4. Lumbar sympathectomy–Lumbar sympathectomy is seldom indicated as the only treatment for patients with occlusion of major arteries in the lower extremities. Sympathectomy is of greatest value (1) for treating patients in the early stage of advanced ischemia whose primary complaint is mild nocturnal rest pain, (2) for drying chronically moist and ulcerated areas between the toes, and (3) for treating patients with reflex sympathetic dystrophy (causalgia). Sympathectomy is ineffective in the management of gangrene of the toes or foot and does not lower the required level for amputation or delay the requirement for amputation. An alternative to operative removal of sympathetic ganglia is percutaneous injection of phenol.

5. Amputation–If intermittent claudication is the only symptom, amputation of the limb will be necessary in only 5% of patients within 5 years and 10% in ten years. Amputation is more likely if patients continue to smoke cigarettes. Of patients who present with ischemic rest pain, however, about 5% require amputation as initial therapy and the majority require amputation within 5 years.

C. Endovascular Therapy: Numerous techniques are available for treating atherosclerosis using devices within blood vessels. Percutaneous transluminal angioplasty (PTA) consists of dilation of a stenotic arterial segment using an inflatable balloon catheter that can be inflated to extremely high pressures without deforming the balloon. The deeper layers of the plaque are cracked and sheared circumferentially away from the media. As the balloon expands, it permanently overstretches the media and adventitia, fracturing atheromatous plaques and ex-

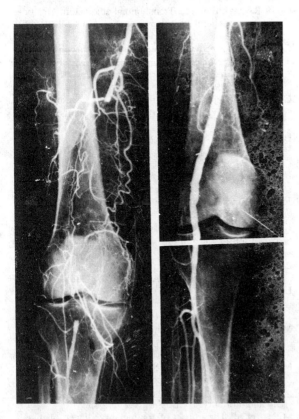

Figure 35–4. *Left:* Femoral arteriogram showing occlusion of the superficial femoral and proximal popliteal arteries. *Right:* Femoral arteriogram showing patency of the femoral and popliteal arteries after endarterectomy.

panding the artery to widen the lumen. Because energy losses associated with a stenosis are inversely proportionate to the fourth power of the radius at that point, small increases in radius can result in substantial increases in blood flow.

PTA may be used as primary therapy or as an adjunct to surgery. The success rate for PTA is highest in the treatment of short stenoses of large proximal arteries. The 1-year success rate is 85% in common iliac disease, 70% in external iliac disease, and only 50% in femoral and popliteal artery disease. Use of PTA with calf vessels is limited. The success rate is inversely related to the length of stenosis, and stenoses longer than ten cm have little chance of remaining patent. In large arteries, the success rate in treating stenoses is about the same as for complete occlusions, but in small vessels the results with stenoses are better.

The initial failure rate of PTA is ten–20%. Other complications include disruption of the artery, false aneurysm formation, dissection of an atherosclerotic plaque, and distal embolization. Local thrombosis with acute ischemia of the extremity is unusual. Since disease can be expected to recur in many cases, the patient should be closely followed using noninvasive tests. Repeat PTA may be indicated for recurrent disease.

Preliminary investigations exploring the utility of lasers in obliterating (vaporizing) atherosclerotic plaques were promising. Coronary artery lesions have been successfully treated using this technique. There have been numerous complications, however, including perforation of the vessel wall or myocardium, vessel thrombosis, and aneurysm formation. Reports indicate that for peripheral vascular disease only 50% of patients benefit from laser angioplasty, and all of these require concomitant balloon angioplasty. At present, only two laser angioplasty devices are approved by the FDA and available for clinical use: a bare-tipped and a metal-tipped delivery system.

Atherectomy is an endovascular procedure in which plaque is removed piecemeal by a cutting or rotating catheter, leaving a portion of the media and arterial wall behind. In theory, removing the plaque should be more effective than angioplasty in treating stenosis, and it does not produce thermal injury as does laser angioplasty. Simpson, Kensey, and TEC atherectomy catheters each have unique characteristics, but all debulk lesions with an intraluminal cutting device. The short-term results of atherectomy are satisfactory, but restenosis is a major problem.

Endovascular stents have been recommended as a way to decrease the frequency of acute occlusion and restenosis after the above techniques. Balloon-expandable (Palmaz) and self-expanding (Wallstent) stents are currently available. Both decrease acute arterial spasm, avoid overdilation, act as a scaffold to prevent intimal dissection, and prevent ingrowth of the myointimal tissue that causes restenosis. Although poor long-term results have been reported for coronary artery stents, the initial results of iliac, femoral, and renal artery stents have been satisfactory.

Agee JM et al: The risk of axillofemoral bypass grafting for acute vascular occlusion. J Vasc Surg 1991;14:190.

Ahn SS et al: Removal of focal atheromatous lesions by angioscopically guided high-speed rotary atherectomy: Preliminary experimental observations. J Vasc Surg 1988;7:292.

Andros G et al: Bypass grafts to the ankle and foot. J Vasc Surg 1988;7:785.

Clowes AW, Reidy MA: Prevention of stenosis after vascular reconstruction: Pharmacologic control of intimal hyperplasia: A review. J Vasc Surg 1991;13:885.

Dahlberg PJ, Frecentese DF, Cogbill TH: Cholesterol embolism: Experience with 22 histologically proven cases. Surgery 1989;105:737.

Dalman R et al: Simultaneous operative repair of multilevel lower extremity occlusive disease. J Vasc Surg 1991;13:211.

Donaldson JC, Mannick JA, Whittemore AD: Causes of graft failure after in situ saphenous vein bypass grafting. J Vasc Surg 1991;15:113.

Fahal AH, McDonald AM, Marston A: Femorofemoral bypass in unilateral iliac artery occlusion. Br J Surg 1989;76:22.

Graor RA, Whitlow PL: Transluminal atherectomy for occlusive peripheral vascular disease. J Am Coll Cardiol 1990;15:1551.

Gooding GAW et al: Lower extremity vascular grafts placed for peripheral vascular disease: Prospective evaluation with duplex Doppler sonography. Radiology 1991;180:379.

Guenther RW et al: Iliac and femoral artery stenoses and occlusions: Treatment with intravascular stents. Radiology 1989;172:725.

Harris HW et al: Saphenous vein bypass to pedal arteries: An aggressive strategy for foot salvage. Arch Surg 1989;124:1232.

Hiatt WR et al: Benefit of exercise conditioning for patients with peripheral arterial disease. Circulation 1990;81:602.

Joffre F, Rousseau H, Puel J: Arterial stenting. J Intervent Radiol 1989;4:155.

Krupski WC et al: Comparison of cardiac morbidity between aortic and infrainguinal operations. J Vasc Surg 1992;15:354.

Leather RP et al: Resurrection of the in situ saphenous vein bypass: 1,000 cases later. Ann Surg 1988;208:435.

Lindgard F et al: Conservative drug treatment in patients with moderately severe chronic occlusive peripheral arterial disease. Circulation 1989;80:1549.

Mangano DT et al: Dipyridamole thallium scintigraphy as a preoperative screening test: A re-examination of its predictive potential. Circulation 1991;84:493.

McCann RL, Clements FM: Silent myocardial ischemia in patients undergoing peripheral vascular surgery: Incidence and association with perioperative cardiac morbidity and mortality. J Vasc Surg 1989;9:583.

Mills J et al: The impact of routine surveillance of distal bypass grafts with duplex scanning: A study of 379 reversed vein grafts. J Vasc Surg 1990;12:379.

Quam JP et al: Duplex and color Doppler sonographic evaluation of vasculogenic impotence. AJR Am J Roentgenol 1989;153:1141.

Rapp JH et al: "Angiography" by magnetic resonance imaging: Detailed vascular anatomy without radiation or contrast media. Surgery 1989;105:662.

Rosenthal D et al: Thermal laser-assisted balloon angioplasty of the superficial femoral artery: A multicenter review of 602 cases. J Vasc Surg 1991;14:152.

Rutherford RB et al: Factors affecting the patency of infrainguinal bypass. J Vasc Surg 1988;8:236.

Sanborn TA et al: Peripheral laser-assisted balloon angioplasty: Initial multicenter experience in 219 peripheral arteries. Arch Surg 1989;124:1099.

Strandness DE JR: *Duplex Scanning in Vascular Disorders.* Raven Press, 1990.

Taylor LM JR et al: Present status of reversed vein bypass grafting: Five-year results of a modern series. J Vasc Surg 1990;11:193.

Taylor LM et al: The incidence of perioperative myocardial infarction in general vascular surgery. J Vasc Surg 1992;15:52.

van den Dungen JJAM, Boontje AH, Kropveld A: Unilateral iliofemoral occlusive disease: Long-term results of the semiclosed endarterectomy with the ringstripper. J Vasc Surg 1991;14:673.

Walsh DB et al: The natural history of superficial femoral artery stenosis. J Vasc Surg 1991;14:299.

Wengerter KR et al: Prospective randomized multicenter comparison of in situ and reversed vein infrapopliteal bypasses. J Vasc Surg 1991;13:189.

Veith FJ et al: Six year prospective multicenter randomized comparison of autologous saphenous vein and expanded polytetrafluoroethylene grafts in infrainguinal arterial reconstructions. J Vasc Surg 1986;3:104.

White RA et al: Initial human evaluation of argon laser-assisted vascular anastomoses. J Vasc Surg 1989;9:542.

Wilson SE et al: Percutaneous transluminal angioplasty versus operation for peripheral arteriosclerosis: Report of a prospective randomized trial in a selected group of patients. J Vasc Surg 1989;9:1

ACUTE OCCLUSION OF MAJOR PERIPHERAL ARTERIES

Sudden occlusion of a previously patent artery supplying an extremity is a dramatic event characterized by the abrupt onset of severe distal ischemia, with pain, coldness, numbness, motor weakness, and absent pulses. Tissue viability depends on the extent to which flow is maintained by collateral circuits or surgical intervention. The clinical manifestations are those of ischemia of nerves, muscle, and skin. When ischemia persists, motor and sensory paralysis, muscle infarction, and cutaneous gangrene become irreversible in a matter of hours. A line of demarcation develops between viable and nonviable tissue. Flow in the distal arteries is reduced progressively by propagating intraluminal thrombus, and surgical restoration of blood flow to the ischemic portion of the extremity eventually becomes impossible.

Acute major arterial occlusion may be caused by an embolus, thrombosis, or trauma. Embolic occlusion usually results from dislodgment of a blood clot into the bloodstream. The heart is the source of embolus in 80–90% of episodes. The clot most frequently originates from the left atrium in patients with arterial fibrillation or from mural thrombus in patients with recent myocardial infarction. Prosthetic heart valves may be the source of emboli, although this is uncommon with chronic systemic anticoagulation and use of tissue valves. Septic emboli may emanate from infective endocarditis. Emboli may arise from clots within aneurysms anywhere in the aortofemoral system; popliteal aneurysms that cause emboli have a particularly poor prognosis. Ulceration in atherosclerotic plaques can lead to dislodgment of platelets, thrombus, or debris. Miscellaneous infrequent sources of emboli include cardiac tumors (including cardiac myxoma), and paradoxic emboli (venous thrombi migrating through a patent foramen ovale).

Sudden thrombosis of an atherosclerotic peripheral artery may be difficult to differentiate clinically from embolic occlusion. The usual mechanism is hemorrhagic dissection beneath an atherosclerotic plaque. These patients have preexisting atherosclerotic stenosis and low blood flow, which predisposes to stagnation and thrombosis. Differentiation between embolic and thrombotic occlusions is based on the clinical setting and a history of long-standing symptoms.

Traumatic occlusion may be due to numerous causes, eg, contusion or laceration by a bone after a fracture or dislocation, penetrating injuries, and more commonly in recent years—as a complication of arterial catheterization or PTA. Intra-arterial injection of drugs of abuse is an increasingly frequent cause of acute arterial occlusion.

Clinical Findings

Acute arterial occlusion is characterized by the five *P*s: *pain, pallor, paralysis, paresthesia,* and *pulselessness.* Severe sudden pain is present in 80% of patients, and its onset usually indicates the time of vessel occlusion. Pain is absent in some patients because of prompt onset of anesthesia and paralysis.

Pallor appears first but is replaced by mottled cyanosis after a few hours as deoxygenated blood gradually suffuses the extremity. Cutaneous hypesthesia slowly progresses to anesthesia. It is important to separate perception of light touch from that of pressure, pain, and temperature, because the larger fibers serving these latter functions are relatively less susceptible to hypoxia. The onset of motor paralysis heralds impending gangrene. If changes persist beyond 12 hours, limb salvage is unlikely. Tense swelling with acute tenderness of a muscle belly—a common occurrence in the gastrocnemius following superficial femoral artery occlusion—generally denotes irreversible muscle infarction. Skin and subcutaneous tissues have greater resistance to hypoxia than nerves and muscles, which demonstrate irreversible histologic changes after 4–6 hours of ischemia.

The level of demarcation of ischemic changes suggests the site of arterial occlusion. Since collaterals always supply the tissues just beyond the occlusion, the demarcation is as follows:

Site of Occlusion	Line of Demarcation
Infrarenal aorta	Mid abdomen
Aortic bifurcation and common iliac arteries	Groin
External iliacs	Proximal thigh
Common femoral	Lower third of thigh
Superficial femoral	Upper third of calf
Popliteal	Lower third of calf

If collateral flow increases, it becomes evident by return of warmth and pinkness of the skin and a lessening of the sensory deficit. When reversible ischemia has been severe and protracted at the onset, normal sensory function may not return. When collateral flow has reached its maximum, the signs and symptoms are those of chronic occlusion of the involved artery.

Treatment & Prognosis

A. Embolism and Thrombosis: Immediate anticoagulation by intravenous heparin slows the propagation of thrombus and allows time for assessment of adequacy of collateral flow and preparation for operation if indicated. When embolus cannot be differentiated from thrombosis, arteriography should be performed if it can be done without delaying therapy. Diagnosis of acute embolic occlusion is based upon an abrupt block of the artery with little accompanying arterial disease; conversely, acute thrombosis is associated with extensive atherosclerosis and an established collateral network. The operative treatment of the average embolus differs from that of preexisting atherosclerosis. Although some surgeons recommend nonoperative management with anticoagulation as the sole therapy for acute arterial ischemia, this approach is not widely favored. Nonoperative management is best reserved for some emboli to major arteries in the upper extremities, where collateral circulation is outstanding, and for some in the lower extremities when skin color improves or neural function returns within 3 hours after occlusion. If the initial ischemia recedes, the decision for removal of the embolus is based upon an estimate of the disability that will be produced by chronic occlusion of the involved artery. Chronic occlusion of the axillary or brachial arteries is usually well tolerated, whereas chronic occlusion of lower extremity vessels causes claudication at best.

If advanced ischemia persists or is profound, the embolus must be removed. Embolectomy may be performed through an arteriotomy at the site of the embolus or, most commonly, by extraction with a balloon (Fogarty) catheter inserted through a proximal arteriotomy. Successful embolectomy requires removal of the embolus and the "tail" of thrombus that extends distally or proximally from it. If operation is not performed within the first few hours, the ramifications of this thrombus into arterial branches usually cannot be extracted and revascularization is impossible. Intraoperative infusion of thrombolytic agents is an important adjunct to embolectomy when thrombus has propagated. Late thrombectomy (after 12 hours) is successful only when propagation of thrombus has been arrested by collateral blood flow reentering the vessel distal to the embolus. Fasciotomy is normally required after prolonged acute ischemia to treat compartment syndrome. Renal insufficiency—the so-called myonephrotic syndrome—should be anticipated after reperfusion of ischemic muscle. Treatment consists of vigorous hydration and alkalinization of the urine. Recently, administration of free radical scavengers has been helpful in this disorder.

Moribund patients with embolic disease should not be treated surgically. Patients with clearly irreversible limb ischemia should undergo amputation without an attempt at revascularization, because revascularization subjects the patient to the serious hazards of the reperfusion syndrome caused by recirculation of acidotic hyperkalemic venous blood.

Many patients present late, when it is difficult to ascertain the cause of occlusion. Initial therapy should consist of anticoagulation. The arterial anatomy should be defined by arteriography. Treatment options include continuation of anticoagulants, thrombolytic therapy with streptokinase or urokinase, arterial embolectomy, or arterial reconstruction. Intravenous thrombolytic therapy is effective but is associated with a high rate of complications. A safer, more effective regimen involves selective intra-arterial infusion of lower doses of streptokinase, urokinase, or alteplase (recombinant human tPA) directly into the clot. This activates thrombus plasminogen more efficiently, protects the drug from circulating antibodies and inhibitors, and lowers complication rates.

B. Traumatic Arterial Occlusion: Traumatic arterial occlusion must be corrected within a few hours to avoid development of gangrene. Repair of arterial injury is usually performed in conjunction with repair of other injuries. The general principles are described in Chapter 13.

Clason AE et al: Morbidity and mortality in acute lower limb ischaemia: A 5-year review. Eur J Vasc Surg 1989; 3:339.

Friedl HP et al: Ischemia-reperfusion in humans: Appearance of xanthine oxidase activity. Am J Pathol 1990;136: 491.

Kitts D, Bongard FS, Klein SR: Septic embolism complicating infective endocarditis. J Vasc Surg 1991;14:480.

Krupski WC, Feldman RA, Rapp JH: Human tissue-type

plasminogen activator is an effective agent for thrombolysis of peripheral arteries and bypass grafts. J Vasc Surg 1989;10:491.

Pan XP et al: Identification of aortic thrombus by magnetic resonance imaging. J Vasc Surg 1989;9:801.

Parent FN et al: Fibrinolytic treatment of residual thrombus after catheter embolectomy for severe lower limb ischemia. J Vasc Surg 1989;9:153.

Sicard GA et al: Thrombolytic therapy for acute arterial occlusion. J Vasc Surg 1985;2:65.

Takolander R, Lannerstad O, Bergqvist D: Peripheral arterial embolectomy: Risks and results. Acta Chir Scand 1988;154:567.

Tawes RL et al: Acute limb ischemia: Thromboembolism. J Vasc Surg 1987;5:901.

Treiman GS et al: An effective treatment protocol for intraarterial drug injection. J Vasc Surg 1990;12:440.

PERIPHERAL MICROEMBOLI

Recurrent microemboli to the small arteries in the extremities can arise from sources already described as well as from ulcerated atheromas. The peripheral aneurysms most commonly implicated are in the popliteal and subclavian arteries. The mural thrombus in the wall of popliteal aneurysms is particularly susceptible to fragmentation with flexion of the knee joint. Subclavian aneurysms are almost always associated with an anomalous cervical rib that compresses the artery, and they develop as extensions of the poststenotic dilatation. The source of atheromatous microembolization is almost always a lesion in the aorta-iliac-femoral portions of the arterial tree.

When a microembolus occludes a digital artery, the patient experiences sudden pain, cyanosis, and coldness or numbness in the affected digit. These changes characteristically improve over several days, only to reappear perhaps in a different area of the hand or foot. This clinical entity has been called **blue toe syndrome,** or **trash foot.** The sudden onset of pain and purple discoloration of a toe in the presence of palpable pulses—the "three *P*s" of this syndrome—is recognized as a potentially limb-threatening arterial problem. With each succeeding episode, recovery is slower and less complete.

Suddenness of onset differentiates peripheral atheroembolism from other causes of blue toes, such as vasculitis, thromboangiitis obliterans, trauma, or chronic ischemia. It is important to remember that a patent proximal artery to serve as a conduit for the embolus is required for occurrence of this syndrome. With embolic occlusion of distal arteries, a normal blood supply is present in adjacent tissue segments. Unless this difference is recognized and the lesion of origin corrected, survival of the foot or hand may be in peril from recurrent microemboli that progressively occlude additional arteries.

Once discovered, the source of microemboli must be removed by appropriate valvular or arterial reconstruction. Sympathectomy aids in recovery of the hand or foot from ischemia. Chronic anticoagulation may be necessary, particularly with valvular disease.

Dollmatch BL et al: Blue toe syndrome: Treatment with percutaneous atherectomy. Radiology 1989;172:799.

Rosman HS et al: Cholesterol embolization: Clinical findings and implications. J Am Coll Cardiol 1990;15:1296.

SMALL ARTERY OCCLUSIVE DISEASE

Obstructing lesions may occur in arteries less than 3 mm in diameter (eg, the radial, ulnar, tibial, or peroneal arteries), most commonly in patients with diabetes mellitus, vasculitis, or thromboangiitis obliterans (Buerger's disease). Hand, foot, or digital ischemia can result from these conditions, and amputation is often required.

Differentiation of occluded arterial segments from vasoconstrictive disorders can best be accomplished in the upper extremity by the **Allen test.** This is done by having the patient make a tight fist while the examiner occludes the radial and ulnar arteries at the wrist and asks the patient to open and close the hand rapidly. With the hand in a relaxed position, patency of the radial artery can be determined by releasing the radial artery and noting the return of color. This maneuver is then repeated for the ulnar artery. The extremity is made ischemic by compressing the proximal artery while the hand is exercised. When the extremity has become pale, the artery is released and the pattern of return color is observed. In a person with normal arteries and normal sympathetic tone, a vivid flush appears almost simultaneously in all areas of the hand. Patients with excess sympathetic tone will have a diffusely delayed return of color. When small artery occlusion is present, there will be a prolonged delay in reperfusion of the cutaneous area supplied by the occluded arteries.

DIABETIC VASCULAR DISEASE

Arterial disease in patients with diabetes mellitus is more diffuse and more severe than in nondiabetics. Advanced disease often affects both large and medium-sized arteries, and even the smaller arteries (especially those in the calf) may be involved. In nondiabetic patients, atherosclerosis at the bifurcation of the popliteal artery and tibioperoneal trunk usually extends into the tibial vessels for only a short distance. In diabetic patients, however, the tibioperoneal vessels frequently contain irregular atherosclerotic changes as far down as the ankle, and the vessels may be heavily calcified. All diabetics have thickened capillary basement membranes at the microcirculatory level.

Diabetic patients also have a high incidence of

neuropathy and are therefore more apt to injure themselves. Neuropathy is also responsible for loss of tone of intrinsic foot muscles that leads to subluxation of the metatarsal phalangeal joints, ultimately resulting in a "rocker-bottom" foot. Thus, ulceration is prone to occur because of altered foot architecture and diminished sensation. Neurotrophic ulcers over the first metatarsophalangeal joint are termed "malperforans ulcers." Such wounds are particularly susceptible to infection because of white blood cell dysfunction in diabetics. Additionally, inflammatory cells and some bacteria elaborate substances that act as procoagulants.

THROMBOANGIITIS OBLITERANS

Thromboangiitis obliterans **(Buerger's disease)** is characterized by multiple segmental occlusions of small arteries in the extremities distal to the brachial and popliteal arteries. In contrast to atherosclerosis, which involves the intima and inner media, thromboangiitis obliterans is manifested by infiltration of round cells in all three layers of the arterial wall. Healing of the arterial wall lesion is associated with fibrous obliteration of the lumen in segmental fashion. Migratory phlebitis is frequently present. The disease occurs almost exclusively in young cigarette-smoking men.

Many patients with Buerger's disease have specific cellular immunity against arterial antigens, specific humoral antiarterial antibodies, and elevated circulatory immune complexes. HLA typing can differentiate such patients from patients with atherosclerosis and from normal individuals. The role of cigarette smoking is unclear; it is probably facilitative rather than causative. Symptoms consist of slowly developing digital pain, cyanosis, and coldness, progressing eventually to necrosis and gangrene. Claudication in the muscles of the foot may be the first symptom.

Examination shows an irregular pattern of digital ischemia. The Allen test (see above) demonstrates delayed filling of affected digital arteries and rapid filling in adjacent vessels.

A precise diagnosis can only be made by microscopic examination showing the typical segmental vasculitis with infiltration of lymphocytes into all layers of the vessel wall. Arteriographic findings are distinctive but not pathognomonic. The artery proximal to the occlusions characteristically is tapered, and the arterial wall is smooth and devoid of irregular atherosclerotic plaques. The configuration resembles a dunce cap.

It is essential that the patient stop smoking to avoid progression of the disease. Sympathectomy decreases arterial spasm and is useful in some patients. Amputation is indicated for persistent pain or gangrene and can be performed adjacent to the line of demarcation with satisfactory primary healing.

The disease may become dormant if the patient can stop smoking, but this is unfortunately difficult to achieve in many who ultimately develop gangrene of additional digits.

Anderson CB, Munn JS: Cutaneous ulcers on the diabetic foot. In: *Current Therapy in Vascular Surgery,* 2nd ed. Ernst CB, Stanley JC (editors). BC Decker, 1991.

Irwin ST et al: Blood flow in diabetics with foot lesions due to "small vessel disease." Br J Surg 1988;75:1201.

Ohta T, Shionoya S: Fate of the ischaemic limb in Buerger's disease. Br J Surg 1988;75:259.

RARE DISORDERS CAUSING LOWER LIMB ISCHEMIA

Popliteal Artery Entrapment Syndrome

A rare cause of popliteal artery stenosis or occlusion occurs as a result of an anomalous course of the popliteal artery. The popliteal artery normally passes between the two heads of the gastrocnemius muscle as it enters the lower leg. In the entrapment syndrome, the artery passes medial to the medial head of the gastrocnemius, causing compression of the popliteal artery when the knee is extended. Fibrous thickening of the intima occurs at the site of compression and gradually progresses to total occlusion. Poststenotic dilatation of the artery may occur with mural thrombus and distal embolization.

Symptoms vary from simple calf claudication to those of more severe ischemia depending upon the adequacy of collateral channels and the extent of distal or proximal clot propagation. Popliteal artery entrapment should be considered when a young, otherwise healthy patient presents with calf claudication. Until the artery becomes occluded, the only finding is a decrease in strength of the pedal pulses, most evident with the knee in extension. Arteriograms, in addition to revealing a zone of stenosis or occlusion in the distal third of the popliteal artery, show medial deviation of the popliteal artery beginning in the middle third. CT scans and MRI images can be used to confirm the diagnosis. Treatment consists of division of the medial head of the gastrocnemius muscle and resection and graft replacement of the diseased arterial segment. Lumbar sympathectomy is often performed as well.

Cystic Degeneration of the Popliteal Artery

Arterial stenosis is produced by a mucoid cyst in the adventitia, usually located in the middle third of the artery. Calf claudication is the most common symptom, and the only finding is decrease in the strength of the peripheral pulses. Rarely, a mass can be palpated. Arteriography shows a sharply localized zone of popliteal stenosis with a smooth concentric tapering having an hourglass appearance. Ultrasound or CT scans can be used to demonstrate the cyst within the vessel wall. The stenosis may be missed on conventional anteroposterior films and may appear only on lateral exposures. Evacuation of the cyst may relieve the stenosis, but because of the possibility of recurrence, local arterial excision and graft replacement may be required occasionally.

Jay GD et al: Clinical and chemical characterization of an adventitial popliteal cyst. J Vasc Surg 1989;9:448.

Melliere D et al: Adventitial cystic disease of the popliteal artery: Treatment by cyst removal. J Vasc Surg 1988; 8:638.

Schurmann G et al: The popliteal artery entrapment syndrome: Presentation, morphology and surgical treatment of 13 cases. Eur J Vasc Surg 1990;4:223.

ARTERIAL ANEURYSMS

Arterial dilatations (aneurysms) may be classified according to etiology (eg, degenerative, inflammatory, mechanical, congenital, dissecting); shape (eg, saccular, fusiform); location (eg, central, peripheral, splanchnic, renal, cerebral); or structure (eg, true, false). A **true aneurysm** is dilatation of an artery to more than twice normal size, with stretching and thinning of all vessel wall layers. Atherosclerotic aneurysms are true aneurysms. Dilatation is associated with elongation of the artery. A **false aneurysm** or **pseudoaneurysm** is a pulsatile hematoma not contained by the vessel wall layers but confined by a fibrous capsule. False aneurysms are caused by disruption of the vessel wall or the anastomotic site between graft and vessel, with containment of blood by surrounding tissue.

Atherosclerotic aneurysms are found, in descending order of frequency, in the distal abdominal aorta, the iliac arteries, the popliteal artery (Figure 35–5), the common femoral artery, the arch and descending portions of the thoracic aorta, the carotid arteries, and other peripheral arteries. As the aneurysm enlarges, mural thrombus is deposited on its interior surface because of eddy currents and stagnant flow. The functional lumen of the artery may remain unchanged and may appear relatively normal on arteriograms—a factor that limits the usefulness of angiography in diagnosis.

Recent studies suggest that aneurysm formation may not always be due to atherosclerosis but may be a separate arterial disease. Studies of families with a history of aneurysm and studies of mice with a predilection to aneurysm formation have identified abnormalities in copper metabolism and pyridinoline

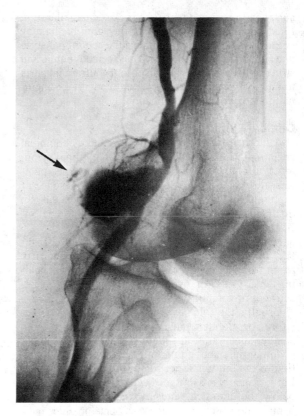

Figure 35–5. Arteriogram showing aneurysm of the popliteal artery (arrow).

cross-linkage of arterial collagen. Increased collagenase and elastase activity in early aneurysmal dilatation has also been described. These abnormalities are not yet accepted as the cause. At present, most aneurysms are still considered to be a manifestation of atherosclerosis.

INFRARENAL ABDOMINAL AORTIC ANEURYSMS

Abdominal aortic aneurysms may be present in 2% of the elderly population, and the incidence appears to be increasing. There is a 19% incidence in first-degree relatives of patients with aortic aneurysms. The abdominal aorta is the most common site of atherosclerotic aneurysms and also the most dangerous site; aneurysms here are much more likely to rupture than are aneurysms of smaller peripheral arteries.

Most aneurysms of the abdominal aorta involve the segment of the aorta between the takeoff of the renal arteries and the aortic bifurcation but may include variable portions of the common iliac arteries. The reasons for this remain speculative, but contributory factors include increased turbulence, decreased turnover in the smooth muscle cells of the infrarenal aorta, and increased tension per elastic lamellar unit. In addition, the nourishment of the aortic media may be important because in humans the abdominal aorta does not have vasa vasorum. Thus, hemodynamic and structural factors may predispose the infrarenal aorta to aneurysmal degeneration. Rupture with exsanguination is the major complication.

Clinical Findings

A. Symptoms and Signs: An intact abdominal aneurysm rarely produces more than minimal symptoms, although the patient may be aware of a painless, throbbing mass. Severe pain in the absence of rupture characterizes the rare inflammatory aneurysm that is surrounded by 2–4 cm of perianeurysmal inflammatory reaction.

Heart failure may occur owing to aortocaval fistulas; gastrointestinal hemorrhage or obstruction may result from duodenal erosion or stretching by expanding aneurysms; or pyelonephritis may develop because of ureteral obstruction by an aneurysm.

Usually, the sole physical finding is a palpable fusiform or globular pulsatile abdominal mass. With smaller aneurysms, this mass is centered in the upper abdomen just above the umbilicus, the normal location of the infrarenal portion of the abdominal aorta. Larger aneurysms bulge distally into the abdomen below the umbilicus and proximally into the space behind the rib cage. In obese patients or older individuals in whom aortas become tortuous, physical examination is not reliable. The aneurysm may be slightly tender to palpation. Severe tenderness is found in inflammatory aneurysms, after rupture has occurred, or if the aneurysm has recently expanded.

B. Imaging Studies: Plain films of the abdomen in anteroposterior, lateral, and oblique projections reveal calcification in the outer layers of most atherosclerotic abdominal aneurysms. This allows assessment of their size and proximal extent. CT scans provide valuable information about aneurysm architecture and have been used to predict aneurysm expansion rates. Aortograms are not needed preoperatively in all cases but should be obtained for the following indications: (1) suspected suprarenal involvement; (2) symptoms of visceral angina suggesting mesenteric arterial insufficiency; (3) evidence on ultrasound scans of a horseshoe or pelvic kidney; (4) suspected renovascular disease; (5) unexplained impairment of renal function; and (6) clinical evidence of coexistent occlusive disease.

Ultrasound is the most useful investigation for measuring the size and position of aneurysms of the infrarenal aorta. In all cases of groin false aneurysms after Dacron graft placement, ultrasound evaluation of the abdominal aorta and graft should be done to assess the proximal anastomosis. More recently it has become possible to detect perigraft collections of blood or fluid, and ultrasound should be part of the evaluation of suspected graft infection. CT scan and MRI can also be used for these purposes but are more expensive than ultrasound examination.

Treatment

The expansion rate of aneurysms of the abdominal aorta is variable and unpredictable in individual patients. Most aneurysms continue to enlarge and will eventually rupture if left untreated. Average expansion rates for abdominal aortic aneurysms are 0.4 cm per year. Rate of expansion and risk of rupture correlate with diastolic blood pressure, initial aneurysm diameter, and degree of obstructive pulmonary disease. The size of the aneurysm correlates best with the risk of rupture. About 40% of aneurysms 6 cm or more in diameter will rupture if untreated, and the average survival of an untreated patient is 17 months. In contrast, 20% of aneurysms less than 6 cm in diameter will rupture, and patient survival averages 34 months. Thus, surgery is recommended for all aneurysms 6 cm or greater in size, but smaller aortic aneurysms can also rupture. Operation is mandatory for any aneurysm, regardless of size, that is symptomatic, tender, or enlarging rapidly on sequential ultrasound examinations.

Operation consists of replacing the aneurysmal segment with a synthetic fabric graft. Tubular or bifurcation grafts of Dacron or polytetrafluoroethylene (PTFE) are preferred. The proximal anastomosis is usually made to the aorta above the aneurysm—the so-called neck— and below the origin of the renal arteries. The site of the distal anastomosis is determined by the extent of aneurysmal involvement of the iliac arteries. In most circumstances, the iliac arms of a bifurcated graft are anastomosed to the distal ends of the transected common iliac arteries (Figs 35–6 and 35–7).

Abdominal aortic aneurysms in high-risk patients may be treated by thrombosis of the aneurysm induced by outflow obstruction while limb perfusion is maintained by axillofemoral bypass. Adequacy of thrombosis is assessed by CT scan. While this approach would seem to combine a minimal operation with elimination of the risk of rupture, the operative mortality rate is ten%, and rupture may still occur despite adequate thrombosis. This method should be used only in patients who could not survive resection. Preliminary studies have investigated intraluminal endovascular grafts placed by percutaneous techniques.

Prognosis

Elective infrarenal abdominal aneurysmectomy has a 4% operative death rate and a 5–10% rate of complications, such as bleeding, renal failure, myocardial infarction, stroke, graft infection, limb loss, bowel ischemia, and impotence. A very rare complication is paraplegia due to sacrifice of an abnormally distally situated accessory spinal artery. Malignant tumors are encountered unexpectedly in about 4% of

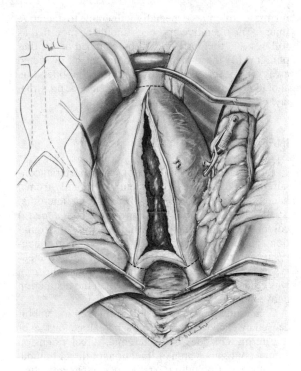

Figure 35–6. Exposure of an infrarenal abdominal aortic aneurysm. Arterial clamps are placed at the neck of the aneurysm below the left renal vein and on the common iliac arteries.

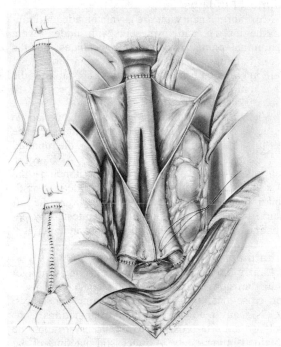

Figure 35–7. Replacement of an aortic aneurysm with a synthetic bifurcation graft. The laminated clot within the aneurysm has been removed and the outer wall is closed over the graft.

cases. Treatment of coincident gallstones is controversial; some authors recommend combined aneurysmectomy and cholecystectomy. The advent of laparoscopic cholecystectomy has led to a staged approach in most cases. The long-term results of aneurysmectomy are excellent: the graft failure rate is low, and false aneurysm formation at the anastomosis is rare. The long-term survival of these patients is determined principally by the presence or absence of disease in other vascular beds, which may lead to myocardial infarction and stroke—the principal causes of death.

SUPRARENAL AORTIC ANEURYSMS

Aneurysms of the segment of aorta between the diaphragm and the renal arteries are rare and are usually associated with similar changes in the thoracic and infrarenal aorta. More commonly, the entire thoracic and abdominal aorta becomes dilated (thoracoabdominal aneurysms). The risk of rupture of the suprarenal segment is not appreciable until the diameter exceeds 7 cm. Symptoms are rare unless rupture occurs.

Aneurysms proximal to the renal arteries cannot be palpated. They should be suspected when chest films show dilatation of the descending thoracic aorta. The size and extent of suprarenal aneurysms are best assessed using CT scan with contrast medium.

Resection and graft replacement of the upper abdominal aorta is an operation of far greater magnitude and risk than operations on the infrarenal aorta. A thoracoabdominal approach is usually necessary, and provisions must be made for reimplantation of the celiac axis and the superior mesenteric and renal arteries. At this time, the risks of operation for asymptomatic aneurysms less than 7 cm in diameter at this level are probably greater than the risk of rupture. Paraplegia, renal failure, and bowel ischemia are much more common after repair of these aneurysms than after repair of infrarenal aortic aneurysms.

RUPTURED AORTIC ANEURYSMS

With increasing size, lateral pressure within the aneurysm may eventually lead to spontaneous rupture of the aneurysmal wall. Although immediate exsanguination may ensue, there is usually an interval of several hours between the first episode of bleeding, a self-limited extravasation into the subadventitia or periaortic tissue, and later retroperitoneal rupture.

Clinical Findings

Most aortic aneurysms are asymptomatic until rupture begins. The patient presents with sudden severe abdominal pain that occasionally radiates into the back. Faintness or syncope results from blood loss. Pain may lessen or faintness may disappear after the first hemorrhage, only to reappear and progress to shock if bleeding continues.

When bleeding remains contained in the periaortic tissue, a discrete, pulsatile abdominal mass can be felt. In contrast with an intact aneurysm, the ruptured aneurysm at this stage is usually tender. As bleeding continues—usually into the retroperitoneum—the discrete mass is replaced by a poorly defined mid-abdominal fullness, often extending toward the left flank. Shock becomes profound, manifested by peripheral vasoconstriction, hypotension, and anuria.

Treatment & Prognosis

Laparotomy must be performed as soon as intravenous fluids have been started and blood has been sent for cross-matching. There is no time for x-rays, ECGs, scans, blood tests, or other examinations. Control of the aorta proximal to the aneurysm must be obtained immediately. A successful outcome of the operation is related to the patient's condition on arrival, the promptness of diagnosis, and the speed of operative control of bleeding and blood replacement. The death rate is about 60–80%, but rates below 20% have been reported. Major factors responsible for improved survival are *immediate* operation with rapid proximal aortic control, avoidance of a left thoracotomy for clamping the aorta above the diaphragm, avoidance of technical errors, and expeditious completion of the operation. Without operation, the outcome is uniformly fatal.

INFLAMMATORY ANEURYSMS

Inflammatory aneurysms are true atherosclerotic aneurysms that elicit a unique inflammatory response adjacent to the external calcified layer of the aneurysmal wall. In contrast to retroperitoneal fibrosis, the inflammation is usually confined to the anterior aorta and iliac arteries. The patient complains of abdominal pain and tenderness over the aneurysm. One-fourth of patients have some degree of ureteral obstruction. Ultrasound or CT scanning demonstrates the characteristic thick wall and confirms the diagnosis. Characteristic pathologic changes include infiltration of the aortic wall by lymphocytes, plasma cells, and occasional multinucleated giant cells and lymphoid follicles with germinal centers. The inflammatory reaction tends to be prominent around the vasa vasorum.

Inflammatory aneurysms are easily recognized at operation by the dense shiny white fibrotic reaction that envelopes the adjacent viscera, especially the duodenum, left renal vein, and inferior vena cava, making these structures especially vulnerable to operative injury. The operative approach should be modified as follows: (1) the aorta should be clamped at the diaphragm; (2) the duodenum should not be dissected away from the aneurysm; and (3) the operation should be performed within the lumen after proximal and distal control has been achieved.

INFECTED ANEURYSMS

An infected aneurysm develops after bacterial contamination of a preexisting aneurysm, usually from a hematogenous source. This differs from microbial aortitis, in which virulent bacteria (often *Salmonella*) colonize the aorta and cause false aneurysm formation and rupture. The confusing term "mycotic aneurysm" is commonly used to denote infected aneurysms in general, not just fungal infections. The term was coined by Osler at the time when the distinction between bacteria and fungi was unclear.

Contamination may result from septic emboli caused by bacterial endocarditis, hematogenous seeding during episodes of bacteremia, direct extension from a contiguous area of infection, or direct trauma. Streptococci (including *Streptococcus pneumoniae*), *Haemophilus, Staphylococcus, Escherichia coli,* other gram-negative organisms, and fungi have all been implicated. The chances of rupture are far greater with gram-negative than gram-positive infections. The survival rate of patients with gram-positive infections is about 70%—in contrast to only 25% in patients with gram-negative organisms.

Mycotic organisms may involve practically every major artery, but aortic involvement is most common. The typical case presents with a rapidly enlarging, tender pulsatile mass that may feel warm. Fever is invariably present, and half of patients have positive blood cultures. Angiography of these patients may show a saccular false aneurysm in which the infection has caused excessive wall necrosis that is likely to rupture.

Treatment consists of excision and extra-anatomic bypass grafting. A prolonged course of antibiotics should be given.

Allardice JT et al: High prevalence of abdominal aortic aneurysm in men with peripheral vascular disease: Screening by ultrasonography. Br J Surg 1988;75:240.

Blair RH, Resnik MD, Polga JP: CT appearance of mycotic abdominal aortic aneurysms. J Comput Assist Tomogr 1989;13:101.

Brophy CM et al: Age of onset, pattern of distribution, and histology of aneurysm development in a genetically predisposed mouse model. J Vasc Surg 1988;8:5.

Cambria RP et al: Transperitoneal versus retroperitoneal approach for aortic reconstruction: A randomized prospective study. J Vasc Surg 1990;11:314.

Crawford ES, Beckett WC, Green MS: Juxtarenal infrarenal

abdominal aortic aneurysm: Special diagnostic and therapeutic considerations. Ann Surg 1986;203:661.

Dobrin PB: Elastin, collagen, and some mechanical aspects of arterial aneurysms. J Vasc Surg 1989;9:396.

Golden MA et al: Evolving experience with thoracoabdominal aortic aneurysm repair at a single institution. J Vasc Surg 1991;13:792.

Innocenti C, Defringne JO, Limet R: Aortic surgery in the presence of cholelithiasis: Should simultaneous cholecystectomy be performed? J Chir (Paris) 1989;127L:159.

Johansen K et al: Ruptured abdominal aortic aneurysm: The Harborview experience. J Vasc Surg 1991;13:240.

Johnston KW: Multicenter prospective study of nonruptured abdominal aortic aneurysm: Part II. Variables predicting morbidity and mortality. J Vasc Surg 1989; 9:437.

Krupski WC et al: Utility of computed tomography for surveillance of small abdominal aneurysms. Arch Surg 1990;125:1345.

Nevitt MP et al: Prognosis of abdominal aortic aneurysms: A population-based study. N Engl J Med 1989;321:1009.

Nora JD et al: Concomitant abdominal aortic aneurysm and colorectal carcinoma: Priority of resection. J Vasc Surg 1989;9:630.

Ouriel K et al: An evaluation of new methods of expressing aortic aneurysm size: Relationship to rupture. J Vasc Surg 1992;15:12.

Powell J, Greenhalgh RM: Cellular, enzymatic, and genetic factors in the pathogenesis of abdominal aortic aneurysms. J Vasc Surg 1989;9:297.

Richardson JW, Greenfield LJ: Natural history and management of iliac aneurysms. J Vasc Surg 1988;8:165.

Roger VL et al: Influence of coronary artery disease on morbidity and mortality after abdominal aortic aneurysmectomy: A population-based study. J Am Coll Cardiol 1989;14:1245.

Shah DM et al: Treatment of abdominal aortic aneurysm by exclusion and bypass: An analysis of outcome. J Vasc Surg 1991;13:15.

Sterpetti AV et al: Inflammatory aneurysms of the abdominal aorta: Incidence, pathologic, and etiologic considerations. J Vasc Surg 1989;9:643.

Tilson MD: Status of research on abdominal aortic aneurysm disease. J Vasc Surg 1989;9:367.

Trairatvorakul P, Sriphojanart S, Sathapatayavongs B. Abdominal aortic aneurysms infected with Salmonella: Problems of treatment. J Vasc Surg 1990;12:16.

Webster MW et al: Ultrasound screening of first-degree relatives of patients with an abdominal aortic aneurysm. J Vasc Surg 1991;13:9.

FEMORAL & POPLITEAL ANEURYSMS

The popliteal artery is the site of peripheral arterial aneurysms in 70% of cases. The next most common site is the femoral artery, but this is unusual. Thrombosis, peripheral embolization, and claudication are the presenting manifestations. Unlike aortic aneurysms, rupture is rare. Occlusion results from fragmentation of the mural thrombus lining the aneurysmal sac, an event that may be due partly to the mobility of the adjacent hip or knee. Thrombus may occlude the lumen of the aneurysm or embolize downstream into smaller arteries in the leg or foot.

Clinical Findings

A. Symptoms and Signs: Until progressive stenosis or thrombosis occurs, symptoms are usually minimal or absent. The patient is aware of a throbbing mass when the aneurysm is in the groin, but popliteal aneurysms are usually undetected by the patient. In most patients, the first symptom is produced by the ischemia of acute arterial occlusion. The pathologic findings range from rapidly developing gangrene to only moderate ischemia that slowly lessens as collateral circulation develops. Symptoms from recurrent embolization to the leg are often transient; sudden ischemia may appear in a toe or part of the foot, followed by slow resolution, and the true diagnosis may be elusive. Recurrent ischemic episodes due to occlusion of small arteries in the leg in patients over age 50 are almost always embolic in origin. Rarely, popliteal aneurysms will produce symptoms by compressing the popliteal vein or tibial nerve.

Palpation of local arterial enlargement is generally adequate for diagnosis. Since popliteal aneurysms are bilateral in 50% of cases, the diagnosis of thrombosis of a popliteal aneurysm is often aided by the palpation of a pulsatile aneurysm in the contralateral popliteal space. One-third of patients with bilateral popliteal aneurysms have abdominal aortic aneurysms.

B. Imaging Studies: Arteriography may not demonstrate the aneurysm accurately, because mural thrombus reduces the apparent diameter of the lumen. Nevertheless, arteriography is advised—especially when operation is considered—to define the status of the arteries distal to the aneurysm.

Gray scale ultrasound is the best investigation to confirm the diagnosis of peripheral aneurysm, to measure its size and configuration, and to demonstrate mural thrombus.

Treatment

Immediate operation is indicated when acute thrombosis has caused pregangrenous ischemia. Early operation is indicated for recurrent peripheral embolization. The evidence is unclear regarding the advisability of routine operation in the absence of symptoms, but operation is usually recommended if the external diameter of the aneurysm exceeds three times the normal arterial diameter at that site or if a large amount of thrombus is present within the aneurysm.

The standard surgical treatment for both femoral and popliteal aneurysms has been resection with graft replacement. Recently, however, popliteal aneurysms have been satisfactorily managed by exclusion and bypass graft with saphenous vein. If exclusion rather than resection is performed, the geniculate "feeder" arteries within the aneurysm must be ligated or progressive enlargement can still occur.

Prognosis

The long-term patency of bypass grafts for femoral and popliteal aneurysms depends on the adequacy of the outflow tract. Late graft occlusion is less common than in similar operations for occlusive disease.

Dawson I et al: Popliteal artery aneurysms: Long-term follow-up of aneurysmal disease and results of surgical treatment. J Vasc Surg 1991;13:398.

Lilly MR et al: The effect of distal arterial anatomy on the success of popliteal aneurysm repair. J Vasc Surg 1988;7:653.

Shortell CK et al: Popliteal artery aneurysms: A 25 year experience. J Vasc Surg 1991;14:283.

Walsh JJ et al: Vein compression by arterial aneurysms. J Vasc Surg 1988;8:465.

EXTRACRANIAL CAROTID ARTERY ANEURYSMS

Aneurysms of the extracranial carotid arteries are rare but may occur at any point along the course of the vessels. True aneurysms of the carotid are usually the result of atherosclerosis but occasionally may be caused by cystic medial necrosis, Marfan's syndrome, or fibromuscular dysplasia. False aneurysms may occur rarely after carotid endarterectomy or as a result of trauma or infection. Pharyngeal abscess was a frequent cause of false aneurysms of the carotid artery in the preantibiotic era.

Clinical Findings

A. Symptoms and Signs: Most patients present with a pulsatile neck mass. A coiled or redundant carotid or subclavian artery is the commonest cause of this type of mass and must be differentiated from aneurysm. On occasion, a carotid aneurysm protrudes into the oropharynx, where it produces symptoms of dysphagia. Pain from the aneurysm may radiate to the angle of the jaw. About 30% of patients will have had a transient neurologic event before presentation. Rupture, which is most common with false aneurysms, may occur into the oropharynx, ear canal, or soft tissues of the neck.

B. Imaging Studies: Arteriography is necessary to plan the operation. Two types of atherosclerotic aneurysms are seen: fusiform and saccular. False aneurysms assume bizarre shapes, depending on location and containment by neck tissues.

Duplex ultrasound can differentiate redundant and coiled arteries from aneurysms and should be used as the initial test in patients who present electively. The spectral analysis component of duplex Doppler is useful in demonstrating coexistent occlusive disease. In the assessment of false aneurysms, it is useful to delineate the extent of the lesion, which may not be apparent from arteriography.

Treatment

Most accessible true aneurysms should be resected and replaced with a graft of autogenous tissue. All false aneurysms should be repaired. Some extensive aneurysms require carotid ligation, which is safe if carotid back pressure is greater than 65 mm Hg. An OPG-GEE test should be performed preoperatively for such patients; if the value is low, a superficial temporal-to-middle cerebral bypass may be required at the time of internal carotid ligation.

Gewertz DL, Krupski WC: Aneurysms of the carotid and vertebral arteries. In: *Current Surgical Therapy,* 4th ed. Cameron J (editor). Mosby Year Book, 1992.

Jebara VA et al: Mycotic aneurysms of the carotid arteries—case report and review of the literature. J Vasc Surg 1991;14:215.

Carotid Body Tumors

The normal carotid body is a 3- to 6-cm nest of chemoreceptor cells of neuroectodermal origin located on the posterior medial side of the carotid bifurcation. It responds to a decrease in oxygen tension, an increase in blood acidity, and an increase in CO_2 tension or an increase in blood temperature by causing an increase in blood pressure, cardiac rate, and the depth and rate of respiration. Thus, the carotid body serves to correct hypoxia and its effects.

Tumors of the carotid body have been called cervical chemodectomas, paragangliomas, glomus tumors, and nonchromaffin paragangliomas. Histologically, the tumors resemble the normal carotid body. While the tumor is capable of metastatic behavior, this only occurs in about ten% of cases. Extension into local structures is the most common complication.

Almost all cases present as slow enlargement of an asymptomatic cervical mass. Rarely, the tumor causes hypertension by secreting catecholamines. A history of slow enlargement is frequently elicited. There is no predilection for either sex. Bilaterality is common when the tumor is familial. The incidence of carotid body tumors is increased in oxygen-deprived individuals (eg, cyanotic heart disease; chronic hypoxia of high altitude).

A solitary midlateral pulsatile neck mass that is firm and rubbery should always suggest carotid body tumor. Because it is attached to the underlying artery, the mass is more mobile in the horizontal than the vertical plane. Bruits are present over the mass in about half of cases. Rarely, cranial nerve dysfunction occurs from tumor extension.

Angiography shows a characteristic tumor blush at the carotid bifurcation, with wide separation of the internal and external carotid arteries (Figure 35–8). Noninvasive studies are of little value. Percutaneous needle biopsy or incisional biopsy is inaccurate and dangerous because of the risk of serious hemorrhage.

Complete excision—the preferred treatment—occasionally requires arterial reconstruction when the

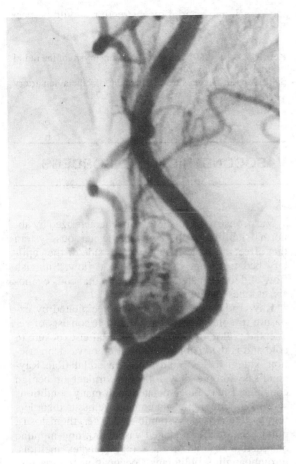

Figure 35–8. Carotid body tumor.

lesion is large and complex. Radiation therapy and chemotherapy have no value. Preoperative angiographic embolization of large tumors decreases vascularity and improves the safety of operative resection. The incidence of cranial nerve injury from operative removal of carotid body tumors is about 40% and is higher with larger masses and prior attempts at resection.

Hallett JW et al: Trends in neurovascular complications of surgical management for carotid body and cervical paragangliomas: A fifty-year experience with 153 tumors. J Vasc Surg 1988;7:284.

Smith RF, Shetty PC, Reddy DJ: Surgical treatment of carotid paraganglioma presenting unusual technical difficulties. J Vasc Surg 1988;7:631.

VISCERAL ARTERY ANEURYSMS

Splenic Artery Aneurysms

Splenic artery aneurysms are second in frequency to aneurysms of the aortoiliac system among intra-abdominal aneurysms. Aneurysms of the splenic artery account for more than 60% of splanchnic artery aneurysms. Women are affected four times more commonly than men and often during childbearing years. Arterial fibrodysplasia and portal hypertension also predispose to formation of splenic artery aneurysms. Rupture, the major complication, has been reported in 25% of cases but rarely occurs with lesions smaller than 2–3 cm in diameter. Rupture during pregnancy tends to occur in the third trimester and is associated with 75% maternal death rate and 90% fetal death rate. Diagnosis is most often made from plain x-ray films of the abdomen, showing concentric calcification in the upper left quadrant.

Operation is indicated for patients with symptomatic aneurysms, pregnant women with splenic artery aneurysms, and patients who are good operative risks and whose aneurysm is greater than 3 cm in diameter.

Hepatic Artery Aneurysms

Hepatic artery aneurysms account for 20% of splanchnic artery aneurysms. They usually present with rupture into the peritoneal cavity, biliary tree, or a nearby viscus. Rupture into the biliary tree producing hemobilia is as frequent as intraperitoneal rupture. The symptomatic triad of intermittent abdominal pain, gastrointestinal bleeding, and jaundice strongly suggests the diagnosis and is present in about one-third of patients. Surgery is usually required for control of bleeding. If the common hepatic artery is involved, the artery may be safely ligated. Aneurysms in other portions of the artery usually require vascular reconstruction.

Superior Mesenteric Artery Aneurysms

Sixty percent of superior mesenteric artery aneurysms are mycotic, and most of the rest are atherosclerotic. The aneurysm may involve the origin or branches of the artery. The presenting findings include nonspecific abdominal pain and a mobile pulsatile abdominal mass. Rupture is one cause of "abdominal apoplexy." Radiologic evaluation, except for arteriography, is unrewarding, since the lesion is rarely calcified.

Operative therapy includes ligation, endoaneurysmorrhaphy, or replacement with a segment of autogenous vessel. For branch aneurysms, bowel resection is often the best choice.

RENAL ARTERY ANEURYSMS

This uncommon aneurysm occurs in less than 0.1% of the population and is strongly associated with hypertension. The aneurysm is usually saccular and located at a primary or secondary bifurcation of the renal arteries. Women are affected slightly more frequently than men.

Most aneurysms are asymptomatic and are discovered on plain abdominal films or during investigation of hypertension. Renovascular hypertension, which occurs in 30% of patients, may be due to turbulent flow within an aneurysm, associated arterial stenosis, dissection, arteriovenous fistula formation, thromboembolism, or compression of adjacent arterial branches. Spontaneous rupture of renal artery aneurysms is rare except during pregnancy, and although a kidney may be lost, death is uncommon. Emboli from the aneurysm to the distal renal vessels occur rarely.

Most small renal artery aneurysms should be managed nonoperatively. Blood pressure should be controlled, and CT scans or digital subtraction angiography should be performed every 2 years. Operation is indicated in women of childbearing age, patients with associated renal artery disease, and patients with large aneurysms. Although most renal artery aneurysms can be repaired in situ, ex vivo repair is occasionally required.

Gelabert HA, Busuttil RW: Celiac, hepatic, and splenic aneurysms. In: *Current Therapy in Vascular Surgery,* 2nd ed. Ernst CB, Stanley JC (editors). BC Decker, 1991.
Martin RS III et al: Renal artery aneurysm: Selective treatment for hypertension and prevention of rupture. J Vasc Surg 1989;9:26.
Melliere D et al: Visceral artery aneurysm: When to operate. J Mal Vasc 1989;14:206.
Salo JA et al: Aneurysms of the hepatic arteries. Am Surg 1989;55:705.
Stanley JC et al: Clinical importance and management of splanchnic artery aneurysms. J Vasc Surg 1986;3:837.

UPPER EXTREMITY ANEURYSMS

Subclavian Artery Aneurysms

Subclavian artery aneurysms are rare; most supraclavicular pulsatile masses represent tortuous vessels. Pseudoaneurysms due to injections by drug addicts are being reported with increasing frequency.

A true subclavian artery aneurysm is usually due to exaggerated poststenotic dilatation in a patient with cervical rib syndrome or thoracic outlet syndrome. The most common manifestations result from emboli to the fingers. Treatment consists of resection of the first rib or a cervical rib (if present) and division of the scalenus anterior muscle. The aneurysm should be resected and replaced by an autogenous or prosthetic graft. Cervical sympathectomy should be performed for distal ischemia.

Radial Artery False Aneurysms

The incidence of radial artery false aneurysms has increased as a result of increasing use of radial artery catheters. Occasionally, the aneurysm is infected. If the Allen test is normal, treatment consists of excision. If the ulnar collaterals are insufficient to preserve viability of the hand, excision, mobilization of the vessel, and arterial reconstruction should be performed.

Kerr DC, Duffey TP: Traumatic false aneurysm of the radial artery. J Trauma 1988;28:1603.
Salo JA et al: Diagnosis and treatment of subclavian artery aneurysms. Eur J Vasc Surg 1990;4:271.

VASOCONSTRICTIVE DISORDERS

Vasoconstrictive disorders are characterized by abnormal lability of the sympathetic nervous system that affects the arterial and venous side of the capillary bed to reduce cutaneous blood flow. Sluggish flow of deoxygenated blood causes cutaneous cyanosis, coldness, numbness, and pain.

Raynaud's syndrome can be precipitated by exposure to cold or emotional stress. It consists of sequential pallor, cyanosis, and rubor after exposure to cold and is the visible manifestation of vasoconstriction, sluggish flow, and reflex vasodilatation. Raynaud's syndrome may follow a virulent or benign course and may be associated with many conditions such as immunologic and connective tissue disorders (eg, scleroderma, systemic lupus erythematosus, polymyositis, drug-induced vasculitis); non-immune obstructive arterial disease (eg, diabetes mellitus, thromboangiitis obliterans); occupation trauma (eg, vibration injury, cold injury); and other disorders (eg, cold agglutinins, chronic renal failure, neoplasia).

The classic differentiation of Raynaud's syndrome into a benign "disease" and a virulent "phenomenon" is confusing. It is more appropriate to distinguish an occlusive lesion from the purely vasoconstrictive variety. If the underlying cause is an unrelenting disorder (eg, collagen vascular disease), cervical sympathectomy has no lasting effect. If the cause is transient or manageable (eg, emboli), sympathectomy may be of value. All patients with Raynaud's syndrome should avoid cold exposure, tobacco, oral contraceptives, beta-adrenergic blocking agents, and ergotamine preparations. Intra-arterial injections of reserpine provide relief of symptoms for a few weeks. Long-term therapy with guanethidine and prazosin has occasionally been effective. Calcium channel blockers and transdermal prostaglandins may also help. A double-blind placebo-controlled study showed that ketanserin lessened symptoms of Raynaud's syndrome.

Acrocyanosis is a common chronic, benign vasoconstrictive disorder related to Raynaud's syndrome that is largely restricted to young females. It is characterized by persistent cyanosis of the hands and feet. Numbness and pain accompany its more severe form.

The changes disappear with exposure to a warm environment. Examination in a cool room shows diffuse symmetric cyanosis, coldness, and occasionally hyperhidrosis of hands and feet. Cyanosis of the skin of the calf, thigh, or forearm usually displays a reticulated pattern and has been called **livedo reticularis** and **cutis marmorata.** The peripheral pulses may diminish in the cold but return to normal with rewarming. The Allen test may show a normal response, but in patients with particularly intense vasoconstriction, color return will be slow but even (as compared to the uneven return in patients with scleroderma and thromboangiitis obliterans).

SCLERODERMA

Scleroderma is a connective tissue disease characterized pathologically by fibrosis due to increase and swelling of collagenous tissue, fragmentation and swelling of the elastic fibers in the cutis, and arterial intimal thickening. It may present as a multisystem disease with changes in the lung, kidney, gastrointestinal tract, muscle, and central nervous system. It occurs more frequently in women, and its first manifestations usually appear between ages 25 and 50.

Its most common form involves first the skin and vasculature of the fingers, hands, and forearms. The skin becomes thickened and taut. Flexion of the fingers is limited by the tightness of the overlying skin. The muscles in the forearm develop woody induration.

Symptoms in the early stages consist of progressive coldness and occasional numbness of the fingers. Intermittent episodic blanching of one or more fingers is frequent. With increasing ischemia, one or more of the terminal phalanges become painful and tender. Atrophy and ulceration of the fingertips, with exquisite tenderness, follow. At this stage, cutaneous fibrosis of the hands and fingers is usually far advanced. Gangrene of the ends of the fingers is the terminal ischemic event.

Vascular examination in the early phases may show only chronic cyanosis and coldness of the hands and fingers. Coincident with the development of skin changes, pallor and atrophy of the fingertips appear. Attempts at finger flexion cause blanching of the knuckles. The Allen test shows slow return of color starting in the proximal hand and progressing in an uneven fashion into the fingers.

Treatment is palliative at best, since there is no way to halt the progression of pathologic change. Sympathectomy is rarely of value. Systemic corticosteroid therapy occasionally slows progression. Finger amputation is necessary once gangrene has developed.

Brotzu G et al: The importance of presynaptic beta receptors in Raynaud's disease. J Vasc Surg 1989;9:767.

Carter SA, Dean E, Kroeger EA: Apparent finger systolic pressures during cooling in patients with Raynaud's syndrome. Circulation 1988;77:988.

Coffman JD et al: International study of ketanserin in Raynaud's phenomenon. Am J Med 1989;87:264.

Edwards JM, Portter JM: Diagnosis of upper extremity vasospastic disease. In: *Current Therapy in Vascular Surgery,* 2nd ed. Ernst CB, Stanley JC (editors). BC Decker, 1991.

Nilsson H et al: The effect of calcium entry blocker nifedipine on cold-induced digital vasospasm: A double-blind crossover study versus placebo. Acta Med Scand 1987;221:53.

CAUSALGIA

The pathophysiology of posttraumatic pain syndromes remains poorly understood. A number of terms are used to refer to the same condition, including causalgia, posttraumatic sympathetic dystrophy, reflex sympathetic dystrophy, Sudeck's atrophy, shoulder-hand syndrome, traumatic neuralgia, and Mitchell's causalgia. Causalgia occurs with equal frequency in the upper and lower extremities and in men and women. The initial injury may be a missile wound, fracture, crush injury, or laceration.

The most distinctive and dramatic feature of the syndrome is the almost unendurable pain that occurs. It is a burning pain involving the entire hand or foot. The slightest stimuli can produce sudden increase in the severity of pain (eg, a breeze from an open window, the touch of clothing, or a step on the stair).

Increased sympathetic nervous system activity characterizes this syndrome. Vasomotor changes in the foot or hand are marked, and vasoconstriction is a prominent feature. The extremity becomes cold, cyanotic, and moist.

Initial management consists of diagnostic sympathetic block with local anesthetic agents. This is successful in relieving pain in the majority of cases. If the patient has long-lasting relief after the block, blocking should be repeated, as this alone will result in permanent cure in about a third of patients. Surgical sympathectomy is indicated for those patients who have short-lived pain relief after sympathetic blockade.

Olcott C IV et al: Reflex sympathetic dystrophy: The surgeon's role in management. J Vasc Surg 1991;14:488.

Scintigraphic patterns of the reflex sympathetic dystrophy syndrome of the lower extremities. Clin Nucl Med 1989;14:657.

THORACIC OUTLET SYNDROME

The term thoracic outlet syndrome refers to the variety of disorders caused by abnormal compression of arterial, venous, or neural structures in the base of the neck. Numerous mechanisms for compression have been described, including cervical rib, anomalous ligaments, hypertrophy of the scalenus anticus muscle, and positional changes that alter the normal relation of the first rib to the structures which pass over it. Patients often describe a history of cervical trauma.

Symptoms rarely develop until adulthood. For this reason, it has been assumed that an alteration of normal structural relationships which occurs with advancing years is the primary factor. Even anomalous cervical ribs seem well tolerated during childhood and adolescence.

Inclusion of these syndromes in discussions of vascular disease originates from a former view that many of the symptoms were the result of intermittent compression of the subclavian or axillary arteries. This assumption was reinforced by the frequent finding that certain postural manipulations could produce depression of the radial pulse. The present view holds that whereas transient circulatory changes may indeed occur, the primary cause of symptoms in most patients is intermittent compression of one or more trunks of the brachial plexus. Thus, neurologic symptoms predominate over those of ischemia or venous compression.

Clinical Findings

A. Symptoms and Signs: Symptoms consist of pain, paresthesias, or numbness in the distribution of one or more trunks of the brachial plexus (usually in the ulnar distribution). Most patients associate their symptoms with certain positions of the shoulder girdle. These may occur from prolonged hyperabduction, as in house painters, hairdressers, and truck drivers. Others may relate their symptoms to the downward traction of the shoulder girdle produced by carrying heavy objects. Numbness of the hands often wakes the patient from sleep. On physical examination, motor deficits are rare and usually indicate severe compression of long duration. Muscular atrophy may be present in the hand. The radial pulse can be weakened by abduction of the arm with the head rotated to the opposite side (**Adson's test**), though pulse reduction by this maneuver often occurs in completely asymptomatic persons. Light percussion over the brachial plexus in the supraclavicular fossa produces peripheral sensations (**Tinel's test**) and reproduces the symptoms in patients with chronic neurologic impingement. A bruit is commonly heard over the subclavian artery above the center of the clavicle with abduction of the arm. Occlusion of the subclavian vein with upper extremity edema is a frequent complication of thoracic outlet syndrome.

B. Diagnosis: Thoracic outlet compression must be differentiated from other disorders that mimic this condition (eg, carpal tunnel syndrome and cervical disk disease). While cervical x-rays and peripheral nerve conduction studies do not confirm the diagnosis of thoracic outlet syndrome, they are valuable to elucidate other possibilities. Arteriograms may demonstrate subclavian or axillary artery stenosis when the arm is in abduction. This finding can occur in normal individuals and is not diagnostic, but poststenotic dilation of the artery is distinctly abnormal and indicates a definite lesion.

Treatment

Most patients benefit from postural correction and a physical therapy program directed toward restoring the normal relation and strength of the structures in the shoulder girdle. Surgical techniques for decompression of the thoracic outlet are reserved for patients who have not responded after 3–6 months of conservative treatment. Some surgeons prefer transaxillary first rib section, while others prefer a supraclavicular approach. With either operation, the anterior scalene muscle should be excised.

Cormier JM et al: Arterial complications of the thoracic outlet syndrome: Fifty-five operative cases. J Vasc Surg 1989;9:778.

Green RM, McNamara J, Ouriel K: Long-term follow-up after thoracic outlet decompression: An analysis of factors determining outcome. J Vasc Surg 1991;14:739.

Reilly LM, Stoney RJ: Supraclavicular approach for thoracic outlet decompression. J Vasc Surg 1988;8:329.

ARTERIOVENOUS FISTULAS

Arteriovenous fistulas may be congenital or acquired. Abnormal communications between arteries and veins occur in many diseases and may affect vessels of all sizes. Their effects depend upon their size. In congenital fistulas, the systemic effect is often not great, because the degree of communication, though diffuse, is small. Larger acquired fistulas enlarge rapidly. Cardiac dilatation and failure result when shunting is excessive, prolonged, or untreated.

Congenital fistulas are often noted in infancy or childhood. When a limb is involved, muscle mass or bone length may be increased. Arteriovenous malformations frequently involve the brain, visceral organs, or lungs. Gastrointestinal hemorrhage may occur.

Pulmonary lesions cause polycythemia, clubbing, and cyanosis.

Acquired fistulas result from injuries that produce artificial connections between adjacent arteries and veins and may be the result of trauma or disease. Penetrating injuries are the most common cause, but fistulas are sometimes seen after blunt trauma. Iatrogenic arteriovenous fistulas after arteriography are becoming increasingly common. Connective tissue disorders (eg, Ehlers-Danlos syndrome), erosion of an atherosclerotic or mycotic arterial aneurysm into adjacent veins, communication with an arterial prosthetic graft, and neoplastic invasion are other causes. A rare but dramatic cause of atraumatic arteriovenous fistula is combined injury to the aorta and inferior vena cava or to the iliac arteries and veins during surgical excision of a herniated nucleus pulposus by the dorsal approach.

Clinical Findings

A. Symptoms and Signs: The time of onset and the presence or absence of associated disease should be determined. A typical continuous machinery murmur can be heard over most fistulas and is often associated with a palpable thrill and locally increased skin temperature. Proximally, the arteries and veins dilate and the pulse distal to the lesion diminishes. There may be signs of venous insufficiency and coolness distal to the communication on the involved extremity. Tachycardia occurs in some patients as a feature of increased cardiac output. When the fistula is occluded by compression, the pulse rate slows **(Branham's sign).**

B. Imaging Studies: MRI may assume an important role in the evaluation and follow-up of peripheral arteriovenous malformations. Precise delineation of arteriovenous fistulas can only be done with appropriate arteriograms. Selective catheter injection techniques have permitted accurate radiologic diagnosis.

Treatment

Not all arteriovenous connections require treatment. Small peripheral fistulas may be observed and frequently will never cause difficulties. Some are surgically inaccessible.

The indications for intervention include hemorrhage, expanding false aneurysm, severe venous or arterial insufficiency, cosmetic deformity, and heart failure.

Most fistulas are now managed by embolization under radiographic control. The embolic material used includes blood clot, glass beads, Gelfoam, and muscle. A number of centers have reported good results with arteriovenous malformations in various parts of the body. Arteriovenous malformations of the head and neck and of the pelvis appear particularly well suited for this form of therapy.

Surgical options include quadruple ligation of all four feeding limbs, amputation of the extremity, en bloc resection of the fistula, and repair of the fistula by reconstruction of the involved arteries and veins. Oversewing the defects in the artery and vein is curative for postarteriography fistulas.

Congenital arteriovenous fistulas are amenable to surgical management only when en bloc resection of all tissue involved in the fistula can be accomplished. When the fistulous connections involve substantial portions of an extremity, local arterial ligation is invariably followed by recurrence, and only temporary palliation can be expected. Amputation may be a last resort to control unmanageable peripheral fistulas.

Prognosis

The results of therapy vary according to the extent, location, and type of fistula. In general, traumatic fistulas have the most favorable prognosis. Congenital fistulas are more difficult to eradicate, because of the numerous arteriovenous connections usually present. These fistulas have a high propensity for recurrence, and most surgeons are reluctant to operate unless the surgical indications are urgent.

Bryant RS, Russell EJ, Curtin JW: Combined treatment of arteriovenous malformations by transarterial microembolization and surgery. Am Surg 1988;54:637.

Lie JT: Pathology of angiodysplasia in Klippel-Trenaunay syndrome. Pathol Res Pract 1988;183:747.

Pearce WH et al: Nuclear magnetic resonance imaging: Its diagnostic value in patients with congenital vascular malformations of the limbs. J Vasc Surg 1988;8:64.

Schonbach B, Schlosser V: Pathogenesis and changes in the aetiology of arterio-venous fistulae. Eur J Vasc Surg 1990;4:233.

Stain S et al: Selective management of nonocclusive arterial injuries. Arch Surg 1989;124:1136.

Widlus DM et al: Congenital arteriovenous malformations: Tailored embolotherapy. Radiology 1988;169:511.

CEREBROVASCULAR DISEASE

Essentials of Diagnosis

- Episodic motor and visual dysfunction; stroke; ataxia and sensory dysfunction.
- Cervical arterial bruits or pulse deficits, or blood pressure differences in the arms.
- Arteriograms showing arterial stenosis, occlusion, or ulceration.

General Considerations

Symptoms of cerebrovascular disease are most often the result of emboli and less often the result of hypoperfusion. About 80% of patients with occlusive cerebrovascular disease have an atherosclerotic lesion in a surgically accessible artery in the neck or mediastinum (Figs 35–9, 35–10, and 35–11) that is the cause of symptoms. Less commonly, symptoms may be due to arterial emboli originating in the heart, fibromuscular disease, arterial dissection, or Takayasu's (giant cell) arteritis.

Cerebral infarction occurs when the blood supply is decreased below a critical level; this causes cellular death within minutes. This event is manifested by a fixed or advancing neurologic deficit. It can result from local arterial thrombosis, cerebral embolization, hemorrhage, or sudden decrease in cardiac output.

Embolization is the most common mechanism of cerebral infarction from carotid lesions. The atherosclerotic plaque ulcerates, and atheromatous debris or blood clot will dislodge to produce infarction when it reaches the brain. Most lesions of this sort occur at the origin of the internal carotid, but the innominate artery and ascending aorta are implicated occasionally.

Characteristically, lesions of atherosclerosis occur along the outer wall of the carotid bulb. Preferential location of advanced disease has been demonstrated in postmortem anatomic specimens, on angiograms of patients with severe carotid stenosis, and in specimens removed during carotid endarterectomy. Low wall shear stress, flow separation, and loss of unidi-

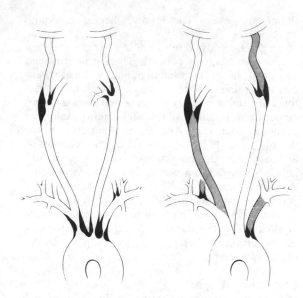

Figure 35–10. Diagram showing common sites of stenosis and occlusion of the extracranial cerebral vasculature.

rectional flow allow for greater interaction of atherogenic particles and vessel walls at this area of the artery.

Neurologic dysfunction without infarction may be produced in two ways: (1) cerebral embolization by small (microembolic) fragments that only temporarily impede arterial flow; and (2) transient reduction in cerebral perfusion short of that required to give irreversible ischemia.

Since most microemboli originate from an ulcerative lesion in the internal carotid artery, neurologic dysfunction is confined to the carotid territory and appears as "short-lived" paresis or numbness of the contralateral arm or leg. This is called a **transient ischemic attack (TIA).** The onset is swift, and most TIAs are brief (minutes). By convention, 24 hours is the arbitrary limit of a TIA. A microembolus to the ophthalmic artery, the first branch of the internal carotid artery, produces a temporary monocular loss of vision called **amaurosis fugax.** Emboli may be visible as small bright flecks (**Hollenhorst plaques**) lodged in arterial bifurcations in the retina. Without treatment, one-third of patients with TIAs will eventually develop permanent neurologic impairment either from dislodgment of a macroembolus or thrombotic occlusion of the internal carotid artery, while 20% of patients with amaurosis fugax will suffer strokes.

Clinical Findings

Patients with cerebrovascular disease may present initially to an internist, family practitioner, neurologist, neurosurgeon, ophthalmologist, or vascular surgeon. Satisfactory management of these patients de-

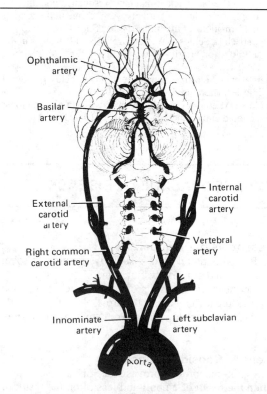

Figure 35–9. Diagram of arterial blood supply to the eyes and brain.

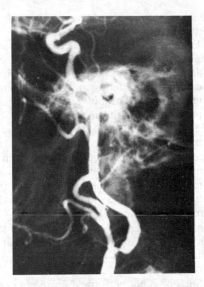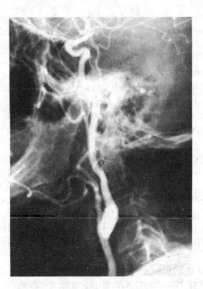

Figure 35–11. **Left:** Preoperative carotid arteriogram showing stenosis of the proximal internal carotid artery. **Right:** Postoperative carotid arteriogram showing restoration of normal luminal size following endarterectomy.

pends on recognition of disease and appropriate referral for further treatment.

A. Symptoms: Patients with cerebrovascular disease can be grouped into five categories based on symptoms at presentation.

1. Asymptomatic disease–An audible bruit heard in the neck may be the only manifestation of cerebrovascular disease. Some evidence supports operative intervention if noninvasive tests are positive and the lesion is highly stenotic. In a controlled randomized prospective series, medically managed patients with severe carotid stenosis suffered twice the number of adverse neurologic events compared with those treated by prophylactic surgery.

2. Transient neurologic or visual episodes–
Most events that occur in the carotid area are caused by emboli from the carotid bifurcation. Symptoms depend upon the site where the embolus has lodged in the brain or eye; size of the embolus, which determines the degree of arterial obstruction; composition of the embolus, which determines the rate of dissolution; and the abundance of collaterals to the target area. Hypoperfusion may also cause transient neurologic and visual attacks.

3. Acute unstable neurologic deficit–Patients in this category have crescendo transient ischemic attacks, stroke in evolution, or waxing and waning neurologic deficits. These patients must be treated urgently, as symptoms will progress to completed stroke.

4. Completed stroke–Intervention is indicated for patients with completed stroke who recover after the initial deficit, because they are at high risk for another stroke and further loss of neural function.

5. Vertebrobasilar disease–Emboli or hypoperfusion of the vertebral and basilar arteries causes drop attacks, clumsiness, and a variety of sensory phenomena. Frequently, the symptoms are bilateral. Vertigo, diplopia, dysphagia, or dysequilibrium occurring *individually* is rarely due to vertebrobasilar disease, but when these symptoms occur in combination the diagnosis becomes more likely.

B. Signs: Auscultation of the carotid and subclavian arteries usually suggests the diagnosis of major vessel stenosis and may delineate the sites of hemodynamically significant disease. Pulse deficits are unusual in the neck but common in the arms. The following lesions may exist without clinical signs: (1) occlusion of the internal carotid artery, (2) high-grade (> 90%) stenosis, (3) occlusion and stenosis of the vertebral arteries, and (4) ulceration without stenosis of any vessel.

1. Palpation–In the neck, only the pulse of the common carotid artery can be felt directly. The status of pulses of the superficial temporal artery and the axillary artery reflects the patency of the external carotid artery and the subclavian artery, respectively.

2. Bruits–A bruit localized to one artery indicates a stenosis at or proximal to the point where it can be heard. A bruit with maximal intensity high in the neck indicates stenosis at the common carotid bifurcation. Bruits caused by stenosis at the origin of the vertebral artery are most prominent over the lower portion of the trapezius muscle at the back of the neck. Bruits due to proximal subclavian stenosis are most audible above the midpoint of the clavicle and are transmitted into the axilla. Innominate artery stenosis produces a bruit heard along the full length of the right common carotid and right subclavian arteries. Cardiac murmurs are loudest over the precordium and radiate along the subclavian and proximal common carotid arteries.

3. Brachial blood pressures—A discrepancy between the blood pressures in the two arms indicates arterial stenosis or occlusion proximal to the brachial artery on the side of reduced pressure. Most commonly, the origin of the left subclavian artery is stenosed.

C. Noninvasive Tests: The most useful noninvasive test for the diagnosis of extracranial carotid artery disease is duplex ultrasound analysis, which combines high resolution B-mode imaging and range-gated Doppler spectral flow analysis. Imaging demonstrates plaque morphology, whereas Doppler analysis determines the degree of stenosis rapidly and accurately. New color-flow duplex devices have further improved the utility of this technology.

D. Imaging Studies: Cerebral arteriography is indicated in patients with symptomatic cerebrovascular disease who are candidates for surgery, although some surgeons will base decisions on noninvasive imaging studies alone. Surgery is indicated if the lesion causing symptoms can be corrected anatomically. Studies should provide extracranial and intracranial views of the carotid and vertebrobasilar systems. Intravenous digital subtraction angiography (DSA) sometimes demonstrates the cerebrovascular anatomy, but it has not supplanted intra-arterial injections as a means of showing the details of lesions. Intra-arterial DSA has permitted use of minimal amounts of dye and small catheters, so that outpatient arteriography is now performed in many centers.

Treatment

The objective of treatment for cerebrovascular disease is to prevent stroke and TIAs. This is accomplished by improving blood flow or removing a source of microemboli. The NASCET (North American Symptomatic Carotid Endarterectomy Trial) study proved that operation is superior to medical management for patients with symptoms produced by carotid stenoses of 80% or more.

Medical therapy consists of anticoagulation and antiplatelet drugs. Oral anticoagulants only variably reduce the incidence of TIAs, do not reduce the risk of completed strokes, and are associated with serious bleeding complications. There have been 4 large cooperative prospective studies of the efficacy of antiplatelet agents for preventing strokes conducted in the USA, Canada, and France. Of these, only the French study concluded that aspirin prevented strokes, although the others found that when the endpoints of stroke, TIA, and death are combined, aspirin was beneficial. A randomized trial comparing another antiplatelet agent, ticlopidine hydrochloride, with aspirin for the prevention of stroke in high-risk patients showed that ticlopidine was somewhat more

effective than aspirin, but the risks of side effects were greater.

Endarterectomy is the preferred technique for the removal of atherosclerotic lesions at the common carotid bifurcation, in the orifices of the right vertebral and subclavian arteries, and in the innominate artery (Figure 35–12). The left vertebral artery is difficult to approach through the neck, and obstruction at its orifice is more easily managed by transplanting the vertebral artery to the side of the adjacent left common carotid artery. Obstruction at the origin of the left common carotid artery would require an open thoracotomy for endarterectomy. However, thoracotomy and its risks can be avoided by dividing the common carotid low in the neck and transplanting it to the left subclavian artery. Alternatively, a prosthetic graft can be placed from the subclavian to the common carotid artery beyond the stenosis (subclavian-carotid bypass).

Surgery is not performed for recent completed cerebral infarction, because restoration of normal blood flow and arterial pressures to an infarcted area may cause hemorrhage into the infarct or increase edema.

The **subclavian steal syndrome** is characterized by the development of neurologic symptoms upon exercise of the upper extremity. Anatomically, there is a proximal subclavian stenosis or occlusion, with reversal of flow through the vertebral artery (ie, the vertebral artery serves as a collateral to supply blood to the arm). While this *anatomic* arrangement is often demonstrated on angiograms, the clinical syndrome is very rare. Symptoms of effort fatigue in the involved extremity are more common than neurologic complaints. Management consists of bypass grafting from the common carotid to the subclavian artery distal to the lesion (Figure 35–13).

There continues to be considerable debate about the correct approach to management of patients with coexistent **coronary and carotid atherosclerosis.** The priorities appear clear in two groups. The patient with symptomatic carotid stenosis whose coronary artery disease is asymptomatic should undergo carotid operation. Similarly, if the patient has an asymptomatic bruit from noncritical carotid stenosis and symptomatic heart disease, the coronary arteries should take precedence. It is the group of patients with symptoms in both vascular distributions for whom the answer is still not clear. Satisfactory results have been achieved with combined carotid and coronary procedures in some centers. There is increasing evidence that the combined procedure is associated with an increased death rate and increased cerebral and cardiac complications over staged procedures, and it is recommended that closely spaced staged procedures be performed whenever possible.

Other Causes of Cerebrovascular Symptoms

Primary disease of the extracranial arteries other than atherosclerosis is rare.

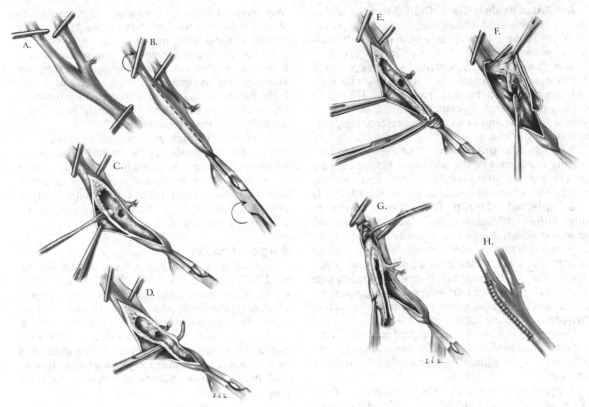

Figure 35–12. Technique of carotid endarterectomy. The common, internal, and external carotid arteries are occluded *(A),* and a longitudinal arteriotomy is created *(B).* Plaque is removed *(C–F)* with careful attention to achieve a smooth end point *(G).* The arteriotomy is closed, using continuous suture technique *(H).*

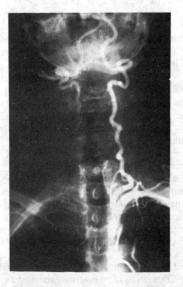
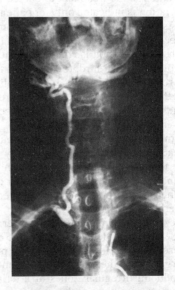

Figure 35–13. *Left:* Arteriogram showing selective injection of the left subclavian artery. There is antegrade flow in the ipsilateral vertebral artery and retrograde flow in the contralateral vertebral artery. *Right:* A later film in this sequence shows filling of the right subclavian artery by retrograde flow in the right vertebral artery. There is proximal occlusion of the right subclavian artery causing the subclavian steal syndrome.

A. Takayasu's (Giant Cell) Arteritis: Takayasu's arteritis is an obliterative arteriopathy principally involving the aortic arch vessels that often affects young women. Until recently, operative treatment of nonspecific arteritis was disappointing, but there has been a resurgence of optimism for various arterial reconstruction procedures. High-dose corticosteroids and cyclophosphamide have been shown to arrest and in some cases reverse the progress of the disease.

B. Dissecting Aneurysms of the Aorta: Dissecting aneurysms of the aorta may extend into the arch branches, producing obstruction and cerebral symptoms. These are discussed in Chapter 19, Part I.

C. Internal Carotid Dissection: Dissection originating in the internal carotid artery and localized to its extracranial segment occurs as an acute event that may narrow or obliterate the internal carotid lumen. The primary lesion is an intimal tear at the distal end of the carotid bulb. It may follow contusion of the neck or, more commonly, severe hypertension. Dissection may also develop spontaneously, most frequently in young adults.

Cerebral symptoms are the result of ischemia in the ipsilateral hemisphere. Localized cervical tenderness adjacent to the angle of the mandible is a frequent finding.

Arteriography shows a characteristic pattern of tapered narrowing at or just beyond the distal portion of the carotid bulb. The lumen beyond this point may be obliterated or may persist as a barely visible narrow shadow. This gives rise to a faint "string" of contrast visible above the top of the cap. If the lumen persists, it resumes a normal caliber beyond the bony foramen.

Anticoagulation is the treatment of choice for this disorder. Operation is indicated only for patients with recurrent TIAs. In most patients, the intramural clot will be resorbed, restoring a normal lumen. In the rare case in which the dissection is confined to the surgically accessible proximal third, this segment may be resected and replaced with a graft. If the involvement is longer and the TIAs are believed to result from embolization and if the carotid back pressure exceeds 65 mm Hg, proximal ligation is indicated.

D. Fibromuscular Dysplasia: Fibromuscular dysplasia is a nonatherosclerotic angiopathy of unknown cause that affects specific arteries, chiefly in young women. Symptoms of cerebrovascular disease can occur when the carotid artery is affected. It is usually bilateral and involves primarily the middle third of the extracranial portions of the internal carotid artery. Several pathologic variants of the disease have been described, but in most of them the primary lesion is overgrowth of the media in a segmental distribution, producing irregular zones of arterial narrowing. The most common result is a series of concentric rings, producing the radiologic appearance of a *string of beads* in a long internal carotid artery. An uncommonly loud bruit high in the neck may be the only physical finding on vascular examination, although about one-third of patients are hypertensive because of renal artery involvement.

The prevalence of fibromuscular dysplasia and the portion of patients who develop symptoms are not known. Once symptoms develop, transient neurologic events are the most common manifestation. However, more than 20% of patients have had a stroke by the time of presentation.

Because of the high incidence of neurologic disability, the lesion should be corrected surgically whenever possible. Use of graduated arterial dilators has given excellent results and is currently the procedure of choice. Percutaneous transluminal angioplasty has been employed, but the risk of causing embolization appears high.

Surgical Results

Late restenosis or occlusion is uncommon after carotid endarterectomy or graduated dilation. The side effects of cerebrovascular operations consist mainly of neurologic deficits, which occur in about 2% of patients. The operative death rate for all extracranial cerebrovascular operations is less than 1%. Transient cranial nerve injury, which occurs during about 20% of operations, may cause tongue weakness, hoarseness, mouth asymmetry, earlobe numbness, and dysphagia.

Caracci BF et al: Asymptomatic severe carotid stenosis. J Vasc Surg 1989;9:361.

Early TF et al: Spontaneous carotid dissection: Duplex scanning in diagnosis. J Vasc Surg 1991;14:391.

Effeny DJ: Fibromuscular disease of the carotid artery. In: *Current Therapy in Vascular Surgery,* 2nd ed. Ernst CB, Stanley JC (editors). BC Decker, 1991.

Forsell C et al: Long term results after carotid artery surgery. Eur J Vasc Surg 1988;2:93.

Graham JM, Miller T, Stinnett DM: Spontaneous dissection of the common carotid artery: Case report and review of the literature. J Vasc Surg 1988;7:811.

Hass WK et al: A randomized trial comparing ticlopidine hydrochloride with aspirin for the prevention of stroke in high-risk patients. N Engl J Med 1989;321:501.

Hertzer NR et al: Surgical staging for simultaneous coronary and carotid disease: A study including prospective randomization. J Vasc Surg 1989;9:455.

Hertzer NR: Carotid endarterectomy: A crisis in confidence. J Vasc Surg 1988;7:611.

Lansfeld M, Gray-Weale AC, Lusby RJ: The role of plaque morphology and diameter reduction in the development of new symptoms in asymptomatic carotid arteries. J Vasc Surg 1989;9:548.

Londrey GL et al: Does color-flow imaging improve the accuracy of duplex carotid evaluation. J Vasc Surg 1991;13:659.

Mattle HP et al: Evaluation of the extracranial carotid arteries: Correlation of magnetic resonance angiography, duplex ultrasonography, and conventional angiography. J Vasc Surg 1991;13:838.

Norris JW, Zhu CZ: Stroke risk and critical carotid stenosis. J Neurol Neurosurg Psychiatry 1990;53:253.

North American Symptomatic Carotid Endarterectomy Trial Collaborators: Beneficial effect of carotid endarterectomy in symptomatic patients with high-grade stenosis. N Engl J Med 1991;325:445.

Nunn DB: Carotid endarterectomy in patients with territorial transient ischemic attacks. J Vasc Surg 1988;8:447.

Perler BA, Burdick JF, Williams GM: Progression to total occlusion is an underrecognized complication of the medical management of carotid disease. J Vasc Surg 1991;14:821.

Robbs JV, Human RR, Rajaruthnan P: Operative treatment of non-specific aortitis (Takayasu's arteritis). J Vasc Surg 1986;3:605.

Taylor LM, Loboa L, Porter JM: The clinical course of carotid bifurcation stenosis as determined by duplex scanning. J Vasc Surg 1988;8:255.

Thompson JE: Carotid endarterectomy for asymptomatic carotid stenosis: An update. J Vasc Surg 1991;13:669.

Whisnant JP et al: Duration of cigarette smoking is the strongest predictor of severe extracranial artery atherosclerosis. Stroke 1990;21:707.

RENOVASCULAR HYPERTENSION

Essentials of Diagnosis

- Severe hypertension.
- Declining renal function.
- Suspicion of renal artery involvement.

General Considerations

More than 23 million people in the USA have hypertension, and renovascular disease is the cause in 2–7% of cases. Atherosclerosis of the aorta and renal artery is present in two-thirds of patients with renovascular disease, and fibromuscular dysplasia is present in most of the rest. Less common causes of hypertension include renal artery emboli, renal artery dissection, hypoplasia of the renal arteries, and stenosis of the suprarenal aorta.

Atherosclerosis characteristically produces stenosis at the orifice of the main renal artery. The lesion usually consists of an atheroma that originates in the aorta and extends into the renal artery. Less commonly, the atheroma arises in the renal artery itself. Renal artery stenosis is more common in males over age 45 years and is bilateral in over 90% of cases.

Fibromuscular dysplasia usually involves the middle and distal thirds of the main renal artery and may extend into the branches (Figure 35–14). It is bilateral in 50% of cases. The arterial stenoses are caused by concentric rings of hyperplasia that project into the arterial lumen. Fibromuscular dysplasia occurs mainly in women, with onset of hypertension usually occurring before age 45 years. It is the causative disorder in 10% of children with hypertension. Developmental renal artery hypoplasia, coarctation of the

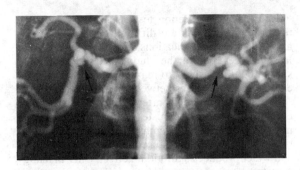

Figure 35–14. Renal arteriogram showing bilateral fibromuscular hyperplasia of the renal arteries (arrows).

aorta, and Takayasu's aortitis are the vascular causes of hypertension in childhood.

Hypertension due to renal artery stenosis results from kidney response to hypoperfusion. Cells of the juxtaglomerular complex secrete renin, which acts on circulating angiotensinogen to form angiotensin I, which is rapidly converted to angiotensin II by angiotensin-converting enzyme (ACE). This octapeptide constricts arterioles, increases aldosterone secretion, and promotes sodium retention. Blood pressure increases in an attempt to overcome renal hypoperfusion. As renovascular hypertension becomes established, pathologic changes occur in the kidneys and other organs, and hypertension becomes volume-dependent.

Clinical Findings

A. Symptoms and Signs: Most patients are asymptomatic, but irritability, headache, and emotional depression are seen in a few. Persistent elevation of the diastolic pressure is usually the only abnormal physical finding. A bruit is frequently audible to one or both sides of the midline in the upper abdomen. Other signs of atherosclerosis may be present when this is the cause of the renal artery disease.

Other clues to the presence of renovascular hypertension include absence of a family history of hypertension; early onset of hypertension (particularly during childhood or, in women, during early adulthood); marked acceleration of the degree of hypertension; resistance to control with antihypertensive drugs; and rapid deterioration of renal function.

B. Diagnostic Studies: Divided urinary excretion studies, which were used to indicate which of the two kidneys was the cause of hypertension, have largely been discarded, because of the frequency of false-negative results when both renal arteries are diseased.

Selective renin determinations from renal vein blood samples are suggestive of the diagnosis if the ratio of the renin from the involved kidney to that of the uninvolved one exceeds 1.5. This is called the renal vein renin ratio (RVRR).

Like urinary excretion tests, selective renal vein renin determinations are difficult to reproduce. All antihypertensive medications must be discontinued at least 1 week before the study, and sodium intake should be diminished (to maximize renin output and exaggerate differences between the kidneys).

When bilateral renal artery disease exists, however, this value may be misleading, because both kidneys produce renin. Systemic serum renin determinations are of little value, since the retention of sodium and water produces a dilutional effect. Only in malignant hypertension are systemic renin concentrations uniformly elevated.

Captopril and enalapril inhibit ACE and cause a precipitous drop in blood pressure in patients with renin-dependent hypertension. Renal function may also deteriorate. The combination of provocative testing with a converting enzyme inhibitor and RVRR determinations increases the accuracy of diagnosis of surgically correctable renovascular hypertension. Captopril renal scintigraphy may help to establish the diagnosis.

Duplex ultrasound scanning may also be useful in the diagnosis of renovascular disease. In experienced hands, the overall agreement of duplex findings and angiography is over 90%. Preliminary studies using MRI have been promising.

C. Imaging Studies: Intravenous urography with rapid injection and rapid sequence exposure is a common screening test that also depends upon comparison of the two kidneys. The ischemic kidney has delayed appearance of dye in the calices and hyperconcentration in the later films as water is extracted by the tubules. The nephrogram phase may show a small kidney on the affected side.

Renal arteriography is the only method that delineates the obstructive lesion. Since atherosclerotic disease most often involves the origins of the renal arteries, a midstream aortogram is preferable to selective renal artery catheterization. Renal arteriography should be performed if the diastolic blood pressure exceeds 110 mm Hg, other clinical criteria are consistent with renovascular hypertension, and long life is otherwise expected. Deteriorating renal function is another indication for arteriography.

The improved imaging associated with DSA usually provides an accurate initial assessment of patients with suspected renovascular disease and is useful in follow-up after surgical reconstruction. The investigation can be done in the outpatient department.

Treatment

A. Surgical Treatment: Primary surgical treatment consists of revascularization of the renal artery. The indications for arterial reconstruction are influenced by the extent of disease in the renal arteries, the degree of associated arterial disease, the response to medical control of hypertension, the patient's life ex-

pectancy, and the anticipated morbidity associated with operation. Nephrectomy should be considered when arterial repair is impossible or especially hazardous and the disease is unilateral.

Endarterectomy is effective in the management of atherosclerotic lesions and is most easily accomplished by a transaortic approach. When there is extensive intimal degeneration in the aorta (eg, associated aneurysmal disease in the aorta), a fabric bypass graft may be used as a side arm from the aortic prosthesis.

Arterial replacement is the preferred method of treatment in patients with fibromuscular dysplasia of the renal artery. Autologous grafts using a segment of saphenous vein or hypogastric artery are advised (Figure 35–15). Instrumental dilation of the diseased renal artery may be effective in relieving stenosis in selected patients.

Obstructive lesions in the secondary branches of the renal artery due to fibromuscular dysplasia were originally considered to be inoperable. Extracorporeal techniques have recently been developed that appear in most instances to overcome the technical difficulties. These require removal of the kidney from the abdomen, continuous cold perfusion of its vascular tree, and microvascular techniques for arterial replacement. The kidney is then either returned to a site near its original position or transplanted to the ipsilateral iliac fossa.

B. Percutaneous Transluminal Angioplasty: Percutaneous transluminal angioplasty has a 90% immediate success rate in patients with fibromuscular dysplasia, and 1 year later about 60% of patients remain cured. Results are not as long-lasting in renal atherosclerosis, however, as restenosis occurs in more than half of treated patients. If lesions occur at some distance from the aorta, results are superior to

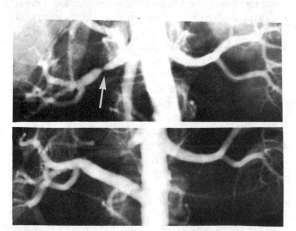

Figure 35–15. *Top:* Preoperative renal arteriogram of a patient with stenosis of the mid portion of the right renal artery (arrow). *Bottom:* Postoperative renal arteriogram after renal artery bypass with an autograft of the hypogastric artery.

those achieved with angioplasty of primarily aortic lesions.

Prognosis

Operations for revascularization of the renal artery are successful in lowering blood pressure in over 90% of patients with fibromuscular hyperplasia. Operation for atherosclerotic stenosis results in improvement or cure in about 60%.

Baert AL et al: Percutaneous transluminal renal angioplasty: Initial results and long-term follow-up in 202 patients. Cardiovasc Intervent Radiol 1990;13:22.

Beebe HG et al: Results of renal artery balloon angioplasty limit its indications. J Vasc Surg 1988;8:300.

Berkowitz HD, O'Neil JA: Renovascular hypertension in children: Surgical repair with special reference to the use of reinforced vein grafts. J Vasc Surg 1989;9:46.

Cohen JR, Birnbaum E: Coarctation of the abdominal aorta. J Vasc Surg 1988;8:160.

Hansen KJ et al: Magnetic resonance imaging: A reliable test for the evaluation of proximal atherosclerotic renal arterial stenosis. J Vasc Surg 1991;13:311.

Libertino JA et al: Changing concepts in surgical management of renovascular hypertension. Arch Intern Med 1988;148:357.

Meier GH et al: Captopril renal scintigraphy: An advance in the detection and treatment of renovascular hypertension. J Vasc Surg 1990;11:770.

Messina LM et al: Real revascularization for recurrent pulmonary edema in patients with poorly controlled hypertension and renal insufficiency: A distinct subgroup of patients with arteriosclerotic renal artery occlusive disease. J Vasc Surg 1992;15:73.

NHLBI Summary Report: Diagnosis and management of renovascular disease. J Vasc Surg 1986;3:453.

O'Mara CS et al: Simultaneous aortic reconstruction and bilateral renal revascularization: Is this a safe and effective procedure? J Vasc Surg 1988;8:357.

Sang CN et al: Etiologic factors in renovascular fibromuscular dysplasia: A case-control study. Hypertension 1989;14:472.

Tollefson DFJ, Ernst CB: Natural history of atherosclerotic renal artery stenosis associated with aortic disease. J Vasc Surg 1991;14:327.

van Bockel JH et al: Extracorporeal renal artery reconstruction for renovascular hypertension. J Vasc Surg 1991; 13:101.

CHRONIC GASTROINTESTINAL ISCHEMIA SYNDROMES

Essentials of Diagnosis

- Postprandial pain.
- Fear of eating.
- Weight loss.
- Epigastric bruit.

General Considerations

The celiac axis, the superior and inferior mesenteric arteries, and the two internal iliac arteries are the principal sources of blood supply to the stomach and intestines. The anatomic collateral interconnections between these arteries are numerous and may become quite large. Single or even multiple occlusions are generally well tolerated, because collateral flow is readily available (Figure 35–16).

Chronic stenosis or occlusion of the celiac or superior mesenteric arteries is caused by atherosclerosis or external compression by ligamentous or neural bands. When atherosclerosis is the cause, the usual lesion is a collar or thickened intima that begins in the aorta itself and extends into the orifice of the visceral artery. Associated atherosclerosis in the aorta and its other branches is frequent.

Visceral ischemia due to external compression of the celiac artery, or median arcuate ligament syndrome, has been diagnosed most often in women age 25–50. The existence of this syndrome is controversial.

Clinical Findings

The principal complaint is postprandial abdominal pain, which has been labeled abdominal or visceral angina. Pain characteristically appears 15–30 minutes after the beginning of a meal and lasts for an

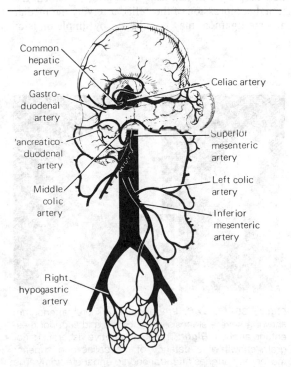

Figure 35–16. Visceral arterial circulation and interconnections.

hour or longer. Pain is occasionally so severe and prolonged that opiates are required for relief. Pain occurs as a deep-seated steady ache in the epigastrium, occasionally radiating to the right or left upper quadrant. Weight loss results from reluctance to eat, although mild degrees of malabsorption occur. Thus, gastrointestinal absorption studies are not helpful. Diarrhea and vomiting have been described. An upper abdominal bruit may be heard in over 80% of patients.

Arteriography in the anteroposterior and especially the lateral projections demonstrates both the arterial lesion and the patterns of collateral blood flow (Figure 35–17). Patients should be well hydrated before angiography, since this procedure can precipitate osmotic diuresis with dehydration, vascular occlusion, and bowel infarction.

Treatment

When the obstruction is atherosclerotic, surgical revascularization of the superior mesenteric and celiac axes may be performed by either endarterectomy or graft replacement (Figure 35–17). During endarterectomy, a sleeve of aortic intima and the orifice lesions in the celiac or superior mesenteric arteries are removed. The operation is performed by a retroperitoneal approach to the aorta through a left thoracoabdominal incision. Alternatively, a Dacron graft may be brought from the lower thoracic aorta to the celiac axis or superior mesenteric artery—an operation that is performed from within the abdomen. External compression of the celiac artery by the median arcuate ligament may be relieved by simple division of the ligament in 50% of cases, but simultaneous arterial reconstruction produces the best results.

Prognosis

Surgery for atherosclerotic visceral artery insufficiency almost always results in relief of symptoms if a technically adequate operation is accomplished. If operation is not performed, death will occur from inanition or massive bowel infarction.

Patients with median arcuate ligament compression respond favorably to operation in the majority of instances; however, some of these patients are not improved even though a technically adequate operation is performed.

Bowersox JC et al: Duplex ultrasonography in the diagnosis of celiac and mesenteric artery occlusive disease. J Vasc Surg 1991;14:780.

Rheudasil JM et al: Surgical treatment of chronic mesenteric arterial insufficiency. J Vasc Surg 1988;8:495.

Sitges-Serra A et al: Mesenteric infarction: An analysis of 83 patients with diagnostic studies in 44 cases undergoing a massive small bowel resection. Br J Surg 1988; 75:544.

Van Dongen RJAM: Renal and intestinal artery occlusive disease. World J Surg 1988;12:777.

INTRA-ARTERIAL INJECTIONS

Intra-arterial injections are being seen more frequently among intravenous drug abusers. Brachial and femoral injections are most frequent. Iatrogenic intra-arterial injections are still seen occasionally. The patient experiences severe burning pain in the affected arterial distribution, followed by intense vasoconstriction and in many cases thrombosis with gangrene of digits or of the entire extremity. In lesser insults, after the period of vasospasm, the extremity becomes swollen and discolored. When intra-arterial injection is recognized, if the needle is still in place, the artery should be copiously irrigated with heparinized saline. Intra-arterial reserpine may be useful to alleviate vasospasm. The patient usually presents late. Infection, pseudoaneurysm formation, and chemical endarteritis are late complications. Various regimens have been advocated—anticoagulants, sympathectomy, dextran, corticosteroids—with mixed results. At present, cervical sympathetic block followed by heparinization is the recommended immediate management.

MacIlroy MA et al: Infected false aneurysms of the femoral artery in intravenous drug addicts. J Rev Infect Dis 1989; 11;587.

Saroyan RM, Sendowski J, Kerstein MD: Vascular injury

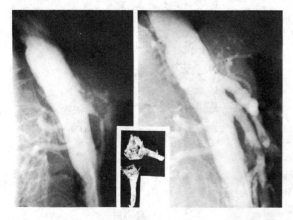

Figure 35–17. *Left:* Preoperative visceral arteriogram showing severe stenosis of the celiac and superior mesenteric arteries. *Right:* The postoperative visceral arteriogram shows wide patency of the celiac and superior mesenteric arteries after transaortic endarterectomy. The inset shows the atherosclerotic stenotic lesions removed by endarterectomy.

secondary to drug abuse. In: *Current Therapy in Vascular Surgery,* 2nd ed. Ernst CB, Stanley JC (editors). BC Decker, 1991.

Welch GH, Reid DB, Pollock JG: Infected false aneurysms in the groin of intravenous drug abusers. Br J Surg 1990; 77:330.

REFERENCES

Bergan JJ, Yao JST (editors): *1991 Year Book of Vascular Surgery.* Year Book, 1991.

Bernhard VM, Towne JB (editors): *Complications in Vascular Surgery.* Quality Medical Publishing, 1991.

Bongard R, Wilson SF, Perry MO (editors): *Vascular Injuries in Surgical Practice.* Appleton & Lange, 1991.

Brewster DC (editor): *Common Problems in Vascular Surgery.* Year Book, 1989.

Ernst CB, Stanley JC (editors): *Current Therapy in Vascular Surgery-II.* BC Decker, 1991.

Greenhalgh RM, Mannick JA, Powell JT: *The Cause and Management of Aneurysms.* Saunders, 1990.

Levin ME, O'Neal LW (editors): *The Diabetic Foot,* 4th ed. Mosby, 1988.

Moore WS (editor): *Vascular Surgery: A Comprehensive Review,* 3rd ed. Grune & Stratton, 1991.

Negus D (editor): *Leg Ulcers: A Practical Approach to Management.* Butterworth Heinemann, 1991.

Rutherford RB (editor): *Vascular Surgery,* 3rd ed. Saunders, 1989.

Sanders RJ, Haug CE (editors): *Thoracic Outlet Syndrome: A Common Sequela of Neck Injuries.* Lippincott, 1991

Wilson SE et al (editors): *Vascular Surgery: Principles and Practice.* McGraw-Hill, 1987.

Veith FJ (editor): *Current Critical Problems in Vascular Surgery.* Grune & Stratton, 1990.

Zarins CK, Gewertz BL: *Atlas of Vascular Surgery.* Churchill Livingstone, 1989.

36

Amputation

William C. Krupski, MD, Harry B. Skinner, MD, PhD, & David J. Effeney, MB, BS, FRACS

Amputation may be the only practical treatment for a limb severely affected by trauma, infection, tumor, or the end stages of ischemia. The immediate aims of amputation are (1) removal of diseased tissue, (2) relief of pain, (3) performance of surgery that will permit primary healing of the wound, and (4) construction of a stump and provision of a prosthesis that will permit useful function.

As the average age of the population has risen, the incidence of peripheral arterial disease and diabetes mellitus has increased. More than 90% of the 65,000 amputations performed in the USA each year are for ischemic or infective gangrene. Sixty to 80% of lower extremity amputations are performed for vascular and infectious complications of diabetes mellitus, and 15–50% of diabetic amputees will lose a second leg within 5 years. Other indications for amputations are nondiabetic infection with ischemia (15–25%), ischemia without infection (5–10%), osteomyelitis (3–5%), trauma (2–5%), and frostbite, tumors, neuromas, and other miscellaneous causes (5–10%).

Mortality rates have progressively declined in the past decade to about 5–10% for lower extremity amputations. Predictably, the more proximal the amputation, the higher the death rate, which is 30% after above-knee amputation and 5% after below-knee amputation. About 50% of deaths are caused by cardiovascular diseases.

Level of Amputation

Amputation should be performed at the level at which healing is most likely to be complete but which will also permit the most efficient use of the limb following rehabilitation. The benefit of more predictable healing in a proximal amputation must be weighed against the greater potential for successful rehabilitation and ease in walking that can be achieved with a distal amputation.

Decisions are based on adequacy of blood flow, extent of tissue necrosis, and location of tumor. In the upper extremities, circulatory impairment is rare. In the lower extremities, in which impairment is more likely to occur, the circulatory status at different levels may be determined by measurement of the peripheral pulses and the capillary refill time and by noting the presence of rubor, the condition of the skin, and

the presence of ischemic atrophy. At present, no single measurement of blood flow can reliably predict the best level of healing. The best predictions are based on clinical assessment by an experienced surgeon, assisted by one of the several techniques for determining amputation level. In patients with distinct lines of demarcation (eg, with gangrene) and in those with tumors, the amount of tissue that must be removed is usually more obvious.

As long a limb as possible should be preserved, in order to maintain the most nearly normal ambulation with the least energy expenditure. Compared with normal walking, energy expenditure is increased 10–40% with a below-knee prosthesis, 50–70% with an above-knee prosthesis, and 60% with crutches. One obvious way to reduce energy cost is to reduce the cadence. The average speed of ambulation for a normal adult is 4.8 km/h, compared with 3.2 to 4 km/h for a below-knee amputee and 2.4 km/h for an above-knee amputee.

Techniques for determining the level of amputation are as follows:

A. Measurement of Blood Pressure: In addition to clinical assessment, measurement of blood pressure in the thigh, ankle, and toes with a Doppler ultrasound device and pneumatic cuffs is a most useful technique for determining the level of amputation. Readings are not accurate enough, however, to be the sole basis for decision. Segmental blood pressures are fallible, and blood pressure in the ankle is an unreliable guide to healing in the foot if the tibial vessels are calcified and cannot be compressed by the cuff. This is particularly common in patients with diabetes mellitus. The notion that above-knee amputation is mandatory if the blood pressure in the ankle is below 60 mm Hg has proved to be mistaken. This technique does not adequately demonstrate collateral circulation, and healing is common even when ankle pressures are extremely low or undetectable. Absence of an arterial flow signal in the popliteal space, however, reliably predicts that below-knee amputation will fail to heal.

B. Xenon Xe 133 Studies: Skin clearance of xenon Xe 133 may help to indicate the level of healing. A small amount of xenon Xe 133 dissolved in saline is injected intradermally at different levels, and wash-out rates, a function of blood flow, are determined by a gamma camera interfaced to a minicomputer. Success rates for primary below-knee amputations are approximately 97% when skin blood flow is greater than 2.6 mL/min/100 g tissue, 80% when flow is between 2 and 2.6 mL/min/100 g tissue, and less than 50% when flow is less than 2 mL/min/100 g tissue. Measurement of blood flow using xenon 133 allows assessment of several potential levels of amputation at once. Disadvantages of this technique include complexity of equipment, invasiveness, and variability of results. The precision of the injection technique is highly technician-dependent, because xenon 133 is highly fat-soluble and a deep injection will yield erroneous results. Because of this—and because the test is expensive, time-consuming, and cumbersome—the test has not been widely adopted.

C. Oxygen Tension Measurements: Transcutaneous measurement of oxygen tension (using a modified Clark-type oxygen electrode) is another guide to healing. A transcutaneous PO_2 of zero indicates that healing will be unsatisfactory at that site, whereas a PO_2 above 40 mm Hg indicates that good healing is likely. Intermediate values do not correlate closely with the degree of healing. Transcutaneous PO_2 measurement is noninvasive and very reproducible. Disadvantages of the technique are the expense of the equipment and the time required for examination (about 30 minutes per site). In addition, it is important to heat the skin to 44 °C, which causes a temperature dependent microstructural change in the lipid phase of the stratum corneum from solid to liquid.

D. Laser Doppler Measurements: The laser Doppler, which measures velocity of flow in the skin microcirculation, reliably indicates poor healing when no flow is detected, but other predictions are not possible with this instrument. When the predictive value of laser Doppler is compared with that of transcutaneous O_2, the latter is more accurate.

E. Skin Fluorescent Studies: Measurement of skin fluorescence with a fluorometer after intravenous injection of fluorescein dye predicts healing with 80% accuracy, about twice the accuracy of Doppler pressure measurements in the ankle. Fluorometers are now commercially available to provide objective numerical values.

F. Skin Perfusion Pressure Measurements: Photoelectrically measured skin perfusion pressure predicts healing with 80% accuracy. A blood pressure cuff placed over a photoelectric detector connected to a plethysmograph measures the minimal external pressure required to prevent skin reddening after blanching. A skin perfusion pressure of at least 20 mm Hg is required for healing.

G. Skin Temperature: Infrared thermography has been correlated with skin blood flow. Oishi has reported a 94% positive predictive value for amputation healing by directly measuring skin temperature;

however, the negative predictive value was only 11%.

H. Arteriography: Arteriography, used primarily to assess feasibility of vascular reconstruction, is of little value in selecting the amputation site because findings do not correlate with circulation to the skin.

Preparation for Amputation

No pharmacologic treatment can forestall amputation; however, patients must be adequately prepared for operation. Diabetes mellitus, heart failure, and infection should be controlled. Material from sites of potential infection should be cultured and appropriate antibiotics administered preoperatively. In the presence of infection or a necrotic tumor, the first step should be a debriding (guillotine-type) amputation, continued antibiotics, and repeated dressing changes. A definitive amputation with primary closure of the wound can be performed 5–7 days later.

Protein-calorie malnutrition affects the healing of amputation sites, and serum albumin levels and total lymphocyte counts correlate with success rates. Assuming that the amputation level is appropriate, healing occurs in 80% of patients when serum albumin is at least 3.5 g/mL and total lymphocyte count is at least 1500 cells/μL, but in less than 30% of patients when values are lower.

Urgent or Emergency Amputation

A. Acute Arterial Occlusion: Arterial flow can be restored surgically in most patients with acute arterial occlusion, but when flow cannot be restored and the limb is dead, urgent or emergency amputation is required. The degree of urgency is determined by the extent of ischemia, the mass of ischemic muscle, the amount of pain, and the presence of systemic toxicity and infection. If there is little ischemic or necrotic tissue, amputation may be deferred until demarcation between viable and nonviable tissue becomes evident; this usually takes a day or two. This allows for maximum development of collateral circulation and increases the chances that a limited amputation will heal. When circulatory improvement stops or if toxicity develops, amputation should be performed promptly. The more extensive the tissue destruction, the greater the risk of serious toxicity when amputation is delayed. Findings of toxicity include deterioration of vital signs, mental confusion, myoglobinuria, renal failure, and sepsis, which mandate emergency amputation.

B. Injury: In patients with massively injured or crushed extremities, early amputation may greatly shorten the time required for successful rehabilitation. There are several scoring systems for determining the advisability of immediate amputation after major extremity trauma. The most popular is designated MESS (Mangled Extremity Severity Score). In brief, severe major nerve injury in conjunction with bone, soft tissue, and vascular injury warrants consideration of primary amputation, because a neurologically useless leg is not worth salvaging.

SPECIFIC TYPES OF AMPUTATIONS

LOWER EXTREMITY AMPUTATIONS

The treatment objectives for patients with lower extremity vascular disease are relief of pain and preservation of gait. Amputation should not be considered synonymous with *failure* of therapy, nor should it be thought of as *destructive* surgery. Instead, it is a means of achieving the same objectives as arterial surgery but in circumstances when the extent of tissue loss precludes preservation of a functional limb.

Lower extremity amputations are made most commonly at one of the following levels: toe (which may be extended to include resection of the metatarsal), transmetatarsal, below-knee, and above-knee. The other most common amputation levels (Syme's amputation, knee disarticulation, and hip disarticulation) are usually used to treat conditions other than vascular disease.

1. TOE & RAY AMPUTATION

Toes are the most frequently amputated parts of the body. Over two-thirds of amputations in diabetics involve the toes and forefoot. The indications include gangrene, infection, neuropathic ulceration, and osteomyelitis limited to the middle or distal phalanx. For dry, uninfected gangrene of one toe, **autoamputation** may be allowed to occur. During this process, epithelialization occurs beneath the eschar, and the toe spontaneously detaches, leaving a clean stump at the most distal site. Although preferable in many patients, autoamputation sometimes requires months to complete.

Contraindications to toe amputation include indistinct demarcation, infection at the metatarsal level, dependent rubor, and ischemia of the forefoot.

Ray or wedge amputation includes removal of the toe and metatarsal head; occasionally, two adjacent toes may be amputated by this method. Good blood supply is required. As with toe amputation, there is little cosmetic deformity and a prosthesis is not required. Ray amputation of the great toe leads to unstable weight bearing and some difficulty with ambulation.

The extents of toe and ray amputations are shown in Figure 36–1. For distal resections, a circular incision is made at the midpoint of the proximal phalanx, and the phalanx is resected at about its midpoint. If it

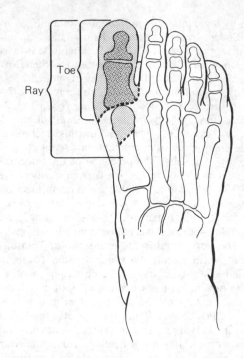

Figure 36–1. Toe and ray amputation.

is necessary to remove the entire phalanx or to excise the distal portion of the metatarsal, the incision is extended proximally over the metatarsal, and the bone is divided behind the metatarsal head. Not uncommonly, the incision must be left open to heal by second intention.

Complications that may require a higher amputation include infection, osteomyelitis of remaining bone, and nonhealing of the incision.

2. TRANSMETATARSAL AMPUTATION

Transmetatarsal forefoot amputations preserve normal weight bearing. The principal indication is gangrene of several toes or the great toe, with or without soft tissue infection or osteomyelitis. The gangrene should have spread beyond a level that could be treated by a two-ray amputation; there must be no evidence of spreading infection within the foot; and the plantar skin must be healthy. Patients who do not meet these criteria require a higher amputation.

The incision creates a generous plantar flap (Figure 36–2). There is no dorsal flap. On the plantar surface, the incision is continued medially to laterally just proximal to the metatarsophalangeal crease. The metatarsal bones are divided, and the tendons are pulled down and transected as high as possible.

Transmetatarsal amputation produces an excellent functional result. Walking requires no increase in energy expenditure, and the gait is usually smooth. A

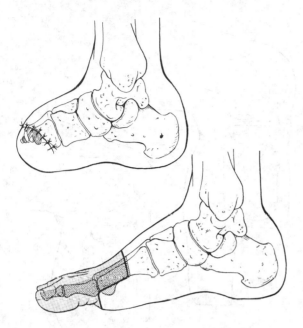

Figure 36–2. Transmetatarsal amputation.

prosthesis is not mandatory, but to achieve optimal gait, the shoes must be modified. Lamb's wool or custom-molded foam can be used to fill the toe portion of the shoe. A spring steel shank in the sole of the shoe approximates the action of the longitudinal foot arch during the toe-off phase of walking.

Open transmetatarsal amputations are occasionally necessary in the presence of infection. After the wound has contracted, a split-thickness skin graft may be used for skin coverage. The prosthetic fitting and rehabilitation of these patients are delayed and more difficult, since preservation of the skin graft becomes a primary concern. An ankle-foot orthosis may be necessary.

Chopart's amputation (transtarsal amputation of the forefoot) is an unpopular procedure because it produces an imbalance in the remaining muscles of the foot. This results in equinovarus deformity of the foot, with a tender scar and unsatisfactory weight bearing.

3. SYME'S AMPUTATION

Syme's amputation is a modification of disarticulation through the ankle joint. Trauma of the forefoot with good vascularity of the heel and ankle are the chief indications for this procedure. Spreading infection in the spaces of the foot, gangrene involving the heel pad, advanced ischemia of the foot, and a neurotropic foot with absence of heel sensation are contraindications to Syme's amputation.

Syme's amputation is the most technically de-

manding lower extremity amputation, and strict attention to surgical detail is crucial for success. The incision is shown in Figure 36–3. During the operation, particular attention must be paid to preserving the posterior tibial vessels, which supply the heel pad and inferior margins of the wound. The calcaneus must be dissected from the heel pad with great care in order to avoid injury to the soft tissues of the heel flap. The malleoli are resected flush with the joint surface, and the bones are trimmed so there are no pressure points. These last steps may be delayed for 6–8 weeks and performed as a second-stage procedure.

Syme's amputation produces an end-bearing stump and leaves a lower extremity only several inches shorter than normal, thus allowing the patient to walk short distances without a prosthesis. A prosthesis is not essential, and the patient can wear a cup slipper around the house. A cosmetic prosthesis employs a lightweight foot with a plastic shell into which the amputated limb fits. It is more difficult to fit than a conventional below-knee prosthesis. Walking speed is decreased, but energy consumption is increased very little.

4. BELOW-KNEE AMPUTATION

The below-knee amputation is the second most common amputation for vascular disease or infection of the lower extremity. Primary healing can be expected in 80–100% of cases (Table 36–1). In most cases, the infection or gangrene is confined to the foot but extends beyond a level that would permit lesser procedures. If gangrene or ulceration is present at the level of the proposed skin incision, if a stroke has paralyzed the extremity, or if there is a severe flexion contracture or arthritis of the knee, above-knee amputation would usually be recommended.

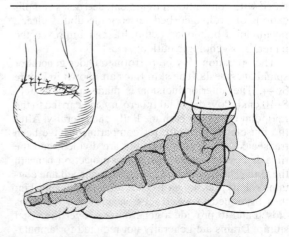

Figure 36–3. Syme's amputation.

Table 36–1. Healing of below-knee amputations.

Selection Method	Patients	% Healed
Clinical examination	38/46	83
Doppler systolic pressure		
30 mm Hg + calf >65 mm Hg	27/27	100
Popliteal >50 mm Hg	36/36	100
Xenon 133 clearance		
MEAN = 3.1 mL/100 g tissue/min	23/26	88
>2.6 mL/100 g tissue/min	35/36	97
Tc PO$_2$		
0 mm Hg	0/3	89
>0< 40 mm Hg	17/19	100
>40 mm Hg	51/51	100
Laser Doppler	8/8	100
Fluorescein dye	23/27	85
Photoelectric skin blood pressure		
>20 mm Hg	26/31	84

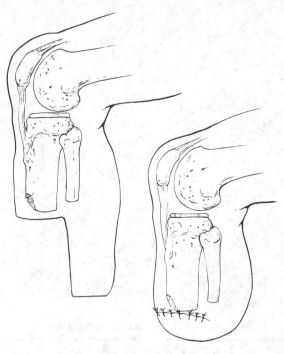

Figure 36–4. Below-knee amputation.

A debriding guillotine amputation of the foot is indicated prior to definitive below-knee amputation whenever severe infection is present. This removes the primary source of infection and allows proximal lymphatic channels to be cleared of bacteria, greatly increasing the chances of success of a subsequent definitive below-knee amputation.

The chances for success have been enhanced by making a long posterior flap and applying a rigid dressing that can be used for early ambulation with a temporary adjustable prosthesis. The blood supply to a posterior flap is generally better than the supply to an anterior flap or to sagittal flaps, because the sural arteries (which supply the gastrocnemius and soleus muscles) arise high on the popliteal artery, an area not often diseased, whereas the more distal popliteal artery or tibial arteries are often diseased, especially in diabetics.

The use of immediate postoperative prostheses provides two advantages: (1) a rigid dressing and (2) early ambulation. The rigid dressing controls edema, improves healing, prevents joint contractures, and protects from trauma. Early ambulation decreases hospital stay, increases rates of rehabilitation compared with conventional treatment, decreases complications of prolonged bed rest (eg, decubitus ulcers, pneumonia, pulmonary emboli), and improves the patient's psychologic outlook.

The operation may be performed under general or spinal anesthesia. The skin flaps are shown in Figure 36–4. The anterior incision is made approximately 8–10 cm below the tibial tuberosity and carried to the midpoint of the leg both medially and laterally. After the muscles of the anterior compartment have been transected, the fibula and tibia are divided, and the tibia is beveled to avoid a sharp projection beneath the skin. The posterior flap is wedge-shaped and contains soleus muscle, gastrocnemius muscle, and skin; it is fashioned to avoid tension when the wound is closed and to provide a generous pad over the distal stump. Drains are generally not required for amputations performed for vascular disease, because bleed-

ing is minimal, but they are often necessary for amputations performed for trauma or tumor.

Ninety percent of unilateral and 75% of bilateral below-knee amputees learn to walk independently. Success depends greatly upon the quality of the rehabilitation program and the preoperative ambulatory status. Less than 15% of patients who are nonambulatory before amputation are successfully rehabilitated.

5. ABOVE-KNEE AMPUTATION

Above-knee amputation should be performed when blood flow is inadequate for healing at a lower level; when the patient is unable to walk because of other debilitating disease; or when serious infection precludes lower amputation. The chief advantage of above-knee amputation is greater likelihood of healing, and the chief disadvantage is a lower rate of subsequent ambulation–only 40% of unilateral above-knee amputees can be expected to walk again. When one of the bilateral lower extremity amputations is at the above-knee level, only 10% of such amputees can walk. Thus, below-knee amputation should be performed whenever possible.

Above-knee amputation may be performed at several levels. Knee disarticulation is a distal above-knee amputation; the patient is left without a functional knee. Through-the-knee amputation is technically more demanding than above-knee amputation at a higher level. When fashioning an above-knee stump, one should preserve as long a lever arm as possible; amputation in the lower thigh is preferable to amputation in the mid or upper thigh. Like the below-knee amputation, a successful above-knee amputation may require a preliminary debriding amputation at a lower level.

The technique is straightforward. Short anterior and posterior flaps, sagittal flaps, or a circular incision may be used. The bone is divided slightly higher than the skin and soft tissue to avoid tension when the wound is closed. A rigid dressing suitable for use with a prosthesis is fitted in the immediate postoperative period in most patients, but it is more cumbersome and less efficacious than a rigid dressing used at lower levels.

6. HIP DISARTICULATION

Most dysvascular patients requiring high amputations can be successfully treated with above-knee amputation. Hip disarticulation is reserved for the few dysvascular patients in whom above-knee amputation fails or who have tumors of the thigh or lower femur. Life-threatening infection that cannot be controlled by hip disarticulation is almost uniformly fatal.

An anterior racket-shaped incision or a long posterior flap can be developed to cover the large defect created by a hip disarticulation. In the presence of vascular insufficiency, the flaps may have to be modified to achieve a closure that heals primarily. The muscles, nerves, and capsule of the hip joint are incised, and the disarticulation is completed by division of the ligamentum teres.

Most of these patients cannot be rehabilitated, but vigorous efforts should be made to rehabilitate selected well-motivated individuals, especially young patients who have undergone operation for tumor.

7. HEMIPELVECTOMY

Hemipelvectomy (hindquarter amputation) is reserved for patients with malignant tumors of the lower extremity or pelvis that cannot be removed by lesser procedures. The classic operation involves removal of the entire lower extremity and varying amounts of the innominate bone (Figure 36–5). If the iliac bone is removed completely, the procedure is termed radical; in conservative hemipelvectomy, part of the iliac bone attached to the sacrum is left in place. Internal hemipelvectomy is the procedure in which the innominate bone and surrounding musculature are removed and the lower extremity is preserved.

The incision for hemipelvectomy is determined by the site of the tumor. For posteriorly placed tumors,

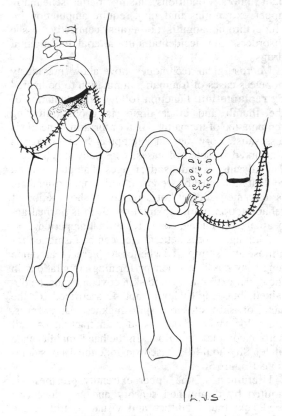

Figure 36–5. Hemipelvectomy.

an anterior flap of skin, subcutaneous tissue, and fascia lata based on the femoral vessels is appropriate. Alternatively, quadriceps muscle can be used for a myocutaneous flap. Rectus abdominis island flaps and thigh flaps based on the femoral vessels have also been used to close the defect after a hindquarter amputation. In some cases, a combination of Marlex mesh and skin graft may be applied over such defects.

The operative mortality rate for hindquarter amputation is about 3%, but complications occur in about 50% of cases. Five-year survival rates depend on the kind of tumor and stage of disease at the time of operation. The 5-year survival rate is 75% after hemipelvectomy for fibrosarcomas and chondrosarcomas; few patients with malignant melanoma are alive after 5 years.

UPPER EXTREMITY AMPUTATIONS

The indications for amputation of upper extremities are considerably different from those of lower extremities, because advanced atherosclerosis is largely confined to the latter. Upper extremity amputations are most often performed for severe trauma or malignant tumors. Conditions causing arterial ischemia in upper extremities that may require amputation include thromboangiitis obliterans, connective tissue disorders, and accidental intra-arterial injection of drugs.

Microsurgical techniques now allow previously hopeless cases of traumatic amputation to be treated by **replantation.** Function following replantation of the thumb and other digits is good; following replantation of the palm, wrist, or forearm, function is less satisfactory, but an attempt at limb salvage is warranted in selected cases, especially in children. The advantages and disadvantages of amputation and replantation must be weighed: with amputation, there is a cosmetic defect but a relatively short period of rehabilitation; with replantation, there is normal appearance but a long, costly rehabilitation period.

Although a prosthetic device can be fashioned for almost any stump, it is better to preserve as much length as possible when performing amputations in the upper extremity. Good skin coverage must be obtained, but length should not be sacrificed for the sake of skin closure; split-thickness skin grafts, musculocutaneous flaps, and skin traction can all help in complex situations. In the hand, maintenance of length should be based on functional considerations (Figure 36–6).

Usefulness of the upper extremity prosthesis is limited by diminished sensory and proprioceptive feedback; thus, auditory and visual control of the prosthesis is required. Limited "gadget tolerance" and high costs due to low demand reduce the availability of electric-powered prostheses. Prostheses

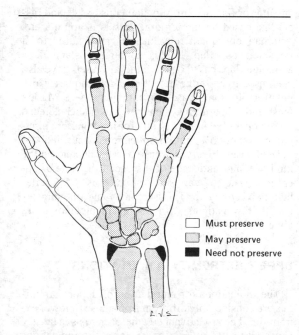

☐ Must preserve
▨ May preserve
■ Need not preserve

Figure 36–6. Amputation in the hand.

with elbow joints and terminal devices activated by body power are generally more acceptable to amputees.

Traumatic amputations do not have to be treated definitively at the initial debridement. Expectant management will permit questionably viable tissues to demarcate and thereby allow maximal preservation of length. When deciding whether to amputate an injured extremity, the physician should assess the status of five structures: skin, tendons, nerves, bones, and joints. If three or more are compromised, amputation is usually favored over attempts at preserving the part.

1. WRIST DISARTICULATION

After amputation below the elbow, only about 50% of the ability to perform pronation and supination can be transmitted to a prosthesis, because of the bulk of the proximal forearm and the length of the remaining radius and ulna. The more proximal the amputation, the less pronation and supination is possible. Amputations through the wrist permit the most pronation and supination and provide for better prosthetic control than higher amputations do.

2. FOREARM AMPUTATION

Even if only a short stump can be achieved, forearm amputation is preferable to above-elbow amputation. As much muscle function as possible should be preserved to maximize control of a prosthesis. Several innovative reconstructive procedures are available that allow upper arm muscles to assist in controlling a prosthesis when a very short stump precludes pronation and supination by forearm muscles.

3. ABOVE-ELBOW AMPUTATION

Every effort should be made to preserve length. Even if a very high amputation is necessary, the head of the humerus should be spared, since it serves as a support for a prosthesis and maintains shoulder width.

4. FOREQUARTER AMPUTATION

Malignant tumor is the usual indication for forequarter amputation. The operation is easiest if done from a posterior approach, but the location and size of the mass may require an anterior approach (Figure 36–7). A thoracotomy or partial neck dissection may be necessary to resect the tumor completely. After the wound has healed, a Silastic foam shoulder cap held

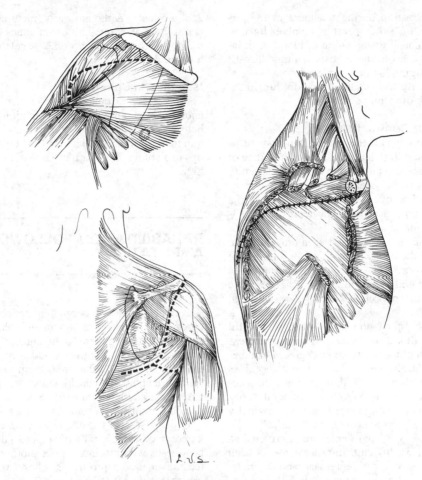

Figure 36–7. Forequarter amputation.

in place with straps provides a cosmetically acceptable shoulder.

COMPLICATIONS OF AMPUTATION

Nonhealing

A nonhealing stump, most often the result of insufficient blood supply or errors in surgical technique, usually requires higher amputation. While some centers report nonhealing in 30% of patients, in specialized centers this rate is about 5%. Lower rates than this can be achieved by performing high amputation in every marginal case, but many patients would then have a shorter stump than necessary and less rehabilitative potential.

Analysis of patients with failed amputations does not reveal any predominant cause, assuming that an appropriate level was selected. Patients with diabetes mellitus have no special predisposition to poor healing. There is some evidence that patients with hemoglobin levels above 13 g/dL heal less well than patients with lower values; this has led some surgeons to advise isovolumetric hemodilution in patients with marginally ischemic tissues.

Infection

Infection rates in amputation stumps average 15% and are highest when distal sepsis exists at the time of amputation. This can be decreased substantially by preliminary guillotine amputations and administration of antibiotics in infected cases. Stump hematomas predispose to infection. If the amputation stump becomes infected, the wound must be opened promptly, and a higher amputation is often required.

Thromboembolism

The amputee is at great risk for venous thrombosis (15%) and pulmonary embolism (2%) postoperatively because (1) amputation often follows prolonged immobilization during treatment of the primary disease and (2) the operation involves ligation of large veins, causing stagnation of blood, a situation that predisposes to thrombosis. If immediate-fit prosthetic techniques are not employed, an additional period of inactivity follows the operation, further increasing the risk of thromboembolism.

Pain & Flexion Contracture

Flexion contracture of the knee or hip may occur rapidly if the distal limb has been a constant source of pain, in which case it is natural to draw the extremity up in a flexed position. Measures to prevent contracture are indicated preoperatively, and application of a rigid dressing postoperatively decreases the incidence of this complication.

Persistent pain in a stump and phantom limb pain are common. If the cause of pain is stump ischemia, higher amputation is the treatment. A neuroma in a stump can be treated by injection of a local anesthetic or excision of the neuroma. Causalgia responds to sympathectomy.

Phantom limb pain is the sensation that a painful limb is present after amputation. Most amputees experience this phenomenon to some degree. Hypotheses concerning etiology include the gate theory (loss of sensory input decreases self-sustaining neural activity of the gate, causing pain), the peripheral theory (nerve endings in the stump represent parts originally innervated by the severed nerve), and the psychologic theory (hostility, guilt, and denial are interpreted as pain). Treatment is difficult; improvement has been reported using tricyclic antidepressants and the transcutaneous electrical nerve stimulation (TENS) apparatus. The incidence and severity of phantom limb pain are increased if there has been prolonged ischemia before amputation and decreased if postoperative rehabilitation has been rapid.

SPECIAL PROBLEMS OF AMPUTEES

Increased Mortality Rate

Five-year survival for all lower extremity amputees is less than 50%, compared with 85% for an age-matched population. Diabetic amputees have only a 40% 5-year survival. Two-thirds of all deaths are due to cardiovascular disease.

Fractures in Stumps

Because their gait is relatively unstable, amputees are at increased risk for falls that may lead to fractures. About 3–5% of amputees experience fractures at some time, principally of the distal femur and hip. The diagnosis of fracture is overlooked or delayed in

25% of cases. Although most fractures can be successfully treated, one-half of amputees who were ambulatory before injury become wheelchair-bound afterward.

Ischemia in Stumps

Progressive vascular disease results in ischemia of about 8% of above-knee amputations and 1% of below-knee amputations. Operations are often required to improve arterial flow when gangrene develops in a stump. The mortality rate of this condition is high.

REHABILITATION FOLLOWING AMPUTATION

Patients about to undergo amputation must be prepared for a course of treatment and rehabilitation directed at returning them to the highest possible level of function. For patients bedridden by vascular disease, an amputation that frees them to move around the house should be considered a success. For young amputees, anything short of return to full function should be considered something of a failure.

In the past, geriatric amputees were rarely rehabilitated: In one report, 60% of amputees discarded their prostheses within 6 months; in another, most amputees never used a prosthesis. These would be unacceptable statistics today.

The longer the interval between amputation and the start of rehabilitative efforts, the less the chance of success. Immediate postoperative prostheses and vigorous early rehabilitation programs have markedly improved the outlook to the point where almost all below-knee amputees can now be made ambulatory early in the postoperative period, compared with 60% treated with more conservative techniques. Immediately fitting a prosthesis after surgery shortens the interval between operation and rehabilitation from an average of 128 days to 31 days.

The length of the stump correlates well with regaining the ability to walk. Cardiopulmonary disease and physical weakness make walking an overwhelming effort for some patients; this emphasizes the importance of preserving as long a stump as possible, so that walking will require the least possible amount of energy.

All below-knee amputees and most above-knee amputees should receive an immediate-fit prosthesis. Patients are seen preoperatively by the prosthetist and the therapist responsible for gait training. A plaster cast is applied to the stump in the operating or recovery room immediately after the operation, and a pylon with a prosthetic foot is attached to the cast.

Use of the prosthesis and gait training begin on the first or second postoperative day. Patients perform upper extremity strengthening exercises and learn techniques for transferring from bed to chair and for care of the stump. Balancing in the upright position is a prerequisite for walking, and this begins with simple activities such as standing beside a wheelchair and walking with the support of parallel bars. The first rigid dressing is removed 10–14 days postoperatively. However, should the patient experience undue pain, unexplained fever, or leukocytosis, the wound must be inspected immediately. If wound healing is satisfactory, a second plaster cast is applied at 2 weeks, at which time patients living nearby may be discharged from the hospital. Skin staples are not removed for at least 4 weeks, during which time the wound remains encased in the plaster cast. The second rigid dressing is removed at the end of 1 month, and during this time the patient continues twice-daily physical therapy sessions and individual efforts at rehabilitation. The patient is allowed to bear increasing amounts of weight on the rigid dressing, until by the end of 1 month, 60–80% of the body weight may be borne on the amputated side.

After the second rigid dressing is removed, a plaster cap is fashioned for the patient to wear when not using the prosthesis. Fabrication of an intermediate prosthesis is begun immediately; use of this prosthesis should begin within 5 weeks after amputation. Another 2-week period of rehabilitation is usually required before the patient is proficient enough to take the prosthesis home full-time. Fitting of a permanent prosthesis is delayed for 6 months to allow for complete maturation (ie, shrinkage and molding) of the stump.

Early prosthetic fitting techniques have also been used with success for patients with upper extremity amputations. The kinds of prostheses available have increased remarkably over the last decade, and cosmetically acceptable, functional, powered prostheses are now available for most of these patients.

Successful rehabilitation of amputees is dependent upon a team approach. The referring physician, surgeon, prosthetist, physical therapist, nurse, social worker, family, and–most importantly–the patient must participate enthusiastically in order to maintain an effective program. While good surgical judgment and technique may result in a satisfactory stump, only the cooperation of all team members will result in optimal functional results. Indeed, from a practical standpoint, most patients identify more with their physical therapists and prosthetists than with their surgeons once they progress beyond the immediate postoperative period. Finally, the patient must be motivated to care for the stump and the contralateral extremity and to play an active role in rehabilitation.

PROSTHESES

The patellar tendon-bearing prosthesis is used for 90% of lower extremity amputees. It provides total contact with the residual limb, avoiding excessive pressure in any one area. A cuff suspension strap above the knee maintains close contact between the limb and prosthesis. The solid ankle cushion heel (SACH) prosthesis, the most frequently prescribed foot used for above-knee and below-knee prostheses, is rugged and adequately simulates ankle motion at heel-strike and toe-off. It is a good initial foot even for the younger, more athletic individual who may go on to a newer, dynamic energy-storing foot after becoming accustomed to the SACH foot.

The most commonly prescribed above-knee prosthesis is the total-contact suction socket. For older, dysvascular amputees, a single-axis constant function knee or single-axis "stabilizing" (friction lock) knee is best because it is lightweight. Younger, more athletic above-knee amputees can tolerate heavier prostheses with hydraulic or pneumatic knees, which permit changes in cadence.

More efficient prostheses requiring less energy are constantly being developed. Components fashioned from new types of plastics, fiberglass casting tapes, and carbon fiber polymers allow construction of ultra-lightweight strong and durable prostheses. They are often easier to fabricate than conventional wood or plastic laminated prostheses and are useful both in elderly amputees (who have less energy) and in young amputees who want to participate in sports.

Gait Analysis

The gait of both above-knee and below-knee amputees is markedly different from normal gait. The forward velocity of walking is significantly lower in amputees and is lower in above-knee than below-knee amputees. The time-distance parameters of velocity, cadence, strike length, and gait cycle are 1 SD below normal in below-knee amputees and 2 SD below normal in above-knee amputees. The normal symmetry of walking is not present, as has been documented by measurements of single-limb support time and motion analyses of the lower extremities, head, arms, and trunk. This asymmetry of motion increases the excursion of the center of mass during each gait cycle and thereby increases the amount of energy used in ambulation.

LONG-TERM CARE FOLLOWING AMPUTATION

Patients who have undergone amputation require periodic checks of the prosthesis and stump, physical therapy, and in many cases psychologic support for life. Shrinkage of the stump requires replacement of the initial prosthesis after about 6 months and again 1 year after amputation. Thereafter, well-made below-knee prostheses should have a useful life of approximately 2 years. Patients must be educated to care for the stump, with utmost attention to cleanliness, and shown how to protect areas of pressure, trauma, or insensitivity.

Following amputation for vascular disease, symptoms in the opposite leg should be anticipated and reported promptly, and ulcers or other changes in the stump should be brought to the attention of the physician as early as possible.

REFERENCES

Behar TA, Burnham SJ, Johnson G Jr: Major stump trauma following below-knee amputation: Outcome and recommendations. J Cardiovasc Surg 1991;32:753.

Clyne CA: Selection of level for lower limb amputation in patients with severe peripheral vascular disease. Ann R Coll Surg Engl 1991;73:148.

Endean ED et al: Hip disarticulation: Factors affecting outcome. J Vasc Surg 1991;14:398.

Finn HA, Simon MA: Limb-salvage surgery in the treatment of osteosarcoma in skeletally immature individuals. Clin Orthop 1991;262:108.

Fisher DF et al: One-stage versus two-stage amputation for wet gangrene of the lower extremity: A randomized study. J Vasc Surg 1988;8:428.

Francis HI et al: The Syme amputation: Success in elderly diabetic patients with palpable foot pulses. J Vasc Surg 1990;12:237.

Harris KA et al: Rehabilitation potential of elderly patients with major amputations. J Cardiovasc Surg 1991;32:463.

Houghton A et al: Rehabilitation after lower limb amputation: A comparative study of above-knee, through-knee and Gritti-Stokes amputations. Br J Surg 1989;76:622.

Jany RS, Burkus JK: long-term follow-up of Syme amputations for peripheral vascular disease associated with diabetes mellitus. Foot Ankle 1988;9:107.

Klasen HJ, ten Duis HJ: Traumatic hemipelvectomy. J Bone Joint Surg [Am] 1989;71:291

Kram HB, Appel PL, Shoemaker WC: Comparison of transcutaneous oximetry, vascular hemodynamic measurements, angiography, and clinical findings to predict the success of peripheral vascular reconstruction. Am J Surg 1988;155:551.

Kram HB, Appel PL, Shoemaker WC: Multisensor transcutaneous oximetric mapping to predict below-knee amputation wound healing: Use of a critical Po_2. J Vasc Surg 1989;9:796.

Kumar VP, Pho RW: A technique for digital replantation. J Hand Surg 1989;14:128.

Leonard JA Jr, Andrews KL: Rigid removable dressings, immediate postoperative prostheses, and rehabilitation of the amputee. In: Current Therapy in Vascular Surgery, 2nd ed. Ernst CB, Stanley JC (editors). BC Decker, 1991.

Light JT Jr, Rice JC, Kerstein MD: Sequelae of limited amputation. Surgery 1988;103:294.

Lind J, Kramhoft M, Bodtker S: The influence of smoking on complications after primary amputations of the lower extremity. Clin Orthop 1991;266:227. London PS: Amputations of the upper limb. Ann R Coll Surg Engl 1991;73:143.

Miller N et al: Transmetatarsal amputation: The role of adjunctive revascularization. J Vasc Surg 1991;13:705.

Moore WS, Malone JM (editors): Lower Extremity Amputation. Saunders, 1989.

Oishi CS, Fronek A, Golbranson FL: The role of non-invasive vascular studies in determining levels of amputation. J Bone Joint Surg [Am] 1988;70:1520.

Raviola CA et al: Cost of treating advanced leg ischemia: Bypass graft vs. primary amputation. Arch Surg 1988;123:495.

Rubin JR, Marmen C, Rhodes RS: Management of failed prosthetic grafts at the time of major lower extremity amputation. J Vasc Surg 1988;7:673.

Ruckley CV, Stonebridge PA, Prescott RJ: Skewflap versus long posterior flap in below-knee amputations: Multicenter trial. J Vasc Surg 1991;13:423.

Sarin S et al: Selection of amputation level: A review. Eur J Vasc Surg 1991;5:611.

Schwartz ME et al: Above-knee amputation in patients with prior hip surgery: A caveat. J Vasc Surg 1990;11:480.

Stebbings WS, Wood RF: Amputations in diabetics. Ann R Coll Surg Engl 1991;73:170.

Stern PH: Occlusive vascular disease of lower limbs: Diagnosis, amputation surgery and rehabilitation: A review of the Burke experience. Am J Phys Med Rehab 1988;676:145.

Sweetnam R: The diminishing role of amputation in the management of malignant tumours of bone. Ann R Coll Surg Engl 1991;73:165.

Taylor LM Jr et al: Limb salvage vs amputation for critical ischemia: The role of vascular surgery. Arch Surg 1991;126:1251.

Tunis SR, Bass EB: The use of angioplasty, bypass surgery, and amputation in the management of peripheral vascular disease. N Engl J Med 1992;326:415.

van den Broek TAA et al: Photoplethysmographic selection of amputation level in peripheral vascular disease. J Vasc Surg 1988;8:10.

Vollmar JR et al: Aneurysm of the abdominal aorta and leg amputation: Chance coincidence or pathogenic correlation? Dtsch Med Wochenschr 1988;113:1795.

Wagner WH et al: Noninvasive determination of healing of major lower extremity amputation: The continued role of clinical judgement. J Vasc Surg 1988;8:703.

Veins & Lymphatics

37

Jerry Goldstone, MD

I. THE VEINS

Functional & Surgical Anatomy

There are three anatomically and functionally distinct sets of veins draining the lower extremities.

A. Superficial Veins: The subcutaneous veins, superficial to the muscular fascia, consist of the greater and lesser saphenous veins on the anteromedial and posterior aspects of the legs, respectively. The two systems communicate freely with each other as well as with the deep veins, and each ends by joining the deep system. The greater saphenous vein is constant in its position at the ankle, just anterior to the medial malleolus, where it is quickly and easily exposed for emergency intravenous cannulation. These superficial veins play an important thermoregulatory function. The anatomy of the other veins is also quite variable. Up to 33% of people have a double greater saphenous vein.

B. Deep Veins: These are the intra- and intermuscular veins, which accompany the named arteries within the musculofascial compartments of the lower extremity and usually are given the same name. They often run as paired venae comitantes below the knee. About 90% of the venous return from the lower extremities normally flows in these veins.

C. Communicating Veins: The communicating veins perforate the deep muscular fascia to connect the superficial and deep venous systems. The valves in the perforating veins direct the flow of blood from the superficial to the deep veins. These veins are more numerous in the distal portion of the leg and ankle and more numerous on the medial side in a plane just posterior to the tibia.

The valves are the most distinctive and important feature of the venous capacitance system. They first appear in venules of about 1 mm in diameter, particularly in the limbs. These valves permit the flow of blood only toward the heart. They are more prominent in the veins of the legs than in those of the arms and are found in both the deep and superficial venous systems of the legs. They are also prominent in the communicating vessels that connect the superficial and deep leg veins. These bicuspid valves direct blood flow from distal to proximal and from superficial to deep, except in the perforating veins of the hands, feet, and forearms, in which flow is from deep to superficial. The venae cavae and the hepatic, portal, splenic, renal, pulmonary, mesenteric, cerebral, and superficial head and neck veins have no valves or possess only functionally incompetent intimal folds.

In humans, when the body is erect, the effective zero level of venous pressure is in the right atrium. The hydrostatic pressure in a vein on the dorsum of the foot is equal to the distance from the right atrium to the foot—about 100 cm H_2O. The more dependent a vein, the higher the hydrostatic pressure and the thicker the vein wall. This is why the greater saphenous vein can be used so readily as an arterial substitute. The thin-walled structure of veins permits them to change their shape from flat to ovoid to circular as flow increases and allows for marked increases in flow with minimal change in venous pressure gradient (compliance system). The valves in the veins of the leg do not by themselves dissipate the hydrostatic pressure of the column of blood between heart and foot. But muscular action, by compressing the deep veins, forces blood toward the heart, since the valves prevent backflow. With muscular relaxation, the pressure in the deep veins drops and they again fill with blood. The more frequent and powerful the muscular movements, the more efficient is this venous pump. With walking, the pressure in the veins on the dorsum of the foot falls to about 30 cm H_2O from the resting venous pressure of approximately 100–120 cm H_2O (Figure 37–1). The fall in venous pressure is maintained until the exercise is halted, and pressure returns slowly to the preexercise level (Figure 37–2).

Knowledge of the above anatomic and physiologic facts allows for a better understanding of the disturbances produced by the venous diseases described below. For example, the basic pathophysiologic mechanism responsible for the postphlebitic state is walking venous hypertension, as shown in Figure 37–2.

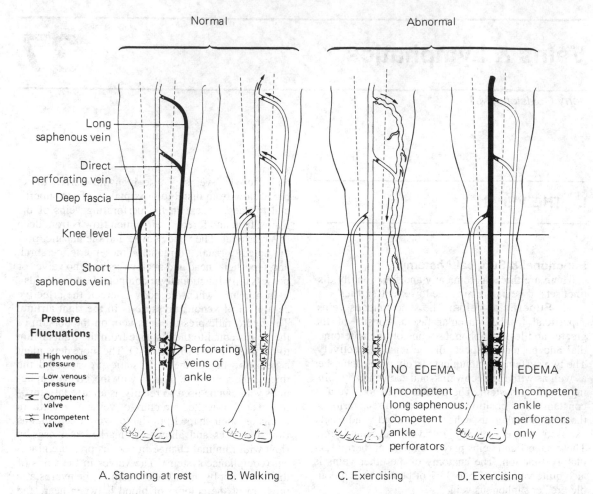

Figure 37–1. Normal venous physiology during standing *(A)* and walking *(B)* and abnormalities during exercise *(C, D)*. Pressure in the superficial veins is diminished (if the valves are competent) by the pumping action of the muscles, which facilitates venous return to the heart *(B)*. When the proximal valves are incompetent, the superficial veins become varicose, but competence of the valves in the distal communications maintains the integrity of the muscle pump, and pressure remains low in the superficial veins even during exercise *(C)*. If the valves of the leg communicators are incompetent, the muscle pump is ineffective even when the valves in the thigh are competent, and the venous pressure at the ankle remains high even during exercise *(D)*. This produces edema, diapedesis of red cells, poor tissue nutrition, and, ultimately, ulceration (postphlebitic syndrome).

DISEASES OF THE VENOUS SYSTEM

VARICOSE VEINS

Essentials of Diagnosis

- Dilated, tortuous superficial veins in the lower extremities, usually bilateral.
- Symptoms may be absent or may consist only of fatigue, aching discomfort, and slight swelling.
- Symptoms relieved by leg elevation.

- Pigmentation, ulceration, and edema of the lower leg suggest secondary varicose veins.

General Considerations

It is estimated that 10–20% of the world's population have varicose veins in the lower extremities. They are more common in women, and the prevalence increases with age. Although varicose means dilated, varicose veins are elongated and tortuous as well. They are most common in the lower extremities but also occur in other areas, such as the spermatic cord (varicocele), esophagus (esophageal varices), and anorectum (hemorrhoids).

On the basis of predisposing causes, varicose veins

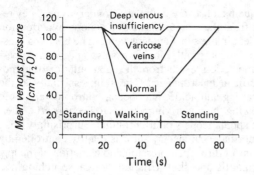

Figure 37–2. Ambulatory venous pressure. Responses of venous pressure measured in a vein on the dorsum of the foot during standing and walking. During standing, venous pressure is that of a hydrostatic column extending from the right atrium to the foot. With contraction of calf muscles, venous pressure falls rapidly and returns to normal slowly after exercise stops. The postphlebitic state is characterized by little if any fall in pressure with exercise and a rapid return to normal (walking venous hypertension). Patients with primary varicose veins show a response between these two extremes. (See text for details.)

are divided into two classes: primary and secondary. Primary varicose veins are associated with normal deep veins. Secondary varicose veins, on the other hand, are a complication of deep venous disease or arteriovenous fistula.

The cause of **primary, or simple, varicose veins** remains obscure. There are two major theories, neither of which satisfactorily explains all cases. Because venous valvular incompetence is the dominant clinical finding in saphenous varicosity and the factor that largely determines the clinical course and rate of progression, it has been postulated that the fundamental abnormality is sequential incompetence of the valves, either in the main saphenous trunks or in the communicating veins. Incompetent valves cause higher pressure at the subjacent valve and localized dilatation of the affected venous segment. The alternative "weak wall" theory assumes an inherited weakness of the vein wall, producing venous dilatation even with normal pressures and secondary failure of valvular competence. Heredity has been incriminated as an important risk factor for varicose veins, but only about 50% of patients have a positive family history, so the weakness is probably not inherited but due to postnatal factors.

Varicose veins are more common in patients with diverticular disease of the colon and correlate well with the low-roughage diet consumed in "developed" countries. The presumed etiologic link is obscure. Aggravating factors associated with an increased incidence of varicose veins are female sex, parity, constricting clothing, prolonged standing, marked obesity, and consumption of estrogens (oral contraceptives).

Secondary varicosities are those that develop following damage or obstruction to the deep veins. Recanalization of the thrombosed deep veins leaves the valves incompetent, and this loss of valve sufficiency leads to reflux and places an unusual strain on the superficial veins, which have little external support because of their location relative to the deep fascia of the leg. Secondary varicosities thus progressively develop because of the increased venous pressure and flow transmitted from the deep to the superficial veins via incompetent perforating veins. Obstruction of the inferior vena cava or iliac veins can result in secondary varicosities in the lower extremities. An example of this is suprapubic varicosities, which represent residual collateral veins that develop with iliofemoral thrombosis. An arteriovenous fistula may also lead to regional varicose veins. Klippel-Trenaunay syndrome—one form of congenital arteriovenous malformation—is associated with extensive varicosities of the lower extremities, usually in atypical locations (eg, lateral), and absence or maldevelopment of the deep veins.

Clinical Findings

Some patients have extremely severe varicose veins and no symptoms, whereas others have severe symptoms from small varices. The commonest symptoms are aching, swelling, heaviness, cramps, itching, and cosmetic disfigurement. Aching, usually described as a dull, heavy, bursting sensation, is particularly apt to occur after prolonged standing and is relieved by elevation of the leg or by the use of an elastic stocking. Symptoms usually become more severe as the day progresses. The swelling that occurs with primary varicose veins is mild and usually involves the feet and ankles only. It resolves completely on elevation of the leg in bed overnight. In women, symptoms are often more severe in the few days just prior to menses. The symptoms of simple, primary varicose veins are rarely severe, and most patients seek medical advice for cosmetic reasons or because they are concerned about the future of the leg.

Secondary varicose veins due to chronic deep venous insufficiency often cause more severe symptoms. Progression to ankle ulcers is relatively common, whereas this complication is rare with primary varicosities. Hemorrhage, sometimes of serious magnitude, may be induced by traumatic rupture of a varix or may be spontaneous. Dry skin and scaling dermatitis with pruritus may be seen over prominent varices, especially at the ankle. Although varicose veins may be tender, it must be emphasized that severe pain or disability should never be ascribed to primary varicose veins but should stimulate a search for primary musculoskeletal, arterial, or chronic deep venous disease.

The general physical examination may reveal predisposing causes of varicosities or conditions that would modify treatment. Inspection of the standing patient readily reveals dilated, elongated, and tortuous subcutaneous veins of the thigh and leg. If the veins are less obvious because of edema or obesity, palpation and percussion along the course of the greater saphenous vein (Schwartz test) is a useful diagnostic maneuver. Mild pitting edema of the ankles and slight pigmentation of the skin are common, especially just above the medial malleolus.

The Brodie-Trendelenburg test is a useful maneuver to test the valvular competence of the perforating veins and those in the greater saphenous system. With the patient supine, the leg is elevated until all the blood is drained from the superficial veins. The saphenous vein is then compressed in the thigh and the patient stands up; the varices are observed for 30 seconds, and the tourniquet is then removed. Normally, gradual filling of the superficial veins occurs from below after the patient stands, and when the tourniquet is removed, filling continues to be gradual. If the veins fill rapidly from below, the valves in the perforating veins are incompetent and the varices are being filled from the deep system. The location of the incompetent communicating veins can be determined by placing multiple tourniquets around the leg and thigh and observing which venous segment fills. To determine competency of the valve at the saphenofemoral junction, the tourniquet around the thigh is removed after 30 seconds. If blood refluxes rapidly into the greater saphenous system, the valves above this level are incompetent. Saphenofemoral valve incompetence can also be detected by demonstrating reverse flow in the saphenous system with a Doppler probe. The short saphenous vein can be tested in a similar manner by compressing it in the popliteal fossa with a tourniquet, but the long saphenous system should be occluded as well to facilitate interpretation.

Careful palpation along the superficial dilated veins will often identify perforating veins, a bulge below each incompetent valve, or defects in the fascia they traverse. In general, perforating veins are more frequent in the lower leg just posterior to the tibia, and are more common medially than laterally.

Differential Diagnosis

When ulceration, brawny induration, and marked hyperpigmentation are present, one can be reasonably certain that deep venous insufficiency exists and that the varicose veins are secondary. Otherwise, they are usually primary. A thrill and bruit over the extremity suggest that an arteriovenous fistula is the cause. If present, sources of extrinsic venous compression are usually obvious in the inguinal and retroperitoneal areas.

Complications

Complications from varicose veins are much more frequent and severe with the secondary type. They result from the venous stasis and venous hypertension present in the subcutaneous veins. The elevated pressure bursts small blood vessels, and skin hyperpigmentation results from the accumulation of hemosiderin in macrophages. The skin, especially at the distal leg and ankle, may become atrophic and thin, allowing the underlying varices to become eroded either spontaneously or after trauma. Surprisingly brisk hemorrhage can occur, but it is readily controlled by means of direct compression and elevation of the leg. Dermatitis and skin irritation can cause itching and severe excoriation from scratching. The affected skin is quite susceptible to cellulitis. Superficial thrombophlebitis, a frequent complication of varicose veins, is discussed further, below.

Treatment

Treatment of varicose veins should relieve discomfort, prevent or ameliorate the complications of venous stasis, improve the appearance of the extremity, and, if possible, eliminate the cause of the varicosities to prevent progression of the disease. The severity and cause of the venous insufficiency determine the type of therapy recommended. About one-third of patients with simple varicose veins require no therapy at all or only commonsense advice about taking care of their legs.

A. Nonoperative Management: Nonoperative management can improve venous return and reduce pressure in varicose superficial veins. Walking should be encouraged, and prolonged sitting and standing should be forbidden. The patient should be instructed to elevate the leg as frequently as possible to reduce venous pressure. Properly fitted elastic stockings will compress the superficial veins and prevent reflux of blood from the deep to the superficial veins via incompetent perforators, prevent edema, and assist the muscular pumping action of the calf. The stockings should extend from the distal metatarsals to just below the knee, because this is where the varicosities are most severe and because stockings that include the thigh always slip downward unless supported by a garter. Elastic stockings relieve symptoms, conceal the veins, and prevent further deterioration. Elastic bandages can also be used for compression but must be applied carefully to avoid a tourniquet effect.

Elastic support combined with periodic elevation and exercise is the treatment of choice for most patients with uncomplicated varicose veins and gives excellent relief of symptoms when the varicosities are mild or when the patient is elderly or refuses surgery.

B. Compression Sclerotherapy: Veins can be eliminated either by sclerotherapy or by surgery. The two methods are often complementary. Sclerotherapy, as now used, obliterates and produces permanent fibrotic obliteration of collapsed veins—unlike earlier injection procedures, which attempted to induce thrombosis of the varices. With the patient recumbent and the vein collapsed, small amounts (0.5 mL) of sclerosing solution (3% sodium tetradecyl sulfate) are injected into each varix with a fine-gauge needle. Isolation of the injected segment is maintained by digital pressure; thereafter, continuous pressure on the veins is maintained for 1–2 weeks with elastic bandages. This prevents thrombosis and allows a fibrous union to form between the two walls of the collapsed vein. Multiple sites can be injected at the initial visit and others subsequently. This method of treatment is generally performed as an outpatient procedure and is much less expensive than surgical therapy. Complications are few, and when injection is successful, it offers the best cosmetic result of any available method. Extravasation necrosis of the skin is the most serious local complication and can cause poor cosmetic results. The short-term results of injection sclerotherapy are as good as operation, but long-term follow-up favors surgery. Injection sclerotherapy is best reserved for small unsightly veins, dilated superficial veins, lower leg perforators, and recurrent or persistent veins after operation. Sclerotherapy at or above the knee tends to be unsatisfactory. With incompetence of the main long or short saphenous vein, the only effective treatment is surgery.

C. Surgical Therapy: A minority of patients will require surgical therapy for one of the following indications: (1) severe symptoms; (2) very large varices, even if asymptomatic; (3) attacks of superficial phlebitis; (4) hemorrhage from a ruptured varix; (5) ulceration from venous stasis (usually in conjunction with deep venous insufficiency); or (6) cosmetic reasons. Surgical treatment entails removal of the varicose veins and ligation of incompetent perforating branches. For secondary varicosities with deep venous insufficiency, surgical removal is usually only an adjunct to the conservative measures outlined above.

The results of vein stripping depend upon the thoroughness of the procedure. Incompetent superficial and perforating veins must all be identified and marked preoperatively. This is best done the evening before operation, using an ink or dye that will not wash off during the surgical scrub. The operation, performed under general or regional anesthesia, involves ligation of the greater saphenous vein and its tributaries at its junction with the common femoral vein in the groin. The entire saphenous vein is then removed by passing an intraluminal stripper from the exposed saphenous vein at the ankle to the divided end in the groin and avulsing the entire vein. Since most of the visible varicosities are actually tributaries of the main trunk, they can be eliminated either through multiple small incisions or by later sclerotherapy. Once the main channels have been removed, however, most of the tributaries will thrombose. Subfascial ligation of the incompetent perforat-

ing branches via separate small incisions is important, since they often communicate with tributaries of the main trunk rather than the main trunk itself. Less extensive operations that spare the main greater saphenous vein are appropriate for cosmetic treatment of asymptomatic small varicosities. Varicosities of the lesser saphenous systems are removed through incisions behind the lateral malleolus and just below the popliteal fossa.

Postoperatively, the legs are supported with elastic bandages for approximately 6 weeks. Elevation of the legs in bed minimizes postoperative swelling. Walking is encouraged, but sitting and standing are forbidden.

Results & Prognosis

After surgical treatment, varicosities recur in about 10% of patients. The most common causes of recurrence are failure to ligate all the tributaries of the greater saphenous system at the saphenofemoral junction and failure to ligate the incompetent perforators. Some recurrences may be due to progression of the initial pathologic process. Symptomatic relief can be expected in nearly all cases if the symptoms were in fact due to the varicose veins. Cosmetic results can be similarly gratifying.

Beaglehole R: Epidemiology of varicose veins. World J Surg 1986;10:898.

Clarke GH et al: Venous wall function in the pathogenesis of varicose veins. Surgery 1992;111:402.

Gloviczki P et al: Klippel-Trenaunay syndrome: The risks and benefits of vascular interventions. Surgery 1991; 110:469.

Hobbs JT: Varicose veins. Br Med J 199 1;303:707.

Jamieson C: The management of varicose veins. Practitioner 1989;233:578.

Keith LM Jr, Smead WL: Saphenous vein stripping and its complications. Surg Clin North Am 1983;63:1303.

Nehler MR, Moneta GL: The lower extremity venous system: Part I. Anatomy and normal physiology. Perspect Vasc Surg 1991;4:104.

Tremblay J, Lewis EW, Allen PT: Selecting a treatment for primary varicose veins. Can Med Assoc J 1985;133:20.

Wilkinson Jr GE, MacLaren IF: Long term review of procedures for venous perforator insufficiency. Surg Gynecol Obstet 1986;163:117.

VENOUS THROMBOSIS & THROMBOPHLEBITIS

Essentials of Diagnosis

- Clinical manifestations may be absent.
- Swelling, pain, erythema, warmth, discomfort, calf tenderness, and a positive Homans sign may be present.
- Fever, tachycardia, elevated sedimentation rate.
- Pulmonary embolism, usually without signs or symptoms in the leg.

General Considerations

Thrombophlebitis and pulmonary embolism are common, sometimes fatal complications of venous thrombosis in surgical patients. Up to 600,000 patients with deep venous thrombosis are hospitalized annually in the United States.

With insight that has withstood the test of many experiments, Virchow postulated in 1856 that venous thrombosis was related to three factors (Virchow's triad): (1) abnormalities in the vein wall (inflammation), (2) alterations in blood flow (stasis), and (3) alterations in the blood (hypercoagulability) (Table 37–1). Although much still remains to be learned, it is useful to think of thrombosis as a response of blood to injury and then attempt to identify the injurious agents. Most episodes are probably multifactorial.

Some understanding of primary hemostasis, coagulation, and the functions of the venous wall is required to appreciate the pathophysiology and treatment of this disease (Figure 37–3). Venous thrombi (red thrombi) are composed principally of erythrocytes trapped in a fine fibrin mesh with few platelets. Arterial thrombi, on the other hand, are composed of large aggregates of platelets trapped in fibrin strands with very few red cells (white thrombi), suggesting a different mechanism of formation.

A. Flow Stasis: It is generally assumed that stasis of blood flow and pooling of blood in the veins of the lower extremities predispose to venous thrombosis. For example, postoperative bed rest and inactivity are associated with decreased velocity of flow in the femoral vein, and the incidence of venous thrombosis increases with periods of immobility. Experimentally, however, stasis alone does not produce thrombosis, although by protecting activated procoagulants from circulating inhibitors and fibrinolysins and from clearance by the liver, it predisposes to spontaneous venous thrombosis.

B. Hypercoagulability: Thrombophlebitis is

Table 37–1. Pathogenesis of venous thrombosis.

Abnormal vein wall
Varicose veins
Previous thrombophlebitis
Trauma to vein wall (intravenous cannulations)
Inflammatory process around veins (especially pelvic)
Venous stasis
Bed rest
Prolonged positions of dependency of legs
Restriction of leg motion (casts, debility, postoperative pain)
Congestive heart failure
Compression of veins by tumor
Pressure from pillows under knees
Decreased arterial flow (shock)
Hypercoagulability of blood
Trauma (surgery, childbirth, injury)
Hyperviscosity (polycythemia)
Cancer
Use of oral contraceptives
Deficiency of antithrombin III, protein S, and protein C

rare among patients with congenital coagulation deficiencies. In postoperative patients, the plasma concentrations of clotting factors rise, and the peak corresponds in time to the peak incidence of thromboembolism. These two observations tend to implicate hypercoagulability, a state in which activated coagulation factors, normally absent, are present intravascularly or where there is decreased activity of naturally occurring anticoagulants. Hypercoagulability remains difficult to define and detect in the laboratory, although most physicians accept its role in the genesis of thromboembolic disease (Table 37–1). The postpartum state, for example, is associated with increased plasma levels of fibrinogen, prothrombin, and other coagulation factors and decreased fibrinolysin. Use of oral contraceptives also appears to cause hypercoagulability, and thromboembolic complications are several times more common in women who take these hormones than in those who do not. Pathologic thrombosis can also be caused by deficiencies in certain plasma proteins that normally inhibit thrombus formation, such as antithrombin III, protein C, protein S, and heparin cofactor II. Deficiencies in these proteins can be congenital or acquired. Patients with antithrombin III deficiency are predisposed to venous thrombosis, pulmonary embolism, and, rarely, arterial thrombosis. circulatory shock is another condition in which thromboembolic complications are increased in association with hypercoagulability.

C. Changes in the Vessel Wall: Damage to the intima explains certain forms of venous thrombosis such as those due to catheters, infection, and external compression, but there has been no conclusive evidence of an abnormal intima preceding the majority of deep venous thromboses. It has been shown experimentally that minor breaches in the endothelium expose underlying collagen and lead to platelet aggregation, degranulation, and thrombus formation. Decreased fibrinolytic activity due to decreased endothelial production of plasminogen or plasminogen activators has been associated with recurrent episodes of thrombosis. It seems certain that most venous thromboses develop in the absence of inflammation of the vein wall (phlebothrombosis) and that the thrombotic process itself initiates the inflammatory reaction recognized clinically as thrombophlebitis.

Pathogenesis of Venous Thrombosis (Table 37–1)

In a given patient, the cause of venous thrombosis may be difficult to pinpoint, but the following general factors in pathogenesis are accepted: Venous thrombi may develop on normal endothelium. The process usually begins in the venous sinuses in the muscles of the legs and in the valve cusps; both are localized areas of relative stasis that allow accumulation of activated clotting factors. Platelets play an important role in the early phases of thrombus formation and

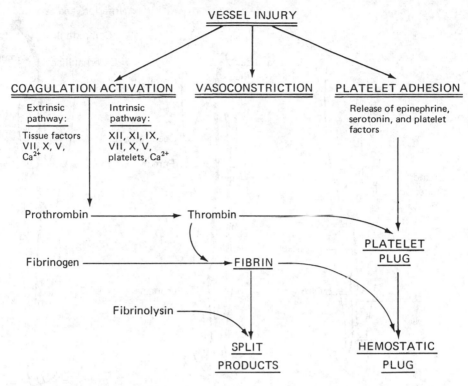

Figure 37–3. Factors involved in arrest of hemorrhage. Injury to the blood vessel wall initiates a series of reactions that arrest hemorrhage. The exposed subendothelial collagen initiates formation of the platelet plug (primary hemostasis). The coagulation system is activated, leading to production of fibrin, which interacts with the platelet plug to form a hemostatic plug. These relationships are also involved in spontaneous thrombus formation, although the inciting event is usually not identifiable.

trigger the coagulation process. As the platelet aggregate grows, procoagulants are released, the venous lumen becomes compromised, and local stasis and hypercoagulability sustain the process. In addition, the platelet nidus creates turbulent flow, which augments platelet aggregation. Once initiated, however, coagulation is the dominant process and produces retrograde and prograde thrombosis.

Clinical Findings

A. Symptoms and Signs: The clinical spectrum varies greatly from no symptoms to severe pain and systemic signs of inflammation. Most patients complain of aching discomfort and tightness in the involved calf or thigh. The pain is aggravated by muscular exercise, and the involved leg may feel stiff. Swelling varies from minimal to massive. In some cases the onset is rapid and associated with tachycardia, anxiety, and fever.

The location of the thrombus determines the location of the physical findings. The most frequent site of thrombus formation is the calf, especially the venous sinuses of the soleus muscle and the posterior tibial and peroneal veins (Figure 37–4). Swelling in

these cases involves the foot and ankle but may be slight or even absent. Calf pain and tenderness are usually prominent but may also be absent.

Femoral vein thrombosis, which is frequently associated with calf thrombosis, produces pain and tenderness in the distal thigh and popliteal region. Swelling is more prominent than with calf vein thrombosis alone and extends to the level of the knee. Thrombi involving the iliofemoral venous segment produce the most dramatic manifestations, often with massive swelling, pain, and tenderness of the entire lower extremity. **Phlegmasia cerulea dolens** is the most severe form of iliofemoral thrombosis. It causes such marked obstruction of venous outflow that cyanosis develops. It can progress to venous gangrene. **Phlegmasia alba dolens** is another variant characterized by arterial spasm and a pale, cool leg with diminished pulses.

There may be tenderness to palpation along the course of any of the involved veins. With deep venous thrombosis in the calf, active dorsiflexion of the foot often produces calf pain (Homans' sign), but diagnostically this is an unreliable test. Tenderness of the calf when the muscles are compressed against the

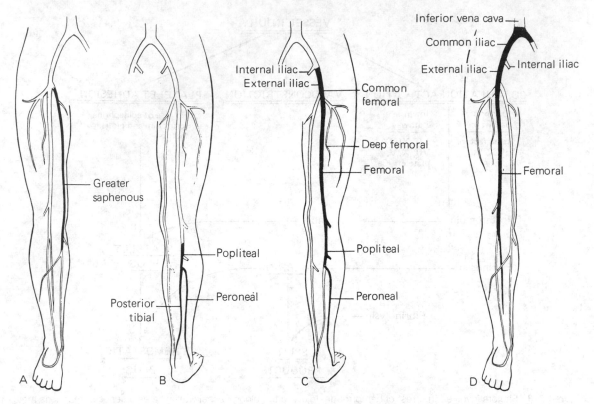

Figure 37–4. Common patterns of venous thrombosis. **A:** Superficial thrombophlebitis. **B:** The most common form of deep thrombophlebitis. **C** and **D:** Deep thrombophlebitis from the calf to the iliac veins. These patterns produce phlegmasia alba dolens or, if more complete, phlegmasia cerulea dolens. The usual locations of thrombosis in milk leg are shown in **C.** (Reproduced, with permission, from Haller JA Jr: *Deep Thrombophlebitis: Pathophysiology and Treatment.* Saunders, 1967.)

tibia may be a manifestation of thrombosis of the deep veins. This finding is also unreliable but may be the first clue to deep venous thrombosis.

Differences in the circumference of the affected extremity compared to the unaffected one are often detectable only with a measuring tape; swelling is one of the most reliable diagnostic signs. The superficial veins are sometimes visibly dilated, and if the inflammatory component is significant, there may be increased local warmth and erythema.

B. Diagnostic Tests: The diagnosis of deep venous thrombosis by clinical examination is incorrect in about half of cases, principally because about half of patients with this condition have no physical signs and because the physical signs that are present are nonspecific. An objective diagnostic test should be used before subjecting a patient to anticoagulation.

1. Ascending phlebography–With the patient standing but not bearing weight on the extremity being examined, radiopaque contrast medium is injected into a vein on the dorsum of the foot. Fluoroscopy and serial x-rays can opacify calf, popliteal, femoral, and iliac veins in one or more views. The four cardinal signs of thrombosis are constant filling defects, abrupt termination of the dye column, nonfilling of the entire deep venous system or portions thereof, and diversion of flow (Figure 37–5). Not all veins in the lower extremities can be visualized by this method—notably the sinuses of the calf muscles, where thrombosis usually begins, and the deep femoral vein, which is opacified in only 50% of patients. Even so, phlebography demonstrates over 90% of thrombi and is considered the most accurate method of detection. If properly performed, a negative venogram essentially rules out venous thrombosis of the lower extremities. Because it is impractical to repeat phlebography at frequent intervals and because venous thrombosis will occasionally develop in the calf after venography, the procedure is unsatisfactory for screening. Venography using radioisotopes (radionuclide venography) instead of contrast medium is a simpler method that appears to be accurate and reliable in detecting major vein occlusion and is being more widely used in many hospitals. Both types of venography can be performed on outpatients.

2. Ultrasound–The hand-held, continuous-wave Doppler ultrasound probe can distinguish between flow and stasis in a major vein and indicate whether

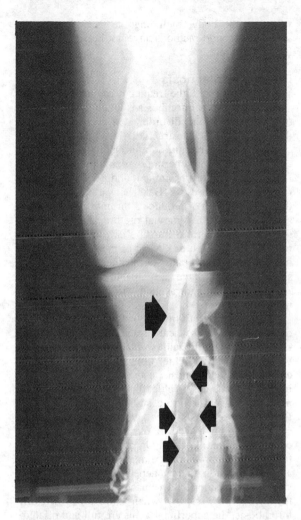

Figure 37–5. Contrast venogram of leg showing multiple intraluminal filling defects *(arrows)*.

the vein is patent or obstructed. Except for the muscular and deep femoral veins, all the major deep veins of the lower limb can be evaluated by Doppler ultrasound. Small thrombi are not revealed, since they produce insignificant obstruction. One component of the test involves briefly squeezing the calf or thigh and listening for the augmented flow in the femoral vein that normally follows. Theoretically, a thrombus might be broken loose if the leg is squeezed too vigorously, though this is a rare occurrence. When the iliofemoral veins are thrombosed, normal respiratory fluctuations in flow are abolished. This can also be detected by ultrasound techniques. False-negative results can occur with thrombi that only partially obstruct the vessel lumen and when extensive collateral venous flow is present. Nevertheless, Doppler ultrasound is a simple and rapid method of searching for large occlusive thrombi and is accurate 80–85% of the time. It is insensitive to isolated calf vein thrombosis and cannot be relied upon as a screening method to detect early disease in this area. The examination is inexpensive and noninvasive and can be repeated frequently, but it is highly operator-dependent.

3. Duplex ultrasound–This method combines real time B-mode ultrasound imaging with Doppler flow analysis. Contemporary instruments also employ color flow imaging, which permits determination of flow direction and turbulence and detects partially occlusive thrombi. B-mode criteria of thrombosis include incompressibility of veins under the ultrasound probe, visible thrombus (echogenicity), and lack of venous distention with Valsalva's maneuver. When combined with Doppler criteria of vein obstruction, duplex ultrasound is very accurate in detecting major above-the-knee axial vein thrombosis (sensitivity and specificity rates are 90–100%). Most duplex errors are in below-the-knee veins, where specificity is only 75%. Isolated iliac vein thrombosis may not be detectable by B-mode imaging but should be correctly diagnosed by the Doppler signals.

In recent years, the duplex scan (with or without color flow) has become the standard test for diagnosis of deep venous thrombosis in symptomatic patients. Its accuracy is superior to that of other noninvasive methods and approaches that of venography. But duplex venous scanning is time-consuming, moderately expensive, and requires considerable technician time and skill.

4. Plethysmography–Deep inspiration slows venous flow, so that if the leg veins are patent, the volume and pressure of their blood rise during inspiration and fall during expiration. Plethysmography measures changes in volume of the extremity resulting from obstruction of venous outflow. **Electrical impedance plethysmography** involves calculation of the amount of blood in the leg based upon changes in conductivity and electrical resistance. This technique can detect iliac, femoral, and popliteal thrombi, the most important sources of pulmonary emboli. As with ultrasound, impedance plethysmography is less accurate for examining the calf and is insensitive to partially occluding thrombi, but a positive test will be correct in at least 90% of patients. As with other methods that depend upon venous obstruction, impedance plethysmography may be negative when proximal vein thrombosis is associated with well-developed collateral vessels. Cooperation of the patient is essential for the respiratory maneuvers and may be difficult to obtain in the immediate post-operative period. The **phleborrheograph,** a sophisticated and expensive instrument consisting of multiple strain-gauge plethysmographs, appears to be very sensitive and accurate in detecting venous obstruction (thrombosis) in the calf, thigh, and pelvis but has been found to be relatively insensitive in asymptomatic patients.

5. Radioactive fibrinogen–Because circulating

fibrinogen becomes incorporated into newly forming thrombi, the thrombi can be detected by external scanning over the veins if the fibrinogen is labeled with a radioactive material such as 125 I. Routine screening with this method has shown that deep venous thrombosis occurs in as many as 30–60% of patients following general surgical procedures and in 50% of patients undergoing orthopedic or neurosurgical operations. Clinical signs of venous thrombosis are present in only 5–10% of these cases. The thrombosis most often begins during the operation. About 90% of postoperative thrombi detected by this method are confined to the calf and are probably not dangerous, but about 20% of these calf thrombi extend into the popliteal or femoral veins, where they produce clinical signs and potentially significant emboli. Radioactive fibrinogen seems sensitive enough to detect small thrombi in venous sinuses of the soleus muscle or the posterior tibial and peroneal veins. At present, this is the most sensitive test for venous thrombosis and is theoretically the best screening method, but it will not detect preexisting thrombi that are not actively incorporating fibrinogen, and it cannot detect femoral, iliac or pelvic thromboses. Its use in diagnosis is limited, because it requires 12–24 hours to complete. The results with radioactive fibrinogen correlate closely with contrast venography, and false-positive and false-negative tests are rare. One of the advantages of the radioactive fibrinogen test is that it can be repeated daily and the progress of the thrombi followed after a single dose of radioactive fibrinogen. Nevertheless, it is rarely used as a clinical test because of its limitations and the availability and accuracy of duplex scans.

6. Venous pressure measurements–The physiology of the deep veins has been discussed earlier in this chapter. With deep venous thrombosis, the walking venous pressure in the veins on the dorsum of the foot is abnormally elevated. Pressure measurement, however, will not distinguish acute from chronic deep venous thrombosis and therefore has relatively little clinical usefulness in diagnosing acute venous thrombosis.

7. Other tests–Several blood tests have been developed to detect intravascular coagulation, including measurement of fibrinopeptide A, circulating fibrin monomer complexes, and serum fibrin degradation products. Measurement of the degradation product fragment E is a sensitive test for venous thromboembolism, but the procedure is still too complicated for practical clinical diagnosis. All of these blood tests lack specificity and for that reason have not proved to be clinically useful.

Monoclonal antibody-labeled platelets and fibrin have recently been introduced as thrombus-imaging agents. Early results in humans have confirmed experimental studies showing the ability of these agents to localize venous thrombi. It is hoped that this technique will eventually be able to detect thrombi anywhere in the body, including the trunk and brain, where ultrasound methods have not been as successful as elsewhere.

Differential Diagnosis

As already noted, the frequency of clinical diagnosis of deep venous thrombosis is much lower than the true incidence of this disorder. Leg swelling could be due to lymphatic obstruction, but this is usually chronic and the edema nonpitting. It may be more acute if cellulitis is superimposed, but in this case, inflammation is more prominent and a wound is often present. Synovial cysts (Baker's cyst) can compress the popliteal vein or produce a thrombophlebitis-like syndrome by acute synovial rupture with extravasation of synovial fluid into the calf **(pseudothrombophlebitis syndrome)**. Most of these patients have inflammatory arthropathy of the knee with knee effusion, and may have a palpable popliteal mass. Arthrography and ultrasound will establish the correct diagnosis.

Contusion of a calf muscle or rupture of the tendon of the plantaris muscle can produce a swollen, painful calf and may be difficult to differentiate from deep venous occlusion. Acute onset of symptoms during exercise and ecchymosis in the calf point to muscle injury. In some cases, phlebography or duplex scanning may be required to establish the true diagnosis. Bilateral swelling of the lower extremities, while sometimes seen in deep venous thrombosis, is usually of cardiac or renal origin. Occasionally it is difficult to distinguish an arterial from a venous occlusion. In arterial occlusion, there is generally more pain and no swelling, the superficial veins are not distended, and they refill very slowly when emptied. In venous thrombosis, the superficial veins are full and dilated. Sensation in the extremity usually disappears promptly in acute arterial occlusion, whereas it usually persists in acute thrombophlebitis. Duplex scanning is of greatest use in demonstrating a patent venous system when venous thrombosis cannot be differentiated from other entities, so that unnecessary anticoagulation and hospitalization can be avoided. A normal venous duplex examination performed by a competent sonographer is strong evidence against the presence of major venous occlusion and can be relied upon nearly as much as a negative venogram.

Complications

A. Chronic Venous Insufficiency: This complication, discussed in detail later, usually follows iliofemoral thrombophlebitis but not thrombosis confined to the leg.

B. Varicose Veins: Secondary varicose veins may develop as collaterals when the deep venous system is occluded.

C. Venous Gangrene: Gangrene due to massive venous thrombosis may occur in phlegmasia cerulea dolens without associated arterial thrombosis. This is a rare condition but is often fatal when it does occur. Venous thrombectomy in phlegmasia cerulea dolens is strongly indicated, since it may prevent gangrene.

D. Pulmonary Embolism: Pulmonary embolism occurs when a thrombus becomes dislodged from its attachment to the venous wall and is carried into the pulmonary arteries. This is discussed in detail below.

Prevention

The incidence of postoperative deep venous thrombosis and pulmonary embolism can be reduced by employing a suitable prophylactic regimen. Nevertheless, pulmonary embolism is the most common preventable cause of death following major operations. Patients with predisposing factors (Table 37–2) comprise a high-risk group in whom the following preventive measures should be considered:

A. Physical Measures to Reduce Venous Stasis: Active leg exercises (quadriceps, plantar flexion), leg elevation, and the use of elastic stockings improve femoral venous blood flow and reduce the incidence of deep venous thrombosis, especially in elderly patients. Early ambulation after surgery and avoidance of prolonged bed rest also promote venous return. Prolonged sitting and standing should be avoided because they cause venous stasis. Adequate postoperative hydration minimizes hemoconcentration and increased blood viscosity. During operative procedures, galvanic stimulation to produce contraction of calf muscles, intermittent external calf compression with a pneumatic sleeve or boot, and the use of motorized foot maneuvers all diminish the incidence of formation of calf thrombi. Of these methods, the pneumatic boots have been the most widely tested and clinically successful. They are nearly as effective as anticoagulants and free from their side effects. Passive measures that promote venous drainage, such as elevating the foot of the bed 15–20 degrees, should also be employed. All of these methods lessen stasis and lower the incidence of venous thrombosis except in high-risk patients undergoing operation for malignant disease. Brief regular periods of walking during long automobile or airplane trips should be encour-

Table 37–2. Risk factors for development of venous thrombosis.

Cancer
Oral contraceptive use
Operations on hips or pelvis
High blood viscosity (polycythemia)
Obesity
Varicose veins
Obstructed venous return
Lack of movement
Childbirth or pregnancy
Previous history of deep vein thrombosis
Old age (over 60)
Prolonged or complex surgical procedures

aged, for venous thrombosis may occur in such settings even in active healthy adults.

B. Anticoagulation: Controlled trials strongly suggest that prophylactic anticoagulation in high-risk patients markedly decreases the incidence of postoperative deep venous thrombosis and pulmonary thromboembolism. The following agents have been studied:

1. Prothrombin depressants–The vitamin K antagonists (warfarin and phenindione derivatives) are effective prophylactic agents when anticoagulation is initiated before and maintained for several days after operation. With careful control of dosage, operation is safe and hemorrhagic complications are infrequent and seldom serious. Warfarin is more effective than mini-dose heparin in patients undergoing hip operation. The use of these agents is less popular in the United States than in Europe.

2. Platelet function suppressants–The use of these agents is based on the observations that platelet deposition behind venous valve cusps is often the first event in the development of a venous thrombus and that platelet aggregation is relatively unaffected by conventional anticoagulants. Infusions of dextran 40 or dextran 70 during and after surgery reduce the incidence of thromboembolism. The mechanism of action of dextran is complex but includes plasma volume expansion, reduced platelet adhesiveness, coating of platelet and red cell surfaces (increased electronegativity), and copolymerization with fibrin, making it more susceptible to fibrinolysis. Among the side effects of dextran infusions are congestive heart failure, acute renal failure, and allergic reactions. The bleeding complications can be avoided if the dose is limited to less than 1 L/d. Aspirin has been shown to be of prophylactic value in hip surgery, but dipyridamole has been found ineffective. Sulfinpyrazone reduces the incidence of idiopathic recurrent venous thrombosis, but its value as a prophylactic agent in surgical patients is unproved.

3. Heparin–Several good clinical trials using iodine ^{125}I-fibrinogen scanning have shown the efficacy and safety of low-dose (mini) heparin in preventing deep venous thrombosis. The usual regimen is 5000 units subcutaneously 2 hours preoperatively and every 8–12 hours postoperatively for several days. This dose does not significantly prolong the coagulation time as measured by the standard laboratory tests (APTT, Lee-White). The beneficial effect is thought to be through enhancement of a natural inhibitor of activated factor X. Bleeding complications (wound hematoma) and transfusion requirements are only slightly increased with this regimen. Low-dose heparin is much less effective in patients undergoing prostate and hip surgery. Addition of the vasoconstrictor dihydroergotamine to the heparin regimen appears to potentiate the prophylactic benefits of heparin alone in these high-risk patients, but this combination of agents is currently not commercially available in the United States.

Low-molecular-weight heparins are a new class of anticoagulants derived from standard unfractionated heparin. They produce equally effective anticoagulation with less risk of bleeding complications than standard heparin. They inhibit activated factor X but have little effect on the partial thromboplastin time. Several such agents have been used in Europe, and some are being tested in the United States. They appear to be effective for prophylaxis after general surgery as well as hip surgery.

Heparin prophylaxis is contraindicated in operations where even minimal bleeding could be disastrous (brain or eye surgery), but intermittent pneumatic calf compression is an effective alternative. In general, heparin is easier to control than the prothrombin depressants.

Treatment of Deep Venous Thrombosis

The objectives of treatment are to prevent formation of additional thrombi, to prevent growth and embolization of existing thrombi, and to minimize venous valve damage.

A. Bed Rest and Elevation: The patient should be confined to bed with the feet elevated 15–20 degrees above the level of the heart. Since it takes 7–8 days for experimental thrombi to become firmly adherent to vein walls, it is common practice to continue bed rest for about this long after the onset of symptoms. Elevation reduces the edema and pain, and the resulting increased venous flow inhibits formation of new thrombus. Application of elastic bandages or stockings to the leg is indicated because they also increase the velocity of venous flow. Bed rest should be continued until the swelling, pain, and tenderness have resolved. Graduated ambulation with elastic support is then permitted, but standing and sitting are forbidden, because the accompanying rise in venous pressure aggravates edema and discomfort. The use of elastic support and limitations on sitting and standing are required for 3–6 months until recanalization and collateralization develop. Continuous warm moist dressings on the involved leg provide symptomatic relief in the acute phase.

B. Drug Treatment: Unless there are specific contraindications, anticoagulants should be administered. The goals are to prevent propagation of the original thrombus, avert the development of new thrombi, and prevent pulmonary embolization of thrombi. By allowing natural fibrinolysis to operate unopposed, anticoagulation may also hasten dissolution of the thrombus.

1. Heparin–Heparin, an acid mucopolysaccharide, inhibits thrombus formation by neutralizing thrombin, by blocking the formation of thromboplastin, and by inhibiting the platelet release reaction. It is of proved benefit in the treatment of deep venous thrombosis and in the prevention of pulmonary em-

bolism. Heparin therapy should be started as soon as the diagnosis of deep venous thrombosis has been confirmed. Since it is not absorbed from the gastrointestinal tract, it must be given either intravenously or subcutaneously, but the intravenous method is clearly more effective. Bleeding complications are reduced if dosage is regulated according to one of the coagulation tests such as the whole blood clotting time (Lee-White), activated partial thromboplastin time (APTT) or activated clotting time (ACT). Recurrent episodes of thrombosis and embolism are minimized by administering sufficient heparin by the continuous intravenous route to maintain the APTT at least at 1½ times control. Since the amount of heparin required to achieve any desired degree of anticoagulation may vary from day to day, the degree of anticoagulation should be monitored daily by one of these tests. Bleeding complications are lowest if the heparin is given by continuous intravenous infusion. An initial dose of 100 units/kg body weight should be given intravenously and subsequent doses determined by laboratory tests. The anticoagulant effects of intravenous heparin are immediate. Most patients will initially require 1000–2000 heparin units per hour to achieve adequate anticoagulation. If bolus therapy is selected, the drug should be given every 4 or 6 hours and the test of coagulation performed 1 hour before the next scheduled dose. For acute thrombophlebitis, heparin has traditionally been continued for 7–10 days, the time required for thrombi to become firmly adherent to the vein walls; but a 5-day course of heparin has been shown to be as effective in a randomized prospective clinical trial. If at the end of this time leg pain and tenderness persist, heparin should be continued until they resolve. If pulmonary embolism has occurred, larger doses of heparin should be given and heparin should be continued for an additional 7–10 days (total of 1–3 weeks). The incidence of recurrent pulmonary embolism during standard intravenous heparin therapy is less than 5%. Bleeding, the major complication, occurs in 5–10% of patients, and is most likely to occur in fresh surgical wounds or in the gastrointestinal or genitourinary tract and usually indicates that too much heparin has been administered. Bleeding may also be the first sign of an undiagnosed neoplastic or ulcerated lesion. Protamine sulfate, a heparin inhibitor, can be given if hemorrhage is significant. Drugs such as aspirin that inhibit platelet aggregation should be used cautiously in heparinized patients, because the combination seriously interferes with primary hemostasis as well as coagulation. Thrombocytopenia may occur during heparin administration. Its onset may be within hours or days after heparin is started, and it may be persistent and severe and associated with severe hemorrhage or recurrent thrombosis or thromboembolism. It is due to a heparin-induced antiplatelet antibody that causes platelet aggregation. Therefore, platelet counts should be obtained before and during heparin therapy. Intramuscular injections should be avoided, because of the danger of local hemorrhage at the injection site. As noted earlier, low-molecular-weight heparins may be associated with reduced bleeding complications and are being evaluated clinically.

2. Oral anticoagulants—Coumarin derivatives (most commonly warfarin) block synthesis in the liver of at least four vitamin K-dependent clotting factors: prothrombin, factor VII, factor IX, and factor X. For this reason, the anticoagulant effects are delayed until existing clotting factors are cleared from the circulation.

Since oral anticoagulants are not as effective as heparin and their onset of action is slow, they are best reserved for prophylaxis (see above) of deep venous thrombosis or for long-term anticoagulation after heparin treatment has been discontinued. After acute deep venous thrombosis, oral anticoagulation should be continued for at least 3 months, since this is the time required for development of venous collaterals and is also the time during which most recurrences of thrombosis occur. After pulmonary embolism, 6 months of anticoagulation is indicated. Because oral anticoagulants also inhibit synthesis of the anticoagulant proteins C and S and because protein C has a very short half-life, there is a period of relative hypercoagulability during the first few days of warfarin therapy. Warfarin should not be started until the first or second day of heparin therapy, and the heparin should be discontinued only after the prothrombin time has been at therapeutic levels for a few days. Because interaction occurs between the coumarin derivatives and many other drugs (eg, barbiturates, nonsteroidal anti-inflammatory agents, some antibiotics, H_2 receptor blockers, etc), patients taking oral anticoagulants must be carefully monitored. The therapeutic range for oral anticoagulant therapy has become controversial. It is now believed that the usual dose sufficient to increase the prothrombin time to 2–2.5 times the control value is excessive and that an equal antithrombotic effect can be achieved with a prothrombin time of 1.35–1.6 times control. The use of the International Normalized Ratio (INR), which accounts for variations in activity of reagents used in prothrombin tests, has been advocated by British and European hematologists but has yet to be endorsed by the vast majority of North American institutions or medical journals. The recommended anticoagulant intensity for treatment of deep vein thrombosis using this system is an INR of 2.0–3.0. Many laboratories are now reporting INR values along with prothrombin time results. With these treatment regimens, recurrent thromboembolic events occur in < 2% and bleeding complications in 5–10% of patients so treated. Excessive prolongation of the prothrombin time can be treated by administration of vitamin K. Self-administered, low-dose heparin therapy is being used by some as an alternative to warfarin in the long-term management of thromboembolic disorders and ap-

pears to be associated with fewer bleeding complications.

3. Other medications—Fibrinolytic activators (urokinase, streptokinase) lyse fresh intravascular thrombi, but bleeding complications are more common than with conventional anticoagulants, especially in fresh surgical wounds. Fibrinolytic agents produce rapid clearance of the occluded veins and may preserve competency and function of venous valves better than heparin therapy. This could limit or prevent development of postphlebitic syndrome, which is the major attractiveness of lytic therapy. Preservation of normal venous function in about 40% of patients has been documented in several studies employing streptokinase or urokinase. However, these agents offer no advantages over heparin for recurrent venous thrombosis or thrombosis that has been present for more than 72 hours. Tissue plasminogen activator produced by recombinant gene technology appears to be more specific for thrombus and more rapid in action than other lytic agents, but so far it has not been shown to be more effective. A coagulant fraction (ancrod) prepared from the venom of the Malayan pit viper attacks fibrinogen and produces intravascular defibrination. It seems effective for deep venous thrombosis but is not superior to heparin. Fibrinolytic and defibrinating agents will undoubtedly receive much attention in the future, as they have several theoretic advantages over conventional anticoagulants.

C. Operative Procedures: The vast majority of patients with acute venous thrombosis are satisfactorily managed medically. In a small percentage, however, operation is necessary.

1. Venous thrombectomy—This operation involves incising the common femoral vein in the groin and extracting the clots. The goals are (1) to prevent the postphlebitic syndrome, (2) to prevent pulmonary embolism, and (3) in phlegmasia cerulea dolens, to prevent venous gangrene. In massive iliofemoral venous thrombosis, successful thrombectomy will rapidly relieve acute venous stasis and the inflammatory reaction and may save the limb when impending venous gangrene exists. It is most likely to be successful if performed within the first 24 hours after onset of symptoms. In about two-thirds of patients, postoperative phlebograms reveal reocclusion of the involved segments, so that the ultimate value of this procedure remains unproved. Construction of a temporary small arteriovenous fistula improves long-term venous patency.

2. Venous interruption—The rationale of venous interruption is the prevention of recurrent and potentially fatal pulmonary embolism by trapping the thrombus in the peripheral venous segment. In patients with a single pulmonary embolus treated with anticoagulants, the fatal pulmonary embolism rate is only about 1–2%. Therefore, surgical treatment should be reserved for the unusual patient who fails to respond to anticoagulant therapy or who has specific contraindications to its use. Ligation of the superficial femoral vein just before its junction with the common femoral vein prevents embolization from distal muscular and deep veins and rarely is followed by chronic venous insufficiency. Obviously, it does not protect against emboli arising central to the point of ligation. Ligation of the common femoral vein is almost always followed by chronic venous insufficiency. With the realization that most fatal pulmonary emboli arise from iliac or pelvic veins, venous interruption in the extremities has given way to techniques that trap emboli in the inferior vena cava. Ligation of the inferior vena cava prevents fatal pulmonary embolism, and the operative death rate is low (about 5%). The incidence of significant venous insufficiency of the legs following vena caval ligation varies greatly and is probably more closely related to the extent of preexisting venous disease than to the caval interruption itself. The lower extremity sequelae are minimized by procedures such as plication or clipping, which only partially occlude the lumen and create a sieve through which blood flows unimpeded but which prevents passage of clot. Ligation of the left ovarian or spermatic vein should be performed concomitantly, particularly when there is pelvic vein thrombosis. These direct approaches have largely been replaced by a variety of intraluminal devices that can be implanted via a femoral or jugular venous cutdown or percutaneously and have a much lower complication rate than do direct operations on the vena cava. Each of these devices is designed to trap large emboli while preserving inferior vena cava flow and patency. They are made in a variety of shapes and are associated with a decreased incidence of both extremity edema and recurrent thrombophlebitis (Figure 37–6). The Greenfield filter is the most commonly used of these devices. Recent studies indicate that it is 97% effective in preventing recurrent pulmonary embolism and has an equally high patency rate.

The indications for venous interruption are (1) patients in whom anticoagulation therapy is clearly contraindicated; (2) recurrent pulmonary embolism despite adequate anticoagulation; (3) multiple small pulmonary emboli creating chronic pulmonary insufficiency or pulmonary hypertension; (4) septic emboli refractory to a combination of antibiotic and anticoagulant therapy; and (5) patients who have undergone pulmonary embolectomy. The safety and efficacy of the Greenfield filter has led some to advocate that it be used prophylactically in high-risk patients who have not had a pulmonary embolism. Patients with large free-floating iliac vein thrombi are one example. When emboli arise from septic pelvic thrombophlebitis, the cava should be ligated, not compartmentalized, although the Greenfield filter has been effective in some septic cases. After caval ligation, as many as 5–10% of patients develop recurrent

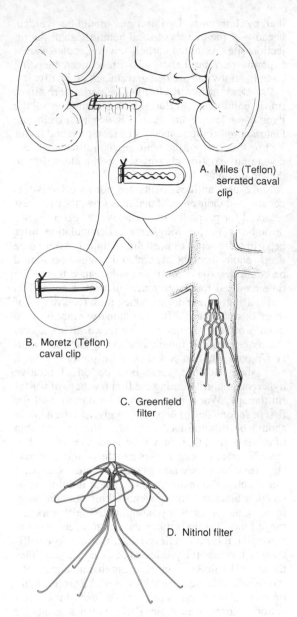

Figure 37–6. Surgical prevention of pulmonary embolism. Large emboli can be trapped by partial interruption of the inferior vena cava. **A:** Serrated Teflon (Miles) clip. **B:** Smooth Teflon (Moretz) clip. These should be placed just distal to the renal veins, and the gonadal veins should be ligated. **C:** Greenfield filter. **D:** Nitinol filter.

emboli transported in collateral veins around the caval ligature or arising in the venous cul-de-sac between the caval ligature and renal veins. Other possible sources are the right atrium and upper extremities.

Barnes RW et al: Perioperative asymptomatic venous thrombosis: Role of duplex scanning versus venography. J Vasc Surg 1989;9:251.

Braverman SJ, Battey PM, Smith RB: Vena cava interruption. Am Surg 1992;58:188.

Browse NL: Prevention of postoperative deep vein thrombosis. Brit J Surg 1988;75:835.

Cambria RP et al: Heparin fails to suppress intimal proliferation in experimental vein grafts. Surgery 1992;111:424.

Colditz GA, Tuden RL, Oster G: Rates of venous thrombosis after general surgery: Combined results of randomised clinical trials. Lancet 1986;2:143.

Collins R et al: Reduction in fatal pulmonary embolism and venous thrombosis by perioperative administration of subcutaneous heparin. N Engl J Med 1988;318:1162.

Comerota AJ et al: Venous duplex imaging: Should it replace hemodynamic tests for deep venous thrombosis? J Vasc Surg 1990;11:53. Cronan JJ: Contemporary venous imaging. Cardiovasc Intervent Radiol 1991;14:87.

Cronan JJ, Dorfman GS: Advances in ultrasound imaging of venous thrombosis. Semin Nucl Med 1991;21:297.

Engesser L et al: Hereditary protein S deficiency: Clinical manifestations. Ann Intern Med 1987;106:677.

Freed JA: Hypercoagulability: Should every patient with venous thrombosis be tested? Postgrad Med 1991;90: 157.

Ginsberg JS, Hirsh J: Anticoagulants during pregnancy. Annu Rev Med 1989;40:79.

Graor RA et al: Comparison of cost-effectiveness of streptokinase and urokinase in the treatment of deep vein thrombosis. Ann Vasc Surg 1987;1:524.

Grossman ZD: Monoclonal antibodies and thromboembolism. J Thorac Imag 1989;4:62.

Harris WH et al: Prophylaxis of deep-vein thrombosis after total hip replacement: Dextran and external pneumatic compression compared with 1.2 or 0.3 gram aspirin daily. J Bone Joint Surg [Am] 1985;67:57.

Hirsh J, Turpie AGG: Use of plasminogen activators in venous thrombosis. World J Surg 1990;14:688.

Hirsh J: Heparin. N Engl J Med 1991;324:1565.

Hirsh J: Oral anticoagulation drugs. N Engl J Med 1991;324:1865.

Hirsh J: Rationale for development of low-molecular-weight heparins and their clinical potential in the prevention of postoperative venous thrombosis. Am J Surg 1991;161:512.

Hommes DW et al: Subcutaneous heparin compared with continuous intravenous heparin administration in the initial treatment of deep vein thrombosis: A meta-analysis. Ann Intern Med 1992;116:279.

Huisman MV et al: Management of clinically suspected acute venous thrombosis in outpatients with serial impedance plethysmography in a community hospital setting. Arch Intern Med 1989;149:511.

Hull RD et al: Continuous intravenous heparin compared with intermittent subcutaneous heparin in the initial treatment of proximal-vein thrombosis. N Engl J Med 1986;315:1109.

Hull RD et al: Heparin for 5 days as compared with 10 days in the initial treatment of proximal venous thrombosis. N Engl J Med 1990;322:1260.

Hull RD et al: Subcutaneous low-molecular-weight heparin compared with continuous intravenous heparin in the treatment of proximal vein thrombosis. N Engl J Med 1992;326:975.

Inada K et al: Effects of intermittent pneumatic leg compression for prevention of postoperative deep venous thrombosis with special reference to fibrinolytic activity. Am J Surg 1988;155:602.

Killewich LA et al: Diagnosis of deep venous thrombosis: A prospective study comparing duplex scanning to contrast venography. Circulation 1989;79:810.

Killewich LA et al: Spontaneous lysis of deep venous thrombi: Rate and outcome. J Vasc Surg 1989;9:89.

Leyvraz PF et al: Prevention of deep vein thrombosis after hip replacement: Randomised comparison between unfractionated heparin and low molecular weight heparin. Br Med J 1991;303:543.

Markel A et al: Pattern and distribution of thrombi in acute venous thrombosis. Arch Surg 1992;127:305.

Mayberry JC et al: The influence of elastic compression stockings on deep venous hemodynamics. J Vasc Surg 1991;13:91.

National Institutes of Health Consensus Development Conference Statement: Prevention of venous thrombosis and pulmonary embolism. Vol 6, No. 2, 1986.

Neglén P et al: Iliofemoral venous thrombectomy followed by percutaneous closure of the temporary arteriovenous fistula. Surgery 1991;110:493.

Parker-Williams J, Vickers R: Major orthopaedic surgery on the leg and thromboembolism: Prophylaxis now or negligence claims later. Br Med J 1991;303:531.

Parsons RE et al: Distinction of age differences in thrombi by ultrasonic tissue characterization. Surg Forum 1991; 42:337.

Plate G et al: Long-term results of venous thrombectomy combined with a temporary arterio-venous fistula. Eur J Vasc Surg 1990;4:483.

Porteous MJ Lef et al: Thigh length versus knee length stockings in the prevention of deep vein thrombosis. Brit J Surg 1989;76:296.

Prandoni P et al: Comparison of subcutaneous low-molecular-weight heparin with intravenous standard heparin in proximal deep-vein thrombosis. Lancet 1992;339:441.

Prins MH, Hirsh J: A critical review of the evidence supporting a relationship between impaired fibrinolytic activity and venous thromboembolism. Arch Intern Med 1991;151:1721.

Reasbeck PG et al: Incidence of deep venous thrombosis after major abdominal surgery in Brisbane. Brit J Surg 1988;75:440.

Rogers LQ, Lutcher CL: Streptokinase therapy for deep vein thrombosis: A comprehensive review of the English literature. Am J Med 1990;88:389.

Rohrer MJ et al: Extended indications for placement of an inferior vena cava filter. J Vasc Surg 1989;10:44.

Rollins DL et al: Origin of deep vein thrombi in an ambulatory population. Am J Surg 1988;156:122.

Samlaska CP, James WD: Superficial thrombophlebitis: II. Secondary hypercoagulable states. J Am Acad Dermatol 1990;23:1.

Schaub RG et al: Early events in the formation of a venous thrombus following local trauma and stasis. Lab Invest 1984;51:218.

Siderov J: Streptokinase vs heparin for deep vein thrombosis: Can lytic therapy be justified? Arch Int Med 1989; 149:1841.

Silver D: An overview of venous thromboembolism prophylaxis. Am J Surg 1991;161:537.

Warkentin TE, Kelton JG: Heparin induced thrombocytopenia. Annu Rev Med 1989;40:31.

Wheeler HB, Anderson FA Jr: Prophylaxis against venous

thromboembolism in surgical patients. Am J Surg 1991; 161:507.

White RH et al: Diagnosis of deep-vein thrombosis using duplex ultrasound. Ann Intern Med 1989;111:2979.

PULMONARY THROMBOEMBOLISM

Essentials of Diagnosis

- Can occur in almost any clinical setting, but most common in elderly, immobilized, sick, or traumatized persons.
- History and clinical findings of deep venous thrombosis often absent.
- Large pulmonary embolus: Sudden onset of dyspnea and anxiety, with or without substernal pain. Signs of acute right heart failure and circulatory collapse may follow shortly afterward.
- Pulmonary infarction: Less severe dyspnea, pleuritic pain, cough, hemoptysis, and peripheral x-ray density in the lung are characteristic.
- Diagnosis suggested by ventilation-perfusion lung scan but established only by pulmonary angiogram.

General Considerations

Pulmonary thromboembolism is common and can occur in almost any clinical setting. It is estimated that 630,000 cases of pulmonary embolism occur annually in the USA, accounting for about 200,000 deaths, making this the third most frequent cause of death. Nonfatal attacks are three to five times more frequent than fatal ones. About one-fourth to one-half of cases of fatal pulmonary embolism occur in patients with an otherwise good prognosis. Elderly, immobilized, sick, or traumatized patients have the highest incidence of pulmonary embolization, and the incidence increases in direct proportion to the duration of the illness and the age of the patient. Embolization is uncommon in healthy young patients. Heart disease is the major risk factor, and deep venous thrombosis of the legs is the most common precursor, though only 30–40% of patients have clinical signs and symptoms of deep vein thrombosis. Other factors affecting incidence include cardiac failure, recent surgical procedures, oral contraceptive use, and blood group A. Bed rest and reduced exercise are associated with a twofold or greater increase in incidence. There is also a high risk of pulmonary embolism during pregnancy and the puerperium.

Most clinically significant pulmonary emboli arise from the iliac and femoral veins. While smaller veins such as those in the calf may become thrombosed, they rarely cause serious clinical manifestations. Only thrombi produced in veins the size of the iliac and femoral veins are large enough to produce emboli with major clinical sequelae. In most patients, the emboli involve lobar arteries in each lung. *Pulmonary embolism and infarction are not synonymous.*

Less than 10% of pulmonary emboli produce infarction. Infarcts are generally located peripherally in the lungs, most often in the lower lobes. The development of an infarct appears related to occlusion of a pulmonary artery in association with chronic lung disease, infection, or congestive heart failure. A true infarct cannot be produced in the normal lung, since complete ligation of the pulmonary artery does not lead to pulmonary infarction. Pulmonary emboli may result from tumor embolization (especially from renal cell carcinoma) of the lungs. Cardiac tumors arising in the right atrium and right ventricle may also cause extensive pulmonary embolization. Thromboemboli can also originate in other systemic veins, such as in axillary-subclavian venous thrombosis.

Occlusion of the pulmonary artery affects the airways, the pulmonary vasculature, the right and left heart, and the bronchial circulation. Thus, many factors are involved in the physiologic responses to pulmonary emboli. Reflex changes, probably secondary to microembolization, may cause tachypnea, pulmonary hypertension, and systemic hypotension. The clinical findings of pulmonary embolism are principally manifestations of mechanical occlusion of the larger pulmonary arteries. The hemodynamic consequences are increases in pulmonary arterial resistance, pulmonary arterial pressure, and right ventricular work. The hemodynamic impact is related to both the immediate preembolic cardiopulmonary status and the extent of embolization. In the absence of preexisting cardiopulmonary disease, the degree of cardiovascular impairment is roughly proportionate to the extent of the obstruction. When cardiorespiratory impairment is severe, however, even minor pulmonary emboli may cause serious cardiorespiratory sequelae. Vasoactive amines—which probably arise from the emboli—as well as prostaglandins appear to contribute to the physiologic response.

Clinical Findings

A. Symptoms and Signs: The clinical manifestations of pulmonary embolism may be similar to many other cardiorespiratory disorders. Many patients have underlying cardiac disease, and dyspnea and tachypnea are the most frequent clinical findings. The more classic signs—hemoptysis, pleural friction rub, gallop rhythm, cyanosis, and chest splinting—are present in only 20% of patients. Clinical signs of venous thrombosis occur in only one-third of patients. Dyspnea is present in 75%, chest pain in 65%, hemoptysis in 25%, altered mental status in 25%, and the triad of dyspnea, chest pain, and hemoptysis in 15%. Sixty percent have tachycardia, and only 10% have an accentuated P_2, 10% cyanosis, and 8% a pleural friction rub. Chest pain of several types may occur, the most common being a dull substernal tightness. Chest pain is frequent with massive but uncommon with lesser emboli.

The most common physical findings are tachypnea

and tachycardia, which are often transient. Sustained tachycardia and tachypnea, particularly when marked, usually indicate massive embolism. Other findings are due to bronchoconstriction. A friction rub, when present, is most commonly heard over the lung bases, because the lower lobes are the most frequent location. A temperature of 37.7–38.3 °C (100–101 °F) is common. A wide, almost fixed splitting of the second heart sound is an ominous finding, since it develops only in patients with marked right ventricular compromise.

Sudden onset of atrial fibrillation in a patient without preexisting cardiac disease should suggest pulmonary embolism, as should the sudden worsening of congestive heart failure. Acute cardiopulmonary disorders such as myocardial infarction, dissecting aortic aneurysm, and pneumothorax are often confused with massive embolism, since they cause substernal discomfort, dyspnea, tachycardia, and electrocardiographic changes.

B. Laboratory Findings:

1. Blood tests–Specific serum enzyme changes may be helpful, although they are seldom conclusive. The triad of elevated LDH and bilirubin and normal AST may be present, but in the presence of massive embolism and acute cardiovascular changes, this combination is not particularly useful. A more rapid means of diagnosis is clearly necessary.

2. Arterial blood gases–Arterial blood gas analysis is frequently helpful, and if arterial hypoxemia is not present, pulmonary embolism is very unlikely. Hypoxemia is nonspecific, however, and, like many of the other findings, may be transient. An increased arterial-alveolar PCO_2 difference may aid in the diagnosis of pulmonary embolism, but it is difficult to measure and is also nonspecific.

C. Imaging Studies:

1. Chest x-ray–Roentgenographic examination of the chest may be normal. With massive pulmonary embolism, there is usually no evidence of congestion, and the peripheral lung fields are blanched because of diminished blood flow. Later, typical wedge-shaped peripheral infiltrates with or without effusion may appear. There is, however, no pathognomonic radiologic sign of pulmonary embolism on the plain chest film, and a reliable diagnosis depends on pulmonary arteriogram or radioactive perfusion scan.

2. Pulmonary perfusion scans–Radioisotope scanning is performed with intravenously injected macromolecules of human serum albumin labeled with ^{99m}Tc or ^{131}I. This procedure delineates the distribution of pulmonary arterial blood flow and reveals areas of decreased perfusion. Lesions present on the plain chest film, such as pneumonitis, atelectasis, emphysematous bullae, or neoplasm, regularly demonstrate a defect on scan (false-positive scan). Therefore, such abnormal areas must be excluded from consideration by a simultaneous plain chest x-ray or ventilation scan (or both). The pulmonary perfusion scan is useful in substantiating the clinical impression of pulmonary embolism before treatment is started. It can be repeated with minimal discomfort to the patient and is the best means of following resolution of pulmonary embolic disease. A perfusion scan with multiple (more than two to four) segmental or lobar defects is interpreted as high probability, whereas subsegmental or nonsegmental perfusion defects are considered low probability for pulmonary embolism. High-probability perfusion scans are very specific for pulmonary embolism and correlate well with pulmonary angiograms. The same is true for low-probability or normal perfusion scans, which exclude significant pulmonary embolism from the differential diagnosis.

3. Ventilation scanning–Sensitivity of perfusion scans can be increased by adding a ventilation scan. ^{133}Xenon ventilation scanning, which demonstrates the distribution of inhaled gas, helps in interpreting the perfusion scan, since it allows differentiation of underperfused and underventilated areas. Typically, a pulmonary embolus produces a defect on perfusion scan in an area of normal ventilation, although ventilation defects are commonly seen in association with the perfusion defect in submassive embolism. Reported figures suggest that pulmonary embolism is present in over 95% of patients with a high probability perfusion scan and a ventilation-perfusion mismatch.

4. Pulmonary arteriography–A selective pulmonary arteriogram is the only definitive method to establish the diagnosis. The potential seriousness of the disease and the significant risks of treatment justify the use of angiography whenever the diagnosis is in reasonable doubt. Arteriography is extremely reliable if performed within 48 hours of the clinical episode. The diagnosis is established by demonstration of unequivocal obstruction or filling defects in the pulmonary arterial tree (Figure 37–7). This most often involves lobar segmental branches. Occasionally, total obstruction of a main pulmonary artery is found, usually in association with severe symptoms.

D. Electrocardiography: About 15% of patients with pulmonary embolism have acute electrocardiographic changes. The most common abnormalities are T-wave inversion and ST segment depression, the result of myocardial ischemia from decreased cardiac output and arterial pressure, and increased right ventricular pressure. Most often the electrocardiographic changes are nonspecific.

Differential Diagnosis

Differential diagnosis includes pneumonia, myocardial infarction, congestive heart failure, angina pectoris, atelectasis, lung abscess, tuberculosis, pulmonary neoplasm, viral pleuritis, asthma, and pericarditis.

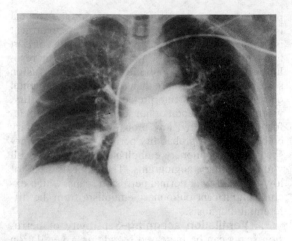

Figure 37-7. Pulmonary angiogram showing extensive bilateral embolic obstruction of pulmonary arteries.

Prevention

Prevention of deep venous thrombosis and pulmonary embolism is discussed on p 777.

Patients with recurrent emboli despite adequate therapy should be considered for placement of a vena cava filter as described in the section on Venous Thrombosis, above.

Treatment

A. Medical Treatment: In patients with a normal or low-probability lung scan and no evidence of venous thrombosis, it is safe to assume that pulmonary embolism is not present and that anticoagulation is not necessary. Anticoagulation can be instituted on the basis of a high-probability scan except in patients with significant contraindications to anticoagulation or those in whom the clinical course strongly opposes the diagnosis of pulmonary embolism. Once the diagnosis of pulmonary embolism is confirmed, a bolus of heparin (eg, 10,000 units) should be given intravenously. Heparin should be given by continuous intravenous infusion for 7–10 days. Oral anticoagulants should be started within a few days of heparinization. Heparin should be discontinued 4–5 days after a one-stage prothrombin time of 1.3–1.6 times the control (INR of 2.0–3.0) has been reached. Oral anticoagulants are continued for 3–6 months. Details of anticoagulant therapy can be found on p 778. The patient's legs should be elevated and kept continuously in this position. Results of the Urokinase Pulmonary Embolism Trial indicate that urokinase combined with heparin significantly accelerated the resolution of pulmonary thromboemboli at 24 hours compared with heparin alone, though no significantly better clinical outcomes were observed. Thrombolytic therapy may be indicated for patients who develop shock or right heart failure as well as those with severe pulmonary

hypertension who may die if additional emboli occur. The following regimens are equally effective: urokinase, 4400 IU/kg intravenously as initial dose, followed by 4400 IU/kg/h for 12 hours; streptokinase, 250,000 IU intravenously over 30 minutes, followed by 100,000 IU/h for 24 hours; and recombinant tissue plasminogen activator (alteplase), 90–100 mg intravenously over 6–7 hours. Heparin should be given after the thrombolytic infusion is completed. Bleeding is the major complication associated with thrombolytic therapy. It occurs most commonly at sites of instrumentation but can occur at sites of recent stroke or operation, so lytic therapy should not be used within 21 days of such events. Streptokinase has the additional complication of pyrogenicity and allergy.

B. Surgical Treatment: In selected patients with massive embolism, thoracotomy and removal of the embolism may be lifesaving. In most candidates for embolectomy, more than half of the pulmonary arterial system is occluded with emboli. An important exception is the patient with preexisting cardiac or respiratory insufficiency. The principal indication for pulmonary embolectomy is refractory hypotension despite maximal resuscitation in a patient who has massive embolism proved by lung scan or pulmonary arteriogram and who has had no response or has a contraindication to thrombolytic therapy. Most patients previously thought to require embolectomy actually respond favorably to heparinization, vasopressors, and inotropic agents. If pulmonary embolectomy is necessary, it must be done using cardiopulmonary bypass. One recent series reported a 77% survival rate. A transvenous method for removing pulmonary emboli using a large suction catheter (Greenfield catheter) inserted through the femoral vein has given promising results. This technique, which is much simpler and less stressful to the patient, may be preferable to surgical embolectomy.

Prognosis

The natural history of pulmonary embolism is one of progressive resolution with return of blood flow through previously occluded arteries. Slight thickening of the endothelium at the embolic site is often the only evidence of a previous lesion. The embolic material is removed both by macrophages and by in situ thrombolysis. Of the more than 600,000 symptomatic episodes of clinical pulmonary embolism in the USA each year, approximately 11% result in death within 1 hour. If the diagnosis is not made, about 30% of untreated patients die, the majority as a result of recurrent embolism. Most patients survive an attack of pulmonary embolism, because the magnitude of pulmonary arterial obstruction is nonlethal at the outset and the emboli begin to decrease (lyse) almost immediately. In those who survive long enough for the diagnosis to be established and adequate therapy to be instituted, death due to pulmonary embolism is uncommon. The acute prognosis is largely determined by the presence of associated disease, particularly cardiac and respiratory insufficiency. Evidence of partial resolution of pulmonary embolic obstruction can be detected by lung scanning or arteriography within a few days of the initial episode, and complete resolution may occur as early as 14 days, although it usually takes longer. The hemodynamic improvement correlates with the degree of resolution of pulmonary vascular obstruction, with return to normal or near-normal pulmonary and cardiac function within several weeks. Complete resolution of the obstruction is the usual course. Extensive and repeated pulmonary emboli can produce chronic respiratory insufficiency with pulmonary hypertension and right ventricular failure **(cor pulmonale),** a condition for which there is no effective therapy. With appropriate therapy, the prognosis of patients with pulmonary embolism is excellent and is mainly determined by the associated disease.

Anderson DR, Levine MN: Thrombolytic therapy for the treatment of acute pulmonary embolism. Can Med Assoc J 1992;146:1317.

Biello DR: Radiological (scintigraphic) evaluation of patients with suspected pulmonary thromboembolism. JAMA 1987;257:3257.

Goldhaber SZ et al: Randomized controlled trial of recombinant tissue plasminogen activator versus urokinase in the treatment of acute pulmonary embolism. Lancet 1988;2:203.

Grassi C: Inferior vena cava filters: Analysis of five currently available devices. AJR Am J Roentgenol 1991; 156:813.

Greenfield L: Assessment of vena cava filters. J Vasc Intervent Radiol 1991;2:425.

Hull RD et al: Pulmonary embolism in outpatients with pleuritic chest pain. Arch Intern Med 1988;148:838.

Juni JE, Alavi A: Lung scanning in the diagnosis of pulmonary embolism: The emperor redressed. Semin Nucl Med 1991;21:281.

Marder VJ, Sherry S: Thrombolytic therapy: Current status. (2 parts.) N Engl J Med 1988;318:1512, 1585.

McCann RL, Sabiston CD: Current management of venous thromboembolic disease. Brit J Surg 1989;76:113.

Moran KT, Jewell ER, Persson AV: The role of thrombolytic therapy in surgical practice. Brit J Surg 1989;76: 298.

Palevsky HI: The problems of the clinical and laboratory diagnosis of pulmonary embolism. Semin Nucl Med 1991;21:276.

PIOPED Investigators: Value of ventilation/perfusion scan in acute pulmonary embolism: The prospective investigation of pulmonary embolism diagnosis. JAMA 1990; 263:2753.

Rosenthal D et al: Massive pulmonary embolism: Triple-armed therapy. J Vasc Surg 1989;9:261.

Stein PD et al: Clinical, laboratory, roentgenographic, and electrocardiographic findings in patients with acute pulmonary embolism and no pre-existing cardiac or pulmonary disease. Chest 1991;100:598.

Stein PD et al: Complications and validity of pulmonary angiography in acute pulmonary embolism. Circulation 1992;85:462.

SUPERFICIAL THROMBOPHLEBITIS

Essentials of Diagnosis

- Pain, tenderness, and induration along course of a superficial vein.
- Palpable "cord" corresponding to course of vein.
- Absence of significant extremity swelling.
- Identifiable source of infection often present in proximity.

General Considerations

Because of their subcutaneous position, thromboses of superficial veins are usually easily recognized. In the upper extremities, intravenous catheters and drug abuse are the most common causes. In the lower extremities, thrombosis may be associated with varicose veins, thromboangiitis obliterans, or a neighboring bacterial infection. There is often a history of trauma. Recurrent or migratory superficial thrombophlebitis may be an early manifestation of abdominal cancer (Trousseau's sign) or other systemic illness, including immune arteritides and hypercoagulable states.

Clinical Findings

Superficial venous thrombosis is almost always accompanied by pain, induration, heat, tenderness, and erythema along the course of the involved vein. The patient may be febrile and have leukocytosis. The involved veins may feel like cords or ovoid nodules. The process most commonly involves the long saphenous vein and its tributaries and tends to remain localized. The inflammatory reaction may take 2–3 weeks to subside, and the thrombosed vein may be palpable for a much longer time. There is no associated edema of the extremity as a whole unless the process is extensive and the patient ambulatory.

Differential Diagnosis

Superficial thrombophlebitis can be confused with acute bacterial cellulitis, lymphangitis, and other acute inflammatory lesions. The distribution of the process along the course of the superficial veins should help in making this distinction. It is frequently confused with deep thrombophlebitis, but the edema associated with the latter condition is not present, and indurated superficial venous cords are not present in deep venous thrombosis. Sometimes, the two may coexist when the superficial phlebitis extends into the deep system via the communicating veins or at the saphenofemoral junction. When chills and high fever are present, suppuration has most likely developed in the involved vein **(septic thrombophlebitis).** *Staphylococcus aureus* is the most frequently cultured organism.

Treatment

In the absence of associated deep venous involvement, treatment is symptomatic and includes analgesics for pain, nonsteroidal anti-inflammatory agents, local heat, elastic compression bandages, and continued ambulation. Bed rest and anticoagulation are not necessary. When inflammation in the saphenous vein is progressing toward the saphenofemoral junction, involvement of the deep venous system, and subsequent pulmonary embolism is possible, and ligation and division of the saphenous vein are indicated. This can be done under local anesthesia. If the vein is varicosed, many would recommend that it be removed. Resolution of the process is usually prompt following surgical therapy. If there is concomitant deep venous involvement, anticoagulation and bed rest should be instituted. When the involved vein is infected (septic thrombophlebitis), high doses of antibiotics should be given, and the involved segment should be excised to avoid persistent bacterial seeding of the bloodstream and a high incidence of septic complications.

Prognosis

The course is ordinarily short and uncomplicated. Pulmonary emboli are rare, because the inflammation produces firm adherence of the clot to the vein wall. Recurrent superficial phlebitis is an indication for venous stripping.

Hammond JS, Varas R, Ward CG: Suppurative thrombophlebitis: A new look at a continuing problem. South Med J 1988;81:969.

Husni EA, Williams WA: Superficial thrombophlebitis of lower limbs. Surgery 1982;91:70.

Samlaska CP, James WD: Superficial thrombophlebitis: II. Secondary hypercoagulable states. J Am Acad Dermatol 1990;23:1.

AXILLARY-SUBCLAVIAN VENOUS THROMBOSIS

Essentials of Diagnosis

- History of repetitive or unusual muscular activity of upper extremity.
- Swelling of entire upper extremity.
- Collateral venous pattern over anterior chest wall.
- Swelling and pain made worse by exercise.
- Obstruction of vein at thoracic outlet as shown by phlebography.

General Considerations

Thrombosis of the axillary and subclavian veins accounts for only 2–3% of all cases of deep venous thrombosis. This low incidence is thought to be due to the shorter course that the blood travels in the upper extremity and the absence of venous stasis because of the frequent movements of the arms.

When axillary vein thrombosis does occur, it frequently is in association with predisposing factors such as congestive heart failure, metastatic tumor in the axilla, indwelling venous catheters (dialysis,

hyperalimentation, chemotherapy, cardiac pacemakers), or external trauma. Many cases are spontaneous but preceded by exercise of the extremity during sports participation or occupational activities that produce direct or indirect injury to the vein (effort thrombosis or Paget-Schroetter syndrome). Injury is thought to result at the thoracic outlet, where the axillary and subclavian veins may be compressed by nearby structures, most often in the costoclavicular space, between the clavicle and the first rib. The thrombosis is actually due to chronic compression of the axillary or subclavian vein.

Clinical Findings

Pain and swelling appear within 24 hours after the inciting event, most often following some type of unusual effort or strain. Males outnumber females (4:1), and the right side is affected more commonly than the left (2:1). The swelling usually involves the entire arm and is nonpitting. The pain is usually described as an aching sensation with a feeling of tightness, often most severe in the axilla. A prominent collateral venous pattern is usually visible over the shoulder and anterior chest wall, and the breast may be enlarged on the side of involvement. The extremity may be cyanotic. Only one-third of patients have a palpable tender cord in the axilla.

Diagnosis

In most cases, the diagnosis can be made on the basis of the signs and symptoms alone. Dilated superficial veins on the anterior chest wall may be shown best by infrared photography. Pressure in the antecubital veins is high and rises further with muscular exercise (normally, venous pressure drops with exercise). Duplex ultrasound can document the presence of an obstructing thrombus in the affected vein. Phlebographic demonstration of thrombotic occlusion of the deep veins is often necessary to confirm the diagnosis. Obstruction is most frequently seen in the region where the vein crosses the first rib, and a collateral venous network bypassing this obstruction can usually be visualized. This supports the etiologic theory of compression of the vein in the costoclavicular space, between the clavicle and the first rib.

Complications

Complications of axillary vein thrombosis are few, but prolonged disability is not rare. Venous gangrene, the counterpart of phlegmasia cerulea dolens in the lower extremity, develops rarely. Pulmonary embolism is seen in 12% of patients—more than has generally been thought.

Treatment

Most patients with primary axillary or subclavian venous thrombosis recover rapidly from the acute symptoms with no therapy other than rest and elevation of the arm. Anticoagulation should be instituted to prevent progression of the thrombus and embolization and to foster development of collaterals. The anticoagulation regimen is the same as described earlier for deep leg vein thrombosis.

Many surgeons now recommend early thrombolytic therapy in order to restore patency and to identify the presence and site of extrinsic venous compression. This is especially important with effort-induced thrombosis and is successful in over 80% of patients. It has largely obviated the need for thrombectomy. Since extraluminal compression of the axillary or subclavian vein is the cause of most of the thromboses, consideration should be given to relieving the cause of venous compression to prevent both rethrombosis and future symptoms. The site of the most severe compression is usually in the costoclavicular space, which should be enlarged by resection of the first rib and the subclavius and anterior scalene muscles. The transaxillary approach has been most popular, but if the vein needs direct repair (patch, etc), a supraclavicular exposure is necessary.

Prognosis

Although rapid recovery from the initial symptoms occurs in most patients, residual symptoms occur in 60–85% of those treated conservatively. Even though the acute swelling and pain subside within a few days to weeks, most patients have persistent or recurrent swelling, numbness, tingling, easy fatigability, and episodes of recurrent superficial phlebitis. Symptoms tend to be precipitated by exercise. The incidence of late symptoms is markedly reduced by early thrombectomy or thrombolysis and surgical relief of venous narrowing.

Ameli FM et al: Consequences of "conservative" conventional management of axillary vein thrombosis. Can J Surg 1987;30:167.

Kunkel JM, Machleder HI: Treatment of Paget-Schroetter syndrome. Arch Surg 1989;124:1153.

Linblad B, Tengborn L, Bergqvist D: Deep vein thrombosis of the axillary-subclavian veins: Epidemiologic data, effects of different types of treatment and late sequelae. Eur J Vasc Surg 1988;2:161.

Molina JE: Surgery for effort thrombosis of the subclavian vein. J Thorac Cardiovasc Surg 1992;103:341.

CHRONIC DEEP VENOUS INSUFFICIENCY (Postphlebitic Syndrome)

Essentials of Diagnosis

- History of previous deep vein thrombosis may be absent.
- Edema, hyperpigmentation, brawny induration, and dermatitis of distal leg and ankle.
- Ulceration, especially above the medial malleolus.
- Secondary superficial varicose veins.

General Considerations

The principal late complication of deep vein thrombosis is chronic venous stasis, and most patients with serious problems have originally had iliofemoral thrombophlebitis. It is rare to develop significant late symptoms after isolated calf vein thrombosis. There is persistent obstruction from incomplete recanalization of the thrombosed veins, destruction of the venous valves, and reflux of blood through incompetent perforator veins—all contributing to a high pressure in the distal veins. When the patient is standing at rest, pressure in a dorsal foot vein is normal in the postphlebitic leg, but with exercise the pressure fails to drop, because the valves are incompetent. The sustained high pressure combined with disordered interstitial fluid clearance results in the postphlebitic syndrome, which consists of edema, stasis dermatitis, and ulceration of the distal leg (Figure 37–1). Although it is generally agreed that venous ulceration results from a failure to lower the venous pressure with exercise, the pathogenesis has been elusive. Current theories include impairment of microcirculation, the presence of pericapillary fibrin cuffs and other causes of impaired tissue oxygenation, and trapping of white cells during dependency. It is estimated that the postphlebitic syndrome affects 0.5% of the population of the USA and accounts for a loss of 2 million working days annually.

Clinical Findings

A. Edema: Subcutaneous edema primarily involving the distal leg and ankle is usually the first manifestation of chronic venous insufficiency. At first, it accumulates during the day and disappears at night during recumbency. Orthostatic edema is usually present for some time before the more serious manifestations of the syndrome appear, and the increased tissue pressure resulting from the accumulation of edema fluid is one of the main factors in the evolution of the syndrome.

B. Dermatitis and Hyperpigmentation: The brownish pigmentation occurs at the ankle, consists of hemosiderin in macrophages, and represents destroyed blood pigment from extravasated red blood cells. Melanocytic reaction also contributes to pigmentary changes. A pruritic eczematous reaction (stasis dermatitis) is common and may lead to neurodermatitis from prolonged scratching.

C. Induration: With long-standing edema, fibrosis develops in the subcutaneous tissues and reduces elasticity of the skin (lipodermatosclerosis). Low-grade, often clinically insignificant bacterial infection may contribute to these changes, which ultimately make the swelling refractory to recumbency.

D. Ulceration: Ulceration is the major complication that causes the patient to seek medical attention. Approximately half of venous ulcers are associated with incompetent perforating veins in the region of the ankle. Ulceration is rarely a manifestation of primary varicose veins but is virtually always associated with incompetence of the popliteal venous valve. Stasis ulcers are most often just proximal or distal to the medial malleolus and often develop at sites of minor trauma or skin infections. Induration, scarring, and secondary bacterial infection all impair healing and make recurrences common if healing does occur. The natural history of venous ulceration is cyclic healing and recurrence unless something definitive is done to correct the high venous pressure at the ankle. Causes of leg ulcers are given in Table 37–3.

E. Pain: Whether there is ulceration or just swelling, the dull pain of venous ulcers is relieved by recumbency and elevation of the foot. In general, arterial ischemic ulcers are more painful than venous ulcers; the pain is made worse by elevation of the leg; and arterial ulcers are less often located at the medial malleolus. Arterial ulcers may extend to or through the fascia, whereas venous ulcers are shallow.

Treatment

The primary goal of therapy is control of the persistent venous hypertension and avoidance of edema. This is readily accomplished in most patients with custom-fitted, heavy-duty, knee-length elastic stockings. Intermittent periods of leg elevation and avoidance of prolonged sitting and standing should be advised. There is usually no need for elastic support above the knee, because the complications of venous insufficiency practically never extend this high. The elastic support must be used indefinitely.

Of primary importance to healing of venous stasis ulcers is the elimination of edema. If the ulcers are small and recent and edema has been controlled, treatment can be instituted on an outpatient basis by providing support to the tissues with a well-fitted, semirigid, boot-like dressing (Gelocast, Unna paste boot, or Gauztex). The boot is reapplied at intervals of 1–2 weeks. After the ulcer has healed, the boot is discarded in favor of heavy-duty elastic stockings. Large ulcers often require hospitalization for bed rest, elevation of the leg, and local wound care, but healing may be slow. Local treatment of the ulcer consists of moist dressings, which should be changed several times daily. Granulation tissue develops, and exudate decreases as the surface infection is controlled. Antibiotics are usually unnecessary except in rare cases when infection is spreading and the patient is febrile.

If the ulcers cannot be controlled by conservative management or if they are large, surgery is indicated. Split-thickness skin grafts may be applied directly to a clean granulating ulcer, or the ulcer may be excised and a skin graft applied primarily. Recurrences are common if nothing is done to treat the diseased veins. The initial operation should include ligation and stripping of the greater saphenous vein and ligation of incompetent perforators in the region of the ulcer. If the lesser saphenous system is involved, it should be removed as well. Contrary to what has been taught

Table 37–3. Classification of chronic leg ulcers.

Vascular
  Arterial
    Atherosclerosis obliterans
    Thromboangiitis obliterans
    Arteriovenous fistula
    Collagen vascular disease (polyarteritis nodosa)
    Hypertension
    Raynaud's disease
  Venous
    Chronic deep venous insufficiency
    Varicose veins
    Postinjection reaction
  Lymphatic: Chronic lymphedema
Infective
  Bone
    Chronic osteomyelitis
    Adherent fracture site
  Pyogenic
  Synergistic gangrene (Meleney's ulcer)
  Miscellaneous
    Syphilis
    Tuberculosis
    Tropical diseases (leishmaniasis)
    Fungal diseases
Systemic-metabolic
  Ulcerative colitis
  Diabetes mellitus
  Sickle cell anemia
  Avitaminosis
Neoplastic
  Primary skin tumor
    Kaposi's sarcoma
    Melanoma
    Squamous cell carcinoma
  Leukemia
  Metastatic
Traumatic
  Radiation
  Thermal burns
  Decubitus
  Insect bites
Neurotrophic
  Cord lesions
  Peripheral neuropathies
    Trauma
    Diabetes
    Tabes dorsalis
    Alcoholism

in the past, removal of secondary varicosities of the saphenous system, except in rare instances, does not impair venous return from the extremity.

When ulceration recurs in spite of these measures, more radical surgical procedures are indicated. The most successful of these is ligation of all of the perforating veins. The perforators that are invariably associated with recurrent ulceration are more easily located and more readily ligated in the subfascial plane than by attempts at individual ligation in the scarred, indurated subcutaneous tissue. They are best approached through a single long posterior midline incision that extends through the fascia, creating two full-thickness flaps. The exposed perforating veins are ligated as they pass from the muscle to penetrate the fascia. Even after this procedure, recurrent ulceration occurs in as many as 10% of patients. As no operation eliminates the venous hypertension, elastic support is required indefinitely after all these procedures.

Rarely, after many years, a chronic ulcer may undergo malignant transformation **(Marjolin's ulcer),** a change that is not always easy to recognize. Therefore, intractable ulcers should be biopsied to check for tumor.

Bypass of an obstructed iliac or femoral vein (or both) with a vein graft has resulted in prolonged symptomatic relief in a number of patients. The procedure is most applicable for localized venous obstruction due to extrinsic compression of the vein. There has been increasing interest in and success with direct venous valve repair or transplantation, since any competent valve in the deep venous system will restore a limb to a compensated condition and allow healing of stasis ulceration. At the present time, these operations are being performed only on patients with severe symptoms and recurrent ulceration.

Prognosis

Recurrent thrombophlebitis is frequent and requires prophylactic measures such as elastic support, periodic elevation of the legs, and avoidance of stasis-producing activities.

Browse NL: The etiology of venous ulceration. World J Surg 1986;10:938.

Coleridge Smith PD et al: Causes of venous ulceration: A new hypothesis. Br Med J 1988;296:1726.

Cornwall JV, Dore CJ, Lewis JD: Leg ulcers: Epidemiology and aetiology. Br J Surg 1986;73:693.

Gilliland EL, Wolfe JHN: Leg ulcers. Br Med J 199 1;303: 776.

Jessup G, Lane RJ: Repair of incompetent venous valves: A new technique. J Vasc Surg 1988;8:569.

Kohler TR, Strandness DE: Noninvasive testing for the evaluation of chronic venous disease. World J Surg 1986; 10:903.

Raju S, Fredericks R: Hemodynamic basis of stasis ulceration: A hypothesis. J Vasc Surg 1991;13:491.

Raju S, Fredericks R: Valve reconstruction procedures for non-obstructive venous insufficiency: Rationale, techniques, and results in 107 procedures with 2–8 year follow-up. J Vasc Surg 1988;7:301.

Wilson NM, Rutt DL, Browse NL: Repair and replacement of deep vein valves in the treatment of venous insufficiency. Br J Surg 1991;78:388.

Young JR, Terwoord BA: Stasis ulcer treatment with compression dressing. Cleve Clin J Med 1990;529.

THE SWOLLEN LEG

Edema consists of increased interstitial fluid resulting from an imbalance between the filtration pressure in proximal capillaries and the absorptive osmotic pressure at the venous end of the capillaries. Venous, lymphatic, or systemic causes can produce chronic edema of the lower extremity. The peripheral

Table 37–4. Causes of swollen leg.

Venous
- Postphlebitic syndrome
- Extrinsic compression
  - Tumor
  - Retroperitoneal fibrosis
  - Compression by iliac artery
- Trauma
  - Surgical ligation, plication, clip
  - Wound
- Arteriovenous fistula

Lymphatic
- Primary lymphedema
  - Congenital lymphedema
  - Lymphedema praecox
  - Lymphedema tarda
- Secondary lymphedema
  - Infection (filariasis)
  - Neoplasia
  - Radiation
  - Insect bites
  - Surgical excision
  - Motor paralysis (disuse)

Systemic
- Congestive heart failure
- Cirrhosis
- Nephrosis
- Myxedema
- Drugs, hormones
- Hypoproteinemia

lymphatics serve as the major route whereby large protein molecules that have escaped from the vascular compartment are removed and returned to the circulation. Failure to remove interstitial proteins, the major pathophysiologic abnormality in lymphedema, produces an osmotic force that perpetuates water retention (edema). In chronic venous insufficiency, edema is principally a consequence of abnormally high net fluid filtration resulting from elevated venular pressure. The lymphatics still remove extracellular protein, so venous edema is characteristically low in protein. In either case, edema means that lymph formation has exceeded lymph resorption. Whatever the cause, long-standing edema produces similar patterns of secondary inflammation and fibrosis.

The causes of chronic leg edema are listed in Table 37–4. If systemic causes can be excluded or if the swelling is unilateral, the disease must be local, and the major diagnostic problem is to decide whether the origin is venous or lymphatic. The distinction can be based on clinical findings in most cases, but special procedures such as venography and lymphangiography are occasionally required.

Baumeister RG, Suida S: Treatment of lymphedemas by microsurgical lymphatic grafting: What is proved? Plast Reconstr Surg 1990;85:64.

Bergan JJ, Yao JST (editors): *Venous Disorders.* Saunders, 1991.

Cooney TG, Reuler JB: The swollen leg. West J Med 1985; 142:405.

Norberg B: The swollen leg. (Editorial.) Acta Med Scand 1988;224:1. O'Brien BM et al: Long-term results after microlymphatico-venous anastomoses for the treatment of obstructive lymphedema. Plast Reconstr Surg 1990; 85:562.

II. THE LYMPHATICS

Surgical Anatomy

Phylogenetically, the lymph vessels are modified veins. Histologically, the lymphatic capillaries are blind endothelial tubes which differ from vascular capillaries mainly in that they are highly permeable to macromolecules. The major function of the lymphatics appears to be the removal of macromolecules. The larger lymphatics have smooth muscle walls and endothelial valves that permit flow only in a central direction. Lymph nodes are interspersed in the course of larger lymphatics and serve a filtrative, phagocytic, and immunologic function. Total lymph flow entering the subclavian veins in humans is 2–4 L daily and contains 75–200 g of protein. Venous obstruction, vasodilatation, muscular exercise, and increased capillary permeability all increase the rate of lymph flow.

The lymphatic capillaries form a superficial plexus in the superficial dermis, a deep plexus in the deeper dermis, and in the extremities, a subfascial plexus within the muscular compartments. Normally, tissue fluid collected in dermal lymphatics drains into subcutaneous lymphatics which accompany superficial veins and which drain into regional lymph nodes. The larger lymph channels tend to travel with the major blood vessels. As with the veins, active or passive contraction of skeletal muscles plays an important role in the movement of lymph, and the lymphatic valves determine the direction of flow.

Lymphangiography

Organic dyes injected into the skin are rapidly picked up by the subdermal or superficial dermal lymphatics, which can then easily be recognized by their color. This allows cannulation of the lymphatics and injection of radiopaque contrast media. X-rays (lymphangiograms) reveal normal lymphatics as slender vessels of uniform diameter that branch as they proceed centrally. Lymphangiography is not practiced as widely as arteriography or venography, because the technique is difficult and the complication rates relatively high. It is nevertheless often helpful in identifying the cause of a chronically swollen lower extremity and can differentiate primary from secondary lymphedema. Lymphangiography can also be used to detect abnormal lymph nodes in the retro-

peritoneum or mediastinum in the evaluation of patients with lymphomas. Since the contrast medium used for lymphangiography may produce a temporary diffusion barrier when it reaches the lungs, preliminary pulmonary function testing is advisable so that the test can be avoided in patients with significant pulmonary disability.

Lymphoscintigraphy

Lymphoscintigraphy involves injection of a small amount of technetium 99m-labeled antimony trisulfide colloid into the second interdigital space and then imaging the extremity with a gamma camera. Normal and delayed transport of lymph can be determined. Visual interpretation of the imaged pattern of lymphatic anatomy together with estimation of appearance time of the colloid in the regional lymph nodes shows whether the lymphatic system is normal or abnormal. Patients with edema due to chronic venous insufficiency have normal or enhanced lymph transport, whereas in lymphedema there are abnormal patterns. This method is simple, has no adverse side effects, and can be performed on an outpatient basis.

LYMPHEDEMA

Essentials of Diagnosis

- Progressive swelling of one or both lower extremities, often without antecedent history.
- Nonpitting edema.
- Recurrent episodes of lymphangitis and cellulitis.
- Edema does not respond to leg elevation.

General Considerations

Lymphedema is an abnormal collection of interstitial lymph fluid due to either a congenital developmental abnormality of lymphatics or secondary lymphatic obstruction. It has multiple causes (Table 37–4), but the pathophysiologic mechanism—obstruction of lymphatics—is similar in all.

Clinical Findings

Primary lymphedema may be present at birth (**congenital lymphedema**) but more often becomes manifest in the teens or twenties (**lymphedema praecox**). **Milroy's disease** is chronic hereditary lymphedema with onset at or near birth. In a small percentage of cases, it develops after age 35 (**lymphedema tarda**). It is caused by developmental abnormalities of the lymphatics, either hypoplasia (55%), varicose dilatation (24%), or aplasia (14%), although some authors consider the lymphatic obstruction to be an acquired event. Whatever the anatomic cause, the functional result is lymphatic obstruction and increased pressure. The lymph vessels dilate, their valves become incompetent. Since the valves are essential to maintain the central direction of flow, incompetency aggravates lymph stasis. The resulting inability to remove subcutaneous protein stimulates fibrosis and further obstruction. The protein-rich fluid is also prone to bacterial infection. In primary lymphedema, the abnormalities are usually confined to the tissues superficial to the deep muscle fascia.

Lymphedema praecox, predominantly a disease of females, begins at puberty or during adolescence. The first symptom, spontaneous swelling, starts as a puffiness about the foot or ankle made worse by long periods of activity. It may be unilateral or bilateral. The edema usually progresses up the leg slowly, with the entire limb becoming involved over a period of months or years. Gradually, the swelling becomes more marked, and elevation and bed rest become less effective for its control. Originally soft and pitting, the edema gradually becomes resistant to pressure, subcutaneous tissue hypertrophies, and the limb becomes permanently enlarged, unsightly, and uncomfortable. The patient experiences a dull, heavy sensation but no actual pain unless infection occurs. About half of patients with primary lymphedema eventually develop bilateral involvement.

Secondary lymphedema, in contrast to primary idiopathic lymphedema, is due to some definable extralymphatic process. Neoplastic obstruction of lymph vessels is the most frequent cause and is usually a result of prostatic carcinoma in men and lymphoma in women. Surgical removal of lymphatics— eg, during radical mastectomy or radical groin dissection—is also a common cause. In some cases, recurrent lymphangitis and cellulitis with progressive obliteration of the lymphatic vessels are the presumed causes. Subsequent attacks tend to occur with increasing frequency, producing more severe degrees of edema. In some parts of the world, filariasis is the most common cause of lymphedema; lymphangiograms will demonstrate the point of lymphatic obstruction.

Complications

The skin becomes thickened and hyperkeratotic. Recurrent cellulitis and lymphangitis are the most frequent complications and usually follow minor injuries to the affected extremity. The patient experiences swelling, erythema, pain, and systemic signs and symptoms. The infection tends to spread rapidly up the involved lymphatics, producing visible red streaks in the skin from the foot to the groin. *Streptococcus* is the most frequent causative organism.

Another late complication is **lymphangiosarcoma,** an uncommon neoplasm that arises from lymphatic endothelium. It is almost always associated with lymphedema, most commonly postmastectomy lymphedema of the upper extremity. The tumor appears as multiple blue, red, or purple macular or papular lesions in the skin or subcutaneous tissue that may coalesce to form a large ulcerating mass. Lymphangiosarcoma spreads rapidly and has an extremely poor prognosis.

Differential Diagnosis

Because it is soft, pitting, and bilateral, lower extremity edema from systemic diseases such as congestive heart failure, cirrhosis, or nephrosis is relatively easy to differentiate from lymphedema. The major difficulty in differential diagnosis is to distinguish between lymphedema and the edema of chronic deep venous insufficiency. In contrast to that of venous disease, the swelling of lymphedema is usually painless. Lymphedema is firm, rubbery, and nonpitting and decreases little if at all with overnight elevation. The edema of chronic deep venous insufficiency is soft and pitting initially but later may become firm and is associated with secondary pigmentation, dermatitis, ulceration, and varicosities. Recurrent cellulitis and lymphangitis are much more common in lymphedema. However, lymphedema may exist in the postphlebitic limb, and differentiation on clinical grounds is therefore not always possible. Phlebograms or lymphangiograms are occasionally useful in such cases.

Treatment

The objectives of treatment are to control edema and prevent recurrent infection. The best results are obtained when treatment is instituted early in the course of the disease, before fibrosis develops and the health of the skin and subcutaneous tissue becomes impaired.

A. Nonoperative Management: Most patients with early lymphedema can be managed adequately without operation. The main objective of treatment is to rid the limbs of as much edema as possible and maintain the reduction permanently. Measures to reduce lymph formation are important. These include elevation of the foot of the bed by 15 cm and elevation of the feet and ankles at intervals during the day. External compression should be provided with custom fitted, heavy-duty elastic stockings worn from the moment of arising until retiring at night. The patient should not be measured for the stockings until maximal reduction of swelling has been accomplished. If compression of the thigh is required, the stocking should be supported by a waist belt and garter or a leotard. Sequential air compression devices that milk edema fluid from the extremity are quite helpful in some patients with mild to moderate lymphedema. These are suitable for outpatient and home use. Dietary sodium must be restricted and diuretics occasionally prescribed when the edema is being actively treated. It is essential that the patient be instructed regarding hygiene to prevent minor foot injuries or infections, which are prone to cause severe cellulitis. If recurrent lymphangitis and cellulitis are otherwise not preventable, long-term prophylactic antibiotics are indicated, using a drug effective against the most prevalent invasive organism, usually one of the streptococci.

B. Surgical Treatment: Only a small number

(16%) of patients develop disease severe enough to require surgical treatment. The reasons for surgery are (1) impaired function of the extremity due primarily to its excessive size and weight; (2) pain; (3) recurrent episodes of cellulitis and lymphangitis; (4) development of lymphangiosarcoma; and (5) desire to improve cosmetic appearance. Since most patients are young women, aesthetic considerations may be important; however, this should rarely be the sole basis for surgical treatment, because the cosmetic result is not a normal-appearing extremity. Excisional procedures remove the skin and lymphedematous subcutaneous tissues and usually require resurfacing of the extremity with extensive skin grafts. Variations of this technique are the procedures most frequently performed for lymphedema, but results are only moderately good because of scarring, sensory loss in the skin, and recurring swelling, especially in the foot.

Physiologic procedures attempt to improve lymph drainage by correcting lymphatic obstruction. Some procedures transfer normal lymphatic channels from a healthy area to a lymphedematous one. The **Thompson procedure** folds a longitudinal flap of beveled dermis beneath the muscles along the medial and lateral aspects of the extremity to allow connections to form between blocked superficial dermal lymphatics and the normal deep lymphatic system. Clinical and cosmetic results have been good, although the establishment of new channels of lymphatic communication has not been documented. Omental pedicle flaps used for this purpose have not been successful in most instances, but an enteromesenteric bridge technique has demonstrated lymphatic connections between inguinal lymph nodes and the bowel with long-term clinical success.

Recent developments in microvascular surgery have led to several new procedures to facilitate lymph drainage. These include axial pattern and myocutaneous flaps and lymphatic-lymphatic and lymphaticovenous anastomoses and microlymphatic bypass. Although early results have been encouraging, long-term good to excellent results documented by physiologic studies have been achieved in only about 25% of patients.

Prognosis

The natural history of lymphedema is one of gradual but steady progression of swelling, progressive disability imposed on the patient by the heavy, clumsy extremity, and recurrent episodes of infection. Some limbs become so large that specially made trousers and shoes are required. Fortunately, most patients can be greatly benefited by strict adherence to the therapeutic program. In severe cases, the cosmetic deformity may produce psychologic problems that interfere with therapy. Insufficient experience with the currently used operations makes it impossible to predict their long-term efficacy.

Borel Rinkes IH, deJongste AB: Lymphangiosarcoma in chronic lymphedema: Reports of three cases and review of the literature. Acta Chir Scand 1986;152:227.

Browse NL: The diagnosis and management of primary lymphedema. J Vasc Surg 1986;3:181.

Browse NL, Stewart G: Lymphoedema: Pathophysiology and classification. J Cardiovasc Surg 1985;26:91.

Christenson JT, Hamad MM, Shawa NJ: Primary lymphedema of the leg: Relationship between subcutaneous tissue pressure, intramuscular pressure, and venous function. Lymphology 1985;18:86.

Collins SP et al: Abnormalities of lymphatic drainage in lower extremities: A lymphoscintigraphic study. J Vasc Surg 1989;9:145.

Gloviczki P et al: Non-invasive evaluation of the swollen extremity: Experience with 190 lymphoscintigraphic examinations. J Vasc Surg 1989;9:683.

Golueke PJ et al: Lymphoscintigraphy to confirm the clinical diagnosis of lymphedema. J Vasc Surg 1989;10:306.

Hadjis NS et al: The role of CT in the diagnosis of primary lymphedema of the lower limb. AJR 1985;144:361.

Kinmonth JB: *The Lymphatics: Surgery, Lymphography, and Diseases of the Chyle and Lymph Systems,* 2nd ed. Arnold, 1983.

Lewis JM, Wald ER: Lymphedema praecox. J Pediatr 1984;104:641.

Richmond DM, O'Donnell TF Jr, Zelikovski A: Sequential pneumatic compression for lymphedema: A controlled trial. Arch Surg 1985;120:1116.

Savage RC: The surgical management of lymphedema. Surg Gynecol Obstet 1985;160:283.

Smeltzer DM, Stickler GB, Schirger A: Primary lymphedema in children and adolescents: A follow-up study and review. Pediatrics 1985;76:206.

Stewart G et al: Isotope lymphography: A new method of investigating the role of the lymphatics in chronic limb edema. Br J Surg 1985;72:906.

Wolfe JH: The prognosis and possible cause of severe primary lymphoedema. Ann R Coll Surg Engl 1984;66:251.

Zelikovski A, Haddad M, Reiss R: The "Lympha-Press" intermittent sequential pneumatic device for treatment of lymph-edema; Five years of clinical experience. J Cardiovasc Surg 1986;27:288.

REFERENCES

Bergan JJ, Yao JST (editors): *Venous Disorders.* Saunders, 1991.

Browse NL, Burnand KG, Thomas ML (editors): *Diseases of the Veins: Pathology, Diagnosis, and Treatment.* Arnold, 1988.

Criado E, Johnson G Jr: Venous disease. Curr Probl Surg 1991;28:338. Ernst CB, Stanley JS (editors): *Current Therapy in Vascular Surgery,* 2nd ed. BC Decker, 1991.

Hirsch J, Hull R: *Venous Thromboembolism: Natural History, Diagnosis, and Management.* CRC Press, 1987.

Strandness DE Jr, Thiele BL: *Selected Topics in Venous Disorders: Pathophysiology, Diagnosis, and Treatment.* Futura, 1981.

Subcommittee on Reporting Standards in Venous Disease, Ad Hoc Committee on Reporting Standards, Society for Vascular Surgery, North American Chapter, International Society for Cardiovascular Surgery: Reporting standards in venous disease. J Vasc Surg 1988;8:172.

Yao JST, Pearce WH (editors): *Technologies in Vascular Surgery.* Saunders, 1992.

38

Neurosurgery & Surgery of the Pituitary

DIAGNOSIS & MANAGEMENT OF DEPRESSED STATES OF CONSCIOUSNESS

Julian T. Hoff, MD

Definitions

The clinical definition of consciousness ranges from alert wakefulness to deep coma. An **alert,** wakeful patient responds immediately and appropriately to all stimuli. A **stuporous** patient responds only when aroused by vigorous stimulation. **Coma** implies failure to respond to stimulation. Most cases of depressed states of consciousness lie between these extremes and are best categorized by accurate descriptions of their responses to specific stimuli—eg, auditory, visual, and tactile (touch or pain).

The Neurologic Examination

The most reliable index for assessing the level of consciousness at any moment is the patient's response to external stimuli (ie, how quick and how accurate are the patient's responses to questions, to touch, to pain, etc?). Brain stem reflexes also allow an accurate estimate of the level of consciousness— pupillary responses to light, corneal reflexes, oculocephalic and caloric responses, cough and gag reflexes, pattern of breathing, etc. Motor activity of the extremities, either spontaneous or induced by the examiner's stimulus, provides assessment of the entire neuraxis. Does the patient move the extremities purposefully, equally, and briskly, or is there failure to move at all? Which extremities do not move? Nonpurposeful or reflex movement of the arms and legs may also establish the level of neuraxis function, though less reliably (eg, decorticate or decerebrate posturing).

Depressed consciousness may occur abruptly (eg, cerebral concussion) or gradually (eg, barbiturate overdose), often with fluctuations in the level of consciousness (eg, waxing-waning consciousness associated with subdural hematoma). Accurate and re-

peated examinations will establish not only the level of consciousness but also its changing course. The urgency of diagnosis depends largely upon the rate of change in the patient's course as determined by repeated examinations.

Diagnostic Possibilities

Depressed states of consciousness may be due to many causes. Trauma is usually obvious, both on the history and on examination of the patient. **Metabolic disorders** (eg, diabetes mellitus, uremia, poisoning, electrolyte imbalance, hypoxia) may similarly alter the state of consciousness. In addition to an accurate history and physical examination, laboratory investigations are required to establish a diagnosis of metabolic coma.

Patients with **intracranial neoplasms** may be alert, comatose, or at any level of consciousness in between. A progressive, unrelenting history is a valuable criterion of this initial diagnosis. **Central nervous system infections** (eg, encephalitis, meningitis) are usually accompanied by systemic signs of infection and a progressively worsening course. Cerebral abscess, on the other hand, behaves more like an expanding neoplasm than a fulminating infection.

Vascular occlusions (emboli, thrombosis) usually cause abrupt neurologic deficits without grossly impaired consciousness, whereas cerebral hemorrhage typically causes abrupt coma with profound neurologic deficits. Conversely, subarachnoid hemorrhage may occur without any alteration of wakefulness. **Degenerative diseases** are usually slowly progressive, dementing illnesses that dull consciousness but characteristically do not produce coma.

Diagnostic Tools

Laboratory and radiographic tests help to establish the clinical diagnosis. Routine examinations should include a complete blood count, urinalysis, plasma glucose, blood urea nitrogen, and serum electrolytes.

Urine and blood for toxicologic study are essential if poisoning is a possibility. Skull and cervical spine films and chest x-ray are obvious aids after trauma. Cerebrospinal fluid analysis is an essential step toward diagnosis of meningitis or subarachnoid hemorrhage. Lumbar puncture is rarely helpful in the assessment of head trauma and probably is contraindicated during the initial workup after injury.

Although most patients are unconscious for a single reason, some may have combined or additive reasons. A severe head injury may have been caused by abrupt coma induced by cerebral hemorrhage in a hypertensive patient, or a diabetic patient with glioblastoma multiforme may be in coma from an insulin overdose and not from the expanding neoplasm. The physician must be aware of these possible—though uncommon—complexities.

The administration of intravenous hypertonic glucose (50%, 50 mL) is occasionally diagnostic but should be done only after blood has been taken for glucose measurement and before an intravenous glucose drip has been started.

Most patients with depressed consciousness should undergo CT scanning or MRI to establish the presence or absence of an intracranial mass lesion. Appropriate therapy depends on the early recognition of the specific intracranial problem.

Management

Protection of the airway and control of shock are fundamental principles of management of patients with depressed consciousness. Most complications of coma can be attributed to failure to follow these basic rules. Responsive patients with good cough reflexes can often protect their own airways. Other patients, usually stuporous or comatose, require endotracheal intubation or tracheostomy in order to (1) reduce the likelihood of aspiration of gastric contents and (2) ensure unrestricted gas exchange (Po_2, Pco_2).

Adequate tracheal suctioning, frequent changes in position, pulmonary physiotherapy, and intermittent positive pressure breathing help maintain good pulmonary function once the airway is secure.

Shock must be controlled. If it is due to hypovolemia, blood and fluids must be given intravenously. In the absence of trauma, other causes of hypotension must be sought and treated specifically (eg, gram-negative sepsis).

A nasogastric tube (to sample ingested drugs, to remove gastric contents that might be aspirated into the lungs, etc), intravenous cannulas to administer drugs and fluids, and an indwelling bladder catheter to assess fluid balance are necessary steps in the early management of comatose patients.

ELEVATED INTRACRANIAL PRESSURE

The skull contains brain, cerebrospinal fluid, and blood (Figure 38–1). At normal intracranial pressures of 10–15 mm Hg (120–180 mm H_2O), these three components maintain volumetric equilibrium. Increased volume of one component will elevate intracranial pressure unless the volume of the other two components decreases proportionately (Monro-Kellie doctrine). Because compensatory volumetric changes have physical and physiologic limits, the ability of the skull's contents to maintain normal pressure can be exceeded by a change of volume that is either too fast or too great.

The compensatory properties of the intracranial contents follow a pressure-volume exponential curve (Figure 38–2). Increased volume of any of the three components can be accommodated to a certain point without change in intracranial pressure. Once that critical volume is reached, however, additional volume increase produces an increase in intracranial pressure.

Increased intracranial pressure exerts its deleterious effect (1) by distorting and shifting the brain as pressure gradients develop, and (2) by reducing the effective perfusion pressure of the brain (cerebral perfusion pressure [CPP] = blood pressure [BP] minus intracranial pressure [ICP]). Common examples of a significant volumetric change in one or more of the three normal intracranial components are cerebral edema (brain), hydrocephalus (cerebrospinal fluid), and cerebral venous occlusion (blood).

An intracranial mass (eg, tumor, hematoma) represents a fourth component, and its presence initiates compensatory adjustments of the other three: (1) Intracranial vessels are compressed, reducing the amount of intracranial blood; (2) cerebrospinal fluid volume is reduced by increased absorption or reduced production (at high intracranial pressure); and (3) intracranial bulk is reduced by brain creeping out of adjacent foramina (eg, transtentorial herniation, tonsillar herniation). Children with expandable skulls have an additional compensatory mechanism to accommodate expanding intracranial volume and are thereby partially protected from extreme rises of intracranial pressure.

Clinical Findings

Most brain insults, whether from trauma, ischemia, poisoning, or other sources, are accompanied by raised intracranial pressure. Following head trauma, intracranial pressure may rise quickly to very high levels as a result of vascular congestion, extravasation, and cerebral edema. Intracranial pressure may also rise substantially when a neoplasm occupies the intracranial cavity. Intracranial hypertension may occur after cerebrovascular occlusions (stroke), during central nervous system infections, and following cerebral hypoxia. Intracranial pressure by itself is rarely a clinical problem when coma is the result of a metabolic disorder (eg, uremia, hepatic coma).

A. Specific Signs of Raised Intracranial Pressure: While any of the following clinical signs may result from causes other than raised intracranial pressure, most will appear during raised intracranial pressure if the elevation is severe or prolonged.

1. Cardiovascular—Blood pressure elevation

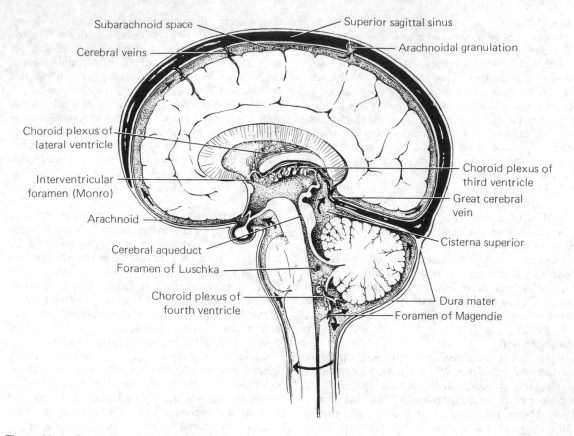

Figure 38–1. Circulation of cerebrospinal fluid. (Redrawn from original drawings by Frank H. Netter, MD, that first appeared in Ciba *Clinical Symposia,* © 1950, Ciba Pharmaceutical Co. Reproduced with permission.)

accompanied by bradycardia and respiratory slowing classically results from raised intracranial pressure. This "Cushing response," however, usually appears only when intracranial hypertension is severe.

2. Gastrointestinal–Hemorrhage from gastric ulcerations (Cushing's ulcer) may accompany raised intracranial pressure.

3. Pulmonary–Hemorrhagic pulmonary edema may result from severe elevation of intracranial pressure as well as from other brain insults. The lung lesion is the end product of a pathophysiologic sequence mediated by the sympathetic nervous system. Few patients survive this hemodynamic storm of neurogenic origin unless intracranial pressure is reduced.

4. Neurologic–Papilledema, abducens nerve paresis (unilateral occasionally; bilateral often), and depressed consciousness are the most common signs associated with generalized intracranial pressure elevations. Loss of visual acuity may occur as a late consequence of optic nerve atrophy.

B. Specific Syndromes: Specific syndromes may appear when intracranial pressure is raised by the presence of an intracranial mass.

1. Transtentorial herniation–A laterally

placed supratentorial mass may push the uncus and hippocampus medially into the tentorial incisure. The oculomotor nerves, the cerebral peduncles, the cerebral aqueduct, and the midbrain (containing the reticular formation) are vulnerable to compression from the displaced temporal lobe. Transtentorial herniation may then appear clinically (Table 38–1).

2. Tonsillar herniation–Herniation of the cerebellar tonsils into the foramen magnum causes compression of the medulla. The hallmark of medullary compression is respiratory failure: slow and irregular breathing followed by apnea. Earlier signs of herniation are nuchal rigidity, intermittent opisthotonos, and depressed gag and cough reflexes. Consciousness may be retained until the patient becomes severely hypoxic.

Although raised intracranial pressure usually becomes obvious clinically, it may go undetected for months. Patients with benign intracranial hypertension (pseudotumor cerebri) often have no symptoms despite severe papilledema and intracranial hypertension. Similarly, patients with obstruction of cerebrospinal fluid pathways may tolerate intracranial pressure elevation for weeks or months without

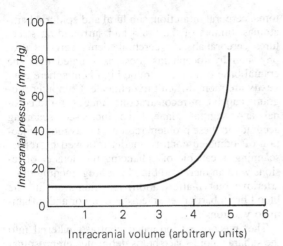

Figure 38–2. Change in intracranial pressure with changes in intracranial compartment volume. The figures along the abscissa represent units of volume.

developing overt clinical signs. Failing mentation may provide the only clue to progressive hydrocephalus in the latter circumstance.

Treatment

A. Specific Treatment: Management of specific causes of raised intracranial pressure is effective treatment. Removal of intracranial masses, shunting of obstructed cerebrospinal fluid, and removal of toxins (eg, lead, in lead encephalopathy) are examples of specific forms of treatment.

B. Nonspecific Treatment: When raised intracranial pressure as such must also be managed, the following nonspecific measures are useful:

1. Control of respiration–Accumulation of CO_2 (PaCO$_2$ > 40 mm Hg) will increase cerebral

blood flow and raise intracranial pressure. A therapeutic goal is maintenance of PaCO$_2$ in the range of 30–40 mm Hg.

2. Control of body temperature–Hypothermia reduces cerebral metabolism and lowers intracranial pressure. Hyperthermia increases intracranial pressure. Thus, fever must be controlled.

3. Osmotic diuretics–Mannitol, urea, or glycerin can reduce intracranial pressure by cerebral dehydration.

4. Corticosteroids–These agents reduce or prevent cerebral edema, thereby helping to control intracranial pressure.

5. Cerebrospinal fluid drainage–Reduction of cerebrospinal fluid volume by repeated spinal taps or by shunting may control raised intracranial pressure from pseudotumor. Ventricular drainage of cerebrospinal fluid reduces intracranial pressure transiently in severe head injury and in patients with obstructive hydrocephalus.

6. Bony decompression–This nonspecific method of reducing intracranial pressure may be employed when other measures fail.

Crockard A, Hayward R, Hoff JT: *Neurosurgery: The Scientific Basis of Clinical Practice,* 2nd ed. Blackwell, 1992.

Youmans J: *Neurological Surgery,* 3rd ed. Saunders, 1990.

NEURODIAGNOSTIC PROCEDURES

Michael S. Edwards, MD

PLAIN RADIOGRAPHS

Plain radiographs of the skull and spine provide only preliminary information, although the presence of abnormal intracranial calcification or bony changes may assist in diagnosis and planning of subsequent neurodiagnostic tests. Pineal calcification, present in 59% of adults over 20 years of age, should be evaluated for displacement from the midline. A careful search for fractures should be performed in all patients with a significant history of head trauma.

ULTRASOUND

High-resolution ultrasound (3.5–7.5 MHz) can image intracranial and spinal anatomy when an acoustic window (bony defect) is present. Because this technique is noninvasive, does not involve x-rays, and can be performed with portable equipment, it has found wide application in the evaluation of intracranial anatomy in infants with open fonta-

Table 38–1. Clinical manifestations of tentorial herniation.

Compressed Structure	Clinical Manifestation
Cranial nerve III	Ipsilateral mydriasis
Midbrain: physiologic (functional) transection	Decerebrate rigidity
Reticular formation	Coma
Ipsilateral cerebral peduncle	Contralateral hemiparesis
Contralateral cerebral peduncle	Ipsilateral hemiparesis (false localizing sign)[1]
Cerebral aqueduct (of Sylvius)	Headache and vomiting due to acute hydrocephalus
Posterior cerebral artery	Contralateral hemianopia (false localizing sign)[1]

[1]This sign is the consequence of herniation and does not indicate the localization of the primary process; in this sense, the sign falsely localizes the primary lesion.

nelles. In the neonatal intensive care unit, ultrasound is the standard technique for evaluating the premature infant for intraventricular hemorrhage and ventricular size. Ultrasound examination of the infant spine can delineate normal and abnormal anatomy. Intraoperative ultrasound is being used to help position the ventricular catheter during shunting for hydrocephalus and to locate subcortical intracranial lesions (eg, tumor, cyst, abscess) at the time of craniotomy. Obstetric ultrasound is used to evaluate fetal intracranial and spinal anatomy and to diagnose central nervous system anomalies such as anencephaly, hydrocephalus, and myelomeningocele.

RADIONUCLIDE IMAGING

Short half-life gamma-emitting isotopes such as technetium Tc 99m pertechnetate or indium In 113m diethylenetriamine pentaacetic acid (DTPA) are excluded by the intact blood-brain barrier. The isotope will cross defects in the blood-brain barrier caused by tumor or vascular accident, which appear as an area of increased "radiolabeling" on the gamma camera photograph. Intravenous injection of the isotope as a bolus followed by rapid-sequence imaging gives qualitative information about extracranial carotid artery and supratentorial cerebral blood flow.

Isotope cisternography can give qualitative information about cerebrospinal fluid flow and absorption characteristics. Indium In 113m DTPA is injected into the subarachnoid space via ventricular, lumbar, or lateral cervical puncture, followed by scanning at intervals of up to 48 hours. This technique is useful for the evaluation of hydrocephalus, cerebrospinal fluid shunt function, and cerebrospinal fluid fistulas.

Injection of xenon 133 into the carotid artery followed by special scanning techniques can give quantitative measurements of regional cerebral blood flow. Positron scanning is a newer, more accurate technique using inhalation of krypton 77 to measure cerebral blood flow. The first method requires puncture or catheterization of the carotid artery, and the latter requires specialized computer equipment; these requirements have prevented their widespread use.

COMPUTERIZED TOMOGRAPHY
(CT Brain Scan)

Computerized tomography of the brain is about 100 times more sensitive than conventional radiographs. The technique is based on computer analysis of the absorption of finely collimated x-ray photons that pass through the skull and brain from numerous angles. A cross-sectional image (Figure 38–3A and 38–3B) is reconstructed by computer calculation.

Lesions that can be identified with a high degree of accuracy by CT scanning include intracerebral hema-

toma, cerebral infarction, subdural and epidural hematomas, tumors of the brain and surrounding structures, cerebral abscess, cerebral edema, cerebral atrophy, and hydrocephalus. Lesions situated near the cranial base or in the extreme high hemisphere convexity are more difficult to delineate. Computer programs capable of reconstructing images in the coronal and sagittal plane have increased scanning accuracy in these problem regions. Intravenous injection of iodinated contrast media followed by repeat scanning is capable of enhancing the density of lesions with an increased blood pool (eg, meningioma, arteriovenous malformation) or alteration in the blood-brain barrier (eg, metastatic tumor and inflammatory lesions).

The injection of iodinated contrast material into the subarachnoid space helps delineate cerebrospinal fluid-containing lesions from normal cerebral tissues.

MAGNETIC RESONANCE IMAGING

Magnetic resonance imaging (MRI) has revolutionized neurodiagnosis and is superior to CT scanning for obtaining images of the brain and spinal cord. Images can be obtained in any plane without the interference of artifacts from bone. MRI is particularly sensitive for lesions in the posterior fossa-foramen magnum and in the spinal cord. For congenital intraspinal lesions, MRI has replaced myelography as the initial diagnostic procedure. MRI is now the preferred modality for screening patients for disease of the central nervous system. The use of paramagnetic contrast agents has dramatically improved the sensitivity and specificity of MRI.

Magnetic resonance angiography delineates the major extracranial and intracranial vessels. The ability to delineate intracranial vascular lesions noninvasively is useful in screening for aneurysms, arteriovenous malformations, vascular occlusive disease, and vasculitis. With continued advances, this technique will supplant routine diagnostic angiography for screening purposes.

MYELOGRAPHY

Myelography is the radiographic study of the spinal canal and its contents with various contrast agents. Most frequently, a water-soluble nonionic positive contrast material is injected into the subarachnoid space via a lumbar or cervical puncture. The contrast material, which is hyperbaric, mixes with cerebrospinal fluid and is manipulated within the spinal canal by tilting the patient to various angles. The flow of contrast material is monitored by fluoroscopy, and radiographs are taken in desired projections to record and preserve with more detail the areas of interest. Since this agent is absorbed, re-

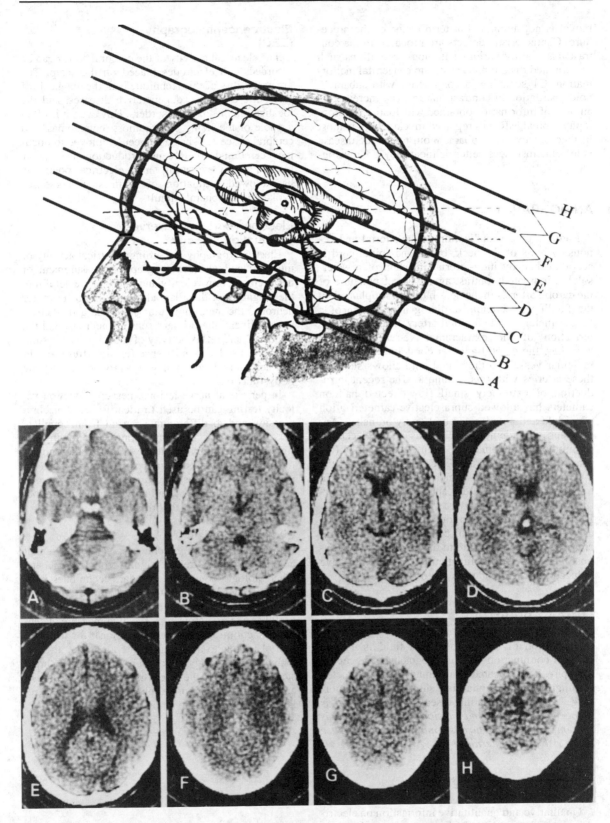

Figure 38–3. Normal CT scan. **Top:** Tomographic planes used in CT scan. Lines define the planes (perpendicular to the page) cut by the CT scanner; letters correspond to the computed projection at **bottom.** (Reproduced, with permission, from Taveras JM, Wood EH: *Diagnostic Neuroradiology,* 2nd ed. Williams & Wilkins, 1976.)

moval is not attempted at termination of the procedure. Characteristic defects are produced in the contrast material by various pathologic conditions such as herniated disk, tumor, cyst, and congenital malformation. CT scanning in conjunction with subarachnoid instillation of contrast material can increase the amount of information obtained with routine myelography. Spinal MRI has replaced myelography in most instances. However, subarachnoid metastatic disease is in some instances better delineated by CT myelography.

ANGIOGRAPHY

Radiographic visualization of the arterial and venous systems of the neck, brain, and spinal cord is accomplished by intra-arterial injection of a water-soluble iodinated contrast agent. Direct puncture of the carotid arteries in the neck has been supplanted by the Seldinger technique utilizing introduction of a long catheter via the femoral artery. Selective catheterization of the extracranial vessels and their branches, the carotid and vertebral arteries, and the radicular vessels to the spinal cord allows study of these arteries with this technique. The recent introduction of extremely small flow-directed balloon catheters has allowed supraselective catheterization of middle and anterior cerebral artery branches. Angiography can demonstrate occlusion, displacement (eg, tumor, hematoma), the diameter of vessels (eg, spasm), abnormalities of the vessel wall (eg, arteritis, atherosclerosis), and abnormal vasculature (in tumor). It is the only study capable of fully characterizing aneurysms and arteriovenous malformations. Digital subtraction angiography (DSA) permits the use of smaller amounts of contrast material and decreases radiation exposure to the patient. Newer contrast materials and careful attention to technique have reduced the rate of side effects to less than 1%.

LUMBAR PUNCTURE

Evaluation of the cerebrospinal fluid is usually done in conjunction with myelography or encephalography. It is indicated as a primary test in suspected meningitis or encephalitis, subarachnoid hemorrhage, and demyelinating disease. *If the patient is suspected of having a mass lesion or if papilledema is present, lumbar puncture is contraindicated because of the risk of fatal herniation.*

ELECTRICAL STUDIES

Qualitative and quantitative information on electrical potentials generated by brain, nerves, and muscle can be obtained by noninvasive techniques.

Electroencephalography (EEG)

The electrical activity of the cerebral cortex can be recorded with electrodes placed on the scalp. The greatest utility of this technique is in the diagnosis of metabolic disorders, degenerative diseases, and the localization of seizure disorders. However, it is often capable of localizing brain tumors, hematomas, and cerebral abscess. It has also been employed to document cerebral death. Recent introduction of computer techniques for averaging small electrical potentials has allowed evaluation of brain stem responses evoked by peripheral stimuli.

Electromyography & Nerve Conduction Velocity

Electromyography (recording electrical activity of muscles) and electroneurography (measurement of nerve conduction velocity and latency) are helpful in the diagnosis of disorders affecting the lower motor neurons, the neuromuscular junction and skeletal muscle fibers, the primary sensory neurons, and the volitional and reflex activity of muscles. These studies can be used to identify specific and diffuse peripheral nerve involvement as well as to localize the site of dysfunction.

In peripheral nerve lesions, nerve conduction velocity testing can be used to identify areas of compression and to differentiate partial from complete nerve injury as well as regeneration. Following peripheral nerve injury, evidence of denervation potentials in muscles does not appear for 14–21 days. In psychogenic weakness and upper motor neuron disease, electromyography and nerve conduction velocity testing disclose no abnormalities.

Evoked Potentials

Computer averaging techniques can extract small amplitude stimulus-related signals from the EEG and other biologic potentials. Standard techniques have been developed to record these potentials, evoked by auditory, somatosensory, and visual stimuli, that are useful as a quantitative and objective measure of sensory function (eg, hearing and vision); for localization of lesions to a particular site along the afferent pathway from receptor to cerebral cortex (eg, brain stem tumors, multiple sclerosis, spinal cord lesions); and for insight into normal physiologic processes related to maturation and aging.

CRANIOCEREBRAL TRAUMA

Lawrence H. Pitts, MD,
& Russ P. Nockels, MD

Among central nervous system disorders, craniocerebral trauma is second only to stroke as a cause of death. Traumatic injury is the leading cause of death in persons below age 45, and head injury constitutes a major portion of deaths in this group. Approximately 500,000 head injuries, accounting for the loss of 70,000 lives, occur each year in the USA. Craniocerebral trauma produces severe disability and imposes a huge financial and psychologic burden on the patient, the patient's family, and society.

Sudden blows to the head may cause rapid movement of the skull and enclosed brain. The brain may be compressed or stretched, or parts of the brain may move relative to other parts of the brain, skull, or dural structures such as the falx or tentorium. These events can result in areas of focal brain injury remote from the site of impact and can cause brain concussion, contusion, or laceration.

Pathology

Craniocerebral trauma can involve scalp, skull, or brain in any combination.

A. Scalp: Scalp lacerations are common and are important chiefly as sources of significant hemorrhage or infection. Thick scalp with its overlying hair provides a cushion for the skull and brain; blunt trauma commonly causes stellate burst lacerations. Numerous arterial and venous anastomoses contribute to brisk bleeding but also to effective healing. Most of these vessels lie in the subcutaneous fat immediately superficial to the galea, the dense fibrous tissue that makes the scalp stiff and unyielding.

B. Skull: A variety of skull injuries may follow blunt trauma:

1. Simple skull fractures–Linear, nondisplaced vault fractures are common and require no specific treatment but are important as markers of the significant force that was delivered to the head. The patient must be carefully observed for 12–24 hours for possible neurologic deterioration secondary to intracranial hematoma.

2. Depressed skull fractures–These usually occur as a result of low-velocity injuries such as blows by small objects. The inner table of the skull invariably suffers greater damage than the outer table. These injuries may result in dural or brain laceration, and if the depression is greater than the thickness of the skull or if it involves the posterior wall of the frontal sinus, surgical elevation may be required.

3. Compound fractures–These are fractures in which the overlying scalp has been lacerated. Proper treatment is essentially the same as with simple fractures and includes adequate wound debridement and closure of the laceration.

4. Basal skull fractures–These exceedingly common fractures are diagnosed largely on clinical grounds. As with linear fractures involving the vault of the skull, basal fractures are important as markers of the severity of injury. In addition, they may cause cerebrospinal fluid leakage, with the attendant risk of meningitis or brain abscess formation. Cerebrospinal fluid leaks usually result from fractures into the paranasal sinuses or mastoid air cells with laceration of the overlying dura and loss of cerebrospinal fluid into the nose or ears. Basilar skull fractures also may injure cranial nerves that course through the skull base.

BRAIN INJURY

Primary injury results at the time of impact; secondary injury is progressive brain damage arising as a consequence of hematoma or edema formation, or ischemia or hypoxic damage leading to later and progressive neurologic deficit.

The brain may be injured directly under the site of impact (coup injuries) or, in some instances, diagonally opposite to the point of impact (contrecoup injuries). Because of the rough surface of the floor of the frontal and temporal fossae, the anterior and interior portions of the frontal and temporal lobes are in particular jeopardy. Abrupt movement of the brain within the skull causes contusion of these areas.

Types of Injury

A. Concussion: Concussion is a clinical diagnosis and is manifested by temporary dysfunction that is most severe immediately after injury and clears within 24 hours. It may be accompanied by a variety of autonomic abnormalities, including bradycardia, hypotension, and sweating. Loss of consciousness often but not invariably accompanies concussion. Amnesia for the event is common, and variable degrees of temporary lethargy, irritability, and memory dysfunction are hallmarks of cerebral concussion. Because concussion is not a fatal injury, data from pathologic examination (necropsy) are sparse; there is either no demonstrable damage or only minor inflammation of the white matter.

B. Cerebral Contusion: Cerebral contusion can be demonstrated by CT scan as small areas of hemorrhage in the cerebral parenchyma. Contusions usually produce neurologic deficits that persist for longer than 24 hours. Extravasation of red cells into gray and white matter can be demonstrated in fatal cases. Craniocerebral trauma is the most common cause of subarachnoid hemorrhage, and blood is present in the cerebrospinal fluid in many patients (although *lumbar puncture should not be done after a head injury*).

Focal neurologic deficits may include weakness, speech disorders, memory or affect abnormalities, or, rarely, visual dysfunction. Cerebral contusion may resolve with the disappearance of neurologic deficits, or focal or global deficits may persist. Blood-brain barrier defects and cerebral edema are common with cerebral contusion.

C. Laceration: Even without skull fracture, if sufficient force is delivered to the skull, the brain may be lacerated as a result of rapid movement and shearing of brain tissue. The pia and arachnoid overlying the surface of the brain may be torn, and accompanying laceration of blood vessels results in intracerebral hemorrhage. Focal neurologic deficits are the rule, and a neurologic deficit will often be permanent, although considerable improvement can occur with time.

Diagnosis

Triage of head-injured patients must be accurate and rapid. Injuries can range from minor impact without loss of consciousness to severe coma-producing fatal head injury. Successful management demands careful data gathering so that a rational course can be planned.

A. History: Valuable information can be gathered from observers of the injury and should include the cause of the injury and an estimate of the severity of the blow, the presence of early neurologic abnormalities such as seizures, weakness, or speech disorders, and documentation of any loss of consciousness. Subsequent management may depend on such sequences of events as a seizure preceding a fall as opposed to a fall with subsequent seizure after head injury. A history of alcohol or drug ingestion will affect the diagnostic evaluation. A history of a preexisting central nervous system disorder can substantially alter conclusions based on the neurologic examination. A history of medical disorders such as diabetes and insulin usage or myocardial disease may also affect initial therapy in unexplained loss of consciousness with or without head injury.

Amnesia for the specific injury is common even in minor head injuries. There may be both retrograde amnesia (forgetting events before the injury) and anterograde amnesia (forgetting the injury and subsequent events), particularly if there has been loss of consciousness. Amnesia for 24 hours or more following the injury is a mark of significant head injury and an adverse prognostic sign. However, amnesia for a brief period before and after the injury has no particular significance.

Severe headache, particularly a unilateral one, may indicate an expanding intracranial mass and warrants careful sequential examinations and, possibly, additional diagnostic tests. Severe occipital headache may be caused by an odontoid fracture.

B. Physical Examination: The initial examination should be rapid and systematic. Attention must be directed to assessment of other major injuries, particularly spinal, chest, or abdominal, because injuries to these organ systems may severely worsen any neurologic damage. Hypoxia, shock, hypo- or hyperglycemia, depressant effects of narcotics, and unstable spine injuries must be recognized immediately and appropriately treated. Only then can the neurologic examination be performed safely.

Examination of the scalp must be meticulous. Large lacerations are easy to recognize, but hair may disguise additional scalp injury that, unless properly debrided and closed, can cause subgaleal abscess formation. Penetrating wounds of the scalp and skull may be missed entirely, but unless they are properly recognized and treated, they may contribute to brain abscess formation.

Subgaleal hemorrhage can cause irregularities of the scalp that suggest skull fractures when in fact no fracture is present. Fractures may at times be palpated through lacerations, and if compound depressed fractures are present, they will need surgical treatment. Basal skull fractures may be recognized by the presence of a hemotympanum (blood noted medial to the tympanic membrane), cerebrospinal fluid otorrhea or rhinorrhea, or bilateral ecchymoses confined to the orbits and not extending out over the supraorbital or malar eminences in the acute phase (raccoon eyes). Fresh bleeding from an ear is also indicative of basal skull fracture more laterally placed in the temporal bone, unless there is evidence of a penetrating injury of the ear or the tympanic membrane has been ruptured by the concussive effects of an explosion.

Because facial injuries often occur along with head injuries, careful attention must be given to orbital fractures with extraocular muscle entrapment. Unstable midfacial fractures must also be excluded; they can be detected by attempts to move the upper teeth manually. Injuries to the nose, pharynx, or soft tissue of the anterior neck may also be present and can lead to respiratory embarrassment if not recognized and treated.

The purpose of the baseline neurologic evaluation is to determine "where the patient is and where he or she is going." It must include a rapid categorization of hemispheric and brain stem function so that changes in subsequent examinations will indicate improvement or deterioration of the patient and help direct further management. The scheme listed below is particularly valuable in that it can be repeated by various observers at different times and reliably indicate change in the patient's status. The sum of eye opening, motor response, and verbal response scores is known as the Glasgow Coma Score, a system widely used to evaluated head-injured patients.

1. Eye opening–This in part replaces "level of consciousness" and is graded by the patient's ability to open the eyes to an appropriate stimulus, including pain if necessary. The grades are (1) no eye opening,

(2) eye opening to painful stimulus, (3) eye opening to verbal stimulus, and (4) spontaneous eye opening.

2. Best motor response–This describes the patient's movement ability and is graded as (1) no movement to painful stimulus, (2) responds with abnormal extension of the upper extremities (formerly "decerebrate"), (3) stereotyped flexion at the elbow of one or both upper extremities (formerly "decorticate"), (4) complicated and variable response of the arms or legs to a painful stimulus, (5) localizes a painful stimulus to the supraorbital rim, and (6) follows commands.

3. Best verbal response–This is a measure of the patient's ability to speak as well as the content of speech. The patient (1) makes no verbal response, (2) makes unintelligible noises, (3) speaks a few words, (4) gives confused answers, or (5) is oriented. In each case the *best* response is recorded even if a painful stimulus is required to elicit that response.

4. Eye signs–Pupillary reactivity to light and size (in millimeters) should be recorded. A "direct" light response (light shined in one eye with that pupil constricting) indicates function, both of the optic nerves transmitting light reception to the brain and the oculomotor nerve conducting parasympathetic pupillary constrictor fibers. A "consensual" reflex (light shined in one eye with the contralateral pupil constricting) should also be noted. A blind eye would give no pupillary constriction to direct testing but would give constriction with consensual testing.

Extraocular eye movement gives a measure of the integrity of the medial longitudinal fasciculus (MLF), a fiber tract running the length of the midbrain and upper pons, that carries information for coordinating eye movement. If spontaneous conjugate eye movements are present, the MLF is intact. Eye movements can be elicited by oculocephalic ("doll's eyes") testing. This is done with rapid rotation of the head to one side. The eyes temporarily remain fixed in space but with head rotation appear to move away from the direction of the turning if the MLF is intact. *Caution: The doll's eyes maneuver should not be done unless a cervical fracture has been excluded.* Oculovestibular (caloric) testing can be done if the tympanic membrane is intact and the external canal is free of blood and wax. Ice water is instilled into the external auditory canal, and after a short delay, the eyes will begin to drift toward the cold ear and have a rapid nystagmus component away from the cold ear if this response is intact. Up to 50 mL of ice water may be required in patients with markedly depressed brain stem function.

Partial or complete ptosis with incomplete or complete closure of one eyelid can be assessed in an awake patient but cannot be determined accurately in comatose patients.

Papilledema may arise with increased intracranial pressure but often does not become evident for 6 hours or more after head injury. Subhyaloid hemorrhages (extravasation of small pools of blood between the retina and the hyaloid membrane) often occur with sudden increases in intracranial pressure such as with head injury or rupture of an intracranial aneurysm.

Conjugate deviation of both eyes to one side usually indicates a lesion of the frontal lobe on that side (adversive fields). Spontaneous nystagmus indicates damage to the cerebellum or vestibular connections. Skew deviation of the eyes occurs in injuries to the brain stem; local damage to the orbit or to the ocular muscles also may produce deviation of one eye.

5. Lower brain stem examination–Lower pontine and medullary function can be assessed by the type of irregular respiratory pattern, presence or absence of gag reflex to stimulation of the hypopharynx, and cough reflex to tracheal stimulation.

6. Motor pattern–Development of a hemiparesis can result from either hemispheric or upper brain stem injury or both. With sufficient damage, a paresis may progress to abnormal flexor or extensor posturing. This posturing was formerly thought to represent direct brain stem involvement, but more recent evidence shows that hemispheric injury can also result in flexor or extensor posturing.

7. Transtentorial herniation–There is a triad of signs that suggests pressure on the upper midbrain resulting from an expanding supratentorial mass lesion. First, there is a progressive third nerve palsy with loss of medial rectus function and sluggish or absent constriction to light by the pupil, which is usually dilated more than 6 mm. The third nerve palsy is almost always present on the same side as the largest supratentorial mass lesion. If pressure on the brain stem is severe, both pupils may become unreactive. Second, asymmetric motor findings also are present with transtentorial herniation, with either a hemiparesis or abnormal posturing of the limbs that is worse on the side contralateral to the mass lesion. In about 25% of patients, the worst motor findings are ipsilateral to the mass lesion ("Kernohan's notch" phenomenon), with the cerebral peduncle opposite the side of the mass lesion being compressed against the free edge of the tentorium. Third, midbrain compression causes lethargy or progressive coma because of depressed mesencephalic reticular activating system function.

Diagnostic Procedures

A. Lumbar Puncture: *Lumbar puncture should not be done when head injury is an obvious or very likely diagnosis.* An abnormal lumbar puncture, with either bloody or xanthochromic fluid or elevated cerebrospinal fluid pressures, does not localize or define an intracranial abnormality. Conversely, a normal lumbar puncture does not exclude the possibility of an intracranial hematoma. The only indication for a lumbar puncture is suspected meningitis. *There is no other role for lumbar puncture in the management of head injury.*

B. Imaging Studies:

1. Skull x-rays–Anteroposterior and lateral skull x-ray films can be valuable in managing head injury. Fracture of the skull vault is usually obvious; if it crosses a major vascular groove, the risk of epidural hemorrhage increases. Basal fractures can be seen in less than 10% of patients. However, air-fluid levels in the sphenoid or frontal sinuses are strongly suggestive of basal fractures. Depressed fractures can often be identified by the double density of bone along the fracture line, indicating overriding of the fractured elements. Lateral x-ray films of the cervical spine should be taken routinely in head-injured patients to rule out unstable neck fractures.

2. Computerized tomography (CT scan)–CT scans have revolutionized the diagnosis of cerebral lesions in head-injured patients. CT scans are noninvasive, except for the injection of a water-soluble iodine contrast material when indicated. They can demonstrate skull fractures, extracerebral and intracerebral hematomas, areas of contusion, and cerebral edema and can accurately demonstrate the size and location of the cerebral ventricles, whose diminished size or shifts are indications of local mass lesions. The newest equipment requires that patients be immobilized for only 2–10 seconds at a time and can avoid artifacts that may obscure cerebral lesions.

3. Magnetic resonance imaging (MRI)–Although MRI has some advantages over CT scans (eg, some traumatic lesions such as subdural hematoma have the same density as brain on CT scans; brain edema is more easily seen on MRI), it is not often used to study acute head injury, because it takes about 45 minutes to obtain MRI scans and because the patient is more inaccessible and not easily manipulated during scanning. MRI is more sensitive in demonstrating small lesions and is most valuable in the chronic recovery phase.

4. Cerebral angiography–Angiography has a limited role in craniocerebral trauma, primarily to evaluate vascular injury in the neck or at the skull base.

5. Ultrasonography–Equipment now available makes it possible to obtain sonograms through openings in the skull, either through bur holes or craniotomy defects (before or during surgery) or via the anterior fontanelle in infants. However, lesions cannot be imaged as accurately on sonograms as on CT scans.

Differential Diagnosis

In the absence of an adequate history, unconsciousness may result from a wide variety of structural or metabolic lesions. Most head injury is attended by some abnormality of the scalp such as abrasions or subgaleal hematomas. However, in a few patients there is no external evidence of injury, and a variety of causes must be considered.

Coma, hemiplegia, and eye deviation plus evidence of chronic hypertension (funduscopic changes, cardiomegaly) suggest a hypertensive intracerebral hematoma. Obtundation, fever, and a stiff neck suggest meningitis, either bacterial or perhaps chemical, from spontaneous subarachnoid hemorrhage. These constitute the only indication for lumbar puncture; if focal findings are present, the lumbar puncture should be preceded by a CT scan. If cerebral infection is clinically likely, antibiotics can be started before diagnostic studies. Diabetic, renal, or hepatic causes of coma can be diagnosed with appropriate blood tests.

Complications

Primary cerebral injuries cause cell death or dysfunction on impact. Because many of these injuries are the result of traffic accidents, only strict enforcement of traffic laws, use of lap and chest restraints in automobiles, and use of helmets on two- or three-wheeled vehicles will decrease the number of primary cerebral injuries. Secondary injuries arise as a result of brain and body changes after the impact.

A. Hemorrhage: Head injury can cause bleeding into the epidural, subdural, or subarachnoid spaces or intracerebrally into brain tissues. Epidural and subdural hematomas are discussed below.

Impact between brain and adjacent bone can result in vascular disruption and focal hemorrhage into the cortex or subcortical white matter. This may cause local brain cell death and often results in marked local cerebral edema. Even without a definite intracerebral hematoma, areas of contusion can create a mass effect and even herniation in severe cases. Subarachnoid hemorrhage is common and occasionally impedes cerebrospinal fluid drainage, requiring shunting procedures in a few patients.

Subdural hygromas are accumulations of cerebrospinal fluid, or cerebrospinal fluid mixed with a small amount of blood. They arise when fluid escapes through a tear in the arachnoid into the subdural space. They can create a focal mass effect and may have to be evacuated through bur holes.

B. Traumatic Vascular Malformations: A carotid cavernous fistula may arise if the cavernous portion of the carotid artery is lacerated by a fracture of the sphenoid bone, causing a major arteriovenous communication. Symptoms may be delayed for a month or more following injury and are often heralded by progressive retro-orbital pain followed by chemosis and proptosis of one or both eyes. Papilledema and engorgement of the retinal veins are usually present. These lesions generally can be cured.

C. Cerebrospinal Fluid Leak: Basal skull fractures involving paranasal sinuses may result in cerebrospinal fluid rhinorrhea or otorrhea, which is indicated by a mixture of clear fluid and blood coming from the nose or ear. Cerebrospinal fluid leak may not be readily apparent soon after the injury. Measurements of the glucose content of the fluid are inaccurate because both nasal secretions and blood contain sufficient amounts of glucose to give a positive test. When a drop of fluid is placed on filter paper, a double ring ("halo test") will appear if cerebrospinal fluid is mixed with blood; blood alone usually gives a single red circle. Because cerebrospinal fluid otorrhea or rhinorrhea may be accompanied by meningitis or brain abscess formation, leakage of the fluid must be stopped. If meningitis occurs, the most likely causative organisms are *Haemophilus influenzae, Streptococcus pneumoniae,* or other streptococci, all of which are common inhabitants of the paranasal sinuses.

D. Cranial Nerve Palsy: The olfactory nerves can be torn at the cribriform plate; traumatic anosmia seldom resolves. *Immediate* optic nerve loss following head injury is almost always permanent; however, if *progressive* loss of vision develops, optic nerve decompression or administration of corticosteroids may result in partial recovery of vision. Palsies of the third, fourth, and sixth cranial nerves usually improve, although partial deficits may persist. Facial nerve palsies after temporal bone fracture may require decompression and repair of the injured seventh cranial nerve. Delayed facial palsies are more common and usually resolve without operation. Lower cranial nerve palsies are uncommon.

E. Posttraumatic Syndrome: A variety of nonspecific complaints are common after head injury, the most prominent of which are headache, dizziness, easy fatigability, and poor memory. Diminished ability to concentrate and emotional lability may also occur. While these symptoms might seem psychologic, electronystagmography and formal mental testing will often reveal some organic basis. Psychologic testing has revealed significantly impaired mental function in many patients. Reassurance, mild sedatives, or medical treatment for dizziness may improve the patient's symptoms until they resolve, usually within weeks to months after surgery.

F. Posttraumatic Epilepsy: Patients may develop seizures shortly after injury, but these early seizures are generally of no consequence. However, an estimated 3–6% of patients who lose consciousness after head injury develop a more chronic seizure disorder. The presence of a subdural or epidural hematoma can cause up to a 30% incidence of posttraumatic seizures, and penetrating injuries of the brain with severe head injury may increase the frequency of seizure to as high as 50%. The use of prophylactic anticonvulsants (eg, phenytoin, 300 mg/d for adults) can prevent seizures while the patient is on medication but probably does not alter the frequency of seizures after anticonvulsants are discontinued.

Treatment

A. Emergency Treatment: Head-injured patients require immediate emergency treatment, including maintenance of an airway and restoration of blood pressure. Unconscious patients should be intubated to prevent hypoxia, hypercapnia, and aspiration. Shock must be vigorously treated with intravenous fluids while possible sources of hemorrhage in the chest or abdomen are being sought.

B. General Treatment: Patients who are comatose or who show rapid neurologic deterioration demand immediate intervention. At most institutions, CT scan precedes surgery. At some centers, exploratory bur holes are made or craniotomy is undertaken without intracranial studies.

Hyperventilation (PCO_2 = 25 mm Hg) can rapidly lower intracranial blood volume and intracranial pressure. Extreme hyperventilation (PCO_2 < 25 mm Hg) should be avoided because it may cause ischemia. Hyperosmotic agents (mannitol, 0.5–1 g/kg body weight intravenously) will dehydrate normal brain within 15–20 minutes and will lower intracranial pressure. Until corticosteroids have been shown to improve outcome from severe head injury, they should not be used routinely in management of craniocerebral trauma.

Antibiotic treatment should be initiated in patients with contaminated compound wounds, but there is no proof of efficacy in patients with basal skull fracture with or without cerebrospinal fluid leak.

Status epilepticus is uncommon following head injury. However, in severe head injury, anticonvulsant therapy should be initiated soon after injury with a loading dose of phenytoin (15 mg/kg body weight intravenously) and continued for at least 1 week. Phenobarbital will increase a patient's lethargy and make the neurologic examination more difficult to interpret.

Progressive neurologic deterioration is an indication for further diagnostic tests or exploratory surgery.

C. Specific Treatment:

1. Scalp wounds–Bleeding usually can be controlled by a simple pressure dressing or, in the case of arterial bleeding, by firm finger pressure along the edges of the wound. A hemostat can be attached to the galea and allowed to hang down to hold the galea firmly against the skin to compress the bleeding vessels. At least 2 inches should be shaved circumferentially around the wound before repair. Simple scalp lacerations should be debrided and closed primarily, using monofilament vertical mattress sutures that penetrate the scalp deeply enough to close the galea as part of the primary closure.

2. Depressed skull fractures–Depressed bone fragments must often be elevated surgically if the depression is equal to or greater than the thickness of the skull, usually 5 mm or more. Unless surgery is required by a deteriorating condition, depressed fractures overlying the dural sinuses are not elevated because of the risk of major hemorrhage.

3. Compound skull fractures–Debridement and closure should be effected in less than 12 hours to lower the risk of subgaleal or intracranial infection. Emergency treatment consists of applying a sterile compression dressing. The wound should not be closed, and no attempt should be made to remove any foreign body protruding from the wound until the patient is in the operating room and all preparations have been made for craniotomy. This assumes that the patient arrives at or is transferred to a hospital with complete neurosurgical facilities.

Prognosis

Thirty to 50 percent of severe head injuries are fatal despite intensive management. Few patients become independent who still show abnormal motor posturing after 3 days. The prognosis in children is much better, and prolonged coma may be followed by a normal outcome. Abnormal physical findings may be permanent after a severe head injury, but many patients are able to adjust to these deficits. Emotional disturbances and psychiatric disorders resulting from head injury are more refractory to therapy.

EPIDURAL HEMATOMA

An epidural hematoma (Figure 38–4) occurs as a result of skull fracture and laceration of a meningeal vessel, usually the posterior branch of the middle meningeal artery. All skull fractures are accompanied by *small* epidural hematomas, usually venous in origin and arising from the diploic space. When the dura is stripped from the inner table of the skull adjacent to a fracture and arterial bleeding from a lacerated meningeal artery begins filling the space, the dura is further stripped, and a large extradural mass that causes se-

vere brain compression may occur. Occasionally, the space is filled with venous blood, most commonly when fracture lines cross the superior sagittal or transverse sinuses, the venous collection arising either from laceration of the sinuses or venous tributaries to the sinuses.

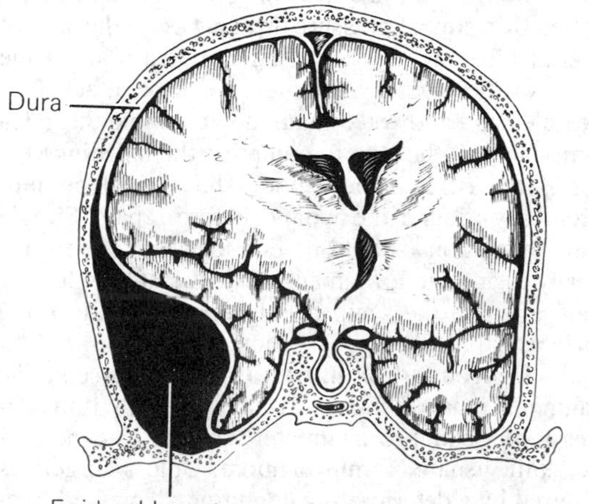

Epidural hematomas may occur after minor head injury. There may be no loss of consciousness or only a transient concussive state with rapid return of normal brain function. Epidural hematomas also may accompany more severe head injury with skull fracture. Only one-third of patients with epidural hematomas will have a classic "lucid interval," with a definite period of essentially normal brain function following impact, before the expanding epidural hematoma causes progressive loss of consciousness and focal neurologic deficits. Epidural hematomas are most common lateral to the temporal lobes where the skull is thinnest and the meningeal vessels are numerous. With expansion of the hematoma, there is medial compression of the temporal lobe that causes a contralateral hemiparesis and eventual transtentorial herniation as the medial temporal lobe compresses midbrain structures at the tentorial incisure.

As many as one-third of patients with epidural hematoma do not present to a physician until the onset of coma. The death rate from epidural hematomas approaches 30–50% in some series, chiefly because of a delay in recognition of the expanding intracranial hematoma. Therefore, admission for observation is justified for head-injured patients who lose consciousness for 2 minutes or more or if skull x-rays show a new fracture.

Extradural hematomas may be seen in the posterior fossa and are most reliably demonstrated on CT scan or vertebral angiography.

SUBDURAL HEMATOMAS

Subdural hematomas are the most common intracranial mass lesions that result from head injury (Figure 38–5). Most subdural hematomas are the result of torn bridging veins that drain blood from cerebral cortex to major overlying dural sinuses. They may go unrecognized for a time or may accompany devastating primary cerebral injury in patients who are unconscious from the time of injury; these patients have a high death rate.

Subdural hematomas may be small at onset of symptoms if there is marked accompanying cerebral edema. In an elderly patient with a "brain smaller than the skull," a hematoma may become quite large before neurologic symptoms or signs appear.

Subdural hematomas are often classified according to the length of time between injury and onset of symptoms.

Figure 38–4. Epidural hemorrhage. (Reprinted from *Hosp Med* [Oct] 1965;1:9, by permission of the authors and Wallace Laboratories.)

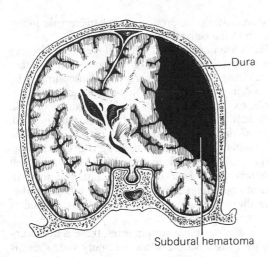

Figure 38–5. Subdural hemorrhage. (Reprinted from *Hosp Med* [Oct] 1965;1:9, by permission of the authors and Wallace Laboratories.)

Acute Subdural Hematomas

These present within 24 hours after injury. The death rate is higher in acute subdural hematomas than in any other category of closed head injury. There is often associated severe brain contusion or laceration, which leads to progressive cerebral edema and cerebral injury even after the acute subdural hematoma is recognized and removed. Although most acute subdural hematomas are venous in origin, laceration of cortical arteries occasionally gives rise to a more rapidly evolving hematoma. Early evacuation of these mass lesions is mandatory, although the death rate remains above 75% for patients with the combination of extrinsic brain compression and intrinsic brain damage.

Subacute Subdural Hematomas

These present between 1 and 14 days after injury. The symptoms are related to progressive brain compression and usually include severe headache, papilledema, and focal neurologic deficits, including hemiparesis or dysphasia.

Chronic Subdural Hematomas

These hematomas are discovered with progressive neurologic deficits that occur later than 2 weeks following head injury. In some instances, the initial head injury is completely forgotten, and patients may be evaluated for possible brain tumors or dementias such as Alzheimer's disease. Headache is common, and focal neurologic deficits may appear; dementia and increasing lethargy usually cause the patient to be brought in for medical evaluation.

The initial hemorrhage may be relatively small or may occur in elderly patients with large ventricles or a dilated subarachnoid space. Membranes deriving from dura mater and arachnoid encapsulate the hematoma, which remains clotted for 2–3 weeks and then gradually liquefies. The patient may have no symptoms for prolonged periods, only to become symptomatic when the hematoma enlarges by additional bleeding into the cavity from friable blood vessels in the capsule.

Chronic subdural hematomas are most common in infants and in adults over 60 years of age. Because of the slow and insidious development of symptoms, the patient's behavior may be attributed to a psychiatric rather than physical cause. Chronic subdural hematomas are bilateral in 20% of patients and are best demonstrated with CT or MRI scans or radionuclide brain scan, all of which will accurately demonstrate the lesion. The liquefied chronic subdural hematoma usually can be removed adequately by bur holes placed over the cavity.

Bennett BR, Jacobs LM, Schwartz RJ: Incidence, costs, and DRG-based reimbursement for traumatic brain injured patients: A 3-year experience. J Trauma 1989;29:556.

Coonan TJ: The management of acute severe head injury. Can J Anaesth 1989;36:S26.

Gennarelli TA et al: Mortality of patients with head injury and extracranial injury treated in trauma centers. J Trauma 1989;29:1193.

Grahm TW et al: Civilian gunshot wounds to the head: A prospective study. Neurosurgery 1990;27:696.

Levi L et al: Diffuse axonal injury: Analysis of 100 patients with radiological signs. Neurosurgery 1990;27:429.

Lighthall JW, Dixon CE, Anderson TE: Experimental models of brain injury. J Neurotrauma 1989;6:83.

Marion DW, Darby J, Yonas H: Acute regional cerebral blood flow changes caused by severe head injuries. J Neurosurg 1991;74:407.

Miller JD et al: Ischemic brain damage in a model of acute subdural hematoma. Neurosurgery 1990;27:433.

Rogers MC, Kirsch JR: Current concepts in brain resuscitation. JAMA 1989;261:3143.

Rosenthal BW, Bergman I: Intracranial injury after moderate head trauma in children. J Pediatr 1989;115:346.

Sosin DM, Sachs JJ, Holmgreen P: Head injury-associated deaths from motorcycle crashes: Relationship to helmet use laws. JAMA 1990;264:2395.

Thompson RS, Rivara FP, Thompson DC: A case-control study of the effectiveness of bicycle safety helmets. N Engl J Med 1989;320:1362.

SPINAL CORD INJURY

Russ P. Nockels, MD,
& Lawrence H. Pitts, MD

Despite recent advances, acute spinal cord injury remains the most devastating of all survivable traumas. Each year, 15,000 new spinal cord injuries occur in the USA as a result of motor vehicle accidents, falls, sports injuries, and various other types of accident. From the time of injury to death, the average cost of care of one patient exceeds $500,000, and the annual cost for acute and chronic care of spinal cord-injured patients is estimated to be $3 billion. Although these injuries necessarily impose a dramatic change in the patients' lives, in some countries as many as 75% of paraplegics and 25% of quadriplegics return to gainful employment. The finding that treatment with methylprednisolone (30 mg/kg intravenously) benefits patients when used within 8 hours after spinal cord injury has provided new hope that future pharmacologic therapies may further diminish neurologic deficits.

Principles of Management

Transection of the spinal cord almost never accompanies spinal cord injury in humans. Strict adherence to the following principles is therefore imperative to protect surviving spinal tissue: First, the injury must be recognized. Second, care must be exercised to prevent further damage ("secondary" injury) and to detect deteriorating neurologic function so that corrective measures can be taken. Third, the patient must be maintained in optimal condition to allow the greatest possible nervous system repair and recovery. Fourth, evaluation and rehabilitation of the patient must be actively pursued to maximize the function of surviving but dysfunctional nervous tissue. These principles must be followed in order to diminish the economic, social, and emotional cost of spinal cord injury.

Posttraumatic instability of the bony spine is discussed elsewhere. Here we will discuss injury to the spinal cord and nerve roots. Injuries of bony and neural elements of the spine often coexist, and the treatment of both should be coordinated to ensure the best possible outcome.

Etiology & Classification

In general, injury to the spinal cord follows compression or severe angulation of the vertebral spine. In rare instances, severe hypotension will lead to cord infarction, or axial distraction of elements of the vertebral column will result in a stretch injury of the cord. Most cord injuries follow subluxation with or without rotation of adjacent vertebral bodies that compress the cord between dislocated bone. Less often, axial compression of the spine will crush or wedge a vertebral body, and either bone or intervertebral disk fragments can be extruded into the spinal canal and compress the spinal cord or the anterior spinal artery. Another injury, seen usually in older patients with degenerative arthritis of the cervical spine, involves neck hyperextension with infolding of the ligamentum flavum located in the spinal canal posterior to the cord. The spinal cord is trapped between arthritic bony spurs anteriorly and the ligamentum flavum posteriorly, producing a characteristic injury known as the **central cord syndrome.**

Early after spinal cord injury, there is a temporary loss of function with little or no demonstrable pathologic change. Progressive necrosis, caused in part by the posttraumatic accumulation of vasoactive eicosanoids, oxygen free radicals, and by-products of lipid peroxidation, is the usual result of injury to the cord. Loss of the "blood-cord barrier" causes edema and increased tissue pressure that, along with cord hemorrhage, limit the blood supply, with the result that cell ischemia may further damage the cord. The distribution of cord edema, hemorrhage, and infarction dictates the neurologic symptoms and signs elicited at the time of evaluation.

In *complete* spinal cord injuries, there is no voluntary nervous function below the injury site. There is an initial phase of spinal shock, a loss of *all reflexes* below the injured segment, including bulbocavernosus, cremasteric, anal contraction to perianal stimulation, and deep tendon reflexes. This phenomenon may be temporary because of ionic and blood flow changes at the injury site. In *incomplete* spinal cord injuries, some function is present below the injury site, accounting for a much more favorable overall prognosis. Cord function may improve rapidly as spinal shock clears, or function may improve slowly in the months or years after injury.

The sites of damage within the cord and nerve root will determine what function is lost and what remains:

(1) Anterior cord syndrome: Damage to spinothalamic tracts and corticospinal tracts with relatively intact dorsal columns and preservation of touch and position sense, often related to injury to the spinal artery.

(2) Brown-Séquard's syndrome: A lesion involving the spinal cord extensively on one side of the midline results in ipsilateral motor weakness and loss of proprioception and contralateral loss of pain perception below the level of injury.

(3) Central cord syndrome: Hemorrhagic necrosis of the central portions of the cervical spinal cord often follows a brief concussive injury. Because distal leg and sacral motor and sensory fibers are located most peripherally in the cervical cord, the perianal sensation and some lower extremity movement and sensation may be preserved.

(4) Nerve root injury: This can occur at the level of vertebral body dislocation. Direct root compression may be relieved by reduction of the dislocation or by removal of fractured bone or disrupted disk.

(5) Conus medullaris compression: Injuries at the thoracolumbar region may cause injury to nerve cells of the tip of the spinal cord, descending corticospinal fibers, and lumbosacral nerve roots with a mixed upper motor neuron and lower motor neuron dysfunction.

(6) Cauda equina syndrome: This syndrome

may arise from bony dislocation or disk extrusions in the lumbar or sacral regions, with compression of lumbosacral nerve roots below the conus medullaris. Bowel and bladder dysfunction as well as leg numbness and weakness occur commonly in this syndrome.

Evaluation of Spinal Cord Injury

A. Physical Examination: Evaluation and initial treatment must be started at the scene of the injury. Early recognition of a spine or spinal cord injury will dictate preventive measures to preserve remaining neurologic function. Patients suspected to have spinal cord injuries must be immobilized with rigid cervical collars and backboards. At the receiving medical facility, care must be taken to treat hypoventilation, hypoxia, and hypercapnia (found with high cervical cord injuries), shock and hypothermia (secondary to loss of sympathetic nerve function with cervical injuries), paralytic ileus with abdominal sequestration of fluid, and bladder distention.

Until x-rays show otherwise, the examiner should assume that any comatose patient has an unstable spine fracture, although the combination of head and spinal cord injury is uncommon. Concern about combined injury *must not delay resuscitation* of hypotension and hypoventilation. If the patient is awake, a history should be taken as soon as possible, including information about the specific nature of the injury and what pain or neurologic symptoms followed. Complaints of numbness and weakness should be noted carefully. Severe headache, particularly occipital pain, is common with odontoid fracture or hangman's fracture (bilateral fracture of the C2 pedicles). To assess weakness, the patient is asked to move hands and feet spontaneously and against resistance. Sensory testing of the extremities, anterior trunk, neck, and face should then be done. Palpation of the spine by sliding the hands under the patient with minimal spine movement can reveal focal bone tenderness or deformity. Deep tendon reflexes must be evaluated in arms and legs; depression or absence of these reflexes will help localize the level of injury (Figure 38–6). Absence of abdominal reflex contraction to skin stimulation of the lower abdomen will localize a lesion in the T9–11 region. Absence of the cremasteric reflex (contraction of scrotal musculature in response to pinching of the medial thigh) indicates a lesion in the T12–L1 region of the cord. An intact bulbocavernosus reflex (anal sphincter contraction to penile or clitoral compression or downward pressure on the bladder trigone by a Foley catheter balloon when the catheter is gently pulled) indicates that sacral motor and sensory pathways are present; absence of the bulbocavernosus reflex is consistent with spinal shock or with sacral spinal cord or nerve root injury.

When the patient must be transferred to an x-ray table or bed, the transfer should be done with a fireman's carry, with at least three people *on each side* of the patient, with a fourth person, who directs the move, keeping the head in a *neutral position* by gentle axial traction (4–7 kg) applied with one hand on the chin and the other on the occiput.

B. Imaging Studies: Along with the physical examination, x-rays are essential for the evaluation of spine injuries. The lateral film is the most informative and should be examined for alignment of the anterior and posterior aspects of adjacent vertebral bodies and for angulation of the spinal canal at any level. Para- or prevertebral soft tissue masses usually indicate hemorrhage into these areas from fractures or ligamentous disruption. Anteroposterior spine films of the thoracic region and other levels permit assessment of lateral displacement of the vertebral bodies or widening or disruption of the pedicles. Oblique views in the cervical and lumbar regions will demonstrate facet fractures or dislocations. Frontal and lateral tomography can further identify bony abnormalities, but this procedure requires movement of the patient onto special tables for study.

MRI gives excellent views of the spine, disks, and spinal cord and is the diagnostic procedure of choice in patients with spinal cord injuries. CT scanning provides superior visualization of the bony spine and extraspinal soft tissue and provides additional insights into the management of spinal injury. Instillation of intrathecal metrizamide can outline the spinal cord and demonstrate cord compression.

Treatment

Emergency resuscitation of the spinal cord-injured patient parallels that of any major trauma, with the modification that spine alignment must be scrupulously maintained. Immediately after recognition of spinal cord injury, patients should be given 30 mg/kg of methylprednisolone intravenously followed by a continuous infusion of 5.4 mg/kg/h for 24 hours. Adequate blood pressure and ventilation are critical. Patients with cervical cord injuries maintain ventilation only with diaphragmatic activity; if paralytic ileus with abdominal distention occurs—or if the patient tires—initial adequate ventilation may deteriorate, and the patient will become hypoxic and require intubation and mechanical ventilation. After loss of spinal cord sympathetic pathways, blood pressure may be lower than normal. If urinary output is inadequate after catheterization, patients with mild hypotension will respond to low doses of pressor agents, but these should be used only after unsuspected sources of hemorrhage in the chest or abdomen have been excluded.

Unstable cervical fractures should be managed initially with external immobilization. Skeletal fixation with Gardner-Wells tongs or halo traction can be achieved in most emergency rooms, or halter traction can be used temporarily. Thoracic and lumbar fractures are managed by keeping the patient in a neutral

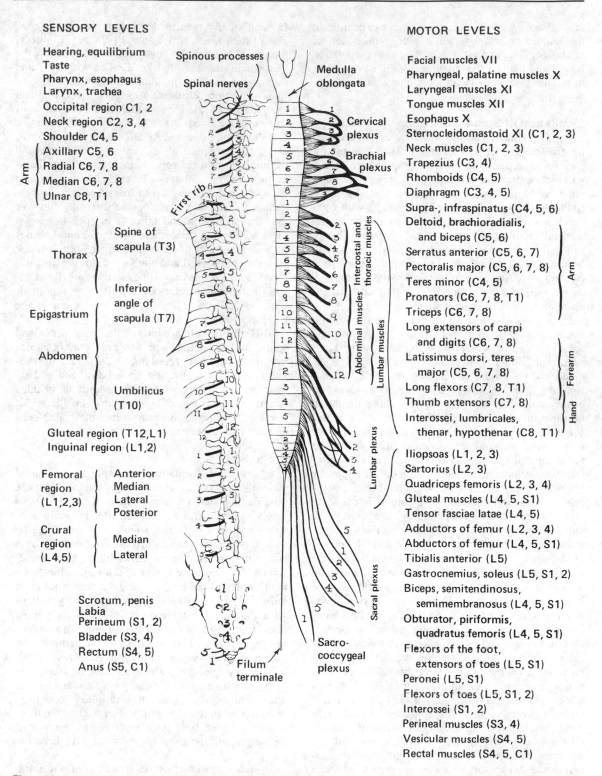

SENSORY LEVELS

Hearing, equilibrium
Taste
Pharynx, esophagus
Larynx, trachea
Occipital region C1, 2
Neck region C2, 3, 4
Shoulder C4, 5

Arm
- Axillary C5, 6
- Radial C6, 7, 8
- Median C6, 7, 8
- Ulnar C8, T1

Spinous processes
Spinal nerves
Medulla oblongata
First rib

Thorax
- Spine of scapula (T3)
- Inferior angle of scapula (T7)

Epigastrium

Abdomen
- Umbilicus (T10)

Gluteal region (T12, L1)
Inguinal region (L1, 2)

Femoral region (L1, 2, 3)
- Anterior
- Median
- Lateral
- Posterior

Crural region (L4, 5)
- Median
- Lateral

Scrotum, penis
Labia
Perineum (S1, 2)
Bladder (S3, 4)
Rectum (S4, 5)
Anus (S5, C1)

Filum terminale

Cervical plexus
Brachial plexus
Intercostal and thoracic muscles
Abdominal muscles
Lumbar muscles
Lumbar plexus
Sacral plexus
Sacro-coccygeal plexus

MOTOR LEVELS

Facial muscles VII
Pharyngeal, palatine muscles X
Laryngeal muscles XI
Tongue muscles XII
Esophagus X
Sternocleidomastoid XI (C1, 2, 3)
Neck muscles (C1, 2, 3)
Trapezius (C3, 4)
Rhomboids (C4, 5)
Diaphragm (C3, 4, 5)
Supra-, infraspinatus (C4, 5, 6)
Deltoid, brachioradialis, and biceps (C5, 6)
Serratus anterior (C5, 6, 7)
Pectoralis major (C5, 6, 7, 8)
Teres minor (C4, 5)
Pronators (C6, 7, 8, T1)
Triceps (C6, 7, 8)
Long extensors of carpi and digits (C6, 7, 8)
Latissimus dorsi, teres major (C5, 6, 7, 8)
Long flexors (C7, 8, T1)
Thumb extensors (C7, 8)
Interossei, lumbricales, thenar, hypothenar (C8, T1)

Arm
Forearm
Hand

Iliopsoas (L1, 2, 3)
Sartorius (L2, 3)
Quadriceps femoris (L2, 3, 4)
Gluteal muscles (L4, 5, S1)
Tensor fasciae latae (L4, 5)
Adductors of femur (L2, 3, 4)
Abductors of femur (L4, 5, S1)
Tibialis anterior (L5)
Gastrocnemius, soleus (L5, S1, 2)
Biceps, semitendinosus, semimembranosus (L4, 5, S1)
Obturator, piriformis, quadratus femoris (L4, 5, S1)
Flexors of the foot, extensors of toes (L5, S1)
Peronei (L5, S1)
Flexors of toes (L5, S1, 2)
Interossei (S1, 2)
Perineal muscles (S3, 4)
Vesicular muscles (S4, 5)
Rectal muscles (S4, 5, C1)

Figure 38–6. Motor and sensory levels of the spinal cord. (Reproduced, with permission, from deGroot J, Chusid JG: *Correlative Neuroanatomy*, 20th ed. Appleton & Lange, 1988.)

position, "logrolling" as necessary for skin care or pulmonary management. Oscillating beds also improve skin and pulmonary care.

Operative management of spinal cord injury must take into account two major considerations: **decompression** and **stability.** Realignment of the spinal canal can be achieved by proper application of traction, postural adjustment, and spine manipulation done by experienced physicians. Surgical exploration for bony realignment may be necessary in some patients. Surgery may also be indicated if bone or a foreign body is in the spinal canal or if the injury is followed by a *progressive* neurologic deficit that may be the result of a spinal epidural or subdural hematoma. Management of spine instability may include spinal fusion with metal plates and screws in combination with bone fusion.

The primary causes of death after cord injury are potentially avoidable. Renal failure following repeated urinary tract infections is best prevented by carefully performed intermittent bladder catheterization, which often can be done by the patient. Decubitus ulcers form easily over bony prominences in anesthetic areas and can be prevented with intermittent turning of patients and rotatory beds.

Optimal chronic care of patients with spinal cord injuries must include prevention or treatment of medical and surgical problems. Rehabilitation also requires emotional support and patient education for the activities of daily living and job retraining. The team approach provided by spinal cord injury centers has been very successful and has shown that hospital stays can be shortened and costs lowered. Ultimately, the patient finds a balance between acceptance of the loss and hope that spinal function will slowly improve.

Bailes JE, Maroon JC: Management of cervical spine injuries in athletes. Clin Sports Med 1989;8:43.

Blight A: Mechanical factors in experimental spinal cord injury. J Am Paraplegia Soc 1988;11:26.

Bracken MB et al: A randomized controlled trial of methylprednisolone or naloxone in the treatment of spinal cord injury. N Engl J Med 190;322:1405.

Bromley I: The quality of rehabilitation. Paraplegia 1989;27:249.

DeVivo MJ et al: Cause of death for patients with spinal cord injuries. Arch Intern Med 1989;149:1761.

Fesmire FM, Luten RC: The pediatric cervical spine: Developmental anatomy and clinical aspects. J Emerg Med 1989;7:133.

Nockels RP, Young W: Pharmacologic treatment of acute spinal cord injury. J Neurotrauma 1992;9(Suppl 1):5211.

Waxman SG: Demyelination in spinal cord injury. J Neurol Sci 1989;91:1.

Weingarden SI et al: A new approach to catastrophic injury: Spinal cord injury patients. Paraplegia 1989;27:314.

TRAUMATIC PERIPHERAL NERVE LESIONS

Nicholas M. Barbaro, MD,
& Michael S. Edwards, MD

Peripheral nerves contain sensory or motor axons (or both), most of which are myelinated. Each axon is surrounded by fine collagen fibers, the endoneurium. Groups of axons called fasciculi are bound together by the perineurium, which consists of Schwann cells and fine collagen fibrils. The epineurium, made of thicker collagen fibrils, surrounds the fasciculi. This layer is thought to elaborate the fibroblastic reaction that is the primary cause of fibrosis subsequent to nerve injury.

The four major causes of nerve injury are laceration, contusion, stretch, and compression. Less commonly, nerves may be injured inadvertently when an injection is given. Irrespective of cause, localized injuries fall into one of three categories: neurotmesis, axonotmesis, and neurapraxia. In **neurotmesis** (eg, nerve laceration), axons and endoneurial tubes are disrupted. The proximal nerve end first swells and then, to a variable degree, undergoes retrograde degeneration. Subsequently, a neuroma develops, composed of connective tissue and a tangle of regenerating axons. The axons in the distal end die (wallerian degeneration), the endoneurial tubes shrink, collagen is deposited, and an end-bulb glioma forms. In **axonotmesis,** there is wallerian degeneration, but because the endoneurial tubes are retained, effective axonal regeneration can occur unless it is impeded by a connective tissue fibroblastic reaction (neuroma in continuity). In **neurapraxia,** there is temporary failure of conduction without loss of axonal continuity.

Clinical Findings

In neurologic diagnosis, the history suggests the type of pathology while the neurologic examination localizes the lesion. A standard neuroanatomy textbook should be available for review of specific motor and sensory innervation and possible anatomic variations. A complete neurologic examination must be done, with emphasis on the nerves involved. Motor, sensory, and reflex deficits must be correlated to determine severity and distribution of involvement. The sensory findings are the least reliable because of overlap from adjacent uninjured nerves. Electromyography and nerve conduction studies establish a baseline for monitoring subsequent recovery but are not helpful until 2–3 weeks after an acute injury.

Differential Diagnosis

An accurate history and a meticulous examination are the key elements. The history will help differentiate traumatic neuropathies from those of infectious origin (diphtheria, mumps, influenza, malaria, syphilis, typhoid, typhus, dysentery, tuberculosis, gonorrhea) or toxic or metabolic origin (diabetes, rheumatic fever, gout, leukemia, vitamin deficiency, polyarteritis nodosa, drug reaction, heavy metals, carbon monoxide).

Complications

Pain resulting from nerve injury (neuropathic pain) can be caused by neuroma formation, by involvement of the sympathetic nervous system (causalgia, or sympathetically maintained pain), or by alterations in peripheral and central processing of sensory information. Painful neuromas produce pain when pressure is applied locally. Causalgic pain is burning and dysesthetic and is associated with hyperpathia and trophic skin and joint changes. Early aggressive treatment of causalgia is essential to avoid permanent disability. Local anesthetic blocks of the peripheral and sympathetic nerves may be helpful in diagnosing and treating these problems. Medical management includes tricyclic antidepressants, anticonvulsants (carbamazepine), or sympathetic blocking agents. Surgical treatment includes neurolysis, resection of the neuroma away from sites of mechanical trigger, sympathectomy, electrical stimulation of the spinal cord, and other pain-relieving procedures involving the central nervous system.

Treatment

The choice of treatment depends on the nature of the nerve injury. Early exploration and repair should be used for clean lacerations. When associated injuries are present (major arterial laceration, shock) or when there is gross contamination, it is better to tag the nerve endings with nonabsorbable suture to prevent excessive retraction and to facilitate subsequent repair. Such injuries should be approached within 10 days if the patient's condition warrants. Patients with nerves injured by stretch or contusion should be followed for clinical signs of recovery. If no recovery is seen within 3 months, exploration is indicated. Intraoperative electrical studies help distinguish between axonotmetic injuries in the process of recovery (compound nerve action potential present) and those with no evidence of recovery. Recovering nerves should be left intact, but in those with no evidence of function, the damaged segment should be resected. Although this approach sometimes results in exploration when the nerves would have recovered spontaneously, initiation of early repair is important in nerve that will not recover. Because nerve regeneration is relatively slow (1 inch per month) and because intraneural fibrosis eventually prevents axonal growth (approximately 18 months), waiting too long may eliminate the chance for recovery.

The techniques of nerve anastomosis depend on whether the primary nerve endings are in close prox-

imity; if so, epineurial repair should be performed with microscopic magnification and fine (8-0 or finer) suture. Nerve repair must be done without tension. If the gap between endings is too long for primary repair, nerve grafts (usually sural) should be used in an interfascicular repair.

Some lesions resulting from contusion or compression are improved by neurolysis. The same is true of some injection neuropathies (depending upon the substance injected).

Prompt institution of physical therapy for improvement of muscle function and maintenance of joint range of motion is indicated. The denervated portion of the limb is subject to muscle atrophy and fibrosis, joint stiffness, motor end-plate atrophy, and trophic skin changes. The longer the denervation persists, the less likely it is that a good functional result will ultimately be achieved. Physical therapy is the best means of minimizing the complications of denervation.

Prognosis

Only careful grading of sensorimotor function following injury will allow accurate evaluation of recovery, especially after surgical repair. Intraoperative factors such as axial orientation of fasciculi, proper coaptation, suture material, hemostasis, and especially suture line tension determine the outcome. In axonotmetic and neurotmetic injuries, regeneration occurs at a rate of 1 inch per month. Thus, improvement may not be noted for many months, and the patient must be psychologically prepared. Recovery of function should proceed smoothly from proximal to distal; maximum recovery may take 3–4 years. Factors that adversely affect the return of function are the type of nerve injured (mixed), the age of the patient, proximal nerve injury, large nerve defect, and associated tissue injury.

Patients must understand that their role in treatment is an active one, and their motivation must be maintained. Early rehabilitation is important to maintain full joint range of motion while awaiting functional return. Later, physical therapy will help maximize the return of useful function. Neurologic recovery is often incomplete, and the use of tendon transfers may be helpful as a means of improving the functional outcome.

Kline DG, Hudson AR: Acute injuries of peripheral nerves. In: *Neurological Surgery,* 3rd ed. Youmans JR (editor). Saunders, 1990.

BRAIN TUMORS

Michael S. Edwards, MD

Essentials of Diagnosis

- Headache.
- Progressive neurologic deficit.
- Convulsions, focal or generalized.
- Increased intracranial pressure.
- Organic mental changes.

General Considerations

Although by custom tumors are considered either benign or malignant, all brain tumors are malignant in the sense that they may lead to death if not treated. Brain tumors cause specific signs of localizing value by compressing or invading neighboring structures. Most brain tumors, either by virtue of their bulk, by production of cerebral edema, or by obstruction of the flow of cerebrospinal fluid, eventually produce increased intracranial pressure, which may have no localizing value.

Approximately 35,000 new intracranial neoplasms are diagnosed each year, half of which are metastatic from outside the central nervous system. The incidence of primary central nervous system tumors increased from 2.4 cases per 100,000 in the years 1973–1982 to 3.3 cases per 100,000 in 1986. In children, brain tumors are the second most common cancer-related cause of death; in adolescents and young adults between 15 and 34, brain tumors are the third leading cancer-related cause of death. However, most central nervous system tumors occur in patients over age 45, with the peak incidence found in the seventh decade of life.

In adults, 70% of primary brain tumors arise above the tentorium cerebelli; the other 30% originate in the infratentorial compartment (ie, posterior fossa). In children, the incidence is the reverse. The age and distribution of intracranial tumors are given in Figures 38–7 and 38–8. The frequency of major tumor types is listed in Table 38–2.

Meningiomas and nerve sheath tumors are more common in females than in males; most glial tumors—particularly medulloblastomas—have a predilection for men, and pineal tumors occur almost exclusively in young men. Other primary tumors afflict the sexes equally.

Tumors of Neuroglial Cells

Because of different systems of classification for brain tumors, the term glioma can apply to various histologic types of tumors. Gliomas account for 40–50% of all intracranial tumors—both primary and metastatic—encountered at all ages of life. Astrocytomas and oligodendrogliomas are widely distributed throughout the brain but are found mainly in the white matter, where astrocytes and oligodendrocytes predominate. Ependymomas arise from ependymal cells that line the ventricular walls and central canal, their most frequent site of origin. Medulloblastomas (primitive neuroectodermal tumor of childhood; PNET) presumably originate from a fetal cell residing in the cerebellum; on rare occasions, supratentorial occurrences have been noted.

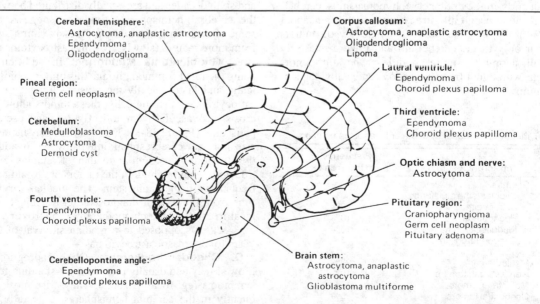

Figure 38–7. Distribution of intracranial tumors in children. (Reproduced, with permission, from Burger PC, Vogel FS: *Surgical Pathology of the Nervous System and Its Coverings.* Wiley, 1976.)

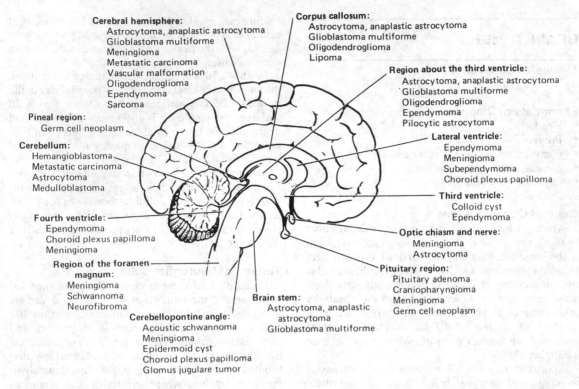

Cerebral hemisphere:
  Astrocytoma, anaplastic astrocytoma
  Glioblastoma multiforme
  Meningioma
  Metastatic carcinoma
  Vascular malformation
  Oligodendroglioma
  Ependymoma
  Sarcoma

Pineal region:
  Germ cell neoplasm

Cerebellum:
  Hemangioblastoma
  Metastatic carcinoma
  Astrocytoma
  Medulloblastoma

Fourth ventricle:
  Ependymoma
  Choroid plexus papilloma
  Meningioma

Region of the foramen magnum:
  Meningioma
  Schwannoma
  Neurofibroma

Cerebellopontine angle:
  Acoustic schwannoma
  Meningioma
  Epidermoid cyst
  Choroid plexus papilloma
  Glomus jugulare tumor

Corpus callosum:
  Astrocytoma, anaplastic astrocytoma
  Glioblastoma multiforme
  Oligodendroglioma
  Lipoma

Region about the third ventricle:
  Astrocytoma, anaplastic astrocytoma
  Glioblastoma multiforme
  Oligodendroglioma
  Ependymoma
  Pilocytic astrocytoma

Lateral ventricle:
  Ependymoma
  Meningioma
  Subependymoma
  Choroid plexus papilloma

Third ventricle:
  Colloid cyst
  Ependymoma

Optic chiasm and nerve:
  Meningioma
  Astrocytoma

Pituitary region:
  Pituitary adenoma
  Craniopharyngioma
  Meningioma
  Germ cell neoplasm

Brain stem:
  Astrocytoma, anaplastic astrocytoma
  Glioblastoma multiforme

Figure 38–8. Distribution of intracranial tumors in adults. (Reproduced, with permission, from Burger PC, Vogel FS: *Surgical Pathology of the Nervous System and Its Coverings.* Wiley, 1976.)

A. Astrocytomas: These slow-growing neoplasms predominate in the third and fourth decades in adults and occur most frequently in the frontal, parietal, and temporal lobes. In children, they arise most frequently in the optic nerve, hypothalamus, cerebellum, and pons. Of all astrocytomas in children, about 40% are cystic and 60% noncystic. Cystic tumors occur only in the cerebellum and leave a relatively small neoplastic mural nodule; noncystic tumors occur with equal frequency above and below the tentorium.

Table 38–2. Frequency of major types of brain tumors.

Intracranial Tumors[1]	Frequency of Occurrence
Gliomas	50%
Glioblastoma multiforme	50%
Astrocytoma	20%
Ependymoma	10%
Medulloblastoma	10%
Oligodendroglioma	5%
Mixed	5%
Meningiomas	20%
Nerve sheath tumors	10%
Metastatic tumors	10%
Congenital tumors	5%
Miscellaneous tumors	5%

[1] Exclusive of pituitary tumors.

B. Anaplastic Astrocytoma: This group of tumors is more malignant than the well-differentiated astrocytoma but less malignant than glioblastoma multiforme. They most frequently occur in the fifth and sixth decades and are equally distributed between the cerebral hemispheres. Evidence suggests that some of these tumors arise by progressive immaturity from more mature (slowly growing) astrocytomas.

C. Glioblastoma Multiforme: In addition to being the most common glioma, this tumor is biologically and histologically the most malignant of the astrocytomas. Histologically, these tumors show necrosis, neovascularity, mitotic figures, and pseudopalisading (Figure 38–9). These tumors may metastasize along the cerebrospinal fluid pathways. In adults, the distribution is similar to that of anaplastic astrocytoma, but in children the tumors are found most frequently in the brain stem. The median survival time from the date of diagnosis after treatment with local irradiation and chemotherapy is approximately 52 weeks, as opposed to a median survival of 2–5 years for anaplastic astrocytomas.

D. Oligodendroglioma: Oligodendrogliomas grow slowly and usually produce long-standing focal symptoms (eg, focal seizures). They arise most frequently in the cerebral hemispheres, especially the frontal lobes. They occur most commonly in adults; over 90% have calcification visible on plain x-ray.

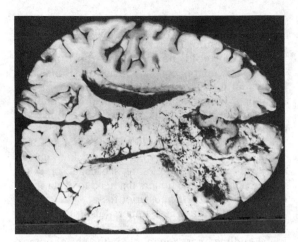

Figure 38–9. Axial gross cross section of glioblastoma multiforme. (Reproduced, with permission, from Burger PC, Vogel FS: *Surgical Pathology of the Nervous System and Its Coverings*. Wiley, 1976.)

Oligodendrogliomas vary in aggressiveness from low-grade minimal (type A) to those with malignant features (type D). The prognosis depends on the degree of aggressiveness.

E. Ependymoma: Most ependymomas are slowly growing, well-circumscribed neoplasms. They are uncommon in adults. Ependymomas situated in the cerebral hemispheres (40%) may extend intracerebrally and are equally distributed through all age groups. Ependymomas situated in the fourth ventricle occur most frequently in the first decade and constitute the largest single category (90%) of infratentorial ependymomas. The infratentorial ependymomas produce clinical and radiographic signs of increased intracranial pressure by obstruction of the cerebrospinal fluid pathway. The prognosis is markedly improved if total resection can be accomplished.

F. Choroid Plexus Papilloma: These papillomas are embryologically related to the ependyma, usually grow slowly, and are most common in children (first decade). Malignant variants (clinoid plexus carcinomas) occur and carry a very poor prognosis. The most frequent site is the fourth ventricle (> 50%), followed by the left lateral ventricle. They are capable of producing hydrocephalus either by producing ventricular obstruction or by causing overproduction of cerebrospinal fluid.

G. Medulloblastoma: Medulloblastoma is essentially restricted to the cerebellum. More than half occur in the second half of the first decade, and one-third occur in adolescence and early adulthood (age 15–35). It is the most common tumor of childhood. Histologically highly malignant, medulloblastomas tend to occur in the vermis in children and in the cerebellar hemispheres of adolescents and adults. They have an extreme propensity to seed throughout the cerebrospinal fluid pathways and on rare occasions spread outside the central nervous system. These tumors are highly radiosensitive, and—depending on the stage of tumor—between 20% and 80% are curable with aggressive craniospinal radiation therapy or chemotherapy, or both.

Nonglial Tumors

These tumors arise from various tissues. They are biologically benign and compress rather than invade adjacent brain.

A. Meningiomas: Meningiomas are slowly growing globular tumors; because of their slow rate of growth, they often reach enormous size before producing symptoms. Meningioma is a tumor of adulthood, with fewer than 2% occurring in children. Meningiomas originate from meningothelial cells that occur in greatest abundance in the arachnoid villi, which correlates well with their site of occurrence. They are most commonly found along the superior sagittal sinus (parasagittal); over the free convexity and falx; along the sphenoid wing; beneath the frontal lobes (olfactory groove and tuberculum sellae); within the posterior fossa (cerebellopontine angle and foramen magnum) and the optic nerve; and in the ventricle (Figure 38–10). They classically arise from a broad base along the dura, may invade bone, and derive most of their blood supply from the external carotid circulation (eg, middle meningeal artery).

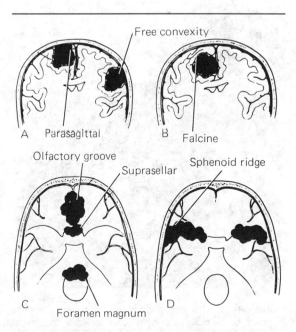

Figure 38–10. Distribution of meningiomas. **A:** Parasagittal and free convexity. **B:** Falx. **C:** Olfactory groove, tuberculum. **D:** Posterior fossa. (Reproduced, with permission, from Burger PC, Vogel FS: *Surgical Pathology of the Nervous System and Its Coverings*. Wiley, 1976.)

When the tumor is small, complete removal results in cure in over 90% of patients.

B. Nerve Sheath Neoplasms: These benign tumors originate from Schwann cells and have a predilection for sensory nerves, especially the eighth nerve (ie, acoustic neuroma), followed much less frequently by the fifth nerve (Figure 38–11). Schwannomas of the eighth nerve primarily arise from the superior or inferior vestibular portion in the internal auditory canal. As the tumor grows, it expands the internal auditory canal and extends into the cerebellopontine angle, compressing the pons, cerebellum, and cranial nerves. Bilateral schwannomas of the eighth cranial nerves are diagnostic of type 2 neurofibromatosis. However, the vast majority of patients harboring acoustic schwannomas have no stigmas of this disease.

C. Craniopharyngiomas: These tumors are believed to originate from squamous cell rests found in the infundibular stalk. Over half develop within the first and second decades. These tumors extend from the sella turcica to involve the optic nerves, hypothalamus, and third ventricle, with resultant visual loss, endocrine dysfunction, and obstruction of cerebrospinal fluid flow. Craniopharyngiomas may be partly solid and cystic, or largely cystic, containing fluid resembling "machinery oil." Those presenting during childhood usually reveal calcification on plain x-ray,

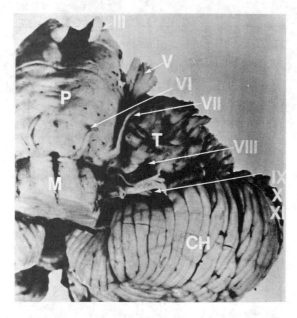

Figure 38–11. The schwannoma and its milieu. T, tumor; P, pons; M, medulla; III, oculomotor nerve; V, trigeminal nerve; VI, abducens nerve; VII, facial nerve; VIII, acoustic nerve with tumor; IX, X, XI, glossopharyngeal, vagus, and spinal accessory nerves. (Reproduced, with permission, from Burger PC, Vogel FS: *Surgical Pathology of the Nervous System and Its Coverings.* Wiley, 1976.)

which is a much less frequent finding in adult patients. Total excision is the goal of surgery.

D. Congenital Tumors:

1. Epidermoid tumors ("pearly tumors")– These cystic tumors contain a mass of desquamated epithelium produced by stratified squamous epithelial lining. Intracranially they occur off the midline, most frequently in the parasellar region and cerebellopontine angle.

2. Intracranial dermoid tumors–Similar to the epidermoid tumor, these cysts contain skin appendages such as hair follicles or sebaceous or sweat glands. They are rare tumors that tend to occur in the midline, especially the posterior fossa.

3. Teratomas–These tumors (also rare) are derived from all three germ layers. They tend to occur in the midline, most commonly in the pineal or third ventricular region.

4. Chordomas–These tumors are derived from embryonic rests of notochord. Intracranial occurrence is usually along the clivus. Although they grow slowly and are histologically benign, they are locally invasive and difficult to remove surgically. High-LET radiation therapy decreases the recurrence rate.

5. Pineal region tumors–The most common neoplasm of this region is derived from primitive germ cells and is morphologically similar to the testicular seminoma and ovarian dysgerminoma. Most germinomas become symptomatic in the second and third decades, and men are much more commonly affected than women. Similar germinomas originating in the suprasellar (hypothalamic) region have been incorrectly termed "ectopic pinealomas." The germinomas are exquisitely radiosensitive but have the capability of spreading along cerebrospinal fluid pathways.

6. Metastatic tumors–Carcinoma of the lung in men and carcinoma of the breast in women account for 61% of all cerebral metastases. These are distantly followed by genitourinary carcinoma, buccal cavity and pharynx carcinoma, gastrointestinal cancer, and malignant melanoma. Most lesions are located in the supratentorial compartment, especially in the distribution of the middle cerebral artery. Only 30% are solitary and amenable to surgery. Marked cerebral edema surrounding a small metastatic focus is not uncommon. Metastatic tumors may invade the meninges and produce a "carcinomatous meningitis."

Clinical Findings

Symptoms produced by brain tumors are largely related to their histologic characteristics, rate of growth, and location. The clinical manifestations may be divided into two broad categories: generalized signs and symptoms, and focal symptoms and signs.

A. Generalized Signs and Symptoms: Generalized symptoms and signs are usually caused by increased intracranial pressure from tumor mass, obstruction of the cerebrospinal fluid pathways, associated cerebral edema, obstruction of venous drainage, or obstruction of cerebrospinal fluid absorption mechanisms, but rarely, they are caused by increased cerebrospinal fluid production (eg, choroid plexus papilloma).

Headache and nausea and vomiting are the most common first symptoms of increased intracranial pressure. Characteristically, headache is diffuse and worse in the early morning, occasionally causing early awakening. In the absence of papilledema, the headache overlies the tumor in 60% of patients. Increased intracranial pressure may lead to papilledema, usually bilateral. However, its absence does not rule out brain tumor or increased intracranial pressure.

When a tumor compresses the optic nerve as it enters the optic foramen, it can isolate the nerve from the effects of increased pressure. As a result, the disk remains flat and tends to become atrophic (pale). The contralateral disk that is not isolated shows evidence of papilledema, known as Foster Kennedy syndrome; it is most common with medial sphenoid wing or tuberculum sella meningioma but has been described also with frontal gliomas. Visual loss may result from long-standing papilledema with secondary optic atrophy but is more often due to direct pressure from tumor (ie, focal symptoms and signs).

Personality change, easy fatigability, listlessness, and a tendency to withdrawal from social contacts are most often seen with rapidly growing infiltrating tumors (eg, glioblastoma multiforme) involving the frontal lobes or corpus callosum. With progression of the tumor or increased intracranial pressure, personality change may give way to alteration in the state of consciousness leading to stupor and coma.

Generalized seizures are the presenting symptom in 15% of adults and 30% of children with brain tumors. Slowly growing tumors and lesions situated in proximity to the sensorimotor cortex are more likely to produce seizures. In children, before closure of the sutures, progressive enlargement of the head and bulging of the anterior fontanelle are seen with increased intracranial pressure.

B. Focal Signs and Symptoms: Focal signs and symptoms are due to interference with the function of the local area of the brain (ie, localized findings). Contralateral motor or sensory impairment is associated with lesions in the posterior frontal lobe (motor) or anterior parietal (sensory) lobe. Tumors located in the dominant hemisphere produce disorders of communication (aphasia), and nondominant hemisphere lesions may produce apraxia. Hemispheric tumors involving the optic tract (anterior temporal) or optic radiations (posttemporal, parietal, occipital) produce contralateral homonymous hemianopia. Incongruous defects point to lesions proximal to the geniculate ganglion tract, in contradistinction to congruous defects seen in lesions of the optic radiations and cortex. Generalized seizures are of little localizing value unless preceded by a well-defined aura or followed by postictal palsy.

Focal seizures of the temporal lobe may produce olfactory aura (uncinate fits), visual aura (well-formed images), or psychomotor seizures. Tumors involving the frontal lobe produce contralateral motor activity, whereas tumors confined to the parietal lobe produce sensory symptoms. Occipital lobe seizures produce poorly organized visual hallucinations (eg, flickering lights). Tumors situated along the floor of the frontal fossa (eg, subfrontal meningioma) often grow to massive proportions before producing symptoms of mental deterioration and signs of anosmia and optic atrophy. Sellar and parasellar tumors may involve the optic nerve, chiasm, or tract (visual loss), the hypothalamus (endocrine disturbances), or the third ventricle (hydrocephalus). Intraventricular tumors usually present with symptoms and signs of increased intracranial pressure and contralateral motor signs. Tumors involving the pineal region produce symptoms and signs of increased intracranial pressure, limitation of upward gaze, and dilated, sluggishly reactive pupils (Parinaud's syndrome). Posterior fossa tumors produce the following characteristic patterns: Brain stem neoplasms cause multiple cranial nerve palsies (usually fifth to seventh) and long tract motor and sensory signs but produce increased intracranial pressure only late in their course. Tumors of the cerebellum involving the vermis produce axial signs (truncal ataxia), whereas tumors involving the hemispheres produce appendicular signs (limb ataxia, hypotonia, and incoordination), often with associated hydrocephalus; fourth ventricular tumors often produce only hydrocephalus by obstructing cerebrospinal fluid outflow.

Extrinsic tumors of the cerebellopontine angle tend to involve the fifth, seventh, and eighth cranial nerves in association with cerebellar hemisphere deficits and, in later stages, hydrocephalus through deformity of the fourth ventricle.

Differential Diagnosis

Because brain tumors can cause focal neurologic signs and increased intracranial pressure, many conditions may be simulated by a brain tumor.

In infants and adolescents, unexplained seizures usually herald the onset of idiopathic epilepsy. In adults, the onset of seizures is often the first manifestation of a brain tumor. Vascular malformations, degenerative diseases, subdural hematoma and empyema, brain abscess, encephalitis, meningitis, congenital hydrocephalus, and toxic states may mimic tumor.

The advent of MRI—especially with the use of paramagnetic contrast agents—has revolutionized neurodiagnosis. In conjunction with a good history and neurologic examination, most of the above conditions can be differentiated from brain tumor. In addition, lesions can be well localized, and, occasionally, a histologic diagnosis can be made. Vascular lesions are still best characterized by angiography. Magnetic resonance angiography is becoming an increasingly sensitive noninvasive screening and diagnostic tool. Infective processes usually require lumbar puncture. It is complementary to MRI, especially in defining calcified lesions.

Again, the history, neurologic examination, and CT or MRI brain scans are capable of differentiating brain tumor from other causes of increased intracranial pressure.

Complications

Missed or late diagnosis may lead to irreversible brain damage, which is all the more tragic in the case of a favorably situated benign tumor. Injudicious lumbar puncture may precipitate fatal temporal lobe or tonsillar herniation.

The advent of CT brain scanning and MRI has decreased surgical complication by allowing more precise preoperative planning of tumor resection and earlier diagnosis of postoperative complications. It has also provided a safe, noninvasive means of following patients for tumor recurrence following subtotal tumor resection or chemotherapy with or without radiation therapy.

The major objectives of treatment are (1) total removal when feasible, especially extra-axial tumors (meningiomas, nerve sheath tumors, craniopharyngiomas, colloid cysts, dermoid and epidermoid tumors) and cerebellar hemangioblastoma; (2) subtotal removal to relieve symptoms and prolong life when the location, size, and vascularity preclude total extirpation; and (3) protection of eloquent brain from damage due to treatment. With the exception of cystic cerebellar astrocytomas containing a mural nodule, glial tumors in the cerebral hemispheres and cerebellum are rarely curable by surgery alone. Subtotal resection of tumor sparing eloquent brain (eg, the dominant rolandic area) followed by postoperative radiation therapy consisting of 5000–6000 cGy delivered over 5–6 weeks affords temporary palliation. Patients harboring medulloblastoma and germinoma with positive cerebrospinal fluid cytology require irradiation of the entire central nervous system, including the spinal axis, because of the propensity of these tumors to seed along the cerebrospinal fluid pathways. Chemotherapy increases survival time in these patients. Because of the severe side effects associated with surgery, tumors of the brain stem (midbrain pons and thalamus) and pineal region are best treated by cerebrospinal fluid shunting (when associated with hydrocephalus) followed by radiation therapy.

Metastatic tumors should be treated by whole-brain irradiation, because approximately 70% are multiple. Solitary lesions and radioresistant tumor metastases should be extirpated surgically when feasible and followed with whole-brain irradiation.

Corticosteroids have been shown to be of benefit in alleviating symptoms and signs by decreasing peritumoral edema associated with primary and metastatic lesions. Preoperative treatment with corticosteroids appears to cause a decrease in surgical morbidity.

Chemotherapy has been used with increasing success for recurrent malignant gliomas and medulloblastomas and pineal germ cell tumors.

A recently concluded national cooperative study of patients harboring malignant gliomas (anaplastic astrocytomas and glioblastomas) established the value of postoperative radiation therapy and the added benefit (measured by survival) of combined radiation therapy and chemotherapy (carmustine).

Prognosis

The average postoperative survival in years for primary and metastatic brain tumors is depicted in Figure 38–12.

Patients with surgically removable tumors can be cured; these patients include the majority with meningiomas and nerve sheath tumors, epidermoids, colloid cysts, and small craniopharyngiomas and many with cerebellar astrocytomas and hemangioblastomas. Although low-grade gliomas are not highly radiosensitive, long survival is possible when operation and radiation therapy are combined. Some glioblastomas appear to be radiosensitive, but survival beyond 18 months is uncommon. For medulloblastomas treated by operation and radiation therapy, the 5-year survival rate is 40–60%.

Bonnin JM, Rubinstein LJ: Astroblastomas: A pathological study of 23 tumors, with a postoperative follow-up in 13 patients. Neurosurgery 1989;25:6.

Challa VR: Cerebral edema associated with intracranial tumors. (Editorial.) Surg Neurol 1987;27:68.

Chang T et al: CT of pineal tumors and intracranial germ-cell tumors. AJNR 1989;10:1039.

Choksey MS et al: Computed tomography in the diagnosis of malignant brain tumours: Do all patients require biopsy? J Neurol Neurosurg Psychiatry 1989;52:821.

Chuang S, Harwood-Nash D: Tumors and cysts. Neuroradiology 1986;28:463.

DeAngelis LM et al: The role of postoperative radiotherapy after resection of single brain metastases. Neurosurgery 1989;24:798.

Deck MD: Computed tomography and magnetic resonance imaging of the skull and brain. Clin Imaging 1989;13:95.

Edwards MSB et al: Pineal region tumors in children. J Neurosurg 1988;68:689.

Freidberg SR: Tumors of the brain. Clin Symp 1986;38:2.

Garfield J: Present status and future role of surgery for malignant supratentorial gliomas. Neurosurg Rev 1986; 9:23.

Higer HP, Pedrosa P, Schuth M: MR imaging of cerebral tumors: State of the art and work in progress. Neurosurg Rev 1989;12:91.

Hoffman HI, Epstein F (editors): Disorders of the Developing Nervous System: Diagnosis and Treatment. Blackwell, 1986.

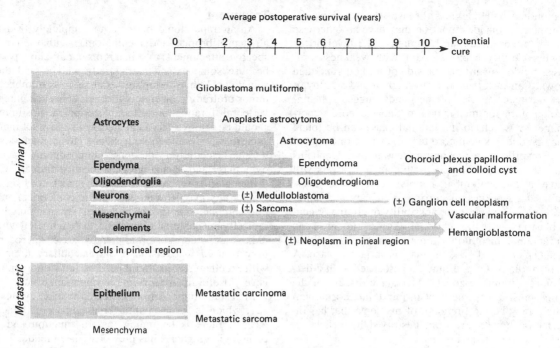

Figure 38–12. Average postoperative survival for patients harboring primary and metastatic intracranial neoplasms. The vertical thickness of the bars illustrates the relative frequency of the lesions. (Modified from Burger PC, Vogel FS: *Surgical Pathology of the Nervous System and Its Coverings.* Wiley, 1976.)

Jiddane M et al: Intracranial malignant lymphoma: Report of 30 cases and review of the literature. J Neurosurg 1986;65:592.

Kelly PJ: Stereotactic biopsy and resection of thalamic astrocytomas. Neurosurgery 1989;25:185.

Laws ER Jr et al: The neurosurgical management of low-grade astrocytoma. Clin Neurosurg 1986;33:575.

Maleci A: Immunotherapy of malignant gliomas. J Neurosurg Sci 1989;33:77.

McLaurin RL et al (editors): *Pediatric Neurosurgery,* 2nd ed. Saunders, 1989.

Ortega JA et al: The effectiveness of chemotherapy for treatment of high grade astrocytoma in children: Results of a randomized trial. A report from the Childrens Cancer Study Group. J Neurooncol 1989;7:165.

Ostertag CB: Stereotactic interstitial radiotherapy for brain tumors. J Neurosurg Sci 1989;33:83.

Warnick RE, Edwards MSB: Pediatric brain tumors. Curr Probl Pediatr 1991;21:129.

TUMORS OF THE SPINAL CORD

Harold Rosegay, MD

The clinical diagnosis of spinal cord tumor should be considered when signs and symptoms localize an intraspinal lesion. These may consist of pain or numbness in a root distribution, Brown-Séquard's syndrome, a sensory level or suspended band of hypalgesia, or weakness and muscle atrophy with loss of the appropriate deep tendon reflexes. In cases in which long tract findings such as spasticity and loss of proprioception predominate, a search for signs of segmental anterior or posterior horn cell loss may indicate the upper level of involvement. Horner's syndrome, when present in conjunction with other signs or symptoms of cord involvement, is helpful in localization. If, in addition, the history is one of progression, and if bladder or bowel function has been impaired, the suspicion of a mass lesion takes precedence over other possibilities. However, valuable time is lost if one expects and waits for the full picture, since decompensation of function begun by compression will accelerate because of the added effect of spinal cord ischemia. Intramedullary tumors may grow to large size while producing only mild sensory loss with sacral sparing, or localized weakness with mild long tract signs.

Certain spinal cord tumors occur in clinical settings that should increase the suspicion of their presence. For example, signs and symptoms of thoracic cord involvement in a middle-aged woman should raise the probability of meningioma. If there is a history of Recklinghausen's disease, one must consider neurofibroma, meningioma, ependymoma, or multiple tumors as likely possibilities. A mass in the posterior mediastinum seen on chest x-ray may have an intraspinal dumbbell extension. A patient with lymphoma or Hodgkin's disease who develops impairment of bladder function may have an otherwise asymptomatic extradural implant at the level of the conus. Cervico-occipital pain with weakness progressing downward on one side of the body and then upward on the other, with nystagmus and atrophy of the intrinsic muscles of the hands, suggests meningioma of the foramen magnum. Subarachnoid hemorrhage for which no intracranial cause can be found may be due to spinal cord tumor, and the rare patient with papilledema or communicating hydrocephalus and elevated cerebrospinal fluid protein levels will have a thoracolumbar neoplasm. Kyphoscoliosis, pain, and weakness occurring in infancy and childhood should suggest the possibility of glioma or neuroblastoma. If the child is known to have an intracranial medulloblastoma or an ependymoblastoma, meningeal seeding may have taken place. A hairy mole or fat pad may be associated with a dermoid or lipomeningocele. Metastatic disease of the spine must always be kept in mind. Intercostal neuralgia may be the first sign of myeloma that has invaded the bone marrow and destroyed the pedicle adjacent to the affected root.

Imaging Studies

On plain x-rays of the spine, one may see the following changes consistent with tumor: destruction of bone or erosion or widening of the pedicles, scalloping of the posterior surfaces of the vertebral bodies, and enlargement of the intervertebral foramina. Calcification is sometimes seen with meningiomas. In general, destructive bony changes are due to metastatic tumor, whereas the more localized erosions are seen with neurofibroma, epidermoid tumor, and ependymoma. Neurofibroma has a predilection for the C1–2 interlaminar space and is shown by marked thinning of the posterior arches. If a thoracic neurofibroma is suspected, one should check for deviation of the mediastinal pleural reflection at the involved level, which is indicative of a dumbbell tumor. CT scans of the spine may differentiate between extramedullary tumors, syrinx, hemangioblastoma, and lipoma but not between astrocytoma or ependymoma. Myelography was once the definitive test, but MRI with gadolinium enhancement has superseded it as the examination of choice. Occasionally, angiography may provide information of diagnostic value (eg, in hemangioblastoma).

Tumors are distributed along the spinal axis as follows (in order of decreasing frequency): thoracic, lumbar, cervical, and sacral. About two-thirds of primary tumors are extramedullary-intradural and are benign (meningioma, neurofibroma, epidermoid), a fact that makes early diagnosis imperative in order to prevent irreversible loss of function. The common intramedullary tumors, for which treatment is less satisfactory, are astrocytoma, ependymoma, hemangioblastoma, and lipoma.

Treatment

An attempt should be made to completely excise all neurofibromas and meningiomas with their respective attachments to spinal roots or dura; however, because some extend extradurally and beyond the spinal canal, this attempt may fall short. A dumbbell tumor protruding discretely through a thoracic intervertebral foramen into the posterior mediastinum should be removed through a curved paraspinal incision that will allow both laminectomy and costotransversectomy to be done. Intramedullary ependymomas and hemangioblastomas that can be demarcated from the surrounding spinal cord after myelotomy may be removed with microsurgical and microbipolar techniques. Infiltrating gliomas may be radically but subtotally resected and then treated with radiation and corticosteroid therapy. Laser microsurgery is used in excision of intramedullary tumors with excellent results. Intraoperative ultrasonography is very useful for localization of tumor and cyst.

Metastatic tumors may be treated with x-ray therapy, which is to be administered on an emergency basis if there is beginning loss of function and a pathologic diagnosis has previously been made. The indications for operation are as follows: (1) rapid progressive loss of function; (2) radioresistant tumors; (3) unverified masses with the possibility of another diagnosis, such as an abscess; (4) recurrence following radiation therapy; and (5) progression in spite of radiation and corticosteroid therapy. Radiation therapy may be used in conjunction with operation. Radiation therapy alone should be used to relieve pain when function is good and there is no bony compression. Lesion-directed surgical approaches have improved the outcome of operation for metastatic disease. Thus, when a metastatic tumor lies anterior to the spinal cord and involves the vertebral body, it is to be approached by anterior vertebrectomy or wide posterolateral laminectomy. This allows not only decompression but also stabilization to be done. Chemotherapy may be a useful adjunct to radiotherapy in the treatment of lymphoma, including Hodgkin's disease.

Cooper PR, Epstein F: Radical resection of intramedullary spinal cord tumors in adults: Recent experience in 29 patients. J Neurosurg 1985;63:492.

Epstein F, McCleary EL: Intrinsic brain-stem tumors of childhood: Surgical indications. J Neurosurg 1986;64: 11.

Grem JL, Burgess J, Trump DL: Clinical features and natural history of intramedullary spinal cord metastasis. Cancer 1985;56:2305.

Modic MT, Masaryk T, Paushter D: Magnetic resonance imaging of the spine. Radiol Clin North Am 1986;24: 229.

Sundaresan N et al: Treatment of neoplastic epidural cord compression by vertebral body resection and stabilization. J Neurosurg 1985;63:676.

TUMORS OF PERIPHERAL NERVES

Nicholas M. Barbaro, MD,
& Charles B. Wilson, MD

Essentials of Diagnosis

- A mass along the course of a peripheral nerve.
- Evidence of motor or sensory dysfunction confined to a single peripheral nerve.
- Pain distributed along a single peripheral nerve.

General Considerations

Peripheral nerve tumors may be removable or diffusely invasive. The most common of the former type is the nerve sheath tumor, variously called perineurial fibroblastoma, neurilemmoma, or schwannoma. These tumors may displace a major portion of the nerve to one side and often can be totally or almost totally excised. They may be found in patients with neurofibromatosis more often than in the general population. In patients with neurofibromatosis and at puberty, these tumors may become malignant, metastasizing to other portions of the body and invading surrounding tissues.

The true schwannoma—a tumor that consists of unequivocally verifiable Schwann cells (fortunately rare)—has a high potential for cancer, particularly in patients with neurofibromatosis.

The neurofibroma is characterized by general neoplastic activity within the nerve sheath. In any histologic preparation, a wide spectrum of connective tissue and endoneurial cells intermixed with axons will be seen. These diffuse growths usually cannot be excised without resecting a segment of the nerve involved; at times they may spread in a plexiform fashion along all of a nerve's branches. Neurofibromas are almost invariably found in patients with neurofibromatosis.

Nerve sheath tumors may be less than 1 mm in diameter and may grow to substantial size—eg, as extensive as the entire sciatic nerve in the thigh. They may be excruciatingly painful even early in development, or may become gigantic before being noted—especially, for example, when deep in an extremity. Growth activity is often associated with puberty.

Clinical Findings

The symptoms and signs are those of peripheral nerve dysfunction, either irritative or paralytic. The nature and distribution of this dysfunction show that it is related to a specific nerve rather than tracts in the cord or cerebral disease. Sensory disturbances or muscular atrophy may be noted. Nerve conduction tests and precise electromyography may be of assistance. MRI is effective in the diagnosis of peripheral nerve neoplasms.

Differential Diagnosis

Peripheral neuropathies, including those that are the result of pressure (entrapment), may mimic peripheral nerve tumors, but a tumor that produces symptoms is usually large enough to be palpated. Nerve tumors may occur anywhere along the course of the nerve, whereas entrapment occurs at characteristic locations. Generalized sensitivity along the nerve pathway is more common in neuritis than it is in dysfunction secondary to a primary tumor mass.

Treatment & Prognosis

The operative approach to peripheral nerve tumors depends on the type of lesion. Schwannomas can almost always be removed with little permanent increase in the preoperative neurologic deficit. Typically, a microscopic approach is used, with attention to separating the lesion from surrounding normal nerve fascicle. Complete resection is curative in these benign lesions. In cases of invasive malignant schwannomas, amputation of the extremity may be advisable unless the cancer is so advanced that the likelihood of long-term survival is slight under any circumstances. Neurofibromas cannot usually be resected without loss of function in the parent nerve. For this reason, true neurofibromas should be biopsied to be sure that they are not malignant.

In patients with neurofibromatosis, the growths are often multiple, and removal of these tumors is confined to those causing clinical signs and symptoms such as pain or sensorimotor loss. In this entity, tumors that do not cause apparent clinical dysfunction should be left alone unless there is exceptional cosmetic deformity or they are subject to repeated trauma or irritation.

Because most peripheral nerve tumors either are completely removable or are slowly growing lesions confined to a single nerve, the overall prognosis is good. However, moderate disability can be produced by unresectable lesions on major nerves. In addition, patients with neurofibromatosis may have multiple lesions including those in the craniospinal axis, which can produce progressive and severe neurologic deficits. Malignant peripheral nerve tumors can be fatal if they are not treated aggressively in their early stages.

Ariel TM: Tumors of the peripheral nervous system. Semin Surg Oncol 1988;1:7.

Mann FA et al: Magnetic resonance imaging of peripheral nerve sheath tumors: Assessment by a numerical visual fuzzy cluster analysis. Invest Radiol 1990;25:1238.

Riccardi VM: Neurofibromatoses. Neurol Clin 1987;5:337.

PITUITARY TUMORS

Charles B. Wilson, MD

Essentials of Diagnosis

- Hypopituitarism, ie, hyposecretion of one or more pituitary tropic hormones.
- Syndrome of pituitary hypersecretion: acromegaly and gigantism, Cushing's disease, amenorrhea-galactorrhea.
- Visual impairment; typically, bitemporal hemianopia.
- Suprasellar expansion detected by MRI.

General Considerations

In the past, pituitary adenomas were classified according to staining patterns seen with light microscopy; the three types (chromophobe, eosinophilic, and basophilic) did not correspond closely with the clinical syndromes of pituitary hypersecretion—eg, chromophobe adenomas could produce hypopituitarism, Cushing's disease, acromegaly, and amenorrhea-galactorrhea. Subsequently, electron microscopic identification of typical secretory granules and immunocytologic demonstration of the specific hormones contained within secretory granules have been correlated with elevations of specific hormones in blood as determined by radioimmunoassay. Consequently, the term "chromophobe" is meaningless and should be dropped, and pituitary tumors should be classified as endocrine-active or endocrine-inactive (Table 38–3).

Table 38–3. Classification of pituitary adenomas.

	Secretory Product	Clinical Syndrome
Endocrine-active[1]		
Somatotropic	Growth hormone (GH)	Acromegaly (adult), gigantism
Corticotropic	Adrenocorticotropic hormone (ACTH)	Cushing's disease, Nelson's syndrome[2]
Prolactinoma	Prolactin (PRL)	Amenorrhea-galactorrhea, impotence
Thyrotropic	Thyroid-stimulating hormone (TSH)	Hyperthyroidism
Gonadotropic	Follicle-stimulating hormone (FSH), luteinizing hormone (LH)	Behave as endocrine-inactive
Endocrine-inactive		
	Alpha subunit	Hypopituitarism

[1]Some tumors secrete more than one hormone, most often GH-PRL and ACTH-PRL.
[2]After adrenalectomy.

Pituitary adenomas are classified by size: microadenomas are tumors with a diameter of less than 1 cm, whereas all larger tumors are macroadenomas.

Clinical Findings

Endocrine-active adenomas produce the characteristic syndromes listed in Table 38–3, and the larger tumors, by compressing the normal anterior pituitary, may cause a mixed endocrine picture of oversecretion accompanied by hypopituitarism. Microadenomas are discovered in patients with one of the pituitary hypersecretory syndromes; because secretion may not be proportionate to size, endocrine-active adenoma is diagnosed by endocrine testing and confirmed radiographically, primarily with MRI. The endocrinopathy of endocrine-inactive adenomas is pituitary hypofunction—GH, FSH, and LH secretion being affected early and TSH and ACTH late. Diabetes insipidus, a result of direct hypothalamic involvement, is rarely caused by pituitary tumors. Although pituitary adenomas may extend out of the sella to produce huge intracranial masses before affecting the function of suprasellar structures, typically the initial clinical manifestation of macroadenomas is visual impairment caused by the upward extension of the tumor (suprasellar extension) that compresses the optic nerves and chiasm. In 90% of patients with visual involvement, the pattern is some variation of bitemporal hemianopia.

Acromegaly and gigantism are readily recognized. Cushing's *syndrome* is caused by adrenal hypercortisolism; Cushing's *disease* is that form of hypercortisolism produced by an ACTH-secreting pituitary adenoma. Following bilateral adrenalectomy, the same pituitary adenoma produces Nelson's syndrome.

Hyperprolactinemia is the most frequent cause of amenorrhea and galactorrhea, and most young women with this clinical presentation harbor a prolactin-secreting microadenoma. The tumor is less common in men but causes impotence and decreased libido when present.

Differential Diagnosis

For endocrine-active adenomas, the diagnosis is established by laboratory tests of pituitary function, including assessment of target organ responsiveness to available hypothalamic releasing factors. With the exception of some patients with Cushing's disease, MRI of the sella will confirm the diagnosis of an intrasellar mass.

Current MRI with coronal and sagittal views will identify all but the smallest (< 2 mm) intrasellar tumors and any extrasellar extensions of tumor. Other masses—eg, craniopharyngioma and giant aneurysms—can mimic endocrine-inactive pituitary adenomas, but MRI should differentiate these conditions from pituitary adenoma.

Cushing's syndrome (adrenal hypercortisolism)

has several causes that can be established by appropriate studies. Hyperprolactinemia can result from administration of certain drugs (eg, phenothiazines), and it may accompany other endocrine disorders such as hypothyroidism.

Treatment

Prolactin-secreting macroadenomas should be treated by transsphenoidal microsurgical removal; certain massive tumors require craniotomy, but this approach is rarely needed. For microadenomas, microsurgical transsphenoidal removal achieves excellent results in patients desiring pregnancy. Nonsurgical therapy involves indefinite administration of bromocriptine in conjunction with contraceptive measures and careful follow-up. Bromocriptine has been administered to patients with large prolactin-secreting adenomas to reduce the size of the tumor preoperatively in an effort to increase the likelihood of surgical cure.

Acromegaly and **Cushing's disease** are treated initially by operation (transsphenoidal), with radiation therapy being used for tumors that cannot be removed completely. Nonsecreting (endocrine-inactive) tumors are treated by operation followed in some cases by radiation therapy.

Galway AB et al: Gonadotroph adenomas in men produce biologically active follicle-stimulating hormone. J Clin Endocrinol Metab 1990;71:907.

Kovacs K, Horvath E: *Atlas of Tumor Pathology,* second series, fascicle 21. Armed Forces Institute of Pathology, 1986.

Littley MD et al: Hypopituitarism following external radiotherapy for pituitary tumours in adults. Q J Med 1989; 70:145.

Mampalam TJ, Tyrrell JB, Wilson CB: Transsphenoidal microsurgery for Cushing disease: A report of 216 cases. Ann Intern Med 1988;109:487.

Molitch ME: Management of prolactinomas. Annu Rev Med 1989;40:225.

Munari C et al: Long term results of stereotactic endocavitary beta irradiation of craniopharyngioma cysts. J Neurosurg Sci 1989;33:99.

Newton DR et al: Gadolinium DTPA-MR imaging of pituitary adenomas, AJNR 1989;10:949.

Newton DR et al: Gd-DTPA-enhanced MR imaging of pituitary adenomas. AJNR 1989;10:949.

Oppenheim DS, Klibanski A: Medical therapy of glycoprotein hormone-secreting pituitary tumors. Endocrinol Metab Clin North Am 1989;18:339.

Peck WW et al: High-resolution MR imaging of pituitary microadenomas at 1.5 T: Experience with Cushing disease. AJR 1989;152:145.

Peillon F et al: Receptors and neurohormones in human pituitary adenomas. Horm Res 1989;31:13.

Ross DA, Wilson CB: Results of transsphenoidal microsurgery for growth hormone-secreting pituitary adenoma in a series of 214 patients. J Neurosurg 1988;68:854.

Rush SC, Newall J: Pituitary adenoma: The efficacy of radiotherapy as the sole treatment. Int J Radiat Oncol Biol Phys 1989;17:165.

Samaan NA et al: Multiple endocrine syndrome type I. Clinical, laboratory findings, and management in five families. Cancer 1989;64:741.

Scotti G et al: MR imaging of cavernous sinus involvement by pituitary adenomas. AJNR 1988;9:657; AJR 1988;151:799.

Shillito J Jr: Treatment of craniopharyngioma. Clin Neurosurg 1986;33:533.

Wang C et al: Long-term treatment of hyperprolactinaemia with bromocriptine: Effect of drug withdrawal. Clin Endocrinol (Oxf)1987;27:363.

Wass JA et al: The treatment of acromegaly. Clin Endocrinol Metab 1986;15:683.

Weiss MH: Treatment options in the management of prolactin-secreting pituitary tumors. Clin Neurosurg 1986; 33:547.

Wilson CB: A decade of pituitary microsurgery: The Herbert Olivecrona Lecture. J Neurosurg 1984;61:814.

Wilson CB: Endocrine-inactive pituitary adenomas. Clin Neurosurg 1992;38:10.

Wilson CB: Role of surgery in the management of pituitary tumors. Neurosurg Clin North Am 1990;1:139.

PEDIATRIC NEUROSURGERY

Julian T. Hoff, MD,
& Michael S. Edwards, MD

Most neurosurgical problems in infancy and childhood are due to four causes: congenital malformations, neoplasms, infections, and trauma. Trauma has been discussed elsewhere in this chapter and will not be considered in this section.

Congenital Malformations

Congenital malformations occur in the nervous system more frequently than in any other organ system and are exceeded only by prematurity as a cause of death in infants. In most cases, no specific cause can be demonstrated, although a number of teratogenic factors have been recognized: (1) Maternal infections, eg, rubella, toxoplasmosis, cytomegalic inclusion disease, and syphilis. (2) Drugs ingested by the mother during a critical period of gestation, eg, thalidomide, LSD, methotrexate. (3) Ionizing radiation (x-rays, radioisotopes) to the mother. (4) Maternal anesthesia. (5) Systemic disease, electrolyte imbalance, and dietary deficiencies.

Even the "genetic" anomalies such as spina bifida, anencephaly, and Down's syndrome probably result from a complicated interplay of genetic predisposition and various intrauterine factors.

The gross structural neonatal abnormalities that can be repaired surgically include malformations of the skull or spine, incomplete formation of the neural tube, disturbances of cerebrospinal fluid circulation and absorption, and vascular malformations.

A. Malformations of the Skull or Spine:
Craniosynostosis is defined as premature closure of
one or more cranial sutures, producing deformity of
the skull. The frequency is 0.4:1000, and most cases
are spontaneous in occurrence. Primary craniosynostosis, which is frequently present at birth, must
be differentiated from the secondary approximation
and fusion of sutures in microcephaly and that which
sometimes follows operative procedures on the skull
or shunting to reduce increased intracranial pressure.
Some forms of craniosynostosis may result from con-
straints to the developing fetal head (eg, sagittal synostosis). In actuality, these are skull deformations
rather than malformations.

Compensatory growth of the craniosynostotic skull
occurs parallel to the plane of the fused suture. When
the process involves two or more sutures, growth and
development of the brain are affected, particularly
during the first year of life when the brain ordinarily
triples its weight.

In order of diminishing incidence, the following
malformations occur: fusion of the sagittal suture results in a long, narrow head (scaphocephaly); of both
coronal sutures, a broad, shortened head with flattened forehead (brachycephaly); and unilateral coronal or lambdoid (plagiocephaly); and of the metopic
suture, a vertical midline prominence of the forehead
(trigonocephaly).

Treatment consists of wide excision of the fused
suture. This should be done as early as possible (before significant cranial deformity is present).

Numerous other skeletal anomalies involve the
base of the skull and cervical spine with various signs
related to compression of the cerebellum, medulla,
spinal cord, or adjacent nerves.

Craniofacial anomalies such as **hypertelorism**
and **coronal synostosis** can be corrected by various
osteoplastic techniques at the skull base, in addition
to excision of fused sutures in the fronto-orbital area.

Basilar impression—upward displacement of the
cervical spine into the base of the skull—results in
reduced capacity of the posterior fossa and stenosis of
the foramen magnum.

Arnold-Chiari malformation—a small posterior
fossa with caudal displacement of the cerebellum and
medulla through the foramen magnum into the cervical canal—is often associated with hydrocephalus or
myelomeningocele.

Klippel-Feil deformity—improper segmentation
and fusion of elements of the cervical spine—is associated with abnormalities of the spinal cord.

Atlanto-occipital fusion—fusion of the atlas to
the foramen magnum is sometimes seen.

Diastematomyelia—bony spicule projecting
through the middle of the spinal canal to divide the
meninges and spinal cord into two compartments—is
usually accompanied by other skeletal anomalies.

B. Incomplete Formation of the Neural Tube:
Such defects originate during the third and fourth
week of fetal life; they may be small and concealed or
exposed and involve large areas of spinal cord, meninges, spine, overlying muscles, and skin. The most
frequently involved anatomic level is the lumbosacral
area; the least frequently involved is the thoracic
area.

Spina bifida occulta is a defect in fusion of the
spinous processes and laminas that is present in many
children. Although isolated spina bifida occulta involving the laminae of the vertebrae only is usually of
no consequence, cases that involve multiple levels
and those associated with skin abnormalities (eg,
hemangioma, patches of hair, dermal sinus, or subcutaneous lipoma) may produce neurologic dysfunction
if the spinal cord is tethered. MRI is the diagnostic
procedure of choice for all patients. In newborn infants, spinal ultrasound can assist in determining the
position of the conus medullaris and associated spinal
cord anomalies. Surgical correction of the tethered
cord usually halts progression of symptoms in most
patients and may improve neurologic and urologic
function in up to 25% of patients.

Meningocele consists of herniation of the meninges through a spina bifida without abnormality of the
spinal cord or nerve roots.

Myelomeningocele (spina bifida aperta) is protrusion of nerve roots or cord elements along with the
meninges. It occurs at least ten times more often than
simple meningocele and always causes some degree
of neurologic deficit. Findings range from mild
weakness and slight sphincteric disturbance to complete sensory and motor paralysis below the lesion
and no control of bowel or bladder function. Hydrocephalus is associated with at least 80% of lumbosacral myelomeningoceles; Arnold-Chiari malformation type II is always present and may cause brain
stem dysfunction or hydromyelia.

Encephalocele with cranium bifidum is a much
less common midline protrusion of the meninges
through the skull. It is usually occipital or at the base
of the nose.

Treatment of all such defects includes early repair
of the meningeal lesion to prevent meningitis, to preserve maximal neurologic function, and to facilitate
nursing care. Supportive appliances should be provided if paralysis is present. Early recognition and
control of hydrocephalus are essential.

Improved means of treating such problems have
increased the number of children who survive and
have greatly improved their condition. Musculoskeletal abnormalities require close attention to prevent
contractures, joint dislocation, and deformities and to
provide as much physical independence as the neurologic deficit and level of intelligence permit. Urologic problems, also either congenital or paralytic,
represent the greatest threat to life after the second
year of age, usually from chronic pyelonephritis.

**C. Disturbances of Cerebrospinal Fluid Cir-
culation and Absorption:** A large proportion of the

cerebrospinal fluid originates in the choroid plexus of the lateral and fourth ventricles, passes through the internal channels and out the foramina of the fourth ventricle into the subarachnoid spaces, along the spinal cord, and thence over the cerebral hemispheres to be absorbed through the arachnoid villi into the venous circulation. Hydrocephalus, the "backing up" of flow and dilatation of the ventricles, results from two processes: (1) an obstruction to cerebrospinal fluid absorption; and (2) rarely, overproduction of cerebrospinal fluid secondary to a choroid plexus papilloma. Obstruction may occur anywhere along the cerebrospinal fluid pathways (eg, interventricular foramen [of Monro], cerebral aqueduct [of Sylvius], outlet foramina of the fourth ventricle, the arachnoid villi associated with the sagittal sinus).

Obstruction of the cerebral aqueduct is the most frequent cause of congenital hydrocephalus. Obstruction of the outlet foramina of the fourth ventricle (Dandy-Walker malformation) may produce hydrocephalus or may be associated with aqueductal stenosis. Small gliomas in critical locations along the cerebral aqueduct may produce obstruction to cerebrospinal fluid flow as their only manifestation. Interventricular hemorrhage secondary to prematurity or infections often cause gliosis (scarring) of the aqueduct or the outlet of foramina of the fourth ventricle, with similar results.

Scarring (arachnoiditis) in the basal cisterns or over the cerebral convexities may result from meningitis, intracranial hemorrhage, meningeal carcinomatosis, or, rarely, tumors blocking the foramen magnum or basal cisterns. Spinal cord tumors have been associated with raised intracranial pressure, which presumably is caused by increased levels of protein in cerebrospinal fluid. In rare instances, hydrocephalus may develop in association with spinal cord tumors.

Management has been facilitated by the use of new diagnostic tests (eg, CT scanning and MRI with and without contrast material, cerebrospinal fluid analysis, and isotopic cerebrospinal fluid flow studies) to determine the site and cause of hydrocephalus resulting from abnormality in absorption of cerebrospinal fluid. Procedures that divert the flow of cerebrospinal fluid are the most common form of management. Although stereotactic third ventriculostomy has recently been used with some success in selected patients, avoiding the need for a shunting procedure, most cases of hydrocephalus are treated with ventriculoperitoneal or ventriculoatrial shunts. When hydrocephalus is caused by obstruction distal to the basal cisterns, lumbar subarachnoid peritoneal shunting may be effective. In the rare instance of cerebrospinal fluid overproduction resulting from choroid plexus papilloma, removal of the tumor may be curative. In about 40% of cases, cerebrospinal fluid diversion is complicated by shunt malfunction (obstruction, infection, dislodgment) over a 7-year follow-up period.

D. Vascular Malformations: Collections of abnormal blood vessels, ranging in size from a large mass to a microscopic crypt, usually provide a direct arteriovenous shunt. The involved vessels have thin walls with defective muscular and elastic layers and thus frequently bleed. The hemorrhage may be minimal or massive. It is usually not fatal in children but is often repeated during later life. Other symptoms include epileptic seizures and intellectual deterioration because of ischemia of the cortex. A loud bruit can be heard over the cranium in some infants with large lesions. The diagnosis is suggested by the history and confirmed by bloody cerebrospinal fluid, skull x-rays, CT scan, MRI, MR angiography, and cerebral angiography. Treatment varies depending on the symptoms, the age and condition of the patient, and on the size and location of the malformation. Interventional neuroradiologic procedures can be used to reduce the size and thus allow safer excision. Total excision is preferred if feasible, but it should not be attempted if it would produce a severe neurologic deficit. Recently, focused irradiation using the Linac scalpel—a gamma knife—has been successful in treating small lesions in eloquent regions of the brain.

A saccular aneurysm at the bifurcation of the arteries that form the circle of Willis is a frequent cause of subarachnoid hemorrhage in the young adult but is rare in children or infants. Aneurysm of the great cerebral vein (of Galen) is more common in the pediatric patient. During infancy, severe congestive heart failure as the result of high-output cardiac failure is the most common presentation. In children and adolescents, obstruction of the aqueduct, producing hydrocephalus and subarachnoid hemorrhage, and the usual modes of presentation.

Neoplasms

Neoplasms of the central nervous system are the most common solid tumors of childhood (3.3:100,000), exceeded in frequency only by neoplastic disease of the hematopoietic system. Twenty percent of pediatric neural tumors are located in the spinal cord and 80% in the brain. Of the latter, 60% are in the posterior fossa and 40% in the supratentorial area (Table 38–4).

A. Brain Tumors: Brain tumors produce symptoms (1) by occupying space, obstructing spinal fluid pathways, or both, thereby increasing intracranial pressure; and (2) by directly invading or compressing neural tissues.

In infants and children, the symptoms and signs of increased intracranial pressure are vomiting, headache, papilledema, mental dysfunction, personality changes, and abducens nerve palsy. Symptoms and signs of direct brain involvement are ataxia, incoordination, nystagmus, weakness of extremities, seizures, and head tilt to the side of the lesion (cerebellar).

The objective of treatment is always total removal of the neoplasm, but in childhood this is possible with

Table 38–4. Types of central nervous system tumors in children.

Cell Type	Incidence	Supraten-torial	Posterior Fossa
Medulloblastoma	30%	...	Midline cerebellum
Astrocytoma	30%	Occasional	Cerebellar hemisphere
Ependymoma	10%	Rare	Fourth ventricle
Pontine glioma	10%	...	Pons
Craniopharyngioma	4%	Suprasellar	...
Dermoid tumors and teratoma	3%	Rare	Rare
Other liomas	8%	Uncommon	Uncommon

only a few tumors (cerebellar astrocytoma, hemangioblastoma, dermoid cyst, craniopharyngioma, unilateral optic nerve glioma). The remaining tumors are partially resected, cerebrospinal fluid pathways are reopened or bypassed, and radiation therapy or chemotherapy is given postoperatively.

B. Spinal Cord Tumors: Spinal cord tumors are uncommon, and early diagnosis is most important. This group includes congenital tumors such as dermoids, teratomas, and neurofibromas; gliomas such as astrocytomas and ependymomas; medulloblastomas, which seed from primary brain tumors; and extradural metastatic tumors such as neuroblastomas and lymphosarcomas.

The manifestations of spinal cord tumors usually include pain in the spine, weakness of the legs or disturbances of gait, torticollis or scoliosis, impairment of bowel or bladder function, numbness of one or more limbs, local tenderness, and paravertebral muscle spasm.

Plain films of the spine are abnormal in 65% of children with spinal cord tumor. Electromyography will differentiate diffuse peripheral nerve and muscle disorders. MRI with paramagnetic contrast agents is the diagnostic test of choice.

Treatment begins with operative biopsy followed by total removal if possible. For tumors that are radiosensitive and clearly cannot be excised—or those that are obviously metastatic—radiation therapy or chemotherapy (or both) is the treatment of choice.

Edwards MSB, Hoffman HJ: (editors): *Cerebral Vascular Disease in Children and Adolescents.* Williams and Wilkins, 1989. Youmans J: *Neurological Surgery,* 3rd ed. Saunders, 1990.

INTRACRANIAL ANEURYSMS

Lawrence H. Pitts, MD,
& Donald A. Ross, MD

Essentials of Diagnosis

- Evidence of intracranial hemorrhage: abrupt onset of headache, stiff neck, impairment of consciousness, seizures, cardiopulmonary abnormalities, etc.
- Evidence of an expanding intracranial mass: progressive cranial nerve, long tract, hemispheric, cerebellar, or brain stem deficits.
- Demonstration of an aneurysmal sac by angiography, CT scan, or MRI.

General Considerations

An aneurysm may be defined as a localized dilatation of a blood vessel secondary to an abnormality of the vessel wall. Intracranial aneurysms may be divided into five types: "berry" or saccular, arteriosclerotic, mycotic, traumatic, and dissecting. Saccular aneurysms most commonly involve the vessels of the circle of Willis or basilar artery (Figure 38–13), vary in size from a few millimeters to 5 cm in greatest diameter, are smoothly or irregularly globoid, and are thought to arise from an acquired degenerative condition that can be aggravated by disorders causing loss of connective tissue strength. The other types are more variable in location and shape, are acquired secondary to other conditions, and in general have a poorer prognosis.

Intracranial aneurysms may be incidental findings at autopsy in as many as 5% of patients. They may present clinically by rupture and subsequent intracranial hemorrhage or by mass effects on neighboring structures; they also may be discovered occasionally in patients being evaluated for another complaint. Approximately 60% of aneurysmal rupture during life occurs in women; below age 40, however, the incidence of rupture is slightly greater in men. Most aneurysms are diagnosed in patients between the ages of 40 and 60 and are a rare finding in children. There is an increased incidence of intracranial saccular aneurysms in patients with polycystic kidney disease.

Approximately 20% of patients with ruptured aneurysms will die before arriving at a hospital, and another 20% will die from rebleeding or the effects of vasospasm. Outcome in the 60% of survivors depends on a number of factors.

Saccular aneurysms arise at branching points or at curves in arteries and usually point in the direction of blood flow. In order of frequency, the location of saccular aneurysms that bleed during life are (1) the anterior cerebral-anterior communicating artery complex; (2) the internal carotid-posterior communicat-

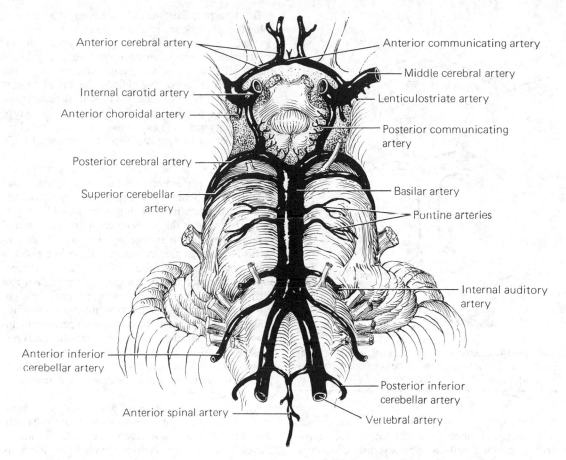

Figure 38–13. Circle of Willis and principal arteries of the brain. (Reproduced, with permission, from deGroot J, Chusid JG: *Correlative Neuroanatomy,* 20th ed. Appleton & Lange, 1988.)

ing artery junction; (3) the middle cerebral artery; (4) the vertebral-basilar artery system; (5) the bifurcation of the internal carotid artery; and (6) the distal anterior cerebral artery (Figure 38–14). Multiple aneurysms occur in 14–34% of patients, are five times more common in women than in men, and may be associated with hypertension, polycystic kidneys, coarctation of the aorta, Ehlers-Danlos syndrome, arteriovenous malformations, pseudoxanthoma elasticum, moyamoya disease, and head trauma. Aneurysms larger than 2.5 cm are considered to be "giant" aneurysms, which constitute about 5% of most series.

Intracranial aneurysms rupture during periods of rest in one-third of patients, during general activity in another one-third, and during activities associated with increased blood pressure (sexual intercourse, lifting, straining at stool) in the final one-third. Hypertension and tobacco smoking may predispose patients to subarachnoid hemorrhage. Subarachnoid hemorrhage is the usual result of the rupture of an aneurysm, which is second only to trauma as the cause.

An intraparenchymal hematoma may result occasionally, or a subarachnoid hemorrhage may rupture into the ventricular system—especially subarachnoid hemorrhage from anterior communicating artery aneurysms. Subdural hematomas are a rare finding.

Clinical Findings

A. Symptoms and Signs: The severity of clinical symptoms is usually related directly to the amount and site of bleeding. Before rupture, up to 48% of patients may experience warning symptoms such as an unusual headache or transient neurologic deficit. Moderate hemorrhages produce the classic picture of sudden, severe headache accompanied by meningismus, photophobia, nausea and vomiting, and prostration. More severe episodes may produce neurologic deficits, impaired consciousness, coma, or death. Patients with subarachnoid hemorrhage are assigned a clinical grade according to a widely used system introduced by Hunt and Hess (Table 38–5).

Patients harboring an intracranial aneurysm may also present with symptoms of an intracerebral mass

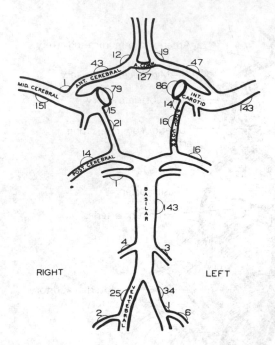

Figure 38–14. Location of intracranial aneurysms in 1023 cases. (Reproduced, with permission, from McDonald CA, Korb B: *Arch Neurol Psychiat* 1939;42:298.)

effect. Aneurysms may press on adjacent cranial nerves, nuclei, or fiber tracts and cause focal neurologic deficits. One well-described syndrome involves the sudden appearance of unilateral pupillomotor dysfunction secondary to pressure on the third cranial nerve by an aneurysm that arises from the posterior communicating artery. Giant aneurysms are often associated with symptoms of an enlarging mass and may produce visual loss, focal cerebral ischemia, or other deficits.

Table 38–5. The Hunt-Hess scale.

Category[1]	Criteria
Grade I	Asymptomatic, or minimal headache and slight nuchal rigidity
Grade II	Moderate to severe headache, nuchal rigidity, no neurologic deficit other than cranial nerve palsy
Grade III	Drowsiness, confusion, or mild focal deficit
Grade IV	Stupor, moderate to severe hemiplegia, possibly early decerebrate rigidity and vegetative disturbances
Grade V	Deep coma, decerebrate rigidity, moribund appearance

[1]Serious systemic disease such as hypertension, diabetes, severe arteriosclerosis, chronic pulmonary disease, and severe vasospasm seen on angiography result in placement of the patient in the next less favorable category. (Reproduced, with permission, from Hunt WE, Hess RM: Surgical repair as related to time of intervention in the repair of intracranial aneurysms. J Neurosurg 1968;28:14.)

B. Imaging Studies: CT scanning is a safe and reliable technique for confirming subarachnoid hemorrhage. Subarachnoid, intraparenchymal, or intraventricular blood can be visualized easily in almost all cases of aneurysm rupture, and the distribution of blood may indicate the site of hemorrhage. When contrast agents are used, the aneurysm itself may on occasion be seen. Complications of ruptured aneurysms such as hydrocephalus, cerebral infarction, or rebleeding can also be diagnosed by CT scanning.

Angiography is the essential diagnostic procedure and must be performed in all cases of spontaneous subarachnoid hemorrhage unless there is a compelling contraindication. Angiography should be performed as soon as the patient's condition permits and need not be done on an emergency basis for two reasons: First, angiography performed within 8 hours following rupture may increase the risk of rebleeding; and second, aneurysms may be very small and difficult to detect unless the angiogram is of the highest quality—ie, the angiogram must be obtained under optimum conditions by an experienced angiography team rather than by an inexperienced crew present on off-hours. Even under optimum conditions, in 15–30% of patients with subarachnoid hemorrhage no aneurysm can be demonstrated despite repeat angiography.

MRI may demonstrate an aneurysm as a signal void, but MRI does not demonstrate acute subarachnoid hemorrhage as sensitively as does CT scanning. Developing techniques of dynamic MRI angiography have demonstrated some aneurysms clearly and may be used more widely in the future.

C. Lumbar Puncture: Subarachnoid hemorrhage may be confirmed by the presence of bloody or xanthochromic cerebrospinal fluid. Because some patients with subarachnoid hemorrhage may deteriorate dramatically because of herniation syndromes or rebleeding that occurs after cerebrospinal fluid is withdrawn, CT scanning and angiography remain the diagnostic procedures of choice.

Treatment

A. Medical Treatment: Nonoperative treatment is designed to prevent rebleeding and vasospasm. The risk of rebleeding is highest in the first several days after the initial rupture and amounts to a 4% rate of rebleeding in the first day to a rate of approximately 20% by the first 2 weeks. The mortality rate associated with rebleeding is 40%. While the initial rupture of an aneurysm is somewhat related to the presence of chronic hypertension, the incidence of rebleeding is definitely increased by hypertension. Blood pressure is maintained within normal ranges with sedation, bed rest, and the judicious use of antihypertensive medication. Anticonvulsants are used to prevent seizure-related alterations in blood pressure.

Vasospasm is the relentless narrowing of cerebral

vessels that follows subarachnoid hemorrhage in 20–30% of patients and may lead to cerebral ischemia or frank infarction. Despite intensive research, the cause of cerebral vasospasm is not clearly understood. The incidence of vasospasm is related to the amount of blood in the subarachnoid space seen on CT scans and is most likely to occur within 3–10 days after the initial rupture. Surgical manipulation during this period may increase the risk of vasospasm. The incidence of irreversible ischemic injury related to vasospasm is increased by the use of antifibrinolytic agents, which should be administered only in the early posthemorrhage period until surgery can be performed. Current therapy for prevention and treatment of vasospasm includes maintaining a high circulating blood volume with colloid and crystalloid solutions to keep central venous pressure elevated to 7–14 cm of water, strictly avoiding hypotension and hypoxia, and inducing hypertension or cerebral vasodilation using aminophylline and isoproterenol in symptomatic patients. Recently, the calcium channel blocking agent nimodipine has been shown to reduce the effects of vasospasm-induced cerebral ischemia.

B. Surgical Treatment: Surgery is performed to permanently prevent the rupture or expansion of an aneurysm. Depending on the size, shape, and location of the aneurysm, these objectives may be achieved by clipping the neck of the aneurysm, wrapping the fundus with reinforcing materials, isolating the aneurysm by proximal and distal clipping of the parent vessel, or ligating a major feeding vessel or by an intravascular technique that uses detachable balloons or glue.

Choice of the optimum time for surgery is still controversial. While early surgery reduces the risk of rebleeding and its high mortality rate, it may increase the risk of vasospasm and subsequent ischemic injury. Some surgeons prefer not to operate on the swollen, inflamed tissues present soon after subarachnoid hemorrhage. Conversely, delaying surgery allows inflammation to subside and reduces the risk of induced vasospasm but puts the patient at risk of rebleeding before surgery is performed. The most common approach has been to operate early on patients with good neurologic status and to delay operation in patients with significant deficits until recovery is observed and the period of risk for induced vasospasm has passed. With the introduction of efficacious therapy for vasospasm, more patients will probably undergo early surgery.

Prognosis

If the aneurysm is treated successfully, long-term outcome depends on damage caused by initial and subsequent hemorrhage and on the appearance of delayed complications such as vasospasm and hydrocephalus. Of the 60% of patients who survive either the initial rupture or rebleeding, approximately 20% will have disabling neurologic deficits and 40% will

have a good recovery, although the latter patients may have deficits of memory and high cognitive function that can be demonstrated by careful examination. If the aneurysm is not operated upon, the risk of rebleeding is 50% over the 6-month period after the initial rupture and about 3% per year thereafter. An unruptured aneurysm carries a risk of rupture of 1–3% per year.

Ausman JI et al: Management of cerebral aneurysms: Further facts and additional myths. Surg Neurol 1989;32:21.

Chyette D, Reilly J, Tilson MD: Morphometric analysis of reticular and elastin fibers in the cerebral arteries of patients with intracranial aneurysms. Neurosurgery 1990;26:939.

Dorsch NW et al: Timing of surgery for cerebral aneurysms: A plea for early referral. Med J Aust 1989; 150:183,187.

Ingall TJ et al: Has there been a decline in subarachnoid hemorrhage mortality? Stroke 1989;20:718.

Newell DW et al: CT infusion scanning for the detection of cerebral aneurysms. J Neurosurg 1989;71:175.

Pickard JD et al: Effect of oral nimodipine on cerebral infarction and outcome after subarachnoid hemorrhage: British aneurysm nimodipine trial. Br Med J 1989; 298:636.

Sacco RL et al: Subarachnoid and intracerebral hemorrhage: Natural history, prognosis, and precursive factors in the Framingham study. Neurology 1984;34:847.

Schievink WI et al: Circumstances surrounding aneurysmal subarachnoid hemorrhage. Surg Neurol 1989;32:266.

Stebbens WE: Etiology of intracranial berry aneurysms. J Neurosurg 1989;70:823.

Strother CM et al: Thrombus formation and structure and the evolution of mass effect in intracranial aneurysms treated by balloon embolization: Emphasis on MR findings. AJNR 1989;10:787.

Todd NV et al: Outcome following aneurysm wrapping: A 10-year follow-up review of clipped and wrapped aneurysms. J Neurosurg 1989;70:831.

Verwej RD, Wijdicks EFM, van Gijn J: Warning headache in aneurysmal subarachnoid hemorrhage. Arch Neurol 1988;45:1019.

Wilson FM, Jaspan T, Holland IM: Multiple cerebral aneurysms: A reappraisal. Neuroradiology 1989;31:232.

VASCULAR MALFORMATIONS
(Arteriovenous Malformations)

Charles B. Wilson, MD

Essentials of Diagnosis

- Seizures, often focal.
- Spontaneous subarachnoid or intracerebral bleeding.
- Normal blood pressure and intracranial bleeding at a younger age than intracranial bleeding from aneurysm and hypertension.

- Progressive ischemic neurologic deficit caused by a "steal" into an arteriovenous shunt or stagnation secondary to venous outflow restriction.
- Cranial bruit, subjective or objective.
- Brain scan often suggests diagnosis.
- Cerebral angiography characteristically diagnostic, but some malformations are not shown.
- Intraspinal arteriovenous malformations are uncommon and are manifested usually by myelopathy but rarely by subarachnoid hemorrhage.

General Considerations

Although once believed to be neoplastic, arteriovenous malformations are now recognized as congenital lesions. The basic abnormality is a more or less direct connection between arteries and veins without an interposed capillary network. Afferent and efferent vessels are dilated but otherwise normal, and they lead to and from a tangle of malformed channels containing arterial blood; because the malformation receives blood at arterial pressure, spontaneous bleeding or progressive expansion may result. If flow through the low-resistance malformation is high, the arteriovenous shunt may steal blood from the surrounding brain with consequent ischemic neurologic deficits; closure (excision) of the malformations will restore normal perfusion to the uninvolved brain.

Arteriovenous malformations come in all sizes; the largest occupy one or more lobes, and the smallest may measure no more than a few millimeters. The large malformations characteristically involve the cortex and extend inward toward the subjacent ventricle, and as a rule the initial manifestation is a seizure. Small malformations are more likely to present with spontaneous hemorrhage, either into the subarachnoid space or into the brain parenchyma, with resultant neurologic deficit.

As a group, patients harboring arteriovenous malformations will bleed at an earlier age than patients harboring aneurysms. In our recent series with an age range of 16 months to 79 years, fully one-third presented in the third decade. In the absence of a blood dyscrasia, spontaneous intracranial bleeding in a child or young adult is the hallmark of an arteriovenous malformation. The death rate following an initial bleeding episode is in the range of 10–15%, clearly lower than with ruptured aneurysms. Having bled, an arteriovenous malformation carries the liability of rebleeding at an estimated 4–5% risk annually. For the patient presenting with seizures, the risk of bleeding at a later date is 1–2% per year.

Clinical Findings

A focal seizure without bleeding may cause temporary postictal neurologic deficits. The patient with a high-flow arteriovenous shunt will be suspected of harboring a brain tumor until an arteriovenous malformation is shown by MRI and confirmed by angiography.

Bleeding into the subarachnoid space produces the characteristic picture of headache, stiff neck, confusion and obtundation, low-grade fever, glycosuria, and leukocytosis. Intraparenchymal bleeding can cause a minor or major neurologic deficit related to the size and location of the hematoma.

Differential Diagnosis

Seizures can be caused by a wide range of structural and biochemical disorders and are therefore only suggestive of arteriovenous malformation. Most malformations will be detected by CT or MRI brain scans, and in almost all cases angiography will be diagnostic. When the history suggests intracranial bleeding, the initial study should be a CT brain scan: all but the smallest malformations exhibit contrast enhancement, and the location and size of hematomas can be established. The next procedure is angiography, which will be diagnostic in all but the smallest lesions. The differential diagnosis includes the conditions listed in the preceding section on aneurysms.

Cryptic vascular malformations are being detected in increasing numbers largely through MRI. These malformations are not visible angiographically, have a typical appearance on MR images, and present clinically because of seizures, bleeding, or progressive neurologic deficit. They are treated with surgical removal.

Treatment

The ideal treatment is excision of the arteriovenous malformation and removal of any associated hematoma. Improved microsurgical techniques have broadened the indications for operation, and any readily accessible malformation that can be removed without creating a significant neurologic deficit should be considered for excision. Some malformations cannot be removed with reasonable risk, and some of these can be treated by techniques for intracranial embolization, such as injection of rapid-setting polymers via catheterization of feeding arteries and focused irradiation (radiosurgery).

Prognosis

With some exceptions, seizures can be controlled by anticonvulsant medication. Because the lesion is present at birth, there is a lifelong risk of the serious complications of bleeding and neurologic deficits. On the other hand, some malformations remain asymptomatic and are detected only after death from other causes.

Abe M, Kjellberg RN, Adams RD: Clinical presentations of vascular malformations of the brain stem: Comparison of angiographically positive and negative types. J Neurol Neurosurg Psychiatry 1989;52:167.

Barnwell SL et al: Complex dural arteriovenous fistulas. Results of combined endovascular and neurosurgical treatment in 16 patients. J Neurosurg 1989;71:352.

Biondi A, Scialfa G: Morphological and blood flow MR findings in cerebral vascular malformations. J Neuroradiol 1988;15:253.

Chyatte D: Vascular malformations of the brain stem. J Neurosurg 1989;70:847.

Colombo F et al: Linear accelerator radiosurgery of cerebral arteriovenous malformations. Neurosurgery 1989;24:833.

Kahl W et al: arteriovenous malformations in childhood: Clinical presentation, results after operative treatment and long-term follow-up. Neurosurg Rev 1989;12:165.

Kemeny AA, Dias PS, Forster DM: Results of stereotactic radiosurgery of arteriovenous malformations: An analysis of 52 cases. J Neurol Neurosurg Psychiatry 1989;52:554.

Loeffler JS et al: Stereotactic radiosurgery for intracranial arteriovenous malformations using a standard linear accelerator. Int J Radiat Oncol Biol Phys 1989;17:673.

Raybaud CA, Strother CM, Hald JK: Aneurysms of the vein of Galen: Embryonic considerations and anatomical features relating to the pathogenesis of the malformation. Neuroradiology 1989;31:109.

Vascular malformations in the brainstem. Lancet 1989;2:720.

Wilson CB: Cryptic vascular malformations. Clin Neurosurg 1992;38:49.

MOVEMENT & PSYCHOPATHOLOGIC DISORDERS RESPONSIVE TO SURGERY

John E. Adams, MD,
& Nicholas M. Barbaro, MD

PARKINSON'S DISEASE

Parkinson's disease is the most common of various disorders of movement and posture. However, such disorders are not clear-cut entities but constitute a spectrum of abnormal postures, states of muscle tone, and movements varying from hypotonic flaccidity to extreme muscular contraction and from akinesia (inability to initiate movement) to relentless violent movements capable of producing exhaustion and death.

Clinical Findings

Parkinson's disease is characterized by three main disturbances in movement and posture: tremor, rigidity, and bradykinesia or akinesia. The tremor is characteristically of the pill-rolling type that begins in the distal upper extremities and progresses proximally as time passes. It is usually abolished by voluntary movement. Rigidity involves both the agonist and antagonist muscles of the extremity and, when severe, literally immobilizes the arm or leg. The bradykinesia or akinesia is represented by a gradually worsening

stooped posture, shuffling gait, festination, or a tendency to fall forward; poverty of speech to the point where the voice becomes only a whisper; difficulty in swallowing, etc.

Treatment

In its early stages, parkinsonism is treated medically and is primarily the concern of the internist or neurologist. Levodopa is very effective in the treatment of the akinetic aspects of the disease, although it may have little effect on tremor. It has now largely been replaced by carbidopa/levodopa (Sinemet), a combination product that decreases the often disabling nausea and vomiting from levodopa and provides higher concentrations of dopamine in the brain. Patients with tremors as their predominant symptom frequently do not respond and are the best candidates for operative treatment. Operative treatment of tremor in medically unresponsive patients should be done relatively early, before the tremor becomes incapacitating.

Stereotaxic surgery is a technique for reaching subcortical or deeper intracerebral structures via electrodes or probes that are guided to the site by a three-dimensional coordinate system attached to the skull. This technique allows creation of subcortical lesions with minimal trauma to overlying cortex. In patients with Parkinson's disease, the lesion is made by most surgeons in the ventrolateral nucleus of the thalamus, but some surgeons prefer to place the lesion in the ansa lenticularis (campotomy). At present, most surgeons make a small lesion (5 mm in diameter) in the ventrolateral nucleus just anterior to the posterior ventrolateral nucleus of the thalamus. If correctly placed, this lesion will effectively stop a tremor in the contralateral hand and arm in well over 80% of cases. Rigidity is likewise improved. The disabling hypokinetic symptoms of parkinsonism are not benefited by such a thalamotomy and at times may even be made worse.

A recent innovative surgical treatment for all manifestations of Parkinson's disease, which is now undergoing clinical trial, consists of the transplantation of adrenal medullary tissue and, more recently, fetal substantia nigra cells into the caudate nucleus. These approaches are highly experimental but can be considered to have possible clinical significance and merit.

Other movement disorders that will respond to a lesion in the same thalamic area are dystonia musculorum deformans, essential cerebellar tremors, hemiballismus, tardive dyskinesia, and chorea. Stereotaxic destruction of the dentate nucleus has been used effectively in the treatment of such disabling conditions as choreoathetosis.

Backlund E-O et al: Transplantation of adrenal medullary tissue to striatum in parkinsonism: First clinical trials. J Neurosurg 1985;62:169.

Laitenen LV: Brain targets in surgery for Parkinson's disease: Results of a survey of neurosurgeons. J Neurosurg 1985;62:349.

Madrazo I et al: Open microsurgical autograft of adrenal medulla to the right caudate nucleus in two patients with intractable Parkinson's disease. N Engl J Med 1987;316:831.

EPILEPSY

Epilepsy may be defined as an uncontrolled paroxysmal discharge of an aggregate of neurons within the brain. These neurons are most frequently within the cerebral cortex but may be subcortical. The unrestrained discharge may remain focal, or it may spread to adjacent areas of cortex and may ultimately involve both hemispheres as well as diencephalic and brain stem structures. Loss of consciousness (complex seizures) during or at the onset of the seizure indicates involvement of diencephalic structures in the abnormal electrical discharge. A discharging focus in the motor area will produce a seizure initiated by clonic contractions of the appropriate portion of the body (face, hand, arm, etc). It is obvious, therefore, that the clinical manifestations of seizure discharges are quite variable and may involve essentially all body systems. For practical purposes, however, any epilepsy that is focal in origin constitutes the basis for the surgical treatment of the disease.

Only medically refractory cases are treated surgically. About 15–20% of epileptic patients cannot be controlled by medical therapy and are candidates for surgical excision of the epileptogenic focus if it can be localized and is accessible. Most of these patients have seizures (complex partial) that originate in a single temporal lobe, although approximately 15% have seizures of frontal lobe origin. Recordings from surgically implanted electrodes are now commonly employed in all major centers treating epilepsy by surgical excision of the focus.

The majority of surgical procedures in the treatment of intractable epilepsy consist of excision of the focus when that is feasible. This treatment is effective in approximately 80% of cases, especially with seizures of temporal lobe onset. Surgical section of part or, at times, the entire corpus callosum is being used in patients with disabling drop attacks (akinetic seizures) with good control in approximately 75% of cases.

Cerebral dominance and epilepsy surgery. (Editorial.) Lancet 1986;2:1318.

Dodrill CB et al: Multidisciplinary prediction of seizure relief from cortical resection surgery. Ann Neurol 1986;20:2.

Engel J (editor): Surgical Treatment of the Epilepsies. Raven Press, 1987.

Marino R Jr: Surgery for epilepsy: Selective partial microsurgical callosotomy for intractable multiform seizures:

Criteria for clinical selection and results. Appl Neurophysiol 1985;48:404.

Spencer SS: Surgical options for uncontrolled epilepsy. Neurol Clin 1986;4:669.

PSYCHIATRIC DISORDERS

Small, carefully placed stereotaxic lesions have replaced the much more disabling and destructive frontal lobotomy in the treatment of certain psychiatric disturbances. Patients with obsessive compulsive behavior can be dramatically improved by small lesions in the cingulum. In rare instances, a severe anxiety neurosis that cannot be managed by more conservative methods will be improved by small lesions placed in the white matter just anterior to the dorsal medial thalamic nucleus or more anteriorly in the frontal orbital white matter.

Criticism of this form of surgical treatment of severe behavior disorder is based upon the misconception that these procedures are analogous to the now discredited prefrontal lobotomy with the attendant often severe alterations in the patient's human character. Such alterations do not result from the more restricted and precise stereotaxic surgical lesion.

PAIN

Nicholas M. Barbaro, MD

Pain has been defined as "an unpleasant sensory and emotional experience associated with actual or potential tissue damage, or described in terms of such damage." This definition takes into account that pain is a well-recognized signal of damage and, as such, an important symptom of numerous diseases. Pain resulting from injury to the nervous system (neuropathic pain) may not indicate tissue damage and thus may not be a useful sensory phenomenon; rather, it may constitute a pathologic process in itself. The above definition of pain also takes into account the emotional aspects of pain, which can be all-consuming for a patient, and suggests the importance of psychologic factors in evaluation and treatment.

Patients with pain can be divided into two groups: those with diseases that limit life expectancy, such as malignant tumors (malignant or cancer pain); and those with normal life expectancy (chronic benign pain). For practical purposes, patients expected to live 2 years or less are put into the malignant pain group. The medical and surgical management of these two groups is very different.

In general, the approach to treating pain begins with an attempt to diagnose the cause. The natural history of the underlying problem must also be considered. For example, pain in a recently operated region is expected to resolve with wound healing. When possible, the source of the pain should be treated directly (eg, removal of a herniated disk, treatment of a primary tumor). If the pain cannot be treated directly or if the source of the pain is unknown, efforts are made to treat the pain as such.

MALIGNANT PAIN

The main goal in treating patients with malignant pain is to reduce suffering during a terminal illness. Therapies that might be inappropriate in patients with normal life expectancies can be considered. Opioids, for example, can be used in high doses unless excessive sedation, respiratory depression, severe constipation, or other significant adverse effects occur. Any dose that relieves pain and maximizes useful function can be used. Other medications, such as tricyclic antidepressants and nonsteroidal anti-inflammatory agents, may provide additional relief. When medical management fails to reduce the pain sufficiently, surgical treatment is indicated. Surgical management of malignant pain involves two approaches: (1) epidural or intrathecally administered morphine and (2) ablation to interrupt pain transmission.

The spinal cord contains opioid receptors which, when activated by locally administered morphine, produce rather profound pain relief. Temporary percutaneous catheters can be used to test this therapy; if significant pain relief is demonstrated, prolonged spinal administration of morphine is indicated. This can be accomplished by implanting a subcutaneous reservoir attached to an epidural or intrathecal catheter; morphine can be injected into the reservoir by the patient or caregiver. Although this technique provides useful pain relief, it is impractical because repeated skin punctures are required and there is a risk of infection. If the patient's life expectancy is more than a few months, implantation of an infusion pump is recommended. Newer pumps provide many convenient features such as percutaneous programmability and allow several weeks of treatment before refilling is required. Spinal morphine is most effective for midline and multifocal pain problems, such as sacral pain associated with prostate tumors, pelvic pain from carcinoma of the cervix, and multifocal bone pain from widely metastatic disease. Unilateral focal pain may respond to such treatment, but other techniques offer excellent pain relief without the inconvenience associated with pumps, such as refilling.

Cancer pain that is unilateral and focal may be treated with cordotomy, creating a lesion in the spinothalamic tract designed to interrupt pain transmission. An open cordotomy, which requires laminectomy, produces excellent analgesia and can be done in the thoracic region for leg pain. Percutaneous cordotomy using a radiofrequency needle is done at the C1–2 level. This is less traumatic for the patient and may produce analgesia in both the arm and the leg. Bilateral high cervical cordotomy is not recommended because of the risk of respiratory depression.

Other ablative techniques for treating cancer pain are used relatively rarely. These include midline myelotomies, rhizotomies (open or percutaneous), and neurectomies.

POSTOPERATIVE PAIN

Some pain is experienced by nearly every patient after invasive surgical procedures. The amount and duration of pain varies with the type of procedure, with the individual patient, and with many other factors, including the rapidity of healing and associated complications such as infection. The fact that pain is expected after surgical procedures does not mean it should not be treated aggressively. Reducing postoperative pain not only lessens the most unpleasant aspect of the procedure for the patient, it also reduces the incidence of other types of morbidity, such as pneumonia and deep vein thrombosis. For these reasons, appropriate doses of opioids and other pain-reducing drugs such as anti-inflammatory agents are an essential part of postoperative care.

The treatment of postoperative pain has improved substantially in recent years. These improvements include the use of epidural or intrathecal opioids and the use of long-acting nerve blocks at the end of a procedure. In addition, new delivery techniques such as patient-controlled analgesia, in which the patient self-administers small incremental doses of opioid analgesic, reduce overall postoperative pain and actually decrease the amount of analgesic required during the postoperative period.

CHRONIC BENIGN PAIN

Patients with a life expectancy longer than 2 years who have pain that cannot be eliminated by treating the underlying cause are considered to have chronic benign pain. Such patients should be evaluated by a team of individuals experienced in pain treatment (pain clinic), including specialists in anesthesiology, psychology, psychiatry and neurology or neurosurgery, physical therapy, and pharmacology. This multidisciplinary approach takes into account the multifactorial cause of long-standing pain.

The medical management of such patients is beyond the scope of this chapter. In general, drugs with little or no potential for addiction or significant dependence should be used. The use of opioids to treat chronic benign pain is controversial; long- acting drugs on a time-contingent rather than pain-contingent schedule are preferred, and short-acting opioids should be avoided. Anticonvulsant and tricyclic antidepressant drugs may be effective and are best administered by physicians with experience in their use.

When medical management fails to reduce pain adequately, surgical treatment can be considered. Ablative techniques such as rhizotomy (cutting of nerve roots), neurectomy, and cordotomy are inappropriate in these cases except as noted below. Techniques of neuromodulation that do not cause neural injury should be used instead.

Neuromodulation techniques take advantage of the capacity of the nervous system to reduce the access of painful stimuli to higher central nervous system centers. Transcutaneous electrical nerve stimulation, the least invasive of these techniques, uses skin electrodes to activate the large fibers in peripheral nerves. This selective activation reduces the ability of nociceptive fibers (A δ and C) to activate spinal neurons, which transmit pain signals to higher centers. This technique is limited by the inability to stimulate large painful areas and by the inconvenience of wearing electrodes for long periods.

A more invasive approach to neuromodulation involves direct or percutaneous implantation of electrodes into the spinal canal to electrically stimulate the dorsal columns. Spinal cord or dorsal column stimulation is most effective for pain in the extremities, such as pain after nerve injury, peripheral neuropathies, and sympathetic dystrophy. In patients with ischemic pain, spinal cord stimulation not only reduces the pain but may also improve blood flow in the involved extremities as well.

The most invasive neuromodulation technique is the implantation of brain-stimulating electrodes to reduce severe pain that has not responded to other techniques. Electrodes are placed stereotactically either in the midbrain periaqueductal gray matter or in the thalamus. Thalamic stimulation is useful for neuropathic pains, while periaqueductal gray stimulation appears to be more useful for "nociceptive pain, such as severe spinal pain.

SPECIFIC PAIN SYNDROMES

1. TRIGEMINAL NEURALGIA

Trigeminal neuralgia is an episodic lancinating facial pain that conforms to one—or perhaps two—divisions of the trigeminal nerve. It is more common in elderly patients except when seen as a manifestation of multiple sclerosis, and is slightly more common in women. The mainstay of treatment is the anticonvulsant drug carbamazepine; other anticonvulsant medications are less effective. Patients who do not re-

spond to medical management may be treated with a percutaneous or open surgical procedure. Percutaneous approaches involve placing a needle through the foramen ovale at the skull base. The trigeminal nerve is then partially damaged with glycerol, a mildly toxic alcohol, a radiofrequency-induced heat lesion, or by balloon compression of the trigeminal ganglion. The percutaneous approaches are minimally invasive and require very short hospitalization, but the recurrence rate is higher than with an open approach, and patients are left with some loss of facial sensation, perhaps including protective corneal sensation.

Many cases of trigeminal neuralgia are caused by irritation of the trigeminal nerve at the brain stem by blood vessels, such as the superior cerebellar and anterior inferior cerebellar arteries. This syndrome can often be cured by moving the offending vessel away from the nerve. When the trigeminal nerve is exposed and such a neurovascular relationship cannot be demonstrated, partial rhizotomy (nerve sectioning) can provide excellent pain relief.

2. PAIN AFTER AMPUTATION

A variety of pain syndromes may follow limb amputation. Most patients experience sensory phenomena in the amputated limb. In a minority of cases, these so-called phantom sensations are painful. Phantom limb pain is described as a continuous pain, as if fingernails were digging into the palm or the limb were being twisted into painful postures. Some patients have painful neuromas at the cut ends of peripheral nerves; the pain is usually electrical and occurs each time the stump is pressed. Injury to the cutaneous nerves may cause painful skin sensitivity in the stump. Medications such as tricyclic antidepressants and anticonvulsants may be effective in these cases, but opioids usually are not. Surgical options include revision and burying of painful neuromas and, in refractory cases, spinal cord or brain stimulation.

3. SPINAL NERVE ROOT AVULSION PAIN

Injuries that radically displace the head and shoulder can avulse the spinal nerves from the spinal cord. This commonly occurs after motorcycle accidents in which the head and shoulder are rapidly and severely distracted. This type of brachial plexus injury is not surgically reparable and usually is not painful. In some cases, however, the pain is severe; typically, it is a burning pain and may include a phantom-like pain sensation. When such pain is refractory to medical management, it can be alleviated in 80% of cases by a dorsal root entry zone lesion. In this procedure, the spinal cord is exposed, and the region where dorsal roots formerly entered the spinal cord is identified. Lesions are made either with small needles (radiofrequency) or with a laser. Care must be taken to avoid damaging nearby spinal tracts.

4. SPINAL CORD INJURY PAIN

Most patients with severe spinal cord injury experience some pain. In some cases, it is severe and requires specific medical treatment. Pain after spinal cord injury may occur at the border zone between normal and abnormal sensation or may affect large areas of the body with little or no sensory function. The former may be treated with the dorsal root entry zone procedure described above; lesions are created at the region immediately above and below the spinal cord injury. More diffuse spinal cord injury pain is very difficult to treat and does not respond well to any surgical procedures.

SUMMARY

Pain is a common and complex sensory experience. When possible, treatment of the underlying primary disease should be attempted. In many cases, this is not possible, either because there is no effective treatment (malignancy, spinal cord injury) or because no specific source of pain is identified. Such cases should be managed by a team that includes medical, surgical, and psychologic specialists.

Barbaro NM: Studies of PAG/PVG stimulation for pain relief in humans. In: *Pain Modulation*. Progress in Brain Research, vol 77. Fields H, Besson JM (editors). Elsevier, 1988.

Bowsher D: Neurogenic pain syndromes and their management. Br Med Bull 1991;47:644.

Fields H: *Pain*. McGraw-Hill, 1987.

Gybels JM, Sweet WH: Neurosurgical treatment of persistent pain: Physiological and pathological mechanisms of human pain. Pain Headache 1989;11:1.

North R: Spinal cord stimulation for chronic, intractable pain: Superiority of "multichannel" devices. Pain 1991; 44:119.

INTERVERTEBRAL DISK DISEASE

Philip R. Weinstein, MD,
& Julian T. Hoff, MD

Anatomic Considerations

A. The Intervertebral Disk: The intervertebral disk has three parts: the circumferential annulus, which consists of dense fibrous tissue and is very strong; the central nucleus, which consists of fibrocartilage and has little tensile strength but great elasticity; and the vertebral body end-plates, which are cartilaginous and form the interface between bone and disk above and below each joint. Fibrocartilage may be fragmented acutely or may degenerate gradually with time. It heals poorly because of limited blood supply. Nutrient arteries atrophy with age beginning in the second decade. The nucleus contains approximately 80% water at birth; it gradually dehydrates and loses its elasticity with age. The annulus, however, has more capacity to heal and is buttressed by thick anterior and posterior longitudinal ligaments that add strength.

Intervertebral disk disease may occur at any level from C2 to L5. The midcervical and lower lumbar areas are affected most often. Thoracic disk disease is uncommon.

B. The Spinal Cord and Nerve Roots: Knowledge of the anatomic and physiologic relationships of the spinal cord, nerve roots, vertebrae, and neural foramina is useful for understanding the principles for diagnosis of intervertebral disk disease.

The cervical spinal cord occupies about half of the cross-sectional area of the normal spinal canal, is centrally placed, and moves rostrally and caudally a few millimeters during flexion and extension of the neck. Anteroposterior and lateral motion is restricted by the tethering effect of the intradural dentate ligaments.

The spinal cord terminates as the conus medullaris at L1–2. Posterior and anterior nerve roots emerge from the conus separately, passing within the lumbar sac to their respective intervertebral foramina, where they exit from the spinal canal. The roots join to form a peripheral nerve within the neural foramen. Sacral nerve roots are medial and central within the lumbar sac, adjacent to the filum terminale, the pia-arachnoid structure that anchors the conus to the caudal end of the spinal canal.

In the neck, the C1 root emerges from the spinal canal above the C1 vertebra; the C2 root emerges below C1. Thus, the nerve root that emerges from the spine between the C5 and C6 vertebrae is the C6 root. C8 emerges between C7 and T1, and the T1 root emerges below the pedicle of the T1 vertebra crossing through the T1–T2 foramen.

Sensation around the deltoid area is basically related to the C5 root; sensation in the thumb and possibly in the finger is a C6 root function. Sensation in the third and fourth fingers is a C7 root function, whereas the fifth finger is supplied by C8. Biceps muscle strength and the biceps tendon reflex require an intact C6 root; triceps reflex and strength are dependent upon the C7 root. Intrinsic muscles of the hand allowing abduction and adduction of the fingers are innervated by C8 and T1.

Lumbosacral nerve roots carry on the same relationships to the vertebrae determined by emergence of the T1 nerve root below the T1 vertebra. That is, the L4 nerve root emerges below the L4 pedicle, and the S1 root emerges below S1.

Each root (eg, L4) passes laterally toward the neural foramen as it descends within the spinal canal. It crosses the adjacent intervertebral disk (eg, L4–5) at the extreme lateral edge of the disk after exiting the spinal canal below the pedicle of the L4 vertebra inferolaterally. The nerve root (eg, L5) that descends to the next lowest foramen passes across the same intervertebral disk (eg, L4–5) more medially, in a location that is more vulnerable to diseases involving the disk.

The sensory distribution of L5 is on the medial aspect of the foot and the great toe. S1 sensation is experienced over the lateral aspect of the foot, the fifth toe, and the sole of the foot. Pain or sensory deficit in those dermatomal areas implies involvement of either L5 or S1 fibers. Plantar flexion is primarily an S1 motor function; dorsiflexion of the foot is an L5 function. Knee extension by the quadriceps muscle group is subserved primarily by the L3 and L4 motor roots. The ankle jerk is primarily dependent upon the S1 root, whereas the knee jerk depends upon L3 and L4. The L5 fibers may contribute to both reflexes or to neither one.

The sensory distribution of the remaining sacral roots S2–5 is in the "saddle" area over the buttocks and on the soles of the feet. Voluntary motor control of the urinary bladder and anal sphincters is subserved by the S2–4 nerve roots. Thus, the cauda equina syndrome, a rare complication of massive extrusion of a lumbar disk, is associated with sensory loss over the perineal area and buttocks and with urinary and fecal incontinence.

CERVICAL DISK SYNDROME

Essentials of Diagnosis

Subjective:
* Pain in the suboccipital, cervical, interscapular, thoracic, and shoulder areas radiating into the upper extremities.
* Discomfort aggravated by neck movement.
* Pain, paresthesias, and dysesthesias in the cervical dermatomes.

Objective:
* Straightening of cervical lordosis, limitation of cervical movements, and paraspinous muscle spasm.
* Weakness, fasciculations, muscle atrophy, depression of deep tendon reflexes, and dermatome sensory change in the upper extremities.
* Spasticity, weakness, and extensor plantar sign in the lower extremities.
* Spastic bladder.
* Radiologic evidence of narrowed disk spaces, formation of osteophytes, and spinal stenosis.
* Myelographic, CT, or MRI evidence of extradural cervical cord or root displacement or compression, often at multiple levels.

General Considerations

If the cervical intervertebral disk ruptures and extrudes through the annulus and posterior longitudinal ligament, adjacent neural structures may be compressed. Compression of the spinal cord may result in paraplegia or quadriplegia, depending on the segment involved, whereas compression of a spinal root may cause weakness and sensory loss in structures of the upper extremity innervated by it. The severity of the clinical syndrome depends upon the site and severity of compression by the displaced disk fragment. Often, intrinsic disruption of the disk occurs, but the adjacent ligaments hold, preventing complete extrusion of the fragmented disk. The annulus may separate from its attachment to the vertebral body margin or tear sufficiently to allow the disk to bulge into the spinal canal or foramina. Thus, neural structures also may be compressed by protrusion of an injured or degenerated disk.

After trauma or spontaneously, the annulus may rupture and the nucleus may herniate into the spinal canal or neural foramen acutely. Often, however, the nucleus does not extrude but simply becomes desiccated and progressively degenerates, losing its biomechanical function and elasticity. The disk space gradually narrows, the joint becomes looser, and the cartilaginous end-plates of the adjacent vertebra touch, stimulating reactive osteogenesis. Bony spurs develop at the joint in reaction to the increased mobility and stress. If a bony spur (osteophyte) forms in the neural foramen, the nerve root passing through may be chronically irritated and compressed. If the osteophyte forms within the spinal canal, spinal cord compression may result in the development of myelopathy with signs and symptoms of impaired cord function. Formation of osteophytes around the joints of vertebrae is termed **spondylosis.**

Cervical spondylosis is common and may even be "normal" in aging persons. Radiographic evidence of cervical spondylosis exists in 85% of people over 65 years of age. It may not be associated with symptoms of cord or root compression, however, unless the neural canal or foramina are narrowed. Developmental reduction of canal dimensions may contribute to the appearance of symptoms that are the result of entrapment of neural elements.

Clinical Findings

A. Symptoms and Signs: The onset of symptoms and signs of an extruded disk fragment may be acute or insidious. Acute symptoms may follow trauma or be unrelated to injury. Neck and radicular pain radiating down the arm occur simultaneously, but spinal cord symptoms are rare. There is usually limitation of neck motion, tenderness over the brachial nerves, and straightening of the normal cervical lordosis. Decrease in a deep tendon reflex (biceps or triceps jerk) is common with or without weakness in the muscles supplied by the compressed root. With foraminal osteophytes, episodes of cervical discomfort may recur over many months or years before radicular symptoms occur. Interscapular aching and suboccipital headaches are common associated complaints that may be explained as episodes of sequential radiation of referred skeletal pain. The signs and symptoms of cervical spondylosis are those of progressive cervical radiculopathy and, in advanced cases, spastic paraparesis with mild to moderate sensory deficit in the lower extremities as well as a cervical dermatome pattern. Neck and arm pain may or may not be present along with some limitation of cervical spine movement.

B. Imaging Studies: Plain x-rays may be normal except for straightening of the cervical lordosis. The lateral view may demonstrate narrowing of one or more disk spaces. X-rays may show osteophyte formation at the appropriate neural foramen in association with disk narrowing. This is usually best seen on oblique views. In cervical spondylosis, there is usually x-ray evidence of osteophytes and disk narrowing at several levels, and in most cases with neurologic symptoms and signs, the sagittal diameter of the cervical spinal canal is also congenitally narrowed. When the diameter of the canal is 10 mm or less, clinically significant spinal cord compression can be expected to occur.

MRI is now being used with increasing success as the initial diagnostic study for patients with cervical radiculomyelopathy. Subarachnoid cerebrospinal fluid spaces, spinal cord, nerve roots, and vertebral structures can be visualized without injection of contrast material, but resolution of anatomic details may not always be as clear as obtained with CT scanning.

CT scans of the spine are useful for evaluating the diameter of the canal and the foramina in patients with cervical spine stenosis. Osteophytes and post-traumatic deformities of the vertebral bodies and facet joints can be identified; soft tissue lesions such as displaced disk or hypertrophied ligaments and joint capsules that may cause compression of neural elements in patients with spondylosis are less well visualized in the cervical and thoracic areas.

Following acute disk herniation, myelography may show a small ventral extradural defect obliterating the nerve root cuff. In cervical spondylosis, the myelogram shows bar-like ventral defects at the disk space, usually at several levels and sometimes associated with apparent widening of the cord shadow on the anteroposterior projection if the spinal diameter is narrowed. CT scanning in conjunction with myelography provides images of the relationship between vertebral and neural elements in the axial plane. With contrast material demonstrating the size and configuration of the subarachnoid space, compression or atrophy of the cervical cord and roots can be clearly visualized and the lesions identified.

Differential Diagnosis

Cervical disk disease must be differentiated from traumatic and inflammatory disease affecting the soft tissues and joints of the neck and pectoral girdle, such as subdeltoid or subacromial bursitis and cervical and shoulder sprains. Nerve entrapment syndromes in the upper extremities such as cervical rib and scalenus anticus syndrome, carpal tunnel syndrome, and tardy ulnar palsy may also cause neck and arm pain, weakness, and numbness. Other conditions that must be considered include coronary insufficiency and angina pectoris; neoplasms of the pulmonary apex (eg, Pancoast tumors), primary peripheral or central nervous system tumor of the brachial plexus, cervical cord, or cervicomedullary junction; fractures, dislocations, or subluxations of the cervical spine; and inflammatory disease of the cervical theca such as arachnoiditis, sarcoidosis, and Pott's disease. The condition that is most difficult to distinguish from cervical radiculopathy is brachial neuritis, an idiopathic inflammatory disease that affects the brachial plexus.

The disorder that most frequently mimics cervical disk disease is invasion of the cervical spine by metastatic tumor. Biopsy and surgical decompression or radiation therapy are indicated as emergency procedures, especially when a pathologic fracture or epidural mass lesion threatens spinal cord function.

Complications

Permanent damage to the nerve roots and spinal cord may occur, with loss of motor and sensory function. This is particularly true in cervical stenosis and spondylosis, in which both direct pressure on the spinal cord and compression of its vascular supply may produce a severe, progressive irreversible myelopathy with spastic paraplegia or quadriplegia that does not respond to surgical decompression. Such patients are also vulnerable to acute onset of paraparesis or quadriparesis initiated by relatively mild cervical hyperextension injuries sustained during a fall or motor vehicle accident.

Treatment

A. Medical Measures: Initially, cervical disk disease should be treated medically unless there is evidence of spinal cord compression or radicular motor loss in an extremity from severe neural compression. Medical therapy for patients suffering from radiculitis includes immobilization of the neck and application of mild traction with the cervical spine in a neutral position. This is best achieved with continuous or interrupted (2 hours) halter cervical traction. Analgesics, tranquilizers, muscle relaxants, and local heat are frequently used in combination with traction. The weight used generally ranges from 4 to 6 kg, depending on the size of the patient.

B. Surgical Treatment: There are two methods of treating cervical disk disease surgically: (1) posterior decompression of the nerve roots, spinal cord, or both; and (2) anterior decompression of nerve roots, spinal cord, or both, with or without fusion. The choice is based on consideration of a particular patient's anatomic lesions as demonstrated with MRI, CT, or myelography. It may be necessary to use both an anterior and a posterior approach in separate stages if satisfactory recovery is not observed within 3–6 months after the initial operation.

Prognosis

Seventy-five percent of patients will recover following an adequate trial (10–14 days) of medical therapy, even though some continue to have cervical or interscapular discomfort or mild paresthesias. In some patients, radicular or myelopathic symptoms recur upon return to full activity. Although many patients with cervical disk disease can be managed symptomatically for years with intervals of cervical traction and a cervical collar, others eventually require surgical therapy. For the 25% who do not respond to conservative therapy, operation is required. Even after surgery, symptoms may reappear, perhaps because of residual or recurrent disease at the same or adjacent disk levels. In some instances, reevaluation for additional surgery is indicated.

Improvement follows operative treatment of a cervical disk in approximately 80% of patients. Surgical treatment of cervical spondylosis with myelopathy results in improvement in 60% of cases and arrest of progression in many of the remainder.

THORACIC DISK DISEASE

Although the disorder is rare, knowledge of thoracic disk disease is essential, because it is associated with significant deficit when it does occur. Occasionally, the nucleus of a thoracic disk extrudes into the spinal canal as a result of forceful trauma. Because the thoracic canal is small in relation to the spinal cord within it, severe cord compression often results from disk rupture. The onset of paraplegia is often abrupt, and paralysis may be permanent. More often, however, osteophyte formation due to a degenerated thoracic disk accounts for spinal canal narrowing. The occurrence of cord compression is then more gradual and progressive.

Treatment for ruptured thoracic disk associated with intractable pain or disabling neurologic deficit is primarily surgical and consists of removal of the offending disk or spur by the anterior thoracotomy or posterolateral transpedicular approach. Posterior decompression is the least effective approach in the thoracic area and has the highest risk of complications.

LUMBAR DISK SYNDROME

Essentials of Diagnosis

- History of back injury or stress or a discrete episode of spontaneous onset.
- Low back pain.
- Pain aggravated by activity and relieved by bed rest.
- Signs of root compression, associated with the onset of radicular radiation to the legs, eg, sciatica.
- Abnormal straight leg-raising test.
- Neurologic findings variable; usually mild.

General Considerations

If the nucleus of a lumbar intervertebral disk extrudes through the annulus and elevates or tears the posterior longitudinal ligament, lumbosacral nerve roots may be displaced or compressed. Sensory loss, dermatomal pain, motor loss in the myotomes innervated by those roots, and loss of the knee and ankle tendon jerks may result. The severity of the syndrome produced depends upon the site and severity of nerve root compression. Occasionally, the entire cauda equina may be compressed, resulting in paraplegia and loss of motor and sensory function below the lesion, including bowel and bladder sphincter control. Disk rupture may occur in the midline, compressing centrally placed sacral nerve roots preferentially, without involvement of laterally placed lumbar roots at the level of herniation.

Disruption of a lumbar disk may occur without extrusion of the nucleus. In that event, elasticity of the joint is reduced and mobility is increased. The annulus may bulge without tearing. As time passes, osteophytes form around the degenerated disk and may encroach upon the spinal canal and foramina. Lumbar spondylosis, a condition common in the elderly, is the end result. Stenosis of the lumbar canal and foramen may also present as a developmental defect, aggravating the compressive effects of degenerative disk disease and spondylosis.

Clinical Findings

Over 90% of problems arise from the L4–5 and L5–S1 intervertebral areas, with most of the remainder at L3–4. Lumbar disk disease rarely involves higher levels.

A. Symptoms and Signs: Although pain is usually acute when associated with frank herniation, it may also be chronic. There may be back pain, leg pain, or both. The radiation of low back pain into the buttock, posterior thigh, and calf is usually the same with disease at the L4–5 or L5–S1 interspaces. This radiating pain may be aggravated by coughing, sneezing, or the Valsalva maneuver. Bending or sitting accentuates the discomfort, whereas lying down characteristically relieves it. Most commonly, the back pain is described as deep, aching, and constant (lumbago) with a sharp shooting element traveling from the buttock down the leg posteriorly to the foot or toes (sciatica). Sometimes pain and paresthesias radiate to the groin (L3), medial thigh (L4), big toe (L5), or little toe (S1).

Palpation of the paravertebral area and the buttock (less frequently, over the vertebral spines) reveals tenderness at the affected disk level or over the sciatic notch. Palpation of the sciatic nerve in the popliteal fossa may also elicit tenderness or referred pain. The paravertebral musculature may be in spasm, and reactive scoliosis may be present. Straight leg raising produces back or leg pain that may be accentuated with further stretching of the sciatic nerve (by ankle dorsiflexion). Pain produced when the leg opposite the affected side is raised is highly suggestive of disk extrusion.

Weakness of the anterior calf musculature (with the extensor hallucis longus being the first affected) is a common finding, especially with L4–5 disk herniation and L5 radiculopathy. Foot drop can occur in advanced cases. Weakness of the gastrocnemius suggests L5–S1 disease. Weakness of the quadriceps may occur with L3–4 herniation. Atrophy may be present in cases of long-standing radiculopathy. Comparison of knee and ankle reflexes is important. Depression of the ankle jerk is common with L5–S1 disease but is also present in a significant number of cases of L4–5 disease. The knee jerk may be depressed in L3–4 disease.

Sensory patterns are variable. Numbness or paresthesias in the legs are present in fewer than one-third of patients. Rarely, bowel and bladder sphincter dysfunction is reported. Hypesthesia on the dorsum of the foot is common; sensory deficit on the little toe and the lateral surface of the foot is more frequent with L5–S1 disease, and deficit on the big toe and medial aspect of the foot is more frequent with L4–5 disease.

B. Imaging Studies: Plain films of the lumbosacral spine should be taken to identify congenital or acquired skeletal abnormalities. Narrowing of the disk spaces occurs with equal frequency in symptomatic and asymptomatic patients and therefore has no diagnostic value.

MRI scans are useful to image the thecal sac, disks, and vertebral elements. Thoracolumbar tumors can be excluded and, in some instances, peridural scar tissue can be distinguished from recurrent disk herniation in postoperative patients by administration of a paramagnetic contrast agent that enhances signal intensity in scar or granulation tissue but not disk. When certain imaging parameters are selected, the cerebrospinal fluid can be demonstrated, and the need to inject contrast material into the lumbar or cervical subarachnoid space is eliminated. Lumbar puncture is not necessary. MRI of the lumbar spine is rapidly replacing both myelography and CT as the initial diagnostic procedure of choice.

CT scanning of the lumbar spine usually provides adequate diagnostic information if disk protrusion or rupture has occurred. Because the neural canal is larger in the lumbar area, soft tissue lesions as well as spinal canal stenosis may be identified. Sagittal and coronal section reconstruction of axial scans may provide images showing the longitudinal configuration of the lumbar thecal sac. In patients with an appropriate history of disk rupture and a neurologic deficit that correlates anatomically with the level of abnormality shown on the CT scan, myelography may not be necessary. However, if more than one level is involved or if previous disk disease has been treated surgically, CT scanning without myelography will not provide sufficient diagnostic information.

Myelography is diagnostic in 80–90% of cases and is important in localizing the disease and ruling out intraspinal tumors. Enough radiopaque contrast material to cover the lower disk spaces in the semi-upright position is injected into the subarachnoid space, and posteroanterior, lateral, and oblique pictures are then taken. By adjustment of the patient's position, the contrast material is shifted to opacify the lower thoracic cord and conus in order to eliminate the possibility of more rostral compression of the lumbosacral nerve roots by tumor or disk. False-positive and false-negative results may occur.

C. Special Examinations: Electromyography may demonstrate denervation of the muscles in the appropriate nerve root distribution and can be used as an adjunct to neurologic examination when diagnosis is difficult. Electromyography alone is not diagnostic of disk rupture.

Although rarely indicated in current practice, discography may demonstrate an abnormal disk. Radiopaque contrast material is injected under fluoroscopic control into the disk space. Degenerated and extruded disks may be identified. Internal disruption or degeneration of the annulus without dislocation of the nucleus into the neural canal can be demonstrated by discography. Such information can often be obtained with MRI without injection of contrast material.

Differential Diagnosis

Back pain with radiation to the leg has many causes: (1) bony abnormalities such as spondylolisthesis, spondylosis, spinal stenosis, or Paget's disease; (2) primary and metastatic tumors of the cauda equina or the pelvic region; (3) inflammatory disorders, including abscess in the epidural space or retroperitoneal lumbosacral plexus, postinfectious or posttraumatic arachnoiditis, and rheumatoid spondylitis; (4) degenerative lesions of the spinal cord and peripheral neuropathies; and (5) peripheral vascular occlusive disease.

Treatment

A. Medical Measures: A trial of medical treatment is indicated in all patients who do not demonstrate progressive weakness or sphincter dysfunction.

This consists initially of bed rest with application of hot packs to the pain site, anti-inflammatory medications, analgesics, and skeletal muscle relaxants. Pelvic traction that partially immobilizes the patient helps relieve muscle spasm. Physical therapy and graded exercise are indicated in chronic cases or after an acute episode subsides. A corset or back brace provides external support and allows patients to return to activity earlier. A body cast or plastic jacket may be required in cases where chronic pain is relieved by immobilization.

B. Surgical Treatment: Surgical treatment is indicated in patients with progressive neurologic deficits and chronic disabling pain. Acute onset of symptoms associated with weakness or sphincteric disturbance must be treated with urgent decompression.

A simple laminotomy and foraminotomy is made posteriorly at the appropriate interspace, with care to protect the nerve root and dura. Microsurgical technique allows adequate exposure through a smaller fascial incision that reduces muscle dissection. If disk extrusion has occurred, the surgeon attempts to remove this piece and diligently searches for other extruded portions. When herniation without extrusion has occurred, the surgeon makes a window in the ligament and annulus and removes all accessible degenerated material from the intervertebral space. Some surgeons recommend that a fusion be done primarily or as a secondary procedure in chronic back pain cases where preoperative immobilization has relieved symptoms. Total diskectomy through bilateral laminotomies can be followed by interbody fusion that replaces the disk with iliac crest bone grafts for relief of intractable discogenic pain syndromes and stabilization of the intervertebral joint.

Transcutaneous injection of enzymes (eg, chymopapain, collagenase) into lumbar disks has been used in the past to dissolve fibrocartilage or collagen material to relieve pain and radiculopathy without surgery. Needle placement is guided by fluoroscopy. Although satisfactory results were reported in 60–80% of patients, complications related to nerve root injury, transverse myelitis, and systemic anaphylaxis occurred. Patients with fragments of disk material that detach and extrude into the spinal canal are unlikely to benefit from such treatments. Percutaneous aspiration of degenerated disk material through an ultrasonic nucleotome cannula inserted into the intervertebral space has recently been attempted as a safer method for relieving painful in situ disk protrusions. Fragmentation and excision of pieces of degenerated fibrocartilage can also be accomplished through a fiberoptic arthroscopic cannula using microsurgical instruments under fluoroscopic control. Further studies are in progress to evaluate long-term results with these techniques.

Prognosis

With medical treatment, most patients improve sufficiently to return to full activity. Lumbar disk syndrome may recur intermittently with stress or exertion. Recurrences may again be treated surgically, often successfully.

About 10–20% of patients require surgical management. The best results are obtained in patients with extrusion of disk material and acute radiculopathy. Those with chronic poorly localized discogenic pain and no neurologic deficit are less likely to benefit from diskectomy. If joint instability is demonstrated at one or two levels, spinal fusion with or without diskectomy may be indicated.

Thus, if the syndrome has resulted from an extruded disk fragment and is accompanied by an unequivocally positive radiographic study that correlates with clinical findings, 85% of patients will recover completely after surgical treatment. If the syndrome is not associated with a ruptured disk and a positive scan or myelogram, intensive physiotherapy for postural correction and strengthening of spinal support musculature is indicated. Emotional and economic factors, including litigation and compensation for injury, play an important role in outcome regardless of whether treatment is medical or surgical.

Bell GR, Simeone FA: The pathophysiology of disc degeneration. In: *Neurosurgery: The Scientific Basis of Clinical Practice.* Hayward R, Hoff JT (editors). Blackwell, 1985.

Hoff J, Hood T: Anterior operative approaches for benign extradural cervical lesions. In: *Neurological Surgery: A Comprehensive Reference Guide to the Diagnosis and Management of Neurosurgical Problems.* Youmans JR (editor). Saunders, 1990.

Hoff JT: Cervical disc disease and cervical spondylosis. In: *Neurosurgery.* Wilkins RH, Rengachary SS (editors). McGraw-Hill, 1985.

Hudgins WR: Posterior micro-operative treatment of cervical disc disease. In: *Neurological Surgery: A Comprehensive Reference Guide to the Diagnosis and Management of Neurosurgical Problems,* 3rd ed. Youmans JR (editor). Saunders, 1990.

Perot PL Jr: Thoracic disc disease. In: *Neurosurgery.* Wilkins RH, Rengachary SS (editors). McGraw-Hill, 1985.

Simeone FA: Lumbar disc disease. In: *Neurosurgery.* Wilkins RH, Rengachary SS (editors). McGraw-Hill, 1985.

SURGICAL INFECTIONS OF THE CENTRAL NERVOUS SYSTEM

Mark L. Rosenblum, MD

BRAIN ABSCESS

Essentials of Diagnosis

- History of predisposing factors such as sinusitis, otitis, systemic infection (especially pulmonary or cardiac), congenital cyanotic heart disease, or brain damage from trauma or surgery.
- Headache, localized neurologic signs, seizures.
- Positive CT or MRI brain scan.
- Acute or subacute course (days to weeks).

General Considerations

In patients with normal immune systems, brain abscesses usually occur secondary to a focus of infection outside the central nervous system. These sources include infections of the paranasal sinuses, middle ear, lungs, and heart. Congenital cyanotic heart disease and other arteriovenous fistulas, and open cranial wounds from trauma or surgical procedures are predisposing factors for abscess formation; however, in 20% of patients, no cause can be identified. The organisms most commonly responsible for infections are *Streptococcus, Staphylococcus,* and *Bacteroides,* although abscesses have been reported as a result of infection with almost every known bacterium. Anaerobic organisms are found in 50% and multiple microbes in 30% of cultures from abscesses; 20% are sterile.

Abscesses arising from frontal and ethmoid sinusitis usually occur in the frontal lobes, whereas those arising from middle ear disease occur in the posterior temporal lobe or cerebellum. Hematogenous abscesses are usually found in a distribution proportionate to the size of the brain regions.

Immunosuppressed patients and patients with AIDS are predisposed to brain abscesses caused by fungi and protozoal infections. As many as 5% of AIDS patients will develop *Toxoplasma* abscesses, which are usually multiple and can be diagnosed by successful presumptive treatment with antitoxoplasma antibiotics or brain biopsy.

Clinical Findings

A. Symptoms and Signs: The usual presenting symptoms are headache, focal neurologic deficits, and seizures, each of which occur in 50% of patients. Because of the effects of increased intracranial pressure, the onset of decreased sensorium, drowsiness, confusion, and stupor may be delayed. Approximately 50% of patients have low-grade fever (37.5–38 °C [99.5–100.4 °F]).

B. Laboratory Findings: Blood studies usually show mild polymorphonuclear leukocytosis and an elevated sedimentation rate. *Lumbar puncture should not be performed with suspected abscess unless CT scan or MRI shows only a small mass or no mass.* When cerebrospinal fluid is examined, the pressure, white cell count, and protein levels are usually elevated, but bacteria are rarely cultured.

C. Imaging Studies: Skull films may show evidence of mastoiditis, sinusitis, or a pineal shift. CT scan shows a discrete mass with a smooth, symmetric contrast-enhancing ring, low-density center, and variable surrounding edema. MRI with enhancement shows an abscess wall similar to the CT scan; edema surrounding the abscess is readily demonstrated as increased signal on T2 weighted images.

D. Special Examinations: Electroencephalography may show a high-voltage, slow-wave focus.

Differential Diagnosis

Brain abscess must be differentiated from brain tumor, cerebral infarction, resolving intracranial hemorrhage, subdural empyema, extradural abscess, and encephalitis.

Complications

The major complications of brain abscess are rupture into the ventricles or subarachnoid space, obstruction of cerebrospinal fluid pathways, and transtentorial herniation, because of the mass effect of the abscess and the reactive brain swelling.

Treatment

A. Medical Treatment: Before starting antibiotic therapy, obtain cultures of blood, nasopharyngeal secretions, sputum, urine, or draining material from paranasal sinuses or wounds, as may be indicated by the suspected source of infection. Culture of the cerebrospinal fluid should only be performed when symptoms of meningitis are present as indicated above. Whenever possible, antibiotics should not be started prior to abscess aspiration, since doing so preoperatively results in cultures that frequently do not grow out organisms.

Vancomycin and a third-generation cephalosporin are started when the diagnosis is made; if staphylococcal infection is a possibility, nafcillin (16 g daily) is given also. If a penicillin-sensitive organism is identified, it is instituted at a dosage of 16–20 million units daily. As soon as the organism is identified, specific antibiotics that are cytotoxic and can cross the blood-brain barrier are instituted if that is possible. *Toxoplasma* abscesses will usually respond to treatment with pyrimethamine and sulfadiazine. Treatment of fungal abscesses relies on the use of agents such as amphotericin B, but the results have been discouraging.

Since new antibiotics with improved activity and ability to cross the blood-brain barrier are being developed every year, the reader is referred to the infectious disease literature for the most recent updates.

If there is an extracerebral focus of infection (sinus, mastoid, wound, etc), it should be drained surgically.

B. Surgical Treatment: Surgical treatment consists of excision of the abscess or aspiration through a bur hole. CT-guided stereotaxic aspiration, performed under local anesthesia, is the procedure of choice for most abscesses, especially small, deep abscesses or diseases found in patients who are poor candidates for surgery. If craniotomy for abscess removal is planned, it should be performed 2 weeks after the initiation of the local infectious process, if possible, to improve the chance of total abscess removal. An open operation can be delayed for 2 weeks only if the patient has a known predisposing factor, a CT scan that suggests the presence of an abscess, is alert and either clinically stable or improving with antibiotic therapy, if the abscess is small (less than 3 cm in diameter), and if there is little associated mass effect. Aspiration of the abscess may be necessary if the organism is not otherwise identifiable and is essential if the patient deteriorates or if CT scans show an increase in abscess size. After the organism is identified, antibiotics are adjusted appropriately. Corticosteroids are given only when there is significant mass effect from the abscess and surrounding edema, both of which may put the patient at significant risk. Anticonvulsants should be used. An operation is performed at 2 weeks in all but high-risk patients who harbor small lesions in eloquent regions of the brain or in patients who are clinically stable or improving and show a reduced lesion on serial CT or MRI scans. An abscess will occasionally resolve with antibiotic treatment alone, as shown by serial CT or MRI scans, but this approach should be reserved for patients with very small lesions or for situations in which a bleeding diathesis is present. In addition, in patients with multiple abscesses, small lesions can be followed with antibiotics after the organism has been identified by aspiration of the largest lesion. The decision to treat with antibiotics alone requires frequent follow-up visits, with CT or MRI scans and treatment planning by a neurosurgeon who is ready to operate whenever the patient's condition deteriorates.

Postoperative CT or MRI scans are done for early detection and management of complications such as hemorrhage and recurrent abscess.

Hainer SJ et al: Cranial and intracranial infections. In: *Neurological Surgery: A Comprehensive Reference Guide to the Diagnosis and Management of Neurosurgical Problems,* 3rd ed. Youmans JR (editor). Saunders, 1990.

Mampalam TJ, Rosenblum ML: Management of bacterial brain abscesses. Contemp Neurosurg 1988;10(20):1.

Mampalam TJ, Rosenblum ML: Trends in the management of bacterial brain abscesses: A review of 102 cases over 17 years. Neurosurgery 1988;23:451.

Rosenblum ML, Levy RM, Bredeson DE (editors): *AIDS and the Nervous System.* Raven Press, 1988.

Rosenblum ML, Mampalam TJ, Pons VG: Controversies in the management of brain abscesses. Clin Neurosurg 1986;33:603.

LESS COMMON PYOGENIC INFECTIONS

Epidural Abscess

Epidural abscess in the cranial or spinal epidural space produces focal neurologic deficit by pressure on the underlying neural tissues. In the cranium, it is usually secondary to adjacent osteomyelitis or subgaleal empyemas caused by metastatic infections, head trauma, or cranial operations. In the spine, epidural abscesses are usually metastatic from a remote infection in the pelvis or lower extremities, or from bacteremia usually caused by urinary tract infection.

Treatment consists of immediate drainage of the pus and appropriate treatment of the primary infection with antibiotics. Operations should also be performed on the primary focal sites of infection.

Subdural Abscess

Subdural abscess or empyema, a serious complication of (usually) frontal sinusitis, progresses rapidly and has a high death rate. Immediate surgical drainage and antibiotic therapy are indicated.

Cerebral Thrombophlebitis

Cerebral thrombophlebitis is a rare complication of meningitis, epidural and subdural abscesses, and thrombophlebitis of facial veins. The lateral, cavernous, and superior sagittal sinuses are most commonly involved, producing neurologic deficit by venous infarction. Treatment is with specific antibiotics. If marked cerebral edema is associated, treatment with glucocorticoids, diuretics, and mannitol should be considered.

CLOSED DISK SPACE INFECTIONS FOLLOWING REMOVAL OF LUMBAR INTERVERTEBRAL DISK

Closed disk space infection is seen in approximately 1–3% of patients following lumbar laminectomy with diskectomy and is thought to be due to pyogenic infection confined to the disk space. Symptoms usually occur 1–2 weeks or longer after operation. Preoperative sciatica has usually resolved when the patient complains of severe pain localized in the back and thighs, aggravated by any motion. The patient may run a low-grade fever or be afebrile; the white count may be normal or slightly elevated. The erythrocyte sedimentation rate is usually over 50 mm/h. Radiographic signs usually appear in 4 weeks and consist of destruction of the vertebral end-plates and narrowing and eventual bony fusion of the disk space.

Treatment consists of immobilization and analgesics. A needle biopsy of the interspace should be performed before antibiotic therapy is planned; antibiotics should be given for 4–6 weeks.

TUBERCULOSIS OF THE SPINE
(Pott's Disease)

Tuberculous infections of the brain and spine are seen most frequently in patients living in developing countries. The spinal cord dysfunction usually seen with far-advanced vertebral tuberculous lesions progresses rapidly to paraplegia or quadriplegia within a few weeks. The thoracic cord is most commonly involved, followed by the cervical cord and the lumbar cord segments. Radiographically, there is usually destruction of one or more intervertebral disks, apposi-

tion of the adjacent vertebral bodies, and destruction of one or more vertebral bodies. Soft tissue swelling is usually evident around the affected area, and a soft tissue mass of varying size is commonly present. A total extradural type block may be seen myelographically 1–2 levels below the obvious bony changes.

Treatment consists of (1) ethambutol, rifampin, and isoniazid; (2) surgical drainage of the abscess via an anterior or lateral approach and fusion if necessary; and (3) immobilization of the affected area. Laminectomy has little place in the treatment of Pott's disease.

Chowdhary UM, Marwah S, Sankarankutty M: Surgical treatment of dorsal and lumbar spinal tuberculosis. J R Coll Surg Edinb 1985;30:386.

LaBerge JM, Brant-Zawadzki M: Evaluation of Pott's disease with computed tomography. Neuroradiology 1984; 26:429.

Shivaram U et al: Spinal tuberculosis revisited. South Med J 1985;78:681.

REFERENCES

Adams RD, Victor M: *Principles of Neurology,* 4th ed. McGraw-Hill, 1989.

Burger PC, Vogel FS: *Surgical Pathology of the Nervous System & Its Coverings,* 2nd ed. Wiley, 1982.

Hoff JT (editor): *Goldsmith's Practice of Surgery: Neurosurgery.* Harper & Row, 1981.

Jennett B: *An Introduction to Neurosurgery,* 4th ed. Mosby, 1983.

Joynt RJ: *Clinical Neurology,* rev ed. Lippincott, 1990.

Russell DJ, Rubinstein LJ: *Pathology of Tumours of the Nervous System,* 5th ed. Williams & Wilkins, 1989.

Youmans JR (editor): *Neurological Surgery: A Comprehensive Reference Guide to the Diagnosis and Management of Neurosurgical Problems,* 3rd ed. 6 vols. Saunders, 1990.

Otolaryngology–Head & Neck Surgery*

Lee D. Rowe, MD

Otolaryngology is a regional surgical specialty devoted to diseases of the head and neck. An understanding of head and neck anatomy, physiology, and pathology is necessary to manage diverse disorders of head and neck structures, ranging from hearing and communication impairments to disorders calling for facial plastic and reconstructive surgery.

EAR

SOUND PHYSICS

Sound waves travel as alternating compressions and rarefactions of the elastic medium through which they are transmitted (sound travels in air at 1100 ft/s [about 336 m/s]). Sound waves exhibit several physical characteristics, including amplitude and frequency, that are related to the subjective psychoacoustic attributes of loudness and pitch. The intensity range of human hearing is great—the most intense tone that can be perceived as sound is several million times louder than the faintest detectable one.

The auricle serves to localize sound in space and to amplify sound waves impinging on the tympanic membrane through the resonance capabilities of the external auditory canal. Sound waves strike the tympanic membrane and produce in-and-out vibrations that transmit sound energy to the ossicular chain. The tympanic membrane protects the round window from simultaneous sound exposure by interposing an air-filled middle ear space. With a large perforation of the tympanic membrane, sound simultaneously strikes the round window and the tympanic membrane, decreasing the energy transmitted to the oval window.

Acoustic energy at the tympanic membrane is transformed by the malleus, incus, and stapes into energy within the oval window perilymph. Sound is amplified by the lever mechanism of the ossicular chain and also as a function of the large ratio of the tympanic membrane area to the area of the small stapes footplate. Therefore, the middle ear and ossicular system act as an efficient device for transferring acoustic energy from one elastic medium (air) to another medium of different impedance (fluid).

Movement of the stapes footplate produces a traveling wave in the scala vestibuli perilymph that is propagated along the basilar membrane of the cochlea from the base to the apex and down the scala tympani to the round window. Vibration of the basement membrane produces a shearing movement between the tectorial membrane and the hairs of the hair cells, generating electrical activity within the cochlea and auditory nerves. The point of maximal displacement of the basilar membrane is dependent upon the frequency (or pitch) of the wave. High-frequency tones cause maximal displacement near the base of the cochlea, and low-frequency tones cause maximal stimulation near the apex.

Cochlear frequency encoding involves depolarization of afferent neurons that synapse in the cochlear nuclei in the brain stem. The attendant perception of loudness and pitch depends upon the total number of neurons activated and their frequency specificities. The central auditory pathway is a complex system with many crossovers and relay stations to the auditory cortex.

CLINICAL AUDIOLOGY

Audiology is the study of hearing and disorders in sound recognition. Sound carried by air to the ear and perceived in the normal way represents hearing by **air conduction.** Tests of hearing by air conduction provide information about the patency of the external auditory canal, the efficiency of sound transmission by the tympanic membrane and the ossicular chain, and the integrity of the cochlea, acoustic nerve, and central auditory pathway. A defect in the auditory system from the external auditory canal to but not including the cochlea produces a conductive hearing

---

*Tumors of the head and neck are discussed in Chapter 15.

loss and raises the intensity threshold for perception of sound. The term **conductive hearing loss** applies only to air conduction. Otitis media with effusion is the most common cause of conductive hearing loss in children. Other causes include ceruminous impactions in the external auditory canal, large tympanic membrane perforations, ossicular chain discontinuities from trauma or infection, otosclerosis, and temporal bone neoplasms involving the external auditory canal or middle ear.

If the sound source is placed on the skull or teeth, the vibration will directly stimulate the cochlear perilymph and bypass the external and middle ear. **Bone conduction** hearing tests thus examine the integrity of the cochlea, eighth nerve, and central auditory pathway. Bone conduction hearing losses are secondary to lesions of the sensory (cochlea) and neural (acoustic nerve) components of the auditory system and are designated **sensorineural** hearing losses. The most common cause of sensorineural hearing loss is aging (presbycusis), which is associated with progressive loss of outer hair cells within the organ of Corti and neural degeneration. However, noise exposure (especially industrial noise), ototoxic drugs including neomycin and other aminoglycosides, temporal bone fractures, labyrinthine infections, and arterial insufficiency may also produce sensorineural hearing disorders. Composite or mixed losses have both conductive and sensorineural elements.

Hearing is clinically evaluated by a careful history and physical examination that includes tuning fork testing, whispered voice assessment, and audiometric analysis. Because of the importance of hearing in speech acquisition and intellectual maturation, it is critical to diagnose disorders early. By noting the verbal responses to spondaic words or phrases (eg, football, hot dog, childhood, heartbreak—taking care to sustain the accent on both syllables), the examiner can grossly establish the level of hearing loss in each ear. The degree of loss may be estimated from Table 39–1 by determining the voice level at which the words are no longer perceived.

It is important to provide masking (noise) by rubbing the tragus or hair in front of the ear not being tested when the loud whispered level is reached. Otherwise, sound or speech may cross over to the nontested ear, yielding a false result.

Further characterization of the type of hearing loss requires the use of tuning forks to differentiate a conductive from a sensorineural defect. In the **Weber test,** placement of a 512-Hz tuning fork on the skull in the midline or on the teeth stimulates both cochleas simultaneously. If the patient has a conductive hearing loss in one ear, the sound will be perceived loudest in the affected ear (ie, it will lateralize). When a unilateral sensorineural hearing loss, the tone is heard in the unaffected ear. The **Rinne test** compares air conduction (AC) with bone conduction (ie, AC > BC) in one ear, and commonly utilizes the 256- and 512-

Table 39–1. Estimation of hearing loss by voice test.*

Examiner's Voice Level	Decibel Equivalent	Degree of Loss
Soft whispered voice (inaudible to examiner)	20 dB	Mild
Moderate whispered voice (just audible to examiner)	35 dB	Mild to moderate
Loud whispered voice	40–50 dB	Moderate
Soft spoken voice	60 dB	Moderate to severe
Moderately loud spoken voice	70–80 dB	Severe
Loud spoken voice	90–120 dB	Very severe to totally deaf

*The degree of hearing loss may be estimated by determining the voice level at which the patient understands the examiner's voice. If the patient hears the examiner's whispered voice distinctly, hearing is probably normal.

Hz tuning forks. Sound stimulation by air in front of the pinna is normally perceived twice as long as sound placed on the mastoid tip (ie, AC > BC). With conductive hearing loss, the duration of air conduction is less than bone conduction (ie, BC > AC; negative Rinne test). In the presence of sensorineural hearing loss, the duration of both air conduction and bone conduction are reduced; however, the 2:1 ratio remains the same (ie, AC > BC; positive Rinne test). The results of these two tuning fork tests are synthesized to determine the type of hearing loss.

Further quantification of the type and degree of hearing loss and the ability to hear and understand speech requires pure tone audiometry, speech reception threshold testing, and speech discrimination analysis. An audiometer is an electronic device capable of delivering pure sound frequencies by both air and bone conduction from 125 to 8000 Hz at intensities ranging from 0 to 110 decibels (dB) in 5-dB steps. The decibel is a logarithmic ratio of two sound pressure levels (SPL) or intensities that are related to a reference intensity, measured in dynes per square centimeter. The threshold intensity of sound perception in a normal individual is 0–20 dB within the speech frequencies (500–3000 Hz). The ear has the greatest sensitivities between these frequencies, because the tympanic membrane and ossicular chain transmit sound most efficiently in this range. Pure tone audiometry in such a person will demonstrate at all frequencies normal thresholds for both air and bone conduction (Figure 39–1). On the other hand, a conductive hearing loss raises the threshold for sound perception in air. With air conduction hearing loss of 60 dB, for example, the threshold is 1000-fold greater than normal (Figure 39–2). Sensorineural hearing losses result in equal increases in the threshold for air conduction and bone conduction and produce a characteristic audiogram (Figure 39–3).

Speech perception can be evaluated by presenting the patient with a list of spondaic words (eg, football, wineglass) at an intensity corresponding to 50% com-

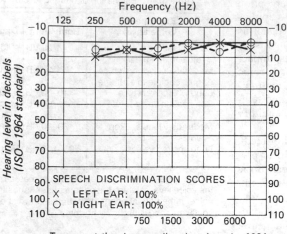

Air Conduction
○ Right ear (red)
✕ Left ear (blue)
△ Right ear with _____ dB
    masking in left
☐ Left ear with _____ dB
    masking in right
Bone Conduction
> Right ear (red)
< Left ear (blue)
▶ Right ear with _____ dB
    masking in left
◀ Left ear with _____ dB
    masking in right
↓ No response at maximum
    limits of audiometer

To convert the above readings based on the 1964 ISO reference thresholds to readings based on the 1951 ASA reference thresholds, subtract the following (rounded) difference in dB:

125	250	500	1000	2000	4000	8000
10	15	15	10	10	5	10

Figure 39–1. Normal hearing.

prehension. The resulting speech reception threshold (SRT) should approximate the average hearing levels for the speech frequencies of 500, 1000, and 2000 Hz. These frequencies are extremely important for understanding conversation in English and fall within the 300- to 3000-Hz transmission range of the telephone. The ability to discriminate speech is ascertained by presenting a list of 50 phonetically balanced monosyllabic words (eg, dog, cat, hat), 30–40 dB above the speech reception threshold. The percentage of words the patient repeats correctly is called the discrimination score and should normally be between 90% and 100%. In conductive hearing loss, the discrimination score is normal; in sensorineural hearing losses, the discrimination score decreases with progressive cochlear and neuronal impairment.

Because the previous tests require a voluntary response, they are of little use if age or illness prevents the patient from performing the required tasks. For example, infants with a high risk of hearing loss (eg, congenital rubella) are unable to give voluntary responses; therefore, an objective method of determining auditory thresholds is necessary to fully evaluate a suspected hearing loss. Evoked response or brain

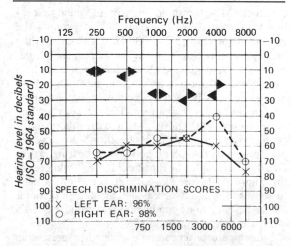

Figure 39–2. Bilateral severe conductive hearing loss due to otosclerosis.

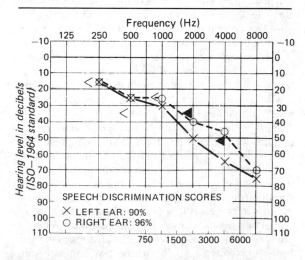

Figure 39–3. Bilateral high-frequency sensorineural hearing loss.

stem audiometry measures electrical responses to sound stimuli (clicks) from the acoustic nerve, cochlear nuclei, and inferior colliculi from the surface of the scalp and the mastoid prominence or ear lobe of the test ear. These techniques are particularly useful in evaluating patients with suspected sensorineural hearing losses secondary to acoustic neuroma, cerebellopontine angle tumor, or a brain stem lesion. Brain stem evoked response audiometry (BSERA) is especially important in newborn nurseries for identifying infants at risk of hearing impairment. These include low-birth-weight infants (< 1500 g), infants with low Apgar scores, infants with hyperbilirubinemia (> 20 mg/dL) or neonatal meningitis, or infants with the TORCH (toxoplasmosis, rubella, *Chlamydia*) complex (Table 39–2). Accordingly, a protocol for audiologic screening of at-risk newborn infants (Table 39–3) is indicated using BSERA. If hearing loss is identified, habilitation should begin by age 6 months.

Audiological screening of newborn infants who are at risk for hearing impairment. ASHA Monogr 1989;31:89.

Osguthorpe JD, Melnick W (editors): Clinical audiology. Otolaryngol Clin North Am 1991;24:233.

Warren MP: The auditory brainstem response in pediatrics. Otolaryngol Clin North Am 1989;22:473.

CONDUCTIVE HEARING LOSS

1. OTITIS MEDIA WITH EFFUSION

Otitis media with effusion is the leading cause of hearing loss in childhood. More than 30% of all children have had three or more episodes of otitis media by their second birthday. The term "nonsuppurative otitis media" denotes a broad range of middle ear effusions characterized by an inflammatory exudate and various amounts of mucus. Several distinct types are recognized: (1) serous otitis media—a sterile, pale, low-viscosity transudate; (2) secretory otitis media—a chronic "glue" ear with infiltration of lymphocytes, histiocytes, plasma cells, leukocytes, and

Table 39–2. High-risk criteria for hearing loss.[1]

1. Family history of childhood hearing impairment
2. Congenital perinatal infection, eg, cytomegalovirus, rubella, herpes, toxoplasmosis, syphilis
3. Anatomic malformation of the head or neck
4. Birthweight <1500 g
5. Hyperbilirubinemia at level exceeding indications for exchange transfusion
6. Bacterial meningitis, especially *Haemophilus influenzae*
7. Severe asphyxia, including infants with Apgar scores of 0–3 who fail to start spontaneous respiration by 10 minutes and those with hypotonia persisting to 2 hours of age

[1]Joint Committee on Infant Hearing, 1982.

Table 39–3. Protocol for screening infants at risk for hearing loss.

1. Newborn infants with no risk factors are not screened unless the parent is concerned about auditory behavior or speech and language development. Parents of infants not at risk are to be given information and education.
2. Infants at risk are screened by ABR prior to discharge. Parents of at-risk infants are to be given information and education.
   a. Infants who pass the screening procedure are provided with follow-up as needed for medical and developmental consideration.
   b. Infants who pass the screening procedure but are at risk for progressive hearing impairment are monitored audiologically and managed as needed.
   c. Infants who fail the screening procedure are evaluated, given follow-up, and provided with a management system.

markedly increased glandular production of mucus; and (3) aerotitis media secondary to barotrauma or direct temporal bone injury. Chronic otitis media with effusion is unsterile in 50% of cases; *Haemophilus influenzae,* pneumococcus, *Moraxella catarrhalis,* and *Streptococcus pyogenes* are the organisms most often found. Although many factors may be implicated, including rhinoviruses, upper respiratory bacteria, and inflammatory mediators of arachidonic acid metabolism, the common denominator appears to be auditory tube (eustachian tube) dysfunction. The physiologic role of the auditory tube is to protect the middle ear from nasopharyngeal secretions, clear middle ear secretions into the nasopharynx, and, more importantly, ventilate the middle ear space. Auditory tube dysfunction develops from barotrauma when the nasopharyngeal pressure exceeds middle ear pressure during rapid descent in an airplane or from adenoidal hypertrophy that produces lymphatic obstruction of the auditory tube. In addition, over half of children with cleft palate deformities manifest auditory tube dysfunction secondary to malfunction of the tensor veli palatini muscle.

If auditory tube function is compromised—as it frequently is in young children—early diagnosis and treatment are critical to prevent impairment of speech development. On physical examination, the tympanic membrane is retracted, the short process of the malleus is extremely prominent, and the light reflex is frequently lost. Pneumatic otoscopy discloses marked reduction of tympanic membrane mobility, and a characteristic yellow or amber color is often seen in the middle ear space.

Unfortunately, otoscopy is not a reliable method of assessing middle ear effusions. Impedance audiometry (tympanometry) is a more accurate means of diagnosing otitis media with effusion. The overall compliance of the tympanic membrane and middle ear system, which varies inversely with its impedance, is measured by delivering to the tympanic membrane a continuous 220-Hz tone signal via a sealed probe tip and recording the amount of energy reflected from the surface. The pressure in the external auditory canal is varied—from +400 mm H_2O to −400 mm H_2O—and the reflected energy is recorded. The resultant tympanogram correlates well with the presence or absence of effusion. A normal type A tympanogram is characterized by a peak compliance at 0 mm H_2O pressure; the absence of a peak of maximal compliance is commonly encountered in middle ear effusions (type B tympanogram). By contrast, type C tympanograms exhibit a peak of maximal compliance of less than −100 mm of H_2O and are chiefly associated with a retracted tympanic membrane with or without effusion.

Initial management of otitis media with effusion consists of identifying the cause. In adults, a malignant neoplasm of the nasopharynx such as carcinoma or lymphoma should be carefully excluded. Unilateral hearing loss secondary to otitis media with effusion is a common manifestation of obstruction of the auditory tube by tumor. Allergy and enlargement of the adenoids may play a causative role in children. Conservative treatment with sympathomimetic amines and antihistamines is often attempted first, though there is no evidence that they alter the clinical course. Nonoperative therapy also includes antibiotics, autoinflation (Valsalva's maneuver), and control of etiologic factors (nasal infections, sinusitis, allergy, etc). Many consultants would start with a course of amoxicillin and if this fails use trimethoprim-sulfamethoxazole, cefaclor, or amoxicillin-clavulanic acid. Alternative antibiotics include cefuroxime and cefixime. Failure of medical treatment necessitates surgical intervention with myringotomy and insertion of ventilating tubes (Figure 39–4). Usually this is defined as 3 months of chemoprophylaxis with amoxicillin-clavulanate potassium. Current indications for sustained middle ear ventilation with tubes include (1) significant conductive hearing loss; (2) persistent tympanic membrane atelectasis and negative middle ear pressure of less than 150 mm H_2O; (3) prevention of recurrent acute otitis media refractory to prophylactic antibiotic therapy; (4) cleft palate; or (5) impending cholesteatoma. Approximately 80% of intubated patients respond after one insertion and require no further treatment. Adenoidectomy, which is recommended for children requiring more than one set of myringotomy tubes, reduces recurrent middle ear infections, since chronically infected adenoids obstruct the auditory tube and serve as a persistent source of infection in the middle ear. Otitis media-prone children carry nontypable *H influenzae* at an unusually high rate.

Giebink GS et al: A controlled trial comparing three treatments for chronic otitis media with effusion. Pediatr Infect Dis J 1990;9:33.

Roland PS et al: Otitis media: Incidence, duration and hear-

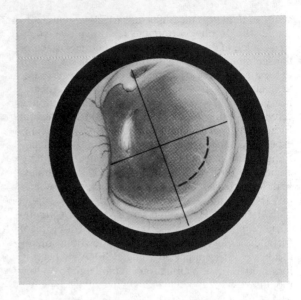

Figure 39–4. Site of myringotomy.

ing status. Arch Otolaryngol Head Neck Surg 1989; 115:1049.

Sade J, Luntz M: Adenoidectomy in otitis media: A review. Ann Otol Rhinol Laryngol 1991;100:226.

Skinner DW, VanHasselt CA, Tsao SY: Nasopharyngeal carcinoma: modes of presentation. Ann Otol Rhinol Laryngol 1991;100:544.

Takahashi H et al: Transtympanic endoscopic findings in patients with otitis media with effusion. Arch Otolaryngol Head Neck Surg 1990;116:1186.

Ziegler AM et al: Rhinovirus in otitis media with effusion. Ann Otolaryngol Rhinol Laryngol 1990;99:451.

2. CHRONIC OTITIS MEDIA

The long-term sequela of chronic auditory tube dysfunction is chronic otitis media, which involves chronic perforation of the tympanic membrane that may or may not be associated with recurrent acute suppuration, destruction of the ossicular chain, or both. The perforation of the tympanic membrane may take two forms: (1) a central (or safe) perforation, in which a remnant of the tympanic membrane is interposed between the rim of the perforation and the annulus of the tympanic membrane (Figure 39–5); and (2) a marginal (or dangerous) perforation, in which the annulus of the tympanic membrane has been destroyed, primarily in the posterosuperior quadrant. In the former case, the middle ear is usually dry; in the latter, suppuration commonly occurs. The pars flaccida is frequently involved in marginal perforations, and central perforations are restricted to the pars tensa. However, suppuration may develop in either situation as a result of the introduction of staphylococci or gram-negative rods (commonly *Pseu-*

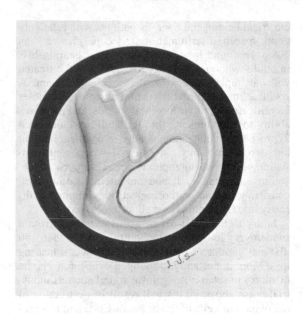

Figure 39–5. Perforation of eardrum.

domonas aeruginosa, *Staphylococcus aureus,* and Enterobacteriaceae) via the auditory tube or external auditory canal. Foul-smelling otorrhea characteristic of anaerobic streptococcal infection should be treated by vacuum drainage of the external auditory canal and instillation of neomycin plus polymyxin otic drops with or without an oral quinolone such as ciprofloxacin, norfloxacin, or ofloxacin. Quinolones are avoided, however, in children and infants. Alternative therapy may be instituted with gentamicin drops plus clindamycin orally. Some clinicians add metronidazole to this regimen. In recalcitrant cases, parenteral azlocillin, ticarcillin, or ceftazidime may prove beneficial if no cholesteatoma is present. Intravenous ciprofloxacin may also be considered in adults.

Complications of chronic otitis media such as seventh nerve paralysis, labyrinthitis, petrositis (Gradenigo's syndrome) or intracranial suppuration are less frequently associated with central perforations than with marginal ones. If squamous epithelium migrates into the middle ear or mastoid, a keratinizing aural cholesteatoma develops. The desquamating epithelium produces bone-destroying collagenase and tends to remain infected. The associated middle ear inflammation interferes with the tenuous blood supply to the stapes and the long process of the incus, resulting in ossicular destruction with a conductive hearing loss of 50–60 dB. White amorphous debris is often observed in the pars flaccida. Computed tomography of the temporal bone may show an unsuspected large radiolucent defect secondary to bone destruction. If untreated, a cholesteatoma may progressively destroy the ossicular chain and erode into the inner ear, producing profound hearing loss.

Bacterial invasion of the cranium from an infected cholesteatoma may occur as a result of osteitis, thrombophlebitis, bony erosion, or along a preformed pathway such as the oval or round windows, perilymphatic duct, or endolymphatic duct. In the preantibiotic era, the onset of severe temporoparietal headache and nuchal rigidity in a patient with chronic otitis media was an ominous sign. The most common intracranial complication of chronic otitis media is meningitis, secondary to either pneumococcus or another streptococcal organism. Additional potential problems include epidural abscess, temporal lobe abscess, cerebellar abscess, lateral sinus thrombosis, subdural empyema, and otitic hydrocephalus. Fortunately, these complications are now rare and can be prevented by early surgical treatment of chronic otitis media and cholesteatoma. Management includes drainage, mastoidectomy, and penicillin or clindamycin (for anaerobic bacteria) and ceftazidime (for *Pseudomonas, Staphylococcus,* and most gram-negative species) as initial agents.

Simple central tympanic membrane perforations are repaired by grafting the tympanic membrane with temporalis fascia or canal wall skin. In the absence of cholesteatoma, associated ossicular discontinuity is repaired with an autogenous homograft or alloplastic materials to reestablish the sound-transforming capability of the middle ear. With advanced middle ear and mastoid disease and associated cholesteatoma, more radical surgery is required. In a radical mastoidectomy, the remnants of the tympanic membrane, ossicles, and cholesteatoma are removed and the mastoid air cells, antrum, and middle ear are converted into an open cavity that is periodically inspected and cleaned. If the cholesteatoma lies above and superficial to the tympanic membrane and middle ear ossicles, either an intact canal wall mastoidectomy or modified radical mastoidectomy is performed. The primary goal of each is to eradicate infection and provide a temporal bone free of cholesteatoma.

Cusimano F, Cocita VC, D'Amico A: Sensori-neural hearing loss in chronic otitis media. J Laryngol Otol 1989;103:158.

Levine BA et al: Sensori-neural hearing loss in chronic otitis media: Is it clinically significant? Arch Otolaryngol Head Neck Surg 1989;115:814.

Nunez DA, Browning GG: Risk of developing an otogenic intracranial abscess. J Laryngol Otol 1991;104:468.

Sheehy JL, Shelton C: Tympanoplasty: to stage or not to stage. Otolaryngol Head Neck Surg 1991;104:339.

Schwaber MK, Pensak ML, Bartels LJ: The early signs and symptoms of neuro-otologic complications of chronic suppurative otitis media. Laryngoscope 1989;99:373.

Tos M et al: Tympanosclerosis of the middle ear: Late results of surgical treatment. J Laryngol Otol 1990; 104:685.

3. OTOSCLEROSIS

In otosclerosis, a localized disease of the otic capsule, new spongy bone replaces normal bone, producing ankylosis or fixation of the stapes footplate. The resulting conductive hearing loss starts insidiously in the third and fourth decades of life and progressively involves both ears in 80% of individuals. Otosclerosis is an inherited disease, more common in whites, with an incidence of approximately 12% in temporal bone series. Bilateral otosclerosis is present more commonly in women. In adults with normal-appearing tympanic membranes, it is the most common cause of progressive conductive hearing loss. The hearing loss may be treated in selected cases by microsurgical removal of the stapes and reconstruction with a metallic prosthesis (3.75–4.50 mm in length) crimped over the long process of the incus. The medial end of the prosthesis is placed over vein or fascia inserted in the oval window. Alternatively, a small hole is created in the footplate of the stapes (stapedotomy) and a Teflon wire or platinum ribbon prosthesis (4.25 × 0.5 mm) inserted. Argon, KTP, and CO_2 lasers can be used for small-fenestra stapedotomy. Stapedectomy or stapedotomy corrects the conductive hearing loss in most patients and may cause partial or total sensorineural hearing loss in fewer than 1% of patients.

Bartels L: KTP laser stapedotomy: Is it safe? Otolaryngol Head Neck Surg 1990;103:685.

Horn KL, Gherini S, Griffin GM Jr: Argon laser stapedectomy using an endo-otoprobe system. Otolaryngol Head Neck Surg 1990;102:193.

Hueb MM et al: Otosclerosis: University of Minnesota, temporal bone collection. Otolaryngol Head Neck Surg 1991;105:396.

Lesinski SG, Palmer A: Lasers for otosclerosis: CO_2 vs. argon and KTP-532. Laryngoscope 1989;99:1.

Pederson CB, Felding JU: Stapes surgery: Complications and airway infection. Ann Otol Rhinol Laryngol 1991; 100:607.

SENSORINEURAL HEARING LOSS

Disorders affecting the cochlea and auditory neurons distort the perception of sound, producing a sensorineural hearing loss. The deficit is generally greater in the higher frequencies and is associated with decreased speech discrimination scores (ie, ability to understand complex speech is impaired).

The most common cause of sensorineural hearing loss is **presbycusis,** a gradual deterioration that starts after 20 years of age in the highest frequencies and often involves all speech frequencies by the sixth and seventh decades. The impaired hearing stems from degenerative changes in the hair cells, auditory neurons, and cochlear nuclei. Tinnitus (ringing in the ear) is a common complaint. Sound amplification with an electrical hearing aid benefits patients with relatively good speech discrimination (a score greater than 60%). Profound bilateral sensorineural hearing loss in adults who are postlingually deaf may be treated with an implanted device, the cochlear implant. A cochlear implant provides sound awareness, enables identification of environmental sounds, and improves ability to communicate through auditory clues such as prosody, rhythm, and intensity. A cochlear implant has two components: an external component, consisting of a small microphone, speech processor, decoding unit, and coil; and an internal component, consisting of one or more electrodes implanted directly into the cochlea as well as a receiver.

Injury to the inner ear or acoustic trauma from a sudden very loud noise (ie, painful, greater than 140 dB) may produce a permanent sensorineural hearing loss. More importantly, prolonged exposure (8 hours or more) to intense nonpainful sound such as industrial noise above 90 dB will result in destruction of the outer hair cells of the organ of Corti and a sensorineural hearing loss that characteristically affects perception at 4000 Hz. These patients may also experience tinnitus. Further noise exposure should be prevented with ear protectors (earmuffs or earplugs) and a hearing conservation program initiated at work.

Additional causes of sudden sensorineural hearing loss include diabetes mellitus, cochlear artery insufficiency, aminoglycosides, ototoxic diuretics (eg, ethacrynic acid), tumors of the vestibular nerve (vestibular schwannoma) or cerebellopontine angle, perilymph fistulas, trauma, autoimmune inner ear disorders, congenital inner ear malformations, multiple sclerosis, and AIDS. Rubella in the first trimester of pregnancy, Rh incompatibility, birth trauma, hyperbilirubinemia, prematurity, congenital syphilis, meningitis, or congenital anomalies are often associated with defective hearing, and infants at risk should be tested immediately with brain stem evoked response audiometry. Unfortunately, over 90% of infants with congenital sensorineural hearing loss have no known risk factors. Hearing loss in these children is caused by a non-X-linked recessive mutation and is associated with no obvious physical abnormalities. If profound hearing loss antedates the acquisition of speech, oral communication is severely impaired. These children might be candidates for a cochlear implant.

In cases of sudden sensorineural hearing loss when no cause can be identified, viruses such as mumps, measles, influenza, and adenoviruses are the most likely cause. Laboratory testing, which is essential to determine the cause, may include a complete blood count, erythrocyte sedimentation rate, determination of rheumatoid arthritis factor and antinuclear antibody levels, quantitative serum immunoglobulin levels, FTA-ABS, fasting blood sugar, cholesterol, triglyceride, and thyroid function tests. In addition, MRI with gadolinium testing should be done. Prednisone (60 mg daily for 9 days and then tapering over 5 days) may be beneficial in preventing permanent hearing loss.

Brookhouser PE, Worthington DW, Kelly WJ: Severe versus profound sensori-neural hearing loss in children: Implications for cochlear implantation. Laryngoscope 1990;100:349.

Cohen NL, Hoffman RA: Complications of cochlear implant surgery in adults and children. Ann Otol Rhinol Laryngol 1991;100:708.

National Institutes of Health consensus development conference statement on cochlear implants. Arch Otolaryngol Head Neck Surg 1989;115:31.

Fenton K, Veton J, Balkany TJ: Status of cochlear implantation in children. J. Pediatr 1991;118:1.

Hughes GB, Sismanis A, House JW: Is there a consensus in perilymph fistula management? Otolaryngol Head Neck Surg 1990;102:111.

Roush J, Rauch SD: Clinical application of an implantable bone conduction hearing device. Laryngoscope 1990; 100:281.

Webb RL et al: Surgical complications with a cochlear multiple-channel intracochlear implant: Experience at Hannover and Melbourne. Ann Otol Rhinol Laryngol 1991;100:131.

Yoon TH et al: Histopathology of sudden hearing loss. Laryngoscope 1990;100:707.

OTALGIA

Ear pain may be caused by a primary disorder of the ear or may be referred from structures with a common sensory innervation. Inflammation of tissues innervated by the fifth cranial nerve—including the nose, paranasal sinuses, nasopharynx, mandible, and salivary glands—may produce otalgia. Inflammatory lesions of the oropharynx, the larynx, and the base of the tongue are commonly associated with otalgia. Unfortunately, however, neoplastic lesions do not produce otalgia until they are significantly advanced.

Inflammation of the external auditory canal (otitis externa) is commonly caused by bacteria (*Proteus mirabilis, Pseudomonas* sp, staphylococci), and occasionally by otomycoses *(Aspergillus niger, Candida albicans)*. Predisposing causes are water immersion, high humidity, instrumentation in the external auditory canal, and ceruminous impaction. Patients complain of otalgia, pruritus, otorrhea, and decreased hearing and intermittent blockage of the canal. Pain on traction of the pinna or tragus differentiates otitis externa from acute otitis media. Hyperemia, edema, and otorrhea are seen on inspection of the external auditory canal. Treatment consists of early precise debridement, topical broad-spectrum antibiotics (eg, polymyxin B, bacitracin, neomycin), and hydrocortisone to reduce canal wall inflammation. In neomycin-sensitive individuals, topical 2% aqueous acetic acid is effective. Contact with water should be avoided, and dry heat hastens resolution. Diabetics

are particularly at risk of developing *Pseudomonas* invasive otitis externa. If untreated, invasive otitis externa can progressively involve the underlying skin, cartilage, or bone, leading eventually to osteomyelitis of the skull, multiple cranial nerve palsies, and death. Patients with invasive otitis externa are treated with immediate debridement and an intravenous semisynthetic penicillin such as ticarcillin, mezlocillin, piperacillin, or azlocillin, and an aminoglycoside (tobramycin or amikacin) for 4–6 weeks. Monotherapy with ceftazidime has proved effective in some cases. Two quinolones—ciprofloxacin (available for intravenous use) and ofloxacin—administered orally are effective for invasive *Pseudomonas* otitis externa. Most clinicians would switch to oral antibiotics only when pain, drainage, and granulation tissue are substantially decreased. When gallium (which is picked up by granulocytes) scans become negative, antibiotics can be discontinued.

Inflammation that progresses to involve the auricular appendage may result in **perichondritis** and then **chondritis** with cartilaginous necrosis. Perichondritis or chondritis of the pinna may also follow auricular trauma and hematoma, frostbite or surgical drainage of a furuncle of the external auditory canal. It is manifested by edema, erythema, and tenderness of the pinna. Treatment consists of a systemic antistaphylococcal penicillin or, as an alternative, cephalothin or clindamycin and incision and drainage of any hematoma or abscess. Cotton soaked in an antiseptic solution (eg, povidone-iodine) is placed within the recesses of the auricle, and a mastoid dressing is applied. Failure to adequately drain an auricular hematoma or abscess will result in a "cauliflower ear" deformity secondary to cartilaginous destruction and fibrosis.

Chandler JR: Malignant external otitis and osteomyelitis of the base of the skull. Am J Otolaryngol 1989;10:108.

Kimmelman CP, Lucente FE: Use of ceftazidime for malignant external otitis. Ann Otol Rhinol Laryngol 1989;98:721.

Schuller DE, Dankle SD, Strauss RH: A technique to treat wrestler's auricular hematoma without interrupting training or competition. Arch Otol Head Neck Surg 1989;115:202.

Zikk D et al: Oral ofloxacin therapy for invasive external otitis. Ann Otolaryngol Rhinol Laryngol 1991;100:632.

Acute Otitis Media

Acute suppurative otitis media is a very common problem in pediatric and family practice, with otalgia the most common ear complaint in childhood. Twenty percent of children under 8 years of age experience at least one episode. The peak prevalence is between 6 and 11 months of age. Recurrence is common, especially if the initial episode occurs during the first 12 months of life. Viruses may produce otitis media, but suppuration is predominantly caused by bacteria, especially *Streptococcus pneumoniae, H in-*

fluenzae, anaerobes, and *M catarrhalis. S pyogenes* (group A) or *S aureus* is also seen. *H influenzae* (non-type B) infection occurs more commonly in the age group under 5 years. In the newborn, gram-negative infections with *Escherichia coli, Klebsiella pneumoniae, P aeruginosa,* and *P mirabilis* predominate.

The presenting clinical signs and symptoms are variable: In adults, otalgia and a conductive hearing loss are most common; infants may exhibit only fever, lethargy, or irritability. Commonly, the tympanic membrane is red, bulging, and extremely painful. Spontaneous perforation of the tympanic membrane with purulent otorrhea and hemorrhage is often present in infants when first seen by a physician. Prompt antibiotic therapy hastens resolution of the disease and prevents the development of temporal bone and intracranial complications. Topical vasoconstrictors such as phenylephrine should be instilled into the nasal cavities, and systemic vasoconstrictors, including ephedrine, pseudoephedrine, or phenylpropanolamine, may be prescribed to improve auditory tube function. In nonallergic patients over 6 weeks of age, amoxicillin is recommended, and erythromycin and sulfisoxazole may be used in penicillin-allergic individuals. Patients who fail to respond probably have an infection caused by β-lactamase-producing *H influenzae* type B and should be given trimethoprim-sulfamethoxazole, cefaclor, cefuroxime, or cefixime. In infants under 1 month of age, therapy must also be directed against gram-negative enteric organisms. In infants with impending otologic or intracranial complications such as meningitis, labyrinthitis, or lateral sinus thrombosis, ampicillin plus gentamicin or tobramycin (or amikacin) in areas where gentamicin resistance is encountered is recommended. In children over 4–6 weeks of age, *H influenzae* type B is the most common cause of meningitis. Because of this organism's high resistance to ampicillin and rare resistance to chloramphenicol, ceftazidime or ceftriaxone is recommended. Early administration of dexamethasone in children with meningitis in a dosage of 0.15 mg/kg four times a day for 4 days may lower the incidence of severe hearing loss. Myringotomy is indicated to relieve severe pain unresponsive to narcotics, or to identify antibiotic-resistant organisms. The development of sudden facial paralysis is an indication for emergency myringotomy. The incision should be made in the posteroinferior quadrant, midway between the umbo and the annulus. For children with recurrent acute otitis media, chemoprophylaxis is begun with amoxicillin, 20 mg/kg, or sulfisoxazole, 50 mg/kg, given once a day in seasons of frequent upper respiratory tract illnesses. Children who continue to have episodes of otitis media in spite of adequate chemoprophylaxis should undergo tympanostomy tube placement.

Alho OP et al: Is a child's history of acute otitis media and respiratory infection already determined in the antenatal and perinatal period? Int J Pediatr Otorhinolaryngol 1990;19:129.

Arola M, Ziegler T: Respiratory virus infection as a cause of prolonged symptoms in acute otitis media. J. Pediatr 1990;116:697.

MacRae DL, Ruby RRF: Recurrent meningitis secondary to perilymph fistula in young children. J Otolaryngol 1990;19:222.

Trujillo H et al: Bacteriology of middle ear fluid specimens obtained by tympanocentesis from 111 Columbian children with acute otitis media. Pediatr Infect Dis J 1989;8:361.

Acute Mastoiditis

Acute mastoiditis is a complication of acute otitis media and develops as a result of pus retention in the mastoid. It is most likely caused by *S pneumoniae,* with *S pyogenes* and *S aureus* also commonly seen. The destruction of bony septa results in a coalescence of mastoid air cells and subsequent erosion of the cortices of the mastoid process of the temporal bone. Otalgia, aural discharge, and fever are characteristically seen 2–3 weeks after an episode of acute suppurative otitis media, and examination reveals severe mastoid tenderness, lateral displacement of the pinna, or postauricular mastoid swelling secondary to subperiosteal abscess. Ceftriaxone with or without metronidazole is given, and if a subperiosteal abscess develops, the mastoid and its air cells must be surgically drained. Alternative antibiotic choices include imipenem or chloramphenicol plus vancomycin or nafcillin. A complete mastoidectomy though a postauricular incision includes exenteration of the infected bone and pus and inspection of the dura of the posterior and middle cranial fossa to exclude epidural abscess.

Farrior J: Complications of otitis media in children. S Med J 1990;83:645.

Rogers M et al: Emergency presentation of coalescent mastoiditis. Am J Emerg Med 1989;7:413.

Foreign Bodies in the Ear

Foreign bodies of the external auditory canal frequently traumatize the epithelium and may also perforate the tympanic membrane or disrupt the ossicular chain, producing a conductive hearing loss. Oval or round window injury may cause a concomitant sensorineural hearing loss. All kinds of objects are inserted into the external canal, especially by children. In addition, insects such as cockroaches may enter the canal, attaching their pincers to the tympanic membrane. Most foreign bodies can be removed with a right-angled hook or forceps if they are not lodged significantly medial to the isthmus of the external auditory canal. Gentle expulsion of nonvegetable matter with a soft rubber syringe—similar to the removal of cerumen—is effective. In young children or adults with firmly embedded objects, a general anesthetic is necessary to avoid injuring the tympanic membrane or ossicular chain. Insects may be suffocated by instilling mineral oil into the external auditory canal.

TINNITUS

Tinnitus is the subjective sensation of noise in the ear or head not of psychogenic origin. Tinnitus is extremely common, affecting an estimated 40 million Americans. Tinnitus is reported by patients as a constant or intermittent buzzing, ringing, or humming sound. Tinnitus is experienced by patients with presbycusis, noise-induced hearing loss, ceruminous impaction, and otitis media (acute and chronic). Exposure to ototoxic drugs, endolymphatic hydrops (Meniere's disease), and vestibular schwannoma (acoustic neuroma) are other causes. Highly vascular lesions of the temporal bone may elicit pulsatile tinnitus; examples are glomus jugulare or tympanicum tumors (non-chromaffin-producing neoplasms of paraganglionic cell origin). Aneurysms or arteriovenous malformations are rare causes of true tinnitus. Comprehensive management includes assessment of hypertension, blood lipids, thyroid function, and allergy and informing patients of factors that aggravate tinnitus, including stress, caffeine, nicotine, and aspirin. Treatment is determined by the primary disease, but since most cases are caused by presbycusis, effective therapy is often unavailable. Attempts at symptomatic relief have included diuretics, antihistamines (eg, dexchlorpheniramine maleate), anticonvulsants (eg, clonazepam), tranquilizers (eg, alprazolam), and antidepressants (eg, nortriptyline). Masking of tinnitus with frequency-specific hearing aids or extraneous noise such as a radio or stereo—especially before sleep—may be helpful in motivated patients. Biofeedback therapy has been used successfully in anxious patients. Recent success has been reported with an electrical radiofrequency transmitter transmitting audiofrequencies across the skin. Other modalities, including acupuncture, psychotherapy, and hypnotherapy, have given inconsistent results and are not recommended.

Axelsson A, Ringdal A: Tinnitus: A study of its prevalence and characteristics. Br J Audiol 1989;23:53.
Neher A: Tinnitus: The hidden epidemic. Ann Otolaryngol Rhinol Laryngol 1991;100:327.
Shulman A: Electrodiagnostics, electrotherapeutics and other approaches to the management of tinnitus. *AAO–HNS Instructional Courses,* vol 2. Mosby, 1989.

TEMPORAL BONE FRACTURES

Fractures of the skull base from blunt trauma commonly involve the temporal bone. Hemorrhagic otorrhea, ecchymosis of the postauricular area (Battle's sign), and disturbances in cochlear or vestibular function may be encountered. Eighty percent of fractures of the temporal bone are longitudinal to the petrous ridge; the remainder are transverse or perpendicular. Longitudinal fractures are chiefly secondary to parietal blows with the fracture line extending across the floor of the middle cranial fossa and through the roof of the external auditory canal, rupturing the tympanic membrane. The incudostapedial joint is frequently disrupted and requires tympanoplastic reconstruction. The labyrinth is often spared, and only 35% of patients develop a sensorineural hearing loss. Twenty percent of patients develop delayed seventh nerve paralysis caused by ischemia and compression rather than neural disruption.

Transverse fractures, on the other hand, are caused by a blow to the occiput and are associated with a higher death rate. The fracture may involve the foramen magnum, pass through or near the jugular foramen, and cross the internal auditory canal to reach the foramen lacerum or spinosum. Often the fracture line will splinter to reach the medial wall of the inner ear. The tympanic membrane remains intact, with a blue-black hemotympanum, and cerebrospinal fluid rhinorrhea is not uncommon. In 38–50% of cases, the seventh nerve is lacerated, resulting in immediate facial paralysis. In addition, disruption of the membranous labyrinth leads to complete loss of cochlear-vestibular function and subsequent sensorineural hearing loss and vertigo.

If there is a cerebrospinal fluid leak, it is treated with head elevation, fluid restriction, and diuretics. In 85% of cases, the leak stops by 7 days, and no repair is necessary. If the leak continues beyond several weeks, surgical repair is necessary. The development of progressive facial paralysis and loss of electrical stimulability of the facial nerve requires immediate neuronal decompression of the facial (fallopian) canal. If the nerve has been anatomically disrupted, debridement and end-to-end anastomosis or nerve grafting will be necessary.

NEOPLASMS OF THE EXTERNAL & MIDDLE EAR

Squamous and **basal cell carcinomas** are the most common tumors of the pinna, occurring in sun-exposed individuals. Small lesions may be removed by V-wedge excision or radiation therapy. Tumors invading the cartilage require wide surgical excision. Squamous cell or basal cell carcinomas arising in the external auditory canal require wide excision for the best chance of cure. High-resolution CT is critical for defining surgical limits. En bloc resection of the external auditory canal is possible for lesions not involving the middle ear or mastoid, whereas more invasive tumors require parotidectomy, temporal bone resection, and, for tumors extending beyond the temporal bone, skull base surgery. Radiation therapy is reserved for neoplasms that cannot be resected and is used in combination with surgery for more advanced lesions. Squamous cell carcinomas arising in the middle ear should be treated by resection of the temporal bone if feasible or radiotherapy if they cannot be excised.

Glomus jugulare and **glomus tympanicum** tumors are vascular neoplasms that usually arise from the jugular bulb and tympanic plexus, respectively. Both tumors spread cephalically and posteriorly into the middle ear and mastoid. Both are non-chromaffin-producing paragangliomas and are histologically the same as carotid body tumors, the most common chemodectomas of the neck. In addition, a **glomus vagale** neoplasm arising in the skull base and neck may extend superiorly into the cranial vault. The natural history of these tumors is one of slow, progressive growth and gradual invasion of the jugular foramen and its nerves (cranial nerves IX, X, XI) as well as cranial nerves VII, XII, and VIII. The overall incidence of central nervous system invasion is less than 20%.

The principal manifestation of a tumor of the middle ear is conductive hearing loss, and pulsatile tinnitus is often present if the tumor is highly vascular. Brown's sign may be present (pulsation of the tympanic membrane that is inhibited by positive pressure applied to the tympanic membrane by a pneumatic otoscope). Thin-section, high-resolution CT scanning in combination with gadolinium-enhanced MRI is used to delineate the extent of tumor. Angiography is used for preoperative assessment of tumors requiring embolization. The treatment of choice is lateral cranial base surgical removal if the lesion does not involve the carotid siphon and has not spread by distant metastases. Small glomus tympanicum tumors may be cured by total surgical removal. When intracranial extension is present, a neurosurgical approach is required 2 weeks before the otologist's second-stage procedure. Radiotherapy causes tumor shrinkage but not eradication and is best combined with surgical excision of the tumor.

Bundgaard T et al: Treatment of glomus tumors: A retrospective survey. Clin Otolaryngol 1989;14:155.

Jackson CG et al: Conservation surgery for glomus jugulare tumors: The value of early diagnosis. Laryngoscope 1990;100:1031.

Korzeniowski S, Pszon J: The results of radiotherapy in cancer of the middle ear. Int J Radiol Oncol Biol Phys 1990;18:63.

Phelps PD, Cheeseman AD: Imaging jugulotympanic glomus tumors. Arch Otolaryngol Head Neck Surg 1990;116:940.

Shih L, Crabtree JA: Carcinoma of the external auditory canal: An update. Laryngoscope 1990;100:1215.

Spector JG: Management of temporal bone carcinomas: A therapeutic analysis of two groups of patients in long term follow up. Otolaryngol Laryngol Head Neck Surg 1991;104:58.

CONGENITAL DEFORMITIES OF THE EAR

Lop ear, the most common congenital deformity of the auricle, is the result of failure of development of the antihelical fold or excessive protrusion of the conchal cartilage. Treatment consists of otoplasty, which is the surgical creation of an antihelical fold or reduction of conchal cartilage projection, or both. Treatment before 5 or 6 years of age, when the auricle is three-fourths adult size, avoids ridicule of the child by peers.

Preauricular cysts and sinus tracts are common unilateral or bilateral congenital defects found anterior to the upper helix or tragus. They develop following incomplete fusion of the auricular hillocks. Many subsequently become infected, requiring complete excision, which may be hazardous because of ramification of the sinus tracts near facial nerve branches. More severe congenital deformities of the auricle are less common. Microtia, with stenosis of the external auditory canal, and complete atresia of the auricle and external auditory canal are unusual, occurring in about one in 20,000 births. Deformities frequently associated with developmental anomalies of the middle ear produce profound conductive hearing loss. Initial treatment requires first establishing the presence of adequate hearing in the opposite ear. If hearing in the opposite ear is normal, surgical repair is not recommended, because the potential risk to the seventh nerve, which takes an anomalous course through the temporal bone, is too great. If there is profound conductive hearing loss on both sides, however, surgical reconstruction of the middle ear is indicated if feasible; if not, bilateral bone conduction hearing aids should be used. Auricular reconstruction for severe microtia or complete atresia is a challenging cosmetic surgical problem, often requiring soft tissue flaps and autogenous cartilaginous grafts, and should be done prior to middle ear reconstruction.

Schuknecht HF: Congenital aural atresia. Laryngoscope 1989;99:908.

VESTIBULAR SYSTEM

The vestibular system serves to maintain balance, posture, and spatial orientation in concert with vision and peripheral proprioception. Loss of two of these three sensory modalities is severely incapacitating.

The vestibular end organs are dynamic structures that respond to linear acceleration (saccule and utricle) and to angular acceleration (semicircular canals). Angular acceleration of the head displaces endolymph and deflects hair cell cupulae in the cristae. Hair cell deflection results in either an increase or decrease in neuronal impulses to the vestibular nuclei. Because the six semicircular canals are arranged in three pairs with one member of a pair (right) lying in a plane parallel to the plane of the other member (left), differences in acceleration between the right and left side of the body are monitored in the vestibular nuclei. Normally, when a person is resting or moving at a constant rate, sensory input from the paired horizontal semicircular canals and two pairs of posterior and superior semicircular canals is balanced. Angular acceleration with subsequent hair cell deflection results in unilateral increased vestibular output and increased muscle tone in the extraocular and skeletal muscles, maintaining balance, posture, and spatial orientation. Failure of the vestibular apparatus to sustain the organism's balance produces vertigo, nystagmus, falling, and past pointing. Sudden unilateral diminution of function in the vestibular system, in Meniere's disease, perilymph fistula, acute labyrinthitis, or temporal bone fracture, causes an imbalance of neuronal information arriving in the temporal lobe cortex. The cortical interpretation is constant motion or vertigo aggravated by head movement. Similarly, neuronal imbalance arriving at the extraocular motor nuclei and reticular formation produces rapid nystagmus, nausea and vomiting, and parasympathetic discharge. In response to overwhelming vestibular disequilibrium, the cerebellum inhibits vestibular nuclei, but only incompletely. Ultimately, restoration of balance will require (1) functional repair of the diseased end organ, requiring hours or days; (2) central nervous system suppression of the normally functioning side requiring months; or (3) generation of new neuronal output in the hypofunctioning labyrinth.

CLINICAL ASSESSMENT OF THE DIZZY PATIENT

Nowhere in medicine and surgery is a carefully taken history more important than in evaluating patients with dizziness. Nonvertiginous or extravestibular dizziness is far more common than otogenic or true vertiginous imbalance. The sensation of lightheadedness or syncope points to a different cause than the perception of the room spinning around. The clinical evaluation of the vestibular system includes examination of cerebellar function (gait, Romberg, two-step Fukuda, finger-to-nose, dysdiadochokinesis, and dysmetria testing) and the cranial nerves and observation of spontaneous or positional nystagmus. Because visual fixation with the eyes open may suppress nystagmus, it is important to record eye movements with electronystagmography. This is a technique for recording changes in the corneoretinal potential with skin electrodes and an electronic apparatus. Spontaneous, positional, and positioning nystagmus may be recorded to determine whether the vertigo is peripheral or central in origin.

Additional information is obtained with the Hallpike caloric stimulation test. Caloric stimulation of the labyrinth via the tympanic membrane induces convection currents within the horizontal semicircular canal, producing cupular deflection in one direction with 30 °C water and in the opposite direction with 44 °C water. With the patient supine and the head elevated 30 degrees, irrigation of the external auditory canal with cold water (30 °C) produces the rapid component of nystagmus to the opposite side; warm water (44 °C) produces nystagmus to the same side. The mnemonic device is COWS (cold to the opposite and warm to the same). Decreased vestibular response to caloric stimulation (canal paresis) indicates a vestibular end organ, vestibular nerve, or brain stem lesion.

Brookler KH: Electronystagmography, 1990. Neurol Clin 1990;8:235.

Brookler KH: Benign paroxysmal positional vertigo. Am J Otolaryngol 1990;11:233.

Brookler KH, Rubin W: The dizzy patient: Etiologic treatment. Otolaryngol Head Neck Surg 1990;103:693.

Brown J: A systematic approach to the dizzy patient. Neurol Clin North Am 1990;8:209.

MENIERE'S DISEASE

Meniere's disease, or endolymphatic hydrops, is characterized by a tetrad of symptoms of unknown cause: episodic vertigo, fluctuating sensorineural hearing loss, aural fullness, and tinnitus. The tinnitus is usually low-pitched and roaring. The hearing loss is more severe in the lower frequencies, frequently progresses over many years, and remains confined to one ear in most patients. The attacks are associated with nausea, vomiting, and prostration. Pathologically, there is generalized dilatation of the membranous labyrinth that includes the scala media and endolymphatic sac and is associated with occasional membrane breaks and intermingling of endolymph and perilymph. Circulating immune complexes may be involved in the pathogenesis of Meniere's disease.

Patients with severe hydrops should be treated with diuretics, salt restriction, a low-caffeine diet, and labyrinthine sedatives such as diazepam, 5 mg three times daily, to prevent recurrent attacks. Antihistamines such as meclizine, dimenhydrinate, and cyclizine are used to reduce the severity of vertigo. Associated vertigo, nausea, and emesis are controlled without antiemetics by combining the synergistic effects of a cholinergic antagonist (scopolamine) and an adrenergic agonist (dextroamphetamine).

Surgical treatment is currently reserved for patients with severe incapacitating vertigo or tinnitus or to prevent further deterioration of hearing. In patients with useful hearing, decompression of the endolymphatic sac and insertion of a shunt between the membranous labyrinth and subarachnoid space improves symptoms in over half of cases. Vestibular neurectomy through either a middle cranial fossa or retrolabyrinthine approach may conserve hearing. With severe loss of hearing and speech discrimination, a total transmastoid labyrinthectomy is used, which relieves vertigo in over 80% of patients. In patients with bilateral Meniere's disease who are incapacitated with vertigo, hearing can be preserved and a chemical labyrinthectomy accomplished with daily intramuscular streptomycin titrated gradually over 1 week to avoid oscillopsia.

Amedee RG, Norris CH, Risey JA: Selective chemical vestibulectomy: Preliminary results with human application. Otolaryngol Head Neck Surg 1991;105:107.

Hebbar GG, Rask-Andersen H, Linthicum FH: Three-dimensional analysis of 61 human endolymphatic ducts and sacs in ears with and without Meniere's disease. Ann Otol Rhinol Laryngol 1991;100:219.

Kemink JL: Transmastoid labyrinthectomy: Reliable surgical management of vertigo. Otolaryngol Head Neck Surg 1989;101:5.

Khetarpal U, Schuknecht HF: Temporal bone findings in a case of bilateral Meniere's disease treated by parental streptomycin and endolymphatic shunt. Laryngoscope 1990;100:407.

Schuknecht HF, Suzuka Y, Zimmermann C: Delayed endolymphatic hydrops and its relationship to Meniere's disease. Ann Otol Rhinol Laryngol 1990;99:843.

Shea JJ: Perfusion of the inner ear with streptomycin. Am J Otolaryngol 1989;10:150.

ACOUSTIC NEUROMA

Acoustic neuromas account for about 8% of intracranial tumors and arise twice as often from the vestibular division of the eighth nerve as from the auditory division. They develop in one per 100,000 individuals yearly. Growth varies according to the patient's age. Although acoustic neuromas account for about 80% of all cerebellopontine angle neoplasms, other lesions in the cerebellopontine angle may produce a nearly identical clinical picture. These include meningiomas, primary cholesteatomas, metastatic tumors, and aneurysms. Acoustic neuromas, which are derived from Schwann cells, initially produce a high-frequency sensorineural hearing loss. Tinnitus is less common, and true vertigo is unusual. However, unsteadiness or balance disorders may develop as the tumor enlarges. Hallpike caloric testing commonly reveals canal paresis on the affected side. The acoustic reflex is frequently absent, and CT scan of the brain will reveal a contrast-enhanced lesion at the porus acusticus. Gadolinium-enhanced MRI is superior to CT in evaluation of suspected acoustic neuroma. If the MRI is negative and a small intracanalicular tumor is suspected, air-contrast CT should be performed.

Management of acoustic neuromas depends on the tumor's size and growth rate, the patient's age, and the state and prognosis of bilateral hearing. For patients under 65, small intracanalicular tumors (within the internal auditory canal) may be surgically removed through the transmastoid labyrinthine route if no useful hearing remains; a middle cranial fossa approach is utilized to preserve serviceable hearing. Both routes maintain the integrity of the facial nerve. Larger tumors (> 3 cm) are removed via a suboccipital craniotomy; huge ones can only be removed via a combined suboccipital and translabyrinthine approach if the facial nerve is to be preserved. For patients over age 65 with slowly growing tumors, surgical removal may not be required.

Baldwin DL et al: Hearing conservation in acoustic neuroma surgery via the posterior fossa. J Laryngol Otol 1990;104:463.

Kemink JL et al: Operative management of acoustic neuromas: The priority of neurological function over complete resection. Otolaryngol Head Neck Surg 1991;104:96.

Millen SJ, Daniels DL, Meyer GA: Gadolinium-enhanced magnetic resonance imaging of temporal bone lesions. Laryngoscope 1989;99:257.

Shelton C et al: Middle fossa acoustic tumor surgery: Results in 106 cases. Laryngoscope 1989;99:405.

LABYRINTHITIS

Acute suppurative labyrinthitis may develop as a complication of acute otitis media or meningitis. The microorganisms responsible for acute otitis media gain access to the inner ear via the oval and round windows, and microorganisms in the meninges enter through the cochlear aqueduct. The clinical manifestations are severe vertigo and a sudden profound sensorineural hearing loss, frequently followed by facial paralysis. Immediate surgical management with labyrinthectomy and radical mastoidectomy is necessary to prevent meningitis. In addition, certain viruses, including mumps, measles, influenza, and adenoviruses, that invade the inner ear may cause endolymphatic labyrinthitis and sudden profound sensorineural hearing loss. In the prenatal period, rubella, virus may attack the developing otic capsule and produce a severe congenital sensorineural hearing loss.

GERIATRIC DYSEQUILIBRIUM

There are many vestibular disorders in the elderly, including vascular disease with ischemia (vertebral basilar insufficiency) or infarction, endolymphatic hydrops, and benign paroxysmal positional vertigo. In addition, degenerative changes and loss of statoconia, vestibular epithelium, vestibular nerves, Scarpa's ganglion, and cerebellum occur with aging. The resulting dizziness and falls that are common among persons over age 65 are usually caused by central discoordination, but positional vertigo not uncommonly plays a central role. The disorder is characterized by episodic vertigo precipitated by a sudden change in position, such as turning to the side or rolling over in bed. The morbidity and mortality associated with falls in the elderly are substantial and increase with age.

Bloom J, Katsarkas A.: Paroxysmal positional vertigo in the elderly. J Otolaryngol 1989;18:96.

Grad A, Baloh RW: Vertigo of vascular origin: Clinical and electronystagmographic features in 84 cases. Arch Neurol 1989;46:281.

Jenkins JA et al: Dysequilibrium of aging. Otolaryngol Head Neck Surg 1989;100:272.

Nadol JB Jr, Schuknecht HF: Pathology of peripheral vestibular disorders in the elderly. Am J Otolaryngol 1990;11:213.

FACIAL NERVE

FACIAL PARALYSIS

Paralysis of the seventh nerve immobilizes the muscles of facial expression: The eye fails to close, the forehead does not wrinkle (as opposed to central or supranuclear facial paralysis with forehead sparing), and the angle of the mouth droops, so the patient drools. Peripheral seventh nerve paralysis suggests serious disease, such as tumor of the cerebellopontine angle, acoustic neuroma, facial nerve neuroma, neoplasm of the middle ear, or parotid gland neoplasm. Acute otitis media, temporal bone fracture, and chronic otitis media with or without cholesteatoma may produce facial paralysis. Other causes include surgical trauma, Guillain-Barré syndrome, Lyme disease, AIDS, and herpes zoster oticus (Ramsay Hunt's syndrome). When the cause is unknown, the condition is known as Bell's palsy. Although Bell's palsy is the commonest cause of peripheral seventh nerve paralysis, the pathogenesis is mysterious. Current theories implicate vascular ischemia and compressive edema within the facial canal as the cause of neurapraxia and cessation of axoplasmic flow. There is evidence that Bell's palsy is part of a viral cranial polyneuropathy which usually resolves in 6–12 weeks.

All patients with facial paralysis should have a thorough history and physical examination. In addition, CT scan of the temporal bones and gadolinium-enhanced MRI should be obtained. The latter frequently demonstrates gadolinium enhancement in Bell's palsy, herpes zoster oticus, facial neuromas, and vestibular schwannomas. The following special diagnostic tests should be performed: pure tone audiometry, speech reception thresholds, and speech discrimination; glucose tolerance test to rule out diabetes mellitus; and site-of-lesion testing. Site-of-lesion testing includes the Schirmer test of lacrimation (absent lacrimation indicates a lesion proximal to the geniculate ganglion), and stapedius muscle reflex testing utilizing impedance audiometry (an intact stapedius reflex indicates a lesion distal to the horizontal portion of the facial nerve). Finally, nerve excitability testing over the peripheral branches and main trunk of the seventh nerve is often used to predict the success of surgical intervention. If neuronal function is completely lost, nerve excitability testing fails to elicit a motor twitch in the corresponding facial muscle at the same threshold as the uninvolved side. Ordinarily, this phenomenon is observed 72 hours after the initial injury. Progressive deterioration in nerve response carries a poor prognosis and necessitates surgical decompression of the nerve to the level of the lesion (ie, above or below the geniculate ganglion, the latter requiring a transmastoid approach and the former a middle cranial fossa approach combined with the transmastoid route).

The initial medical management of Bell's palsy is controversial. Approximately 70% of patients recover completely, but the prognosis for complete recovery falls to 10% in the presence of dry eye. Early treatment with corticosteroids (eg, 60–80 mg of prednisone daily with gradual tapering over 7–10 days) is felt by some experts to hasten resolution of edema and improve the outcome (ie, prevent permanent paralysis or synkinesis). In patients with herpes zoster oticus, acyclovir may prove useful. Nonpregnant adults with facial paralysis secondary to Lyme disease are best treated with tetracycline. Phenoxymethyl penicillin, benzathine penicillin G, erythromycin, ceftriaxone, or cefuroxime may be used as substitutes.

Rehabilitation of the paralyzed face exhibiting no recovery is a challenging problem. Unilateral facial paralysis is unlikely to recover if a year has passed since the injury and no voluntary motion is noted. Nerve crossover procedures using a hypoglossal to seventh nerve anastomosis are recommended for restoring resting facial tone. For traumatic lesions, immediate neural repair or interposition grafting of the damaged segment with a greater auricular or sural nerve graft may be efficacious. Occasionally, decompression of the facial nerve combined with rerouting through the temporal bone is sufficient. Finally, neuromuscular transfer techniques utilizing either temporalis or masseter muscle pedicles are effective for facial reanimation in selected cases.

Grundfast KM et al: Diverse etiologies of facial paralysis in children. Int J Pediatr Otorhinolaryngol 1990;19:223.

Harrison DH: Current trends in the treatment of established unilateral facial palsy. Ann R Coll Surg Engl 1990; 72:94.

May M, Sobol SM, Mester SJ: Hypoglossal facial nerve interpositional jump graft for facial reanimation without tongue atrophy. Otolaryngol Head Neck Surg 1991;104: 818.

Schwaber MK et al: Gadolinium enhanced magnetic resonance imaging in Bell's palsy. Laryngoscope 1990;100: 1264.

Smith IM et al: Facial weakness: A comparison of clinical and photographic methods of observation. Arch Otolaryngol Head Neck Surg 1991;117:906.

Ylikoski J: Pathological features of the facial nerve in patients with facial palsy of varying etiology: Light and electronmicroscopic study. J Laryngol Otol 1990;104: 294.

NOSE & PARANASAL SINUSES

NASAL FOREIGN BODIES

Nasal foreign bodies are common in children, who frequently place pebbles, beads, seeds, buttons, or paper into the nares. A severe inflammatory reaction ensues, especially with organic matter, and this is associated with a foul-smelling unilateral nasal discharge. Chronic foreign bodies may encrust with calcium and magnesium to form rhinoliths. Removal of a foreign body requires topical vasoconstrictors such as phenylephrine and topical anesthesia with lidocaine or cocaine. General anesthesia may be needed in uncooperative children.

NASAL VESTIBULITIS

Inflammation of the nasal vestibule may assume two forms: a localized acute furunculitis or a chronic diffuse dermatitis. Acute staphylococcal furunculitis of the pilosebaceous follicles in the vestibule may develop into a spreading cellulitis of the tip of the nose. Treatment includes hot soaks and systemic penicillinase-resistant penicillin. Incision and drainage of a localized abscess is rarely necessary, since the majority of cases will drain spontaneously. Diffuse nasal vestibulitis is treated with antibiotic ointment containing polymyxin B, bacitracin, and neomycin. Early treatment of all acute infections of the nose, paranasal sinuses, and face is important to prevent the occurrence of retrograde thrombophlebitis and cavernous sinus thrombosis.

ACUTE RHINITIS

Acute rhinitis (coryza, common cold) is often secondary to infection with respiratory viruses, including rhinoviruses, coronaviruses, and papillomaviruses. It is associated with sneezing, watery rhinorrhea, tearing, malaise, and headache. Examination of the nasal mucous membrane reveals hyperemia, edema, and watery mucosal discharge. Later, the secretions may become thick and yellow-green in color. Tenderness to palpation over the paranasal sinuses may be found. Nonnarcotic analgesics such as aspirin, decongestants, and antihistamines as well as fluids and rest will alleviate symptoms. Topical vasoconstrictors such as oxymetazoline and phenylephrine provide symptomatic relief. Antibiotic therapy is not necessary unless secondary bacterial invasion occurs. The condition usually resolves within 5–10 days. Ultimately, antiviral therapy may be needed for control of the common cold.

Akerlund A et al: Nasal decongestant effect of oxymetazoline in the common cold: An objective dose response study in 106 patients. J Laryngol Otol 1989;103:743.

Jackson RT: Mechanisms of action of some commonly used nasal drugs. Otolaryngol Head Neck Surg 1991;104:433.

ALLERGIC RHINITIS

Antigens inhaled and deposited on the mucous membrane of the nasal cavities of hypersensitive individuals elicit an IgE-mediated rhinitis. This perennial or seasonal disorder is often associated with additional respiratory allergies such as asthma, chronic laryngitis, or tracheobronchitis. Allergens such as animal danders, molds, dust, and pollens are commonly implicated, and sensitivity to them may be confirmed by skin testing or radioallergosorbent testing (RAST). Allergic rhinitis is characterized by sneezing, watery rhinorrhea, tearing, dysosmia, and nasal obstruction. The mucous membrane appears edematous and pale, with a thin discharge. Individuals with chronic allergic rhinitis commonly develop nasal polyps and acute or chronic sinusitis. Polyps may arise from the middle meatal region at the sinus ostia and appear as pale gray, glistening edematous masses within the nasal cavity. Occasionally, a large antrochoanal polyp arises from the maxillary sinus ostia in conjunction with chronic maxillary sinusitis and presents as a long pedunculated mass in the nasopharynx. Treatment requires removal of the polyp and drainage of the maxillary sinus.

Treatment is started with an antihistamine (Table 39–4). Topical steroids in the form of beclometha-

Table 39–4. Oral antihistamines for allergic rhinitis.

Drug	Usual Adult Dose
Alkylamines	
Brompheniramine maleate	4 mg every 4–6 hours
Chlorpheniramine maleate	4 mg every 4–6 hours
Dexchlorpheniramine maleate	2 mg every 4–6 hours
Triprolidine hydrochloride	2.5 mg every 4–6 hours
Ethanolamines	
Carbinoxamine maleate	4–8 mg every 4–6 hours
Clemastine fumarate	1.34–2.68 mg every 12 hours
Diphenhydramine hydrochloride	20–50 mg every 4–6 hours
Ethylenediamines	
Pyrilamine maleate	25–50 mg every 6–8 hours
Tripelennamine hydrochloride	25–50 mg every 4–6 hours
Phenothiazines	
Promethazine	12.5 mg every 12 hours or 25 mg at bedtime
Others	
Azatidine maleate	1–2 mg every 12 hours
Cyproheptadine hydrochloride	4 mg every 6–8 hours
Phenindamine tartrate	25 mg every 4–6 hours
Terfendadine	60 mg every 12 hours

sone dipropionate, triamcinolone acetonide, or flunisolide or the use of topical cromolyn sodium delivered intranasally is effective in reducing or eliminating symptoms in some patients. These nasal sprays are given in concert with saline nasal rinses. Rarely, oral glucocorticoids or intramuscular steroids are employed. Desensitization immunotherapy with stimulation by IgG-blocking antibodies is reserved for patients who fail these simpler measures. Finally, surgical removal of nasal polyps associated with allergic rhinitis combined with surgical drainage of obstructed maxillary and ethmoid sinuses is performed for severe nasal obstruction and chronic sinusitis unresponsive to medical therapy.

Howarth PH: Allergic rhinitis: A rational choice of treatment. Respir Med 1989;83:179.

Naclerio RM: Allergic rhinitis. N Engl J Med 1991;325:860.

Nuutinen J et al: Terfenadine with or without phenylpropanolamine in the treatment of seasonal allergic rhinitis. Clin Exp Allergy 1989;19:603.

Perkins JA, Blakeslee DB, Andrade P: Nasal polyps: A manifestation of allergy. Otolaryngol Head Neck Surg 1989;101:641.

Skoner DP et al: Nasal physiology and inflammatory mediators during natural pollen exposure. Ann Allergy 1990;65:206.

RHINITIS MEDICAMENTOSA

Misuse or abuse of intranasal vasoconstrictors (eg, phenylephrine, cocaine) may lead to mucosal edema, hyperemia, and watery rhinorrhea. The resulting nasal obstruction is severe, prompting the individual to increase the use of topical decongestants and thus perpetuate the cycle. Successful treatment requires complete cessation of intranasal medications for 2–3 weeks, and an oral decongestant such as pseudoephedrine must be used. A short course of systemic corticosteroid therapy or the gradual substitution of topical steroids for topical decongestant therapy seems to assist the withdrawal process. Unfortunately, a new complex of nasal septal perforation, palatal retraction, pharyngeal wall ulceration, and nasal collapse secondary to cocaine abuse that mimics midline granuloma does not respond to this management. Invariably, these lesions are colonized with *S aureus* and require intravenous antistaphylococcal penicillin and, in rare cases, external beam radiation therapy.

Becker GD, Hill S: Midline granulomas due to illicit cocaine use. Arch Otolaryngol Head Neck Surg 1988;114:90.

Dutsh HL, Millard DR: A new cocaine abuse complex. Arch Otolaryngol Head Neck Surg 1989;115:235.

VASOMOTOR RHINITIS

Vasomotor rhinitis results from hyperreactivity of parasympathetic control of the nasal vasculature and glands. The vasomotor reaction is characterized by vascular engorgement, mediated by the release of acetylcholine (a powerful vasodilator) at parasympathetic nerve endings. This commonly occurs in response to changes in external temperature and humidity and is not caused by allergens. Exposure to inhalant irritants such as tobacco smoke and industrial pollutants may provoke parasympathetic activity. There is often a history of trauma. The patient complains of nasal obstruction, sneezing, and watery rhinorrhea. Systemic decongestants such as pseudoephedrine and phenylpropanolamine give some relief. Antihistamines help combat the problem through their anticholinergic action. Corticosteroid nasal spray is occasionally effective, while the use of intranasal cromolyn sodium may benefit the patient by preventing the release of mediators from mast cells. Septoplasty to correct traumatic nasal septal obstruction with or without bilateral partial inferior turbinectomy is successful in relieving nasal airway obstruction.

PARANASAL SINUSITIS

Inflammation of the paranasal sinuses is commonly precipitated by an acute upper respiratory tract infection of viral origin. Edema of the nasal mucosa produces obstruction of the sinus ostia, resulting in secondary bacterial invasion and localized pain, tenderness, and headache exacerbated by changes in position and barometric pressure. Other symptoms that commonly occur are auditory tube dysfunction with otalgia, rhinorrhea, nasal congestion, postnasal discharge, and sometimes anosmia in adults. Microorganisms responsible for acute sinusitis are most often *S pneumoniae, M catarrhalis,* and *H.* Because β-lactamase production is common among strains of *Haemophilus influenzae* and particularly *Moraxella catarrhalis,* therapy with amoxicillin with clavulanic acid, cefuroxime, doxycycline, clarithromycin, or trimethoprim-sulfamethoxazole is preferred initial management of acute sinusitis. In persons allergic to penicillin, erythromycin plus a sulfonamide is recommended. Therapy also includes oral decongestants, antihistamines for patients who have a substantial component of allergic rhinitis, immunotherapy with IgE desensitization, and corticosteroids in the form of topical nasal sprays, systemic agents, or both.

Endoscopic sinus surgery is indicated for patients with persistent facial pain, headache, or nasal congestion and those who fail to respond to aggressive medical management. CT scans should be obtained in the axial and coronal planes to evaluate the persistence of chronic sinusitis and the presence of sinus abnormalities such as nasal septal deformity, pneumatization of the middle turbinates (concha bullosa), inferior turbinate hypertrophy, or substantial obstruction of the osteomeatal complex. Because the flow of mucus in the sinuses is toward the natural osteum, relief of obstruction of the osteomeatal complex (hiatus semilunaris and ethmoid infundibulum) is indicated to restore drainage from the sinuses and prevent persistent symptoms. Reestablishment of ethmoid and maxillary sinus ventilation and elimination of foci of ethmoid disease are necessary for success. The introduction of the nasal endoscope combined with articulating video cameras and video imaging allows removal of just enough mucosa to restore drainage. The commonest site of infection in chronic sinusitis is the anterior ethmoid air cells. Endoscopic sinus surgery is most effective in controlling localized disease, recurrent acute sinusitis, and sinusitis secondary to anatomic obstruction, particularly in patients with no previous sinus surgery or in those who have a maxillary sinus mycetoma. The prognosis is unfavorable in patients with immunodeficiencies, immotile cilia syndrome, severe allergy, triad asthma with nasal polyposis and aspirin sensitivity, multiple prior operations, diffuse severe polypoid disease, or polyposis with diffuse extramucosal fungal infection.

Patients undergoing successful endoscopic sinus surgery show the greatest improvement with respect to resolution of facial pain. Frequently, simultaneous septoplasty and partial inferior turbinectomies is necessary for adequate exposure and endoscopic drainage of the sinuses. Patients with opacification of the sphenoid sinus have a poorer outcome, whereas those who have no purulent drainage or reformation of polypoid mucosa postoperatively have a dramatic resolution of facial pain, nasal obstruction, postnasal discharge, rhinorrhea, and improvement in their history of recurrent asthma. If maxillary sinus disease remains after this approach, a Caldwell-Luc procedure through an incision in the gingival labial sulcus may be necessary. For patients who have persistent ethmoid disease, external ethmoidectomy is indicated via a Lynch incision midway between the dorsum of the nose and the medial canthal ligament of the eye.

Complications of acute sinusitis are rare in infancy and childhood. Acute maxillary sinusitis and, more commonly, ethmoiditis may be complicated by orbital cellulitis and abscess formation. The progressive development of chemosis, scleral erythema, proptosis, and ophthalmoplegia points to orbital infection and potential intracranial invasion. A CT scan with contrast enhancement will detect an orbital abscess and eliminate other causes of unilateral proptosis. Treatment consists of intravenous ceftriaxone or vancomycin plus aztreonam or chloramphenicol. In patients developing an orbital abscess, drainage through a Lynch incision must be performed early to avoid serious intracranial complications such as meningitis, epidural abscess, subdural abscess, cerebral abscess, and cavernous sinus thrombosis. Several factors in pediatric sinusitis are critical: (1) Chronic purulent rhinosinusitis in children has an immunologic or anatomic origin; (2) children under age 7 with nasal polyposis and chronic sinusitis must be considered to have cystic fibrosis until proved otherwise; (3) sinusitis exacerbates asthma; (4) atopic children are more likely to develop sinusitis; and (5) allergy must be suspected in the 3- to 5-year age group, particularly when the symptoms include eczema, colic, and a history of parental allergy.

Acute frontal sinusitis is more common in adults and frequently occurs following nasal trauma involving the nasal frontal duct. In the adolescent, it is the major source of orbital infection. In cases refractory to medical management, treatment consists of trephination of the anterior floor of the frontal sinus in the medial portion of the eyebrow. Chronic frontal sinusitis unresponsive to medical treatment and development of a mucocele are additional indications for operation. Endoscopic removal of frontal sinus mucoceles is now possible. A mucocele results from mucosal membrane duplication and obstruction of the sinus osteum secondary to chronic infection or trauma. It gradually enlarges to destroy the frontal bone and encroach upon the orbit or anterior cranial fossa. In large mucoceles of the frontal sinus that cannot be approached endoscopically, a bicoronal incision with an osteoplastic flap is used to excise and obliterate the sinus with fat or muscle. Finally, if patients have persistent postendoscopic drainage with facial pain, headache, or recurrent asthma, a repeat CT scan is indicated.

Calhoun KH et al: CT evaluation of the paranasal sinuses in symptomatic and asymptomatic populations. Otolaryngol Head Neck Surg 1991;104:480.

Davis WE et al: Middle meatus antrostomy: Patency rates and risk factors. Otolaryngol Head Neck Surg 1991; 104:467.

Jorgensen JH et al: Antimicrobial resistance among respiratory isolates of *Haemophilus influenzae, Moraxella catarrhalis,* and *Streptococcus pneumoniae* in the United States. Antimicrobial Agents Chemother 1990;34:2075.

Levine HL: Functional endoscopic sinus surgery: Evaluation of surgery and follow up of 250 patients. Laryngoscope 1990;100:79.

Maniglia AJ et al: Intracranial abscesses secondary to nasal, sinus and orbital infections in adults and children. Arch Otolaryngol Head Neck Surg 1989;115:1424.

Matthews BB et al: Endoscopic sinus surgery: Outcome in 155 cases. Otolaryngol Head Neck Surg 1991;104:244.

Orobello PW et al: Microbiology of chronic sinusitis in children. Arch Otolaryngol Head Neck Surg 1991;117:980.

EPISTAXIS

The nasal cavity is a common site of spontaneous hemorrhage. The blood supply to the nose is derived from both the external and internal carotid artery systems. In 90% of cases, the epistaxis originates in the anterior nasal septum in the rich vascular plexus (Kiesselbach's plexus) in Little's area. The terminal septal branches of the anterior and posterior ethmoidal arteries arising from the internal carotid artery (via the ophthalmic artery) anastomose in this area, along with branches from the superior labial artery (via the external facial) and the sphenopalatine artery (via the internal maxillary artery). Both originate from the external carotid artery system. Because of their location, vessels on the anterior septal mucosa are readily susceptible to trauma from nasal picking, drying, crusting, and infection. Severe caudal septal deformities may lead to mucosal drying over the point of deflection, causing spontaneous hemorrhage.

Mild epistaxis from the anterior septum is readily controlled with digital pressure for 5–10 minutes. Persistent hemorrhage requires topical cocainization and cauterization with a silver nitrate applicator or electrocautery (Figure 39–6). If hemorrhage is still not controlled, ¼-inch gauze packing impregnated with petrolatum should be placed atraumatically in the nasal cavity. Bleeding associated with leukemia, uremia, hepatic failure, coagulopathies, or hereditary hemorrhagic telangiectasia (Rendu-Osler-Weber syndrome) should be treated with absorbable gelatin

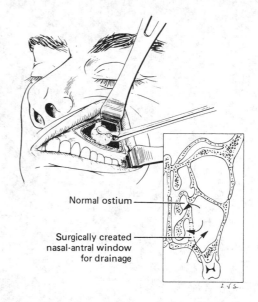

Figure 39–6. Cauterization to control bleeding in Kiesselbach's area.

sponge (Gelfoam) soaked in topical thrombin, oxidized regenerated cellulose (Surgicel), or microfibrillar collagen hemostat (Avitene Hemostat) inserted into the nasal cavity for 4–5 days. Treatment of the underlying coagulopathy, leukemia, uremia, or liver disorder is obviously important. Moderate long-term success in hemorrhagic hereditary telangiectasia has been achieved with estrogen derivatives and septal dermoplasty. Septal dermoplasty involves removing the diseased mucosa together with subepithelial telangiectasias and replacing it through a lateral rhinotomy with a skin graft. The YAG laser is currently used in recalcitrant cases for photocoagulation of nasal hemorrhagic telangiectasias.

Posterior epistaxis from the terminal branches of the sphenopalatine and internal maxillary arteries is more serious and is frequently associated with hypertension, diabetes, or major systemic vascular disorders. Successful treatment requires the use of both anterior and posterior packing, inserted with topical 4% cocaine anesthesia. The posterior pack is made by tying folded 4 × 4 gauze squares to the end of a catheter that has been passed transnasally and brought out through the mouth. Two strings are tied to the pharyngeal end of the catheter and brought out through the nares. They are then tied over an anterior nasal pack and bolster (Figure 39–7). The remaining third string is brought out through the mouth and taped to the cheek, where it can be grasped and removed in 4–5 days. This technique, however, is extremely uncomfortable, lowers arterial oxygen saturation, and may induce dysrhythmias or an acute myocardial infarction in patients with severe cardiovascular disease. Because toxic shock syndrome has been re-

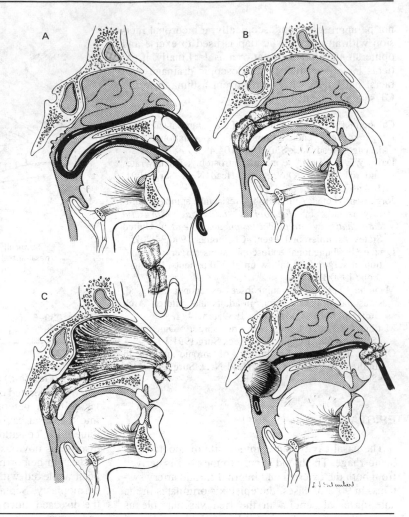

Figure 39–7. Packing to control bleeding from the posterior nose. **A:** Catheter inserted and pack attached. **B:** Pack drawn into position as catheter is removed. **C:** Strip tied over a bolster to hold pack in place with anterior pack installed "accordion pleating" style. **D:** Alternative method using balloon catheter instead of a gauze pack.

ported with the use of nasal packs, patients are started on intravenous cephalothin. Therefore, transantral ligation of the internal maxillary artery, sphenopalatine artery, and descending palatine artery via a Caldwell-Luc approach is advocated in selected patients. Ligation of the internal maxillary artery may also be necessary in some situation where adequate nasal packing fails to control hemorrhage.

Guarisco JL, Graham HD III: Epistaxis in children: Causes, diagnosis and treatment. Ear Nose Throat J 1989;68:522.

Levine HL, Mehta A: Management of nasal mucosal telangiectasias: Operative techniques. Otolaryngol Head Neck Surg 1991;2:173.

Rebeiz EE, Parks S, Shapshay SM: Management of epistaxis in hereditary hemorrhagic telangiectasia with neodymium:yttrium-aluminum garnet laser photocoagulation: Operative techniques. Otolaryngol Head Neck Surg 1991;2:177.

Stevens HE: Epistaxis. Can Fam Physician 1990;36:757.

Padgham N: Epistaxis: Anatomical and clinical correlates. J. Laryngol Otol 1990;104:308.

NASAL TRAUMA

Nasal fractures are the most common fractures of the maxillofacial skeleton and frequently are associated with septal fractures and epistaxis. Clinical findings commonly include periorbital edema and ecchymosis, displacement of the bony dorsum to the right with depression of the left nasal bone (secondary to a right hook), crepitus, and, occasionally, laceration of the dorsum. In severe facial trauma, because the other facial bones are often broken, the entire facial skeleton should be x-rayed.

Early reduction under local anesthesia before significant swelling appears produces an excellent result. Elevation with a periosteal elevator, combined with laterally applied digital pressure, is usually effective. An external plaster of Paris splint or commercially available splint is applied and removed in 1 week. It may be necessary to reduce severely impacted nasal bones with Walsham forceps, one blade placed intranasally and the other extranasally. If the nasal fracture is encountered after severe edema has developed, it is better to postpone reduction for several days to allow resolution of edema. In children, the facial skeleton heals so fast that fracture must be reduced within 4–5 days to avoid malunion. Malunion in adults is treated by rhinoplasty and often concomitant septoplasty to repair the deviated nasal septum.

Complications of nasal trauma include septal hematoma and abscess formation, septal perforation, septal deviation, and cerebrospinal fluid rhinorrhea secondary to fracture of the cribriform plate, the roof of the ethmoid sinus, the posterior table of the frontal sinus, or the sphenoid sinus.

A septal hematoma is a collection of blood underneath the mucoperichondrium or mucoperiosteum of the septum. Physical examination discloses a bulging red septum, and nasal obstruction is usually complete and bilateral. Unless the hematoma is immediately incised and drained, a staphylococcal abscess may develop that results in cartilaginous necrosis and saddle nose deformity. Intravenous nafcillin, oxacillin, cefazolin, or clindamycin should be given to prevent cavernous sinus thrombosis and meningitis.

A septal deviation, especially along the nasal floor, produces varying degrees of nasal obstruction, depending upon the severity of deflection into the nasal cavity. The caudal end of the septum may be deflected into the nasal vestibule, causing obstruction or external deformity. Nasal septoplasty through a caudal submucoperichondrial incision is used to reconstruct and straighten the septum.

Septal perforations are repaired only if complicated by persistent epistaxis, crusting with nasal obstruction, or, rarely, whistling. The repair involves use of a temporalis fascial or perichondrial graft and advancement of two bipedicled mucoperichondrial flaps to cover the defect. Alternatively, a pedicled upper lip mucosal flap may be used.

Fractures of the nasal bones, nasoethmoidal region, and frontal region may occur in association with a dural defect and cerebrospinal fluid rhinorrhea. This provides a potential route for ascending infection and meningitis. The dural defect may communicate with the nasal cavity via the ethmoidal, frontal, or sphenoidal sinuses or the cribriform plate. A basilar skull fracture with an intact tympanic membrane may also present with cerebrospinal fluid rhinorrhea.

The diagnosis should be suspected by finding watery rhinorrhea with an increased glucose content and may be confirmed by CT scan following subarachnoid instillation of metrizamide or, more recently, iohexol (Omnipaque) intrathecal injection. The source of cerebrospinal fluid leak may be demonstrated in many cases by placing fluorescein dye (0.5 mL of 5% solution) in the lumbar subarachnoid space. Thirty minutes later, the nose can be endoscopically examined to determine the fistula site: frontal sinus, sphenoid sinus, roof of the ethmoid (fovea ethmoidalis), cribriform plate, or middle ear (via the auditory tube). Cerebrospinal fluid appears as a yellowish-green fluid, and a Wood lamp is not necessary. If this fails to demonstrate the leak, CT scan combined with metrizamide introduced into the subarachnoid space may be useful. Five milliliters of isosmolar metrizamide is inserted into the lumbar space with the patient positioned head down. After 2 minutes, coronal CT sections can be obtained with the patient in the prone position.

Acute posttraumatic cerebrospinal fluid rhinorrhea is treated conservatively, with bed rest in the semisitting position, fluid restriction, lumbar drain, and diuretics. The patient should avoid straining, blowing the nose, sneezing, or vigorous coughing. Indications for surgery are persistent cerebrospinal fluid leakage of more than 6 weeks' duration, recurrent meningitis, pneumoencephalos, or intermittent leakage.

Small defects of the cribriform plate, fovea ethmoidalis, and sphenoid sinus are successfully repaired through an external ethmoidectomy incision using a variety of septal or middle turbinate mucoperiosteal flaps. Alternatively, an endoscopic approach using fascia, muscle, fascia lata, or fibrin glue can be used. Fibrin glue, composed of 10% calcium chloride and topical thrombin, added to cryoprecipitate in separate syringes, becomes gelatinous when combined and effectively seals the leak. The fibrin glue will last about 7–10 days and then dissolve. In all cases, the graft or glue is held in position by an absorbable packing such as Gelfoam. Small defects of the posterior table of the frontal sinus are best managed by a bicoronal incision, osteoplastic flap approach, and obliteration of the frontal sinus with abdominal fat. Large defects will necessitate anterior fossa craniotomy and repair.

Other soft tissue facial injuries and fractures of the zygoma, maxilla, orbit, and mandibles are discussed in Chapter 45.

Eviatar A, Myssiorek D: Repair of nasal septal perforation with tragal cartilage and perichondrium graft. Otolaryngol Head Neck Surg 1989;100:300.

Fairbanks DNFM: Nasal septal perforations: Operative techniques. Otolaryngol Head Neck Surg 1991;2:194.

Stankiewicz JA: Endoscopic intranasal closure of cerebral spinal fluid fistulas, operative techniques. Otolaryngol Head Neck Surg 1991;2:206.

Stankiewicz J: Cerebral spinal fluid fistula and endoscopic sinus surgery. Laryngoscope 1991;101:250.

CONGENITAL NASAL MALFORMATIONS

Congenital malformations of the nose and its appendages are unusual. Facial clefts, such as cleft lip and palate or a bifid nose, commonly result from genetic or teratogenic factors operating in the second month of fetal life. Although atresia and stenosis of the anterior nares are rare, they should be suspected in any infant who has difficulty breathing. Bilateral bony posterior choanal atresia is more commonly the cause of congenital neonatal respiratory impairment. Because they are obligatory nasal breathers during the first several weeks of life, newborns develops apnea and cyanosis when crying stops and the mouth is closed. The definitive diagnosis is confirmed by inability to pass a catheter transnasally.

Initial treatment includes either an oral endotracheal tube or McGovern nipple, followed by early transnasal or transpalatal correction of the atresia. The atretic plate can be successfully removed transnasally with diamond burs or the CO_2 laser. The surgically created posterior choana is kept patent with a 16F or 18F polyvinylchloride (Portex) endotracheal tube that is removed in 6–8 weeks. Unilateral choanal atresia, on the other hand, is usually not diagnosed until later in childhood or early adulthood and is associated with unilateral nasal obstruction or rhinorrhea. Repair is best performed when the nasal cavities and hard palate have reached adult size.

Other congenital lesions that may produce nasal obstruction include nasal gliomas, encephaloceles, meningoceles, and teratomas (dermoids, teratoids, true teratomas, and epignathi). Nasal gliomas are composed of neural and glial elements. Similarly, meningoceles and encephaloceles that have intracranial connections through the cribriform plate, fovea ethmoidalis, or sphenoid bone may present as a nasal mass that may be mistaken for a nasal polyp. Not infrequently, these heterotopic brain elements are seen as a mass on the nasal dorsum that is frequently confused with a midline dermoid cyst. CT scans or MRI of the anterior cranial fossa and cribriform plate must be obtained to rule out intracranial connections. Treatment of heterotopic brain elements with an intracranial connection requires a combined craniotomy and transfacial approach. If the diagnosis remains in doubt, frontal craniotomy is performed before transfacial excision to avoid development of cerebrospinal fluid rhinorrhea and meningitis.

Morgan DW, Bailey CM: Current management of choanal atresia. Int J Pediatr Otorhinolaryngol 1990;19:1.

Morgan DW, Evans JNG: Developmental nasal anomalies. J Laryngol Otol 1990;104:394.

NEOPLASMS OF THE NOSE & PARANASAL SINUSES

Benign neoplasms of the nasal cavities and paranasal sinuses are rare. The most common benign lesions are of epithelial origin: the exophytic squamous papilloma and inverting papilloma. **Exophytic papillomas** arise primarily at the mucocutaneous junction within the nasal vestibule and should be excised with a small margin of normal tissue. **Inverting papillomas,** on the other hand, emerge almost exclusively from the lateral nasal wall as bulky vascular lesions with a marked tendency to invade and destroy bone. In 10–15% of cases, squamous cell carcinoma arising in the same anatomic area has been found. Wide surgical excision through a lateral rhinotomy approach is necessary to prevent local recurrence.

Malignant neoplasms of the nasal cavity and paranasal sinuses represent 0.2–0.3% of all cancers and 3% of all malignant tumors of the upper aerodigestive tract. Squamous cell carcinomas are the most common malignant neoplasms of the nasal cavities and paranasal sinuses. On the sun-exposed skin of the nasal tip and dorsum, basal cell carcinoma is more common. Early lesions are removed by local excision, using a MOHS (microscopically oriented histologic surgical) technique. More advanced carcinomas necessitate wide local excision of underlying bone and cartilage with flap reconstruction.

Squamous cell carcinoma most frequently arises in the maxillary sinus and presents with unilateral nasal obstruction; foul-smelling, bloody rhinorrhea; and headache. Preoperative evaluation includes axial and coronal CT views. MRI is better for distinguishing tumor from inflammatory disease in the sinuses. Treatment consists of combined external beam radiation therapy and partial or total maxillectomy with or without orbital exenteration, depending upon the presence or absence of orbital invasion. Other neoplasms arising in the nose and paranasal sinuses include lymphoma, adenoid cystic carcinoma, mucoepidermoid carcinoma, olfactory neuroblastoma, a variety of mesenchymal cancers, and adenocarcinoma. Adenocarcinomas tend to occur in the ethmoid air cells and may follow long-term exposure to wood dust or prior radiation therapy for bilateral retinoblastoma. Fortunately, primary carcinomas of the frontal, ethmoid, and sphenoid sinuses are extremely rare. Treatment requires combined radiation therapy and radical pansinusectomy for resectable lesions. A combined intracranial transfacial approach with skull base surgery is necessary when the dura is involved.

Karim AB et al: Ethmoid and upper nasal cavity carcinoma: Treatment results and complications. Radiol Ther Oncol 1990;19:109.

Phillips PP et al: The clinical behavior of inverting papilloma of the nose and paranasal sinuses. Laryngoscope 1990;100:463.

Ward BE et al: Carcinoma arising in oncocytic Schneiderian papilloma. Am J Surg Pathol 1990;14:364.

ORAL CAVITY

WHITE LESIONS OF THE ORAL CAVITY

The mucous membrane resembles the skin in that individual cells arise from the germinal layer and mature, but they do not keratinize. Mechanical, thermal, and chemical (eg, alcohol; nicotine, including smokeless tobacco products) trauma may lead to thickening of the germinal layer and later development of a nonnucleated keratinized layer that appears as gray-white nonulcerated plaques on the oral cavity mucosa (leukoplakia). Because the histologic appearance varies considerably and 6% of these lesions exhibit malignant transformation, biopsy is indicated to rule out early carcinoma. The treatment is surgical excision of small lesions with a knife or with a CO_2 or KTP laser and avoidance of further exposure to irritants. Laser excision has a lower recurrence rate plus the advantages of better precision, bloodless field, excellent tissue healing, and less pain and discomfort.

Lichen planus, although primarily a dermatologic disorder, may involve any mucous membrane exposed to trauma or chronic irritation such as tobacco—eg, the buccal mucosa frequently develops white papules or striae from repetitive biting. Hyperkeratosis, acanthosis, and subepithelial edema complete the histologic picture. Topical triamcinolone is often useful for associated submucosal inflammation. In some cases, this may undergo malignant degeneration into squamous cell carcinoma.

Finally, ill-fitting dentures may elicit white, raised folds of tissue in the gingivolabial sulcus that histologically consist of fibrous tissues proliferation and overlying epithelial hyperplasia. An inflammatory papillary hyperplasia on the hard palate may occur as a result of improperly fitting dentures. These polypoid lesions are hyperemic, soft, and mobile. Surgical removal is necessary, followed by denture readjustment.

Ernster VL et al: Smokeless tobacco use and health effects among baseball players. JAMA 1990;264:218.
Katz RW, Brahim JS, Travis WD: Oral squamous cell carcinoma arising in a patient with long-standing lichen planus: A case report. Oral Surg Oral Med Oral Pathol 1990;70:282.
Kaugar GE, Mehailescu WL, Gunsolley JC: Smokeless tobacco use in oral epithelial hyperplasia. Cancer 1989;64:1527.

1. INFLAMMATORY DISEASES OF THE GINGIVA

Inflammation of the gums (gingivitis) frequently develops as a result of poor oral hygiene, heavy smoking, and lowered resistance. **Acute necrotizing ulcerative gingivitis** (Vincent's gingivitis) is due to an overgrowth of the normal oral bacterial symbionts. Clinically, it is characterized by painful hemorrhagic gums, ulceration, and a yellow-gray gingival pseudomembrane. Treatment consists of topical hydrogen peroxide, proper oral hygiene with removal of plaque and tartar at the teeth margin, and oral penicillin.

Although not limited to the gingivae, recurrent **aphthous stomatitis** (canker sores) frequently presents on the gingivae as round or ovoid, discrete, erythematous macules 2–20 mm in diameter that rapidly indurate but do not vesiculate (unlike herpetic lesions). They may elicit enough pain to interfere with mastication and speaking. Tetracycline solution, 250 mg held in the mouth for 20 minutes four to six times a day, and an analgesic, dyclonine 0.5%, plus diphenhydramine elixir are effective treatment. Alternative therapy includes an emollient paste such as 0.1% triamcinolone acetonide in sodium carboxymethyl cellulose. The application of silver nitrate to the ulcerating base is also useful. The cause is uncertain, but evidence suggests that severe recurrent aphthous stomatitis may respond to oral colchicine.

Trauma to a tooth may provoke inflammation of the periodontal membrane (**acute periodontitis**), rendering it tender to touch. If the traumatic stimulus is removed, the inflammation resolves. Recurrent gingivitis coupled with poor dental hygiene may cause chronic periodontitis, pyorrhea, and regression of the periodontal ligament from the neck of the tooth. The gingival sulcus deepens, pockets form between the roots of the teeth and the surrounding gingivae, and debris and tartar accumulate. Mild periodontitis is characterized by gingival erythema, edema, tenderness, and hemorrhage. Severe periodontitis is associated with gingival necrosis, halitosis, and loss of unstable teeth. Unless the cycle is broken, periapical abscess formation and tooth devitalization will continue. Frequent flossing and regular professional dental care are recommended.

Hartsfield CD Jr: Recurrent aphthous ulcer: An effective method of self treatment. Gen Dentistry 1990;38:194.
Lamey PJ, Louis MAO: Oral medicine in practice: Burning mouth syndrome. Br Dent J 1989;167:197.

2. HERPETIC STOMATITIS

Herpetic lesions of the oral cavity are divided into primary and recurrent labial herpes. Both are caused by herpes simplex virus and present as small vesicles that rupture, yielding a yellow-white superficial ulcer surrounded by a red halo. They are usually located on the labial and buccal mucosa, gingivae, and tongue. In severe cases, the gingivae are edematous and bleed readily. Although the primary disease is self-limiting, virus may be reactivated by physical trauma and endogenous stress. Treatment is supportive, including topical anesthetics in solution or troche form. If herpetic stomatitis occurs as part of a disseminated infection, parenteral acyclovir is indicated.

3. CANDIDIASIS

Oral candidiasis (thrush) is caused by the yeast-like fungus *C albicans* and characterized by a white membranous lesion closely adherent to the mucous membrane that bleeds and ulcerates when it sloughs. It also occurs in a hyperplastic form that cannot be removed, an erythematous or atrophic form, and as angular cheilitis. *Candida* is normally a part of the oral biota but may become pathogenic after prolonged administration of antibiotics; radiation therapy to the cavity or pharynx; immunotherapy for carcinoma, leukemia, or lymphoma; or immune deficiency associated with corticosteroid therapy, diabetes, hepatic disease, etc. In addition, candidiasis along with oral hairy leukoplakia (nontender; caused by Epstein-Barr virus) is identified in patients with AIDS. Other local causative factors include xerostomia, smoking, smokeless tobacco, and mechanical changes in the oral environment. Oral nystatin or miconazole is effective treatment. For immunocompromised hosts who develop systemic candidal infections, amphotericin B is recommended. Ketoconazole administered orally is the drug of choice for chronic mucocutaneous candidiasis. The treatment of chronic mucocutaneous candidiasis may also include immunologic therapy with thymic transplants and infusion of lymphocytes from immunocompetent donors. Severely immunocompromised patients may benefit from the protracted use of prophylactic fluconazole. Chlorhexidine rinses have proved useful in treating oral candidiasis in children with leukemia.

Budt Z, Jorgenson E: Etiology, pathogenesis, therapy and prophylaxis of oral yeast infections. Acta Odontol Scand 1990;48:61.

Epsteine JB: Oral and pharyngeal candidiasis: Topical agents for management and prevention. Postgrad Med 1989;85:257.

Holmstrup P, Axel T: Classification and clinical manifestations of oral yeast infections. Acta Odontol Scand 1990;48:57.

CONGENITAL ORAL CAVITY MALFORMATIONS*

1. TORUS PALATINUS & TORUS MANDIBULARIS

Torus palatinus, a common developmental abnormality of the oral cavity, consists of a bony exostosis of varying size and shape in the midline of the palate. Clinically, it may interfere with the proper fitting of dentures and require surgical removal. It must be distinguished from tumors of the minor salivary glands and fissural cysts of the palate.

Torus mandibularis, like its palatal counterpart, is a bony exostosis usually situated on the lingual surface of the mandible, adjacent to the cuspid and first bicuspid teeth. It is asymptomatic until an attempt is made at fitting a denture.

2. MACROGLOSSIA

Isolated macroglossia is rare and may be seen in cretinism, Down's syndrome, and acromegaly. It may also be caused by lymphangiomatous invasion of the tongue. Relative macroglossia is encountered in the Pierre Robin syndrome (micrognathia and cleft palate). The relatively large tongue may obstruct the upper airway, necessitating insertion of an oral airway or tongue-lip adhesion. The tongue base is sutured over an anterior neck button to assist in anterior displacement of the tongue. These measures are only necessary until the oral cavity enlarges enough to accommodate the tongue. Rarely is tracheotomy necessary.

3. ANKYLOGLOSSIA

Tongue-tie or partial ankyloglossia is manifested by an abnormally short and thick lingual frenulum. Various degrees of ankyloglossia occur, ranging from mild restriction with only a mucous membrane band to those in which both the frenulum and the underlying fibers of the genioglossus muscle are markedly fibrosed. Rarely, complete ankyloglossia with fusion of the tongue to the floor of the mouth may be encountered. Limitation of movement of the tongue tip results in malocclusion with an anterior "open bite" deformity, early prognathism, and swallowing and speech difficulties. Children with severe ankyloglossia meeting any of these criteria require frenulectomy, genioglossus myotomy, and mucous membrane closure with multiple Z-plasties.

---

*Cleft lip and cleft palate are discussed in Chapter 44

4. RANULA

A ranula is a transparent retention cyst in the floor of the mouth arising from the sublingual salivary glands. The cyst enlarges gradually, penetrating the deep structures of the floor of the mouth above the mylohyoid muscle. It should be excised if it is small; marsupialization is necessary for large cysts, owing to their multiple ramifications.

SALIVARY GLANDS

CHRONIC SIALADENITIS*

Chronic or recurrent bacterial parotitis may develop as a result of antecedent acute suppuration or viral inflammation. More commonly, however there is a history of ductal obstruction. Recurrent bacterial invasion of the parotid gland leads to destruction and fibrosis of acini with ductal ectasia. The subsequent decrease in salivary flow creates a cycle of ascending sialadenitis, ductal ectasia, acinar atrophy, and obstructive fibrosis. Clinically, the patient complains of recurrent parotid pain and swelling, typically while eating. Initial treatment should be conservative, utilizing sialagogues (lemon balls or chewing gum), adequate oral hydration to stimulate salivary flow, and amoxicillin and clavulanic acid. In patients with recalcitrant disease, an extended course of clindamycin, cefoxitin, nafcillin, or vancomycin plus metronidazole may be necessary. Superficial parotidectomy is recommended if prolonged conservative management fails.

Martinez-Madrigal F, Mecheau C: Histology of the major salivary glands. Am J Surg Pathol 1989;13:879.

SIALOLITHIASIS

Salivary gland stones are both a cause and a consequence of chronic sialadenitis. In addition, they may produce acute suppurative sialadenitis. The stones are composed of inorganic calcium and sodium phosphate salts that are deposited in the duct on an organic nidus of mucus or cellular debris. Eighty to ninety percent of salivary calculi occur in the submandibular gland and may lead to complete acute obstruction of the gland, with most stones occurring in the ducts rather than the gland itself. The patient complains of painful swelling, especially with meals, and may report extrusion of gravel from the duct.

The diagnosis is confirmed by palpation of a stone or by demonstration of decreased salivary flow from the duct. Soft tissue films may reveal a radiodense stone, and CT sialography may disclose complete or partial filling defects in the ductal system with retention of dye on evacuation films. Treatment consists of intraoral removal of stones that are close to the duct orifice by ductal dilation and massage. Stones in the hilum of the submandibular gland necessitate excision of the gland; parotid sialoliths are managed in a similar fashion.

SALIVARY GLAND TRAUMA

Injuries to the salivary glands may be intraoral or extraoral, blunt or lacerating. The parotid gland is most commonly injured along with associated structures, including the facial nerve, Stensen's duct, soft tissues, mandible, or zygoma. Laceration of the parotid duct may occur with a facial laceration posterior to the anterior edge of the masseter muscle and results in simultaneous injury to the buccal branch of the facial nerve. The severed duct is repaired over a small polyethylene catheter using fine interrupted sutures. The associated seventh nerve injury is repaired by anastomosing the cut ends with 10-0 monofilament suture. All lacerations in the parotid gland region must be examined for seventh nerve injury. Injury may occur either to the main trunk proximal to the pes anserinus or to one of the branches within the parotid gland. Facial injuries anterior to a vertical line from the lateral canthus of the eye generally do not require exploration, and the nerve will regenerate spontaneously. However, some surgeons advocate microscopic repair to offer a better chance of complete recovery without the development of synkinesis (mass movement of the face). If injury to the nerve is suspected, each of the five major branches is assessed by observing voluntary movements and responses to nerve excitability testing. If transection of the facial nerve is likely, exploration and precise repair through a parotidectomy incision with the operating microscope is crucial. The greater auricular or sural nerve may be used as a cable graft for avulsed segments of the facial nerve. An exception to this approach would be an extensively contaminated wound such as a shotgun injury. In this situation, it is better to explore and debride the wound, tag the proximal and distal branches of the injured nerve with metal clips, and delay nerve repair until wound healing is more complete. This should be performed within 30 days after injury to achieve the best results.

May M, Sobol SM, Mester SJ: Managing segmental facial nerve injuries by surgical repair. Laryngoscope 1990; 100:1062.

*Acute parotitis is discussed in Chapter 4.

PHARYNX

PHARYNGITIS

Acute pharyngitis is usually caused by viruses (especially the adenoviruses and rhinoviruses) or group A beta-hemolytic *Streptococcus.* Clinically, erythema, edema, and occasional membrane formation are present, and the patient complains of pain on swallowing. In bacterial pharyngitis, the white count and fever are higher and cervical adenopathy is more marked. Pneumococci, *H influenzae, M catarrhalis, Neisseria gonorrhoeae,* and coagulase-positive staphylococci are occasionally the primary pathogens. Pharyngeal cultures are obtained, and penicillin is started pending the results.

One must differentiate acute bacterial pharyngitis from diphtheritic pharyngitis and infectious mononucleosis. *Corynebacterium diphtheriae* is a potentially lethal bacterium in a nonimmunized host. Characteristic features are odynophagia, fever, and the development of a gray pseudomembrane on the oropharynx associated with a fetid odor. The membrane bleeds easily when removed and may gradually involve the larynx, producing acute upper airway obstruction. Infectious mononucleosis may mimic diphtheria, exhibiting faucial arch edema, a pharyngeal pseudomembrane, and laryngeal edema. A positive heterophil agglutination or Monospot test, absolute lymphocytosis, generalized lymphadenopathy, and hepatosplenomegaly differentiate this disease from diphtheria. Tonsilloadenoidal hyperplasia may be so marked as to obstruct the upper airway, necessitating intubation and tonsilloadenoidectomy.

Acute tonsillitis secondary to group A beta-hemolytic streptococcal infection commonly occurs in children under 10 years of age and may occasionally present in epidemic form. Clinically, pyrexia, odynophagia, referred otalgia, and malaise predominate. The usual signs of viral upper respiratory tract infection—cough, coryza, and conjunctivitis—are absent. The tonsils appear hyperemic and edematous, with or without a purulent exudate filling the tonsillar crypts that coalesces to form a yellow-white pseudomembrane. A 7- to 10-day course of penicillin is adequate therapy. An alternative choice is erythromycin in patients allergic to penicillin. Clindamycin is indicated for those who do not respond to these drugs.

Chronic tonsillitis may follow acute or subacute episodes of tonsillitis, especially in older children, and is associated with recurrent odynophagia, cough, and findings of tonsillar enlargement, debris in tonsillar crypts, and cervical lymphadenitis. There is increasing evidence that *H influenzae* plays a major role in this disorder as well as in the pathogenesis of tonsillar hypertrophy. In addition, *S aureus* has become more prominent, along with actinomycetes. In view of the high incidence of β-lactamase-producing organisms, amoxicillin with clavulanic acid, clindamycin, or an antistaphylococcal penicillin is recommended. Tonsillectomy is indicated if there are five or more documented episodes of acute tonsillitis per year.

Acute tonsillitis may in some instances extend beyond the tonsillar tissue into the space between the anterior and posterior tonsillar pillars or into the soft palate, producing a **peritonsillar abscess.** Physical examination reveals an edematous, bulging, anterior tonsillar pillar with medial displacement of the soft palate and uvula. Immediate therapy includes incision and drainage of the abscess through the anterior tonsillar pillar or needle aspiration, intravenous penicillin or clindamycin, hydration, and antipyretics followed by either immediate tonsillectomy or an interval tonsillectomy in 6 weeks. The advantages of immediate tonsillectomy in carefully selected patients include complete abscess drainage without recurrence, rapid relief of symptoms, greater technical simplicity with less hemorrhage, less severe illness, and shorter hospitalization.

Pulmonary hypertension, cor pulmonale, and congestive heart failure (Noonan's syndrome) secondary to chronic hypoxia have been reported in young children with hyperplasia of Waldeyer's ring. More recently, chronic hypersomnolence and periodic apnea have been recognized in patients with upper airway obstruction secondary to tonsilloadenoidal hyperplasia. During sleep, these patients experience periods of cessation of nasal-oral air flow of longer than 10 seconds, persistent chest wall movement, and subsequent hypoxia and hypercapnia. The obstructive sleep apnea syndrome is characterized by frequent arousals during sleep and more subtle clinical findings such as weight loss, behavioral disturbances, and enuresis. Tonsillectomy and adenoidectomy are indicated to relieve upper respiratory tract obstruction.

Isolated adenoidal hypertrophy secondary to physiologic enlargement of the adenoids or chronic viral nasopharyngitis may produce nasal airway obstruction. These children exhibit chronic rhinorrhea, mouth breathing, dental abnormalities, an elongated face, and snoring during sleep. Adenoidectomy is curative.

The obstructive sleep apnea syndrome in adults (Pickwickian syndrome) is commonly seen in obese middle-aged men and spans a wide range of severity. It is characterized by loud, stertorous snoring. Snoring is caused by high-frequency oscillation of the soft palate, resulting in intermittent narrowing of the pharyngeal airway. An estimated 25% of the adult male population and 15% of the adult female population snore every night. The degree of severity of airway obstruction is ascertained by obtaining a polysomnogram that measures the number, frequency, and duration of apneic episodes, degree of arterial oxygen saturation, presence of cardiac arrhythmias associated with apnea, and degree of daytime impairment. There are many forms of treatment, including behavioral, surgical, medical, and mechanical, some of which can be used in combination. In mild sleep apnea, behavioral treatment—particularly weight reduction—is sufficient. Alcohol consumption should be reduced at nighttime, and sedative medications that can worsen sleep apnea should be avoided. Mechanical treatment is the best choice for many patients. Nasal continuous positive airway pressure (CPAP) is given by a silicone mask over the nose that is attached by tubing to an air pump. It acts as a pneumatic splint to maintain the patency of the airway. If this is not tolerated, the upper airway obstruction can be corrected with either a uvulopalatal pharyngoplasty (UPPP) and tonsillectomy or, in severely obstructed patients, a tracheotomy. Patients who respond to uvulopalatal pharyngoplasty generally have collapse limited to the upper part of the pharynx, not to the lower part.

Anand VK, Ferguson PW, Schoen LS: Obstructive sleep apnea: A comparison of continuous positive airway pressure and surgical treatment. Otolaryngol Head Neck Surg 1991;105:382.

Fairbanks DNF: Uvulopalatal pharyngoplasty: Complications and avoidance strategies. Otolaryngol Head Neck Surg 1990;102:239.

Lockhart R, Parker GS, Tammy TA: Role of quinsy tonsillectomy in the management of peritonsillar abscess. Ann Otol Rhinol Laryngol 1991;100:569.

Principato JJ: Upper airway obstruction and craniofacial morphology. Otolaryngol Head Neck Surg 1990;104:881.

Rosenfeld RM, Green RP: Tonsillectomy and adenoidectomy: Changing trends. Ann Otol Rhinol Laryngol 1990;99:187.

Timon CI et al: Changes in tonsillar bacteriology of recurrent acute tonsillitis: 1980 vs. 1989. Respir Med 1990;84:395.

BENIGN NEOPLASMS OF THE PHARYNX*

The most common benign tumor of the nasopharynx is the juvenile angiofibroma, a highly vascular, nonencapsulated, invasive neoplasm with a propensity to occur in adolescent males. Onset of clinical signs and symptoms may be at any time from 7 to 21 years of age. Epistaxis occurs in 75% of cases in addition to nasal obstruction and rhinorrhea. Anosmia is common. Preoperative digital subtraction angiography and CT scanning should be performed to evaluate the blood supply and anatomic extent of the tumor. The major blood supply is from the internal maxillary artery. Preoperative embolization of the

*Malignant lesions of the pharynx are discussed in Chapter 15.

tumor and estrogen therapy markedly decrease blood loss at surgical resection. For lesions confined to the nasopharynx, a transpalatal approach is satisfactory. Larger tumors with involvement of the nasal cavity, maxillary, ethmoid, or sphenoid sinus require a lateral rhinotomy via transpalatal or Caldwell-Luc approach (or both) for complete excision. Although these neoplasms are only moderately responsive to radiation therapy, such therapy is often the treatment of choice for orbital or intracranial invasion.

PHARYNGEAL FOREIGN BODIES

Irregular foreign bodies entering the pharynx are likely to lodge in the lingual or palatine tonsils, valleculae, or piriform sinuses. Smooth round or ovoid objects commonly lodge at the opening to the esophagus or cricopharyngeus muscle, especially in children. Dysphagia, odynophagia, or aphagia may result. In a young child or infant, drooling is a characteristic sign. Dyspnea, wheezing, or persistent cough may develop secondary to compression of the larynx or trachea. If the esophagus is penetrated by a sharp object such as a pin or fish bone, subcutaneous emphysema can be palpated in the neck. Foreign bodies lodging more distally in the esophagus such as at the level of the aortic arch, left main bronchus, or gastroesophageal junction generally do not produce early symptoms.

Chest x-ray, anteroposterior and lateral neck films, and occasionally a barium swallow are necessary to delineate the site of a foreign body. Foreign bodies of the palatine and lingual tonsils are removed directly with a curved hemostat; objects located in the hypopharynx or esophagus require direct laryngoscopy or esophagoscopy under general anesthesia.

LARYNX

The larynx has four functions: (1) protection of the lower airway, (2) phonation, (3) respiration, and (4) fixation of the chest. Laryngeal dysfunction can therefore lead to abnormalities such as aspiration, weak cry, hoarseness, stridor, and poor cough. These problems point to laryngeal dysfunction and should prompt an inspection of the larynx with a laryngeal mirror (indirect laryngoscopy) or fiberoptic nasopharyngolaryngoscopy (NPL) during phonation and deep inspiration. Cinefluoroscopy with barium sulfate allows assessment of the competency of the larynx during swallowing. Neoplasms and traumatic lesions of the larynx are effectively evaluated by CT scan or MRI. In any individual with hoarseness of more than 2–3 weeks' duration, the larynx should be inspected as described above. If the larynx cannot be inspected in this way, transnasal fiberoptic laryngoscopy or direct laryngoscopy under general anesthesia is required. A specimen of larynx is obtained at direct laryngoscopy for biopsy examination for suspected neoplasms.

FOREIGN BODIES OF THE LARYNX & TRACHEOBRONCHIAL TREE

In children, a variety of objects, including seeds beans, pins, and tiny toys, may be aspirated into the tracheobronchial tree. In adults, meat is the most common cause of obstruction and is associated with a number of factors: (1) large, poorly chewed pieces of food; (2) elevated blood alcohol; and (3) upper and lower dentures. The development of a "café coronary" is frequently confused with a myocardial infarction.

Foreign bodies entering the tracheobronchial tree must pass (1) the epiglottis, (2) the upper laryngeal inlet, (3) the false cords (ventricular bands), (4) the true vocal cords, and (5) the cough reflex. If a foreign body lodges in the larynx, there is immediate pain and laryngospasm, dyspnea, and inspiratory stridor proportionate to the degree of upper airway obstruction. The voice may be hoarse or aphonic.

If partial airway obstruction is present and the victim can exchange air and cough, no attempt should be made to move the foreign body at that time. If the victim is aphonic, unable to cough or exchange air, and is clutching his or her neck, complete airway obstruction is present. If equipment is not at hand for emergency tracheotomy or cricothyrotomy, two manual maneuvers are recommended for relieving foreign body airway obstruction: (1) a series of four back blows are delivered with the heel of the hand over the spine between the shoulder blades, and (2) a series of four manual thrusts are administered to the upper abdomen or lower chest. Finally, if the foreign body remains in the larynx or pharynx after these maneuvers, manual removal with the finger probe may be successful.

In the conscious adult patient with adequate air exchange, indirect laryngoscopy supplemented with anteroposterior and lateral x-rays of the neck and chest will confirm the position of the foreign body. Removal of a laryngeal foreign body necessitates general anesthesia and a laryngoscope and alligator forceps. Foreign bodies in the tracheobronchial tree also require general anesthesia and open bronchoscopy with forceps removal.

The reaction of the tracheobronchial tree to a foreign body depends upon the degree of obstruction and the physical nature of the foreign body. For example, a bean acts as a ball valve, rising with expiration and occluding the distal airway on inspiration.

Vegetable matter produces a violent bronchitis that may be associated with chronic suppurative pneumonitis; nonobstructive metallic objects may remain within the tracheobronchial tree for an extended period with little tissue damage.

Tracheal foreign bodies produce inspiratory and expiratory wheezing. With distally located objects, three different patterns may occur: (1) partial (bypass valve) bronchial obstruction, in which the foreign body permits the passage of air during both inspiration and expiration; (2) expiratory check valve obstruction, where ingress of air is minimally impeded but egress is checked, resulting in obstructive emphysema; and (3) stop valve obstruction, in which no air enters the subjacent lung, resulting in atelectasis. Radiographic evaluation is invaluable. The recommended protocol includes anteroposterior and lateral neck and chest films, inspiratory and expiratory films, and, in selected cases, fluoroscopy and decubitus films. Currently, open (rigid) bronchoscopy is the standard way to remove foreign bodies of the tracheobronchial tree. Flexible fiberoptic bronchoscopy is reserved for removing peripheral foreign bodies in patients on mechanical ventilators or in patients with cervical or maxillofacial trauma.

Hayashi AH et al: Management of foreign body bronchial obstruction using endoscopic laser therapy. J Pediatr Surg 1990;25:1174.

Hollinger LD: Diagnostic endoscopy of the pediatric airway. Laryngoscope 1989;99:346.

Limper AH, Prakash UBS: Tracheobronchial foreign bodies in adults. Ann Intern Med 1990;112:604.

Mu L, He P, Sun D: The causes and complications of late diagnosis of foreign body aspiration in children. Arch Otolaryngol Head Neck Surg 1991;117:876.

Puhakka H et al: Tracheobronchial foreign bodies: A persistent problem with pediatric patients. Am J Dis Child 1989;143:543.

LARYNGEAL TRAUMA

Trauma to the larynx and trachea may occur from iatrogenic causes (prolonged endotracheal intubation or inappropriate tracheotomy, laryngotomy or cricothyrotomy) or extrinsic injuries (automobile accidents, neck blows, strangulation, etc). The passenger in the front seat of an automobile is particularly vulnerable to hyperextension injury of the neck. This results in compression of the larynx, hyoid bone, and upper trachea between the dashboard and the cervical spine. Injuries of the larynx are less common in children because of the higher position of the larynx in the neck and the resulting protection provided by the mandible. Severe laryngotracheal injury may occur, however, in children riding bicycles, motor bikes, snowmobiles, etc, who strike a horizontal cable or fall against the handlebars.

The most common injury to the larynx is vertical

fracture of the thyroid cartilage with or without fracture of the cricoid cartilage. Because the cricoid cartilage is the only complete cartilaginous ring in the respiratory tract, its functional integrity is critical in maintaining a patent airway. An unreduced fracture of the cricoid may result in subglottic stenosis. Associated injuries of the pharynx, trachea, esophagus, soft tissues, and neurovascular structures of the neck are common. Escape of air into the mediastinum may produce tension pneumothorax.

Clinical findings in laryngotracheal trauma include (1) subcutaneous emphysema or crepitus, (2) dysphonia, (3) loss of the laryngeal prominence (Adam's apple), (4) dysphagia, (5) odynophagia, (6) stridor, (7) hemoptysis, and (8) cough.

Conservative treatment with cool mist, intravenous fluids, cefazolin, and parenteral corticosteroids will suffice for laryngeal soft tissue edema without significant airway obstruction or impaired vocal cord mobility. CT scanning is done to evaluate the laryngeal skeleton for fracture and determine the subsequent course of treatment. It is not performed in patients with an obvious penetrating wound who will require immediate tracheotomy and exploration. More severe laryngotracheal injury requires endotracheal intubation or tracheotomy. In an emergency, an endotracheal or tracheotomy tube may be introduced through an open laryngotracheal wound. Ideally, tracheotomy should be performed after the airway is controlled by intubation or open bronchoscopy. However, this may not be possible in cases of complete laryngotracheal separation. If a high tracheotomy or a cricothyrotomy has been performed, it should be revised as soon as possible to the third or fourth tracheal ring to prevent vocal cord paralysis and subglottic stenosis. Open reduction and stabilization of all cartilaginous, mucosal, and soft tissue defects with internal fixation and a soft stent is done immediately if the patient's general condition permits. This is recommended within 24 hours. Late laryngeal stenosis may be successfully treated in some patients with the CO_2 laser. Ultimately, the following factors affect wound healing within the larynx and trachea and determine the success or failure of therapy: (1) mechanical loss of lumen-supporting structures, (2) loss of blood supply to cartilaginous structures, (3) presence of chondritis, and (4) degree of progressive fibrosis and stenosis.

Jurkovich GJ: Treatment dilemmas in laryngotracheal trauma. J Trauma 1988;28:1439.

Reece GP, Shatney CH: Blunt injuries of the cervical trachea: Review of 51 patients. South Med J 1988;81:1542.

Schaefer SD: The treatment of acute external laryngeal injuries. Arch Otolaryngol Head Neck Surg 1991;117:35.

Schaefer SD: Use of CT scanning in management of the acutely injured larynx. Otolaryngol Clin North Am 1991;24:31.

Weymuller EA, Bishop MJ: Problems associated with prolonged intubation in the geriatric patient. Otolaryngol Clin North Am 1990;23:1057.

PEDIATRIC AIRWAY OBSTRUCTION

Airway obstruction at birth or in the first several months of life is commonly secondary to congenital and neoplastic disorders. At birth, immediate differentiation must be made between respiratory depression with cyanosis, shallow and slow respirations, and respiratory tract obstruction producing tachypnea, stridor, and suprasternal and subcostal retractions.

Stridor (noisy breathing) is the most prominent symptom and is an expression of partial respiratory tract obstruction secondary to external compression or partial occlusion within the airway. The character and intensity of stridor depend upon the site and degree of obstruction and the airflow velocity and pressure gradient across the point of obstruction. Obstruction at the level of the true vocal cords produces high-pitched inspiratory stridor. By contrast, stridor that occurs chiefly during expiration and is lower in pitch is commonly associated with tracheal obstruction. The quality of the cry remains normal in most infants with airway obstruction who do not have a laryngeal lesion. A weak or absent cry at birth suggests neurogenic vocal cord impairment. In addition to evaluating the cry and breathing patterns, the physician should also assess swallowing function in all infants with stridor. Mediastinal tumors and vascular rings producing extrinsic esophageal and tracheal compression cause feeding difficulties and failure to thrive. The presence of recurrent pneumonitis and aspiration suggests a laryngeal lesion of tracheoesophageal fistula. All infants with stridor should have an anteroposterior and lateral chest film and barium swallow followed by endoscopy.

Newborns & Small Infants

The most common cause of infantile stridor is laryngomalacia, or congenital flaccid larynx. During inspiration, there is extreme infolding of the omega-shaped epiglottis and aryepiglottic folds owing to inadequate cartilaginous support. The supine position or head flexion aggravates the stridor, whereas patency of the airway is improved by the prone position and head extension. The stridor gradually resolves in most infants within 2–3 months. Endoscopic inspection is necessary in infants with persistent or progressive stridor.

Congenital subglottic stenosis is the second most frequently encountered laryngeal lesion and may become evident several weeks or more after birth, following an upper respiratory tract infection. Because the subglottic region is the narrowest point in the upper respiratory tract, a small amount of edema will critically narrow this conduit. In those instances where stenosis is severe, a tracheotomy followed by either expectant waiting or dilation may be necessary. Although controversy exists concerning the surgical correction of subglottic stenosis, a variety of techniques are available. These include anterior laryngotracheal decompression (cricoid split); laryngotracheal reconstruction with auricular cartilage, nasal septal, costal, or thyroid cartilage; pedicled hyoid bone interposition graft; laser excision of the stenosis; or long-term tracheotomy to allow laryngeal growth.

Progressive laryngeal stridor and a croup-like illness in the first several months of life suggest a lesion simulating subglottic stenosis—the **subglottic hemangioma.** The neoplasm is a soft compressible, bluish tumor below the level of the true vocal cords that is frequently poorly delineated from surrounding tissue. There is a 2:1 female to male preponderance, and 50% of the lesions are associated with cutaneous hemangiomas. The lateral neck film confirms the presence of a localized subglottic soft tissue mass.

Mechanical airway obstruction is treated with tracheotomy; however, early therapy with systemic corticosteroids may decrease the need for tracheotomy. Hemangiomas producing severe airway obstruction that do not respond to corticosteroids or regress spontaneously should be surgically removed. Because they are so vascular, these lesions are best controlled with the neodymium:YAG laser.

Drake AF et al: Lateral cricoid cuts as an adjunctive measure to enlarge stenotic subglottic airway. An anatomic study. Int J Pediatr Otorhinolaryngol 1989;18:129.

Montgomery WW, Montgomery SK: Manual for use of Montgomery laryngotracheal and esophageal prosthesis. Ann Otol Rhinol Laryngol Suppl 1990;150:2.

Larger Infants & Children

Supraglottitis is an acute inflammatory disorder of the larynx secondary to infection with H influenzae type B that affects the epiglottis, aryepiglottic folds, arytenoids, and ventricular bands (Table 39–5). There is usually no prodromal phase, and dysphagia, odynophagia, and shortness of breath rapidly progress to drooling, inspiratory stridor, and a muffled but clear voice. The disease affects principally children 2–6 years of age. Most children are extremely toxic, with fever, tachycardia, and tachypnea. The child sits erect, anxious and increasingly exhausted, drooling, and hungry for air. Lateral neck films confirm the diagnosis and reveal massive edema of the epiglottis (Figure 39–8).

Immediate control of the airway is mandatory and lifesaving. Children are given 100% humidified oxygen and taken immediately to the operating room, where rapid halothane and oxygen anesthetic induction is followed by atraumatic peroral endotracheal intubation. Pharyngeal blood cultures are obtained, and an intravenous line is started. A course of parenteral antibiotics consisting of (1) ampicillin and chloramphenicol, (2) cefuroxime, (3) cefotaxime, or (4) ceftriaxone is initiated pending culture and sensitivity reports. Many consultants today prefer

Table 39–5. Laryngotracheobronchitis and supraglottitis.

Laryngotracheobronchitis	Supraglottitis
Onset and history Relatively slow in onset as the terminal event of a 4- or 5-day respiratory tract infection	Rapid in onset and progression, advancing to severe airway obstruction within 6–8 hours. Usually no antecedent respiratory infection.
Etiology Usually viral but may be bacterial	Usually bacterial (*Haemophilus influenzae*) but may be viral
Symptoms Stridor, barking cough, sometimes hoarseness	Stridor preceded by severe sore throat and dysphagia (drooling)
X-ray findings Narrowing of the subglottic airway ("steeple sign")	Enlarged epiglottis on soft tissue lateral to the pharynx and larynx (thumbprint sign)
Treatment Early: Moist oxygen, corticosteroids, antibiotics, and nebulized epinephrine Late: Endoscopic intubation with or without tracheostomy	Immediate moist oxygen and early establishment of an airway by endoscopic intubation. This is followed by administration of intravenous antibiotics.

ceftriaxone. If a history of penicillin allergy is obtained, aztreonam or chloramphenicol alone is begun. Direct laryngoscopy is performed to rule out other potential causes of acute laryngeal obstruction. Direct inspection of the larynx reveals a cherry-red swollen epiglottis. At this time, the endotracheal tube is changed to a nasotracheal tube (1–2 sizes smaller than normal). Within 36–48 hours, the infant in generally afebrile and coughing around the tube during suctioning and may be successfully extubated.

By contrast, **acute laryngotracheobronchitis** is a viral illness that is far more common than acute supraglottitis (Table 39–5). This illness occurs chiefly in late autumn and winter, with parainfluenza (types 1, 2, 3) and influenza A and B viruses accounting for most cases. The principal lesion is subglottic edema, with a variable component of tracheobronchial inflammation. Infants 3 months to 3 years of age are principally affected, exhibiting a 2:1 female to male ratio. The symptoms of barking cough, hoarseness, inspiratory and expiratory stridor, and substernal retractions are frequently preceded by an insidious upper respiratory tract illness lasting 1–7 days. In contrast to children with supraglottitis, the infant appears sick but not toxic. Anteroposterior neck films confirm the clinical impression of marked subglottic narrowing and assist in excluding aerodigestive tract foreign bodies, mediastinal tumors, laryngotracheal neoplasms, and vascular compression of the trachea (Figure 39–9). Initial treatment includes high humidification, oxygenation, hydration, and parenteral cor-

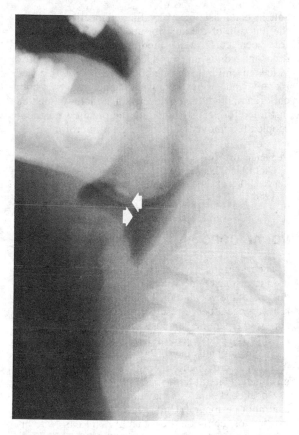

Figure 39–8. Lateral neck film in child with acute supraglottitis. Note the enlarged epiglottis (arrows).

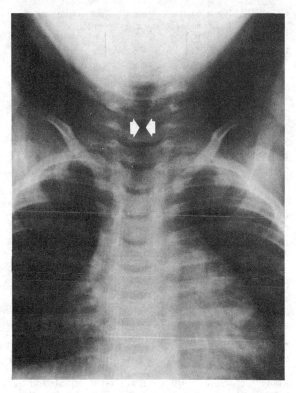

Figure 39–9. Anteroposterior chest film in infant with laryngotracheobronchitis. Marked narrowing of the subglottic space is seen (arrows).

ticosteroids. Cefuroxime is recommended if the disease is complicated by pneumonia. Racemic epinephrine is administered by nebulizer, decreasing airway obstruction within 10–30 minutes after administration, with the effect waning after 2 hours. Patients with progressive hypoxia, cyanosis, hypercapnia, and increasing tachypnea and tachycardia who do not respond to medical management should be intubated. Tracheotomy is performed after 3–4 days of intubation if significant subglottic stenosis associated with prolonged intubation with an inflamed larynx. The only difference between adult and pediatric tracheotomy is that in children, a vertical incision of the trachea is used and no cartilage is excised.

Kairys SW et al: Steroid treatment of laryngotracheitis: A meta analysis of the evidence from randomized trials. Pediatrics 1989;83:683.

Losek JD et al: Epiglottitis: Comparison of signs and symptoms in children less than two years and older. Ann Emerg Med 1990;19:55.

Skolnik NS: Treatment of croup. Am J Dis Child 1989; 143:1045.

Super DM et al: A prospective randomized double blind study to evaluate the effect of dexamethasone in acute laryngotracheitis. J Pediatr 1989;115:323.

LARYNGEAL PAPILLOMAS

Laryngeal papillomas are thought to be caused by the human papovavirus. They may occur as early as 1 year of age but are more common in the second or third year. There is an association between laryngeal and respiratory tract papillomas in infants less than age 2 when there is a maternal history of genital condylomas and laryngeal papilloma. Neither cesarean section nor prepartum treatment of human papillomavirus lesions will always protect against neonatal acquisition of human papillomavirus. They present initially with hoarseness and may multiply rapidly to obstruct the airway. Papillomas recur promptly after surgical excision and may be implanted in the trachea or distal bronchi by mechanical trauma. CO_2 laser excision of papillomas with the operating microscope appears to be associated with less risk of laryngeal stenosis and perhaps a decrease in the rate of recurrence. Since the laser bronchoscope has become available, it is easier to cure papillomas in the trachea than in the larynx. Alpha interferon is currently being evaluated as adjunctive therapy to reduce the growth rate of papilloma.

Cole RR, Myer CM III, Cotton RT: Tracheotomy in children with recurrent respiratory papillomatosis. Head Neck Surg 1989;11:226.

Quincey RE, Hall D, Croft DB: Laryngeal papillomatosis: Analysis of 113 patients. Clin Otolaryngol 1989;14:217.

Smith EM et al: Perinatal vertical transmission of human papilloma virus and subsequent development of respiratory tract papillomatosis. Ann Otol Rhinol Laryngol 1991;100:479.

LARYNGITIS

Acute laryngitis often occurs in association with a general viral upper respiratory tract infection predominantly caused by rhinoviruses, respiratory syncytial virus, and adenoviruses. However, if hoarseness persists for longer than several days, the possibility of secondary bacterial invasion by *M catarrhalis, H influenzae,* or *S pneumoniae* must be considered. Hoarseness, cough, and odynophagia are often quite marked, with minimal edema or erythema of the true vocal folds. Treatment includes voice rest, hydration, humidification, and oral cefuroxime, cefaclor, amoxicillin and clavulanic acid, or erythromycin plus a sulfonamide.

Chronic laryngitis, on the other hand, is related to many factors, including voice misuse, inhalation of irritants, gastroesophageal reflux, and chronic allergies. Pathologically, fluid accumulates in the subepithelial space of the vocal cords (Reinke's space). In some individuals, large sessile **polyps** may develop and occupy the entire vocal cord or portion thereof. The voice is severely compromised, having a hoarse and breathy character. In adults, polyps and chronic laryngitis are managed by voice rest, avoidance of chronic irritants, and speech therapy. Microdirect laryngoscopy and surgical excision with microforceps or the CO_2 laser are necessary for polyps not responding to conservative management. In patients with gastroesophageal reflux, nocturnal heartburn, chronic throat pain, and cough are common complaints. The diagnosis of posterior laryngitis in these patients secondary to reflux is confirmed by esophagogastroduodenoscopy, direct laryngoscopy, and 24-hour pH monitoring. Treatment with ranitidine, 150 mg orally twice a day for 12 weeks, suffices in most cases.

McNally PR: Evaluation of gastroesophageal reflux as the cause of idiopathic hoarseness. Dig Dis Sci 1989;34:1900.

Wilson JA et al: Gastroesophageal reflux and posterior laryngitis. Ann Otol Rhinol Laryngol 1989;98:405.

VOCAL NODULES

Misuse of the voice, particularly shouting or roaring in a very high or very low tone of voice, will result in condensation of hyaline connective tissue at the junction of the anterior and middle thirds of the true vocal cords. Vocal nodules occur in both children and adults and produce a hoarse and breathy voice. In children, most nodules regress with voice therapy, and surgical removal is unnecessary. In both children and adults, however, voice therapy must be instituted for persistent nodules before they are endoscopically removed with the laser or microforceps.

Benjamin B, Croxson G: Vocal nodules in children. Ann Otol Rhinol Laryngol 1987;96:530.

Lancer JM et al: Vocal nodules: a review. Clin Otolaryngol 1988;13:43.

VOCAL CORD PARALYSIS

The recurrent laryngeal nerves of the vagus nerves are the primary innervators of the abductors and adductors of the vocal folds. Isolated injury of the recurrent laryngeal nerve results in paralysis of the vocal cord in the paramedian position on one side, 2–3 mm lateral to the laryngeal midline. Combined injury of the recurrent and superior laryngeal nerves paralyzes the vocal cord in the intermediate position, several millimeters lateral to the paramedian position.

Vocal cord paralysis may be unilateral or bilateral, central or peripheral. Unilateral left vocal cord paralysis is most common. Less than 20% of cases are bilateral. Thyroidectomy is by far the most common cause of bilateral vocal cord paralysis. Central causes include brain stem and supranuclear lesions and account for only 5% of all cases. Supranuclear or cortical causes of vocal cord paralysis are exceedingly rare, owing to the bilateral crossed neural innervation to the brain stem medullary centers in the nucleus ambiguus. The most frequent central cause is vascular insufficiency or a stroke affecting the brain stem. Congenital central lesions are usually secondary to Arnold-Chiari malformation or brain stem dysgenesis and are often associated with additional cranial neuropathies.

Most cases of peripheral vocal cord paralysis are secondary to thyroidectomy or nonlaryngeal neoplasms, including bronchogenic, esophageal, and thyroid carcinoma. Other less common lesions causing paralysis of the vocal cord include tumors of the deep lobe of the parotid gland, carotid body tumors, glomus jugulare and vagale tumors, and neurogenic neoplasms of the tenth nerve and jugular foramen. External penetrating wounds to the neck or prolonged endotracheal intubation may also traumatize the recurrent laryngeal nerve, producing vocal cord paralysis. Finally, toxic neuropathy and idiopathic causes account for a few cases.

In adults, unilateral recurrent laryngeal nerve paralysis generally produces hoarseness and a weak, breathy voice with varying amounts of aspiration.

The normal vocal cord may cross the midline to approximate the paralyzed vocal cord in the paramedian position. In children, varying degrees of inspiratory stridor may also be present. Bilateral vocal cord paralysis is commonly associated with inspiratory stridor, shortness of breath, and dyspnea on exertion.

Diagnostic assessment of vocal cord paralysis includes indirect laryngoscopy, examination of the head and neck for neoplasms, chest x-ray, CT scan of the base of skull to upper mediastinum, thyroid scan, upper gastrointestinal series, and endoscopic evaluation of the aerodigestive tract.

Management of unilateral vocal cord paralysis due to lesions of the recurrent laryngeal nerve includes the injection of Teflon paste or Gelfoam under local anesthesia into the paralyzed vocal cord, mobilizing it medially. Medialization is valuable in the therapy of aspiration and results in dramatic improvement in voice quality. Other injection options for glottic insufficiency include bovine collagen, injectable fat, and Gelfoam. Medialization of the paralyzed cord may also be accomplished externally via a thyroidotomy and placement of a Silastic wedge implant inside the thyroid cartilage in a small pocket deep to the paralyzed vocal cord. In the past, bilateral paramedian vocal cord paralysis was commonly managed by permanent tracheotomy. More recently, arytenoidectomy through an endolaryngeal approach using the CO_2 laser has been used. This procedure may be complicated by loss of adequate voice production and exacerbation of aspiration. Attempts to treat bilateral abductor vocal cord paralysis with nerve-muscle transposition of the ansa hypoglossi nerve and the omohyoid muscle to the posterior cricoarytenoid muscle have met with qualified success. This reinnervation technique attempts to provide inspiratory neuronal input to the sole abductor of the vocal cord, the posterior cricoarytenoid muscle. Direct anastomosis of the ansa cervicalis to the recurrent laryngeal nerve may reinnervate the larynx and allow the tracheostomy tube to be removed.

Crumley RL: Teflon vs. thyroplasty vs. nerve transfer: A comparison. Ann Otol Rhinol Laryngol 1990;99:759.

Crumley RL: Muscle transfer for laryngeal paralysis. Arch Otolaryngol Head Neck Surg 1991;117:1113.

Green DC, Berk EGS, Graves MD: Functional evaluation of ansa cervicalis nerve transfer for unilateral vocal cord paralysis: Future directions for laryngeal reinnervation. Otolaryngol Head Neck Surg 1991;104:453.

Woo P et al: Functional staging for vocal cord paralysis. Otolaryngol Head Neck Surg 1991;105:440.

LARYNGEAL NEOPLASMS

Most malignant epithelial neoplasms of the larynx are squamous cell carcinomas, ranging from well-differentiated to undifferentiated cell types. Alcohol and tobacco abuse are common predisposing factors. Cancer of the larynx affects chiefly men in a 9:1 ratio to women. Any patient who complains of persistent hoarseness, odynophagia, "a lump in the throat," or a change in voice quality should be examined promptly by indirect laryngoscopy or flexible nasopharyngolaryngoscopy. Precancerous laryngeal lesions appearing as leukoplakia or erythroplasia often evolve into carcinoma and should be biopsied to rule out carcinoma in situ or invasive carcinoma. Additional findings that arouse suspicion of laryngeal carcinoma include persistent localized edema or ulceration, irregular epithelium, and a paralyzed vocal cord.

Suspicious epithelial lesions of the true vocal cords are treated surgically by removing the entire vocal cord epithelium or by laser excision. Fortunately, true vocal cord carcinomas tend to be well-differentiated, to grow slowly, and to metastasize late, because of the limited lymphatic drainage of the cords. As a result, cervical metastases are infrequent, and fixation of the vocal cord is an unusual early clinical finding. Glottic cancers without vocal cord fixation are successfully treated by irradiation (5500–6500 cGy in 5–7 weeks through a limited field). Total laryngectomy is necessary for vocal cord fixation and should include radical neck dissection followed by postoperative radiation therapy if cervical nodes are palpable.

Supraglottic carcinomas more often manifest local invasion and lymph node metastasis. As many as 50% of patients present with palpable metastases in jugular lymph nodes owing to the rich lymphatic drainage from this region. CT or MR imaging is obtained before endoscopic staging of tumors to look for occult metastases and delineate the extent of tumor invasion. Unfortunately, the patients seek care late, because the tumor does not interfere with phonation and breathing until it is relatively large. Spread to the base of the tongue and hypopharynx is common. For tumors that stop 5 mm above the anterior commissure, that do not involve the true vocal cords, and that do not extend 5 mm above the vallecula, a horizontal supraglottic laryngectomy combined with postoperative radiation therapy may preserve the vocal cords and phonation. The objectives of this operation and other procedures that preserve the larynx are to provide an adequate surgical margin, prevent aspiration, and conserve speech and the airway. This procedure is contraindicated in old and debilitated patients or those with severe chronic obstructive pulmonary disease. Radiation therapy to the neck is given routinely after surgery to treat clinically inapparent lymph node metastases or as an adjunct to radical neck dissection for palpable metastases.

True subglottic carcinomas are uncommon (< 5% of all laryngeal carcinomas). However, subglottic extension across the true vocal cord from a transglottic carcinoma is not unusual. When this occurs, lymphatic spread to the jugular chain, paratracheal, and tracheoesophageal lymph nodes may be rapid. Total laryngectomy is necessary for these tumors and other far-advanced laryngeal carcinomas. Irradiation is used as primary therapy for patients who reject laryngectomy. A method of speech rehabilitation is preoperatively discussed with each patient and may include esophageal speech, artificial larynx, or surgical restoration. Excellent vocal restoration is achieved with insertion of a valved silicone prosthesis in a fistula created between the posterior tracheal wall and the anterior esophageal wall. By manually occlusion of the tube after inhalation, air is diverted into the hypopharynx, and the intact pharyngeal resonators and oral articulators assist in speech formation. Periodic follow-up examinations of the remainder of the aerodigestive tract are mandatory for the rest of the patient's life, because of the high incidence of second or even third primary carcinomas.

Bocca E: Surgical management of supraglottic cancer and its lymph node metastases in a conservative perspective. Ann Otol Rhinol Laryngol 1991;100:261.

Casiano RR et al: Laser cordectomy for T1 glottic carcinoma: a ten year experience and videostroboscopic findings. Otolaryngol Head Neck Surg 1991;104:831.

DeRienzo DP, Greenberg SD, Fraire AE: Carcinoma of the larynx, changing incidence in women. Arch Otolaryngol Head Neck Surg 1991;117:681.

Pellitteri PK et al: Radiotherapy. The mainstay in the treatment of early glottic carcinoma. Arch Otolaryngol Head Neck Surg 1991;117:297.

Recher G et al: Italian experience of voice restoration after laryngectomy with tracheoesophageal puncture. Ann Otol Rhinol Laryngol 1991;100:206.

Rothfield RE, Myers EN, Johnson JT: Carcinoma in situ and microinvasive squamous cell carcinoma of the vocal cords. Ann Otolaryngol Rhinol Laryngol 1991;100:793.

INFLAMMATORY NECK MASSES*

Acute suppurative lymphadenitis usually occurs in infants and children with viral upper respiratory tract infections. In adults with AIDS, it may initially present with painful lymphadenopathy in the neck. Bacterial lymphadenitis commonly develops secondary to infection with group A streptococci, S aureus, or mouth anaerobes and may evolve into a deep neck abscess forming a lateral neck mass. These abscesses are most commonly mixed infections, with anaerobic organisms predominating. Mixed infections are synergistic, and β-lactamase production is common.High fever and leukocytosis characterize this complication. Deep neck abscesses may develop in the prevertebral, sublingual, submandibular, submental, or retropharyngeal spaces as well as in the lateral neck region. Abscesses of the neck are compartmentalized by two of the three envelopes of the deep cervical fascia: the superficial, middle, and deep layers. Infections may spread from one space to another or extend downward into the mediastinum. In addition, cellulitis or abscess formation in the retropharyngeal space or sublingual space (Ludwig's angina) can obstruct the airway. Infection around the carotid sheath may also produce serious hemorrhage by necrosis of the great vessels and their branches.

Patients with deep neck infections should be hospitalized immediately. An intravenous antistaphylococcal penicillin or clindamycin, ceftazidime, or aztreonam is used. Preoperative localization of the abscess is performed with CT scanning. MRI may be superior to CT in some cases. The airway should be controlled with an endotracheal tube or tracheostomy before the abscess is incised and drained. The surgical approach to a deep neck abscess depends on the space involved. Proximal control of the carotid artery should be obtained. The lateral pharyngeal space is approached through an incision parallel to the anterior border of the sternocleidomastoid muscle. Most retropharyngeal abscesses are drained intraorally. Submandibular abscesses are approached through an incision 2 cm below the inferior border of the mandible.

Chronic granulomatous infections, which may involve the cervical lymph nodes, include tuberculosis, cat-scratch disease, infections with atypical mycobacteria, and occasionally actinomycosis. Tuberculous adenitis commonly develops following pulmonary tuberculosis and usually responds to triple-drug chemotherapy. Persistently enlarged or suppurative nodes should be excised. Atypical mycobacterial adenitis, on the other hand, is seldom associated with pulmonary disease, and routine tuberculin skin tests are either negative or weakly positive. In contrast to tuberculous adenitis, these atypical infections do not respond well to chemotherapy alone and frequently must be excised. Neck masses may result from intravenous cervical drug abuse. S aureus is the most common pathogen, and treatment with incision and drainage and intravenous nafcillin or cephalothin is recommended.

Finally, actinomycosis may present as an abscess with multiple draining sinuses near the angle of the mandible, discharging pus with characteristic sulfur granules. Often there is underlying dental disease or osteomyelitis of the adjacent bone. Long-term (3–4 weeks) intravenous penicillin in high doses is necessary; surgical excision should be reserved for persistent disease.

de Marie S et al: Clinical infections and nonsurgical treatment of parapharyngeal space infections complicating throat infection. Rev Infect Dis 1989;11:975.

---

*See also Chapter 15, Tumors of the Head and Neck.

Gianoli GJ et al: Retropharyngeal space infection: Changing trends. Otolaryngol Head Neck Surg 1991;105:92.

Hawkins DB, Austin JR: Abscesses of the neck in infants and young children: A review of 112 cases. Ann Otol Rhinol Laryngol 1991;100:361.

Yuh WTC et al: Magnetic resonance imaging and computed tomography in pediatric head and neck masses. Ann Otol Rhinol Laryngol 1991;100:54.

ACQUIRED IMMUNE DEFICIENCY SYNDROME IN OTOLARYNGOLOGY

Because of AIDS, the otolaryngologist is encountering previously rare diseases more often. Examples include cranial and cervical herpes zoster, oral hairy leukoplakia, and oral candidiasis. There are many similarities between AIDS and primary immunodeficiency disorders, including ataxia-telangiectasia, common variable immunodeficiency disease, Wiscott-Aldrich syndrome, and severe combined immunodeficiency disease. As immunosuppressed patients survive longer, they are beginning to manifest cancers such as lymphomas and squamous cell carcinomas in addition to Kaposi's sarcoma.

The most common manifestations of AIDS in the head neck region are sinusitis and postnasal discharge. In the mouth, Kaposi's sarcoma may occur, primarily on the hard palate. Lymphoma and oral candidiasis are also common. Hairy leukoplakia, a nontender lesion caused by the Epstein-Barr virus, is frequently seen with major aphthous ulcers. In the cervical region, Kaposi's sarcoma, lymphoma, and *Mycobacterium avium-intracellulare* infections are also encountered.

The otologic manifestations of AIDS are primarily hearing loss, otalgia, otorrhea, vertigo, and tinnitus. Sensorineural hearing loss is the most common finding, with the loss greater in high frequencies. Most commonly, Kaposi's sarcoma presents as a flat lesion involving the auricle. Kaposi's sarcoma of the ear canal is easily managed with the argon laser. *Pneumocystis carinii* granuloma of the ear canal is treated by resection and sulfonamide drugs. There is no evidence of increased external ear canal fungal infection in AIDS. However, serous otitis media due to auditory tube dysfunction secondary to benign lymphoid hyperplasia is frequent.

The herpes zoster oticus syndrome (Ramsay Hunt's syndrome) is associated with facial paralysis, vertigo, and hearing loss. Ototoxic drugs used in the treatment of AIDS include acyclovir (which produces vertigo), trimethoprim-sulfamethaxosole (which produces vertigo and tinnitus), and zidovudine (which causes vertigo and hearing loss). The human immune deficiency virus may alter the natural course of latent syphilis, and patients may present with otosyphilis that is difficult to treat because of the poor vascularity of the otic capsule and its isolation from cerebrospinal fluid. Early treatment with zidovudine (AZT) may help control progression of the disease. Treatment for Kaposi's sarcoma and non-Hodgkin's lymphoma is combination chemotherapy or chemotherapy plus erythropoietic support drugs.

Corey JP, Seligman I: Otolaryngology problems in the immune compromised patient: An evolving natural history. Otolaryngol Head Neck Surg 1991;104:196.

Volberding PA et al: Zidovudine in asymptomatic human immunodeficiency virus infection: A controlled trial in persons with fewer than 500 CD4 positive cells per cubic millimeter. N Engl J Med 1990;322:941.

REFERENCES

Bluestone CD, Casselbrant ML (editors): Workshop on epidemiology of otitis media. Ann Otol Rhinol Laryngol 1990;(Suppl 149):1.

Bluestone CD, Klein JO (editors): Workshop on the role of anaerobic bacteria infections of the upper respiratory tract–head and neck. Ann Otol Rhinol Laryngol 1991; 100(Suppl 154):1.

Friedman M (editor): Endoscopic sinus surgery. Otolaryngol Clin North Am 1989;22.

Friedman EM, Healy GB (editors): Pediatric otolaryngology. Otolaryngol Clin North Am 1989;22.

Goycoolea MV (editor): Otitis media. Otolaryngol Clin North Am 1991;24.

Kimmelman CP (editor): Nasal obstruction. Otolaryngol Clin North Am 1989;22.

Koopman CF, Moran WB (editors): Sleep apnea. Otolaryngol Clin North Am 1990;23.

Mattox DE (editor): Management of facial nerve disorders. Otolaryngol Clin North Am 1991;24.

Osguthorpe JD, Melnick W (editors): Clinical audiology. Otolaryngol Clin North Am 1991;24.

Paparella NM, Maniglia AJ (editors): Otology: Current concepts and technology. Otolaryngol Clin North Am 1989;22.

Parisier SC, Edelstein DR (editors): Cholesteatoma. Otolaryngol Clin North Am 1989;22.

Parkin JL (editor): Lasers in otolaryngology. Otolaryngol Clin North Am 1990;23.

Sisson GA, Pelzer HG (editors): Head neck diseases in the elderly. Otolaryngol Clin North Am 1990;23.

Wigan DME: *Endoscopic Surgery of the Paranasal Sinuses and Anterior Skull Base.* Thieme, 1990.

40

The Eye & Ocular Adnexa

Khalid F. Tabbara, MD

EXAMINATION OF THE EYE

Evaluation of the eye and its adnexa requires a good history, physical examination of the eyes, and assessment of visual function. The history should include general information about the patient's age, occupation, and health status as well as ocular complaints. Occasionally, special examinations may be required to identify specific ocular disorders or to establish the presence of associated systemic disease.

The basic office equipment required for a routine eye examination by a nonophthalmologist includes the following: (1) a hand-held flashlight, (2) a binocular magnifying loupe, (3) an ophthalmoscope, (4) a visual acuity chart, and (5) a tonometer.

The basic medications required for an eye examination are (1) a local anesthetic such as proparacaine 0.5% or tetracaine 0.5%; (2) fluorescein strips; and (3) dilating drops, such as phenylephrine 2.5% or tropicamide 1%.

Visual Acuity Testing

Central visual acuity should be part of the routine examination of the eye in all patients. The Snellen chart is most commonly used. The patient faces the test chart at a distance of 6 meters (20 feet). The patient is tested by occluding one eye at a time and reading the chart with the unoccluded eye. Visual acuity corresponds to the smallest line the patient can read and is recorded as 20/20, 20/30, 20/40, 20/50, etc. The patient who is unable to read the large letters at the top of the chart should be moved progressively closer until the characters can be read, whereupon the distance between the patient and the chart should be recorded. If the patient wears eyeglasses for distance, the visual acuity should be repeated with the glasses on and the results recorded as uncorrected vision and corrected vision. Preschool children or illiterates should be properly instructed and then tested with the illiterate E chart.

Visual Field Testing (Perimetry)

Visual field testing (perimetry) is used to examine the central and peripheral visual fields. The technique is performed separately for each eye. It is used to measure the function of the retina, the optic nerve and the intracranial visual pathway. Because perimetry relies on subjective patient responses, the results will depend on the patient's alertness and cooperation. Several methods are used to assess visual field functions, including the tangent screen, Goldmann perimetry, and computerized automated perimetry.

Tonometry

Tonometry measures intraocular pressure. The two most common instruments are the Schiotz tonometer and applanation tonometer. The Schiotz tonometer measures the amount of corneal indentation produced by a preset amount of weight or force. The softer the eye, the less force is required to indent the cornea, and this is measured on a scale. The normal intraocular pressure varies between 10 and 20 mm Hg.

Inspection of Anterior Segment & Adnexa

Inspection of the external ocular structures—lids, conjunctiva, cornea, sclera, and lacrimal apparatus—should include everting the upper eyelids for inspection of the conjunctival surface with the patient looking down. The exposed surfaces are inspected for anatomic defects, foreign bodies, lacerations, inflammation, discharge, tearing, dryness, or other abnormalities. In patients who are unconscious or in coma, the degree of lid closure and the presence of Bell's phenomenon—upward position of the cornea during sleep—are significant findings. Corneal sensation and reflexes in each eye should be noted before any anesthetic drops are used. With the aid of a hand-held flashlight and magnifying loupe or with a biomicroscope (slit lamp), the eye and adnexa can be inspected.

A direct ophthalmoscope focused on the ocular surface may provide some magnification. In addition, considerable detail of the ocular surface can be observed using a +20 diopter lens and a hand-held flashlight. The depth of the anterior chamber should be noted by shining a light across the eye.

Assessment of Pupillary Functions

Examination of the pupils should be performed before any dilating drops are instilled. In hospitalized patients and those with neurologic disorders, pupils should be dilated with discretion and only with short-acting mydriatics. Both direct and consensual light reflexes of the pupils should be assessed. The size of the pupil should be noted, and any differences between the size of the right and left pupil should be recorded and described.

Eye Movements

Ocular motility should be assessed in different directions of gaze. In examining eye movements, one should note random movements, the position of the eyes in primary gaze, the alignment of the eyes and whether there are deviations or latent nystagmus, the convergence of the eyes, and ductions in the cardinal positions of gaze. Oculocephalic reflexes may be tested, and the response to forced eyelid closure or Bell's phenomenon should be noted. Light reflection ("reflex") is at the same point in each eye when the eyes are straight.

Whenever indicated, optokinetic and caloric stimulation of the external ear canal should be performed.

Ophthalmoscopy

Ophthalmoscopy is important for the diagnosis of both ocular and systemic conditions. It can be critical in neurologic and neurosurgical contexts. In most instances, the optic nerve head can be clearly seen without dilating the pupils. In hospitalized patients with neurologic and neurosurgical disorders, dilation of the pupils should be avoided, because the pupillary reflexes are abolished by dilation, and they are important for initial or follow-up assessment of certain neurologic conditions. In exceptional cases when doing so does not jeopardize neurologic follow-up and care, short-acting mydriatics such as phenylephrine 2.5% can be used to dilate the pupils.

SYMPTOMS & SIGNS OF OCULAR DISORDERS

Visual disturbances or decrease in visual acuity may be due to a number of ocular and systemic diseases.

Decrease in Visual Acuity

Decrease in visual acuity may be unilateral or bilateral, painful or painless, and persistent or transient. The duration of the decrease in visual acuity is important. Was the change noted recently? Was it gradual or sudden? Was it binocular or monocular? Was it discovered accidentally? Unilateral acute painful loss of vision may be due to angle-closure glaucoma, endophthalmitis, or uveitis. Painless unilateral loss of vision may be due to ischemic optic neuropathy, optic neuritis, central retinal artery or vein occlusion, retinal detachment, vitreous hemorrhage, or retinal hemorrhages. Transient painless acute loss of vision in one eye may be due to migraine or amaurosis fugax. Bilateral acute loss of vision may be due to

pituitary abnormality, ophthalmic migraine, conversion reaction, or intracranial vascular occlusion.

Disturbances in Vision

Disturbances in vision may consist of image distortion, photophobia, color change, spots before the eyes, visual field defects, night blindness, momentary loss of vision, or haloes around lights. Distortion of normal shapes is most often due to astigmatism or macular lesions. Photophobia is commonly due to corneal inflammation, iritis, ocular albinism, or aniridia. Changes in color (chromatopsia) such as yellow vision are due to retinal lesions or the use of systemic medications such as digoxin. Spots before the eyes are reported by patients with vitreous opacities or in association with intraocular inflammation. Visual field defects may be due to lid edema, retinal and optic nerve lesions, lesions in the visual pathway, or cortical abnormalities. Night blindness may be congenital, such as in patients with retinitis pigmentosa, or acquired—eg, as a result of vitamin A deficiency, glaucoma, optic atrophy, cataract, or retinal degeneration. Transient loss of vision may imply impending cerebrovascular accident or partial occlusion of the internal carotid artery. Haloes around lights or bright objects are suggestive of acute angle-closure glaucoma. Incipient cataract may also cause haloes around light sources.

Double Vision (Diplopia)

Double vision can be constant or intermittent and may occur suddenly in certain positions of gaze or only at certain distances. It is important to differentiate between horizontal diplopia and vertical diplopia, because the nerve pathways are different. Monocular diplopia occurs in lenticular changes, macular lesions, malingering, or conversion reactions. Binocular double vision is most often due to misalignment of the eyes from extraocular muscle dysfunction or neurologic abnormalities.

Ocular & Orbital Pain

Ocular pain may result from corneal lesions, inflammations, increase in intraocular pressure, anterior uveitis, cyclitis, scleritis, or optic neuritis. Other causes of pain from the ocular adnexa may result from inflammations of the orbit or tumors in the orbit. Dacryocystitis may also cause severe pain. Pain may arise from infections of the meibomian glands and the glands of Zeis and Moll.

Redness of the Eye

Acute redness (injection) of the eye not associated with trauma may be due to conjunctivitis, acute anterior uveitis, acute angle-closure glaucoma, corneal infection, or corneal erosion (Table 40–1). Subconjunctival hemorrhage may also present as a red eye. Conjunctivitis is the most frequent cause of red eye and can be due to bacterial, chlamydial, viral, or

Table 40–1. Differential diagnosis of common causes of inflamed eye.

	Acute Conjunctivitis	Acute Iritis[1]	Acute glaucoma[2]	Corneal Trauma or Infection
Incidence	Extremely common	Common	Uncommon	Common
Discharge	Moderate to copious	None	None	Watery or purulent
Vision	No effect on vision	Slightly blurred	Markedly blurred	Usually blurred
Pain	None	Moderate	Severe	Moderate to severe
Conjunctival injection	Diffuse; more toward fornices	Mainly circumcorneal	Diffuse	Diffuse
Cornea	Clear	Usually clear	Steamy	Change in clarity related to cause
Pupil size	Normal	Small	Moderately dilated and fixed	Normal
Pupillary light response	Normal	Poor	None	Normal
Intraocular pressure	Normal	Normal	Elevated	Normal
Smear	Causative organisms	No organisms	No organisms	Organisms found only in corneal ulcers due to infection

[1]Acute anterior uveitis.
[2]Angle-closure glaucoma.

allergic causes. Nonspecific irritation by exogenous agents or a foreign body may also cause redness of the eye.

Discharge

Ocular discharge may be noted as watery, mucopurulent, purulent, or chronic crusting of the lid margins. When the discharge is watery and not associated with redness or pain, it may be due to excessive formation of tears or obstruction of the lacrimal passages. Watery discharge with photophobia, pain, or irritation may be due to keratitis or keratoconjunctivitis. Purulent discharge is a sign of bacterial infection or severe inflammation of the conjunctival surface. Mucopurulent discharge may be due to infections with bacterial organisms (eg, *Haemophilus* spp). When the discharge forms mucoid strings, it is characteristic of allergic disorders involving the conjunctiva.

Swelling of the Eyelids

Swelling of the eyelids may be unilateral or bilateral. In unilateral swelling, the patient may suffer from infection of the glands of Meibom, Zeis, or Moll; bilateral swelling may indicate blepharitis or allergic dermatitis. Systemic diseases associated with water retention, hyperthyroidism, or hypothyroidism may also be associated with swelling or puffiness of the eyelids.

Displacement of the Eyes

Forward displacement of the eyes (exophthalmos, proptosis) may be due to abnormalities of the thyroid glands or to tumors of the orbit.

Squint

Squint is due to misalignment of the eyes due to muscle imbalance and may be in the form of tropia (manifest squint) or phoria (latent squint). Ocular deviations may be lateral (exotropia) or medial (esotropia) and upward (hypertropia) or downward (hypotropia).

Leukocoria

A white pupil in a child may signify a serious eye disorder. The most frequent causes of leukocoria is congenital cataract, which requires urgent management to prevent amblyopia. Other causes of leukocoria include retinoblastoma, retrolental fibroplasia (retinopathy of prematurity), toxocariasis, persistent hyperplastic primary vitreous, vitreous hemorrhage, retinal detachment, retinal dysplasia, incontinentia pigmenti, Coats's disease, and Norrie's disease.

DISEASES OF THE EYE & ADNEXA

ACUTE HORDEOLUM

Acute hordeolum (sty) is a common infection of the glands of the eyelids involving the glands of Zeis or Moll (external hordeolum). The meibomian glands may be infected, leading to internal hordeolum. The usual causative agent is *Staphylococcus aureus.*

Acute hordeolum is characterized by pain, swelling, and redness of the eyelid. A large hordeolum is rarely associated with a preauricular lymph node. Hordeolum may form an abscess in the eyelid.

If pus is localized and pointing out to the skin or conjunctiva, treatment consists of making a local horizontal (skin) or vertical (conjunctiva) incision. If there is no evidence of abscess formation, the patient can be discharged with instructions to apply warm compresses three times daily and to use topical antibiotics such as erythromycin or bacitracin ophthalmic ointment twice daily for 5–7 days.

CONJUNCTIVITIS

Acute conjunctivitis is the most frequent cause of red eye. Infectious causes include bacterial, viral, chlamydial, fungal, and parasitic agents. Less common causes of conjunctivitis include chemical irritation, allergy, hypersensitivity to topical medications, vitamin A deficiency, dry eye syndrome, and injury.

Clinical Findings
A. Symptoms and Signs: Patients with conjunctivitis complain of irritation, a foreign body sensation, and conjunctival discharge. One or both eyes may be affected. In patients with bacterial conjunctivitis, the eyelids may be stuck together in the morning. Examination reveals conjunctival hyperemia with purulent or mucopurulent discharge and variable degrees of lid swelling.

B. Laboratory Findings: If bacterial conjunctivitis is suspected, conjunctival swabs and scrapings should be taken for culture on blood agar and chocolate agar and for staining with Gram's and Giemsa's stains.

Treatment
Treatment of patients with allergic conjunctivitis consists of topical decongestants such as naphazoline 0.1% and an H_1 receptor blocker or disodium cromoglycate 2% eye drops four times daily. In severe cases of allergic conjunctivitis, topical corticosteroids may be used under the surveillance of an ophthalmologist. In patients with suspected bacterial conjunctivitis and until laboratory reports are received, topical broad-spectrum antibacterial agents can be prescribed, eg, sulfacetamide 10% eye drops or ciprofloxacin 0.3% eye drops four to six times daily during the day plus erythromycin or tetracycline ophthalmic ointment at bedtime.

CORNEAL ULCERS

Corneal infections leading to ulceration maybe due to bacteria (including chlamydiae), viruses, fungi, or protozoa. The most serious infection of the cornea is caused by *Pseudomonas* spp.

Clinical Findings
A. Symptoms and Signs: Patients with corneal ulcers complain of pain, photophobia, and blurring of vision. Patients develop conjunctival hyperemia and chemosis, with ulceration of the cornea and whitish or yellowish infiltration. Hypopyon (pus in the anterior chamber) may be present in cases due to bacterial or fungal infections.

B. Laboratory Findings: Laboratory studies include culture and cytologic inspection of corneal scrapings.

Treatment
Corneal ulceration is a serious condition that should be managed carefully and followed closely. The most severe and devastating infection of the cornea is caused by *Pseudomonas aeruginosa.* Specific topical and subconjunctival antibiotics should be given on an empirical basis until the results of culture and sensitivity tests are reported, and specific antimicrobial treatment should then be given. Central corneal ulcers may leave corneal scars, causing loss of vision. Patients so affected may require penetrating keratoplasty (corneal graft).

Patients wearing contact lenses should be advised to stop wearing them. Patients using topical corticosteroids should stop using them.

DACRYOCYSTITIS

Dacryocystitis is a common infection of the lacrimal sac. It may be acute or chronic and occurs most often in infants and in persons over age 40 years. It is usually unilateral and always secondary to obstruction of the nasolacrimal duct.

Normally, the nasolacrimal ducts open spontaneously during the first month of life. Occasionally, failure of canaliculization of one or both ducts leads to obstruction of the nasolacrimal ducts and secondary dacryocystitis.

The cause of nasolacrimal duct obstruction is usually unknown, but trauma to the nose or infection may be responsible. In infants, dacryocystitis leading to obstruction may be due to *Haemophilus influenzae,* staphylococci, or streptococci. In patients with trachoma, nasolacrimal and canalicular obstruction is common. The cause of acute dacryocystitis in adults is usually *Staphylococcus aureus* or betahemolytic streptococci. In chronic dacryocystitis, *Streptococcus pneumoniae* is a common cause.

Clinical Findings
A. Symptoms and Signs: Acute dacryocystitis is characterized by pain, swelling, tenderness, and redness in the tear sac area; pus may be expressed. In chronic dacryocystitis, tearing and discharge are the principal signs. Mucus or pus may be expressed from the tear sac.

B. Laboratory Findings: Pus can be expressed from the upper or lower puncta and should be examined by Gram's stain and culture and sensitivity testing.

Treatment

A. Adults: Acute dacryocystitis responds well to systemic antibiotic therapy, but recurrences are common if the obstruction is not surgically relieved.

B. Infants: When ductal obstruction is due to failure of canaliculization in the first month of life, forceful massage of the tear sac is indicated, and topical antibiotics should be instilled in the conjunctival sac four or five times daily. If this is not successful after a few weeks, probing of the nasolacrimal duct is indicated regardless of the infant's age. The probe should be passed through the upper canaliculus.

ORBITAL CELLULITIS

Orbital cellulitis is manifested by an abrupt onset of swelling and redness of the lids, accompanied by proptosis and fever. It is usually caused by staphylococci or streptococci. Immediate treatment with systemic antibiotics is indicated to prevent abscess formation and rapid increase in the orbital pressure, which may interfere with the blood supply to the eye. The response to antibiotics is excellent, but surgical drainage may be required if an abscess forms.

PTERYGIUM

Pterygium is a fleshy, triangular encroachment of the conjunctiva onto the nasal side of the cornea and is usually associated with excessive exposure to wind, sun, sand, and dust. Pterygium may be either unilateral or bilateral. There may be a genetic predisposition, but no hereditary pattern has been described. Excision is indicated if the growth threatens vision by approaching the pupillary area.

Treatment is by superficial excision. After excising large or recurrent pterygia, autologous conjunctival tissue transplantation is indicated. A thin layer of conjunctiva is obtained from the upper bulbar conjunctiva and sutured to the area where the pterygium was removed. This leads to rapid restoration of anatomic integrity of the epithelial surface and may prevent further recurrences. Patients should be advised to wear sunglasses out of doors.

CATARACT

Cataract is an opacity in the lens that may lead to decrease in vision when it occupies the visual axis. Cataract is the leading cause of curable blindness in the world.

There are three types: (1) congenital cataract, (2) cataract associated with other disorders, and (3) age-related (senile) cataract. Some cataracts are rapidly progressive, while others may show slow progression.

1. CONGENITAL CATARACT

Congenital cataract may be genetically determined or may be caused by intrauterine factors that interfere with normal development of the lens. Intrauterine viral infections (the most common is rubella), for example, can lead to congenital cataract.

Congenital cataract may be unilateral or bilateral and complete or incomplete. Dense cataract present at birth is an indication for urgent operative management to prevent amblyopia. Extracapsular posterior extraction with central posterior capsulectomy and limited anterior vitrectomy is recommended for congenital cataract. Preservation of the posterior capsule and zonule is important for future implantation of intraocular lenses. If the cataract is aspirated, leaving the posterior capsule intact, the posterior capsule becomes opaque, requiring discission at a later stage. Correction with soft contact lenses can be started immediately after surgery. Posterior chamber intraocular lenses may be implanted when the child is older.

Epikeratophakia is a new form of refractive corneal surgery for the correction of hyperopia that can be used following cataract extraction. Epikeratophakia utilizes a corneal tissue lenticule—obtained in lyophilized form from a commercial source and frozen and lathed—sutured onto the surface of the recipient cornea after removal of the corneal epithelium. The parameters required to order such a lenticule are similar to those required in ordering a contact lens, including the refractive power of the eye and the corneal curvature. The lathed corneal tissue eventually becomes repopulated by keratocytes from the patient's cornea and exists as an extension of the normal corneal tissue, increasing the dioptric power of the cornea. It is possible to exchange or replace failed epigrafts.

Restoration of binocular vision in very young children is seldom achieved after operation in cases of unilateral congenital cataracts.

2. CATARACTS ASSOCIATED WITH OTHER DISORDERS

Several systemic conditions may be associated with cataracts. Examples are diabetes mellitus, galactosemia, hypocalcemia, myotonic dystrophy, Down's syndrome, cutaneous disorders such as atopic dermatitis, systemic drugs, or eye drops (corticosteroids). Other disorders of the eye may also be associated with cataracts, such as retinal detachment or chronic uveitis. Physical, mechanical, and thermal injury or ionizing radiation may also lead to cataract.

The treatment of such cataracts is similar to that of senile cataract.

3. SENILE CATARACT (Age-Related Cataract)

Senile cataract—due to aging of the lens—is the most common type. The rate of progression is variable. Diagnosis is by slit lamp examination. In advanced cataract, a white opacity may be seen in the pupillary area upon gross inspection.

Treatment

Once the cataract leads to visual impairment, treatment is by surgical removal of the lens. Clinical trials of agents that may delay or prevent the formation of cataracts are under way, but no pharmacologic means of prevention is available at present.

Cataract surgery can be done in three different ways. All three methods give excellent results, with complete restoration of visual acuity. In cases where intraocular lenses are contraindicated, such as in certain forms of uveitis, optical correction can be achieved with eyeglasses or contact lenses.

A. Intracapsular Lens Extraction: Intracapsular extraction removes the lens entirely within its capsule either by forceps or a cryoprobe. This procedure cannot be performed on children or young adults be-

cause of the adhesion between the lens and the vitreous.

B. Extracapsular Extraction: (Figure 40–1.) Extracapsular cataract extraction is the most widely used procedure at present. The anterior capsule of the lens is removed; the nucleus of the cataract is expressed; and the residual cortical material is aspirated from the eye. The posterior capsule is left intact, and a polymethylmethacrylate (PMMA) intraocular lens is placed in the capsular bag, which restores vision. In 25–35% of patients undergoing extracapsular cataract extraction, the posterior capsule may become opacified. This is treated by Nd:YAG laser capsulotomy. If such a laser is not available, surgical incision of the opaque posterior capsule is required.

C. Phacoemulsification: Phacoemulsification is a modification of the extracapsular cataract extraction procedure whereby the nucleus of the cataract is fragmented by a probe oscillating at ultrasonic frequency and simultaneously aspirating nuclear fragments from the eye. The advantage of phacoemulsification is that the incision can be as small as 3 mm, and the patient is quickly rehabilitated. The cortical material is removed by irrigation and aspiration, and the incision can be widened to 6 mm to place the posterior chamber intraocular lens in the capsular bag.

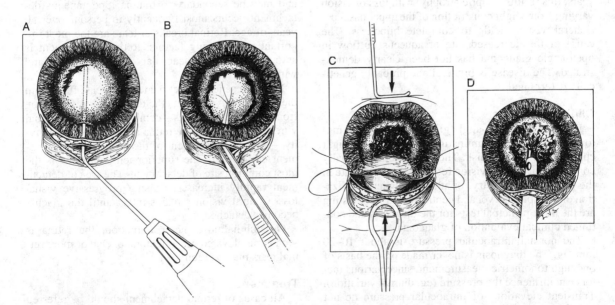

Figure 40–1. Extracapsular cataract extraction. **A:** Performing a circular anterior capsulotomy. **B:** Removal of the excised anterior capsule of the cataract. **C:** Expression of the nucleus of the cataract. **D:** Removal of the remaining cortical material by irrigation and aspiration.

ANGLE-CLOSURE GLAUCOMA
(Acute Glaucoma)

About 1% of people over age 35 have anatomically narrow anterior chamber angles. In such patients, if the pupil dilates spontaneously or is dilated with a mydriatic or cycloplegic agent, the angle will close and an attack of acute glaucoma is thus precipitated. For this reason, it is a wise precaution to estimate the depth of the anterior chamber angle before instilling these drugs.

Acute angle-closure glaucoma is manifested by an acute onset of pain, headache, and blurring of vision. Some patients develop nausea and vomiting. The eye is red, the cornea is hazy, and the pupil is moderately dilated and does not react to light. Intraocular pressure is elevated.

The attack is aborted by the use of topical pilocarpine eye drops, intravenous acetazolamide, and an intravenous hyperosmotic agent such as mannitol. Definitive treatment consists of peripheral iridectomy and establishment of a communication between the posterior and anterior chambers. This can be achieved by argon laser or Nd:YAG laser peripheral iridectomy. If laser equipment is not available or the patient is uncooperative, surgical peripheral iridectomy can be done.

OPEN-ANGLE GLAUCOMA
(Chronic Simple Glaucoma)

In open-angle glaucoma, the intraocular pressure is consistently elevated. Over a period of months or years, this results in optic atrophy, with loss of vision varying from slight constriction of the upper nasal peripheral visual fields to complete blindness. The cause of the decreased rate of aqueous outflow in open-angle glaucoma has not been clearly demonstrated. The disease is bilateral and probably genetically determined.

Clinical Findings

Patients with open-angle glaucoma have no symptoms initially. On examination, there may be slight cupping of the optic disk. The visual fields gradually constrict, but central vision remains good until late in the disease. Tonometry, ophthalmoscopic visualization of the optic nerve, and central visual field testing are the three principal tests for the diagnosis and continued clinical evaluation of glaucoma.

The normal intraocular pressure is about 10–20 mm Hg. The diagnosis is never made on the basis of one high tonometric measurement, since various factors can influence the pressure (eg, diurnal variation). Transient elevations of intraocular pressure do not constitute glaucoma for the same reason that periodic or intermittent elevations of blood pressure do not constitute hypertensive disease. All persons over age 20 should have tonometric and ophthalmoscopic examinations every 3–5 years. The examination may be performed by the general physician, internist, or ophthalmologist. If there is a family history of glaucoma, annual examination is indicated.

Treatment

Most patients can be controlled with beta-blockers (eg, timolol maleate, 0.25–0.5%, 1 drop in each eye twice daily) or miotics (eg, pilocarpine, 1–2%, 1 drop in each eye three or four times daily). Oral carbonic anhydrase inhibitors—eg, acetazolamide—to decrease the rate of aqueous production are used in patients with persistently high intraocular pressures not under control. Epinephrine eye drops, 0.5–2%, 1 drop in each eye twice daily, may be used. (*Caution:* Epinephrine is contraindicated if the anterior chamber angle is narrow.)

Argon laser trabeculoplasty can be helpful in decreasing the intraocular pressure in some patients. In those with uncontrolled pressures despite all the above measures, surgery is indicated. The most common filtering procedure is trabeculectomy. The success of this procedure has been improved by the use of intraoperative application of mitomycin to inhibit the fibrosis and closure of the filtering channels. In certain types of glaucoma such as neovascular glaucoma or aphakic glaucoma with failed filtering procedures, setons can be used.

RETINAL DETACHMENT

Detachment of the retina is usually spontaneous and may be secondary to trauma. Spontaneous detachment occurs most frequently in persons over 50 years of age. Retinal breaks or tears are the most important predisposing factors. Retinal detachment is associated with intracapsular cataract surgery and with myopia.

In the presence of a retinal tear or break, fluid from the vitreous cavity enters the defect and transudation from choroidal vessels—combined with abnormal vitreous traction on the retina and the force of gravity—leads to detachment of the retina from the pigment epithelium. The superior temporal area is the most common site of detachment. The area of detachment rapidly increases, causing progressive visual loss. Central vision remains intact until the macula becomes detached.

On ophthalmoscopic examination, the retina is seen as an elevated gray membrane. One or more retinal tears may be seen.

Treatment

All cases of retinal detachment should be referred immediately to an ophthalmologist. If the patient must be transported a long distance, the head should be positioned so that the detached portion of the retina will recede with the aid of gravity. For example, a patient with a superior temporal retinal detachment in the right eye should lie supine with the head turned to the right. Position is less important for a short trip.

Retinal detachment is a true emergency if the macula is threatened. If the macula is detached, permanent loss of central vision usually occurs even though the retina is eventually successfully reattached by surgery. Treatment consists of closure of retinal tears by cryosurgery or scleral buckling (or both). This produces an inflammatory reaction that causes the retina to adhere to the choroid. The laser is of value in a limited number of cases of minimal detachment. The laser creates an inflammatory adhesion between the choroid and the retina. Its main use is in the prevention of detachment by sealing small retinal tears before detachment occurs.

In uncomplicated retinal detachment with a superior retinal tear and healthy vitreous, pneumoretinopexy may be performed. The procedure consists of injection of air or certain gases into the vitreous cavity through the pars plana, and the patient is then positioned to augment sealing of the retinal hole and spontaneous reabsorption of the subretinal fluid.

About 85% of uncomplicated cases can be cured with one operation; an additional 10% will need repeated operations; and the remainder never reattach. The prognosis is worse if the macula is detached, if there are many vitreous strands, or if the detachment is of long duration.

Without treatment, retinal detachment almost always becomes total in 1–6 months. Spontaneous detachments are ultimately bilateral in 20–25% of cases.

STRABISMUS

Any child under age 7 with strabismus should be seen without delay to prevent amblyopia and to treat it at an early stage. In adults, the sudden onset of strabismus usually follows head trauma, intracranial hemorrhage, or brain tumor. About 3% of children are born with or develop strabismus. In descending order of frequency, the eyes may deviate inward (esotropia), outward (exotropia), upward (hypertropia), or downward (hypotropia). If a child is born with straight eyes but has inherited "weak fusion," strabismus may develop.

Clinical Findings

Children with frank strabismus first develop diplopia. They soon learn to suppress the image from the deviating eye, and the vision in that eye therefore fails to develop. This is the first stage of amblyopia. Most cases of strabismus are obvious, but if the angle of deviation is small or if the strabismus is intermittent, the diagnosis may be missed.

Amblyopia due to strabismus can be detected by routine visual acuity examination of all preschool children. Visual acuity testing with an illiterate E card is best done by age 4.

Treatment
(Figure 40–2)

The objectives in treatment of strabismus are to achieve good visual acuity in each eye; straight eyes, for cosmetic purposes; and coordinate function of both eyes. The best time to initiate treatment is at about age 6 months. If treatment is delayed beyond this time, the child will favor the straight eye and suppress the image in the other eye; this results in failure of visual development (amblyopia) in the deviating eye.

If the child is under age 6 years and has an amblyopic eye, vision may be improved by occluding the good eye. At age 1 year, patching may be successful within 1 week; at 6 years, it may take a year to achieve the same result, ie, to equalize the visual acuity in both eyes. Surgery is usually performed after the visual acuity has been equalized.

The prevention of blindness by these simple diagnostic and treatment procedures is one of the most rewarding experience in medical practice.

Surgery for correction of strabismus consists of weakening or strengthening the extraocular muscles. For correction of exotropia, the lateral rectus muscle is weakened by recession. The muscle is detached at its insertion and then resewn posteriorly to the sclera at a distance not to exceed 8 mm from the original insertion while the medial rectus is cut at its insertion and a part of the muscle not to exceed 6 mm is resected. The muscle is sutured to its original insertion. The amount of recession and resection and the number of extraocular muscles resected or recessed is de-

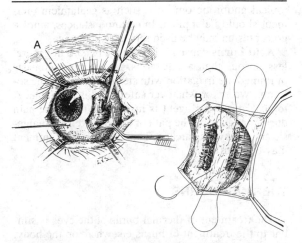

Figure 40–2. A: Exposure of an extraocular muscle in surgery for strabismus. **B:** Recession of the muscle behind its original insertion followed by suturing to the sclera with absorbable suture.

termined by the degree of ocular deviation (squint). In patients with esotropia, the medial rectus is recessed and the lateral rectus is resected. For vertical deviation, the vertical muscles are recessed, resected, tucked, or weakened by disinsertion (eg, inferior oblique muscle).

OCULAR BURNS

CHEMICAL BURNS

Apart from the history, the diagnosis of chemical eye burns is usually based on the presence of swelling of the eyelids and marked conjunctival hyperemia and chemosis. The limbus may show blanched patchy areas and conjunctival sloughing, especially in the interpalpebral area. There is usually corneal stromal haze and diffuse edema, with wide areas of epithelial cell loss and corneal ulcerations. Defects in the cornea can be better visualized with the instillation of fluorescein.

Alkali burns of the eye are a serious injury because tiny particles in the conjunctival fornices may cause progressive damage. Patients are managed by instilling a topical anesthetic agent and then promptly irrigating copiously with isotonic saline solution. Double eversion of the eyelid should be performed to look for and remove material lodged in the fornix. This can be easily done by using a forceps or moist cotton applicator. A lid speculum is placed after the instillation of tetracaine 0.5% eye drops, and the eye is irrigated with saline. Topical dilating drops such as atropine 1% or homatropine 5% are instilled, and a topical antibiotic ointment such as gentamicin ointment should be applied. In certain instances, autologous plasma may be used topically in the eye.

Acid burns cause rapid damage but are in general less serious than alkali burns. Management consists of immediate irrigation with sterile isotonic saline solution, water, or whatever safe liquid is available. A topical anesthetic agent is instilled to minimize pain during irrigation. The patient is then given an analgesic and the eye is patched. Topical antibiotic ointment may be instilled.

THERMAL BURNS

The treatment of thermal burns of the eyes is similar to the treatment of burns elsewhere on the body. Systemic analgesia should be provided. Topical anesthetic agents such as proparacaine 0.5% or tetracaine 0.5% is used to minimize pain during manipulation. In cases of burns involving the cornea, topical dilating drops such as atropine 1% or homatropine 5% are instilled. The eye is patched.

BURNS DUE TO ULTRAVIOLET RADIATION

Injuries to the corneal epithelium by ultraviolet rays may be mild or severe. This is referred to as actinic keratitis, snow blindness, welder's arc burn, or flash burn, depending on the source of ultraviolet radiation. Patients present with severe pain and photophobia. The examination reveals diffuse punctate staining of the cornea, seen with fluorescein staining and magnification of a cobalt blue light.

A topical antibiotic such as gentamicin ointment is instilled, and the eye is patched.

OCULAR TRAUMA

Ocular trauma may be classified as penetrating or nonpenetrating. Trauma can lead to reduced vision or loss of vision. Eye injuries are common in spite of the protection afforded by the bony orbit. The use of safety goggles at work and safety belts or air bags in the car would prevent most serious injuries to the eye.

Clinical Evaluation

A careful history of the injury should be obtained from the patient or someone who knows what happened. Visual acuity should be measured with and without glasses. The eyelids, conjunctiva, cornea, anterior chamber, iris, lens, vitreous, and fundus should be inspected for lacerations, breaks, or hemorrhage. Search for corneal lesions such as abrasions can be performed by instilling fluorescein dye and examining the eye using a cobalt blue light under magnification. X-ray examination is helpful in looking for fractures of the orbital bones and trying to rule out radiopaque foreign bodies. CT scan is performed when available. Patients with severe injuries should have immediate ophthalmic consultation. Further damage can be caused by manipulation, which for that reason should be avoided.

PENETRATING OR PERFORATING INJURIES

Penetrating or perforating ocular injuries require immediate careful attention and prompt surgical repair to prevent functional loss. Penetrating injuries are those that result from sharp pointed objects or flying small missiles entering the globe but not interrupting the continuity of the coats (sclera)—ie, the coats of the eye are spontaneously reapproximated after entry; perforating injuries result in rupture of the globe—ie, the coats are not spontaneously reapproximated—and sometimes loss of ocular contents.

Many facial injuries—especially those occurring in automobile accidents—are associated with penetrating ocular trauma. Some injuries may be concealed and inapparent because of eyelid swelling or because the patient's other injuries have dominated the attention of the emergency room staff. Such injuries, if not promptly attended to or adequately managed by an ophthalmologist, may lead to loss of vision. Accurate records and a description of how the injury occurred should be obtained. The eye and ocular adnexa should be examined, including vision testing and testing of ocular motility. *Do not apply pressure on the globe.* X-ray examination and CT scan are performed to rule out fractures of orbital bones or the presence of intraocular foreign bodies.

Penetrating injuries may lead to disruption of the outer coats of the eye such as the cornea or sclera with or without prolapse of the intraocular contents and uveal tissue. Proper management of lacerations can prevent further prolapse of ocular contents.

Perforating injuries are those resulting in complete anatomic disruption of the sclera or cornea. Careful repair and approximation of corneal and scleral lacerations should be performed in the operating room. Metallic intraocular foreign bodies can often be removed with a magnet at the time of suturing of the corneal or scleral lacerations. The major objectives in management of ocular penetrating or perforating injuries are to relieve pain, preserve or restore vision, and achieve good cosmetic results. Pain relief may be achieved by the administration of morphine, 2–4 mg intravenously or subcutaneously, or meperidine, 50–75 mg intramuscularly as needed. Sedatives such as diazepam, 5 mg, may be given orally as required.

The injured eye should be covered gently with sterile gauze or an eye pad, but no pressure should be applied. Parenteral broad-spectrum antibiotics such as cefazolin or gentamicin should be given. Antiemetics—chlorpromazine, 25 mg by deep intramuscular injection every 4–6 hours—should be given to patients who are vomiting to prevent further injury.

LACERATIONS OF THE OCULAR ADNEXA

Lacerations of the eyelids and the periorbital skin should be carefully evaluated and inspected. Superficial laceration of the skin can be sutured by approximation. In cases of deep eyelid lacerations, intraocular or orbital damage should be ruled out. The skin of the eyelids has good elasticity, is loosely attached to underlying tissue, and in adults is frequently present in surplus quantities. This facilitates the development of flaps and grafts. Small linear skin lacerations may be easily sutured and the wound secured with interrupted 7-0 silk suture. Because of the good blood supply, the sutures may be removed in 3–4 days. In deep lacerations of the eyelids, the wound divides the orbicularis muscle parallel to its fibers. Only skin sutures are generally required, but when the muscle fibers are transversely divided they should be approximated with absorbable sutures using 7-0 Vicryl or Dexon sutures. The skin can be approximated with fine silk or nylon sutures. In patients with lacerations resulting in round or oval losses of skin, the skin is undermined and the laceration approximated. In larger defects, reconstruction with flaps may be required. Flaps used in reconstruction of the eyelids are advancement flaps, rotational flaps, transposition flaps, island flaps, and Z-plasty flaps.

In large defects, when flaps cannot be used, free skin grafts may be obtained from behind the ear or from the skin of the inner upper arm.

The main problem that complicates suturing of the lower eyelid is retraction or eversion from vertical tension, which for that reason should be avoided.

BLUNT TRAUMA TO THE OCULAR ADNEXA & ORBIT
(See Table 40–2.)

Contusions of the eyeball and ocular adnexa may result from blunt trauma. The outcome of such an injury cannot always be determined, and the extent of damage may not be obvious upon superficial examination. Careful eye examination is needed, along with x-ray or CT scan.

BLOWOUT FRACTURE OF THE FLOOR OF THE ORBIT

Blowout fracture of the floor of the orbit is associated with enophthalmos, double vision in primary position or in upper gaze, limitation of ocular movement in upper gaze, hypotropia, and decreased or absent sensation over the maxillary area. X-ray or CT scan of the orbit shows orbital floor displacement.

The management of patients with blowout fractures of the orbital floor should be carefully assessed by an ophthalmologist and otolaryngologist because of potential fractures of the maxilla or zygoma.

CORNEAL & CONJUNCTIVAL FOREIGN BODIES

Patients may give a history of working with high-speed tempered steel tools, or drilling, or hammering against a hard object. There may be no history of trauma to the eye, and the patient may not be aware of

Table 40–2. Types of ocular injury associated with blunt trauma.

Eyelids	Ecchymosis, swelling, laceration, abrasions, conjunctival or sub-conjunctival hemorrhages.
Cornea	Edema, lacerations.
Anterior chamber	Hyphema, recession of angle, secondary glaucoma.
Iris	Iridodialysis, iridoplegia, rupture of iris sphincter.
Ciliary body	Hyposecretion of aqueous humor.
Lens	Cataract, dislocation.
Vitreous	Vitreous hemorrhage.
Ciliary muscle	Paralysis.
Retina	Commotio retinae, retinal edema, choroidal breaks in Bruch's membrane, choroidal hemorrhage.

a foreign body. In most cases, however, the patient complains of foreign body sensation in the eye or under the eyelid.

A corneal foreign body can be seen with the aid of a loupe and diffuse light. Conjunctival foreign bodies often become embedded in the conjunctiva under the upper eyelid; the lid must be everted to facilitate inspection and removal. Sterile fluorescein should be instilled to visualize small foreign bodies not readily visible with the naked eye or loupe. A topical anesthetic such as proparacaine 0.5% or tetracaine 0.5% is applied. Some loose foreign bodies can be removed with a moist cotton applicator, while superficial foreign bodies can be removed with the tip of a hypodermic needle. Topical prophylactic antibiotic ointment should be instilled, eg, gentamicin or erythromycin. The eyes should be covered overnight.

OCULAR TUMORS

Tumors of the eye and its related adnexal structures can be recognized and diagnosed early because they are visible and cause local disfigurement, changes in color, interference with vision, or displacement of the globe. In children, ocular tumors such as retinoblastoma affecting visual function may lead to squint or leukocoria. Tumors of the eye may be primary, affecting only the ocular or adnexal tissues; or secondary to metastasis of malignant tumors from other organs. In the eye, the most frequent site of metastasis is the choroid, and the tumors that most frequently metastasize to the eye are carcinoma of the breast in women and carcinoma of the lung in men.

The history of growth of the lesion is extremely

important, as well as recent changes in its size or appearance. Excisional biopsy of lesions of the skin or conjunctiva is indicated if cancer is suspected.

LID TUMORS
(Figure 40–3)

Benign Tumors of the Eyelids

The most frequent benign tumors of the eyelids are **melanocytic nevi.** Excision is indicated for cosmetic reasons. Xanthelasmas represent lipid deposits in histiocytes in the dermis of the skin of the eyelid. In such patients, serum lipid and serum cholesterol levels should be determined. Treatment is indicated for cosmetic reasons and consists of simple excision. Recurrences are common.

Hemangiomas of the eyelids are of two types: capillary and cavernous. **Capillary hemangiomas** consist of dilated capillaries and proliferation of endothelial cells. The lesions appear as bright red spots. They may show rapid growth in the neonatal period but later undergo involution and subside spontaneously. **Cavernous hemangiomas,** on the other hand, are venous channels in the subcutaneous tissue. They

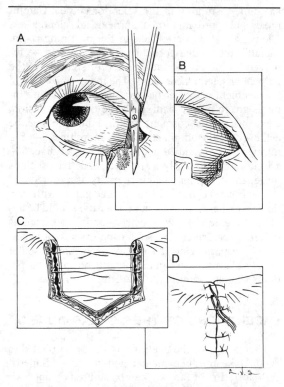

Figure 40–3. Tumor of the left lower eyelid involving the lid margin. **A:** Two vertical incisions are made. **B:** The defect after removal of the tumor. **C:** Suturing of the tarsus and orbicularis with absorbable sutures. **D:** Approximation of skin with interrupted 6-0 silk sutures.

appear bluish in color and are distended. Treatment of hemangiomas in infancy and early childhood is not indicated unless the lesion causes interference with vision, which may lead to amblyopia. Low-dose oral steroids or local injection of steroids may cause rapid involution of capillary hemangiomas. Surgical excision may be required. Radiation is not recommended because it leads to excessive scarring of the eyelid.

Other benign tumors of the eyelids include verrucae and molluscum contagiosum. These lesions are caused by viruses.

Malignant Tumors of the Eyelids

Squamous cell carcinoma has a tendency to grow slowly and painlessly. It begins as a small lesion covered by a layer of keratin. The lesion may erode, causing an ulcer with hyperemic edges. It may enlarge to form a fungating mass and may invade the orbital cavity. Early excision may result in cure. If early treatment is not provided, squamous cell carcinoma may spread via the lymphatic system to the preauricular and submandibular lymph nodes.

Basal cell carcinoma begins as a slowly growing, locally invasive tumor forming the so-called rodent ulcer with raised nodular borders. Inner canthal basal cell carcinoma may invade the structures of the inner canthus and the orbit. Treatment should include complete excision to prevent recurrences.

Malignant melanomas of the eyelids are similar to malignant melanomas of the skin elsewhere on the body.

CONJUNCTIVAL TUMORS

Benign tumors of the conjunctiva include melanocytic nevi (pigmented or nonpigmented), papillomas, granulomas, dermoid tumors, and lymphoid hyperplasia. Malignant tumors of the conjunctiva include carcinoma, malignant melanoma, and, rarely, lymphoma. Carcinoma of the conjunctiva arises frequently at the limbus or the inner canthus in the exposed area of the bulbar conjunctiva. Early in the course of the disease, the lesion may resemble pterygium. The tumor is slightly elevated, with a gelatinous surface, and may spread over the corneal surface. The growth of this lesion is slow. Treatment is by excisional biopsy.

INTRAOCULAR TUMORS

Benign Intraocular Tumors

Melanocytic nevi of the iris, ciliary body, or choroid are common. No treatment is required for these lesions. Retinal angioma may be seen in patients with phacomatoses (eg, Bourneville's disease). Choroidal hemangioma is another less frequently encountered benign intraocular tumor.

Malignant Intraocular Tumors

Malignant intraocular tumors include malignant melanoma, retinoblastoma, and a rare tumor of the ciliary body known as dictyoma or medulloepithelioma.

Malignant melanoma is most common. It typically occurs in the fifth or sixth decade and is almost always unilateral. The most frequent site is the choroid, but malignant melanoma may occur also in the ciliary body or iris. Malignant melanomas of the choroid may cause decrease in vision and may undergo necrosis, leading to intraocular inflammation. Histopathologic examination shows spindle-shaped cells with or without prominent nuclei and large epithelioid tumor cells. Intraocular malignant melanomas may spread directly through the sclera by local invasion.

The first step in diagnosis is to suspect the lesion. Malignant melanomas can be seen by ophthalmoscopy.

Treatment of malignant melanoma of the choroid consists of enucleation or radiotherapy, using radioactive plaques or charged particles. Extension outside the eye may require exenteration of the orbit. Patients with small melanomas—less than 10 mm in diameter—can be observed by serial photography of the fundus. Similarly, small melanomas of the iris that have not invaded the iris root can be safely followed and observed until growth is documented. If there is growth of the iris tumor, treatment is by local iridectomy. If the iris malignant melanoma invades the root and ciliary body, it can be removed surgically by iridocyclectomy.

Retinoblastoma is a rare but life-threatening condition in childhood. It is the most frequent intraocular malignant tumor in children. Most patients with retinoblastoma present in the first or second year of life. Patients may present with leukocoria or squint. Retinoblastoma may be multifocal and arise from the embryonic cone cells of the photoreceptor layer. It may appear sporadically or may be familial. It may be nodular and multifocal and grows slowly to fill the intraocular space and undergo necrosis, leading to calcific deposits. Tumor cells may seed on the iris and in the anterior chamber, causing fluffy whitish exudates.

Spontaneous cure of retinoblastoma has been reported. The treatment of choice is enucleation. Other therapeutic modalities include radiotherapy, cryotherapy, and chemotherapy.

ORBITAL TUMORS

Orbital tumors may be of two types: those arising from orbital tissues (primary orbital tumors) and those invading the orbit from adjacent structures (secondary orbital tumors). Primary orbital tumors include benign tumors such as dermoid cysts, hemangiomas, lipomas, fibromas, osteomas, chondromas, neurofibromas, and lacrimal gland tumors. Malignant tumors of the orbit include rhabdomyosarcoma, adenocarcinoma of the lacrimal gland, and lymphomas. Invading tumors include malignant melanoma and retinoblastoma from the intraocular structures and malignant melanomas and carcinomas from the skin of the eyelids and conjunctiva. Metastatic lesions may reach the orbit from the lung or breast. Neuroblastoma may also metastasize to the orbit in children. Meningiomas of the cranial nerves may invade the orbit through the optic canal.

Treatment and prognosis in all cases depend on the type of tumor.

REFERENCES

Duane TD, Jaeger EA (editors): *Clinical Ophthalmology,* vol 1. Harper & Row, 1986.

Ellis PP: *Ocular Therapeutics and Pharmacology,* 7th ed. Mosby, 1985.

Gittinger JW, Asdourian GK: *Manual of Clinical Problems in Ophthalmology.* Little, Brown, 1988.

Gold DH, Weingeist TA (editors): *The Eye in Systemic Disease.* Lippincott, 1990.

Hedges TR: *Consultation in Ophthalmology.* Mosby, 1986.

Hersh PS: *Ophthalmic Surgical Procedures.* Little, Brown, 1988.

Hodges E, Tabbara KF: Orbital cellulitis: Review of 23 cases from Saudi Arabia. Br J Ophthalmol 1989;73:205.

Morrison JC, Robin AL: Adjunctive glaucoma therapy: A comparison of apraclonidine to dipivefrin when added to timolol maleate. Ophthalmology 1989;96:3.

Newell FW: *Ophthalmology: Principles and Concepts,* 6th ed. Mosby, 1986.

Ragge NK, Easty D: *Immediate Eye Care.* Wolfe, 1990.

Shingleton BJ, Hersh PS, Kenyon KR (editors): *Eye Trauma.* Mosby Year Book, 1991.

Tabbara KF: Eye emergencies. In: *Current Emergency Diagnosis & Treatment,* 3rd ed. Ho MT, Saunders CE (editors). Appleton & Lange, 1990.

Tabbara KF, Hyndiuk RA: *Infections of the Eye.* Little, Brown, 1986.

Vaughan D, Asbury T, Tabbara KF (editors): *General Ophthalmology,* 12th ed. Appleton & Lange, 1989.

Waltman SR et al: *Surgery of the Eye.* 2 vols. Churchill Livingstone, 1988.

Urology

41

James F. Donovan, Jr., MD, & Richard D. Williams, MD

EMBRYOLOGY OF THE GENITOURINARY TRACT

Embryologically, the genital and urinary systems are intimately related. Associated anomalies are commonly encountered.

The Kidneys

The kidneys pass through three embryonic phases (Figure 41–1): (1) The **pronephros** is a vestigial structure without function in human embryos that, except for its primary duct, disappears completely by the fourth week. (2) The pronephric duct gains connection to the **mesonephric tubules** and becomes the mesonephric duct. While most of the mesonephric tubules degenerate, the mesonephric duct persists bilaterally; where it bends to open into the cloaca, the ureteral bud develops from it and starts to grow cranially to meet the metanephric blastema. (3) This forms the **metanephros**, which is the final phase. The metanephros develops into the kidney. During cephalad migration and rotation, the metanephric tissue progressively enlarges, with rapid internal differentiation into the nephron and the uriniferous tubules. Simultaneously, the cephalad end of the ureteral bud expands within the metanephros to form the renal pelvis and calices. Numerous outgrowths from the renal pelvis develop, branch and rebranch, and finally connect the differentiating metanephric tissue to the calices, establishing continuity between the secreting and collecting ducts.

The Bladder & Urethra

Subdivision of the cloaca (the blind end of the hindgut) into a ventral (urogenital sinus) and a dorsal (rectum) segment is completed during the seventh week and initiates early differentiation of the urinary bladder and urethra. The urogenital sinus receives the mesonephric duct and gradually absorbs its caudal end, so that by the end of the seventh week the ureteral bud and mesonephric duct have independent openings. The former migrates upward and laterally. The latter moves downward and medially, and the structure in between (the trigone) is formed by the absorbed mesodermal tissue, which maintains direct continuity between the two tubes (Figure 41–2).

The fused müllerian ducts also meet the urogenital sinus at Müller's tubercle. The urogenital sinus above Müller's tubercle differentiates to form the bladder and the part of the prostatic urethra proximal to the seminal colliculus in the male or the bladder and the entire urethra in the female (Figure 41–3). Below Müller's tubercle, the urogenital sinus differentiates into the distal part of the prostatic urethra and the membranous urethra in the male or the distal vagina and vaginal vestibule in the female. The rest of the male urethra is formed by fusion of the urethral folds on the ventral surface of the genital tubercle. In the female, the genital folds remain separate and form the labia minora.

The prostate develops at the end of the 11th week as several groups of outgrowths of urethral epithelium both above and below the entrance of the ejaculatory duct (distal vas deferens). The developing glandular element (seminal colliculus) incorporates the differentiating mesenchymal cells surrounding it to form the muscular stroma and capsule of the prostate. The seminal vesicles form as duplicate buds from the distal end of the mesonephric duct (vas deferens).

The Gonads

Each embryo is anatomically bisexual initially; the development of one set of sex primordia and the gradual involution of the other are determined by the genetic sex of the embryo and differential secretion of numerous hormones. Gonadal differentiation begins during the seventh week (Figure 41–3). If the gonad develops into a testis, the germinal epithelium progressively grows into radially arranged, cord-like seminiferous tubules. If it develops into an ovary, it becomes differentiated into a cortex and a medulla; the cortex later differentiates into ovarian follicles containing ova.

The testes remain in the abdomen until the seventh month and then pass through the inguinal canal to the scrotum, guided by the primary attachment to the gubernaculum. The ovary, which is attached to ligaments, undergoes internal descent to enter the pelvis.

Lack of complete testicular descent is known as cryptorchidism; descent to an abnormal site is known as testicular ectopia. In the male, the genital duct sys-

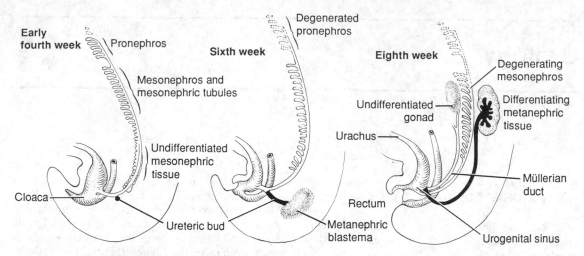

Figure 41–1. Schematic representation of the development of the nephric system. Only a few of the tubules of the pronephros are seen early in the fourth week, while the mesonephric tissue differentiates into mesonephric tubules that progressively join the mesonephric duct. The first sign of the ureteral bud from the mesonephric duct is seen. At 6 weeks, the pronephros has completely degenerated and the mesonephric tubules start to do so. The ureteral bud grows dorsocranially and has met the metanephric blastema. At the eighth week, there is cranial migration of the differentiating metanephros. The cranial end of the ureteral bud expands and starts to show multiple successive outgrowths (renal calices).

tem develops from the mesonephric duct, which differentiates into the epididymis, vas deferens, seminal vesicles, and ejaculatory ducts. In the female, the genital duct system develops from the müllerian ducts, which fuse at their caudal ends and differentiate into the uterine tubes, the uterus, and the proximal two-thirds of the vagina.

The external genitalia start to differentiate by the eighth week. The genital tubercle and genital swellings develop into the penis and scrotum in the male and the clitoris and labia majora in the female.

With the breakdown of the urogenital membrane in the seventh week, the urogenital sinus achieves a separate opening on the undersurface of the genital tubercle. The expansion of the infratubercular part of the urogenital sinus will form the vaginal vestibule and the distal part of the vagina. The two folds on the undersurface of the genital tubercle unite in the male to form the penile urethra; in the female, they remain separate to form the labia minora.

Rabinowitz R: Congenital anomalies. In: *Adult and Pediatric Urology.* Gillenwater JY et al (editors). Mosby Year Book, 1991.

ANATOMY OF THE GENITOURINARY TRACT: GROSS & MICROSCOPIC

The Kidneys

The kidneys lie retroperitoneally in the posterior abdomen and are separated from the surrounding renal fascia (Gerota's fascia) by perinephric fat. The renal vascular pedicle enters the renal sinus; the vein is anterior to the artery, and both are anterior to the renal pelvis. The renal artery divides just outside the renal sinus into anterior and posterior branches that undergo further subdivisions with variable extents of distribution. They are end arteries and thus result in segmental infarction when occluded. The venous tributaries anastomose freely and usually drain into one renal vein.

The Renal Parenchyma

The renal parenchyma consists of more than 1 million functioning units (nephrons) and is divided into a peripheral cortex containing secretory elements and a central medulla containing excretory elements. The nephron starts as Bowman's capsule, which surrounds the glomerulus and leads to elongated proximal and distal convoluted tubules with the loop of Henle in between, ending in a collecting duct that opens into a minor calix at the tip of a papilla.

The Renal Pelvis & Calices

The renal pelvis and calices are within the renal sinus and function as the main collecting reservoir. The pelvis, which is partly extrarenal and partly intrarenal (but occasionally is totally extra- or intrarenal), branches into three major calices that in turn branch into several minor calices. These calices are directly related to the tips of the medullary pyramids (the papillae) and act as a receiving cup to the collecting tubules. The pelvicaliceal system is a highly mus-

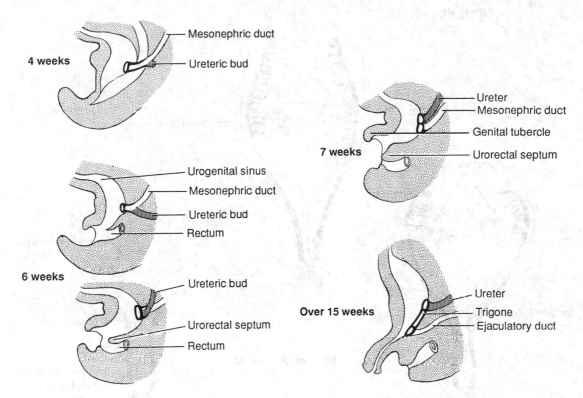

Figure 41–2. The development of the ureteral bud from the mesonephric duct and their relationship to the urogenital sinus. The ureteral bud appears at the fourth week. The mesonephric duct distal to this ureteral bud will be gradually absorbed into the urogenital sinus, resulting in separate endings for the ureter and the mesonephric duct. The mesonephric tissue that is incorporated into the urogenital sinus will expand and form the trigonal tissue. The mesonephric duct will form the vas deferens in the male and Gartner's duct (if present) in the female.

cular structure; the fibers run in many directions and are directly continuous from the calices to the pelvis, allowing synchronization of contractile activity.

The Ureter

The ureter connects the renal pelvis to the urinary bladder. It is a muscularized tube; its muscle fibers lie in an irregular helical arrangement and function primarily in peristaltic activity. Ureteral muscle fibers are directly continuous from the renal pelvis cranially to the vesical trigone distally.

The blood supply to the renal pelvis and ureters is segmental, arising from the renal, gonadal, and vesical arteries—with rich subadventitial anastomoses.

The Bladder

The bladder is primarily a reservoir with a meshwork of muscle bundles that not only change from one plane to another but also branch and join each other to constitute a synchronized organ. Its musculature is directly continuous with the urethral musculature and thus functions as an internal urethral sphincteric mechanism in spite of the lack of a true circular sphincter.

The ureters enter the bladder posteroinferiorly through the ureteral hiatus; after a short intravesical submucosal course, they open into the bladder and become continuous with the trigone, which is superimposed on the bladder base though deeply connected to it.

The Urethra

The adult female urethra is about 4 cm long and is muscular in its proximal four-fifths. This musculature is arranged in an inner longitudinal coat that is continuous with the inner longitudinal fibers of the bladder and an outer circular coat that is continuous with the outer longitudinal coat of the bladder. These outer circular fibers comprise the sphincteric mechanism. The striated external sphincter surrounds the middle third of the urethra.

In the male, the prostatic urethra is heavily muscular and sphincteric. The membranous urethra is within the urogenital diaphragm and is surrounded by the striated external sphincter. The penile urethra is poorly muscularized and traverses the corpus spongiosum to open at the tip of the glans.

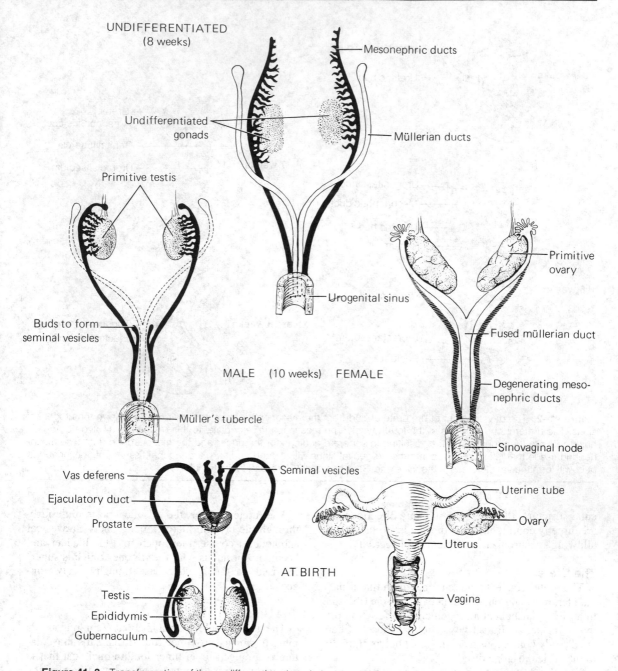

Figure 41–3. Transformation of the undifferentiated genital system into the definitive male and female systems.

The Prostate

The prostate surrounds the proximal portion of the male urethra; it is a fibromuscular, cone-shaped gland about 2.5 cm long and normally weighing about 20 g. It is traversed from base to apex by the urethra and is pierced posterolaterally by the ejaculatory ducts from the seminal vesicles and vas deferens that converge to open at the verumontanum (seminal colliculus) on the floor of the urethra.

The prostatic glandular elements drain through about 12 paired excretory ducts that open into the floor of the urethra above the verumontanum. The prostate is surrounded by a thin capsule, derived from its stroma, which is rich in musculature, and part of the urethral musculature and the sphincteric mechanism. A rich venous plexus surrounds the prostate, especially anteriorly and laterally. Its lymphatic drainage is into the hypogastric, sacral, obturator, and external iliac lymph nodes.

The Testis, Epididymis, & Vas

The testis is a paired organ surrounded by the tunica albuginea and subdivided into numerous lobules by fibrous septa. The extremely convoluted seminiferous tubules gather to open into the rete testis, where they join the efferent duct and drain into the epididymis. The epididymis drains into the vas deferens, which courses through the inguinal canal into the pelvis and is joined by the duct from the seminal vesicle before opening into the prostatic urethra on either side of the verumontanum.

Arterial supply is via the spermatic, vas deferential, and external cremasteric arteries. Venous drainage is through the pampiniform plexus, which drains into the internal spermatic veins; the right spermatic vein joins the vena cava and the left joins the renal vein.

Testicular lymphatics drain into the lumbar lymph nodes; the right primarily into the interaortocaval area, the left into the para-aortic area, both just below the renal vessels.

McNeal JE: The prostate gland: Morphology and pathobiology. Monogr Urol 1988;9(3):36.

Redman JF: Anatomy of the genitourinary system. In: *Adult and Pediatric Urology.* Gillenwater JY et al (editors). Mosby Year Book, 1991.

Tisher CC, Madsen KM: Anatomy of the kidney. In: *The Kidney.* Brenner BM, Rector JC (editors). Saunders, 1991.

PHYSIOLOGY OF THE GENITOURINARY TRACT

The Kidneys

The kidneys maintain and regulate homeostasis of body fluids by the following mechanisms:

A. Glomerular Filtration: This is dependent on glomerular capillary arterial pressure minus plasma colloid osmotic pressure plus Bowman's capsular resistance. The resultant glomerular filtration pressure (about 8–12 mm Hg) forces protein-free plasma through the capillary filtering surface into Bowman's capsule. Normally, about 130 mL of plasma is filtered every minute through the renal circulation; the entire volume of plasma recirculates through the kidney and is subjected to the filtration process once every 27 minutes.

B. Tubular Reabsorption: About 99% of the filtered volume will be reabsorbed through the tubules, together with all the valuable constituents of the filtrate (chlorides, glucose, sodium, potassium, calcium, and amino acids). Urea, uric acid, phosphates, and sulfates are also reabsorbed to varying degrees. The process of reabsorption is a combination of active and passive transport mechanisms. Reabsorption of water and electrolytes is under the control of adrenal, pituitary, and parathyroid hormones.

C. Tubular Secretion: This helps (1) to eliminate certain substances and thus maintain their plasma levels and (2) to exchange valuable ions from the filtrate for less desirable ions in the plasma (eg, a sodium ion from the urine for a hydrogen ion in the plasma). Failure of adequate secretory function leads to the acidosis commonly encountered in chronic renal disease.

The Ureteropelvicaliceal System

This system is one continuous tubular structure with adequate musculature that is imperceptibly in motion from one segment to the other to maintain anatomic continuity and physiologic synchrony at various levels. Waves of peristaltic contractions start from the calices and proceed in antegrade fashion toward the urinary bladder. These peristaltic waves occur at a rate of about 5–8/min, involve a 2- to 3-cm segment at a time, and usually proceed at the velocity of 3 cm/s. Frequency, amplitude, and velocity are influenced by urine output and flow rate. Ureteral filling is primarily passive; ureteral emptying is primarily active, which is essential to urine transport across points of resistance (eg, ureterovesical junction) and to prevent retrograde flow.

The Ureterovesical Junction

The ureterovesical junction allows free flow of urine from the ureter to the bladder and at the same time prevents retrograde flow. The continuity and the specific muscular arrangement of the intravesical ureter and the trigone provide a muscularly active valvular mechanism that can efficiently adapt itself to the variable phases of bladder activity during filling and voiding.

Progressive bladder filling leads to firm occlusion of the intravesical ureter against retrograde urine flow and to increased resistance to antegrade flow resulting from trigonal stretching. During voiding, trigonal contraction completely seals the intravesical ureter against any antegrade or retrograde flow of urine.

The Urinary Bladder

The urinary bladder functions primarily as a reservoir that can accommodate variable volumes without increasing its intraluminal pressure. When the bladder reaches full capacity, the detrusor muscle voluntarily contracts uniformly and maintains its contraction until the bladder is completely empty. Funneling of the bladder outlet with progressive downward movement of the dome ensures complete emptying.

The vesical sphincteric mechanism is primarily a smooth muscle sphincter in the male prostatic urethra and in the proximal four-fifths of the female urethra. There is no purely circular sphincteric entity, but there are abundant circularly oriented muscle fibers that are directly continuous with the outer coat of the detrusor muscles. The sphincter has the same nerve supply as—and reacts simultaneously with—the detrusor. It maintains urethral closure by its passive tone, yet when it shares detrusor contraction it does not hinder voiding.

There is another voluntary striated sphincter that is part of the urogenital diaphragm and surrounds the mid urethra in the female and the membranous urethra in the male. It is not essential for continence, though it adds to urethral resistance. Its pathologic irritability or spasticity can lead to obstructive manifestations.

Benigni A et al: Functional implications of decreased renal cortical atrial natriuretic peptide binding in experimental diabetes. Circ Res 1990;66:1453.

Diamond JR: Effects of dietary interventions on glomerular pathophysiology. Am J Physiol 1990;258:F1.

Ihle BU et al: The effect of protein restriction on the progression of renal insufficiency. N Engl J Med 1989;321:1773.

McDougal WS: *The Diagnosis, Management, and Pathophysiology of Acute Renal Failure.* AUA Update Series 1985;Vol 4: Lesson 7.

Walser M, Drew HH, LaFrance NJ: Creatinine measurements often yield false estimates of progression in chronic renal failure. Kidney Int 1988;34:412.

DEVELOPMENTAL ANOMALIES OF THE GENITOURINARY TRACT

Genitourinary tract anomalies occur in over 10% of the population. The severity varies from lesions incompatible with life to insignificant findings detected during diagnostic studies done for unrelated reasons. The anatomic abnormalities are often not intrinsically harmful, yet they may predispose to infection, stone formation, or chronic renal failure.

RENAL ANOMALIES

Bilateral absence of the kidneys is rare and is commonly associated with oligohydramnios, Potter facies, and pulmonary hypoplasia. It occurs more often in males and results in death shortly after birth. Unilateral renal agenesis is seen more often but is not usually associated with illness. **Renal agenesis** is thought to be due to both lack of a ureteral bud and lack of subsequent development of the metanephric blastema. The bladder trigone is absent on the side affected. Because adrenal gland development is unrelated to kidney development, both adrenals are usu-

ally present in the normal position. Rarely, more than two kidneys are seen, a condition clearly dissimilar to ureteral duplication, as described later.

Abnormal ascent of the metanephros leads to an **ectopic kidney,** which may be unilateral or bilateral. Lumbar, pelvic, and the less common thoracic and crossed ectopic varieties are seen. Ectopic kidneys are associated with genital anomalies in 10–20% of cases. Fusional abnormalities, which are also due to failure of normal ascent, include fused pelvic kidneys and **horseshoe kidneys** (the most common), which are typically fused at the lower poles. Intravenous urography typically establishes the diagnosis. The relationship of the kidneys to the psoas muscles is abnormal: instead of an oblique orientation with the medial border of the kidney parallel to the psoas muscle, the kidneys are vertical and the medial border intersects and crosses the psoas muscle (Figure 41–4). These latter conditions predispose to recurrent infection and calculi in 10–20% of patients and is associated with an increased incidence of ureteropelvic junction obstruction due to compression by one of many anomalous arteries. Failure of rotation during ascent results in "malrotated" kidneys and is rarely significant.

Polycystic Kidneys

Parenchymal anomalies include a variety of cystic and dysplastic lesions. Polycystic kidney disease is hereditary and bilateral. The infantile form is autosomal recessive and leads to progressive renal failure and short life expectancy without dialysis or transplantation. The cause is **tubular ectasia,** a disorder of the renal medulla in which dilated collecting tubules and medullary cysts are seen.

The adult form is autosomal dominant. It is much more common than the infantile form, being the third leading cause of end-stage renal disease in adults. Large kidneys are seen, with cysts of varying sizes in the collecting tubules. Renal cysts are thought to be due to failure of union of the collecting tubules and convoluted tubules. Cysts may also be present in the liver and pancreas, and cerebral arterial aneurysms may occur. Cystic enlargement exerts pressure on normal parenchyma, leading to its gradual destruction.

The diagnosis is often made during a workup for hypertension or uremia discovered in the third to sixth decades. Hematuria with or without flank pain is a common finding. An intravenous urogram will reveal the enlarged kidneys, with marked elongation of the calices, which are compressed by large cysts (Figure 41–5). Ultrasonography or CT scan will readily make the diagnosis.

Surgery is rarely warranted. Therapy is medical and ultimately includes hemodialysis. Renal transplantation is often indicated, though potential family donors must be carefully screened to determine whether they have the same disorder.

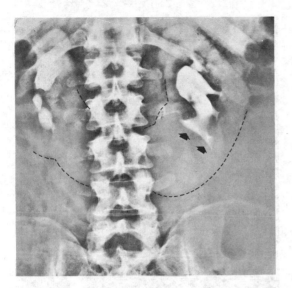
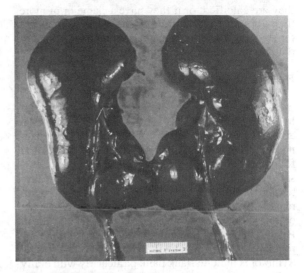

Figure 41–4. **A:** Excretory urogram showing horseshoe kidney with expansion of left side of isthmus and compression of lower left caliceal system. The surgical diagnosis was adenocarcinoma. **B:** Gross pathology of horseshoe kidney.

Medullary Sponge Kidney

Medullary sponge kidney results from collecting tubular ectasia (see Polycystic Kidneys) and is associated with recurrent urolithiasis and an increased incidence of infection in 50% of patients. The lesion is often bilateral and may involve all of the calices. Intravenous urograms reveal dilated collecting tubules as a "blush" in the renal papilla. The symptoms are of pyelonephritis or urolithiasis. Microscopic hematuria is common. Specific antibiotics should be given for documented infections, and prophylactic therapy for renal stones should be recommended, based on the results of metabolic stone evaluation.

Simple Renal Cysts

Simple renal cysts are common (approximately 50% after age 50) and are thought to arise from tubu-

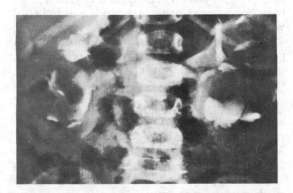

Figure 41–5. Polycystic kidneys. Excretory urogram in a child, showing elongation, broadening, and bending of the calices around cysts. Good renal function.

lar dilatation. They may be solitary or bilateral and multiple. They rarely have pathologic significance except in the differentiation from solid renal masses. (See Renal Adenocarcinoma, p 923.)

Renal Dysplasia

In renal dysplasia, multicystic kidneys are present. These are usually unilateral, nonfunctioning, and associated with unilateral ureteral atresia. They are often discovered in infancy as a palpable flank mass. They do not predispose to other pathologic conditions, and in the classic case with typical features no treatment is necessary. They may require differentiation from renal tumors. Bilateral renal dysplasia is rare and generally results in renal failure early in childhood. There is often associated lower urinary tract obstruction, such as posterior urethral valves or **prune belly syndrome** (absence of abdominal musculature, cryptorchidism, and functional bladder outlet obstruction). Studies of dysplastic kidneys in utero have documented regression or resorption of the affected renal unit. Thus, without prenatal ultrasound, these patients would be diagnosed as having unilateral renal agenesis.

Renal Vascular Abnormalities

Multiple renal arteries occur in 15–20% of patients and are significant only when they cause ureteropelvic junction obstruction. Congenital **renal artery aneurysms** are infrequent; they are differentiated from acquired lesions by their location at the bifurcation of the main renal artery or at a distal branch point. The lesions are usually asymptomatic, but they can cause hypertension. They require surgical treatment only if hypertension is uncontrolled, if they are calcified, or if they have a diameter of more than 2.5 cm. **Congenital arteriovenous fistulas** are rare but may result in hematuria, hypertension, or cardiac failure necessitating operative treatment.

Renal Pelvis Anomalies

Ureteropelvic junction obstruction is one of the more common causes of hydronephrosis in childhood. The condition may result from anomalous renal arteries or intrinsic stenosis of the junction. The diagnosis is not uncommonly made when gross hematuria follows minor trauma. Renal ultrasound provides a safe screening technique in patents suspected of ureteropelvic junction obstruction. Intravenous urography will suggest the diagnosis, and diuretic renal scan or retrograde pyelography, or both, will confirm it. Bilaterality is not uncommon, and the condition may require surgical repair if symptomatic or severe. Symptoms include flank pain, particularly with orally induced diuresis.

Avni EF et al: Multicystic dysplastic kidney: Natural history from in utero diagnosis and postnatal followup. J Urol 1987;138:1420.

Hashimoto BE, Filly RA, Callen PW: Multicystic dysplastic kidney in utero: Changing appearance on US. Radiology 1986;159:107.

Regan JB, Benson RC: Congenital renal arteriovenous malformations. J Urol 1986;136:1184.

Williams RD: Anomalies of the urinary tract. In: *Cecil Textbook of Medicine.* Wyngaarden JB (editor). Saunders, 1992.

URETERAL ANOMALIES

Congenital Obstruction of the Ureter

Congenital obstruction of the ureter may be due to ureterovesical and ureteropelvic junction obstruction or to neurologic deficits such as sacral agenesis or myelomeningocele. Functional ureteral obstruction—also known as **megaureter** or **ureteral achalasia**—is not uncommon (Figure 41–6). Symptoms are renal pain during oral diuresis or those resulting from pyelonephritis. Excretory urograms depict dilatation above the obstruction. There is usually no reflux on cystography. Vesicoureteral reflux may accompany ureteropelvic obstruction in 10% of cases; otherwise, vesicoureteral reflux is uncommonly associated with megaureter. Milder forms without symptoms or significant hydronephrosis are the rule and do not require treatment. When treatment is necessary, it consists of division of the ureter just proximal to the obstruction, with reimplantation of the ureter into the bladder.

Duplication of Ureters

Bifurcation of the ureteral bud results in incomplete ureteral duplication, commonly in the mid or upper ureter. An accessory ureteral bud leads to complete ureteral duplication (Figure 41–7A, right kidney) draining one renal unit. This represents the most common ureteral anomaly; it occurs more often in females. The presence of more than two ureters on each side is not common, but bilaterality of ureteral duplication is. Usually, all of the duplicated ureters enter the bladder; the ureter draining the upper pole of the kidney enters closest to the bladder neck (due to its later reabsorption into the bladder). Because of this relationship, the ureter draining the lower pole has a short intramural tunnel and an inadequate surrounding musculature and is thus prone to vesicoureteral reflux. The ureter draining the upper pole may be ectopic (again because of its late absorption) and thus empty into the bladder neck, urethra, or genital structures (vagina or vestibule in the female and seminal vesicle or vas deferens in the male [Figure 41–7A, left kidney]). The ureter draining the upper pole is prone to obstruction whether ectopic or orthotopic (within the bladder), in which case ureterocele is a common cause of obstruction. Duplication becomes significant when hydronephrosis or pyelonephritis occurs. The diagnosis is made by intravenous urography (Figure 41–7B). Ureteral reimplantation to prevent recurrent infection is necessary in some cases. An anastomosis between the upper pole renal pelvis and the lower pole ureter is an alternative in selected cases. The upper pole of the kidney and its ureter may require removal if obstruction is severe.

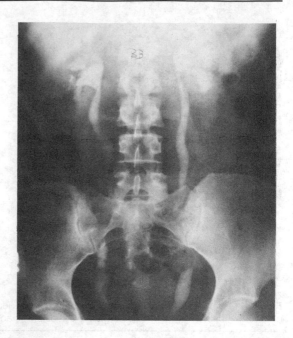

Figure 41–6. Excretory urogram showing bilateral megaureter.

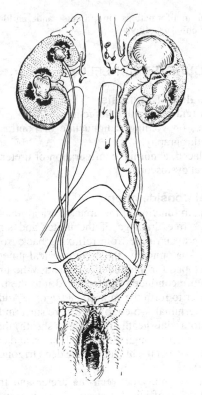
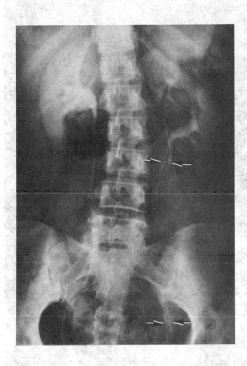

Figure 41–7. **A:** Duplication of ureters and ectopic ureteral orifice. Complete duplication with obstruction to one ureter with ectopic orifice on left. The ureter with the ectopic opening always drains the upper pole of the kidney. **B:** Excretory urogram showing left complete ureteral duplication.

Ectopic Ureteral Orifice

Ureteral ectopia can occur in the absence of duplication and drain into any of the abnormal positions mentioned above. If the orifice lies proximal to the external urinary sphincter, no incontinence ensues, but vesicoureteral reflux is common. Should it drain into the vagina or at the vestibule, there is continuous leakage of urine apart from voiding. Most ectopic orifices involve the ureter draining the upper pole of a duplicated system, and most are observed in the female. Hydroureteronephrosis of the involved segment is the rule.

An ectopic orifice may be seen beside the urethral orifice or in the roof of the vagina on endoscopy. Intravenous urograms will reveal hydroureteronephrosis, usually involving the upper renal segment. Cystography may show reflux into the ectopic orifice. If the hydronephrotic segment is only moderately damaged, the ureter can be divided and reimplanted into the bladder. Usually, however, heminephroureterectomy is necessary.

Ureterocele

A ureterocele is a ballooning of the distal submucosal ureter into the bladder. This structure commonly has a pinpoint orifice and therefore leads to hydronephrosis. If large enough, it may obstruct the vesical neck or the contralateral ureter. It is most common in females with ureteral duplication and always involves the ureter draining the upper renal pole.

Symptoms are usually those of pyelonephritis or obstruction. Intravenous urograms may show a negative shadow in the bladder cast by the ureterocele (Figure 41–8). The ureter and renal calices may reveal marked dilatation or no excretory function at all. A cystogram may show reflux into the ipsilateral lower pole ureter.

Small, slightly obstructive or nonobstructive ureteroceles need no treatment. Larger ones with significant renal caliceal dilatation seen in early childhood require transvesical excision and reimplantation of one (if not duplicated) or both ipsilateral ureters into the bladder. Folding or reduction ureteroplasty may be necessary to permit reimplantation and establishment of antireflux. Partial or total nephrectomy may be necessary in cases associated with severe obstruction.

Ehrlich RM: The ureteral folding technique for megaureter surgery. J Urol 1985;134:668.

Fredrich U et al: Ultrastructure of the distal ureter with con-

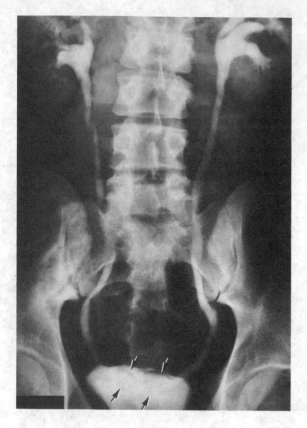

Figure 41–8. Ureterocele. Excretory urogram showing bilateral space-occupying lesions in the bladder caused by ureteroceles (arrows).

genital malformations in infants and children. Z Kinderchir 1987;42:94.

VESICOURETERAL REFLUX

Essentials of Diagnosis
- Recurrent urinary tract infections.
- Reflux on voiding radionuclide or contrast cystourethrography.
- Displaced, abnormal configuration of ureteral orifices at cystoscopy.

General Considerations

The main function of the ureterovesical junction is to permit free drainage of the ureter and simultaneously prevent urine from refluxing back from the bladder. Anatomically, the ureterovesical junction is well equipped for this function, because the ureteral musculature continues uninterrupted into the base of the bladder to form the superficial trigone. Additionally, the terminal 4–5 cm of ureter are surrounded by a musculofascial sheath (Waldeyer's sheath) that follows the ureter through the ureteral hiatus and continues in the base of the bladder as the deep trigone (Figure 41–9).

Direct continuity between the ureter and the trigone offers an efficient, muscularly active, valvular function. Any stretch of the trigone (with bladder filling) or any trigonal contraction (with voiding) leads to firm occlusion of the intravesical ureter, thus increasing resistance to flow from above downward and sealing the intravesical ureter against retrograde flow (Figure 41–10).

Etiology & Classification

Vesicoureteral reflux may be classified as follows: (1) Primary reflux due to developmental ureterotrigonal weakness. (2) Secondary obstructive reflux due to infravesical obstruction, neuropathic dysfunction,

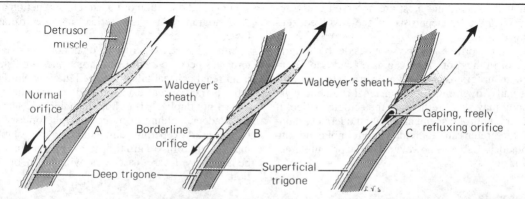

Figure 41–9. Vesicoureteral reflux. The length and fixation of the intravesical ureter and the appearance of the ureteral orifice depend upon the muscular development and efficiency of the lower ureter and its trigone. **A:** Normal structures. **B:** Moderate muscular deficiency. **C:** Marked deficiency results in a golf hole distortion of the submucosal ureter.

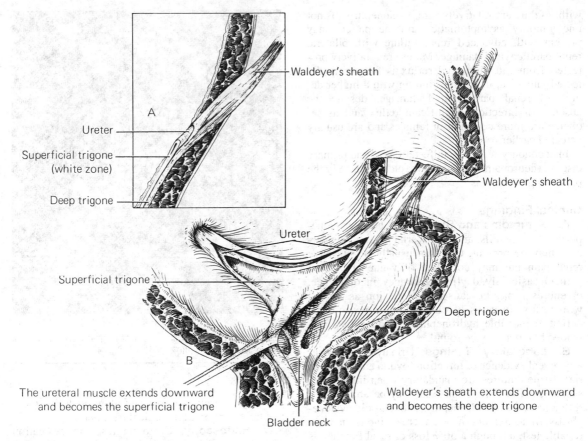

Waldeyer's sheath

A

Ureter

Superficial trigone
(white zone)

Deep trigone

Waldeyer's sheath

Ureter

Superficial trigone

Deep trigone

B

The ureteral muscle extends downward
and becomes the superficial trigone

Waldeyer's sheath extends downward
and becomes the deep trigone

Bladder neck

Figure 41–10. Normal ureterotrigonal complex. **A:** Side view of ureterovesical junction. Waldeyer's muscular sheath invests the juxtavesical ureter and continues downward as the deep trigone, which extends to the bladder neck. The ureteral musculature becomes the superficial trigone, which extends to the verumontanum in the male and stops just short of the external meatus in the female. **B:** Waldeyer's sheath is connected by a few fibers to the detrusor muscle in the ureteral hiatus. This muscular sheath, inferior to the ureteral orifices, becomes the deep trigone. The musculature of the ureters continues downward as the superficial trigone. (Adapted from Tanagho EA, Pugh RCB: Br J Urol 1963;35;151.)

iatrogenic causes, and inflammation, especially specific infection (eg, tuberculosis). (3) Secondary congenital reflux due to ureteral anomalies—ectopic orifices, duplicated ureters, or ureterocele.

Primary reflux is by far the most common type and is consistently associated with some degree of congenital muscular deficiency in the trigone and terminal ureter. The severity of reflux is proportionate to the degree of this muscular deficiency.

Secondary reflux is relatively rare. In most such cases, there is also an underlying muscular deficiency, especially in cases of inflammation. Aside from specific infections (tuberculosis, schistosomiasis), nonspecific infections rarely lead to significant reflux unless there is an underlying muscular deficiency and a marginally competent valve.

Reflux is harmful to the upper urinary tract for the following reasons: (1) It increases postvoiding residual urine in the bladder, enhancing bacterial growth

and causing risk of infection. (2) It allows bacteria free access from the bladder to the kidney. (3) It permits the transmittal of high intravesical pressure to the kidneys, leading to interstitial extravasation of urine. (4) It functionally increases the load of urine to be transported by the ureter, thus leading to stasis, dilatation, and tortuosity. (5) It can result in stone formation or secondary ureteropelvic junction obstruction.

Reflux is the most common cause of pyelonephritis and is found in about 50% of children presenting with urinary tract infection. It is present in over 75% of patients with radiologic evidence of chronic pyelonephritis and is responsible for end-stage renal disease in a large percentage of patients requiring chronic dialysis or renal transplantation.

In primary reflux, the child usually presents with symptoms of pyelonephritis or cystitis. Vague abdominal pain is not uncommon. Renal pain and pain with voiding are relatively rare. Pyelonephritis is not uncommonly asymptomatic, and the patient may present with advanced renal failure with bilateral renal parenchymal damage. Males are relatively protected from infection, and reflux is frequently detected late as an incidental finding with a higher degree of renal parenchymal damage, despite the absence of infection. Significant reflux and its sequelae are more common in females and are usually detected earlier.

In secondary reflux, manifestations of the primary disease (neuropathic, obstructive, etc) are usually the presenting symptoms.

Clinical Findings

A. Symptoms and Signs: With acute pyelonephritis, fever, chills, and costovertebral angle tenderness may be present. Children usually do not have renal pain but may complain of vague abdominal pain. Occasionally, daytime frequency, incontinence, or enuresis may be caused by infection associated with reflux. In cases of obstruction or neuropathic deficit, a palpable hydronephrotic kidney or a distended bladder may be found.

B. Laboratory Findings: Urinalysis will usually reveal evidence of infection (pyuria and bacteriuria). Urine cultures are mandatory when infection is suspected. Renal function tests may be abnormal if reflux has caused hydronephrosis or chronic pyelonephritis. Measurement of serum creatinine is the most reliable test, although a 50% loss of renal function is required before a rise in creatinine is evident.

C. Imaging Studies: Until recently, intravenous urograms were indispensable for determining the degree of renal scarring and caliceal and ureteral dilatation and for measurement of renal size. Currently, radioisotopic scanning with technetium Tc 99m DTPA and DMSA provides similar information as well as accurate differential renal function data with somewhat less overall risk to the patient. Ultrasound can provide accurate measurement of renal size and demonstrate the presence of renal scarring and ureteral or cal i ceal dilatation. In mild cases, there may be no abnormality visible in the upper urinary tract, or only mild distal ureteral dilatation may be seen.

The most useful study to conclusively diagnose reflux continues to be voiding cystourethrography (Figure 41–11). Currently, radionuclide voiding studies are as accurate and perhaps more desirable in young children. Either a contrast or radionuclide voiding study is mandatory in the evaluation of recurrent urinary tract infections. Either study may reveal secondary causes of reflux, such as **posterior urethral valves** in young males, ectopic ureteral orifices, or spastic external sphincter syndrome in young females. In some cases with mild urinary reflux, however, radiologic evidence may be difficult to demonstrate except with repeated attempts to do so. Voiding cystourethrography or radioisotope voiding cystogra-

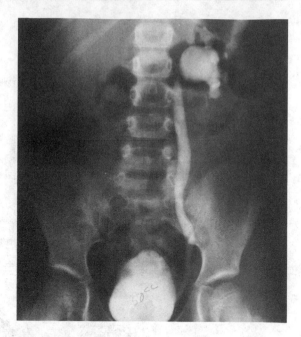

Figure 41–11. Voiding cystourethrogram showing total left vesicoureteral reflux.

phy may be useful for routine follow-up during medical treatment or after surgical treatment.

D. Endoscopy: Cystourethroscopic evaluation of trigonal development and the position and configuration of the ureteral orifices may help in determining the cause, prognosis, and treatment (surgical or nonsurgical), though it is not necessary in all cases. The incompetent ureterovesical orifice is usually displaced laterally and superiorly and may be widely open.

Differential Diagnosis

Ureteral stasis and distal ureteral dilatation may be present in conditions of intravesical obstruction or neurologic bladder lesions causing trigonal hypertrophy. Functional ureteral obstruction may allow reflux as well. Finally, although much controversy exists, there is some evidence to support the concept that a spastic striated external sphincter syndrome (perhaps with a neurologic basis, psychologic basis, or both) can cause similar findings and lead to recurrent urinary tract infections.

Treatment

In primary reflux, the initial steps should be treatment of infection, elimination of urethral obstruction, and evaluation of the degree of trigonal ureteral muscular deficiency and the chances of reversibility. Not every refluxing orifice requires surgical repair. The improvement in voiding dynamics achieved by conservative management may be all that is needed. If infection is controlled by long-term antibiotic prophylaxis, reflux may never recur (one-third of cases). In another one-third, advanced ureteral or pyelonephritic changes occur together with severe ureteral orifice deformity, indicating the need for operation. Many of the remaining one-third of cases will come to surgical repair after repeated conservative attempts to control urinary tract infection and stop progression of the renal damage have proved inadequate.

In obstructive secondary reflux (eg, posterior urethral valves), release of obstruction may cure reflux. Occasionally, surgical reimplantation is still required. In neuropathic reflux, intermittent catheterization for control of infection may allow return of valvular competence. However, many cases will require surgical repair (reimplantation) of the ureterovesical junction. In congenital secondary reflux, ectopic orifices, duplication with ureterocele, and other congenital malformations, reimplantation is generally required.

The aim of surgery is to excise the muscularly weak terminal ureter, provide proper ureterotrigonal fixation, and give adequate posterior support to provide an intravesical ureter about 2.5 cm long. One of three methods is used in most cases. In **suprahiatal repair (Politano-Leadbetter procedure),** a new ureteral hiatus is developed about 2.5 cm above the original one, and the ureter, after passing through a submucosal tunnel, is sutured to the cut edge of the trigone at the level of the original orifice. In **infrahiatal repair (Hutch-Paquin procedure),** the original hiatus is maintained, and after the weak terminal ureter is discarded, the ureter is advanced through a 2.5-cm submucosal tunnel to end closer to the internal meatus. More recently, a totally extravesical ureteral advancement procedure **(extravesical ureteroplasty)** reportedly achieves results similar to those achieved with the methods described above with a shorter hospitalization stay and convalescence.

Recently, the use of Teflon paste or collagen gel injections has received attention. With proper placement beneath the ureteral orifice under endoscopic vision, the Teflon paste acts to bolster the deficient antireflux mechanism and may obviate the need for more extensive surgery in a significant number of cases. Concern regarding late sequelae of Teflon (eg, migration, possible carcinogenesis) are under study.

Prognosis

The long-term prognosis is excellent for patients with mild to moderate reflux successfully treated with antibiotic prophylaxis. There are few instances of recurrent infection or renal insufficiency. Patients with more significant reflux or persistent urinary tract infections will benefit from surgical repair; the success rate is approximately 95% (cessation of reflux, clearance of renal infection, and absence of obstruction). Unfortunately, for patients with advanced disease (irreversible ureteral decompensation and

chronic pyelonephritis, which is now thought to be a self-perpetuating immune complex process), the prognosis is less favorable. These patients account for a significant proportion of patients with end-stage renal disease who ultimately require chronic dialysis, renal transplantation, or both.

Dodat H, Takvorian P: Treatment of vesicoureteral reflux in children by endoscopic injection of Teflon: Review of 2 years of experience. Eur Urol 1990;17:304.

Kangarloo H et al: Urinary tract infection in infants and children evaluated by ultrasound. Radiology 1985; 154:367.

Leonard MP et al: Endoscopic injection of glutaraldehyde cross-linked bovine dermal collagen for correction of vesicoureteral reflux. J Urol 1991;145:115.

Leonidas JC et al: Sonography as a substitute for excretory urography in children with urinary tract infection. AJR Am J Roentgenol 1985;144:815.

Puri P, Giuney EJ: Endoscopic correction of vesicoureteric reflux secondary to neuropathic bladder. Br J Urol 1986; 58:504.

BLADDER ANOMALIES

Anomalies of the bladder are infrequent and include the following: (1) **agenesis,** or complete absence, which results in a persistent cloaca; (2) bladder **duplication,** which may be complete, with separate ureteral openings drained by duplicated urethras, or incomplete, with a septum or hourglass deformity; and (3) **urachal anomalies,** which in the most severe forms appear as a patent opening at the umbilicus and are usually associated with some form of bladder outlet obstruction. In less severe forms, a **urachal diverticulum** may be present at the dome of the bladder or a **urachal cyst** along the course of the partially obliterated urachus. These latter conditions may cause abdominal pain and umbilical or bladder infection requiring surgical treatment. Occasionally, adenocarcinoma develops in a urachal remnant (see Tumors of the Bladder, p 929).

Failure of cloacal division results in a persistent cloaca. Incomplete division is more frequent (though still rare) and results in a rectovesical, rectourethral, or rectovestibular fistula (usually with imperforate anus or anal atresia).

Exstrophy of the Bladder

Exstrophy of the bladder is the most severe bladder anomaly—the result of a complete ventral defect of the urogenital sinus and the overlying inferior abdominal wall musculature and integument (Figure 41–12A). The lower central portion is devoid of skin and muscle. The anterior bladder wall is absent, and the posterior wall is contiguous with surrounding skin. Urine drains onto the abdominal wall, the rami of the pubic bones are widely separated (Figure 41–12B), and the open pelvic ring may affect gait. In

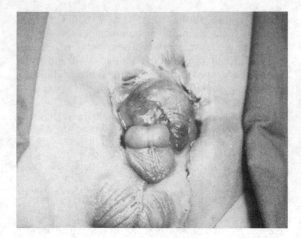

Figure 41–12A. Photograph of male patient with bladder exstrophy.

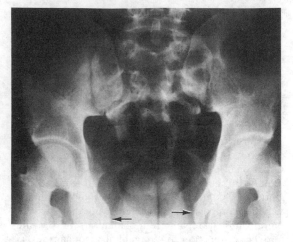

Figure 41–12B. Roentgenogram of pelvis with widely separated pubes (arrows) in patient with exstrophy.

males, the penis is epispadiac, resulting from development of the genital primordia more caudal than normal. The exposed bladder mucosa tends to be chronically inflamed. Hydronephrosis from ureterovesical occlusion is common. Late development of squamous cell carcinoma of the untreated bladder was common.

Currently, the favored treatment is bladder salvage, which includes closure of the bladder with or without pelvic osteotomies in the newborn period. Phalloplasty and urethral reconstruction may be performed at a later time after growth and some degree of physical maturation. Ureteral obstruction or vesicoureteral reflux may develop and require ureteral reimplantation. The closed bladder is apt to have a small capacity, and incontinence is often a complication. Good results have been observed in more than half of all patients treated, with preservation of renal function and continence.

Kramer SA, Jackson IT: Bilateral rhomboid flaps for reconstruction of external genitalia in epispadias ex s trophy. Plast Reconstr Surg 1986;77:621.

Oesterling JE, Jeffs RD: The importance of a successful initial bladder closure in the surgical management of classical bladder ex s trophy: Analysis of 144 patients treated at the Johns Hopkins Hospital between 1975 and 1985. J Urol 1987;137:258.

Prune Belly Syndrome

Prune belly (Eagle-Barrett) syndrome is a complex anomaly of the lower urinary tract and abdomen consisting of absence of the abdominal muscles, bilateral cryptorchidism, ureteral dilatation and reflux, and an enlarged, poorly functioning bladder and proximal urethra. The cause is not known but may be marked intra-abdominal distention in utero. One must screen for and treat high-grade vesicoureteral reflux in order to preserve renal function. The syndrome is variable in its degree of phenotypic expression.

Congenital Neurovesical Dysfunction

Congenital neurovesical dysfunction frequently accompanies a posterior myelomeningocele and sacral agenesis, with associated spinal abnormalities. Both conditions may result in incontinence and recurrent urinary infection with late sequelae (ureteral reflux and pyelonephritis).

PENILE & URETHRAL ANOMALIES

Hypospadias

Hypospadias is the most common urethral anomaly in males and occurs in one in 300 births. It results from failure of fusion of the urethral folds on the undersurface of the genital tubercle. The urethral meatus is ventrally displaced on the shaft of the penis. The severity of hypospadias is variable; the meatus may appear from the glans to the perineum (but never proximal to the bulbous urethra). With more proximal displacement, chordee—ventral curvature of the penile shaft—necessitates excision of the fibrous, malformed corpora spongios a which, if left untreated, would preclude straight erections and normal intercourse (Figure 41–13). The midscrotal hypospadiac penis may resemble female external genitalia with an enlarged clitoris and labia. Sexual assignment in these latter infants requires rapid and complete study by hormone and chromosome analysis.

A few patients may have a rudimentary uterus and vagina (**pseudohermaphroditism**). The urinary sphincters are normal.

The incidence of cryptorchidism accompanying

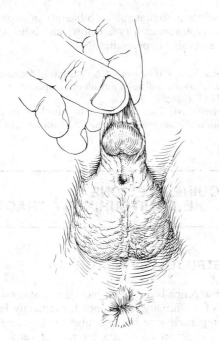

Figure 41–13. Hypospadias, penoscrotal type. Redundant dorsal foreskin that is deficient ventrally; ventral chordee.

this anomaly is high. In hypospadias with the meatus positioned proximal to the corona, the prepuce is abnormal—not forming a complete cylinder due to a ventral defect. Circumcision should not be done in these patients, as the prepuce can be used later in surgical repair.

The degree of hypospadias dictates the need for repair. If the opening is glandular or coronal (85% of patients), the penis is usually functional both for micturition and procreation, and repair is done primarily for cosmetic reasons. Openings that are more proximal on the shaft require correction to allow voiding while standing, normal erection, and proper sperm deposition during intercourse. Surgical plastic repair of hypospadias is currently accomplished by a variety of highly successful one-stage operations and should be completed prior to school age.

Epispadias

Epispadias is a rare congenital anomaly that is almost always associated with bladder exstrophy. When it occurs alone, it is considered a milder degree of the exstrophy complex.

The urethra opens on the dorsum of the penis, with deficient corpus spongiosum and loosely attached corpora cavernosa. If the defect is extensive, it may extend to the bladder neck, causing incontinence. The pubic bones are separated, as in exstrophy. Marked dorsiflexion of the penis is usually present.

Treatment consists of correction of penile curvature, reconstruction of the urethra, and reconstruction of the bladder neck in incontinent patients.

Urethral Strictures

Congenital urethral strictures are rare but when present are most common in the fossa navicularis (just proximal to the meatus) and in the bulbomembranous urethra. Commonly, these strictures are thin diaphragms that may respond to simple dilation or to direct vision internal urethrotomy. Rarely is open surgical repair necessary. Congenital urethral strictures in girls and meatal stenosis in boys are very uncommon. When the latter does occur, it appears to be acquired, as it is seen only in circumcised boys.

Urethral Diverticulum

Urethral diverticula are common congenital lesions. In males, they are nearly always in the pendulous or bulbous urethra. They are often associated with an obstructive flap of the urethral mucosa (anterior urethral valve)—thought to represent incomplete closure of the urethral folds. Treatment by endoscopic unroofing is usually successful, though most diverticula are small and require no therapy. In females they occur in adult life and are usually manifested by irritative symptoms and recurrent infection. The cause is unknown, but the disorder is most likely congenital. Treatment is usually by transvaginal excision. Diverticula may occasionally harbor stones or tumors.

Posterior Urethral Valves

Posterior urethral valves are the most common obstructive urethral lesion in newborn and infant males. They consist of obstructive folds of mucosa, seen only in males, which originate at or are attached at some point to the verumontanum in the prostatic urethra. The embryologic derivation is indefinite. They are partially obstructive and thus lead to variable degrees of back pressure damage to the urinary bladder and upper urinary tract. Progressive renal damage may occur as a result of early obstruction at the ureterovesical junction because of trigonal hypertrophy and later development of reflux. Dilatation and obstruction of the prostatic urethra are always present. Spontaneous urinary ascites from the kidneys is often seen in neonates. This clears when the obstruction is relieved.

Manifestations consist of difficult voiding, a weak urinary stream, and a midline lower abdominal mass that represents a distended bladder. In some cases, the kidneys are palpable. Urinary incontinence and urinary tract infection may occur. Laboratory findings include elevated serum urea nitrogen and creatinine and evidence of urinary infection. Intravenous urograms show evidence of bladder thickening and trabeculation, hydroureter, and hydronephrosis. Demonstration of urethral valves on a voiding cystourethrogram establishes the diagnosis, as does endoscopic identification of valves.

Posterior urethral valves must be differentiated from neuropathic dysfunction, tumors, and meatal stenosis. If meatal stenosis and phimosis are excluded, any lower urinary tract obstructive disorder in a newborn or young boy should be considered posterior urethral valves until proved otherwise.

Treatment consists of destruction of the valves by endoscopic fulguration or resection, which can be accomplished through a perineal urethrotomy or suprapubic cystostomy tract (transvesical antegrade) in neonates and young boys or in a retrograde fashion transurethrally in older males. Vesical drainage by percutaneous cystostomy may be required to improve impaired kidney function and may provide access for transvesical antegrade valve ablation. Bilateral ureteral reimplantation may be needed for a persistently obstructed or refluxing ureterovesical junction, though these changes may correct themselves after the valves are destroyed.

The prognosis depends upon the original degree of kidney damage and the success of efforts to prevent or treat infection. In cases seen early, the prognosis is quite favorable.

Barakat AV, Seikaly MG, Der Kaloustian VM: Urogenital abnormalities in genetic disease. J Urol 1986;136:778.

Mitchell ME, Kulb TB: Hypospadias repair without a bladder drainage catheter. J Urol 1986;135:321.

Warshaw BL et al: Prognostic features in infants with obstructive uropathy due to posterior urethral valves. J Urol 1985;133:240.

Zaontz MR, Firlit CF: Percutaneous antegrade ablation of posterior urethral valves in infants with small caliber urethras: An alternative to urinary diversion. J Urol 1986;136:247.

SCROTAL & TESTICULAR ANOMALIES*

Testicular Torsion

Neonatal testicular torsion (extravaginal torsion) is an extremely rare condition that occurs due to faulty scrotal fixation. The entire tunica vaginalis is twisted. Even when detected immediately following birth, this condition results in an infarcted testicle. Current studies suggest that early removal of the infarcted testicle may prevent functional damage in the opposite testicle. Intravaginal testicular torsion in adolescents is described later in this chapter.

Scrotal Lesions

Congenital scrotal lesions include hypoplasia of

---

*Undescended testicles (cryptorchidism) and hydroceles in infants are discussed in Chapter 46.

the scrotum (unilateral or bilateral) in association with cryptorchidism (see below) and bifid scrotum with extensive hypospadias.

Anderson JB, Williamson GCN: The fate of the human testes following unilateral torsion of the spermatic cord. Br J Urol 1986;58:698.

Hadziselimovic F et al: Testicular histology in children with unilateral testicular torsion. J Urol 1986;136:208.

ACQUIRED LESIONS OF THE GENITOURINARY TRACT

OBSTRUCTIVE UROPATHY

Obstruction is one of the most important abnormalities of the urinary tract, since it eventually leads to decompensation of the muscular conduits and reservoirs, back pressure, and atrophy of renal parenchyma. It also invites infection and stone formation, which cause additional damage and can ultimately end in complete unilateral or bilateral destruction of the kidneys.

Both the level and the degree of obstruction are important to an understanding of the pathologic consequences. Any obstruction at or distal to the bladder neck may lead to back pressure affecting both kidneys. Obstruction at or proximal to the ureteral orifice leads to unilateral damage unless the lesion involves both ureters simultaneously. Complete obstruction leads to rapid decompensation of the system proximal to the site of obstruction. Partial obstruction leads to gradual progressive muscular hypertrophy followed by dilatation, decompensation, and hydronephrotic changes.

Etiology

Acquired urinary tract obstruction may be due to inflammatory or traumatic urethral strictures, bladder outlet obstruction (benign prostatic hyperplasia or cancer of the prostate), vesical tumors, neuropathic bladder, extrinsic ureteral compression (tumor, retroperitoneal fibrosis, or enlarged lymph nodes), ureteral or pelvic stones, ureteral strictures, or ureteral or pelvic tumors.

Pathogenesis

Regardless of its cause, acquired obstruction leads to similar changes in the urinary tract, which vary depending on the severity and duration of obstruction.

A. Urethral Changes: Proximal to the obstruction, the urethra dilates and balloons. A urethral diverticulum may develop, and dilatation and gaping of the prostatic urethra and ejaculatory ducts may occur.

B. Vesical Changes: Early, the detrusor and trigonal thickening and hypertrophy compensate for the outlet obstruction, allowing complete bladder emptying. This change leads to progressive development of bladder trabeculation, cellules, saccules, and, finally, diverticula. Subsequently, bladder decompensation occurs and is characterized by the above changes plus incomplete bladder emptying (ie, postvoid residual urine). Trigonal hypertrophy leads to secondary ureteral obstruction owing to increased resistance to flow through the intravesical ureter. With detrusor decompensation and residual urine accumulation, there is stretching of the hypertrophied trigone, which appreciably increases ureteral obstruction. This is the mechanism of back pressure on the kidney in the presence of vesical outlet obstruction (while the ureterovesical junction maintains its competence). Catheter drainage of the bladder relieves trigonal stretch and improves drainage from the upper tract.

Λ very late change with persistent obstruction (more frequently encountered with neuropathic dysfunction) is decompensation of the ureterovesical junction, leading to reflux. Reflux aggravates the back pressure effect on the upper tract by transmitting abnormally high intravesical pressures and favors the onset or persistence of urinary tract infection.

C. Ureteral Changes: The first change noted is a gradual increase in ureteral distention. This increases ureteral caliber and stimulates hyperactive ureteral contraction and ureteral muscular hypertrophy. Because the ureteral musculature runs in an irregular helical pattern, stretching of its muscular elements leads to lengthening as well as widening, causing the dilated ureter to assume a tortuous, serpiginous course, weaving back and forth across the relatively straight course of the ureteral vessels, which are unaffected by the ureteral obstruction. This is the start of ureteral decompensation, where tortuosity and dilatation become apparent. These changes progress until the ureter becomes atonic, with infrequent, ineffective, or completely absent peristalsis.

D. Pelvicaliceal Changes: The renal pelvis and calices, subjected to increased volumes of retained urine, distend. First, the pelvis shows evidence of hyperactivity and hypertrophy, and then progressive dilatation and atony. The calices show similar changes to a variable degree, depending on whether the renal pelvis is intrarenal or extrarenal. In the latter, caliceal dilatation may be minimal in spite of marked pelvic dilatation. In the intrarenal pelvis, caliceal dilatation and renal parenchymal damage are maximal. The successive phases seen with obstruction are rounding of the fornices, followed by flattening of the papillae and finally clubbing of the minor calices.

E. Renal Parenchymal Changes: With continued pelvicaliceal distention, there is parenchymal compression against the renal capsule and, more importantly, compression of the arcuate vessels results in a marked drop in renal blood flow leading to parenchymal ischemic atrophy. With increased intrapelvic pressure, there is progressive dilatation of the collecting and distal tubules, with compression and atrophy of tubular cells.

Clinical Findings
A. Symptoms and Signs: The findings vary according to the site of obstruction.

1. Infravesical obstruction–Infravesical obstruction (eg, due to urethral stricture, benign prostatic hypertrophy, bladder neck contracture) leads to difficulty in initiation of voiding, a weak stream, and a diminished flow rate with terminal dribbling. Burning and frequency are common associated symptoms. A distended or thickened bladder wall may be palpable. Urethral induration due to stricture, benign prostatic hypertrophy, or cancer of the prostate may be noted on rectal examination. Meatal stenosis and impacted urethral stones are readily diagnosed by physical examination.

2. Supravesical obstruction–Renal pain or renal colic and gastrointestinal symptoms are commonly associated. Supravesical obstruction (eg, due to ureteral stone, ureteropelvic junction obstruction) may be completely asymptomatic when it develops gradually over a period of months. An enlarged kidney may be palpable. Costovertebral angle tenderness may be present.

B. Laboratory Findings: Evidence of urinary tract infection, hematuria, or crystalluria may be seen. Impaired renal function may be noted in cases of bilateral obstruction. Postrenal azotemia (serum changes reflecting impaired renal function due primarily to obstruction) is suggested by elevation of serum urea nitrogen and serum creatinine with a ratio greater than 10:1.

C. Imaging Studies: Radiologic examination is usually diagnostic in cases of stasis, tumors, and strictures. Dilatation and anatomic changes occur above the level of obstruction whereas distal to the obstruction, the configuration is usually normal. This helps in localizing the site of obstruction. Combined antegrade imaging by intravenous urograms and retrograde imaging by ureterograms or urethrograms is sometimes needed to demonstrate the obstructed segment. In supravesical obstruction, demonstration of stasis and delayed drainage is essential to establish and quantitate the severity of obstruction.

1. Antegrade urography–Antegrade urography via percutaneous needle or tube nephrostomy is valuable when the obstructed kidney fails to excrete the radiopaque material on excretory urography. The Whitaker test requires percutaneous catheter access to the collecting system above the site of suspected obstruction. This permits fluid introduction into the renal pelvis and simultaneous measurement of urine flow rate and pressures in the bladder and renal pelvis, thus providing a quantitative assessment of the degree and severity of obstruction. The fluid transport can be measured and the degree of obstruction estimated by the use of a pressure monitor.

2. Ultrasonography–This will reveal the degree of dilatation of the renal pelvis and calices and allows for diagnosis of hydronephrosis even in the prenatal period.

3. Isotope studies–A technetium Tc 99m DMSA scan portrays the degree of hydronephrosis as well as renal function. Use of diuretics during the scan can provide information similar to that obtained with the Whitaker test.

4. CT scan–This may be of value in revealing the degree and site of obstruction as well as the cause in many cases. The use of contrast agents will allow estimation of residual renal function.

Complications

The most important complication of urinary tract obstruction is renal parenchymal atrophy as a result of back pressure. Obstruction also predisposes to infection and stone formation, and infection occurring with obstruction leads to rapid kidney destruction.

Treatment

The first goal of therapy is relief of the obstruction (eg, catheterization for relief of acute urinary retention). Definitive therapy often requires operation. Simple urethral stricture may be managed by dilation or internal urethrotomy (incision of the stricture under direct vision through the resectoscope). However, urethroplasty (open surgical graft of skin or bladder mucosa to replace urethral diameter) may be required. Benign prostatic hyperplasia and obstructing bladder tumors classically require excision.

Impacted ureteral stones must either be removed or bypassed by a catheter if it is thought that they may pass spontaneously.

Ureteral or ureteropelvic junction obstruction requires surgical repair. Renal stones may be removed instrumentally via percutaneous nephrostomy or by irrigation through a tube placed directly into the kidney.

Preliminary drainage above the obstruction is sometimes needed to improve kidney function. Occasionally, intestinal urinary diversion or permanent nephrostomy is required. If damage is advanced, nephrectomy may be indicated.

Prognosis

The prognosis depends on the cause, site, duration, and degree of kidney damage and renal decompensation. In general, relief of obstruction leads to improvement in kidney function except in seriously damaged kidneys, especially those destroyed by inflammatory scarring.

Claesson G et al: Experimental obstructive hydronephrosis in newborn rats: XI. A one-year followup study of renal function and morphology. J Urol 1989;142:1602.

Coptcoat MJ, Watkinson L, Duff P: Monitoring of upper urinary tract pressures in the ambulatory patient. Br J Urol 1988;61:465.

Kekomaki M et al: Correlates of diuretic renography in experimental hydronephrosis. J Urol 1989;141:391.

Piepsz A et al: Long-term followup of separate glomerular filtration rate in partially obstructed kidneys: Experimental study. Scand J Urol Nephrol 1988;22:327.

URETEROPELVIC JUNCTION OBSTRUCTION

Stenosis of the renal pelvis outlet is commonly due to congenital narrowing of the junction or compression by anomalous vessels. However, the lesion may be acquired. Presentation is similar in either case, with abrupt onset of flank pain usually following ingestion of large amounts of fluids.

The diagnosis is made by intravenous urography, which reveals hydronephrosis with a dilated renal pelvis and thin renal cortex. Occasionally, patients present with intermittent hydronephrosis and normal urograms except during attacks of pain when x-rays show typical obstruction. These patients generally have a normal renal parenchyma. Retrograde ureteropyelography is usually needed in patients with chronic moderate to severe obstruction to determine the extent of the lesion and to provide assurance that the distal ureter is normal (Figure 41–14). Marked obstruction may make it difficult to determine whether kidney function is surgically salvageable. In these cases, it may be necessary to perform either (1) differential radioisotope renography with use of a diuretic during the study or (2) percutaneous nephrostomy with flow measurement through the pelvic junction (Whitaker test) and differential creatinine clearance collection.

Severe obstruction with minimal remaining renal function is best treated by unilateral nephrectomy. I f renal function is adequate (> 10% of total renal function or > 10 mL/min creatinine clearance) , surgical repair of the stenosis, either by creation of a renal pelvis flap or by resection of the stenotic area and reanastomosis, is warranted. Recently, the use of percutaneous nephroscopy with endopyelotomy, incising the strictured ureteropelvic junction, offers an alternat iv e method of therapy. The surgical results are excellent in terms of functional preservation and relief of symptoms, but dilation of the calices may persist .

URETERAL STENOSIS

Acquired ureteral stenosis is less common than the congenital types. Causes include (1) ureteral injury (surgical, traumatic, radiation therapy), (2) compression of the ureter by lymph nodes harboring cancer,

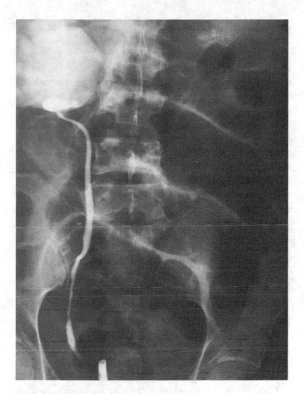

Figure 41–14. Retrograde ureteropyelogram showing right ureteropelvic junction obstruction.

(3) prolonged compression by an anomalous blood vessel, (4) tuberculous or bilharzial ureteritis, (5) retroperitoneal fibrosis, (6) aneurysm of the aorta following aortofemoral bypass grafts, (7) ureteropelvic obstruction secondary to reflux, (8) occlusion of the ureterovesical junction by infiltrating cancer of the bladder or cervix, and (9) functional obstruction of the ureterovesical junction secondary to hypertrophy of the trigone developing from obstruction distal to the bladder neck.

Symptoms are usually those of obstruction to urine flow from the kidney, though many cases are asymptomatic. An unsuspected lesion is often discovered on excretory urography.

Therapy consists of treatment of the cause, eg, resection of the stenosed segment with end-to-end anastomosis. Endoscopy-guided ureteral dilation or ureteral stents may be beneficial for postoperative ureteral stricture or following injury due to radiation therapy.

RETROPERITONEAL FIBROSIS
(See also Chapter 22.)

One or both ureters may be compressed by a chronic inflammatory process, usually of unknown cause, which involves the retroperitoneal tissues of the lumbosacral area. Patients treated for migraine with methysergide may develop this fibrosis. Sclerosing Hodgkin's disease and fibrosis from metastatic cancer have also been implicated. Symptoms include renal pain, low backache, and those associated with uremia. Some patients present with complete anuria. Urinary infection is unusual. If both ureters are obstructed, the serum creatinine is elevated.

Excretory urograms show hydronephrosis and a dilated ureter down to the point of obstruction. The ureters are displaced medially in the lumbar area. Retrograde ureterograms show a long segment of ureteral stenosis, though a catheter passes easily through the ureter. Sonograms and CT scans may demonstrate fibrous plaques with proximal hydroureteronephrosis. If the patient is anuric, indwelling ureteral catheters or percutaneous nephrostomy should be done. When the patient's condition has improved, definitive therapy can be accomplished. If methysergide is suspected to be the causative agent, fibrosis may subside when the drug is discontinued. These patients may benefit from administration of corticosteroids. Chronic indwelling ureteral stents have also been used successfully. If these methods fail, ureterolysis must be performed to free the ureter from the fibrous plaque. The involved ureter should be dissected from the plaque, moved to a lateral position, and wrapped with omentum to prevent recurrent entrapment.

BENIGN PROSTATIC HYPERPLASIA

Essentials of Diagnosis
- Prostatism: nocturia, hesitancy, slow stream, terminal dribbling, frequency.
- Residual urine.
- Acute urinary retention.
- Uremia in advanced cases.

General Considerations
The cause of benign prostatic enlargement (BPH) is not known but is probably related to hormonal factors. By upsetting the mechanism for opening and funneling the vesical neck at the time of voiding, hyperplasia of the prostate causes increased outflow resistance. Consequently, a higher intravesical pressure is required to accomplish voiding, causing hypertrophy of the vesical and trigonal muscles. This may lead to the development of bladder diverticula—outpocketings of vesical mucosa between the detrusor muscle bundles. Hypertrophy of the trigone causes excessive stress on the intravesical ureter, producing functional obstruction and resulting in hydroureteronephrosis in late cases. Stagnation of urine can lead to infection; the onset of cystitis will exacerbate the obstructive symptoms. The periurethral and subtrigonal prostate enlargement produces the most significant obstruction.

The prostate in young men has an anatomic capsule like an apple peel. In men with prostatic enlargement, there is a thick "surgical" capsule similar to an orange peel, composed of peripherally compressed true prostatic tissue. This permits intracapsular enucleation of the enlarged periurethral glands (Figure 41–15).

Clinical Findings

A. Symptoms and Signs: Typically, the patient notices hesitancy and loss of force and caliber of the stream. He may also be awakened by the urge to void several times at night (nocturia). Postvoid dribbling ("terminal dribbling") is particularly disturbing. The complication of infection increases the degree of obstructive symptoms and is often associated with burning on urination. Acute urinary retention may supervene. This is associated with severe urgency, suprapubic pain, and a distended, palpable bladder.

The size of the prostate rectally is not of diagnostic importance, since there is a poor correlation between the size of the gland and the degree of symptoms and amount of residual urine.

B. Laboratory Findings: Urinalysis may reveal evidence of infection. Residual urine is commonly increased, and a timed urinary flow rate will be decreased. The serum creatinine may be elevated in cases with prolonged severe obstruction.

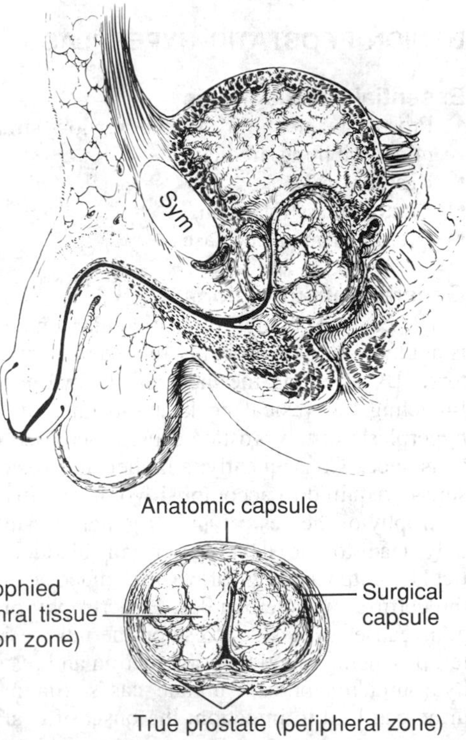

C. Imaging Studies: Excretory urograms are often normal and are thus not required. In late-stage cases, the study may show hydroureteronephrosis if severe obstruction is present. This almost always resolves after prostatectomy. The enlarged gland may cause an indentation in the inferior surface of the bladder, which may result in a "J-hook" deformity of the distal ureter. The postvoiding film may reveal varying amounts of residual urine. Renal ultrasound examination may obviate the need for urograms. Pelvic ultrasound can also accurately predict the amount of residual urine.

D. Endoscopic Examination: The presence of residual urine may be documented if the patient is catheterized immediately after voiding. Endoscopy will reveal secondary vesical changes (eg, trabeculation) and enlargement of the periurethral prostatic glands.

Differential Diagnosis

Neuropathic bladder may produce a similar syndrome. A history suggesting a neuropathic difficulty may be obtained. Neurologic deficit involving S2–4 is particularly significant.

Cancer of the prostate also causes symptoms of vesical neck obstruction. Symptoms and signs of osseous metastases may also be present. Typically, the cancerous gland is stony hard. Serum prostate-specific antigen may be slightly elevated in patients with benign prostatic hypertrophy, but if it is over 10 ng/mL, cancer should be suspected (normal is < 4 ng/mL by Hybritech assay). Serum acid phosphatase is elevated in advanced cases. Serum alkaline phosphatase is usually increased if the tumor has spread to bone.

Acute prostatitis may cause symptoms of obstruction, but the patient is septic and has infected urine. The prostate is exquisitely tender.

Urethral stricture diminishes the caliber of the urinary stream. There is usually a history of gonorrhea or local trauma. A retrograde urethrogram will show the stenotic area. A stricture blocks the passage of an instrument or catheter.

Complications

Obstruction and residual urine lead to vesical and prostatic infection and occasionally pyelonephritis; these may be difficult to eradicate.

The obstruction may lead to the development of bladder diverticula. Infected residual urine may contribute to the formation of calculi.

Functional obstruction of the intravesical ureter, caused by the hypertrophic trigone, may lead to hydroureteronephrosis.

Treatment

The indications for operative management are im-

Figure 41–15. Benign prostatic hyperplasia. The enlarged periurethral glands are enclosed by the surgical capsule. The true prostate has been compressed.

pairment of or threat to renal function and bothersome symptoms. Because the degree of obstruction progresses slowly in most patients, conservative treatment (watchful waiting) may be adequate. Drugs that relax the prostatic capsule and internal sphincter (α-adrenergic blocking agents) or decrease the volume of the prostate (5α-reductase inhibitors or antiandrogens) have been tried with some success. Further study is required to determine their relative effectiveness.

A. Conservative Measures: Treatment of chronic prostatitis may reduce symptoms. The resolution of a complicating cystitis will usually afford some relief. In order to protect vesical tone, the patient should be cautioned to void as soon as the urge develops. Forcing fluids over a short time causes rapid vesical filling, decreasing vesical tone; this is a common cause of sudden acute urinary retention. These conservative measures are of only temporary help—if any—in patients with prostatic hyperplasia.

Controversy surrounds choices in the treatment of benign prostatic hyperplasia. No treatment may be appropriate in patients who complain of mild to moderate prostatism. Recent interest has focused on nonoperative medical therapy, including α-sympatholytic agents, which relax the internal (bladder neck) sphincter and prostatic capsule; 5 α-reductase inhibitors, which block conversion of testosterone to dihydrotestosterone (the androgen active in promoting prostate growth); antiandrogens; and hyperthermia.

Catheterization is mandatory for acute urinary retention. Spontaneous voiding may return, but a catheter should be left indwelling for 3 days while detrusor tone returns. If this fails, surgery is indicated.

B. Surgical Measures: There are four classic approaches used in prostatectomy: transurethral, retropubic, suprapubic, and perineal. The transurethral route is preferred in patients with glands weighing under 50 g because morbidity rates are lower and the hospital stay is shorter. Larger glands may require open surgery, depending on the preference of the urologist. The death rate is low in each procedure (1–2%). Potency is at greatest risk when the transperineal exposure is used, but impotence occasionally results following transurethral resection of the prostate.

Two recent alternative approaches to the treatment of benign prostatic hypertrophy include (1) transurethral balloon dilatation of the prostate (TUBD) and (2) transurethral incision of the prostate (TUIP). Balloon dilatation requires insertion of a balloon catheter positioned in the prostatic urethra with fluoroscopic and endoscopic guidance. Once placed in the prostatic urethra, the balloon is inflated under manometric control and left in place for 5–10 minutes. Treatment appears to disrupt the prostatic capsule and expansion-decompression of the ade-

noma. TUIP requires incision of the prostate at the bladder neck up to the verumontanum, allowing expansion of the entire prostatic urethra. This procedure is especially effective when the primary point of obstruction is caused by a "median bar" (subtrigonal benign hyperplasia).

Prognosis

Most patients with marked symptoms receive considerable relief following surgical treatment; however, those with milder forms may benefit from drug or dilatation therapy.

URETHRAL STRICTURE

Acquired urethral strictures in males may be due to external trauma or to prior instrumentation (most common). Strictures may be inflammatory, due to gonorrhea, tuberculous urethritis, or schistosomiasis, or may rarely be a complication of cancer. The common presenting symptoms are dysuria, weak stream, splaying of the urinary stream, urinary retention, and urinary tract infection. Evidence of scarring due to trauma or induration and perineal fistula may be seen. Urethral calibration reveals the degree of narrowing. A retrograde urethrogram will delineate the site and degree of stricture.

Urethral stricture must be differentiated from bladder outlet obstruction due to prostatism, impacted urethral stones, urethral foreign bodies, and tumors.

Treatment consists of transurethral direct vision internal urethrotomy (incision of the stricture). Successful results are obtained in 75% of patients. For long dense strictures or those failing to respond to internal urethrotomy, open surgical repair is indicated. This is probably best achieved by the transpubic route if the lesion involves the membranous urethra. If the mid urethra is involved, the perineal approach is indicated; if the distal urethra is involved, the penile approach is appropriate. End-to-end anastomosis is satisfactory, but a one-stage inlay patch, tube, or pedicle graft of preputial skin is currently favored for most strictures. An indwelling stainless steel mesh cylinder has been used successfully to expand and maintain urethral caliber following incision.

Arrighi HM et al: Symptoms and signs of prostatism as risk factors for prostatectomy. Prostate 1990;16:254.

Branen GE, Bush WH, Lewis GP: Endopyelotomy for primary repair of ureteropelvic junction obstruction. J Urol 1988;139:29.

Clayman RV et al: Ureteronephroscopic endopyelotomy. J Urol 1990;144:246.

Fowler FJ et al: Symptom status and quality of life following prostatectomy. JAMA 1988;259:3018.

Higgins PM et al: Non-operative management of retroperitoneal fibrosis. Br J Surg 1988;75:573.

Kramolowsky EV, Tucker RD, Nelson CMK: Management

of benign ureteral strictures: Open surgical repair or endoscopic dilation? J Urol 1989;141:285.

Lang EK, Glorioso LW III: Antegrade transluminal dilation of benign ureteral strictures: Long-term results. AJR Am J Roentgenol 1988;150:131.

Lepor H, Knapp-Maloney G, Sunshine H: A dose titration study evaluating terazosin, a selective, once-a-day α-blocker for the treatment of symptomatic benign prostatic hyperplasia. J Urol 1990;144:1393.

Milroy EJG et al: A new treatment for urethral strictures. Lancet 1988;1:1424.

Nielsen HO: Transurethral prostatotomy versus transurethral prostatectomy in benign prostatic hypertrophy: A prospective randomized study. Br J Urol 1988;61:435.

Nielsen KK et al: The intraprostatic spiral: New treatment for urinary retention. Br J Urol 1990;65:500.

Sapozink MD et al: Transurethral hyperthermia for benign prostatic hyperplasia: Preliminary clinic results. J Urol 1990;143:944.

URINARY TRACT INFECTIONS

Urinary tract infection is the second most common type of infection in humans and is encountered in a large segment of patients seen by urologists.

These infections are caused by a variety of pyogenic bacteria, and the pathologic tissue response is not specific to the offending organism. The most common organisms are gram-negative bacteria, particularly *Escherichia coli.* Less common are *Enterobacter aerogenes, Proteus vulgaris, Proteus mirabilis, Pseudomonas aeruginosa,* and *Streptococcus faecalis.*

Owing to the short length of the female urethra and bacterial colonization of the introitus, ascending infection is a common occurrence in young girls and in sexually active women. In males, ascending infection is usually a consequence of urethral instrumentation. In any case, infection will be confined to the bladder if the ureterovesical junctions are competent. Otherwise, ascending infection can reach the kidney, leading to pyelonephritis (see below).

Descending or hematogenous infection is relatively uncommon. When it occurs, it is usually in association with local urinary tract disorders—most commonly, obstruction and stasis; less commonly, trauma, foreign bodies, or tumors.

Lymphatic spread occasionally occurs from the large bowel or from the cervix and adnexa in the female through the perivesical and periureteral lymphatics.

Direct extension to the urinary bladder of nearby inflammatory processes—eg, appendiceal abscess, enterovesical fistula, or pelvic abscess—may occur.

Predisposing Factors

Infection is usually initiated or sustained by predisposing factors. Predisposing systemic factors include diabetes mellitus, immunosuppression, and malnutrition; these disorders probably favor urinary tract infection by interfering with normal bladder and body defense mechanisms. Predisposing local factors include organic or functional obstruction, stasis (residual urine), vesicoureteral reflux, foreign bodies (especially catheters and stones), tumors or necrotic tissue, and trauma (especially to the kidneys).

Classification of Urinary Tract Infection

Urinary tract infection is classified as (1) upper urinary tract infection (most commonly, acute or chronic pyelonephritis or infection due to renal abscess); (2) lower urinary tract infection (cystitis of urethritis, including gonorrheal urethritis); or (3) genital infection (prostatitis, epididymitis, seminal vesiculitis, or orchitis).

Urologic Instrumentation or Surgery & Urinary Tract Infection

In the absence of urinary tract infection, surgery of the upper urinary tract rarely requires prophylactic antibacterial therapy. In the presence of infection, one attempts to sterilize the system before operation. If stenting or tube drainage is required and there are no symptoms of infection, colonization by urea-splitting organisms such as *P mirabilis* or *Klebsiella pneumoniae* does not call for antibacterial therapy until the stent or tube is to be removed. Urine culture is obtained approximately 24 hours before removal, and *specific* antibacterial therapy is started at that time. With lower urinary tract surgery, the situation is different: Even when the urine is sterile, antibacterial therapy is advised before operations involving the urethra and the bladder, especially for women in whom contamination from vaginal organisms is likely. Men undergoing prostatectomy for obstructive prostatism often have urinary tract infection, particularly when catheter drainage is used preoperatively. In such cases, or when there is preexisting prostatitis, antimicrobial therapy is necessary before and after surgery to prevent bacteremia.

In the presence of urinary tract infection, any urethral instrumentation poses a threat of bacteremia—more apt to occur in males than in females. Appropriate antibacterial coverage should be instituted before manipulation.

When the urinary tract cannot be sterilized, effective serum levels of antibiotic (eg, aminoglycoside plus ampicillin) should be achieved before instrumentation.

A. Principles of Catheterization: After a short-term single catheterization, the rate of infection is 1–5%. However, in certain patients—pregnant women, elderly or debilitated patients—and in the presence of urologic disease, the risk is much higher. An indwelling catheter often leads to colonization, especially in women. The incidence is proportionate to the duration of catheterization and reaches approximately 95% after 5 days.

Strict aseptic technique is of critical importance in catheterization. Proper cleansing of the genitalia is essential. Iodophor preparations may be used for cleaning the vaginal introitus or the glans and meatus. Many of the common urinary tract pathogens are present in normal colonic flora, and these organisms often gain access to the urinary tract of catheterized patients. Cross-contamination of urinary catheters (passive transmission of bacteria from patient to patient on the hands of hospital personnel) is a frequent mode of transfer of resistant organisms. Measures directed to the prevention of catheter cross-contamination are essential. Closed catheter drainage is probably the best way to reduce cross-contamination. Antibacterial cleansing of the external meatus and perineum twice daily has been advocated, though its effectiveness is doubtful.

With sterile technique during catheterization and a closed drainage system, most catheters can be kept sterile for 48–72 hours. In a closed drainage system, an added airlock or one-way valve preventing reflux of urine from the collecting bag to the draining tubes also helps prevent infection. The general principles are as follows: (1) Indwelling catheters should be used only when absolutely necessary. (2) Catheters should be inserted with strict aseptic technique. (3) A closed drainage system, preferably with a one-way valve, is advisable. (4) Nonobstructed, dependent drainage is essential. (5) Unnecessary irrigation of the system should be avoided. (6) If the catheter is needed for a prolonged period, it should be changed every 2–3 weeks to minimize encrustation and stone formation. (7) The urine of catheterized patients should be cultured before manipulation. (8) Catheterized patients with asymptomatic catheter colonization should be given antibiotics just before the catheter is removed—not during the period of catheterization unless symptomatic infection occurs.

B. Antibacterial Therapy: The choice of antibiotics depends on the type of organism and its sensitivity, as determined by urine cultures. For uncomplicated infection, adequate urine concentrations of the antibiotic determine efficacy, but in cases of bacteremia and septic shock, serum concentrations are crucial. Commonly used oral medications are sulfonamides, nitrofurantoin, ampicillin, trimethoprim-sulfamethoxazole, nalidixic acid, and oxytetracycline. For parenteral therapy, aminoglycosides and cephalosporins are effective against the most common organisms, ie, *P mirabilis, E aerogenes,* and *P aeruginosa.*

ACUTE PYELONEPHRITIS

Essentials of Diagnosis

- Chills, fever, and flank pain.
- Frequency and urgency of urination; dysuria.
- Pyuria and bacteriuria.
- Bacterial growth on urine cultures.

General Considerations

Except in the presence of stasis, foreign bodies, trauma, or instrumentation, pyelonephritis is an ascending type of infection. Pathogenic organisms usually reach the kidney from the bladder via an incompetent ureterovesical junction.

Clinical Findings

A. Symptoms and Signs: In acute attacks, pain is present in one or both flanks. Young children commonly present with poorly localized abdominal pain; irritative lower urinary tract symptoms may be present. Chills and fever are common. Severe infection may produce hypotension, peripheral vasoconstriction, and acute renal failure. Gross hematuria is not common.

B. Laboratory Findings: Pyuria and bacteriuria are consistent findings. Leukocytosis with a shift to the left is common. Urine culture identifies the organism.

C. Imaging Studies: In acute attacks, only minimal changes such as delayed visualization and poor concentrating ability are noted on intravenous urography. Renal or ureteral calculi may be seen on plain abdominal x-rays. Chest x-ray may show a mild ipsilateral pleural effusion.

Differential Diagnosis

Pneumonia, acute cholecystitis, or splenic infarction can be confused with pyelonephritis. Acute appendicitis will sometimes cause pyuria and microhematuria. Any acute abdominal illness such as pancreatitis, diverticulitis, or intestinal angina can simulate pyelonephritis. Appropriate chest x-rays and urinalysis will usually make the distinction.

Complications

If the diagnosis is missed in the acute stage, the infection may become chronic. Both acute and chronic pyelonephritis lead to progressive renal damage.

Treatment

Specific antibiotic therapy should be given to eradicate the infecting organism after proper identification and sensitivity determination. Symptomatic treatment is indicated for pain and irritative voiding symptoms. Adequate fluid intake to assure optimum urinary output is required. Failure to simultaneously identify and treat predisposing factors (eg, obstruction) is the principal cause of failure to respond to therapy, leading to chronic pyelonephritis.

Prognosis

The prognosis is good with adequate treatment of both the infection and its predisposing cause, depending on the degree of preexisting renal parenchymal damage.

EMPHYSEMATOUS PYELONEPHRITIS

Emphysematous pyelonephritis is a form of acute pyelonephritis secondary to a gas-producing bacteria (most often *E coli*). It is commonly seen in diabetic patients with upper urinary tract obstruction. The diagnosis is made by the usual signs of acute pyelonephritis and by the presence of gas in the renal collecting system and parenchyma seen on plain films of the abdomen or on an intravenous urogram. The condition is life-threatening, with a mortality rate of greater than 40%. Operative treatment, including nephrectomy and drainage, is indicated if a rapid response to antibiotics is not obtained.

CHRONIC PYELONEPHRITIS

Chronic pyelonephritis is the result of inadequately treated or recurrent acute pyelonephritis. The diagnosis is primarily made by x-ray, since patients rarely have signs or symptoms until late in the course, when they develop chronic flank pain, hypertension, anemia, or renal failure. Pyuria is not a consistent finding. Because chronic pyelonephritis may be a progressive local immunologic response initiated by bacteria long since eradicated, urine cultures are commonly sterile. Early cases may have no findings on intravenous urography, whereas late cases will reveal small kidneys with typical caliceal deformities (clubbing), with evidence of peripheral scarring and a thin cortex. Voiding cystourethrography often reveals reflux. Complications include hypertension, stone formation, and chronic renal failure.

Antibiotic treatment is not helpful in these patients unless ongoing infection can be documented. The prognosis depends on the status of renal function but is generally not good, particularly when the disease is contracted in childhood. Progressive deterioration of renal function usually occurs.

Xanthogranulomatous pyelonephritis is a form of chronic pyelonephritis seen most frequently in middle-aged diabetic women. The disease is usually unilateral and is associated with prolonged obstructing nephrolithiasis. Patients often have symptoms similar to those of acute pyelonephritis but have an enlarged kidney with calculi and a mass often indistinguishable from tumor. *Proteus* species are common causative agents. Histologic examination may confirm the diagnosis following nephrectomy performed because of unrelenting symptoms.

PAPILLARY NECROSIS

This disorder consists of ischemic necrosis of the renal papillae or of the entire pyramid. Excessive ingestion of analgesics, sickle cell trait, diabetes, obstruction with infection, and vesicoureteral reflux with infection are common predisposing factors.

The symptoms are usually those of chronic cystitis with recurring exacerbations of pyelonephritis. Renal pain or renal colic may be present. Azotemic manifestations may be the presenting symptoms. In acute attacks, localized flank tenderness and generalized toxemia may occur. Laboratory findings consist of pyuria, occasionally glycosuria, and acidosis. Impaired kidney function is shown by elevated serum creatinine and urea nitrogen. Intravenous urography usually shows impaired function and poor visualization in advanced cases. Evidence of ulceration, cavitation, or linear breaks in the base of the papillae and radiolucent defects due to sloughed papillae may be seen; the latter may become calcified. Retrograde urograms may be needed for proper imaging if kidney function is markedly impaired.

Preventive measures consist of proper management of diabetic patients with recurrent infections and avoidance of chronic use of analgesic compounds containing phenacetin and aspirin.

Intensive antibacterial therapy may be needed, though it is commonly unsuccessful in eradicating infection. Little can be done surgically except to remove obstructing papillae and correct predisposing factors (eg, reflux, obstruction) if identified.

In severe cases, the prognosis is poor. Renal transplantation may be required.

RENAL ABSCESS

While renal abscess is occasionally due to hematogenous spread of a distant staphylococcal infection, most abscesses are secondary to chronic nonspecific infection of the kidney, often complicated by stone formation. The onset may be acute, with high fever, but occasionally low-grade fever and general malaise are the presenting symptoms. Localized costovertebral angle tenderness and a palpable flank mass may be present. A mass may be evident on intravenous urograms, DTPA scans, sonograms, CT scans, or renal angiograms. If the abscess is due to hematogenous spread, the urine will not contain bacteria unless the abscess has broken into the pelvicaliceal system. More frequently, gram-negative organisms are found, as would be expected in light of the preponderance of ascending infection.

If organism sensitivity can be established by appropriate tests (blood and urine cultures and sensitivity tests), treatment with the proper antibiotic is indicated. Many cases have responded to percutaneous drainage and irrigation with antibiotic solutions. Surgical drainage or even heminephrectomy may be necessary.

When the abscess is found to be secondary to chronic renal infection, nephrectomy is usually indicated because of advanced destruction of the kidney.

PERINEPHRIC ABSCESS

Abscess between the renal capsule and the perirenal fascia most often results from rupture of an intrarenal abscess into the perinephric space. *E coli* is the most common causative organism. The pathogenesis usually begins with severe pyonephrosis secondary to obstruction, as with renal or ureteral calculi. Clinical findings are similar to those of renal abscess. A pleural effusion on the affected side and signs of psoas muscle irritation are common. Abdominal plain films may show obliteration of the psoas muscle shadow, and an intravenous urogram may show poor concentration of contrast medium and hydronephrosis.

Treatment involves prompt drainage of the abscess and use of appropriate systemic antibiotics. Percutaneous drainage with local antibiotic irrigations is often successful; however, open surgical drainage is necessary if percutaneous drainage is incomplete.

CYSTITIS

Cystitis is more common in females and is usually an ascending infection. In males, it usually occurs in association with urethral or prostatic obstruction, prostatitis, foreign bodies, or tumors. The urinary bladder is normally capable of clearing itself of infection unless an underlying pathologic process interferes with its defensive mechanisms.

In the acute phase, the principal symptoms of cystitis are dysuria, frequency, urgency, and hematuria; low-grade fever and suprapubic, perineal, and low back pain may be present. In chronic cystitis, irritative symptoms are usually milder.

Evidence of prostatitis, urethritis, or vaginitis may be present. Laboratory findings, in addition to hematuria, consist of bacteriuria and pyuria. Leukocytosis is not common. Urine culture identifies the organism. Cystoscopy is not advisable in the acute phase. In chronic cystitis, evidence of mucosal irritation may be present.

In any documented recurrent lower urinary tract infection (particularly in males), a complete urologic workup is indicated. Instrumentation is contraindicated in the acute phase, but cystoscopy is essential to identify the predisposing factor in chronic or recurrent bacterial cystitis.

Specific antibacterial therapy is given according to sensitivity testing of recovered organisms (*E coli* in > 80% of cases). Sterilization of urine should usually be followed by a variable period of continuous antibiotic therapy (depending upon the predisposing factor or the chronicity and recurrence of the disease). Prolonged suppressive medication is usually indicated in cases associated with voiding dysfunction.

In women with recurrent postcoital cystitis, premedication (eg, sulfonamides, nitrofurantoin) on the night of intercourse and the following day in addition to immediate postcoital voiding will prevent recurrences.

PROSTATITIS

Acute Prostatitis

Acute prostatitis is a severe acute febrile illness caused by ascending coliform bacteria which frequently colonize the male urethra. Symptoms include high fever; chills; low back and perineal pain; and urinary frequency and urgency, with diminished stream or retention. On examination, the prostate is extremely tender, swollen, and warm to the touch. A fluctuant abscess may be palpable. The prostate must be examined cautiously, because vigorous palpation may cause acute septicemia. Laboratory findings include pyuria, bacteriuria, and leukocytosis.

Transurethral manipulation by catheter or cystoscopy should be avoided; urinary retention should be treated by introducing a percutaneous suprapubic tube. Treatment with systemic antibiotics (aminoglycosides and ampicillin-cephalosporin) should be started immediately and should be adjusted later when results of culture and sensitivity tests are known. Treatment with oral antibiotics for several weeks after the initial phase has subsided is necessary to eradicate the bacteria completely. A prostatic abscess usually requires open perineal drainage or transurethral unroofing. The prognosis is good if treatment is thorough and prompt.

Chronic Prostatitis

Chronic prostatitis is a common and complex problem. With differential diagnosis including urethritis, bacterial and nonbacterial prostatitis, prostatodynia, and seminal vesiculitis, assigning the correct diagnosis may challenge even the expert. The symptoms are varied and include suprapubic pain, low back pain, orchialgia, dysuria at the tip of the penis, and urinary frequency and urgency. The urinalysis may be normal. There may be a clear white urethral discharge. Prostate examination may reveal a soft, boggy prostate.

Expressed prostatic secretions may contain numerous leukocytes (> 15 per high-power field) in clumps as well as macrophages. Cultures of urine are usually sterile, but cultures of expressed prostatic secretions are usually positive in bacterial prostatitis. *Chlamydia* may be an offending organism, particularly in males under age 35. Determination of the site of infection may require differential cultures. The first part of the voided urine stream is collected as VB$_1$ and the midstream specimen as VB$_2$. The prostate is then massaged to obtain expressed prostatic secretions (EPS), and the postmassage urine is collected as VB$_3$. The differential leukocyte and bacterial counts from each of these specimens can help localize the site of infection. If VB$_1$ has high levels of leukocytes and bacteria relative to the other specimens, urethritis is likely; if VB$_2$ has high levels, a site above the bladder neck is likely; and if the EPS, VB$_3$, or both, have high counts, prostatitis is likely.

Treatment depends on culture results, but if there is no bacterial growth on culture, tetracycline, 250–500 mg four times a day for 14 days, is often curative. Many authors recommend trimethoprim-sulfamethoxazole, 400 mg/80 mg twice a day for 10 days, as an acceptable alternative. Surgical treatment for prostatitis is rarely indicated or helpful. Some patients improve following discontinuation of caffeine and alcohol, and a few respond to repeated prostatic massage. Patients with no evidence of bacterial infection or obstructive findings and those who have recurrent pelvic pain in association with voiding dysfunction (eg, intermittent or weak urinary stream) may be given α-adrenergic blocking agents such as prazosin, 1–2 mg/d, to relieve sphincter spasms and symptoms. Psychologic consultation may be warranted in some of these patients but is seldom accepted by them.

ACUTE EPIDIDYMITIS

Acute epididymitis is most commonly a disease of young males, caused by bacterial infection ascending from the urethra or prostate. The disease is less common in older males, but when it does occur, it is most often due to infection secondary to urinary tract obstruction or instrumentation.

The symptoms are sudden pain in the scrotum, rapid unilateral scrotal enlargement, and marked tenderness that extends to the spermatic cord in the groin and is relieved by scrotal elevation **(Prehn's sign).** Fever is present. An acute hydrocele may result, and secondary orchitis with a swollen, painful testicle may occur. Laboratory studies reveal pyuria, bacteriuria, and marked leukocytosis.

Epididymitis must be differentiated from torsion of the testis, testicular tumor, and tuberculous epididymitis. A technetium Tc 99m pertechnetate scan reveals increased uptake with epididymitis but decreased uptake with torsion. Scrotal ultrasound will distinguish between the solid mass of a testicular tumor and an enlarged, inflamed epididymis and can also identify epididymal or testicular abscess, which will require operative treatment.

In cultured aspirates from inflamed epididymides, men under age 35 tend to show chlamydiae; in men older than 35, *E coli* is most common. Epididymal aspiration for culture is not required routinely, however. Pyuria with a negative urine culture suggests the presence of chlamydial infection in both prostate and epididymis. (See also Tuberculosis, below.)

Treatment consists of bed rest, scrotal elevation, and antibiotics (usually tetracycline in men under age 35 and trimethroprim-sulfamethoxazole, ampicillin, or cephalosporin in those over age 35). Nonresponders may require parenteral aminoglycosides. In some patients, pain is relieved by scrotal hypothermia, and consideration should be given to infiltration of the spermatic cord by 1% bupivacaine. Some clinicians recommend giving nonsteroidal anti-inflammatory drugs such as ibuprofen or indomethacin to aid in pain relief. In most instances, prompt treatment will result in rapid resolution of pain, fever, and swelling. Patients must refrain from exertion for 1–3 weeks.

Exacerbations can be controlled by treating the predisposing factor. Chronic epididymitis rarely resolves completely; it has no consequences except, occasionally, sterility in bilateral cases. Rarely, epididymectomy is necessary.

TUBERCULOSIS

Tuberculosis is a commonly missed genitourinary infection that should be considered in any case of pyuria without bacteriuria or in any case of urinary tract infection that does not respond to treatment.

Genitourinary tuberculosis is always secondary to pulmonary infection, though in many cases, the primary focus has healed or is in a quiescent form. Infection occurs via the hematogenous route. The kidneys and (less commonly) the prostate are the principal sites of urinary tract involvement, though any part of the genitourinary system can be affected.

Pathology

Renal tuberculosis usually starts as a tuberculoma that gradually enlarges, caseates, and finally ulcerates, break ing into the pelvicaliceal system. Caseation and scarring are the principal pathologic features of renal tuberculosis. In the ureter, tuberculosis usually leads to stricture, periureteritis, and mural fibrosis.

In the bladder, the infection is characterized by areas of hyperemia and a coalescent group of tubercles, followed by ulcerations around the involved ureteral orifice. Bladder wall fibrosis and contracted bladder are the end results.

Urethral involvement in the male is uncommon but when present leads to urethral stricture, usually in the bulbous portion. Periurethral abscess and fistula are possible complications.

Genital tuberculosis may involve the prostate, seminal vesicles, and epididymides, either separately or in association with renal involvement. Tubercle formation with later caseation and fibrosis is the basic pathologic feature. The prostate becomes enlarged, with palpable nodules and an irregular consistency. The affected seminal vesicle is fibrotic and distended. Induration and thickening of the epididymis and beading of the vas deferens are characteristic findings. The testicles are rarely involved.

Clinical Findings

A. Symptoms and Signs: The patient commonly presents with lower urinary tract irritation, usually with pyuria. Less common manifestations are hematuria, renal pain, and renal colic.

B. Laboratory Findings: "Sterile" pyuria is the rule, but 15% of cases have secondary bacterial infection (eg, *E coli*). *Mycobacterium tuberculosis* can be identified on an acid-fast stain of the centrifuged sediment of a 24-hour urine specimen or by culture of the first morning urine collected on three successive days (positive in 90% of cases).

C. Imaging Studies: Radiologic findings that suggest genitourinary tuberculosis include motheaten, caseous cavities or bizarre, irregular calices. Strictures in straight, rigid, moderately dilated ureters and a contracted bladder with vesicoureteral reflux are all suggestive evidence.

Treatment

A. Medical Treatment: Tuberculosis must be treated as a systemic disease. Once the diagnosis is established, medical treatment is indicated regardless of the need for surgery. Whenever possible, medical treatment should be continued for at least 3 months before operation.

Specific triple-drug therapy should be given to eradicate the infecting organism. This might include ethambutol, 1.2 g/d orally; isoniazid (INH), 5 mg/kg/d orally in divided doses; and rifampin, 600 mg/d orally as a single dose. Pyridoxine, 100 mg/d orally in divided doses, will counteract the vitamin B_6 depletion effect of INH. This regimen has usually been given for 2 years, though recent studies have shown that 6 months of treatment is adequate.

B. Surgical Measures: If medical therapy fails to cure a unilateral lesion, nephrectomy may be necessary. However, this is rare. In bilateral disease that has seriously damaged one kidney and is in an early stage in the other, unilateral nephrectomy may be considered; in localized polar lesions, partial nephrectomy may be done.

In unilateral epididymal involvement, epididymectomy plus contralateral vasectomy is indicated to prevent descent of the infection from the prostate to that organ; bilateral epididymectomy should be done if both sides are involved.

For a severely contracted bladder, augmentation enterocystoplasty will increase vesical capacity.

Prognosis

In a high percentage of cases, cure is obtained by medical means. Unilateral renal lesions have the best prognosis.

Chawla JC, Clayon CL, Stickler DJ: Antiseptics in the long-term urological management of patients by intermittent catheterization. Br J Urol 1988;62:289.

Corriere JN: Avoiding "overkill" in diagnosing and treatment of lower urinary tract infections. Urology 1988;32 (Suppl):17.

Lang EK: Renal, perirenal, and pararenal abscesses: Percutaneous drainage. Radiology 1990;174:109.

Nasu Y: The virulence factor of *E coli* in genitourinary tract infections. Nippon Hinyokika Gakkai Zasshi 1988; 32:17.

Rajkumar S et al: Trimethoprim in pediatric urinary tract infection. Child Nephrol Urol 1989;9:77.

Sheinfeld J et al: Association of the Lewis blood-group phenotype with recurrent urinary tract infections in women. N Engl J Med 1989;320:773.

Shurbaji MS et al: Immunohistochemical detection of chlamydial antigens in association with cystitis. Am J Clin Pathol 1990;93:363.

Smith AD: Management of iatrogenic ureteral strictures after urological procedures. J Urol 1988;140:1372.

Stamm WE: Protocol for diagnosis of urinary tract infection: Reconsidering the criterion for significant bacteriuria. Urology 1988;32:6.

Stapleton A et al: Postcoital antimicrobial prophylaxis for recurrent urinary tract infection: A randomized, double-blind, placebo controlled trial. JAMA 1990

VanCangh PJ et al: Endoureteropyelotomy: Percutaneous treatment of ureteropelvic junction obstruction. J Urol 1989;141:1317.

CALCULI

RENAL STONE

Essentials of Diagnosis

- Flank pain, hematuria, pyelonephritis, previous stone passage.
- Costovertebral tenderness.
- Red cells in urine.
- Stone visualized on urography, ultrasonography, or CT scan.

General Considerations

Most stones are composed of calcium salts (oxalate, phosphate) or magnesium-ammonium phosphate—the latter secondary to urea-splitting organisms. Most calcium stones are idiopathic (idiopathic hypercalciuria). In patients with hyperparathyroidism or those who ingest large amounts of calcium or vitamin D or are dehydrated or immobilized, hyper-calciuria promotes stone formation.

The less common metabolic stones, cystine and uric acid, usually form secondary to hypersecretion of these substances or to a defect in urinary acidifica-tion. Owing to the radiodensity of sulfur, cystine stones are radiopaque, whereas uric acid stones are radiolucent. Stones that obstruct the ureteropelvic junction or ureter lead to hydronephrosis and infec-tion.

Clinical Findings

A. Symptoms and Signs: If the stone acutely obstructs the ureteropelvic junction or a calix, moder-ate to severe renal pain will be noted, often accompa-nied by nausea, vomiting, and ileus. Hematuria is common. Symptoms of infection, if present, will be exacerbated. Nonobstructing calculi are usually pain-less. This includes staghorn calculus, which may form a cast of all calices and the pelvis. In the symp-tomatic patient, there may be costovertebral angle tenderness and a quiet abdomen. Infection secondary to obstruction may lead to high fever and abdominal muscle rigidity.

B. Laboratory Findings: With acute infection, leukocytosis is to be expected. Urinalysis may reveal red and white blood cells and bacteria. A pH of 7.6 or higher implies the presence of urea-splitting organ-isms. A pH consistently below 5.5 is compatible with the formation of uric acid or cystine stones. If the pH is fixed between 6.0 and 7.0, renal tubular acidosis should be considered as a cause of nephrocalcinosis. Crystals of uric acid or cystine in the urine are sug-gestive. A 24-hour urine collection for calcium may reveal hypercalciuria, which is observed with hyperparathyroidism, idiopathic hypercalciuria, and disseminated osseous metastases.

The output of calcium, phosphate, and urate for a 24-hour period may be determined. Increases in cal-cium and phosphate plus hypercalcemia (and hypo-phosphatemia) suggest the presence of hyperpara-thyroidism. Radioimmunoassay for parathyroid hor-mone is helpful in patients suspected of having hyperparathyroidism. Excessive urinary uric acid is compatible with uric acid stone formation.

A qualitative test for urinary cystine should be part of the routine evaluation. If levels are elevated, a 24-hour quantitative measurement should be made. Hyperchloremic acidosis suggests renal tubular aci-dosis with secondary renal calcifications. Total renal function will be impaired only if the stones are bilat-eral, and particularly if infection is a complication.

C. Imaging Studies: About 90% of calculi are radiopaque (calcium, cystine). Excretory urography is necessary to verify their location within the excre-tory tract and also affords a measure of renal function (Figure 41–16). An acutely obstructed kidney may show only increasing density of the renal shadow without significant radiopaque material in the calices. A nonopaque stone (uric acid) will be seen as a radio-lucent defect in the opaque contrast media. Calculi larger than 1 cm cast a specific acoustic shadow on ultrasonography. CT scans without contrast agents also show the precise location of calculi within the kidney, and stone density will aid in distinguishing stone from clot or tumor. Plain x-ray of the skeletal system may identify Paget's disease, sarcoidosis, or prolonged immobilization responsible for hyper-calciuria.

D. Stone Analysis: If a stone has previously been passed or if one is recovered, its chemical com-position should be analyzed. Such information may be useful when planning a preventive program.

Differential Diagnosis

Acute pyelonephritis may begin with acute renal pain mimicking that of renal stone. Urinalysis reveals pyuria, and urograms fail to reveal a calculus.

Renal adenocarcinoma may bleed into the tumor,

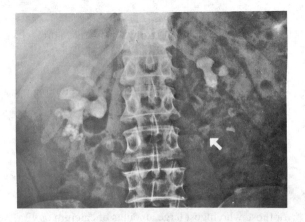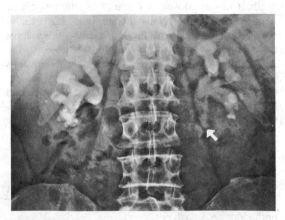

Figure 41–16. Bilateral staghorn calculi and left upper ureteral stone. **Left:** Plain film. Arrow points to ureteral stone. **Right:** Excretory urogram showing bilateral impaired function.

causing acute pain mimicking that of an obstructing stone. Urograms make the differentiation.

Transitional cell tumors of the renal pelvis or calices will mimic uric acid stone; both are radiolucent. CT scan or ultrasound will reveal the stone.

Renal tuberculosis is complicated by stone formation in 10% of cases. Pyuria without bacteriuria is suggestive. Urography reveals the moth-eaten calices typical of tuberculosis.

Papillary necrosis may cause renal colic if a sloughed papilla obstructs the ureteropelvic junction. Excretory urography will settle the issue.

Renal infarction may cause renal pain and hematuria. Evidence of a cardiac lesion, nonfunction of the kidney on urography, and exclusion of the presence of calculus help in differentiation. Infarction is established by angiography or radiosotopic renography.

Complications

Acting as a foreign body, a stone increases the probability of infection. However, primary infection may incite stone formation. A stone lodged in the ureteropelvic junction leads to progressive hydronephrosis. A staghorn calculus, as it grows, may destroy renal tissue by pressure, and the infection that is usually present also contributes to renal damage.

Prevention

An effective preventive regimen depends upon stone analysis and chemical studies of the serum and urine.

A. General Measures: Ensure a high fluid intake (3–4 L/d) to keep solutes well diluted. This measure alone may decrease stone-forming potential by 50%. Combat infection, relieve stasis or obstruction, and advise the patient to avoid prolonged immobilization. For calcium stone formers, stop vitamin D supplements and foods and medications containing calcium salts.

B. Specific Measures:

1. Calcium stones–Remove the parathyroid tumor, if present. Reduce dairy products (milk, cheese) in the diet. Calcium in the diet should be less than 400 mg/d. Dietary sodium may promote calcium absorption, and restriction to 100 meq/d may be helpful. Limitation of proteins and carbohydrates may also reduce hypercalciuria.

Oral orthophosphates are effective in reducing the stone-forming potential of urine. Thiazide diuretics such as hydrochlorothiazide, 50 mg twice daily, decrease the calcium content in urine by 50%. If hyperuricosuria is coincident with calcium urolithiasis, then allopurinol and urinary alkalinization can reduce the formation of urate crystals, which may act as a nidus for calcium crystallization.

For a patient with primary absorptive hypercalciuria, cellulose sodium phosphate (Calcibind) can be given. This substance will combine with calcium in the gut to prevent absorption.

2. Oxalate stones (calcium oxalate)–Prescribe phosphate or a thiazide diuretic (see above) and limit calcium intake. Elimination of excessive oxalate in coffee, tea, colas, leafy green vegetables, and chocolate may also be helpful. Vitamin C in excess of 3–5 g will be metabolized in some individuals to oxalate and thus should be avoided.

3. Magnesium-ammonium-phosphate stones–These stones are usually secondary to urinary tract infection due to bacteria that produce urease (primarily *Proteus* species). Eradication of the infection will prevent further stone formation but is nearly impossible when stones are present. After all calculi (or as many as possible) have been removed, prevention of stone growth is best accomplished by urinary acidification, long-term use of antibiotics, and, perhaps, use of acetohydroxamic acid, a urease inhibitor that maintains an acid urinary pH and may potentiate antibiotic action.

4. Metabolic stones (uric acid, cystine)–These substances are most soluble at a pH of 7.0 or higher. Give sodium-potassium citrate solution, 4–8 mL four times orally daily; monitor the urine pH with a paper indicator. For uric acid stone formers, limit purines in the diet and give allopurino. Patients with mild cystinuria may need only urinary alkalinization, as described above. For severe cystinuria, giving penicillamine, 30 mg/kg/d orally, will reduce urinary cystine to safe levels. Penicillamine should be supplemented with pyridoxine, 50 mg/d orally. Propionyl glycine preparations have been used with similar results and fewer side effects in Europe.

Treatment

A. Conservative Measures: Intervention is not required for small nonobstructive, asymptomatic caliceal stones. Hydration and dietary management may be sufficient to prevent growth of existing or new calcium stones in patients without metabolic abnormalities. Those with identifiable metabolic disorders may benefit from the specific measures described previously. Patients with primary renal tubular acidosis and secondary stones can be treated with hydration and urinary alkalinization.

B. Percutaneous Intervention (Endourology): In selected patients with symptomatic or large pelvic stones, percutaneous stone removal may be successful. A percutaneous tract enters the renal collecting system through an appropriate calix (**percutaneous nephrostomy**). The tract is subsequently dilated, and endoscopic extraction of the stones (**percutaneous nephroscopy and percutaneous nephrolithotomy**). Pulverization by means of ultrasonic, electrohydraulic, or laser probes passed through the nephrostomy tract may also be useful. Residual infection stones may be dissolved by percutaneous irrigation with hemiacidrin. For cystine and uric acid stones, alkaline or other irrigants that increase the specific crystal solubility may be used (eg,

N-acetyl-L-lysine or propionyl glycine for cystine stones). Specific antibiotic treatment for infection must be given before irrigation to prevent sepsis.

Success with these endourologic methods approaches 100%. The advantages over surgical procedures include no incision, use of local anesthesia in many cases, and rapid recovery and return to employment. Disadvantages include the occasional need for multiple treatments to completely remove the calculi and the uncommon occurrence of significant hemorrhage.

C. Extracorporeal Shock Wave Lithotripsy (ESWL): With this technique, patients are positioned in the path of shock waves focused on the renal calculi with the aid of fluoroscopy or ultrasound (Figure 41–17). General or regional anesthesia or, in selected patients, local anesthesia is required. The shock waves (generally > 1500 are given) pulverize the stones, and the small particles pass spontaneously over 2–5 days. Results to date have been excellent. Calcium stones and magnesium-ammonium-phosphate stones have been treated successfully. Because of the physical properties of the crystal lattice, ESWL is not as effective in fragmenting cystine stones. Ra-

diolucent uric acid stones, which can be "visualized" using contrast via intravenous pyelography or retrograde ureteropyelography, are amenable to ESWL treatment. Staghorn calculi are amenable to a combined approach: percutaneous nephrolithotomy to remove the major bulk of the stone followed by ESWL to pulverize any inaccessible fragments. Fewer than 10% of patients treated with ESWL have required subsequent endourologic or surgical treatment.

Recently, the necessity for submerging the patient in a water bath for transmission of the shock waves has been obviated by construction of a membrane coupling device applied directly to the skin overlying the kidney. A variety of devices now effectively pulverize stones using less energy and thus can be used with only intravenous sedation; an increased number of pulses are required to obtain the same results as before. Some newer instruments use ultrasound instead of x-ray for stone localization.

D. Open Surgical Removal of Stones: Endourologic intervention and ESWL have markedly decreased the indications for open surgery. Rarely, both percutaneous nephrolithotomy and ESWL will be contraindicated, and open nephrolithotomy will be necessary. The goal of any approach is to remove all stone fragments, and the approach chosen must allow for intraoperative localization by radiography or ultrasonography. Incisions into the renal pelvis (pyelolithotomy) or the renal parenchyma (radial nephrotomy or anatrophic nephrolithotomy) may be required for complete stone removal. Instillation of a mixture of thrombin and calcium into the kidney causes the fragments to become trapped in a dense clot which is removed through a pyelotomy incision (coagulum pyelolithotomy). Operative nephroscopy allows a full view of all the calices and removal of all fragments. "Bench" surgery with autotransplantation of the kidney may be required in some instances. Rarely, poorly functioning kidneys containing symptomatic stones require nephrectomy.

Prognosis

The recurrence rate of renal stone is high unless sufficient attention is paid to measures for prevention of stone formation. The danger of recurrent stone is progressive renal damage due to obstruction and infection.

URETERAL STONE

Essentials of Diagnosis

- Severe ureterorenal colic.
- Hematuria.
- Nausea, vomiting, and ileus.
- Stone visible on excretory urography.

General Considerations

Ureteral stones originate in the kidney. When

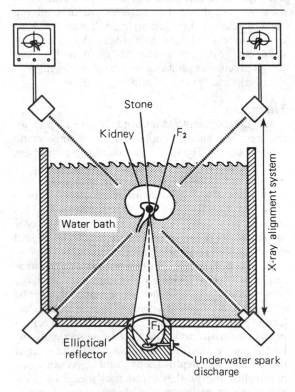

Figure 41–17. Extracorporeal shock wave lithotriptor. An underwater spark is produced that results in shock wave propagation. The shock wave is focused by an elliptical reflector, and the force of the shock is concentrated at the kidney stone, which has been positioned in F_2 (second focal point) with the aid of fluoroscopy.

symptoms occur, ureteral obstruction is implicit and renal function endangered. Complicating infection may occur. Most ureteral stones pass spontaneously.

Clinical Findings

A. Symptoms and Signs: The onset of pain is usually abrupt. Pain is felt in the costovertebral angle and radiates to the ipsilateral lower abdominal quadrant. Nausea, vomiting, abdominal distention, and gross hematuria are common. When the stone approaches the bladder, symptoms mimic cystitis. If the kidney is infected, acute ureteral obstruction exacerbates the infection.

The patient is usually in such agony that only parenteral narcotics will give relief. Costovertebral angle tenderness and guarding may be evident. Absence of bowel sounds and abdominal distention signify ileus. Fever may occur as a result of complicating renal infection.

B. Laboratory Findings: Laboratory findings are the same as for renal stone.

C. Imaging Studies: Excretory urograms are essential. Plain films may reveal an opacity in the region of the ureter. Confirmation of ureteral location requires demonstration of confluence of stone and ureteral contrast (Figure 41–18). Excretory urograms with oblique films are diagnostic. This procedure depicts the degree of obstruction and the size and position of the stone, information that permits selection of

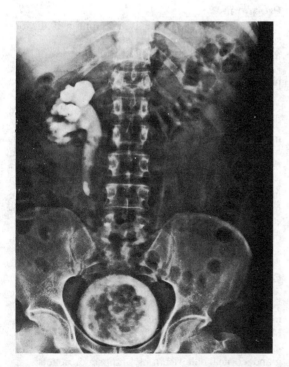

Figure 41–18. Excretory urogram showing right ureteral stone causing hydronephrosis. Large irregular filling defect from unsuspected vesical neoplasm.

appropriate treatment. A radiolucent stone will appear as a filling defect within a proximally dilated ureter—indistinguishable from a ureteral tumor or blood clot by intravenous urography. CT scan will discriminate between stone and tumor or clot density. Cystoscopy, ureteral catheterization, retrograde urography, and ureteroscopy may also be helpful.

Differential Diagnosis

A tumor of the kidney or renal pelvis may bleed, and passage of a blood clot may cause ureteral colic. Urograms may reveal a radiolucent area in the ureter surrounded by the radiopaque urine. A CT scan without contrast agents will reveal no radiopacity.

A primary tumor of the ureter may cause obstructing pain and hematuria. The urogram will reveal the ureteral filling defect, often with secondary obstruction. A CT scan will differentiate a stone from tumor. Urinary cytologic study may reveal malignant transitional cells.

Acute pyelonephritis may cause pain as severe as that seen with stone. Pyuria and bacteriuria are found but do not rule out stone. Stone is absent on urography.

A sloughed papilla traversing the ureter may cause colic and will produce a urogram compatible with uric acid stone. Papillary sloughs should be evident, however.

Complications

If obstruction from the ureteral stone is prolonged, progressive renal damage may ensue. Bilateral stones may cause anuria, requiring immediate drainage of the proximal collecting system with indwelling ureteral catheters or percutaneous nephrostomy.

Infection may supervene, but many renal infections are iatrogenic, ie, introduced at the time of stone manipulation.

Prevention

See Renal Stone.

Treatment

A. General Measures: Most ureteral stones pass spontaneously—particularly those less than 0.5 cm in diameter. Once the diagnosis has been established, analgesics should be given and the patient hydrated. Periodic plain films should be taken to follow the progress of the stone and interval renal ultrasound studies obtained to assess the degree of hydronephrosis. The urine should be strained until the stone passes in order to recover the calculus for analysis.

B. Specific Measures: If the stone causes intractable pain, progressive hydronephrosis, or acute infection, it should be removed. Obstructing stones in the upper two-thirds of the ureter can often be successfully treated by simultaneous ureteral catheterization and manipulation of the stone back to the renal pelvis followed by ESWL or percutaneous nephrolithotomy as described above. Ureteroscopy permits ultrasonic or laser fragmentation and stone basket retrieval under direct vision. Retrograde basket extraction under fluoroscopic control may be used to remove small distal ureteral stones. Open surgical removal (ureterolithotomy) is only occasionally required for ureteral stones. ESWL has been applied to ureteral stones in the proximal ureter but is more problematic in the distal ureter owing to bone interference with imaging.

Prognosis

About 80% of ureteral stones pass spontaneously. Periodic plain films of the abdomen or excretory urograms will portray progress of the stone and warn of ensuing renal damage that would prompt operative intervention.

VESICAL STONE

Primary vesical calculi are rare in the USA but are common in Southeast Asia and the Middle East. The cause is probably dietary. Secondary stones usually complicate vesical outlet obstruction with residual urine and infection; 90% of those affected are men. Other causes of bladder stasis such as neurogenic bladder and bladder diverticula also promote vesical stone formation. They are common in vesical schistosomiasis or in association with radiation cystitis. Foreign bodies in the bladder may act as nuclei for the precipitation of urinary salts. Most stones contain calcium; some are composed of uric acid.

Clinical Findings

A. Symptoms and Signs: Symptoms of bladder neck obstruction are elicited. There may be sudden interruption of the stream and urethral pain if a stone occludes the bladder neck during voiding. Hematuria is common. Vesical distention may be noted; evidence of urethral stricture or an enlarged prostate is usually found.

B. Laboratory Findings: Pyuria and hematuria are almost always present.

C. Imaging Studies: Vesical calculi arc usually radiopaque. Excretory urograms will reveal that the stones are intravesical; residual urine is usually depicted on the postvoiding film. If nonopaque areas are noted, CT scan or ultrasound will differentiate between stones and vesical tumors or blood clots, but direct vision endoscopically is preferred.

D. Instrumental Examination: Inability to pass a catheter or sound into the bladder signifies urethral stricture. Catheterization may demonstrate residual urine. Cystoscopy will visualize the stones and may reveal an obstructing prostate.

Differential Diagnosis

A pedunculated vesical tumor may suddenly occlude the vesical neck during voiding. Excretory urograms, pelvic ultrasound CT scan, ultrasound, or cystoscopy leads to definitive diagnosis.

Extravesical opacifications may simulate stones on a plain film. Excretory urograms, CT scan, or cystoscopy will make the differentiation.

Complications

Acting as foreign bodies, bladder stones exacerbate urine infection and foil antibiotic therapy given for the purpose of sterilizing the urine. Stones obstructing the urethra must be removed.

Prevention

Prevention requires relief of the primary obstruction, removal of the stones, and sterilization of the urine.

Treatment

A. General Measures: Analgesics should be given for pain and antimicrobials for control of infection until the stones can be removed.

B. Specific Measure: Small stones can be removed or crushed transurethrally (**cystolitholopaxy**). Larger stones are often disintegrated by transurethral electrohydraulic lithotripsy (shock wave generating probe), or may require suprapubic transvesical removal (vesicolithotomy). The obstructive lesion must also be corrected.

Prognosis

Recurrent vesical stone is uncommon if the obstruction and infection are treated.

NEPHROCALCINOSIS

Nephrocalcinosis is a precipitation of calcium in the tubules, parenchyma, and, occasionally, the glomeruli. It always causes renal functional impairment, often severe. Stones may be found in the calices and pelvis. The common causes are primary hyperparathyroidism, excessive milk-alkali or vitamin D intake, and hyperparathyroidism secondary to severe renal damage associated with hyperchloremic acidosis, renal tubular acidosis, or sarcoidosis. Calcifications may also be seen in the skin, lungs, stomach, spleen, and corneas or around the joints.

Clinical Findings

A. Symptoms and Signs: There are no specific symptoms. In childhood, the patient may merely fail to thrive. Stones or sand may be passed. The complaints are usually those of the primary disease. Physical examination may reveal an enlarged parathyroid gland, corneal calcifications, and pseudorickets.

B. Laboratory Findings: The urine may be infected. In renal tubular acidosis, the pH is fixed between 6.0 and 7.0. Urinary calcium is high in hyperparathyroidism, both primary and secondary. Tests of renal function are depressed; uremia is common. Hypercalcemia and hypophosphatemia are seen with primary hyperparathyroidism; secondary hyperparathyroidism may be associated with a low serum calcium and an elevated serum phosphate. Hyperchloremic acidosis and hypokalemia accompany renal tubular acidosis.

C. Imaging Studies: A plain x-ray will reveal punctate calcifications in the papillae of the kidneys. Caliceal or pelvic stones may also be noted. The pattern of calcification may have to be differentiated from renal tuberculosis and medullary sponge kidney.

Complications

Complications include renal damage caused by the calcifications and renal and ureteral calculi. Chronic renal infection may complicate the primary disease.

Treatment & Prognosis

The primary cause should be treated, if possible (eg, parathyroidectomy). Discontinue vitamin D, give a low-calcium diet, and force fluids. With hyperchloremic acidosis, alkalinize the urine with potassium citrate. Osteomalacia requires administration of vitamin D and calcium even though nephrocalcinosis is present.

If nephrocalcinosis is secondary to primary renal disease, the outlook is poor. If the cause is correctable and renal function is fairly good, the prognosis is more favorable.

Danielson BG: Drugs against kidney stones: Effects of magnesium and alkali. In: *Urolithiasis and Related Clinical Research.* Schwille PO et al (editors). Plenum, 1985.

Dobbins JW: Nephrolithiasis and intestinal disease. J Clin Gastroenterol 1985;7:21.

Ettinger B et al: Chlorthalidone reduces calcium oxalate calculus recurrence but magnesium hydroxide does not. J Urol 1988;139:679.

Fellstrom B: Allopurinol treatment in urolithiasis. In: *Urolithiasis and Related Clinical Research.* Schwille PO et al (editors). Plenum, 1985.

Gautier JR et al: Pulsed dye laser in the treatment of 325 calculi of the urinary tract. Eur Urol 1990;18:6.

Kahnowski RJ et al: Combined percutaneous and extracorporeal shock wave lithotripsy for staghorn calculi: An alternative to anatrophic nephrolithotomy. J Urol 1986; 135:679.

Kramolowsky EV, Loening SA: Extracorporeal shock wave lithotripsy: Noninvasive treatment for urinary stones. Postgrad Med 1986;79:69.

Lingeman JE, Woods JR, Toth PD: Blood pressure changes following extracorporeal shock wave lithotripsy and other forms of treatment of nephrolithiasis. JAMA 1990;263:1789.

Ljunghall S, Fellstrom B, Johannson G: Prevention of renal stones by a high fluid intake? Eur Urol 1988;14:381.

Pak CYC et al: Correction of hypocitraturia and prevention of stone formation by combined thiazide and potassium citrate therapy in thiazide-unresponsive hypercalciuric nephrolithiasis. Am J Med 1985;79:284.

Pak CYC, Peterson R: Successful treatment of hyperuricosuric calcium oxalate nephrolithiasis with potassium citrate. Arch Intern Med 1986;146:863.

Pak CYC: Medical management of nephrolithiasis in Dallas: Update 1987. J Urol 1988;140:461.

Preminger GM, Pak CYC: Eventual attenuation of hypocalciuric response to hydrochlorothiazide in absorptive hypercalciuria. J Urol 1987;137:1104.

Winfield HN, Clayman RV: *Complications of Percutaneous Removal of Renal and Ureteral Calculi, Parts I and II.* World Urology Update Series, Vol 2, Lesson 38, 1985.

Winfield HN et al: Monotherapy of staghorn calculi: A comparative study between percutaneous nephrolithotomy and extracorporeal shock wave lithotripsy. J Urol 1988;139:895.

GENITOURINARY TRACT TRAUMA

INJURIES TO THE KIDNEY

Essentials of Diagnosis

- History or evidence of trauma, usually local.
- Hematuria.
- Flank mass.
- Failure to opacify the kidney or extravasation of urine on excretory urography.

General Considerations

Renal injury is uncommon but potentially serious and often accompanied by multisystem trauma. The most common causes are athletic, industrial, or automobile accidents. The degree of injury may range from contusion to laceration of the parenchyma or division of the renal pedicle.

Clinical Findings

A. Symptoms and Signs: Gross hematuria following trauma means injury to the urinary tract. Pain and tenderness over the renal area may be significant but could be due to musculoskeletal injury. Hemorrhagic shock may result from renal laceration and lead to oliguria. Nausea, vomiting, and abdominal distention (ileus) are the rule. Physical examination may reveal ecchymosis or penetrating injury in the costovertebral angle or flank. Extravasation of blood or urine may produce a palpable flank mass. Other injuries should be sought.

B. Laboratory Findings: Serial hematocrit determinations will give clues to persistent bleeding. Hematuria is to be expected, but the absence of hematuria does not exclude renal injury (as in renal vascular injury).

C. Imaging Studies: A plain film may reveal obliteration of the psoas shadow; this suggests the presence of a retroperitoneal hematoma or urinary extravasation. Bowel gas may be displaced from the area. Evidence of transverse vertebral process fractures or rib fracture may be noted. Excretory urograms may show a normal kidney if it is mildly contused or may show extravasation of contrast if the kidney is lacerated. Nonfunction suggests injury to the vascular pedicle. The excretory urogram should demonstrate that the contralateral kidney is normal. Retrograde urograms are seldom necessary. CT scan is frequently helpful in assessing the extent of renal injury and may be used in place of excretory urography in appropriate cases. If renal vascular damage is suspected and the patient's condition is stable, preoperative renal angiography should be performed to facilitate planning of renovascular reconstruction. In special circumstances, selective renal artery embolization may control bleeding.

Differential Diagnosis

Bony fractures or contusion of soft tissues in the region of the kidney may cause confusion. Hematuria might be secondary to vesical injury. The absence of a perirenal mass on normal urograms or CT scans would rule out significant renal trauma.

Complications

A. Early: The most serious complication is continued perirenal hemorrhage, which may be fatal. Serial hematocrit, blood pressure, and pulse determinations are essential. Evidence of an enlarging flank mass implies persistent bleeding. In most cases, bleeding stops spontaneously, probably as a result of tamponade by the perirenal fascia. Delayed bleeding 1 or 2 weeks later is rare. Infection of the perirenal hematoma may occur.

B. Late: Ultrasound should be obtained 1–3 months after surgery to look for progressive hydronephrosis from ureteral obstruction. The blood pressure should be checked at regular intervals, because hypertension may be a late sequela.

Treatment

Treat shock and hemorrhage with fluids and transfusion. Most patients with blunt renal trauma stop bleeding and heal spontaneously. Bed rest is indicated until hematuria resolves. If bleeding persists, laparotomy is indicated.

Penetrating renal trauma requires exploration. Lacerations may be sutured, the collecting system closed, and urinary extravasation drained. Nephrectomy or partial nephrectomy may be necessary to remove devitalized tissue and secure the collecting system.

Late complications may occur. Perinephric abscess should be drained. Hypertension due to renal ischemia requires vascular reconstruction or nephrectomy.

Prognosis

Most injured kidneys heal spontaneously, though the patient must be examined at intervals for the onset of hypertension due to renal ischemia or progressive hydronephrosis due to secondary ureteral stricture. Many patients with genitourinary trauma have associated injuries. In most cases, death is due to associated injury rather than renal injury.

INJURIES TO THE URETER

Essentials of Diagnosis

- Anuria or oliguria; prolonged ileus or flank pain following pelvic operation.
- Onset of urinary drainage through wound or vagina.
- Demonstration of urinary extravasation or ureteral obstruction by urography.

General Considerations

Most ureteral injuries are iatrogenic in the course of pelvic surgery. Ureteral injury may occur during transurethral bladder or prostate resection or ureteral manipulation for stone or tumor. Ureteral injury is rarely a consequence of penetrating trauma. Unintentional ureteral ligation during operation on adjacent organs may be asymptomatic, though hydronephrosis and loss of renal parenchyma will result. Ureteral division leads to extravasation and ureterocutaneous fistula.

Clinical Findings

A. Symptoms: If the ureteral injury is not recognized at surgery, the patient may complain of flank and lower abdominal pain on the injured side. Ileus and pyelonephritis may develop. Later, urine may drain through the wound (or vagina following transvaginal surgery). Wound drainage may be evaluated by comparing urea and creatinine levels found in the drainage fluid to serum levels: urine exhibits very high urea and creatinine levels when compared to serum. Intravenous administration of 5 mL of indigo carmine will cause the urine to appear blue-green; therefore, drainage from a ureterocutaneous fistula becomes blue, while serous drainage remains yellow. Anuria following pelvic surgery means bilateral ureteral ligation until proved otherwise. Peritoneal signs may occur if urine leaks into the peritoneal cavity.

B. Laboratory Findings: Microscopic hematuria is usually found but may be absent. Tests of renal function are normal unless both ureters are occluded.

C. Imaging Studies: Excretory urograms may show evidence of ureteral occlusion. Extravasation of radiopaque fluid may be seen in the region of the ureter. Retrograde ureterography will depict the site and nature (occlusion or division) of the injury.

Ultrasonography will reveal hydroureter and hydronephrosis or a fluid mass representing urinary extravasation. Radionuclide scanning will show delayed excretion, with an accumulation of counts in the pelvis and renal parenchyma resulting from ureteral obstruction. Although urinary extravasation is detected, anatomic specificity for site of injury is not clearly define.

Differential Diagnosis

Ureteral injury may mimic peritonitis if urine leaks into the peritoneal cavity. Excretory urography will reveal the ureteral involvement.

Oliguria may be due to dehydration, transfusion reaction, or bilateral incomplete ureteral injury. A survey of fluid and electrolyte intake and output, including serial body weights, should prove definitive. Total anuria implies bilateral ureteral injury and indicates the need for immediate urologic investigation.

Vesicovaginal and ureterovaginal fistulas may be confused. Methylene blue solution instilled into the bladder will stain the drainage of a vesicovaginal fistula. Cystoscopy may show the vesical defect. Retrograde ureterography should reveal a ureteral fistula.

Complications

These include urinary fistula, ureteral obstruction or stenosis with hydronephrosis, renal infection, peritonitis, and uremia (with bilateral injury).

Prevention

Before operation for large pelvic masses, which may cause dislocation of the ureters, catheters should be placed in the ureters to facilitate their identification at surgery.

Treatment

A. Injury Recognized at Surgery:

1. Ureteral division–Repair of a ureter inadvertently cut during surgery consists of anastomosis of the ends over an indwelling stent (**ureteroureterostomy**), reimplanting the ureter into the bladder if the injury is juxtavesical (**neoureterocystostomy**), or anastomosing the proximal segment of divided ureter to the side of the contralateral ureter (**transureteroureterostomy**). The area of repair must be drained.

2. Ureteral resection–Repair of a ureter from which a segment has been removed requires interposition of a ureteral substitute or mobilization of the proximal and distal ureter and urothelium to provide a tension - free anastomosis. In extreme cases, autotransplant of the kidney to the pelvis may be necessary.

B. Injury Discovered After Surgery: Early reoperation is recommended. Depending on the findings, the following procedures may be utilized: ureteroureterostomy, neoureterocystostomy, and transureteroureterostomy. If a long segment of ureter is not viable, an intestinal ureter may be constructed. If hydronephrosis is advanced or if sepsis develops,

percutaneous nephrostomy should precede repair. When the patient's condition is stable, definitive repair can be accomplished. Nephrectomy may be indicated if the contralateral kidney is normal and there is a contraindication to transureteroureterostomy.

Prognosis

In cases of iatrogenic injury, the results are best if the injury is recognized at the time of surgery. Late repair, if severe periureteral fibrosis has developed, is less likely to afford a good outcome.

INJURIES TO THE BLADDER

Essentials of Diagnosis

- History of trauma (including surgical or endoscopic).
- Fracture of the pelvis.
- Suprapubic pain and muscle rigidity.
- Hematuria.
- Extravasation shown on cystogram.

General Considerations

The most common cause of vesical injury is an external blow over a full bladder. Rupture of the organ is seen in 15% of patients with pelvic fracture. The bladder may be inadvertently opened during pelvic surgery or injured by cystoscopic maneuvers, eg, transurethral resection of vesical tumor. If the injury is intraperitoneal, blood and urine will extravasate into the peritoneal cavity, producing signs of peritonitis. If it is extra peritoneal, a mass will develop in the pelvis.

Clinical Findings

A. Symptoms and Signs: There is usually a history of hypogastric or pelvic trauma. Hematuria and suprapubic pain are expected. Associated injury may cause hemorrhagic shock. There is suprapubic tenderness and guarding. Intraperitoneal extravasation causes peritoneal signs, while extraperitoneal extravasation results in formation of a pelvic mass.

B. Laboratory Findings: A falling hematocrit reflects continued bleeding. Hematuria is expected in patients who are able to void. A patient who cannot void should be catheterized unless pelvic fracture (and urethral injury) is suspected and blood is noted at the urethral meatus.

C. Imaging Studies: A plain film may reveal fracture of the pelvis. An extraperitoneal collection of blood and urine may displace the bowel gas laterally or out of the pelvis. If bladder trauma is suspected, cystography should precede excretory urography. Extravasation is most reliably demonstrated by a postdrainage cystogram film. If one suspects urethral trauma, a retrograde urethrogram should precede catheter insertion. The excretory urogram may suggest the diagnosis of bladder perforation but by itself is insufficient to exclude bladder injury. As in the case of renal injury, CT scan may provide necessary information and obviate the need for cystography.

Differential Diagnosis

Renal injury is also associated with trauma and usually presents with hematuria. Excretory urograms show changes compatible with trauma; the cystogram is negative.

Injury to the membranous urethra can mimic extraperitoneal rupture of the bladder. A urethrogram will reveal the site of injury. Urethral disruption is a contraindication to urethral catheterization.

Complications

Extraperitoneal extravasation may lead to pelvic abscess. Intraperitoneal extravasation will cause delayed peritonitis, oliguria, and azotemia.

Treatment

Treat shock, hemorrhage, and other life-threatening injuries. Marked extraperitoneal extravasation should be drained, the bladder decompressed by either a suprapubic or urethral catheter, and appropriate antibiotics administered. Small extraperitoneal extravasations are treated nonoperatively by urethral catheter.

Intraperitoneal extravasation of bladder urine requires celiotomy, bladder closure, and bladder catheter drainage. Other injuries are sought.

Prognosis

Early diagnosis minimizes morbidity and mortality rates. The prognosis depends chiefly upon the severity of associated injuries.

INJURIES TO THE URETHRA

Membranous Urethra

Injury to the membranous urethra is usually a consequence of pelvic fracture and thus is associated with hemorrhage and multi-organ injury. The mechanism of injury is blunt trauma and deceleration resulting in shearing forces applied to the prostate and urogenital diaphragm. Penetrating injuries result from external missiles or laceration by bone fragments acting as secondary projectiles.

If the urethral disruption is incomplete, the patient may be able to void, and hematuria would be inevitable. Urethral injury is suspected if blood is expressed from the urethral meatus. In cases of complete avulsion, extravasation causes a suprapubic mass. Rectal examination may reveal a nonpalpable or upwardly displaced prostate.

X-ray reveals a fractured pelvis; urethrography delineates any extravasation, and cystography identifies an associated bladder injury (Figure 41–19). An immediate excretory urogram should be obtained in all cases to assess kidney and ureteral function.

Treatment must be coordinated with care of associ-

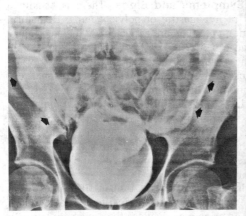
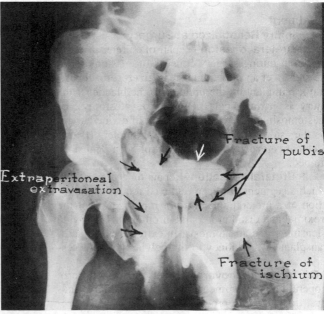

Figure 41–19. Vesical injuries. *Left:* Retrograde cystogram showing intraperitoneal extravasation. Note radiopaque material in both lumbar gutters. *Right:* Retrograde cystogram showing extraperitoneal rupture of the bladder secondary to fracture of the pelvis.

ated injury. Once a membranous urethral injury with urinary extravasation has been identified, suprapubic cystostomy should be performed either at the time of celiotomy or percutaneously with fluoroscopic control before placement of external pelvic fixation. Definitive urethral repair may be delayed until the patient has recovered from the acute injury and pelvic fractures have healed. Occasionally, when urethral disruption is incomplete, late repair is unnecessary.

Late sequelae are urethral stricture, impotence, and incontinence. Urethral stricture must be identified by retrograde urethrography and may be treated by transurethral urethrotomy (incision of scar tissue). Impotence due to injury of nerves to the corpora cavernosa that course adjacent to the membranous urethra may resolve without treatment during the year following injury. In patients who are not so fortunate, vasoactive injection therapy may be successful or a penile prosthesis may be inserted. Vascular injury of the hypogastric or pudendal arteries may cause impotence following trauma. Cavernosometry and arteriography will confirm the diagnosis; appropriate treatment may include vascular reconstruction. Incontinence is unusual, and treatment depends upon the neurologic status of the patient. Medical or surgical therapy is utilized to increase bladder capacity and bladder outlet resistance.

Bulbous Urethra

The bulbous urethra may be injured as a result of instrumentation or, more commonly, falling astride an object (straddle injury). Urethral contusion may cause a perineal hematoma without injury to the urethral wall. Laceration will lead to urinary extravasation.

Perineal pain and some urethral bleeding are to be expected. Sudden swelling in the perineum may develop following attempted urination. Examination reveals a perineal mass; swelling due to extravasation of blood and urine involves the penis and scrotum and may spread onto the abdominal wall.

If the patient can void well and the perineal hematoma is small, no treatment is necessary. If urethrography reveals significant extravasation, suprapubic cystostomy should be performed. Minor injury without extravasation (contusion, compression by hematoma) may be managed by careful insertion of a urethral catheter (Figure 41–20).

The only serious complication is stricture, which requires internal urethrotomy or surgical repair.

Pendulous Urethra

External injury to this portion of the urethra is not common, since the penis is so mobile. The erect organ, however, is vulnerable. Most trauma to this area is secondary to instrumentation or sex play. As a

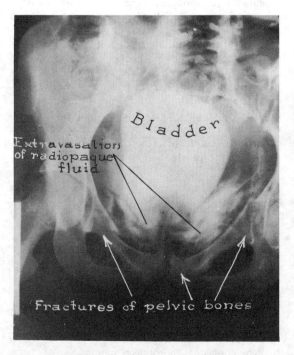

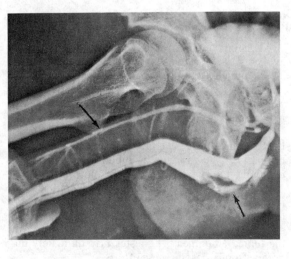

Figure 41–20. Injury to the membranous urethra. **Left:** Retrograde cystogram showing periprostatic extravasation; laceration of membranous urethra with fracture of pelvis. **Right:** Oblique urethrogram showing extravasation in region of bulbous urethra. Pressure injection caused radiopaque solution to enter venous system. (This is the mechanism for emboli if oily lubricants are injected into the urethra.)

rule, these injuries are mild, although a few may be complicated by stricture.

Urethral bleeding and penile swelling are to be expected. A urethrogram will reveal the site and severity of injury.

If voiding is normal, no treatment is required. A large hematoma may require drainage. If significant injury is present, a suprapubic tube should be inserted and delayed surgical repair performed after swelling and inflammation have resolved.

INJURIES TO THE PENIS

Mechanisms of penile injury include penetration, blunt trauma to the erect penis during sexual activity (eg, fracture of corpora cavernosa), avulsion of skin (also known as "power takeoff injury"), and amputation. Pendulous urethral injury is rare (discussed above).

Tourniquet injury is also uncommon; the circumferential compression may be due to a rubber band, a steel ring, string, or a hair and may be exacerbated by subsequent erection. The tourniquet may have been applied unintentionally, but child abuse cases have been reported in which the penis has been ligated as punishment for enuresis.

Treatment includes assessment and care of urethral injuries if present. Removal of tourniquet, skin grafting of avulsion injuries, and primary closure of corporal lacerations are principles of therapy. The amputated penis may be acutely reimplanted using microsurgical techniques.

INJURIES TO THE SCROTUM & TESTIS

Avulsion of the skin may require a skin graft. If the avulsion is severe, involving the skin and dartos muscle, then the testes should be implanted in the subcutaneous tissue of the thigh. Scrotal reconstruction is performed at a later time, using skin flaps with placement of the testes into the neoscrotum.

Penetrating trauma rarely injures the mobile testes. Lacerations should be explored, debrided, and closed primarily. If hemorrhage into the tunica vaginalis is noted, drainage is indicated.

Blunt trauma to the testes may cause contusion or rupture. Rupture of the tunica albuginea may be demonstrated by ultrasonography. In cases of rupture, scrotal exploration allows debridement and closure of the tunica albuginea. The testes may ultimately undergo atrophy despite these efforts.

Bertini JE, Corriere JN: The etiology and management of genital injuries. J. Trauma 1988;18:1278.

Chiou RK et al: Endoscopic treatment of posterior urethral obliteration: Long-term followup and comparison with transpubic urethroplasty. J Urol 1988;140:508.

Corriere JN, Sandler CM: Mechanisms of injury, patterns of extravasation, and management of extraperitoneal bladder rupture due to blunt trauma. J Urol 1988;139:43.

Federle MP, Brown TR, McAninch JW: Penetrating renal trauma: CT evaluation. J Comput Assist Tomogr 1987; 11:1026.

Horton CE, Dean JA: Reconstruction of traumatically acquired defects of the phallus. World J Surg 1990;14:757.

Husmann DA, Morris JS: Attempted nonoperative management of blunt renal lacerations extending through the corticomedullary junction: The short-term and long-term sequelae. J Urol 1990;143:682.

Mee SL et al: Radiographic assessment of renal trauma: A 10-year prospective study of patient selection. J Urol 1989;141:1095.

Monstrey SJM et al: Renal trauma and hypertension. J Trauma 1989;29:65.

TUMORS OF THE GENITOURINARY TRACT*

Tumors of the genitourinary tract are among the most common neoplastic diseases found in adults. Prostate cancer, for example, is the most common cancer in males (23%); renal and bladder cancer account for approximately 9% of all malignant tumors in adults. Even though excellent diagnostic methods are available, nearly half of all genitourinary tumors are not found until regional or distant spread has occurred. Advances in diagnosis and treatment of genitourinary tract tumors have occurred in recent years, and the prognosis has improved in conditions such as Wilms' tumor, testicular cancer, and, recently, bladder cancer. The mainstay of diagnosis continues to be physical examination, complete urinalysis, intravenous urography, and cystoscopy whenever indicated. Curative treatment of these tumors continues to be surgical in most instances.

PRIMARY MALIGNANT RENAL TUMORS

1. RENAL ADENOCARCINOMA (Renal Cell Carcinoma)

Essentials of Diagnosis
- Painless gross or microscopic total hematuria.
- Solid renal parenchymal mass on intravenous urography with nephrotomograms, renal ultrasound, or abdominal CT scan.
- Paraneoplastic syndromes common.

---

*Wilms' tumor is discussed in Chapter 46.

General Considerations

Malignant tumors of the kidney account for approximately 6% of all tumors in adults. Most often the diagnosis is suspected because of microscopic hematuria or manifestations of metastases such as pathologic fractures or superficial skin nodules. The cause is unknown, though a hormonal influence is suspected, as the disease occurs in males three times more commonly than in females. The cell of origin appears to be in the proximal convoluted tubule, as determined by morphologic and cell surface antigen homology; thus, 90% of these tumors are adenocarcinomas. The tumor metastasizes commonly to the lungs (30%), adjacent renal hilar lymph nodes (25%), ipsilateral adrenal (12%), opposite kidney (2%), and bones (mainly long bones).

There are numerous conditions that predispose to renal cell cancer, including adult polycystic kidney disease, von Hippel-Lindau syndrome (cerebellar hemangioblastomas, retinal angiomatosis, and bilateral renal cell carcinoma), and acquired renal cystic disease developing in patients with end-stage renal disease. Paraneoplastic syndromes are common in renal cell carcinoma and are often what suggests the diagnosis, yet they rarely have prognostic significance. These syndromes include hypercalcemia, erythrocytosis (but not polycythemia), hypertension, fever of unknown origin, anemia, and hepatopathy (**Stauffer's syndrome**). Renal cell carcinoma has a predilection for producing occlusive tumor thrombi in the renal vein and the inferior vena cava (particularly from the right), manifested by signs of acute scrotal varicoceles and lower extremity edema. This phenomenon occurs in approximately 12% of patients. Occasionally, the tumor thrombus reaches up through the inferior vena cava to the right atrium.

Clinical Findings

A. Symptoms and Signs: Painless gross or microscopic hematuria throughout the urinary stream ("total hematuria") occurs in 60% of patients. The degree of hematuria is not necessarily related to the size or stage of the tumor. Although a triad of hematuria, flank pain, and a palpable flank mass suggests renal cell carcinoma, fewer than 10% of patients will so present. Both pain and a palpable mass are late events occurring only with tumors that are very large or invade surrounding structures or when hemorrhage into the tumor has occurred. Symptoms due to metastases may be the initial complaint (eg, bone pain, respiratory distress).

B. Laboratory Findings: Microscopic urinalysis will reveal hematuria in most patients. The erythrocyte sedimentation rate may be elevated but is nonspecific. Elevation of the hematocrit, prothrombin time, and levels of serum calcium, alkaline phosphatase, and transaminase occur in less than 10% of patients. These findings nearly always resolve with curative nephrectomy and thus are not usually signs of metastases. Anemia unrelated to blood loss occurs in 10–15% of patients, particularly those with advanced disease.

C. Imaging Studies: The diagnosis of renal cell carcinoma is often made by intravenous urography performed as an initial step in the workup of hematuria, an enigmatic metastatic lesion, or suspicious laboratory findings (Figure 41–21). Ultrasonography and CT scan often reveal incidental renal masses. Plain abdominal x-rays may reveal a calcified renal mass, but only 20% of renal masses contain demonstrable calcification. (Twenty percent of masses with peripheral calcification are malignant; over 80% with central calcification are malignant.) The initial technique for workup of hematuria is intravenous urography with nephrotomography; intravenous urography alone will define only 75% of renal mass lesions. Differentiation of the most common renal mass (ie, a simple benign cyst) can be made by the finding of a radiolucent center with a thin wall and a sharp interface between the mass and the renal cortex (the typical "beak sign" of a cortical cyst).

1. Ultrasonography–Further definition of all renal masses seen on intravenous urography is required. Abdominal ultrasonography can define the mass as a benign simple cyst or a solid mass in 90–95% of cases (Figure 41–22D). Previously, cytologic study of aspirated fluid was considered necessary to confirm the presence of simple cysts, but ultrasound techniques are accurate enough in all but a few equivocal cases to obviate such studies. Abdominal ultrasound can also identify a vena caval tumor thrombus.

2. Isotope scanning–Occasionally, a renal mass will be suspected on intravenous urography but is equivocal or not seen on ultrasound. In these cases, a renal cortical isotope scanning agent such as technetium Tc 99m DMSA will be helpful. Isotope scans

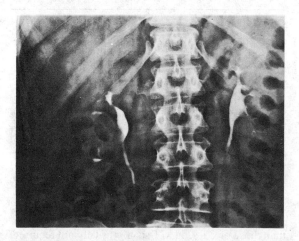

Figure 41–21. Adenocarcinoma of the kidney. Excretory urogram. Distortion of the pelvis and the middle and lower calices of the right kidney. The left kidney is normal.

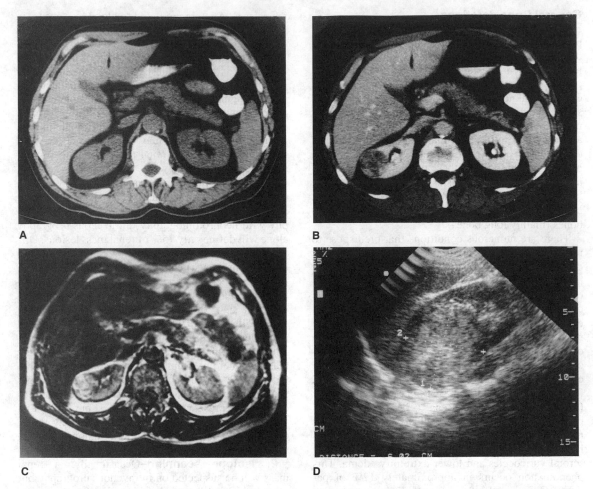

Figure 41–22. *A:* Nonenhanced CT scan showing renal cell carcinoma in the right kidney. The mass, which is difficult to identify, is lateral to the lower pole of the kidney. *B:* Contrast-enhanced CT scan in the same patient clearly shows heterogeneous enhancement of the tumor. *C:* T1-weighted magnetic resonance image (MRI) delineates an obvious mass in the same patient without contrast injection. *D:* Renal ultrasound shows a solid mass within the renal parenchyma of the left kidney in another patient.

of a renal tumor or cyst will show an area of decreased uptake, whereas an area of increased uptake indicates a renal "pseudotumor" or a hypertrophied column of Bertin.

3. CT scan–CT scan is now the diagnostic procedure of choice when a solid renal mass is noted on ultrasound. CT scan accurately delineates renal cell carcinoma in over 95% of cases. Over 80% of tumors are enhanced by iodinated contrast medium, reflecting their high vascularity (Figures 41–22A and 22B). Because of the high accuracy of CT scan, renal angiography is indicated only when CT scan is equivocal (Figure 41–23). The accuracy of angiography is lower (80%) and the morbidity rates and cost higher than those of CT scan. CT scan is usually not required for diagnosis of renal cysts; these lesions do not concentrate contrast agents.

CT scan is also helpful in local staging and can re-

veal tumor penetration of perinephric fat; enlargement of local hilar lymph nodes, indicating metastases; or tumor thrombi in the renal vein or inferior vena cava. Occasionally, an inferior venacavogram may be required to determine the presence and extent of these thrombi.

4. Magnetic resonance imaging (MRI)–MRI holds great promise, particularly in the staging of renal masses (Figure 41–22C). It is the most accurate noninvasive means of detecting renal vein or vena caval thrombi. With the further refinement of pulse sequencing and the use of paramagnetic contrast agents, MRI may become the primary technique for staging solid renal masses.

D. Other Diagnostic or Staging Techniques: Isotopic bone scanning, chest x-ray, and CT scan of the chest can be used to examine the most common sites of metastases and are necessary before deter-

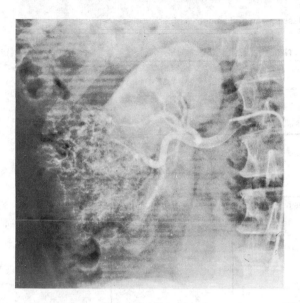

Figure 41–23. Adenocarcinoma of the kidney. Selective renal angiogram showing marked vascularity of mass in lower portion of right kidney typical of malignant tumor.

mining treatment. Cystoscopic examination with or without retrograde pyelograms is rarely necessary. There are no useful tumor markers for renal cell carcinoma. Occasionally, aspiration cytology of the mass can be useful in an enigmatic case. Previously, such procedures were discouraged because of fear of disseminating the tumor along the needle tract, but this has proved to be rare, and the technique is safe. The diagnosis is most often made by noninvasive means, and needle aspiration is required only in indeterminate cases (< 10%).

Differential Diagnosis

A variety of lesions in the retroperitoneum and kidney other than renal cysts may simulate renal cancer. These include lesions due to hydronephrosis, adult polycystic kidney disease, tuberculosis, xanthogranulomatous pyelonephritis, angiomyolipoma, or adrenal cancer and retroperitoneal lipomas, sarcomas, or abscesses. In general, the radiographic and ultrasonographic techniques described above should make the differentiation. Hematuria may be caused by renal, ureteral, or bladder calculi; renal pelvis, ureteral, or bladder tumors; or many other benign conditions usually delineated by the studies described. Cystoscopy is obligatory in hematuric patients with a normal intravenous urogram to rule out disease of the bladder and to determine the source of the hematuria.

Complications

Occasionally, patients may present with acute flank pain secondary to hemorrhage within a tumor or colic secondary to obstructing ureteral clots. Tumor in the renal vein or vena cava may cause a varicocele or lower extremity edema associated with proteinuria. Pathologic fractures due to osteolytic metastases in long bones are common, as are symptomatic brain metastases.

Treatment

Staging is the key to designing the treatment plan (Table 41–1). Patients with disease confined within the renal fascia (Gerota's fascia) or limited to nonadherent renal vein or vena caval tumor thrombi (stages I, II, and IIIA) are best treated by radical nephrectomy. This involves en bloc removal of the kidney and surrounding Gerota's fascia (including the ipsilateral adrenal), the renal hilar lymph nodes, and the proximal half of the ureter. Para-aortic node dissection has not been beneficial and is not recommended. Nephrectomy has not been associated with improved survival rates in patients with gross nodal involvement or multiple distant metastases (stages IIIB, IIIC, and IV), and the procedure is not recommended unless patients are symptomatic or a promising therapeutic protocol is being studied. Patients with solitary pulmonary metastases have benefited from joint surgical removal of both the primary lesion and the metastatic lesion. Preoperative arterial embolization in patients with or without metastases does not improve survival rates, though it may be helpful in patients with symptomatic but nonresectable primary lesions. Radiation therapy is of little benefit except for symptomatic bone metastases. Medroxyprogesterone for metastatic renal cell carcinoma has given an equivocal 5–10% response rate of short duration. Vinblastine has also had a response rate of approximately 20%, again of minimal duration. There are no other cytotoxic chemotherapeutic agents of benefit. Immunotherapy with BCG, immune RNA, and thymosin fraction V has been tried with only limited responses in each case. Alpha interferon (IFN-α) has had a 15–20% response rate. Other interferons, alone (IFN-β or IFN-γ) or in combination with chemotherapeutic agents, have been less effective than IFN-α. Recently, adoptive immunotherapy—using lymphocytes (lymphokine-activated killer [LAK] cells) from exposure of patient's own peripheral blood lymphocytes to interleukin-2 (IL-2) in vitro followed by reinfusion into the patient along with systemic IL-2 infusion—has shown up to 33% objective response rates in early studies. The IL-2 causes a profound capillary leak syndrome and substantial toxicity. Subsequent studies showed only a 16% response rate. Studies using lymphocytes isolated from the patient's own tumor (tumor-infiltrative lymphocytes [TIL]) and expanded in IL-2 in vitro followed by reinfusion of the TIL and systemic IL-2 have shown some promise, but clinical studies are incomplete. Finally, early clinical trials of combined IL-2 and IFN-α show a 30% response rate and extended survival, but confirmatory studies are necessary.

Table 41–1. Conventional and TNM staging classification and prognosis of renal cell cancer.

Conventional Stage	T	N	M	Five-year Survival (%)
I. Tumor confined by renal capsule	T_1 (small tumor with minimal caliceal distortion) T_2 (large tumor with caliceal deformity)			60–70
II. Tumor extension to perirenal fat or ipsilateral adrenal but confined by Gerota's fascia	T_{3a}			50–65
IIIa. Renal vein or inferior vena cava involvement	T_{3b} (renal vein involvement) T_{3c} (renal vein and caval involvement below the diaphragm) T_{4b} (caval involvement above the diaphragm)	N_0 (nodes negative)	M_0 (lack of distant metastases)	50–60 (renal vein) 25–35 (vena cava)
IIIb. Lymphatic involvement	T_{1-3}	N_1 (single homolateral regional node involved) N_2 (multiple regional, contralateral or bilateral nodes involved) N_3 (fixed regional nodes) N_4 (juxtaregional nodes involved)		15–35
IIIc. Combination of IIIa and IIIb	T_{3-4}	N_{1-4}		15–35
IVa. Spread to contiguous organs except ipsilateral adrenal	T_{4a}	N_{0-4}		0–5
IVb. Distant metastases	T_{1-4}	N_{0-4}	M_1	0–5

Prognosis

Patients with localized renal cancer (stages I, II, and IIIA) treated surgically have 5-year survival rates of approximately 70%, whereas rates for those with local nodal extension or distant metastases are 30% and less than 10%, respectively. Most patients who present with multiple distant metastases succumb to disease within 15 months (Table 41–1).

2. RENAL SARCOMA

Renal sarcomas include rhabdomyosarcoma, liposarcoma, fibrosarcoma, and leiomyosarcoma; the latter is the most common, though all are very uncommon. Sarcomas are highly malignant and are usually detected at a late stage and thus have a poor prognosis. The diagnostic approach is similar to that of renal cell carcinoma. The histology of the lesion is rarely suspected preoperatively. These tumors have a tendency to surround the renal vasculature and do not exhibit neovascularity on arteriography.

Treatment is surgical, with wide local excision; however, local recurrence and subsequent distant metastases are the rule. There is no therapy of proved benefit for metastatic disease.

SECONDARY MALIGNANT RENAL TUMORS

Metastases to the kidney often develop from primary tumors of distant sites, most commonly the lung, stomach, and breast. It is rare for the diagnosis to be made before autopsy; this suggests that renal metastasis is a late event. There are usually no symptoms, though microscopic hematuria occurs in 10–20% of cases. Intravenous urograms may be normal, since the tumors are located peripherally in the parenchyma. Contiguous spread of a tumor adjacent to the kidney is not infrequent (eg, tumors of the adrenal, colon, and pancreas and retroperitoneal sarcomas). Tumors such as lymphoma, leukemia, and multiple myeloma may also infiltrate the kidney. Routine radiologic, hematologic, and chemical examinations should demonstrate the primary tumor in most cases.

BENIGN RENAL TUMORS

Renal Adenoma

Renal adenoma is the most common benign solid parenchymal lesion. Tumors less than 3 cm in diameter have been considered benign and those larger than 3 cm malignant; however, small lesions are not histologically distinguishable from renal adenocarcinomas, and the biology cannot be predicted preoperatively. These tumors should be considered malignant and should be treated by total excision.

Renal Oncocytoma

Renal oncocytoma is a subtype of adenoma. The tumors are generally asymptomatic, unassociated with the paraneoplastic syndromes often encountered in patients with renal adenocarcinoma. There commonly is a central stellate scar in these tumors that produces a typical spoke-wheel pattern on angiography. However, because neither this nor any other diagnostic finding is specific enough to exclude malignancy preoperatively, radical nephrectomy is most often performed for these lesions.

Mesoblastic Nephroma

Mesoblastic nephroma is a benign congenital renal tumor seen in early childhood, which must be distinguished from the highly malignant nephroblastoma, or Wilms' tumor (see Chapter 46). Unlike Wilms' tumor, mesoblastic nephroma is commonly diagnosed within the first few months of life. Histologically, it is distinguished from Wilms' tumor by cells resembling fibroblasts or smooth muscle cells and by the lack of epithelial elements. The prognosis is excellent; complete surgical resection is curative, and neither chemotherapy nor radiotherapy is required.

Angiomyolipoma

Angiomyolipoma is a benign hamartoma seen most often in adults with tuberous sclerosis (adenoma sebaceum, epilepsy, and mental retardation). It is often detected following spontaneous retroperitoneal hemorrhage. The tumors may be quite large and are commonly multiple and bilateral. CT scan defines these tumors; a negative CT number is seen in areas of fat within the mass. Occasionally, an angiomyolipoma will elude diagnosis preoperatively and will require nephrectomy. However, asymptomatic patients with small (< 5 cm) tumors and typical findings on CT scan of fat within the tumor do not require surgery, as the prognosis is excellent without treatment.

Other Benign Renal Tumors

Other benign renal tumors include the following: (1) **fibroma,** a renal parenchymal capsular or perinephric fibrous mass; (2) **lipoma,** an adipose deposit within or around the kidney, often perihilar or within the renal sinus; (3) **leiomyoma,** a common retroperitoneal tumor that may arise from the renal capsule or renal vascular walls; and (4) **hemangioma,** which is occasionally found to be the elusive cause of hematuria. Hemangiomas are generally quite small, and the diagnosis is confirmed by angiography or direct vision of the lesion in the renal collecting system. Because these and other benign tumors are infrequent, the final diagnosis is generally made by the pathologist after the kidney is removed.

TUMORS OF THE RENAL PELVIS & CALICES

Essentials of Diagnosis

- Gross or microscopic hematuria.
- Radiolucent filling defect in the renal pelvis or the calices on intravenous urography.
- Malignant cells on urine cytologic study.

General Considerations

In over 90% of cases, tumors involving the collecting system of the kidney are urothelial transitional cell carcinomas. Less than 5% of tumors in this location are squamous carcinomas (often in association with chronic inflammation and stone formation) or adenocarcinomas. The cause of transitional cell carcinoma of the upper urinary tract is similar to that of epithelial tumors in the ureter or bladder; there is a strong association with cigarette smoking and exposure to industrial chemicals. Excessive use of phenacetin-containing analgesics and the presence of Balkan nephritis are also predisposing factors.

Clinical Findings

A. Symptoms and Signs: Gross or microscopic painless hematuria occurs in over 70% of patients. The lesions are usually asymptomatic unless bleeding causes acute flank pain secondary to obstructing clots. Presenting symptoms are often due to metastases to bone, the liver, or the lungs. Physical examination is not usually helpful.

B. Laboratory Findings: Microscopic hematuria on urinalysis is the rule. Pyuria is not seen. Cytologic examination of voided urine specimens may be diagnostic in high-grade tumors. Urine obtained from the ureter by retrograde catheterization or by brushing with specialized ureteral instruments can improve the diagnostic accuracy of cytologic examinations. There are no commonly associated paraneoplastic syndromes or diagnostic tumor markers in transitional cell carcinoma.

C. Imaging Studies: The diagnosis is commonly made on intravenous urography and confirmed by retrograde pyelography, which reveals a radiolucent filling defect in the renal pelvis or calices (Figure 41–24). Renal ultrasound or CT scan can be used to rule out calculus. CT scan is also useful in local staging of the tumor. Transitional cell carcinoma is usually avascular on arteriography, and for that reason the study is not diagnostically useful. The tumors metastasize to the lungs, liver, and bone, so chest films, CT scan of the lungs and liver, and a bone scan are useful to determine the presence of metastases. Transitional cell carcinoma tends to be multifocal in the urinary tract, involving the opposite kidney (1–2%), ureter, or bladder (40–50%). Surveillance of these potential sites is important; careful scrutiny of the opposite kidney and ureter on intravenous urography and of the bladder at cystoscopy is important.

D. Endoscopic Findings: Cystoscopy is necessary when gross hematuria is present to determine the location of the bleeding. Retrograde pyelography and ureteral cytologic studies or brushing as described above can be useful, though mildly abnormal cytologic findings may occur in patients with upper tract inflammation or calculi. Rigid or flexible ureteroscopes can be used to view the upper ureter and renal pelvis directly. Biopsy of upper tract lesions is possible through these instruments. Although percutaneous approaches to the renal collecting system have been perfected, their use for diagnosis or treatment of suspected transitional cell carcinoma in routine cases is not recommended, because of the possibility of spreading tumor cells outside the kidney.

Differential Diagnosis

A variety of conditions may mimic transitional cell carcinoma of the renal pelvis, including calculi, sloughed renal papillae, tuberculosis, and renal cell carcinoma with pelvic extension of the tumor. These

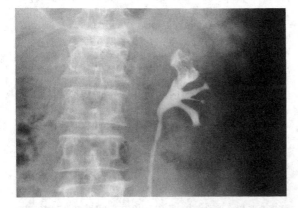

Figure 41–24. Retrograde pyelogram showing transitional cell carcinoma of left upper pole collecting system.

can usually be ruled out by the diagnostic studies described above.

Complications

Occasionally, bleeding may be severe enough to require immediate nephrectomy. Infection may develop, particularly when there is obstruction and hydronephrosis, requiring prompt use of systemic antibiotics.

Treatment

Renal transitional cell carcinoma is treated by nephroureterectomy (perifascial nephrectomy and removal of the entire ureter, down to and including the ureteral orifice within the bladder). Recently, transureteral or percutaneous endoscopic techniques for resection of selected low-grade lesions has been described. High recurrence rates and the potential for local tumor spread would argue against this approach except in unusual circumstances (renal insufficiency or solitary kidney). Para-aortic lymphadenectomy has not been shown to improve survival rates and is not recommended. Because 50% of these patients will develop transitional cell carcinoma of the bladder, cystourethroscopy must be performed postoperatively; it is usually done quarterly during the first year, twice the second year, and then annually.

Prognosis

Because most of these tumors are low-grade and noninvasive, the 5-year tumor-free survival rate is higher than 90% for lesions treated with complete removal of the ipsilateral upper urinary tract. Survival rates are much lower for lesions that invade the renal parenchyma or are of histologic grade III or higher. A poor prognosis is associated with tumors having histologic features of squamous carcinoma or adenocarcinoma. These tumors are mildly radiosensitive, but pre- or postoperative radiotherapy has not been particularly helpful. Metastatic lesions are particularly problematic, and survivors are rare. Chemotherapy combinations, which have shown benefit in transitional cell carcinoma of the bladder (methotrexate, cisplatin, and vinblastine [CMV] or, with the addition of doxorubicin [Adriamycin], M-VAC) may also be efficacious in transitional cells carcinoma of the upper urinary tract.

TUMORS OF THE URETER

Essentials of Diagnosis

- Gross or microscopic hematuria.
- Radiolucent filling defect in the ureter on intravenous urography or retrograde pyelography.
- Malignant cells on urine cytologic study.

General Considerations

Ureteral tumors are rarely benign, but benign

fibroepithelial polyps do occasionally occur within the ureter. More than 90% of ureteral tumors are transitional cell carcinomas. The cause is unknown, but tobacco smoking and exposure to industrial chemicals are known to be associated. Ureteral transitional cell carcinoma is often found in association with renal pelvis transitional cell carcinoma and slightly less often with bladder transitional cell carcinoma. The lesions develop in persons age 60–70 and are twice as common in men as in women. More than 60% of these tumors occur in the lower ureter.

Clinical Findings

A. Symptoms and Signs: Gross or microscopic hematuria is the rule (80% of cases). Because ureteral tumors grow slowly, they may not cause symptoms even though they completely obstruct the kidney. Occasionally, gross hematuria may cause acute obstruction because of clots. The initial presentation may be due to symptomatic metastases to bone, lungs, or liver. Extensive mid and lower ureteral tumors may be palpable.

B. Laboratory Findings: Urinalysis commonly reveals hematuria. There are no biochemical markers specific to the diagnosis, though patients with metastases may have abnormal liver function tests or anemia. Serum creatinine levels may be elevated with complete unilateral obstruction in elderly patients. Cytologic studies of voided urine or ureteral urine or brush studies may be diagnostic.

C. Imaging Studies: The diagnosis may be made on intravenous urography, though the tumor often obstructs the ureter completely, so that cystoscopy and retrograde pyelography are required for definition of the lesion. These studies often reveal a filling defect in the ureter (classically described as a "goblet sign") (Figure 41–25). The ureter is dilated proximal to the lesion. CT scan is useful in ruling out nonopaque calculi and perhaps in abdominal tumor staging. Arteriography is of little value. Chest x-ray, CT scans, and bone scans are helpful in determining the presence of metastases.

D. Endoscopic Findings: Cystoscopy is necessary when gross hematuria is present to determine the site of bleeding. Retrograde pyelography may then be necessary. Ureteroscopy may provide a direct view of the tumor and access for biopsy.

Differential Diagnosis

Nonopaque calculi, sloughed renal papillae, blood clots, or extrinsic compression by retroperitoneal masses or nodes may all produce signs, symptoms, and x-ray findings similar to those with ureteral tumors. The radiographic, cytologic, and endourologic studies listed above should make the distinction, but surgical exploration will be required occasionally.

Treatment

Most ureteral transitional cell carcinomas are not

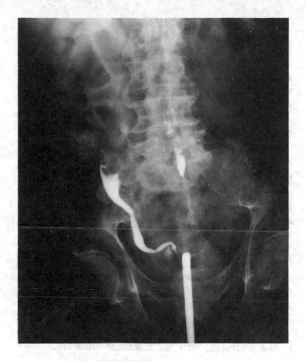

Figure 41–25. Retrograde ureterogram showing "negative" shadow caused by transitional cell carcinoma of the obstructed lower right ureter and the typical "goblet sign."

associated with metastases and can be definitively treated with nephroureterectomy. Selected patients with noninvasive low-grade lesions may be treated by segmental ureteral resection with end-to-end anastomosis (ureteroureterostomy). In selected patients with low-grade tumors and renal insufficiency or solitary kidney, an endoscopic transureteral resection can be considered. Para-aortic lymphadenectomy has not been helpful. Pre- or postoperative radiation therapy appears to be of no benefit. As with renal pelvis and bladder transitional cell carcinoma, cystoscopy should be performed periodically postoperatively. Patients with metastases are rarely helped by removal of the primary tumor. These tumors are generally not responsive to chemotherapy, though the recent observation that a small series of metastatic ureteral cancer patients treated with CMV (cisplatin, methotrexate, and vinblastine) showed a 60% response rate has raised hopes that this combination may result in durable remissions and long-term survival.

Prognosis

The 5-year survival rate for patients with low-grade noninvasive lesions treated surgically approaches 100%. Those with high-grade or invasive lesions have a poorer prognosis, and those with metastases have a 5-year survival rate of less than 10%.

TUMORS OF THE BLADDER

Essentials of Diagnosis
- Gross or microscopic hematuria.
- Malignant cells on urine cytologic study.
- Cystoscopic visualization of the tumor.
- Histologic confirmation of the lesions.

General Considerations
Vesical neoplasms account for nearly 2% of all cancers and are the second most common cancer of the genitourinary tract. Males are affected twice as often as females. More than 90% of tumors are transitional cell carcinomas, while a few are squamous cell carcinomas (associated with chronic inflammation, as in bilharziasis) or adenocarcinomas (often seen at the dome of the bladder in patients with a urachal remnant).

Most transitional cell carcinomas are superficial (not invasive into the bladder wall) when recognized, and over 80% remain so even when they recur. Twenty percent of recurrent tumors will become invasive. Eighty percent of patients who present with invasive disease will not have had prior superficial tumors.

The cause of transitional cell carcinoma is unknown; there is a strong association with chronic cigarette smoking and exposure to chemicals prevalent in dye, rubber, leather, paint, and other chemical industries. Common use of artificial sweeteners such as cyclamates and saccharin was thought to be related to bladder tumor development, but recent reports have found little evidence to substantiate this.

The treatment and prognosis depend entirely on the degree of anaplasia (grade) and the depth of penetration of the bladder wall or beyond (Table 41-2). Most of these tumors develop on the trigone and the adjacent posterolateral wall; thus, ureteral involvement with obstruction is common. Tumors tend to be multifocal within the bladder. Approximately 5% of patients develop upper urinary tract transitional cell carcinoma as well.

Clinical Findings
A. Symptoms and Signs: Gross hematuria is a common finding, though the finding of microscopic hematuria is often what leads to the diagnosis. Patients with diffuse superficial tumors, particularly carcinoma in situ, may have urinary frequency and urgency. Occasionally, large necrotic tumors become secondarily infected, and patients exhibit symptoms of cystitis. Pain secondary to clot retention, tumor extension into the pelvis, or ureteral obstruction may occur but are not frequent presenting complaints. When both ureters are obstructed, azotemia with attendant secondary symptoms may be the finding that serves as an occasion for diagnostic studies.

External physical examination is not generally revealing, though occasionally a suprapubic mass may be palpable. Rectal examination may reveal large tumors, particularly when they have invaded the pelvic side walls. Thus, bimanual examination is a necessary part of staging evaluation.

B. Laboratory Findings: Microscopic hematuria is the only consistent diagnostic finding. Patients with bilateral ureteral obstruction may have azotemia and anemia. Liver metastases may cause elevation of serum transaminases and alkaline phosphatase. There are no paraneoplastic syndromes or tumor markers consistently present in patients with transitional cell carcinoma. Urinary and serum CEA levels may be elevated but are not specific for transitional cell carcinoma and thus are not helpful.

C. Imaging Studies: Small bladder tumors will not be seen on intravenous urography, but larger tumors will usually produce filling defects in the bladder (Figure 41-26). Ureteral obstruction with hydroureteronephrosis may be seen as well. Invasion of the bladder wall may be predicted in patients with asymmetry or marked irregularity of the bladder wall. Noninvasive lesions seen on intravenous urography tend to be exophytic within the bladder, without evidence of bladder wall distortion.

Ultrasonography by external, transrectal, or (recently) transurethral routes can accurately define moderate-sized bladder tumors and can often depict deep invasion. Vesical angiography is of little benefit in the diagnosis or staging of bladder neoplasms.

Pelvic CT scan can diagnose bladder tumors, but the study is too expensive and too inaccurate to use

Table 41-2. Treatment and prognosis of bladder tumors related to stage of disease.

Conventional Stage	TNM Stage	Tumor Involvement	Treatment	Five-Year Survival (%)
O	T_a	Mucosa only	Transurethral resection	85–90
A	T_1	Submucosal invasion (lamina propria)	Transurethral resection and intravesical chemotherapy	60–80
B_1	T_2	Superficial muscle invasion	Total cystectomy and pelvic lymphadenectomy	50–55
B_2	T_{3a}	Deep muscle invasion		30–50
C	T_{3b}	Perivesical fat invasion		30–40
D_1	$T_{3-4}N_+$	Regional lymph node invasion	Systemic chemotherapy	6–35
D_2	$T_{3-4}M_1$	Distant metastases		0–10

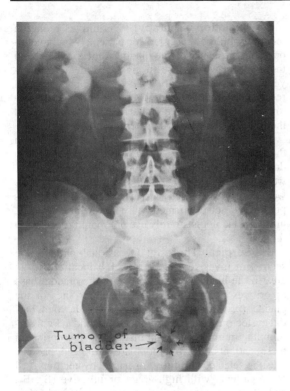

Figure 41–26. Excretory urogram showing space-occupying lesion (transitional cell carcinoma) on the left side of the bladder. The upper tracts are normal.

routinely. CT scan can be useful for staging, but the depth of bladder wall penetration and delineation of tumor deposits in adjacent nonenlarged lymph nodes are not accurately defined. Bipedal lymphangiography can depict tumor deposits in high iliac or para-aortic nodes, but nodes more likely to be involved (internal iliac and obturator nodes) may not be shown. In patients with nodal metastases suspected on lymphangiography or CT scans, fine-needle aspiration and cytologic studies may confirm the diagnosis and eliminate the need for surgical exploration. MRI is helpful in the pelvis, where motion artifacts are minor and the scant pelvic fat is just enough to provide organ differentiation. However, the information is not superior to that obtained with CT at present.

D. Urinary Cytologic Studies: Transitional cell tumors shed neoplastic cells into the urine in large numbers. Low-grade tumor cells may not appear abnormal on cytologic examination, but higher-grade tumor cells can be detected by cytologic study. These studies are most useful in checking for recurrence of transitional cell carcinoma. Flow cytometry (differential staining of DNA and RNA within urine cells to measure the amount of nuclear protein and thus the relative number of aneuploid [abnormal] cells) has been used to screen patients with some success. This

technique may be useful for early diagnosis of recurrence.

E. Endoscopic Findings: Cystoscopy is mandatory in any adult patient with unexplained hematuria and a normal intravenous urogram. Many transitional cell carcinomas will not be seen on intravenous urography. Cystoscopic examination should detect nearly all tumors in the bladder (Figure 41–27). Only a few patients will have carcinoma in situ (superficial high-grade tumor) that is not visible. Any tumor seen should be biopsied. Superficial-appearing tumors can be diagnosed and removed transurethrally at the same time. The entire bladder, including the bladder neck, should be routinely scrutinized in all patients with microscopic hematuria. In patients without visible tumor and no other causes of hematuria, random biopsies may be diagnostic of carcinoma in situ. A bimanual examination should be done during cystoscopy in all patients with transitional cell carcinoma to be certain that the bladder is not fixed, signifying extensive extravesical extension.

F. Staging: Therapy depends on the stage of the tumor as seen on histologic sections and examinations for metastases. Table 41–2 sets forth the stage, treatment, and prognosis of patients with transitional cell carcinoma of the bladder. The histologic grade of the tumor is also important in determining treatment and prognosis, but in general, low- and high-grade histologic characteristics tend to occur in low- and high-stage tumors, respectively.

As previously discussed, CT scan, MRI, or both may be helpful in predicting the stage of the tumor. Isotope bone scanning, chest x-ray, and CT scan will eliminate the possibility of bone or pulmonary metastases and should be done before determining therapy in patients with invasive lesions.

The absence of blood group antigens on tumor cell membranes may predict subsequent tumor invasion,

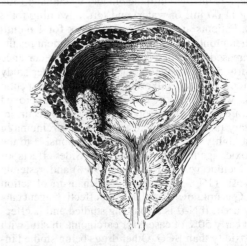

Figure 41–27. Transitional cell (papillary) carcinoma of the bladder with minimal invasion of the bladder wall.

but techniques for determining this are not universally available. It is not yet known whether this finding is reliable enough to serve as a basis for recommending prophylactic ablative surgery in patients without ABO(H) antigens on tumor cell surfaces in the absence of bladder wall invasion.

Treatment

A. Transurethral Resection, Fulguration, and Laser Therapy: Endoscopic transurethral resection of superficial and submucosally invasive low-grade tumors can be curative. Nevertheless, because the tumor recurs in more than 50% of patients, cystoscopy should be performed periodically. Quarterly examinations are recommended during the first year following tumor resection, every 6 months during the second year, and annually thereafter. Periodic urinary cytologic examinations can be helpful as well. Intravenous urography is recommended yearly for the first 3–5 years but is not mandatory. Recurrent small tumors without obvious invasion may be treated by fulguration only, though biopsy is recommended to document the stage and grade.

Neodymium:YAG lasers have been used for desiccation of low-grade, low-stage tumors. There is as yet no proved advantage to this approach except that patients can be treated under local anesthesia as outpatients. Biopsies for diagnosis and staging are still required, however. An approach currently undergoing study involves using photosensitizing agents (eg, hematoporphyrin derivative [Hpd]), which are preferentially taken up by tumors when given systemically. Selective wavelengths of laser light (630 nm) directed to the bladder transurethrally in patients previously given Hpd can selectively destroy tumor cells and perhaps adjacent premalignant cells as well.

B. Intravesical Chemotherapy: A variety of chemotherapeutic agents have been used in patients with recurrent low-grade, low-stage (O–A) tumors. Thiotepa is instilled into the bladder by catheter (30–60 mg in 60 mL of water) and left indwelling for 2 hours. Patients are treated once a week for 1 month and then monthly for up to 2 years. Treatment results in decreased frequency of recurrence or no recurrence in nearly 50% of patients. Other agents under study are mitomycin and doxorubicin. Immunotherapeutic drugs, which include the recently FDA-approved BCG, are effective in prophylaxis (60%) of recurrent papillary tumors and curative (70%) in carcinoma in situ, a highly malignant lesion less responsive to the cytotoxic agents described above. Side effects of BCG include vesical irritability (90%) and systemic BCG-osis (1%). Although the mechanism of action of BCG is unknown, it is the most effective agent currently used. IFN-α is also being studied and is effective (nearly 50% of cases) for carcinoma in situ, with less toxicity than BCG. Other drugs being studied include IL-2, tumor necrosis factor, and various interferon inducers.

C. Radiation Therapy: Definitive radiation therapy should be reserved for patients who have inoperable muscle-invasive bladder cancer localized to the pelvis or who refuse surgical treatment, as the 5-year survival rate is only 30%. In some patients with recurrence after radiation therapy, "salvage cystectomy" can be curative (in at least 30% of cases), though surgical morbidity rates are high.

Much controversy surrounds the use of radiation therapy preoperatively. Some workers have claimed a down-staging effect with 2000 cGy given over 1 week or 4000 cGy given over 3–4 weeks. The studies were poorly controlled, however, and subsequent reports have not confirmed these findings. Currently, urologic oncologists rarely use preoperative radiation therapy.

D. Surgical Therapy: Occasional patients are seen with invasive lesions (B_1, B_2) localized to an area in the bladder well away from the bladder base or orifices and without tumor in other sites of the bladder (proved by multiple biopsies) or beyond. Partial cystectomy (removal of the tumor and a 3-cm surrounding margin of normal bladder) is appropriate in these patients. Such tumors are rare, and patients must be selected carefully for partial cystectomy. All other patients with high-grade or invasive (B_1, B_2, and C) lesions without distant spread or a fixed pelvis on bimanual examination are best treated by cystectomy and pelvic lymph node dissection. This includes removal of the bladder and the prostate in males. Removal of the entire urethra may be necessary in selected patients with tumors at the bladder neck or in the prostate or in those with diffuse carcinoma in situ in the bladder. In females, the uterus, the urethra, and the anterior vaginal wall are removed. Urinary diversion is required and is usually accomplished by creation of an ileal diversion. Recently, continent cutaneous urinary diversions requiring intermittent catheterization rather than cutaneous bag drainage have become popular. Variations of small bowel pouches (**Koch procedure**) or ileocolonic pouches (**Indiana or Mainz procedures**) are most often used. The basic principles are large-volume reservoirs with detubularization of bowel to maintain low intrapouch pressures and construction of an intussuscepted or plicated ileal segment to provide cutaneous continence. In selected cases, continent internal diversions utilizing bowel configurations similar to those described above with attachment to the intact urethra in males is gaining popularity. Urethral recurrence of tumors is a concern (5–10%) with this procedure.

E. Systemic Chemotherapy: Chemotherapy in the form of CMV (cisplatin, methotrexate, vinblastine) or M-VAC (CMV plus doxorubicin [Adriamycin]) has been used precystectomy (neoadjuvant) or postcystectomy (adjuvant) for muscle-invasive tumors or as treatment of metastatic urothelial cancer. The neoadjuvant series all show an approximate 60% downstaging from clinical to pathologic stage and a

30% rate of complete tumor eradication. As with the prior preoperative radiation studies, however, there is no evidence as yet that these results will eventuate in a higher long-term survival rate. A randomized trial of cystectomy alone versus neoadjuvant chemotherapy and cystectomy is now in progress to answer this important question. Adjuvant chemotherapy may be useful, but few patients have been studied and no definitive prospective randomized trials comparing adjuvant versus no adjuvant treatment have been reported. Several reports of efficacy with either CMV or M-VAC for treatment of metastatic disease have shown a 60% overall objective response rate with a 30% complete response rate. A few long-term survivors with apparent cure have been reported, and either of these regimens thus appears to be a definite advance in the treatment of urothelial cancer. These results have caused a few investigators to study chemotherapy alone or in combination with radiation to attempt bladder salvage in patients with invasive bladder cancer. To date, these studies are incomplete, but they appear to show unacceptable recurrence rates; thus, neither regimen is currently recommended.

Prognosis

Approximately half of the low-grade superficial tumors will be controlled by transurethral surgery or intracavitary use of chemotherapeutic agents (Table 42–2). Following radical cystectomy, the 5-year survival rate varies with the extent, stage, and grade of the tumor but averages about 30–55%. The complications of urinary diversion (ureteral obstruction with hydronephrosis, pyelonephritis, and nephrolithiasis) also influence the outcome.

CARCINOMA OF THE PROSTATE

Essentials of Diagnosis

- Palpable rock-hard nodule in the prostate on rectal examination.
- Histologic confirmation on needle biopsy.
- Osteoblastic bone metastases and elevated serum acid phosphatase in advanced cases.

General Considerations

In adult males, prostate cancer is the most common neoplasm (after skin cancer) and the most common cause of death due to cancer. The tumor is more prevalent in black males than any other group in the USA. The tumor rarely occurs before age 50, and the incidence increases with age such that in the eighth decade, more than 60% of men have prostate cancer (at autopsy). In most of these older men, however, the disease is not clinically apparent; only 10% of men over age 65 develop clinical evidence of the disease. Ninety-five percent of tumors are adenocarcinomas. The tumor arises primarily in the peripheral zone

(70%), an area that differs in embryologic derivation from the periurethral zone, which is the site of formation of benign prostatic hyperplasia. Thus, the causes of the two diseases are considered to be different; they may occur simultaneously but are not related. The cause of prostate cancer is unknown, but many factors appear to be involved, including genetic, hormonal, dietary, and perhaps environmental carcinogenic influences.

Screening

Recent advances in transrectal ultrasound (TRUS) and prostate-specific antigen (PSA) monitoring have allowed for enhanced detection of nonpalpable tumors. Much controversy currently exists over whether men over age 50 should be encouraged to undergo screening. There is as yet little evidence that screening will improve survival rates of men with prostate cancer. Despite this lack of data, the realities of clinical practice are that the combination of digital rectal examination and serum PSA monitoring is the most effective screening protocol.

Clinical Findings

A. Symptoms and Signs: Incidental or stage A carcinoma of the prostate presents no physical signs (it is nonpalpable) and is only diagnosed by the pathologist when prostate tissue is removed as treatment for symptomatic bladder outlet obstruction presumed to be caused by benign prostatic hyperplasia or is found by TRUS or PSA monitoring. Patients with stage B or higher disease have a hard nodule on the prostate that can be felt during rectal examination (Table 41–3). In over 60% of these men, the cancer causes obstructive symptoms, urinary retention, or urinary infection (Figure 41–28). Nearly 50% of patients present with evidence of metastases, including weight loss, anemia, bone pain (commonly in the lumbosacral area), or acute neurologic deficit in the lower limbs.

B. Laboratory Findings. Patients with extensive metastases may have anemia due to bone marrow replacement by tumor. Those with bilateral ureteral obstruction secondary to trigonal compression by tumor may exhibit azotemia and uremia. Serum acid phosphatase is usually elevated in patients with bone metastases. Much controversy has surrounded the use of radioimmune assays for acid phosphatase, but recent data have shown the enzymatic acid phosphatase assay (particularly the thymolphthalein monophosphate method) to be nearly as sensitive, more specific, and certainly less expensive than radioimmune assays, so the enzymatic assays are still indicated. Bone marrow acid phosphatase has been shown to be falsely positive in numerous conditions and is thus not useful. Serum acid phosphatase can be falsely elevated by vigorous prostate examination and urethral instrumentation, and serum studies should be drawn before such intervention. Serum

Table 41–3. Treatment and prognosis of prostate cancer related to tumor stage.

Conventional Stage	TNM Stage	Clinical Findings	Treatment	Fifteen-Year Survival (%)
A₁	T₁ₐ	Nonpalpable tumor; incidental finding at prostatectomy (low-grade cancer seen in <5% of prostate).	Observation	Normal
A₂	T₁ᵦ	Same as above except tumor is high-grade or >5% of prostate is involved, or both.	Total prostatectomy with pelvic lymphadenectomy	30–45
B₁	T₂ₐ	Localized nodule 1–1.5 cm in diameter in one lobe.		50–60
B₂	T₂ᵦ	Tumor is ≥ 1.5 cm in diameter or in more than one lobe.		35–45
C	T₃, T₄	Periprostatic extension.	Irradiation with or without pelvic lymphadenectomy	20–30
D	N₊ or M₊	Pelvic lymph node involvement or distant metastases.	Hormonal therapy (orchiectomy or LHRH/antiandrogen) when symptomatic. Irradiation for isolated bone pain.	0–10

acid phosphatase is elevated in approximately 75% of patients with metastases to bone; such patients without elevated levels tend to have poorly differentiated cancers. Serum alkaline phosphatase is often elevated in patients with bone metastases but not in those with localized disease. Prostate-specific antigen (PSA) has recently been shown to be elevated in the serum of approximately 60% of men with prostate cancer, but it cannot be used to definitively determine localized versus metastatic disease. PSA appears to be most helpful in following patients after treatment, as levels fall to almost nil with complete response and rise early (as much as 6 months before serum acid phosphatase) when tumor recurs. Note that neither acid phosphatase nor PSA alone can be used for screening

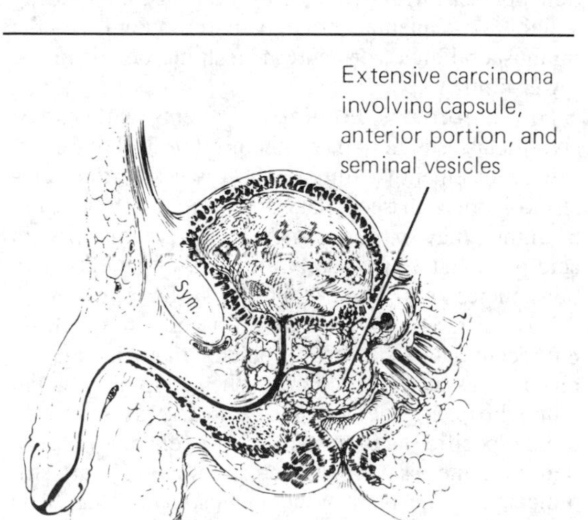

patients for prostate cancer, since normal men with benign prostatic hypertrophy can have false-positive levels (10–30%) and up to 30% of men with cancer will have false-negative levels.

C. Imaging Studies: Transrectal ultrasound (TRUS) using a 7-MHz probe has become the most accurate diagnostic imaging study, revealing typical hypoechoic peripheral zone lesions in 70% of patients with palpable lesions (Figure 41–29). Because some prostate cancers are not hypoechoic and not all hypoechoic lesions are cancer, TRUS alone for screening for prostate cancer is not recommended in the general population. An intravenous urogram may reveal urinary retention or distal ureteral obstruction. Extensive lesions may exhibit a ragged-edged filling defect in the bladder base. A chest x-ray may help in identifying the uncommon lung metastases but more often shows typical osteoblastic metastases in the thoracic spine or ribs. An abdominal x-ray may reveal metastases in the lumbosacral spine or ilium. A CT scan of the pelvis may show an enlarged prostate and large pelvic or para-aortic lymph nodes; however, the study is rarely accurate for staging and is not routinely recommended. Pedal lymphangiography can show defects in large common iliac or para-aortic lymph nodes involved with tumor but rarely delineates the obturator and internal iliac nodes accurately. The lymphangiogram or CT (or both) is most useful in patients with high-grade lesions, who are likely to have pelvic lymph node metastases. Fine-needle aspiration and cytologic studies of abnormal nodes may provide important staging data and perhaps obviate staging laparotomy. MRI appears to be more helpful in pelvic staging of prostate cancer than is CT scan, but like CT it is incapable of differentiating intraprostatic lesions (Figure 41–30). Magnetic resonance spectroscopy has recently shown differences in phosphocreatine/ATP and citrate/lactate ra-

Extensive carcinoma involving capsule, anterior portion, and seminal vesicles

Figure 41–28. Advanced carcinoma of prostate; trabeculation of bladder wall.

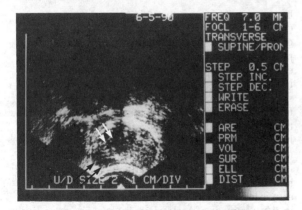
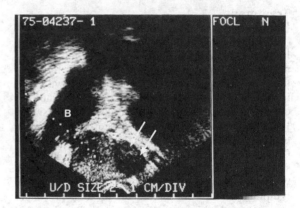

Figure 41–29. Transrectal ultrasound of the prostate. **A:** Transaxial plane. Transition zone is shown at short arrows and hypoechoic prostate cancer in the peripheral zone at long arrows. **B:** Sagittal plane, showing large hypoechoic prostate cancer at arrows. (B = bladder.)

tios in benign versus malignant prostate cancer and thus may be useful for diagnosis in the future. Recently, a monoclonal antibody, Cyt-356, has been coupled with a radioisotope for diagnosis of soft tissue and bone metastases. The early results are encouraging, but definitive studies are yet to be completed.

D. Biopsy: The diagnosis is established by needle biopsy performed either transperineally or transrectally. TRUS-guided transrectal biopsies are quite accurate for diagnosis when typical hypoechoic areas are identified. In patients with nonpalpable disease (stage A), the diagnosis is made by the pathologist after transurethral prostatectomy. Transurethral biopsy is not usually recommended for palpable lesions, however. Transrectal needle aspiration and cytologic studies are highly accurate, though an expert cytologist is required to interpret the findings and histologic grading is not possible with this method.

E. Staging: Rectal examination can provide initial staging in patients with palpable tumors (Table 41–3). Needle biopsy is confirmatory, and histologic grading can fairly accurately predict the metastatic potential of the tumor. Normal levels of serum acid phosphatase and a normal isotopic (technetium Tc 99m) bone scan will rule out bone metastases. A lymphangiogram or pelvic CT scan may be useful to define pelvic lymphadenopathy in patients with high-grade lesions, but pelvic lymphadenectomy is the most reliable procedure for pelvic staging. Recently the laparoscopic approach to pelvic lymph node dissection has provided the same prognostic information as the open surgical procedure with less morbidity and a markedly reduced hospital stay. This approach is useful in patients with high-grade or high-stage lesions, those considered for radical perineal prostatectomy, or those considered for radiation therapy either externally or by interstitial placement. Cystoscopy is not required except in large lesions suspected to involve the bladder neck and trigone.

Differential Diagnosis

Nodules caused by benign prostatic hyperplasia may be difficult to distinguish from cancer; benign nodules are usually rubbery, whereas cancerous nodules have a much harder consistency. Fibrosis following a prior prostatectomy or secondary to chronic prostatitis may be associated with lesions indistinguishable from cancerous nodules and require biopsy for definition. Occasionally, phleboliths or prostatic calculi on the surface of the prostate may be confusing; however, TRUS can be helpful in the differentiation and for biopsy guidance.

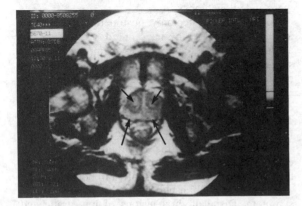

Figure 41–30. T2-weighted MRI in the transaxial plane showing transition zone at short arrows and peripheral zone at long arrows, with hypointense area in right posterior zone of prostate cancer.

Treatment
(Table 41–3)

A. Curative Therapy: Patients with low-grade, low-stage incidental lesions (stage A_1) have a prognosis similar to patients without cancer of the prostate, and require observation only. Patients with clinical stage A_2, B_1, or B_2 lesions are candidates for curative therapy. The pendulum has recently swung from radiation therapy back toward total prostatectomy as the procedure of choice in these patients. Complete staging, including pelvic lymph node dissection, is important, so that appropriate candidates will be selected. Patients with grossly positive pelvic lymph nodes are not candidates for total prostatectomy. Recent advances in surgical technique have led to a low incidence of incontinence (1–4%) and preservation of potency in up to 80% of patients. Alternative procedures include external-beam pelvic irradiation plus interstitial radiation (with ^{125}I, ^{198}Au, or ^{192}Ir). The 15-year results of radiotherapy are nearly as good as those of total prostatectomy in patients with localized disease.

Patients with stage C cancer are best treated with external-beam radiation therapy, but when the lesion is large, palliation only is expected.

B. Palliative Therapy: Patients with metastatic disease cannot be cured, but significant palliation can be offered. Androgen deprivation therapy in the form of oral estrogen (diethylstilbestrol, 3 mg/d) or bilateral orchiectomy is effective in 70–80% of symptomatic patients. Choice of therapy depends on patient preference (many patients find castration unacceptable) or coexistent disease (eg, estrogens have numerous side effects—about 25%—including congestive heart failure, thrombophlebitis, and myocardial infarction, and thus should not be used except in selected patients). These hormonal treatments are not additive, and use of both treatments simultaneously has no advantages over use of either alone. Controversy continues concerning whether to treat asymptomatic patients at the time of diagnosis or to wait until symptoms develop. Because either approach is palliative only and there are no definitive studies to show survival advantages with early treatment, it is recommended that treatment be withheld until symptoms occur except in patients who cannot accept a no-treatment philosophy. Studies using luteinizing hormone-releasing hormone (LHRH) agonists have shown efficacy comparable to estrogen or orchiectomy, with reduced side effects. The drug must be given by monthly injection and is expensive. A recent national study showed that if an LHRH agonist is used, concomitant administration of an antiandrogen (flutamide) improves survival with early treatment as compared to the LHRH alone (7 months difference). Currently, studies to determine if orchiectomy plus an antiandrogen is more effective than orchiectomy alone are in progress.

Patients in whom hormonal therapy has failed can be treated by aminoglutethimide or ketoconazole (both of which inhibit adrenal androgen production) or oral corticosteroids for short-term relief of bone pain. Radiation therapy for symptomatic bone lesions can be helpful, as can local irradiation for an obstructing or bleeding prostate tumor. Recently, a bone-seeking radioisotope (^{186}Re) appears to have some efficacy in therapy of bone metastases. On occasion, transurethral prostatectomy will be required to relieve bladder outlet obstruction. Chemotherapy has not shown dramatic results, though cyclophosphamide, doxorubicin, and cisplatin have all produced minor objective responses in some patients. Enthusiasm is building for suramin, a growth factor inhibitor in the treatment of metastatic disease, but definitive studies have not been reported.

Prognosis

Radical prostatectomy cures 50–60% of the patients suitable for that operation, but its use should be limited to those with a reasonable life expectancy (Table 41–3). Only about 20–30% of patients with prostatic cancer are amenable to curative therapy when their disease is discovered. Careful annual rectal examination to check for suspicious areas of induration and perhaps serum PSA monitoring should be performed in all men at high risk over age 50 if this cure rate is to be improved.

SARCOMA OF THE PROSTATE

Sarcoma of the prostate is rare. Half of all cases occur in boys under age 5. The tumor is highly malignant and metastasizes to the pelvic and lumbar lymph nodes, lungs, liver, and bone. Symptoms of urinary tract obstruction are present. The prostate is enlarged. Cystography or excretory urography may show superior displacement of the bladder or encroachment of the tumor into the bladder. Endoscopy will reveal the mass and allow biopsy.

Total prostatocystectomy, postoperative radiotherapy, and chemotherapy have cured a few cases in adults. In children, combination chemotherapy with surgery for residual tumor has shown increasing success. The tumor is relatively radioresistant.

TUMORS OF THE URETHRA

Malignant tumors of the urethra are rare. The disease is more common in females than in males. Squamous cell types are seen most often in both sexes.

In females, urethral bleeding is the most common symptom. Distal urethral lesions of low grade and without extension can be treated by radiotherapy or wide local excision. Extensive or proximal lesions are best treated by preoperative irradiation and anterior exenteration (removal of the bladder, uterus, adnexa, and urethra with the anterior vaginal wall), including pelvic lymphadenectomy and urinary diversion. The prognosis is excellent for distal lesions without extension, but 5-year survival rates are less than 50% for those with proximal lesions.

In males, the lesion is most commonly in the bulbomembranous urethra and is associated with a history of chronic urethral strictures, often secondary to gonorrheal infection. Patients present with urethral bleeding, a weak urinary stream, and a perineal mass. The diagnosis is made by urethroscopy and biopsy. Distal penile lesions can be treated by partial or total penectomy. Lesions in the bulbous urethra or more proximal lesions require extensive surgical resection, including en bloc removal of the penis, urethra, prostate, bladder with overlying pubis, and pelvic lymph nodes and urinary diversion. Preoperative radiation therapy (2000–4000 cGy) is recommended, although too few patients have been treated to determine the benefit. In both males and females with distal lesions, groin lymphatics may be involved, but node dissection is required only when gross disease is palpable. Five-year survival rates are 60% for distal urethral tumors but less than 40% for the more common proximal lesions.

Primary irradiation—other than to distal lesions in the female—is rarely helpful. Patients with metastatic disease may respond to methotrexate or cisplatin alone or in combination, but objective remissions are usually of short duration.

TUMORS OF THE TESTIS

Essentials of Diagnosis

- Painless, firm mass within the testicle in a man aged 18–40.
- Elevated serum levels of the beta subunit of human chorionic gonadotropin (hCG$_\beta$), alpha-fetoprotein (AFP), lactic dehydrogenase (LDH), or all three.
- Enlarged retroperitoneal nodes on abdominal CT scan.
- Palpable abdominal mass in advanced cases.

General Considerations

Most testicular tumors are malignant germ cell tumors. Non-germ cell tumors such as Sertoli cell tumors and Leydig cell tumors are rare and usually benign. Germ cell tumors are categorized as either seminomatous (35%) or nonseminomatous (embryonal, 20%; teratocarcinoma, 38%; teratoma, 5%; choriocarcinoma, 2%). Cryptorchidism predisposes to testicular cancer, with the incidence increasing inversely with the level of testicular descent (ie, testicles remaining in the abdomen have a much higher incidence of cancer). Metastases first develop in the retroperitoneal nodes; right-sided tumors metastasize primarily to the interaortocaval region just below the renal vessels, and left-sided tumors primarily to the

left para-aortic area at the same level. Distant spread is to supraclavicular areas (left, primarily) and the lungs. Just under 50% of patients have metastases when first seen.

Clinical Findings

A. Symptoms and Signs: Testicular tumors present as a painless firm mass within the testicular substance. They often have been present for several months before the patient seeks consultation. Occasionally (10%) a hydrocele will be present, obscuring palpation of the mass. A few patients have spontaneous bleeding into the mass, causing pain. Patients with high serum levels of hCG may have gynecomastia. Patients with extensive abdominal metastases may present with abdominal pain, anorexia, and weight loss. Examination may reveal palpable retroperitoneal nodes when spread is extensive, or palpable supraclavicular nodes, particularly on the left side.

B. Laboratory Findings: In general, testicular tumors do not alter the usual laboratory parameters, but serum tumor markers are diagnostically helpful. Patients with extensive retroperitoneal metastases may have bilateral ureteral obstruction that causes azotemia and anemia.

Serum lactic dehydrogenase (LDH), particularly isoenzyme I, is elevated in approximately 60% of patients. hCG$_\beta$, a particularly sensitive marker, is a glycoprotein produced by 65% of nonseminomatous testicular tumors but only 10% of seminomas. The alpha subunit of the molecule is identical to luteotropic hormone (LH), but the beta subunit is unique to testicular tumors in adult males. There is cross-reactivity in some assays between the alpha and beta subunits; treated patients who develop modest elevations should have simultaneous assay of LH to be certain the marker detected is hCG$_\beta$. Urinary hCG$_\beta$ studies have been even more sensitive than serum levels but are useful only in selected patients with suspected early recurrences.

Alpha-fetoprotein (AFP) is elevated in 70% of patients with nonseminomatous testicular cancer but is not elevated in patients with seminoma. Patients in whom histologic study has shown seminoma but in whom serum AFP is elevated should be suspected of having nonseminomatous elements in the primary specimen or metastatic lesions.

Approximately 85% of patients demonstrate elevation of one of these markers at presentation. Serum levels decrease when the tumor is completely removed or regresses. Markers are used mainly to follow tumor regression or predict recrudescence, as even minute amounts of tumor may cause serum elevations.

C. Imaging Studies: An intravenous urogram, though not essential, may reveal deviated or obstructed ureters secondary to retroperitoneal metastases. Lymphangiography may show enlarged retroperitoneal nodes with intranodal filling defects, but there are many false-positive and false-negative results. Abdominal CT scan will define enlarged lymph nodes in approximately 90% of cases when they are present. Chest x-ray and CT scan will detect most pulmonary metastases.

Scrotal ultrasound is useful for identifying the typical hypoechoic lesion in the testicle when there are equivocal physical findings. Regardless of the findings on ultrasound, however, a young man with an intratesticular mass on palpation requires surgical definition of the mass.

Differential Diagnosis

Testicular masses in men age 18–40 are almost always malignant and should be treated accordingly. Confusion can occur with scrotal hydroceles, cord hydroceles, epididymal masses or cysts, or epididymitis. Most of these can be differentiated from masses within the testicle by palpation, but if not, transillumination or scrotal ultrasound (or both) is usually helpful. Hydrocele aspiration with a fine needle may be helpful, but care must be exercised not to puncture the mass and thus spread tumor cells.

Treatment
(Table 41–4)

Inguinal orchiectomy with high ligation of the cord at the internal ring is proper initial treatment for all kinds of testicular cancer. Rarely is incisional biopsy of the testicle advisable. Recommendations for further therapy (retroperitoneal dissection, chemotherapy, radiation therapy) are then based on the pathologic findings. A staging workup, including measurement of serum markers, chest x-ray and CT scan, and abdominal CT scan, is done to determine the extent of disease. Lymphangiography may be considered but is useful chiefly in patients with pure seminoma or those who are candidates for expectant management (which is acceptable only if there is no evidence of metastases).

A. Nonseminomatous Tumors: Following orchiectomy, retroperitoneal lymph node dissection is recommended for all patients with nonseminomatous testicular cancer except in the presence of bulky abdominal or distant metastases. Patients with pure

choriocarcinoma are an exception and usually do not have retroperitoneal surgery, because the disease in such cases is invariably systemic and requires multiagent chemotherapy. The extent of lymphadenectomy depends on the testicle involved but in general includes para-aortic and paracaval nodes from the renal vessels down to the aortic bifurcation and along the external iliac artery to the internal inguinal ring on the involved side. Seminal emission can be preserved; loss of this function was previously a complication of retroperitoneal lymph node dissection because of interruption of autonomic nerves crossing the aorta and near the aortic bifurcation.

Because of the associated morbidity, some have proposed that retroperitoneal lymph node dissection be withheld after orchiectomy in patients with normal serum markers and no evidence of retroperitoneal nodal disease on abdominal CT scan and lymphangiography who have no findings of distant metastases on chest x-ray and CT scan. The rationale was that only 20% of these patients will develop recurrent disease, which could then be treated when it appeared. This approach should be discussed with the patient but is not usually recommended.

Patients with any nonseminomatous cell type who have extensive retroperitoneal or chest metastases are best treated after orchiectomy by multiagent chemotherapy followed by excision of persistent masses. Combination chemotherapy with cisplatin, vinblastine, and bleomycin gives a 70% cure rate even in stage III patients. Recent studies have shown that etoposide (VP-16) can replace vinblastine with equal efficacy and less toxicity. Patients who do not respond may be treated with ifosfamide, doxorubicin, or both, with some expectation of success.

B. Seminoma: In the absence of extensive distant spread, patients with pure seminoma should be treated with external-beam radiation therapy (2500 cGy) to the abdomen following orchiectomy. In the presence of bulky abdominal disease or more distant metastases, survival rates are better with multiagent chemotherapy (described above) given initially in lieu of radiation therapy. Patients with substantial residual tumor after chemotherapy may benefit from surgical removal of the remaining tumor.

Table 41–4. Treatment and prognosis of testicular cancer related to tumor stage.

Conventional Stage	TNM Stage	Clinical Findings	Treatment	Five-Year Survival (%)
I	T_1	Confined to testicle	Inguinal orchiectomy; retroperitoneal lymphadenectomy (irradiation for seminoma)	> 95
IIA	N_1–N_{2a}	< 6 microscopic nodes		> 90
IIB	N_{2b}	> 6 microscopic nodes		> 85
IIC	N_3	Bulky abdominal nodes	Orchiectomy and chemotherapy followed by resection of residual disease	≈ 70
III	M_+	Distant metastases		

Prognosis

The prognosis for the various stages of testicular cancer is outlined in Table 41–4. Even in the presence of metastases, many of these patients can be cured. The only exception is patients with choriocarcinoma, who still have a poor survival rate (35% at 5 years) despite extensive chemotherapy.

Johnson DE et al: Surveillance alone for patients with clinical stage I nonseminomatous germ cell tumors of the testis: Preliminary results. J Urol 1984;131:491.

TUMORS OF THE PENIS

Cancer of the penis is a rare disease occurring in the fifth to sixth decades. The cause is uncertain. The disease is rarely seen in circumcised men. The lesion commonly is on the glans penis or foreskin. Early cases may exhibit a painless red, velvety lesion, but most often the lesion is an exophytic nodular or wart-like growth with secondary infection. The initial diagnosis is made by a generous incisional biopsy of the lesion, which reveals squamous cell carcinoma in over 95% of cases. The tumors tend to metastasize to superficial or deep inguinal nodes, though the attendant infection may cause enlarged, tender nodes, which may be difficult to differentiate from metastatic cancer.

The differential diagnosis includes syphilitic chancre, soft chancre due to *Haemophilus* infection, and simple or giant condyloma. Biopsy will usually differentiate between these conditions.

Small noninfiltrating lesions can be treated with fluorouracil cream, external-beam radiation, or laser therapy. However, close follow-up is mandatory in patients so treated. Larger lesions not involving deep structures are treated by partial penile amputation at least 2 cm proximal to the lesion, leaving enough of the penis for adequate direction of the urinary stream. Deeply infiltrating lesions require total penectomy, with formation of a perineal urethrostomy.

Palpable inguinal nodes should be treated by antibiotics for 6 weeks following treatment of the primary lesion to eliminate infection. Persistently palpable nodes will require bilateral ilioinguinal lymphadenectomy. Prophylactic node dissection has not been associated with increased survival rates in patients without palpable nodal involvement. Even those who undergo delayed node dissection when the nodes become palpable can be cured. Radiation therapy for palpable nodes or as prophylaxis for nonpalpable nodes has not been as effective as surgical treatment.

Patients with distant metastases (to the lungs or bone) have a poor prognosis, though cisplatin and methotrexate have shown objective but not durable responses. Five-year survival rates for patients with noninvasive lesions localized to the penis are 80%; for those with inguinal node involvement, 50%; and for those with distant metastases, nil.

Andriole GL et al: Transrectal ultrasonography in the diagnosis and staging of carcinoma of the prostate. J Urol 1988;140:758.

Bukowski RM et al: Interleukin-2 in metastatic renal cell carcinoma: A southwest oncology group study. J Natl Cancer Inst 1990;82:143.

Dreicer R et al: Perioperative methotrexate, vinblastine, doxorubicin and cisplatin (M-VAC) for poor risk transitional cell carcinoma of the bladder: an Eastern Cooperative Oncology Group pilot study. J Urol 1990;144:1123.

Cooner WH et al: Prostate cancer detection in a clinical urological practice by ultrasonography, digital rectal examination and prostate specific antigen. J Urol 1990;143:1146.

Coplen DE et al: Long-term follow-up of patients treated with 1 or 2, 6-week courses of intravesical bacillus Calmette-Guérin: Analysis of possible predictors of responses free of tumor. J Urol 1990;144:652.

Drago JR: The role of new modalities in the early detection and diagnosis of prostate cancer. CA 1989;39:326.

Duchesne GM et al: Orchidectomy alone for stage 1 seminoma of the testis. Cancer 1990;65:1115.

Dunphy CH et al: Clinical stage I nonseminomatous and mixed germ cell tumors of the testis: A clinicopathologic study of 93 patients on a surveillance protocol after orchiectomy alone. Cancer 1988;63:1202.

Fallon BF, Williams RD: Renal cancer associated with acquired renal cystic disease and chronic renal failure. Semin Urol 1989;4:228.

Freuhauf JP, Myers CE, Sinha BK: Synergistic activity of suramin with tumor necrosis factor alpha and doxorubicin on human prostate cancer cell lines. J Natl Cancer Inst 1990;82:1206.

Glashan RW et al: A randomized controlled study of intravesical alpha-2b-interferon in carcinoma in situ of the bladder. J Urol 1990;144:658.

Goldfarb DA et al: Magnetic resonance imaging for assessment of vena caval tumor thrombi: A comparative study with venacavography and computerized tomography scanning. J Urol 1990;144:1100.

Hanks GE: Radical prostatectomy or radiation therapy for early prostate cancer: Two roads to the same end. Cancer 1988;61:2153.

Hricak H et al: The value of magnetic resonance imaging in the diagnosis and staging of renal and pararenal neoplasms. Radiology 1985;154:709.

Jewett MAS et al: Retroperitoneal lymphadenectomy for testis tumor with nerve sparing for ejaculation. J Urol 1988;139:1220.

Kinney P et al: Phase II trial of interferon-beta-serine in metastatic renal cell carcinoma. J Clin Oncol 1990;8:881.

Klein FA, White FK: Flow cytometry deoxyribonucleic acid determinations and cytology of bladder washings: Practical experience. J Urol 1988;139:275.

Lange PH, Fraley EE: Controversies in the management of low volume stage II nonseminomatous germ cell testicular cancer. Semin Oncol 1988;15:324.

Logothetis CJ et al: A prospective randomized trial comparing MVAC and CISCA chemotherapy for patients with metastatic urothelial tumors. J Clin Oncol 1990;8:1050.

Marshall FF: Creation of an ileocolic bladder after cystectomy. J Urol 1988;139:1264.

Maxon HR III et al: Re-186(Sn) HEDP for treatment of painful osseous metastases: Initial clinical experience in 20 patients with hormone-resistant prostate cancer. Radiology 1990;176:155.

McNeal JE et al: Zonal distribution of prostatic adenocarcinoma: Correlation with histologic pattern and direction of spread. Am J Surg Pathol 1988;12:897.

Motzer RJ, Bosl GJ, Geller NL: Advanced seminoma: The role of chemotherapy and adjunctive surgery. Ann Intern Med 1988;108:513.

Niedhart JA: Interferon therapy for the treatment of renal cancer. Cancer 1986;57(Suppl):1696.

Oesterling JE et al: The management of renal angiomyolipoma. J Urol 1986;135:1121.

Oesterling JE: Prostate specific antigen: A critical assessment of the most useful tumor marker for adenocarcinoma of the prostate. J Urol 1991;145:907.

Rifkin MD et al: Comparison of magnetic resonance imaging and ultrasonography in staging early prostate cancer: Results of a multi-institutional cooperative trial. N Engl J Med 1990;323:621.

Rosenberg SA: The adoptive immunotherapy of cancer using the transfer of activated lymphocytic cells and interleukin-2. Semin Oncol 1986;13:200.

Rosenberg SJ, Williams RD: Photodynamic therapy of bladder carcinoma. Urol Clin North Am 1986;13:435.

Scher HI et al: Neoadjuvant M-VAC (methotrexate, vinblastine, doxorubicin, and cisplatin) effect on the primary bladder lesion. J Urol 1988;139:470.

Shipley WU, Kaufman SD, Prout GR Jr: The role of radiation therapy and chemotherapy in the treatment of invasive carcinoma of the urinary bladder. Semin Oncol 1988;15:390.

Shortliffe L: Immune modifiers in genitourinary cancers. In: Advances in Urologic Oncology, vol 1. Williams RD (editor). Macmillan, 1987.

Skinner DG, Liekobsky G, Boyd SD: Continent urinary diversion: A 5-year experience. Ann Surg 1988;208:337.

Steinberg GD et al: Family history and the risk of prostate cancer. Prostate 1990;17:337.

Thuroff JW et al: 100 cases of Mainz pouch: Continuing experience and evolution. J Urol 1988;140:283.

Wahle SM et al: CMV chemotherapy for extensive urothelial carcinoma. World J Urol 1988;6:158.

Williams RD: Intravesical interferon alfa in the treatment of superficial bladder cancer. Semin Oncol 1988;15:10.

Williams RD: Magnetic resonance imaging/spectroscopy and positron emission tomography. In: Adult and Pediatric Urology. Gillenwater JY et al (editors). Mosby Year Book, 1991.

Williams RD: Problems in Urology: Controversies in Prostate Cancer Management. Lippincott, 1990.

Williams RD: Renal, perirenal, and ureteral neoplasms. In: Adult and Pediatric Urology. Gillenwater JY et al (editors). Mosby Year Book, 1991.

Winfield HN et al: Urological laparoscopic surgery. J Urol 1991; 146:941.

NEUROPATHIC (NEUROGENIC) BLADDER

Myoneural Anatomy

The urinary bladder and its involuntary sphincter develop and differentiate from the tubular urogenital sinus. The differentiation of the encasing mesenchymal cells forms the musculature of the detrusor and urethral sphincter.

Innervation

The innervation of the bladder and its involuntary sphincter is via the autonomic nervous system. The parasympathetic supply to the bladder and the sphincter is via the pelvic nerves, which arise from S2–4. These fibers also carry the stretch sensory receptors to the same spinal cord center (S2–4).

The sensory supply for pain, touch, and temperature is carried via the sympathetic fibers arising from the thoracolumbar segments (T11–L2).

Motor and sensory supply of the trigone is via the thoracolumbar sympathetic fibers.

The striated external sphincter, as well as the entire urogenital diaphragm, receives its motor and sensory innervation from the somatic fibers arising from S2–4 (via the pudendal nerve).

It is clear that the S2–4 segment is the origin of the motor supply to the bladder musculature, to the involuntary sphincter, and to the striated external sphincter. The trigone is the only structure that is partly independent in its innervation. This is why segment S2–4 is called the spinal cord center for micturition. It is located at the level of the T12 and L1 vertebral bodies. There are connections between the spinal cord center and the midbrain and cerebral cortex. Through these connections, inhibition and control of the spinal cord reflexes can be maintained. Any injury above the level of the T12 vertebral body will leave the spinal cord center intact, leading to an **upper motor neuron lesion;** injuries at the spinal cord center or below will lead to a **lower motor neuron lesion.**

Myoneurophysiology

The primary functions of the urinary bladder are to act as a reservoir, maintain urinary continence, and prevent vesicoureteral reflux. Intact myoneural elements are essential for these functions. The primary reservoir function is possible through the particular detrusor muscle arrangement and because of the accommodation phenomenon. The normal bladder can accommodate volumes up to 400 mL without increasing intravesical pressure. Bladder fullness is perceived through increases in intravesical pressure.

Until this happens, no perception of the actual volume in the bladder is apparent.

Distention and stretch initiate detrusor activity that can be controlled and inhibited by the high cortical centers or can be allowed to progress to active detrusor contraction and voiding. Normally during voiding, detrusor contraction continues until the bladder is completely empty unless voiding is voluntarily interrupted or inhibited.

Before voiding begins, the pelvic floor and the striated external sphincter relax, the bladder base descends, and the bladder outlet assumes a funnel shape. As a result, urethral resistance decreases. This is followed by detrusor muscle contraction and a rise in intravesical pressure to 20–40 cm of water, which results in a urine flow of about 15–30 mL/s. When the bladder is completely empty, the pelvic floor and striated external sphincter contract, elevating the bladder base, increasing urethral pressure, and ending voiding. Intact nerve pathways are essential for these synchronized activities to occur.

Cystometry

Cystometry is a simple method for testing the above functions and gives the following information: bladder capacity, extent of accommodation, the ability to sense bladder filling and temperatures, and the presence of an appropriate and effective detrusor muscle contraction. In addition, residual urine can be measured at the same time. The apparatus for performing simple water cystometry and a normal cystometrogram is shown in Figures 41–31 and 41–32A.

Uroflowmetry

Uroflowmetry is the measurement of urine flow rate. If detrusor contraction is properly coordinated with sphincter relaxation, then the outlet resistance will fall as the bladder pressure increases, and the flow rate will be adequate. Normally, the flow rate is 20–25 mL/s in males and 25–30 mL/s in females. Any flow rate below 15 mL/s suggests obstruction or dysfunction. A flow rate under 10 mL/s is definitely pathologic.

Urethral Pressure Profiles

Urethral pressure profiles measure and record sphincteric activity to determine the efficiency of the sphincteric elements around the urethral canal. Pressure profiles detect any weakness or hyperactivity in either component: the internal or the external voluntary sphincter.

Classification & Clinical Findings

Neuropathic bladder can be divided into two main groups depending on the site of the lesion in relation to the spinal cord center (S2–4): (1) upper motor neuron lesions (above the spinal cord center) and (2) lower motor lesion lesions through the spinal cord center or its efferent and afferent divisions.

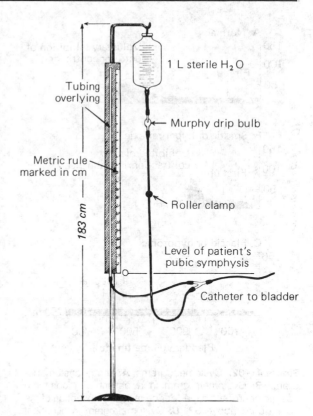

Figure 41–31. Cystometry. A simple water manometer apparatus.

A. Upper Motor Neuron Lesions (Spastic): Lesions above the voiding reflex arc are most commonly due to trauma. Although the reflex arc is intact, it lacks the inhibitory control of the higher centers. Both motor and sensory fibers are usually involved. Accommodation is lost, and uninhibited detrusor contractions may occur. The bladder outlet is usually funneled. The striated external sphincter and pelvic floor are spastic. Although detrusor contractions can generate abnormally high intravesical pressure, they are not effective in producing adequate urine flow because of the spastic external sphincter and are not sustained. Thus, there is always residual urine. Bladder capacity is reduced. Detrusor contraction and mass reflexes can be initiated from certain trigger areas.

There is marked detrusor thickening and hypertrophy. Trigonal hypertrophy initially leads to functional obstruction at the ureterovesical junction; later, decompensation of the ureterovesical valve increases renal back pressure, leading to renal damage.

Figure 41–32B is a typical cystometrogram of a spastic upper motor neuron lesion.

B. Lower Motor Neuron Lesions (Flaccid): Any lesion involving the spinal cord center (S2–4), cauda equina, sacral roots, or their peripheral nerves

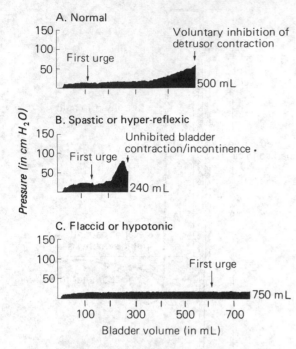

Figure 41–32. Cystometrograms. **A:** Normal cystometrogram. **B:** Cystometrogram in a patient with complete spastic neuropathic bladder caused by transection of the spinal cord above S2. **C:** Cystometrogram in a patient with flaccid neuropathic bladder caused by a myelomeningocele.

leads to atonic, or flaccid, lower motor neuron changes. Trauma is the most common cause, but tumors, ruptured intervertebral disks, and meningomyelocele may also cause this type of neuropathic bladder. Both motor and sensory fibers are usually affected. Damage of stretch receptors results in loss of sense of fullness. Accordingly, bladder capacity progressively increases.

Detrusor contractions are primarily on a myogenic basis, because the bladder has lost its connection to the spinal cord center (Figure 41–32C). These contractions are usually weak and unsustained. In spite of diminished outflow resistance (funneled bladder neck and flaccid external sphincter), flow rates are inadequate and bladder emptying is incomplete, resulting in large amounts of residual urine. Bladder and trigonal hypertrophy develop but are less apparent because of the overstretching. Trigonal hypertrophy, a result of bladder stretch due to residual urine, leads to functional obstruction of the ureterovesical junction. Decompensation and reflux occur relatively late in comparison to spastic upper motor neuron lesions.

Differential Diagnosis

Cystitis, interstitial cystitis, and organic obstruction are occasionally confused with neuropathic bladder, but associated neurologic lesions usually make the diagnosis of neuropathic bladder easy. Psychosomatic disturbances can cause spasm of the external sphincter, incomplete voiding, retention, or incontinence.

Complications

Common complications include urinary tract infection, stone formation, and incontinence. The most serious consequences of these lesions are the hydrodynamic back pressure on the kidneys, hydronephrosis, infection, decompensation of the ureterovesical junction, and loss of renal function.

Treatment

Immediately following spinal cord injury, there is a shock phase that may last a few weeks to 2–3 years. The average time is 2–3 months. The bladder is completely dissociated from nervous control and thus has no sensation and is completely inactive.

Treatment is aimed at avoiding the aforementioned complications in the hope of partial or complete recovery. During the shock phase, continuous closed drainage or, preferably, intermittent (every 4–6 hours) aseptic catheterization should be instituted until bladder activity is restored.

Control of infection and maintenance of a high fluid intake are important. Dietary measures and early mobilization are helpful in prevention of stone formation.

A. Spastic Neuropathic Bladder: In the spastic neuropathic lesion, bladder rehabilitation is the therapeutic goal. Attaining a functional bladder depends upon mobilizing residual urine and increasing the bladder capacity.

Residual urine volume can be decreased by reducing urethral resistance by several methods: transurethral prostatectomy, division of the external sphincter, pudendal nerve manipulation (ablation or electrical stimulation), or alpha-blocker pharmacologic therapy (prazosin).

Functional capacity can be increased (1) by control and prevention of bladder infection, (2) by decreasing detrusor instability with an anticholinergic-parasympatholytic drug (oxybutynin), and (3) by operative augmentation with small or large intestine (enterocystoplasty).

Conversion to a flaccid lower motor neuron lesion can be achieved by cord rhizotomy or subarachnoid injection of absolute alcohol. The storage function of the bladder is preserved, and the patient can be managed by clean intermittent catheterization.

Supravesical urinary diversion may be called for in patients with upper tract deterioration due to ureterovesical valve decompensation and in female incontinence. Male incontinence is controlled by a condom catheter. Implantation of an artificial sphincter serves that purpose in either sex.

B. Flaccid Neuropathic Bladder: Function of

the flaccid bladder can be improved by measures that facilitate complete emptying; these include voiding by Credé's maneuver (suprapubic pressure), transurethral resection of the bladder neck to reduce outlet resistance, and timed voiding or timed clean intermittent catheterization. An indwelling urethral catheter or suprapubic cystostomy is required in a few cases, but chronic intubation should be avoided if possible.

Suprapubic urinary diversion (ureterostomy, ileal or colon conduit, etc) can circumvent decompensation of the ureterovesical junction if deterioration of upper tracts occurs. Attempts are being made to improve the quality of detrusor contraction by means of electrodes implanted in the bladder wall or sacral cord. The early results are encouraging. Implantable prosthetic sphincters may also afford good urinary control.

Prognosis

Ureterovesical junction decompensation and persistent infection are the most serious consequences of neuropathic bladder. Spastic neuropathic bladders cause renal deterioration more rapidly than lower motor neuron lesions. When diversion is required, proper timing of the operation is essential for preservation of kidney function.

Dairiki Shortliffe LM et al: Treatment of urinary incontinence by the periurethral implantation of glutaraldehyde cross-linked collagen. J Urol 1989;141:538.

Frost F et al: Intrathecal baclofen infusion: Effect on bladder management programs in patients with myelopathy. Am J Phys Med Rahabil 1989;68:112.

Herzog AR et al: Methods used to manage urinary incontinence by older adults in the community. J Am Geriatr 1989;37:339.

Nanninga JB, Frost F, Penn R: Effect of intrathecal baclofen on bladder and sphincter function. J Urol 1989;142:101.

Noll F et al: Intermittent catheterization versus percutaneous suprapubic cystostomy in the early management of traumatic spinal cord lesions. Paraplegia 1988;26:4.

Tanagho EA, Schmidt RA: Electrical stimulation in the clinical management of the neurogenic bladder. J Urol 1988;140:1331.

Webster GD, Kreder KJ: Voiding dysfunction following cystourethropexy: Its evaluation and management. J Urol 1990;144:670.

OTHER DISEASES & DISORDERS OF THE GENITOURINARY TRACT

SIMPLE RENAL CYST

A simple renal cyst is usually unilateral and solitary but may be multiple and bilateral. The cause of this disorder is unclear. The cyst can compress and destroy adjacent parenchyma. Cysts contain fluid that resembles (but is not) urine. Most are diagnosed in patients after the fourth decade. Occasionally, what appears to be a simple cyst may, in fact, be a papillary cystadenocarcinoma—an uncommon form of renal cancer with both solid and cystic components. In those cases, however, ultrasound will usually demonstrate a complex mass with both cystic and solid components.

Flank pain may be a presenting symptom, though most renal cysts are found incidentally on urography done for other purposes. A mass may be felt in the flank or upper quadrant and must be distinguished from tumor. Urinalysis and tests of renal function are normal. Excretory urograms reveal a mass that distorts adjacent calices. Nephrotomography shows a radiolucent mass (in contradistinction to tumor). If the CT scan or ultrasound reveals an equivocal cystic mass, cyst aspiration may be performed, the fluid submitted for cytologic examination, and the cyst filled with contrast material to delineate its wall. A simple cyst must be distinguished from adenocarcinoma of the kidney; ultrasonography or CT scan usually makes that distinction.

Complications are rare, but bleeding into or infection of a cyst may occur.

If the diagnosis of cyst is established, surgery is not necessary unless the lesion causes pain or endangers renal function. Simple percutaneous aspiration with instillation of 95% ethanol may suffice. If sclerosis fails, operative excision may be performed.

RENAL ARTERY ANEURYSM

Aneurysm of the renal artery is relatively rare. It results from weakening of the artery wall by arteriosclerosis, poststenotic dilatation, intimal or perimedial fibroplasia, or trauma. If the aneurysm causes stenosis of the artery, hypertension may ensue secondary to ischemia and activation of the renin-angiotensin system. A plain abdominal x-ray may reveal a ring-like calcification in the wall (Figure 41–33). Angiography or CT scan is diagnostic.

Surgery is indicated in the following situations: (1) secondary renal ischemia and hypertension, (2) dissecting aneurysm, (3) aneurysm associated with pain or hematuria, (4) anticipation of pregnancy, (5) aneurysm coincident with significant stenosis, (6) radiographic evidence of incomplete calcification or increase in size on serial films, and (7) aneurysm containing thrombus with evidence of distal embolization. If the aneurysm ruptures, emergency nephrectomy may be necessary.

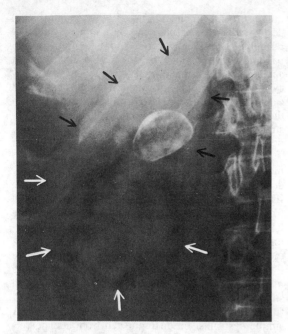

Figure 41–33. Intrarenal aneurysm of renal artery. Plain film showing calcified structure over the right renal shadow.

RENAL INFARCTION

The common causes of renal artery occlusion include emboli due to subacute infective endocarditis, atrial or ventricular thrombi, arteriosclerosis, polyarteritis nodosa, trauma, and, in the neonate, umbilical artery catheterization. Multiple emboli are common and lead to patchy renal ischemia. Occlusion of a main renal artery will cause renal infarction.

The patient may suffer from flank pain, or the lesion may be silent. Hematuria is common. Excretory urograms may reveal no excretion of radiopaque material or may only opacify a portion of the kidney. With complete occlusion of the main renal artery, a ureteral catheter will drain no urine, yet the retrograde urogram will reveal normal anatomy. Renal angiography or digital subtraction angiography makes the diagnosis by revealing occlusion of the artery or arterioles; a renal scan will show similar findings. CT scan after the intravenous injection of radiopaque medium will show no concentration in the ischemic area. Ureteral stone may mimic renal infarction, but urograms, CT scan, or angiograms will distinguish one from the other. Following renal infarction, hypertension may develop secondary to renal ischemia; it may later resolve spontaneously.

If the diagnosis is made promptly (within 5–8 hours), thrombectomy or endarterectomy should be considered. Otherwise, anticoagulation therapy should be instituted (eg, heparin). Thrombolytic therapy (eg, streptokinase) may be used to lyse the clot. If permanent hypertension develops, definitive treatment of the arterial occlusion or nephrectomy should be performed.

RENAL VEIN THROMBOSIS

Thrombosis of the renal vein affects both infants and adults and can be either acute or chronic. In children, thrombosis may be caused by severe dehydration (eg, due to ileocolitis and diarrhea or the nephrotic syndrome). In adults, it may be secondary to renal infection, ascending thrombosis of the vena cava, or caval occlusion due to tumor thrombus. There is usually flank pain and a palpable distended kidney. If renal vein thrombosis is secondary to infection, the patient is septic and urinalysis reveals pus cells and bacteria. In noninfectious cases, the urine may reveal microhematuria and mild proteinuria. The patient with bilateral involvement is azotemic. Nephrotic syndrome may develop. Excretory urograms show delayed opacification in an enlarged kidney. The calices are elongated. Later, the kidney may become atrophic. Renal angiography reveals stretching and bowing of arterioles. Selective renal venography will demonstrate the thrombus (Figure 41–34).

Treatment should attempt to eliminate the underlying cause whenever possible. If the diagnosis of unilateral infected renal vein thrombosis can be established, nephrectomy should be performed. In bi-

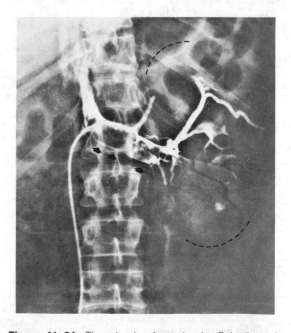

Figure 41–34. Thrombosis of renal vein. Selective left renal venogram showing almost complete occlusion of vein. Veins to lower pole failed to fill. Note large size of kidney.

lateral disease, anticoagulant or thrombolytic therapy (or both) is required.

VESICAL FISTULAS

Vesical fistulas may be congenital or acquired. Congenital fistulas usually involve the urachus. Acquired fistulas may be iatrogenic or due to trauma, tumor, or inflammation.

The most common types of vesical fistulas are vesicovaginal, vesicointestinal, and vesicocutaneous. Vesicovaginal fistulas are commonly secondary to gynecologic trauma; rarely, they occur as a complication of infiltrating cervical carcinoma. Vesicointestinal fistulas are most often due to inflammatory bowel disease: Crohn's disease, diverticulitis, and appendicitis. Cystostomy in the presence of bladder outlet obstruction, bladder cancer, or foreign body may result in vesicocutaneous fistula.

Diagnostic maneuvers include cystoscopy, conventional cystography, barium enema or barium swallow, and CT scan with contrast infusion. Oral charcoal may be useful for detecting a urinary intestinal fistula, as the granules can be seen in spun urine under the microscope.

Therapy for vesicovaginal fistula requires surgical closure, with placement of an omental flap between the bladder and the vagina. For vesicointestinal fistula, the primary intestinal lesion must be resected and the bladder closed. An indwelling urethral catheter is necessary during the healing period.

INTERSTITIAL CYSTITIS

This lesion is most commonly found in middle-aged women. Urinary frequency both day and night is most often accompanied by suprapubic pain with bladder distention. The cause is uncertain, though some suggest an autoimmune collagen disease while others have documented the presence of mast cells and mast cell mediators (histamine and prostaglandin) in bladder biopsy specimens of affected patients.

The diagnosis is based on the history and the results of cystoscopy under general anesthesia. Cystoscopy reveals a small-capacity bladder and punctate hemorrhage following forceful distention. Biopsy may reveal lymphocytic infiltration, mast cell infiltration, and submucosal fibrosis. In patients suspected of having interstitial cystitis, one must rule out carcinoma in situ; urine cytologic study precedes cystoscopy and random bladder biopsy.

Treatment of established cases of interstitial cystitis often fails. Response has been obtained with hydraulic bladder overdistention, intravesical treatment with 50% DMSO, 0.4% oxychlorosene sodium, or sodium pentosanpolysulfate. Systemic corticosteroids have their proponents as well. Some patients require operative augmentation of bladder capacity by enterocysto plasty or, rarely, permanent urinary diversion.

URINARY STRESS INCONTINENCE

Involuntary loss of urine during stress (coughing, sneezing, or physical strain) is a common complaint of postmenopausal women. The cause is related to pelvic relaxation with age, resulting in descent of the trigone and proximal urethra. There is obliteration, of the urethrovesical angle, which normally provides resistance at the bladder outlet. The diagnosis is made by the history and physical examination. When the bladder is full, the patient should be asked to cough while in both the supine and upright positions, producing incontinence. Digital pressure applied to the paraurethral tissues in an anterior direction through the vagina will reestablish the urethrovesical angle and prevent stress incontinence (Marshall's test).

Treatment in patients with normal bladder function and low residual urine is operative. This can be accomplished by retropubic urethrovesical resuspension either using the Marshall-Marchetti-Krantz procedure or the Stamey modification of the Pereyra procedure. New approaches include the use of Teflon paste injection into the periurethral tissues, resulting in increased urethral outflow resistance. Patients with mild symptoms may be helped by oxybutynin chloride or ephedrine (or both).

FEMALE URETHRITIS & PERIURETHRITIS

Urethritis in the female may be acute or chronic. Acute urethritis can be gonorrheal in origin. Chemical urethritis is occasionally acquired from exposure to soap or bath oils. Chronic urethritis is a common problem in females, since the female urethra is exposed to pathogenic bacteria because of its anatomic location. Urethral trauma, instrumentation, and increase in the number of pathogenic organisms lead to infection and overt urethritis. Urethritis usually precedes cystitis.

Hormonal changes associated with menopause cause vaginal and urethral mucosal changes, leading to irritative symptoms and increased susceptibility to inflammation.

Urethritis usually causes irritative voiding symptoms similar to those of cystitis and, occasionally, functional obstructive symptoms. Examination may reveal urethral discharge, marked tenderness, or congested everted mucosa at the external meatus. Induration of the urethra may be associated with vaginitis and cervicitis. Endoscopy may reveal obstruction, mucosal congestion, and inflammatory polyps. Urethral calibration rarely reveals obstruction. Spasm of the external sphincter may be noted.

Treatment is directed to the underlying cause. Estrogen cream or diethylstilbestrol suppositories are indicated for senile vaginitis. Surgical treatment consists of urethral dilation and opening and draining infected periurethral ducts. Alpha-blockers (prazosin) given orally may also help decrease urethral resistance. Correction of vaginitis, cervicitis, and cervical erosions helps in ameliorating symptoms.

FEMALE URETHRAL CARUNCLE

Urethral caruncle, commonly seen after menopause, represents granulomatous overgrowth of the posterior lip of the external meatus. The caruncle is tender and causes pain with intercourse and urination. The primary concern is exclusion of urethral cancer. Treatment is complete excision.

FEMALE URETHRAL DIVERTICULUM

Urethral diverticulum in the female commonly presents as recurrent lower urinary tract infection. It should be suspected whenever urinary infection fails to resolve with treatment. Symptoms are urinary dribbling and cystic swelling in the anterior vaginal wall during voiding. If diverticulum is suspected, it can usually be identified during panendoscopy and opacified by contrast on a voiding cystourethrogram while occluding the external meatus. These lesions occasionally contain stones.

Treatment consists of transvaginal diverticulectomy, taking care to preserve the urethral sphincter.

SPERMATOCELE

Spermatocele is a retention cyst of a tubule of the rete testis or the head of the epididymis. The cyst is distended with a milky fluid that contains sperm. Located at the superior pole of the testis and caput epididymidis, the spermatocele is soft and fluctuant and can be transilluminated.

No treatment is needed unless the spermatocele is painful, in which case surgical excision may be performed.

VARICOCELE

Varicocele is due to incompetent valves in the testicular vein, permitting transmission of hydrostatic venous pressure; distention and tortuosity of the pampiniform plexus results. Varicocele is on the left side in 90% of cases, presumably because of venous drainage of the left testes to the left renal vein, causing increased retrograde venous pressure.

Mild varicoceles are commonly asymptomatic, but a dragging scrotal sensation may be noted. Varicocele may lead to infertility in some men (see Male Infertility).

Asymptomatic varicocele is best untreated unless it is a suspected factor in male infertility. Treatment then consists of operative ligation of the spermatic vein at or above the internal inguinal ring, which can be done open or laparoscopically. In recurrent varicocele, transfemoral catheterization and occlusion or ablation of the spermatic vein may be performed with a detachable balloon or sclerosing agents. The technical success rate is high.

TORSION OF THE SPERMATIC CORD

Torsion of the spermatic cord (intravaginal torsion) is most common in adolescent boys. A twist in the spermatic cord interferes with testicular blood supply. If torsion is complete, testicular infarction may occur within 4–6 hours. The cause is unknown, but an underlying anatomic abnormality (spacious tunica vaginalis, loose epididymotesticular connection, undescended testis) is usually present.

Clinical findings consist of precipitous onset of lower abdominal and scrotal pain and scrotal swelling. There may be a history of previous attacks in young adolescents. The testis is swollen, tender, and retracted. The pain is not relieved by testicular support. The cord above the swelling is normal. The cremasteric reflex is absent on the affected side.

Torsion must be differentiated from orchitis, epididymitis, and pain due to testicular trauma. Technetium Tc 99m pertechnetate scan *may* differentiate orchitis-epididymitis from testicular torsion if performed early in the course of symptoms: the former will demonstrate increased blood flow, in contrast to the ischemic pattern of torsion. If the diagnosis cannot be established by examination and history, exploration is required.

Torsion of the spermatic cord is a surgical emergency! Recent evidence suggests that the infarcted testicle may incite an immune reaction to antigenic sperm, which are otherwise privileged. Normally, sperm are isolated from the immune system by the "blood-sperm" barrier. Once the antisperm immune response is in effect, infertility may result. Thus, the infarcted testes should be removed to minimize immune stimulation. Contralateral orchiopexy is always necessary because of frequent bilateral involvement —ie, the "bell clapper" deformity (lack of fixation of the cord structures by the testicular mediastinum) —and the high incidence of recurrent torsion and infertility in bilateral cases.

TORSION OF TESTICULAR APPENDAGES

The epididymis and the testicle often have a vestigial remnant of embryologic ducts known as an appendix testis or appendix epididymidis. These structures can undergo spontaneous infarction usually in young boys, causing acute testicular pain and swelling that may be difficult to differentiate from testicular torsion. Occasionally, the infarcted appendage can be seen through the scrotal wall as a "blue dot" sign on the scrotum. This sign is only visible early in the course, prior to hydrocele formation and onset of scrotal edema. Scrotal ultrasound occasionally delineates the enlarged appendage and a normal testicle, establishing the diagnosis. In most cases—and certainly in equivocal ones—immediate scrotal exploration and removal of the infarcted appendage is required to rule out testicular torsion. Although the appendages often occur bilaterally, appendiceal torsion does not; thus, removal of the opposite appendage is not indicated.

MALE INFERTILITY*

Male infertility accounts for 30–50% of infertile couples (10–15% of marriages). Both partners should be evaluated for causes of infertility.

The causes of male infertility include the following: congenital anomalies (genetic, such as Klinefelter's syndrome; or developmental, such as absent vas deferens), trauma (both testicular, resulting in atrophy; and neurologic, resulting in erectile or ejaculatory dysfunction), infections (either systemic or reproductive organ specific), endocrine disorders (pituitary insufficiency, androgen deficiency), acquired anatomic abnormalities (varicocele, vasectomy), drug side effects (nitrofurantoin, estrogens, antineoplastic agents).

Diagnosis

The most important aspect of infertility evaluation is the history, which uncovers the cause in many patients. The physical examination is no less important and may reveal small testicles, a varicocele, or absence of the vas deferens.

A. Semen Analysis: Semen analysis is essential in evaluation of male factor infertility. At least three samples should be analyzed, since values may vary over time and with the method of collection. The specimen is produced by masturbation after 3 days of ejaculatory abstinence and collected in a clean widemouth container and examined within 2 hours. Determination of the volume, pH, liquefaction, sperm

count, viability, abnormal forms, and motility constitutes a complete analysis. Normal values include volume of more than 2 mL, 20 million sperm per milliliter, 60% motile sperm, and 60% normal oval sperm heads. Timed videomicroscopic measurement of sperm velocity is a more precise measurement of motility.

B. Hormone Studies: Patients with no sperm in the ejaculate (azoospermia) or very low counts (oligospermia) should have serum FSH, LH, prolactin, and testosterone levels measured. Patients with elevated prolactin levels should be investigated for pituitary tumor; those with markedly elevated FSH levels probably have primary testicular abnormalities.

C. Testicular Biopsy: Testicular biopsies are indicated in azoospermic patients to distinguish obstructive versus parenchymal disease. Testicular biopsy should be performed in patients with unexplained oligospermia to establish a histologic diagnosis, to assess prognosis, and to direct treatment. If the serum FSH is more than two times normal, one may presume the presence of severe and irreversible testicular damage without confirmatory testis biopsy.

Vasography requires injection of contrast material into the vas. The purpose of this study is to delineate obstruction of the vas, epididymis, seminal vesicle, or ejaculatory duct. Vasography is used in patients who are azoospermic and have no evidence of retrograde ejaculation while demonstrating normal spermatogenesis on testicular biopsy. Seminal fructose levels should be obtained before operative exposure of the vas. Absence of fructose would indicate obstruction of the ejaculatory duct, and if this diagnosis is confirmed by vasography, the obstructing tissue may be resected by transurethral methods.

D. Other Diagnostic Studies: The **sperm penetration assay,** performed by incubation of sperm with hamster eggs whose zona pellucida has been enzymatically removed, offers an objective method of determining the ability of sperm to penetrate the ovum. **The cervical mucus penetration test** compares sperm motility in cervical mucus with a known standard. Although these two important parameters of sperm function can be evaluated, neither test alone can establish the cause of male factor infertility.

Antisperm antibodies can be measured in the serum of either the male or female partner, or in the seminal fluid. This assessment is indicated when spontaneous sperm agglutination or decreased sperm motility is noted on semen analysis. If antisperm antibodies are found, immunosuppressive therapy in the form of steroids may be effective in reducing agglutination (clumping) and increasing motility. Another method of treating autosperm antibodies is in vitro sperm washing with immunobeads coated by anti-human antibody. The sperm not bound by antibody remain in the supernatant and can be used for intrauterine insemination.

---

*Female infertility is discussed in Chapter 42.

Studies to detect a nonpalpable varicocele include **venous Doppler, scrotal thermography, venography,** and, more recently, **ultrasound with color Doppler.** Physical examination is the most effective method of detecting clinically significant varices. Venography is reserved for patients with recurrent varices, since identification of collateral venous channels would direct choice of therapy.

Transrectal ultrasound is used to support the diagnosis of ejaculatory duct obstruction in the azoospermic patient. Absence of the seminal vesicles or distention due to distal obstruction can be identified. This study should be preceded by measurement of fructose in the ejaculate (lack of fructose suggests obstruction of the ejaculatory duct) and examination of postejaculate urine (to determine the presence of sperm, suggesting retrograde ejaculation).

Treatment

A. Nonoperative Treatment: Primary male infertility may be caused by hypogonadotropic hypogonadism, diagnosed by demonstrating low serum levels of FSH, LH, and testosterone. Spermatogenesis may be stimulated by administration of hCG followed by FSH. Isolated absence of either FSH or LH is rare; the LH deficiency is overcome by administration of testosterone, and lack of FSH is treated by administration of menotropins (Pergonal). Hyperprolactinemia may contribute to male infertility and would be treated with bromocriptine.

Infection of the reproductive organs should be treated when found during evaluation of male infertility. Infection may cause infertility immediately by several mechanisms: decreased spermatogenesis due to hyperthermia, immune interaction with sperm causing agglutination and decreased motility, as well as later sequelae such as obstruction of the ejaculatory tract. Pyospermia suggests the diagnosis, and treatment should be designed to eliminate the common pathogens: *Neisseria gonorrhoeae, Chlamydia trachomatis,* and *Ureaplasma urealyticum* (all are sensitive to tetracycline).

If antisperm antibodies are found in either partner, steroids may be used to suppress the immune system. One must use steroids with caution and after thoroughly discussion of possible side effects with the patient; acne, hypertension, gastrointestinal bleeding, and avascular necrosis of the hip have been reported with steroid administration. Response to treatment is assessed by repeat semen analysis and measurement of antisperm antibodies in the patient's serum. Sperm washing in an attempt to remove cytotoxic antibodies may improve motility and decrease clumping; washed semen may then be instilled into the uterus (artificial insemination of the husband's semen; AIH) or used in conjunction with in vitro fertilization techniques.

Retrograde ejaculation or lack of seminal emission—usually due to spinal cord injury or sympathetic nerve injury during retroperitoneal surgery leading to bladder neck (ie, internal sphincter) incompetence—can be treated with α-adrenergic drugs or antihistamines to reestablish internal sphincter function and antegrade ejaculation. Alternatively, alkalinized postejaculate urine can be collected and centrifuged and the concentrated sperm instilled into the female partner's uterus.

Other medications under investigation include clomiphene and tamoxifen. Currently, these drugs are used empirically to treat idiopathic oligospermia; responses have been favorable in 8–66% of cases.

B. Operative Therapy: Ligation of varicocele will yield pregnancy in 30–50% of patients. Several approaches are available, including inguinal and retroperitoneal. Recently, laparoscopic varix ligation has been reported with markedly reduced postoperative time to recovery. Transvenous occlusion of the spermatic vein by balloon is useful especially in cases of recurrent varicocele.

Obstruction of the epididymis-vas system may be amenable to vasovasostomy or vasoepididymostomy. Currently, these procedures are performed with the aid of the operating microscope, and patency is established in 50–90%.

Obstruction of the ejaculatory ducts is rare. When this diagnosis is made, transurethral resection of the ducts may establish patency.

C. Other Methods: Other methods undergoing evaluation include the following: artificial insemination with husband's sperm (AIH), gamete intrafallopian transfer (GIFT), and in vitro fertilization (IVF). In cases of male factor infertility not amenable to treatment, artificial insemination by donor sperm is available.

PRIAPISM

Priapism is a rare disorder in which prolonged, painful erection occurs, usually not associated with sexual stimulation. The blood in the corpora cavernosa becomes hyperviscous but not clotted. About 25% of cases are associated with leukemia, metastatic carcinoma, sickle cell anemia, or trauma. In most cases, the cause is uncertain.

If the erection does not subside, needle aspiration of the sludged blood of the corpora followed by lavage should be performed. Delayed or unsuccessful treatment may result in impotence. Unsuccessful treatment calls for the Winter procedure, in which a biopsy needle is passed through the glans into one of the corpora. A piece of tunica albuginea is removed, creating a fistula between corpora cavernosa and corpus spongiosum. This simple procedure is highly successful, and potency is usually maintained. Other procedures include cavernosal-glandular shunt, cavernosal-spongiosum shunt, and saphenous vein-cavernous shunt. If priapism persists, impotence results.

In sickle cell anemia, hydration and hypertransfusion often give relief and should constitute initial therapy.

PEYRONIE'S DISEASE
(Plastic Induration of the Penis)

Fibrosis of the dorsal covering sheaths of the corpora cavernosa occasionally occurs without known cause in men over age 45. The fibrosis will not permit the involved surface to lengthen with erection, thus leading to dorsal chordee. The disorder may be due to vasculitis in the connective tissues. Palpation of the penile shaft reveals a raised, firm plaque dorsally. There is an association with Dupuytren's contracture.

Controversy exists regarding treatment. Expectant therapy or medical treatment, including vitamin E and aminobenzoic acid, may limit or cure the disease in half of patients. Operative therapy is necessary for patients who do not respond or for impotent patients. In the potent patient, a Nesbit procedure—excision of an ellipse of tunica albuginea from the ventral convex aspect of the shaft and suture closure—or plaque excision and dermal grafting has been used successfully. If the patient is impotent, insertion of a penile prosthesis is the procedure of choice.

PHIMOSIS & PARAPHIMOSIS

Phimosis—inability to retract the foreskin to expose the glans—may be congenital but is more often acquired. At birth, the foreskin cannot be easily retracted, but by age 3, the prepuce becomes pliant and the glans can be exposed and cleansed. If the foreskin is then retractable, circumcision is not necessary. Acquired phimosis is usually a result of chronic and recurrent bacterial balanitis (infection of the prepuce), common in patients with diabetes or balanitis xerotica obliterans. These patients are best treated by circumcision.

Paraphimosis is the inability to reduce a previously retracted foreskin. The prepuce becomes fixed in the retracted position proximal to the corona. With prolonged retraction, lymphedema of the prepuce exacerbates the condition and increases the circumferential pressure of the shaft proximal to the glans. Manual reduction can usually be accomplished using the index fingers to pull the prepuce distally while pushing the glans into the prepuce. If this measure fails, the preputial cicatrix may be incised (dorsal slit) and the foreskin reduced with relative ease. Circumcision may be performed as an elective procedure once the edema has subsided.

CONDYLOMATA ACUMINATA

Condylomata acuminata are wart-like lesions that occur on the penis, scrotum, urethra, and perineum in men and the vagina, cervix, and perineum in women. They are caused by human papillomavirus and are usually transmitted by sexual contact. Pain and bleeding are common presenting complaints. Warts outside the urethra can be treated with excision, application of podophyllum resin, liquid nitrogen, or CO_2 laser. Urethroscopy is needed to determine the proximal extent of lesions in the urethra. Intraurethral fulguration, CO_2 laser treatment, injection of fluorouracil solution, or IFN-α can be curative.

IMPOTENCE

Impotence is the inability to obtain and sustain an erection satisfactory for sexual intercourse.

Causes of Impotence

Causes can be grouped into the following categories: neurologic, vascular, endocrine, systemic, pharmacologic, and psychologic. Treatment is directed accordingly.

A. Neurologic: Reflex erections are mediated by the afferent fibers of the pudendal nerve and efferent fibers of the parasympathetic outflow (S2–S4). Psychogenic erections are initiated via cerebral centers. Specific neurologic diseases that may cause impotence may be congenital (spina bifida), acquired (cerebrovascular accident, Alzheimer's disease, multiple sclerosis), iatrogenic (electroshock therapy), neoplastic (pituitary or hypothalamic tumors), traumatic (cord compression), infectious (tabes dorsalis), and nutritional (vitamin deficiency).

B. Vascular: Vascular causes of impotence may be cardiac (anginal syndromes, congestive failure), aortoiliac disease (Leriche's syndrome, atherosclerosis, other embolic phenomena), microangiopathy (diabetes, radiation injury), and abnormal venous drainage.

C. Endocrine: The accepted endocrine causes of impotence are hypogonadism, hyperprolactinemia, pituitary tumors, hypothyroidism, Addison's disease, Cushing's syndrome, acromegaly, and testicular feminizing syndrome.

D. Pharmacologic: Impotence is a common and often unsuspected complication of many therapeutic and illicit drugs. Major groups that may cause sexual dysfunction are the following: major tranquilizers, antidepressants, antianxiety agents, anticholinergic drugs, antihypertensives, and many drugs with abuse potential. One should recognize that virtually all antihypertensives (including diuretics) can be associated with impotence or ejaculatory dysfunction. Drugs with abuse potential include alcohol (both as a direct affect and secondary to cirrhosis) and cocaine.

E. Psychogenic: Up to 50% of cases of impotence are related to psychogenic factors. Establishing an organic cause of impotence is important in choosing appropriate therapy. Factors that indicate a psychogenic cause are the following: selective erectile dysfunction (episodic, normal nocturnal erections, normal erections with masturbation), sudden onset, associated anxiety or external stress, affect disturbances (anger, anxiety, guilt, fear), and patient convinced of an organic cause.

Diagnosis

The history and physical examination suggest the cause in most cases. Confirmatory tests are necessary to ensure an appropriate choice of therapy.

In investigating a possible neurologic cause of impotence, the neurologic examination should include review of systems with respect to bladder and bowel function. More invasive studies would include a cystometrogram with bethanechol supersensitivity testing, electromyography of the external urethral sphincter, and bulbosphincteric reflex latency.

Vascular impotence is suggested by signs of peripheral vascular disease as well as a history of atherosclerotic heart disease. Noninvasive diagnostic testing is performed by Doppler penile-brachial index. A penile blood pressure to brachial blood pressure ratio less than 0.6 suggests a vascular cause. Venous leak requires cavernosography and cavernosometry. Arteriography is rarely required but may be indicated in patients with a history of pelvic trauma.

Endocrine evaluation mandates measurement of serum testosterone and prolactin; many investigators would include assessment of follicle-stimulating and luteinizing hormones. Routine automated chemical screening may suggest other hormonal abnormalities that require additional testing. These studies should also detect systemic disease capable of causing impotence: cirrhosis, renal failure, scleroderma, and diabetes.

Psychogenic impotence may be established by nocturnal penile tumescence monitoring or outpatient snap-gauge cuffs. Additional testing includes one of the following: Minnesota Multiphasic Personality Inventory, DeRogatis Sexual Function Inventory, and Walker Sex Form.

Treatment

A. Nonoperative Treatment: In patients without arterial-vascular causes of impotence, papaverine or phentolamine (or both) or prostaglandin E_1 intracorporal injections offer a nonoperative means of restoring sexual function. Intractable psychogenic impotence may also respond to this treatment.

Endocrine disturbances responsible for impotence include hypotestosteronemia and hyperprolactinemia. Testosterone deficiency is treated by replacement therapy using a depot testosterone intramuscular injection every 2–3 weeks. Hyperprolactinemia is currently treated by bromocriptine therapy; the patient should be evaluated to assess the presence of a pituitary tumor.

Pharmacologic causes of impotence require altering medical treatment to ameliorate or eliminate secondary impotence. The ability to change medications depends upon the severity of the underlying disease.

Psychogenic impotence is treated by a trained sex therapist, and response may be anticipated in a majority of cases. The importance of eliminating organic causes of impotence before embarking upon psychologic therapy is obvious: the best psychologic methods applied to organic impotence will not resolve the dysfunction but will serve to frustrate both the therapist and patient.

B. Operative Treatment: Penile prosthesis insertion is currently the most common operative method for treatment of impotence. Two categories of prosthesis are in use: semirigid and inflatable. The semirigid prostheses are composed of a rigid shaft and a flexible hinge at the penile-pubic junction or a malleable soft metal case within the prosthesis; the erection is constant and is satisfactory to effect vaginal penetration, but the penile circumference is not equal to that of a natural erection.

Inflatable prostheses offer erections more similar in size to those experienced by the patient prior to the onset of impotence when compared to those achieved by semirigid prostheses. Two types of inflatable prostheses are available: the standard inflatable prosthesis consists of two corporal inflatable rods, a reservoir situated in the retropubic space, and a pump placed in the scrotum; the new inflatable rods combine the simplicity of two corporal rods with the sophistication of a self-contained pump and reservoir system (Flexi-Flate and Hydroflex), permitting the convenience of inflation and deflation without tubing and multiple components.

Satisfactory results are achieved in 85% of patients. Complications common to both types of prostheses are infection and erosion of skin or urethra. The inflatable prostheses are also at risk for mechanical failure of the pump, tubing or reservoir leak, and aneurysm or rupture of the corporal cylinders.

Arterial revascularization of the penile arteries has met with limited success. Aortoiliac reconstruction improves erectile function in only 30% of cases. Microsurgical revascularization of the penile arteries (dorsal artery of the penis or deep corporal arteries) is successful in 60% of patients. While these methods avoid the risks of prosthetic infection and offer the advantage of reestablishing the natural physiologic mechanisms of erection, the mediocre success rate (when compared with the results of prosthetic insertion) would suggest that microsurgical penile revascularization be reserved for carefully selected cases.

Allen R, Brendler CB: Snap-gauge compared to a full nocturnal penile tumescence study for evaluation of patients with erectile impotence. J Urol 1990;143:51.

Bassi P et al: Therapeutic aspects of intrarenal artery aneurysms. Eur Urol 1988;14:99.

Bradley WE: New techniques in evaluation of impotence. Urology 1987;29:383.

Donovan JF, Winfield HN: Laparoscopic varix ligation. J Urol 1992;147:77.

Fisch H et al: Gonadal dysfunction after testicular torsion: Luteinizing hormone and follicle-stimulating hormone response to gonadotropin releasing. J Urol 1989;139: 961.

Gelet A et al: Percutaneous treatment of benign renal cysts. Eur Urol 1990;18:248.

Hanno PM, Wein AJ: Medical treatment of interstitial cystitis (other than RIMSO-50/Elmiron). Urology 1987;29 (Suppl):22.

Hansen SW, Berthelsen JG, von der Maase H: Long-term fertility and Leydig cell function in patients treated for germ cell cancer with cisplatin, vinblastine and bleomycin versus surveillance. J Clin Oncol 1990;8:1695.

Horton CE, Sadove RC, Devine CJ: Peyronie's disease. Ann Plast Surg 1987;18:122.

Krebs HB, Helmkamp BF: Does the treatment of genital condylomata in men decrease the treatment failure rate of cervical dysplasia in the female sexual partner? Obstet Gynecol 1990;76:660.

Lakin MM et al: Intracavernous injection therapy: Analysis of results and complications. J Urol 1990;143:1138.

Molina L et al: Diluted epinephrine solution for the treatment of priapism. J Urol 1989;141:1127.

Salgarello G et al: Transvenous sclerotherapy of the gonadal veins for treatment of varicocele: Long-term results. Angiology 1990;41:427.

Sarr MG et al: Enterovesical fistula. Surg Gynecol Obstet 1987;164:41.

Silber SJ et al: Congenital absence of the vas deferens: The fertilizing capacity of human epididymal sperm. N Engl J Med 1990;323:1788.

Stackl W, Hasun R, Marberger M: Intracavernous injection of prostaglandin E_1 in impotent men. J Urol 1988;140: 66.

Turner TT: On the development and use of alloplastic spermatoceles. Fertil Steril 1988;49:226.

Vessey SG, Rivett A, O'Boyle PJ: Teflon injection in female stress incontinence: Effect on urethral pressure profile and flow rate. Br J Urol 1988;62:39.

REFERENCES

Brenner BM, Rector FC Jr (editors): *The Kidney,* 4th ed. Saunders, 1991.

Carson CC, Dunnick NR: *Endourology.* Churchill Livingstone, 1985.

Crawford ED, Das S: *Current Genitourinary Cancer Surgery.* Lea & Febiger, 1990.

Davidson AJ: *Radiology of the Kidney.* Saunders, 1985.

Droller MJ: *Surgical Management of Urologic Disease: An Anatomic Approach.* Mosby Year Book, 1992.

Gillenwater J et al (editors): *Adult and Pediatric Urology,* 2nd ed. Mosby Year Book, 1991.

Hinman F Jr: *Atlas of Urologic Surgery.* Saunders, 1989.

Javadpour N (editor): *Principles and Management of Testicular Cancer.* Thieme-Stratton, 1985.

Kelalis PP, King LR, Belman AB (editors): *Clinical Pediatric Urology,* 2nd ed. Saunders, 1985.

Leaf A, Cotran RS: *Renal Pathophysiology,* 3rd ed. Oxford Univ Press, 1985.

Rifkin MD: *Diagnostic Imaging of the Lower Genitourinary Tract.* Raven Press, 1985.

Seldin DW, Giebisch G (editors): *The Kidney: Physiology and Pathophysiology.* Raven Press, 1985.

Skinner DG, Leiskovsky G: *Diagnosis and Management of Genitourinary Cancer.* Saunders, 1988.

Tauxe WN, Dubovsky EV: *Nuclear Medicine in Clinical Urology and Nephrology.* Appleton-Century-Crofts, 1985.

Vander AJ: *Renal Physiology,* 3rd ed. McGraw-Hill, 1985.

Walsh PC et al (editors): *Campbell's Urology,* 6th ed. Saunders, 1992.

Zawada ET Jr, Sica DA: *Geriatric Nephrology and Urology.* PSG Publishing Co., 1985.

Zingg EJ, Wallace DMA: *Bladder Cancer.* Springer-Verlag, 1985.

42

Gynecology

Edward C. Hill, MD

CONGENITAL ANOMALIES OF THE FEMALE REPRODUCTIVE SYSTEM

Congenital defects of the female reproductive system arise as a result of abnormal embryologic development of the müllerian ducts and urogenital sinus. The most common defects are imperforate hymen, septate or double vagina, transverse septum of the vagina, congenital absence of the vagina, and duplication defects of the uterus. Although most such defects are idiopathic, some result from in utero exposure to teratogenic agents such as diethylstilbestrol or androgenic progestins during the first 4½ months of fetal development.

An adequate physical examination will detect or at least arouse a suspicion of defective development. Careful examination of genitalia in the newborn is especially important. Errors have been made in gender assignment because of casual examinations. If the disorders are not discovered until later in life, examination under anesthesia and exploration of the uterus with a sound will often provide additional valuable information. Excretory urography should always be done, because one-third to one-half of cases are associated with anomalies of the urinary tract such as absent kidney, horseshoe kidney, and duplication of the collecting system. Injury to the urinary tract can result from failure to recognize associated urinary tract anomalies during corrective surgery.

Congenital anomalies of the genitourinary tract must be distinguished from primary amenorrhea caused by endocrine disorders, leiomyomas of the uterus, and ovarian tumors. Errors in diagnosis have resulted in unnecessary surgery, particularly when a preoperative diagnosis of leiomyoma uteri is made in a case of uterus didelphys or bicornuate uterus. Imaging techniques and laparoscopic examination may be of considerable value in evaluation of the patient with a suspected anomaly of the genitourinary tract.

Minor anomalies of the reproductive tract require only explanation and reassurance. For example, a small vaginal septum, bicornuate uterus, or even complete uterus didelphys usually will not interfere with coital or reproductive function and will cause no significant symptoms.

IMPERFORATE HYMEN

Imperforate hymen is often not recognized until puberty, when, despite the appearance of menstrual symptoms, bleeding fails to occur. Examination at this time will reveal a bulging, imperforate hymen. Rectal examination may demonstrate a large, cystic pelvic mass representing a distended vagina (hematocolpos) and even a cystically enlarged uterus (hematometra). Urinary obstruction has been reported as a result of a large hematocolpos from accumulation of menstrual fluid behind an imperforate hymen.

Imperforate hymen is treated by cruciate incisions (hymenotomy) or laser excision of the mucous membrane, releasing the trapped menstrual discharges and correcting the hematocolpos and hematometra. Antibiotics should be given when there is significant hematocolpos and hematometra in order to prevent secondary infection.

DUPLICATION OF THE VAGINA

Duplication of the vagina may occur with or without a single or double uterus. There may be a double vagina, a double cervix, and a single uterus. The duplication may be only partial and may take the form of a longitudinal septum, in which case excision may be required if soft tissue dystocia occurs in labor. Complete duplication of the vagina usually requires no treatment.

Occasionally, the duplication takes the form of a rudimentary vagina that fails to communicate with the second vagina or the outside. This may result in formation of a hematocolpos at menarche, with an apparent paravaginal cystic mass as a presenting sign. The finding of old blood upon incising such a tumor should lead to the correct diagnosis. A separate cervix and corpus will be found at the top of this space. Marsupialization of the rudimentary vagina with the primary vagina is the usual method of management.

TRANSVERSE SEPTUM OF THE VAGINA

A transverse vaginal septum usually is incomplete. If imperforate, it may be mistaken for congenital absence of the vagina.

Transverse vaginal septa are treated by excision.

ABSENCE OF THE VAGINA

Absence of the vagina usually is associated with absence of the uterus. Often, there is a very small lower vagina, representing that portion that develops from the urogenital sinus. The condition is commonly not recognized until the physician is consulted because of primary amenorrhea in a teenager.

Congenital absence of the vagina is managed by construction of an artificial vagina. This should be deferred until the patient has a desire and a need for a functioning vagina. A variety of techniques have been described, but those utilizing skin grafts placed in an artificially created channel between the bladder and the rectum have been the most widely used. Amnion membrane has been used successfully in lieu of split-thickness skin graft. Artificial vaginas can be constructed by using tissues from the labia majora or isolated segments of the large intestine.

Construction of an artificial vagina will allow girls to develop satisfactory social and sexual relationships.

In a well-motivated patient, congenital absence of the vagina may be corrected by nonoperative dilation and elongation of the vulvar vestibule. Particular success has been reported by Ingram using a bicycle seat stool and graduated Lucite dilators. Should this approach fail, the condition is managed by surgical construction of an artificial vagina.

DUPLICATION DEFECTS OF THE UTERUS

Duplication defects of the uterus are most often detected in the course of investigation for habitual abortion or for repeated premature labor. They may vary from a simple midline septum in a single uterus to complete duplication of the corpus and cervix. Uterine anomalies of this type can often be detected during the third trimester of pregnancy because of the characteristic abdominal outlines of the uterine fundus and persistent malpresentations of the fetus. Manual exploration of the uterine cavity immediately postpartum will demonstrate a uterine septum or a double horn. Hysterosalpingography is essential to an accurate diagnosis.

If there is a history of repeated fetal loss due to abortions or premature labor, the surgical correction of uterine anomalies is warranted in the hope of improving fertility. The classic operation for bicornuate uterus is that described by Strassman in which the horns are incised transversely anterior to the insertion of the uterine tubes and then closed in a longitudinal direction. The septate uterus is corrected either by excising a midline wedge, removing the septum, or merely incising the septum and suturing the margins, thus constructing a single cavity. Subsequent pregnancies after operations for such uterine anomalies should be delivered by cesarean section in order to avoid the risk of uterine rupture in labor. Ideally, this is done approximately 10 days before the expected date of confinement, since the risk of rupture increases with approaching term and with labor. Resection of the septum using a hysteroscope under laparoscopic control has been reported to have encouraging results. The method avoids laparotomy, and subsequent pregnancies may be delivered vaginally without the risk of uterine rupture.

When uterine anomalies are responsible for a poor obstetric history with high fetal wastage, one can expect significant improvement following surgical correction. Fortunately, most patients with abnormalities of the uterus have no significant obstetric problems and require no therapy.

CERVICAL & VAGINAL ABNORMALITIES ASSOCIATED WITH PRENATAL EXPOSURE TO DIETHYLSTILBESTROL (DES)

Women exposed in utero to stilbestrol and other related nonsteroidal estrogens have characteristic changes in the cervix and vagina. Careful inspection and palpation will reveal these changes. The cervical anomalies may present as circular sulci on the exocervix or recessed areas around the external os. There may be a complete covering of the exocervix by columnar epithelium, giving it the so-called "eroded" appearance, or it may present as a "pseudopolyp." Often there is an anterior cervical protuberance that has been described as a "cock's comb."

The vaginal changes take the form of surface or cystic adenosis, fibrous bands, mucosal membranes or elevations, narrowing at the apices, and obliteration of the fornices. Unusual configurations of the endometrial cavity, described as T-shaped or box-like, have been found.

Over two-thirds of patients thus exposed will show one or more of these changes. There is a relationship between exposure to nonsteroidal estrogens in utero and the subsequent development of clear cell carcinoma of the vagina or cervix, but thus far the risk of cancer seems to be small—in the range of less than 1:1000. There may be an increased incidence of cervical and vaginal intraepithelial squamous neoplasia in exposed women.

Careful follow-up examinations of the DES-exposed female population are indicated, with examinations and Papanicolaou smears annually for those in whom pelvic examination reveals no abnormalities and two or three times a year if vaginal or cervical anomalies such as those described above are found.

Daly DC, Maier D, Sotoalbors C: Hysteroscopic metroplasty: Six years' experience. Obstet Gynecol 1989;73: 201.

Ingram JM: Nonsurgical technique corrects vaginal agenesis and stenosis. Contemp Obstet Gynecol (March) 1982;19:46.

March CM, Israel R: Hysteroscopic management of recurrent abortion caused by septate uterus. Am J Obstet Gynecol 1987;156:834.

Robboy SJ et al: Increased incidence of cervical and vaginal dysplasia in 3,980 diethylstilbestrol-exposed young women: Experience of the National Collaborative Diethylstilbestrol Adenosis Project. JAMA 1984;252:2979.

Robboy SJ et al: Normal development of the human female reproductive tract and alterations resulting from experimental exposure to diethylstilbestrol. Hum Pathol 1982;13:190.

Tridenti G et al: Uterus didelphys with an obstructed hemivagina and ipsilateral renal agenesis in teenagers: Report of three cases. Am J Obstet Gynecol 1988;159: 882.

INFECTIONS OF THE FEMALE REPRODUCTIVE SYSTEM

BACTERIAL & SPIROCHETAL INFECTIONS

1. CHANCROID

Chancroid is an acute ulcerative (soft chancre) lesion of the vulva with secondary involvement of the inguinal and femoral lymph nodes caused by *Haemophilus ducreyi*. It is transmitted through coitus and has an incubation period of 2–14 days. The lesion first appears as a papule that rapidly becomes a large pustule. This breaks down, ulcerates, and forms satellite lesions. The regional nodes become enlarged and painful, and chills, fever, and malaise develop. Leukocytosis is usually present. The diagnosis is confirmed by finding the organism in a smear of the exudate, although a culture may be required.

The skin test of chancroid (suspension of the organism) becomes positive within 3–5 weeks of an acute infection and remains positive for life. It is therefore of limited value.

Erythromycin, 500 mg orally four times daily, or trimethoprim-sulfamethoxazole double strength (160 mg/800 mg) one tablet orally twice daily, is the drug of choice. Therapy should be continued for a mini-mum of 10 days or until ulceration and adenopathy have subsided.

Large, painful, fluctuant buboes may be aspirated but prompt antibiotic therapy usually allows prompt regression.

Schmid GP et al: Chancroid in the United States: Reestablishment of an old disease. JAMA 1987;258:3265.

2. SYPHILIS

The primary lesion of syphilis in women is often a transient, painless, small ulcer on the cervix or the labia. Because this lesion does not take the usual classic form of a chancre, it is often overlooked. The disease is usually transmitted by coitus and is due to the spirochete *Treponema pallidum,* which can be recognized by darkfield examination of serum obtained from the lesion. Most often, however, the diagnosis is based on a positive serologic test. the fluorescent *Treponema* antibody absorption test may be helpful in identifying the false-positive VDRL reaction.

Penicillin is the antibiotic of choice. Primary syphilis is treated with benzathine penicillin G, 2.4 million units intramuscularly. Secondary and latent syphilis should receive more vigorous antibiotic therapy by repetition of the injection after 1 week. Tetracycline or erythromycin can be used in the patient allergic to penicillin.

3. GONORRHEA

Neisseria gonorrhoeae is transmitted by sexual intercourse. It may involve the lower genital tract as a suppurative process involving the Bartholin glands, Skene's ducts, or the cervix. Only in prepubertal girls does it involve the vaginal mucosa, since cornified squamous epithelium of the adult vagina resists infection. After infecting the lower tract, it may spread via the endometrial surface, following a menstrual period, to the uterine tubes, where it produces acute salpingitis, sometimes leading to pelvic peritonitis, tubo-ovarian abscess, chronic salpingitis, and tubal obstruction with bilateral hydrosalpinx. The incidence of subsequent sterility is high.

If the infection involves only the lower tract, there may be no or few symptoms unless a Bartholin abscess develops, in which case there is a large, painful swelling in the posterior aspect of the labium majus. Acute gonorrheal cervicitis is seen as a mucopurulent exudate from an inflamed cervix. With tubal involvement, which is almost always bilateral, there is lower abdominal pain of a colicky nature, malaise, and fever. There may be signs of acute peritonitis with tenderness, and ileus. The white blood cell count and the sedimentation rate are moderately elevated. Gonorrheal proctitis may be an accompaniment, producing perianal irritation, occasional diarrhea, and purulent exudate in the stool.

Pain in the right upper quadrant of the abdomen is an unusual manifestation due to spread of infection in a cephalad direction up the right "peritoneal gutter." Violin-string adhesions between the liver and parietal peritoneum may result. Pain and tenderness may closely simulate the findings in acute cholecystitis (Fitz-Hugh and Curtis syndrome).

The diagnosis of gonorrhea is made by finding the typical gram-negative intracellular diplococci in smears or in anaerobic culture (Thayer-Martin V.C.N. medium). Disease of the upper tract and the pelvic peritoneum must be distinguished from acute appendicitis, ovarian cysts, tubal pregnancy, endometriosis, diverticulitis, tuberculous salpingitis, and pedunculated leiomyomas of the uterus. Laparoscopy may be necessary for definitive diagnosis. In large numbers of suspected cases of pelvic inflammatory disease, laparoscopic examination has demonstrated that errors in diagnosis, both positive and negative, are frequent.

Although acute salpingitis may begin as a pure gonococcal infection, secondary invaders including *Chlamydia trachomatis* and aerobic and anaerobic bacteria, complicate the process, producing a polymicrobial infection. Single-agent therapy carries a 20% failure rate. Outpatient treatment of mild acute salpingitis consists of probenecid, 1 g orally, followed by doxycycline, 100 mg twice daily for 10–14 days, along with one of the following: (1) cefoxitin, 2 g intramuscularly; (2) amoxicillin, 3 g orally; (3) ampicillin, 3.5 g orally; (4) aqueous procaine penicillin, 4.8 million units intramuscularly at two sites.

Patients with more severe degrees of salpingitis should be hospitalized and treated with cefoxitin, 2 g intravenously every 6 hours, and doxycycline, 100 mg intravenously every 12 hours. This is continued for at least 48 hours beyond fever defervescence. Oral doxycycline, 100 mg twice daily, is then administered for 10 days.

An important part of the treatment regimen is examination and treatment of male sex partners.

Anaerobic infection with *Bacteroides fragilis* should be strongly suspected in the patient who fails to respond to the regimen outlined above. With appropriate anaerobic culture techniques, these organisms can frequently be recovered from soft tissue infection sites. *B fragilis* is not susceptible to penicillin at easily maintained therapeutic levels and is insensitive to the cephalosporins and aminoglycosides. The current drugs of choice are chloramphenicol and clindamycin. *Chlamydia trachomatis* may also infect the uterine tubes, either alone or in association with gonorrheal salpingitis. Both chlamydiae and gonococci may produce the Fitz-Hugh and Curtis syndrome.

Bartholin's abscess should be incised and drained. Marsupialization or excision of Bartholin cysts may be required if the duct remains obstructed and the cyst is large or symptomatic. Tubo-ovarian abscesses that are unresponsive to intensive antibiotic therapy likewise require incision and drainage. This can usually be accomplished through the vagina via the culde-sac. Tuboplastic procedures are performed for the relief of sterility in chronic tubal obstruction. Chronic salpingo-oophoritis often requires total abdominal hysterectomy and bilateral salpingo-oophorectomy.

Judson FN: Management of antibiotic-resistant *Neisseria gonorrhoeae.* Ann Intern Med 1989;110:5.

Kahn JG et al: Diagnosing pelvic inflammatory disease: A comprehensive analysis and considerations for developing a new model. JAMA 1991;266:2594.

Peterson HB et al: Pelvic inflammatory disease: Key treatment issues and options. JAMA 1991;266:2605.

Rice PA, Schachter J: Pathogenesis of pelvic inflammatory disease. JAMA 1991;266:2587.

Teisala K, Heinonen PK, Punnonen R: Transvaginal ultrasound in the diagnosis and treatment of tuboovarian abscess. Br J Obstet Gynaecol 1990;97:178.

Tyrrel RT, Murphy FB, Bernardino ME: Tuboovarian abscesses: CT-guided percutaneous drainage. Radiology 1990;175:87.

Washington AE, Cates W Jr, Wasserheit JN: Preventing pelvic inflammatory disease. JAMA 1991;266:2574.

Washington AE et al: Assessing risk for pelvic inflammatory disease and its sequelae. JAMA 1991;266:2581.

4. TUBERCULOSIS

Because of increased immigration to the United States from areas where tuberculosis is still endemic and because of reactivation of old tuberculosis in AIDS patients, the incidence of pulmonary tuberculosis in the United States is rising. Tuberculous infection of the uterine tubes with secondary involvement of the endometrium (and rarely of the cervix) accounts for 5–10% of cases of salpingitis. It is usually secondary to tuberculous infection elsewhere, such as in the lung and urinary tract, so an increase in its incidence can be expected.

The process may be asymptomatic, with infertility the only complaint. Symptoms, when they occur, are lower abdominal pain, low-grade fever, weight loss, fatigue, and menstrual irregularities. There may be palpable adnexal masses.

The diagnosis may be made when a granulomatous lesion is found in the endometrium in the course of dilation and curettage performed for menstrual irregularity. The acid-fast organisms are difficult to demonstrate in histologic sections, and culture of endometrial tissue or the menstrual discharge often is necessary for confirmation. Chest x-ray, sputum studies, and acid-fast smears and cultures of the urine should be performed as well.

Combination antibiotic therapy is effective. Because concomitant pulmonary infection is frequent, treatment is best conducted in cooperation with a pulmonary disease physician. A 6-month regimen consists of at least 2 months of daily administration of isoniazid 300 mg, rifampin 600 mg, and pyrazinamide, 20–35 mg/kg, in two divided doses. This is followed by isoniazid and rifampin daily or twice weekly for 4 months. Ethambutol, 15–25 mg/kg/d, or streptomycin, 1 g intramuscularly daily, should be added if resistance to isoniazid is suspected or if advanced or life-threatening disease exists. Total abdominal hysterectomy with bilateral salpingo-oophorectomy is indicated if there is an adnexal mass in a woman over 40 years of age or if there is persistent pelvic pain, persistent infection, or poor patient compliance.

Charles D: Pelvic tuberculosis: Not gone, but sometimes forgotten. Contemp Ob/Gyn July 1991;97.
Schaeffer G: Female genital tuberculosis. Clin Obstet Gynecol 1976;19:223.
Sutherland AM: Postmenopausal tuberculosis of the female genital tract. Obstet Gynecol 1982;59(6 Suppl):54S.
Sutherland AM: Surgical treatment of tuberculosis of the female genital tract. Br J Obstet Gynaecol 1980;87:610.

5. GRANULOMA INGUINALE

Infection with *Calymmatobacterium granulomatis* is seen in the USA most often in the southern states. The disease is transmitted through sexual intercourse and begins as a small vulval papule that then becomes a small area of beefy-red granulomatous tissue. This process spreads superficially and eventually involves the entire perineum, extending into the inguinal areas. Secondary infection is a common complication.

The symptoms are pain, burning, itching, and discharge from the involved area. Smears or biopsies stained with Wright's stain or hematoxylin-eosin stain will show the characteristic Donovan inclusion bodies within large mononuclear cells.

Treatment is with tetracycline, 500 mg orally four times daily for 1 week and then 250 mg four times daily for an additional 2 weeks.

6. CHLAMYDIAL INFECTIONS

Chlamydia trachomatis produces a variety of infections in humans. These organisms are obligate intracellular bacteria that require the oxidative phosphorylation mechanism of the host cell for replication. In addition to causing conjunctivitis and pneumonitis in the newborn—infections acquired in the birth canal—they are the etiologic agent of lymphogranuloma (lymphopathia) venereum, "nonspecific" urethritis in the male, and cervicitis-salpingitis in the female.

Lymphogranuloma venereum (LGV), caused by *C trachomatis* types L_1–L_3, is transmitted by coitus and is manifested initially as a small vulvar vesicle 1–3 weeks after exposure. This disappears but is followed 2–3 weeks later by inguinal lymphadenitis, which progresses to bubo formation and eventually to tissue breakdown and ulceration. The perirectal lymphatics are similarly affected. Healing leads to inguinal scarring, rectal and vaginal stricture, and vulvar elephantiasis.

Diagnosis is made by isolating an LGV strain of *C trachomatis* from pus aspirated from a bubo, by positive LGV complement fixation test, or by a microimmunofluorescent or counterimmunoelectrophoresis test. The latter two tests are not widely available.

Tetracycline, 1 g orally four times daily for 3 weeks, is the treatment of choice. Sulfisoxazole, 1 g orally four times daily for 3 weeks, is also effective. Rectal stricture may require dilation or even colostomy if it causes bowel obstruction.

Nongonococcal urethritis, cervicitis, and salpingitis. *C trachomatis* is the cause of the most commonly sexually transmitted disease in the United States, being two to five times more prevalent than *N gonorrhoeae*. It is responsible for the urethral syndrome, mucopurulent cervicitis, acute salpingitis, and the Fitz-Hugh and Curtis syndrome. Like *N gonorrhoeae,* the organism gains access to the uterine tubes from the endocervix via ascending infection of the endometrium. Transmission to a newborn infant in passage through an infected birth canal may cause inclusion conjunctivitis or pneumonia.

Because isolation of the organism by culture is technically difficult, the diagnosis of lower genitourinary tract infection is often one of exclusion. A monoclonal antibody fluorescence test is helpful in making the diagnosis.

C trachomatis urethritis and cervicitis are best treated with tetracycline, 500 mg orally four times daily for 7 days. Sexual partners should be treated concurrently to prevent reinfection.

Holmes KK: The *Chlamydia* epidemic. JAMA 1981;245:1718.
Schacter J: Chlamydial infections. West J Med 1990;153:523.
Sweet RL et al: The occurrence of chlamydial and gonococcal salpingitis during the menstrual cycle. JAMA 1986;255:2062.

7. *GARDNERELLA VAGINALIS* VAGINITIS

This disorder is also called bacterial vaginosis because of absence of inflammation and problems associated with demonstrating the etiologic agent, a small pleomorphic variably gram-staining coccobacillus, which is probably sexually transmitted. *Gardnerella* may be the cause of up to 50% of cases of vaginitis. The only symptom usually is a malodorous thin grayish-white discharge. The typical fish-like odor is due to the release of amines from the synergistic action of G vaginalis and anaerobic bacteria in the vaginal flora. The odor is markedly enhanced by the addition of 10% potassium hydroxide to the discharge (positive "sniff test"). A finding of "clue cells" on a wet mount specimen from the vagina confirms the diagnosis. The most effective therapy is metronidazole, 500 mg orally every 12 hours for 7 days. Because the organisms causing bacterial vaginosis are not sexually transmitted, male sex partners do not require concurrent treatment. Less effective therapeutic agents are triple-sulfonamide cream intravaginally, doxycycline, and ampicillin.

Moi H et al: Should male consorts of women with bacterial vaginosis be treated? Genitourin Med 1989;65:263.

8. CERVICITIS

Essentials of Diagnosis

- Leukorrhea.
- Intermenstrual bleeding may occur.
- Sense of pelvic heaviness and backache.
- Dyspareunia.
- Cervix may show old, healed obstetric lacerations and appear elongated and enlarged.
- Cervical eversion or ectopy is common.

General Considerations

Acute cervicitis is caused by acute gonorrheal infection or occurs in association with trichomonal or candidal vaginitis (see below). Chronic cervicitis (very common) usually results from the trauma of cervical effacement and dilatation during vaginal delivery. This condition is frequently seen by the pathologist on cervical biopsy or hysterectomy specimens from multiparous individuals and probably is of little clinical significance in most instances. *Chlamydia trachomatis* as a cause of cervicitis is receiving more attention recently and may be present in many cases of chronic cervicitis previously though to be nonspecific and related to vaginal delivery. Like *Neisseria gonorrhoeae,* this organism infects primarily the columnar epithelial cells of the cervix. It has also been established as a cause of chronic nonspecific urethritis in males.

Clinical Findings

A. Symptoms and Signs: In acute cases, the cervix is acutely inflamed and there is a purulent exudate; gonorrhea should be suspected. Chronic cervicitis may be mild and asymptomatic. In symptomatic cases, a copious vaginal discharge is the most common presenting complaint. In severe, deep-seated infections, there may be a low-grade pelvic cellulitis

(parametritis), with a sense of heaviness in the pelvis, low backache, and dyspareunia. Postcoital bleeding may be present. The cervix appears distorted by old, healed obstetric lacerations and is reddened, boggy, and edematous. Nabothian cysts are frequently seen and are due to obstruction of the cervical tunnels, clefts, and crypts lined by mucus-secreting columnar epithelium. Endocervical and ectocervical polyps are commonly present.

B. Laboratory Findings: Cytologic smears demonstrate numerous pus cells and may show epithelial dysplasia. Cervical biopsy shows a leukocytic infiltrate in the subepithelial stroma and often squamous metaplasia and cystic dilatation of the glandular spaces. A gram-stained smear from a patient with acute gonorrheal cervicitis will often show the typical diplococci. Anaerobic cultures are often required for diagnosis in chronic cases. Chlamydial infections can be detected using fluorescein-conjugated monoclonal antibodies or an enzyme immunoassay (Chlamydiazyme test).

Differential Diagnosis

Cervical ectopy (columnar endocervical type mucus-secreting epithelium on the portio vaginalis of the cervix) should not be confused with cervicitis. Cervical ectopy is a self-limited disorder found in a significant number (up to 60%) of younger women. The cervical mucosa appears red, granular, and angry and bleeds on contact. It is gradually replaced by squamous epithelium through the process of metaplasia and becomes the normal tissue of the so-called transformation zone of the cervix. Cervical ectopy was at one time called cervical erosion, which is a misnomer.

Early cervical cancer may present similar symptoms and signs and must be excluded before treatment proceeds. A negative cytologic smear does not rule out malignant disease. Multiple, representative punch biopsies from the transformation zone of the cervix are required.

Complications

Infertility may result from chronic cervical inflammation, which produces an environment unfavorable to penetration of the cervical mucus by spermatozoa.

Treatment

Acute gonorrheal cervicitis is best treated with penicillin. Tetracycline or kanamycin may be used in penicillin-resistant cases or in individual who are allergic to penicillin. Tetracycline is also the agent of choice in suspected chlamydial cervicitis. Treatment of nonspecific cervicitis is indicated even in asymptomatic cases because of the possible relationship between chronic cervicitis and carcinoma of the cervix. Mild degrees of cervicitis can be treated effectively with office cauterization, either chemically, with 20% silver nitrate solution on cotton-tipped applicators, or by light radial cauterization with the nasal-tipped thermal cautery or electrocautery. For the deeply involved, deformed cervix, hospitalization is required for electroconization of the cervix under anesthesia. Trachelorrhaphy (plastic repair) of the obstetrically deformed cervix may be necessary in an occasional patient with secondary infertility due to chronic cervicitis. Cryosurgery (freezing) of chronic cervicitis has been used recently with good results.

Cervical polyps usually can be removed in the office. These should be examined by a pathologist for evidence of cancer.

Prognosis

Cure of acute cervicitis can usually be accomplished within a few days. Chronic cervicitis usually is more resistant and may require several weeks or months of treatment.

Kovacs GT et al: Microbiological profile of the cervix in 1,000 sexually active women. Aust N Z J Obstet Gynaecol 1988;28:216.

VIRAL INFECTIONS

1. CONDYLOMATA ACUMINATA (Venereal Warts)

Venereal warts are usually multiple papules caused by the human papillomavirus (HPV). Recent evidence has associated certain types (types 16 and 18) with squamous cell neoplasia of the vulva, vagina, and cervix. On the skin of the perineum, lesions are more apt to be papillary and acuminate (sharp-pointed), whereas on the mucous membranes of the vagina and cervix, lesions are most often flat and difficult to recognize without colposcopy. Vulvar lesions are often associated with vaginal discharge and irritation. Biopsy of representative areas will determine if there is an associated intraepithelial neoplastic process.

Treatment of isolated vulvar lesions is with podophyllum resin applied topically in 25% solution of compound tincture of benzoin or trichloroacetic acid. Patient application of 0.5% podofilox, a purified and less toxic drug than crude podophyllum resin, is also effective. Interferon therapy is useful in persistent disease. Vaginal and cervical lesions are treated with electrocoagulation, cryotherapy, or laser vaporization. Topical fluorouracil is used to treat extensive vaginal involvement and as maintenance therapy after ablation by one of the physical modalities.

Examination and treatment of male consorts is an important part of the treatment regimen. As with the female vagina and cervix, penile lesions frequently are not apparent without the use of acetic acid and the colposcope.

Bergeron C et al: Multicentric human papillomavirus infections of the female genital tract: Correlation of viral types with abnormal mitotic figures, colposcopic presentation, and location. Obstet Gynecol 1987;69:736.

Gall SA, Constantine L, Konkol D: Therapy of persistent human papillomavirus disease with two different interferon species. Am J Obstet Gynecol 1991;164:130.

Greenberg MD et al: A double-blind, randomized trial of 0.5% podofilox and placebo for the treatment of genital warts in women. Obstet Gynecol 1991;77:735.

Krebs HB: Treatment of vaginal condylomata acuminata by weekly topical application of 5-fluorouracil. Obstet Gynecol 1987;70:68.

Krebs HB, Schneider V: Human papillomavirus-associated lesions of the penis: Colposcopy, cytology and histology. Obstet Gynecol 1987;70:299.

Meisels A, Morin C: Human papillomavirus and cancer of the uterine cervix. Gynecol Oncol 1981;12:S111.

Nash JD, Burke TW, Hoskins WJ: Biologic course of cervical human papillomavirus infection. Obstet Gynecol 1987;69:160.

Schneider A et al: Human papillomaviruses in women with a history of abnormal Papanicolaou smears and in their male partners. Obstet Gynecol 1987;69:554.

Winkler B et al: Koilocytotic lesions of the cervix: The relationship of mitotic abnormalities to the presence of papillomavirus antigens and nuclear DNA content. Cancer 1984;53:1081.

2. HERPES GENITALIS

Herpes genitalis is caused by herpesvirus hominis type 2 and is sexually transmitted. It is characterized by the appearance of clusters of small, painful, erythematous vesicular lesions on the vulva. Examination may also demonstrate these in the vagina and on the portio vaginalis of the cervix. The vesicles often proceed to ulceration; with coalescence, large, painful ulcers of the vulva, vagina, and cervix may develop. Healing occurs within 2 weeks, but recurrences are common.

The diagnosis can be made cytologically by finding characteristic "ground glass" inclusions in mononucleated or multinucleated giant cells from the squamous epithelium or by culturing the virus.

There appears to be a relationship between herpes genitalis and carcinoma of the cervix, since antibodies to herpesvirus hominis type 2 have been found significantly more often in women with cervical cancer than in matched control groups. Virus particles have also been found in tumor cells. Whether this is merely a coincidental factor transmitted sexually or an etiologic relationship has not yet been established.

Oral acyclovir, 200 mg orally five times daily for 10 days, is useful in the treatment of primary infections. With frequent recurrent episodes, chronic suppressive therapy in the form of 200 mg three times daily for 6 months may be necessary.

Primarily palliative treatment can be given with topical anesthetic agents such as lidocaine and moist compresses of Burow's solution. Secondary bacterial infection may require treatment with antibiotics.

Because of the risk of severe systemic disease in infants delivered vaginally, a patient with an acute infection near term should be delivered by cesarean section. Herpes genitalis is to be distinguished from herpes gestationis, a relatively rare blistering disease of pregnancy and the puerperium that imposes a risk to the fetus which is unknown at present.

TRICHOMONAS VAGINALIS VAGINITIS

Trichomonas vaginalis vaginitis is caused by a motile flagellated protozoon that produces a vaginal inflammation characterized by a profuse, thin, foamy, yellowish discharge, local burning, and itching. The diagnosis is made by finding the organism in a wet mount smear from the vagina.

Treatment with metronidazole, 250 mg orally three times daily for 7 days, is usually successful. A dose of 2 g in 1 day has also been effective, but gastrointestinal side effects such as nausea are more frequent. It may be necessary to treat the patient's sexual partner at the same time in order to prevent recurrent infections. Numerous topical agents are available for use in the vagina, and until the teratogenicity of metronidazole has been ruled out, the drug should not be used in a pregnant patient.

CANDIDIASIS

Candida albicans, a yeast, is the cause of candidal vaginitis, seen often in diabetics, pregnant patients, and women using oral contraceptives. Candidal infections also occur as a complication of antibiotic therapy, with suppression of the normal bacteria flora and overgrowth by yeast organisms. Candidal vaginitis and vulvitis are characterized by intense itching and inflamed skin and mucosa. Frequently there is a clinging, cheesy-white exudate, although this finding may be absent. Intense pruritus is the primary symptom. The diagnosis is made by finding spores or mycelia on a wet mount smear preparation to which a few drops of 10% potassium hydroxide are added or by culturing the organism on Nickerson's medium.

Office treatment consists of cleansing the vagina of the curd-like exudate and applying a 2% aqueous solution of gentian violet. Miconazole is the antifungal treatment of choice; give one 200-mg suppository vaginally each night at bedtime for three nights plus topical cream to the vulva twice daily for 2 weeks.

MENSTRUAL DISORDERS

AMENORRHEA

Amenorrhea may be primary (delay of menarche beyond age 17) or secondary (cessation of menstrual function of several months' or years' duration occurring after the development of normal cyclic menstruation). True primary amenorrhea may be due to an abnormality in function or disease of the ovary, pituitary, or hypothalamus. Congenital anomalies of the uterus and vagina as a cause of primary amenorrhea are discussed above.

Clinical Findings
A. Primary Amenorrhea:
  1. **Congenital anomalies** (p 950).
  2. **Ovarian agenesis and dysgenesis (Turner's syndrome)–**
     a. Short stature.
     b. Webbing of neck.
     c. Cubitus valgus.
     d. Infantile external genitalia.
     e. Absent sex chromatin on buccal smear.
     f. Most have a chromosomal karyotype of 45,X/46,XX or 45,X/46,XX/47,XXX.
  3. **Female pseudohermaphroditism–**
     a. Usually secondary to congenital adrenal hyperplasia (21-hydroxylase deficiency).
     b. Masculinization of external fetal female genitalia related to in utero exposure to 19-nor (androgenic) progestins given to mother.
  4. **True hermaphroditism–**
     a. Ambiguous external genitalia with enlarged clitoris and urogenital sinus into which vagina and urethra open.
     b. Normal breast development.
     c. Menstruation may occur.
     d. Sex chromatin present in buccal smear.
     e. Chromosomal karyotype usually 46,XX (46,XY in 12% of cases).
     f. Ovarian and testicular tissue combined in a single gonad (ovotestis) or separate ovary and testis.
  5. **Androgen insensitivity (testicular feminization) syndrome–**
     a. Female habitus with relatively large hands and feet.
     b. Normal breast development.
     c. Scant or absent pubic and axillary hair.

d. Normal external genitalia.

e. Hypoplastic vagina ending in a short, blind pouch.

f. Absent or rudimentary uterus and tubes.

g. Sex chromatin absent in buccal smear.

h. Chromosomal Karyotype is 46,XY.

i. Gonads are testes that lie in abdomen, pelvis, or inguinal canal.

6. Resistant ovary syndrome–

a. Chromosomal karyotype 46,XX.

b. Phenotypic female.

c. Elevated gonadotropin levels.

d. Normally developed follicles on ovarian biopsy.

e. Failure of ovarian follicles to respond to large doses of human gonadotropins.

B. Secondary Amenorrhea:

1. Pregnancy–

a. Signs and symptoms of pregnancy.

b. Positive chorionic gonadotropin.

2. Menopause–

a. Hot flashes.

b. Familial history of early menopause.

c. Elevated pituitary gonadotropin.

3. Psychogenic–

a. Traumatic experience or psychologic disturbance.

b. Usually temporary (less than 6 months).

4. Following oral contraceptives.

5. Polycystic ovary (Stein-Leventhal) syndrome–

a. Oligomenorrhea or amenorrhea.

b. Obesity.

c. Hirsutism.

d. Ovaries may or may not be enlarged bilaterally.

e. Normal high LH.

f. Elevated unbound testosterone.

6. Pituitary insufficiency or failure (depressed pituitary gonadotropins)–

a. Following traumatic labor or delivery (Sheehan's syndrome).

b. Pituitary tumors (headache and visual disturbances).

7. Resistant ovary syndrome–

a. Under 30 years of age.

b. See Primary Amenorrhea, above (pg 6).

8. Intensive exercise (runner's syndrome).

Treatment

A. Primary Amenorrhea:

1. Congenital anomalies–Primary amenorrhea due to obstruction of the passage of menstrual blood can be corrected surgically.

2. Ovarian agenesis and dysgenesis–

a. Cyclic estrogen-progestin therapy to simulate normal menstrual cycle and develop secondary sex characteristics.

b. Plastic surgery if webbing of neck is severe.

3. Female pseudohermaphroditism–

a. Cortisone acetate to suppress abnormal adrenal steroidogenesis.

b. Mineralocorticoid therapy and other treatment as for Addison's disease.

c. Surgical correction of abnormal sex organs.

4. True hermaphroditism–Surgical removal of contradictory sex organs and reconstruction of those compatible with sex in which patient has been reared.

5. Androgen insensitivity syndrome–

a. Excision of gonads.

b. Cyclic estrogen therapy.

c. Construction of artificial vagina.

6. Resistant ovary syndrome–Pregnancy has been reported during or following estrogen replacement therapy.

B. Secondary Amenorrhea:

1. Pregnancy–Obstetric care.

2. Menopause–Replacement estrogen therapy given cyclically to relieve menopausal symptoms.

3. Psychogenic–

a. Usually self-limited.

b. Cyclic estrogen-progestin therapy in the anxious patient.

4. Following oral contraceptives–Same as for psychogenic amenorrhea.

5. Polycystic ovary (Stein-Leventhal) syndrome–

a. Ovulation induction with clomiphene citrate or human gonadotropin.

b. Estrogen-dominant oral contraceptives or spironolactone to suppress androgens.

c. Laparoscopic ovarian stromal reduction by "drilling" or "branding" if no response to above.

6. Pituitary insufficiency or failure–

a. Replacement therapy (corticosteroids, thyroid, estrogens).

b. Treatment of pituitary tumors.

7. Resistant ovary syndrome–See Primary Amenorrhea, above (pg 6).

Bullen BA et al: Induction of menstrual disorders by strenuous exercise in untrained women. N Engl J Med 1985;312:1349.

Burke KD, Lin TJ: A systematic laboratory approach to amenorrhea. Female Patient 1987;12:43.

Coulam CB, Graham ML II, Spelsberg TC: Androgen insensitivity syndrome: Gonadal androgen receptor activity. Am J Obstet Gynecol 1984;150:531.

Daniell JF, Miller W: Polycystic ovaries treated by laparoscopic laser vaporization. Fertil Steril 1989;51:232.

Luciano AA et al: Hyperprolactinemia and contraception: A prospective study. Obstet Gynecol 1985;65:506.

Reindollar RH et al: Adult-onset amenorrhea: A study of 262 patients. Am J Obstet Gynecol 1986;155:531.

Ronkainen H et al: Physical exercise-induced changes and season-associated differences in the pituitary-ovarian function of runners and joggers. J Clin Endocrinol Metab 1985;60:416.

Simon JA et al: Characterization of recombinant DNA derived-human luteinizing hormone in vitro and in vivo: Efficacy in ovulation induction and corpus luteum support. JAMA 1988;259:3290.

Sumioki H et al: The effect of laparoscopic multiple punch resection of the ovary on hypothalamic-pituitary axis in polycystic ovary syndrome. Fertil Steril 1988;50:567.

ABNORMAL UTERINE BLEEDING

Abnormal uterine bleeding may occur at any age. In the newborn it is frequently related to removal of the infant at birth from the influence of maternal estrogen, which has produced endometrial proliferation in the baby's uterus. During the reproductive years, it may occur as **hypermenorrhea,** excessive or prolonged bleeding at the normal time of menstruation; **polymenorrhea,** bleeding that occurs more frequently than every 3 weeks; or **intermenstrual bleeding,** which occurs during the interval between normal menstrual periods.

Hypermenorrhea may be due to such organic conditions as uterine leiomyoma, endometrial polyps, and blood dyscrasias, or it may be related to a functional disturbance such as irregular shedding of the endometrium, presumably resulting from faulty regression of the corpus luteum of the ovary. Polymenorrhea may be related to early ovulation with a shortened proliferative phase, which frequently is secondary to hypothyroidism. One of the most frequently encountered problems is the completely acyclic and sometimes heavy and prolonged bleeding of the anovulatory patient, leading to so-called **dysfunctional uterine bleeding.** This condition is seen most often in adolescents and in premenopausal women and is due to a failure in regular ovulatory function by the ovaries. The endometrium is proliferative in type at a time in the menstrual cycle when it would show secretory changes if ovulation had occurred. In many instances there is, after a period of time, the development of endometrial hyperplasia, of either the cystic glandular or adenomatous pattern, owing to the prolonged stimulus of estrogen on the endometrium without the modifying influence of progesterone. Intermenstrual bleeding may be due to the slight drop

in estrogen titer associated with ovulation, in which event it occurs quite regularly at about mid cycle. Other causes of intermenstrual bleeding that occurs at any time are polyps, submucous leiomyomas, blood dyscrasias, genital tuberculosis, and cancer of the cervix, uterine corpus, or uterine tube. Complications of pregnancy should not be overlooked as a cause of abnormal bleeding in women of reproductive age.

Postmenopausal bleeding (vaginal bleeding occurring a year or more after menopause) is due to cancer in about 40% of cases. The exogenous administration of estrogenic substance, including their use in cosmetic preparations, is another important cause of this type of abnormal bleeding. Atrophic changes, polyps, trauma, blood dyscrasias, hypertensive cardiovascular disease, and estrogen-producing tumors of the ovary are less frequent causes. The bleeding may be represented by a scant brownish vaginal discharge, or it may be frank, profuse, bright-red bleeding. Because it looms so large in the etiology of postmenopausal bleeding, cancer should be considered the cause until proved otherwise.

Clinical Findings

In the assessment of any type of menstrual disorder, the following points should be considered:

(1) Careful documentation of the menstrual history and a record of the temporal relationship of the abnormal bleeding to the menstrual cycle are necessary. A special menstrual calendar kept by the patient or a basal body temperature graph can be very helpful.

(2) A history of hormonal medication or cosmetics containing hormones.

(3) A general history and physical examination may lead to the correct diagnosis of hypothyroidism, blood dyscrasia, genital tuberculosis, etc.

(4) A carefully performed pelvic examination will often reveal vaginal, cervical, uterine, or adnexal disease.

(5) Cytologic examination is essential in all patients, and the specimen should be collected prior to the introduction of lubricating jelly into the vagina.

(6) A complete blood count and measurement of red cell indices will reflect the degree of iron deficiency secondary to acute or chronic blood loss. Additional blood studies may be necessary when blood dyscrasias are suspected.

(7) Thyroid function studies may be indicated.

(8) Endometrial biopsy is often required to establish the cause of abnormal menstrual bleeding. Biopsy should be done at an appropriate time in the menstrual cycle, eg, after the 16th day of the cycle if anovulatory bleeding is suspected, or on the fourth or fifth day if the working diagnosis is irregular shedding of the endometrium.

(9) Hysteroscopy may help establish the cause.

Endometrial suction with the Vabra aspirator or biopsy using a small curette such as the Novak or Randall instrument can be accomplished in an office setting. Full-scale dilation and curettage under anesthesia is recommended in cases of cervical stenosis or when endometrial polyps, submucous myomas, or uterine cancer is suspected. A fractional technique (separate curettage of the endocervix and endometrial cavity; each specimen submitted individually) and cervical biopsies are recommended if cancer is suspected.

Treatment

Acute, massive blood loss should be treated by recording the central venous pressure, placing the patient in the Trendelenburg position, and replenishing the circulating blood volume with intravenous fluids and whole blood transfusions.

Dilation and curettage is the most effective method of controlling uterine bleeding.

In chronic blood loss due to hypermenorrhea produced by leiomyomas, total menstrual suppression may be achieved by the continuous administration of an estrogen-progestin preparation (see section on endometriosis). The oral administration of iron may obviate blood transfusion in the preparation of the patient for a definitive surgical procedure.

After organic causes have been excluded, dysfunctional bleeding due to chronic anovulation is treated with cyclic progestin therapy (medroxyprogesterone acetate, 10 mg/d for 10 days every 4 weeks). In teenagers, control of acute heavy bleeding may be achieved through the use of combination oral contraceptives (one pill four times a day for 1 week). Complete sloughing of the endometrium will follow. On the fifth day of this new cycle, a low-dose cyclic oral contraceptive is started and continued for 3 months. Intravenous conjugated estrogen, 25 mg every 4 hours, has been used also to control acute bleeding. Such a regimen must be followed by administration and subsequent withdrawal of progestin.

Severe, intractable bleeding of a dysfunctional nature may require hysterectomy, but this is rare. In the absence of other causes, hypermenorrhea associated with ovulatory cycles can be effectively managed with meclofenamate sodium, 100 mg three times daily for 6 days, or less if menstruation ceases. Hysteroscopic endometrial ablation by Nd:YAG laser or electrosurgical resection may avoid hysterectomy in the premenopausal patient with intractable bleeding.

Postmenopausal bleeding of nonneoplastic cause may require estrogen therapy if it is due to atrophic changes. Curettage is curative if the bleeding is due to endometrial polyps. Endometrial carcinoma is a contraindication to estrogen therapy and is treated by total abdominal hysterectomy and bilateral salpingo-oophorectomy with or without preoperative radiation therapy.

Loffer FD: Hysteroscopy with selective endometrial sampling compared with D&C for abnormal uterine bleeding: The value of a negative hysteroscopic view. Obstet Gynecol 1989;73:16.

Lomano JM: Dragging technique versus blanching technique for endometrial ablation with the Nd:YAG laser in the treatment of chronic menorrhagia. Am J Obstet Gynecol 1988;159:152.

Magos AL, Baumann R, Turnbull AC: Transcervical resection of endometrium in women with menorrhagia. Br Med J 1989;298:1209.

ADENOMYOSIS & ENDOMETRIOSIS

ADENOMYOSIS

Essentials of Diagnosis

- Multiparous patient 35–50 years of age.
- Hypermenorrhea, polymenorrhea, or intermenstrual bleeding with dysmenorrhea or dyspareunia.
- Uterus slightly to moderately enlarged, symmetric, and globular.
- May be tender to palpation, particularly in premenstrual phase of cycle.

General Considerations

Adenomyosis—formerly called "internal endometriosis"—occurs when fingers of endometrium extend into the myometrium to a depth greater than two low-power microscopic fields. It may be a focal or a diffuse process and not infrequently involves the entire thickness of the myometrium. The pathogenesis is not known, but the theory of direct growth of the basal layer of endometrium into the myometrium is widely accepted. Estrogen has been implicated as a stimulus to the development of adenomyosis, and the symptomatic improvement that occurs with the onset of menopause supports this concept. The disease is seen most often in the decade preceding menopause.

Clinical Findings

A. Symptoms and Signs: The preoperative diagnosis of adenomyosis is very difficult, and the diagnosis is usually not made until pathologic examination is made of a uterus that has been removed because of hypermenorrhea, polymenorrhea, or intermenstrual bleeding occurring just prior to menses. Because it may be associated with endometriosis (see next section), there may be an acquired dysmenorrhea and dyspareunia. The condition should be suspected if one or more of these symptoms occurs in a multiparous woman aged 35–50. Examination will reveal a slightly to moderately enlarged, symmetric, mobile uterus with a finely granular external surface.

B. Special Examinations: Hysterography or

MRI may be helpful in confirming the clinical diagnosis.

Differential Diagnosis

Adenomyosis must be distinguished principally from leiomyomas of the uterus. The symptoms may be quite similar, but the palpatory findings should enable a careful observer to make the correct diagnosis. Hysterography or MRI is necessary in doubtful cases.

An analogous condition, endolymphatic stromal myosis (stromal endometriosis, low-grade stromal sarcoma), although histologically benign, clinically behaves as a low-grade cancer. In this condition, connective tissue cells resembling those of the endometrial stroma infiltrate the lymphatic and venous spaces of the myometrium. This process may extend into the vessels of the broad ligament, in which event local recurrence is possible following hysterectomy. Metastases to the ovary, peritoneal surfaces, and lung have been reported, but only rarely. This disease, usually of the postmenopausal years, is very rare and should not be confused with adenomyosis.

Other disorders that may be confused with adenomyosis are chronic subinvolution of the uterus (benign, idiopathic uterine hypertrophy), endometriosis, chronic salpingitis, and cancer of the endometrium.

Treatment

Total hysterectomy with or without bilateral salpingo-oophorectomy is curative. Hormonal therapy—estrogen alone, progesterone alone, or estrogen-progesterone combinations—has not been successful and has actually caused exacerbations of symptoms. If the symptoms are not severe and more serious conditions such as endometrial carcinoma or submucous leiomyomas have been excluded, symptomatic treatment in anticipation of the menopause constitutes rational therapy.

Prognosis

Adenomyosis is self-limited process that undergoes spontaneous regression, becoming asymptomatic after the menopause.

Kilkku P, Erkkola R, Gronroos M: Nonspecificity of symptoms related to adenomyosis: Prospective comparative survey. Acta Obstet Gynecol Scand 1984;63:229.

ENDOMETRIOSIS

Essentials of Diagnosis

- History of progressive dysmenorrhea and dyspareunia.
- Patient (often nulligravid and infertile) 20–40 years of age.
- Symptoms of rectal or bladder pain at menses, rarely with blood in feces or urine at the time of menstruation.
- Tender, shotty nodules in cul-de-sac.
- Enlarged, adherent ovary.
- Constricting lesion of large intestine on barium enema.
- Typical findings at peritoneoscopy (laparoscopy or culdoscopy).

General Considerations

In endometriosis, functioning endometrial tissue is present in ectopic sites other than the myometrium (see Adenomyosis, above). The areas most often involved are the ovaries, the uterine tubes, the serosal surface of the uterus, the cul-de-sac peritoneum, the uterosacral ligaments and rectovaginal septum, the sigmoid colon, the pelvic peritoneum, and the small intestine (Figure 42–1). Cancer may develop in areas of endometriosis. Ectopic endometrium has been found in the umbilicus, in abdominal scars, and (rarely) in the breasts, the extremities, the pleural cavity, and the lungs.

The histogenesis of endometriosis involves three different mechanisms: (1) Sampson's theory of retro-

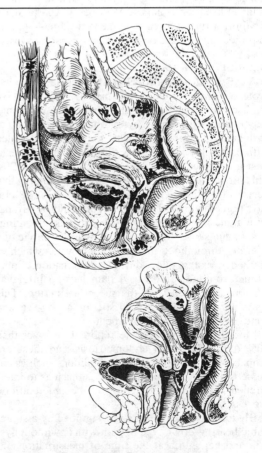

Figure 42–1. Endometriosis.

grade menstruation and implantation; (2) müllerian metaplasia of coelomic epithelium; and (3) lymphatic and venous dissemination. Retrograde menstruation through the uterine tubes is common, and most cases of endometriosis probably develop as a result of this phenomenon. Bits of menstrual endometrium implant on the surface of the ovaries and fall by gravity into the cul-de-sac (pouch of Douglas), where they implant and respond to the cyclic hormonal influences of the menstrual cycle, shedding and bleeding at the time of menstruation. Conditions favoring retrograde passage of menstrual discharge, eg, cervical stenosis, uterine retroflexion, congenital anomalies such as vaginal atresia and bicornuate uterus, and uterotubal insufflation—particularly in the menstrual or premenstrual phase of the cycle—predispose to endometriosis.

Endometriosis is primarily a disease of women in the higher socioeconomic levels and is uncommon in black women. It occurs only after the onset of regular menstruation, sometimes in teenage girls, but it is rarely encountered in patients with anovulatory cycles.

Endometriosis is commonly associated with infertility, but it is not known which comes first. It becomes quiescent during pregnancy and hormonally induced pseudopregnancy. Multiparity—particularly if childbearing starts early in menstrual life—appears to protect against the development of endometriosis.

Clinical Findings

A. Symptoms and Signs: Endometriosis has protean manifestations. Some patients with extensive disease with large, bilateral ovarian endometriomas may remain essentially asymptomatic, whereas other with small peritoneal implants may be incapacitated with pain. Characteristically, the disease is first manifest as dysmenorrhea developing in the 20s or 30s. This progresses, with increasing severity, to pain that occurs only with menstruation but also during several days preceding menses, often accompanied by dyspareunia and rectal tenesmus. There may be a continuous, vague sense of lower abdominal and pelvic discomfort throughout the menstrual cycle, which is markedly exaggerated during menstruation. Some women complain of low back pain and of painful defecation associated with the menstrual period. This symptom is quite characteristic of cul-de-sac and rectovaginal septum involvement.

Menstrual aberrations are reported in fewer than 50% of patients with endometriosis, and these are probably related to associated conditions such as endometrial polyps or leiomyomas as much as to interference with ovarian function by the endometriotic process.

Bladder involvement may be signified by a suprapubic bearing-down type of pain with or without dysuria and hematuria at the time of menstruation. Involvement of the bladder mucosa is quite rare. If an endometriotic implant involves the peritoneum overlying the ureter, the resulting tissue reaction may produce hydroureter and hydronephrosis with flank and lower abdominal pain.

Implants on the sigmoid colon or rectum may produce signs of partial obstruction of the large bowel, recurring with the menstrual periods.

Occasionally, rupture of a large ovarian endometrial cyst presents symptoms of an acute abdominal emergency with all the signs and symptoms of peritonitis.

B. Pelvic Examination: Rectovaginal bimanual pelvic examination is vital to the detection of pelvic endometriosis, since this is the only way the cul-de-sac, the area of the uterosacral ligaments, and the posterior wall of the uterine corpus can be adequately palpated. Moreover, the ovaries, when they are involved, frequently are prolapsed and adherent to the posterior leaf of the broad ligament lateral to the cul-de-sac and are best felt by the rectal finger. An examination performed during the days just preceding the menstrual period is most likely to provide the best opportunity for palpation of the characteristic shotty nodules in the pouch of Douglas, since this is the stage of the menstrual cycle when they are under the full stimulus of the ovarian hormones.

Bilateral, tender, fixed ovarian cystic masses 5–10 cm in diameter are significant findings.

C. Special Examinations: Laparoscopic examination is often quite helpful in establishing a diagnosis of endometriosis when the patient's symptoms are suggestive but the signs are minimal or absent. A finding of characteristic raspberry or blueberry implants of ectopic tissue or the powder-burn marks of scarred endometrium is diagnostic. Laparotomy is occasionally necessary.

D. Classification: A clinically useful classification of endometriosis is as follows:

1. **Mild–**
    a. Scattered pelvic implants other than on uterus, tubes, and ovaries; no scarring.
    b. Rare superficial implants on ovaries.
    c. No significant adhesions.
2. **Moderate–**
    a. Multiple implants or small endometriomas (< 2 cm) involving one or both ovaries.
    b. Minimal periovarian or peritubal adhesions.
    c. Scattered implants with scarring on other structures.
3. **Severe–**
    a. Large ovarian endometriomas (> 2 cm).
    b. Significant periovarian or peritubal adhesions.
    c. Tubal obstruction.
    d. Obliteration of cul-de-sac.
    e. Bowel or bladder adhesions.

Differential Diagnosis

Endometriosis may mimic chronic salpingitis with bilateral tubo-ovarian masses, ovarian carcinoma, twisted ovarian cyst, appendicitis, ectopic pregnancy, diverticulitis, and carcinoma of the rectosigmoid colon. A detailed history, a carefully performed physical examination, and the use of diagnostic x-ray and laparoscopy or culdoscopy will be helpful in the differential diagnosis. Biopsy of suspicious lesions of the intestine prior to resection will be helpful in avoiding needless bowel resection when endometriosis simulates carcinoma of the gastrointestinal tract.

Complications

Infertility is a common problem in patients with endometriosis and occurs in about three-fourths of women with this disease. It may be the only presenting complaint.

Bowel obstruction does not develop often, but it may occur when there is intestinal involvement by endometrial implantation involving either the small or large bowel. A mechanical ileus may result from the numerous dense adhesions that form as a result of the inflammatory reaction in response to cyclic bleeding from peritoneal implants.

Rupture of a large endometrial cyst of the ovary usually produces an acute, widespread peritoneal reaction with signs and symptoms of an acute surgical emergency.

Scarring around the ureter may cause obstruction, with the development of hydroureter and hydronephrosis, and this may explain many cases of idiopathic hydronephrosis seen in women during the reproductive years.

Ovarian carcinoma has been known to develop in endometriomas and usually takes the form of endometrioid adenocarcinoma. Adenoacanthomas and endometrial stromal sarcomas have been reported, but these are rare.

Prevention

Early, repeated pregnancy appears to prevent the development of endometriosis.

Assuming that retrograde passage of endometrial tissue through the uterine tubes is the primary method of implantation, one should avoid repeated injections into the endometrial cavity, such as gas insufflation for determination of tubal patency or the introduction of radiopaque media for the purpose of x-ray delineation of the uterine cavity and tubal lumen (hysterosalpingography), particularly at or near the menstrual period.

The early diagnosis and treatment of menstrual obstruction (dilation of the cervix, hymenotomy, metroplasty, and the correction of fixed retroversion) may help to prevent or delay the development of endometriosis.

There is suggestive evidence that long-term contraceptive pill users are less likely to develop endometriosis, particularly if the pill contains a small amount of estrogen in combination with a potent progestin. Regular physical exercise, particularly if begun during adolescence and continued during the adult years, also reduces the risk.

Treatment

Therapy may be medical, surgical, or a combination of both methods. Treatment should be tailored to fit the circumstances with respect to the age of the patient, her symptoms, her desire for children, and the extent of the disease. Therapy may vary, therefore, from mere observation, reassurance, and analgesia if necessary, to complete surgical removal of the uterus, tubes, and ovaries.

A conservative approach is recommended for the patient who is symptom-free or only mildly symptomatic, with minimal pelvic findings such as slightly tender cul-de-sac nodules. Regular examinations should be carried out at intervals of not more than 6 months. Evidence of progression of the disease—in the form of either increasing symptomatology, infertility, or the development of pelvic masses—requires more specific treatment.

A. Medical Treatment: The induction of anovulation and amenorrhea has been successful in bringing about regression in a high percentage of patients with endometriosis. This may be accomplished in several ways:

1. Danazol–This synthetic androgen derived from ethisterone has been found to be effective in the medical treatment of endometriosis. It acts by suppressing the secretion of gonadotropins, thus achieving medical castration. It is given in doses of 200–800 mg daily and continued without interruption for 6–9 months. Drawbacks are expense and androgenic side effects.

2. Progestins–Norethynodrel, norethindrone, hydroxyprogesterone caproate, and medroxyprogesterone are the agents most commonly used. They are most often used in combination with an estrogen (to prevent breakthrough bleeding). One such combination—norethynodrel, 2.5 mg, with mestranol, 0.1 mg, may be given in the following schedule: 2.5 mg/d for 1 week, 5 mg/d for 1 week, and 10 mg/d for 2 weeks, increasing by 2.5 mg *each time there is breakthrough bleeding.* The production of a pseudopregnancy state through hormonal therapy is maintained for 6–12 months and is effective in about 80% of patients. It is useful as a preoperative adjunct for 6 weeks to soften areas of scarred endometriosis and to make the surgical procedure somewhat easier. The most frequent indication for the prolonged use of these compounds is recurrent endometriosis following a conservative operation. Sides effects are nausea, breast tenderness, fluid retention, and breakthrough bleeding.

3. GnRH analogues–The analogs of gonadotropin-releasing hormone administered continuously rather than periodically have been used to bring about artificial menopause and arrest the progress of endometriosis. This approach must be considered experimental at this time.

Hormonal therapy is not indicated in patients with unproved endometriosis or uterine leiomyomas or in individuals with a history of breast cancer, thrombophlebitis, pulmonary embolus, or liver disease.

B. Surgical Treatment: The surgical approach to endometriosis may be designed to improve fertility, prevent further progression of the disease with preservation of the ovaries, or cure the disease by removal of the uterus and the adnexal structures.

1. Conservative surgery–Preservation of childbearing function by removal or cauterization of implants, freeing up of tubal adhesions, presacral neurectomy for the relief of pain, and uterine suspension is indicated in the young woman who desires to have children. It is not recommended in the patient with extensive endometriosis involving the intestines. Laparoscopic surgery on an ambulatory basis may eliminate the need for laparotomy.

2. Modified radical surgery–This involves the removal of the uterus, excision or fulguration of endometrial implants, and preservation of the ovaries. This approach may be considered in the younger woman who has no desire to retain her childbearing function but is not near the menopause. It carries the risk of recurrence, but without the uterus the risk is small.

3. Definitive surgery–This requires the removal not only of the uterus but of the tubes and ovaries as well. Since endometriosis is dependent upon ovarian function for its continued growth and development, total hysterectomy and bilateral salpingooophorectomy should be done in patients with extensive disease, particularly those with bowel involvement. It is critically important not to mistake bowel implants for cancer. Unnecessary abdominoperineal resections have been performed in young women for unrecognized endometriosis. Provided there has been a preoperative bowel preparation, bowel implants can be locally resected.

Oral estrogen replacement therapy in the form of diethylstilbestrol, 0.25–0.5 mg/d, ethinyl estradiol, 0.02–0.05 mg/d, or conjugated estrogens, 0.625–1.25 mg/d, interrupting the cycle for 5–7 days each month, may be given without danger of exacerbating the endometriotic process. The use of estrogen-progestin combinations is not recommended.

Barbieri RL: Etiology and epidemiology of endometriosis. Am J Obstet Gynecol 1990;162:565.

Cedars MI et al: Treatment of endometriosis with a long-acting gonadotropin-releasing hormone agonist plus medroxyprogesterone acetate. Obstet Gynecol 1990; 75:641.

Henzl MR et al: Administration of nasal nafarelin as compared with oral danazol for endometriosis: A multicenter double-blind comparative clinical trial. N Engl J Med 1988;318:485.

Jenkins S, Olive DL, Haney AF: Endometriosis: Pathogenetic implications of the anatomic distribution. Obstet Gynecol 1986;67:335.

Kane C, Drouin P: Obstructive uropathy associated with endometriosis. Am J Obstet Gynecol 1985;151:207.

Keye WR Jr, Dixon J: Photocoagulation of endometriosis by the argon laser through the laparoscope. Obstet Gynecol 1983;62:383.

Schlaff WD et al: Megestrol acetate for treatment of endometriosis. Obstet Gynecol 1990;75:646.

Weed JC, Ray JE: Endometriosis of the bowel. Obstet Gynecol 1987;69:727.

TUBAL PREGNANCY

Essentials of Diagnosis

- Cramping, colicky, or steady lower abdominal pain.
- Missed period or menstrual irregularity.
- Vaginal bleeding.
- Tender adnexal mass.
- Signs of intraperitoneal bleeding (culdocentesis).
- Slight uterine enlargement.

General Considerations

Ectopic pregnancy occurs once in every 150–200 pregnancies. In patients with documented histories of salpingitis, the rate is one per 24 pregnancies. IUD users also have an increased risk of ectopic pregnancy, with an incidence of one in 23 pregnancies in one series. Induced abortions may also increase the risk of subsequent ectopic pregnancy. The ectopic pregnancy rate in the USA more than doubled during 1970–1978, apparently owing to increased incidence of pelvic inflammatory disease. Other contributing factors to the rise in the number of ectopic pregnancies are the increased use of IUDs and the rising number of induced abortions. The uterine tube is the most frequent site of an ectopic pregnancy (95%), and the ampulla is the section usually involved. Interstitial (cornual) pregnancies are infrequent but significant because profuse, exsanguinating intraperitoneal bleeding occurs at the time of rupture. Ectopic pregnancies are seen also in the peritoneal cavity (abdominal pregnancy), ovary, and cervix; because they are extremely rare, only tubal pregnancy will be discussed here.

Tubal pregnancy is the result of implantation of the fertilized ovum into the wall of the uterine tube, an event probably related to a delay in the transfer of the egg through the tubal lumen. Preexisting disease affecting the tubes (salpingitis, appendicitis, endometriosis, and pelvic operation, particularly tuboplastic procedures and partial salpingectomy for sterilization) predisposes to tubal pregnancy, but tubal pregnancy is not infrequent in patients with no such history.

With implantation of the ovum, there is vascular engorgement and trophoblastic invasion, with resultant weakening of the wall of the uterine tube. Rupture of the tube frequently follows, often with massive bleeding into the peritoneal cavity. The ovum, on the other hand, may separate from the implantation site, pass into the lumen of the tube, and then be extruded through the fimbriated extremity into the peritoneal cavity, together with a considerable amount of blood (tubal abortion). In either event there may be sufficient acute blood loss to produce the clinical picture of hypovolemic shock.

Regardless of the implantation site, uterine enlargement with decidual change in the endometrium occurs because of the influence on the uterus of pregnancy levels of estrogen and progesterone.

Clinical Findings

The symptoms and signs of tubal pregnancy are extremely variable, and this disease is not infrequently overlooked or misdiagnosed because of the atypical clinical picture.

A. "Classic" Findings: Classically, in a ruptured tubal pregnancy the history is of one or two missed menstrual periods, with accompanying presumptive symptoms of pregnancy (tender breasts, urinary frequency, nausea). Mild to moderate vaginal bleeding then ensues, followed, after an interval of a few days, by the onset of unilateral lower abdominal pain—at first cramping or colicky and then steady, becoming generalized through the lower abdomen. Referred shoulder pain results from irritation of the diaphragm by the intraperitoneal blood. Syncope often occurs as a result of hypotension.

Examination reveals a pale, cold, clammy, apprehensive patient with a rapid, thready pulse and hypotension. The abdomen is tender throughout, with rigidity and rebound tenderness. These findings are often more pronounced on the affected side. Rarely, there is a bluish discoloration around the umbilicus (Cullen's sign). Dark blood from the cervical canal is often present in the vagina. Marked tenderness throughout the entire abdomen can be elicited, and displacement of the cervix digitally produces considerable discomfort in the abdomen. The uterus is slightly to moderately enlarged and soft. A tender adnexal mass may be palpated, and there is often a feeling of fullness in the cul-de-sac. Culdocentesis reveals nonclotting blood in the peritoneal cavity.

Hemoglobin and hematocrit are below normal values, and moderate leukocytosis is present. The pregnancy test may or may not be positive. Radioimmunoassay for the beta subunit of hCG is very sensitive and may prove helpful in the diagnosis of suspected ectopic pregnancy.

B. "Atypical" Findings: The majority of tubal pregnancies (60–85%) do not fit this typical picture and manifest themselves in more subtle ways. There may be no history of menstrual irregularity or presumptive symptoms of pregnancy. The abdominal pain may be mild and vague. Physical findings often are confusing, with some pelvic tenderness but no palpable adnexal mass. The uterus may or may not be enlarged and softened. Slow hemorrhage into the peritoneal cavity may circumvent the clinical picture of surgical shock. A gradually falling hematocrit may be the only real clue to bleeding. For these reasons, tubal pregnancy often is a diagnostic enigma, and it is necessary to be alert to the possibility and to properly investigate suspected cases.

Culdocentesis is particularly helpful in proving the presence of free blood in the peritoneal cavity, but it may be negative in an unruptured tubal pregnancy or if a blood clot obstructs the lumen of the needle. The combination of pelvic ultrasonography and serial qualitative βhCG assays with a sensitivity of 25 mIU/mL has markedly improved the accuracy of diagnosis of unruptured ectopic pregnancy. The ovisac may be detected as early as at 5 weeks of gestational age.

A decidual cast from the uterus passed through the vagina or curettings that demonstrate decidua but no evidence of trophoblast on careful pathologic examination are suggestive of ectopic pregnancy. Laparoscopy may help establish the correct diagnosis.

Differential Diagnosis

Early intrauterine pregnancy with or without threatened abortion and salpingitis are the conditions most often confused with ectopic pregnancy. The cramping pain of a threatened or inevitable intrauterine abortion is usually suprapubic rather than unilateral. There is no adnexal structure suggestive of tubal pregnancy; little pain is present in the adnexal area or on cervical motion; and culdocentesis shows no blood in the peritoneal cavity. An intrauterine ovisac may be detected on pelvic sonography. Laparoscopy reveals normal adnexal structures. Acute appendicitis may simulate a tubal pregnancy on the right side. A diagnosis of appendicitis is suggested by nausea and vomiting of acute onset, absence of a significant menstrual history or vaginal bleeding, a higher white blood cell count, and culdocentesis negative for blood but perhaps productive of a small amount of fluid that has a high white blood cell count. Acute salpingitis, particularly when the symptoms and signs are more pronounced on one side, may be confused with ectopic pregnancy. In this condition, there is usually some evidence of bilateral disease. There are no symptoms or signs of pregnancy, and culdocentesis may show inflammatory elements rather than blood in the peritoneal cavity. A corpus luteum cyst of the ovary with rupture and bleeding into the peritoneal cavity may closely simulate a ruptured tubal pregnancy and often requires laparotomy for the differential diagnosis. Laparoscopy may be diagnostic.

Complications

The complications of tubal pregnancy are those of shock due to hemorrhage, infection, and sterility.

Prevention

Prompt diagnosis and treatment of unruptured ectopic pregnancy will prevent the often massive intraperitoneal hemorrhage associated with rupture. Unruptured ectopic pregnancy must be considered whenever a patient is presumed to be pregnant and an adnexal mass is palpated which is thought to be separate from the ovary on that side. Only prompt investigation regarding the nature of the mass will circumvent the possibility of a ruptured tubal pregnancy.

Treatment

Ideally, treatment is surgical, with excision of the implant and preservation of the uterine tube before rupture occurs. With a high index of suspicion, a positive hCG assay, and a sonogram demonstrating an adnexal structure that resembles a small cyst and an empty uterus, the diagnosis of unruptured ectopic pregnancy can be made with reasonable certainty.

Fimbrial expression of the unruptured pregnancy, salpingostomy, and even salpingectomy are surgical techniques available to the experienced laparoscopist that avoid the need for laparotomy. With tubal preservation techniques, persistence of trophoblastic activity may occur and should be monitored postoperatively by following serial β-hCG titers. Systemic methotrexate is being used for the nonsurgical management of unruptured tubal pregnancy (and for persistent trophoblastic activity following salpingostomy or fimbrial expression) but must be considered experimental at the present time.

Ruptured tubal pregnancy with hemodynamic shock is a surgical emergency! Immediate transfusion and operation are imperative. The surgical procedure usually performed is unilateral salpingectomy or salpingo-oophorectomy. Hysterectomy should be considered in patients with a known recent benign cervical smear whose vital signs are stable and who have obvious inflammatory destruction or surgical loss of both tubes.

Prognosis

The prognosis is good if the diagnosis is made promptly and appropriate therapy given. Death may result from hemorrhage or infection in neglected cases.

American College of Obstetricians and Gynecologists: *Ectopic Pregnancy.* Technical Bulletin No. 126. ACOG, 1989.

Henderson SR: Ectopic tubal pregnancy treated by operative laparoscopy. Am J Obstet Gynecol 1989;160:1462.

Lundorff P et al: Persistent trophoblast after conservative treatment of tubal pregnancy: Prediction and detection. Obstet Gynecol 1991;77:129.

Pansky M et al: Nonsurgical management of tubal pregnancy: Necessity in view of changing clinical appearance. Am J Obstet Gynecol 1991;164:888.

Pauerstein CJ et al: Anatomy and pathology of tubal pregnancy. Obstet Gynecol 1986;67:301.

Stock RJ: Persistent tubal pregnancy. Obstet Gynecol 1991;77:267.

Stovall TG et al: Methotrexate treatment of unruptured ectopic pregnancy: A report of 100 cases. Obstet Gynecol 1991;77:749.

Stovall TG, Ling FW, Gray LA: Single-dose methotrexate for treatment of ectopic pregnancy. Obstet Gynecol 1991;77:754.

INCOMPETENCE OF PELVIC SUPPORT
(Uterine Prolapse, Cystourethrocele, Rectocele, Enterocele, Prolapsed Vagina After Hysterectomy)

Essentials of Diagnosis

- Parous woman.
- Complaints of "bearing down" or "falling out" sensation in the pelvis, mass protruding from vaginal introitus, urinary stress incontinence, and difficulty in evacuating rectum.
- Physical findings of defective perineal body, bulge of anterior vaginal wall with loss of urethrovesical angle, bulge of posterior vaginal wall due to defect in rectovaginal septum or hernia sac between rectum and vagina (enterocele), descent of uterus in pelvis, and protrusion of vagina (following hysterectomy).

General Considerations

An understanding of pelvic floor relaxation with its sequelae of cystourethrocele, rectocele, enterocele, and uterine (or vaginal) prolapse requires a thorough knowledge of the anatomic relationship of the pelvic viscera and their supporting tissues. Almost invariably, these conditions result initially from stretching and tearing of the connective tissues of the pelvis during delivery. The supporting structures are weakened, and this is followed by the slow, insidious additional loss of strength brought about by the gravitational forces of the erect position over the years and the sudden, intermittent increases of pressure from above (intra-abdominal pressure) associated with lifting, coughing, straining, sneezing, etc. Finally comes the additional insult of loss of tone due to the hormonal withdrawal associated with the menopause.

These conditions are rarely seen in nulligravidas, in whom they are thought to be related to congenital anomalies (spina bifida occulta).

The levator ani muscle forms the basic portion of the floor of the pelvis. It is trough-shaped and perforated in its thickened, central portion (pubococcygeus) by the urethra, vagina, and rectum—the genital hiatus. The fascia covering the superior surface of this muscle is continuous with the endopelvic fascia as well as the cardinal and uterosacral ligaments supporting the uterus. The fascia covering the inferior surface of the levator ani muscle is in continuity with that of the obturator internus and the urogenital diaphragm (Figure 42–2). The bladder, upper vagina, and rectum all rest horizontally upon and are supported by the fused posterior portion of the pelvic floor, the levator plate. The urogenital diaphragm (triangular ligament) bridges that portion of the perineum anterior to the ischial tuberosities, between the descending rami of the pubis. It is composed of the deep transverse perineal muscle and its investing superficial and deep fascia and is penetrated by the urethra and the vagina. It forms a secondary but less important support for these structures.

In obstetric injuries to the pelvic floor there is often damage to the investing endopelvic fascia and the supporting ligaments of the uterus as well as a widening of the genital hiatus and a downward inclination of the levator plate so that combinations of anatomic defects often are encountered rather than a single one—ie, prolapse of the uterus in combination with cystourethrocele, rectocele, and enterocele.

Stress incontinence is involuntary loss of urine from the urethra with increases in intra-abdominal pressure such as occur with coughing, straining, sneezing, laughing, etc. It can be demonstrated clinically during pelvic examination by asking the patient to cough. Stress incontinence should be carefully distinguished from another common type of involuntary loss of urine, ie, urgency incontinence. The latter condition usually is related to inflammatory conditions in and around the bladder trigone, producing bladder irritability, and the patient experiences the loss of urine with bladder filling and the desire to void. The two conditions may occur simultaneously. Surgical correction of stress incontinence may produce a temporary urgency incontinence until the postoperative inflammatory reaction subsides. Other types of urinary incontinence such as the overflow type of neuropathic bladder must also be recognized.

Anatomically, the bladder and urethra are supported by the muscles of the pelvic floor and the endopelvic fascia. The intraluminal hydrostatic pressure relationships are all-important to an understanding of the mechanism of stress incontinence and its correction. In the nulliparous woman, the proximal urethra is held high and is subjected to the same intra-abdominal pressure changes as those affecting the bladder. Thus, with coughing, straining, sneezing, etc, the greater "closure pressure" of the proximal

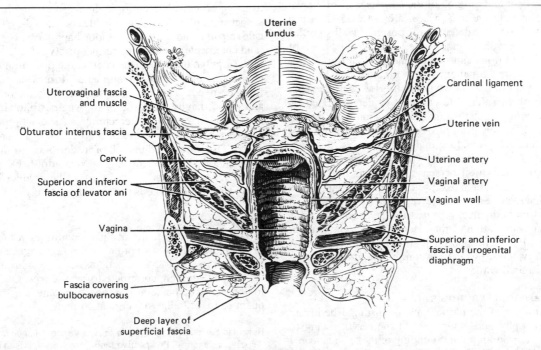

Figure 42–2. Ligamentous and fascial support of pelvic viscera. (Redrawn from original drawings by Frank H Netter, MD, that first appeared in Ciba *Clinical Symposia,* Copyright © 1950. Ciba Pharmaceutical Co. Reproduced with permission.)

urethra (50–135 cm water) over that of the bladder (10–60 cm water) is maintained, and the patient remains continent. In the multipara with pelvic floor relaxation, however, descent of the posterior wall of the bladder neck and urethra produces a funneling effect (loss of the posterior urethrovesical angle). The proximal urethra no longer maintains a higher closing pressure with stress, and incontinence occurs. Most operations for the correction of urinary stress incontinence are designed to elevate the urethrovesical junction and proximal urethra, restoring the increased "closure pressure" of the urethra over the hydrostatic pressure within the bladder during stress.

A cystocele of significant degree may be present without stress incontinence, and the overzealous surgeon may, in correcting the cystocele, straighten out the posterior angle, produce a funneling of the bladder neck and urethra, and thus cause an iatrogenic stress incontinence.

Clinical Findings

Mild degrees of pelvic floor relaxation are found in many multiparous women without significant symptoms. Prolapse of the uterus varies in degree depending upon the level of the uterus in the pelvis. In first-degree prolapse, the cervix does not protrude through the vaginal introitus. Second-degree prolapse is manifest by the presence of the cervix outside the vagina, whereas in third-degree prolapse (procidentia) the entire uterus comes through the introitus covered by the everted vagina.

Descent and bulging of the anterior wall of the vagina indicate the presence of a cystocele, whereas a similar anatomic defect in the posterior wall signifies that a rectocele or enterocele (or both) exists. All of these conditions can be demonstrated during examination with the patient in the lithotomy position by asking her to bear down or strain. However, the existence of an enterocele can best be demonstrated by performing a rectovaginal examination with the patient in the standing position. The hernia is felt between the rectal and vaginal fingers.

The symptoms of pelvic floor incompetence are a dragging sensation or sense of "falling out" of the pelvic organs, a mass protruding from the vagina (which may be a cystocele, rectocele, cervix, or all 3), stress incontinence, repeated urinary tract infections due to sacculation of the bladder and a large amount of residual urine, and difficulties in defecation, occasionally requiring digital compression of the posterior vaginal wall.

Differential Diagnosis

Prolapse of the uterus must be distinguished from hypertrophy and elongation of the cervix owing to chronic inflammation. Sounding of the cervical canal to the level of the internal os will confirm the diagnosis.

Urethral diverticula may simulate cystocele and produce a bulge of the anterior vaginal wall. The diverticulum is usually palpable as a discrete mass, and pressure against the mass often expresses purulent material from the urethral meatus. Endoscopic and urethrocystographic examinations confirm the diagnosis. Urodynamic studies are helpful in distinguishing true stress urinary incontinence from the urge incontinence of an unstable bladder (detrusor dyssynergia) and the overflow incontinence of neuropathic bladder.

Treatment

The asymptomatic patient requires no treatment, and it is best to defer therapy in such a patient or one with only mild symptoms until she requests correction for the relief of symptoms.

A. Nonoperative Treatment: The postmenopausal woman with mild to moderate anatomic defects may become symptom-free after the administration of estrogen—either topically, in the form of creams or suppositories, or systemically, by oral tablets or intramuscular injections of a long-acting estrogen preparation. Programmed, active exercises of the pelvic floor musculature (Kegel exercises) may prove helpful in relieving symptoms of mild degree.

Pessary support of the descending pelvic structures will provide temporary relief of symptoms and is useful in the surgical high-risk patient.

B. Surgical Treatment: The operation performed most often for the correction of pelvic floor relaxation with multiple anatomic defects is vaginal hysterectomy with anterior colporrhaphy (urethral suspension, plication of the bladder neck, and cystocele repair) and posterior colporrhaphy (rectocele [and enterocele] repair with perineoplasty).

Retropubic urethral suspension is the operation of choice for severe stress incontinence. It may be performed in combination with vaginal hysterectomy and colporrhaphy. Prolapse of the vagina following abdominal or vaginal hysterectomy is a special problem requiring resuspension of the vagina to the presacral fascia (an abdominal procedure) or to the sacrospinous ligament (a vaginal operation). Occasionally, a colpocleisis operation is the best choice in the elderly patient who is not sexually active.

Prognosis

The surgical correction of these conditions results in complete relief of symptoms and no recurrence of the defect in about 85% of patients. Obesity, chronic cough, and straining contribute to recurrences. Overlooking an enterocele at the time of repair is a frequent cause of failure of surgical correction.

Bergman SA et al: Primary stress urinary incontinence and pelvic relaxation: Prospective randomized comparison of three different operations. Am J Obstet Gynecol 1989;161:97.

Fantl JA et al: Urinary incontinence in community-dwelling

women: Clinical, urodynamic, and severity characteristics. Am J Obstet Gynecol 1990;162:946.

Low JA et al: The unstable urethra in the female. Obstet Gynecol 1989;74:69.

Raz S et al: Four-corner bladder and urethral suspension for moderate cystocele. J Urol 1989;142:712.

FISTULAS

URINARY TRACT FISTULAS

Urinary tract fistulas are of several varieties: vesicovaginal (most common), ureterovaginal, and urethrovaginal. They occur most often as a result of accidental injury to the urinary tract at the time of pelvic surgery or because of ischemic necrosis resulting from an impaired blood supply. The latter can occur either following radiation therapy for carcinoma of the reproductive organs (especially the cervix) or following prolonged impaction of the fetal head during labor.

Total abdominal hysterectomy is the operation most often complicated by the development of vesicovaginal fistula, which may also occur as a result of tumor invasion of the vesicovaginal septum.

Clinical Findings

A. Symptoms and Signs: Constant urinary incontinence is the cardinal symptom. Urine can usually be seen coming through an opening in the vagina. In vesicovaginal and ureterovaginal fistulas, the vaginal ostium is at or near the vault closure, whereas the urethrovaginal fistula opens along the anterior wall of the vagina. If the urethrovaginal fistula involves the distal urethra, the patient may remain continent and lose urine into the vagina only at the time of voiding.

A communication between the urinary bladder and the vagina can be demonstrated by instilling sterile milk or a dye (methylene blue or indigo carmine) into the bladder via a catheter and watching it come through into the vagina on speculum examination. If leakage of urine into the vagina cannot be colored in this fashion, the defect probably is ureteral and can be demonstrated by giving the patient methylene blue tablets by mouth and finding a blue stain on a cotton pledget placed in the vagina.

B. Urologic Examination: Cystoscopy and x-ray studies of the urinary tract will localize the urinary tract opening of the fistulous tract. Occasionally, the fistulous tracts are branching or multiple.

Prevention

Fistulas caused by urinary tract injury can be pre-vented by skillful surgical technique. The surgeon should be alert for injuries, and if they occur, they should be repaired at the time of operation.

Treatment

Urinary tract fistulas rarely close spontaneously. They must be repaired surgically, but sufficient time should elapse (4–6 months) to allow for resolution of edema and inflammatory reaction. Otherwise, attempts at repair are doomed to failure. The use of cortisone as an anti-inflammatory agent has been recommended to shorten this waiting period. Urinary tract infections should be treated with appropriate urinary antiseptic agents before surgical correction.

Ureterovaginal fistulas are repaired by performing a ureteroureterostomy or by implanting the severed ureter into the bladder (ureteroneocystostomy).

The abdominal (suprapubic) and vaginal approaches are used to repair vesicovaginal fistulas, and a number of techniques are available (layered closure, partial colpocleisis). Regardless of the method used, the principles of repair are the same: meticulous technique, using fine suture material; approximation of broad surfaces without tension; and maintenance of bladder decompression postoperatively until healing can occur.

Radiation fistulas are more complex because of tissue ischemia. They may require the introduction of a new blood supply provided by bulbocavernosus or gracilis myocutaneous flaps for successful repair.

Hoskins WJ et al: Repair of urinary tract fistulas with bulbocavernosus myocutaneous flaps. Obstet Gynecol 1984;63:588.

RECTOVAGINAL FISTULAS

Rectovaginal fistulas are most often a result of obstetric injury, surgical procedures, cervical cancer, radiation therapy, or inflammatory bowel disease. The symptoms are those of incontinence of flatus or feces through the vagina. The vaginal ostium usually can be demonstrated by speculum examination, and a probe passed through the fistulous tract can be palpated by the rectal finger.

Low rectovaginal fistulas near the vaginal introitus should be repaired after the surrounding inflammatory reaction and edema have subsided. This may require 3–4 months. Those found high in the vagina—particularly fistulas resulting from radiation therapy—are often best managed with an initial diverting colostomy which is then closed 2–3 months after a successful repair.

Before surgical repair of a rectovaginal fistula, the bowel should be prepared with a low-residue diet, enteric antibiotics, and cleaning enemas.

Those fistulas that are related to inflammatory bowel disease carry a very poor prognosis and usually will not heal when repair is attempted unless the disease is clearly in remission. Ileostomy and abdominoperineal resection are necessary in patients whose symptoms are unacceptable despite medical management. Fistulas that occur as a result of cancer are not amenable to surgical repair. A diverting colostomy may give the patient considerable comfort.

Elkins TE et al: The use of modified Martius graft as an adjunctive technique in vesicovaginal and rectovaginal fistula repair. Obstet Gynecol 1990;75:727.

TUMORS OF THE FEMALE GENITAL TRACT

BENIGN TUMORS OF THE VULVA & VAGINA

1. HIDRADENOMA

Hidradenomas are small, discrete, firm, mobile structures in the subcutaneous tissues of the labia or perianal region. These sweat gland tumors are benign but may be mistaken for a cancer because of an adenomatous microscopic pattern.

Treatment consists of local excision.

2. SEBACEOUS CYSTS

Sebaceous cysts are small, raised, discrete, white cystic structures in the skin of the labia majora or minora that contain white sebaceous material. They may become infected, producing small abscesses.

Most sebaceous cysts require no therapy. If they cause discomfort, simple excision is indicated.

3. BARTHOLIN CYST

Bartholin cysts cause swelling deep in the tissues of the posterior portion of the labium majus. The cysts vary in size from 1 cm in diameter to several centimeters. The larger masses tend to bulge into the vestibule of the vulva and the lower vagina. They may be asymptomatic or may produce local pressure symptoms and dyspareunia. Secondary infection occurs frequently, producing a large, painful abscess.

Bartholin's abscesses with surrounding cellulitis should be treated with antibiotic therapy followed by incision and drainage. Symptomatic cysts and low-grade abscesses should be either marsupialized (in

order to retain the mucus-secreting gland) or surgically excised.

4. GARTNER DUCT CYSTS

These occur as small round or fusiform cystic swellings, often bilateral, beneath the mucosa of the anterolateral wall of the vagina. They arise from remnants of the vaginal portion of the mesonephric (wolffian) duct and contain a clear serous fluid. They are usually asymptomatic and are discovered in the course of a routine physical examination. Occasionally, they reach 5–6 cm in size.

Small, asymptomatic cysts require no therapy. Larger masses should be surgically excised.

5. ENDOMETRIOSIS

Small, bluish, cystic elevations of the vaginal mucosa representing ectopic endometrial tissue are seen most often in the posterior fornix (as an extension of cul-de-sac endometriosis) or in episiotomy scars.

Vaginal endometrial implants are treated by local excision or fulguration. (See Endometriosis, above.)

6. CYSTIC ADENOSIS

Multiple small submucosal cysts of the vagina may represent persistent müllerian (paramesonephric duct) remnants. In utero exposure to diethylstilbestrol should be suspected. Unless there are signs of cancer (Papanicolaou smears, iodine staining, and selected punch biopsy), the cysts require no specific treatment.

CARCINOMA OF THE VULVA

Essentials of Diagnosis
- Patient in postmenopausal age group.
- Long history of vulval irritation with pruritus, local discomfort, and slightly bloody discharge.
- Early lesions may appear as chronic vulval dermatitis.
- Late lesions appear as a lump in the labium, a large cauliflower growth, or a hard ulcerative area in the vulva.
- Biopsy is necessary to make the diagnosis.

General Considerations
The vast majority (90–95%) of vulval cancers are squamous cell carcinomas, and these tumors represent about 5% of all cancers of the female reproductive tract. Human papillomavirus (HPV) plays a role in etiology. In situ squamous cell carcinoma occurs frequently in premenopausal women (20–25% of vul-

var carcinomas). A definite relationship to invasive cancer has not yet been established. Other types of vulval cancer are Bartholin gland carcinoma (adenocarcinoma), Paget's disease of the vulva, basal cell carcinoma, malignant melanoma, and metastatic carcinoma from the cervix, endometrium, ovary, or elsewhere. Rarely, sarcomas are found arising primarily in the vulval soft tissues.

Squamous cell carcinoma is frequently associated with leukoplakia (50–70%), which, in the vulva, is considered a premalignant change only when associated with epithelial dysplasia.

The area most often involved is the labium majus. The clitoris is the second most often involved.

Metastasis to the regional lymph nodes (inguinal, femoral, iliac, and obturator) occurs in about 35–60% of invasive lesions. Because of bilateral lymph drainage, the nodes on the contralateral side may be involved (Figure 42–3). There is a high incidence of second primary cancers in these patients, particularly in the cervix, endometrium, and breast. Cancer of the vulva should be classified and clinically staged according to the recommendations of the Cancer Committee of the International Federation of Gynecology and Obstetrics (Table 42–1).

Clinical Findings

In situ squamous cell carcinoma (Bowen's disease) of the vulva may be seen in women age 25–40 years as small, slightly raised or papillary (resembling condylomas) white, red, or brownish patches of skin or mucosa. One-third of lesions are solitary, and two-thirds are multiple. The early invasive lesion is a small, elevated, superficial papillary or ulcerated lesion with underlying subcutaneous induration. Late cancers present either as large, fungating, infected tumors or as shallow ulcers with indurated margins. The larger the primary lesion, the greater the chance of lymph node involvement; but palpatory evidence is misleading, as regional node enlargement may be related to secondary infection in these tumors. Furthermore, metastatic disease in the lymph nodes may not be palpable. There may be submucosal spread of the tumor cephalad to involve the vagina and urethra, or there may be involvement of the posterior vulva with invasion of the anus and rectum.

All suspicious lesions should be examined frequently by biopsy.

Differential Diagnosis

Chronic hypertrophic and atrophic skin conditions may or may not be associated with vulval cancer. Multiple biopsies are necessary to establish the correct diagnosis. Granulomatous venereal lesions of the vulva may be clinically suspicious, and biopsy of the involved area is mandatory. The complement fixation test may be helpful, but it must be remembered that

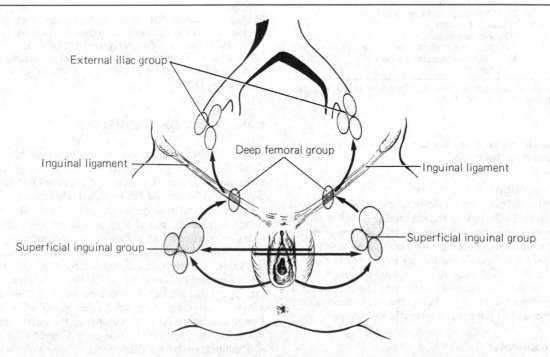

Figure 42–3. Diagram of lymphatic drainage of vulva, showing capacity for bilateral node involvement. (From Way S: Carcinoma of the vulva. In: *Progress in Gynecology,* vol 3. Meigs JV, Sturgis SS [editors]. Grune & Stratton, 1957.)

Table 42–1. Staging of carcinoma of the vulva.[1]

Cases should be classified as carcinoma of the vulva when the primary site of the growth is in the vulva. Tumors present in the vulva as secondary growths from either a genital or extragenital site should be excluded from registration, as should cases of malignant malenoma. (See also carcinoma of the vagina.)

FIGO Nomenclature

Stage 0	Carcinoma in situ.
Stage I	Tumor confined to vulva—2 cm or less in diameter. Nodes are not palpable or are palpable in either groin, not enlarged, mobile (not clinically suspicious of neoplasm).
Stage II	Tumor confined to the vulva—more than 2 cm in diameter. Nodes are not palpable or are palpable in either groin, not enlarged, mobile, (not clinically suspicious of neoplasm).
Stage III	Tumor of any size with (1) adjacent spread to the urethra and any or all of the vagina, the perineum, and the anus, and/or (2) nodes palpable in either or both groins (enlarged, firm, and mobile, not fixed but clinically suspicious of neoplasm).
Stage IV	Tumor of any size (1) infiltrating the bladder mucosa or the rectal mucosa or both, including the upper part of the urethral mucosa, and/or (2) fixed to the bone or other distant metastases. Fixed or ulcerated nodes in either or both groins.

TNM Nomenclature

1.1	Primary Tumor (T)	
	TIS, T1, T2, T3, T4	
	See corresponding FIGO stages.	
1.2	Nodal Involvement (N)	
	NX	Not possible to assess the regional nodes.
	N0	No involvement of regional nodes.
	N1	Evidence of regional node involvement.
	N3	Fixed or ulcerated nodes.
	N4	Juxtaregional node involvement.
1.3	Distant Metastasis (M)	
	MX	No assessed.
	M0	No (known) distant metastasis.
	M1	Distant metastasis present.
		Specify _____

[1]*Annual Report on the Results of Treatment in Gynecological Cancer.* FIGO, Vol 20, 1988.

granulomatous disease and cancer of the vulva may occur simultaneously.

Prevention

Simple excision of lesions that show epithelial dysplasia will prevent the subsequent development of invasive carcinoma. Likewise, the discovery and removal of intraepithelial carcinoma of the vulva is effective prophylaxis for the invasive form of the disease. Toluidine blue in 1% solution applied to the vulval skin and mucosa and then decolorized with 1% acetic acid solution has been effective in determining the extent of the neoplastic epithelial change.

Treatment

Carcinoma in situ (Bowen's disease), if localized, may be treated by wide excision or laser vaporiza-

tion. Skinning vulvectomy with split-thickness skin grafting is done for diffuse, multifocal disease.

Radical vulvectomy with bilateral inguinofemoral and iliac-obturator lymph node dissection is the most widely accepted treatment for invasive carcinoma of the vulva. Ipsilateral lymph node dissection alone is acceptable if the primary lesion is localized to one side away from the midline and the removed nodes are negative to frozen section examination. Radiation therapy is required for inoperable lesions.

Prognosis

Adequate surgery is effective in a high percentage of patients, even when there is evidence of spread to the inguinal and femoral nodes. When the nodes are not involved, 5-year cure rates of 86% are reported, and a 50% salvage rate is possible in the presence of lymph node involvement if the surgical procedure has been adequate.

Brinton LA et al: Case-control study of cancer of the vulva. Obstet Gynecol 1990;75:859.

Burrell MO et al: The modified radical vulvectomy with groin dissection: An eight-year experience. Am J Obstet Gynecol 1988;159:715.

Carson LF: Human papillomavirus DNA in adenosquamous carcinoma and squamous cell carcinoma of the vulva. Obstet Gynecol 1988;72:63.

Cavanagh D et al: Invasive carcinoma of the vulva: Changing trends in surgical management. Am J Obstet Gynecol 1990;163:1007.

Hacker NF et al: Individualization of treatment for stage I squamous cell vulvar carcinoma. Obstet Gynecol 1984; 63:155.

Hoffman JS, Kumar NB, Morley GW: Prognostic significance of groin lymph node metastases in squamous carcinoma of the vulva. Obstet Gynecol 1985;66:402.

Sedlis A et al: Positive groin lymph nodes in superficial squamous cell vulvar cancer. Am J Obstet Gynecol 1987:156:1159.

CARCINOMA OF THE VAGINA

Carcinoma in situ of the vagina occurs either as a direct extension of the process from the portio vaginalis of the cervix or as a separate area in a "neoplastic field." It should be suspected whenever carcinoma in situ or invasive carcinoma of the vulva or cervix is present, and it may appear in the vagina many months or years after successful treatment of either of these two conditions. Carcinoma in situ of the vagina is most often diagnosed by cytologic examination and by biopsy of Schiller-positive areas of the vagina that are Schiller-positive, ie, those that do not take up the iodine stain after application of Lugol's solution. As in carcinoma of the cervix and vulva, human papillomavirus is an etiologic factor.

Treatment is by local excision of involved areas when they are few and small. Radiation therapy, electrocautery, laser therapy, and topical fluorouracil have been used; failure rates are 25–50%. Extensive involvement of the vaginal mucosa may require vaginectomy with complete colpocleisis in the elderly, sexually inactive patient or with skin graft construction of an artificial vagina in the patient who wishes to retain coital function.

Invasive squamous cell carcinoma of the vagina, arising primarily from the vagina, is an unusual lesion, most cancers of the vagina being extensions from an epidermoid carcinoma of the cervix. The lesion is most often ulcerative, with a cauliflower configuration being less common. There is a firm induration surrounding the ulcerative lesion, and these are easily palpated, whereas a small, soft papillary lesion may be missed. The upper third of the vagina is the site in about 75% of patients. In many cases the only symptom is a bloody vaginal discharge, and the diagnosis is made by biopsy.

Treatment is by radiation therapy or radical surgery. Unfortunately, these tumors grow rapidly and insidiously, and in over 50% of patients they have penetrated the vaginal wall at the time of the initial examination. Involvement of the bladder and rectum is common. As a result, the overall 5-year survival figures are in the range of 20–30%.

Adenocarcinoma of the vagina has occurred in teenage girls, apparently arising in areas of vaginal adenosis (probably müllerian duct remnants). There appears to be a relationship between the appearance of this tumor in these young patients and the administration of diethylstilbestrol to their mothers during the fetal life of the patient.

The classification and staging of carcinoma of the vagina is outlined in Table 42–2.

Metastatic carcinoma of the vagina is much more common than primary carcinoma, the most frequent sources being the cervix, vulva, bladder, urethra, rectum, endometrium, and ovary.

Rare primary tumors of the vagina are sarcoma (mixed mesodermal tumors, including sarcoma botryoides of infants, fibrosarcoma, leiomyosarcoma, hemangiosarcoma), adenocarcinoma arising from mesonephric (Gartner's) duct or müllerian duct remnants, embryonal carcinoma, and malignant melanoma. Radical surgical removal offers the best hope of cure for the majority of these neoplasms.

Manetta A et al: Primary invasive carcinoma of the vagina. Obstet Gynecol 1990;76:639.

Skinberg H et al: Human papillomavirus DNA in invasive carcinoma of the vagina. Obstet Gynecol 1990;76:432.

Spirtos NM et al: Radiation therapy for primary squamous cell carcinoma of the vagina: Stanford University experience. Gynecol Oncol 1989;35:20.

TUMORS OF THE UTERINE TUBE (Adenocarcinoma)

Benign tumors of the uterine (fallopian) tubes are very rare. Primary carcinoma of the tube is the most common malignant lesion, but it is rarely encountered, constituting less than 1% of female reproductive cancers.

Postmenopausal vaginal bleeding is the usual presenting complaint. There may be a history of intermittent, profuse, serous, yellow or bloody vaginal discharge (hydrops tubae profluens). An adnexal mass may or may not be palpable.

The diagnosis of primary carcinoma of the uterine tube is rarely made preoperatively. Total abdominal hysterectomy and bilateral salpingo-oophorectomy constitute the treatment of choice in operable lesions. Tumors that are inoperable yet are confined to the pelvic structures should receive radiation therapy—followed by operation if there is a favorable response as judged by increased mobility and diminution in tumor size. Radical hysterectomy and bilateral pelvic lymph node dissection have been advocated as possibly a more curative procedure than simple hysterectomy and bilateral salpingo-oophorectomy.

If the disease is confined to the tube, the prognosis is quite good. Unfortunately, most of these tumors are advanced at the time of discovery, and the overall 5-year cure rate is in the range of 10–20%.

The early use of the laparoscope or the CT scanner may be of aid in the earlier diagnosis of this disease and should be considered in any postmenopausal woman with a vague adnexal mass, particularly if it is accompanied by a watery discharge or postmenopausal bleeding.

Eddy GL et al: Fallopian tube carcinoma. Obstet Gynecol 1984;64:546.

Podratz KC et al: Primary carcinoma of the fallopian tube. Am J Obstet Gynecol 1986;154:1319.

Table 42–2. Staging of carcinoma of the vagina.[1]

Preinvasive carcinoma	
Stage 0	Carcinoma in situ, intraepithelial carcinoma.
Invasive carcinoma	
Stage I	The carcinoma is limited to the vaginal wall.
Stage II	The carcinoma has involved the subvaginal tissue but has not extended to the pelvic wall.
Stage III	The carcinoma has extended to the pelvic wall.
Stage IV	The carcinoma has extended beyond the true pelvis or has involved the mucosa of the bladder or rectum. A bullous edema as such does not permit allotment of a case to stage IV.
Stage IVA	Spread of the growth to adjacent organs.
Stage IVB	Spread to distant organs.

[1]*Annual Report on the Results of Treatment of Gynecological Cancer.* FIGO, Vol 20, 1988.

CANCER OF THE CERVIX

Essentials of Diagnosis

- May be asymptomatic.
- Vaginal discharge.
- Intermenstrual bleeding.
- Suspicious or positive cytologic examination.
- Biopsy diagnosis is essential.

General Considerations

Carcinoma of the cervix is now the second most common invasive cancer in the female reproductive tract.

Early sexual activity, promiscuity, parity, and chronic inflammation are predisposing factors. Herpesvirus hominis type 2 and human papillomavirus (HPV) have been found to be frequently associated with cervical cancer, and there is increasing evidence of a strong relationship with HPV infections, particularly types 16 and 18. Dysplasia of the cervical epithelium is probably a precursor, beginning with mild degrees of dysplasia (CIN I) and progressing to moderate (CIN II) and then severe (CIN III; carcinoma in situ). Eventually, a clone of malignant cells breaks through the basement membrane to produce early stromal invasion (stage IA1).

The majority of cervical cancers are squamous cell (85%); the remainder consist of adenocarcinomas, mixed carcinomas (adenosquamous), and rare sarcomas (mixed mesodermal tumors, lymphosarcomas).

The earliest squamous cell carcinoma is confined to the epithelial layers (carcinoma in situ, intraepithelial carcinoma, preinvasive carcinoma), and it is thought that the disease remains confined to the mucous membrane for several years before invading the subjacent stroma. Carcinoma in situ occurs most frequently during the decade between 30 and 40 years of age, whereas invasive carcinoma is encountered most often in women between 40 and 50.

Following penetration of the basement membrane and involvement of the cervical stroma, the disease spreads by direct contiguity to the vagina and the adjacent parametrium, and via the lymphatic channels (which are abundant in this area) to the regional lymph nodes of the pelvis (iliac and obturator) and to the periaortic lymph nodes.

Estimating the extent of the malignant process is extremely important in determining the mode of therapy and in estimating the prognosis. This is judged clinically and is defined according to the Clinical Classification of the International Federation of Gynecology and Obstetrics, as shown in Table 42–3.

It is known from an examination of surgical specimens that the probability of lymph node metastasis increases according to the local extent of the disease, being approximately 15% in stage I, 30% in stage II, and 45% in stage III. About 80% of patients with stage IV cancer have lymph node involvement.

Table 42–3. Clinical stages in cancer of the cervix.[1]

Preinvasive carcinoma		
Stage 0		Carcinoma in situ, intraepithelial carcinoma.
Invasive carcinoma		
Stage I		Carcinoma strictly confined to the cervix (extension to the corpus should be disregarded).
	IA	Preclinical carcinomas of the cervix, diagnosed only by microscopy.
	IA1	Minimal stromal invasion.
	IA2	Lesions measurable microscopically. Depth of invasion should be no more than 5 mm from the basement membrane, either surface or glandular, and horizontal spread no greater than 7 mm.
	IB	Lesions greater in dimension than stage IA2 whether seen clinically or not. Vascular space involvement should not alter the stage but should be specifically recorded so as to determine whether it should affect treatment decisions in the future.
Stage II		Carcinoma extends beyond the cervix but has not extended onto the pelvic wall. Carcinoma involves the vagina but not the lower third.
	IIA	No obvious parametrial involvement.
	IIB	Obvious parametrial involvement.
Stage III		Carcinoma has extended onto the pelvic wall. On rectal examination, there is no cancer-free space between the tumor and the pelvic wall. The tumor involves the lower third of the vagina. All cases with hydronephrosis or nonfunctioning kidney.
Stage IV		Carcinoma that has extended beyond the true pelvis or clinically involves the mucosa of the bladder or rectum.
	IVA	Spread of growth to adjacent organs.
	IVB	Spread to distant organs.

[1]*Annual Report on the Results of Treatment in Gynecological Cancer.* FIGO, Vol 20, 1988.

Clinical Findings

A. Carcinoma in Situ: Carcinoma in situ does not cause symptoms. However, the majority of patients with this condition have an area of redness (erythroplakia) on the portio vaginalis of the cervix that is indistinguishable from chronic cervicitis. In fact, the two conditions often coexist. Fifteen to 20% of patients with carcinoma in situ have no visible lesion. Cytologic examination (Papanicolaou) of a representative specimen collected from the squamocolumnar junction (transformation zone) of the cervix will demonstrate severely dysplastic or frankly malignant cells in 95% of women with this stage of disease.

The Schiller test, using Lugol's solution (see above), is often helpful in demonstrating areas of abnormal epithelium, even in a cervix that appears normal on gross inspection, because the lack of glycogen in these cells makes them unable to take up the stain. The test is not specific for neoplasm, since area of ectopy, cervicitis, atrophy, and dysplasia are also iodine-negative. A sharply demarcated border of nonstaining is more suggestive of epithelial neoplasia.

Colposcopic examination of the cervix may define areas of dysplasia and carcinoma in situ and should be done in all women who have abnormal (dysplastic or malignant) epithelial cells unrelated to an inflammatory condition. This method is based primarily upon changes that occur in the capillary vascular pattern of the cervix associated with epithelial proliferation.

Punch biopsy is required in all cases in which there is a visible area of redness, an iodine-negative area, or an urea of colposcopic abnormality. A knife cone biopsy and curettage should be done when cytologic examination reveals moderate or severe dysplasia, carcinoma in situ, or perhaps invasive carcinoma and (1) if colposcopy is not available and there is no visible lesion and no iodine-nonstaining area; (2) when colposcopy reveals no abnormalities of the exocervix or when an abnormal transformation zone is seen that extends into the endocervical canal; (3) when a colposcopically directed punch biopsy reveals microinvasive carcinoma; or (4) when colposcopically directed biopsies fail to explain the abnormal cytologic findings.

B. Invasive Carcinoma: With the exception of early stromal involvement, invasive carcinoma of the cervix usually produces symptoms. Intermenstrual or postcoital bleeding is often the first symptom. A watery vaginal discharge, occasionally blood-streaked, may be the only symptom. Pain is a manifestation of far-advanced disease. In most patients with invasive cancer, inspection of the cervix reveals an ulcerated or papillary lesion of the cervix that bleeds on contact. The cytologic examination almost always demonstrates exfoliated malignant cells, though it should be remembered that false-negative Papanicolaou smears are more frequent in the face of invasive carcinoma than in intraepithelial neoplasia. Biopsy usually reveals the invasive nature of the lesion. An occasional endocervical, endophytic lesion will produce enlargement of the cervix without becoming evident on the portio vaginalis.

Differential Diagnosis

Chronic cervicitis can be distinguished from cancer of the cervix only by multiple negative cytologic and biopsy examinations. Polyps of the cervix should be examined by a pathologist to exclude malignant change. The new Bethesda system of reporting cervical cytology, shown in Table 42–4, will help to distinguish benign intraepithelial condylomatous changes, previously reported as mild dysplasia, from early cervical intraepithelial neoplasia.

Complications

The complications are those caused by spread of the disease or occurring secondary to treatment. Obstruction of the ureter, resulting in hydroureter, hydronephrosis, and uremia, occurs with advancing disease. Bilateral obstruction of the ureters leads to failure of kidney function and death.

Involvement of the iliac and obturator lymph

Table 42–4. The 1988 Bethesda system for reporting cervical/vaginal cytologic diagnoses.[1]

EPITHELIAL CELL ABNORMALITIES

Squamous Cell

Atypical squamous cells of undetermined significance (recommended follow-up and/or type of further investigation: specify)

Squamous intraepithelial lesion (SIL) (comment on presence of cellular changes associated with HIV if applicable)

Low-grade, encompassing:
Cellular changes associated with HPV
Mild (slight) dysplasia (CIN I)
High-grade, encompassing:
Moderate dysplasia (CIN II)
Severe dysplasia (CIN III)
Carcinoma in situ (CIN III)

Squamous cell carcinoma

Glandular cell

Presence of endometrial cells in one of the following circumstances:
Out of phase in a menstruating woman
In a postmenopausal woman
No menstrual history available

Atypical glandular cells of undetermined significance (recommended follow-up and/or type of further investigation: specify)
Endometrial
Endocervical
Not otherwise specified

Adenocarcinoma
Specify probable site of origin: endocervical, endometrial, extrauterine
Not otherwise specified

Other epithelial malignant neoplasm: specify

[1]Report of National Cancer Institute Workshop, Bethesda, MD, December 12 and 13, 1988. Published in JAMA 1989;262:931.

nodes may lead to lymphatic obstruction, with lymphedema of the lower extremity.

The lumbosacral plexus may become infiltrated by tumor, causing pain in the low back, hip, and leg.

Vesicovaginal and rectovaginal fistulas occur as a result of tumor involvement of these structures or as complications of radiation therapy. A cloaca may result from massive slough of necrotic tumor tissue. Widespread metastases to lung, liver, brain, and bone may occur.

Complications of radiation therapy such as cystitis, colitis, and proctitis are not uncommon but are usually only transitory problems in modern treatment centers. Castration is an unavoidable complication of radiation therapy. Severe radiation damage to the bladder and rectum may result in hemorrhage, fistulas, and strictures. Radiation necrosis of the cervix and diffuse radiation pelvic fibrosis are rare complications.

The complications of surgery are hemorrhage, infection, thromboembolism, and fistula (ureterovaginal, vesicovaginal, rectovaginal) formation.

Prevention

Invasive cancer of the cervix can be prevented by detecting and properly treating chronic cervicitis, cervical dysplasia, and carcinoma in situ of the cervix. Annual cytologic and pelvic examinations, with appropriate therapy, have proved to be effective in the prevention of this disease.

Treatment

The proper treatment of cervical cancer requires individualization of therapy for each patients according to the clinical circumstances. Cervical epithelial dysplasia is destroyed by cauterization or cryosurgery or by laser therapy.

A. Carcinoma in Situ: Carcinoma in situ and lesser degrees of cervical intraepithelial neoplasia are best treated by eradication of the entire transformation zone. This can be accomplished by cauterization, cryotherapy, laser vaporization, cone biopsy, electrosurgical loop excision, or trachelectomy. Hysterectomy may be done if there is another indication for removing the uterus. Regardless of the procedure, close follow-up is necessary in order to ensure that treatment has indeed been adequate.

B. Invasive Carcinoma: In general, invasive carcinoma is best treated by irradiation under the cooperative management of a radiotherapist and a gynecologist experienced in the treatment of cancer. Both internal sources (radium or cesium) and external sources (x-ray, 60 Co, betatron, linear accelerator) should be employed. Radical hysterectomy may be indicated in certain cases of early (stage IB, IIA) disease in young women or invasive carcinoma complicating pregnancy. Recurrent or persistent cancer following radiation therapy may require pelvic exenteration.

Prognosis

The earlier the disease is treated, the better the prognosis. Carcinoma in situ is almost 100% curable. The prevalence of invasive carcinoma of the cervix is decreasing, partly as a result of detection and treatment in the intraepithelial stage of the disease. The best results in stage I cancer of the cervix approach a 90% 5-year survival rate. For stage II, the figure drops to 60%; for stage III, to 30%; and for stage IV, to less than 10%.

Benedet JL et al: The results of cryosurgical treatment of cervical intraepithelial neoplasia at one, five, and ten years. Am J Obstet Gynecol 1987;157:268.

Burghardt E et al: Prognostic factors and operative treatment of stages IB to IIB cervical cancer. Am J Obstet Gynecol 1987;156:988.

Chu J, White E: Decreasing incidence of invasive cervical cancer in young women. Am J Obstet Gynecol 1987;157:1105.

McIndoe GAH et al: Laser excision rather than vaporization: The treatment of choice for cervical intraepithelial neoplasia. Obstet Gynecol 1989;74:165.

Nash JD, Burke TW, Hoskins WJ: Biologic course of cervical human papillomavirus infection. Obstet Gynecol 1987;69:160.

Paavonen J et al: Significance of mild cervical cytologic atypia in a sexually transmitted disease clinic population. Acta Cytol 1989;33:831.

Ramirez EJ et al: Cervical conization findings in women with dysplastic cervical cytology and normal colposcopy. J Reprod Med 1990;35:359.

Schneider A et al: Human papillomaviruses in women with a history of abnormal Papanicolaou smears and in their male partners. Obstet Gynecol 1987;69:554.

Shy K et al: Papanicolaou smear screening interval and risk of cervical cancer. Obstet Gynecol 1989;74:838.

LEIOMYOMAS OF THE UTERUS

Essentials of Diagnosis

- Often asymptomatic.
- Palpable, irregular enlargements of the corpus
- Abnormal uterine bleeding (hypermenorrhea or intermenstrual bleeding).
- Vague pelvic discomfort or pressure on neighboring pelvic organs (urinary frequency, constipation).
- Enlargement of uterine cavity (sounding).
- MRI and sonography.
- Laparoscopy (peritoneoscopy) may be useful in difficult diagnostic cases.

General Considerations

Leiomyomas of the uterus are found in approximately 20% of all white women and 50% of black women. The cause is not known. Most are asymptomatic. They probably arise from the smooth muscle of the myometrium, and they grow in response to the stimulus of estrogen, as evidenced by an increased growth rate during pregnancy and a cessation of growth with the menopause. They are usually multiple and, depending upon the direction of growth, may remain within the myometrium (intramural), distend the external surface of the uterus (subserous), or come to lie beneath the endometrium (submucous). Other types of myomas are intraligamentous (between the leaves of the broad ligament), parasitic (detached from the uterus and deriving blood supply from other abdominal organs), and cervical. Myomas may vary in size from tiny "seedlings" to massive tumors filling the entire abdomen and pelvis.

On cut section, leiomyomas are well-circumscribed, solid tumors with a pseudocapsule of compressed myometrium and a pearly-gray whorled appearance.

Leiomyomas are subject to various degenerative

changes, probably as a result of interference with the blood supply to various segments of the tumor: hyaline and cystic degeneration, calcification, carneous degeneration (during pregnancy), and, rarely, malignant change (sarcoma).

Clinical Findings

A. Symptoms and Signs: The majority of leiomyomas produce no symptoms and are discovered in the course of a routine pelvic examination. Symptoms, when they occur, are those of an enlarging tumor—abdominal distention, discomfort, urinary frequency, constipation, and hypermenorrhea. Submucous myomas may cause intermenstrual bleeding; at times alarmingly profuse. They may also become pedunculated and protrude through the cervix.

Palpation of the uterus reveals an irregularly enlarged structure that, if large enough, may be felt on abdominal examination. It is usually nontender, but it may become painful in the event of carneous degeneration or torsion of the pedicle of a pedunculated subserous myoma.

A rapidly growing myoma suggests the possibility of sarcomatous change within the tumor (leiomyosarcoma).

B. Laboratory Findings: Anemia may result from acute or chronic blood loss.

C. Imaging Studies: X-rays may demonstrate the typical calcifications, but sonography and magnetic resonance imaging are more accurate in defining leiomyomas without calcifications. Hysterography or exploration of the uterine cavity with a curette will define submucous tumors.

Differential Diagnosis

Enlargement of the uterus by a large, soft myoma (cystic degeneration) may mimic the pregnant uterus or vice versa. A history of amenorrhea suggests pregnancy, as does the appearance of any of the presumptive signs of pregnancy such as secondary breast changes, Montgomery follicles, and a positive Chadwick or Hegar sign. A pregnancy test should be done in all suspected cases. Pregnancy may occur in a myomatous uterus.

Solid ovarian tumors and pedunculated subserous myomas pose a problem in differential diagnosis. In ovarian neoplasm there is a distinct separation between the adnexal mass and the uterus. If examination (under anesthesia if necessary) does not provide sufficient information to allow differentiation, sonography, CT scan, or laparoscopy may be helpful.

Complications

Hemorrhage from a submucous myoma or prolonged hypermenorrhea often results in secondary iron deficiency anemia. Rapid growth of myomas and degenerative changes may occur in women taking oral contraceptives. Torsion of the pedicle of a pe-

dunculated subserous myoma may result in necrosis and present the picture of an acute abdominal emergency.

Infertility may be secondary to myomas. Abortion, premature labor, prolonged labor, and postpartum hemorrhage due to uterine atony are encountered in pregnancy complicated by myomas. These tumors infrequently obstruct the birth canal, producing a soft tissue dystocia.

Treatment

Small, asymptomatic myomas require no therapy. Examination every 6 months to observe the rate of growth is recommended. If treatment is made necessary by symptoms or because of infertility, myomectomy should be done in the young woman who desires preservation of childbearing function. Hysterectomy is the treatment of choice in most patients with symptoms or in the asymptomatic woman who harbors a rapidly growing myoma. Myomectomy usually requires laparotomy and, in terms of postoperative complications, is more hazardous than hysterectomy. Nonsurgical therapy in the form of GnRH analogues has been useful in shrinking the size of leiomyomas and may be employed in symptomatic women wishing to preserve fertility and those approaching the menopause.

Prognosis

Myomectomy may not cure the condition, and the risk of recurrence should be accepted by the patient before the physician proceeds with the operation. Hysterectomy is curative.

Hendee WR: Magnetic resonance imaging of the abdomen and pelvis: Council on Scientific Affairs report. JAMA 1989;261:420.

Miller NF, Ludvici PP: On the origin and development of uterine fibroids. Am J Obstet Gynecol 1955;70:720.

Moskovitz B, Marut EL: Uterine fibroids and the role of GnRH analogues. Female Patient 1988;13:81.

ENDOMETRIAL CARCINOMA

Essentials of Diagnosis

- Postmenopausal bleeding.
- Uterus frequently not enlarged.
- Uterine enlargement and pain are signs of advanced disease.
- Vaginal cytology fails to detect a high percentage of cases.
- Endometrial biopsy or curettage is required to confirm the diagnosis.

General Considerations

Endometrial carcinoma is primarily a disease of postmenopausal women, with a peak incidence in the decade from 55–65 years of age. It also occurs in premenopausal women, particularly those with pro- longed anovulation. Evidence suggests that pro- longed unopposed (by progesterone) estrogen stimu- lation of the endometrium may be a predisposing factor in the development of endometrial carcinoma. The prolonged use of exogenous estrogens in postmenopausal women increases the risk of endo- metrial cancer about seven times. The coincidence of obesity, hypertension, and diabetes in many patients with this disease is indicative of an underlying endo- crine disorder. The peripheral conversion of endoge- nous androstenedione to estrone in relatively large amounts has been implicated as a cause of this dis- ease. Although cancer of the endometrium has been produced in laboratory animals through the continu- ous administration of estrogen, there is no conclusive evidence that estrogens cause cancer in women.

Benign cystic hyperplasia progressing to adenoma- tous hyperplasia and then adenomatous hyperplasia with anaplasia and, finally, neoplasia has been dem- onstrated as a preliminary sequence in a number of patients with endometrial carcinoma.

Carcinoma of the endometrium probably has an in situ (intraepithelial) first stage, followed by invasion of the surrounding endometrial stroma before the un- derlying myometrium is involved. Fortunately, deep myometrial penetration, extension, beyond the cor- pus of the uterus, lymph node involvement, and dis- tant metastases occur relatively late in the disease, so that most lesions are detected early. This is especially true if the lesion is well differentiated histologically. Anaplastic tumors and the papillary serous, clear cell, and squamous cell variants, on the other hand, are much more aggressive.

Endometrial cancer is now staged surgically as shown in Table 42–5. Because a small number of poor-risk patients are treated primarily with radiation therapy rather than surgery, these patients should be staged clinically as before. The fact that clinical stag- ing is used should be stated.

Clinical Findings

Postmenopausal bleeding is the primary symptom and should be considered to be caused by cancer until proved otherwise. About 40% of women with vaginal bleeding following the menopause will have repro- ductive tract cancer, and in the vast majority of these cases the cancer is endometrial. Cervical stenosis with pyometra or hematometra is highly suggestive of endometrial carcinoma. Pain is not a common symptom, but there may be mild uterine cramping, particularly if there is any degree of stenosis of the cervix. Vaginal cytology is positive in 40–80% of cases. Endometrial biopsy will almost always detect an endometrial carcinoma, as will cytologic sampling of the endometrial cavity also. Curettage, first of the endocervix and then of the endometrial cavity, with careful examination under anesthesia is considered the most definitive method of diagnosing and clini-

Table 42–5. Staging for carcinoma of the corpus uteri.[1]

Stage	IA	G123	Tumor limited to endometrium
	IB	G123	Invasion to less than one-half the myometrium
	IC	G123	Invasion to more than one-half the myometrium
Stage	IIA	G123	Endocervical glandular involvement only
	IIB	G123	Cervical stromal invasion
Stage	IIIA	G123	Tumor invades serosa and/or ad- nexa, and/or positive peritoneal cy- tology
	IIIB	G123	Vaginal metastasis
	IIIC	G123	Metastases to pelvic and/or para- aortic lymph nodes
Stage	IVA	G123	Tumor invasion of bladder and/or bowel mucosa
	IVB		Distant metastases, including intra- abdominal and/or inguinal lymph nodes

Histopathology: Degree of differentiation–

Cases of carcinoma of the corpus should be classi- fied (or graded) according to the degree of histo- logic differentiation as follows:

G1	5% or less of a nonsquamous or nonmorular solid growth pattern
G2	6–50% of a nonsquamous or non- morular solid growth pattern
G3	More than 50% of a nonsquamous or nonmorular solid growth pattern

Notable nuclear atypia, inappropriate for architec- tural grade, raises the grade of a grade 1 or grade 2 tumor by 1.

In serous adenocarcinomas, clear cell adenocarci- nomas, and squamous cell carcinomas, nuclear grading takes precedence.

Adenocarcinomas with squamous differentiation are graded according to the nuclear grade of the glandu- lar component.

[1]International Federation of Gynecology and Obstetrics: An- nual report on the results of treatment in gynecological cancer. Int J Gynecol Obstet 1989;28:189.

cally staging the disease. Myometrial involvement is suspected if the corpus is enlarged. Magnetic reso- nance imaging may be helpful in defining myome- trial penetration.

Differential Diagnosis

Other causes of postmenopausal and inter- menstrual bleeding such as vaginitis, cervicitis, pol- yps, cervical cancer, and hormonal therapy must be considered. (See section menstrual disorders, above.)

Complications

Endometrial carcinoma that is histologically poorly

differentiated may disseminate relatively early in the course of the disease. Metastatic spread to the vagina, regional pelvic and para-aortic lymph nodes, ovaries, lungs, brain, and bone may occur.

The most frequent site of recurrence following treatment for endometrial carcinoma is the vaginal vault.

Prevention

There is presumptive evidence that cyclic progesterone therapy will reduce the possibility of endometrial carcinoma in the anovulatory patient as well as in the postmenopausal women receiving estrogen replacement therapy. Detection and adequate therapy of the precursors of the disease (polyps, hyperplasia, and carcinoma in situ of the endometrium) will prevent the subsequent development of endometrial carcinoma.

Treatment

Total hysterectomy and bilateral salpingo-oophorectomy are recommended in the patient with a well-differentiated tumor in a small uterus without cervical involvement.

Total abdominal hysterectomy and bilateral salpingo-oophorectomy is definitive therapy for endometrial carcinoma. Washings of the peritoneal cavity for cytologic examination should be obtained at the time. If the tumor involves more than 50% of the myometrial thickness and is grade 2 or 3—or if there is evidence of gross adnexal or pelvic lymph node metastases—pelvic and para-aortic lymph node dissection should be done. Stage IIB disease is treated in a similar fashion. Adjuvant radiation therapy is administered to those with nodal disease and to those with deep myometrial involvement.

The application of multiple small-dose radium capsules (Heyman packing technique) to the endometrial cavity, supplemented by intravaginal radium and full pelvis external therapy, is the treatment of choice in patients who are considered poor surgical risks. Stage II disease is treated with preoperative intracavitary and full pelvis external radiation therapy followed by total abdominal hysterectomy and bilateral salpingo-oophorectomy. Radical hysterectomy with bilateral pelvic lymph node dissection can be used in selected patients who are in good general condition.

Disseminated endometrial carcinoma is treated with large-dose progestin therapy (hydroxyprogesterone caproate, medroxyprogesterone or megestrol), which produces satisfactory remission of the metastatic disease in about 35% of cases, particularly in patients with tumors that are positive for progesterone receptors. Subjective improvement is noted in the majority of patients so treated. Cisplatin or carboplatin, doxorubicin, and cyclophosphamide are given to those with absent receptors and disseminated disease.

Prognosis

Five-year survival rates of 70–90% are recorded in stage I disease. This drops to 60% in stage II. Histologic undifferentiation, deep myometrial penetration, and absence of estrogen and progesterone receptors all worsen the prognosis.

de Cicco Nardone F: Hormone receptor status in human endometrial adenocarcinoma. Cancer 1989;64:2572.

Doering DL et al: Intraoperative evaluation of depth of myometrial invasion in stage I endometrial adenocarcinoma. Obstet Gynecol 1989;74:930.

Feuer GA, Canalog A: Endometrial carcinoma: Treatment of positive para-aortic nodes. Gynecol Oncol 1987; 27:104.

Hricak H et al: Endometrial carcinoma staging by MR imaging. Radiology 1987;162:297.

Mannel RS et al: Management of endometrial cancer with suspected cervical involvement. Obstet Gynecol 1990; 75:1016.

Moore DH et al: Morbidity of lymph node sampling in cancers of the uterine corpus and cervix. Obstet Gynecol 1989;74:180.

Torrisi JR: Postoperative adjuvant external-beam radiotherapy in surgical stage I endometrial carcinoma. Cancer 1989;64:1414.

Varia M et al: Primary radiation therapy for medically inoperable patients with endometrial carcinoma: Stages I–II. Int J Radiat Oncol Biol Phys 1987;13:11.

SARCOMAS OF THE UTERUS

Uterine sarcomas are relatively rare. They may arise in preexisting leiomyomas, from the myometrium itself, or from the endometrial stroma. Mixed tumors (carcinosarcoma, mixed mesodermal tumors) containing both epithelial and connective tissue malignant cells are also encountered.

Sarcomas of the uterus metastasize via the bloodstream and lymphatics and spread by contiguity. The lungs are a frequent site of metastatic disease.

In patients in whom the tumor is confined to the pelvic organs, treatment consists of total hysterectomy and bilateral salpingo-oophorectomy with individualized postoperative radiation or chemotherapy (or both) for those with deep myometrial invasion.

The outlook for patients with uterine sarcoma is variable. Leiomyosarcomas with more than ten mitoses per ten high-power fields carry a poor prognosis, with recurrence within 5 years in about two-thirds of patients. Approximately 70% of patients with between five and nine mitoses per ten high-power fields are cured. About 40% of patients with malignant mixed müllerian tumors survive.

Doxorubicin (Adriamycin) has been reported to be effective in the treatment of some leiomyosarcomas. High-dose progestin therapy will bring about complete resolution of metastatic low-grade endometrial sarcoma in some patients. Unresectable or recurrent malignant mixed mesodermal tumors may respond to vincristine, cyclophosphamide, and dactinomycin.

Covens AL et al: Uterine sarcoma: An analysis of 74 cases. Am J Obstet Gynecol 1987;156:370.

Leibson S et al: Leiomyosarcoma in a series of hysterectomies performed for presumed uterine leiomyomas. Am J Obstet Gynecol 1990;162:968.

O'Connor DM, Norris HJ: Mitotically active leiomyomas of the uterus. Hum Pathol 1990;21:223.

Rose PG, Boutselis JG, Sachs L: Adjuvant therapy for stage I uterine sarcoma. Am J Obstet Gynecol 1987;156:660.

Silverberg SG et al: Carcinosarcoma (malignant mixed mesodermal tumor) of the uterus: A Gynecologic Oncology Group pathologic study of 203 cases. Int J Gynecol Pathol 1990;9:1.

OVARIAN TUMORS

Essentials of Diagnosis

- Adnexal mass palpated during pelvic examination.
- Rupture of a cyst or a twisted pedicle may produce symptoms of an acute abdominal emergency.
- Abdominal distention and symptoms of pressure on surrounding organs are manifestations of a large tumor or of ascites resulting from peritoneal seeding.
- Abdominopelvic CT scanning and ultrasonography often are helpful. Because the ovaries are a frequent metastatic site for bowel cancer, x-ray studies of the small and large intestine are indicated when ovarian cancer is suspected.
- Laparoscopy is often useful.
- Paracentesis with cytologic examination of ascitic fluid.
- Chest x-ray will demonstrate pulmonary disease and pleural fluid.
- Culdocentesis with cytologic examination of a small amount of peritoneal fluid (which is present under normal circumstances) may detect very early lesions.

General Considerations

Because of their complex embryologic and histogenetic development, the ovaries are a source of a greater variety of tumors, both benign and malignant, than any other organ in the body. Ovarian tumors may be frankly benign, frankly malignant, or somewhere in between; they may be solid or cystic, or there may be mixed types; and they may be functional (producing sex steroids) or nonfunctional. Of greatest clinical significance is the fact that whether benign or malignant, they are often clinically silent until late in the course of their development.

Benign cysts of the ovary may be functional (follicle or corpus luteum cysts) or proliferative (dermoid, serous, and mucinous cystadenomas). The more frequent solid benign tumors are fibromathecomas, fibroadenomas, and the Brenner tumors. Endometriosis is a frequent cause of cystic enlargement of the ovary (see section on endometriosis, above).

The common malignant tumors are serous and mucinous cystadenocarcinoma, endometrioid carcinoma, and undifferentiated solid adenocarcinoma. Less common are the hormone-producing neoplasms: granulosa-theca cell tumors, Sertoli-Leydig cell tumors, and adrenal cell rest tumors. These have variable degrees of malignancy. Rarely encountered are tumors of germ cell origin, ranging from the dysgerminoma, the homolog of the testicular seminoma, to the highly malignant teratocarcinoma, immature teratoma, and endodermal sinus tumor. Metastatic carcinoma from the gastrointestinal tract (Krukenberg's tumor), breast, pancreas, and kidney must always be considered as a possible diagnosis whenever there is bilateral malignant disease of the ovaries.

Follicle cysts result from failure of a number of developing ovarian follicles to undergo atresia (regression) during the second half of the menstrual cycle. Usually they appear as multiple cystic structures filled with clear serous fluid, but they may be single. Rarely do they cause the ovary to become larger than 6–7 cm in diameter.

Corpus luteum cysts likewise do not become very large. They are single cysts and result from failure of the corpus luteum to regress; they often contain an amber or brown serous fluid, or they may be filled with blood.

Dermoid cysts (benign cystic teratomas) are common, comprising about 20% of all ovarian tumors in mature women. Occasionally, they are bilateral (8–15%). They may vary from a few millimeters to more than 20 cm in diameter, and the external appearance is one of a smooth, glistening, thick-walled, pearly-gray cyst. When opened, they are found to contain a thick sebaceous material and hair. Occasionally, bone structures and teeth are found. In fact, almost any tissue may be found on microscopic examination. A rare but interesting type is the benign cystic teratoma composed largely of thyroid tissue (struma ovarii), which, if functional, may give rise to hyperthyroidism. Current thinking regarding the histogenesis of these tumors is that they develop from an autofertilization of haploid germ cells. Malignant change is rarely encountered in dermoid cysts, but where it occurs most such tumors are squamous cell carcinomas.

Serous, endometrioid, and mucinous cystic tumors (cystomas, cystadenomas, cystadenocarcinomas) arise from the surface epithelium of the ovary, derived from the primitive coelomic epithelium. Approximately 85–90% of ovarian cancers arise from these cells, and the tumor type depends on the direction of cellular differentiation. The serous variety is the most common (20% of benign tumors and 40% of malignant tumors). They may become very large—particularly those of the mucinous type—and may fill and distend the entire abdomen. They may be unilocular or multilocular. If they contain small papillary excrescences, the likelihood of cancer is greater. Although mucinous tumors of a benign type are about as frequent as the serous variety, malignant mucinous tumors are less common (10% of ovarian cancers). Endometrioid carcinomas are the second most frequent variety (24% of ovarian cancers). A 50% risk of ovarian cancer has been documented in patients with a family history of two first-degree relatives with the disease. An increased risk has also been observed in women from families with a background of bowel cancer.

Granulosa-theca cell and **Sertoli-Leydig cell tumors** arise from the ovarian stroma. They frequently retain the ability to secrete sex hormones (estrogen, androgen), producing the systemic effects associated with these steroids—feminization or masculinization, as the case may be. The granulosa-theca cell tumors are the most frequent of the hormonally active tumors, constituting about 4–6% of ovarian cancers. About two-thirds are benign in their clinical behavior. Sertoli-Leydig cell tumors are rare and usually manifest themselves first by producing defeminization (amenorrhea, atrophy of the breast) and then masculinization (deepening of the voice, hirsutism, clitoral hypertrophy). Like granulosa-theca cell tumors, the majority are benign, the reported incidence of cancer being about 20%.

The staging of ovarian cancer recommended by the International Federation of Gynecology and Obstetrics is shown in Table 42–6.

Clinical Findings

Functional cysts of one or both ovaries are a frequent finding on routine pelvic examination of young women in the reproductive age group. In general, these are nonneoplastic and cause no symptoms. They rarely become larger than 8 cm in diameter and usually regress without treatment. Torsion of the pedicle with consequent strangulation may occur, producing abdominal pain of sudden onset, nausea and vomiting, a tender abdominopelvic mass, peritoneal irritation, slight fever, and moderate leukocytosis. Dermoid cysts are particularly apt to twist in this fashion. Because they are usually filled with sebaceous material and may contain tooth structures, these may be diagnosed by x-ray.

Any enlargement of the ovary in women of menopausal or postmenopausal age should be regarded as malignant until proved otherwise. Nodularity of an ovarian tumor (palpated on pelvic examination) is presumptive evidence of cancer, as is associated ascites also. Although ultrasonography or CT scanning may be helpful, it is often impossible to determine the benign or malignant nature of an ovarian tumor until laparotomy. Papillarity of the external surface, adherence to surrounding structures, and peritoneal implants are signs of cancer. Psammoma bodies seen on

Table 42–6. Staging for carcinoma of the ovary.[1]

Staging of ovarian carcinoma is based on findings at clinical examination and by surgical exploration. The histologic findings are to be considered in the staging, as are the cytologic findings as far as effusions are concerned. It is desirable that a biopsy specimen be taken from suspicious areas outside of the pelvis.

Stage	I	Growth limited to the ovaries.
	IA	Growth limited to one ovary; no ascites present containing malignant cells. No tumor on the external surface; capsule intact.
	IB	Growth limited to both ovaries; no ascites present containing malignant cells. No tumor on the external surface; capsules intact.
	IC[2]	Tumor classified as either stage IA or IB but with tumor on the surface of one or both ovaries or with ruptured capsules; or with ascites containing malignant cells or with positive peritoneal washings.
Stage	II	
	IIA	Growth involving one or both ovaries, with pelvic extension.
	IIB	Extension and/or metastases to the uterus and/or tubes.
	IIC[2]	Extension to other pelvic tissues. Tumor either stage IIA or IIB but with tumor on the surface of one or both ovaries; or with capsules ruptured; or with ascites containing malignant cells or with positive peritoneal washings.
Stage	III	
		Tumor involving one or both ovaries with peritoneal implants outside the pelvis and/or positive retroperitoneal or inguinal nodes. Superficial liver metastasis. Tumor is limited to the true pelvis but with histologically proved malignant extension to small bowel or omentum.
	IIIA	Tumor grossly limited to the true pelvis with negative nodes but with histologically confirmed microscopic seeding of abdominal peritoneal surfaces.
	IIIB	Tumor of one or both ovaries with histologically confirmed implants of abdominal peritoneal surfaces, none exceeding 2 cm in diameter; nodes are negative.
	IIIC	Abdominal implants > 2 cm in diameter and/or positive retroperitoneal or inguinal nodes.
Stage	IV	
		Growth involving one or both ovaries with distant metastases. Pleural effusion containing malignant cells. Parenchymal liver metastases.

[1]International Federation of Gynecology and Obstetrics: Annual report on the results of treatment in gynecological cancer. Int J Gynecol Obstet 1989;28:189.
[2]It should be noted whether rupture of the capsules was spontaneous or caused by the surgeon and if the source of malignant cells was peritoneal washings or ascites.

x-ray may arouse suspicion of a papillary process. If there is any doubt at the time of surgery, the tumor should be removed without spilling its contents into the peritoneal cavity and should be submitted to a pathologist in the operating room for gross examination and frozen-section microscopic analysis of any suspicious areas. These cystic enlargements may represent simple cysts, serous or mucinous cystadenomas, or cystadenocarcinomas with serous, mucinous, endometrioid, or mesonephric duct epithelium.

Solid enlargements of the ovary may be benign. Fibroma-thecoma tumors of the ovary comprise about 5% of benign ovarian neoplasms. They are smooth, rounded, firm, mobile masses, usually unilateral and relatively small. An infrequent accompaniment of these solid, benign ovarian tumors is the development of ascites and right-sided hydrothorax (Meigs' syndrome). The ascites in these benign tumors is believed to be related to fluid seepage from the tumor into the peritoneal cavity, with subsequent transfer to the pleural cavity via the diaphragmatic lymphatics.

Tumors with solid as well as cystic areas palpated at the time of pelvic examination are highly suggestive of cancer, and the diagnosis is virtually certain if there are, in addition, nodulations in the cul-de-sac, an upper abdominal mass (omental cake), and ascites.

Differential Diagnosis

Ovarian enlargements must be distinguished from pedunculated uterine myomas, hydrosalpinx, tubal tuberculosis, diverticulitis, tumors of the colon, pelvic kidney, retroperitoneal tumors, and metastatic disease from distant sites. In most instances the correct diagnosis can be made if an accurate medical history is obtained, a careful physical examination performed, and judicious use made of ancillary diagnostic procedures such as CT scanning, ultrasonography, cytologic examination, and laparoscopy. Laparotomy is often required in order to establish the nature (malignant or benign) of an ovarian mass and, if the mass is malignant, to accurately assess (by clinical staging) the extent of disease. Any ascitic fluid should be submitted for cytologic examination. If ascites is not present, submit washings from the peritoneal cavity (saline or Ringer's solution). All peritoneal surfaces, parietal as well as visceral, including the undersurface of the diaphragm and the omentum, should be carefully inspected and palpated for evidence of metastases. Involvement of the pelvic and para-aortic lymph nodes also should be noted (Table 42–6).

Prevention

Bilateral salpingo-oophorectomy at the time of hysterectomy for benign uterine disease in women over age 40 and after childbearing function has been completed in younger women with strong family histories is advocated by many to prevent the possible development of ovarian cancer. Estrogen replacement should be given to forestall menopausal symptoms, osteoporosis, and atherosclerosis. The detection and removal of potentially malignant ovarian tumors (serous cystadenoma, granulosa-theca cell tumors, dysgerminomas, Sertoli-Leydig cell tumors) may prevent the development of ovarian cancer, particularly if both ovaries are removed. Problems arise

when one encounters such neoplasms in young women who wish to retain their childbearing potential. In such patients, a conservative approach with very careful follow-up examinations utilizing CA 125 (see below) and ultrasound testing is probably best.

Treatment

Cystic enlargements of the ovary suspected to be physiologic (follicle and corpus luteum cysts) require only repeat examinations at intervals of 4–6 weeks to ascertain that they are regressing.

Many benign neoplasms can be treated by simple excision, conserving the ovary. Dermoid cysts, endometriomas, simple serous cysts, and para-ovarian cysts (broad ligament cysts arising from mesonephric duct remnants) can be managed in this fashion. The proper management of ovarian neoplasms obviously requires an intimate knowledge of the gross appearance of ovarian tumors.

Cystadenomas and solid tumors of the ovary should, in younger women, be removed by unilateral salpingo-oophorectomy. The tumor should be opened in the operating room, and frozen-section examination of any solid or papillary areas should be done before the incision is closed.

Total hysterectomy and bilateral salpingo-oophorectomy are indicated in women who are approaching the menopause, in those who are older, or in those who have bilateral disease or evidence of peritoneal spread.

When the disease extends beyond the ovaries into the pelvis or abdomen (stage II or III), abdominal hysterectomy and bilateral salpingo-oophorectomy are done if surgically feasible. The omentum is removed, as it frequently contains microscopic or macroscopic metastatic disease. If complete removal of all gross tumor is not possible, remove as much as possible in order to reduce the tumor load. Radiation therapy or chemotherapy (or both) is then given. An antigen, CA 125, detectable in the serum, serves as a tumor marker and as a guide to the effectiveness of therapy. A second-look operation may be indicated following therapy.

Chemotherapy may take the form of combinations such as platinum compounds and cyclophosphamide. These agents are toxic, and close attention—particularly to hematopoietic and kidney function—must be maintained during treatment. Although these drugs are not curative, long-term remissions have occasionally been achieved with their use.

Small bowel obstruction due to tumor occasionally requires surgical treatment, but this should not be done in a patient in the terminal stage of the disease.

Prognosis

The outlook for patients with benign ovarian neoplasms is excellent. The prognosis for those with malignant disease is related primarily to histologic grade and extent of disease. Because 70% of such cancers are stage III or IV at the time of initial diagnosis, the overall cure rate for ovarian cancer is no more than 30%. For stage IA disease, however, 5-year survival rates of 80–85% can be achieved.

Andolf E, Jörgensen C, Östedt B: Ultrasound examination for detection of ovarian carcinoma in risk groups. Obstet Gynecol 1990;75:106.

Buchsbaum HJ et al: Surgical staging of carcinoma of the ovaries. Surg Gynecol Obstet 1989;169:226.

Dembo AJ et al: Prognostic factors in patients with stage I epithelial ovarian cancer. Obstet Gynecol 1990;75:263.

Lynch HT et al: Hereditary carcinoma of the ovary and associated cancers: A study of two families. Gynecol Oncol 1990;36:48.

Rubin SC et al: Serum CA 125 levels and surgical findings in patients undergoing secondary operations for epithelial ovarian cancer. Am J Obstet Gynecol 1989;160:667.

Scully RE: *Tumors of the Ovary and Maldeveloped Gonads.* Armed Forces Institute of Pathology Fascicle 16, 1979.

Sevelda P, Schemper M, Spona J: CA 125 as an independent prognostic factor for survival in patients with epithelial ovarian cancer. Am J Obstet Gynecol 1989;161: 1213.

Sevelda P, Dittrich C, Salzer H: Prognostic value of the rupture of the capsule in stage I epithelial ovarian cancer. Gynecol Oncol 1989;35:321.

Sparks JM, Varner RE: Ovarian cancer screening. Obstet Gynecol 1991;77:787.

Speroff T et al: A risk-benefit analysis of elective bilateral oophorectomy: Effect of changes in compliance with estrogen therapy on outcome. Am J Obstet Gynecol 1991;164:165.

Vasilev SA et al: Serum CA 125 levels in preoperative evaluation of pelvic masses. Obstet Gynecol 1988;71:751.

HYDATIDIFORM MOLE & CHORIOCARCINOMA

Essentials of Diagnosis

- Presumptive symptoms of pregnancy.
- Vaginal bleeding.
- Uterus disproportionately large for duration of pregnancy.
- Absence of fetus.
- Passage of grape-like vesicles.
- High serum or urine levels of hCG.

General Considerations

Hydatidiform mole represents hydropic changes in the placental villi of a pregnancy that is developing in the absence of an embryo (blighted ovum). The swelling of the villi is related to the absence of a fetal circulation and is often accompanied by varying degrees of trophoblastic proliferation. There is a tendency to myometrial penetration that may progress to frank, deep invasion of the uterine wall (chorioadenoma destruens, or invasive mole), and a small percentage (about 2–3%) of hydatidiform moles are

followed by development of the highly malignant choriocarcinoma.

The frequency of hydatidiform mole is about 1:2000–1500 pregnancies in the USA and about 1:650–240 pregnancies in the Far East and Mexico. Hydatidiform mole is also more common in women over 40 years of age.

Trophoblastic disease should be staged for the purpose of determining optimal treatment and prognosis (see Table 42–8).

Clinical Findings

The usual picture is one of a presumed threatened abortion, with a missed menstrual period, nausea, breast changes, and urinary frequency followed by vaginal bleeding. This may go on for several weeks with little or no abdominal pain. Examination reveals a disproportionately large uterus for the duration of the pregnancy in about 50% of cases. There may be bilateral cystic enlargement of the ovaries (theca lutein cysts). Preeclampsia may develop in women with large moles, and molar pregnancy should be suspected in any patient who develops hypertension, edema, and proteinuria in the first half of pregnancy. Anemia is common.

Serum and urinary hCG levels are unusually high and persist at high levels beyond the 12th week, when in normal pregnancy there is usually a significant drop. X-ray studies are helpful, and the absence of a fetal skeleton in a pregnancy longer than 16 weeks in duration is suggestive of molar pregnancy. Amniography (transabdominal injection of radiopaque material) has been largely replaced by ultrasound (B scan), which is diagnostic.

In many cases, the diagnosis is not made until the patient spontaneously aborts the molar pregnancy. All therapeutic abortion specimens should be carefully examined for the presence of hydatidiform mole.

Differential Diagnosis

Threatened abortion is the diagnosis most often entertained in the presence of a mole. Multiple pregnancy must be considered because it may produce unusually high levels of chorionic gonadotropin. If a fetal skeleton is visible on x-ray (at 16 weeks) or if a fetal heartbeat can be heard, the patient almost certainly does not have a mole.

Complications

About 15% of moles become locally invasive (chorioadenoma destruens), which carries the danger of hemorrhage owing to penetration of the vascular uterine wall or pelvic infection from perforation.

Two to three percent of moles are followed by choriocarcinoma, a highly malignant tumor. Although this cancer may occur after normal pregnancy, abortion, or ectopic pregnancy, about half of cases develop from an antecedent hydatidiform mole.

Metastases are found in the lungs, liver, central nervous system, bone, vagina, and vulva. High-risk metastatic gestational trophoblastic disease exists if (1) the duration of disease is longer than 4 months; (2) there are liver or brain metastases; (3) the βhCG titer is over 100,000 mIU/mL; or (4) it follows a full-term pregnancy.

Treatment

Once the diagnosis of a molar pregnancy has been established, the uterus should be emptied. This is done by dilation and curettage if the uterus is smaller than a 12–week pregnancy. Larger moles are better evacuated by suction with the simultaneous administration of oxytocin solution intravenously; this is then followed by careful curettage to ensure complete removal of the molar tissue. All specimens are examined pathologically for evidence of proliferative activity of the trophoblast, which serves as an index to the probability of malignant change.

Lutein cysts of the ovaries, which occur in about a third of molar pregnancies, will regress following removal of the mole and should not be surgically excised.

All patients with hydatidiform mole should be examined weekly following evacuation of the uterus for the possible development of chorioadenoma destruens or choriocarcinoma. Chest x-rays should be obtained at monthly intervals. Patients should be given effective contraceptive advice and advised not to become pregnant for at least a year. Weekly serum gonadotropin levels should be obtained, using beta subunit radioimmunoassays of hCG, until the titer is normal for 3 weeks; thereafter monthly levels are determined until the titer is normal for 6 months. It may take as long as 14–16 weeks for hCG to reach normal levels following molar evacuation. A plateau or disappearance of the hormone followed by a later reappearance, particularly with rising titers, is strongly suggestive of choriocarcinoma or invasive mole if pregnancy can be ruled out.

Methotrexate, a chemotherapeutic agent that competes with folic acid in cellular metabolism, has been very effective in controlling not only invasive moles but choriocarcinoma as well. It is given in courses of 15–25 mg/d for 5 days. It is an extremely cytotoxic agent and is preferably given by someone skilled in its use (see Chapter 48). Dactinomycin has been found to be equally effective as and less toxic than methotrexate. High-risk gestational trophoblastic disease is treated with combination chemotherapy: methotrexate, dactinomycin, and cyclophosphamide or chlorambucil. Cisplatin, vinblastine, bleomycin, and etoposide have been employed in resistant cases.

Prognosis

The prognosis for cure in hydatidiform mole and chorioadenoma destruens is excellent. Before the anticancer drugs became available, the outlook for choriocarcinoma was very poor. Five-year remission rates in the range of 80% of better are now being reported. In fact, if adequate treatment is initiated within 3 months of apparent onset, the figure is close to 100% if metastatic disease is limited to the lungs or pelvis and the initial hCG titer is less than 100,000 IU/24 h. A relatively poor prognosis exists in patients with one or more of the following: (1) initial hCG titer in excess of 1 million IU/24 h; (2) metastatic disease involving the central nervous system, liver, or gastrointestinal tract; (3) duration of disease of more than 4 months without treatment; (4) metastatic choriocarcinoma following a term pregnancy; or (5) resistance of the disease to single-agent chemotherapy.

Curry SL et al: Hormonal contraception and trophoblastic sequelae after hydatidiform mole: A Gynecologic Oncology Group study. Am J Obstet Gynecol 1989;160:805.

Hunter V et al: Efficacy of the metastatic survey in the staging of gestational trophoblastic disease. Cancer 1990; 65:1647.

Mortakis AE, Braga CA: "Poor prognosis" metastatic gestational trophoblastic disease: The prognostic significance of the scoring system in predicting chemotherapy failures. Obstet Gynecol 1990;76:272.

Rice LW et al: Persistent gestational trophoblastic tumor after partial hydatidiform mole. Gynecol Oncol 1990; 36:358.

Theodore C et al: Treatment of high-risk gestational trophoblastic disease with chemotherapy combinations containing cisplatin and etoposide. Cancer 1989;64:1824.

CORRECTION OF INFERTILITY DUE TO TUBAL ABNORMALITIES

A married couple may be considered infertile if a pregnancy does not occur after 1 year of normal coital activity without contraceptives. About 15% of marriages are infertile, and in approximately 40% of these there is a significant male factor (low sperm count, impaired motility, or anomalous forms). Chronic salpingitis is the single most common cause of sterility in women, although endometriosis and peritubal adhesions from previous appendicitis (with rupture) may be causative factors. Desire to reverse previous tubal sterilization is becoming a more common reason for tubal surgery.

Clinical Findings

There may or may not be palpable adnexal lesions. If chronic tubal disease is suspected, a hysterosalpingogram should be obtained. This may reveal an obstruction at the cornu, hydrosalpinx, fimbrial occlusion, or peritubal adhesions. If an oil contrast medium is used, the procedure itself may enhance fertility. Laparoscopy with the passage of a dye through a uterine cannula while the uterine tubes are under vision is an excellent diagnostic method and has largely replaced other methods of further investigation.

Treatment

Transvaginal tubal catheterization or probing by individuals trained in this technique may avoid the need for more elaborate procedures to relieve tubal obstruction. Tuboplasty operations are designed to reestablish tubal patency. These surgical procedures are more successful if the obstruction is localized and there is little damage to the uterine tube as a whole (fimbrial adhesions, previous tubal ligation). Reestablishment and maintenance of tubal patency have been more successful with the development of microsurgical techniques and the use of inert plastic materials for splinting and protecting the tube from adhesions during the healing process. Salpingolysis, reimplantation of the tube into the uterus, end-to-end anastomosis, and fimbrial salpingostomy are the operations usually performed. Preoperative, intraoperative, and postoperative administration of dexamethasone and promethazine is useful in prevention of postoperative pelvic adhesions following operations for infertility, as is the intraperitoneal instillation of 32% dextran 70 at the time of the operation.

In vitro fertilization as well as fertilization and transfer of a surrogate ovum is an alternative when tubal obstruction cannot be remedied.

Prognosis

An overall pregnancy incidence of about 20% is reported following tuboplasty, but about one in ten of these is a tubal pregnancy. The best results (26%) are achieved following cornual reimplantation when the remainder of the tube is anatomically and physiologically normal. Conception rates in excess of 50% can be achieved in the surgical correction of the simpler forms of tubal sterilization.

Boyers SP, DeCherney AH: Human in vitro fertilization and embryo transfer: An overview. In: *The 1987 Year Book of Obstetrics and Gynecology.* Year Book, 1987.

Kitchin JD III, Nunley WC Jr, Bateman BG: Surgical management of distal tubal occlusion. Am J Obstet Gynecol 1986;155:524.

Lang EK, Dunaway HE Jr, Roniger WE: Selective osteal salpingography and transvaginal catheter dilatation in the diagnosis and treatment of fallopian tube obstruction. AJR Am J Roentgenol 1990;154:735.

Thurmond AS, Rösch J: Nonsurgical fallopian tube recanalization for treatment of infertility. Radiology 1990; 174:371.

ENDOSCOPY IN GYNECOLOGY

The development of fiberoptics has stimulated the use of three techniques for the visualization of the internal organs of reproduction above the portio vaginalis of the cervix: culdoscopy, laparoscopy, and hysteroscopy. The first utilizes the knee-chest position and can be performed with either local or conduction (caudal or spinal) anesthesia. Laparoscopy is usually performed with the patient in the Trendelenburg position or in the dorsal recumbent position under general anesthesia. Hysteroscopy may be performed at the time of laparoscopy, though it can be done as an outpatient procedure using meperidine or diazepam plus paracervical block. The first two techniques depend upon the introduction of a pneumoperitoneum, atmospheric air usually being used in culdoscopy and either CO_2 or N_2O in laparoscopy. Hysteroscopy uses CO_2, dextran or dextrose; however, the new contact hysteroscope does not require distention. In addition to the diagnostic value of these techniques, they also allow for certain operative and manipulative procedures. Each method has its advantages and disadvantages and its proponents and opponents.

Culdoscopy can be performed under local anesthesia after preoperative sedation. Although CO_2 or N_2O pneumoperitoneum can be used, air is usually allowed to enter the peritoneal cavity through a posterior vaginal fornix/cul-de-sac puncture. Visualization is carried out transvaginally, and the view of the pelvic organs is somewhat more restricted than that seen through the laparoscope. The procedure is contraindicated whenever a lesion such as endometriosis, chronic salpingitis, or a tumor occupies the cul-de-sac. It cannot be done in the presence of vaginal atresia. Because of these limitations, it has been largely replaced by laparoscopy.

Laparoscopy has the disadvantage of requiring endotracheal anesthesia and operating room facilities. It affords a better view of the pelvic contents and allows a greater variety of manipulative and minor operative procedures than does culdoscopy. Laparoscopic cauterization and sectioning of the uterine tubes has become a widely accepted method of female sterilization. It can be done under local anesthesia in selected patients. The most significant complication is injury to the small intestine. It is contraindicated in patients with cardiac or respiratory insufficiency, abdominal hernias, large abdominal tumors, or advanced pregnancy and in patients with a likelihood of disseminated abdominal cancer. Previous abdominal surgery is not an absolute contraindication, and the procedure can be done safely in patients with abdominal surgical scars provided certain safeguards are observed in the induction of the pneumoperitoneum and the placement of the trocar through the anterior abdominal wall. Open laparoscopy, a modification of the original technique, allows examination of such patients with less risk of injury to the viscera. The field of operative laparoscopy is gradually being expanded to include many pelvic operations previously requiring laparotomy. It does require extensive training and experience.

Hysteroscopy, using CO_2, dextran, or dextrose to distend the endometrial cavity, has allowed more accurate diagnosis of intrauterine disorders such as submucous leiomyomas, endometrial and endocervical polyps, and intrauterine synechiae (Asherman's syndrome). It has also been advocated for the staging of endometrial carcinoma and has been useful in the localization and removal of misplaced and embedded IUDs. It has also been used to remove uterine septa and to treat intractable uterine bleeding. Contraindications to the procedure are acute and chronic upper genital tract infections, profuse bleeding, cervical stenosis, and recent uterine perforation.

Daly DC, Maier D, Sotoalbors C: Hysteroscopic metroplasty: Six years' experience. Obstet Gynecol 1989;73:201.

DeCherney AH, Diamond MP: Laparoscopic salpingostomy for ectopic pregnancy. Obstet Gynecol 1987; 70:948.

Grainger DA et al: Ureteral injuries at laparoscopy: Insights into diagnosis, management and prevention. Obstet Gynecol 1990;75:839.

Loffer FD: Hysteroscopy with selective endometrial sampling compared with D&C for abnormal uterine bleeding: The value of a negative hysteroscopic view. Obstet Gynecol 1989;73:16.

Loffer FD: Removal of large symptomatic growths by the hysteroscopic resectoscope. Obstet Gynecol 1990; 76:836.

March CM, Israel R: Hysteroscopic management of recurrent abortion caused by septate uterus. Obstet Gynecol 1987;156:834.

Nezhat C, Nezhat FR: Safe laser endoscopic excision or vaporization of peritoneal endometriosis. Fertil Steril 1989;52:149.

Paterson-Brown S et al: Laparoscopy as an adjunct to decision making in the "acute abdomen." Br J Surg 1986; 73:1022.

Perry CP, Upchurch JC: Pelviscopic adnexectomy. Am J Obstet Gynecol 1990;162:79.

Spirtos NM et al: Laparoscopy: A diagnostic aid in cases of suspected appendicitis. Its use in women of reproductive age. Am J Obstet Gynecol 1987;156:90.

Vancaillie TG: Electrocoagulation of the endometrium with the ball-end resectoscope. Obstet Gynecol 1989;74:425.

REFERENCES

Buchsbaum HJ, Walton LA (editors): *Strategies in Gynecologic Surgery.* Springer-Verlag, 1986.

Droegemueller W et al: *Clinical Gynecology.* Mosby, 1987.

Garcia CR, Mikutaa JJ, Rosenblum NG: *Current Therapy in Surgical Gynecology.* Mosby, 1986.

Kase NG, Weingold AB (editors): *Principles and Practice of Clinical Gynecology.* Wiley, 1983.

Rosenwaks Z, Benjamin F, Stone ML (editors): *Gynecology: Principles and Practice.* Macmillan, 1987.

Sanders RC, James AE Jr (editors): *The Principles and Practice of Ultrasonography in Obstetrics and Gynecology,* 3rd ed. Appleton-Century-Crofts, 1985.

Sanz LE (editor): *Gynecologic Surgery.* Medical Economics, 1988.

Orthopedics

43

David S. Bradford, MD, Robert S. Pashman. MD, Serena S. Hu, MD, Lorraine J. Day, MD, Peter G. Trafton, MD, Howard A. Cohen, MD, & James O. Johnston, MD

A Note on Terminology

The specialized vocabulary of orthopedics facilitates communication between experienced practitioners, but for the uninitiated, the terminology may seem impenetrable. In general, the use of eponyms to describe fractures or deformities is best avoided by the student and nonorthopedist. Although well-entrenched eponyms are included in this chapter, it is often less confusing to use anatomic terms. A few conventional terms will be defined to simplify this task.

Varus and **valgus** are descriptive terms frequently used in the characterization of angular musculoskeletal deformities. They refer to the direction of the apex of the deformity in relation to the midline of the body. If the apex points away from the midline, the deformity is varus. If the apex is directed toward the midline, the deformity is valgus. Knock-knees are an example of valgus deformity; the entire lower limb is abnormally angulated, with the apex of the deformity (the knee) pointing toward the midline. In bowlegs, the angle of deformity points away from the midline; this condition is called varus knees or genu varum. Similar designations apply to angular deformities of the elbow (cubitus varus or valgus) and the hip (coxa vara or valga).

When a long bone such as the femur or humerus is fractured, the limb may be visibly deformed. The relationship between the main fracture fragments, or the **alignment,** can be characterized by describing the angular deformity. In this case, the fracture itself constitutes the apex of the deformity and may be designated as varus or valgus. The fracture is said to be **comminuted** if the bones are fragmented. If the main bony fragments are widely separated, the fracture is **displaced.**

If there is a wound overlying the fracture through which the fracture is exposed or through which it may have communicated with the external environment, the fracture is described as **open.** This is a critical aspect of skeletal injury, as the likelihood of fracture contamination must be urgently addressed by surgically cleaning the wound. In this way, the surgeon strives to minimize infection of the fracture and thus avoid the potentially catastrophic consequences. A fracture of the femur produced by high-energy impact, such as that sustained in a motorcycle accident, might well be found to be "an open, comminuted midshaft femoral fracture, with wide displacement and severe valgus deformity."

Joint dislocations also warrant immediate treatment. Vascular structures spanning the joint may be torn at the time of injury or may be temporarily occluded by stretch deformation resulting from malalignment of the joint. Any description of a dislocation should include the status of pulses distal to the joint. If the vessels are torn, early repair is often required to restore circulation. If the vessel is occluded by stretch, the joint must be promptly returned to its proper alignment to reestablish distal blood flow. The maneuver to restore proper alignment of a joint or fracture is called **reduction.**

Joint or fracture reduction may be performed by **open** (surgical) or **closed** (nonsurgical) techniques. A dislocation or fracture is described as **unstable** if there is a high likelihood of further deformation. Following reduction, unstable fractures or dislocations may be stabilized by closed or open technique. Closed techniques involve traction, casts, or splint; open techniques involve surgical application of hardware to secure fixation of the fragments. The surgical management of an unstable fracture or dislocation is therefore described as "open reduction and internal fixation."

FRACTURES & JOINT INJURIES*

FRACTURES & DISLOCATIONS OF THE SPINE
(Figure 43–1)

The spinal column can be viewed as a segmented semiflexible long bone with both a weight-bearing

---

*Injuries of the hand are discussed in Chapter 45.

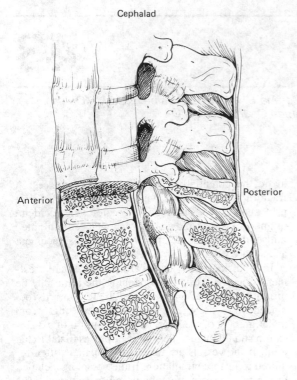

Cephalad

Anterior

Posterior

Figure 43–1. Anatomy of the spine.

function, which requires stability, and a mobility function, which tends to compromise stability. Mobility is greatest in the cervical spine, least in the thoracic spine, and intermediate in the lumbar spine.

The spine also protects the spinal cord from trauma. In the cervical and thoracic spine, the spinal canal contains the spinal cord, nerve roots, and spinal nerves as they exit from the neural foramina. During development, the spinal cord does not grow as rapidly longitudinally as the spine, so the terminal segment of the spinal cord (conus medullaris) ends near the lower border of the first lumbar vertebra. The dural sac distal to the lumbar vertebra 1 (L1) contains the spinal nerves for all the segments from L2 through sacral 5 (S5). One nerve pair exits at each appropriate spinal segment. The spinal cord cannot spontaneously recover from a functionally **complete** injury (no voluntary nervous function below the injury site). However, spinal nerves at or below (cauda equina) will recover from functionally complete injuries if they have not been transected and if initial compression by bone fragment, angulation, disk material, etc, has been relieved. Complete spinal cord injury above the level of L2 persisting for over 24 hours or after recovery from spinal shock is predictably permanent. **Spinal shock** is defined as temporary loss of reflex activity in the spinal cord at and below the level of injury. The occasional references to apparent

recovery are probably cases where spinal shock masked an incomplete lesion.

Fracture healing follows the same sequence in the spine as in the extremities. The deeply buried anatomic site of the spinal column and the proximity of the spinal cord permit fewer reduction and immobilization procedures, particularly if a sensory deficit secondary to spinal cord or cauda equina injury is present. External immobilization devices such as casts or braces may cause pressure ulceration on insensitive skin.

Most fractures and dislocations in the spinal column are the result of compression forces or, less often, extension forces. Except for gunshot wounds, direct trauma to the spine is rarely the mechanism of injury. Knowing the mechanism of injury frequently helps in designing the treatment plan. For example, flexion and compression injuries are usually best reduced and maintained with extension and traction forces.

The most common spine fracture is anterior compression injury to the vertebral body at or near the thoracolumbar junction (Figure 43–2). These fractures are usually stable and seldom accompanied by spinal cord injury. They require only accurate diagnosis to exclude the possibility of instability, followed by symptomatic treatment and ambulation as early as comfort permits. A corset or brace is used for protection from recurrent hyperflexion for 3–6 weeks. This type of injury is most common in persons of middle age or older and may occur following minor trauma in patients with osteoporosis. Adolescent patients or young adults with moderately severe but stable compression fractures may require 6 weeks

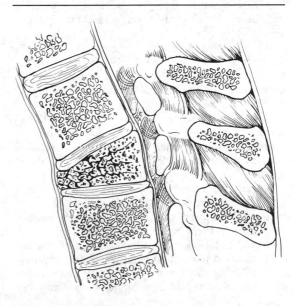

Figure 43–2. Anterior compression fracture. Note lack of neural canal involvement.

of recumbency in extension. An extension body cast or brace is then used for an additional 6 weeks to limit the degree of angulation secondary to settling at the fracture site.

Spinal cord injury patients, particularly quadriplegics, carry a significant risk of pulmonary embolism, gastrointestinal bleeding, pulmonary insufficiency secondary to intercostal muscle paralysis, hypotension, and paralytic ileus. In addition, bowel and bladder dysfunction are present in patients who have lost sphincter control.

Classification of Injury

A. Classification of Bony Injury: The spinal column consists of three components that contribute to its stability. (1) the vertebral bodies. (2) the posterior elements (pedicles, laminae, spinous process, and interlocking paired facets at each level), and (3) the ligamentous and musculoaponeurotic sleeves attached to the bone. In general, an injury disrupting only one of the three components will be relatively stable if protected, whereas if all three components are disrupted, the spinal column will be significantly unstable at the level of injury with risk of reinjury to the spinal canal contents. If injury is present in two of the components, the degree of instability will lie between these extremes. For example, the common mild anterior compression fracture at the thoracolumbar junction of the vertebral body is stable, whereas anterior dislocation of the cervical vertebrae is quite unstable. In the latter injury, there is complete anterior displacement of the facets, disruption of the posterior elements, rupture of the interspinous ligaments and the capsule of the facet joints, and disruption of the entire annulus fibrosus with or without a small fracture of the anterior vertebral body beneath the dislocation.

B. Classification of Neurologic Injury: Patients with fracture or dislocation of the spine must have a thorough initial neurologic examination that is adequately recorded. The patient must be reassessed at intervals as the clinical situation demands. Patients with spinal injury fall into one of three categories.

1. No neurologic deficit.

2. Complete neurologic deficit at the level of injury–These patients have no sensation or voluntary motor function below the level of injury. In the first hours after significant spinal cord injury, spinal shock produces complete flaccid paralysis. This usually terminates in less than 24 hours, accompanied by return of muscle tone and reflex activity below the level of the lesion. The lowest reflex available to the examiner is the bulbocavernosus reflex (contraction of the anal sphincter on compression of the glans penis or clitoris), and the lowest voluntary muscle is the external anal sphincter. After spinal shock subsides, the examiner should not mistake reflex muscle contraction for voluntary muscle activity. The conus medullaris portion of the cord has virtually no long

tract segments, which is why complete cauda equina lesions cause permanent flaccid paralysis.

3. Incomplete neurologic deficit–In these lesions, some function is retained. Most can be subcategorized as anterior cord, posterior cord, central cord, or Brown-Séquard lesions (ipsilateral muscle paralysis and contralateral hypesthesia for pain and temperature). Occasionally, there will be isolated root (spinal nerve) lesions. The category is determined by matching the neurologic deficit to the cross-sectional geography of the spinal cord at the level of injury. The major determinant of severity of spinal cord injury occurs at the time of impact. It is felt that removal of bony or disk fragments from the canal and alignment of an angulated spinal column may increase the possibility of recovery. Brown-Séquard lesions have the highest probability of recovery of significant function. Central cord lesions have a high probability of recovery in the lower extremities but a poor prognosis in the upper extremities. Selection of treatment is based on the severity of injury as categorized by Frankel and associates. Category A includes patients with no motor or neurologic function; B, those with sensory sparing but no significant motor function; C, those with voluntary motor capabilities but insufficient strength for significant functional use (ie, motor units unable to move a part against gravity); D, those who retain functionally useful but less than completely normal motor power; and E, those with complete motor power and sensation.

Clinical Findings

A. History and Physical Examination: Conscious patients will have pain at the fracture site and local tenderness, best elicited by percussion over the spinous processes at the site of injury. Visible external deformity is seldom apparent except in the thoracolumbar spine particularly at or near the thoracolumbar junction. The possibility of neurologic deficit requires a careful search even though gross normal motor power and sensation may be present in all four extremities. Sphincter loss from cauda equina or conus medullaris lesions may involve only the last few sacral segments and is best detected by assessment of active rectal sphincter control and perianal sensation. The important distinction between Frankel categories C and D will be appreciated only if the neurologic examination includes assessment (and recording) of motor power.

Unconscious patients are extremely difficult to classify accurately. A history of trauma as a cause of unconsciousness or a traumatic episode during unconsciousness calls for x-rays of the entire spinal column. The spinal column must be protected if unstable fracture or spinal canal compromise is identified.

B. Imaging Studies: All patients with significant injury and pain in the spinal area require anteroposterior and lateral x-rays of appropriate regions of the spine. Overlying shadows (ribs, transverse processes, visceral soft tissue shadows) frequently make accurate interpretation of fracture configuration difficult. Right and left oblique x-rays or tomography can be of assistance. CT scan provides a way of assessing all components of the spine, including neural canal integrity, and does not require turning of the patient. Myelography is of no prognostic value in the patient with complete spinal cord injury; it is useful in evaluating the extent and site of possible compression of the dural contents in partial lesions.

Complications

Patients with cervical spine injury may have impaired pulmonary function secondary to intercostal muscle paralysis.

Patients with thoracolumbar spine fractures with or without spinal cord injury may have paralytic ileus secondary to sympathetic chain dysfunction. Oral intake should be limited to clear fluids initially, and gastric suction may be necessary if the degree or duration of ileus is significant.

In the acute phase of spinal cord injury, pulmonary embolism is a significant risk. Anticoagulation is usually not advisable, because it may cause bleeding at the site of cord injury. Frequent turning of the patient, passive motion of the lower extremities, and use of elastic stockings are indicated.

Visceral injury may be masked in the paralyzed patient and necessitates careful monitoring of the abdomen and chest for signs of bleeding or organ injury.

Treatment

A. Spine Fractures or Dislocations Without Neurologic Deficit: The goal of treatment is to maintain stability sufficient to protect the cord from pressure resulting from recurrent angulation or displacement of fragments at the fracture site.

1. Stable fractures–Fractures with a stable configuration, such as a common anterior wedge compression, can be managed by the use of a simple neck brace or cervical collar or an extension type brace or corset at the level of the thoracolumbar spine. In the adolescent or young adult patient with anterior compression greater than 50% of normal vertebral height, recumbency for 6 weeks in an extension cast or brace followed by ambulation with an extension brace may prevent a late increase in deformity. In older people, early mobilization is necessary to avoid the complications of prolonged bed rest.

2. Unstable fractures or fracture-dislocations–These injuries require external immobilization (cast or brace), skeletal traction, or reduction and internal fixation. In most cervical spine fractures, skeletal traction in the long axis will achieve adequate reduction and restore canal integrity. If used as definitive treatment, 6–12 weeks of traction in recumbency is required, followed by appropriate bracing for another 6–12 weeks. However, halo-vest or halo-cast immobilization (Figure 43–3) will permit control with earlier ambulation. Ninety-five percent of cervical spine injuries become stable after 3 months of immobilization. If both facet joints are dislocated, traction with guarded manipulation may reduce the dislocation. If the dislocation persists, open reduction and internal fixation are indicated. In the cervical spine, interspinous wiring provides stability. External support postoperatively is usually required.

Thoracolumbar fractures may be reduced by positioning in bed or on a fracture table, followed by protection with a body cast or body brace. Most unstable fractures require 6 weeks of recumbency before ambulation. Open reduction and internal fixation are justified in patients who require early mobilization to prevent complications such as acute respiratory distress syndrome (eg, multiply injured or very elderly patients). In the thoracolumbar spine, skeletal traction (halo-femoral or halo-tibial) will diminish angulation but usually will not reduce the fracture fragments encroaching on the canal. Facet dislocation in the thoracolumbar spine almost always requires open reduction and internal fixation to restore stability. In the thoracolumbar spine, internal fixation is most commonly achieved with Harrington distraction rods. Compression rods are available for use in fractures caused by traction injuries. Shorter segments of spine can be stabilized with a system of pedicle-screw fixation. Metal plates are placed posteriorly, with fixation by screws through the plates into the vertebral pedicle. Such instrumentation is followed by monitored ambulation with the patient in a body jacket or equivalent protection. Some injuries require a longer period of recumbency, even after internal fixation. The

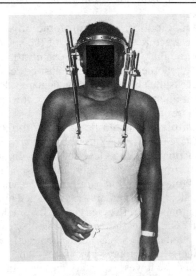

Figure 43–3. Halo cast for immobilization of cervical spine injuries. The halo is attached by metal bars to a well-fitting plaster body jacket. This allows the patient to be ambulatory soon after injury.

segment of injury should be fused by placement of an onlay bone graft; the internal fixative device may be removed after the fracture and graft have healed.

B. Spine Fractures or Dislocations With Neurologic Deficit:

1. Incomplete neurologic deficit–

a. Patients with stable fractures can be treated in the same way as patients with no neurologic abnormalities if angulation is corrected and if CT scan shows no evidence of bone or disk fragments significantly compromising the canal. If a significant degree of canal compromise is demonstrated, consideration of surgical decompression is justified. This can be done either through an anterolateral approach (followed by strut graft) or through a posterior costotransversectomy approach including pedicle removal and Harrington rod fixation for stability.

b. Patients with incomplete neurologic deficit and unstable fracture or fracture-dislocation have the same stability requirements as patients without neurologic deficit. They more often require either internal fixation or continuous traction in recumbency, since many of these patients have a significant neurologic deficit and cannot tolerate plaster casts. Neural canal compromise should be managed as in the preceding paragraph.

2. Complete neurologic deficit–No operative procedure has been devised that will achieve recovery in cases of complete neurologic deficit that has persisted beyond the stage of spinal shock. It is important to prevent significant late deformity for two reasons: (1) because deformity may interfere with rehabilitation training and (2) because it may result in loss of function at a higher level if it causes angulation tension on the roots just above the level of injury. All stable bony injuries are treated in the same way as those that occur in neurologically negative patients except that any brace device that extends below the level of sensory loss carries a risk of pressure ulceration and needs to be properly designed and the skin underneath checked frequently. Patients with unstable injuries of the cervical spine can be managed with continuous traction for 6–12 weeks. Frequent turning either in an ordinary hospital bed or on a turning frame and good skin care are necessary to prevent pressure ulceration.

Relatively early mobilization of patients with cervical spine injuries can be achieved using halo-vest immobilization. In some cervical fractures of the "burst type" with intact posterior elements, surgical replacement of the comminuted body with iliac or fibular strut graft will produce adequate stability for early mobilization of the patient with only a cervical brace for protection (Figures 43–4 and 43–5). In thoracolumbar spine injuries, halo-femoral or halo-tibial traction can minimize the risk of motion at the fracture site, but it makes turning of completely paralyzed patients more difficult. If postural positioning is ineffective in controlling motion in markedly un-

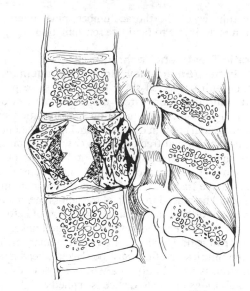

Figure 43–4. "Burst" fracture. Note encroachment on neural canal.

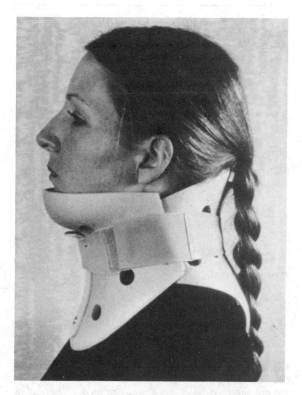

Figure 43–5. Collar for immobilization of stable cervical injuries.

stable injuries of the thoracolumbar spine, internal fixation is desirable to facilitate rehabilitation.

Specific Treatment Techniques

A. Initial (Emergency Room) Management: Patients with suspected spine injuries must be protected from angulatory stress until adequate neurologic and radiologic examination has identified or ruled out spinal column or spinal cord injury. Patients with unstable spinal fractures with or without spinal injury should receive immediate treatment as outlined above. For example, a patient with an unstable cervical spine fracture with or without spinal cord injury should be placed in skeletal traction in the emergency room or equivalent initial contact point before other studies or treatment programs are undertaken.

B. Traction: To be effective in the management of spine injuries, traction must be skeletal; head halter traction is useful only as a temporary device before skull tongs or a halo device is applied.

1. Cervical spine—In the cervical spine, traction is applied to the halo or tongs in the longitudinal axis of the neck and trunk. A halo is a metal ring attached to the skull by four screws drilled into the outer table of the cranium—two anteriorly and two posterolaterally (Figure 43–6). To overcome the weight of the head, 4.5 kg (10 lb) of traction is necessary, and 2.2 kg (5 lb) can be added for each segment below C2. Bilateral facet dislocations (Figure 43–7) with locked facets may require heavier traction, which should be increased by gradual increments under fluoroscopic or radiologic control while the patient is sedated but awake for neurologic monitoring. Some initial mild flexion of the neck with the patient awake and appropriately monitored may be necessary for reduction. The halo device is more effective than tongs, since the direction of traction can be easily adjusted. The halo may be attached to a padded vest or a plaster cast to permit mobilization of some patients.

2. Thoracolumbar spine—In the thoracolumbar spine, halo-femoral or halo-tibial traction is instituted by applying traction both to the halo and to Steinmann pins through either the supracondylar femur bilaterally or the proximal tibial metaphysis bilaterally. Halo-tibial traction may be used for initial control of very unstable thoracolumbar fractures, permitting safe control at the injury site until the neurologic deficit is clarified (by subsidence of spinal shock, signs of recovery, regression, or static state for incomplete lesions) and while the patient is assessed for other injuries. Most unstable thoracolumbar spine fractures are managed with either external cast or brace support or open reduction and internal fixation, depending upon the degree of instability and the presence or absence of sensory deficit.

C. External Support:

1. Cervical spine—The halo vest or halo cast is constructed by connecting the halo to either a plaster body cast or a padded plastic vest. The body cast offers better fixation if properly molded over the iliac crests, but it cannot be used if sensory impairment is present.

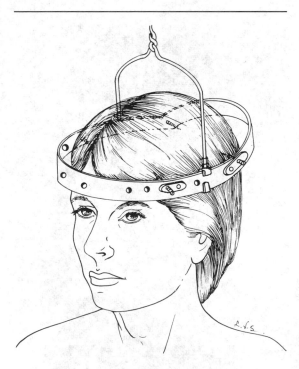

Figure 43–6. Halo device for spinal skeletal traction. Four screw pins are inserted through threaded holes in the halo into the skull. The screw pins have a short point and broad shoulder, so that penetration is no deeper than the outer cortex in normal bone.

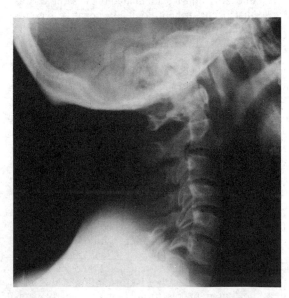

Figure 43–7. Bilateral facet dislocation of the cervical spine.

In stable injuries of the cervical spinal, cervical collars or cervical thoracic braces (4-poster) are adequate.

2. Thoracolumbar spine—In the thoracolumbar spine, cast or brace immobilization for fractures with potential instability must reach from the sternal notch to the symphysis pubis anteriorly and be molded to fit body contours (Figure 43–8). As noted above, if brace support is used in patients with sensory deficit, frequent monitoring for potential pressure necrosis of skin requires that the cast or brace be removable to permit inspection of all body surfaces at appropriately frequent intervals.

Anderson PA, Bohlman HH: Anterior decompression and arthrodesis of the cervical spine: Long-term motor improvement: Part II–Improvement in complete traumatic quadriplegia. J Bone Joint Surg [Am] 1992;74:683.

Beyer CA, Cabanela ME, Berquist TH: Unilateral facet dislocations and fracture-dislocations of the cervical spine: J Bone Joint Surg [Br] 1991;73:977.

Bohlman HH, Anderson PA: Anterior decompression and arthrodesis of the cervical spine: Long-term motor improvement: Part I–Improvement in incomplete traumatic quadriparesis. J Bone Joint Surg [Am] 1992;74:671.

Carl AL, Tromanhauser SG, Roger DJ: Pedicle screw instrumentation for thoracolumbar burst fractures and fracture-dislocations: Spine 1992;17(8 Suppl):S317.

Cybulski GR et al: Complications in three-column cervical spine injuries requiring anterior-posterior stabilization. Spine 1992;17:253.

Denis F, Burkus JK: Shear fracture-dislocations of the thoracic and lumbar spine associated with forceful hyperextension (lumberjack paraplegia): Spine 1992;17:156.

Garvey TA, Eismont FJ, Roberti LJ: Anterior decompres-
sion, structural bone grafting, and Caspar plate stabilization for unstable cervical spine fractures and/or dislocations: Spine 1992;17(10;Suppl):S431.

Gertzbein SD: Scoliosis Research Society: Multicenter spine fracture study. Spine 1992;17:528.

Heary RF et al: Acute stabilization of the cervical spine by halo/vest application facilitates evaluation and treatment of multiple trauma patients: J Trauma 1992;33:445.

Huhn SL, Wolf AL, Ecklund J: Posterior spinal osteosynthesis for cervical fracture/dislocation using a flexible multistrand cable system: Technical note. Neurosurgery 1991;29:943.

Jeanneret B, Magerl F: Primary posterior fusion C½ odontoid fractures: Indications, technique, and results of transarticular screw fixation: J Spinal Disord 1992;5:464.

Kiwerski J: The influence of the mechanism of cervical spine injury on the degree of the spinal cord lesion. Paraplegia 1991;29:531.

Pellise F, Bago J, Villanueva C: Double-level spinal injury resulting in "en bloc" dislocation of the lumbar spine: A case report. Acta Orthop Belg 1992;58:349.

Roy-Camille R et al: Treatment of lower cervical spinal injuries–C3 to C7: Spine 1992;17(10 Suppl):S442.

Saleh J, Raycroft JF: Hyperflexion injury of cervical spine and central cord syndrome in a child: Spine 1992;17:234.

FRACTURES & DISLOCATIONS OF THE PELVIS

Fractures of the pelvis that involve mainly the acetabulum are discussed in the section on traumatic lesions of the hip joint.

Depending on the mechanism and the severity of trauma to the pelvic region, lesions may be limited predominantly to osteoarticular structures or may be complicated by injuries of varying magnitude to adjacent soft tissue structures. These complex injuries may require treatment by surgical specialists in multiple disciplines.

1. AVULSION FRACTURES OF THE PELVIS

Avulsion fractures of the pelvis include those involving the anterior superior and anterior inferior iliac spines, a portion of the iliac crest epiphysis anteriorly, and the apophysis of the ischium. The ischial apophysis may be avulsed indirectly by violent contraction of the hamstring muscles in the older child or adolescent. If displacement is minimal, prompt healing without disability is to be expected. If displacement is marked (ie, > 1 cm), reattachment by open operation is justifiable.

Pruner RA, Johnston CE 2d: Avulsion fracture of the ischial tuberosity: Orthopedics 1990;13:357.

Wootton JR, Cross MJ, Holt KW: Avulsion of the ischial apophysis: The case for open reduction and internal fixation. J Bone Joint Surg [Br] 1990;72:625.

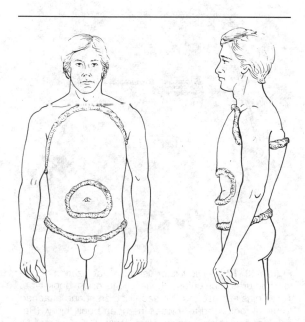

Figure 43–8. Plaster cast for immobilization of thoracolumbar spine fractures.

2. FRACTURE OF THE WING OF THE ILIUM

Isolated fracture of the wing of the ilium without involvement of the hip or sacroiliac joints most often occurs as a result of direct trauma. With minor displacement of the free fragment, soft tissue injury is usually minimal and treatment is symptomatic. Wide displacement of the free fragment may be associated with extensive soft tissue injury and hematoma formation. Healing may be accompanied by ossification of the hematoma with exuberant new bone formation.

3. ISOLATED FRACTURE OF THE OBTURATOR RING

Isolated fracture of the obturator ring, involving either the pubic or the ischial rami with minimal displacement, is associated with little or no injury to the sacroiliac joints. This is also true of minor subluxation of the symphysis pubis. Initial treatment consists of bed rest for a few days followed by ambulation on crutches. As soon as discomfort disappears, unassisted weight bearing may be permitted.

4. COMPLEX FRACTURES & DISLOCATIONS OF THE PELVIC RING

Complex fractures of the pelvic ring are due either to direct violence or to force transmitted indirectly through the lower extremities. When severe and complex fractures of the pelvic ring are suspected, the extent of associated injuries must be determined at once by physical and x-ray examination. Shock due to blood loss may be present. Treatment of the fracture by reduction should not be instituted until the extent of associated injuries has been determined, because treatment of some of those injuries may be more urgent than treatment of the fracture. A careful search must be made for possible injury to the bowel, bladder, ureters, or major blood vessels.

These fractures are of three main types: (1) open book, (2) lateral compression, and (3) vertical shear.

Open book fractures (Figure 43–9) occur from anteroposterior compression and may be associated with minor separation of the symphysis pubis, requiring only a few days of bed rest, or they may consist of gross separation with severe injury to the perineum and urogenital structures. Reduction is obtained by manually compressing the iliac wings or by placing the patient in the lateral position. A hip spica or an external fixator is used to maintain reduction. With an external fixator, two or three fixation pins are placed into each iliac crest under direct vision through a surgical incision. A metal frame is then attached to the pins to maintain reduction of the ante-

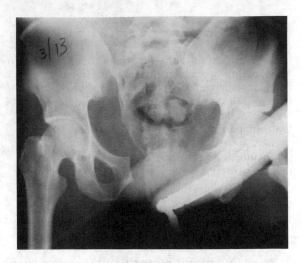

Figure 43–9. Pelvic injury demonstrating open book (symphysis diastasis) and vertical displacement of the hemipelvis.

rior separation (Figure 43–10). Stabilization may be obtained by open reduction and internal fixation by one or two metal plates with screws on the symphysis pubis. An immediate increase in pelvic stability decreases discomfort, facilitates nursing care, may decrease hemorrhage, and may allow earlier mobilization, depending on the seriousness of the injury.

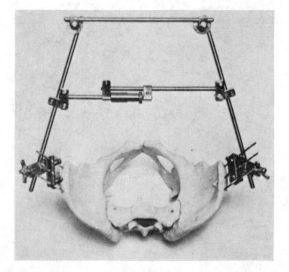

Figure 43–10. Pelvic fixator used for stabilization of pelvic fractures, particularly those of the open book type. Three pins are inserted into each iliac crest and attached to metal rods used to "close" the open book injury. (Reproduced, with permission, from Slatis P, Karaharju EO: External fixation of the pelvic girdle with a trapezoid compression frame. Injury 1975;7:53.)

5. LATERAL COMPRESSION FRACTURES

Lateral force applied to the pelvis causes inward displacement of the hemipelvis through the sacroiliac complex and the contralateral pubic rami. It may be impacted in its displaced position, causing infolding of the hemipelvis with overlapping of the symphysis. Major displacement requires manipulation under general anesthesia by external rotation and traction on the pelvis through the ipsilateral femur. This must be done soon after injury, since disruption of the impacted fragments becomes very difficult after the first few days. After reduction, position is maintained by use of an external fixator or by internal fixation devices. If the fracture is unstable posteriorly, early mobilization is not possible even with an external fixator, but pain is decreased and nursing care is made easier. Adequate fixation often can be obtained by a plate and screws on the symphysis and fixation of the sacroiliac joint if necessary.

6. VERTICAL SHEAR FRACTURE

Anteriorly, the injury may fracture the pubic rami or disrupt the symphysis pubis. Posteriorly, the sacroiliac joint is dislocated, or there is a fracture immediately adjacent to it in the sacrum or the ilium. This injury allows vertical displacement of one hemipelvis in relation to the other. Massive hemorrhage and injury to the lumbosacral nerve plexus are common. Reduction of this highly unstable injury is achieved by longitudinal skeletal traction through the distal femur or proximal tibia. If traction is used as the definitive method of treatment, it must be maintained for a long period—frequently 6–12 weeks. External fixators alone are insufficient to maintain reduction in very unstable vertical shear fractures.

Open reduction and internal fixation are sometimes indicated for these fractures, but these procedures are difficult and there is a significant risk of complications. These procedures should be performed only by a skilled, experienced surgeon thoroughly familiar with the surgical approach and the internal fixation devices.

Massive hemorrhage is the most frequent complication associated with severe pelvic fractures. Application of an external fixator may help to control bleeding even though it cannot completely control vertical displacement. Angiography is helpful in identifying a specific bleeding site, which can then be embolized with sterile Gelfoam or muscle placed through the catheter.

Use of the gravity suit (G suit) to control hemorrhage is still controversial, as no controlled studies are available. If the suit is applied at the scene of the accident, it must be removed in the emergency room to allow for examination. Mechanical ventilation is frequently required, and skin blisters may develop.

The death rate of closed pelvic fractures is 8–15%; in open fractures, it approaches 50%.

Jerrard DA: Pelvic fractures. Emerg Med Clin North Am 1993;11:147.

Pohlemann T et al: Fixation of transforaminal sacrum fractures: A biomechanical study. J Orthop Trauma 1993;7:107.

Rizzo PF et al: Diagnosis of occult fractures about the hip: Magnetic resonance imaging compared with bone-scanning. J Bone Joint Surg [Am] 1993;75:395.

Schafermeyer R: Pediatric trauma: Emerg Med Clin North Am 1993;11:187.

Siegel JH et al: Safety belt restraints and compartment intrusions in frontal and lateral motor vehicle crashes: Mechanisms of injuries, complications, and acute care costs. J Trauma 1993;34:736.

Sinnott R, Rhodes M, Brader A: Open pelvic fracture: An injury for trauma centers. Am J Surg 1992;163:283.

Takahara T et al: Isolated fracture-dislocation of the sacrum: Case report. J Trauma 1993;3;34:600.

INJURIES OF THE SHOULDER GIRDLE

1. FRACTURE OF THE CLAVICLE

Fracture of the clavicle may occur as a result of a direct trauma or indirect force transmitted through the shoulder. Most fractures of the clavicle occur in the middle third. Because of the relative fixation of the medial fragment and the weight of the arm, the distal fragment is displaced downward and toward the midline. The fracture can be seen on anteroposterior x-rays, and occasionally an oblique cephalad projection will give additional information. Injury to the brachial plexus or subclavian vessels is not common but should be sought on physical examination.

Treatment

Fracture of the outer third of the clavicle distal to the coracoclavicular ligaments is comparable to dislocation of the acromioclavicular joint. If the coracoclavicular ligaments are intact and the fragments are not widely displaced, immobilization in a sling and swathe or figure-of-eight dressing is adequate. If the coracoclavicular ligaments have been lacerated and extensive displacement of the main medial fragment is present, treatment is similar to that advocated for acromioclavicular dislocation.

A. Fracture Without Displacement: Treatment is by immobilization in a sling or figure-of-eight dressing for 4–6 weeks (Figure 43–11).

B. Fracture With Displacement or Comminution:

1. Closed reduction–Comminuted fractures of the clavicle with displacement can usually be man-

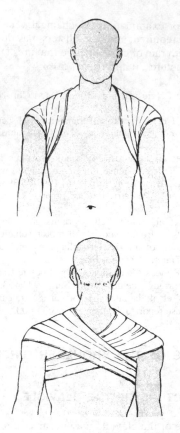

Figure 43–11. Figure-of-eight dressing.

aged successfully by closed reduction. Reduction need not be exact, because excessive callus formation will be partially or completely obliterated in the late stages of the natural healing process. Reduction of fragments may be performed easily, but maintenance of reduction is more difficult. Immobilization must be maintained for 6–8 weeks. Even though the fragments may appear significantly displaced, the incidence of non-union is less than 1% after closed treatment.

2. Open reduction—Open reduction and internal fixation may be justifiable where there is interposition of soft tissue or when the fracture is not reducible and is causing damage to the overlying skin. Fixation may be achieved by use of a metal plate and screws or by a Steinmann pin drilled retrograde through the lateral fragment. The fracture is then reduced, and the pin is driven across the fracture site. Complications of open reduction include infection, migration or breakage of the fixation device (if a pin is used), and an increased incidence of nonunion.

Lewonowski K, Bassett GS: Complete posterior sternoclavicular epiphyseal separation: A case report and review of the literature. Clin Orthop 1992;Aug(281):84.

Martin-Herrero T, Rodriguez-Merchan C, Munuera-

Martinez L: Fractures of the coracoid process: Presentation of seven cases and review of the literature. J Trauma 1990;30:1597.

2. ACROMIOCLAVICULAR DISLOCATION

Dislocation of the acromioclavicular joint may be incomplete or complete. There is often a history of a blow or fall on the tip of the shoulder. The acromial end of the clavicle is displaced upward and backward; the shoulder falls downward and inward. Anteroposterior x-rays should be taken of both shoulders with the patient erect. Displacement is more likely to be demonstrated when the patient holds a 5- to 8-kg (12- to 18-lb) weight in each hand.

Injuries to the acromioclavicular joint can be classified according to the severity of damage done by the force of injury. Type I injury is associated with minor strain to the acromioclavicular ligament; the joint remains stable. Type II injury involves separation of the acromioclavicular ligament with the coracoclavicular ligament remaining intact. The joint may be subluxated, but upward displacement of the clavicle from the acromion is relatively minor. Type III injury generally includes separation of both the acromioclavicular and coracoclavicular ligaments, with marked superior migration of the lateral end of the clavicle (Figure 43–12). The shoulder appears depressed when compared to the opposite normal side.

Treatment

Unreduced acromioclavicular dislocations may cause no disability; however, painful posttraumatic

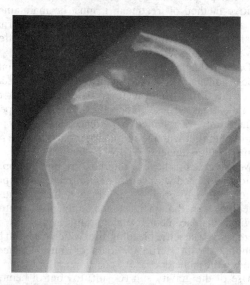

Figure 43–12. Fracture of the distal clavicle and complete dislocation of the acromioclavicular joint. Wide separation of the clavicle from the coracoid process indicates complete tear of the conoid and trapezoid ligaments.

arthritis may require excision of the distal 1–1.5 cm of the clavicle.

Type I and type II injuries may be treated by a sling until acute pain from movement and the weight of the upper extremity has been relieved.

Type III injury is associated with complete dislocation, and treatment is controversial. It is generally agreed that maintenance of reduction and adequate immobilization of this injury by closed methods are difficult. Conservative treatment is available with the help of devices (braces, harnesses, and strapping) for depressing the clavicle and elevating the shoulder. Any device chosen must be worn for 6 weeks, tightly enough to maintain reduction. Patient acceptance of the device may be poor.

Surgical realignment and fixation within 2 weeks after complete dislocation offers the best hope of restoring anatomic alignment. If surgery is deferred longer, the ligaments will have partially healed with elongation, and deformity can be expected to recur when immobilization is discontinued unless the ligaments are reconstructed. Fixation is obtained by Kirschner wires or a Steinmann pin driven across the acromioclavicular joint or by fixation of the clavicle to the coracoid process by means of a screw or wire. Complications include infection, redislocation after hardware removal, and migration of hardware.

Many surgeons treat type III injuries with a sling only. Even though upward displacement of the clavicle continues, the patient may prefer to live with a "bump" rather than a scar from the surgical procedure. There are reports that the results of conservative treatment of type III injuries do not vary greatly from those achieved with operative treatment.

Old and unreduced dislocations with secondary osteoarthritis can be treated by resection of the distal 1–1.5 cm of the lateral clavicle. When gross displacement and marked instability are present, supplementary reconstruction of the damaged coracoclavicular ligament is indicated.

Bannister GC et al: A classification of acute acromioclavicular dislocation: A clinical, radiological and anatomical study. Injury 1992;23:194.

Meislin RJ, Zuckerman JD, Nainzadeh N: Type III acromioclavicular joint separation associated with late brachial-plexus neurapraxia. J Orthop Trauma 1992;6:370.

Richards RR: Acromioclavicular joint injuries. Instr Course Lect 1993;42:259.

Sundaram N, Patel DV, Porter DS: Stabilization of acute acromioclavicular dislocation by a modified Bosworth technique: A long-term follow-up study. [Published erratum appears in Injury 1992;23:359.] Injury 1992;23:189.

Verhaven E, Casteleyn PP, De Boeck H, Handelberg F, Haentjens P, Opdecam P: Surgical treatment of acute type V acromioclavicular injuries: A prospective study. Acta Orthopaedica Belgica 1992;58:176.

3. STERNOCLAVICULAR DISLOCATION

Displacement of the sternal end of the clavicle may occur superiorly, anteriorly, or inferiorly. Retrosternal displacement is less common. Complete dislocation can be diagnosed by physical examination supplemented by anteroposterior and oblique x-rays. Examination by CT scan may be necessary to confirm the diagnosis, especially with retrosternal displacement.

Complete dislocations are generally not difficult to reduce. If a retrosternal dislocation does not reduce with lateral traction applied to the abducted arm, it may be necessary to grasp the medial clavicle with the fingers to dislodge it from behind the manubrium. If this is unsuccessful, the skin can be sterilized and a sterile towel clip used to grasp the medial clavicle and reduce it. Open reduction with repair of torn sternoclavicular and costoclavicular ligaments with or without internal fixation may be required to maintain adequate reduction. Additional protection by external immobilization should be continued for 6–8 weeks while the internal fixation apparatus is in place.

Complications associated with retrosternal dislocation include occlusion of the subclavian artery, pneumothorax, and rupture of the esophagus. Unreduced anterior subluxation is asymptomatic except for a "bump" that may be cosmetically objectionable.

Complications associated with surgical repair of sternoclavicular dislocation include infection, breakage and migration of internal fixation devices, redislocation, and persistent pain. Extraperiosteal resection of the medial portion of the clavicle may be necessary for relief of pain.

Lewonowski K, Bassett GS: Complete posterior sternoclavicular epiphyseal separation: A case report and review of the literature. Clin Orthop 1992;Aug(281):84.

van Holsbeeck M et al: Radiographic findings of spontaneous subluxation of the sternoclavicular. Clin Rheumatol 1992;11:376.

4. FRACTURE OF THE SCAPULA

Fracture of the neck of the scapula is most often caused by a blow on the shoulder or by a fall on the outstretched arm. The main glenoid fragment may be impacted into the body fragment. The treatment of impacted or undisplaced fractures in patients 40 years of age or older should be directed toward the preservation of shoulder joint function, since stiffness may cause prolonged disability. In young adults especially, unstable fractures require arm traction with the arm at right angles to the trunk for about 4 weeks and protection in a sling and swathe for an additional 2–4 weeks. Open reduction is rarely required even for major displaced fragments, except for those involving the articular surface. These fractures are likely to involve only a segment of the articular surface and may be impacted. When major displacement of an articular fragment is present, accurate repositioning and internal fixation are desirable because of the likelihood of secondary glenohumeral osteoarthritis.

Fracture of the acromion, or spine, of the scapula requires reduction only when the displaced fragment is apt to cause interference with abduction of the shoulder. Persistence of an acromial epiphysis should not be confused with fracture.

Fracture of the coracoid process may result from violent muscular contraction or, rarely, may be associated with anterior dislocation of the shoulder joint or with dislocation of the acromioclavicular joint.

When fracture of the body of the scapula is caused by direct violence, fractures of underlying ribs may be present. Eighty-five percent of patients with fracture of the scapula have associated bone and soft tissue injuries, most commonly in the thoracic area. Treatment of uncomplicated fracture should be directed toward the comfort of the patient and the preservation of shoulder joint function.

Ballmer FT, Gerber C: Coracoclavicular screw fixation for unstable fractures of the distal clavicle: A report of five cases. J Bone Joint Surg [Br] 1991;73:291.

Niggebrugge AH et al: Dislocated intra-articular fracture of anterior rim of glenoid treated by open reduction and internal fixation. Injury 1993;24:130.

Nordqvist A, Petersson C: Fracture of the body, neck, or spine of the scapula: A long-term follow-up study. Clin Orthop 1992;Oct(283):139.

5. FRACTURE OF THE PROXIMAL HUMERUS

Fracture of the proximal humerus (Figure 43–13) occurs most frequently during the sixth decade. It is commonly the result of indirect injury such as a fall on the hand with the arm outstretched. Swelling of the shoulder region with visible or palpable deformity and restriction of motion due to pain are the principal clinical features. The precise diagnosis is established by x-rays taken perpendicular to the plane of the scapula and by a lateral view made at a right angle to the former, tangential to the body of the scapula. The transthoracic projection may be inadequate to demonstrate detail because of interference by the ribs and spine. Axillary x-rays are helpful to demonstrate the direction of any displacement of the head of the humerus from the glenoid or infractions involving the articular surfaces of the shoulder joint.

This discussion follows a classification of proximal humeral fractures proposed by Neer that is based on the presence or absence of displacement of the articular surface of the humeral head, greater tuberosity, lesser tuberosity, and shaft.

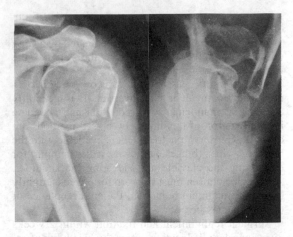

Figure 43–13. Comminuted fracture of the proximal humerus involving the surgical neck and greater tuberosity. The uninjured lesser tuberosity suggests that the articular fragment retains some blood supply.

Undisplaced Fractures of the Proximal Humerus

Undisplaced or minimally displaced fractures of the proximal humerus—with the exception of those of the anatomic neck—require little treatment beyond guarding of the shoulder by the use of a sling until discomfort is tolerable and, subsequently, judicious exercise. Restoration of firm bone continuity occurs in about 8–12 weeks.

Single Fractures of the Proximal Humerus

A. Fracture of the Anatomic Neck: Isolated fracture of the anatomic neck of the humerus is uncommon and may be followed by avascular necrosis of the articular fragment even in the absence of displacement. Healing of fractures in malalignment may cause limitation of shoulder motion. When displacement is the determinant of open operation, primary prosthetic arthroplasty is likely to provide a more satisfactory long-term result than anatomic replacement of the devascularized articular fragment.

B. Fracture of the Surgical Neck: The main fracture cleft is distal to the tuberosities. Minor comminution of the proximal segment can be disregarded if displacement of the tuberosities does not occur. Some angulation is likely to accompany any displacement in the transverse plane of the humerus. The apex of angulation is generally directed anteriorly, but its direction should be accurately determined by biplane x-rays. When angulation greater than 45 degrees occurs in the active person, it should be corrected to avoid subsequent restriction of abduction and elevation. Lesser degrees of deformity do not require manipulation, especially when encountered in elderly persons. Impacted and minimally angulated fractures can be treated by means of a shoulder immobilizer.

When displacement at the fracture site is complete, the free end of the distal fragment lies medially and anteriorly (in relation to the proximal fragment). Neurovascular injury is not a common complication. Closed manipulation is justifiable, but because persistent instability is a frequent complication, impaction or locking of the fragments is desirable if it can be done. If reduction is stable, a Velpeau dressing (Figure 43–14) provides reliable immobilization after correction of anterior angulation. Redisplacement may occur when reduction is not stable or when the arm is immobilized in abduction. Continuous traction by a Kirschner wire through the proximal ulna with the arm at right angle elevation (Figure 43–15) is advisable when the fracture cannot be maintained in reduction by a Velpeau or other dressing. Traction must be continued for about 4 weeks before partial healing provides stability. This closed method of traction treatment is commonly required also for comminuted fractures of the surgical neck. When comminution is not extensive, the fracture that has been adequately reduced by closed reduction may be stabilized by rods or plates and screws. However, the severe osteoporosis associated with these fractures leads to a high rate of failure of internal fixation. With the fragments fixed, the arm is then brought to the side and immobilized either by a sling and swathe or by a plaster Velpeau dressing. Open reduction and internal fixation of uncomplicated fractures of the surgical neck are sometimes required to ensure an adequate functional result.

C. Fracture of the Surgical Neck and Both Tuberosities: This uncommon but serious lesion is generally complicated by displacement of one or all of the component fragments. Separation of the tuberosities and displacement of the shaft provide a mechanism for subluxation or dislocation of the main articular fragment that may occur anteriorly, posteriorly,

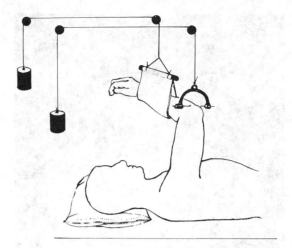

Figure 43–15. Method of suspension of upper extremity with skeletal traction on olecranon.

laterally, or inferiorly. Extensive laceration of the rotator cuff is a part of the injury.

Because of comminution and displacement of the fragments of the proximal segment, satisfactory functional results are unlikely and delay of bone healing probable after any type of closed treatment. Interruption of the blood supply to the humeral head may cause avascular necrosis. Hemiarthroplasty is the best method for preserving some function with minimal discomfort. The prosthesis replaces the articular portion of the proximal humerus and allows the tuberosities to be reattached. The rotator cuff tear should be repaired also. Passive range-of-motion exercises are started on the fourth or fifth day. For a satisfactory outcome, the patient must take part in a rehabilitation program for many months.

Hawkins RJ, Switlyk P: Acute prosthetic replacement for severe fractures of the proximal humerus. Clin Orthop 1993;Apr(289):156.

Jaberg H, Warner JJ, Jakob RP: Percutaneous stabilization of unstable fractures of the humerus. J Bone Joint Surg [Am] 1992;3;74:508.

Moeckel BH et al: Modular hemiarthroplasty for fractures of the proximal part of the humerus. J Bone Joint Surg [Am] 1992;74:884.

6. DISLOCATION OF THE SHOULDER JOINT

Over 95% of all cases of shoulder joint dislocation are anterior, mainly subcoracoid or subglenoid. Posterior dislocations comprise the remainder.

Anterior Dislocation of the Shoulder Joint

Anterior dislocation of the shoulder joint (Figure 43–16) presents the clinical appearance of flattening

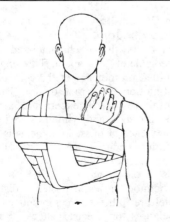

Figure 43–14. Velpeau dressing.

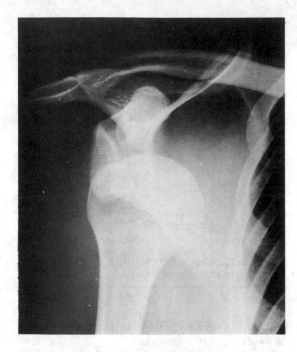

Figure 43–16. Anterior (subcoracoid) dislocation of the shoulder. The humeral head is anterior to the glenoid.

of the deltoid region, anterior fullness, and restriction of motion due to pain. The mechanism producing anterior dislocation is usually a combination of abduction and external rotation. Both anteroposterior and axillary x-rays are necessary to determine the site of the head and the presence or absence of complicating fracture, which may involve either the head of the humerus or the glenoid. Anterior dislocation may be complicated by (1) injury to major nerves arising from the brachial plexus, most commonly the axillary nerve; (2) fracture of the humeral head or neck or greater tuberosity; (3) compression or avulsion of the anterior glenoid; and (4) tears of the capsulotendinous rotator cuff. The most common sequela is recurrent dislocation. Before manipulation, careful examination is necessary to determine the presence or absence of complicating nerve or vascular injury. The examiner should check particularly over the lateral aspect of the arm for sensory changes due to injury of the axillary nerve. The radial pulse should be palpated. With analgesia, reduction can usually be accomplished by simple traction on the arm for a few minutes or until the head has been disengaged from under the coracoid. This may be done by placing the patient prone on the edge of an examining table with an appropriate weight (approximately 2.2 kg [5 lb], depending on the size of the patient) taped to the wrist of the dislocated shoulder. The extremity and the weight should hang free off the edge of the table. It may take 15–20 minutes for reduction to occur. If

reduction cannot be achieved in this way, the surgeon should apply lateral traction manually to the upper arm, close to the axilla, while an assistant continues to exert axial traction on the extremity. This is a modification of **Hippocrates' manipulation,** in which the surgeon exerts traction on the patient's arm while placing an unshod heel in the axilla to provide countertraction and simultaneously force the head of the humerus laterally from beneath the glenoid. More and safer countertraction may be applied by having an assistant hold a folded sheet looped across the front of the patient's chest through the axilla of the dislocated shoulder and then across the back to form an axillary swathe.

If neither of the foregoing techniques proves successful, **Kocher's method** may be useful. This maneuver, however, must be carried out gently, or spiral fracture of the humerus may result. The elbow is flexed to a right angle, and the surgeon applies traction and gentle external rotation to the forearm in the axis of the humerus. The surgeon continues traction to the arm while gentle external rotation about the longitudinal axis of the humerus is applied, using the patient's forearm flexed to a right angle at the elbow as a lever. The maneuver can be completed by shifting the elbow across the anterior chest while traction is continuously exerted and, finally, applying slow internal rotation of the arm until the palm of the affected side rests on the opposite shoulder. If closed reduction with analgesics is still impossible, general anesthesia with complete relaxation is usually successful. If the dislocation is associated with a nondisplaced fracture of the humeral neck, reduction should only be attempted under general anesthesia, so that fracture displacement will be less likely to occur during reduction.

After closed reduction of an initial dislocation, the extremity is placed in a shoulder immobilizer for 1–3 weeks before active motion is begun. Dislocation in an older person or recurrent dislocation in any patient should be reduced and the arm immobilized in a sling for a few days for pain relief only.

Posterior Dislocation of the Shoulder Joint

Posterior dislocation is characterized by fullness beneath the spine of the scapula, flattening of the anterior shoulder, prominence of the coracoid, and restriction of motion in external rotation. This injury is frequently missed even by experienced surgeons unless the specific signs and symptoms are known. The reported incidence of missed diagnosis is as high as 60%. The injury occurs either from direct or indirect force to the anterior shoulder, so that the humeral head is pushed out posteriorly.

Other common causes of posterior dislocation of the shoulder are indirect forces produced with convulsive seizures or electric shock. Routine anteroposterior x-ray of the shoulder may look deceptively normal with posterior dislocation (Figure 43–17), but an axillary view will show the true position of the head in relation to the glenoid. This dislocation may be reduced by the same combination of coaxial and transverse traction as described for anterior dislocation. If the reduction is stable, immobilization in a shoulder immobilizer is sufficient. If there is any doubt about the stability of the reduction, immobilization following an initial episode should be accomplished by a plaster spica, with the arm in 30 degrees of external rotation and the elbow flexed to a right angle. This position should be held for 3–6 weeks before active motion is permitted.

Recurrent & Chronic Dislocations of the Shoulder Joint

Recurrent dislocation of the shoulder is almost always anterior. The incidence of recurrence in younger age groups is as high as 60–80%. In patients over age 40, the incidence drops sharply to 10–15%. Various factors can influence recurrent dislocation. The recurrence rate is inversely proportionate to the severity of the original trauma—ie, the easier the dislocation occurred primarily, the easier it recurs. Immobilization weeks after initial dislocation followed by an aggressive rehabilitation program can reduce the incidence of recurrence. Avulsion of the anterior and inferior glenoid labrum or tears in the anterior capsule remove the natural buttress that gives stability to the arm with abduction and external rotation. Other lesions that impair the stability of the shoulder joint

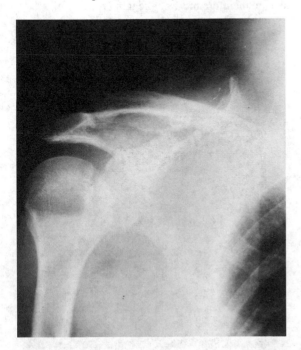

Figure 43–17. Posterior shoulder dislocation visualized on anteroposterior view. The shoulder may look deceptively normal, but note vacant glenoid.

are fractures of the posterior and superior surface of the head of the humerus (or of the greater tuberosity) and longitudinal tears of the rotator cuff between the supraspinatus and subscapularis muscles. Reduction of the acute episodic dislocation is by closed manipulation. Immobilization of a recurrent dislocation does not prevent subsequent dislocation, and it should be discontinued as soon as acute symptoms subside, usually within a few days.

If the patient's history of recurrent anterior dislocation is difficult to evaluate, documentation may consist either of x-rays on several occasions, confirming dislocation, or the presence of a Hill-Sachs lesion, which consists of a wedge-shaped defect or groove in the posterolateral aspect of the humeral head. This lesion can be demonstrated by x-rays taken either in full internal rotation or with the patient supine, the hand of the affected shoulder resting on the head and the elbow pointing straight upward. This defect in the humeral head is caused by repeated compression of the humeral head against the glenoid labrum during dislocation.

Adequate treatment of recurrent dislocation of the shoulder frequently requires surgical repair. Most of the procedures are directed toward repair of the anterior capsular mechanism, subscapularis muscle shortening, or subscapular transfer. These procedures attempt to limit external rotation enough to eliminate dislocation but not enough to restrict functional range of motion.

After operative repair, the shoulder is usually immobilized in a shoulder immobilizer for 3–6 weeks before active motion is begun. Reparative procedures for anterior dislocation are successful in preventing further episodes of dislocation in 90–95% of patients.

Shoulders that have been dislocated for at least 3 weeks are termed chronic unreduced dislocations. Reduction should be attempted by closed manipulation, followed by open reduction if necessary. If the humeral head is severely damaged, replacement with Neer prosthesis may be preferable. Reduction of the dislocation, even though it is performed late, leads to a better result than allowing the shoulder to remain chronically dislocated.

Bankart AS, Cantab MC: Recurrent or habitual dislocation of the shoulder-joint: 1923 [classical article]. Clin Orthop 1993;Jun(291):3.

Glousman RE: Instability versus impingement syndrome in the throwing athlete. Orthop Clin North Am 1993;24:89.

Pollock RG, Bigliani LU: Recurrent posterior shoulder instability: Diagnosis and treatment. Clin Orthop 1993; Jun(291):85.

Post M, Grinblat E: Congenital anteroinferior instability treated by Bankart repair. Clin Orthop 1993;Jun(291):97.

Silliman JF, Hawkins RJ: Classification and physical diagnosis of instability of the shoulder. Clin Orthop 1993; Jun(291):7.

Tibone JE, Bradley JP: The treatment of posterior subluxation in athletes. Clin Orthop 1993;Jun(291):124.

7. ROTATOR CUFF TEARS

The rotator cuff of the shoulder includes four muscles that stabilize the humeral head in the glenoid fossa to allow abduction of the arm by the deltoid. These muscles are the supraspinatus, infraspinatus, teres minor, and subscapularis.

Acute Tears

Complete tears of the rotator cuff occasionally occur in young people as a result of severe trauma. They may be associated with anterior dislocation of the shoulder or fracture of the greater tuberosity. Complete tears involve the full thickness of the tendon (usually the supraspinatus) and expose the humeral head to the deltoid muscle.

Symptoms include pain over the tip of the shoulder, weakness, and inability to abduct the arm. If the tear is complete, discontinuity of the cuff muscles allows the humeral head to ride superiorly out of the glenoid instead of being stabilized for abduction by the deltoid.

To decide whether a tear is complete or incomplete, the painful area can be infiltrated with 8–10 mL of 1% plain lidocaine to eliminate pain alone as a cause for lack of abduction. If the patient can abduct the arm and hold it against some resistance, treatment may consist of wearing a sling for 2–3 weeks followed by progressive resumption of function and rehabilitation.

When severe pain and disability persist, an arthrogram should be performed. If dye appears in the subacromial bursa, the diagnosis of rotator cuff tear is confirmed (Figure 43–18). Surgical repair is performed by direct suture of the defect in most cases. The shoulder is immobilized for 4–6 weeks before progressive exercises are started.

Chronic Tears

Tears may result from minor trauma (a fall on the outstretched hand) or degeneration of the rotator cuff in older patients. These are included in the general category of **supraspinatus syndrome** and are associated with symptoms of pain, muscle atrophy, weakness, tenderness over the tip of the shoulder, and limitation of motion.

Aging of the tendons of the rotator cuff is accelerated by repeated mechanical irritation from impingement between the humeral head and the acromion. Tears of the rotator cuff usually occur in the fifth decade and after, probably as a result of loss of elasticity and degeneration of the tendon in this high-stress area.

Diagnosis is made in the same way as with an acute tear. Arthrography is not indicated in early management, however. It should be remembered that many asymptomatic tears are present in older people. Treatment is directed toward relief of pain, improvement of function, and prevention of atrophy. Rest in a sling for immediate relief of pain followed by pendulum exercises within a few days is successful in 90% of patients with chronic rotator cuff tears. If severe pain and disability persist after conservative treatment, operative repair should be considered. Chronic tears usually have larger residual defects than acute tears and are therefore more challenging to correct.

Anterior acromioplasty performed at the time of

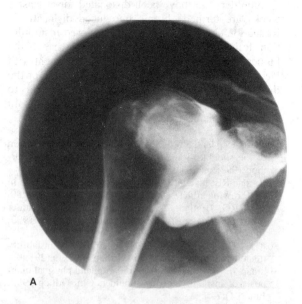
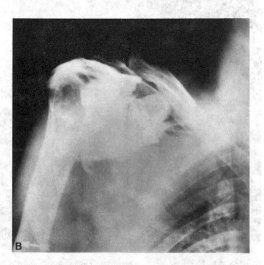

Figure 43–18. *A:* Normal arthrogram of the shoulder. Dye is present in the shoulder capsule only. The rotator cuff is intact. *B:* Abnormal arthrogram. Note that dye is present in the subacromial bursa, revealing a tear in the rotator cuff.

surgical repair will decrease the possibility of future impingement of the rotator cuff.

Burkhart SS: Arthroscopic debridement and decompression for selected rotator cuff tears: Clinical results, pathomechanics, and patient selection based on biomechanical parameters. Orthop Clin North Am 1993;24:111.

Ellman H: Diagnosis and treatment of incomplete rotator cuff tears. Clin Orthop 1990;May(254):64.

Esch JC: Arthroscopic subacromial decompression and postoperative management. Orthop Clin North Am 1993; 24:161.

Post M: Complications of rotator cuff surgery. Clin Orthop 1990;May(254):97.

Snyder SJ: Evaluation and treatment of the rotator cuff. Orthop Clin North Am 1993;24:173.

8. GLENOHUMERAL ARTHRITIS

The shoulder joint is a non-weight-bearing joint and is therefore less commonly involved with arthritis than the joints of the lower extremity. Among the more common causes of arthritis of the shoulder joint are traumatic injuries that cause tears of the rotator cuff, dislocation of the joint, fracture of the articular surface of the humerus or scapula, and rheumatoid arthritis. Examination by x-ray shows the characteristic thinning of the articular cartilage, especially at the site of maximal contact of the apposing surfaces. Osteophytes may be found at the chondrosynovial junction, especially in the region of the inferior head and superior glenoid. Incongruity of the joint surface of the humeral head or of the glenoid cavity due to malhealed intra-articular fracture can cause secondary osteoarthritis. Painful restriction of motion is the main subjective symptom.

Treatment of this sequela is directed primarily toward the relief of pain and secondarily toward preservation or augmentation of range of motion. Before operative treatment is elected, a thorough test of conservative measures is indicated, including physical therapy, analgesics, and nonsteroidal anti-inflammatory drugs.

Fusion of the joint (**arthrodesis**) may be necessary because of antecedent or persistent infection or because of irreparable instability due either to prior destruction of surrounding soft tissues or bone or to denervation of muscles essential for shoulder joint function. This procedure may also be arbitrarily selected by the patient. Bony fusion of the joint eliminates pain from that source but results in disability due to loss of function.

Criteria for a satisfactory result include solid union, relief of pain, restoration of strength in the limb, and some improvement of function of the extremity. Shoulder fusion includes surgical removal of intra-articular debris and any remaining joint cartilage. Internal fixation is generally required. Autogenous iliac crest bone grafting is frequently needed.

An acceptable position for fusion is between 20 and 50 degrees of abduction and about 25 degrees of flexion. The angle of rotation should be individualized to the particular major tasks the patient wishes to perform. Rotation is felt to be the most important determinant of functional success after this procedure. After surgical fusion is performed, the shoulder is immobilized in a spica cast or abduction splint for 3–4 months or until fusion is solid.

Relief of pain is adequate in about 75% of patients. Complications include nonunion, infection, and persistent pain. In patients with rheumatoid arthritis, fusion usually occurs more quickly and results are frequently superior to those achieved in patients with other forms of arthritis.

Barrett WP et al: Nonconstrained total shoulder arthroplasty in patients with polyarticular rheumatoid arthritis. J Arthroplasty 1989;4:91.

McCoy SR et al: Total shoulder arthroplasty in rheumatoid arthritis. J Arthroplasty 1989;4:105.

Shoulder Replacement Arthroplasty

Because of the non-weight-bearing nature of the shoulder joint and other factors, **hemiarthroplasty** by use of a humeral head prosthesis has had good results when performed by an experienced surgeon after careful assessment of indications. Serviceable function and significant relief of pain can be obtained afterward (see section on humeral neck fractures, p 997).

Total shoulder replacement is indicated for severe shoulder disability resulting from involvement of both the glenoid and humeral articular surfaces secondary to rheumatoid arthritis, posttraumatic arthritis, or avascular necrosis. Symptoms include intractable pain and marked limitation of motion and must be severe enough so that shoulder fusion is being considered. The patient must be motivated to carry out a sustained rehabilitation program.

Two types of shoulder prosthetic joints are available: nonconstrained and constrained. The nonconstrained (nonarticulated) type contains separate glenoid and humeral portions and is designed to maintain and reproduce the normal anatomy of the shoulder joint. The constrained (articulated) shoulder prosthesis has a fixed fulcrum with a ball-and-socket design and can be used if there is irreparable rotator cuff damage.

Contraindications to total arthroplasty are active or latent septic arthritis, paralysis of the shoulder musculature, and neuropathic joints.

Following total shoulder replacement, the shoulder is immobilized in a sling or abduction splint (if the rotator cuff has been repaired). Immobilization is continued for 2–3 weeks, but passive exercises are begun 3–6 days postoperatively.

Short-term follow-up shows that 80–85% of patients have significant improvement in pain and motion required for activities of daily living. Complications include dislocation, loosening, and infection. Severe infection may require permanent removal of the prosthesis.

Brostrom LA et al: The Kessel prosthesis in total shoulder arthroplasty: A five-year experience. Clin Orthop 1992; Apr(277):155.

Figgie MP et al: Custom total shoulder arthroplasty in inflammatory arthritis: Preliminary results. J Arthroplasty 1992;7:1.

Kadic MA et al: A surgical approach in total shoulder arthroplasty. Arch Orthop Trauma Surg 1992;111:192.

Zuckerman JD, Cuomo F: Glenohumeral arthroplasty: a critical review of indications and preoperative considerations. Bull Hospital Jt Dis Orthop Inst 1993;(Winter)52:21.

FRACTURES OF THE SHAFT OF THE HUMERUS

Most fractures of the shaft of the humerus result from direct violence, although spiral fracture of the middle third of the shaft occasionally results from violent muscular activity such as throwing of a ball.

X-rays in two planes are necessary to determine the configuration of the fracture and the direction of displacement of the fragments. The shoulder and elbow must be included on the initial x-rays to rule out the possibility of fracture or dislocation involving adjacent joints. Before definitive treatment is initiated, a careful neurologic examination should be done (and recorded) to determine the status of the radial nerve. Injury to the brachial vessels is not common.

Fracture of the Upper Third of the Shaft of the Humerus

Fracture through the metaphysis proximal to the insertion of the pectoralis major is classified as fracture of the surgical neck of the humerus.

Fractures between the insertions of the pectoralis major and the deltoid commonly demonstrate adduction of the distal end of the proximal fragment, with lateral and proximal displacement of the distal fragment. If the fracture occurs distal to the insertion of the deltoid in the middle third of the shaft, medial displacement of the shaft occurs.

Treatment depends upon the presence or absence of complicating neurovascular injury, the site and configuration of the fracture, and the magnitude of displacement. An effort should be made to reduce completely displaced transverse or slightly oblique fractures by manipulation. To prevent recurrence of medial convex angulation and maintain proper alignment, it may be necessary to bring the distal fragment into alignment with the proximal one by bringing the arm across the chest and immobilizing it with a plas-

ter Velpeau dressing. If the ends of the fragments cannot be approximated by manipulation, skeletal traction with a wire through the olecranon may be indicated (Figure 43–15). Traction should be continued for 3–4 weeks until stabilization occurs, after which time the patient can be ambulatory with an external immobilization device. If adequate approximation and alignment of the fragments cannot be obtained by manipulation or traction, internal fixation may be necessary.

Fracture of the Mid & Lower Thirds of the Shaft of the Humerus (Figure 43–19)

Spiral, oblique, and comminuted fractures of the humeral shaft below the insertion of the pectoralis major may be treated by application of a U-shaped coaptation plaster splint with a shoulder immobilizer (Figure 43–20). The coaptation splint may be molded to improve reduction of the fracture. Alignment should be verified on anteroposterior and transthoracic x-rays with the patient standing.

These fractures may also be treated by Caldwell's hanging cast (Figure 43–21), which consists of a plaster dressing from the axilla to the wrist with the elbow in 90 degrees of flexion and the forearm in midposition. The cast is suspended from a bandage around the neck by means of a ring at the wrist. Angulation may be corrected by lengthening or shortening of the suspension bandage. With this technique, the arm must always be dependent to provide traction

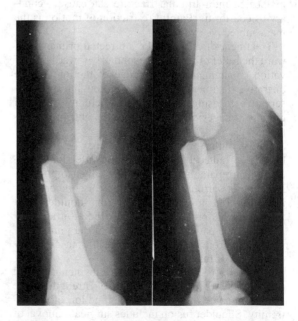

Figure 43–19. Comminuted fracture of the middle third of the humeral shaft complicated by immediate and complete paralysis of the radial nerve.

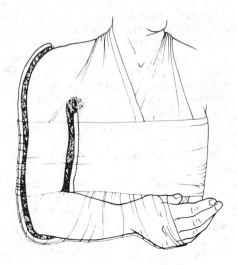

Figure 43–20. Coaptation splint.

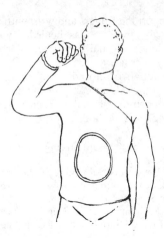

Figure 43–22. Plaster shoulder spica for fracture of humerus.

force. The patient is instructed to sleep in the semireclining position. This is a difficult method of treatment in obese patients. Some believe that this method may cause increased distraction of fragments. When fracture of the shaft of the humerus is associated with other injuries that require confinement to bed, initial treatment may be by overhead skeletal traction. Significant success in the treatment of these fractures has been reported with the use of a prefabricated polypropylene sleeve applied soon after pain and swelling subside.

Fractures of the shaft of the humerus—especially transverse fractures—may heal slowly. If stabilization has not taken place after 6–8 weeks, consideration of internal fixation and bone grafting is justified. If the patient is not a surgical candidate, more secure external immobilization may be obtained with a shoulder spica (Figure 43–22).

About 5–10% of humeral fractures demonstrate radial nerve involvement. Fractures of the distal third of the humerus are especially vulnerable, because the nerve is fixed to the proximal fragment by the intermuscular septum and is more easily injured at the time of displacement (Figure 43–23).

Most radial nerve injuries are the result of stretching or contusion, and function will return in days or months.

If the radial nerve lesion is complete, results may be as good with delayed repair as with primary repair. A proper plan is to reduce and immobilize the frac-

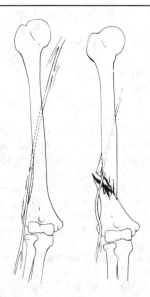

Figure 43–23. Drawing shows the close relationship of the radial nerve to the humerus. There is a significant possibility of injury to the nerve with fracture in the distal third of the humerus.

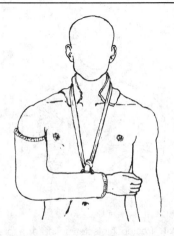

Figure 43–21. Caldwell's hanging cast.

ture and support the fingers and wrist with a dynamic splint until the fracture has healed. By this time, nerve function has usually returned. Early exploration is rarely necessary.

Open reduction of closed fractures may be indicated if arterial circulation has been interrupted or if adequate apposition of major fragments cannot be obtained by closed methods.

Camden P, Nade S: Fracture bracing the humerus. Injury 1992;23:245.

Robinson CM et al: Locked nailing of humeral shaft fractures: Experience in Edinburgh over a two-year period. J Bone Joint Surg [Br] 1992;74:558.

Szyszkowitz R, Schippinger G, Seggl W: Fractures of the humerus. J R Coll Surg Edinb 1990;35(6 Suppl):S27.

INJURIES OF THE ELBOW REGION

1. FRACTURE OF THE DISTAL HUMERUS IN ADULTS

Fracture of the distal humerus is most often caused by indirect violence. The configuration of the fracture cleft and the direction of displacement of the fragments are likely to be typical. Injuries of major vessels and nerves and elbow joint dislocation are apt to be present.

Clinical findings consist of pain, swelling, and restriction of motion. Minor deformity may not be apparent, because swelling usually obliterates landmarks. The type of fracture is determined by x-ray examination.

Examination for peripheral nerve and vascular injury must be made and all findings carefully recorded before treatment is instituted.

Supracondylar Fracture of the Humerus

Supracondylar fracture of the humerus occurs proximal to the olecranon fossa; transcondylar (diacondylar) fracture occurs more distally and extends into the olecranon fossa. Neither fracture extends to the articular surface of the humerus. Treatment is the same for both types.

The direction of displacement of the distal fragment from the midcoronal plane of the arm serves to differentiate the "extension" from the less common "flexion" type. This differentiation has important implications for treatment.

A. Extension Type Fracture: In the extension type of supracondylar fracture, the usual direction of displacement of the main distal fragment is posterior and proximal. The distal fragment may also be displaced laterally and, less frequently, medially. The direction of these displacements is identified easily on biplane x-ray films. Internal torsional displace-

ment, however, is more difficult to recognize. Unless torsional displacement is reduced, relative cubitus varus with loss of carrying angle will persist.

Displaced supracondylar fractures are emergencies. Immediate treatment is required to avoid occlusion of the brachial artery and to prevent or avoid further peripheral nerve injury. If hemorrhage and edema prevent complete reduction of the fracture at the first attempt, a second manipulation will be required after swelling has regressed.

1. Manipulative reduction–Minor angular displacements (tilting) may be reduced by gentle flexion of the elbow under local or general anesthesia, followed by immobilization in a posterior plaster splint in 120–130 degrees of flexion (Figure 43–24). If displacement is marked but normal radial pulsation indicates that circulation is not impaired, closed manipulation under general anesthesia should be done as soon as possible. If radial pulses are absent or weak on initial examination and do not improve with manipulation, an arteriogram is indicated to check for vascular injury. Capillary flush in the nail beds cannot be relied on as the sole indication of competency

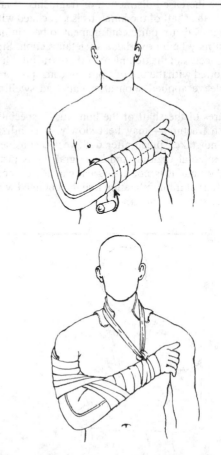

Figure 43–24. Posterior plaster splint for supracondylar fracture.

of deep circulation. After reduction and application of a posterior plaster splint or bivalved cast, the patient should be placed at bed rest, preferably in a hospital, with the elbow up on a pillow and the dressing arranged so that the radial pulse is accessible for frequent monitoring. Swelling can be expected to increase for 24–72 hours. During this critical period, continued observation is necessary so that any circulatory embarrassment which may lead to Volkmann's ischemic contracture can be identified at once. The circular bandage must be adjusted frequently to compensate for initial increase and subsequent decrease of swelling. If during manipulation it was necessary to extend the elbow beyond 45 degrees to restore radial pulses, the joint should be flexed to the optimal angle as swelling subsides to prevent loss of the reduction.

2. Traction and immobilization–In certain instances, supracondylar fractures of the humerus with posterior displacement of the distal fragment should be treated by traction (Figure 43–25): (1) If comminution is marked and stability cannot be obtained by flexion of the elbow, traction is indicated until the fragments have stabilized. (2) If two or three attempts at manipulative reduction have been unsuccessful, continuous traction under x-ray control for 1–2 days is justifiable before further manipulation. (3) If the radial pulse is absent or weak at initial examination and does not improve with manipulation, overhead traction may be necessary to prevent displacement of the fracture and further embarrassment of circulation. (Arteriography may be indicated.) During the early phase of treatment by continuous traction, flexion of the elbow beyond 90 degrees should be avoided, since this may jeopardize circulation.

B. Flexion Type Fracture: Flexion type fracture of the humerus is quite rare. It is characterized by anterior and sometimes also torsional and lateral displacement of the main distal fragment. Treatment is by closed manipulation. A posterior plaster splint is then applied from the axillary fold to the level of the wrist, with the forearm in supination and the elbow in full extension. Elevation is advisable for at least 24 hours or until soft tissue swelling has reached the maximum, after which time the patient may be ambulatory. Immobilization is then continued for 8–12 weeks. When satisfactory reduction cannot be accomplished by closed manipulation, treatment should be by traction with the elbow in full extension until the fragments become stabilized.

If adequate reduction cannot be obtained or maintained by closed manipulation or traction, internal fixation is indicated. Rigid fixation should be achieved to allow for early motion.

Intercondylar Fracture of the Humerus

Intercondylar fracture of the humerus is classically described as being of the T or Y type (or both), according to the configuration of the fracture cleft observed on an anteroposterior x-ray. This fracture is commonly the result of a blow to the posterior aspect of the flexed elbow. Open fracture and other injuries to the soft tissues are frequently present. The fracture often extends into the trochlear surface of the elbow joint, and unless the articular surfaces of the distal humerus can be accurately repositioned, restriction of joint motion, pain, instability, and deformity can be expected.

A. Closed Reduction: If the fragments are not widely displaced, closed reduction may be successful. Since comminution is always present, stabilization is difficult to achieve and maintain by manipulation and external immobilization. Significant displacement requires overhead skeletal traction by means of a Kirschner wire inserted through the proximal ulna. Traction is continued until stabilization occurs. The extremity may then be immobilized in a tubular plaster cast. Complete bone healing usually occurs within 12 weeks.

B. Open Reduction: Open reduction may be indicated if adequate positioning cannot be obtained by closed methods. A requirement for acceptable results of open reduction and internal fixation is that the fragments be sufficiently large so that they can be fixed to one another. Immediate internal fixation may improve alignment of the fragments and may allow early motion of the joint, thereby decreasing subsequent elbow stiffness. However, comminution may be so extensive that satisfactory stabilization cannot be accomplished by current techniques of internal fixation. Under such circumstances, it may be better to abandon open operation and to accept the imperfect results of closed treatment. It is important to remember that the final x-ray appearance of these fractures does not always coincide with the functional results. Posttraumatic arthritis and restriction of joint

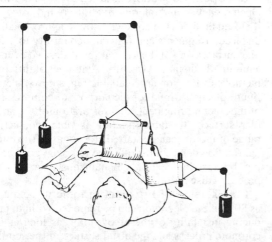

Figure 43–25. Skeletal traction for supracondylar fracture.

motion can occur even if the articular surface is restored anatomically.

Neurovascular injury is quite common in distal humeral fractures, and infection may occur following open reduction. Late complications of injury include limitation of motion (sometimes severe), deformity, and pain.

Fracture of the Lateral Condyle of the Humerus

Fractures of the lateral condyle of the humerus are of two types. One type involves articular and nonarticular components of the condyle and must be differentiated from the second type—fractures of the capitellum.

Undisplaced or minimally displaced fractures of the lateral condyle may be treated with immobilization in a long-arm plaster cast for 6–8 weeks until stable. If the fracture is significantly displaced, closed reduction is rarely successful in maintaining alignment. Open reduction and internal fixation allow anatomic restoration of the articular surface and the possibility of early motion of the elbow.

Fracture of the capitellum is characterized by proximal displacement of the anterior detached fragment and probably occurs as one component of a spontaneously reduced incomplete dislocation of the elbow joint. The lesion is most clearly demonstrated on lateral x-rays. Closed reduction should be attempted by placing the elbow in acute flexion. After reduction, the extremity is immobilized in a posterior plaster splint with the elbow in full flexion to prevent displacement of the small distal fragment.

When accurate reduction cannot be accomplished by closed techniques, open operation may be desirable to avoid subsequent restriction of elbow movement. If the small distal fragment retains sufficient soft tissue attachment to ensure adequate blood supply, it may be fixed to the main fragment in anatomic position by a Kirschner wire. If the articular fragment lacks significant soft tissue bonds, removal is recommended, since avascular necrosis is likely to follow.

Fracture of the Trochlea of the Humerus

Isolated fractures of the trochlea are very unusual. Signs of intra-articular injury, including pain, effusion, restriction of motion, and crepitus, are usually present. The diagnosis is confirmed by x-ray showing a fragment lying on the medial side of the joint. Large fragments may be replaced; smaller fragments are better excised.

Godette GA, Gruel CR: Percutaneous screw fixation of intercondylar fracture of the distal humerus. Orthop Rev 1993;3;22:466.

Holdsworth BJ, Mossad MM: Fractures of the adult distal humerus: Elbow function after internal fixation. J Bone Joint Surg [Br] 1990;72:362.

Letsch R et al: Intraarticular fractures of the distal humerus: Surgical treatment and results. Clin Orthop 1989; Apr(241):238.

Perry CR, Gibson CT, Kowalski MF: Transcondylar fractures of the distal humerus. J Orthop Trauma 1989;3:98.

2. FRACTURE OF THE PROXIMAL ULNA (Olecranon Fractures)

Fracture of the olecranon that occurs as a result of indirect violence (eg, forced flexion of the forearm against the actively contracted triceps muscle) is typically transverse or slightly oblique. Fracture due to direct violence is usually comminuted and associated with other fracture or anterior dislocation of the joint (discussed below). Since the major fracture cleft extends into the elbow joint, treatment should be directed toward restoration of anatomic position to afford maximal recovery of range of motion and functional competency of the triceps.

Treatment

Treatment depends upon the degree of displacement and the extent of comminution.

A. Closed Reduction: Minimal displacement (1–2 mm) can be treated by closed manipulation with the elbow in full extension and immobilization in a plaster cast that extends from the anterior axillary fold to the wrist. X-rays should be taken weekly for 2 weeks after reduction to determine whether reduction has been maintained. Immobilization must be continued for at least 6 weeks before active flexion exercises are begun. Position of the arm in full extension for this length of time keeps the hand far away from the body and makes the extremity quite useless during the time of immobilization. This treatment generally has poor patient acceptance.

B. Open Reduction and Internal Fixation: Open reduction and internal fixation are indicated (1) if closed methods are not successful in approximating displaced fragments and restoring congruity to articular surfaces, or (2) if early motion is desired even in a minimally displaced fracture. A number of different methods of fixation are available (eg, screws, plates, figure-of-eight wires) for the purpose of compression of the fracture fragments and restoration of the articular surface. If stable fixation is obtained, active range of motion can be started at 5–7 days. The internal fixation device must often be removed after healing, because its location subcutaneously on the ulna produces discomfort.

C. Excision of Proximal Fragment: As much as 80% of the olecranon can be removed without producing instability of the elbow joint, as long as the coronoid process and the distal surface of the semilunar notch of the ulna are intact and the triceps is adequately repaired. This procedure is as effective as open reduction and internal fixation and does not require subsequent operation for hardware removal.

Hume MC, Wiss DA: Olecranon fractures: A clinical and radiographic comparison of tension band wiring and plate fixation. Clin Orthop 1992;Dec(285):229.
Maffulli N, Chan D, Aldridge MJ: Overuse injuries of the olecranon in young gymnasts. J Bone Joint Surg [Br] 1992;74:305.
Rowland SA, Burkhart SS: Tension band wiring of olecranon fractures: A modification of the AO technique. Clin Orthop 1992;Apr(277):238.

3. FRACTURE OF THE PROXIMAL RADIUS

Fracture of the head and neck of the radius may occur as an isolated injury uncomplicated by dislocation of the elbow or the proximal radioulnar joint. This fracture is usually caused by indirect force, such as a fall on the outstretched hand, when the radial head is driven against the capitellum. Care must be taken to obtain true anteroposterior and lateral x-rays of the proximal radius as well as of the elbow joint, since minor lesions may be obscured by a change in position from midposition to full supination during exposure of the films.

Treatment

A. Conservative Treatment: Radial head fractures ranging from no displacement to involvement of two-thirds of the head and 2–3 mm of depression can be treated symptomatically, with evacuation of the tense hemarthrosis by aspiration to minimize pain. The extremity may be supported by a sling or immobilized in a posterior plaster splint with the elbow in 90 degrees of flexion. Active exercises of the elbow are to be encouraged within a few days to a week. Recovery of function can take up to 6 weeks. Slight restriction of motion (especially extension) may persist but usually is not functionally significant.

B. Surgical Treatment: When severe comminution involves the entire articular surface or there is a loose fragment in the joint, surgical treatment is indicated. Excision of either the loose fragment or the entire comminuted radial head allows return to satisfactory elbow function. After excision of the head, the radius may migrate proximally, but migration is usually less than 2 mm and rarely causes major symptoms other than a moderate decrease in forearm strength.

If radial excision is indicated, it is best done early unless this will contribute to serious instability of the elbow joint. A silicone radial head replacement arthroplasty may be done primarily to improve stability in an unstable joint or to minimize proximal migration of the radius.

D'souza S, Vaishya R, Klenerman L: Management of radial neck fractures in children: a retrospective analysis of one hundred patients. J Pediatr Orthop 1993;13:232.
Geel CW, Palmer AK: Radial head fractures and their effect on the distal radioulnar joint: A rationale for treatment. Clin Orthop 1992;Feb(275):79.
King GJ, Evans DC, Kellam JF: Open reduction and internal fixation of radial head fractures. J Orthop Trauma 1991;5:21.

4. SUBLUXATION & DISLOCATION OF THE ELBOW JOINT

Dislocation of the Head of the Radius

Isolated dislocation of the radius at the elbow is a rare lesion that implies dislocation of the proximal radioulnar and radiohumeral joints without fracture. It occurs in children over age 5 years or occasionally in adults and must be differentiated from subluxation of the head of the radius. To cause dislocation, injury must be severe enough to disrupt the capsulotendinous support—especially the annular ligament—of the proximal radius. The direction of displacement of the radial head is usually anterior or lateral, but it may be posterior.

Reduction can usually be accomplished by forced supination of the forearm under local or general anesthesia. The extremity should be immobilized for 3–4 weeks with the elbow in flexion and the forearm in supination.

Dislocation of the Elbow Joint Without Fracture (Figure 43–26)

Dislocation of the elbow joint without major fracture is almost always posterior. It usually occurs from a fall on the outstretched hand. Complete backward dislocation of the ulna and radius implies extensive tearing of the capsuloligamentous structures and in-

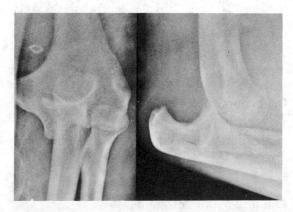

Figure 43–26. Complete posterior dislocation of the elbow joint without fracture or neurovascular injury.

jury to the region of insertion of the brachialis muscle. Biplane x-rays of the highest quality are necessary to determine that no fracture is associated. Peripheral nerve function must be carefully assessed before definitive treatment is instituted. The ulnar nerve is most likely to be injured.

Complete muscle relaxation is necessary to achieve atraumatic reduction. This can be accomplished by sedation, regional block, or general anesthesia and is the choice of the surgeon. Closed reduction can be achieved by axial traction on the forearm with the elbow in the position of deformity. Hyperextension is not necessary. Lateral or medial dislocation can be corrected during traction. As soon as displacement is corrected, the elbow should be fully flexed and extended to make certain reduction has actually occurred. The medial and lateral ligaments should also be tested, as major instability in either plane may require surgical repair. The elbow should then be immobilized in at least 90 degrees of flexion by applying a posterior plaster splint that reaches from the posterior axillary fold to the wrist. The duration of immobilization depends mainly on the stability of the elbow after reduction. The elbow must be x-rayed at 3, 7, and 10 days postreduction in the cast to make certain that reduction is maintained. As swelling decreases, the elbow may redislocate in the cast with minimal pain experienced by the patient. In uncomplicated stable dislocations with intact and stable collateral ligaments and an intact coronoid process, the splint may be removed after 3–4 days and active motion started. There is no place for passive motion or any form of manipulation in the rehabilitation process, as forceful treatment may lead to severe loss of motion and joint stiffness.

Closed reduction should be attempted even if unreduced dislocation has persisted for 2–3 weeks following injury. Open reduction of the persistent dislocation may be successful for up to 2 months after injury. Myositis ossificans of the brachialis muscle is a rare sequela.

Habernek H, Ortner F: The influence of anatomic factors in elbow joint dislocation. Clin Orthop 1992;Jan(274):226.
O'Driscoll SW et al: Elbow subluxation and dislocation: A spectrum of instability. Clin Orthop 1992;Jul(280):186.
Trousdale RT et al: Radio-ulnar dissociation: A review of twenty cases. J Bone Joint Surg [Am] 1992;74:1486.

Dislocation of the Elbow Joint With Fracture

Dislocation of the elbow is frequently associated with fracture. Some fractures are insignificant and require no specific treatment; others demand specialized care.

Fracture of the Coronoid Process of the Ulna

Fracture of the coronoid process of the ulna is the most frequent complication of posterior dislocation of the elbow joint. Treatment requires at least 3–4 weeks of immobilization to obtain stability.

Fracture of the Head of the Radius With Posterior Dislocation of the Elbow Joint

This injury is treated as two separate lesions. The severity of comminution and the magnitude of displacement of the radial head fragments are first determined by x-ray. If comminution has occurred or the fragments are widely displaced, the dislocation is reduced by closed manipulation; the head of the radius is then excised.

If fracture of the head of the radius is not comminuted and the fragments are not widely displaced, treatment is as for uncomplicated posterior dislocation of the elbow joint.

Fracture of the Olecranon With Anterior Dislocation of the Elbow Joint (Figure 43–27)

This very unstable injury usually occurs from a blow to the flexed elbow that drives the olecranon forward. Fracture through the olecranon permits the distal fragment of the ulna and the proximal radius to be displaced anterior to the humerus and may cause extensive tearing of the capsuloligamentous structures around the elbow joint. The dislocation can be reduced by bringing the elbow into full extension, but anatomic reduction of the olecranon fracture by closed manipulation is not likely to be successful, and immediate open reduction is usually indicated. Recovery of function is apt to be delayed and incomplete.

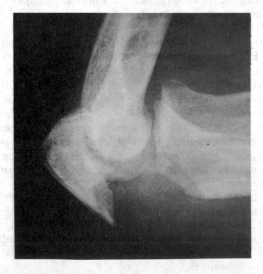

Figure 43–27. Fracture of the olecranon and anterior subluxation of the radius.

5. TOTAL ELBOW ARTHROPLASTY

Severe pain and disabling stiffness may result from rheumatoid arthritis, posttraumatic arthritis, or osteoarthritis. Over the years, nonprosthetic arthroplasties (eg, resection or interpositional soft tissue arthroplasties) have failed to produce consistently good results. Total elbow replacement has been developed in an attempt to provide mobility, stability, and freedom from pain. The joint is replaced with a metal and polyethylene prosthesis, usually with extensions placed into the humeral and ulnar shafts to provide stability. Significant pain relief and some increase in motion result in nearly 80% of patients. Complications are frequent and include dislocation, intraoperative fracture, triceps weakness, loosening, and sepsis. Loosening of the prosthesis sufficient to necessitate revision occurs in 10–15% of patients. Infection is the most serious complication and usually requires removal of the prosthesis.

Kasten MD, Skinner HB: Total elbow arthroplasty: An 18-year experience. Clin Orthop 1993;May(290):177.

Weiss AA, Berman AT, O'Brien J: What are the current indications for total elbow arthroplasty? Report of a case using allograft for TEA. Orthopedics 1993;16:237.

INJURIES OF THE SHAFTS OF THE RADIUS & ULNA

1. FRACTURES OF THE SHAFTS OF THE RADIUS & ULNA

General Considerations

A. Causative Injury: Spiral and oblique fractures are apt to be caused by indirect injury. Greenstick, transverse, and comminuted fractures are commonly the result of direct injury.

B. Radiography: In addition to anteroposterior and lateral films of the entire forearm, including the elbow and wrist joints, oblique views are often desirable. The lateral projection is usually taken with the forearm in midposition (between complete pronation and supination). For the anteroposterior projection, care must be taken to prevent any change in relative supination of the radius; if this happens, the distal radius will be the same in both views.

C. Anatomic Peculiarities: Both the radius and the ulna have biplane curves that permit 180 degrees of rotation in the forearm. If the curves are not preserved by reduction, full rotatory motion of the forearm may not be recovered, or derangement of the radioulnar joints may follow.

Torsional displacement by muscle activity has important implications for manipulative treatment of certain fractures of the radial shaft. The direction of displacement of the distal fragment following fracture of the shaft is influenced by the location of the lesion in reference to muscle insertion. If the fracture is in the upper third (above the insertion of the pronator teres), the proximal fragment will be drawn into relative supination by the biceps and supinator and the distal fragment into pronation by the pronator teres and pronator quadratus. The relative position of the proximal fragment may be determined by comparing the position of the bicipital tubercle on an anteroposterior film with similar projections of the uninjured arm taken in varying degrees of forearm rotation. In fractures below the middle of the radius (below the insertion of the pronator teres), the proximal fragment characteristically remains in midposition and the distal fragment is pronated; this is due to the antagonistic action of the pronator teres on the biceps and supinator.

D. Closed Reduction and Splinting: With fracture and displacement of the shaft of either the radius or the ulna, injury of the proximal or distal radioulnar joints should always be suspected. The presence of swelling and tenderness around the joint may aid in localization of an occult injury when x-rays are not helpful.

Reduction of uncomplicated fractures of the radius and ulna should be attempted. The type of manipulative maneuver depends upon the configuration and location of the fracture and the age of the patient. The position of immobilization of the elbow, forearm, and wrist depends upon the location of the fracture and its inherent stability. Internal fixation allows anatomic alignment and early motion (see Fractures of the Shafts of Both Bones).

Fracture of the Shaft of The Ulna

Isolated fracture of the shaft of the proximal third of the ulna (above the radial insertion of the pronator teres) with displacement is often associated with dislocation of the head of the radius. (See Fracture and Dislocation of the Radius and Ulna.) Reduction of an isolated transverse fracture may be achieved by axial traction followed by digital pressure to correct displacement in the transverse plane. With the patient supine, the hand is suspended overhead, and countertraction is provided by a sling around the arm above the flexed elbow. After the fragments are distracted, transverse displacement is corrected by digital pressure. With the elbow at a right angle and the forearm in midposition, the extremity is then immobilized in a tubular plaster cast extending from the axilla to the metacarpophalangeal joints. During the first month, weekly examination by x-ray is necessary to determine whether displacement has occurred. Immobilization must be maintained until bone continuity is restored (usually in 8–12 weeks).

Fracture of the distal shaft of the ulna is apt to be complicated by angulation. The proximal end of the distal fragment is displaced toward the radius by the pronator quadratus muscle. Reduction can be achieved by the maneuver described above. To prevent recurrent displacement of the distal fragment, the plaster cast must be carefully molded so as to force the mass of the forearm musculature between the radius and ulna in the anteroposterior plane. Care should be taken to avoid pressure over the subcutaneous surfaces of the radius and ulna around the wrist. Healing is slow, and frequent radiologic examination is necessary to make certain that displacement has not occurred. Stabilization by bone healing may require longer than 3–4 months of immobilization.

An oblique fracture cleft creates an unstable mechanism with a tendency toward displacement, and immobilization in a tubular plaster cast is not reliable. Open reduction and rigid internal fixation with bone plates or an intramedullary rod are indicated.

Undisplaced or minimally displaced fracture of the ulna may be treated with a removable forearm fracture brace for a few weeks, followed by an Ace bandage until healing is complete.

Fracture of the Shaft
of the Radius

Isolated closed fracture of the shaft of the radius can be caused by direct or indirect violence; open fracture usually results from penetrating injury. Closed fracture with displacement is usually associated with other injury (eg, fracture of the ulna or dislocation of the distal radioulnar joint). X-rays may not reveal dislocation, but localized tenderness and swelling suggest injury to the distal radioulnar joint.

If the fracture is proximal to the insertion of the pronator teres, closed reduction is indicated. The extremity should then be immobilized in a tubular plaster cast that extends from the axilla to the metacarpophalangeal joints, with the elbow at a right angle and the forearm in full supination (Figure 43–28).

If the fracture is distal to the insertion of the pronator teres, manipulation and immobilization are as described above except that the forearm should be in midrotation rather than full supination. Since injury

to the distal radioulnar joint is apt to be associated with fracture of the radial shaft below the insertion of the pronator teres, weekly anteroposterior and lateral x-ray projections should be taken during the first month to determine the exact status of reduction.

In adults, if stability cannot be achieved, if reduction does not approach the anatomic, or if early joint motion is desired, open reduction and internal fixation with metal plate and screws are recommended, since deformity as a result of displacement of fragments is likely to cause limitation of forearm and hand movements.

Fracture of the Shafts
of Both Bones
(Figure 43–29)

The management of fractures of the shafts of both bones of the forearm is essentially a combination of those techniques that have been described for the individual bones. If both bones are fractured at the same time, dislocation of either radioulnar joint is not likely to occur. If the configuration of the fracture cleft is approximately transverse, stability may be attained by closed methods provided reduction is anatomic or nearly so. Oblique or comminuted fractures are unstable.

Treatment depends in part upon the degree of displacement, the severity of comminution, and the age of the patient.

A. Without Displacement: In adults, fracture of the shaft of the radius and ulna without displacement can be treated by immobilization in a tubular plaster cast extending from the axilla to the metacarpophalangeal joints with the elbow at a right angle and the forearm in supination (fractures of the upper third) or midposition (fractures of the mid and lower

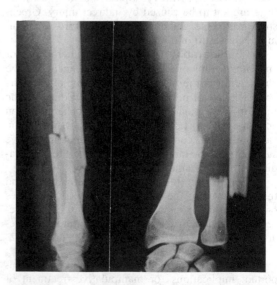

Figure 43–29. Fracture of the lower third of the shafts of the radius and ulna.

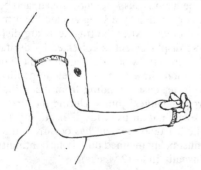

Figure 43–28. Full upper extremity plaster for fracture of both bones of the forearm.

thirds). Immobilization for 16–20 weeks is generally sufficient for restoration of bone continuity. To avoid late angulation or refracture, the elbow should be included in the plaster until the callus is well mineralized (Figure 43–28).

B. With Displacement: Although it is not always possible to correct displaced fractures of both bones of the forearm by closed methods, an attempt can be made to do so if x-ray studies show a configuration whereby stabilization can be accomplished without operation. Most commonly, accurate apposition and stability of fragments cannot be achieved in fractures of both bones. Therefore, open reduction and internal fixation (with bone plate and screws or intramedullary rods) are recommended provided experienced personnel and adequate equipment are available. Persistent displacement of the fragments of one or both bones may be associated with delay of healing, restriction of forearm movements, derangement of the radioulnar joints, and deformity. In fractures in which open reduction is justifiable in the adult, rigid internal fixation is indicated; a technical pitfall to be avoided is the use of a single wire loop or trans-fixation screw, a short bone plate attached with unicortical screws, or small intramedullary wires. If excellent stability is achieved at operation with bone plates, motion of the extremity may be started as soon as the surgical wound is healed.

Duncan R et al: Immediate internal fixation of open fractures of the diaphysis of the forearm. J Orthop Trauma 1992;6:25.

Gibson WK, Timperlake RW: Operative treatment of a type IV Monteggia fracture-dislocation in a child. J Bone Joint Surg [Br] 1992;74:780.

Jones JA: Immediate internal fixation of high-energy open forearm fractures. J Orthop Trauma 1991;5:272

Schuind F, Andrianne Y, Burny F: Treatment of forearm fractures by Hoffman external fixation: A study of 93 patients. Clin Orthop 1991;May(266):197.

2. FRACTURE & DISLOCATION OF THE RADIUS & ULNA

Fracture of the Ulna With Dislocation of the Radial Head (Monteggia's Fracture)

Fracture of the ulna, especially when it occurs near the junction of the middle and upper thirds of the shaft, may be complicated by dislocation of the radial head. This unstable fracture-dislocation, the so-called Monteggia fracture, is categorized commonly under three types. The most common type is anterior dislocation of the radial head with fracture of the ulnar diaphysis with anterior angulation (type I). In type II, posterior dislocation of the radial head is accompanied by posterior convex angulation at the fracture site of the ulna. The type III lesion—lateral dislocation of the radial head with fracture of the ulna in its proximal third, distal to the coronoid process—is rare.

In all types, there is marked pain and tenderness in the forearm and around the elbow, and the patient resists any motion of the elbow joint. Complete neurologic examination of the extremity is indicated, since paralysis of the deep branch of the radial nerve is the most common associated neurologic lesion. Spontaneous recovery is usual, and exploration of the nerve is rarely indicated.

These injuries are usually caused by direct violence to the forearm. The annular ligament may be torn, or the head may be displaced distally from beneath the annular ligament without causing a significant tear. The injured ligament may be interposed between the articular surface of the head of the radius and the capitellum of the humerus or the adjacent ulna.

The diagnosis is confirmed by x-rays of the elbow and forearm in the anteroposterior and lateral planes. Fracture of the ulna is obvious, but dislocation of the radial head is frequently missed. Proper positioning of the x-ray tube in relation to the elbow and the film will improve identification of the radial head dislocation, as will familiarity of the physician with the lesion.

Good results are most readily obtained by rigid internal fixation of the fractured ulna with plate and screws and complete reduction of the dislocated radial head. The radial head can usually be adequately reduced by closed manipulation. Open reduction of the radial head is indicated only when a portion of the annular ligament may be obstructing closed reduction. The extremity should be immobilized in 110 degrees of flexion for 6 weeks to maintain reduction of the radial head. X-rays should be taken 1, 2, and 6 weeks postoperatively to ensure maintenance of reduction.

Fracture of the Shaft of the Radius With Dislocation of the Ulnar Head

In fracture of the shaft of the radius near the junction of the middle and lower thirds with dislocation of the head of the ulna distally (Galeazzi's fracture), the apex of major angulation is usually directed anteriorly while the ulnar head lies volar to the distal end of the radius.

The results of closed treatment are poor, since anatomic alignment is difficult to maintain in plaster. Good results can be obtained by accurate reduction and internal fixation of the fractured radius with plate and screws and immobilization in a long-arm cast with the forearm in full supination for 6–8 weeks. Even though this injury includes complete dislocation of the distal radioulnar joint, Kirschner wire fixation of the joint is not necessary as long as the forearm is immobilized in supination to allow for reduction.

Complications of fracture-dislocations of the radius and ulna are similar to those of forearm fractures in general: infection, malunion, and nonunion.

Dicke TE, Nunley JA: Distal forearm fractures in children: Complications and surgical indications. Orthop Clin North Am 1993;3;24:333.

INJURIES OF THE WRIST REGION

1. SPRAINS OF THE WRIST

Isolated severe sprain of the ligaments of the wrist joint is not common, and the diagnosis of wrist sprain should not be made until other lesions (eg, carpel fractures and dislocations) have been ruled out. If symptoms persist for more than 2 weeks, and especially if pain and swelling are present, x-ray examination should be repeated.

Treatment may be by immobilization with a volar splint extending from the palmar flexion crease to the elbow. The splint should be attached with elastic bandages so that it can be removed at least three times daily for gentle active exercise and warm soaks.

2. COLLES' FRACTURE (Figure 43–30)

Abraham Colles described this fracture as an impacted fracture of the radius 2–3 cm proximal to the wrist joint. Modern usage has extended the term Colles' fracture to include a variety of complete fractures of the distal radius characterized by varying degrees of dorsal displacement of the distal fragment.

The fracture is commonly caused by a fall with the hand outstretched, the wrist in dorsiflexion, and the forearm in pronation, so that the force is applied to the palmar surface of the hand. Colles' fracture is most common in middle life and old age. Avulsion of the ulnar styloid may accompany the distal radius fracture. If the ulnar styloid process is not fractured, the collateral ulnar ligament may be torn. The head of the ulna may lie anterior to the distal fragment of the radius.

Clinical Findings

Clinical findings vary according to the magnitude of injury, the degree of displacement of fragments, and the interval since injury. If the fragments are not displaced, examination soon after injury will demonstrate only slight tenderness and insignificant swelling. Marked displacement produces the classic "silver fork," or "bayonet," deformity, in which a dorsal prominence caused by displacement of the distal fragment replaces the normal convex curve of the lower radius and the ulnar head is prominent on the anteromedial aspect of the wrist. Later, swelling may extend from the fingertips to the elbow.

Complications

Derangement of the distal radioulnar joint is the most common complicating injury. Direct injury to the median nerve by bone spicules is not common. Compression of the nerve by hemorrhage and edema or by displaced bone fragments can occur and may cause all gradations of sensory and motor paralysis. Initial treatment of the fracture by immobilization of the wrist in acute flexion can be a significant factor in aggravation of compression. Persistent compression of the nerve creates classic symptoms of the carpal tunnel syndrome, which may require operative division of the volar carpal ligament for relief.

Treatment

Complete recovery of function and a pleasing cosmetic result are goals of treatment that cannot always be achieved. The patient's age, sex, and occupation, the presence of complicating injury or disease, the severity of comminution, and the configuration of the fracture cleft govern the selection of treatment.

Open reduction of recent closed Colles' fracture is rarely the treatment of choice. Many techniques of closed reduction and external immobilization have been advocated; the experience and preference of the surgeon determine the selection.

A. Minor Displacement: Colles' fracture with minimal displacement is characterized by absence of comminution and slight dorsal impaction. Deformity is barely perceptible or may not be visible even to a trained observer. In the elderly patient, treatment is directed toward early recovery of function. In young

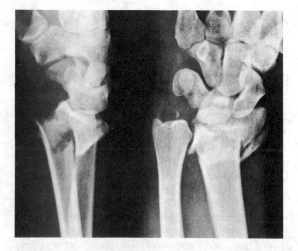

Figure 43–30. Comminuted Colles' fracture in a 58-year-old man. Because of severe comminution, this fracture is unstable.

patients, prevention of further displacement is the first consideration.

Reduction is not necessary. In an elderly patient, the wrist is immobilized for 3–4 weeks in a short-arm cast or volar splint for comfort; then motion is begun.

B. Marked Displacement: (Figure 43–30.) Early reduction and immobilization are indicated. Muscular relaxation of the extremity can usually be attained by systemic analgesia and local anesthesia. Regional block or general anesthesia will give more complete pain relief. Reduction by manipulation is accomplished by applying traction through the grasped injured hand with countertraction to the forearm or humerus. After disimpaction of the fragments, the fracture is reduced by palmar displacement of the distal fragment and ulnar deviation. The wrist is immobilized in this position. Some authors advocate immobilization of the wrist in pronation and some in supination. The latter position is felt to decrease the tension of the brachioradialis and its tendency to redisplace the fracture.

A lightly padded tubular cast or a "sugar tong" splint is preferred. The plaster should extend distally only to the flexion crease on the palmar side (to allow full flexion of metacarpophalangeal joints) and out to the web space of the fingers dorsally (to decrease swelling over the dorsum of the hand). The cast or sugar tong splint may be extended above the elbow, particularly in obese patients, to allow more complete immobilization (Figure 43–31). After the plaster has been applied, x-rays are taken while anesthesia is continued. If x-rays show that reduction is not adequate, remanipulation is carried out immediately.

Immobilization is maintained for 6 weeks, during which time the patient is strongly encouraged to exercise and use the fingers, elbow, and shoulder of the affected extremity. X-ray examination is repeated on the third day and thereafter at weekly intervals during the first 2–3 weeks.

C. Unstable Fractures: If x-rays show extensive comminution with intra-articular extension and involvement of the volar cortex, the fracture is likely to be unstable, and skeletal distraction is probably indicated. This can be accomplished by use of an external fixation device or with skeletal traction pins incorporated in plaster. In either case, pins are drilled into or through the bone above and below the fracture to allow for distraction and manipulation of the fragments to obtain adequate alignment and length. The pins are left in place for 6–8 weeks. Initial reduction may be improved by the use of Chinese fingertraps or weight placed on the traction pins to allow distraction of the fracture fragments.

Postreduction Treatment

Frequent observation and careful management can prevent or minimize some of the disabling sequelae of Colles' fracture. The patient's full cooperation in the exercise program is essential. If comminution is

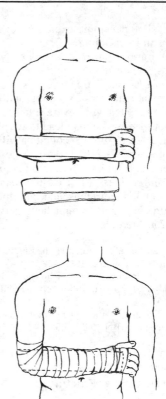

Figure 43–31. "Sugar tong" plaster splint.

marked, if swelling is severe, or if there is evidence of median nerve deficit, the patient should remain under close observation (preferably in a hospital) for at least 72 hours. The extremity should be elevated to minimize swelling, and the adequacy of circulation should be determined at frequent intervals. Active exercise of the fingers and shoulder is encouraged. In order that the extremity be used as much as possible, the plaster should be trimmed in the palm to permit full finger flexion. Increased use of the hand and shoulder will be encouraged if the patient is not allowed to use a sling.

As soon as the plaster is removed, the patient is advised to use the extremity for routine daily activities.

Sequelae

Joint stiffness is the most disabling sequela of Colles' fracture. Derangement of the distal radioulnar joint may be caused by the original injury and perpetuated by incomplete reduction; it is characterized by restriction of forearm movements and pain. Late rupture of the extensor pollicis longus tendon is relatively uncommon. Symptoms of median nerve injury due to compression caused by acute swelling alone usually do not persist more than 6 months. Prolonged symptoms can cause carpal tunnel syndrome. Failure to perform shoulder joint exercises several times daily can result in disabling stiffness.

Shoulder-hand syndrome (reflex sympathetic dystrophy) is an infrequent but severely disabling complication of Colles' fracture. It is characterized by marked pain, tenderness, swelling, and induration of the hand associated with severe stiffness of the fingers and shoulder, which may lead to atrophy and residual contractures. Prompt recognition will allow for effective treatment. Gentle, progressive exercises of the shoulder and hand have been most helpful for relief of pain and stiffness. More controversial methods of treatment include intramuscular injections of lidocaine or corticosteroids, sympathetic nerve blocks, and oral corticosteroids.

Herndon JH: Distal radius fractures: nonsurgical treatment options. Instr Course Lect 1993;42:67.

Kopylov P et al: Fractures of the distal end of the radius in young adults: A 30-year follow-up. J Hand Surg [Br] 1993;18:45.

Roysam GS: The distal radio-ulnar joint in Colles' fractures J Bone Joint Surg [Br] 1993;75:58.

3. SMITH'S FRACTURE (Reverse Colles' Fracture)

Although Smith did not observe an anatomic preparation of this lesion, his description in 1847 placed the fracture of the radius 2–2.5 cm proximal to the wrist joint. The distal fragment is displaced volarly. The ulnar head is prominent dorsally, and there may be derangement of the distal radioulnar joint. This lesion should be differentiated from Barton's fracture-dislocation (see below).

The fracture can be reduced by closed manipulation and immobilized with the wrist in dorsiflexion. Unstable fractures may require initial skeletal distraction (see above for unstable Colles' fracture). Fractures that cannot be reduced adequately by closed methods may require open reduction and bone plating.

van Raay JJ, van der Werken C: External fixation of Smith's fracture: 16 patients followed for 2 years. Acta Orthop Scand 1991;62:284.

4. FRACTURE OF THE RADIAL STYLOID

Forced radial deviation of the hand at the wrist joint can fracture the radial styloid process. A large fragment of the process is usually displaced by impingement against the scaphoid bone. If the fragment is large, it can be displaced farther by the brachioradialis muscle, which inserts into it.

Because the fracture is intra-articular, reduction of large fragments should be anatomic. If the styloid fragment is not displaced, immobilization in a plaster gauntlet for 3 weeks is sufficient. If the fragment is displaced, manipulative reduction should be tried. If the distal, smaller fragment tends to displace but can be apposed by digital pressure, percutaneous fixation can be achieved by a medium Kirschner wire inserted through the proximal anatomic snuffbox so as to transfix both fragments. The wrist is then immobilized in a snugly molded plaster gauntlet for 6 weeks. X-ray examination is repeated every week for 2–3 weeks.

If closed methods fail, open reduction is indicated, since persistent displacement is likely to cause post-traumatic degenerative arthritis relatively early.

5. FRACTURE & DISLOCATION OF THE RADIOCARPAL JOINT (Barton's Fractures)

Dislocation of the radiocarpal joint without injury to one of the carpal bones is usually associated with fracture of the anterior surface of the radius or ulna. Comminuted fracture of the distal radius may involve either the anterior or posterior cortex and may extend into the wrist joint. Subluxation of the carpus may occur at the same time. The most common fracture-dislocation of the wrist joint involves the posterior or anterior margin of the articular surface of the radius.

Anterior Fracture-Dislocation of the Radiocarpal Joint

Anterior fracture-dislocation of the wrist joint is characterized by intra-articular fracture of the volar margin of the carpal surface of the radius. The fracture cleft extends proximally in the coronal plane in an oblique direction, so that the free fragment has a wedge-shaped configuration. The carpus is displaced volarly and proximally with the articular fragment. This uncommon injury should be differentiated from Smith's fracture by x-ray examination.

These fractures tend to be very unstable and frequently require percutaneous fixation with pins or open reduction and internal fixation with a volar bone plate and screws. Immobilization in a short-arm plaster cast or splint is continued for 5–6 weeks. Long-arm support may be necessary.

Posterior Fracture-Dislocation of the Radiocarpal Joint

Posterior fracture-dislocation of the wrist joint (dorsal rim fracture) should be differentiated by x-ray from Colles' fracture. In most cases, the marginal fragment is smaller than in anterior injury and often involves the medial aspect where the extensor pollicis longus crosses the distal radius. If reduction is not anatomic, fraying of the tendon at this level may lead to late rupture.

Treatment is by manipulative reduction as for

Colles' fracture and immobilization for 6 weeks in a short-arm plaster cast with the wrist in neutral position. A tendency to redisplacement requires percutaneous fixation with pins or open reduction and fixation with a bone plate and screws. Prognosis and complications are similar to those described in the section on Colles' fractures.

Mehara AK et al: Classification and treatment of volar Barton fractures. Injury 1993;24:55.

Takami H, Takahashi S, Ando M: Comminuted intraarticular fracture of the distal radius with rotation of the palmar medial articular fragment: Case reports. J Trauma 1992; 32:404.

6. DISLOCATION OF THE DISTAL RADIOULNAR JOINT

The articular disk is the most important structure in preventing dislocation of the distal radioulnar joint. The accessory ligaments and the pronator quadratus muscle play a secondary role. Complete anterior or posterior dislocation implies a tear of the articular disk and disruption of accessory joint ligaments. Tearing of the articular disk in the absence of major injury to the supporting capsular ligaments causes subluxation or abnormal laxity of the joint. Since the ulnar attachment of the articular disk is at the base of the styloid process, x-rays may demonstrate an associated fracture. Widening of the cleft in comparison with the opposite radioulnar joint suggests dislocation even if frank anterior or posterior displacement is not present.

Dorsal dislocation or subluxation is treated by reducing the ulnar head by full supination of the forearm. The arm is placed in an above-the-elbow cast with the elbow in 90 degrees of flexion and the forearm in supination.

Volar dislocation is rare and is usually stable after reduction.

Bruckner JD, Lichtman DM, Alexander AH: Complex dislocations of the distal radioulnar joint: Recognition and management Clin Orthop 1992;Feb(275):90.

Trousdale RT et al: Radio-ulnar dissociation: A review of twenty cases. J Bone Joint Surg [Am] 1992;74:1486.

7. FRACTURES & DISLOCATIONS OF THE CARPUS

Injury to the carpal bones occurs predominantly in men during the most active period of life. Because it is difficult to differentiate these injuries by clinical examination, it is imperative to obtain x-ray films of the best possible quality. The oblique film should be taken in midpronation, the anteroposterior film with the wrist in maximal ulnar deviation. Special views, such as midsupination to demonstrate the pisiform, and carpal tunnel views for the hamate, may be necessary.

Fracture of the Carpal Scaphoid

The most common injury to the carpus is fracture of the scaphoid bone. This fracture should be suspected in any injury to the wrist in men unless a specific diagnosis of another type of injury is obvious. Since 2–5% of these fractures are not visible on the first radiograph, if tenderness on the radial aspect of the wrist is present and fracture cannot be demonstrated, initial treatment should be the same as if fracture were present (see below) and should be continued for at least 2 weeks. Further x-ray examination after 2 weeks may demonstrate an occult fracture.

Three types of carpal scaphoid fracture are distinguished:

(1) Fracture of the tubercle: This fracture usually is not widely displaced, and healing is generally prompt if immobilization in a plaster gauntlet is maintained for 3–4 weeks.

(2) Fracture through the waist: Fracture through the narrowest portion of the bone is the most common type. The blood supply to the proximal fragment is usually not disturbed, and healing will take place if reduction is adequate and treatment is instituted early. If the nutrient artery to the proximal third is injured, avascular necrosis of that portion of the bone may occur. X-ray examination in multiple projections may be necessary to determine displacement of the proximal fragment. If the proximal fragment is displaced, it may be reduced under local anesthesia by radial deviation of the wrist. Immobilization in a plaster gauntlet with the wrist in neutral is necessary. The plaster should extend distally to the palmar flexion crease in the hand and to the base of the thumbnail. If reduction has been anatomic and the blood supply to the proximal fragment has not been jeopardized, adequate bone healing can be expected within 10–12 weeks. However, such healing must be demonstrated by the disappearance of the fracture cleft and restoration of the trabecular pattern between the two main fragments. X-ray examination to verify healing should be repeated 3 weeks after removal of the cast.

(3) Fracture through the proximal third: Fracture through the proximal third of the scaphoid bone is apt to be associated with injury to the arterial supply of the minor fragment. This can be manifested by avascular necrosis of that fragment. If the lesion is observed soon after injury, reduction and immobilization in a plaster gauntlet will promote healing. The plaster gauntlet should be applied snugly and must be changed if it becomes loose. X-rays should be taken every 4–6 weeks to determine the progress of bone healing; it may be necessary to prolong immobilization for 4–6 months. The same criteria of radiographic examination as are used for healing of fractures through the waist are used in fractures of the proximal third. It is advisable to make an additional x-ray examination 3–4 weeks after removal of the cast.

About 95% of carpal scaphoid fractures unite following treatment by standard techniques. If evidence of healing is not apparent after immobilization for 6 months or more, further immobilization will probably not be effective. Poor prognostic factors for healing are displacement during treatment, increasing visibility of the fracture line, and the presence of early cystic changes. If the interval between the time of injury and the establishment of a diagnosis is 3 months or more, a trial of immobilization for 2–3 months may be elected. If obliteration of the fracture cleft and evidence of restoration of bone continuity are not visible in x-rays taken after this trial period, some form of operative treatment will be necessary to initiate bone healing. Bone grafting is most successful. Prolonged immobilization in a plaster gauntlet after bone grafting is necessary before bony continuity is restored.

If avascular necrosis has occurred in the proximal fragment (exhibited by increased radiodensity of the fragment), bone grafting is less likely to be successful. Although excision of the avascular fragment may relieve painful symptoms for a time, the patient usually notes weakness of grasp and discomfort after prolonged use. Posttraumatic arthritis is apt to develop late.

Prolonged failure of bone healing predisposes to posttraumatic arthritis. Bone grafting operations or other procedures directed toward restoration of bone continuity may be successful, but arthritis can cause continued disability. Arthrodesis of the wrist gives the best assurance of relief of pain and a functionally competent extremity in these cases.

Fracture of the Lunate

Fracture of the lunate bone may be manifested by minor avulsion fractures of the posterior or anterior horn. Careful multiplane x-ray examination is necessary to establish the diagnosis. Either of these lesions may be treated by the use of a volar splint for 3 weeks.

Fracture of the body may be manifested by a crack, by comminution, or by impaction. A fissure fracture can be treated by immobilization in plaster for 3 weeks.

One complication of this fracture is persistent pain in the wrist, slight restriction of motion, and tenderness over the lunate bone. X-ray examination can demonstrate areas of sclerosis and rarefaction. Impaction or collapse can be accompanied by arthritic changes surrounding the lunate bone. This x-ray appearance is referred to as Kienböck's disease, osteochondrosis of the lunate bone, or avascular necrosis.

Fracture of the Hamate

Fracture of the hamate bone may occur through the body and is shown on x-ray as a fissure or compression. Fracture of the base of the hamulus is less common and more difficult to diagnose; special projections are necessary to demonstrate the cleft. If the hamulus is displaced, closed manipulation will not be effective. Prolonged pain or evidence of irritation of the ulnar nerve may require excision of the loose fragment.

Fracture of the Triquetrum

Fracture of the triquetrum bone is caused commonly by direct violence and is often associated with fracture of other carpal bones. Treatment is by immobilization in a plaster gauntlet for 4 weeks.

Kerluke L, McCabe SJ: Nonunion of the scaphoid: A critical analysis of recent natural history studies. J Hand Surg [Am] 1993;18:1.

Mody BS et al: Nonunion of fractures of the scaphoid tuberosity. J Bone Joint Surg [Br] 1993;75:423.

Nakamura R et al: Scaphoid non-union: Factors affecting the functional outcome of open reduction and wedge grafting with Herbert screw fixation. J Hand Surg [Br] 1993;3;18:219.

Tiel-van Buul MM et al: Radiography and scintigraphy of suspected scaphoid fracture: A long-term study in 160 patients. J Bone Joint Surg [Br] 1993;75:61.

Traumatic Carpal Instability

Carpal dislocations, fracture-dislocations, and collapse deformities secondary to ligamentous injuries occur by similar mechanisms and have similar tendencies to deform. Dislocation is caused by forced dorsiflexion of the wrist. X-rays of excellent technical quality taken in the anteroposterior and the true lateral projections are necessary. Even with the highest-quality films, the diagnosis may be missed by experienced physicians.

The carpal injury is focused around the lunate and proximal scaphoid, leading to perilunate or transscaphoid perilunate fracture-dislocation. Dislocation may be manifested by dorsal displacement of the capitate bone though the lunate retains contact with the radius. A further degree of injury is manifested by complete displacement of the lunate bone from the radius, so that it comes to lie anterior to the capitate bone and loses its relationship to the articular surface of the radius (Figure 43–32). Most surgeons agree that perilunate and lunate dislocations are two stages of the same injury.

If the lunate is subluxated and the scaphoid is not fractured, a triangular gap between the scaphoid and lunate can often be demonstrated on the anteroposterior x-ray (Figure 43–33). If the scaphoid is fractured, no gap will be present, as the lunate bone and the proximal fragment of the scaphoid retain their relationship. On the lateral x-ray, the scaphoid normally lies at an angle of 45–50 degrees to the longitudinal axis of the radius. With carpal instability, the scaphoid lies in a vertical position (Figure 43–32).

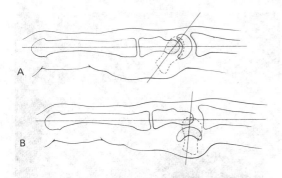

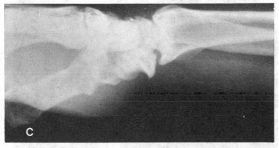

Figure 43–32. A: Normal anatomy of the wrist. Note that the proximal end of the capitate rests in the lunate concavity. A straight line drawn through the metacarpal and capitate into the radius should bisect the lunate. The scaphoid makes an angle of 45 degrees with the long axis of the radius. **B:** Lunate dislocation. Lunate dislocates volarly. The angle between the scaphoid and the long axis of the radius is 90 degrees instead of the normal angle of 45 degrees. **C:** X-ray of perilunate dislocation. Lunate is volarly dislocated.

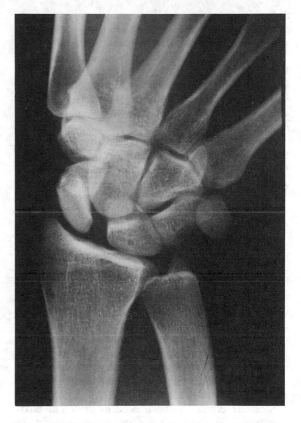

Figure 43–33. Rotatory subluxation. Note the triangular gap between the scaphoid and lunate.

In carpal dislocation without fracture, reduction may be achieved by closed manipulation with a strong longitudinal distraction force assisted by dorsally directed pressure on the palmar dislocated lunate. Follow-up x-rays are then taken. If reduction is adequate, the extremity is immobilized in neutral position for 6 weeks in a plaster cast extending from the elbow to the palmar flexion crease and to the base of the thumb. Repeat x-rays at 1 and 2 weeks postreduction to ensure that reduction has been maintained.

If manipulative reduction is unsuccessful or lost, or if there is fracture of the scaphoid, open reduction and internal fixation with Kirschner wires are indicated. Adequate reduction is confirmed by x-rays showing absence of the triangular gap between the scaphoid and lunate on an anteroposterior film plus proper relationship of the carpal bones on lateral x-ray. In unstable carpal dislocations without fracture, the Kirschner wires are left in place and the wrist is immobilized in a short-arm plaster cast for a minimum of 6 weeks. If scaphoid fracture complicates the dislocation, the wrist is immobilized until the fracture heals.

Failure to recognize and treat this serious injury leads to significant disability from a painful, weak "collapsing wrist."

Lichtman DM et al: Palmar midcarpal instability: results of surgical reconstruction. J Hand Surg [Am] 1993;18:307.

Mody BS, Dias JJ: Carpometacarpal dislocation of the thumb associated with fracture of the trapezium. J Hand Surg [Br] 1993;3;18:197.

Watson H et al: Rotary subluxation of the scaphoid: A spectrum of instability. J Hand Surg [Br] 1993;18:62.

INJURIES OF THE HIP REGION

1. FRACTURE OF THE FEMORAL NECK

Fracture of the femoral neck occurs most commonly in patients over age 50. If displacement has occurred, the extremity is externally rotated and shortened. Motion of the hip joint causes pain. If the fragments are not displaced and the fracture is stable, pain at the extremes of passive hip motion may be the only significant finding. The fact that the patient can actively move the extremity often interferes with prompt diagnosis.

Before treatment is instituted, anteroposterior and lateral films of excellent quality must be obtained. Gentle traction and internal rotation of the extremity while the anteroposterior film is exposed may provide a more favorable relation of fragments to demonstrate the fracture cleft.

Fractures may be classified as stable or unstable. Stable fractures include stress fractures and impacted fractures. The unstable category includes displaced and comminuted fractures.

Stable Fractures of the Femoral Neck

Patients with stress fractures or impacted fractures may have minimal groin pain and may be able to walk with some pain and a limp. No obvious deformity or shortening is apparent on physical examination. A high index of suspicion must be maintained in these patients, as the diagnosis may be difficult to make. If initial x-rays do not reveal the stress fracture, a repeat x-ray made 10–14 days after the injury will show the radiolucent line. An impacted fracture is usually in valgus position. Impaction must be seen on both anteroposterior and lateral films for diagnosis.

Stress fractures can be treated by crutch ambulation to minimize weight-bearing stress. The patient should be instructed not to place the leg in stressful positions or use it for leverage. If the fracture appears to be healing, partial weight bearing may be started at 6 weeks after injury, with progression to full weight bearing when the fracture is healed. Healing usually takes place in 3–6 months.

Impacted fractures may also be treated nonoperatively, but the tendency for displacement is much greater than in stress fractures. Most surgeons prefer to use internal fixation for impacted fractures to allow maintenance of reduction, earlier crutch ambulation, and earlier weight bearing. Multiple screw or pin fixation is frequently the method of choice and should be secure enough to allow weight bearing immediately. Truly impacted fractures treated with internal fixation without disruption of the fracture have healing rates approaching 100%.

Unstable Fractures of the Femoral Neck

Displaced and comminuted femoral neck fractures (Figure 43–34) can be a life-endangering injury, especially in elderly persons. Treatment is directed toward preservation of life and restoration of function to the hip joint. In most cases, reduction and internal fixation are the treatment of choice. Immobilization of this fracture by means of a plaster spica is unreliable. Definitive treatment by skeletal traction requires prolonged recumbency with constant nursing

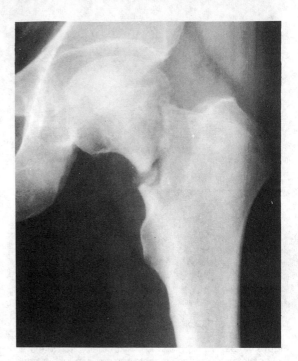

Figure 43–34. Fracture of the neck of the femur. Interposition of a small intermediate fragment and soft tissues prevented adequate reduction by closed manipulation.

care and is associated with more numerous complications than early mobilization. Operative treatment usually consists of internal fixation or primary arthroplasty and should be done as soon as the patient is medically prepared for surgery.

(1) Internal fixation: The goal of internal fixation is to preserve the femoral head fragment by providing a setting for bony healing of the fracture. The objective is to allow the patient as much general physical activity during healing as is compatible with the mechanics of fixation. To permit necessary preoperative evaluation of the patient when internal fixation is elected, initial treatment may be by balanced suspension, skeletal traction, and prompt closed reduction of the fracture. Persistent displacement may cause further compromise of the retinacular blood supply to the articular fragment.

Anatomic or near-anatomic reduction and firm fixation are desirable to provide optimal conditions for bone healing. Comminution at the fracture site, injury to the retinacular blood supply of the capital fragment, excessive stressing of the fracture site, and insecure fixation are some of the factors that lead to failure.

When the fragments are undisplaced or minimally displaced, manipulation is unnecessary. Displacement may be corrected by closed reduction preliminary to fixation or by surgical exposure of the fracture site. Adequate closed reduction is usually obtained by traction and marked internal rotation of the extremity—frequently to 90 degrees. The fixation apparatus may consist of multiple pins applied percutaneously or more elaborate implants that require open operation. After operation, the patient does not require traction and may be mobilized at an early date. If operative fixation is precarious, traction in balanced suspension or immobilization in a plaster spica for 1–4 months may be necessary until preliminary healing gives additional stability.

Depending upon the relative security of fixation, the extent of early weight bearing must be regulated until bone continuity is restored to the point where displacement of fragments is unlikely. Patients may be ambulatory on crutches or with a walker within a few days after operative treatment.

(2) Primary arthroplasty: In selecting primary arthroplasty, the surgeon realizes that the main proximal fragment must be sacrificed because of injury to the blood supply, preexisting disease, or inability to obtain satisfactory reduction of the fracture for internal fixation.

When the acetabulum is undamaged or is not the site of preexisting disease, the commonly accepted technique is hemiarthroplasty using a femoral component (generally of the intramedullary type) that may or may not be stabilized by a grouting substance such as methylmethacrylate. In the rare circumstance when there is concomitant involvement of the acetabulum, total joint replacement may be justified. Primary head and neck resection may be indicated when there is preexisting infection or local tumor.

The most common sequelae of fracture of the femoral neck are redisplacement after reduction and internal fixation, failure of bone healing, and avascular necrosis of the head fragment. Avascular necrosis and associated collapse occur in 15–35% of these patients from interruption of the blood supply to the femoral neck at the time of injury. It is most likely to appear during the 2 years after fracture. Secondary osteoarthritis (posttraumatic arthritis) appears somewhat later and may be complicated by any of the common sequelae mentioned above. The most serious complication of any open operative treatment is infection.

Cummings SR et al: Bone density at various sites for prediction of hip fractures: The Study of Osteoporotic Fractures Research Group. Lancet 1993;341:72.

Eiskjaer S, Ostgard SE: Survivorship analysis of hemiarthroplasties. Clin Orthop 1993;Jan(286):206.

Hinton RY, Smith GS: The association of age, race, and sex with the location of proximal femoral fractures in the elderly. J Bone Joint Surg [Am] 1993;75:752.

Nilsson LT, Johansson A, Stromqvist B: Factors predicting healing complications in femoral neck fractures: 138 patients followed for 2 years. Acta Orthop Scand 1993; 3;64:175.

Parfenchuck TA, Carter LW, Young TR: Ipsilateral fractures of the femoral neck and shaft. Orthop Rev 1993;22:356.

Ragnarsson JI et al: Instability and femoral head vitality in fractures of the femoral neck. Clin Orthop 1993; Feb(287):30.

2. TROCHANTERIC FRACTURES

Fracture of the Lesser Trochanter

Isolated fracture of the lesser trochanter is quite rare but may develop as a result of the avulsion force of the iliopsoas muscle. It occurs commonly as a component of intertrochanteric fracture.

Fracture of the Greater Trochanter

Isolated fracture of the greater trochanter may be caused by direct injury or may occur indirectly as a result of the activity of the gluteus medius and gluteus minimus muscles. It occurs most commonly as a component of intertrochanteric fracture.

If displacement is less than 1 cm and there is no tendency to further displacement (determined by repeated x-ray examinations), treatment may be by bed rest with the affected extremity in balanced suspension until acute pain subsides. As rapidly as symptoms permit, activity can increase gradually to protected weight bearing with crutches. Full weight bearing is permitted as soon as healing is apparent, usually in 6–8 weeks. If displacement is greater than 1 cm and increases on adduction of the thigh, extensive tearing of surrounding soft tissues may be assumed, and open reduction and internal fixation are indicated.

Intertrochanteric (Including Peritrochanteric) Fractures

These fractures occur most commonly among elderly persons, usually after a fall. The cleft of an intertrochanteric fracture extends upward and outward from the medial region of the junction of the neck and lesser trochanter toward the summit of the greater trochanter. Peritrochanteric fracture includes both trochanters and is likely to be comminuted.

It is important to determine whether comminution has occurred and the magnitude of displacement. These fractures may vary from fissure fracture without significant separation to severe comminution into four major fragments: head-neck, greater trochanter, lesser trochanter, and shaft. Displacement may be marked, with obvious extreme rotation and shortening of the extremity more severe than with femoral neck fractures.

These fractures are extracapsular and occur through cancellous bone, which has a good blood supply. Healing occurs in 3–4 months, and lack of healing is uncommon.

Initial treatment of the fracture in the hospital can be by balanced suspension and, when indicated, by the addition of traction. The selection of definitive treatment—closed or operative techniques—depends in part upon the general condition of the patient and the type of fracture. Rates of illness and death are lower when the fracture is internally fixed, allowing for early mobilization. Operative treatment is indicated as soon as the patient is medically able to tolerate surgery.

If the patient is unable to tolerate anesthesia or if the fracture is too severely comminuted to permit internal fixation with good stability, the fracture may be treated by skeletal traction with a Kirschner wire through the proximal tibia. Within 3–4 months, healing is usually sufficient to allow the patient to be out of bed. Long-term traction is associated with many complications, including bedsores, pulmonary complications, deterioration of mental status, and varus position of the fracture.

Open reduction may be done electively or may be mandatory for optimal treatment. Reduction of the fracture can be accomplished by closed techniques, or it can be an integral part of the open operation. Some surgeons do not prefer to anatomically reduce unstable fractures caused by comminution of the medial femoral cortex. It is maintained by some authors that medial displacement of the upper end of the main distal fragment enhances mechanical stability (although it may cause concomitant varus deformity), and this advantageously permits earlier weight bearing and earlier healing. The chief objective of open operation is to provide sufficient fixation of the fragments by a metallic surgical implant so that the patient need not be confined to bed during the healing process.

The fixation most widely used is a sliding screw with a side plate. The screw can slide in the barrel of the side plate, allowing the fracture to impact. A fixed nail and side plate may cause the fracture to be "nailed apart" and contribute to lack of healing. As the fracture impacts, the nail cannot slide and may instead cut through the head of the femur.

Desjardins AL et al: Unstable intertrochanteric fracture of the femur: A prospective randomised study comparing anatomical reduction and medial displacement osteotomy. J Bone Joint Surg [Br] 1993;75:445.

Pitsaer E, Samuel AW: Functional outcome after intertrochanteric fractures of the femur: does the implant matter? A prospective study of 100 consecutive cases. Injury 1993;24:35.

Shaw JA, Wilson S: Internal fixation of proximal femur fractures: a biomechanical comparison of the Gamma Locking Nail and the Omega Compression Hip Screw Orthopaedic Review 1993;22:61.

3. SUBTROCHANTERIC FRACTURE

Subtrochanteric fracture due to severe trauma occurs below the level of the lesser trochanter at the junction of cancellous and cortical bone. It is most common in men during the active years of life. Soft tissue damage is extensive. The direction of the fracture cleft may be transverse or oblique. Comminution occurs, and the fracture may extend proximally into the intertrochanteric region or distally into the shaft.

Closed reduction should be attempted by continuous traction to bring the distal fragment into alignment with the proximal fragment. If comminution is not extensive and the lesser trochanter is not detached, the proximal fragment is often drawn into relative flexion, external rotation, and abduction by the predominant activity of the iliopsoas, gluteus medius, and gluteus minimus muscles.

Prolonged skeletal traction by means of a Kirschner wire inserted through the supracondylar region of the femur (with the hip and knee flexed to a right angle) is necessary (Figure 43–35) if traction treatment is chosen. Thereafter, the extremity is left in this position with an appropriate amount of traction until stabilization occurs, usually in 8–12 weeks. The angle of flexion is then reduced by gradually bringing the hip and knee into extension. After 2–3 months of continuous traction, the extremity can be immobilized in a plaster spica provided stabilization of the fracture has occurred. Weight bearing must not be resumed for 4–6 months or even longer, until bone healing obliterates the fracture cleft.

Interposition of soft tissue between the major fragments may prevent closed reduction. If open reduction of this fracture is anticipated, it should be undertaken early; if treatment is delayed until the third week following injury, the fracture fragments are more difficult to align and extensive bleeding at the fracture site is likely to be encountered.

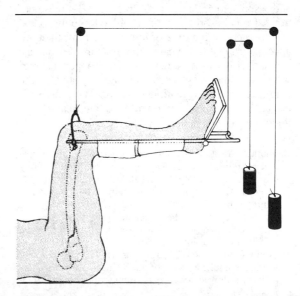

Figure 43–35. Method of suspension of lower extremity with skeletal traction for subtrochanteric fracture.

After open reduction has been performed, internal fixation is required to prevent redisplacement. A variety of devices are available (eg, interlocking nail, Zickel nail, condylocephalic devices, nail with long side plate) that give varying degrees of rotational control, longitudinal alignment, and stability.

The activity status after operation depends upon the adequacy of internal fixation. If fixation is precarious, additional protection with a spica cast or skeletal traction may be necessary until healing is well underway. If fixation is secure and the patient is agile and cooperative, ambulation on crutches (non-weight-bearing or partial weight-bearing) on the affected side may be allowed a few days after the operation.

Karachalios T et al: Reconstruction nailing for pathological subtrochanteric fractures with coexisting femoral shaft metastases. J Bone Joint Surg [Br] 1993;75:119.

Mullaji AB, Thomas TL: Low-energy subtrochanteric fractures in elderly patients: Results of fixation with the sliding screw plate. J Trauma 1993;34:56.

4. TRAUMATIC DISLOCATION OF THE HIP JOINT

Traumatic dislocation of the hip joint may occur with or without fracture of the acetabulum or the proximal end of the femur. It is most common during the active years of life and is usually the result of severe trauma unless there is preexisting disease of the femoral head, acetabulum, or neuromuscular system. The head of the femur cannot be completely displaced from the normal acetabulum unless the ligamentum teres is ruptured or deficient because of some unrelated cause. Traumatic dislocations can be classified according to the direction of displacement of the femoral head from the acetabulum.

Posterior Hip Dislocation (Figure 43–36)

The head of the femur is usually dislocated posterior to the acetabulum while the thigh is flexed, eg, as may occur in a head-on automobile collision when the driver's or passenger's knee is driven violently against the dashboard.

The significant clinical findings are shortening, adduction, and internal rotation of the extremity. Anteroposterior, transpelvic, and, if fracture of the acetabulum is demonstrated, oblique x-ray projections are required. Common complications are fracture of the acetabulum, injury to the sciatic nerve, and fracture of the head or shaft of the femur. The head of the femur may be displaced through a rent in the posterior hip joint capsule, or the glenoid lip may be avulsed from the acetabulum. The short external rotator muscles of the femur are commonly lacerated.

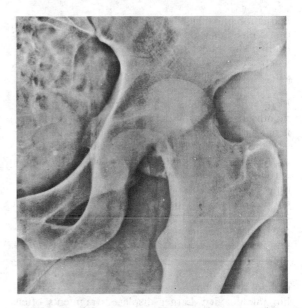

Figure 43–36. Fracture of the head of the femur and posterior dislocation of the hip. Closed reduction was unsuccessful because of the head fragment that was retained in the acetabulum.

Fracture of the posterior margin of the acetabulum can create instability.

If the acetabulum is not fractured or if the fragment is small, reduction by closed manipulation is indicated. General anesthesia provides maximum muscle relaxation and allows gentle reduction. Reduction should be achieved as soon as possible, preferably within the first few hours after injury as soon as the patient's general injury status has been adequately assessed. The main feature of reduction is traction in the line of deformity, followed by gentle flexion of the hip to 90 degrees with stabilization of the pelvis by an assistant. While manual traction is continued, the hip is gently rotated into internal and then external rotation to obtain reduction.

The success of reduction is determined immediately by anteroposterior and lateral x-rays. Interposition of capsule substance or bone fragments will be manifest by widening of the joint cleft. If x-rays are difficult to interpret, CT scan can be helpful in assessing concentricity of reduction. If reduction is adequate, the hip will usually be stable with the extremity in extension and slight external rotation. Stability of the hip should be tested immediately after reduction by motion of the hip in flexion and adduction to assess the maximum limits of stability. A very easy manipulative reduction (eg, the hip "slides in" with very little effort) may suggest major instability and potential for redislocation even though the hip is maintained in traction.

Postreduction treatment may be by immobilization

in traction or balanced suspension or in a plaster spica cast. Since this is primarily a soft tissue injury, sound healing should occur in 4 weeks. Opinion differs on when unsupported weight bearing should be resumed. Some authors believe that disability caused by ischemic osteonecrosis of the femoral head is less likely when complete weight bearing is deferred for 6 months after injury; others believe that early loading is not harmful.

If the posterior or superior acetabulum is fractured, dislocation of the hip must be assumed to have occurred even though displacement is not present at the time of examination. Undisplaced fissure fractures may be treated initially by bed rest and avoidance of full weight bearing for 2 months. Frequent examination is necessary to make certain that the head of the femur has not become displaced from the acetabulum.

Minor fragments of the posterior margin of the acetabulum may be disregarded unless they are in the hip joint cavity. Larger displaced fragments often cannot be reduced adequately by closed methods. If the fragment is large and the hip is unstable following closed manipulation, open operation is indicated. The fragment is then placed in anatomic position and fixed with bone screws or a bone plate and screws.

After the operation, if fixation is tenuous because of severe comminution of the fracture, the patient is placed in bed with the extremity in balanced suspension with 5–8 kg of skeletal traction on the tibial tubercle for about 4–6 weeks or until healing of the acetabular fracture is sound. If fixation is stable, the patient may be allowed out of bed in a few days with progression to ambulation on crutches that is nonweight bearing on the injured side. Full weight bearing is not permitted until healing is complete—a process that takes about 3–6 months.

Anterior Hip Dislocation

In anterior hip dislocation, the head of the femur may lie medially on the obturator membrane, beneath the obturator externus muscle (obturator dislocation), or in a somewhat more superior position, beneath the iliopsoas muscle and in contact with the superior ramus of the pubis (pubic dislocation). The thigh is classically in flexion, abduction, and external rotation, and the head of the femur is palpable anteriorly and distal to the inguinal flexion crease. Anteroposterior and lateral films are required; films prepared by transpelvic projection may be helpful.

Closed manipulation with general anesthesia is usually adequate. Postreduction treatment may be by balanced suspension or by immobilization in a plaster spica with the hip in extension and the extremity in neutral rotation. Active hip motion is permitted after 3 weeks.

Central Dislocation of the Hip With Fracture of the Pelvis

Central dislocation of the head of the femur with fracture of the acetabulum may be caused by crushing injury or by axial force transmitted through the abducted extremity to the acetabulum. Comminution is commonly present. There are usually two main fragments: superiorly, the ilium with the roof of the acetabulum; inferiorly and medially, the remainder of the acetabulum and the obturator ring. Fracture occurs near the roof of the acetabulum, and the components of the obturator ring are displaced inward with the head of the femur. Extensive soft tissue injury and massive bleeding into the soft tissues are likely to be present. Intra-abdominal injury must not be overlooked. Initially, anteroposterior and oblique x-rays are required.

In the absence of complicating injury or immediately after such an injury has received priority attention, closed treatment of the fracture-dislocation by skeletal traction should be tried. For the average adult, approximately 10 kg of force is applied axially to the shaft of the femur, in neither abduction nor adduction, through a Kirschner wire placed in the distal femur or proximal tibia. A trochanteric screw or Kirschner wire and bow may be inserted in the greater trochanter to apply force at a right angle to the direction of axial traction. The extremity is placed in balanced suspension. Progress of reduction is observed by serial portable x-rays until adequate positioning is manifested by relocation of the head of the femur beneath the roof of the acetabulum. Bidirectional traction is maintained for 4–6 weeks. Daily inspection of the trochanteric traction apparatus is necessary to rule out localized infection, because motion of skin and fat around the device predisposes to sepsis. The transverse traction component is gradually diminished under appropriate x-ray control until it can be discontinued. Axial traction is maintained until stabilization of the fracture fragments by early bone healing has occurred, usually 8 weeks after injury. During the next 4–6 weeks, while balanced suspension is continued, gentle active exercises of the knee and hip are encouraged. After discontinuation of balanced suspension, more elaborate exercises designed to aid recovery of maximal hip function are performed frequently during the day. Full and unprotected weight bearing should not be advised until healing is complete, usually in 4 months.

Sequelae are common, and the patient should be warned of their probable occurrence. Anatomic reduction is an unattainable goal in most severely comminuted and widely displaced fractures of this type. Scarring within and around the hip joint, with or without ectopic bone and exuberant callus formation, is incidental to the healing process and can be a significant factor in restriction of motion in varying degrees. Osteonecrosis of the femoral head and secondary osteoarthritis are common sequelae that appear somewhat later.

Indications for open reduction and internal fixation include the presence for free osteochondral fragments in the joint, associated femoral head fracture, instability severe enough to allow chronic dislocation of the femoral head, and incongruity of weight-bearing surfaces. Some authors feel that all displaced acetabular fractures should undergo open reduction and internal fixation, as there is a correlation of anatomic position with prognosis.

Letournel has classified acetabular fractures according to which column of the pelvis is involved. The anterior column comprises the anterior iliac crest, the anterior acetabulum, and the pubic symphysis. The posterior column contains the posterior portion of the acetabulum, the ischial tuberosity, and the great sciatic notch. Fractures may involve one or both columns.

Four radiographic views are necessary to delineate the extent of the fractures: a standard anteroposterior view of the pelvis, an anteroposterior view of the affected hip, and two oblique views taken with the patient rolled 45 degrees toward and away from (respectively) the affected side. Accurate assessment of the fracture fragments allows the surgeon to choose the most appropriate surgical approach. CT scan may give additional information. These complex acetabular fractures are difficult to manage surgically, and the procedure should be performed only by an expert in the technique.

Daum WJ: Traumatic posterior acetabular defects reconstructed with iliac crest autograft: A report of two cases. Clin Orthop 1993;Jun(291):188.

Oransky M, Sanguinetti C: Surgical treatment of displaced acetabular fractures: results of 50 consecutive cases. J Orthop Trauma 1993;7:28.

Roffi RP, Matta JM: Unrecognized posterior dislocation of the hip associated with transverse and T-type fractures of the acetabulum. J Orthop Trauma 1993;7:23.

Schlickewei W et al: Hip dislocation without fracture: Traction or mobilization after reduction? Injury 1993;24:27.

Snorrason F, Karrholm J, Holmgren C: Fixation of cemented acetabular prostheses: The influence of preoperative diagnosis. J Arthroplasty 1993;8:83.

5. TREATMENT OF SEQUELAE OF FRACTURES & DISLOCATIONS OF THE HIP REGION

Sequelae of fractures, dislocations, and fracture-dislocations of the hip region may be due to or modified by the nature of the initial lesion, preexisting local or systemic disease, or the type of treatment that has been given. Some sequelae are unique to one injury, while others are common to the three major categories.

Femoral Neck Fractures

Comminution can make precise reduction difficult or impossible by either open or closed techniques. When comminution is so severe that intimate approximation of major fragments is impossible, fibrous healing or pseudarthrosis is probable. Further complications result from injury to the retinacular blood supply of the proximal articular fragment of the femur, which enhances the likelihood of ischemic necrosis. Preexisting osteopenia due to osteoporosis or other causes is characterized by a reduced volume of cancellous bone at the fracture site available for endosteal healing. Lack of bone substance offers insecure support to an internal fixation apparatus. Infection after the primary surgical procedure may limit or determine the selection of types of reconstructive operations. Excessive physical activity such as unsupported weight bearing prior to bone healing may cause loosening at the interface between the surgical implant and bone or may cause fatigue breakage of the fixation apparatus.

This fracture occurs most commonly in elderly persons but can occur with major trauma in younger people. The incidence of complications (ie, nonunion and avascular necrosis) is as high in the young as in the elderly.

Operations designed to enhance bone healing may be done primarily as prophylaxis or secondarily as corrective procedures. These operations include cancellous or cortical bone grafting; muscle pedicle flap transfers to the fracture site with or without attached bone; supportive or displacement osteotomies with or without internal fixation apparatus; and refixation.

As time passes, either partial or complete ischemic osteonecrosis of the femoral head is likely to complicate or be associated with secondary osteoarthritis. Before infraction or collapse of the superior sector of the head occurs, operations designed to enhance blood supply, such as bone grafting or muscle pedicle flap transfers, have been performed with varying success. The rationale of osteotomy in the trochanteric region for the treatment of osteonecrosis is to place an uninvolved area of the femoral head in contact with the major weight-bearing surface of the acetabulum. Arthrodesis for this condition was used more frequently in the past. Arthroplasty (replacement of the femoral head or the head and acetabulum) provides both mobility and stability. It is currently more popular than head and neck resection, which provides only mobility, or arthrodesis, which provides only stability.

If active infection has been of short duration and apparently has been suppressed, any of the operations mentioned above may be justified if there is reasonable assurance that reactivation of infection can be controlled. Otherwise, head and neck resection or perhaps arthrodesis combined with removal of implants and aggressive adjunctive antimicrobial drug therapy is a more realistic alternative. A tertiary reconstructive procedure such as total hip joint replacement may be feasible at some later date.

Trochanteric Fractures

Undisplaced or anatomically reduced fractures of the trochanteric region that have been firmly fixed and have not been loaded excessively during the phase of restoration of bone continuity are unlikely to exhibit prolonged delay of healing. Comminution and incomplete reduction are factors that do delay healing. Occasionally, especially in younger persons, extensive comminution and marked displacement may be complicated by ischemic necrosis of the femoral head and secondary osteoarthritis.

If the fracture has no intracapsular extension and infection is limited to the fracture site, treatment is as for chronic osteomyelitis. If the internal fixation apparatus is firmly attached and adequately stabilizes an incompletely healed fracture, removal of the implant may be deferred until sound bone healing occurs. The treatment of complicating intra-articular infection is similar to that for femoral neck fractures with pyogenic arthritis.

Traumatic Dislocation of the Hip Joint

Recurrent posttraumatic dislocation of the hip joint uncomplicated by acetabular fracture, fracture of the femoral head, or a neurologic lesion is uncommon and may be anterior or posterior; it is likely to be due to extensive soft tissue dehiscence. Treatment is by repair of the soft tissues. Recurrent or persistent subluxation or dislocation is more commonly due to fracture-dislocation. The precise cause must be determined by physical and x-ray examination. If significant secondary osteoarthritis is not a complication, operative replacement and fixation of displaced acetabular fragments or removal of a minor but offending fragment of the femoral head can correct articular instability. If it is a complication, arthroplasty or arthrodesis will probably give a more favorable long-term result than repair of the fracture followed by tertiary osteotomy (see below).

Persistent infection of the joint after operation for fracture-dislocation requires treatment similar to that for infection complicating femoral neck or trochanteric fractures.

6. OPERATIONS FOR SEQUELAE OF FRACTURES & DISLOCATIONS OF THE HIP REGION

Osteotomy

Osteotomy is usually performed in the predominantly cancellous intertrochanteric region, and the bone fragments are generally stabilized by a fixation device. An indication is correction of torsional or varus deformity. Supportive osteotomy is used to minimize displacing stresses at unhealed fracture sites. Abduction, adduction, or rotational osteotomy has been performed for relief of pain associated with ischemic osteonecrosis of the femoral head or secondary osteoarthritis. Although osteotomy preserves joint motion and provides stability, the prognosis for relief of pain is unpredictable for the individual patient.

Arthrodesis

Arthrodesis may be intra-articular, extra-articular, or a combination of both. Bone grafting to aid fusion and internal fixation to provide support at the coxofemoral relationship are elective supplemental features. Arthrodesis has been a favored operation as an adjunct in the control of chronic hip joint infection. When arthrodesis is bony—although articular pain is relieved and mechanical stability of the joint is ensured—added stress is placed on the lumber spine and knee joint. Pain is a frequent result. The patient must also accept some disability because of loss of hip joint function.

Head & Neck Resection (Girdlestone Arthroplasty)

The indications for resection of the head and neck of the femur for treatment of fractures, dislocations, and fracture-dislocations have been frequently modified. This operation allows motion but causes significant shortening of the extremity and creates instability that usually requires one or two crutches for ambulation. Currently, its chief application is in the treatment of chronic hip joint infection. It is useful occasionally in the treatment of pathologic fracture of the proximal femur due to primary or metastatic tumors. Rarely is osteopenia or destruction of bone from causes other than those mentioned above so extensive that resection is preferable to prosthetic arthroplasty.

Total Hip Joint Replacement

Increasing interest in total hip joint replacement has been generated during the past 15 years both abroad and in the USA. This technique implies substitution of at least the articular surfaces of both the acetabulum and the head of the femur by implants made of metal or plastic. The femoral component is usually made of cobalt-chrome alloy, stainless steel, or titanium. The acetabular constituent is usually made of high-molecular-weight polyethylene.

The main indications for any type of hip arthroplasty are relief of incapacitating pain and restoration or improvement of joint function. The presence of joint sepsis is a contraindication to replacement arthroplasty.

Total hip joint replacement requires removal of the entire head of the femur and part of the femoral neck as well as extensive remodeling of the acetabulum. The femoral head and acetabular components are stabilized in bone either by a "press fit" or poly-methylmethacrylate cement. Total hip joint replacement has wider application in the treatment of sequelae of fracture and fracture-dislocation of the hip joint in the mature adult than in the primary treatment of those lesions. It is useful as a reconstructive procedure in the treatment of failure of the joint without infection. Success rates of over 90% have been reported. Because long term reliability has not been established, the operation should be reserved for patients over age 50 unless specific factors warrant its use in younger persons.

Failure of total hip joint replacement can be caused by recurrent dislocation within the prosthesis complex, loosening of the components at the interface between the bone and the cementing substance, breakage of the femoral component, sepsis, and undetermined causes of disabling pain. The long-term effects of wear of the material and the effect of wear debris on the surrounding tissues have not been determined. Infection is the most serious complication; even if it is promptly discovered and vigorously treated, removal of the device complex may be necessary. Removal of the prosthesis leaves the patient with a severely shortened extremity and an unstable hip and necessitates indefinite use of crutch support for ambulation.

Many attempts have been made to develop prostheses that do not require such extensive removal of bone, so that if failure occurs, major shortening and instability are less likely to develop. The younger the patient, the longer the time the prosthesis will be subjected to loading and wear. Thus, several revision arthroplasties over the patient's lifetime may be needed.

Hemiarthroplasty (Endoprosthesis)

Hemiarthroplasty involves replacement of the femoral head and neck fragment and implies the presence of a normal or nearly normal acetabulum. The procedure is useful when the femoral head is extensively involved with a degenerative process or when treatment is required for unhealed femoral neck fracture. The femoral stem may be stabilized in the femoral canal by a "press fit" or with methylmethacrylate cement. For best results, the patient must be motivated to participate in a vigorous rehabilitation program, and improvement continues over several years. Causes of failure include motion between the implant and cement or bone, acetabular deterioration secondary to wear, and postoperative infection.

Bipolar or Universal Endoprosthesis

These prostheses are intermediate steps between the conventional femoral head prosthesis (endoprosthesis) and the total hip joint prosthesis. The femoral head is removed and replaced with an en-doprosthesis with the stem cemented in the femoral intramedullary canal. A polyethylene liner is fixed in a metallic cup, and the edges of the liner are so fashioned that the socket "snap fits" on the head. The acetabulum is not altered. Motion occurs between the outer surface of the metallic cup and the articular surface of the acetabulum and between the head of the femoral prosthesis and the polyethylene liner. Theoretic advantages of this prosthesis are that there may be less erosion of the acetabulum than with an endoprosthesis alone, and if revision to total hip joint is necessary later, only the cup may have to be replaced. One major disadvantage is that dislocation within the prosthetic complex is virtually impossible to reduce by closed manipulation.

Gebhard JS et al: A comparison of total hip arthroplasty and hemiarthroplasty for treatment of acute fracture of the femoral neck. Clin Orthop 1992;Sep(282):123.

Jalovaara P et al: Treatment of hip fracture in Finland and Sweden: Prospective comparison of 788 cases in three hospitals. Acta Orthop Scand 1992;63:531.

Kim YH, Oh JH, Koh YG: Salvage of neglected unstable intertrochanteric fracture with cementless porous-coated hemiarthroplasty. Clin Orthop 1992;Apr(277):182.

Moeckel BH et al: Modular hemiarthroplasty for fractures of the proximal part of the humerus. J Bone Joint Surg [Am] 1992;74:884.

Parker MJ: Internal fixation or arthroplasty for displaced subcapital fractures in the elderly? Injury 1992;23:521.

7. INFECTIONS ASSOCIATED WITH JOINT REPLACEMENTS

Infections that occur following joint replacement arthroplasty may be due to organisms introduced at surgery or may result from late hematogenous contamination. They are generally more serious than infections that follow fractures, since the implanted prosthesis is intended to be a permanent substitute for a failed joint and not a temporary fixation such as is used for fracture healing. Removal of the prosthesis shortens the limb and produces instability unless arthrodesis is achieved, fusing the adjacent bones to prevent motion. Removal of a prosthetic joint without arthrodesis leaves a so-called "excisional arthroplasty," which may offer an acceptable salvage. Arthroplasty following removal of a total hip prosthesis is often called Girdlestone arthroplasty, after the surgeon who proposed hip joint excision as primary treatment for certain disorders. While such a salvage procedure may be well tolerated, crutches are usually required, and pain is a frequent problem. Furthermore, even removal of all of the implanted material may fail to cure the infection.

Sometimes it is possible to control infection and repeat the prosthetic arthroplasty. However, early failure rates tend to be at least 15%, with significant questions remaining about long-term results following revision arthroplasty for infection. Chronic oral antibiotic treatment—to suppress rather than cure infection—may be a reasonable alternative to removal or replacement of the prosthesis for appropriately selected patients.

Treatment of infected joint replacement operations depends upon the time of occurrence, the virulence of the infecting organism, and the mechanical stability of the prosthesis. Infection must be suspected whenever pain develops following prosthetic arthroplasty. Loosening of the prosthetic components within their bony seats may be due to infection, mechanical failure, or both. Either loosening or infection may cause pain. Relatively avirulent organisms cause infection with a low-grade smouldering course that slowly spreads through the bone adjacent to the prosthesis. Aspiration for culture and sensitivity testing is essential for early diagnosis. Treatment requires surgery and skillful antibiotic management. If the prosthesis is loose, it will require removal, which is necessary for adequate debridement of most chronic infections. All foreign material and infected granulation tissue must be debrided. Viable bone should be preserved. Wound closure over tubes, 4–6 weeks of intravenous antibiotic treatment to achieve adequate serum killing levels (usually 1:8 dilution or more), and adequate mechanical support of the limb are advised. Following removal of a total hip prosthesis, traction may be needed for several weeks. Decisions must be made about whether or not to replace the removed prosthesis and, if replacement is chosen, whether to proceed immediately or defer reimplantation for several weeks or months until the wound is quiescent. Two-stage reimplantation of an infected total hip prosthesis may be more successful than single-stage reimplantation, but this remains controversial. Adding antibiotics to the acrylic cement used to seat prosthetic components is another adjunct that appears to improve the success rate of total hip revision for infection.

Beck-Sague CM et al: Outbreak of surgical wound infections associated with total hip arthroplasty. Infect Control Hosp Epidemiol 1992;13:526.

Fitzgerald RH Jr: Total hip arthroplasty sepsis: Prevention and diagnosis. Orthop Clin North Am 1992;3;23:259.

Schmalzried TP et al: Etiology of deep sepsis in total hip arthroplasty: The significance of hematogenous and recurrent infections. Clin Orthop 1992;Jul(280):200.

FRACTURE OF THE SHAFT OF THE FEMUR

Fracture of the shaft of the femur (Figure 43–37) usually occurs as a result of severe trauma. Indirect violence, especially torsional stress, is likely to cause spiral fractures that extend proximally or, more commonly, distally into the metaphyseal regions. Most are closed fractures; open fracture is often the result

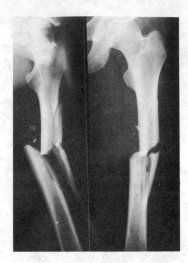

Figure 43–37. Comminuted fracture of the middle third of the femur.

of compounding from within. Extensive soft tissue injury, bleeding, and shock are commonly present.

The most significant features are severe pain in the thigh and deformity of the lower extremity. Surgical shock is likely to be present, as several units of blood may be lost into the thigh with only moderate swelling becoming apparent. Careful x-ray examination in at least two planes is necessary to determine the exact site and configuration of the fracture cleft. The hip and knee should be examined and x-rays obtained to look for associated injury.

Injuries to the sciatic nerve and to the superficial femoral artery and vein are not common but must be recognized promptly. Surgical shock and secondary anemia are the most important early complications. Later complications are essentially those of prolonged recumbency, eg, the formation of renal calculi.

Treatment

A. Closed Treatment: Treatment depends upon the age and medical status of the patient as well as the site and configuration of the fracture. Skeletal traction is generally the most effective form of closed treatment. However, 2–3 months of traction are often required, followed by external plaster or brace support. Fractures of the distal femoral shaft are more amenable to cast-brace treatment. After about 6 weeks in traction, the patient may be placed in a cast-brace (long-leg cast with a hinged knee) to allow early knee motion and progressive weight bearing.

B. Operative Treatment: Most fractures in the middle third of the femur can be internally fixed by an intramedullary rod. Intramedullary fixation of femoral shaft fractures allows early mobilization of the patient (within 2–3 days if the fracture fixation is stable), more anatomic alignment, improved knee function by decreasing the time spent in traction, and a marked decrease in the cost of hospitalization.

The procedure may be performed open or "blind." In open nailing, the fracture site is opened and the nail is driven retrograde from the fracture site into the proximal fragment. The fracture is then reduced and the nail driven across the fracture into the distal fragment. This requires a large incision and major manipulation of the fracture fragments, with significant blood loss.

In "blind" nailing, the fracture is reduced by closed manipulation on the fracture table under fluoroscopic control. An 8- to 10-cm incision is made proximal to the greater trochanter, and the nail is inserted through the trochanteric notch down into the intramedullary canal. The fracture site is not opened. "Blind" nailing decreases the chance of infection by decreasing the amount of soft tissue dissection necessary and by leaving the fracture site closed.

If the fracture is comminuted, interlocking nails can be used to maintain length by increased fixation proximally and distally. These may allow patients early mobilization even with comminuted femoral shaft fractures. If there is extensive soft tissue loss surrounding the fracture, stability of the bone fragments may be achieved with an external fixation device.

Complications of this procedure usually involve technical problems at the time of surgery resulting in malalignment or shortening from choosing a rod that is too short or too narrow. Infection can occur after any open procedure but is very uncommon in "blind nailing." Occasionally, a painful bursa may develop over the proximal end of the nail that causes discomfort when the patient sits or walks. The rod may be removed after healing is complete—usually after 1–1½ years. The healing rate of femoral shaft fractures in general is very high and approaches 100% after "blind" nailing.

Benirschke SK et al: Closed interlocking nailing of femoral shaft fractures: assessment of technical complications and functional outcomes by comparison of a prospective database with retrospective review. J Orthop Trauma 199;7:118.

Hajek PD et al: The use of one compared with two distal screws in the treatment of femoral shaft fractures with interlocking intramedullary nailing: A clinical and biomechanical analysis. J Bone Joint Surg [Am] 1993;3; 75:519.

Parfenchuck TA, Carter LW, Young TR: Ipsilateral fractures of the femoral neck and shaft. Orthop Rev 1993; 22:356.

Wu CC et al: Treatment of segmental femoral shaft fractures. Clin Orthop 1993;Feb(287):224.

INJURIES OF THE KNEE REGION

1. FRACTURES OF THE DISTAL FEMUR

Supracondylar Fracture of the Femur (Figure 43–38)

This comparatively uncommon fracture (at the junction of cortical and cancellous bone) may be transverse, oblique, or comminuted. The distal end of the proximal fragment is apt to perforate the overlying vastus intermedius, vastus medialis, or rectus femoris muscles and may penetrate the suprapatellar pouch of the knee joint to cause hemarthrosis. The proximal end of the distal fragment is usually displaced posteriorly and slightly laterally.

Since the distal fragment may impinge upon the popliteal vessels, circulatory adequacy distal to the fracture site should be verified as soon as possible. Absence or marked diminution of pedal pulsations is an indication for immediate reduction. If pulsation does not return promptly after reduction, an immediate arteriogram or exploration (or both) with appropriate treatment of the vascular lesion is indicated.

A less frequent complication is injury to the peroneal or tibial nerve.

If the fracture is transverse or nearly so, closed manipulation under general anesthesia will occasionally be successful. Stable fractures with minimal displacement can be immobilized in a single plaster hip spica with the hip and knee in about 30 degrees of flexion. Frequent x-ray examination is necessary to make certain that redisplacement has not occurred.

Stable or unstable uncomplicated supracondylar fracture can be treated with skeletal traction if soft tissue interposition does not interfere with reduction.

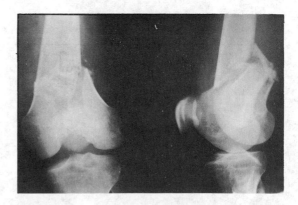

Figure 43–38. Comminuted T fracture of the distal femur. Adequate closed reduction was prevented by interposition of small intermediate fragments between the two main condylar fragments.

Two traction pins may be necessary—one in the distal femur for vertical traction and one in the proximal tibia for longitudinal traction—in order to maintain alignment (Figure 43–39). If adequate reduction cannot be obtained, it may be necessary to manipulate the fragments under general anesthesia, using skeletal traction to control the distal fragment.

Traction must be continued for about 6 weeks or until stabilization occurs. The extremity can then be immobilized in a cast-brace for another 2–3 months until complete healing occurs. This combines support with early motion of the knee to decrease restriction due to scarring and adhesion formation in adjacent soft tissues.

If reduction is inadequate by closed technique or if early motion of the patient and the joint is desired, internal fixation with a condylar nail or screw and side plate or with a supracondylar intramedullary device may be performed.

Intercondylar Fracture of the Femur

This comminuted fracture is classically described as a T (Figure 43–38) or Y fracture according to x-ray configuration of the fragments. Closed reduction is difficult when the proximal shaft fragment is interposed between the two main distal fragments. Maximal recovery of function of the knee joint requires anatomic reduction of the articular components if possible. If alignment is satisfactory and displacement minimal, skeletal traction for 6–10 weeks followed by a cast-brace will be sufficient. If displacement is marked, open reduction and internal fixation of the fragments are indicated to restore articular congruity. A condylar screw and side plate are used to maintain alignment of the articular fragments to each other and to the femoral shaft. Even if the articular fragments are restored to their anatomic positions, posttraumatic arthritis with joint stiffness and pain is common.

Condylar Fracture of the Femur

Isolated fracture of the lateral or medial condyle of the femur is rare. Occasionally, only the posterior portion of the condyle is separated. Injury to the cruciate ligaments or the collateral ligament of the opposite side of the knee often occurs.

The objective of treatment is restoration of anatomic intra-articular relationships. If displacement is minimal, closed reduction can be attempted by manipulation, with a bending stress used in the direction opposite to the apex of angular deformity. If anatomic reduction cannot be obtained by closed manipulation, open reduction and fixation of the minor fragment with two or three bone screws are recommended. The ligaments must be explored and repaired if they are found to be injured.

Butler MS et al: Interlocking intramedullary nailing for ipsilateral fractures of the femoral shaft and distal part of the femur. J Bone Joint Surg [Am] 1991;73:1492.

Foster TE, Healy WL: Operative management of distal femoral fractures. Orthop Rev 1991;20:962.

Shewring DJ, Meggitt BF: Fractures of the distal femur treated with the AO dynamic condylar screw. J Bone Joint Surg [Br] 1992;74:122.

2. FRACTURE OF THE PATELLA

Transverse Fracture of the Patella

Transverse fracture of the patella (Figure 43–40) is the result of indirect violence, usually with the knee in semiflexion. Fracture may be due to sudden voluntary contraction of the quadriceps muscles or sudden forced flexion of the leg when these muscles are contracted. The level of fracture is most often in the middle. The extent of tearing of the patellar retinacula depends upon the degree of force of the initiating injury. The activity of the quadriceps muscles causes displacement of the proximal fragment; the magni-

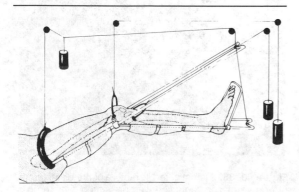

Figure 43–39. Method of suspension of lower extremity with biplane skeletal traction for supracondylar fracture.

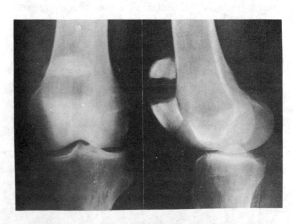

Figure 43–40. Transverse fracture of the patella.

tude of displacement is dependent upon the extent of the tear of the quadriceps expansion.

Swelling of the anterior knee region is caused by hemarthrosis and hemorrhage into the soft tissues overlying the joint. If displacement is present, the defect in the patella can be palpated, and active extension of the knee is lost.

Open reduction is indicated if the fragments are offset or separated more than 2–3 mm. The fragments must be accurately repositioned to prevent early posttraumatic arthritis of the patellofemoral joint. If the minor fragment is small (no more than 1 cm in length) or severely comminuted, it may be excised and the rectus or patellar tendon (depending upon which pole of the patella is involved) sutured directly to the major fragment. If the fragments are approximately the same size, repair by wire cerclage or figure-of-eight wire is preferred.

Accurate reduction of the articular surface must be confirmed by lateral x-rays taken intraoperatively.

Comminuted Fracture of the Patella

Comminuted fracture of the patella is caused only by direct violence. Little or no separation of the fragments occurs, because the quadriceps expansion is not extensively torn. Severe injury may cause extensive comminution of the articular cartilages of both the patella and the opposing femur. If comminution is not severe and displacement is insignificant, immobilization for 8 weeks in a plaster cylinder extending from the groin to the supramalleolar region is sufficient.

Severe comminution requires excision of the patella and repair of the defect by imbrication of the quadriceps expansion. Excision of the patella can result in decreased strength, pain in the knee, and general restriction of activity.

Appel MH, Seigel H: Treatment of transverse fractures of the patella by arthroscopic percutaneous pinning. Arthroscopy 1993;9:119.

Boyd AD Jr et al: Long-term complications after total knee arthroplasty with or without resurfacing of the patella. J Bone Joint Surg [Am] 1993;75:674.

Braun W et al: Indications and results of nonoperative treatment of patellar fractures. Clin Orthop 1993;Apr(289):197.

3. TEAR OF THE QUADRICEPS TENDON

Tear of the quadriceps tendon occurs most often in patients over age 40. Preexisting attritional disease of the tendon is apt to be present, and the causative injury may be minor. The tear commonly results from sudden deceleration, such as stumbling, or slipping on a wet surface. A small flake of bone may be avulsed from the superior pole of the patella, or the tear may occur entirely through tendinous and muscle tissue.

Pain may be noted in the anterior knee region. Swelling is due to hemarthrosis and extravasation of blood into the soft tissues. The patient is unable to extend the knee completely. X-rays may show avulsion of a bit of bone from the superior patella.

Operative repair is recommended for complete tear. If treatment is delayed until partial healing has occurred, the suture line can be reinforced by transplantation of the iliotibial band from the upper area of the tibia.

Rasul AT Jr, Fischer DA: Primary repair of quadriceps tendon ruptures: Results of treatment. Clin Orthop 1993; Apr(289):205.

4. TEAR OF THE PATELLAR LIGAMENT

The same mechanism that causes tears of the quadriceps tendon, transverse fracture of the patella, or avulsion of the tibial tuberosity may also cause tear of the patellar ligament. The characteristic finding is proximal displacement of the patella. A bit of bone may be avulsed from the lower pole of the patella if the tear takes place in the proximal patellar tendon.

Operative treatment is necessary for complete tear. The ligament is resutured to the patella, and any tear in the quadriceps expansion is repaired. The extremity should be immobilized for 8 weeks in a tubular plaster cast extending from the groin to the supramalleolar region. Guarded exercises may then be started.

5. DISLOCATION OF THE PATELLA

Acute traumatic dislocation of the patella should be differentiated from episodic recurrent dislocation, since the latter condition is likely to be associated with occult organic lesions. When this injury occurs alone, it may be due to direct violence or muscle activity of the quadriceps, and the direction of dislocation of the patella is usually lateral. Spontaneous reduction is apt to occur if the knee joint is extended; if so, the clinical findings may consist merely of hemarthrosis and localized tenderness over the medial patellar retinaculum. Gross instability of the patella, which can be demonstrated by physical examination, indicates that injury to the soft tissues of the medial aspect of the knee has been extensive. Recurrent episodes require operative repair for effective treatment.

6. DISLOCATION OF THE KNEE JOINT (Figure 43–41)

Traumatic dislocation of the knee joint is uncommon. It is caused by severe trauma. Displacement may be transverse or torsional. Complete dislocation can occur only after extensive tearing of the supporting ligaments and is apt to cause injury to the popliteal vessels or the tibial and peroneal nerves.

Signs of neurovascular injury below the site of dislocation are an absolute indication for prompt reduction, preferably under general anesthesia, since failure of circulation will undoubtedly result in gangrene of the leg and foot. Axial traction is applied to the leg to obtain reduction. If pedal pulses do not return promptly, patency of the popliteal vessels should be investigated immediately by angiography. Even if pulses do return, angiography is usually indicated to rule out an intimal tear of the vessel. Inadequate assessment and treatment of the vascular injuries can lead to an amputation rate of 50%. If a vascular injury is confirmed, repair should be started as soon as the patient's general status allows. Ischemia of more than 4 hours implies a poor prognosis for limb salvage. Prophylactic fasciotomy of the leg compartments should be performed at the time of vascular repair to eliminate the compartment syndrome caused by postischemic edema.

Anatomic reduction of uncomplicated dislocation should be attempted. If impinging soft tissues cannot be removed by closed manipulation, arthrotomy is indicated. After reduction, repair of the major ligamentous injuries may be performed, but this should not be done if the time and dissection necessary will further jeopardize survival of the limb. The extremity should be immobilized in a plaster cast extending from the inguinal region to the toes, with the knee in slight flexion. A window should be cut in the plaster over the dorsum of the foot to allow for frequent determination of dorsalis pedis artery pulsation. In anteroposterior dislocations, adequacy of reduction should be assessed at frequent intervals during the first 3–4 weeks to rule out posterior subluxation. If subluxation occurs, the knee joint must be reduced and placed in an external fixation device. After 8 weeks of immobilization, the knee can be protected by a long-leg brace. Intensive quadriceps exercises are necessary to minimize functional loss.

Schenck RC Jr, Heckman JD: Injuries of the knee. Clin Symp 1993;45:1.
Tucker JB, Corsetti J, Gregg JR: Arthroscopically assisted proximal quadricepsplasty for patellar instability. Clin Sports Med 1993;12:81.

7. INTERNAL DERANGEMENTS OF THE KNEE JOINT

Internal derangements of the knee joint mechanism may be caused by trauma or attritional disease. Although ligamentous and cartilaginous injuries are discussed separately, they commonly occur as combined lesions.

Arthroscopy and newer techniques of arthrography using single or double contrast media can be valuable adjuncts in establishing a precise diagnosis when the usual diagnostic methods are inconclusive.

Injury to the Menisci

Injury to the medial meniscus is the most frequent internal derangement of the knee joint. The significant clinical findings after acute injury are swelling (due to hemarthrosis) and varying degrees of restriction of flexion or extension. True locking (inability to fully extend the knee) is highly suggestive of meniscal tear. A marginal tear permits displacement of the

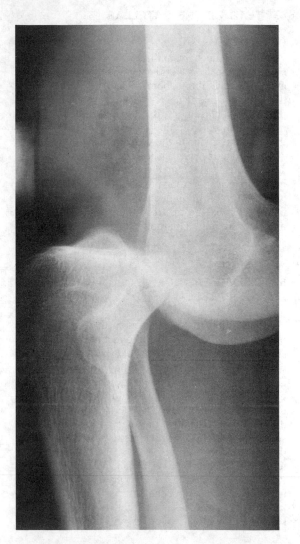

Figure 43–41. Complete dislocation of the knee joint.

medial fragment into the intercondylar region (bucket-handle tear) and prevents either complete extension or complete flexion. Motion may cause pain over the anteromedial or posteromedial joint line. Tenderness can often be elicited at the point of pain. Forcible rotation of the foot with the knee flexed to a right angle may cause pain over the medial joint line. If symptoms have persisted for 2–3 weeks, weakness and atrophy of the quadriceps femoris may be present.

Injury to the lateral meniscus less often causes mechanical blockage of joint motion. Pain and tenderness may be present over the lateral joint line. Pain can be elicited by forcible rotation of the leg with the knee flexed to a right angle. Arthrography is less accurate for diagnosing tears of the lateral meniscus, because of interference by the presence of the popliteus tendon.

Initial treatment may be conservative. Swelling and pain caused by tense hemarthrosis can be relieved by aspiration. The knee may be placed in a removable knee immobilizer for comfort. Younger patients usually prefer to be ambulatory on crutches. As long as acute symptoms persist, isometric quadriceps exercises should be performed frequently throughout the day with the knee in maximum extension (as a "straight leg lift"). Unrestricted activity must not be resumed until complete motion is recovered.

Arthroscopy or exploratory arthrotomy is advisable for recurrent or persistent "locking," recurrent effusion, or disabling pain. Isometric quadriceps exercises are instituted after meniscectomy and gradually increased in frequency. As soon as the patient is able to perform these exercises comfortably, graded resistance maneuvers should be started. Exercises must be continued until all motion has been recovered and the volume and competency of the quadriceps are equal to those of the uninjured side.

Injury to the Collateral Ligaments

The collateral ligaments prevent excursion of the joint beyond normal limits. When the knee is in full extension, the collateral ligaments are taut; in flexion, only the anterior fibers of the tibial collateral ligament are taut.

A. Tibial Collateral Ligament: Forced abduction of the leg at the knee, which is frequently associated with torsional strain, causes injury varying from tear of a few fibers to complete rupture of the ligament. A bit of bone may be avulsed from its femoral or tibial attachment.

A history of a twisting injury at the knee with valgus strain can usually be obtained. Pain is present over the medial aspect of the knee joint. In severe injury, joint effusion may be present. Tenderness can be elicited at the site of the lesion. When only an isolated ligamentous tear is present, x-ray examination may not be helpful unless it is made while valgus stress is applied to the extended knee. Under local or

general anesthesia, the extremities are bound together in full extension at the knee joint, and an anteroposterior film is made with the legs in forced abduction. If the medial joint cleft is 1 cm or more wider than the uninjured side, complete rupture is suggested.

Treatment of incomplete tear consists of protection from further injury while healing progresses. Painful hemarthrosis should be relieved by aspiration. The knee may be immobilized in a splint or a tubular cast extending from the inguinal to the supramalleolar region.

Complete rupture may be surgically repaired or may be treated in a long-leg cast for 6 weeks. Tear of the medial collateral ligament is frequently associated with other lesions, such as tear of the medial meniscus, rupture of the anterior cruciate ligament, or fracture of the lateral condyle of the tibia.

B. Fibular Collateral Ligament: Tear of the fibular collateral ligament is often associated with injury to surrounding structures, eg, the popliteus muscle tendon and the iliotibial band. Avulsion of the apex of the fibular head may occur, and the peroneal nerve may be injured.

Pain and tenderness are present over the lateral aspect of the knee joint, and hemarthrosis may be present. X-rays may show a bit of bone avulsed from the fibular head. If severe injury is suspected, x-ray examination under stress, using local or general anesthesia, is required. A firm, padded nonopaque object about 20–30 cm in diameter is placed between the knees, and the legs are forcibly adducted while an anteroposterior exposure is made. Widening of the lateral joint cleft indicates severe injury.

The treatment of partial tear is similar to that described for partial tear of the medial collateral ligament. If complete tear is suspected, exploration may be justified. The extremity is protected for 6 weeks in a plaster cylinder extending from the inguinal region to the toes.

Injury to the Cruciate Ligaments

The function of the anterior and posterior cruciate ligaments is to restrict anterior and posterior gliding of the tibia when the knee is flexed. If the tibia is rotated internally on the femur, the ligaments twist around themselves and become taut; if the tibia is rotated externally, they become lax.

A. Anterior Cruciate Ligament: Injury to the anterior cruciate ligament is usually associated with injury to the medial meniscus or the tibial collateral ligament. The cruciate ligament may be avulsed with part of the medial tibial tubercle or may rupture within the substance of its fibers.

The characteristic clinical sign of tear of either cruciate ligament is a positive anterior "drawer" sign: The knee is flexed at a right angle and pulled forward; if excessive anterior excursion of the proximal tibia (in comparison with the opposite normal side) can be noted, a tear of the anterior ligament is likely.

Complete recent rupture of the anterior cruciate ligament within its substance can occasionally be repaired with stout sutures. When avulsed, displaced tibial bone is present, and attachment of the fragment in anatomic position by arthrotomy or arthroscopy is necessary. When the fragment of bone is large, displaced, and not treated until several weeks after injury, excision of the fragment and reinsertion of the ligament may be necessary to eliminate the blocking effect of the bone fragment and permit recovery of function. Old tears may require reconstructive procedures.

B. Posterior Cruciate Ligament: Tear of the posterior ligament may occur within its substance or may be manifest by avulsion of a fragment of bone of variable size at its tibial attachment. Tear of the posterior cruciate ligament can be diagnosed by the posterior "drawer" sign: The knee is flexed at a right angle, and the upper tibia is pushed backward; if excessive posterior excursion of the proximal tibia can be noted, tear of the posterior ligament is likely.

Treatment is directed primarily at the associated injuries and maintenance of competency of the quadriceps musculature. Primary repair of tears within the fibers is difficult and of dubious value. Open reduction and fixation of a fragment of tibia with the attached ligament is feasible and is likely to restore functional competency of the ligament.

Aglietti P et al: Patellofemoral problems after intraarticular anterior cruciate ligament reconstruction. Clin Orthop 1993;Mar(288):195.

Andriacchi TP, Birac D: Functional testing in the anterior cruciate ligament-deficient knee. Clin Orthop 1993; Mar(288):40.

De Smet AA et al: Diagnosis of meniscal tears of the knee with MR imaging: Effect of observer variation and sample size on sensitivity and specificity. AJR Am J Roentgenol 1993;160:555.

Markolf KL et al: Direct measurement of resultant forces in the anterior cruciate ligament: An in vitro study performed with a new experimental technique. J Bone Joint Surg [Am] 1990;3;72:557.

Shino K et al: Deterioration of patellofemoral articular surfaces after anterior cruciate ligament reconstruction. Am J Sports Med 1993;21:206.

Stanish WD, Lai A: New concepts of rehabilitation following anterior cruciate reconstruction. Clin Sports Med 1993;12:25.

Ligamentous Reconstruction of the Knee

Knee joint instability may be (1) single plane (medial, lateral, posterior, or anterior), (2) rotatory, or (3) combinations of the two. Repair of ligaments denotes treatment of acute injuries, whereas reconstruction is the term reserved for treatment of ligamentous laxity several months after injury.

Even though numerous types of repair have been described for many types of instability, there is still controversy over whether the long-term results of repair or reconstruction of certain ligamentous injuries are superior to the results of nonsurgical treatment.

Reconstructive procedures to replace the function of the anterior cruciate ligament include use of a portion of patellar tendon introduced through a drill hole in the proximal tibia, passed through the intercondylar notch, and attached to the lateral femoral condyle.

Posterior cruciate function may be restored by use of the medial head of the gastrocnemius, which is detached from the medial femoral condyle, passed through the posterior capsule and intercondylar notch, and attached to the inner surface of the medial femoral condyle.

Most commonly, knee instability is in more than one plane and may require both extra-articular and intra-articular reconstructive procedures. The pes anserinus medially and the iliotibial band laterally are examples of structures that may be used for these extra-articular procedures.

Indications for major reconstruction of knee ligaments depend on the patient's age and activity level and the status of the articular cartilage within the knee. Even though early results of these procedures are frequently excellent, the integrity of the repair tends to deteriorate after 2–5 years.

DiStefano V: Anterior cruciate ligament reconstruction: Autograft or allograft? Clin Sports Med 1993;12:1.

Gillquist J: Repair and reconstruction of the ACL: Is it good enough? Arthroscopy 1993;9:68.

Gomez-Castresana FB, Bastos MN, Sacristan CG: Semitendinosus Kennedy ligament augmentation device anterior cruciate ligament reconstruction. Clin Orthop 1992; Oct(283):21.

Halling AH, Howard ME, Cawley PW: Rehabilitation of anterior cruciate ligament injuries. Clin Sports Med 1993;3;12:329.

Howe JG et al: Anterior cruciate ligament reconstruction using quadriceps patellar tendon graft: Part I: Long-term followup Am J Sports Med 1991;19:447.

Kaplan MJ et al: Anterior cruciate ligament reconstruction using quadriceps patellar tendon graft: Part II: A specific sport review. Am J Sports Med 1991;19:458.

Shelbourne KD, Wilckens JH: Current concepts in anterior cruciate ligament rehabilitation. Orthop Rev 1990;19: 957.

Woo SL, Livesay GA, Engle C: Biomechanics of the human anterior cruciate ligament: Muscle stabilization and ACL reconstruction. Orthop Rev 1992;21:935.

Arthroscopy of the Knee

Arthroscopy is a valuable adjunct to a history, physical examination, and x-ray studies for evaluation of the knee joint. The arthroscope is introduced into the knee joint through a small stab incision and allows examination of most structures inside the knee without major surgical exploration.

Arthroscopy is particularly helpful in the management of the patient with a "problem knee"—significant symptoms but minimal or confusing physical findings. It is also of value in preoperative confirmation of a clinical diagnosis (eg, patients with anterior cruciate tears, meniscal tear, or chondromalacia) and for follow-up evaluation after therapy.

Surgical procedures such as meniscectomy, synovial biopsy, or removal of loose bodies can be performed through the arthroscope with minimal postoperative morbidity compared to open procedures. However, this is a demanding technique and requires considerable experience for good results.

DeHaven KE, Sebastianelli WJ: Open meniscus repair: Indications, technique, and results. Clin Sports Med 1990; 9:577.

Durand A, Richards CL, Malouin F: Strength recovery and muscle activation of the knee extensor and flexor muscles after arthroscopic meniscectomy: A pilot study. Clin Orthop 1991;Jan(262):210.

Lanzer WL, Komenda G: Changes in articular cartilage after meniscectomy. Clin Orthop 1990;Mar(252):41.

Newman AP, Daniels AU, Burks RT: Principles and decision making in meniscal surgery. Arthroscopy 1993;9:33.

Spiers AS et al: Can MRI of the knee affect arthroscopic practice? A prospective study of 58 patients. J Bone Joint Surg [Br] 1993;75:49.

8. FRACTURES OF THE PROXIMAL TIBIA

Fracture of the Lateral Tibial Condyle (Figure 43–42)

Fracture of the lateral condyle, or plateau, of the tibia is commonly caused by a blow on the lateral aspect of the knee with the foot in fixed position, producing an abduction strain. The lateral femoral condyle is driven down into the tibial condyle, causing

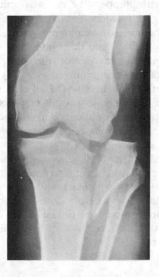

Figure 43–42. Fracture of the lateral condyle of the tibia.

fracture. Hemarthrosis is always present, as the fracture cleft involves the knee joint. Soft tissue injuries are apt to be present also. The tibial collateral and anterior cruciate ligaments may be torn. A displaced free fragment may tear the overlying lateral meniscus. If displacement is marked, fracture of the proximal fibula may be present also.

The objective of treatment is to restore the articular surface and normal anatomic relationships, so that torn ligaments can heal without elongation. In cases of minimal displacement where ligaments have not been extensively damaged, treatment may be by immobilization for 6–12 weeks in a tubular plaster cast extending from the toes in the inguinal region.

Many fractures of the lateral condyle of the tibia, especially comminuted fractures, cannot be reduced adequately by closed methods. If depression of the articular surface exceeds 7–8 mm in younger patients, open reduction is usually indicated.

After elevation of the articular surface, insertion of bone graft may be necessary to maintain alignment. Stabilization with a bolt or multiple bone screws is usually necessary. Weight bearing is resumed after 3 months.

Fracture of the Medial Tibial Condyle

Fracture of the medial condyle of the tibia is caused by the adduction strain produced by a blow against the medial aspect of the knee with the foot in fixed position. The medial meniscus and the fibular collateral ligament may be torn. Severe comminution is not usually present, and there is only one major free fragment.

Treatment is by closed reduction to restore the articular surface of the tibia so that ligamentous healing can occur without elongation. If closed reduction is unsuccessful, open reduction and stabilization with multiple screws may be necessary. After reduction, the extremity is immobilized for 10–12 weeks in a tubular cast extending from the inguinal region to the toes with the knee in full extension. If internal fixation has provided stability, early motion may be started, although weight bearing is not permitted for at least 3 months.

Fracture of Both Tibial Condyles

Axial force, such as may result from falling on the foot or sudden deceleration with the knee in full extension (as during an automobile accident), can cause simultaneous fracture of both condyles of the tibia. Comminution is apt to be severe. Swelling of the knee due to hemarthrosis is marked. Deformity is either genu varum or genu valgum. X-ray examination should include oblique projections.

Severe comminution makes anatomic reduction difficult to achieve by any means and difficult to maintain following closed manipulation alone. Sustained skeletal traction is usually necessary. When stability has been achieved, the extremity can be immobilized for another 4–6 weeks in a tubular plaster cast extending from the toes to the inguinal region with the knee in full extension. Unassisted weight bearing is not permitted for 3–4 months.

If closed methods are not effective, open reduction must be attempted.

Instability and restriction of motion of the knee are common sequelae of this type of fracture. If reduction is not adequate, posttraumatic arthritis will appear early.

Fracture of the Tibial Tuberosity

Violent contraction of the quadriceps muscle may cause avulsion of the tibial tuberosity. When avulsion of the tuberosity is complete, active extension of the knee is not possible.

If displacement is minimal, treatment is by immobilization in a tubular plaster cast extending from the inguinal to the supramalleolar region with the knee in full extension. Immobilization is maintained for 8 weeks or until stabilization occurs.

A loose fragment that has been displaced more than 0.5 cm can be treated either by closed reduction and percutaneous fixation, with plaster immobilization, or by open reduction.

Fracture of the Tibial Eminence

This injury usually occurs in association with comminuted fracture of the condyles. The medial intercondylar tubercle may be avulsed with adjacent bone attached to the anterior cruciate ligament, and injury to that structure is of greater importance. In addition to avulsion of the anterior cruciate ligament, there may also be injury to the tibial collateral ligament and the medial knee joint capsule. Hemarthrosis is always present.

Isolated and undisplaced fracture may be treated by immobilization of the extremity for 6 weeks in a tubular plaster cast extending from the inguinal region to the toes with the knee in slight flexion. The treatment of displaced fracture is the same as that of rupture of the anterior cruciate ligament (see above).

Benirschke SK et al: Immediate internal fixation of open, complex tibial plateau fractures: Treatment by a standard protocol. J Orthop Trauma 1992;6:78.

Honkonen SE, Jarvinen MJ: Classification of fractures of the tibial condyles. J Bone Joint Surg [Br] 1992;74:840.

Mallik AR, Covall DJ, Whitelaw GP: Internal versus external fixation of bicondylar tibial plateau fractures. Orthop Rev 1992;21:1433.

O'Dwyer KJ, Bobic VR: Arthroscopic management of tibial plateau fractures. Injury 1992;23:261.

9. TOTAL KNEE REPLACEMENT

Reconstructive surgery for the arthritic knee has been characterized by the development of total replacement prostheses, each designed to compensate for varying degrees of cartilage, bone, or ligament destruction. Indications for knee replacement include intractable pain (with or without deformity) with x-ray evidence of arthritis, either rheumatoid, posttraumatic, or degenerative. The many designs of implants available vary in the degree to which they constrain knee motion. The unconstrained implants are mainly resurfacing replacements and require intact collateral and posterior cruciate ligaments. A minimum amount of bone is removed from the articular surfaces of the distal femur and proximal tibia and is replaced by metal on the femoral side and polyethylene on the tibial side. The components are cemented in place with polymethylmethacrylate. The largest number of prostheses fall into the semiconstrained category and provide varying amounts of intrinsic stability. Fully constrained prostheses permit motion only in the sagittal plane and are used in joints with severe deformity or major ligamentous laxity. These prostheses require removal of a significant amount of bone to allow room for the device, to correct deformity, and to allow for placement of the intramedullary stems.

Enthusiastic early short-term reports of total knee arthroplasty have been replaced by more thoughtful long-term studies, with reoperation rates of 15% and higher. The most common mechanism of failure has been loosening of the prosthetic components, most often on the tibial side. Factors contributing to loosening include inadequate fixation, less than optimum cementing techniques, and restricted rotation of the prosthesis. Obesity, overactivity, and insufficient bone stock are patient factors contributing to failure.

Patients with preoperative varus deformity appear to have a higher incidence of loosening. Other complications include peroneal nerve palsy, problems with wound healing, and deep infection, which frequently requires removal of the prosthesis and arthrodesis of the knee joint.

Pain relief occurs in 80–90% of patients, and a mild to moderate increase in a range of motion of the knee can be expected. Patients must be motivated to participate in a vigorous rehabilitation program for maximum results.

If osteoarthritis involves one compartment of the joint only, unicompartmental replacement has been successful in elderly patients. In young active patients who have varus deformity of less than 10 degrees, no subluxation, and flexion of 80 degrees or more, high tibial osteotomy to correct varus deformity is advocated.

Cates HE et al: Intramedullary versus extramedullary femoral alignment systems in total knee replacement. Clin Orthop 1993;Jan(286):32.

Edgerton BC, Mariani EM, Morrey BF: Distal femoral varus osteotomy for painful genu valgum: A five-to-11-year follow-up study. Clin Orthop 1993;Mar(288):263.

Skinner HB: Pathokinesiology and total joint arthroplasty. Clin Orthop 1993;Mar(288):78.

Whiteside LA: Correction of ligament and bone defects in total arthroplasty of the severely valgus knee. Clin Orthop 1993;Mar(288):234.

FRACTURE OF THE SHAFTS OF THE TIBIA & FIBULA

Fracture of the shaft of the tibia or fibula occurs at any age but is most common during adolescence and active adulthood. In general, open, transverse, comminuted, and segmental fractures are caused by indirect violence. Fracture of the middle third of the shaft (especially if comminuted) is apt to be complicated by delay of bone healing.

If fracture is complete and displacement is present, clinical diagnosis is not difficult. However, critical local examination is of utmost importance in planning treatment. The nature of the skin wounds that may communicate with the fracture site often suggests the mechanism of compounding, whether it has occurred from within or from without. A small laceration without contused edges suggests that the point of a bone fragment has caused compounding from within. A large wound with contused edges, especially over the subcutaneous surface of the tibia, suggests compounding from without. The presence of abrasions more than 6 hours old, pyoderma, and pre-existing ulcers precludes immediate open treatment of closed fracture. Extensive swelling due to hemorrhagic exudate in closed fascial compartments may prevent complete reduction immediately. Extensive hemorrhagic and edematous infiltration can make difficult satisfactory closure of the subcutaneous tissue and skin incidental to elective open reduction. Neurovascular integrity below the level of the fracture must be verified before definitive treatment is instituted.

X-rays in the anteroposterior and lateral projection of the entire leg, including both the knee and ankle joints, are always necessary, and oblique projections are often desirable. The surgeon must know the exact site and configuration, and the direction of displacement of fragments. Inadequate x-ray examination can lead to an incomplete diagnosis.

1. FRACTURE OF THE SHAFT OF THE FIBULA

Isolated fracture of the shaft of the fibula is uncommon and is usually associated with other injury of the leg, such as fracture of the tibia or fracture-dislocation of the ankle joint. If no other lesion is present, immobilization is for comfort only. This requires 3–4 weeks in a plaster boot (equipped with a walking surface) extending from the knee to the toes or in a removable knee immobilizer. Complete healing of uncomplicated fracture can be expected.

2. FRACTURE OF THE SHAFT OF THE TIBIA

Isolated fracture of the shaft of the tibia is apt to be caused by indirect injury, such as torsional stress. Because of mechanical stability provided by the intact fibula, marked displacement is not apt to occur. Marked overriding suggests a lesion of either tibio-fibular joint.

If the fragments are not displaced, reliable treatment may be given by immobilization in a tubular plaster cast extending from the inguinal region to the toes with the foot in neutral position. The plaster should be changed at appropriate intervals to correct the loosening that will occur as a result of absorption of hemorrhagic exudate and atrophy of the thigh and calf muscles. Immobilization should be continued for at least 16–20 weeks or until healing is demonstrated by x-ray.

If the fragments are displaced, manipulation under anesthesia may be necessary. a long-leg plaster cast is applied as for undisplaced fracture. Alignment should be checked by x-ray frequently during the first 6–8 weeks of treatment, because varus angulation can be a significant problem with isolated tibial shaft fractures. If x-rays do not show satisfactory apposition of fragments, alternative methods of treatment should be used (see below).

3. FRACTURE OF THE SHAFTS OF BOTH BONES IN ADULTS (Figures 43–43, 43–44, 43–45)

Simultaneous fractures of the shafts of the tibia and fibula are unstable and tend to become displaced following reduction. Treatment is directed toward reduction and stabilization of the tibial fracture until healing takes place. For adequate reduction, the fragments must be in contact, and angulation and torsional displacement of the tibial fracture must be corrected.

If reduction by closed manipulation is anatomic, transverse fractures tend to be stable. X-rays must be repeated weekly for the first 4 weeks and then at decreasing intervals to determine whether displacement has recurred. Recurrent angular displacement can be corrected by "cast wedging." This involves dividing the plaster circumferentially and inserting wedges in the appropriate direction. After satisfactory reduction

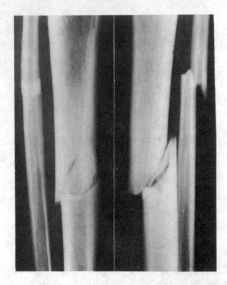

Figure 43–43. Short oblique fracture of the mid diaphysis of the tibia and fracture of the fibular shaft. This fracture is inherently unstable and is likely to become displaced when treated by plaster immobilization alone.

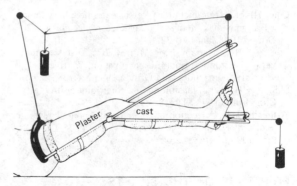

Figure 43–45. Calcaneal skeletal traction and full lower extremity plaster for unstable fracture of the tibia and fibula.

has been obtained and early healing has begun, the long-leg cast may be replaced by a prefabricated functional brace to allow motion of the knee and ankle.

If oblique and spiral fractures are unstable following manipulation and immobilization, internal fixation, percutaneous fixation, or skeletal traction may be required. Percutaneous fixation can be accomplished either by incorporation into the cast of pins or

wires that transfix the major bone fragments or by use of an extraskeletal apparatus called an external fixator. Comminuted fractures with large overlying wounds or major soft tissue loss are frequently best treated by use of an external fixator. This provides fairly rigid fixation of the fracture fragments yet allows for accessibility for wound treatment.

If adequate apposition and correction of the deformity cannot be achieved by closed methods, open reduction and internal fixation are required. Intramedullary rods give excellent fixation in middle-third shaft fractures and can be introduced through the area of the tibial tubercle, proximal to the fracture site, thus allowing the closed fracture to remain "closed." The fracture is reduced and the nail inserted under fluoroscopic control. Segmental fractures can be treated very satisfactorily with interlocking nails that maintain length and proper rotational control, resulting in significantly improved alignment and healing rates superior to those achieved with plaster cast treatment.

Metal plates and screws provide more rigid fixation than intramedullary rods but require more soft tissue dissection, thus increasing the risk of infection and delayed union.

Brumback RJ: Open tibial fractures: Current orthopaedic management. Instr Course Lect 1992;41:101.

Dagher F, Roukoz S: Compound tibial fractures with bone loss treated by the Ilizarov technique. J Bone Joint Surg [Br] 1991;73:316.

Garcia-Cimbrelo E et al: Ilizarov technique: Results and difficulties. Clin Orthop 1992;Oct(283):116.

Piccioni L, Guanche CA: Clinical experience with unreamed locked nails for open tibial fractures. Orthop Rev 1992;21:1213.

Shen WJ, Shen YS: Fibular nonunion after fixation of the tibia in lower leg fractures. Clin Orthop 1993;Feb(287): 231.

Siebenrock KA, Schillig B, Jakob RP: Treatment of complex tibial shaft fractures: Arguments for early secondary intramedullary nailing. Clin Orthop 1993;May(290):269.

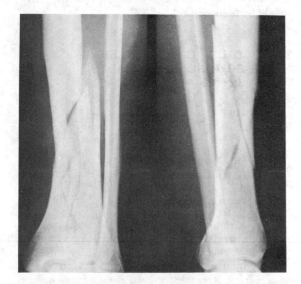

Figure 43–44. Comminuted fracture of the distal diaphysis of the tibia extending into the metaphysis and entering the ankle joint.

Wiss DA, Johnson DL, Miao M: Compression plating for non-union after failed external fixation of open tibial fractures. J Bone Joint Surg [Am] 1992;Oct,74:1279.

ACUTE COMPARTMENT SYNDROME

Compartment syndrome is caused by increased tissue pressure in a closed fascial space compromising circulation to the nerves and muscles within the involved compartment. The fascial compartments of the leg and forearm are most commonly involved. The syndrome can be caused by a fracture with subsequent hemorrhage and edema in the compartment, limb compression or crush, or vigorous exercise. Intracompartmental fluid pressure is increased, leading to ischemia. Severe ischemia for 6–8 hours or more leads to muscle and nerve death, resulting in a useless limb called Volkmann's contracture.

Clinical findings include swelling and palpable tenseness over a muscle compartment. Paresis and pain with stretch of the involved muscle are common findings but are unreliable in an obtunded or comatose patient. Sensory deficit is a more reliable finding and may occur early in the course of compartment syndrome. Contrary to what is commonly asserted, the presence of palpable peripheral pulses does not rule out a damaging increase in intracompartmental pressure, since pressure may be high enough to cause ischemia of muscle and nerve without being high enough to occlude a major artery.

If compartment syndrome cannot be diagnosed clinically, intracompartmental pressure must be measured directly. This is done by placing a large-bore catheter into the compartment using sterile technique. The catheter is connected to a pressure monitor via intravenous tubing filled with sterile saline solution. Compartments with pressures above 30–40 mm Hg should be considered for fasciotomy. Fasciotomy is performed by generous opening of the skin and fascia of the involved compartments. Compartment pressures are rechecked after fasciotomy to ensure that decompression has been achieved. The wounds are usually left open and covered with sterile dressings and are then treated by delayed primary closure or skin grafting 5 days later.

Delay in diagnosis of compartment syndrome for 6–8 hours after onset of ischemia can lead to irreversible death of muscle and nerve.

Cameron SE: Acute compartment syndrome of the triceps: A case report. Acta Orthop Scand 1993;64:107.

Cohen MS et al: Acute compartment syndrome: Effect of dermotomy on fascial decompression in the leg. J Bone Joint Surg [Br] 1991;73:287.

Fakhouri AJ, Manoli A 2d: Acute foot compartment syndromes. J Orthop Trauma 1992;6:223.

Power RA, Greengross P: Acute lower leg compartment syndrome Br Sports Med 1991;25:218.

Roger DJ et al: Compartment pressures of the leg following intramedullary fixation of the tibia. Orthop Rev 1992; 21:1221.

Yoshioka H: Gluteal compartment syndrome: A report of 4 cases. Acta Orthop Scand 1992;63:347.

INJURIES OF THE ANKLE REGION

1. ANKLE SPRAIN

Ankle sprain is most often caused by forced inversion of the foot, as may occur in stumbling on uneven ground. Pain is usually maximal over the anterolateral aspect of the joint; greater tenderness is apt to be found in the region of the anterior talofibular and talocalcaneal ligaments. Eversion sprain is less common; maximal tenderness and swelling are usually found over the deltoid ligament.

Sprain is differentiated from major partial or complete ligamentous tears by anteroposterior, lateral, and 30-degree internal oblique (mortise view) x-ray projections; if the joint cleft between either malleolus and the talus is greater than 4 mm, major ligamentous tear is probable. Occult lesions can be demonstrated by x-ray examination under inversion or eversion stress after infiltration of the area of maximal swelling and tenderness with 5 mL of 1% lidocaine.

If swelling is marked, elevation of the extremity and avoidance of weight bearing for a few days are advisable. The ankle can be supported with Gibney strapping (Figure 43–46) or a cast for 2–3 weeks to relieve pain and swelling. Further treatment may be by warm foot baths and elastic bandages. continue treatment until muscle strength and full joint motion are recovered. Tears of major ligaments of the ankle joint are discussed below.

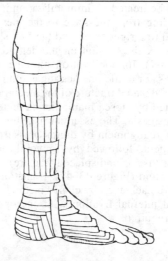

Figure 43–46. Gibney ankle strapping.

Nyska M et al: Radiological assessment of a modified anterior drawer test of the ankle Foot and Ankle 1992; 13(7):400.

Raatikainen T, Putkonen M, Puranen J: Arthrography, clinical examination, and stress radiograph in the diagnosis of acute injury to the lateral ligaments of the ankle. Am J Sports Med 1992;Jan-20:2.

2. FRACTURES & DISLOCATIONS OF THE ANKLE JOINT

Fractures and dislocations of the ankle joint may be caused by direct force, in which case they are apt to be comminuted and open; or by indirect force, which often causes typical lesions (see below).

Pain and swelling are the prominent findings. Deformity may or may not be present. X-rays of excellent technical quality must be prepared in a sufficient variety of projections to demonstrate the extent and configuration of all major fragments. A special oblique (mortise) view is required. This is taken with the foot in 20–30 degrees of internal rotation in order to demonstrate widening of the medial clear space between the talus and the medial malleolus. This confirms lateral shift of the talus, usually caused by rupture of the deltoid ligament or fracture of the medial malleolus.

Fracture of the Medial Malleolus

Fracture of the medial malleolus may occur as an isolated lesion of any part of the malleolus (including the tip) or may be associated with (1) fracture of the lateral malleolus with medial or lateral dislocation of the talus and (2) dislocation of the inferior tibiofibular joint with or without fracture of the fibula. Isolated fracture does not usually cause instability of the ankle joint.

Undisplaced isolated fracture of the medial malleolus should be treated by immobilization in a plaster boot extending from the knee to the toes with the ankle flexed to a right angle and the foot slightly inverted to relax the tension on the deltoid ligament (Figure 43–47). Immobilization must be continued for 6–8 weeks or until bone healing is sound.

Displaced isolated fracture of the medial malleolus can be treated by closed manipulation under general or local anesthesia. The essential maneuver consists of anatomic realignment by digital pressure over the distal fragment, followed by immobilization in a plaster boot (as for undisplaced fracture) until bone healing is sound (Figure 43–47). If anatomic reduction cannot be achieved by closed methods, open reduction and internal fixation with one or two bone screws are required.

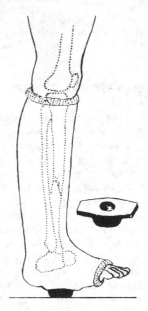

Figure 43–47. Weight-bearing plaster boot.

Fracture of the Lateral Malleolus

Fracture of the lateral malleolus may occur as an isolated lesion or may be associated with fracture of the medial malleolus, tear of the deltoid or posterior lateral malleolar ligament, or avulsion of the posterior tibial tubercle. If the medial aspect of the ankle is injured, lateral subluxation of the talus is apt to be present. The tip of the lateral malleolus may be avulsed by the calcaneofibular and anterior talofibular ligaments. Transverse or oblique fracture may occur. Oblique fractures commonly extend downward and anteriorly from the posterior and superior aspects.

Isolated undisplaced fracture of the lateral malleolus may be treated by a plaster walking boot (Figure 43–47) for 6 weeks. An elastic bandage is worn thereafter until full joint motion is recovered and the calf muscles are functioning normally. If anatomic reduction cannot be achieved by closed methods, additional injury to the medial side of the joint should be suspected and open reduction is required.

Combined Fracture of the Medial & Lateral Malleoli

The combination of external rotation and abduction is the most common mechanism producing ankle fracture. Bimalleolar fractures are often accompanied by displacement of the talus, usually in a medial or lateral direction. In conjunction with dislocation in the coronal plane, concurrent displacement may take place in the sagittal plane, either anteriorly or posteriorly, or in torsion about the longitudinal axis of the tibia.

Bimalleolar fracture may be treated by closed manipulation. Knowledge of the mechanism of injury is necessary to carry out manipulative reduction. The fracture is reduced by placing the ankle in the position reverse to that of the injuring forces—eg, an injury caused by external rotation and abduction should be reduced by internal rotation and adduction. Immobilization in a long-leg cast for 6 weeks and then a short-leg walking cast for 2–4 weeks allows complete healing in most cases.

Radiologic examination may give valuable information regarding the mechanism of injury. If the medial malleolus is fractured in the horizontal plane, the injury was caused by an avulsion mechanism with the talus being displaced laterally. If the fracture of the medial malleolus is vertical, the injury was most probably caused by the talus being driven medially. Open reduction and internal fixation are indicated if x-rays show that perfect anatomic reduction has not been achieved by closed manipulation or if early joint motion is desired. The talus must be positioned anatomically under the tibial plafond, since even slight shift may cause degenerative changes from joint incongruity. The medial malleolus is fixed with a bone screw or Kirschner wires. The lateral malleolus may be fixed with a single screw across the fracture site or with a plate and multiple screws.

Damage to the syndesmotic ligaments between the distal tibia and fibula is demonstrated by distal tibiofibular diastasis. Anatomic reduction must be maintained by a transverse screw placed from the distal fibula into the tibia. It is generally suggested that rigid tibiofibular fixation be removed before unprotected weight bearing is permitted. If the screw is removed before 3 months after injury, tibiofibular diastasis may occasionally recur.

Fracture of the Distal Tibia

Fracture of the distal tibia is usually associated with other lesions.

A. Fracture of the Posterior Margin: Fracture of the posterior margin may involve part or all of the entire posterior half and is apt to be accompanied by fracture of either malleolus and posterior dislocation of the talus. It must be differentiated from fracture of the posterior tibial tubercle, which is usually caused by avulsion with the attached posterior lateral malleolar ligament.

Anatomic reduction by closed manipulation or open reduction is required if the fracture involves more than 25% of the articular surface. The extremity is immobilized in a plaster cast extending from the inguinal region to the toe.

Frequent x-ray examination is necessary to make certain that redisplacement does not occur. The plaster should be changed as soon as loosening becomes apparent. Immobilization must be maintained for 8–12 weeks. Weight bearing must not be resumed until bone healing is sound, usually in about 12 weeks.

B. Fracture of the Anterior Margin: Fracture of the anterior articular margin of the tibia (rare) is likely to be caused by forced dorsiflexion of the foot. If displacement is marked and the talus is dislocated, tears of the collateral ligaments or fractures of the malleoli are likely to be present.

If closed reduction is unsuccessful, open reduction and internal fixation with bone screws or a plate and screws should be done. If comminution is present, the extremity should be immobilized for 12 weeks. Weight bearing should not be permitted until bone healing is sound.

C. Comminuted Fractures: Extensive comminution of the distal tibia ("compression type" fracture [Figure 43–48]) presents a difficult problem of management. The congruity of articular surfaces cannot be restored by closed manipulation, and satisfactory anatomic restoration may be difficult and sometimes impossible even by open reduction. If the fracture is amenable to internal fixation, an attempt should be made to restore the congruity of the articular surface. Extensively comminuted and widely displaced fractures may be best treated by closed manipulation and skeletal traction (Figure 43–45). After traction has been applied and impaction of fragments has been disrupted, displacement in the transverse plane is corrected by manual molding with compression. A tubular plaster cast is applied from the inguinal region to the toes with the knee in 10–15 degrees of flexion and the foot in neutral position. With the extremity immobilized in plaster, continuous skeletal traction can be maintained for 8–12 weeks or until stabilization by early bone healing occurs. An alternative is distraction with pins in the calcaneus and shaft of the tibia. The pins are attached to an external fixator or incorporated in plaster to maintain length.

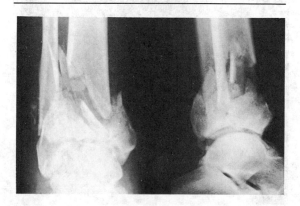

Figure 43–48. Comminuted fracture of the distal tibia and fibula with disruption of the ankle joint. The position achieved by skeletal traction on the calcaneus and closed manipulation is unsatisfactory. Early onset of secondary osteoarthritis is likely.

Healing is likely to be slow. If the articular surfaces of the ankle joint have not been properly realigned, disabling posttraumatic arthritis is apt to occur early. Early arthrodesis may be indicated to shorten the period of disability.

Bonar SK, Marsh JL: Unilateral external fixation for severe pilon fractures. Foot Ankle 1993;14:57.

Etter C, Ganz R: Long-term results of tibial plafond fractures treated with open reduction and internal fixation. Arch Orthop Trauma Surg 1991;110:277.

McFerran MA et al: Complications encountered in the treatment of pilon fractures. J Orthop Trauma 1992;6:195.

Murphy CP, D'Ambrosia R, Dabezies EJ: The small pin circular fixator for distal tibial pilon fractures with soft tissue compromise. Orthopedics 1991;14:283.

Dislocation of the Ankle Joint (Figure 43–49)

A. Complete Dislocation: The talus cannot be completely dislocated from the ankle joint unless all ligaments are torn. This lesion is rare.

B. Incomplete Dislocation: Major ligamentous injuries in the region of the ankle joint are usually associated with fracture.

1. Tear of the deltoid ligament–Complete tear of the talotibial portion of the deltoid ligament can permit interposition of the posterior tibial tendon between the medial malleolus and the talus. Associated injury is usually present, especially fracture of the lateral malleolus with lateral dislocation of the talus.

Pain, tenderness, swelling, and ecchymosis in the region of the medial malleolus without fracture suggest partial or complete tear of the deltoid ligament. If fracture of the lateral malleolus or dislocation of the distal tibiofibular joint is present, the cleft between the malleolus and talus is likely to be widened.

If significant widening is not apparent, x-ray examination under stress is necessary.

Interposition of the deltoid ligament between the talus and the medial malleolus often cannot be corrected by closed manipulation. If widening persists after closed manipulation, surgical exploration is indicated so that the ligament can be removed and repaired by suture.

Associated fracture of the fibula can be treated by fixation with a plate and screws to ensure maintenance of anatomic reduction.

2. Tear of the talofibular ligament–Isolated tear of the anterior talofibular ligament is caused by forced inversion of the foot. X-ray examination under stress may be necessary, using local or general anesthesia. Both feet are forcibly inverted and internally rotated about 20 degrees while an anteroposterior film is exposed. If the tear is complete, the talus will be seen to be axially displaced from the tibial articular surface (talar tilt). Up to 25 degrees of talar tilt has been reported in normal ankles without a history of injury.

Rupture of the anterior talofibular ligaments may be associated with tear of the calcaneofibular ligament. Tear of both ligaments may be associated with fracture of the medial malleolus and medial dislocation of the talus.

Instability of the ankle joint, characterized by a history of recurrent sprains, may result from unrecognized tears of the anterior talofibular ligament.

Recent isolated tear of the anterior talofibular ligament or combined tear of the calcaneofibular ligament should be treated by immobilization for 4 weeks in a plaster boot. Associated fracture of the medial malleolus creates an unstable mechanism. Unless anatomic reduction can be achieved and maintained by closed methods, open reduction of the malleolar fragment is indicated, followed by internal fixation of the fracture and repair of the ligamentous injury.

Eventov I et al: An evaluation of surgical and conservative treatment of fractures of the ankle in 200 patients. J Trauma 1978;18:271.

Toohey JS, Worsing RA: A long-term follow-up study of tibiotalar dislocations without associated fractures. Clin Orthop 1989;(Feb)239:207.

INJURIES OF THE FOOT

1. FRACTURE & DISLOCATION OF THE TALUS

Dislocation of the Subtalar & Talonavicular Joints

Dislocation of the subtalar and talonavicular joints without fracture occasionally occurs. Displacement of the foot can be by either inversion or eversion. Re-

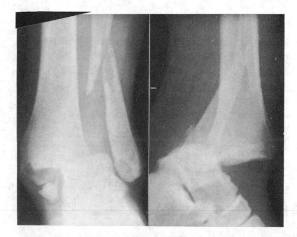

Figure 43–49. Closed fracture of the lower fibular shaft and medial malleolus with dislocation of the inferior tibiofibular and ankle joints. Open reduction and internal fixation are necessary for optimal treatment.

duction by closed manipulation is usually not difficult. Incarceration of the posterior tibial tendon in the talonavicular joint may prevent reduction by closed manipulation. After reduction, the extremity should be immobilized in a plaster boot for 4 weeks.

Fracture of the Talus
(Figure 43–50)

Major fracture of the talus commonly occurs either through the body or through the neck; the uncommon fracture of the head involves essentially a portion of the neck with extension into the head. Indirect injury is usually the cause of closed fracture as well as most open fractures; severe comminution is not commonly present. Compression fracture or infraction of the tibial articular surface may be caused by the initial injury or may occur later in association with complicating avascular necrosis. The proximal or distal fragments may be dislocated.

A. Fracture of the Neck: Forced dorsiflexion of the foot may cause this injury. Undisplaced fracture of the neck can be treated adequately by a non-weight-bearing plaster boot for 8–12 weeks. Dislocation of the body or the distal neck fragment with the foot may complicate this injury. Fracture of the neck with anterior and frequently medial dislocation of the distal fragment and foot can usually be reduced by closed manipulation. Subsequent treatment is the same as that of undisplaced fracture.

Dislocation of the proximal body fragment may occur separately or may be associated with dislocation of the distal fragment. If dislocation of the body fragment is complete, reduction by closed manipulation is not successful, open reduction should be done as soon as possible to prevent or to minimize the extent of the avascular necrosis. The blood supply to the talus enters in the neck area and is likely to be disrupted with dislocation; therefore bone healing is likely to be retarded, and some degree of avascular necrosis is possible.

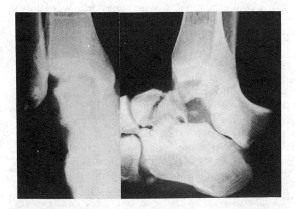

Figure 43–50. Comminuted fracture of the talus with dislocation of the body from the ankle and subtalar joints. Closed reduction is impossible.

Complete dislocation of the neck fragment from the talonavicular and subtalar joints is rare, but if it does happen, avascular necrosis of the fragment may occur even though anatomic reduction is promptly accomplished. If reduction by closed manipulation is not possible, immediate open operation with reduction of the fragment is advisable, since delay may cause necrosis of overlying soft tissues.

B. Fracture of the Body: Closed uncomminuted fracture of the body of the talus with minimal displacement of fragments is not likely to cause disability if immobilization is continued until bone continuity is restored. If significant displacement occurs, the proximal fragment is apt to be dislocated from the subtalar and ankle joints. Reduction by closed manipulation is frequently difficult but is best achieved by traction and forced plantar flexion of the foot. Immobilization in a plaster boot with the foot in plantar flexion for about 8 weeks should be followed by further casting with the foot at a right angle until the fracture cleft has been obliterated by new bone formation as evidenced by x-ray examination. Even though prompt adequate reduction is obtained by either closed manipulation or open operation, extensive displacement of the proximal body fragments may be followed by avascular necrosis. If reduction is not anatomic, delayed healing of the fracture may follow, and posttraumatic arthritis is a likely sequela. If this occurs, arthrodesis of the ankle and subtalar joints may be necessary to relieve painful symptoms.

C. Compression Fracture: Compression fracture or infraction of the dome of the talus from the initial injury (which is likely to have been violent) cannot be reduced. When this lesion occurs as a separate entity or in combination with other fractures of the body, prolonged protection from weight bearing is the major means of preventing the further collapse that is so likely to occur in the area of healing.

Johnson EE et al: Ilizarov ankle arthrodesis. Clin Orthop 1992;Jul(280):160.

Michelson JD et al: Examination of the pathologic anatomy of ankle fractures. J Trauma 1992;32:65.

Raasch WG, Larkin JJ, Draganich LF: Assessment of the posterior malleolus as a restraint to posterior subluxation of the ankle. J Bone Joint Surg [Am] 1992;74:1201.

Swanson TV, Bray TJ, Holmes GB Jr: Fractures of the talar neck: A mechanical study of fixation. J Bone Joint Surg [Am] 1992;3;74:544.

2. FRACTURE OF THE CALCANEUS

Fracture of the calcaneus is commonly caused by direct trauma. Since this fracture is likely to occur as a result of a fall from a height, fracture of the spine at the thoracolumbar junction may also be present. Comminution and impaction are general characteristics. Minor infractions or impactions and fissure fractures are easy to miss on clinical examination, and x-rays must be prepared in multiple projections to demonstrate adequately some fracture clefts.

Various classifications have been advocated. Fractures that are generally comminuted and disrupt the subtalar and calcaneocuboid articulations should be distinguished from those that do not; this differentiation has important implications for treatment and prognosis.

Fracture of the Calcaneal Tuberosity

Isolated fracture of the tuberosity is not common. It may occur in a horizontal or vertical direction.

A. Horizontal Fracture: Horizontal fracture may be limited to the superior portion of the region of the former apophysis and represents an avulsion by the Achilles tendon. Where the superior minor fragment is widely displaced proximally with the tendon, open reduction and fixation with a stout wire suture may be necessary to obtain the most satisfactory functional result.

Further extension of the fracture cleft toward the subtalar joint in the substance of the tuberosity creates the "beak" fracture. The minor fragment may be displaced proximally by the action of the triceps surae. If displacement is significant, reduction can be achieved by skeletal traction applied to the proximal fragment with the foot in plantar flexion. Immobilization is obtained by incorporation of the traction pin or wire in a full extremity plaster with the knee flexed 30 degrees and the foot in plantar flexion. If adequate reduction cannot be accomplished in this way, open reduction is advised.

B. Vertical Fracture: Vertical fracture occurs near the sagittal plane somewhat medially through the tuberosity. Because the minor medial fragment normally is not widely displaced, plaster immobilization is not required but will decrease pain. Comfort can be enhanced by limitation of weight bearing with the aid of crutches.

Fracture of the Sustentaculum

Isolated fracture of the sustentaculum tali is a rare lesion that may be caused by forced eversion of the foot. Where displacement of the larger body fragment occurs, it is lateral. Incarceration of the tendon of the flexor hallucis longus in the fracture cleft has been reported. Generally, this fracture occurs in association with comminution of the body.

Fracture of the Anterior Process of the Calcaneus

Fracture of the anterior process is caused by forced inversion of the foot. It must be differentiated from midtarsal and ankle joint sprains. The firmly attached bifurcate ligament (calcaneonavicular and calcaneocuboid components) avulses a bit of bone. Maximal tenderness and slight swelling occur midway between the tip of the lateral malleolus and the base of

the fifth metatarsal. The lateral x-ray view projected obliquely demonstrates the fracture cleft. The treatment is by a non-weight-bearing plaster boot with the foot in neutral position for 4 weeks.

Fracture of the Body of the Calcaneus

Fracture of the body may occur posterior to the articular surfaces, in general vertical but somewhat oblique plane, without disruption of the subtalar joint. Most severe fractures of the calcaneal body are comminuted and extend into the subtalar and frequently the calcaneocuboid joints. Fissure fractures without significant displacement cause minor disability and can be treated simply by protection from weight bearing, either by crutches alone or in combination with a plaster boot until bone healing is sufficiently sound to justify graded increments of loading.

A. Nonarticular Fracture: Where fracture of the body with comminution occurs posterior to the articular surface, the direction of significant displacement of the fragments attached to the tuberosity is proximal, causing diminution of the subtalar joint angle. Since the subtalar joint is not disrupted, symptomatic posttraumatic degenerative arthritis is not an important sequela even though some joint stiffness persists permanently. Marked displacement should be corrected by skeletal traction applied to the main posterior fragment to obtain an optimal cosmetic result. Success of reduction can be judged by the adequacy of restoration of the subtalar joint angle.

B. Articular Fracture: Articular fractures are of three general types:

1. Noncomminuted–Fracture of the body without comminution may involve the posterior articular facet. Where displacement of the posterior fragment of the tuberosity occurs, the direction is lateral. Fractures of this type with more than minimal displacement should be treated by the method advocated for nonarticular fracture of the body.

2. With minor comminution–In fractures with minor comminution, the main cleft occurs vertically, in a somewhat oblique lateral deviation from the sagittal plane. From emergence on the medial surface posterior to the sustentaculum it is directed forward and rather obliquely laterally through the posterior articular facet. The sustentaculum and the medial portion of the posterior articular facet remain undisplaced with relation to the talus. The body below the remaining lateral portion of the posterior articular facet, together with the tuberosity, is impacted into the lateral portion of the posterior articular facet.

3. With extensive comminution–Fracture with extensive comminution extending into the subtalar joint may involve the calcaneocuboid joint as well as the tuberosity. The multiple fracture clefts involve the entire posterior articular surface, and the facet is impacted into the substance of the underlying body. There are many variants; the clefts may extend across the calcaneal groove into the medial and anterior articular surfaces, and detachment of the peroneal tubercle may be a feature. This serious injury may cause disability in spite of the best treatment, since the bursting nature of the injury may defy anatomic restoration.

Some surgeons advise nonintervention. Displacement of fragments is disregarded. Initially, a compression dressing and splint are applied, and the extremity is elevated for a week or so. After 3–5 days, as the intense pain begins to subside, active exercises should be started, but weight bearing is avoided until early bone healing has taken place. In spite of residual deformity of the heel, varying degrees of weakness of the calf, and discomfort in the region of the subtalar joint (which may be intensified by weight bearing), acceptable functional results can be obtained, especially among vigorous young persons who are willing to put up with the discomforts involved. Pain may persist for 6–12 months.

Other surgeons, notably Hermann and Bohler, advocate early closed manipulation, which can partially restore the external anatomic configuration of the heel region. Open reduction and internal fixation may improve the alignment of the subtalar joint, decreasing the chance of early arthritis.

Persistent and disabling painful symptoms originating in the deranged subtalar joint may require arthrodesis for adequate relief. Concomitant involvement of the calcaneocuboid joint is an indication for the more extensive triple arthrodesis.

Burdeaux BD Jr: The medical approach for calcaneal fractures. Clin Orthop 1993;May(290):96.

Stephenson JR: Surgical treatment of displaced intraarticular fractures of the calcaneus: A combined lateral and medial approach. Clin Orthop 1993;May(290):68.

3. FRACTURE OF THE NAVICULAR

Minor avulsion fractures of the tarsal navicular may occur as a feature of severe midtarsal sprain and require neither reduction nor elaborate treatment. Avulsion fracture of the tuberosity near the insertion of the posterior tibialis muscle is uncommon and must be differentiated from a persistent, ununited apophysis (accessory scaphoid) and from the supernumerary sesamoid bone, or the os tibiale externum.

Major fracture occurs either through the middle in a horizontal or, more rarely, in a vertical plane or is characterized by impaction of its substance. Only noncomminuted fractures with displacement of the dorsal fragment can be reduced. Closed manipulation by strong traction on the forefoot and simultaneous digital pressure over the displaced fragment can restore it to its normal position. If a tendency to redisplacement is apparent, this can be counteracted by temporary fixation with a percutaneously inserted Kirschner wire. Non-weight-bearing immobilization in a plaster cast is required for a minimum of 6 weeks. Comminuted and impacted fractures cannot be anatomically reduced. Some authorities offer a pessimistic prognosis for comminuted or impacted fractures. It is their contention that even though partial reduction has been achieved, posttraumatic arthritis supervenes, and that arthrodesis of the talonavicular and cuneonavicular joints will be ultimately necessary to relieve painful symptoms.

Khan KM et al: Outcome of conservative and surgical management of navicular stress fracture in athletes: Eighty-six cases proven with computerized tomography. Am J Sports Med 1992;20:657.

4. FRACTURE OF THE CUNEIFORM & CUBOID BONES

Because of their relatively protected position in the mid tarsus, isolated fracture of the cuboid and cuneiform bones is rarely encountered. Minor avulsion fractures occur as a component of severe midtarsal sprains. Extensive fracture usually occurs in association with other injuries of the foot and often is caused by severe crushing. Simple classification is impractical because of the complex character and the multiple combination of the whole injury.

Heckman JD, Champine MJ: New techniques in the management of foot trauma. Clin Orthop 1989;(Mar)240:105.

5. MIDTARSAL DISLOCATIONS

Midtarsal dislocation through the cuneonavicular and calcaneocuboid joints or more proximally through the talocalcaneonavicular and calcaneocuboid joints may occur as a result of twisting injury to the forefoot. Fractures of varying extent of adjacent bones are frequent complications. When treatment is given soon after the accident, closed reduction by traction on the forefoot and manipulation is generally effective. If reduction is unstable and displacement tends to recur upon release of traction, stabilization for 4 weeks by percutaneously inserted Kirschner wires is recommended.

Tountas AA: Occult fracture-subluxation of the midtarsal joint. Clin Orthop 1989;Jun(243):195.

6. FRACTURES & DISLOCATIONS OF THE METATARSALS

Fractures of the metatarsals (Figure 43–51) and tarsometatarsal dislocations are likely to be caused by direct crushing or indirect twisting injury to the fore-

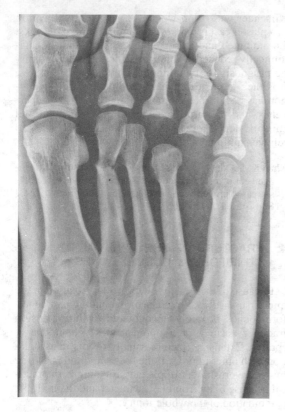

Figure 43–51. Closed fracture of the shaft of the second metatarsal and dislocations of the third and fourth metatarsophalangeal joints.

foot. Besides osseous and articular injury, complicating soft tissue lesions are often present. With severe trauma, circulation may be compromised from injury to the dorsalis pedis artery, which passes between the first and second metatarsal.

Tarsometatarsal Dislocations

Possibly because of strong ligamentous support and relative size, dislocation of the first metatarsal at its base occurs less frequently than similar involvement of the lesser bones. If dislocation occurs, fracture of the first cuneiform is likely to be present also. More often, however, tarsometatarsal dislocation involves the lesser metatarsals, and associated fractures are to be expected. Dislocation is more commonly caused by direct injury but may be the result of stress applied indirectly through the forefoot. The direction of displacement is ordinarily dorsal, lateral, or a combination of both. Direct injuries are frequently complicated by soft tissue damage, open wounds, and vascular impairment.

Attempted closed reduction should not be deferred. Skeletal traction applied to the involved bone by a Kirschner wire or a stout towel clamp can be a valuable aid to manipulation. Even though persistent dis-

location may not cause significant disability, the resulting deformity can make shoe fitting difficult and the cosmetic effect undesirable. Open reduction with Kirschner wire stabilization is a preferred alternative to unsuccessful closed treatment. When effective treatment has been deferred 3 weeks or longer, early healing will prevent satisfactory reduction of persisting displacement by closed techniques. Under such circumstances, it is better to defer open reduction and direct treatment toward recovery of function. Extensive operative procedures and continued immobilization can increase joint stiffness. Reconstructive operations can be planned more suitably after residual disability becomes established.

Complications of this injury include local circulatory disturbance called Sudeck's atrophy and painful degenerative arthritis.

Faciszewski T, Burks RT, Manaster BJ: Subtle injuries of the Lisfranc joint [see comments]. J Bone Joint Surg [Am] 1990;72:1519.
Leenen LP, van der Werken C: Fracture-dislocations of the tarsometatarsal joint, a combined anatomical and computed tomographic study. Injury 1992;23:51.
Mehara AK, Bhan S: Isolated fracture-dislocations of the first tarsometatarsal joint. J Trauma 1992;33:683.

Fracture of the Metatarsal Shafts

Undisplaced fractures of the metatarsal shafts cause no permanent disability unless failure of bone healing is encountered. Displacement is rarely significant where fracture of the middle metatarsals is oblique and the first and fifth are uninjured, since they act as splints. Even fissure fractures should be treated by a stiff-soled shoe (with partial weight bearing) or, if pain is marked, by a plaster walking boot.

Great care should be taken in displaced fractures to correct angulation in the longitudinal axis of the shaft. Persistent convex dorsal angulation causes prominence of the head of the involved metatarsal on the plantar aspect, with the implication of concentrated local pressure and production of painful skin callosities. Deformity of the shaft of the first metatarsal due to convex plantar angulation can transfer the stress of weight bearing to the region of the head of the third metatarsal. After correction of angular displacement, the plaster cast should be molded well to the plantar aspect of the foot to minimize recurrence of deformity and to support the longitudinal and transverse arches.

If reduction is not reasonably accurate, fractures through the shafts near the heads (the "neck") may cause great discomfort from concentrated pressure beneath the head on the plantar surface and reactive skin callus formation. Every effort should be made to correct convex dorsal angulation by disruption of impaction and appropriate manipulation. Closed reduction is best achieved by use of the Chinese fingertrap applied to the toes of the involved metatarsals. The efficacy of closed treatment should be determined without delay; if success has not been achieved with closed treatment, open operation with Kirschner wire fixation should be performed.

Fatigue Fracture of the Metatarsal Shafts

Fatigue fracture of the shafts of the metatarsals has been given various names (eg, march, stress, and insufficiency fracture). Its protean clinical manifestations cause difficulty in precise recognition, even to the point of confusion with osteogenic sarcoma. Commonly, it occurs in active young adults, such as military recruits, who are unaccustomed to vigorous and excessive walking. A history of a single significant injury is lacking. Incipient pain of varying intensity in the forefoot that is accentuated by walking, swelling, and localized tenderness of the involved metatarsal are cardinal manifestations. Depending upon the stage of progress, x-rays may not demonstrate the fracture cleft, and extracortical callus formation may ultimately be the only clue. More striking findings may vary from an incomplete fissure to an evident transverse cleft. Persistent unprotected weight bearing may cause arrest of bone healing and even displacement of the distal fragment. The second and third metatarsals are most frequently involved near the junction of the middle and distal thirds. The lesion can occur more proximally and in other lesser metatarsals. Since weight bearing is likely to prolong and aggravate symptoms, treatment is by protection in either a plaster walking boot or a heavy shoe with the sole reinforced by a steel strut. Weight bearing should be restricted until painful symptoms subside and restoration of bone continuity has been demonstrated by x-ray examination, usually within 3–4 weeks.

Fracture of the Tuberosity of the Fifth Metatarsal

Forced adduction of the forefoot may cause avulsion fracture of the tuberosity of the fifth metatarsal, and where supporting soft tissues have been torn, activity of the peroneus brevis muscle may increase displacement of the avulsed proximal fragment. If displacement of the minor fragment is minimal, adhesive strapping or a stiff-soled shoe is adequate treatment. If displacement is significant, treatment should be by a walking boot until bone healing occurs. Rarely does healing fail to occur. Fracture should be differentiated from a separate ossific center of the tuberosity in adolescence and the supernumerary os vesalianum pedis in adulthood.

Sammarco GJ: The Jones fracture. Instr Course Lect 1993; 42:201.

7. FRACTURES & DISLOCATIONS OF THE PHALANGES OF THE TOES

Fractures of the phalanges of the toes are caused most commonly by direct violence such as crushing or stubbing. Spiral or oblique fractures of the shafts of the proximal phalanges of the lesser toes may occur as a result of indirect twisting injury.

Comminuted fracture of the proximal phalanx of the great toe, alone or in combination with fracture of the distal phalanx, is the most disabling injury. Since wide displacement of fragments is not likely, correction of angulation and support by an adhesive dressing and splint usually suffices. A weight-bearing plaster boot may be useful for relief of symptoms arising from associated soft tissue injury. Spiral or oblique fracture of the proximal phalanges of the lesser toes can be treated adequately by binding the involved toe to the adjacent uninjured member. Comminuted fracture of the distal phalanx is treated as a soft tissue injury.

Traumatic dislocation of the metatarsophalangeal joints and the uncommon dislocation of the proximal interphalangeal joint usually can be reduced by closed manipulation. These dislocations are rarely isolated and usually occur in combination with other injuries to the forefoot.

Daly PJ, Johnson KA: Treatment of painful subluxation or dislocation at the second and third metatarsophalangeal joints by partial proximal phalanx excision and subtotal webbing. Clin Orthop 1992;May(278):164.

8. FRACTURE OF THE SESAMOIDS OF THE GREAT TOE

Fracture of the sesamoid bones of the great toe is rare, but it may occur as a result of crushing injury. It must be differentiated from a bipartite sesamoid. Undisplaced fracture requires no treatment other than a foot support or a metatarsal bar. Displaced fracture may require immobilization in a walking plaster boot, with the toe strapped in flexion. Persistent delay of bone healing may cause disabling pain arising from arthritis of the articulation between the sesamoid and the head of the first metatarsal. If a foot support and metatarsal bar do not provide adequate relief, excision of the sesamoid may be necessary.

FRACTURES THAT FAIL TO UNITE

Prolonged delay in fracture healing is most common in long bone fractures associated with severe soft tissue damage or infection. However, routine closed fractures with minimal displacement occasionally fail to unite for reasons that remain obscure.

The tibia is the long bone most frequently affected by failure or delay of healing. Nonunion of the carpal scaphoid and the femoral neck is not uncommon and is thought to be associated with damage to blood supply of the fractured area at the time of injury.

If a fracture fails to unite in 1½ times the usual healing time for that bone, it can be considered a delayed union, and some means of improving healing should be sought. The standard method has been the use of cancellous bone graft obtained from the iliac crest and placed subperiosteally around the nonunion site. The stable fibrous union of the unhealed bone does not have to be removed for successful healing to occur. If there is instability of the fibrous union or significant malalignment of the fracture, compression plating for rigid fixation, with or without bone graft, has proved successful. After bone grafting, the extremity must again be immobilized in a cast for approximately 3 months to allow the bone graft to mature unless internal fixation provides rigid support.

A newer method of treatment of nonunion utilizes electrical current. Three different methods have been developed: noninvasive, semi-invasive, and totally invasive. In the noninvasive technique, electromagnetic coils are placed at a measured distance on opposite sides of the cast at the fracture site. The coils are attached to a power source for 10–12 hours a day for 3 months. Weight bearing is not allowed on the involved extremity. Immobilization with weight bearing is continued for an additional 3 months after treatment with the coils. The semi-invasive technique uses Kirschner wire electrodes placed percutaneously into the fracture site under sterile conditions in the operating room. The electrodes are attached to a small portable battery incorporated into the cast. The electrodes are left in place for 3 months, after which time immobilization in a weight-bearing plaster cast is continued for an additional 3 months. In the totally invasive technique, both the electrode and the battery are implanted in the involved extremity. Postoperative care is similar to that given following noninvasive and semi-invasive management.

The success rates of bone grafting and all forms of electrical treatment are reported to approach 80%. If the first attempt is unsuccessful, repeat of any of the techniques has a significant chance of success.

Infection at the nonunion site is a contraindication to the use of the semi-invasive or totally invasive types of electrical treatment. Electromagnetic coils, external fixators for rigid immobilization, and bone grafting (from posteriorly in anteriorly infected tibial non-unions) have all been useful in treating infected nonunions.

Cameron HU et al: Repair of nonunion of tibial osteotomy. Clin Orthop 1993;Feb(287):167.

Mody BS et al: Nonunion of fractures of the scaphoid tuberosity. J Bone Joint Surg [Br] 1993;75:423.

Shahcheraghi GH, Doroodchi HR Supracondylar fracture of the femur: closed or open reduction? J Trauma 1993;3; 34:499.

Shen WJ, Shen YS: Fibular nonunion after fixation of the tibia in lower leg fractures. Clin Orthop 1993;Feb(287): 231.

Siebenrock KA, Schillig B, Jakob RP: Treatment of complex tibial shaft fractures: Arguments for early secondary intramedullary nailing. Clin Orthop 1993;May(290):269.

Zwipp H et al: Osteosynthesis of displaced intraarticular fractures of the calcaneus: Results in 123 cases. Clin Orthop 1993;May(290):76.

PEDIATRIC ORTHOPEDICS

CHILDREN'S FRACTURES & DISLOCATIONS

Children are not "small adults," and their skeletal injuries are different from those of adults in several significant ways. The most striking characteristic of immature bone is its potential for growth. Longitudinal growth occurs at the physis, or cartilaginous growth plate. Bones increase in diameter by appositional growth from the periosteum. Injuries can affect normal growth, usually by impeding it. However, growth may be accelerated, especially by femoral shaft fractures in mid childhood. Growth may help correct deformity of some *but not all* children's fractures. Such correction is greatest in young children with much remaining growth. Growth tends to correct angulation in the plane of motion of an adjacent joint but improves varus or valgus deformities only in the very young and does not correct rotational malalignment. Children's bones heal rapidly, and nonunion is exceedingly rare. A child's periosteum is thick and strong. It surrounds a long bone like a sleeve and must be torn to permit displacement of a fracture. Usually the displaced fracture end protrudes through a rent in the periosteum, but the remaining intact portion of the sleeve bridges the fracture area to facilitate reduction and maintenance of alignment.

Any injury in a young child, especially one under 3 years of age, must be considered a sign of possible battered child syndrome (see Chapter 46). State law in all jurisdictions requires that suspected cases be reported to local authorities. Good patient care requires thorough pediatric and social service assessments.

Closed treatment is usually sufficient for children's fractures. Manipulative reduction under general anesthesia may be required for significant displacement. Open fractures, epiphyseal fractures with articular surface displacement, and the very rare fracture that cannot be reduced satisfactorily by closed manipulation are the generally accepted indications for open treatment of fractures in children.

Although children's fractures do heal rapidly and pain soon ceases to interfere with function, it is important to recognize that callus bridging a fracture may deform plastically and angulate if the fracture is loaded too early. Immobilization rarely causes joint stiffness in children, so that casts can and should be left on until union is secure.

Because bone in children is mechanically different from that in adults, there are several unique fracture types in this age group. Immature bone is more porous and fails in compression as well as in tension. The result is the so-called **buckle** or **torus fracture** that occurs near the metaphysis. The distal forearm provides a typical example. This stable injury should be protected in plaster for 3 weeks to control symptoms and prevent further trauma to the weakened bone.

Immature bone is less brittle than that of adults, and children's bones may therefore bend significantly rather than fracture. Two potential injury patterns result. The first is **traumatic bowing,** in which the shaft of a bone is bent. Bowing may produce significant deformity; eg, bowing of the ulna may prevent reduction of an associated displaced fracture of the radius. Depending upon the age of the child, some correction of the deformity can occur, but osteotomy may be required for severe traumatic bowing.

Greenstick fracture, the second fracture type related to the plasticity of children's bones, incompletely disrupts a long bone, so that it fails partially on the tension side but maintains continuity of a portion of the opposite cortex. The periosteum also remains intact on the concave side. Depending upon how much it has been bent, the intact cortex promotes persisting angulation. This can be prevented by briskly "overcorrecting" the deformity, thereby completing the fracture. The remaining periosteum prevents actual reversal of the deformity and facilitates maintenance of reduction. If angulation of a greenstick fracture exceeds 15 degrees, reduction should be carried out as described. Following reduction—or without it if angulation is minimal—the fracture is immobilized in a long plaster cast with three-point molding (Figure 43–52) to keep tension on the intact periosteal hinge during healing.

Colton CL: Pediatric trauma: The last 30 years. Clin Orthop 1989;No. 247:22.
Ogden JA: *Skeletal Injury in the Child.* Lea & Febiger, 1982.
Rang M: *Children's Fractures,* 2nd ed. Lippincott, 1982.
Rockwood CA Jr, Wilkins KE, King RE: *Fractures in Children,* Lippincott, 1984.

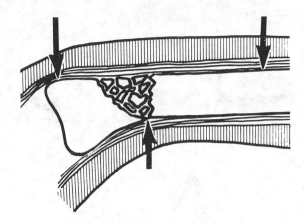

Figure 43–52. Three-point molding of distal radius fracture.

1. GROWTH PLATE FRACTURES (Epiphyseal Fractures, Epiphyseal Separations)

About 15% of children's fractures involve a growth plate—most commonly the distal radius, distal tibia or fibula (or both), and distal humerus.

Classification

Classification of physeal injuries helps to distinguish patterns that may disturb growth and also provides some guidance for treatment. However, it should be recognized that even "benign" injuries of the distal femoral and tibial growth plates can have clinically significant consequences. Naturally, injuries to nearly mature physes have little effect on growth no matter what their type or location.

Physeal injuries are classified according to Salter and Harris (Figure 43–53). A given injury may have different degrees of severity. For example, an apparent type II fracture may have sustained sufficient compression adjacent to the metaphyseal fragment so that a localized area of type V injury is present, with attendant growth abnormality.

A. Type I: Type I injuries have fracture lines that follow the growth plate, separating epiphysis from metaphysis. Unless the periosteum is torn, displacement cannot occur. Without displacement, radiographs appear normal, and only tenderness localized over the physis instead of an adjacent collateral ligament confirms that a growth plate injury has occurred. Healing is rapid, usually within 2–3 weeks. Complications are rare.

B. Type II: In type II injuries, the fracture line separates epiphysis from metaphysis much as in type I injuries but also enters the metaphysis, so that a flake of metaphyseal bone is carried with the epiphysis. This finding is known as the Thurston-Holland sign and is diagnostic of a growth plate injury. Type

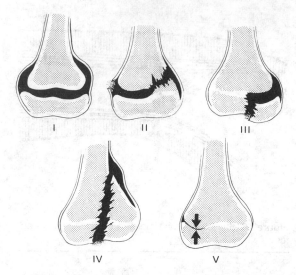

Figure 43–53. Classification of growth plate fractures according to Salter and Harris. Displacement may be more or less apparent and is the only obvious indicator of disruption of the radiolucent cartilaginous growth plate. Note the metaphyseal flake attached to the epiphysis in type II fractures and the articular surface involvement in types III and IV fractures. Radiographs of type V injuries may appear normal, but microscopic crushing of the physis has damaged its ability to grow.

II injuries are the commonest physeal fractures. Gentle closed reduction should achieve satisfactory alignment. Healing is rapid, and growth is rarely disturbed. Type II injuries of the distal ends of femur and tibia may result in impaired growth that should be watched for.

C. Type III: Type III physeal injuries are quite uncommon separations of a portion of the epiphysis along the physis, with the fracture line then passing through the epiphysis to the articular surface. This generally occurs when the growth plate is partially fused. Although growth disturbances are therefore rare, displacement of these injuries disturbs the joint surface and therefore may merit open reduction.

D. Type IV: Type IV fractures potentially interfere with normal growth. The fracture line crosses the physis, separating a peripheral fragment of bone that includes portions of epiphysis, physis, and metaphysis. Because it involves the articular surface, it may compromise normal joint mobility and longevity. Anatomic reduction, maintained until healing, is essential to minimize the after-effects of type IV growth plate fractures. If they are displaced, open reduction and internal fixation are advisable. Very gentle technique is essential, with avoidance of unnecessary periosteal elevation. Fixation is best obtained with fine smooth Kirschner wires that do not cross the physis or do so temporarily through its most central portion, since screw threads and even periph-

ally placed smooth wires can interfere with physeal growth. Unless anatomic reduction is obtained, growth disturbance, nonunion, and joint incongruity are common complications. Even with perfect reduction, growth may be affected, and the prognosis is guarded. The commonest example of type IV injury is fracture of the lateral humeral condyle. If anatomic alignment is not maintained, the fractured lateral condyle fails to unite and makes no further contribution to elongation of the distal humerus. With relative overgrowth of the medial condyle, a progressive cubitus valgus deformity develops. As it becomes stretched around the medial epicondyle, the ulnar nerve develops a "tardy" palsy.

E. Type V: Type V growth plate injuries are due to severe axial loading. Some or all of the physis is so severely compressed that growth potential is destroyed. Since initial radiographs may appear normal, the history of a significant fall with swelling and tenderness over the physis should suggest the possibility of such an injury. Subsequent follow-up radiographs confirm it by demonstrating failure to grow, with premature closure of the physis, or progressive angular deformity from tethering of one side of the growth plate. The outlook for these rare injuries is poor. Progressive angulation can be stopped—if a third or less of the physis is involved—by resecting the bridging bone and filling the defect with autogenous fat or a Silastic spacer. This should allow normal growth to resume. An alternative, which stops growth, is to obliterate any remaining physeal plate. Osteotomy may be required to correct significant angulation. Any resulting leg length inequality may require treatment.

Imaging Studies

Radiographs are essential but may be difficult to interpret. In addition to the usual anteroposterior and lateral views, oblique projections may be helpful to show displacement or a small Thurston-Holland fragment of metaphysis. Localized soft tissue swelling and signs of hemarthrosis should be heeded. Comparison views of the opposite normal limb may be helpful, especially if exactly symmetric projections are obtained. Epiphyseal injuries that are undisplaced may be demonstrated by varus or valgus stress films, which are required for differentiating ligament disruptions from growth plate injuries in skeletally immature children.

Treatment

A. Conservative Treatment: Most fractures involving the physis may be managed nonoperatively. Undisplaced injuries of any type should be protected in plaster casts until healed. A cast for 3–6 weeks is usually sufficient, depending upon the child's age and the site and type of injury. Displaced type I and type II injuries should be treated by gentle closed reduction, followed by immobilization as above. Acceptance of some deformity is better than repeated vigorous attempts to correct it, since these efforts involve a risk of additional damage to the physis.

B. Operative Treatment: Displaced type III and type IV injuries usually require open reduction and internal fixation. Type V injuries should be protected in a cast or splint, but the poor outcome of these fortunately rare injuries cannot be improved by any early treatment.

Prognosis

All injuries that involve physes should be followed long enough to confirm that normal growth has not been disrupted. This may require several years, especially if the child is growing slowly or if interference is slight. If the child sustains a type III or type IV injury or any injury of the distal femoral physis, the parents should be warned of the possibility of altered growth. Close follow-up observation is required after growth plate injuries to permit timely diagnosis and treatment of any resulting growth abnormality. Progressive angular deformity may result from an incomplete bony bridge crossing and tethering one side of the physis. Such bridges can be resected, with interposition of a free fat graft, to restore normal growth. A number of techniques are now available to correct limb length inequality due to complete growth arrest. Traditionally, the most frequent has been epiphyseodesis to stop growth of the contralateral limb. Lengthening techniques are being developed that often permit restoration of the short limb to its normal length.

Paley D: Current techniques of leg lengthening. J Pediatr Orthop 1988;8:73.

Peterson HA: Premature partial physeal closure. J Bone Joint Surg [Br] 1987;69:154.

2. UPPER EXTREMITY FRACTURES & DISLOCATIONS

Proximal Humeral Fractures

An occasional birth injury causes separation of the unossified proximal humeral epiphysis. The child's failure to use the arm raises the possibility of brachial plexus palsy. Such pseudoparalysis resolves quickly, and radiographs in 10 days demonstrate abundant callus, confirming the nature of the original trauma. Older children usually sustain type II epiphyseal fractures. Most are only slightly displaced and can be treated in a sling for 3 weeks. If more displacement is present, manipulation under anesthesia and skin or skeletal traction can improve alignment. There is so much potential for remodeling in the proximal humerus that the best obtainable closed reduction is preferable to open surgery. Deformity, nonunion, and restricted motion are almost never problems for children who sustain proximal humerus fractures.

Supracondylar Fractures of the Humerus

Hyperextension of a child's elbow may cause an undisplaced greenstick supracondylar fracture. There is elbow pain, swelling, and tenderness of both epicondylar ridges. Radiographs confirm swelling and usually show a positive fat pad sign, indicating elbow hemarthrosis. The fracture line is easily missed but may be found where it crosses the olecranon fossa transversely. Careful inspection of a lateral radiograph of the distal humerus shows loss of normal anterior angulation of the capitellum, which may be compared with the other elbow if necessary. Closed reduction is advised if angulation is more than 20 degrees from normal. Whether or not closed reduction is performed, the fracture should be protected for 3 weeks in a long-arm cast or splint, with the elbow flexed above 90 degrees and the arm restrained to the chest with a secure sling or collar and cuff.

Rotation superimposed upon a hyperextended elbow produces a displaced supracondylar fracture of the humerus. A sharp corner of the proximal piece penetrates the periosteum but leaves an intact hinge on the side toward which the distal fragment is displaced. The anteroposterior radiograph shows the direction of displacement and thus the site of the periosteal hinge. Displaced supracondylar fractures of the humerus are serious injuries that threaten the neurovascular status of the involved limb and may result in unsightly deformity if reduction is not accurate. Before radiographs are taken, the elbow should be splinted in moderate extension rather than flexed to a right angle. The wrist pulses and the function of radial, ulnar, and median (including anterior interosseous) nerves should be checked immediately. Ischemia may be present initially or may develop during early treatment. If left to progress, ischemia causes **Volkmann's contracture,** with loss of motor and sensory function and necrosis of some of the forearm flexor muscles. The involved muscles contract as they are replaced by scar, so that the wrist develops a flexion contracture and the fingers become clawed. Irreversible muscle necrosis begins after 4–6 hours of ischemia. Effective treatment requires prompt restoration of arterial flow and, if necessary, reduction of elevated compartmental pressure in the forearm. It is mandatory to recognize the signs of ischemia: pain in the forearm (rather than the elbow) and progressive loss of sensory and motor function. Ischemic pain is usually increased when the involved muscles are stretched, so that pain on extension of the fingers is a danger sign. Pulses may be felt at the wrist, and the skin may appear well perfused in spite of elevated compartmental pressure. Alternatively, the pulses may be diminished or absent without dangerously impaired perfusion as long as the forearm is comfortable and the hand warm and pink, with intact sensation and motion. If elevated compartmental pressures is suspected, prompt measurement of tissue pressures is indicated (see Acute Compartment Syndrome, p 1037). Ischemia with supracondylar fractures may be due to (1) vascular injury, which requires surgical repair; (2) vascular entrapment, which usually resolves with reduction; or (3) compression from marked elbow flexion, in which position the elbow may have been placed to preserve fracture alignment, or from tight casts or bandages.

Prompt reduction of deformity is the next step to restoring normal perfusion and venous drainage. Acute flexion helps maintain closed reduction but is contraindicated if it impairs perfusion of the forearm. Ischemia that develops during treatment must be corrected by release or removal of any constricting bandages and by extension of the elbow as necessary to reestablish arterial flow. Prompt surgical exploration of the brachial artery and forearm musculature may be required if ischemia is evident. Arteriography usually adds little helpful information, and indirect attempts to restore flow (stellate ganglion blocks, anticoagulants, or vasodilators) waste time and are usually not successful.

Supracondylar humerus fractures can usually be managed without open operation. If displacement and soft tissue damage are mild to moderate, closed reduction is done under general anesthesia by manipulating the distal fragment into position and flexing the elbow to hold it. A bandage or cast that leaves the antecubital fossa free is applied, and the arm is secured to the chest to prevent rotation. If the fracture is badly displaced or unstable, if soft tissue swelling is marked, or if the amount of flexion required to hold the reduction obliterates the radial pulse, some other means must be chosen. Overhead skeletal traction with an olecranon pin or screw is effective (Figure 43–15). Dunlop's skin traction with the arm out to the side is less effective. The currently favored approach is to maintain the reduction with pins inserted percutaneously across the fracture with fluoroscopic guidance, following which the elbow can be splinted in sufficient extension to avoid interfering with perfusion.

The "gunstock deformity" of cubitus varus is the commonest late problem after supracondylar fracture. It is caused by inadequate reduction or reduction that is not maintained during healing. Radiographic monitoring is difficult but must be done with care, since correction is much easier and safer before healing has occurred than with a late osteotomy.

Mubarak SJ, Carroll NC: Volkmann's contracture in children: Aetiology and prevention. J Bone Joint Surg [Br] 1979;61:285.

Webb AJ, Sherman FC: Supracondylar fractures of the humerus in children. J Pediatr Orthop 1989;9:315.

Worlock P: Supracondylar fractures of the humerus. J Bone Joint Surg [Br] 1986;68:755.

Subluxation of the Radial Head (Pulled Elbow, Nursemaid's Elbow)

This common minor injury occurs in children under 4 years of age. It is caused by a sudden pull on the extended pronated arm, usually by an adult tugging on a reluctant toddler. The pronated radial head slips partially under the annular ligament the proximal portion of which displaces into the radiocapitellar joint. The distressed child suddenly stops using the arm, which is held flexed and pronated. Tenderness, usually mild, is well localized to the radial head region, and all motions are permitted except supination. After these physical findings are confirmed, the physician performs reduction by firmly supinating the forearm with one hand while the other supports the elbow in 90 degrees of flexion, feeling for a "click" near the radial head just as full supination is achieved. Radiographs, if obtained, are normal. In fact, positioning for elbow films will often reduce the subluxation. Promptly after reduction, the child becomes less apprehensive and soon resumes use of the limb. A sling may be applied for a few days. Recurrence is an occasional complication that may require more formal immobilization.

Other Elbow Region Fractures & Dislocations

It is essential to remember that "sprains" rarely occur and that swelling, tenderness, and difficulty in moving an injured elbow suggest a serious problem. Radiographic interpretation is difficult, because many of the pertinent structures ossify late in childhood. However, precise early diagnosis is necessary to identify several exceptions to the general principle of nonoperative treatment of children's fractures. Surgery is needed for displaced lateral condylar fractures, displaced medial epicondylar fractures, and badly angulated radial neck fractures that resist closed manipulation. Displaced olecranon fractures, if not reduced by elbow extension, will also require internal fixation. Significant distortion of the elbow region by any fracture or dislocation raises the specter of vascular compromise and resulting Volkmann's contracture. Hospitalization for a day or so is advisable if swelling is severe or if parents cannot be relied upon to bring the child in promptly for follow-up visits.

Forearm Fractures

Fractures of the shafts of both the radius and the ulna occur frequently in children. Neurovascular complications, including those due to constricting plasters, are always possible. Initial elevation of the limb and close observation are thus advisable, and children treated as outpatients must be supervised by an observant and informed adult. Forearm fractures in children unite reliably. The commonest problem is malunion with angular or rotational deformity and limited supination-pronation. Closed reduction almost always corrects angulation. Greenstick fractures are reduced as described above. If displacement is complete, general anesthesia is advisable. Direct manipulation or traction can be used to align the fracture. End-on-end reduction is not essential. Side-by-side ("bayonet") apposition is acceptable in a growing child, but angulation must be minimal; the space between radius and ulna must be preserved; and rotational alignment must be correct. Radiographs are repeated weekly for 3 weeks to permit early remanipulation should a potentially unstable fracture displace in plaster. More distal fractures may involve the physis but rarely interfere with growth.

It is important to be aware of the possibility of dislocation of one forearm bone in association with an isolated displaced fracture of the other. With **Monteggia's fracture,** there is dislocation of the radial head at the elbow, associated with a broken or bent ulnar shaft. **Galeazzi's fracture** combines dislocation of the distal radioulnar joint with fracture of the radial shaft. Fracture lines attract attention on radiographs, but dislocations are not as obvious. To avoid missing these injuries, check for tenderness, swelling, and deformity at the wrist and elbow in any patient with trauma to the forearm. Look carefully at radiographs of the wrist and the elbow to ascertain that the normal bony relationships are present. Children with these injuries, unlike adults, can usually be treated successfully with closed reduction of both the fracture and the joint dislocation. Open reduction is required if joint alignment cannot be restored by closed manipulation.

3. LOWER EXTREMITY FRACTURES & DISLOCATIONS

Traumatic Hip Dislocation

In children, traumatic dislocation is more common than fracture of the hip and has fewer complications. Prompt closed reduction under general anesthesia with good muscle relaxation is usually successful. Interposed soft tissue or bone fragments may necessitate open reduction. Following reduction, the hip should be protected for 4–6 weeks until soft tissue healing has occurred. Balanced suspension, traction, or a spica cast may be used. With prompt reduction, avascular necrosis is a rare problem.

Fractures of Proximal Femur

Proximal femur fractures are rare in children. This is fortunate, as displacement and injury to the growth plate and blood supply predispose to frequent complications, such as avascular necrosis, nonunion, and deformity that imperils the hip joint. The strength and resiliency of the proximal femur are such that a fracture in this region can only occur with severe trauma, another factor increasing the likelihood of complications.

Birth fractures, now quite unusual, may displace the proximal femoral epiphysis. Pain and swelling suggest septic arthritis, and the deformity raises fears of dislocation. Aspiration or arthrography yields no pus but demonstrates that the femoral head is located in a normal acetabulum and that deformity is at the neck/shaft junction. Splinting in abduction and flexion, a spica cast, or skin traction will maintain alignment during the 2–3 weeks required for healing. Remodeling may occur with any of these injuries, but nonunion, avascular necrosis, and deformity are possible.

In older children, most hip fractures involve the mid and lower portions of the femoral neck. If there is no displacement, spica cast immobilization maintains alignment during healing, but close radiographic monitoring is required for prompt identification and rectification of any displacement. Displaced fractures of the femoral neck should be treated with three or four small pins, preferably placed short of the physis. Postoperatively, a spica cast is advisable until healing is progressing. Satisfactory results are achieved in half or less of cases, with avascular necrosis, varus malunion, epiphyseal arrest, non-union, and postoperative wound infection the significant complications. Intertrochanteric and subtrochanteric fractures can generally be managed well by use of traction for 3 or 4 weeks, until early fracture stability is present, at which time a 1½ hip spica is applied for 8–12 weeks. Late problems (eg, angular deformity, unequal limb lengths) are rare but do occur.

Heinrich SD et al: Stabilization of pediatric diaphyseal femur fractures with flexible intramedullary nails (a technique paper). J Orthop Trauma 1992;6:452.
Hennrikus WL et al: The function of the quadriceps muscle after a fracture of the femur in patients who are less than seventeen years old. J Bone Joint Surg [Am] 1993;3; 75:508.
Levy J, Ward WT: Pediatric femur fractures: An overview of treatment. Orthopedics 1993;16:183.

Femoral Shaft Fractures

Femoral shaft fractures are fairly common childhood injuries. They often result from significant trauma, so that other injuries may also be present. Radiographs of the hip are required to ensure that fracture or dislocation is not present. The knee should also be x-rayed. Alignment of femoral shaft fracture is achieved with skin or (for older children) skeletal traction or immediate spica application. Rotational alignment should be corrected. Children from 2 to 10 years of age will usually demonstrate transiently stimulated growth of a fractured femur. It is conventional to align their fractures with about a 1-cm overlap to compensate for this overgrowth. Protection must be continued until mature bony callus has developed, a process that takes roughly as many weeks as the child's age in years. So-called Bryant's skin traction, with both legs suspended vertically, may cause severe ischemia and Volkmann's contracture, even of the uninjured leg. This technique is dangerous for children over the age of 2 years. Femoral fractures in children who are closer to maturity are often most effectively managed with intramedullary nailing, especially if there is head trauma or multiple injuries.

Gross RH et al: Cast brace management of the femoral shaft fracture in children and young adults. J Pediatr Orthop 1983;3:572.

Herndon WA et al: Management of femoral shaft fractures in the adolescent. J Pediatr Orthop 1989;9:29.

Skak SV et al: Femoral shaft fracture in 265 children: Lognormal correlation with age of speed of healing. Acta Orthop Scand 1988;59:704.

Splain SH, Denno JJ: Immediate double spica immobilization as the treatment for femoral shaft fractures in children. J Trauma 1985;25:994.

Ziv I et al: Femoral intramedullary nailing in the growing child. J Trauma 1984;24:432.

Distal Femoral Growth Plate Fractures

Fractures of the distal femoral growth plate are potentially serious injuries that cause growth abnormalities in up to 45% of patients. They must be suspected whenever a child sustains a knee injury and are suggested by the finding of an intra-articular fat-fluid line on a cross-table lateral radiograph of the knee. Stress radiographs may be required to demonstrate instability. With marked displacement, the popliteal artery or peroneal nerve may be injured. Treatment must be individualized. Gentle anatomic reduction should be accomplished and reduction should be maintained until healing is secure. A hip spica cast is often required to prevent displacement. If instability is marked, fixation with smooth pins may be required; if open reduction is necessary, such fixation is advisable. The distal femoral epiphysis is responsible for 70% of the growth of the femur and 35% of the growth of the entire lower extremity. Even small disturbances of growth can produce significant limb length inequality if the injured child is young enough. Follow-up of distal femoral growth mechanism injuries should be continued until skeletal maturity is achieved.

Caine D et al: Stress changes of the distal radial growth plate: A radiographic survey and review of the literature. Am J Sports Med 1992;20:290.

Krueger-Franke M, Siebert CH, Pfoerringer W: Sports-related epiphyseal injuries of the lower extremity: An epidemiologic study. J Sports Med Phys Fitness 1992; 32:106.

Meyers MC et al: Delayed treatment of a malreduced distal femoral epiphyseal plate fracture. Med Sci Sports Exerc 1992;24:1311.

Fractures of Tibia & Fibula

Fractures of the tibia and fibula are not unusual in childhood. An occult undisplaced spiral fracture may be the cause of an acute gait disturbance ("toddler's fracture"). Oblique radiographs may reveal this injury. Most are easy to manage and heal rapidly in a long-leg cast. The spectrum of injuries is quite wide, however, so that each must be evaluated carefully and treated according to its particular attributes. Nerve and vessel damage may be present, especially with displaced fractures of the proximal metaphysis. Nearly undisplaced valgus greenstick fractures of the proximal tibia are pernicious causes of deformity. The initial angulation may not be appreciated, or progressive medial overgrowth may follow apparently satisfactory healing. Fractures in this region with any valgus deformity should be *completely* reduced and held extended in a long-leg or single-spica cast molded into varus. In some cases, open reduction may be required to remove interposed soft tissues. Another cause of angular deformity is an intact fibula, which may have been bent by the original injury or may encourage collapse into varus by providing relatively more support to the lateral aspect of the leg. One must critically assess the postreduction and early follow-up radiographs following casting to permit timely treatment of angulation. Rotational alignment requires careful visual comparison with the other limb, as it is not obvious on radiographs.

Briggs TW, Orr MM, Lightowler CD: Isolated tibial fractures in children. Injury 1992;23:308.

Henderson RC, Kemp GJ, Campion ER: Residual bone-mineral density and muscle strength after fractures of the tibia or femur in children. J Bone Joint Surg [Am] 1992;74:211

Hope PG, Cole WG: Open fractures of the tibia in children. J Bone Joint Surg [Br] 1992;74:546.

Oestreich AE, Ahmad BS: The periphysis and its effect on the metaphysis: I: Definition and normal radiographic pattern. Skeletal Radiol 1992;21:283.

Salter RB, Best TN: Pathogenesis of progressive valgus deformity following fractures of the proximal metaphyseal region of the tibia in young children. Instr Course Lect 1992;41:409.

Fractures of Distal Epiphyses of Tibia & Fibula

Fractures of the distal epiphyses of the tibia and the fibula occur frequently in children, often from trauma that would produce ligamentous injury in an adult. Suspicion, physical examination that localizes tenderness to a growth plate, and carefully evaluated radiographs will usually indicate the diagnosis. Additional radiographic views, including stress films, will occasionally be required for confirmation. Salter-Harris type I fractures, type II fractures of the fibula, and undisplaced (within 2 mm of anatomic position) type III and type IV fractures have little risk of growth disturbance. Type II fractures of the distal tibial epiphysis are unpredictable, with a higher risk of growth disturbance that does not correlate well with original displacement. Displaced type III and type IV injuries and comminuted epiphyseal fractures have a 30% chance of growth disturbance.

If displaced, growth plate injuries of the ankle should be treated by gentle closed reduction, usually under anesthesia. If this does not correct displacement, type III and type IV injuries should be treated by open reduction and internal fixation, whereas moderate deformity, especially in the sagittal plane, can generally be accepted in type I and type II fractures. Distal fibular growth plate injuries usually have few complications, but those of the distal tibia should be followed until skeletal maturity is achieved.

Ertl JP et al: Triplane fracture of the distal tibial epiphysis: Long term follow-up. J Bone Joint Surg [Am] 1988;70: 967.

Kling TF Jr et al: Distal tibial physeal injuries in children that may require open reduction. J Bone Joint Surg [Am] 1984;66:647.

Krueger-Franke M, Siebert CH, Pfoeringer W: Sports-related epiphyseal injuries of the lower extremity: An epidemiologic study. J Sports Med Phys Fitness 1992;32: 106.

Landin JP et al: Late results in 65 physeal ankle fractures. Acta Orthop Scand 1986;57:530.

GAIT DISORDERS & LIMB DEFORMITY

Abnormalities of the lower extremities in children are often a source of parental concern and are frequently noticed when the child is first learning to walk. Rotational alignment, indicated by the orientation of the feet to the line of progression, and angulation at the knees are the two commonest areas of concern.

Intoe Gait
(Pigeon Toe)

Children normally walk with their feet externally rotated 10 degrees away from the line of progression. Significant variation occurs from step to step, so that gait must be observed more than just briefly before a reliable conclusion can be made about whether a problem exists. **Metatarsus adductus**—medial deviation of the forefoot at the tarsometatarsal junction—is a deformity occasionally present at birth. If it persists beyond early childhood, gait appears intoed.

Tibial torsion, the relative rotational alignment of the ankle joint axis compared to that of the knee, increases in an outward direction during childhood. The ankle axis is a line connecting the tips of the medial and lateral malleoli. In a very young child whose leg is hanging freely with the knee flexed 90 degrees and the tibia in neutral rotation, the ankle axis is in the same plane as the knee axis. By adulthood, the transmalleolar axis is externally rotated about 20 degrees. Children 1–3 years of age with intoeing will frequently have relative internal tibial torsion, which

almost always corrects spontaneously with growth. Treatment is necessary only if there is significant interference with gait and if spontaneous correction is not occurring. A Denis Browne splint is a metal bar that connects the shoes and holds them in external rotation. It is worn while the child sleeps. This treatment is usually effective. Only rarely, and in children over 8 years of age, must tibial osteotomy be considered.

Excessive **femoral anteversion** is a common finding in older children who walk with their feet turned in. Observation reveals that the whole limb is internally rotated, so that the patella—as well as the foot—points medially. Anteversion refers to the normal anterior inclination of the femoral neck when the distal femur is positioned with the knee axis in a frontal plane. From about 40 degrees in the newborn, femoral anteversion decreases normally to about 15 degrees by adulthood. Excessive femoral anteversion also decreases, often to a normal range, although significant correction is unlikely to occur after age 8 years. Precise measurement of femoral anteversion requires complicated radiographic techniques, but a good clinical determination can be made by internally rotating the extended hip to produce maximal lateral prominence of the greater trochanter. The required amount of internal rotation is roughly equivalent to the degree of femoral anteversion. Significant anteversion is the usual cause of limited external rotation of the extended hip, with associated increase of the range of internal rotation. The normal newborn's hips have an external rotation contracture, presumably the result of intrauterine posture. This diminishes during the first 3 years of life independently of changes in anteversion of the femoral neck. Femoral anteversion can be corrected only by rotational osteotomy. If the limb can be externally rotated beyond neutral, osteotomy is rarely needed.

Angular Deformity of the
Lower Extremities
(Knock-Knees & Bowlegs)

The angle (varus denotes tibia deviated medially, valgus denotes tibia deviated laterally) between femur and tibia in the frontal plane is age-dependent. Bowlegs (genu varum) are normal in the newborn but progress toward valgus, passing through neutral at about age 18 months. Valgus becomes maximal between ages 2 and 3 years, gradually resolving so that the average leg appears straight by age 6 or 7 years. In young children, angular deformity of the knees requires x-ray evaluation (and perhaps measurement of serum calcium, phosphate, and alkaline phosphatase) if it is not symmetric; if it is associated with abnormally short stature; or if it is severe (more than 10 cm between the knees with the ankles touching in genu varum, or more than 10 cm between the ankles with the knees touching in genu valgum). Operative treatment may be considered in severe cases to improve function and appearance and perhaps to decrease the risk of degenerative joint disease in middle age. Angulation can be corrected by stapling one side of a physis to obtain asymmetric growth, or by osteotomy with removal or addition of a wedge of bone.

Pathologic genu varum. It is important to distinguish symmetric infantile bowlegs, which should resolve by age 3–5 years, from varus deformity produced by rickets, **Blount's disease,** or skeletal dysplasias, in which involvement is often bilateral but usually asymmetric. Blount's disease (tibia vara) is a frequently bilateral disorder that has both infantile and adolescent types. Radiologic changes in the medial proximal tibial metaphysis consist of lucency, sclerosis, and fragmentation. Unilateral varus suggests a traumatic origin. In young patients, the metaphyseal-diaphyseal angle of the tibia helps to differentiate between physiologic bowing and infantile tibia vara prior to development of typical radiologic signs. The angle is formed between the line of the lateral tibial cortex and the line of the prominent medial and lateral metaphyseal beaks. A metaphyseal-diaphyseal angle of greater than 11 degrees strongly suggests Blount's disease. Progressive tibia vara should be treated with corrective osteotomy of the proximal tibia and fibula to achieve physiologic valgus alignment of both knees.

Heath CH, Staheli LT: Normal limits of knee angle in white children: Genu varum and genu valgum. J Pediatr Orthop 1993;13:259.

Levine AM, Drennan JC: Physiological bowing and tibia vara. J Bone Joint Surg [Am] 1982;64:1158.

Phillips WA: The child with a limp. Orthop Clin North Am 1987;18:489.

Staheli LT: Torsion: Treatment indications. Clin Orthop 1989;(Oct)247:61.

Staheli LT et al: Lower-extremity rotational problems in children: Normal values to guide management. J Bone Joint Surg [Am] 1985;67:35.

SYSTEMIC DISORDERS AFFECTING BONES & JOINTS IN CHILDREN

1. JUVENILE RHEUMATOID ARTHRITIS

Rheumatoid arthritis is an autoimmune disorder whose exact cause remains elusive. It is a systemic disease that in its most florid form is characterized by rash, fever, and enlargement of lymph nodes and spleen. There are three basic clinical types of juvenile rheumatoid arthritis. **Pauciarticular arthritis** generally involves the knee or the ankle but occasionally the hip or an upper extremity (mainly the elbow or the wrist). One or only a few joints are affected. Insidious onset of swelling, with effusion, synovial thickening, and often flexion contracture, are noted.

Except for possible sedimentation rate elevation, systemic signs are absent. A serious complication of juvenile rheumatoid arthritis, most common in the pauciarticular form, is **iridocyclitis**—inflammation of the iris and ciliary body. This insidious process can lead to glaucoma and blindness if left untreated. Early diagnosis is essential and requires slit lamp examination every 3–6 months in these patients. The outlook for patients with pauciarticular juvenile rheumatoid arthritis is said to be good, but although residual involvement may be minimal, few patients remain truly asymptomatic.

Polyarthritis is characterized by multiple joint involvement and minimal evidence of systemic disease. Fingers and toes, the neck, and the temporomandibular joints are more likely to be involved. The course is persistent, with periods of exacerbation.

Polyarthritis with systemic rheumatoid disease (Still's disease) usually presents with multiple (more than five) involved joints, fever, lymphadenopathy, hepatosplenomegaly, rash, subcutaneous nodules, and pericarditis. The course may be remitting or relentless, causing severe permanent disability.

Inflamed joints develop synovial hypertrophy and pannus, which destroy articular cartilage. The associated hyperemia can stimulate the adjacent physes, with resulting overgrowth, or physeal arrest may occur. Damage to underlying bone and ligament can produce severe deformity and joint subluxation. In polyarthritis, musculoskeletal involvement is more likely to include the cervical spine, typically with spontaneous fusion of the apophyseal joints. Occasionally, C1–C2 instability will occur, as in the adult with rheumatoid arthritis.

When a single joint is inflamed, it is necessary to exclude the differential diagnoses of septic arthritis, foreign body synovitis, and transient synovitis of the hip. Polyarticular juvenile rheumatoid arthritis must be differentiated from rheumatic fever and leukemia. Lyme disease may present as joint inflammation.

Management is initially medical, with anti-inflammatory drugs, rest, splinting, and range-of-motion exercises, followed by strengthening as synovitis resolves and appropriate bracing to minimize deformity and allow function. Synovial biopsy—percutaneously with a needle, via arthroscopy, or with formal arthrotomy—may be helpful for diagnosis, especially to rule out infection. Synovectomy is controversial but may retard the progression of arthritis if medical measures fail. To be successful, it must be done before joint destruction has progressed too far. Contractures may require soft tissue releasing procedures. Osteotomy may be needed to correct bony deformity, and symptomatic destroyed joints can be treated by arthrodesis or arthroplasty. Extensive orthopedic surgery can often be avoided if the pediatrician and the orthopedist cooperate to provide maximal medical control and appropriate use of bracing and physical therapy.

Rydholm U et al: Synovectomy of the knee in juvenile chronic arthritis: A retrospective consecutive follow-up study. J Bone Joint Surg [Br] 1986;68:223.

Senac MO Jr et al: MR imaging in juvenile rheumatoid arthritis. AJR 1988;150:873.

Swann M: Juvenile chronic arthritis. Clin Orthop 1987;No. 219:38.

2. BRACHIAL PLEXUS PALSY

Brachial plexus palsy due to birth injury has three general patterns of involvement: (1) Erb's palsy, involving C5 and C6 roots; (2) Klumpke's paralysis, involving C8 and T1; and (3) whole arm paralysis, where the extent of involvement of individual roots may vary. Erb's palsy is most common and affects the shoulder, with loss of extension, abduction, and external rotation. Also affected are elbow flexion and forearm supination. Spontaneous improvement will occur and will level off by age 1½ years. Initial treatment is directed at maintaining shoulder motion by positioning and passive stretching to prevent the characteristic contracture in adduction and internal rotation. If muscle imbalance persists at the shoulder, the pectoralis major and subscapularis muscles can be lengthened with posterior transfer of the latissimus dorsi and teres major muscles, so that they become external rotators. Humeral osteotomy may be preferable to tendon transfer when the shoulder joint is unstable. These procedures will position the hand where it can best be used, but a normal limb is not achieved.

Boome RS et al: Obstetric traction injuries of the brachial plexus: Natural history, indications for surgical repair and results. J Bone Joint Surg [Br] 1988;70:571.

Jackson ST et al: Brachial-plexus palsy in the newborn. J Bone Joint Surg [Am] 1988;70:1217.

SCOLIOSIS & SPINAL DEFORMITY

The normal spine is straight in the frontal plane, whereas in the sagittal plane it is composed of three curves: cervical lordosis, thoracic kyphosis, and lumbar lordosis. Deviations in normal spinal contours comprise a group of disorders termed spinal deformities, of which idiopathic scoliosis is the most common (Table 43–1). Spinal deformities are clinically important because they may produce pain, difficulty with sitting or ambulating, neurologic compromise, unacceptable cosmesis, and, in advanced cases, cardiopulmonary compromise. Each type of spinal deformity is associated with its own clinical presentation, symptoms, and natural history for progression.

Although scoliosis has been defined as lateral curvature of the spine, it is associated with vertebral ro-

Table 43–1. Classification of spinal deformities.

Scoliosis
  Idiopathic
    a. Infantile (0–3 years)
    b. Juvenile (3–10 years)
    c. Adolescent (> 10 years)
  Neuromuscular
    a. Neuropathic
    b. Myopathic
  Congenital
    a. Failure of formation
    b. Failure of segmentation
  Neurofibromatosis
  Mesenchymal disorders
  Rheumatoid disease
  Trauma
  Extraspinal contractures
  Osteochondrodystrophies
  Infection of bone
  Metabolic disorders
  Related to lumbosacral joint
  Tumors
Kyphosis
  Postural
  Scheuermann's disease
  Congenital
  Neuromuscular
  Myelomeningocele
  Traumatic
  Postsurgical
  Postirradiation
  Metabolic
  Skeletal dysplasias
  Collagen disease
  Tumor
  Inflammatory
Lordosis
  Postural
  Congenital
  Neuromuscular
  Postlaminectomy

tation, which produces the cosmetically unacceptable rib hump. Idiopathic scoliosis is classified according to the age at onset: infantile, juvenile, and adolescent. Scoliosis seen after skeletal maturity is termed adult scoliosis. Progression of idiopathic curves correlates with the magnitude of the curve, the age of the patient at presentation, and the patient's menarcheal status. Nonidiopathic causes of scoliosis must be determined because of their less predictable and generally higher risk for progression (eg, congenital scoliosis, scoliosis associated with neurofibromatosis, and neuromuscular scoliosis).

Clinical Findings

A. Symptoms and Signs: Examination of the patient with spinal deformity should include determination of the patient's overall frontal and sagittal alignment with particular attention to the relationship of the occiput with the sacrum. When the occiput is not centered over the sacrum, the patient is said to be decompensated. Asymmetry of the shoulders and the pelvis may be present with high thoracic and lumbar curves, respectively. The skin should be carefully in-

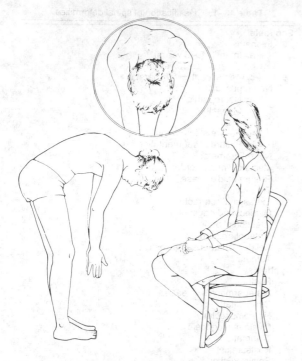

Figure 43–54. Forward bending test. Back is uncovered. Child stands with feet and fingers together, and bends forward 90 degrees, with knees straight. Examiner looks down entire spine for a "hump" (beside the spinous processes) which indicates abnormal vertebral rotation, produced by structural scoliosis. The spine should also be checked from the side for abnormal convexity (sharp angulation) or total kyphosis over 40 degrees.

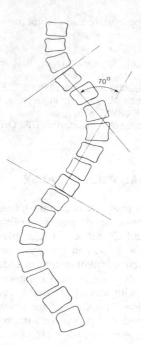

Figure 43–55. The angle of a scoliotic curve equals the angle of intersection of perpendiculars to the end plates of the highest and lowest vertebrae in the curve. This should be measured on a standing posteroanterior radiograph. The same end vertebrae must be used when serial films are checked for increasing curvature.

spected for signs of café au lait spots (neurofibromatosis) or hair patches (spinal dysraphism). The forward bend test (Figure 43–54) detects the rib hump, which correlates with curve magnitude and vertebral rotation. A bowel and bladder history and a complete neurologic examination are mandatory for all patients.

Significant pain or neurologic symptoms are uncommon with idiopathic scoliosis. These findings warrant further investigation to rule out tumor, infection, disk herniation, or other nonidiopathic causes of spinal deformity.

B. Imaging Studies: Patients referred for evaluation of spinal deformities should be examined by standing anteroposterior and lateral radiographs, including the entire spine (3 14 film). If treatment is contemplated, bending films in the direction of each curve convexity will help to determine curve flexibility. Curves are measured according to the Cobb method (Figure 43–55). The vertebrae which are maximally tilted into the concavity of the curve are the end vertebrae. Perpendiculars from their endplates are drawn, and the angle between them determines the curve magnitude. Curves should be mea-

sured from the same vertebrae during each examination for serial comparison.

Patients presenting with neurologic signs or symptoms, left thoracic curves, or rapid progression should be examined by MRI to rule out intraspinal disease.

Treatment of Adolescent Idiopathic Scoliosis

A. Observation: Skeletally immature patients presenting with curves less than 20 degrees or those presenting with curves less than 40 degrees at skeletal maturity should be observed. Adolescent patients should be followed with radiographs at intervals of 4–6 months until the age of skeletal maturity. Curves greater than 20 degrees or with progression of greater than 5 degrees should be referred for treatment to a surgeon experienced in the management of patients with spinal deformity.

B. Bracing: Growing children with curves measuring 20-D40 degrees or documented progression are candidates for brace treatment. Patients with curve apices below T8 can be fitted with polypropylene underarmDtype braces . Higher curves can be controlled only with a cervicoDthoracicDlumbar orthosis (Milwaukee brace). The goal of bracing is to halt progression. LongDterm curve correction is rarely achieved with brace treatment.

The daily duration of brace wear necessary to halt progression is controversial. Although historically braces have been worn for 23–24 hours per day, recent studies have indicated that limited daily brace wear may be equally effective. Generally, patients should be braced until the age of skeletal maturity and then should be gradually weaned.

C. Surgical Treatment: The prevalence of patients with curves greater than 20 degrees is 0.13–0.30%, with few requiring surgery . Patients with progressive curves, curves of 40 degrees or more, and those resistant or nonamenable to brace treatment are should be referred for surgery. Newer surgical techniques include variable hookDrod systems designed to both correct the frontal curve and decrease vertebral rotation while providing secure fixation so that postoperative brace wear is often not needed (Figure 43–56). Instrumentation is accompanied by surgical fusion with bone grafting. Anterior fusion and instrumentation has been developed for certain lumbar curves. The length of the fusion depends on the type of curve treated. The preservation of lumbar motion segments below the fusion has been shown to correlate with a decreased incidence of low back pain in the adult patient.

Bradford DS et al: *Moe's Textbook of Scoliosis and Other Spinal Deformities,* 2nd ed.Saunders, 1987.

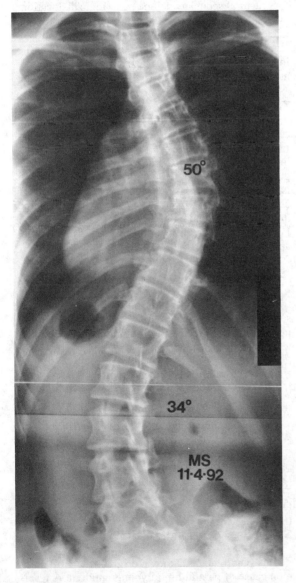 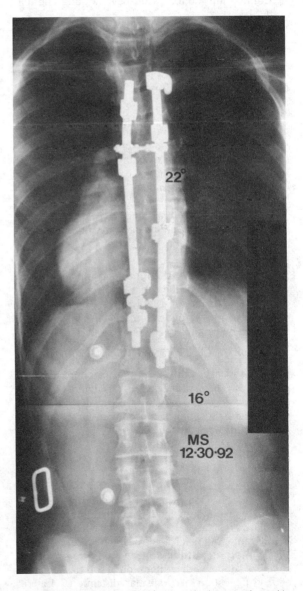

Figure 43–56. **A:** Posteroanterior radiograph of right thoracic idiopathic scoliosis. **B:** After surgical correction with Cotrel-Dubousset instrumentation.

Kehl DK, Morrissy RT: Brace treatment in adolescent idiopathic scoliosis: An update on concepts and technique. Clin Orthop Rel Res 1988;229:34.

Lonstein JE, Carlson JM: The prediction of curve progression in untreated idiopathic scoliosis during growth. J Bone joint Surg [Am] 1984;66:1061.

Rogala EH, Drummond DS, Gurr J: Scoliosis: Incidence and natural history, a prospective epidemiological study. J Bone Joint Surg [Am] 1978; 60:173.

SEPTIC ARTHRITIS OF THE HIP

Essentials of Diagnosis

- Limited hip motion, with local swelling and tenderness.
- Variable signs of systemic illness.
- Purulent exudate in the hip joint, confirmed by aspiration or arthrotomy.

General Considerations

Infection is usually hematogenous and more frequent in infants exposed to invasive measures likely to cause bacteremia. The joint can be primarily involved, or secondary involvement may occur by spread of hematogenous osteomyelitis from the proximal femur. Hip sepsis has also followed penetration of the joint during attempted blood aspiration from the femoral vein.

Staphylococcus aureus and *Streptococcus pyogenes* are the most common causative organisms.

Clinical Findings

A. Symptoms and Signs: Impaired voluntary and reflex motion of the entire involved limb—pseudoparalysis—is the most typical early finding. Fever is unlikely in very young children, but sepsis may be suggested by irritability and failure to thrive. Another focus of infection should increase suspicion. The hip is held flexed in slight abduction and external rotation, with local swelling becoming evident as disease progresses. The area is tender, and attempts to move the hip are resisted and seem especially painful. If pathologic dislocation has occurred, hip asymmetry and instability may be noted.

B. Laboratory Findings: The sedimentation rate is elevated, but the white blood count may be normal. Leukocytes are abundant in the joint fluid, and gram-stained smears of fluid show microorganisms as well. Bone scan may initially be negative, especially in children under 6 months of age, but usually shows increased uptake around the involved joint before radiographic changes become evident.

C. Imaging Studies: The early radiographic signs are subtle, with obliteration of soft tissue planes and a suggestion of "capsular distention." Lateral subluxation and complete dislocation may occur. Decreasing bone density and periosteal erosion or new bone formation occur later. Ultrasound imaging provides an early indication of joint effusion.

Differential Diagnosis

Alternative diagnoses in the neonate are fractures of the femur occurring during birth and acute hematogenous osteomyelitis of the proximal femur that has not yet spread into the hip. Congenital hip dislocation is not painful and limits motion to a lesser extent. In older children, transient synovitis, rheumatoid arthritis, pelvic osteomyelitis, and acute hemarthrosis from hemophilia must also be considered.

Complications

Structural sequelae include pathologic dislocation; avascular necrosis that may cause total and irreversible destruction of the femoral head and neck; and leg length discrepancy, usually due to undergrowth of the involved femur. Chronic persisting infection may also result.

Treatment

Surgical drainage is required as an emergency procedure. Side effects from negative arthrotomy are so few that exploration is warranted if the diagnosis is uncertain. Gram-stained smears of intra-articular pus guide the initial choice of parenteral antibiotic, which is modified if necessary according to the results of culture and sensitivity tests. Suction-irrigation tube drainage will maintain adequate decompression. Postoperatively, traction or a spica cast is used to rest and align the joint.

Course & Prognosis

If the diagnosis is made and surgical drainage performed within a few days of onset, the long-term results are good. Delay and nonoperative treatment are predictably followed by the complications mentioned above.

Hunka L et al: Classification and surgical management of the severe sequelae of septic hips in children. Clin Orthop 1982;No. 171:30.

Wenger DR: Childhood hip sepsis: Improving the yield of good results. Instr Course Lect 1985;34:457.

Wopperer JM et al: Long-term follow-up of infantile hip sepsis. J Pediatr Orthop 1988;8:322.

TRANSIENT SYNOVITIS OF THE HIP (Irritable Hip Syndrome, Toxic Synovitis, "Observation Hip")

This syndrome of unknown origin is the most common cause of painful hip in young children. A respiratory illness often precedes the complaint of pain, which may be localized in the knee, thigh, or hip. The short duration of symptoms, absence of diagnostic radiographic signs, and nearly normal laboratory studies suggest a benign process. Children of any age may be affected, although the average age is 6 years. Perhaps the most important aspect of transient synovitis is to recognize it appropriately and not confuse it with more serious causes of hip joint inflammation.

Clinical Findings

A. Symptoms and Signs: When first seen, the child has rarely been symptomatic for more than a week. Pain in the lower extremity with activity (or even with rest) is the commonest complaint. Limp and refusal to walk are also common. Localization of pain to the hip region is not reliable, and therefore a specific provocative test of hip motion must always be part of the physical examination of a child with lower extremity complaints. The passive range of motion of the hip must be checked and compared carefully with the opposite side. Normally, the child should be able to relax and motion should be free and easy without "guarding," which is especially noticeable on rotation or at extremes of flexion or extension. Low-grade fever may be present, but the child does not appear ill.

B. Laboratory Findings: Although white blood cell count and erythrocyte sedimentation rate may be somewhat elevated, they are usually normal. Bone scan often shows increased activity in the hip joint, without the decreased femoral head uptake suggestive of early avascular necrosis. Hip aspiration, if performed to help clarify a confusing case, reveals clear synovial fluid with a low white cell count, no organisms on gram-stained smears, and negative cultures for all types of organisms.

C. Imaging Studies: Radiographs are essential to rule out other diagnoses. X-rays are usually normal with transient synovitis of the hip. Shadows adjacent to the femoral neck sometimes suggest "hip effusion," but the significance is questionable, since they can be produced by abduction and external rotation of a normal hip. Occasionally, the joint space will be widened.

Differential Diagnosis

Pyogenic or tuberculous sepsis is the primary concern. Legg-Perthes disease (avascular necrosis), slipped capital femoral epiphysis, and, rarely, other forms of inflammatory joint disease, such as rheumatoid arthritis or rheumatic fever, must be considered.

Treatment

Hospitalization is often advisable to ensure that an infection is not missed. The hip is placed at rest in 4–5 lb of Buck's or Russell's skin traction. This almost always relieves symptoms promptly and also helps confirm the diagnosis. A few days of rest may be required to regain normal hip motion. A week or two of protection from weight bearing with bed rest at home or with crutches is usually advised. The child should then be reexamined to make certain that normal hip motion and comfort have been achieved. Anteroposterior and lateral x-rays are repeated in 2–3 months to ensure that avascular necrosis has not developed. Occasionally, signs of systemic reaction are more pronounced or the child continues to guard the hip longer than usual. In such cases, needle aspiration confirmed by arthrogram should be performed to rule out infection.

Prognosis

Recurrent symptoms may develop after release from the hospital and resumption of activity but usually resolve with more rest. Permanent (but usually unnoticeable) limitation of motion is present in about 18% of cases. A small number of patients develop other abnormalities and may represent errors in initial diagnosis.

Hasegawa Y et al: Scintimetry in transient synovitis of the hip in the child. Acta Orthop Scand 1988;59:520.
Landin LA et al: Transient synovitis of the hip: Its incidence, epidemiology, and relation to Perthes' disease. J Bone Joint Surg [Br] 1987;69:238.

CONGENITAL DYSPLASIA & DISLOCATION OF THE HIP

Essentials of Diagnosis

- Mechanical instability of the hip.
- Persistent limitation of abduction.
- Shortening or other asymmetry of the hip if unilateral.
- Widening of buttocks and perineum if bilateral.
- Abnormal gait once walking begins.

General Considerations

Congenital hip dysplasia may be manifested by dislocatability, dislocation, or inadequate joint development that results in early degenerative arthritis of the hip. True dislocation is not necessarily present at birth but develops early in life in some infants with dislocatable hips. The incidence of dislocation is one in 1000 infants. Both hips may be involved. Congenital hip dysplasia is commoner in females and patients with other congenital deformities. It is neither painful nor disabling in children but causes significant symptoms in adults if successful atraumatic closed reduction is not achieved in early childhood. If atraumatic reduction is not possible, surgical release of the obstructing or limiting soft tissues should be performed.

Clinical Findings

A. Symptoms and Signs: The physical signs of congenital hip dislocation are the key to diagnosis. They may be subtle, however, and can be missed by the most experienced examiner. This emphasizes the need for repeated evaluation of the hips during routine "well baby" checks.

1. Dislocatable hip–The examiner attempts to displace the infant's femoral head posterolaterally from the acetabulum by means of the subluxation provocation test (Figure 43–57). In a positive test, the femoral head is felt to displace with a jerk, which is repeated as the femur slides back into the acetabulum upon release of the displacing force. Mechanical instability—not a "click"—is the essential finding. Dislocatability is most easily demonstrated shortly after birth and should resolve within a few days.

2. Dislocated hip–Ortolani described the sign of "snapping" produced by relocation of a dislocated femoral head when the examiner abducts the flexed hip and lifts the greater trochanter anteriorly. This test can appear normal in the presence of congenital hip dysplasia if the soft tissues surrounding the joint are not lax enough to permit reduction. Diagnosis then rests upon other signs: limitation of abduction, asymmetry with apparent shortening, and deeper skin creases (if the dislocation is unilateral). As the child begins to walk, an abnormal gait becomes apparent. Trendelenburg's sign is positive, the contralateral side of the pelvis drooping when the child stands on the affected limb. If dislocation is bilateral, the diagnosis is more challenging. The perineum and buttocks are widened, and abduction limitation is bilateral. Gait is "waddling," and lumbar lordosis is prominent.

B. Imaging Studies: Until the cartilaginous acetabulum, and femoral head become substantially ossified, x-rays may fail to indicate the true condition of the hip joint. Obvious abnormalities must be considered significant, but apparently normal radiographs do not exclude congenital hip dysplasia until a well-ossified femoral head is adequately contained by the acetabulum. Femoral head ossification is usually present by 6 months of age but is often delayed in dislocated hips. Figure 43–58 shows several of the many radiographic relationships that are important for evaluation of the hip joint in infants. In older children, the femoral head should be adjacent to the radiolucent triradiate cartilage that forms the medial wall of the acetabulum. Displacement of the femoral head confirms dislocation. A shallow acetabulum that poorly covers the femoral head is termed dysplastic. Hip arthrography or CT scans help evaluate reduction of the unossified hip joint. Ultrasonography is gaining popularity as a technique for assessing the infant's hip prior to calcification of the cartilaginous joint structures. Congenital hip disease in the adult is shown in Figure 43–59.

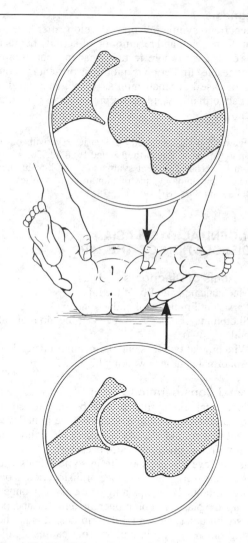

Figure 43–57. *Upper window:* Subluxation provocation test. Holding the thighs of the relaxed infant as illustrated, the examiner stabilizes the pelvis with one hand while gently but firmly trying to displace the opposite femoral head posteriorly out of the acetabulum. Adduction of the thigh aids this maneuver. If mechanical instability of the femoral head is present, a "jerk" will be felt, indicating that the hip is subluxable. *Lower window:* In Ortolani's test, abduction and lifting with the fingers produce a corresponding jerk when the dislocated femoral head slides back into the acetabulum.

Differential Diagnosis

Congenital abduction contracture of the hip is not unusual in neonates. Proximal femoral focal deficiency and congenital coxa vara are rare conditions that produce shortening or instability in the hip region. Pathologic dislocation can occur rapidly in infected hips; the femoral head is displaced from a radiographically normal acetabulum. Hip dislocation may be caused by muscle imbalance in some children with cerebral palsy or myelomeningocele.

Complications

Complications include inability to gain or maintain a stable reduction, avascular necrosis of the femoral

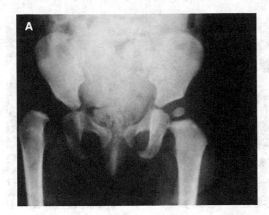

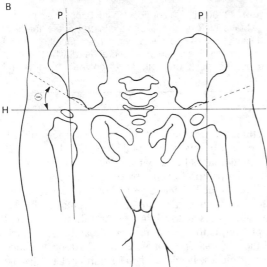

Figure 43–58. ***A:*** X-ray of congenital dislocation of the right hip. ***B:*** Analysis of hip radiographs presupposes adequately exposed films of a properly positioned patient. Hilgenreiner's horizontal line is drawn through both triradiate cartilages (H), and Perkins's vertical line is drawn through the outer margin of each acetabulum (P). If the hip is located, the proximal femoral epiphysis will lie in the inferomedial quadrant formed by the two intersecting lines. Proximal or lateral displacement indicates dislocation. Abnormal acetabular development is suggested by lack of obvious concavity and by an acetabular index (O) greater than 30 degrees.

head following operative or nonoperative treatment, and limitation of motion.

Treatment

A. Dislocatable Hip: Neonates with confirmed dislocatable hips should be treated by means of abduction splinting (Pavlik harness, Frejka cushion, etc) until stability and normal radiographic development are confirmed. It is important to flex the hips and abduct them no more than 60 degrees to avoid

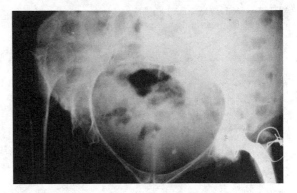

Figure 43–59. Adult with left total hip arthroplasty and persistent dislocation of the right hip caused by bilateral congenital hip dislocations.

interfering with the blood supply, so that avascular necrosis does not occur.

B. Dislocated Hip:

1. Birth to 18 months–In this age group, closed reduction is usually possible. Reduction can be maintained with removable splints as mentioned above if parents are reliable and careful medical supervision continues. A plaster spica cast is often safer. If closed reduction is not possible or cannot be maintained, open reduction is required. X-rays to confirm reduction and its maintenance are essential to any form of treatment.

2. Eighteen months to 4 years–Preliminary traction and open reduction are more likely to be required in this group. If adequate reduction is obtained, more than 90% of patients should have satisfactory results.

3. Older children and adults–Treatment of newly diagnosed congenital hip dysplasia in this age group is difficult. Acetabular remodeling through growth is slight. Mere achievement of a concentric reduction does not ensure a stable pain-free hip. Choices of treatment are operation or no treatment at all. Several osteotomies of the innominate bone have been described for improving acetabular coverage of the femoral head. Pain and limitation of motion will eventually necessitate total hip arthroplasty for many of these individuals.

Bennett JT, MacEwen GD: Congenital dislocation of the hip: Recent advances and current problems. Clin Orthop 1989;No. 247:15.

Davies SJ et al: Problems in the early recognition of hip dysplasia. J Bone Joint Surg [Br] 1984;66:479.

Grill F et al: the Pavlik harness in the treatment of congenital dislocating hip: Report on a multicenter study of the European Pediatric Orthopaedic Society. J Pediatr Orthop 1988;8:1.

Hartofilakidis G et al: Low friction arthroplasty for old untreated congenital dislocation of the hip. J Bone Joint Surg [Br] 1988;70:182.

Malefijt MCD, Hoogland T: Chiari osteotomy in the treatment of congenital dislocation and subluxation of the hip. J Bone Joint Surg [Am] 1982;64:996.

Terjesen T, Bredland T, Berg V: Ultrasound for hip assessment in the newborn. J Bone Joint Surg [Br] 1989; 71:767.

Williamson DM, Glover SD, Benson MKD'A: Congenital dislocation of the hip presenting after the age of three years. J Bone Joint Surg [Br] 1989;71:745.

SLIPPED CAPITAL FEMORAL EPIPHYSIS

During the period of rapid growth in early adolescence, the normal relationship of the femoral head with the femoral neck may become distorted by a shearing displacement through the growth plate—so-called slipped capital femoral epiphysis. The head remains within the acetabulum, while the femoral neck shifts anteriorly and laterally. This displacement may occur rapidly, often in response to minor trauma, or it can be gradual, as indicated by reactive bone formation and remodeling of the femoral neck adjacent to the growth plate. An acute slip may be superimposed upon a gradual, "chronic" one. An acute slip is not a traumatic injury to a normal growth plate but is a "pathologic fracture" through a plate that is abnormally weak. Boys are more likely to be affected than girls. Involvement is bilateral in at least 25% of cases. The condition is progressive and can lead to severe deformity and limitation of hip motion if untreated. Marked deformity may cause early degenerative joint disease and is associated with increased risk of avascular necrosis and chondrolysis, although it is difficult to differentiate between the natural history of the disease and the complications of its treatment.

Clinical Findings

A. Symptoms and Signs: The patient reports pain in the knee or groin, limps, and has limited hip motion, especially flexion, internal rotation, and abduction.

B. Imaging Studies: (Figure 43–60.) Radiographs are diagnostic in all but the most minimal slips. The epiphysis is not centered on the neck, as is normally the case, but is relatively posterior and medial. Since posterior displacement is often more marked, the deformity may not be as evident on the anteroposterior view as on the lateral view. Bony callus, or widening of the metaphysis adjacent to the growth plate, indicates a chronic slip. A significant slip produces a bony prominence on the anterolateral femoral neck, restricting hip motion.

Treatment

Surgical stabilization of the proximal femoral epiphysis is advised. As soon as the diagnosis is made, the patient is hospitalized and placed in skin

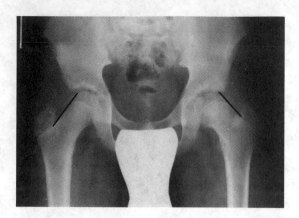

Figure 43–60. Left slipped capital femoral epiphysis. Note that a line extended along the lateral side of the femoral neck misses the capital epiphysis. On the normal right side, this line enters the femoral head, which should overlap the neck on both anteroposterior and lateral views.

traction. An internal rotation strap may help reduce an acute slip; this is preferable to forceful manipulation under anesthesia, which increases the risk of avascular necrosis. In situ pinning of the epiphysis is then performed. The surgeon should make sure that pins do not enter the joint space. Gradual mobilization with protected weight bearing follows. The goal of pinning is to prevent further slip and gain closure of the physis. The opposite side must be watched until it closes, because of the significant risk of its slipping as well. If severe deformity prevents normal motion, a subtrochanteric osteotomy or excision of the bony hump may be considered. Interference with function rather than abnormality on radiograph is the indication for such procedures.

Birch JG: Slipped capital femoral epiphysis: Still an emergency. J Pediatr Orthop 1987;7:334.

Crawford AH: Slipped capital femoral epiphysis. J Bone Joint Surg [Am] 1988;70:1422.

Stambough JL et al: Slipped capital femoral epiphysis: An analysis as to pin placement and number. J Pediatr Orthop 1986;6:265.

LEGG-PERTHES DISEASE (Legg-Calvé-Perthes Disease, Coxa Plana)

Legg-Perthes disease is an uncommon hip affliction that occurs in about one in 2000 children, generally between the ages of 4 and 10. Boys are affected five times as often as girls, who tend to have more severe involvement. About 10–15% of patients have bilateral disease. The process is self-limited and of unknown cause. Its hallmark is avascular necrosis of the capital femoral epiphysis. When avascular necrosis of the femoral head occurs in adults, little potential exists for reconstitution of dead bone; however, the growing child with Legg-Perthes disease is able to completely replace the necrotic bone with new live bone. Some patients achieve normal hip development. Others acquire permanent deformity of the femoral head, with limited motion and degenerative joint disease becoming symptomatic in middle age.

Determinants of Final Outcome

A. Stage of Illness: The earliest signs are an apparent increase in density of the capital epiphysis and thickening of the surrounding cartilage. As revascularization occurs, femoral head density increases, a subchondral crescent-shaped radiolucent fracture appears transiently, and the metaphysis may widen. The epiphysis itself appears irregular and flattened. Gradually, living bone replaces cartilage and fibrous tissue, so that the femoral head is completely ossified. The ultimate shape will depend upon the molding of the malleable head during replacement of the necrotic epiphysis. A spherical head correlates well with good long-term results.

B. Age of Patient: Younger patients have a better prognosis. They are lighter in weight, have more rapid healing of necrotic bone, and have more growth time in which remodeling of residual deformity may occur.

C. Severity of Involvement: Catterall has classified patients with Legg-Perthes disease into four groups, according to the extent of involvement of the epiphysis, from group I, with only the anterior part of the epiphysis involved, to group IV, with involvement of the entire head. The extent of involvement is an indicator of the likelihood that the femoral head will deform and thus helps suggest the outcome for a given patient.

D. The "Head at Risk": Catterall also proposed certain clinical and radiographic criteria for determining whether the femoral head might deform in the course of the disease. The clinical criteria are (1) obesity, (2) decreasing range of motion of the involved hip, and (3) adduction contracture. The radiographic criteria are (1) lateral subluxation of the femoral head, (2) Gage's sign (widening of the lateral part of the growth plate, so that the superior portion of the femoral neck appears convex), (3) calcification lateral to the epiphysis in the cartilaginous femoral head, (4) diffuse metaphyseal reaction, and (5) a horizontal growth plate. Others agree that these signs are helpful indications of which patients are likely to have a poor outcome and might thus benefit from treatment aimed at maintaining a spherical femoral head.

Clinical Findings

A. Symptoms and Signs: Insidious development of limp and sometimes pain in the groin, anterior thigh, or knee eventually brings the patient to a physician. An occasional case presents as acute synovitis. Examination shows antalgic gait, decreased hip motion (especially abduction and internal rotation), and sometimes flexion-adduction contracture. Passive motion is guarded rather than free.

B. Laboratory Findings: Bone scan may help with early diagnosis and assessment of the extent of head involvement.

C. Imaging Studies: Well-exposed radiographs in both anteroposterior and frog-leg lateral views are essential. If synovitis significantly limits hip motion, a period in traction may be required before adequate positioning can be achieved. Findings will depend upon the stage and severity of disease, as discussed above, but initial films usually show increased density and deformity of the femoral head epiphysis, which may be flattened or fragmented (Figure 43–61).

Differential Diagnosis

The early, inflammatory stage of Legg-Perthes disease can be confused with toxic synovitis, septic (including tuberculous) arthritis, and rheumatoid arthritis. The epiphyseal abnormalities are similar to those seen in epiphyseal dysplasias, hypothyroidism, and avascular necrosis from other causes, notably sickle cell anemia, Gaucher's disease, and chronic use of corticosteroid drugs.

Treatment

Rational treatment requires categorization according to stage of disease, extent of head involvement, and congruity of the hip joint at the time of presentation. The mobility of the involved joint must be determined and then followed as an important indicator of prognosis.

A. Observation: Treatment is unnecessary and contraindicated for the following patients: children with involvement of less than half the femoral head,

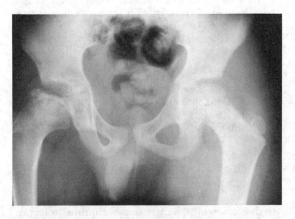

Figure 43–61. X-ray of Legg-Perthes disease, with significant deformity of right femoral head.

young children (under 5 years of age) without "at risk" signs, and children who already show radiologic evidence of healing. If significant deformity exists and insufficient growth time remains for remodeling, only symptomatic treatment is appropriate.

B. Rest and Traction: If joint motion is limited, bed rest and traction are employed to decrease synovitis and muscle spasm. Muscle releasing procedures may be required if contractures have developed. Once the hip is mobilized, containment of the femoral head within the acetabulum is necessary to maintain its spherical shape. If it is allowed to extrude laterally from the acetabulum, it will become deformed.

C. Bracing: Containment can be achieved with bracing, which should be maintained until reossification is under way; an average of 18 months is required.

D. Surgical Treatment: An alternative to prolonged bracing is surgery to reorient the acetabulum or the proximal femur to achieve containment. Both innominate osteotomy and varus proximal femoral osteotomy have advocates. Surgical containment properly achieved appears to be as effective as containment by bracing and to be much more expeditious.

Prognosis

Prolonged follow-up is necessary to determine the outcome. Poor results on x-rays do correlate positively with pain, limited motion, and disability. However, the affected hip may not be symptomatic for years. If Legg-Perthes disease of all degrees of severity is untreated, 55% of patients report good results and 45% report fair and poor results. If group I patients are excluded, the figures can be reversed. Following osteotomy of selected patients with more severe disease, two-thirds or more are reported to have a favorable outcome.

Joseph B: Morphological changes in the acetabulum in Perthes' disease. J Bone Joint Surg [Br] 1989;71:756.

Price CT et al: Behavioral sequelae of bracing versus surgery for Legg-Calvé-Perthes disease. J Pediatr Orthop 1988;8:285.

Salter RB: The present status of surgical treatment for Legg-Perthes disease. J Bone Joint Surg [Am] 1984;66:961.

Stulberg SD et al: The natural history of Legg-Calvé-Perthes disease. J Bone Joint Surg [Am] 1981;63:1095.

Thompson GH et al: Legg-Calvé-Perthes disease: Current concepts and controversies. Orthop Clin North Am 1987;18:617.

FOOT DEFORMITIES IN CHILDREN

Positional deformities of the foot are described with the following specific terms. **Equinus** refers to plantar flexion. **Calcaneus** is the opposite position, or dorsiflexion. **Varus** indicates angulation in the frontal plane, with inversion of the involved part. The forefoot alone may be in varus, or the deformity may be present in the hindfoot as well. **Valgus** is the opposite of varus and implies eversion of the involved part. **Inversion** and **eversion** of the forefoot (metatarsus) describe rotation about the long axis of the foot. **Adduction** of the forefoot is used to differentiate deviation of the metatarsals toward the medial side of the foot, without the rotational component suggested by the term varus.

The goal of treatment of foot deformity is a pain-free, flexible, **plantigrade** foot—ie, a foot whose plantar surface is level with the ground during normal gait.

1. CLUBFOOT

Talipes equinovarus, or clubfoot, is most commonly an idiopathic congenital condition affecting approximately one in 1000 children. It occurs twice as often in boys and is bilateral half the time. There is a familial tendency, with a 5% chance that a sibling will also be affected.

Clinical Findings

A. Symptoms and Signs: In congenital clubfoot, there is more or less rigid inversion of the hindfoot, adduction of the forefoot, and limited dorsiflexion—an equinovarus deformity. While the cause is not certain, the deformity involves medial subluxation of the navicular and calcaneus on the talus. The joints principally involved are thus the subtalar and talonavicular joints. The adjacent ankle and midtarsal joints are affected to a lesser degree. The overlying soft tissues are contracted, and the longer the subluxation remains, the more deformed become the involved bones, which are composed largely of malleable cartilage. Successful treatment requires early reduction of joint subluxations and maintenance of correction throughout growth.

B. Imaging Studies: X-rays are useful primarily for assessing the adequacy of correction rather than for establishing the diagnosis of clubfoot. At birth, only the ossific nuclei of the calcaneus, talus, and metatarsals are present. Navicular ossification does not begin until about age 4. Therefore, radiographs of the newborn foot provide less information than the clinical examination. A good photograph documents the deformity more adequately. By 2–3 months of age, the ossification centers of the talus and calcaneus have elongated sufficiently to indicate their long axes, so that radiographs can provide helpful data about interosseous relationships. An anteroposterior view of a normal foot shows divergence of the talus and calcaneus, the former directed along the first ray and the latter along the fifth ray. In clubfoot, the talus usually points more laterally and may actually appear superimposed upon the calcaneus. On a lateral radiograph of a normal foot in maximal dorsiflexion, the calcaneus is dorsiflexed, so that its axis crosses that of the navicular, and the anterior ends of their shadows overlap. Clubfoot prevents this dorsiflexion and overlapping. Full calcaneal dorsiflexion is a valuable radiographic indicator of adequate treatment.

Treatment

Initial treatment is always nonoperative and should be started as soon as possible, preferably the day the child is born.

A. Manipulation: Gentle manipulation into a corrected position should be done in order to stretch the contracted soft tissues—specifically, to align the calcaneus and navicular relative to the talus. Gentleness is required to avoid tissue trauma and to prevent overcorrection of the forefoot relative to persisting tarsal deformity.

B. Casting: After several minutes of manipulation, a plaster cast is applied and molded to maintain the maximally corrected position. Manipulation and cast application should be repeated weekly.

Casts are advisable for at least 6 months, followed by a Denis Browne bar with attached out flare shoes. Similar shoes are worn when the child begins to walk, but the Denis Browne bar should be continued at night and nap time for several more years. During this time, close follow-up is required, with immediate use of a plaster cast if deformity recurs. Correction achieved by age 7 years is usually permanent. Carefully and conscientiously pursued, nonoperative treatment has been sufficient to correct clubfoot deformity in 35–90% of cases in large series. If satisfactory correction has not been achieved by age 3 months, operative management should be considered.

C. Surgical Treatment: Operations for clubfoot are many and varied. The present trend is toward a single combined procedure to release all of the posteromedial contracted tissues and permit open realignment of the talonavicular and talocalcaneal joints. Temporary percutaneous wire fixation is advocated by some surgeons. Postoperative care requires persistent follow-up and prolonged support in a plaster cast, splints, and special shoes. Satisfactory results from posteromedial release are reported in 75–85% of patients. Triple arthrodesis and other surgical procedures provide salvage for symptomatic patients in whom posteromedial release does not provide good results.

Carroll NC: Congenital clubfoot: Pathoanatomy and treatment. Instr Course Lect 1987;36:117.
Cummings RJ et al: Operative treatment of congenital idiopathic club foot. J Bone Joint Surg [Am] 1988;70:1108.

2. METATARSUS ADDUCTUS

The terms "metatarsus varus" and "metatarsus adductus" are used more or less interchangeably for deformity characterized by medial "hooking" of the forefoot. The adduction is at the tarsometatarsal joint, and the hindfoot is either in neutral position or in valgus. Metatarsus adductus is somewhat commoner than clubfoot and seems to have a stronger familial tendency. The deformity is often quite mobile. If passively correctable, there is an 85% chance of spontaneous correction by age 3 years. No treatment is required if stroking of the lateral border of the foot provokes active correction. Easy passive correction also suggests that treatment is unnecessary. If the forefoot cannot readily be returned to a normal position, restoring a concave lateral border to the foot, treatment is advisable. The surgeon stabilizes the hindfoot with one hand while manipulating the forefoot to correct the deformity with the other hand. A well-molded plaster cast is applied to maintain this position. The cast is changed every 1–2 weeks for 6–8 weeks, followed by night splints for several months. Only a very rare severe deformity will require surgical release or osteotomy and fusion of the tarsometatarsal joints.

Berg EE: A reappraisal of metatarsus adductus and skewfoot. J Bone Joint Surg [Am] 1986;68:1185.
Cook DA et al: Observer variability in the radiographic measurement and classification of metatarsus adductus J Pediatr Orthop 1992;12:86.

3. FLATFOOT

The normal newborn foot appears flat because subcutaneous fat fills the longitudinal arch. This fat deposit recedes over the first 4 years of life to reveal the typical adult appearance of a medial arch under the midfoot, which does not contact the floor with weight bearing. An inadequate bony arch, which permits the medial portion of the midfoot to bear weight, is the essential feature of true flatfoot. This deformity is classified as rigid or flexible.

Rigid flatfoot is identified by the absence of normal mobility of the foot. Obvious deformity with convexity of the sole is present in congenital convex pes valgus, where congenital dorsal dislocation of the talonavicular joint is the cause. Early open reduction is advisable. Rigid flatfoot presenting later in childhood is usually due to coalition of the tarsal bones. Associated episodic foot pain and spasm of the peroneal muscles are typical. Depending on the child's age and symptoms and the site of coalition, resection may be advisable or nonoperative treatment may suffice.

In flexible flatfoot, weight bearing obliterates the medial arch and also produces obvious valgus alignment of the calcaneus. Standing on tiptoes or sitting with the feet hanging free will restore the arch and substantially correct heel valgus. Some patients with flexible flatfoot develop foot pain with weight bearing. Pain may range from minimal to severely incapacitating and is not clearly related to the severity of the deformity.

Treatment of asymptomatic flexible flatfoot in children is controversial. Parents distressed by the foot's appearance or by abnormal shoe wear often request treatment, but there is little evidence that it prevents future symptoms, and many young children with flexible flatfoot have minimal deformity or symptoms in adulthood. The child with painful flexible flatfoot deformity deserves treatment. Exercises to stretch tight gastrosoleus muscle groups or strengthen intrinsic plantar muscles are usually advised, and external support for the mediolongitudinal arch can be provided if necessary by flexible or rigid arch supports or shoe modifications. If nonoperative treatment fails to control symptoms or if deformity precludes use of normal footwear, surgery may be considered. Many procedures have been proposed. If present, an accessory navicular may be excised, with transposition of an abnormally inserted tibialis posterior tendon. Ligament reconstructions, arthrodeses, and osteotomies may be used separately or in combination to attempt restoration of the arch. A major risk of all such procedures is that a flexible deformity will be exchanged for a potentially more painful rigid one.

Chang FM: The flexible flatfoot. Instr Course Lect 1988; 37:109.
Crawford AH et al: Foot and ankle problems. Orthop Clin North Am 1987;18:649.
Marcinko DE, Azzolini TJ, Mariash SA: Enigma of pediatric vertical talus deformity. J Foot Surg 1990;29:452.
Salo JM et al: Congenital flat foot: Different clinical forms. Acta Orthop Belg 1992;58:406.

PAIN SYNDROMES

PAIN SYNDROMES OF THE SHOULDER

1. PAINFUL ARC SYNDROME (Rotator Cuff Tendinitis, Subacromial Bursitis)

Essentials of Diagnosis

- Pain over the anterior or lateral shoulder most marked during abduction.
- Restriction of joint motion.

General Considerations

Inflammation within the glenohumeral joint is the most frequent cause of shoulder pain and limitation of motion. The patient is typically middle-aged. Repeated minor trauma from occupational or sports activity is the cause, and the most common site of inflammation at onset is the rotator cuff, particularly the supraspinatus tendon. The location of the supraspinatus tendon between the greater tuberosity of the humeral head and the overhanging acromion process renders it particularly vulnerable to mechanical compression. Rotator cuff inflammation will often spill over into the subacromial bursa, and subdeltoid soreness frequently radiates along the lateral humerus to the deltoid insertion.

Clinical Findings

Active abduction becomes especially painful when the shoulder moves between 60 and 120 degrees, because the inflamed rotator cuff and overlying bursa are compressed beneath the acromion. Because of this characteristic feature, the condition is known as painful arc syndrome. The range of active abduction may be extended if the patient is instructed to rotate the arms so that the palms face upward. This rotates the greater tuberosity posteriorly, so that the attached rotator cuff tendons pass behind the acromion, resulting in diminished pain with continued abduction.

Treatment

Treatment of rotator cuff tendinitis and subacromial bursitis is with analgesics, such as aspirin or nonsteroidal anti-inflammatory agents (naproxen, ibuprofen), and local application of cold packs. Physical therapy may be useful in preserving full range of motion. Slings and shoulder immobilization should not be used for more than a few days, since capsular adhesions and prolonged stiffness may result. Gentle passive range-of-motion exercises by a therapist or family member should be started as soon as tolerated, followed by active pendulum exercises consisting of circular swinging motions of the dangling arm while leaning forward. Active exercise is gradually increased while passive range of motion is extended with exercises such as pulley-enhanced abduction using a bath towel over a shower curtain rod.

If pain does not respond to oral anti-inflammatory agents, prolonged relief may be obtained by injecting 40 mg of methylprednisolone acetate (or equivalent) and 1–2 mL of lidocaine into the subacromial bursa. The patient should be warned that injection may produce a brief exacerbation of pain before relief is noted and should be provided with analgesic medications. When full function has been recovered, reduction of stressful activities should be advised.

2. CALCIFIC TENDINITIS

Essentials of Diagnosis
- Excruciating shoulder pain.
- Severe restriction of joint motion.

General Considerations
Calcium deposition in the degenerative rotator cuff may lead to a variant form of tendinitis in the shoulder region. Asymptomatic bilateral calcium deposits in the shoulder tissues are a common finding in persons over age 40. The pathogenesis is unclear. The deposits may enlarge or rupture into the subacromial bursa.

Clinical Findings
A. Symptoms and Signs: The presentation of acute calcific tendinitis or bursitis is dramatic, with excruciating pain and severe restriction of shoulder motion. The patient may refuse even the gentlest examination for fear of motion-induced muscle spasm.

B. Imaging Studies: X-rays reveal either focal calcium deposits within the rotator cuff or a large "cap" of calcium overlying the humeral head, which represents dissemination of calcium into the subacromial bursa.

Treatment
Treatment of acute calcific tendinitis includes immediate injection of a corticosteroid and lidocaine solution into the tendon near the calcium deposit or into the bursa if calcium has entered that structure. Multiple needle punctures into the calcium deposit may break up the deposit and provide dramatic relief. Mobilization of the shoulder should proceed as described in the preceding section.

3. BICEPS TENDINITIS

Essentials of Diagnosis
- Localized tenderness over the bicipital groove.
- Pain during supination of the forearm against resistance.

General Considerations
A common inflammatory lesion producing shoulder pain involves the biceps tendon in the bicipital groove. Biceps tendon inflammation usually affects individuals whose occupation involves repetitive biceps flexion against resistance or whose recreational activities include forceful throwing of a ball. Pain is prominent over the anterior aspect of the arm and is aggravated by shoulder motion. Symptoms are worse at night and improve with rest. Deltoid muscle spasm may be present and may limit both active and passive motion.

Clinical Findings
Biceps tendinitis can be distinguished from rotator cuff tendinitis by localization of tenderness to the bicipital groove. Forearm supination against resistance with the elbow flexed at the patient's side elicits extreme tenderness in the region of the bicipital groove when the tendon is palpated near the shoulder. Instability of the tendon in the groove is occasionally manifested by a snapping sensation as the arm is abducted and externally rotated. Subluxation of the tendons can be provoked for diagnostic verification by Yergason's maneuver. The patient actively flexes the elbow against resistance while the physician rotates the humerus externally. An unstable tendon will "pop" out of the groove.

Treatment
Treatment of bicipital tendinitis includes cessation of offending activities and short-term immobilization of the shoulder in a sling; a trial of aspirin or nonsteroidal anti-inflammatory agents; and, occasionally, local injection of corticosteroids. Repeated corticosteroid injections may result in tendon attrition or rupture and should be avoided. Surgery is occasionally required to stabilize a subluxating tendon.

When discomfort has subsided, progressive mobilization in begun with exercises similar to those described in the section on rotator cuff tendinitis.

4. ADHESIVE CAPSULITIS (Frozen Shoulder)

Essentials of Diagnosis
- Diffuse shoulder tenderness.
- Restriction of shoulder joint motion.

General Considerations
A common cause of shoulder pain in middle-aged and elderly patients is adhesive capsulitis, or so-called frozen shoulder. This disorder may complicate other inflammatory shoulder ailments, particularly in individuals immobilized for prolonged periods. It may also occur without any identifiable inciting trauma and has been associated with cardiovascular disease, rheumatoid arthritis, and degenerative cervical spine disease. Though the exact pathogenesis is unknown, the end result is a chronically inflamed, contracted fibrotic capsule densely adherent to the humeral head, the acromion, and the underlying biceps and rotator cuff tendons. Normal bursae are obliterated by scarring.

Clinical Findings
A. Symptoms and Signs: The onset of symptoms is usually gradual and heralded by complaints of diffuse tenderness with disproportionately severe restriction of active and passive motion. Motion is not improved by lidocaine or corticosteroid injection.

B. Imaging Studies: Arthrography reveals a contracted joint capsule and no bursal filling. X-rays may reveal severe osteoporosis of the humeral head.

Treatment

The success of various treatments is difficult to assess, as the natural history of adhesive capsulitis is spontaneous resolution. Subsidence of pain and return of nearly full motion can be anticipated, although the process may persist for 6 months to several years. Efforts to speed return of function have included intensive physical therapy, oral corticosteroids and anti-inflammatory agents, and a procedure called infiltration brisement, which consists of pressure injection of the joint with 50 mL of saline and corticosteroid solution in order to break the adhesions binding the capsule to the surrounding structures.

Clearly, the best treatment of this condition is prevention. Prolonged disuse or immobilization of a painful shoulder must be avoided. Early mobilization is stressed, with initiation of gentle range-of-motion exercises and persistent encouragement and guidance by the physician and the therapist.

Ekelund AL, Rydell N: Combination treatment for adhesive capsulitis of the shoulder. Clin Orthop 1992;Sep(282): 105.
Ozaki J et al: Recalcitrant chronic adhesive capsulitis of the shoulder: Role of contracture of the coracohumeral ligament and rotator interval in pathogenesis and treatment [see comments]. J Bone Joint Surg [Am] 1989;71:1511.

PAIN SYNDROMES OF THE ELBOW

1. TENNIS ELBOW (Humeral Epicondylitis)

Essentials of Diagnosis

- Tenderness over the lateral humeral epicondyle.
- Pain at the elbow with flexion or extension of the wrist.

General Considerations

Though far more common in nonathletes, humeral epicondylitis is commonly termed tennis elbow. This overuse syndrome is uncommon before age 18 years and most frequent in the fourth or fifth decade. Though frequently blamed on faulty backhand motion, tennis elbow is occasionally seen in professional players but is far more common in nonathletes performing activities that require frequent rotary motion of the forearm, such as gardening, use of screwdrivers or wrenches, turning of doorknobs, and even operation of vehicles without power steering.

Clinical Findings

Tennis elbow is characterized by tenderness and

pain at the humeral epicondyle provoked by extension or flexion of the wrist, depending on which epicondyle is involved. The lateral aspect of the elbow is far more often involved, and the origin of the inflamed common extensor muscle is the source of discomfort. Underlying synovitis may accompany the tendinitis. The pain is readily reproduced with traction on the extensor muscles by passive flexion of the fingers and wrist with the elbow extended.

Though the pathogenesis of tennis elbow is unknown, symptoms are usually attributed to inflammation of the origin of the common extensor muscle and, in some cases, to a tear in the origin of the extensor carpi radialis brevis. The tears are thought to be the result of repeated stress on degenerated tendon fibers. Elbow motion remains normal.

Differential Diagnosis

Differential diagnosis includes radial nerve irritation at the elbow, which may often be delineated by electromyography.

Treatment

A. Medical Treatment: Most patients with tennis elbow respond favorably to a brief period of rest and administration of analgesics followed by a program of gradually increasing exercise to strengthen the forearm muscles. Anti-inflammatory drugs or subtendinous injection of soluble corticosteroids with lidocaine may be required in more severe cases. Repeated injections may further weaken tendons and should be avoided.

After the acute symptoms subside, a nonelastic forearm band is prescribed to be worn near the elbow during occupational or recreational activities that aggravate the condition. The band is thought to be effective either because it limits full contraction of the tender muscles or because it slightly alters the position of the extensor tendons. Tennis players are advised to warm up slowly. Changes in the tension of racket strings and racket size or composition may also be of benefit.

B. Surgical Treatment: Some patients with severe or refractory symptoms may require operative treatment. Most surgeons repair the origin of the torn wrist extensor tendon after excision of granulation tissue and any rough subjacent bone. Lengthening of the short wrist extensor has also been advocated, though loss of strength has been reported with this procedure.

2. OLECRANON BURSITIS

Essentials of Diagnosis

- Tenderness and swelling over the olecranon.
- Limitation of elbow flexion.

General Considerations

Olecranon bursitis is a common cause of periarticular elbow pain. Like epicondylitis, this condition is often related to occupational activities, in this case prolonged periods of leaning on the elbow while studying ("student's elbow"), gardening, working on plumbing, or carpentry.

Clinical Findings

A. Symptoms and Signs: The subcutaneous olecranon bursa becomes distended, sometimes to dramatic proportions. The skin of the extensor surface of the forearm may be edematous and pitted. Traumatic bursitis is often only mildly painful despite marked swelling.

B. Laboratory Findings: Because of the tenderness of the skin over the bursa, elbow motion is limited only in extreme flexion. Fluid obtained by aspiration demonstrates a predominance of mononuclear cells, with fewer than 1000 white cells per microliter. Red cells are numerous, and mucin clot formation is poor. Strict aseptic technique is advised during aspiration of the bursa, as superinfection is common after multiple aspirations. Penetration of the inner wall of the cavity must be avoided; in septic olecranon bursitis, penetration may result in inoculation of bacteria into the underlying triceps tendon, leading to disastrous extension of infection into the posterior aspect of the arm.

Differential Diagnosis

Laboratory findings will differentiate septic olecranon bursitis, in which aspiration fluid demonstrates a predominance of PMNs in far greater numbers. Gout may affect the olecranon bursa, but urate crystals are present.

Treatment

Treatment of idiopathic or traumatic olecranon bursitis consists of protecting the bursa from further pressure or irritation. Aspiration and compression dressings may be necessary if symptoms are prolonged. Recurrence is not uncommon. Water-soluble corticosteroid injection may be helpful once infection has been ruled out as a possible cause. Excision of the bursa may be required for rare persistent cases. The bursa must be totally excised and the overlying skin sutured to the olecranon periosteum to ensure obliteration of the space.

Labelle H et al: Lack of scientific evidence for the treatment of lateral epicondylitis of the elbow: An attempted meta-analysis. J Bone Joint Surg [Br] 1992;74:646.

Wittenberg RH, Schaal S, Muhr G: Surgical treatment of persistent elbow epicondylitis. Clin Orthop 1992; May(278):73.

PAIN SYNDROMES OF THE HIP

1. BURSITIS & TENDINITIS OF THE HIP

Essentials of Diagnosis

- Localized tenderness over the greater trochanter.
- Pain with external rotation or abduction of the hip.

General Considerations

Bursitis and tendinitis around the hip are commonly mistaken for intra-articular hip joint disease. Tendinitis of the gluteus medius and minimus at their insertions into the greater trochanter is frequent cause of pain in middle-aged and elderly patients. Inflammation in the region of the tendon insertions usually involves the overlying trochanteric bursa as well, with localized tenderness over the posterolateral trochanteric prominence.

Clinical Findings

Patients present with complaints of hip pain, often most severe in external rotation, with radiation of pain down the lateral aspect of the thigh. Occasionally, there is warmth or erythema of the skin overlying the greater trochanter, and the bursa may feel boggy when palpated.

Differential Diagnosis

Because pain in the buttock and thigh is frequently referred from the lumbar spine, degenerative disk disease and sciatica must be excluded in the workup of trochanteric bursitis. In bursitis, pain is localized with palpation of the trochanteric bursa and straight leg raising is rarely painful. Differentiation of bursitis from intra-articular hip joint disease is also important. Pain from hip joint disease may be referred to the buttock, thigh, or knee but is most commonly felt in the groin. Extreme internal rotation of the hip will often provoke substantial pain in a diseased hip but only slight pain in a hip with bursitis. Forceful percussion with the first over the heel of the extended lower extremity will also aggravate a diseased hip joint but not an inflamed trochanteric bursa.

Treatment

Treatment of the inflamed bursa is symptomatic, with rest and anti-inflammatory medication. Injection of the bursa with a water-soluble corticosteroid and lidocaine often produces lasting relief. If injection therapy is elected, it is helpful to begin with injection of lidocaine alone and leave the needle in place. Pain relief after several moments is further proof of the presence of bursitis. Corticosteroid injection is then made through the same needle. Pain should subside over 48–72 hours, though repeat injection may occasionally be necessary.

2. AVASCULAR NECROSIS OF THE FEMORAL HEAD

Structural deformities may also cause pain in the adult hip joint. Though degenerative arthritis is the usual cause, less common primary deformity of the joint is also encountered.

Avascular necrosis of the femoral head is a disease process that involves the microcirculation within the bone. The most frequent cause of vascular insufficiency within the femoral head is trauma. Hip dislocation and fractures of the femoral neck often result in disruption of the intracapsular retinacular blood vessels that supply the femoral head (Figure 43–62).

A more perplexing entity is so-called primary, or nontraumatic, avascular necrosis. Several systemic diseases have been associated with death of bone within the femoral head, including hypercortisolism (exogenous or endogenous), alcoholism and liver disease, hemoglobinopathy, gout, hyperlipidemia, diabetes, Gaucher's disease, and decompression sickness in divers and caisson workers. Men are more often affected than women.

Though vascular insufficiency within the femoral head is the common denominator among these conditions, the cause has not yet been established. Hypotheses include fat or gas microemboli and interosseous venous hypertension involving the terminal blood vessels within the head. The pathologic process begins with the anoxic death of osteocytes within the avascular area (stage I). The bone remains structurally sound because the mineralized noncellular elements retain their strength. The patient is asymptomatic, and x-rays appear normal. Cell death apparently incites a healing reaction that includes ingrowth of vascular tissues from uninvolved portions of the femoral head. In stage II disease, revascularization proceeds with laying down of new bone by osteoblasts and resorption of anoxic bone by osteoclasts. X-rays show a sclerotic segment within the head. Bone resorption may outstrip new bone formation, with resulting loss of strength. The stress of weight bearing creates microfractures within the weakened healing region. This stage is often accompanied by pain and the appearance of a lucent zone beneath the subchondral bone on x-ray. Typically located in the anterolateral portion of the head, the lucent zone represents segmental collapse of the weakened trabeculae, and there is progressive deformation of the weakened head. This results in further circulatory embarrassment followed by infarction and sequestration of cortical bone in the subchondral area, and, ultimately, death of the overlying joint cartilage. X-rays of stage III (end-stage) avascular necrosis show a flattened sclerotic femoral head with grossly irregular contours and joint space narrowing from loss of articular cartilage on the femoral head.

Clinical Findings

A. Symptoms and Signs: The clinical presentation of nontraumatic avascular necrosis depends upon the stage of disease. Stage I disease—the anoxic phase—is frequently asymptomatic. If pain is present in this stage, it is quite mild and usually exacerbated by internal rotation.

B. Imaging Studies: X-rays show no abnormalities. The patient is frequently reassured that the hip is fine but returns with advanced disease some months later.

During stage II, the revascularization phase, sclerosis or a lucent line appears on x-rays where subchondral collapse has occurred. Pain and limitation of motion are generally mild. Though widely variant rates of progression have been reported, once these x-ray changes are apparent, untreated hips will typically deteriorate further, ultimately reaching stage III collapse with irreversible arthrosis and severe disability. Unfortunately, because of relatively mild symptoms in the early stages of this disease, most patients are diagnosed in the later stages, when treatment is limited to salvage of function rather than arrest of disease.

C. Laboratory Findings: Of particular significance in the management of avascular necrosis is the high incidence of bilaterality—reported in one-third to two-thirds of cases. The stage of involvement is usually more advanced in one hip than in the other, and preradiographic involvement of the opposite "silent" hip must therefore be assessed. This is best ac-

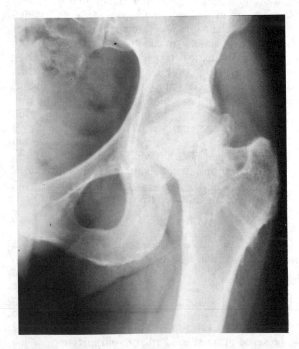

Figure 43–62. Avascular necrosis of the femoral head. Collapse of the femoral head caused by damage to the blood supply from a femoral neck fracture 2 years earlier.

complished with technetium bone scanning (uptake may be diminished in the anoxic stage I hip before any change is apparent on x-ray) or by CT scanning. MRI has recently proved to demonstrate very early changes in fat and bone marrow, making it an excellent diagnostic tool in the early stages of avascular necrosis. In more advanced disease, revascularization is indicated by increased uptake of technetium on bone scan. Intraosseous pressure testing and intraosseous venography may reveal venous hypertension and poor venous drainage of contrast from the affected hip. These techniques are experimental and currently available in relatively few institutions.

Treatment

Treatment of nontraumatic avascular necrosis of the femoral head varies according to the age of the patient and the stage of disease. In the early stages, protection of the involved femoral head from weight-bearing forces may arrest progression of the disease. Variable results have been reported with a surgical procedure involving "core decompression" of involved hips. With this procedure, the abnormally high venous pressure within the avascular femoral head is lowered. A hollow reaming device is introduced into the femoral neck and head to remove a cored column of bone. The patient is then protected with non-weight-bearing ambulation for a minimum of 6 weeks. Preliminary studies indicate that arrest of disease progression may be possible with this technique, particularly if it is performed in the earlier stages.

In patients with limited head involvement, rotation osteotomy of the femoral head and neck may bring normal cartilage and bone weight-bearing position and reduce the weight-bearing forces on the necrotic area. This procedure is technically demanding but has been employed successfully in some centers.

In older patients and those with profound disability, replacement arthroplasty is the procedure of choice. Replacement may involve only the femoral head or may include both the head and the acetabulum, depending upon the extent of cartilage involvement. In younger patients, conservative measures should be exhausted before joint replacement is attempted.

Experiments with electrical stimulation are currently under way. Early indications suggest that healing of avascular bone may be accelerated by electric current generated by external coils worn over the involved hip joint.

Howie DW, Cornish BL, Vernon-Roberts B: The viability of the femoral head after resurfacing hip arthroplasty in humans. corr3;Jun(291):171.

Lafforgue P et al: Early-stage avascular necrosis of the femoral head: MR imaging for prognosis in 31 cases with at least 2 years of follow-up. Radiology 1993;3;187:199.

Sadat-Ali M: Avascular necrosis of the femoral head in sickle cell disease: An integrated classification. Clin Orthop 1993;May(290):200.

Swiontkowski MF et al: The effect of fracture on femoral head blood flow: Osteonecrosis and revascularization studied in miniature swine. Acta Orthop Scand 1993; 3;64:196.

Takatori Y et al: Avascular necrosis of the femoral head: Natural history and magnetic resonance imaging. J Bone Joint Surg [Br] 1993;75:217.

CERVICAL PAIN SYNDROMES

1. CERVICAL STRAIN

Essentials of Diagnosis

- Paraspinous neck pain with or without radiation to the shoulder.
- Limitation of neck rotation.

General Considerations

Neck pain is a common complaint in most outpatient clinics. It has been estimated that at any given time in the general population, one of every ten persons is suffering from neck and arm pain. Taking all ages together, 40% of all persons have suffered from neck and arm pain at some time. In most cases, symptoms are mild and self-limited.

Cervical muscle strain is perhaps the most frequent cause. Patients are usually in the fourth or fifth decade. History reveals that pain arose within 24 hours following an episode of overexertion. Prolonged tension or poor posture may also generate symptoms.

Clinical Findings

A. Symptoms and Signs: Pain is most intense in the paraspinous muscles, within the superior trapezius fibers between the spine and the scapula, or at the periosteal site of muscle attachments in the scapula or occiput. Discomfort is characterized as deep aching or boring, and pain may occasionally radiate to the posterior shoulder or upper arm. Discrete "trigger points"—specific points of deep tenderness—may be present. Spasm within the trapezius, levator scapulae, or paraspinous muscles may be palpable as a firm "knot." The neck is held in a guarded position, with canting of the head. Active and passive motion of the neck is often limited in all planes owing to voluntary splinting of the painful muscles, though rotation away from the afflicted side is most vigorously resisted by the patient. The patient may also complain of headache or dizziness. Reflexes, motor power, and sensation within the upper and lower extremities are normal.

B. Imaging Studies: X-ray examination often reveals flattening of the normal cervical lordosis. Mild or severe degenerative changes may be present, including osteophytes of the vertebral bodies or posterior facets.

Differential Diagnosis

The differential diagnosis includes degenerative or prolapsed disk with or without cervical spondylosis. Cervical disk syndrome is easily distinguished from cervical muscle strain when accompanied by predominant radicular symptoms, including numbness or paresthesias, muscle weakness or wasting, and diminished reflexes. However, acute cervical disk degeneration is often accompanied by symptoms indistinguishable from those of cervical strain. Some authors attribute pain to stretching of the well-innervated posterior annulus or posterior longitudinal ligament by a bulging cervical disk. Whatever the precise anatomic source of pain, distinguishing cervical muscle sprain from early degenerative disk symptoms is of little importance, since both conditions are usually self-limited and require only conservative management.

Treatment

Treatment of acute cervical spine pain consists primarily of rest and immobilization. If pain is severe, traction on the neck may be required to control spasm. Halter traction with 2.5–3.5 kg (5–7 lb) may be used conveniently at home by most patients. Hospitalization is reserved for those who fail to respond to therapy at home. Analgesics and muscle relaxants are prescribed as needed to facilitate rest. Injection of trigger points with 0.5% lidocaine may help to break up spasm. Heating pads may also diminish discomfort.

Severe neck pain often subsides within 1 week. Mobilization may then be facilitated by the use of a soft cervical collar that holds the head in a slightly flexed position. The collar is worn full time initially, and as pain diminishes, the patient is gradually weaned from the collar over a period of 1–2 weeks. Prolonged use of a collar should be avoided, as atrophy of cervical muscles as well as deleterious psychologic dependence may result. When acute pain has subsided, the patient should begin exercises to strengthen cervical muscles and improve posture. Exercises are isometric and may be performed at home after instruction by the therapist. When all pain has resolved, range-of-motion exercises are added to improve flexibility.

Prevention of flare-ups also depends upon maintenance of good posture with avoidance of overhead work, long automobile rides, or prolonged cervical flexion and extension posture. Patients are cautioned to avoid sleeping in the prone position, which places the neck in excessive rotation. A cylindric pillow may help to keep the neck in neutral position during sleep.

Course & Prognosis

The prognosis in cervical pain syndrome not associated with disk degeneration is good if the above measures are undertaken. Symptoms may recur, but early institution of home traction and avoidance of offending activities greatly limit the duration of pain.

2. WHIPLASH INJURY

Essentials of Diagnosis

- Pain in paraspinous muscles radiating to arms.
- Occipital headache.
- Limitation of neck rotation.

General Considerations

A well-known type of soft tissue injury of the neck is the acceleration-extension injury called whiplash. The mechanism is most often a rear-end automobile collision. The trunk of the victim's body is rapidly accelerated by the force of impact and the head is "left behind" because of lack of head contact with the seat. Acute hyperextension overstretches the neck flexors and anterior ligaments, producing fiber tearing. The longus colli and sternocleidomastoid muscles are particularly vulnerable. The cervical sympathetic plexus may also be torn. When acceleration of the car stops, the head recoils into flexion.

Clinical Findings

A. Symptoms and Signs: The symptom complex following whiplash injury is highly variable. Onset of pain may be delayed as long as 24 hours. Pain may be located in the neck, shoulders, or interscapular region and often radiates down the arms. Occipital headache and retro-ocular pain are also frequent sequelae. The presence of numbness in the medial hand and forearm has been attributed to scalenus muscle spasm. Visual blurring may result from stretch injury to the cervical sympathetic plexus, and, rarely, Horner's syndrome may occur. Dysphagia may represent retropharyngeal hematoma or swelling. Vertebral artery spasm occasionally causes tinnitus, dizziness, and vertigo. When the neck is rotated at the time of injury, symptoms are more pronounced on the side toward which the head is turned.

Physical findings are usually attributable to muscle spasm and only rarely to nerve root compression or disk herniation. Spasm is manifested by diminished neck motion and predominant anterior paracervical tenderness to palpation. Posterolateral pain may occur if articular facet joint damage is present. Neurologic examination, including testing of reflexes and muscle strength, is typically normal.

B. Imaging Studies: X-rays are generally unremarkable. Care must be taken to avoid overlooking subtle hyperextension injuries, such as widening of an anterior disk space, avulsion fractures of the anterior vertebral body, retropharyngeal swelling, or fracture of the posterior facet. Loss of cervical lordosis may imply spasm but may also be artifactual. Reversal of cervical lordosis, resulting in an S-shaped (swan-neck) deformity, signifies damage to the posterior joints.

Treatment

Management of acceleration extension sprains is as for other soft tissue injuries (ie, analgesics, rest, and immobilization until pain is controlled, followed by gradual mobilization with cervical collar support). Isometric strengthening exercises are initiated when range of motion returns to normal.

Course & Prognosis

Most patients respond well to conservative measures, though anticipated litigation may complicate management. Many patients become asymptomatic following settlement of lawsuits. Degenerative changes in the cervical spine and minor neck discomfort are more common following whiplash injuries, but persistent pain and prolonged disability are unusual.

3. DEGENERATIVE CERVICAL DISK DISEASE (Cervical Spondylosis)

Essentials of Diagnosis

- Neck pain radiating down the arm.
- Muscle weakness.
- Dermatomal sensory changes.

General Considerations

The degenerative changes typically associated with aging are collectively termed spondylosis of the cervical spine. Men and women are affected equally. Among persons over age 50, radiologic signs of degeneration of the cervical spine are extremely common. It is estimated that by the seventh decade, 75% of individuals demonstrate such degeneration, though most are asymptomatic. Disk degeneration is therefore considered a natural aging phenomenon.

Cervical spondylosis is characterized initially by tears in the posterior annulus, followed by softening and fragmentation of the disk. The weakest area of the annulus is the posterolateral region, which is the commonest site of bulging of the disk. The hydrostatic support provided by the degenerating disk steadily diminishes, and the adjacent vertebral bodies converge. The longitudinal ligaments become lax and are stripped from their bony attachments by the bulging disks. Degenerative calcification of the ligaments produces the familiar bony spurs. The ligamentum flavum also becomes lax and may bulge into the spinal canal. The posterolateral regions of the vertebral bodies become closely approximated and ultimately form an area of friction. These so-called uncoverte-

bral joints of Luschka become increasingly hypertrophic, creating prominent spurs that may ultimately extend across the entire posterior rim of the vertebral body and produce a bony bar projecting into the neural canal.

As the vertebral bodies converge because of loss of disk support, the facet joints become subluxated as the superior facet slides posteriorly. Mechanical dysfunction of the joints results in osteoarthritic degeneration and osteophyte formation. Osteophytes about the facets may project into the intervertebral foramina and impinge upon the exiting nerve roots.

Pathogenesis & Clinical Findings

A. Symptoms and Signs: Clinical symptoms may or may not accompany the degenerative changes of cervical spondylosis. Neurologic compromise may result from nerve root compression (cervical spondylotic radiculopathy) or compression of the cord itself (cervical spondylotic myelopathy). Vertebral artery and radicular artery constriction may also result from osteophyte formation, leading to vertebrobasilar insufficiency or cervical cord ischemia.

1. Cervical spondylotic radiculopathy—Cervical spondylotic radiculopathy results from pressure on a nerve root as it emerges from the cord to pass peripherally through the intervertebral foramen. The prolapsed disk is usually the offending agent, with additional pressure created by edema and by osteophytes projecting from the uncovertebral and facet joints. The onset of symptoms may be acute or insidious. Pain in the neck with radiation into the intrascapular area and arm is the chief complaint.

2. Cervical spondylotic myelopathy—Direct compression of the spinal cord may lead to cervical spondylotic myelopathy. This demyelinating process usually corresponds to the level of a spondylotic ridge that deforms the cord. Degenerative changes in the lateral columns may ascend and descend, and central gray matter necrosis may also occur. Multisegmental lesions may exist, making accurate localization difficult. Intermittent vascular compression by spondylotic osteophytes may cause altered arterial inflow and venous congestion in vessels supplying the cord, contributing to more generalized cord damage and further complicating attempts to localize the disease process. Pressure on the cervical cord may also be attributed to a thickened ligamentum flavum that folds into the canal with cervical extension. When spondylotic osteophytes are present, the cord may be pinched between the osteophytes and the ligamentum flavum during extension. This may be particularly important in cases of myelopathy associated with hyperextension injuries.

The incidence of cervical spondylotic myelopathy is twice as great in men as in women. The onset of symptoms is usually gradual, but an abrupt onset can be associated with extension injuries. The usual age at onset is between 40 and 60 years.

When symptoms of myelopathy come on gradually, the patient usually complains of "numbness" in the arms and legs and often of clumsiness and burning in the hands and difficulty in handling small objects. Walking is difficult. Diffuse, nonlocalized "pins and needles" in the forearm and anterior thigh are also typical. Neck pain may be present or absent, but neck motion is frequently limited. Progression of symptoms is sporadic. Remission is common but incomplete. A few patients demonstrate steadily progressive deterioration leading to spastic paraplegia or quadriplegia.

When myelopathy is precipitated by trauma, symptoms are similar to those described above. Onset is abrupt, and central cord involvement is typical. Limb involvement is usually more symmetric, with more marked weakness in the arms and hands. The acute injury generally subsides, though neurologic deficits frequently persist. Central disk herniation may follow cervical trauma but rarely causes myelopathy.

Physical examination of patients with spondylotic myelopathy is characterized by marked motor findings and relatively few sensory changes. Spasticity is present in the upper and lower extremities. Clonus and hyperreflexia are common though often asymmetric. Long-tract signs, including positive Babinski and Hoffman signs, may be present. Fine motion of the fingers is often lacking, and intrinsic muscle wasting may be profound. Generalized muscle wasting and weakness are less common. Sphincter control is generally preserved, though mild difficulty with micturition is common. Impotence is common. Vibration sensation in the lower extremities may be diminished.

B. Imaging Studies: The roentgenographic changes in cervical spondylosis include narrowing of the disk space, seen most clearly on a lateral projection. Osteophyte formation at the vertebral body margins and in particular at the posterolateral uncovertebral joints is best observed on an anteroposterior projection. Arthritic degeneration of the facet joints with osteophyte formation is best demonstrated in oblique views. The highest incidence of degeneration is observed in segments C5–6 because of the concentration of mechanical forces in this region. C6–7 is the next most common level.

Myelography may demonstrate indentation of the dye column by spondylotic osteophytes projecting into the anterior canal and by an infolded ligamentum flavum during cervical extension. Electromyography may be useful to demonstrate generalized motor impairment resulting from motor neuron involvement.

Differential Diagnosis

A. Cervical Spondylotic Radiculopathy: The syndrome is difficult to distinguish from cervical muscle strain unless there are objective radicular signs, such as muscle atrophy and sensory changes in a dermatomal distribution.

B. Cervical Spondylotic Myelopathy: Differential diagnosis includes spondylotic radiculopathy, spinal tumor, syringomyelia, primary motor neuron disorders, and multiple sclerosis. Radiculopathy is common in association with myelopathy. Upper motor neuron involvement producing spasticity in the extremities distinguishes myelopathy with radiculopathy from isolated radiculopathy, in which pain and weakness in the extremity are limited to the specific neural segment involved. Radiculopathy is aggravated by neck motion and is associated with more profound dermatomal sensory loss. Multiple sclerosis tends to occur in younger patients, with a peak onset between ages 20 and 40 years, and seldom appears for the first time after age 50 years. Though many of the motor signs are similar, onset in multiple sclerosis is usually more abrupt. Cranial nerve palsies are common in multiple sclerosis, as is cerebellar dysarthria, giving rise to characteristic "scanning speech" (speech punctuated by long, regularly occurring pauses). Elevated cerebrospinal fluid IgG levels and abnormal visual evoked responses also accompany multiple sclerosis. Remission in multiple sclerosis is frequently more complete than in spondylotic myelopathy.

Neoplasm of the cervical cord is usually more profound and progressive. The segmental level is more discrete with spinal tumor, and cerebrospinal fluid protein is elevated. Loss of sphincter control is rare in spondylotic myelopathy and extremely common with neoplasms. Myelography often provides definitive evidence of tumor.

Treatment

A. Cervical Spondylotic Radiculopathy: Most patients with acute onset of cervical spondylotic radiculopathy will demonstrate regression of symptoms over 4–6 weeks. Progression to myelopathy is rare, and most patients require only rest, analgesics, and immobilization to control pain. Paresthesias and slight sensory changes may persist after neck and arm pain have subsided. Chronic symptoms may involve an element of nerve root inflammation that may require vigorous anti-inflammatory drug therapy.

If pain persists longer than expected, an extruded fragment of cervical disk may be lying within the intervertebral foramina. In these rare cases, cervical myelography should be performed to accurately localize the site of compression. Only when discrete herniation is documented should surgical decompression be performed, either with foraminotomy performed through a posterior approach or by complete removal of the involved cervical disk and osteophytes through an anterior approach followed by anterior interbody fusion.

B. Cervical Spondylotic Myelopathy: Management of cervical spondylotic myelopathy depends upon the course and severity of symptoms.

1. Medical measures–The management of slowly progressive disease in elderly patients is conservative, and a cervical collar for support is generally sufficient.

2. Surgical treatment–When symptoms are more profound or progressive despite use of a collar and when they occur in younger patients, operative treatment may be necessary. The anterior approach allows removal of spondylotic osteophytes after disk excision and also permits adequate foraminotomy. Anterior interbody fusion following decompression will diminish pathologic intervertebral motion. With multiple-level spondylosis and diffuse canal stenosis, the posterior approach may be elected, with cord decompression by excision of laminae and ligamenta flava at the affected levels. Laminectomy may be combined with opening of the dura and sectioning of the dentate ligaments that tether the sides of the spinal cord to the dura. This permits the cord to slacken and move backward, away from anterior osteophytes.

Course & Prognosis

A. Cervical Spondylotic Radiculopathy: The course is benign. Most cases resolve in 4–6 weeks with conservative management.

B. Cervical Spondylotic Myelopathy: In general, the results of surgical management of spondylotic myelopathy are better when symptoms are mild and of relatively shorter duration. However, complete postoperative resolution of symptoms is rare even in these cases. It is noteworthy that the natural evolution of spondylotic myelopathy will often produce at least partial spontaneous remission. Chronic myelopathy and multiple-level involvement are associated with poor surgical results, particularly in elderly individuals. Overall results appear to have improved with more recent application of anterior decompression and interbody fusion.

Evans RW: Some observations on whiplash injuries. Neurol Clin 1992;10:975.

Poggi JJ et: Cervical spondylolysis. J Spinal Disord 1992;5: 349.

Jonsson H Jr et al: Locking screw-plate fixation of cervical spine fractures with and without ancillary posterior plating. Arch Orthop Trauma Surg 1991;111:1.

LUMBAR PAIN SYNDROMES

1. LOW BACK PAIN

Essentials of Diagnosis

- Paraspinous low back pain aggravated by exertion.
- Radiation of pain into the buttock or thigh.

General Considerations

Low back pain is the cause of much time lost from work in the USA, with about 400,000 workers disabled by back pain each year. It has been estimated that 80% of the population suffers low back pain at some time. All physicians are called on at least occasionally to advise patients with this complaint, and a systematic approach is necessary to differentiate the numerous possible causes. Diagnosis and management can be frustrating, because the exact cause of most low back pain is uncertain and no cure is known. The first task is to identify the relatively few cases with specific causes that can be treated. The less rewarding and more demanding task is to provide long-term guidance and management for patients for whom specific remedies are unavailable.

Clinical Findings

A. Symptoms and Signs: The most common cause of low back pain is mechanical strain. Patients complain of pain related to overexertion. Pain may immediately follow lifting or other forms of exertion or may have a more insidious onset after prolonged physical activity. Many patients in this group demonstrate generally poor conditioning, with poor abdominal muscle tone and poor posture.

Pain from lumbar strain is exacerbated by bending or lifting and relieved by rest. Pain is often described as a deep-seated aching that is dull and somewhat diffuse. Pain is most severe in the lumbosacral area and may radiate into the buttocks. Palpation reveals tenderness in the paraspinous area, with "trigger points" or "knots" in the erector spinae. Spasm of the paraspinous muscles is a common finding, and the patient may have a slight list toward the nonpainful side. Motion is limited by pain.

Physical examination is remarkable for the lack of neurologic involvement. Deep tendon reflexes are present and symmetric. Motor power and sensation in the lower extremities are normal. Rectal tone is normal. The straight leg-raising test is normal. This test is performed with the patient lying supine on the examining table. The examiner lifts the patient's leg, which is extended at the hip and knee. This maneuver passively stretches the sciatic nerve and results in transmission of tension to the lumbosacral roots that contribute to the nerve. The lack of radicular leg pain associated with straight leg raising diminishes the likelihood of spinal nerve compression as the source of symptoms.

B. Imaging Studies: X-ray examination may reveal changes such as lumbar disk space narrowing and osteophytosis or may be entirely normal. Because x-ray signs are nonspecific, many clinicians avoid x-ray studies during the initial evaluation. X-rays should be obtained for persons over age 50, in whom metastatic tumors are more likely, and those under age 20, in whom symptomatic congenital or developmental anomalies may be present. For other patients, x-rays may be obtained during subsequent visits if symptoms do not resolve within weeks.

Treatment

Management of lumbar strain includes analgesics and rest during the acute phase. A firm board beneath the patient's mattress provides support for tender spinal muscles. Abdominal conditioning and spinal muscle strengthening exercises are prescribed only when pain subsides. Typical exercises include bent-knee sit-ups and hamstring and spinal muscle stretching. Lumbosacral corsets with steel stays provide mechanical support for the spine by compressing and reinforcing the flaccid abdominal wall. Proper body mechanics should be discussed with the patient, especially the proper manner of lifting objects while bending the legs rather than the spine. Postural exercises may be useful and most effectively taught by trained physical therapists.

Course & Prognosis

The usual course of lumbar strain is spontaneous remission with time. Relapses of pain are commonly precipitated by stressful activity, though months may pass without symptoms. Some patients complain of constant pain without real remission. Probing inquiry frequently reveals profound depression in these individuals, for whom illness and disability have become dominant elements in their lives. When strain is attributed to working conditions, the clinical course may be complicated by considerations of secondary gain.

Patients who fail to respond to rest and supportive measures must be carefully reexamined to rule out development of neurologic compromise. Those who remain neurologically normal must be encouraged to return to normal activities as rapidly as possible. Prolonged reliance upon analgesics must be discouraged.

2. LUMBAR DISK SYNDROME

Essentials of Diagnosis

- Low back pain radiating into the thigh, leg, and foot.
- Paresthesia in the affected dermatome.

General Considerations

Relapse of low back pain may or may not be associated with leg pain. Patients who present with low back and leg pain frequently recall earlier episodes of postexertional pain limited to the low back. Though specific evidence is lacking, the pattern of leg pain developing secondarily has led many clinicians to attribute the initial episode of localized low back pain to early degeneration of the annulus. With annulus degeneration, the nucleus pulposus bulges into the defect causing further concentration of stress on the damaged fibers. The annulus is richly innervated with pain fibers, and further degeneration tends to be associated with more frequent and more intense episodes of pain. Locking and stiffness characterize the pain-free periods. Degeneration continues with alteration in the collagen structure of both the annulus and the nucleus, culminating in fibrosis and nuclear fragmentation. The shock-absorbing capacity of the nucleus is diminished, and forces are transmitted in a progressively irregular fashion. Fragments of the deteriorating nucleus are pushed outward against or through the weakened annulus, which tends to be weakest at the lateral margin of the posterolongitudinal ligament. The protrusion begins as a posterolateral bulge that causes variable compression and irritation of neural structures.

The contents of the neural tube below the first lumbar segment consist of nerve roots only. Each nerve root emerges below its respective vertebra. The L4–5 and L5–S1 disk levels correspond to the region of maximal mechanical stress in the lumbar spine. Disk protrusions at these levels are likely to involve the portion of the root above the exit at the next lower interspace. Lesions affecting the L5 and S1 nerve roots account for over 90% of disk-mediated nerve root lesions.

Clinical Findings

A. Symptoms and Signs: Sciatica or pain radiating down the leg, is the most common presentation. Presenting complaints of the patient with established discogenic back pain are remarkable for radicular symptoms. Prolonged compression results in nerve root inflammation and pain referred in a dermatomal distribution. The onset of leg pain is usually insidious, but pain may begin acutely when sudden disk herniation follows injury.

Pain is piercing and typically radiates from the thigh into the leg and foot. Activities such as coughing, sneezing, or bearing down during bowel movements increase intra-abdominal pressure, which is directly transmitted to intraspinal structures, provoking or exacerbating pain.

When nerve root compression results from annular bulging, it is often accentuated by prolonged sitting or standing and relieved at least partially by rest. A patient usually prefers to sleep on one side in the fetal position and when sitting prefers a straight-back chair. When disk extrusion occurs, pain may be less responsive to rest.

Compression of nerve roots often produces objective sensory changes early, with paresthesia and loss of sensation detectable in the affected dermatome. With continued root compression, motor weakness may develop. With involvement of the L4 root, the patellar tendon reflex may be diminished and slight quadriceps weakness may be observed. Sensation may be diminished over the medial calf. With involvement of the L5 root, weakness is frequently manifested by loss of strength in great toe dorsiflexion. Pain and numbness are present in the anteromedial leg and foot. First sacral root involvement affects the calf muscles, and the Achilles reflex may be lost on the involved side. Weakness is best demonstrated by the patient's inability to rise on the toes repeatedly. Sensory findings include pain and numbness in the posterolateral leg and foot. Muscle atrophy may accompany sensory and motor changes.

Occasionally, acute posterior midline disk prolapse at the L2–3 level may cause compression of many nerve roots in the cauda equina. This is known as acute cauda equina syndrome. Symptoms include intense leg pain in one or both extremities, with severe muscle weakness or paralysis. Compression of sacral roots results in acute urinary retention. Decompression of the cauda equina is undertaken after myelographic confirmation of the lesion.

B. Diagnostic Tests: With less well defined signs of root compression, several tests may help to detect the presence of lumbar disk disease. The straight leg-raising test is performed by lifting the extended leg of the supine patient. The test produces tension in the lumbosacral roots and frequently reproduces sciatica in the presence of inflamed or irritated lumbosacral roots.

The straight leg-raising test can also be performed on the leg without symptoms. The test is positive if it produces sciatica in the symptomatic leg. Many clinicians believe that a positive test is strong evidence of disk herniation.

Lasègue's test is performed with the patient lying supine. The hip and knee are flexed 90 degrees. The knee is then slowly extended, producing sciatic stretch as in the straight leg-raising maneuver.

C. Imaging Studies: X-ray examination may reveal degenerative changes, such as disk space narrowing and osteophytosis, or results may be entirely normal. A myelogram, CT scan, or MRI will confirm the diagnosis.

Differential Diagnosis

Whether nerve root signs are present or not, the main differential concern with back pain is spinal tumor. The most common extradural tumors in adults are metastatic, most often from carcinoma of the breast in women and the prostate in men. Lung, thyroid, and uterine tumors are less common sources of metastases. Multiple myeloma also frequently involves the spine and often causes pain by weakening of bony structures, causing pathologic fractures. Intradural spinal tumors are less common than metastases in adults and include neurofibromas, meningiomas, and ependymomas. Diagnosis of these slow-growing tumors is often quite difficult, as symptoms may mimic discogenic pain and may appear to improve with conservative measures. Metastatic tumors of bone are often detected on routine x-ray studies.

The history may suggest the possibility of spinal tumor. A history of primary tumors elsewhere should immediately raise this suspicion. The complaint of pain that is more severe at night than during the day is also strongly suggestive of spinal tumor. The reasons for this phenomenon are unclear but may be related to nocturnal increase in cerebrospinal fluid pressure. Persistent bilateral leg pain with no history of back pain also suggests spinal tumor. Myelography with contrast media or CT scan with metrizamide is essential to detect intradural and intramedullary tumors.

Treatment

Management of acute lumbar disk disease is controversial.

A. Conservative Management: If symptoms are produced by bulging rather than by extrusion of the herniated disk, conservative measures such as bed rest, analgesics, and anti-inflammatory medications often result in complete resolution of symptoms.

B. Percutaneous Discectomy: If pain becomes intractable or if neurologic symptoms progress or fail to respond to conservative measures, laminectomy for removal of the herniated disk may be required. Recently, use of a special suction-cutting device has permitted successful percutaneous aspiration of herniated lumbar disks. The so-called **nucleotome** is used under local anesthesia with fluoroscopic placement. The herniated disk must be contained within the annular ligament as demonstrated by preoperative CT scan or MRI (no "free fragments" in the spinal canal). The indications for the technique include failure of conservative measures and a predominance of leg pain (sciatica) over back pain. Percutaneous discectomy has been shown to be effective and safe in well-selected patients and has the advantage of being performed under local anesthesia on an outpatient basis. Complications include disk space infection, nerve root injury, and hematoma formation. Disadvantages include the difficulty of nucleotome placement in the L5–S1 disk space and the contraindication of this technique when free disk fragments are present in the spinal canal.

C. Laminectomy: If free fragments are present in the spinal canal, laminectomy is clearly indicated if pain or neurologic symptoms fail to respond to conservative measures. Complications of laminectomy for disk removal include recurrence of pain due to reherniation of residual disk fragments or scar formation involving the nerve roots; damage of nerve roots, resulting in neurologic deficit; tear of the dura, with resulting dural leak of cerebrospinal fluid; and penetration of the anterior annulus during diskectomy, with damage of the great vessels lying anterior to the spine. Hemorrhage in this situation may be catastrophic owing to difficulty in detection and control.

3. MECHANICAL BACK PAIN
(Facet Syndrome)

Essentials of Diagnosis
- Pain in the low back.
- "Locking" of back during bending.

General Considerations
Persons with long-standing lumbar disk disease may develop numerous degenerative changes in the involved segments (facet syndrome). Collapse of the disk results in abnormal motion both anteriorly between the vertebral bodies and posteriorly between the intervertebral facets. Osteophytes form as a result of abnormal stress on the annulus and the joint capsules of the facets.

Clinical Findings
Symptoms may arise from inflammation surrounding the abnormal facets and generally include diffuse aching that may or may not radiate into the buttock or posterior thigh.

The "mechanical" nature of the pain is reflected by postural discomfort and by "locking" of the low back during stooping or attempts to straighten the back after forward bending. Abnormal motion is the presumed cause of irritation that leads to reflex muscular inhibition and spinal "locking."

Differential Diagnosis
Experimental injection of hypertonic saline into normal facet joints has been noted to cause low back pain associated with sciatica as well as limitation of straight leg raising. These experimentally induced symptoms are eradicated by injection of the facets with lidocaine. These observations make it clear that sciatica without weakness or sensory deficit is insufficient evidence on which to base a diagnosis of nerve root compression.

Treatment
Patients demonstrating symptoms suggestive of facet syndrome may respond well to systemic anti-inflammatory agents or to fluoroscopically guided injection of the lumbar facets with corticosteroids and lidocaine. Lumbar fusion by anterior or posterior techniques has been advocated to eliminate abnormal motion, but results have been inconsistent.

Fischgrund JS, Montgomery DM: Diagnosis and treatment of discogenic low back pain. Orthop Rev 1993;22:311.

Frank A: Low back pain. Br Med J 1993;306:901.

Frymoyer JW: Predicting disability from low back pain. Clin Orthop 1992;Jun(279):101.

Haldeman S, Rubinstein SM: Cauda equina syndrome in patients undergoing manipulation of the lumbar spine. Spine 1992;17:1469.

PAIN SYNDROMES OF THE FOOT

1. MORTON'S NEUROMA

The interdigital nerve to the third and fourth toes is formed by the third digital branch of the medial plantar nerve and a connecting branch from the lateral plantar nerve. In 1876, Morton described a painful condition of the forefoot that he attributed to neuritis of this digital nerve. The symptoms included pain centered around the forth metatarsophalangeal joint and in the third intermetatarsal space. Pain is exacerbated by weight bearing and in some cases is steadily progressive. Neuroma pain is distinguishable from simple structural forefoot pain by the fact that it is constant and not relieved by rest. Structural metatarsalgia is experienced almost exclusively during weight bearing and is relieved by rest.

Interdigital nerve neuroma has been attributed to the course the nerves follow on the way to their destination in the skin of the toes. Each nerve passes beneath the deep intermetatarsal ligament and then changes its course in dorsal direction. The more dorsally situated digital branches then enter adjacent toes to provide cutaneous sensation. Dorsiflexion of the toes produces constant friction along the edge of the intermetatarsal ligament. Friction causes fibrosis and enlargement of the nerve sheath, which in turn increase the potential for impingement. The third and fourth interdigital nerves are most commonly involved. This predilection is attributed to the peculiar mobility of the fourth metatarsal, which is least rigidly anchored at its base. The third and fourth interdigital nerves may be relatively less mobile owing to tethering by the filaments contributed by the lateral plantar nerve. The second and third interdigital nerves are sometimes affected, and the first nerve is only rarely involved.

Clinical Findings
Diagnosis is based on the history and physical examination. The complaint of unremitting pain in the interspaces of the foot is highly suggestive. Palpation of the space reproduces sharp, stabbing pain, as does compression of the interspaces produced by squeezing the forefoot circumferentially. Simple metatarsalgia can be ruled out by a trial of shoe inserts to pad the metatarsals. Neuroma pain will rarely respond to orthotics alone.

Treatment
Intractable neuroma pain in the intermetatarsal space unresponsive to shoe pads requires operative treatment. Treatment consists of excision of the nerve through a longitudinal incision in the dorsal web space. Pressure applied with a finger on the plantar interspace will deliver the neuroma into the dorsal

wound. The neuroma is usually located at the bifurcation into digital branches. The excision must be made well proximal to the intermetatarsal ligament to prevent subsequent adhesion of the cut nerve end and the ligament, with recurrence of pain. Denervation of the digits with sensory loss has proved inconsequential to patients, who usually describe dramatic relief of symptoms immediately after surgery.

2. METATARSALGIA

Essentials of Diagnosis
* Pain beneath the metatarsal heads with weight bearing.
* Plantar callosities.

General Considerations
Metatarsalgia is a descriptive term denoting a group of disorders causing pain beneath the metatarsophalangeal joints. Mechanical factors are perhaps the chief cause. Laxity of the transverse intermetatarsal ligament permits collapse of the transverse metatarsal arch, resulting in loss of the concavity beneath the central metatarsal heads. The normal concentration of weight bearing by the first and fifth metatarsal heads is dispersed, with relatively greater loads delivered to the second and third metatarsals.

Clinical Findings
Plantar keratoses (callosities) form in areas of excessive stress and are particularly common beneath the second metatarsal head. This is in part due to the prominence of the condyle on the fibular aspect of the central metatarsal heads. Constant irritation of hypertrophic callosities results in inflammation and pain with weight bearing. Symptoms vary from intermittent discomfort to severe and disabling pain.

Collapse of the transverse arch may result from laxity of the intermetatarsal ligament. Ligamentous laxity may exist as a congenital deformity or may result from obesity, prolonged standing, injury, or aging. Intramuscular paralysis may also permit collapse of the arch, and shoes that crowd the toes also create abnormal stress concentration beneath the metatarsal heads.

Differential Diagnosis
Diagnosis is easily made if callosities are evident. Reactive keratoses are occasionally mistaken for plantar warts, but the latter are rarely located beneath metatarsal heads. Excision or fulguration of callosities mistaken for warts results in further thinning of the weight-bearing skin and worsening of pain.

Treatment
A. Orthotics: Therapy is directed toward relieving pressure beneath the metatarsal heads by placing felt or rubber pads into the shoe behind the central metatarsal heads. Shoes that comfortably accommodate the padded forefoot are mandatory.

B. Surgical Treatment: In case where pain is intractable despite conservative measures, operative treatment is required. Procedures designed to relieve metatarsal pressure include excision of the plantar condylar prominence, osteotomy to shorten the metatarsal, resection of the metatarsal head, and, in particularly resistant cases, excision of the entire offending metatarsal. The latter procedures may cause increased disability and should be undertaken only after failure of less radical procedures, such as condylectomy.

3. HALLUX VALGUS

Essentials of Diagnosis
* Prominence of the medial first metatarsal.
* Lateral deviation of the great toe.

General Considerations
Hallux valgus is subluxation of the first metatarsophalangeal joint, which results in lateral deviation (valgus) of the great toe and formation of medial bunions. The cause is a topic of controversy, though a number of factors are involved.

Anatomic factors predisposing to hallux valgus include varus alignment of the first metatarsocuneiform joint. The medially directed first metatarsal widens the angle between the first and second metatarsal beyond the normal 5–8 degrees. This so-called metatarsus varus adds mechanical advantages to the adductor hallucis tendon insertion on the proximal phalanx of the great toe, with resulting lateral deviation of the toe. Ligamentous laxity may also aggravate the imbalance.

The most significant extrinsic causative factor in development of hallux valgus is improper footwear. The great predominance of women in all reports of this deformity has been interpreted as a strong indictment of women's shoe styles. Bunching up of the toes in a pointed shoe buckles the first metatarsophalangeal joint by forcing the great toe into a marked valgus deformity. The first metatarsal is levered medialward. With prolonged use of offending footwear, the medial joint capsule becomes attenuated, further lowering the resistance to deformation. The abductor hallucis tendon is pulled plantarward, and its ability to resist great toe adduction is lost. The long flexor and extensor tendons are pulled laterally with the great toe. When the displaced tendons contract, they create a bowstring effect, further exacerbating the deformity.

Clinical Findings
The "bunion" of hallux valgus represents a prominence of the medial first metatarsal head, which results when the great toe becomes progressively later-

ally subluxated. True exostosis is uncommon. The ligamentous structures overlying the medial eminence may be thickened, and an adventitial bursa may form over the prominent medial metatarsal head. Pain from irritation of the bursa and the overlying skin occurs as these tissues are compressed between the shoe and underlying bone.

Treatment

A. Orthotics: Conservative measures for treatment of hallux valgus are centered around selection of footwear of adequate size and appropriate shape to accommodate the deformed forefoot. Frequently, the pain associated with irritation of the bunion can be minimized by this simple measure. Night splints have also been recommended, though hallux valgus may progress despite their use. Only when the deformity significantly interferes with the patient's life-style should surgery be recommended.

B. Surgical Treatment: Many operations have been advocated for the correction of hallux valgus. The main indications for surgery include intractable pain and inability to find comfortable shoes. The elements of surgical correction include excision of the medial prominence of the metatarsal head ("bunionectomy"), release of the deforming adductor hallucis tendon, excision of the lateral sesamoid if it is widely displaced, and reefing of the medial capsular structures to reinforce static resistance to recurrence of the deformity. When the varus deformity of the first metatarsal is excessive, sutures are placed between the capsules of the first and second metatarsal heads or corrective osteotomy of the metatarsal is performed.

Recurrence of the deformity and overcorrection creating hallux varus deformity are the major complications of surgery. Both problems are more apt to occur when correction of severe hallux valgus deformity has been attempted. Adequate vascularity must be confirmed prior to any correction procedure. The complication rates are low when surgery is performed by experienced surgeons. Ambulation is usually possible shortly after surgery. Careful attention must be paid to postoperative dressings, which should immobilize the great toe and thus reinforce the surgical repair.

Coughlin MJ: Treatment of bunionette deformity with longitudinal diaphyseal osteotomy with distal soft tissue repair. Foot Ankle 1991;11:195.

Schoenhaus HD, Cohen RS: Etiology of the bunion. J Foot Surg 1992;31:25.

ARTHRITIC PAIN SYNDROMES

1. OSTEOARTHRITIS

Osteoarthritis has traditionally been described as "wear and tear" joint degeneration attributable to the aging process. Pain due to osteoarthritis constitutes the most common joint complaint for which patients seek medical attention. Primary osteoarthritis affects the articular cartilage of otherwise normal joints. Secondary osteoarthritis occurs as a sequela of trauma, joint disease such as Legg-Perthes disease, or subtle anomalies such as mild acetabular dysplasia resulting in long-standing joint incongruity.

Osteoarthritis is the most common of all arthropathies, affecting roughly 30–50% of the entire population. Heritability has not been demonstrated. Women are more often affected than men, though virtually all persons over age 55 have some x-ray evidence of this disease. Fortunately, less than half of patients with x-ray changes will experience joint symptoms. Onset of symptomatic disease is usually in the sixth decade.

Though the specific inciting agent remains unclear, the earliest histopathologic change in osteoarthritic joints is loss of mucopolysaccharide ground substance in the outermost layers of articular cartilage. As a result, the mechanical properties of the cartilage are altered and resistance to deformation is lowered. The weakened superficial layers of cartilage develop fissures in response to increased deformation by normal loads. This results in uneven distribution of stress transmission to deeper layers of cartilage and to the underlying subchondral bone. This concentration of stress further accelerates cartilage wear with thinning of outer layers and propagation of cracks and fissures in the deeper layers. Cartilage debris within the joint results in low-grade chronic inflammatory synovitis and joint effusion.

If weight bearing or stress loading of the affected joint continues, thinning of the cartilage may progress to eventual full-thickness cartilage loss. The subchondral bone bears progressively greater loads as cartilage destruction evolves. Increased loading of bone stimulates bone remodeling and new bone deposition, manifested by marginal osteophyte formation and sclerosis within the subchondral bone. Microfractures within the overloaded subchondral bone incite a chronic inflammatory response. Replacement of necrotic bone by fibrous tissue results in subchondral cyst formation.

Clinical Findings

A. Symptoms and Signs: Osteoarthritis is a local condition without systemic manifestations. Asymptomatic degenerative joint changes in the hands and spine are common, but weight-bearing joints such as the knee and hip are often stiff and painful, particularly following the activities of the day. Symptoms may be episodic, with long periods of spontaneous remission, or slowly but steadily progressive, resulting in profound disability and intractable pain. Discomfort is characteristically more severe at night, and morning stiffness is minimal. Monarticular osteoarthritis is unusual. Both knees are typically involved, though one usually more extensively than the other. Osteoarthritis of the hip occurs slightly less frequently but is still quite common. Nodular swelling of the distal joints of the fingers (Heberden's nodes) is present in over half of affected individuals, and painful degeneration of the carpometacarpal joint of the thumb and the metacarpophalangeal joint of the great toe is common. The ankle, shoulder, and elbow are rarely involved, and the wrist least frequently of all.

Examination of osteoarthritic joints is remarkable for the absence of inflammatory signs. Effusion, when present, is slight, and redness and warmth are usually absent. Pain with motion is the predominant finding, and crepitation may be palpated with passive motion. Range-of-motion testing reveals limitation of terminal flexion and extension in the involved knee joints and internal rotation in involved hips. More severe limitation is characteristic of more advanced disease. Varus or valgus deformity of the knee may be present, depending upon the predominance of involvement of the medial or lateral joint compartment. Heberden's nodes of the distal interphalangeal joints of the hand are classic findings. These dorsal bony prominences represent marginal osteophytes. Similar degenerative changes of the proximal interphalangeal joints may be present and are known as Bouchard's nodes.

B. Laboratory Findings: Laboratory studies are usually normal.

C. Imaging Studies: X-ray findings are consistent with the histopathologic stage of degeneration. Early changes consist of mild joint space narrowing and minimal osteophyte formation ("spurring") at the periphery of involved joints. More advanced disease is manifested by severe joint space narrowing, marked osteophyte formation at the joint margins, dense sclerosis of subchondral bone, and subchondral cysts. Subluxation and joint space narrowing are often apparent only on weight-bearing films, which should be obtained for both knees and hips.

Treatment

A. External Support Measures: Management of osteoarthritis depends upon the stage of disease. When degeneration in a weight-bearing join is mild, symptoms are significantly relieved by use of external supports such as a cane, crutches, or a walker. Though actual healing of osteoarthritic cartilage is difficult to demonstrate, remission of joint pain is sometimes dramatic when stress is diminished by use of external aids.

B. Medication: Anti-inflammatory drugs are

less effective in osteoarthritis than in rheumatoid arthritis or gout. A trial of nonsteroidal anti-inflammatory drugs is warranted, however, as some patients report considerable relief with their use. Analgesics, hot packs, ultrasound, and massage may also provide symptomatic relief. Physical therapy for joint-strengthening exercises may occasionally be warranted, and weight reduction is beneficial.

C. Surgical Treatment: Joint arthroplasty has revolutionized the management of severe and disabling osteoarthritis. Pain can be reliably eliminated in most patients with hip or knee joint disease, and improvement in joint motion is generally achieved. Because the cemented prosthetic components often loosen over decades of use, total joint arthroplasty has the longest-lasting results in older, less active individuals.

Persons in the fifth and sixth decades may benefit from osteotomy, particularly when arthropathy is moderate. Following surgical realignment of a joint, the load upon the joint may be shifted toward less severely damaged cartilage. Several years of serviceable joint function may be achieved. Joint replacement may be performed late if required, and the likelihood of component failure will be proportionately diminished.

Chang RW et al: A randomized, controlled trial of arthroscopic surgery versus closed-needle joint lavage for patients with osteoarthritis of the knee. Arthritis Rheum 1993;36:289.
Graves SC, Mann RA, Graves KO: Triple arthrodesis in older adults: Results after long-term follow-up. J Bone Joint Surg [Am] 1993;75:355.
Redden JF, Stanley D: Arthroscopic fenestration of the olecranon fossa in the treatment of osteoarthritis of the elbow Arthroscopy 1993;9:14.
Rorabeck CH et al: The Miller-Galante knee prosthesis for the treatment of osteoarthrosis: A comparison of the results of partial fixation with cement and fixation without any cement. J Bone Joint Surg [Am] 1993;75:402.

2. RHEUMATOID ARTHRITIS

Essentials of Diagnosis
- Symmetric erosive polyarthritis with marked inflammatory synovitis.
- Positive rheumatoid factor test.

General Considerations

Rheumatoid arthritis is a systemic connective tissue disorder manifested within the joints by a chronic inflammatory synovitis. Immunologic derangement may well underlie the development of synovitis. Joint symptoms result initially from synovial inflammation and later from invasion of articular and periarticular structures by inflammatory granulation tissue, known as pannus. Compromise of joint function is in part due to enzymatic erosion of cartilage and subchondral bone by the proliferating synovial pannus. Ligamentous stretching by repeated inflammatory joint effusion results in mechanical joint instability, typified by the familiar deformity of the rheumatoid hand. End-stage rheumatoid joint changes may also include marked fibrosis due to replacement of pannus by dense scar tissue.

The cause of rheumatoid arthritis is unknown. Infectious agents have not been found. An underlying immune mechanism is suggested by the presence of IgM antibodies (rheumatoid factor) within the joint fluid and plasma of 80% of rheumatoid arthritis patients. Diminished complement activity within actively inflamed joints and the proliferation of lymphocytes and plasma cells within the synovium are also suggestive. Antigen-antibody complexes appear to activate the complement system and attract neutrophils into the synovial fluid. Phagocytosis of the immune complexes results in release of lysosomal enzymes into the joint. These enzymes may be responsible for the cartilage destruction that characterizes inflammatory arthritis.

Women are affected by rheumatoid arthritis three times more commonly than men. About 0.25–3% of the population is affected, depending upon the criteria employed for diagnosis. The disease commonly appears in young adults, with a peak incidence in the fifth decade. About 15% of patients will have spontaneous remission, usually within the first year. If remission does not occur within 2–3 years, it is unlikely to occur. Another 10% will suffer a rapid malignant course culminating in severe deformity and functional disability. The remaining patients display a chronic course with exacerbations and partial remissions of synovitis lasting for several months.

Clinical Findings

A. Symptoms and Signs: Usually, patients present with pain, stiffness, and swelling in several joints. Symptoms occur in a bilateral and symmetric distribution and often spread from one set of joints to another. About 15% of patients present with monarticular arthritis, predominantly in the knee, but develop more typical polyarthritis within a week. Palindromic rheumatism is an uncommon presentation characterized by recurrent attacks of pain and swelling occurring in only one joint at a time. Morning stiffness is typical of many musculoskeletal complaints but is suggestive of rheumatoid arthritis when it lasts longer than 1–2 hours. Stiffness is often generalized, involving many joints rather than only those which are noticeably inflamed.

Physical findings vary with the extent of disease. Initially, synovitis is the predominant finding, with effusion, warmth, tenderness, and synovial thickening upon palpation. The joints most frequently involved are the metacarpophalangeal, proximal interphalangeal, and metatarsophalangeal joints other than the great toe. Early involvement of the wrist is

helpful in differentiating rheumatoid synovitis from osteoarthritis, which rarely involves this joint. Synovitis typically occurs later in the joints of the lower extremities and midfoot as well as the shoulder, elbow, and upper cervical spine.

Long-standing or recurrent effusion results in capsular distention and, together with pannus invasion of periarticular ligament insertions, may profoundly compromise joint stability. The wrist and metacarpophalangeal joints frequently demonstrate palmar subluxation. Marked ulnar deviation of the fingers is typical of advanced rheumatoid arthritis. Another common instability pattern known as swan-neck deformity consists of hyperextension of the proximal interphalangeal joint coupled with fixed flexion of the distal interphalangeal joint. Limitation of prehension may lead to severe functional disability. A "boutonnière" deformity features buttonhole protrusion of the proximal interphalangeal knuckle through the extensor expansion. This deformity is caused by attrition of the extensor hood overlying the proximal interphalangeal joint, which allows anterior subluxation of the tendons of the intrinsic muscles. The intrinsic tendons then act as proximal interphalangeal joint flexors rather than extensors. A fixed flexion contracture at the proximal interphalangeal joint with distal interphalangeal joint extension is the end result. Fortunately, this common deformity does not affect function and does not critically limit pinch or grasp.

B. Laboratory Findings: Laboratory investigations in the workup of arthritis include serologic tests, synovial fluid analyses, roentgenographic evaluations, and, occasionally, histologic studies. About 80–90% of patients demonstrate IgM rheumatoid factor in sera with latex and sheep cell agglutination tests. Rheumatoid factors are autoantibodies directed against human IgG. Patients with very high titers of IgM rheumatoid factor are more likely to have systemic extra-articular manifestations of rheumatoid disease. Though most rheumatoid factors are of the IgM class, IgG and IgA immunoglobulins may also be present. These antibodies are not routinely measured and may be the cause of some cases of so-called seronegative rheumatoid arthritis, in which symptoms of erosive polyarthritis are present but classic IgM rheumatoid factor is not found in the sera. About 5% of normal individuals and up to 25% of elderly persons may have rheumatoid factor in their sera.

Synovial fluid aspirated during an acute exacerbation of rheumatoid arthritis demonstrates typical inflammatory characteristics, with white cell counts in the range of 500–25,000/μL and 80–90% PMNs. Gram-stained smears and cultures must be performed to rule out infection even when the diagnosis of rheumatoid arthritis is definite, as superinfection is not uncommon. Examination for crystals is likewise mandatory.

Synovial biopsy is rarely indicated but may be useful in inflammatory joint disease of uncertain cause. Though the histologic picture of synovial hyperplasia with plasma cell and lymphocyte infiltration may be present in all forms of chronic inflammatory arthritis, these findings may help to exclude tuberculosis or villonodular synovitis. The presence of a pronounced infiltrate of PMNs suggests bacterial infection.

Acceleration of the erythrocyte sedimentation rate is common in rheumatoid arthritis as well as in other inflammatory arthritides. Though obviously not a specific indicator of rheumatoid disease, the sedimentation rate provides a general index of inflammatory activity and is a useful indicator of response to therapy. A normal rate does not rule out rheumatoid arthritis.

LE cells and antinuclear antibodies are present in virtually all patients with active systemic lupus erythematosus and in about 15% of patients with rheumatoid arthritis. These overlapping populations may be differentiated by screening for antibodies to native DNA. Although such antibodies are found in systemic lupus erythematosus, they are not present in rheumatoid arthritis patients, including those who demonstrate positive antinuclear antibody studies.

C. Imaging Studies: X-ray changes early in the course of rheumatoid arthritis reflect the inflammatory nature of the disease. Osteoporosis is apparent around inflamed joints and represents reabsorption of spongy bone resulting from inflammatory hyperemia. Effusion and synovial thickening may cause joint space widening and displacement of deep soft tissue planes. Rheumatoid nodules are easily visualized.

Later roentgenographic changes mirror the destructive activity of the synovial pannus. Destruction of bone begins at joint margins and initially appears as blurring of the cortical outline. Deep erosions develop later and have an irregular cup-shaped appearance often described as a "rat bite"—as though the bone had been gnawed away. Destruction of articular cartilage results in joint space narrowing. Ligamentous laxity results in subluxation and is apparent on x-ray by joint malalignment.

Common deformities noted in the x-ray evaluation of rheumatoid arthritis include erosive destruction of the distal ulna; diffuse narrowing of radiocarpal, intercarpal, and interphalangeal joint cartilage; and bony destruction involving the second, third, and fourth metacarpophalangeal joint margins. Metacarpophalangeal and metatarsophalangeal subluxation is especially common. A potentially catastrophic form of subluxation occurs between the first and second cervical vertebrae as a result of alar and transverse ligament destruction. About 25% of rheumatoid arthritis patients demonstrate anterior atlantoaxial subluxation, seen on flexion x-rays by a greater than 3 mm widening of the interval between the dens axis and the anterior arch of the atlas. Erosion of the lateral masses and the occipitocervical joints allows settling of the skull downward onto the atlas. About 5%

of rheumatoid arthritis patients demonstrate invagination of the dens axis into the foramen magnum. Clinical manifestations of cervical cord compression include severe neck pain, urinary incontinence, muscle weakness, and paresthesias. Myelopathy may be insidious or may progress rapidly.

Differential Diagnosis

Diagnosis of rheumatoid arthritis is easily made in patients with well-established symmetric erosive polyarthritis, rheumatoid nodules, and a positive rheumatoid factor test. Diagnosis is more difficult in the early phase of the disease, when monarticular arthritis may be present in the so-called seronegative patient and the slowly progressive or palindromic patient. When monarticular arthritis is present, joint aspiration should be performed to rule out septic or crystal-induced arthritis. About 5% of patients with crystal-induced synovitis will present with polyarticular disease, and repeat arthrocentesis may be necessary to confirm the presence of urate or pyrophosphate crystals. Infectious arthritis may also present as polyarticular disease, and gram-stained smears and synovial fluid cultures are mandatory to rule out bacterial sepsis.

Viral arthritis may mimic the early presentation of rheumatoid arthritis. The jaundice of viral hepatitis is often preceded by polyarthralgia and myalgia. Anicteric hepatitis may be distinguishable from early rheumatoid arthritis only by abnormal liver function tests or the presence of hepatitis B surface antigen. The joint symptoms associated with hepatitis should resolve spontaneously after several weeks.

Reiter's syndrome includes polyarthritis as a predominant feature. This syndrome affects primarily men in the third and fourth decades and is often, though not always, preceded by *Shigella* gastroenteritis or, in the classic form, by urethritis, iritis, and conjunctivitis. Other features of this syndrome include sacroiliitis, spondylitis, rash, and aortic insufficiency. Arthritis tends to be asymmetric, and lower limb joints are more commonly involved. Enthesitis, or inflammation at the sites of ligamentous attachment to bone, is characteristic. Achilles tendinitis and plantar fasciitis are common. HLA-B27 antigen is present in about 75% of patients with Reiter's syndrome.

Ankylosing spondylitis also affects principally young men positive on testing for HLA-B27 antigen. Though a few patients present with peripheral arthritis, most complain of low back pain. As the disease progresses, all patients develop sacroiliitis; many develop spondylitis; and one-third to one-half develop peripheral arthritis. Hand involvement is present in less than 10% of cases—a feature that facilitates distinction from rheumatoid arthritis. Arthritis below the cervical region is present in ankylosing spondylitis but is unusual in rheumatoid arthritis. Ankylosing spondylitis is distinguished from Reiter's syndrome by the absence of iritis, urethritis, conjunctivitis, or mucocutaneous lesions.

Systemic lupus erythematosus affects predominantly women and often presents with transient arthralgia and synovitis. The hands and wrists are frequently involved, and early symptoms are often mistaken for rheumatoid arthritis. The erosion of cartilage and subchondral bone that occurs in rheumatoid arthritis is absent in systemic lupus erythematosus; this is the most distinctive difference between the two diseases. Skin rash, photosensitivity, and constitutional symptoms and findings of anti-DNA antibodies help to diagnose systemic lupus erythematosus.

Treatment

The major goals of therapy for rheumatoid and other inflammatory arthritides include suppression and control of synovitis and preservation of joint function. The latter may require the concerted efforts of a physical therapist to guide the patient in performing exercises and using adaptive devices to overcome physical disability.

A. Splinting: When acute polyarthritis is present, rest and splinting of joints often hasten resolution of symptoms and prevent flexion deformity.

B. Medication: Anti-inflammatory drugs help to control symptoms and provide necessary analgesia, but there is no convincing evidence that these agents influence the overall course of rheumatoid arthritis. Aspirin is the standard agent used. An average dose of 4 g/d should be given, producing blood levels of 20 mg/dL. If blood levels are not obtainable, doses may be increased until tinnitus develops and then reduced slightly. Enteric-coated aspirin may produce fewer gastrointestinal side effects.

If gastrointestinal bleeding or aspirin intolerance occurs, many nonsteroidal anti-inflammatory agents may be substituted with equal effectiveness, though at far greater expense to the patient. Ibuprofen, naproxen, sulindac, and zomepirac are currently the most widely prescribed drugs and may cause fewer gastrointestinal side effects. Indomethacin is also effective though perhaps more ulcerogenic. If night pain and morning stiffness are pronounced, a larger dose of medication is prescribed in the evening.

Perhaps the most controversial form of therapy is systemic administration of corticosteroid drugs. Most clinicians prescribe these agents only for patients with uncontrollable progression of arthritis or for elderly patients who may otherwise become wheelchair-dependent. The dose and duration of corticosteroids must be minimized to prevent catabolic side effects and the development of drug dependency. Intra-articular injections of soluble corticosteroids may bring temporary relief of symptoms and permit mobilization of a troublesome joint. Injections should be minimized to prevent corticosteroid-induced cartilage degeneration.

Suppressive agents, including gold salts, penicillamine, and antimalarial drugs, produce long-term suppression or remission of rheumatoid arthritis; the full effects of these agents are not apparent for months. They are administered to prevent or diminish permanent joint damage when arthritis is progressive despite an adequate trial of anti-inflammatory drugs. The action of suppressive agents is not well understood, but controlled studies indicate that about one-third of patients will experience remission of symptoms with these drugs. A 20-week trial is recommended. Dermatitis, stomatitis, proteinuria, thrombocytopenia, and aplastic anemia are side effects associated with gold salts and penicillamine. Use of chloroquine for longer than 2 years may result in corneal deposits or retinopathy. Suppressive drugs have no analgesic effects, and analgesic medication must be given concurrently.

Cytotoxic drugs such as cyclophosphamide may produce improvement of arthritis in otherwise resistant joints. Most patients develop cystitis or alopecia, and the administration of immunosuppressive drugs is therefore of limited use.

C. Surgical Treatment: Surgery in rheumatoid arthritis is reserved for joints that have deteriorated to the point of severely limited function. Functional disability may result from subluxation, such as that commonly affecting the metacarpophalangeal joints, or from mechanical impairment due to cartilage destruction and joint space fibrosis. Synovectomy and tendon transfer may restore function in the subluxated digits with intact joint cartilage. Joint fusion or replacement arthroplasty is necessary to restore motion when cartilage destruction and joint fibrosis are advanced. Hip, knee, metacarpophalangeal, and elbow joints have been successfully restored by replacement arthroplasty. The wrist and interphalangeal joints have been more favorably managed with fusion.

Adolfsson L, Nylander G: Arthroscopic synovectomy of the rheumatoid wrist. J Bone Joint Surg [Br] 1993;18:92.

Boublik M, Tsahakis PJ, Scott RD: Cementless total knee arthroplasty in juvenile onset rheumatoid arthritis. Clin Orthop 1993;Jan(286):88.

Ewald FC et al: Capitellocondylar total elbow replacement in rheumatoid arthritis: Long-term results. J Bone Joint Surg [Am] 1993;3;75:498.

Kirschenbaum D et al:: Arthroplasty of the metacarpophalangeal joints with use of silicone-rubber implants in patients who have rheumatoid arthritis: Long-term results. J Bone Joint Surg [Am] 1993;75:3.

Maric Z, Haynes RJ: Total hip arthroplasty in juvenile rheumatoid arthritis. Clin Orthop 1993;May(290):197.

Niskanen RO et al: Arthrodesis of the first metatarsophalangeal joint in rheumatoid arthritis: Biodegradable rods and Kirschner-wires in 39 cases. Acta Orthop Scand 1993;64:100.

Sorokin R: Management of the patient with rheumatic diseases going to surgery. Med Clin North Am 1993; 77:453.

OSTEOMYELITIS & SEPTIC ARTHRITIS

A broad spectrum of bone infections are grouped under the term osteomyelitis. Pathogenetically, osteomyelitis is best divided into three categories: (1) hematogenous osteomyelitis, (2) osteomyelitis due to direct inoculation of a traumatic or surgical wound, and (3) osteomyelitis due to extension from a contiguous infection, as occurs especially with ischemic, diabetic, and neurotrophic ulcers. Necrotic bone develops progressively in the first stages of acute hematogenous osteomyelitis. In traumatic osteomyelitis, bone necrosis is often produced by the injury itself and is thus present when infection begins. When infectious organisms invade normal bone, necrosis is slow to develop and tends to remain localized to the immediate area. Osteomyelitis is further categorized as acute or chronic and by the specific infecting organism.

Hughes SPF, Fitzgerald RH Jr (editors): *Musculoskeletal Infections.* Year Book, 1986.

ACUTE HEMATOGENOUS OSTEOMYELITIS

Essentials of Diagnosis
- Pain or unwillingness to move limb.
- Localized swelling and tenderness.
- Bacteria or pus in aspirate or biopsy.

General Considerations
Hematogenous osteomyelitis of long bones is an acute infectious disease that is far more common in children than adults. Blood-borne organisms settle in the metaphyseal vascular bed of rapidly growing long bones, where blood flows slowly through a hairpin turn form arteriole to venous lake, just beneath the cartilaginous growth plate. In this region, local defense mechanisms are readily overwhelmed. Bacterial proliferation, inflammation, and resulting edema cause increased intraosseous pressure, blocking local blood flow and resulting in necrosis in the involved area. Under increasing pressure, pus spreads peripherally, penetrating the thin metaphyseal cortex. The periosteal membrane, thick and well-developed in the child, is dissected from underlying bone by the advancing exudate, which continues to spread under the periosteum along the diaphysis. The bone itself becomes devascularized, but the periosteum retains its blood supply and forms a layer of new bone on its inner surface—the involucrum that surrounds a sequestrum of necrotic original bone. Increasing uncon-trolled infection may penetrate the involucrum to "point" as a subcutaneous abscess and become a persistent sinus tract or cloaca through which pus and bits of bony sequestrum are expelled. In very young children (18 months of age or less), this typical pattern of spread is altered, because intraosseous blood vessels pass from the metaphysis to the cartilaginous epiphysis. Therefore, septic arthritis and damage to the epiphysis, with severe growth abnormalities, are more common in this age group. For unknown reasons, spread of infection throughout the entire bone and multiple bone involvement are also more common in very young infants.

Small sterile "sympathetic" joint effusions often occur adjacent to metaphyseal osteomyelitis and should not be confused with septic arthritis, another common pediatric musculoskeletal infection (see p 1092). Aspiration of fluid followed by cell count, gram-stained smear, and cultures readily distinguishes pyarthrosis from sympathetic effusion. It is important to remember that the metaphysis lies within the joint capsule of the hip, shoulder, or ankle. Therefore, these joints can develop septic arthritis by extension of osteomyelitis involving the proximal femur or humerus or the distal tibia.

In about 80% of cases, acute hematogenous osteomyelitis affects the femur, tibia, humerus, or fibula. However, any bone can be affected.

By far the most frequent organism causing acute hematogenous osteomyelitis is *Staphylococcus aureus,* usually the penicillin-resistant type. It is recovered from 80% of children with acute hematogenous osteomyelitis. Group A streptococci and gram-negative rods are also seen occasionally. In neonates, group B streptococci, *S aureus,* and *Escherichia coli* are most frequent. *Salmonella* as well as the more common organisms may cause acute hematogenous osteomyelitis in patients with hemoglobinopathies, especially sickle cell disease.

Before antibiotics became available, acute hematogenous osteomyelitis was associated with a high rate of death and severe illness. For reasons not entirely clear, the disease now often follows a more attenuated course even before treatment and may in fact present as subacute osteomyelitis. Few children appear acutely ill. High fever and significantly elevated white counts are unusual. Localized pain and radiographic findings suggestive more of neoplasia than infection characterize this type of hematogenous osteomyelitis. Subacute osteomyelitis is more common in older children and adults. Somewhat atypical hematogenous osteomyelitis occurs in intravenous drug abusers, with frequent involvement of the spinal, sacroiliac, and sternoclavicular regions.

Acute hematogenous osteomyelitis associated with hemoglobinopathy. The pathogenesis of acute hematogenous osteomyelitis is different in patients with hemoglobinopathy. Bone infarcts, often painful in their own right, result from thromboses caused by the abnormal red cells. The infarcts often occur in the diaphyses of long bones rather than the metaphyses, the usual site for acute hematogenous osteomyelitis. The infarcts become secondarily infected by transient bacteremias. Multiple bone involvement is common. In areas where *Salmonella* is endemic, this pathogen is the dominant infecting organism in patients with hemoglobinopathy.

Clinical Findings

A. Symptoms and Signs: A complete history and physical examination are required to search for possible primary foci of infection. Pain, unwillingness to move or use the involved area, and, occasionally, generalized symptoms of malaise, fever, chills, anorexia, etc, are noted. Patients often describe some recent minor injury. Physical findings include limited use of the limb, sometimes sufficient to justify the term "pseudoparalysis"; local tenderness; and, as the disease progresses local signs of inflammation—swelling, warmth, and erythema. Gentle palpation will localize the precise point of maximal tenderness, where the disease process is likely to be closest to the surface, so that aspiration of subperiosteal or intraosseous pus can be performed. Gentle passive motion of the adjacent joint is usually less painful and guarded than when septic arthritis is present.

B. Laboratory Findings:

1. Aspiration—For patients who present with acute metaphyseal hematogenous osteomyelitis, the point of maximal tenderness should be aspirated with a large-bore needle (14- to 18-gauge) after attempts have been made to obtain pus from just outside the bone, under the periosteum, and inside the cortex, which is usually quite thin in the metaphysis. Aspiration that fails to yield gross pus does not exclude osteomyelitis. Thick pus may not pass through the needle, and aspiration may be erroneously interpreted as negative. Any material aspirated should be gram-stained and cultured, as serosanguineous exudate is not unusual. Needle or open biopsy can establish the diagnosis in questionable cases. Any joint effusion should be aspirated and the fluid examined microscopically and sent for culture in order to diagnose septic arthritis, which may coexist or present a similar clinical picture.

2. Bone scans—Scintigraphy using technetium 99m-labeled phosphate compounds may be valuable, especially if comparison is made between early and delayed images. Scans usually become positive during the first few days. However, scans are not specific, since uptake is also increased by fracture, neoplasia, bone infarct, septic arthritis, and even cellulitis. In septic arthritis, the scan is diffusely positive on both sides of the joint. In cellulitis, increased uptake is usually mild and poorly localized.

Bone scans may be falsely negative with acute hematogenous osteomyelitis. Infants frequently have normal-appearing bone scans. During the early ischemic phase of disease in patients of any age, scans can appear "cold" or normal, and repeat studies should be obtained. *Negative bone scans do not exclude the diagnosis of osteomyelitis and never justify the withholding of treatment if the history and physical findings are clear.*

3. Other studies—Blood cultures should be obtained in any patient with suspected acute hematogenous osteomyelitis, as they are positive in 50% or more of cases. The sedimentation rate is usually elevated. The white blood count may be increased, and an increased percentage of PMNs is common. Cultures should be taken of any suspected primary focus of infection—urine, pharyngeal secretions, sputum, or pus from pyoderma.

C. Imaging Studies: The earliest radiographic signs are those of soft tissue swelling—increased width of soft tissue shadows with loss of normal fat planes. A diffuse haziness is present that is not seen in x-rays of the other limb. Soft tissue swelling is adjacent to the bone rather than outside the deep fascia, as is typical with cellulitis. Evidence of bone involvement—focal, poorly marginated decrease in density and periosteal new bone formation—is not seen until 10–14 days after onset of the disease process. MRI may prove to be a valuable technique for diagnosis of intramedullary infections.

Differential Diagnosis

Other infectious possibilities include septic arthritis, cellulitis, and soft tissue abscesses. Lymphadenitis, as in cat-scratch fever, may cause confusion in rare cases. Leukemia, lymphoma, Ewing's sarcoma, metastatic neuroblastoma, and other neoplastic possibilities must be considered. Trauma—especially the metaphyseal fractures typical of child abuse, metabolic bone disease, and rheumatic fever—will occasionally suggest acute hematogenous osteomyelitis.

Complications

Recurrent infection—chronic osteomyelitis—is the most common complication of acute hematogenous osteomyelitis, occurring in about 20% of large series. Most recurrences are within the first 6–12 months. Multiple foci of infection may be confusing, especially in infants. Septic arthritis may lead to joint destruction. Pathologic fracture can occur in bone weakened by infection, surgery, or both. A potentially disastrous complication in an infant is growth arrest from destruction of the epiphyseal plate. Hyperemia can lead to mild bone overgrowth.

Treatment

A. Antibiotic Therapy: During the first 1–3 days of symptoms, acute hematogenous osteomyelitis usually responds promptly to intravenous administration of appropriate antibiotics in adequate doses. If the history and examination are consistent with hematogenous osteomyelitis, antibiotics should be started even if laboratory tests are not positive. Unless the clinical situation suggests otherwise, begin treatment with a cephalosporin or semisynthetic penicillin effective against *S aureus* as soon as all culture specimens have been obtained. The choice of antibiotic may subsequently be modified according to culture and sensitivity results, clinical response, and serum assays or serum killing levels. Treatment should be continued for at least 6 weeks in order to minimize the possibility of recurrence. Once signs and symptoms of infection have been convincingly resolved, oral antibiotics may be used if well-documented, adequate serum killing levels can be maintained.

B. Surgical Treatment: Surgery to incise and drain the involved area, decompress the intraosseous abscess, and remove any obvious necrotic debris is indicated (1) if gross pus is aspirated, (2) if signs and symptoms fail to resolve after 24–48 hours of antibiotic treatment, or (3) if the history at presentation strongly suggests advanced acute hematogenous osteomyelitis. Decompression rather than extensive debridement is the goal of early surgery. Specimens must be obtained for gram-stained smears, cultures, and sensitivity studies as well as for pathologic examination. Leaving the wound open for delayed closure over tubes permits a second look at the area in a few days to assess adequacy of drainage and debridement. Following incision and drainage of acute hematogenous osteomyelitis, the limb must be protected in a cast, since the bone has been seriously weakened by the operation. The risk of pathologic fracture remains for many weeks, until sufficient bone remodeling has occurred to restore osseous strength.

Course & Prognosis

Because of the less severe symptoms now seen in the early course of disease, delayed diagnosis and inadequate treatment are not unusual. Recurrence rates of 20% or more and crippling complications such as joint destruction, growth arrest, and chronic osteomyelitis justify continued vigilance. Early adequate treatment, including prompt surgery for cases that do not respond to antibiotics alone, decreases the incidence of complications from osteomyelitis.

Demopoulos GA et al: Role of radionuclide imaging in the diagnosis of acute osteomyelitis. J Pediatr Orthop 1988; 8:558.

Jones NS et al: Osteomyelitis in a general hospital: A five-year study showing an increase in subacute osteomyelitis. J Bone Joint Surg [Br] 1987;69:779.

LaMont RL et al: Acute hematogenous osteomyelitis in children. J Pediatr Orthop 1987;7:579.

Mallouh A et al: Bone and joint infections in patients with sickle cell disease. Pediatr Orthop 1985;5:158.

Scoles PV et al: Antimicrobial therapy of childhood skeletal infections. J Bone Joint Surg [Am] 1984;66:1487.

Tang JS et al: Musculoskeletal infection of the extremities: Evaluation with MR imaging. Radiology 1988;166:205.

Vaughan PA et al: Acute hematogenous osteomyelitis in children. J Pediatr Orthop 1987;7:652.

HEMATOGENOUS OSTEOMYELITIS OF THE AXIAL SKELETON IN THE ADULT

The vertebral column is the commonest site of hematogenous osteomyelitis in the adult. The cause is usually urinary tract infection, which spreads via the vertebral venous plexus (Batson's plexus). There is some question about whether infection develops first in the intervertebral disk or the adjacent vertebral body. The disk and both adjacent vertebral end plates quickly become involved. The course is often subacute or chronic, so that the disorder may be confused with other disorders associated with back pain. Pain unrelieved by rest is especially suspicious. Routine radiographs are slow to show signs of infection in the axial skeleton. Important diagnostic signs are a focally positive bone scan, elevated sedimentation rate, and evidence on CT scan of localized periarticular bone destruction with or without adjacent soft tissue abscess. MRI changes may be helpful. Intravenous drug abusers are at risk of developing osteomyelitis of not only the vertebral column but also the sacroiliac and sternoclavicular joints. *Pseudomonas* and *Serratia* are frequent causative organisms of osteomyelitis in drug addicts.

Unlike childhood vertebral osteomyelitis, which is almost always due to *Staphylococcus*, adult spinal infections and infections of the sacroiliac and sternoclavicular joints may be caused by a large number of organisms, with varying antibiotic sensitivities. Infections with pyogenic organisms, tubercle bacilli, *Brucella, Echinococcus*, and various fungi have been reported. Metastatic or primary malignant tumors must occasionally be considered in the differential diagnosis. Therefore, biopsy for culture and histopathologic study is an essential part of management, even if organisms are recovered from the blood or other foci of infection. In addition to routine bacteriologic studies, cultures for mycobacteria and fungi are required. Needle biopsy is usually adequate for this purpose except in the thoracic spine, where posterolateral costotransversectomy or anterior open biopsy is less risky for the spinal cord.

Prolonged administration of appropriately chosen intravenous antibiotics is often sufficient treatment. It is occasionally necessary to drain an associated abscess or debride the infected bone and joint in preparation for arthrodesis using cancellous bone graft. Impairment of the spinal cord or nerve roots should be watched for. An epidural abscess may require emergency drainage via laminectomy; however, a gibbus deformity with anterior compression of the cord can be accentuated by laminectomy, with additional damage to the neural elements. If deformity or infection compromises the cord anteriorly, anterior decompression is necessary.

Gepstein R et al: Management of pyogenic vertebral osteomyelitis with spinal cord compression in the elderly. Paraplegia 1992;30:795.

Lewis M, Grundy D: Vertebral osteomyelitis following manipulation of spondylitic necks: A possible risk. Paraplegia 1992;30:788.

Owen PG, Willis BK, Benzel EC: *Torulopsis glabrata* vertebral osteomyelitis. J Spinal Disord 1992;5:370.

Tehranzadeh J, Wang F, Mesgarzadeh M: Magnetic resonance imaging of osteomyelitis. Crit Rev Diagn Imaging 1992;33:495.

TUBERCULOSIS OF BONES & JOINTS

Essentials of Diagnosis

- Local signs of inflammation, abscess, synovial hypertrophy, or joint destruction on physical examination or radiographs.
- Histologic confirmation of chronic inflammation with caseating granulomas.
- Confirmatory cultures or acid-fast organisms on smear.

General Considerations

Mycobacterium tuberculosis infection of the musculoskeletal system occurs from hematogenous spread and typically involves the vertebral column or a single bone or joint. Foci of infection may be found in the lungs, gastrointestinal tract, or kidneys but are often occult, so that tuberculosis is not always included in the differential diagnosis of an inflammatory arthritic process. Atypical mycobacteria occasionally infect wounds of the extremities, and this possibility should be investigated whenever a chronic ulcer is present on the hand.

Spinal tuberculosis is often mistaken for metastatic cancer, a much commoner disease in the United States. This error should be avoided because of the different treatments involved and the relatively good prognosis for recovery, even with neurologic involvement, when tuberculosis of the spine is properly diagnosed and treated.

Clinical Findings

A. Symptoms and Signs: The onset is usually insidious, with gradually developing limitation of motion and mild pain that is worse at night. With joint involvement, contracture develops, and adjacent muscles become atrophied from disuse. Bone destruction can produce deformity, particularly a sharply angled gibbus resulting from thoracolumbar spine involvement. An abscess may drain spontaneously to produce a sinus. Caseating abscesses, synovial hypertrophy with pannus formation, and rice bodies (small, free white bodies composed of compact masses of fibrin, necrotic synovial villi, or cartilage fragments) are typical findings upon surgical exploration.

B. Laboratory Findings: Recovery of M tuberculosis (or other mycobacteria) from joint fluid, pus, or a tissue specimen is the key to diagnosis. Special culture techniques are required. Histologic findings of caseating necrosis and giant cells may be characteristic but are not specific for the causative organism.

C. Imaging Studies: Soft tissue swelling and joint effusion appear first, followed by decreased bone density, cortical thinning, and enlargement of the medullary canal. With joint involvement, bone density is decreased both proximally and distally. Eventual cartilage destruction leads to joint narrowing. Metaphyseal lesions may develop single or multilocular cystic changes, perhaps with central calcification. The anterior spinal column—vertebral bodies and disks—is the commonest site of skeletal involvement. Decreased vertebral body density, disk narrowing, erosion of end plates on both sides of the involved interspace, and the development of paravertebral abscesses are typical findings. Occasionally, a tuberculous vertebral body may collapse abruptly. Retropulsed bone fragments thus produced may compromise the spinal canal and interfere with spinal cord function. Pyogenic vertebral osteomyelitis may have a similar appearance but tends to progress faster, with more complex disk destruction and more sclerotic bone reaction.

Differential Diagnosis

Other subacute and chronic infections of joints, bones, or the tendon sheath must be considered, in addition to rheumatoid arthritis, gout, and fibrous dysplasia of bone.

Complications

Spinal cord involvement with paralysis from spinal tuberculosis (Pott's disease) is the most serious musculoskeletal complication of this potentially life-threatening systemic infection. Deformity, ankylosis, abscess formation, and sinus tracts are, as mentioned above, other potential complications of untreated skeletal tuberculosis.

Treatment

Early skeletal tuberculosis will usually respond well to appropriate antibiotic treatment. Nutritional support, rest, and immobilization are valuable adjuncts.

A. Medical Treatment: Chemotherapy of osteoarticular tuberculosis relies on systemic administration of drugs. In vitro sensitivity testing helps to indicate which drugs should be used. Resistant strains of pathogens are likely to emerge during treatment with single drugs, and combinations are therefore usually prescribed. Isoniazid, rifampin, pyrazinamide, and ethambutol are currently the most widely used drugs. Typical combinations include at least two of the four. A minimum of 6–9 months of adequate treatment is required.

B. Surgical Treatment: Biopsy is often required to establish the diagnosis and obtain organisms for culture and sensitivity studies. Abscesses should be drained surgically before drainage occurs spontaneously, creating a risk of superinfection. Synovectomy may speed recovery and help preserve function of involved joints and tendon sheaths. Since the development of effective chemotherapy, arthrodesis of involved joints has been required much less frequently for the management of tuberculosis. Significant destructive lesions of the vertebral column have been managed successfully with chemotherapy alone, and this is probably the method of choice in economically underdeveloped parts of the world. Aggressive surgery, with an anterior approach to the spine, drainage of the abscess, and debridement of necrotic bone fragments, provides prompt decompression of the spinal cord if neurologic deficit develops. With adequate antibiotic coverage, bone grafts can be placed in the resulting defect, so that spinal stability is restored earlier. Fusion is more predictable than with chemotherapy alone; the risk of progressive kyphosis is decreased; and the time required for recovery is significantly shortened. If experienced surgeons are available, anterior debridement and fusion of tuberculous vertebral osteomyelitis is advisable when bone destruction is marked or significant abscesses are present. Anterior fusion should be considered seriously for children, who are at greater risk of progressive spinal deformity. Laminectomy is usually contraindicated.

Prognosis

Residual pain and limitation of motion may be problems following tuberculous arthritis of the hip. If the disease is under medical control and has been quiescent for many years, satisfactory results can be achieved with total hip arthroplasty. Pre- and postoperative coverage with antituberculosis drugs may be advisable. Arthroplasty should be reserved for secondary posttuberculous degenerative joint disease and not done while recrudescent tuberculosis of the joint is present.

Martini M et al: Bone and joint tuberculosis: A review of 652 cases. Orthopedics 1988;11:861.

POSTTRAUMATIC OSTEOMYELITIS

When bone is fractured or surgically disrupted, its local blood supply is damaged, and necrosis occurs to a greater or lesser extent, depending upon the amount of damage to bone and soft tissue. In posttraumatic

osseous infections, necrotic bone is present from the onset of disease. In this regard, the infection is similar to chronic osteomyelitis but not to acute hematogenous osteomyelitis, in which necrotic bone develops progressively. Associated hematoma and traumatized soft tissue provide a medium for posttraumatic bone infection. The insertion of foreign material—prosthetic joints, acrylic cement, and metallic fracture fixation hardware—impairs the host's attempts to resist bacterial proliferations.

Clinical Findings

Increasing pain, fever that fails to resolve after fracture or orthopedic surgery, and local signs of wound inflammation—drainage, erythema, progressive swelling—are highly suggestive of posttraumatic infection. The wound must be examined without delay. If drainage is present, gram-stained smears and cultures are required. Deep aspiration or surgical wound exploration may be necessary to obtain representative samples not contaminated with skin flora. Deep infection in a wound due to fracture or osteotomy *must* place the bone at risk of infection. Only surgical exploration will demonstrate the extent of bone involvement and permit appropriate treatment. Sometimes a sterile hematoma causes early postoperative wound drainage. There is considerable risk that this drainage, if it continues, will provide a pathway for wound contamination and infection. Late wound drainage is almost always due to infection. The risk of infection following clean orthopedic surgical procedures is generally under 2%. Infections are exceedingly rare after closed fractures unless they are treated with open surgery. Open fractures, however, are associated with infection rates dependent upon the extent of the original wound and ranging from 1–2% for small relatively clean wounds to over 20% for severe wounds.

Prevention

Prevention is one of the most important aspects of managing posttraumatic wound infections. The basic principles (see Chapter 8) are avoidance of contamination and unnecessary tissue damage, thorough wound debridement and irrigation, minimally traumatic skeletal stabilization, delayed closure of contaminated wounds, and appropriate adjunctive use of antibiotics.

Treatment

Early diagnosis is crucial if infection develops. Prompt appropriate treatment is often rewarded by successful control of the infectious process. Infections that persist or present late, after smoldering for a few weeks, may be harder to control.

Specific treatment of posttraumatic wound infections is operative decompression and debridement. Pus and infected hematoma must be evacuated and necrotic tissue removed. Mature judgment is required to determine how much bone to remove. It is not always easy to tell which bone is necrotic and which can resist infection. Adequate debridement of infected and devitalized tissue is easier when coverage is obtained with muscle pedicle grafts, either moved locally or transplanted from another region of the body with microvascular anastomoses. For restoration of function, adequate bone reconstruction is also essential.

Melissinos EG, Parks DH: Post-trauma reconstruction with free tissue transfer: Analysis of 442 consecutive cases. J Trauma 1989;29:1095.

INFECTED FRACTURES

Infections that develop in fractures are rarely controlled until fracture healing has occurred. It is now generally accepted that rigid immobilization is an important part of treatment of infected fractures. This can be achieved with external skeletal fixation or internal fixation; use of a cast or traction is generally not as successful. Therefore, internal fixation devices that provide stability should not be removed before bone healing has occurred, even though their presence increases the likelihood of recurrent infection. Once the fracture has healed, removal of internal fixation and thorough wound debridement will often result in control of infection. Loose fixation devices do not provide stability and should therefore be removed, since they decrease resistance to infection. Following removal, the fracture must be stabilized with external or internal means as appropriate.

Systemic antibiotics, chosen according to results of culture and sensitivity studies, are helpful adjuncts in surgical wound management. Antibiotic treatment should be extended for as long as each individual case requires; there are no well-defined guidelines for length of treatment. Posttraumatic infections often involve multiple organisms or gram-negative organisms that require toxic antibiotics. Attenuation of infection is often the most that can be hoped for before fracture healing and hardware removal. If an antibiotic with cumulative toxicity is necessary, it may be best to avoid prolonged administration until after hardware can be removed. However, if the infecting organism is sensitive to an oral drug that can achieve satisfactory serum levels without dangerous side effects, suppressive treatment may be continued until the fracture is healed and hardware can be removed.

Burri C: *Post-traumatic Osteomyelitis.* Hans Huber, 1975.
Fleischmann W, Kinzl L: Philosophy of osteosynthesis in shoulder fractures. Orthopedics 1993;16:59.
Johnson KD: Management of open fractures and infections. In: *Orthopaedic Infections.* D'Ambrosia RD, Marier RL (editors). Slack, 1989.
May JW et al: Clinical classification of post-traumatic os-
teomyelitis. (Current Concepts Review.) J Bone Joint Surg [Am] 1989;71:1422.

INFECTED PUNCTURE WOUNDS OF THE FOOT

Although most puncture wounds of the foot respond to local cleansing and tetanus prophylaxis, infection does develop occasionally. The causative organism is frequently *Pseudomonas aeruginosa.* Treatment requires prompt incision and drainage of involved bone or joint tissues and administration of appropriate antibiotics.

OSTEOMYELITIS DUE TO EXTENSION OF ADJACENT SOFT TISSUE INFECTION

Infections that develop in the soft tissues of the fingers or toes can extend into and destroy adjacent bone. Septic arthritis from puncture wounds may have a similar result. Prompt adequate treatment of the initial infection will prevent this complication and avoid the need either for amputation or for joint resection and fusion to salvage some function. A more common form of osteomyelitis due to extension from an established infected site is that which occurs beneath trophic ulcers associated with arterial insufficiency, diabetes mellitus, or neuropathy due to other causes. Such chronic soft tissue ulcers inevitably become infected, usually with a mixture of organisms that frequently includes anaerobes. Persisting infection may spread to involve adjacent bone but usually only its surface, unless septic arthritis develops or the infection is of exceptionally long duration. The possibility of osteomyelitis is raised by radiographs of the involved area. Focal demineralization may be present without bone infection. Cortical erosion and periosteal new bone formation are more suggestive, but only the presence of necrotic sequestered bone is convincing evidence of osteomyelitis. In fact, persistence of such trophic ulcers rarely results from osteomyelitis but instead from inadequate debridement of soft tissues, continuing mechanical trauma, or inadequate blood supply. Treatment should be directed at these factors. Ray resection or amputation may be necessary to achieve soft tissue healing. Superficially involved bone at the base of an ulcer may require only superficial debridement. Prolonged antibiotic treatment is not necessary in such cases if healing is progressing and will be insufficient if it is not.

Joints adjacent to pressure sores (decubitus ulcers) or neurotrophic or ischemic ulcers may develop septic arthritis that is easily overlooked without synovial fluid aspiration or arthrogram. Without adequate joint drainage and debridement, there is little hope for controlling these serious infections.

It is important to be aware of the marked radiographic abnormalities produced by neuropathic joint destruction in diabetes mellitus as well as other causes of peripheral neuropathy. These can be confused with infection or can coexist with it.

Lowen RM et al: *Aeromonas hydrophila* infection complicating digital replantation and revascularization [see comments]. J Hand Surg [Am] 1989;14:714.

Scallion JH et al: Treatment of diabetic foot infections: Wagner classification, therapy, and outcome. Foot Ankle 1988;9:101.

Wagner FW Jr: The diabetic foot. Orthopedics 1987;10: 163.

CHRONIC OSTEOMYELITIS

The foregoing discussions should suggest that there is often no clear division between acute and chronic osteomyelitis. From a practical viewpoint, however, the concept of chronic osteomyelitis is valuable because it emphasizes the persisting, recurring nature of infections involving bone and because it is usually associated with more or less easily definable areas of necrotic bone that harbor the causative microorganisms and thus provide a source for recurrences. If technically possible, removal of sequestered necrotic bone may significantly reduce the risk or severity of recurrent infection. Radiologic signs of chronic osteomyelitis may persist with little or no sign of active disease. However, a flare-up can occur after decades of inactivity. It is therefore reasonable to consider chronic osteomyelitis a disease that is controlled but never really cured. Evaluation of host resistance fractures, local and systemic, is crucial for diagnosis and treatment.

Clinical Findings

A. Symptoms and Signs: Chronic osteomyelitis may recur as apparent cellulitis in the region of previously infected bone or as an obvious soft tissue abscess. This may "point" and rupture to produce a sinus tract that persists or drains periodically. Convincing evidence of chronic osteomyelitis is persisting or recurring wound drainage, which may be serous or purulent.

B. Laboratory Findings: Cultures of a draining sinus usually yield organisms but do not necessarily differentiate pathogens from superficial growth. Tissue biopsy or deep aspiration is necessary for reliable bacteriologic diagnosis, which is the key to appropriate antibacterial therapy. Chronic bone infections may be caused by mycobacteria or fungi, so stains and cultures appropriate for these microorganisms are always required. When tissue is obtained for culture, an adjacent specimen should also be sent for histopathologic study.

C. Imaging Studies: Radiographs demonstrate both destructive and reactive bone changes, with more or less circumscribed areas of lucency, sclerosis, and often periosteal or appositional new bone formation. Involucra may be obvious or may require tomograms or CT scans for demonstration. A sinogram, obtained by gentle injection of iodinated soluble contrast medium (Renografin or Hypaque) will delineate the area of involvement and may indicate the source of recurring infection. Occasionally, a sinus that appears to arise from the pelvis communicates with infection originating in the gastrointestinal or genitourinary tract.

Differential Diagnosis

Chronic osteomyelitis must be differentiated from benign and malignant bone tumor, bone dysplasia, and traumatic lesions, including fatigue fracture.

Complications

Persistence and recurrence are common. Infection may spread systemically or locally. Pathologic fracture may occur, especially after bone debridement. Bone deformity or shortening, nonunion, malunion, and stiffness or ankylosis of adjacent joints may cause significant loss of function. Amputation may be necessary to control infection or to provide a more functional limb than would remain after prolonged infection and repeated surgery. After years of drainage, malignant degeneration may occur in the sinus tract. This should be suspected if increasing pain or drainage develops with long-standing osteomyelitis.

Treatment

A. Conservative Treatment: When chronic osteomyelitis is quiescent, no treatment is necessary, and the patient may live an essentially normal life. Dressing changes alone may be sufficient for minor exacerbations with drainage.

B. Medical Treatment: If symptoms are more severe, rest with elevation of the involved limb, analgesics as needed, and systemic antibiotics are advisable. The choice of antibiotic may be aided by culture and sensitivity test results from prior symptomatic episodes; by aspiration or biopsy of the involved area; or least desirably, by a more or less educated guess at the infecting organism and its antibiotic sensitivities. In the early phases of recurrence, without abscess or sinus tract, these measures alone may produce a prompt, though usually temporary, clinical resolution. The optimal duration of antibiotic treatment for chronic osteomyelitis remains unclear. Some authors recommend only brief usage, during acute exacerbations and surgical procedures. Current opinion among infectious disease experts supports a 4- to 6-week course, though the results of this regimen are not well documented. It is clear that antibiotics are adjuncts to adequate debridement and are not in themselves sufficient treatment. Adjunctive oral antibiotic coverage for at least 6 months appears to be beneficial for treatment of chronic staphylococcal osteomyelitis due to susceptible organisms.

C. Surgical Treatment: Surgical treatment will be necessary if rest and antibiotics do not result in prompt improvement or if significant drainage, bone destruction, or sequestration is evident. Soft tissue abscesses require incision and drainage. The resulting wound may be left open or closed over suction-irrigation tubes. Tubes can be managed in several ways. Continuous flow systems are complicated. Doses of antibiotics delivered by continuous flow may be too large, and toxicity may occur. Scrupulous sterile precautions must be followed with all techniques, and tubes should generally be removed within a few days to minimize the risk of superinfection. The following regimen has been effective: Periodic irrigation is performed with small volumes of antibiotic solution, followed by prolonged suction to prevent fluid accumulation and minimize soft tissue dead space. As a rule, no more than 10–20 mL of solution (eg, 0.1% gentamicin in normal saline) is injected every 12 hours, allowed to stay in the wound for a few hours, and then withdrawn by suction applied to the tube via a three-way stopcock that also permits irrigation. A single tube is used for small wounds, but double tubes may be needed for larger ones (Figure 43–63). Suction-irrigation tube systems are not a substitute for adequate surgical drainage of pus and adequate debridement of poorly vascularized, chronically infected tissue. Neither do they replace systemic antibiotic treatment with appropriate drugs. They do offer an effective means of obtaining early closure of an infected wound that would otherwise require open management.

Removal of bone may be necessary to extract a sequestrum or to unroof an intraosseous abscess. The resulting cavity acts as a "dead space," which fills with hematoma rather than healthy, well-perfused tissue and leaves a potential focus for recurrence. Saucerization and then exteriorization of the cavity may be followed by split-thickness skin grafting or open cancellous bone grafting once the defect is lined with healthy granulation tissue. A better alternative is to fill the defect with a muscle graft, either with its own local blood supply or as a free microvascular transfer. Coverage of adequately debrided chronic osteomyelitis with a well-perfused muscle pedicle appears to be the most effective surgical treatment for significantly symptomatic chronic osteomyelitis. Extensive bone debridement is often required, resulting in a need for bone grafts if function and structural integrity are to be preserved. Free vascularized muscle grafts make adequate debridement and reconstruction possible

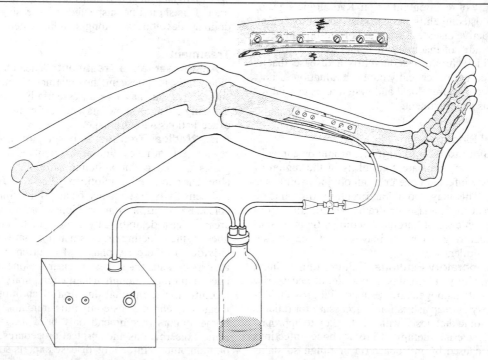

Figure 43–63. Jergesen tube system for periodic suction-irrigation. A tube with several openings near the end is positioned in the area to be drained and brought out obliquely through the soft tissues and skin. The tube is attached to a sterile three-way stopcock and sterile trap bottle. Small volumes of irrigating solution containing antibiotics are injected via the stopcock with sterile technique. The solution is allowed to remain in the wound for a few hours before the stopcock is opened for suction for several more hours. The process is then repeated.

when the involved area is too large to be managed with locally available tissue resources.

Prognosis

Whatever the initial cause, once an infection involving bone has become well-established, with focally necrotic bone and scar tissue and microabscesses scattered through the involved area, the long-term outlook must remain guarded. Although infection may be controlled with adequate debridement and prolonged treatment with antibiotics, there is always a risk of late recurrence, even after many years of quiescence.

Cierney G III, Mader JT: Adult chronic osteomyelitis: An overview. In: *Orthopaedic Infections.* D'Ambrosia RD, Marier RL (editors). Slack, 1989.

Moore JR et al: Free vascularized bone and muscle flaps for osteomyelitis. Orthopedics 1986;9:819.

Tong Y et al: The treatment of chronic hematogenous osteomyelitis. Clin Orthop 1987;(Feb)215:72.

Torholm C et al: Chronic progressive osteoblastic osteomyelitis: A new approach to treatment. J Pediatr Orthop 1988;8:326.

SEPTIC ARTHRITIS

Septic arthritis is an acute or chronic inflammatory joint disease caused by bacteria or fungi. Primary infection is caused by direct inoculation of the joint by trauma, including surgery. Secondary infection occurs hematogenously or by extension from adjacent osteomyelitis. Septic arthritis characteristically involves a single joint. This disease must always be considered in the differential diagnosis of monarticular arthritis.

Occasionally, septic arthritis will develop in a joint already involved by another form of arthritis. This possibility must be considered whenever an arthritic joint "flares" or an arthritic patient becomes systemically ill. Septic arthritis is more common in children and debilitated elderly individuals except when gonococci are the cause. (See also Septic Arthritis of the Hip, p 1057.)

ACUTE SEPTIC ARTHRITIS

Essentials of Diagnosis

- Joint pain.
- Limited motion.
- Joint swelling, effusion, warmth, and tenderness.
- Pus and organisms in synovial fluid aspirate.

General Considerations

Septic arthritis destroys articular cartilage. The initial reaction to joint infection is acute synovitis, with effusion that develops an increasing concentration of PMNs. The fluid tends to coagulate, producing loculations within the joint cavity. Inflammatory cells infiltrate the synovium, and the overlying tissues become edematous. With continuing infection, the cartilage matrix is destroyed, collagen is lost, and chondrocytes are killed. The damaged cartilage is susceptible to mechanical trauma and is eroded at points of loading. Continued infection may destroy synovial and capsular components as well as cartilage and bone. Spread to adjacent bone produces osteomyelitis. Following successful treatment of early infections, there may be no permanent sequelae, but extensive tissue destruction rarely resolves completely. Fibrous or complete bony ankylosis may result, as well as painful postinfectious degenerative arthritis.

Gonococci are probably the commonest cause of septic arthritis at present, at least in sexually active individuals, and must be considered whenever a seemingly sterile pyarthrosis is encountered. *S aureus* is by far the next most common pathogen. Septic joints in children from 6 months to 2 years of age are often due to *Haemophilus influenzae.* Gram-negative bacilli have recently become a more frequent cause of septic joints, especially in adults with chronic debilitating illness. However, almost every bacterial pathogen has been reported to cause septic arthritis, and the clinical presentation is not helpful for determining the causative organism.

Clinical Findings

A. Symptoms and Signs: In acute hematogenous arthritis, the larger joints (knee, hip, elbow, shoulder, and ankle) are more commonly involved. Infections of other organ systems (skin, respiratory tract, genitourinary tract, etc) are possible sources of blood-borne infections. Although infections in adults usually involve only one joint, multiple joint involvement occurs occasionally in children. Any joint may be involved secondarily by spread of a nearby acute or chronic infection. Systemic disease or another serious infection may divert attention from the infected joint. Systemic symptoms usually include fever, chills, and malaise and, occasionally, misleading migratory polyarthralgia. Pain is progressive and accentuated by joint motion. Local tenderness and warmth are accompanied by soft tissue swelling, and an effusion is palpable if the joint is superficial.

B. Laboratory Findings: Examination of joint fluid is crucial. By the time infection is clinically apparent, the fluid is usually turbid or purulent. The white cell count is often over 50,000/L, with more than 90% PMNs. Synovial fluid glucose is decreased, usually to 50 mg/dL below a simultaneously obtained blood glucose level. Gram-stained smears and cultures are essential. The stain will often dictate the choice of first antibiotic pending sensitivity confirmation. Pyarthrosis without visible organisms on a gram-stained smear is usually gonococcal in origin. Culture specimens for this fastidious organism must be conveyed promptly to the bacteriology laboratory for proper plating on a selective medium and incubation in 5% carbon dioxide. The erythrocyte sedimentation rate is almost always elevated, and the white count may be. Blood cultures are sometimes positive even when organisms are not recovered from joint fluid.

C. Imaging Studies: The appearance of significant x-ray findings depends upon the duration and virulence of infection. X-ray changes lag behind the clinical and pathologic process. During the first 2 weeks, the joint capsule may appear distended, the overlying soft tissues swollen, and fat planes obscured. In infants especially, increased intra-articular pressure from effusion may cause widening of the radiologic "joint space," with possible progression to pathologic dislocation. Comparative x-rays of the opposite normal joint can aid in identification of subtle changes. With persistent hyperemia and disuse, demineralization of subchondral bone occurs and extends proximal and distal to the joint. Trabecular detail is progressively lost, and the compact subchondral bone appears accentuated. Destruction of cartilage is reflected by narrowing of the width of the joint space until subchondral bone is in apposition, a finding accentuated by x-rays taken during weight bearing.

Complications

Complications consist of joint destruction, osteomyelitis, and direct or hematogenous spread to other sites. The risk of complication is increased by delayed diagnosis.

Differential Diagnosis

Acute pyogenic arthritis must be differentiated from other acute arthropathies (reactive arthritis, systemic lupus erythematosus, rheumatoid arthritis, gout, pseudogout, neurogenic arthropathy, etc). Hematogenous osteomyelitis (especially of the proximal femur), rheumatic fever, and epiphyseal trauma may mimic acute septic arthritis in childhood. Lyme disease must also be considered.

Acute pyogenic arthritis may complicate almost any type of preexisting joint disease, especially rheumatoid arthritis and neuropathic arthropathy. Concomitant or recent treatment with locally injected or systemic corticosteroids may both predispose to infection and interfere with diagnosis. Polyarthralgia occurs in systemic viral infections and allergic reactions, but the other features of septic arthritis are lacking. Acute infections or inflammations of periarticular structures (eg, septic bursitis and tenosynovitis, osteomyelitis, cellulitis, and acute calcific tendinitis) may be especially difficult to differentiate. Aspiration, examination, and culture of joint fluid are essential to establish or rule out infection of a joint. Occasionally, synovial biopsy is helpful in diagnosing obscure cases of synovitis.

Treatment

A. General Measures: Analgesics and splinting of the involved joint in the position of maximal comfort alleviate pain. Other foci of infection and any coexisting medical conditions must be identified and treated appropriately. Fluid replacement and nutritional support may be required.

B. Specific Measures: Definitive treatment requires drainage of the pyarthrosis and prompt institution of effective antibiotic therapy. The technique of drainage depends upon the joint involved, the stage of infection, and the response of the patient. Although many infected joints can be drained satisfactorily with repeated needle aspiration, the hip—and perhaps other joints that are difficult to aspirate—will require arthrotomy as soon as possible after identification of joint sepsis. Other indications for surgical drainage of septic arthritis are inability to aspirate loculated pus, lack of prompt response to nonoperative management, long-standing infection, and joint infections after surgery or penetrating wounds.

Parenteral antibiotics are indicated for septic arthritis. If organisms are not seen on gram-stained smears and the patient is a previously healthy adult, gonococcal arthritis is an appropriate working diagnosis, and penicillin should be started as outlined below. Children under 4 years of age have a significant incidence of *Haemophilus influenzae* arthritis. Preliminary antibiotic treatment in this age group must be effective against this organism, which also may be difficult to see on gram-stained smears. In adults with negative results on gram-stained smears and a suspected cause of infection other than gonococci, treatment should be started with a cephalosporin or beta-lactamase-resistant penicillin and an aminoglycoside.

When organisms are seen, initial antibiotic therapy should be based on that finding. Culture results and clinical response must subsequently be used to ensure an appropriate antibiotic regimen. Parenteral antibiotics are continued at high doses until inflammation resolves significantly. Ten to 14 days is usually required. An additional 3–4 weeks of oral antibiotic therapy is often advised after parenteral treatment. Briefer treatment usually suffices for gonococcal arthritis. Intravenous penicillin G, 10 million units/24 h, should be continued until significant improvement is achieved. While the response is often prompt, several days of treatment may be required. Once local signs resolve, the antibiotic can be changed to oral ampicillin, 500 mg four times daily, to complete a 7-day course.

Prognosis

Satisfactory results are achieved in 70% or more of patients with septic arthritis if early diagnosis and treatment are provided. Joint destruction—especially of the hip in infants—and joint stiffness in the elderly are the commonest causes of failure. Deaths are rare but may occur in debilitated patients and those who are immunologically suppressed. It is thought that involved joints may be at risk for early degenerative joint disease. Extended follow-up of patients who have been treated for septic arthritis is difficult to obtain, but available studies suggest that satisfactory early results are maintained.

Chaudhuri K et al: Septic arthritis of the shoulder after mastectomy and radiotherapy for breast carcinoma. J Bone Joint Surg [Br] 1993;75:318.

Cristofaro RL et al: Musculoskeletal manifestations of Lyme disease in children. J Pediatr Orthop 1987;7:527.

Dagan R: Management of acute hematogenous osteomyelitis and septic arthritis in the pediatric patient. Pediatr Infect Dis J 1993;12:88.

O'Meara PM et al: Septic arthritis: Process, etiology, treatment outcome. A literature review. Orthopedics 1988; 11:623.

Ostrum RF: *Nocardia* septic arthritis of the hip with associated avascular necrosis A case report. Clin Orthop 1993;Mar(288):282.

Ouzounian TJ et al: Evaluation of musculoskeletal sepsis with indium-111 white blood cell imaging. Clin Orthop 1987;(Aug)221:304.

Parisien JS: Arthroscopic management of pyarthrosis: An overview. Bull Hosp Jt Dis Orthop Inst 1987;47:52.

Rankin KC, Rycken JM: Bilateral dislocation of the proximal humeral epiphyses in septic arthritis: A case report. J Bone Joint Surg [Br] 1993;75:329.

Wilson NI et al: Acute septic arthritis in infancy and childhood: 10 years' experience. J Bone Joint Surg [Br] 1986;68:584.

BONE TUMORS

Primary tumors of bone are relatively uncommon in comparison with secondary or metastatic neoplasms. However, they are of great clinical significance because of the possibility of cancer and because some grow rapidly and metastasize widely. Persistent skeletal pain, localized tenderness, and an enlarging mass with or without limitation of motion of adjacent joints or spontaneous fracture are indications for prompt clinical, x-rays, laboratory, and perhaps biopsy examination. Histologic characteristics generally provide the best information about the nature of the lesion, but they must be correlated with all other related facts. The diagnosis of bone tumors is most precise when made by the clinician, the radiologist, and the pathologist in close consultation.

Mercuri M et al: The management of malignant bone tumors in children and adolescents. Clin Orthop 1991; Mar(264):156.

Simon MA, Finn HA: Diagnostic strategy for bone and soft-tissue tumors. J Bone Joint Surg [Am] 1993;3;75:622.

Operative Technique

There are several surgical approaches to the treatment of bone tumors. With intralesional excision (curettement, debulking), the tumor is entered, but gross as well as microscopic tumor may remain. Excision indicates local removal of a tumor following visualization of the capsule or pseudocapsule to establish the plane of dissection. Tumor cells may be left in the wound even if the capsule is not grossly violated. Wide excision indicates a margin of normal tissue between the capsule or pseudocapsule and the planes of dissection. Radical resection implies removal of the entire anatomic compartment containing the tumor. Amputation may be any of these depending on the margin, but it is usually "wide excision" or "radical resection."

Radiologic Characteristics

A. Benign Characteristics:

1. Cystic expansion of a diaphysis or metaphysis with mature cortex around the area of expansion.

2. The presence of a definable though thin cortical end plate (capsule) around an intraosseous area from which cancellous or cortical bone has been lost, sometimes referred to as a "geographic lesion."

3. No periosteal new bone formation.

B. Malignant Characteristics:

1. Permeative destruction of either cancellous or cortical bone, manifested by gradual transition from a region of gross destruction with loss of bony continuity to region of lesser destruction and normal bone. There is no clear line of demarcation between abnormal and normal bone.

2. Gross bone destruction with cortical defects, manifested by loss of large areas of bony substance without encapsulation.

3. Periosteal or tumor bone formation within the tumor or at its margins. This may be manifested by multiple layers of parallel periosteal reaction (onion-skin formation) or sunburst (spiculated, hair-on-end) linear areas of calcification. The latter generally parallel the expansile direction of the tumor as it breaks through bone.

4. A few metastatic tumors (breast, prostate) incite local reactive new bone formation and are classified as osteoblastic rather than osteolytic tumors (the latter are more common in metastatic cancer).

Grading & Staging

Some tumor categories can be subclassified into varying degrees of malignancy (grading) according to histologic criteria, radiologic appearance, and clinical course. Grade 0 is benign; grade 1 is low-grade malignancy; grades 2 and 3 indicate increasingly higher degrees of malignancy. Grading reflects the biologic behavior of the lesion.

The size of the tumor, the presence or absence of local invasion of adjacent compartments or lymph nodes, and the presence or absence of distant metastases can be combined with the surgical grade to establish stage categories that reflect prognosis. When grading and staging are possible, treatment options may be more realistically chosen.

Among musculoskeletal neoplasms, chondrosarcomas lend themselves to grading, although in tumors occurring secondary to osteochondroma, size is of less significance than with other sarcomas. Grading and staging of soft tissue sarcomas by histologic criteria, intra- or extracompartmental location, and metastatic spread have prognostic value and aid in planning treatment.

In osteogenic sarcoma and Ewing's sarcoma, the prognosis is not easily determined from the histologic pattern, and grading is therefore not as useful as in soft tissue sarcomas or chondrosarcomas.

Enneking WF: A system of staging musculoskeletal neoplasms. Clin Orthop 1986;(Mar)204:9.
Murphy WA Jr: Imaging bone tumors in the 1990s. Cancer 1991;67(4 Suppl):1169.
Sundaram M: Radiographic and magnetic resonance imaging of bone and soft-tissue tumors and myeloproliferative disorders. Current Opin Radiol 1991;3:746.

Biopsy

The possibility of cancer exists in almost every lesion prior to histologic examination. Therefore, the choice of excision and the extent of exposure for biopsy should be planned to avoid unnecessary contamination of tissue planes with tumor cells, which would complicate subsequent local resection. This consideration takes precedence over more standard surgical approaches used for trauma and reconstruction. In the extremities, biopsy incisions should be longitudinal and placed where minimal dissection is needed to reach the tumor. Frozen section guidance should be obtained. This may permit immediate definitive diagnosis and operation. Even when this is not so, the surgeon can be assured that an adequate and representative sample has been examined and may occasionally be forewarned that the lesion is inflammatory rather than neoplastic. For the latter reason, it is also advisable to take appropriate culture specimens of some of the tissue removed at biopsy even though the clinical picture and x-ray appearance may seem typical of a neoplastic lesion.

Chemotherapy

It has recently been shown that adjunctive chemotherapy following appropriate management of the primary lesion has delayed the appearance and lowered the incidence of metastases and lowered the 2-year death rates for osteogenic sarcoma, Ewing's sarcoma, and primary lymphoma of bone. Alterations in drug combinations, dosage, and frequency continue to be made. For this reason, specific protocols for chemotherapy will not be included in this chapter. The reader is referred to reports of the appropriate cancer study groups of the National Cancer Institute for current guidelines.

Radiation Therapy

Radiation therapy combined with chemotherapy has become standard treatment for Ewing's sarcoma and primary lymphoma of bone. Radiation therapy used alone sometimes produced dramatic initial control of primary lesions, but 5-year survival rates for these tumors did not improve significantly until chemotherapy was added.

Radiation therapy plus chemotherapy has a less well defined role in the treatment of primary osteogenic sarcoma. Irradiation alone will produce a temporary response manifested largely by brief cessation of the prior rapid rate of growth. However, even when chemotherapy is added, sufficient control of the primary lesion is not achieved.

Radiation therapy of benign lesions of bone is undesirable if the primary can be controlled surgically, since radiation-induced sarcoma of bone occurs with an incidence of 0.2% in normal bone (ie, in radiation fields in patients treated for other lesions). The risk appears to be greater in growing bone than adult bone. Certain benign but locally aggressive tumors of bone with high local recurrence rates necessitate consideration of radiation therapy if the anatomic location makes the risk of morbidity and death associated with surgical removal unacceptable (spine, skull, or facial bones).

METASTATIC BONE TUMORS

The commonest form of cancer affecting the skeleton is metastatic tumor deposits from primary lesions elsewhere in the body. Eighty percent of these metastatic lesions are from primary carcinomas, particularly of the breast, prostate, lung, kidney, thyroid, pancreas, or stomach, in that order of frequency.

The presenting symptom is usually pain. Pathologic fracture may be present and is more common in the lower than the upper extremity.

The presenting radiologic finding is destruction of bone—usually osteolytic but in the case of breast or prostate metastasis either partly or solely osteoblastic. The size of an individual lesion is usually less than what is seen in primary tumors of bone at the time of first diagnosis.

In a patient with a known primary malignant tumor presenting with a painful lytic lesion of bone, a diagnosis of metastatic deposit can be made with some assurance; but there are individuals in whom the primary is not yet recognized at the time the early metastatic lesion becomes painful. Bone scan or skeletal survey will aid the prebiopsy workup, since there is a high probability of more than one area of skeletal involvement. The most common primary source of solitary skeletal metastases at the time of first diagnosis is carcinoma of the kidney. Therefore, an excretory urogram should be part of the prebiopsy workup of solitary metastases with no obvious primary. Metastases from carcinoma of the kidney are extremely vascular—an important point to remember when planning biopsy.

The treatment of metastatic cancer has two goals: management of the neoplasm and management of the symptoms produced by the local lesion.

Management of the neoplasm at the metastatic site depends upon the type and prognosis in each case but usually involves radiation therapy, chemotherapy, hormone therapy, or a combination of these.

Operative treatment with internal fixation for pathologic fracture is often desirable in long bones, particularly in the lower extremities, so that the patient can remain ambulatory and more comfortable during the months or even years of life that remain. Although less commonly indicated because of the non-weight-bearing function of the upper extremity, internal fixation may be necessary for pain control or to improve the patient's ability to manage crutches. In addition to the usual techniques for fracture fixation, methylmethacrylate supplementation frequently is necessary to substitute for bone loss and possible lack of healing response.

Brage ME, Simon MA: Evaluation, prognosis, and medical treatment considerations of metastatic bone tumors. Orthopedics 1992;15:589.

Habermann ET, Lopez RA: Metastatic disease of bone and treatment of pathological fractures. Orthop Clin North Am 1989;20:469.

Present D, Shaffer B: Disease-associated fractures: Detection and management in the elderly. Geriatrics 1990; 45:48, 59.

Thompson RC Jr: Impending fracture associated with bone destruction. Orthopedics 1992;15:547.

Weinstein JN: Differential diagnosis and surgical treatment of pathologic spine fractures. Instr Course Lect 1992; 41:301.

MYELOMA

In one sense, multiple myeloma is the commonest malignant tumor affecting bone, but since it arises from the hematopoietic marrow, it is not, strictly speaking, a tumor "of bone." Its incidence is about equal to that of all malignant tumors of bone combined. Pain is the principal presenting symptom, and local swelling is uncommon. Pathologic fractures do occur but are not a common initial symptom. The lesions can occur in any bone, but small bone involvement is infrequent. There is a slightly higher incidence in males than females, with peak incidence in the sixth and seventh decades. The bony lesions are manifested radiologically by osteolytic areas of bone destruction, with little or no reactive bone.

As indicated by the term multiple myeloma, there frequently are multiple lesions at the time of initial diagnosis.

The treatment strategy is essentially the same as that outlined above for metastatic tumors.

McCarthy CS, Becker JA: Multiple myeloma and contrast media. Radiology 1992;183:519.

Steiner RM et al: Magnetic resonance imaging of diffuse bone marrow disease. Radiol Clin North Am 1993;31: 383.

MALIGNANT BONE TUMORS

1. OSTEOGENIC SARCOMA

Osteogenic sarcoma is the most common primary malignant tumor of bone, with an incidence of 0.25 cases per 100,000 population per year. It usually occurs in the distal femoral metaphysis, proximal tibial metaphysis, proximal humeral metaphysis, pelvis, and proximal femur, in that order of frequency. Most patients are in the adolescent age group, and males predominate in a 3:2 ratio.

The usual presenting manifestation are pain, tenderness, and swelling near a joint. Some limitation of motion may be present.

X-rays show a permeative destructive lesion in the metaphysis that rarely crosses the epiphyseal plate and is commonly accompanied by periosteal elevation. Periosteal new bone frequently presents in the form of Codman's triangle at the diaphyseal end of the lesion (Figure 43–64). The more central area will show evidence of tumor extension beyond the confines of the cortex and contains sunburst or hair-on-end radially oriented filaments of calcification and bone formation. There is considerable variation in the degree of osteolytic versus osteoblastic activity in these lesions.

The natural history of this tumor is one of relentless growth, early metastases to the lungs, and death if appropriate treatment is not given. Lymphatic involvement is not common. Treatment by resection (usually amputation) of the primary lesion in past years produced a 5-year survival rate of 15–20%. Most deaths occurred in the first 2 years. With adjunctive chemotherapy following amputation or other local complete resection of the tumor, the appearance of pulmonary metastases has been significantly delayed, and the projected 5-year survival rate currently is about 60%. The apparent ability of adjunctive chemotherapy to destroy microscopic metastases suggests that local resection of primary lesions followed by adjunctive chemotherapy may be substituted for amputation. This is still experimental, however, since at this time, 5-year rates for both survival and absence of local recurrence in a suitably functioning limb are not available. Lesions in the pelvis or spine might

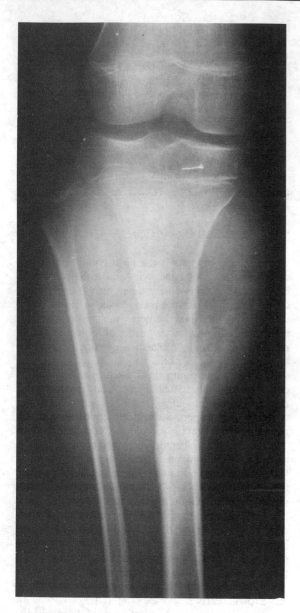

Figure 43–64. Osteosarcoma with Codman's triangle.

have boundaries too close to vital structures and hence will be treated with local excision, adjunctive chemotherapy, and perhaps radiation therapy.

Rare variants of osteogenic sarcoma with a less ominous history are parosteal, periosteal, and central sarcomas. These variants may be more amenable to local resection.

Enneking WF, Springfield D, Gross M: The surgical treatment of parosteal osteosarcoma in long bones. J Bone Joint Surg [Am] 1985;67:125.

Lane JM et al: Osteogenic sarcoma. Clin Orthop 1986;No. 204:93.

Simon MA: Causes of increased survival of patients with osteosarcoma: Current controversies. J Bone Joint Surg [Am] 1984;66:306.

2. PRIMARY CHONDROSARCOMA

The incidence of chondrosarcoma is about half that of osteogenic sarcoma. Most of these tumors are located either in the pelvic girdle, ribs, or shoulder girdle, in that order. The peak incidence is in the late fifth and early sixth decades, with a 2:1 male predominance.

The presenting symptom is usually local discomfort. A visible or demonstrable mass is seldom present.

The x-ray appearance is that of a central slightly expansile radiolucent lesion containing flocculent areas of calcific density in the lower-grade forms of the tumor. High-grade chondrosarcomas may simulate osteogenic sarcoma on x-rays. The tumor occurs commonly in the metaphyseal region when present in long bones but has a predilection for flat bones, as evidenced by the high incidence in the pelvis and ribs and a relatively high incidence in the scapula. The gross pathologic anatomy is that of firm, translucent, usually gritty gray tissue of cartilaginous density with demonstrable fine sediment of calcific density. The natural history is one of continued growth, with a high rate of local recurrence if all tumor is not removed. Metastases to distant sites, particularly the lungs, occur much later than is the case with most other bone sarcomas.

The treatment of chondrosarcoma is individualized in terms of how radical the attempt at surgical removal should be. There is no evidence that x-ray therapy will control the lesion or that chemotherapy will affect the outcome. Complete surgical removal will result in cure at 5 years in almost all grade I tumors and a significant percentage of grade III tumors. When these tumors are graded, it is important to be certain that all of the tumor has been well sampled, since there may be considerable variation in different geographic areas within the tumor.

Gitelis S et al: Chondrosarcoma of bone: J Bone Joint Surg [Am] 1981;63:1248.

Healey JH, Lane JM: Chondrosarcoma. Clin Orthop 1986; No. 204:119.

3. EWING'S TUMOR
(Ewing's Sarcoma)

Ewing's sarcoma occurs with an incidence of 0.1 cases per 100,000 population per year. The male/female ratio is 3:2. The tumor occurs most commonly in the second decade. Patients tend to be slightly younger than those with osteogenic sarcoma.

Ewing's tumor is most common in the extremities, particularly the lower extremities and pelvic girdle. The symptoms and signs are pain, local swelling, and, occasionally, fever, with an elevated white blood count.

The x-ray appearance is that of a permeative destructive lesion, usually in the metaphysis but also in the diaphysis more often than osteogenic sarcoma. Periosteal new bone formation is common. The gross pathologic picture is nonspecific, with neoplastic tissue permeating bone and muscle with a consistency varying from gray firm connective tissue to liquefaction necrosis. The latter has at times mimicked purulence secondary to bacterial infection and may be confused with osteomyelitis. These facts reinforce the general wisdom (see Biopsy, p 1095) of routinely obtaining material both for culture and for histopathologic examination whether the clinical diagnosis is infection or neoplasm.

The early history is one of progressive local growth, early distant metastases, and death if proper treatment is not given. Metastases are most common to the lung but may occur in other tissues (including bone) more frequently than is the case with osteogenic sarcoma. Radiation therapy to the primary tumor combined with multiple-drug chemotherapy has improved the 5-year survival rate to about 60%.

Treatment of Ewing's sarcoma of the pelvis has a significantly higher failure rate following such combination therapy. Hence, anatomically feasible resection or wide excision following initial tumor response to combined treatment should be considered. If the primary tumor is in an expendable bone, wide excision or resection may be considered after an initial course of combined treatment.

Benmeir P et al: Primary and secondary spinal epidural extraskeletal Ewing's sarcoma: Report of two cases and review of the literature. Spine 1991;16:224.

Horowitz ME, Neff JR, Kun LE: Ewing's sarcoma: Radiotherapy versus surgery for local control. Pediatr Clin North Am 1991;3;38:365.

Neff JR: Nonmetastatic Ewing's sarcoma of bone: The role of surgical therapy. Clin Orthop 1986;(Mar)204:111.

O'Connor MI, Pritchard DJ: Ewing's sarcoma: Prognostic factors, disease control, and the reemerging role of surgical treatment. Clin Orthop 1991;Jan(262):78.

Womer RB: The cellular biology of bone tumors. Clin Orthop 1991;Jan(262):12.

4. FIBROSARCOMA

The incidence of fibrosarcoma is about 0.05 cases per 100,000 population per year. Males and females are equally affected. More than half of cases occur in the long bones, and the distal femur and proximal tibia are the commonest sites. The humerus and scapula together have been reported as representing perhaps the second or third most common site. These tu-

mors have been reported in every decade through the ninth but are most common in the third and fourth. If fibrosarcoma in Paget's disease or other preexisting disease is included, the mean age at diagnosis is the mid fifties.

The signs and symptoms are those of pain and, at times, local swelling. The incidence of pathologic fracture is relatively high.

X-rays show a destructive lesion of bone, almost universally osteolytic, with little or no calcification within the tumor mass but with periosteal reactions at the margins, which may be horizontal (onionskin) in character or spiculated (hair-on-end). The periosteal reaction is less prominent than in osteogenic sarcoma. The lesions are usually quite large at first presentation. The gross pathologic anatomy is nonspecific, and the tumor itself consists of tissue of connective tissue density and is seldom accompanied by liquefaction necrosis.

The natural history is one of progressive growth, frequent pathologic fracture, and distant metastases usually to the lung, with death if appropriate treatment is not given. Treatment consists of local removal of the primary tumor, which in most situations requires amputation. Neither radiation therapy nor chemotherapy has been helpful. The 5-year survival rate is 30–35%.

Hudson TM, Stiles RG, Monson DK: Fibrous lesions of bone. Radiol Clin North Am 1993;31:279.

Mercuri M et al: The management of malignant bone tumors in children and adolescents. Clin Orthop 1991; Mar(264):156.

Pennington DG, Marsden W, Stephens FO: Fibrosarcoma of metacarpal treated by combined therapy and immediate reconstruction with vascularized bone graft. J Hand Surg [Am] 1991;16:877.

5. MALIGNANT LYMPHOMA (Reticulum Cell Sarcoma of Bone)

This tumor occurs with an estimated incidence of 0.1 cases per 100,000 population per year. There is a slight (3:2) male predominance. The tumor is commonest between the third and sixth decades. It is relatively rare in the forearm, hand, and foot but otherwise rather universally present in the skeleton.

The usual presenting signs and symptoms are pain, local tenderness, and, occasionally, local swelling.

The x-ray appearance is usually that of a permeative diffuse, destructive lesion with minimal or absent periosteal reaction, even in the case of rather large lesions.

The gross pathologic picture is nonspecific.

If systemic generalized involvement is excluded by appropriate staging, the treatment of choice is radiation therapy, which has a 5-year survival rate of 35–50%. The generalized disease, which may be present with localized symptoms initially, requires combined radiation therapy and chemotherapy and has a reported 5-year survival rate of 23%.

Leeson MC et al: The use of radioisotope scans in the evaluation of primary lymphoma of bone. Orthop Rev 1989; 3;18:410.

BENIGN BONE TUMORS

1. OSTEOCHONDROMA

Osteochondromas (bony exostoses) comprise at least 45% of benign bone tumors. These tend to occur at the metaphyses of long bones but may also occur in the spine and ribs. The most common sites are the distal ends of the femur and the proximal ends of the humerus. The patients are usually under 20 years of age at the time of initial excision. Since these are very slow growing tumors, the time of diagnosis or excision does not coincide with the time of onset.

The x-ray appearance is that of a bony stalk with a cartilaginous cap extending from the metaphyseal region near the epiphyseal plate and usually inclined away from the joint. These lesions rarely enlarge after childhood. The usual reasons for operation are local mechanical problems related to tumor size or perhaps pressure against musculotendinous structures operating in the vicinity. Sarcomatous degeneration occurs in 1% of cases. Thus, sudden increase in size or a change in symptomatology warrants exploration and biopsy.

Multiple congenital osteochondromas (exostoses) occur as a heritable autosomal dominant characteristic. There is usually some growth retardation and bowing deformity of the long bones. The incidence of sarcomatous degeneration is variously reported to be 5–15% in this group, but this may simply reflect the larger number of lesions present.

The treatment of symptomatic lesions is by surgical excision, which should include the entire stalk and its base. Secondary chondrosarcoma requires complete removal (resection, with some anatomic areas requiring amputation).

2. ENCHONDROMA
(Chondroma)

Enchondroma is most common in the hand, including the metacarpals and phalangeals, and next most common in the proximal end of the humerus. It is equally distributed between males and females and represents about 10% of benign tumors. It may occur from the first decade through the seventh, with the mean age in the mid thirties. The x-ray appearance is that of a cystic, slightly expansile lesion in the shaft of a long bone, with some scalloping of the cortex but without periosteal new bone formation. A speckled, calcific series of shadows within the cystic lesion is characteristic. The gross pathology is that of firm, translucent gray-white granular material.

The natural history is one of slow growth and a low incidence of pathologic fracture. Pain is often present. Except for lesions in the clavicle or small bones of the hand or foot, visible or palpable masses are uncommon.

Treatment consists of curettement and bone grafting.

3. GIANT CELL TUMOR OF BONE
(Figure 43–65)

Giant cell tumor is most common around the knee, the sacrum, the distal radius, and the proximal humerus. It occurs with a female/male ratio of 3:2. It is almost never seen before closure of the epiphyseal plate. It tends to be centered in the epiphyseal area and to extend eccentrically beyond the epiphyseal plate boundary. The chief symptom is pain. Pathologic fracture is rare, and the pain usually leads to diagnosis before there is visible or palpable external swelling.

X-rays show a cystic expansion of the involved bone. The area of destruction has a soap bubble appearance, with normal trabeculae and little reactive bone at the margins. Grossly, the lesion is filled with an orange and brown soft tumor mass without calcification. Ninety-eight percent of cases are benign and 2% are malignant, with potential for metastatic spread. The neoplastic portion of the tumor is the mesenchymal stromal cell rather than the giant cell element. Benign giant cell tumor may recur and become malignant.

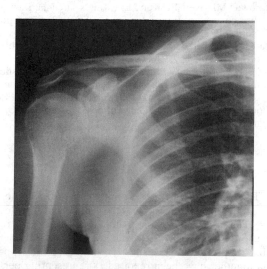

Figure 43–65. Giant cell tumor of proximal humerus.

The natural history, without treatment, consists of continuous growth resulting in an enormous tumor, pathologic fracture, and, at times, necrosis of the overlying skin. Treatment is by operative removal, and complete cure can be expected if the lesion is completely resected. Since it is most common in non-expendable bones, thorough curettement and grafting is the standard initial treatment. This form of treatment carries a risk of recurrence as high as 40%. If tumor recurs, biopsy should be performed again to verify the absence of malignant change. If malignant change has not taken place, resection followed by allograft, arthrodesis, or prosthetic replacement has the greatest probability of preventing recurrence. But curettement, followed by filling the cavity with methylmethacrylate, is not inappropriate.

In addition to a high recurrence rate, this lesion also carries a higher rate of postoperative wound infection than comparable operations in the same anatomic region.

Radiation therapy is probably not justified because of a risk of later postradiation sarcoma—except in the spine or sacrum, where complete surgical removal is not possible.

Eckardt JJ, Grogan TJ: Giant cell tumor of bone. Clin Orthop 1986;(Mar)204:45.
McDonald DJ et al: Giant-cell tumor of bone. J Bone Joint Surg [Am] 1986;68:235.

4. ANEURYSMAL BONE CYST

Aneurysmal bone cyst is most common in the metaphyses of long bones and in the vertebrae, particularly the posterior elements. The peak incidence is in the second decade. The male/female sex incidence is equal. The most common symptoms and signs are pain and swelling. Pathologic fractures are rare.

The x-ray appearance is that of an eccentric metaphyseal lesion containing expansile cysts with septa. A large thin shell portion protrudes beyond the normal confines of the bony anatomy. Grossly, the tumor is a blood-filled cavity with a soft membrane lining the bony margins.

These tumors are locally destructive by expansile growth but do not metastasize.

Treatment consists of operative removal. Radiation therapy is justified only for lesions in areas where local resection (or thorough curettement) is not feasible (eg, the spine). A recurrence rate ranging from 30% to 60% has been reported following curettement. Several factors relating to recurrence are (1) the adequacy of surgical removal; (2) the age of the patient (risk is much greater in patients under age 15); and (3) tumor size (large tumors in young patients have a high recurrence rate). There may also be a correlation between the frequency of mitotic figures and an increased risk of recurrence.

Resection is the treatment of choice where location permits. Some giant cell tumors and some osteogenic sarcomas will have an aneurysmal cystic element, and diagnosis therefore requires a representative sample.

Caso Martinez J et al: En-bloc resection of the distal fibula for aneurysmal bone cyst. Acta Orthop Belg 1993;59:87.
Conway WF, Hayes CW: Miscellaneous lesions of bone. Radiol Clin North Am 1993;31:339.

5. UNICAMERAL BONE CYST (Figure 43–66)

The incidence of unicameral bone cyst in the general population is not clearly defined, since this is a benign lesion with a tendency to be self-limited and possibly self-healing. Most patients are children, usually between the ages of 5 and 15 years, with a slight (3:2) male preponderance. These tumors are usually asymptomatic until pathologic fracture produces pain.

The roentgenographic appearance is that of a multilocular expansile, cystic lesion, principally radiolucent, with its proximal end at or near the epiphyseal plate. The overlying cortex is attenuated, but no periosteal new bone formation is present. The central portion is rarefied, and undisplaced fracture is the most common initial symptom.

Grossly, the cyst is predominantly a fluid-filled space with a thin capsule. The fluid may vary from serous to sanguineous. The lesions are of varying size, from moderately large to small, and are occasionally seen in x-rays taken for other reasons in asymptomatic patients. At first presentation, however, they classically will encompass the entire diameter of the metaphysis. Recognition that these tumors are seen in asymptomatic patients permits the assumption that some are self-healing. Spontaneous regression has been documented following fracture in about 15% of these lesions.

In the past, the usual treatment was curettement and autogenous bone graft to fill the space. The recurrence rate following this treatment varies from 20% to 50% and is reported to be twice as high in patients under age 10 compared to those over age 10. Subtotal resection techniques, with excision of most of the cyst wall including the bony shell, both with or without grafting, have been associated with a recurrence rate of 5–9%, but the number of cases from which these figures are derived is small. If the proximal end of the cyst is in contact with the epiphyseal plate, the cyst is classified as "active"; if the cyst is separated from the plate by normal cancellous metaphyseal bone, it is classified as "latent." Active cysts carry the greater risk of recurrence following curettement and grafting and also (owing to the proximity to the epiphyseal plate) carry a higher risk of damage to the plate at the time of operation. Intracystic injection of methylprednisolone is a safe alternative to surgical treat-

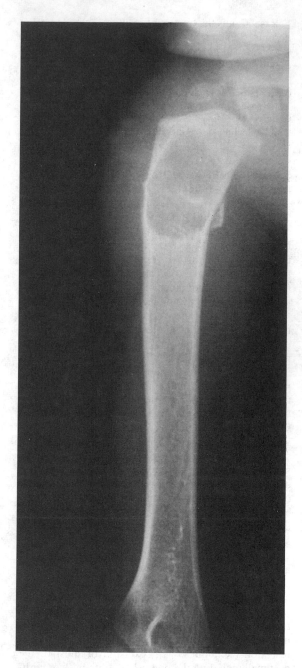

Figure 43–66. Unicameral bone cyst with fracture.

ment of these lesions. Results of this procedure show a recurrence rate of 5–10% with few complications.

Expectant treatment can be offered until the pathologic fracture is healed, at which time needle biopsy should be done. Although details of classification are sometimes difficult with needle biopsy because of the small sample, this procedure will clearly separate the classic cyst from solid tumor lesions simulating unicameral bone cyst. If the mass is identified as cystic,

consideration of operative removal can be postponed (particularly if the patient is under 10 years of age) and the progress of the cyst merely observed. If a second pathologic fracture occurs and the cyst does not show signs of resolution, either curettement with grafting or steroid injection may be tried.

Oppenheim WL, Gallend H: Operative treatment versus steroid injection in the management of unicameral bone cysts. J Pediatr Orthop 1984;4:1.

6. EOSINOPHILIC GRANULOMA

Eosinophilic granuloma is a solitary lytic lesion of bone that is classified with disorders of the reticuloendothelial system and may not be a true neoplasm. It is relatively rare, and the most common site is the skull. The male/female ratio is 3:2 and the peak incidence is between 7 and 8 years of age. Most cases occur before age 30.

Pain is the principal presenting complaint. There is almost never any demonstrable tumor mass on physical examination.

The radiologic appearance is that of a lytic defect, which in long bones frequently expands the shaft and may be accompanied by periosteal new bone formation, usually of the horizontal (onionskin) type. In flat bones, the lesion is also lytic but tends to be flattened to conform to the shape of the host bone.

Grossly, the tissue is soft (sometimes semigelatinous) and gray or yellow. Hemorrhagic areas are occasionally seen.

If the systemic variants of histiocytosis X (Hand-Schüller-Christian disease, Letterer-Siwe disease) are excluded, the lesions are probably self-limited and may run through a rapid growth cycle followed by spontaneous healing. There is evidence that they heal following biopsy with or without bone grafting. Low-dose irradiation has been used (in addition to biopsy) in treatment, particularly for symptomatic spine lesions, but it is more appropriate to merely observe the patient following biopsy in the hope that spontaneous healing will occur. If pathologic fractures are present, they should be treated by cast or fixation.

Mickelson MR, Bonfiglio M: Eosinophilic granuloma and its variation. Orthop Clin North Am 1977;8:933.
Nauert G et al: Eosinophilic granuloma of bone: Diagnosis and management. Skeletal Radiol 1983;10:227.

7. CHONDROBLASTOMA

Chondroblastoma is a relatively rare lesion that characteristically occurs in the epiphysis prior to closure of the epiphyseal plate. This location is a rare site of other primary or secondary tumors in growing bone. Ninety percent of cases occur between the ages of 5 and 25 years. The male/female ratio is 2:1. The epiphyses around the knee and the proximal humerus are the common locations. Pain and joint effusion are common, with associated local tenderness and limitation of motion of the adjacent joints.

The x-ray appearance is that of a lytic lesion in the epiphyseal body or, if the plate is closed, in its former location. The lesions are usually not expansile and seldom as large as giant cell tumors. They rarely extend significantly across the old epiphyseal plate in patients whose physeal lines are closed. The lesions tend to be eccentric in the epiphysis and have a mottled appearance compatible with calcification within the tumor. Pathologic fracture and subperiosteal reaction are uncommon. The gross pathologic anatomy is that of granular tissue of cartilaginous density containing foci of calcification. A chondroblastoma grows slowly and lacks malignant characteristics, although a few cases of metastases have been reported.

The commonest treatment is curettement and bone grafting, since the location frequently does not permit resection. The recurrence rate varies from 10% to 40% in different series. If recurrence develops, recurettement with grafting is still the treatment of choice if the site is one that does not permit resection. There is no evidence that radiation therapy or chemotherapy has any value in these lesions.

Bloem JL, Mulder JD: Chondroblastoma: A clinical and radiological study of 104 cases. Skeletal Radiol 1985;14:1.

REFERENCES

Adams JC, Hamblen, DL: *Outline of Fractures: Including Joint Injuries,* 10th ed. Churchill Livingstone, 1992.

Andersson G, McNeill TW: *Lumbar Spine Syndromes: Evaluation and Treatment.* Springer-Verlag, 1989.

Avioli LV, Krane SM (editors): *Metabolic Bone Disease and Clinically Related Disorders,* 2nd ed. Saunders, 1990.

Bunker TD et al (editors): *Frontiers in Fracture Management.* Aspen, 1989.

Cameron HU: *The Technique of Total Hip Arthroplasty.* Mosby Year Book, 1992.

Clayton ML, Smyth CJ (editors): *Surgery for Rheumatoid Arthritis: A Comprehensive Team Approach.* Churchill Livingstone, 1992.

Crenshaw AH (editor): *Campbell's Operative Orthopaedics,* 8th ed. Mosby Year Book, 1992.

Denaro V: *Stenosis of the Cervical Spine: Causes, Diagnosis, and Treatment.* Springer-Verlag, 1991.

Evarts CM (editor): *Surgery of the Musculoskeletal System,* 2nd ed. Churchill Livingstone, 1990.

Foreman SM, Croft AC: *Whiplash Injuries: The Cervical Acceleration/Deceleration Syndrome.* Williams & Wilkins, 1988.

Green DP (editor): Operative Hand Surgery, 3rd ed. Churchill Livingstone, 1993.

Greenfield GB: *Radiology of Bone Diseases,* 5th ed. Lippincott, 1990.

Huvos AG: *Bone Tumors: Diagnosis, Treatment, and Prognosis,* 2nd ed. Saunders, 1991.

Lewis MM (guest editor): Bone tumors: evaluation and treatment. Orthop Clin North Am 1989;20(3):1.

Lonstein JE et al (editors): *Moe's Textbook of Scoliosis and Other Spinal Deformities,* 3rd ed. Saunders, 1993.

McCarty DJ: *Arthritis and Allied Conditions: A Textbook of Rheumatology,* 11th ed. Lea & Febiger, 1989.

Morrey BF et al (editors): *Joint Replacement Arthroplasty.* Churchill Livingstone, 1991.

Ninfo V, Chung EB, Vavazzana AO (editors): *Tumors and Tumorlike Lesions of Soft Tissue.* Vol 18 in: *Contemporary Issues in Surgical Pathology.* Churchill Livingstone, 1991.

Rockwood CA Jr, Green DP, Bucholz RW (editors): *Rockwood and Green's Fractures in Adults,* 3rd ed. Lippincott, 1991.

Rosenthal DL (guest editor): Metabolic bone disease. Radiol Clin North Am 1991;29(1):1.

Scott WN (editor): *Arthroscopy of the Knee: Diagnosis and Treatment.* Saunders, 1990.

Strobel M et al: *Basic Principles of Knee Arthroscopy: Normal and Pathological Findings Tips and Tricks.* Springer-Verlag, 1992.

Uhthoff HK, Stahl E (editors): *Current Concepts of Diagnosis and Treatment of Bone and Soft Tissue Tumors.* Springer-Verlag, 1984.

Vinken PV et al (editors): *Myopathies.* Vol 62 in: *Handbook of Clinical Neurology.* Elsevier, 1992.

44

Plastic & Reconstructive Surgery

Luis O. Vasconez, MD, & Henry C. Vasconez, MD

The basic principles of plastic surgery are careful analysis of the surgical problem, careful planning of procedures, precise technique, and atraumatic handling of tissues. Alteration, coverage, and transfer of skin and associated tissues are the most common procedures performed. Plastic surgery may deal with closure of surgical wounds, removal of skin tumors, repair of soft tissue injuries or burns, correction of acquired or congenital deformities of the breast, or repair of cosmetic defects. Operations on the head and neck and the hand may require special surgical training.

In the past 2 decades, increased knowledge of anatomy and the development of many new techniques have brought about many changes in plastic surgery. It is now known that in many areas, the blood supply of the skin is derived principally from vessels arising from underlying muscles and larger perforating blood vessels rather than solely from vessels of the subdermal plexus, as was formerly thought. One-stage transfer of large areas of skin and muscle tissue can be accomplished if the axial pedicle of the underlying muscle is included in the transfer. With the use of new microsurgical techniques, musculocutaneous units or combinations of bone, muscle, and skin can be successfully transferred and vessels and nerves less than 1 mm in size can be repaired. These so-called free-flap transplantations are a major advance in the treatment of defects that were previously untreatable or required lengthy or multistaged procedures.

The plastic surgeon, as a member of the craniofacial team, is able to dramatically improve the appearance and function of children with severe congenital deformities. Children of normal intelligence who previously had been social outcasts are now able to lead relatively normal lives. Improved understanding of facial growth and abnormal development and newer diagnostic techniques such as the CT scan, MRI, and the three-dimensional computer-assisted imaging enable the reconstructive surgeon to devise a complex strategy for remodeling the deformed craniofacial skeleton. This may involve remodeling or repositioning of part or all of the cranial vault, the orbits, the mid face, and the mandible.

I. GRAFTS & FLAPS

SKIN GRAFTS

A graft of skin detaches epidermis and varying amounts of dermis from its blood supply in the **donor area** and is placed in a new bed of blood supply from the base of the wound, or **recipient area.** Although the technique is relatively simple to perform and generally reliable, definite considerations about the donor area and adequacy of the recipient area are important. Skin grafting is a quick, effective way to cover a wound if vascularity is adequate, infection is not present, and hemostasis is assured. Color match, contour, durability of the graft, and donor morbidity must be considered.

Types of Skin Grafts

Skin grafts can be either split-thickness or full-thickness grafts (Figure 44–1). Each type has advantages and disadvantages and is indicated or contraindicated for different kinds of wounds (Table 44–1).

A. Split-Thickness Grafts: Thinner split-thickness grafts (0.010–0.015 inch) become vascularized more rapidly and survive transplantation more reliably. This is important in grafting on less than ideal recipient sites, such as contaminated wounds, burn surfaces, and poorly vascularized surfaces (eg, irradiated sites). A second advantage is that donor sites heal more rapidly and can be reused within a relatively short time (7–10 days) in critical cases such as major burns.

In general, however, the disadvantages of thin split-thickness grafts outweigh the advantages. Thin grafts exhibit the highest degree of postgraft contraction, offer the least amount of resistance to surface trauma, and are least like normal skin in texture, suppleness, pore pattern, hair growth, and other characteristics. Hence, they are usually aesthetically unacceptable.

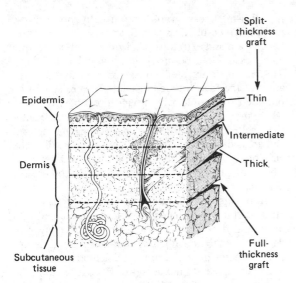

Figure 44–1. Depths of full-thickness and split-thickness grafts.

Thicker split-thickness skin grafts (> 0.015 inch) contract less, are more resistant to surface trauma, and are more similar to normal skin than are thin split-thickness grafts. They are also aesthetically more acceptable but not as acceptable as full-thickness grafts.

The disadvantages of thick split-thickness grafts are relatively few but can be significant. They are less easily vascularized than thin grafts and thus result in fewer successful takes when used on less than ideal surfaces. Their donor sites are slower to heal (requiring 10–18 days) and heal with more scarring than donor sites for thin split-thickness grafts—a factor that may prevent reuse of the area.

Meshed grafts are usually thin or intermediate split-thickness grafts that have been rolled under a special cutting machine to create a mesh pattern. Although grafts with these perforations can be expanded from 1½ to nine times their original size, expansion to 1½ times the unmeshed size is the most useful. Meshed grafts are advantageous because they can be placed on an irregular, possibly contaminated wound bed and will usually take. Also, complications of hemostasis are fewer, because blood and serum exude through the mesh pattern. The disadvantage is poor appearance following healing (alligator hide).

Donor sites for split-thickness grafts heal spontaneously by epithelialization. During this process, epithelial cells from the sweat glands, sebaceous glands, or hair follicles proliferate upward and spread across the wound surface. If these three structures are not present, epithelialization will not occur.

B. Full-Thickness Grafts: Full-thickness skin grafts include the epidermis and all the dermis. They are the most aesthetically desirable of the free grafts since they include the highest number of skin appendage elements, undergo the least amount of contracture, and have a greater ability to withstand trauma. There are several limiting factors in the use of full-thickness grafts. Since no epidermal elements remain to produce epithelialization in the donor site, it must be closed primarily, and a scar will result. The size and number of available donor sites is therefore limited. Furthermore, conditions at the recipient site must be optimal in order for transplantation to be successful.

Areas of thin skin are the best donor sites for full-thickness grafts (eg, the eyelids and the skin of the postauricular, supraclavicular, antecubital, inguinal, and genital areas). Submammary and subgluteal skin is thicker but allows camouflage of donor area scars. In grafts thicker than approximately 0.015 inch (0.038 cm), the results of transplantation are often poor except on the face, where vascularity is so good.

C. Composite Grafts: A composite graft is also a free graft that must reestablish its blood supply in the recipient area. It consists of a unit with several tissue planes that may include skin, subcutaneous tissue, cartilage, or other tissue. Dermal fat grafts, hair transplant grafts, and skin and cartilage grafts from the ear fall into this category. Obviously, composite grafts must be small or at least relatively thin and will require recipient sites with excellent vascularity. These grafts are generally used in the face.

D. Cultured Epithelial Grafts: Epithelial cells can now be cultured in vitro and made to coalesce into sheets that then can be used to cover full-thickness wounds. This technique is presently being used

Table 44–1. Advantages and disadvantages of various types of skin grafts.

Type of Graft	Advantages	Disadvantages
Thin split-thickness	Survive transplantation most easily. Donor sites heal most rapidly.	Fewest qualities of normal skin. Maximum contraction. Least resistance to trauma. Sensation poor. Aesthetically poor.
Thick split-thickness	More qualities of normal skin. Less contraction. More resistant to trauma. Sensation fair. Aesthetically more acceptable.	Survive transplantation less well. Donor site heals slowly.
Full thickness	Nearly all qualities of normal skin. Minimal contraction. Very resistant to trauma. Sensation good. Aesthetically good.	Survive transplantation least well. Donor site must be closed surgically. Donor sites are limited.

in selected patients with extensive burns where donor sites are at a premium. The main disadvantage of cultured grafts is their fragility and the uncertainty of graft take. Therefore, the work of developing artificial dermis made out of a collagen matrix to which one can apply the cultured epithelial layer is a topic of active investigation.

Obtaining Skin Grafts

Instruments used for obtaining skin grafts include razor blades, skin grafting knives (Blair, Ferris Smith, Humby, Goulian), manual drum dermatomes (Padgett, Reese), and electric or air-powered dermatomes (Brown, Padgett, Hall). The electric and air-powered dermatomes are the most widely used because of their reliability and ease of operation. A surgeon, even with only limited experience, can successfully obtain sheets of split-thickness skin grafts, using the electric dermatomes.

The Skin Graft Recipient Area

To ensure survival of the graft, there must be (1) adequate vascularity of the recipient bed, (2) complete contact between the graft and the bed, (3) adequate immobilization of the graft-bed unit, and (4) relatively few bacteria in the recipient area.

Since survival of the graft is dependent upon growth of capillary buds into the raw undersurface of the graft, vascularity of the recipient area is of prime importance. Avascular surfaces that will not generally accept free grafts are tissues with severe radiation damage, chronically scarred ulcer beds, bone or cartilage denuded of periosteum or perichondrium, and tendon or nerve without their paratenon or perineurium, respectively. For these surfaces, a bed capable of producing capillary buds must be provided; in some cases, excision of the deficient bed down to healthy tissue is possible. All unhealthy granulation tissue must be removed, since bacteria counts in granulation tissue are often very high. If bone is exposed, it can be decorticated down to healthy cancellous bone with the use of a chisel or power-driven burr, and a meshed split-thickness skin graft can be applied. If an adequate vascular bed cannot be provided or if the presence of essential structures such as tendons or nerves precludes further debridement, skin or muscle flaps are generally indicated.

Inadequate contact between the graft and the recipient bed can be caused by collection of blood, serum, or lymph fluid in the bed; formation of pus between the graft and the bed; or movement of the graft on the bed.

After the graft has been applied directly to the prepared recipient surface, it may or may not be sutured in place and may or may not be dressed. Whenever the maximum aesthetic result is desired, the graft should be cut exactly to fit the recipient area and precisely sutured into position without any overlapping of edges. Very large or thick split-thickness grafts

and full-thickness grafts will usually not survive without a pressure dressing. In areas such as the forehead, scalp and extremities, adequate immobilization and pressure can be provided by circular dressings. Tie-over pressure stent dressings are advisable for areas of the face, where constant pressure cannot be provided by simple wraparound dressings, or areas where movement cannot be avoided, such as the anterior neck, where swallowing causes constant motion; and areas of irregular contour, such as the axilla. The ends of the fixation sutures are left long and tied over a bolus of gauze fluffs, cotton, a sponge, or other suitable material (Figure 44–2).

Grafts applied to freshly prepared or relatively clean surfaces are generally sutured or stapled into place and dressed with pressure. A single layer of damp or other nonadherent fine-mesh gauze is applied directly over the graft. Immediately over this are placed several thicknesses of flat gauze cut in the exact pattern of the graft. On top of these is placed a bulky dry dressing of gauze fluffs, cotton, a sponge, or other material. Pressure is then applied by wraparound dressings, adhesive tape, or a tie-over pressure stent dressing.

In many cases, it is permissible—and sometimes even preferable—to leave a skin graft site open with no dressing. This is particularly true in slightly infected wounds, where the grafts tend to float off in the purulent discharge produced by the wound. These wounds are best treated with meshed grafts, so that liquid forming between the graft and the wound bed can exude and be removed without disturbing the graft. This treatment can also be used for noninfected wounds that produce an unusual amount of serous or lymphatic drainage, as occurs following radical groin dissections.

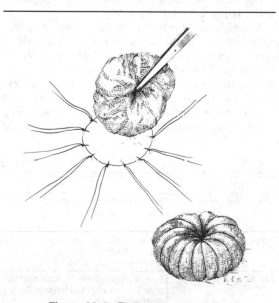

Figure 44–2. Tie-over stent dressing.

In severely ill patients, such as those with major burns, where time under anesthesia must be kept to a minimum, large sheets of meshed split-thickness skin grafts are rapidly applied but not sutured. Skin staples may be used to fix the graft rapidly. Grafts need not be dressed if the area is small, but if the area is large or circumferential, a dressing should be applied. Meshed grafts should generally be covered for 24–48 hours to prevent dryness, since their dermal barrier has been partly disrupted.

Various biologic adhesives, in particular autologous fibrin glue, is being used to immobilize skin grafts. This is especially useful in the face or hands, or areas where bandaging is difficult or cumbersome.

Skin graft dressings may be left undisturbed for 5–7 days after grafting if the grafted wound was free of infection, if complete hemostasis was obtained, if fluid collection is not expected, and if immobilization is adequate. If any one of these conditions is not met, the dressing should be changed within 24–48 hours and the graft inspected. If blood, serum, or purulent fluid collection is present, the collection should be evacuated—usually by making a small incision through the graft with a scalpel blade and applying pressure with cotton-tipped applicators. The pressure dressing is then reapplied and changed daily so that the graft can be examined and fluid expressed as it collects.

The Skin Graft Donor Area

The ideal donor site would provide a graft identical to the skin surrounding the area to be grafted. Since skin varies greatly from one area to another as far as color, thickness, hair-bearing qualities, and texture are concerned, the ideal donor site (such as upper eyelid skin to replace skin loss from the opposite upper eyelid) is usually not found. However, there are definite principles that should be followed in choosing the donor area.

A. Color Match: In general, the best possible color match is obtained when the donor area is located close to the recipient area. Color and texture match in facial grafts will be much better if the grafts are obtained from above the region of the clavicles. However, the amount of skin obtainable from the supraclavicular areas is limited. If larger grafts for the face are required, the immediate subclavicular regions of the thorax will provide a better color match than areas on the lower trunk or the buttocks and thighs. When these more distant regions are used, the grafts will usually be lighter in color than the facial skin in Caucasians. In people with dark skin, hyperpigmentation occurs, producing a graft that is much darker than the surrounding facial skin.

B. Thickness of the Graft and Donor Site Healing: Donor sites of split-thickness grafts heal by epithelialization from the epithelial elements remaining in the donor bed. The ability of the donor area to heal and the speed with which it does depends upon the number of these elements present. Donor areas for very thin grafts will heal in 7–10 days, whereas donor areas for intermediate-thickness grafts may require 10–18 days and those for thick grafts 18–21 days or longer.

Since there is a normal anatomic variation in the thickness of skin, donor sites for thicker grafts must be chosen with the potential for healing in mind and should be limited to regions on the body where the skin is thick. Infants, debilitated adults, and elderly people have thinner skin than healthy younger adults. Grafts that would be split-thickness in the normal adult may be full-thickness in these patients, resulting in a donor site that has been deprived of the epithelial elements necessary for healing.

C. Management of the Donor Site: The donor site itself can be considered a clean open wound that will heal spontaneously. After initial hemostasis, the wound will continue to ooze serum for 1–4 days, depending on the thickness of the skin taken. The serum should be collected and the wound kept clean so that healing can proceed at a maximal rate. The wound should be cared for as described above for clean open wounds in either of two ways.

The more common method is the open (dry) technique. The donor site is dressed with porous sterile fine-mesh or nonadherent gauze. After 24 hours, the dry gauze is changed but the nonadherent gauze is left on the wound and exposed to the air, a heat lamp, or a blow dryer. A scab will form on the gauze and will peel off from the edges as epithelialization is completed underneath. This method has the advantage of simple maintenance once the wound is dry.

The second method is the closed (moist) technique. Studies have demonstrated that the rate of epithelialization is enhanced in a moist environment. In contrast to the dry technique, pain can be reduced or virtually eliminated. Moist-to-moist gauze dressings that require frequent wetting have been replaced by newer synthetic materials. A gas-permeable membrane (OpSite) that sticks to the surrounding skin provides an artificial blister over the wound. Occasionally there is a break in the protective seal covering leakage of serum collected under the membrane. This increases the risk of infection, especially in a contaminated zone. Newer hygroscopic dressings actually absorb and retain many times their weight in water. They are permeable to oxygen yet impervious to bacteria. Infection is still a concern, however, because of occasional exposure of the wound during healing.

Dean SJ, Nieber S, Hickerson WL: The use of cultured epithelial autograft in a patient with idiopathic pyoderma gangrenosum. Ann Plast Surg 1991;26:194. Gallico GG III et al: Cultured epithelial autografts for giant congenital nevi. Plast Reconstr Surg. 1989;84:1.

Leicht P, Siim E, Srensen B: Treatment of donor sites: Duoderm or Omiderm. Burns Incl Therm Inj 1989;15:7.

Nakano M: Clinical application of cultured autologous epithelium to donor sites for split-thickness skin graft. Hokkaido Igaku Zasshi 1990;65:56.

Saltz R, Sierra D, Feldman D: Experimental and clinical applications of fibrin glue. Plast Reconstr Surg 1991;88:1005.

FLAPS

The term "flap" refers to any tissue used for reconstruction or wound closure that retains part or all of its original blood supply after the tissue has been raised and moved to a new location. That part still connected through which the blood supply enters and exits is referred to as the base of the flap. With local skin flaps, a section of skin and subcutaneous tissue is raised from one site and moved to a nearby area, with the base remaining attached at its original location.

Flaps can be classified according to the pattern of blood supply to the skin into random or axial pattern. Flaps can further be classified according to their tissue content into muscle, musculocutaneous, fasciocutaneous, and others.

Random Pattern Flaps

Random pattern flaps consist of skin and subcutaneous tissue cut from any area of the body in any orientation, with no distinct pattern or particular relation to the blood supply of the skin of the flap. Such flaps receive their blood supply from vessels in the subdermal plexus. Although commonly used, this is the least reliable type of flap, and except when cut from facial and scalp skin, the ratio of length to width cannot safely exceed 1.5:1.

Axial Pattern Flaps

The axial pattern flap has a well-defined arteriovenous system running along its long axis. Because of good vascular supply, it can be made comparatively long in relation to width. Foremost among the axial flaps are the deltopectoral and the forehead flaps, which are based on perforating branches of the internal mammary artery and supraorbital and supratrochlear or superficial temporal vessels, respectively. Other axial flaps are the groin flap, based on the superficial circumflex iliac artery; the dorsalis pedis flap, based on the artery of the same name; the radial forearm flap; the scapular flap; the lateral upper arm flap; and various scalp flaps.

Muscle & Musculocutaneous Flaps

Musculocutaneous flaps consist of skin and underlying muscle, which provide reliable coverage with usually one operation. The use of musculocutaneous units has developed as surgeons have gained more knowledge of the way in which blood is supplied to the skin. The technique has revolutionized reconstructive surgery.

The subdermal plexus of vessels from which skin flaps derive their blood supply is augmented or directly supplied in many areas by sizable perforating vessels arising from underlying muscles. Many muscles receive their blood supply from a single axial vessel, with only minor contributions from other sources (Figure 44–3). The skin over these muscles can be completely circumscribed and elevated in continuity with the underlying muscle up to its major vascular pedicle. If the vessels in the pedicle are preserved, the unit can be moved in wide arcs to distant areas of the body while normal or near normal blood flow is continued to the skin island as well as to the muscle. The donor sites of such flaps can often be closed primarily.

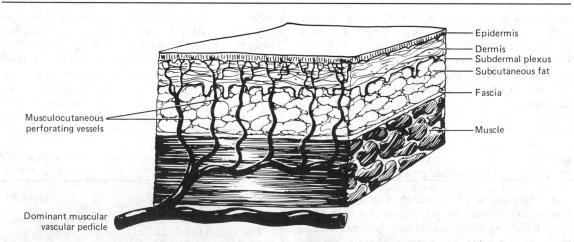

Figure 44–3. Arterial supply to skin from main artery supplying muscles, as occurs in musculocutaneous flaps.

Knowledge of the anatomy of muscles and their nerve and blood supply is necessary for the successful design of musculocutaneous flaps. Although almost any skeletal muscle can be used, muscles with a dominant arterial pedicle and reliable perforating vessels to the skin are most useful.

In addition to their reliability, musculocutaneous flaps sterilize recipient sites that are heavily contaminated with bacteria better than skin flaps do. This is why muscle-containing flaps are the best choice for coverage of wounds caused by radiation or osteomyelitis or those that have a high probability of infection.

The most commonly used muscles and musculocutaneous flaps are the latissimus dorsi, pectoralis major, tensor fasciae latae, rectus femoris, rectus abdominis, trapezius, temporalis, serratus anterior, gluteus maximus, gracilis, and gastrocnemius muscles.

A. Latissimus Dorsi: The latissimus dorsi musculocutaneous unit is supplied by the thoracodorsal vessels. Use of this unit has been widely applied in the one-stage reconstruction of the breast following radical or modified radical mastectomy (see rectus abdominis muscle below). The entire latissimus dorsi muscle can be detached from its origin and transposed to the anterior chest. An island of skin can also be included in the center of the muscle to restore the skin lost on the anterior chest wall. Refinements in technique utilize only enough muscle to carry the skin island, thus leaving intact a good portion of innervated, functional muscle. This unit is also useful for coverage of defects on the anterior chest, shoulder, head and neck, and axilla and even for restoration of flexion of the elbow. It is a popular muscle for free tissue transfer due to its long and relatively large and reliable vascular pedicle.

B. Pectoralis Major: The pectoralis major musculocutaneous unit obtains its vascular supply from the thoracoacromial axis of the subclavian artery just medial to the medial border of the pectoralis minor. It derives a dual blood supply from medial intercostal perforators branching from the internal mammary artery. The entire unit may be transposed medially, especially after disinsertion from the humerus, to cover defects of the sternum, neck, and lower face. Also, an island of skin can be outlined low on the chest and made to reach intraoral defects following cancer excision.

C. Trapezius: The trapezius musculocutaneous unit, based on the descending branch of the transverse cervical artery, is useful for covering defects in the neck, face, and scalp. When skeletonized as an island, the flap will reach the top of the head. When it is used in conjunction with a neck dissection, the transverse cervical artery must be preserved. Functional preservation of shoulder elevation may be accomplished by selectively sparing the transverse, superior fibers of the muscle.

D. Temporalis: The temporalis muscle extends from the temporal fossa to the coronoid process of the mandible. It is supplied by the deep and superficial temporal systems. It is commonly used to fill orbital defects. However, it can cover neighboring cranial, maxillary, palatal and pharyngeal regions.

E. Tensor Fasciae Latae: The tensor fasciae latae musculofascial unit is supplied by the lateral femoral circumflex artery, a branch of the profunda femoris. It has a wide arc of rotation anteriorly and posteriorly. It is elevated with the fascia lata and thus can be used to reconstruct the lower abdominal wall. It has been used to cover defects following excision of osteoradionecrotic ulcers of the pubis or groin. It is also the method of choice for coverage of greater trochanteric pressure ulcers.

F. Rectus Femoris: The rectus femoris, a more robust flap than the tensor fasciae latae with a shorter arc of rotation, has supplanted the latter for reconstruction of the lower abdominal wall and for coverage to postradiation ulcers in the pubis and groin. It has a dual blood supply: a muscular branch from the profunda femoris and an axial branch from the superficial femoral artery to the overlying skin and fascia.

G. Rectus Abdominis: The rectus abdominis is supplied by the deep superior and inferior epigastric vessels that run in the undersurface of the muscle and anastomose with the segmentally arranged intercostal vessels to form the epigastric arcade. These vessels send perforating branches throughout the length of the muscle, perforating the anterior rectus sheath and supplying the overlying skin. The flap, when based on the superior epigastric vessel and including the infraumbilical skin, has become the method of choice for autologous tissue breast reconstruction. In situations of marked deformity such as a radical mastectomy associated with radiation therapy or previous abdominal surgery, reconstruction of the breast can be accomplished reliably with infraumbilical skin and adipose tissue based on both rectus muscles. This superiorly based rectus abdominis musculocutaneous flap involves an abdominoplasty as well as reconstruction of the breast. It is a technically demanding operation but gives a very satisfying result. When based on the deep inferior epigastric vessel and using the supraumbilical skin (the "flag" flap), the flap can cover defects of the abdominal wall, flank and thigh.

H. Gluteus Maximus: The gluteus maximus is useful as a muscle or musculocutaneous unit for covering pressure sores or traumatic defects over the sacrum and ischium. The muscle has a double blood supply from the superior and inferior gluteal arteries to the respective halves of the muscle. In ambulatory patients, it is advisable to perform a function-preserving operation by advancing the muscle medially and preserving its insertion laterally.

I. Gracilis: The gracilis muscle receives its dominant blood supply proximally from the medial femoral circumflex artery. Its arc of rotation makes it an excellent source of coverage for ischial pressure sores and vaginal reconstruction. Other recent uses have included transportation of the muscle alone for repair of a persistent perineal sinus following abdominal-perineal resection.

J. Gastrocnemius: The gastrocnemius musculocutaneous unit is based on either the medial or lateral head of the muscle. Each head is supplied by a sural artery, a branch of the popliteal artery that enters the muscle at its most proximal third near its origin. The flap is most useful to cover defects of the knee and proximal anterior tibia. Coverage of exposed bone in the middle and lower leg, where this unit cannot reach, can be accomplished by use of local muscle flaps such as the soleus. Complex bone and soft tissue injuries of the middle and lower leg are best handled with free muscle flaps.

Fasciocutaneous Flaps

A plexus of vessels is located on top of the muscular fascia and is supplied from vessels that run within the intermuscular septa. These vessels tend to run axially along the fascia, sending perforators to the skin at intervals. Flaps can be designed that are safer than random flaps and that need not contain an entire muscle unit for their transfer. Furthermore, it is possible to make fasciocutaneous or septocutaneous flaps that safely exceed the traditional limits of a 1:1 ratio between length and width. Examples of fasciocutaneous flaps are those overlying the gastrocnemius, quadriceps, and rectus abdominis muscles. Other commonly used flaps are the radial forearm, lateral arm, scapular, and temporalis flaps.

Free Flaps

Free flaps involve tissue transplantation using microvascular surgery. The term is actually incorrect, since the blood supply from the main axial pedicle of the flap is completely detached and then reattached at a distance to recipient vessels near the wound area.

An operating microscope with two viewing binocular lenses, specialized instruments, and swaged-on needles of 60–80 μm are required for microsurgery. 8-0, 9-0, and 10-0 suture is used to anastomose vessels as small as 0.5 mm in diameter.

Examples of free flaps in current use are axial pattern skin flaps, such as groin and scapular flaps, which are used when only skin is needed, and musculocutaneous flaps, such as latissimus dorsi, gracilis, and rectus abdominis flaps, which are used when the bulk and vascularity of muscle are needed. The temporalis fascia may be transferred as a free flap to provide thin, adaptable tissue that can be grafted. This type of flap is useful for facial and ear reconstruction and coverage of tendons where mobility is important.

The vascular pedicle areas of some flaps contain functional nerves, which can also be reattached with microscopic guidance. Examples are inferior gluteal, thigh and tensor fasciae latae flaps, which contain sensory nerves, and serratus anterior and latissimus dorsi flaps, which contain motor nerves. **Sensory flaps** provide protective sensation in critical areas such as the feet or the ischium in paraplegic patients. **Motor flaps** can restore functions such as forearm flexion or facial expression.

Bone and functional joints can be transplanted as free flaps. Flaps from the ribs, fibula, and iliac crest have all been successfully transferred to areas such as the mandible and tibia. The toe-to-thumb transfer is an example of a complex transplantation, that includes bone with a functional joint, tendons and nerves as well as skin.

Chandrasekhar B et al: The inferior trapezius musculocutaneous flap in head and neck reconstruction. Ann Plast Surg 1988;21:201.

Elliott LF, Raffel B, Wade J: Segmental latissimus dorsi free flap: Clinical applications. Ann Plast Surg 1989; 23:231.

Grotting JC et al: Conventional TRAM flap versus free microsurgical TRAM flap for immediate breast reconstruction. Plast Reconstr Surg 1989;83:828.

Hartrampf C Jr: The transverse abdominal island flap for breast reconstruction: A 7-year experience. Clin Plast Surg 1988;15:703.

Hirase Y: Composite reconstruction for chest wall and scalp using multiple ribs-latissimus dorsi osteomyocutaneous flaps as pedicled and free flaps. Plast Reconstr Surg 1991;87:555.

Lamberty BG, Cormach GC: Fasciocutaneous flaps. Clin Plast Surg 1990;17:713.

McCraw J, Arnold P: *Atlas of Muscle and Musculocutaneous Flaps.* Hampton Press, 1987.

Taylor GI, Palmer JH: The vascular territories (angiotomes) of the body: Experimental study and clinical applications. Br J Plast Surg 1987;40:113.

II. PRINCIPLES OF WOUND CARE

There are many types of wounds and many factors to consider when choice of coverage procedure is made. Skin type and color, glandular association, and hair-bearing characteristics must be considered. Avascular wound beds, such as exposed bone, cartilage, or tendon, will not accept skin grafts unless viable periosteum, perichondrium, or paratenon (respectively) is present. Other areas with poor vascularity are joint capsules, radiation-damaged tissue, and heavily scarred tissue. Exposed or implanted alloplastic material cannot be used as a graft bed. Such areas must be covered with tissue that is attached to its own blood supply. Skin flaps can be used but are sometimes inadequate because their blood supply is tenuous and the layer of subcutaneous fat is even less reliably vascular and may not attach to the underlying avascular surface. Muscle or musculocutaneous flaps are generally required for avascular areas.

The coverage tissue may need to have more bulk than the original tissue. Areas such as bony surfaces and prominences, weight-bearing surfaces, densely scarred areas, and areas of potential pressure breakdown may require thick, durable covering. Again, skin grafts or skin flaps may not be of adequate thickness even though they may survive and cover the wound. Musculocutaneous flaps are more successful. Bulkiness may be undesirable in areas such as the scalp, face, neck, or hand. Defects in these areas that for other reasons require a musculocutaneous flap for coverage may need to be debulked in a secondary procedure. Axial skin flaps or free axial pattern flaps may be a better choice than musculocutaneous flaps in some areas.

Contraction begins during the proliferative phase of healing and continues to a large degree in wounds covered only by split-thickness skin grafts. The grafted area may shrink to 50% of its original size, and both the graft and surrounding tissue may become distorted. Splinting of the area for 10 days or longer may favorably alter contraction. Full-thickness skin grafts rich in dermis, attached to a fresh wound bed will considerably reduce contraction and skin flaps will eliminate it altogether. In an orifice or tubular passageway, such as the nasal airway, pharynx, esophagus, or vagina, absence of contraction is critical.

The effects of atrophy and gravity should also be considered when technique of coverage is chosen. A denervated muscle will atrophy up to 60% of its regular size. The muscle tissue in a musculocutaneous flap will atrophy even when the nerve to the muscle is preserved in the pedicle, because the muscle's functional tension is generally not restored. Gravity will cause sagging of any tissue that does not have enough plasticity or muscle dynamics to counteract gravitational pull. Reconstructions in the face often tend to sag.

Wounds at risk for or known to have bacterial contamination also require certain types of coverage (eg, pressure sores, lower extremity defects, and wounds resulting from incision and drainage of abscesses). If the area can be skin grafted, meshed split-thickness grafts are most effective, since bacterial exudate will not collect under these grafts. Musculocutaneous flaps are associated with fewer residual bacteria over time than are random pattern skin flaps. This is probably due to the vastly superior vascularity of musculocutaneous flaps.

Wounds associated with nearby injuries that will probably require further surgery (eg, injuries to tendons or nerves) should be covered with flaps, because the flaps can be incised or undermined to allow for additional surgery. Skin grafts do not have sufficient vascularity to allow for these procedures.

Choice of Coverage

Table 44–2 shows some of the indications for choice of coverage in various types of wounds.

Once a given type of flap is chosen, there are still at least two major considerations in the selection of the exact flap to be used. The most significant consideration is the degree of injury that will occur in the donor area. There is always a trade-off when tissue is taken from one area and used in another. This trade-off is minimal when a well-designed, well-placed skin flap leaves a donor defect that can be closed primarily, but the trade-off is great when the donor defect is as severe as the original wound (eg, skin graft donor sites that become infected or musculocutaneous donor sites that fail to heal).

The patient can often participate in the choice of donor locations and should certainly be made aware of potential donor site scars and complications. The tendency has been to use muscle flaps instead of musculocutaneous flaps to permit easy primary closure of the donor site. The muscle can then be resurfaced with a split-thickness skin graft during the same procedure to give a satisfactory result. This provides for an acceptable donor site scar rather than risking disruption of a tight closure or an otherwise ugly donor site.

The second consideration in selection of a flap is that some or all of the graft or flap may be lost. In general, if the patient's overall condition is poor or the loss of a flap would result in a devastating defect, a very reliable type of flap should be chosen. For example, a microvascular anastomosis can be performed on a leg with one remaining vessel to the foot, but if the anastomosis fails, the vessel may thrombose and the leg may be lost. In this case, a flap that is safer, although more time-consuming to place, may be chosen, such as a cross-leg flap.

Elevation & Transposition of Flaps

Additional considerations in reconstructive surgery involve the technique of elevating and transposing flaps. For random skin flaps, these considerations include proper length-to-width ratio, careful planning to allow for transposition with minimal tension and adjustments at the recipient site, accurate dissection in the subcutaneous plane to avoid injury to the subdermal plexus, and avoidance of folding or kinking of the flap. Surgical technique must be atraumatic, and hemostasis must be achieved. With axial pattern flaps, the surgeon must have knowledge of the important underlying blood vessels as well.

Closure Technique

Closure technique is as important as elevation and transposition technique. Flaps should not be allowed to dry out. The wound bed should be irrigated. Closed-system, nonreactive suction drains are routinely used in both the wound bed and the donor defect for most flaps of any significant size. Suction

Table 44–2. Indications for various types of tissue coverage.

Type of Wound	Type of Coverage	Reason for Choice
Mildly (<10⁵) infected wounds (including burns)	Thin split-thickness or meshed	Difficulty in obtaining successful take of thicker grafts. Donor sites may be re-used sooner.
Significantly (>10⁵) infected wounds (osteomyelitis)	Thin split-thickness or meshed skin grafts or muscle or musculocutaneous flaps	Rich muscle vascular supply can sterilize an infected wound.
Wounds with poorly vascularized surfaces	Thin split-thickness skin grafts or flaps	Difficulty in obtaining successful take of thicker grafts. Flap with intrinsic blood supply may be required.
Small facial defects	Full-thickness skin graft or local flap	Produces best aesthetic result.
Large facial defects	Thick split-thickness skin grafts or flaps	Cannot use full-thickness graft, because of limited size of donor sites.
Full-thickness eyelid loss	Local flap or composite graft	Repair requires more than one tissue element.
Deep loss of nasal tip	Local flap or composite graft	Repair requires thicker tissue than present in split- or full-thickness grafts.
Avulsive wounds with exposed tendons and nerves	Flap	Requires thick protective coverage without graft adherence to tendons and nerves.
Exposed cortical bone or cartilage	Skin or muscle flap	Free grafts will not survive on avascular recipient site.
Wounds resulting from radiation burns	Muscle or musculocutaneous flap	Free grafts will not survive on avascular recipient site. Damaged tissue extends deeper than may be apparent.

evacuates blood or serum that may accumulate and keeps the flap firmly pressed against the wound bed. External pressure is both ineffective and detrimental for these purposes. Sutures should accurately and completely appose skin edges without strangulating the epithelium, particularly on the flap side. Buried half-mattress (flap) sutures are recommended (Figure 44–4). Dressings over flaps should be minimal and should not cause pressure or constriction. Emollient dressings, such as petrolatum gauze, antibiotic ointment, or silver sulfadiazine cream, have been shown to aid in preventing desiccation and subsequent necrosis of areas of marginal vascularity.

After a flap is at least temporarily tacked into its final position, adequacy of vascularity can be determined by intravenous injection of fluorescein dye, 10–15 mg/kg, and examination under ultraviolet light (Wood's light). Areas that fluoresce within 10 minutes following dye injection can be expected to survive. Areas that do not fluoresce usually lack arterial inflow, which may be due to temporary arterial spasm but is often due to insufficient perfusion that will result in necrosis. A good clinical evaluation of the flap on the operating table is usually sufficient. Any sign of mottling or cyanosis or flap congestion that indicates a degree of venous obstruction warrants serious consideration of reexploration.

Excision & Primary Closure

The ideal type of wound closure is primary approximation of the skin and subcutaneous tissues immediately adjacent to the wound defect, producing a fine-line scar and the optimal aesthetic result in skin texture, thickness, and color match.

All excisions and wound closures should be planned with this ideal in mind. Obviously, large lesions cannot be excised and closed primarily. With invasive cancers, such as sarcomas, the primary goal is performance of adequate en bloc resection, with the type of wound closure being of secondary importance. Nevertheless, even larger excisions, such as mastectomies, can be planned with definite consideration for closure and subsequent reconstruction.

In most cases, minimal scars can be achieved only if the line or lines of incision are placed in, or parallel to, the skin lines of minimal tension. These lines lie perpendicular to the underlying muscles. On the face, they are obvious as wrinkles or lines of facial expression that become more pronounced with age, since they are secondary to repeated muscle contraction (Figure 44–5). On the neck, trunk, and extremities, the lines of minimal tension are most noticeable as horizontal lines of skin relaxation on the anterior and posterior aspects of areas of flexion and extension.

So-called Langer's lines, which were determined by cadaver study, probably show the direction of fibrous tissue bundles in the skin and are no longer considered accurate guides for placing skin incisions.

If the lines of expression cannot be followed, the line of incision should (if possible) be placed at the junction of unlike tissues such as the hairline of the scalp and the forehead, the eyebrow and the fore-

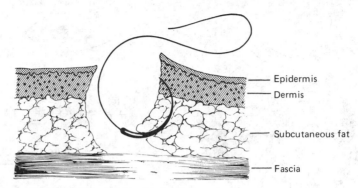

A. The strength of the closure lies in the dermis. Occasionally, the subcutaneous fat is incorporated to obliterate dead space.

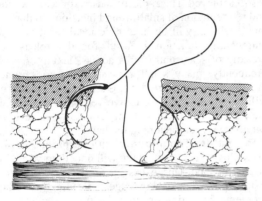

B. The suture is placed so that the knot will lie in the deepest part of the wound. Take care to avoid incorporating the epidermis with this suture, since epithelial cysts will form and result in suture extrusion.

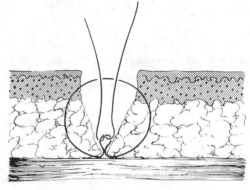

C. The dermal suture is tied just tightly enough to approximate the wound margins. Synthetic absorbable sutures are most commonly used for closure of the dermis.

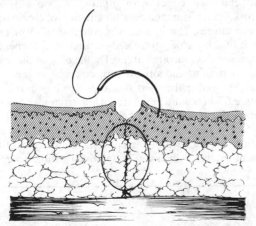

D. After the dermis is approximated, a fine "epidermal" suture is placed to align the wound edges. This suture adds little to the tensile strength of the wound closure.

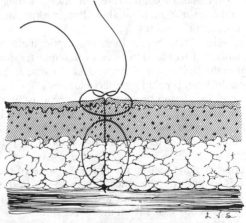

E. The epidermal suture is tied just tightly enough to approximate the epidermal edges of the wound. Since the strength of this closure lies in the dermis, the epidermal suture can be removed after 2–3 days. Skin tapes are often used to support the wound for an additional 7–10 days.

Figure 44–4. Layered cutaneous closure (buried half-mattress [flap] sutures).(Reproduced, with permission, from Ho MT, Saunders CE [editors]: *Current Emergency Diagnosis & Treatment,* 3rd ed. Appleton & Lange, 1990.)

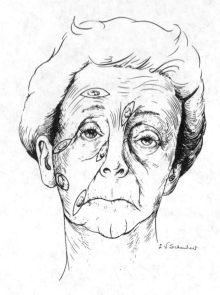

Figure 44–5. Sites of elliptic incisions corresponding to wrinkle lines on the face.

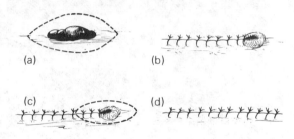

Figure 44–6. Correction of dog-ear.

head, the mucosal and skin junction of the lips, or the areolar and skin margins of the breast. Scars will be partially hidden if incisions are placed in inconspicuous areas such as the crease of the nasal ala and cheek, the auricular-mastoid sulcus, or the submandibular-neck junction. Lines of incision should never purposely cross flexor surfaces such as the neck, axilla, antecubital fossa, or popliteal space or the palmar skin creases of the fingers and hand, because of the risk of contracture formation. A transverse oblique or S incision should be incorporated when crossing these sites.

If a lesion is to be excised, an elliptic incision placed parallel to the skin lines of minimal tension will give the best result if the amount of tissue to be excised does not preclude primary closure.

If the ellipse is too broad or short, a protrusion of skin, commonly called a "dog-ear," will occur at each pole of the wound closure (Figure 44–6). This is most easily corrected by excising the dog-ear as a small ellipse.

A dog-ear may also be present if one side of the ellipse is longer than the other (Figure 44–7). In this case, it may be easier to excise a small triangle of skin and subcutaneous tissue from the longer side.

A. Z-Plasty: One of the most useful and commonly used techniques in primary wound closure is the Z-plasty. The procedure is illustrated in Figure 44–8. The angles formed by the Z-shaped incision are transposed as shown, in order (1) to gain length in the direction of the central limb of the Z or (2) to change the line of direction of the central limb of the Z. Ninety-degree angles would provide the greatest gain in length of the central limb, but smaller angles, such

as 60-degree angles, are usually used, because the incision is easier to close and significant gain in length is still achieved. The Z-plasty is used for scar revision and reorientation of small wound incisions so that the main incision will be in a more ideal location. The lengthening function is used for the release or breakup of scar contractures across flexion creases. Frequently, many small Z-plasties in series rather than one large one are done. Occasionally, incisions will be placed under excessive vertical tension after the release of an underlying contracture, such as Dupuytren's contracture in the hand.

B. Suture Technique: Suture technique in primary closure is important but will not compensate for poorly planned flaps, excessive tension across the incision, traumatized skin edges, bleeding, or other problems. Sometimes even a skillfully executed closure may result in an unsightly scar because of healing problems beyond the control of the surgeon.

The goal of closure is level apposition of dermal and epithelial edges with minimal or no tension across the incision and no strangulation of tissue between sutures. This is usually accomplished by placement of a layer of interrupted or running absorbable sutures in the subcuticular level at the base of the dermis. A running monofilament permanent suture can also be used and pulled out after healing has progressed. This suture prevents tension from forming in the upper dermis and epithelium and also causes the surface planes to be level. The epithelial edges can then be opposed with interrupted or running monofilament sutures, which can be removed within a week

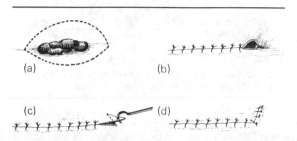

Figure 44–7. Alternative method of correction of dog-ear.

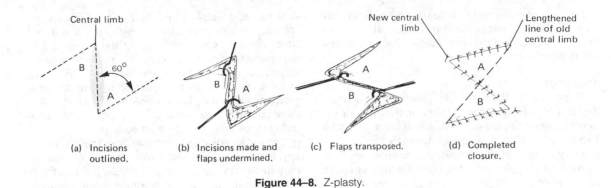

(a) Incisions outlined. (b) Incisions made and flaps undermined. (c) Flaps transposed. (d) Completed closure.

Figure 44–8. Z-plasty.

(within 3–4 days in the face), so the suture tracks can be avoided. Sterile adhesive tape (Steri-Strips) placed across the incision will also prevent surface marks and can be used either primarily or after surface sutures have been removed. Taping will not correct errors in suturing that have resulted in uneven edges or tension across the incision. Tape burns may occur if there is excessive tension or swelling around the incision.

The size and even the type of suture material are less important than careful suture placement and observance of previously mentioned factors. Almost any suture properly placed and removed early enough will provide closure without leaving suture marks. The use of monofilament nylon or polypropylene suture material is advised, however, since these types of sutures cause the fewest reactions of currently available suture materials, excluding stainless steel. Running subcuticular, pullout type monofilament sutures may be left in for up to 3 weeks without causing reactions. Even buried nylon sutures are well tolerated and generally cause fewer problems than braided or absorbable sutures.

Sutures should be removed as soon as possible, depending on the healing characteristics of the skin involved and tension created locally by movement of shearing. The incision should be free of crusts, debris, and bacteria.

Casanova R et al: Clinical evaluation of flap viability with a dermal surface fluorometer. Ann Plast Surg 1988;20: 112.

Jenkins S, Sepka R, Barwick WJ: Routine use of laser doppler flowmetry for monitoring autologous tissue transplants. Ann Plast Surg 1988;21:423.

Swartz WM et al: Direct monitoring of microvascular anastomoses with the 20-MHz ultrasonic doppler probe: An experimental and clinical study. Plast Reconstr Surg 1988;81:149.

Yamamoto Y et al: Development of laserflowgraphy: A comparison between this technique and the 133 xenon clearance method. Jpn J Plast Reconstr Surg 1990; 33:887.

III. SPECIFIC DISORDERS TREATED BY PLASTIC SURGERY

DISORDERS OF SCARRING

HYPERTROPHIC SCARS & KELOIDS

In response to any injury severe enough to break the continuity of the skin or produce necrosis, the skin heals with scar formation. Under ideal circumstances a fine, flat hairline scar will result. The details of wound healing are presented in Chapter 7.

However, hypertrophy may occur, causing the scar to become raised and thickened, or a keloid may form. A keloid is a true tumor arising from the connective tissue elements of the dermis. By definition, keloids grow beyond the margins of the original injury or scar; in some instances, they may grow to enormous size.

The tendency should be resisted to regard all thickened scars as keloids and to label as keloid formers all patients with unattractive scars. Hypertrophic scars and keloids are distinct entities, and the clinical course and prognosis are quite different in each case. The overreactive process that results in thickening of the hypertrophic scar ceases within a few weeks—before it extends beyond the limits of the original scar—and in most cases, some degree of maturation occurs and gradual improvement takes place. In the case of keloids, the overreactive proliferation of fibroblasts continues for weeks or months. By the time it ceases, an actual tumor is present that typically extends well beyond the limits of the original scar, involves the surrounding skin, and may become quite large. Maturation with spontaneous improvement does not usually occur.

Hypertrophic scars and keloids can be differentiated by histopathologic methods. Clinical observation of the course of the scar is also a practical means of differentiation.

Treatment

Since nearly all hypertrophic scars undergo some degree of spontaneous improvement, they do not require treatment in the early phases. If the scar is still hypertrophic after 6 months, surgical excision and primary closure of the wound may be indicated. Improvement may be expected when the hypertrophic scar was originally produced by excessive endothelial and fibroblastic cell proliferation, as is present in open wounds, burns, and infected wounds. However, little or no improvement can be anticipated if the hypertrophic scar followed uncomplicated healing of a simple surgical incision. Improvement of hypertrophic scars across flexion surfaces such as the antecubital fossa or the fingers requires a procedure such as a Z-plasty to change the direction of the scar.

Pressure may help flatten a potentially hypertrophic scar. It is particularly useful for burn scars. A measured elastic garment or face mask (Jobst) is applied to the scarred area and provides continued pressure that causes realignment and remodeling of the collagen bundles. Pressure should be applied early, continuously, and for 6–12 months. Use of intermittent pressure (eg, only at night) or after the hypertrophic scar is established (6–12 months) is of little value.

The treatment of choice for keloids and intractable hypertrophic scars is injection of triamcinolone acetonide, 10 mg/mL (Kenalog-10 Injection), directly into the lesion. This will also help control itching associated with these lesions. In the case of larger lesions, injection is made into more than one site. There is evidence that keloids may respond better to early than to late treatment.

Lesions are injected every 3–4 weeks, and treatment should not be carried out longer than 6 months. The following dosage schedule is used:

Size of Lesion	Dose per Injection
1–2 cm^2	20–40 mg
2–6 cm^2	40–80 mg
6–10 cm^2	80–110 mg

For larger lesions, the maximum dose should be 120 mg. The maximum doses for each treatment for children are as follows:

Age	Maximum Dose
1–2 years	20 mg
3–5 years	40 mg
6–10 years	80 mg

There is a tendency to inject the drug into the scar too often or in too high a dosage—or into the subja-

cent tissue, which may produce too vigorous a response, resulting in excessive atrophy of the skin and subcutaneous tissues surrounding the lesion and in depigmentation of darker skins. Both of these adverse responses may improve spontaneously in 6–12 months, but not necessarily completely. The response varies greatly; some lesions become flat after two or three injections, and some fail to respond at all. Topical corticosteroid therapy is of no value.

Before the advent of corticosteroid injection therapy, surgical excision and radiation therapy were the only methods of treatment of keloids. Both methods are disappointing; surgical resection usually leads to recurrence of a larger lesion; with very few exceptions, radiation therapy produces an unpredictable result and has obvious potential side effects, including neoplastic degeneration. At present, surgical excision is used only in conjunction with intralesional corticosteroid therapy. Excision is usually confined to the larger lesions in which steroid therapy would exceed safe dosages. (The wound is injected at the time of surgery and then postoperatively according to the schedule recommended above.) Care should be taken so that surgical incisions are not extended into the normal skin around the keloid, since the growth of a new keloid may occur in these scars. We have observed that intramarginal excisions yield better results than extramarginal excisions.

Engrav LH et al: A comparison of intramarginal and extramarginal excision of hypertrophic burns scars. Plast Reconstr Surg 1988;81:40.

Muir IF: On the nature of keloid and hypertrophic scars. Br J Plast Surg 1990;43:61.

CONTRACTURES

Contraction is a normal process of wound healing. Contracture, on the other hand, is a pathologic end stage related to the process of contraction. Generally, contractures develop when wounds heal with too much scarring and contraction of the scar tissue results in distortion of surrounding tissues. Although scar contractures can occur in any flexible tissue, such as the eyelids or lips, contractures usually occur across areas of flexion, such as the neck, axilla, or antecubital fossa. The contracted scar brings together the structures on either side of the joint space and prevents active or even passive extension. Exceptions to this pattern of flexion contractures are extension contractures of the toes and MP (metacarpophalangeal) joints of the digits. Contraction is thought to occur via smooth muscle contractile elements in myofibroblasts, but the mechanism is not well understood. In one vertical abdominal scar there may be an area of normal scar formation and an area of hypertrophic scar formation with visible contracture. Contracture can occur in response to the presence of foreign material such as Silastic breast implants. Overall, there is a 10% incidence of some form of breast capsular contracture. Myofibroblasts are thought to play an important role, but the actual cause is not known. Some patients have a soft, excellent result on one side but significant contracture on the other. Experiment and practice with newer types of implants have shown considerable reduction in the contracture rate: For example, the polyurethane coated and textured silicone implants apparently interfere with normal capsule formation thereby leading to less contracture.

The best treatment of contractures is prevention. Incisions should not be made at right angles to flexion creases or should be reoriented by Z-plasties. Wounds in areas of flexion can be covered with flaps or grafted early with thick split-thickness or full-thickness grafts to stop the process of contraction. Such wounds should also be splinted in a position of extension during healing and for 2–3 weeks after healing is complete. Vigorous physical therapy may also be helpful.

Once a contracture is established, stretching and massage are rarely beneficial. Narrow bands of contracture may be excised and released with one or more Z-plasties. Larger areas must be incised from the medial to the lateral axis across the flexion surface and completely opened up to full extension. The resulting defect can be extensive and must be resurfaced with a skin flap or skin graft. In recurrent contractures a fasciocutaneous flap is the treatment of choice. If a skin graft is used, the area must be splinted in extension for approximately 2 weeks after the graft has healed. Less aggressive surgery is likely to result in recurrence.

Achauer GM, Spenler CW, Gold ME: Reconstruction of axillary burn contractures with the latissimus dorsi fasciocutaneous flap. J Trauma 1988;28:211.

SKIN TUMORS*

Tumors of the skin are by far the most common of all tumors in humans. They arise from each of the histologic structures that make up the skin—epidermis, connective tissue, gland, muscle, and nerve elements—and are correspondingly numerous in variety. Skin tumors are classified as benign, premalignant, and malignant.

*Melanoma is discussed in Chapter 47.

BENIGN SKIN TUMORS

The many benign tumors that arise from the skin rarely interfere with function. Since most are removed for aesthetic reasons or to rule out malignancy, they are quite commonly treated by the plastic surgeon. The majority are small and can be simply excised under local anesthesia following the principles of elliptical excision and wound closure discussed above. General anesthesia may be necessary for larger lesions requiring excision and repair by skin grafts or flaps or those occurring in young children.

When the diagnosis is not in doubt, most superficial lesions (seborrheic keratoses, verrucae, squamous cell papillomas) can be treated by simple techniques such as electrodesiccation, curettage and electrodesiccation, cryotherapy, and topical cytotoxic agents.

Seborrheic Keratosis

Seborrheic keratoses are superficial noninvasive tumors that originate in the epidermis. They appear in older people as multiple slightly elevated yellowish, brown, or brownish-black irregularly rounded plaques with waxy or oily surfaces. They are most commonly found on the trunk and shoulders but are frequently seen on the scalp and face.

Since the lesion is raised above the epidermis, treatment usually consists of shave excision.

Verrucae

Verrucae (common warts) are usually seen in children and young adults, commonly on the fingers and hands. They appear as round or oval elevated lesions with rough surfaces composed of multiple rounded or filiform keratinized projections. They may be skin-colored or gray to brown.

Verrucae are caused by a virus and are autoinoculable, which can result in multiple lesions around the original growth or frequent recurrences following treatment if the virus is not completely eradicated. They may disappear spontaneously.

Treatment by electrodesiccation is effective but is frequently followed by slow healing. Repeated applications of bichloroacetic acid, liquid nitrogen, or liquid CO_2 are also effective. Surgical excision is not recommended, since the wound may become inoculated with the virus, leading to recurrences in and around the scar.

Because recurrences are common despite thorough treatment, it is reasonable to delay treatment of asymptomatic lesions for several months to determine if they will disappear spontaneously.

Cysts

A. Epidermal Inclusion Cyst: Although sebaceous cyst is the commonly used term, these lesions more properly should be called epidermal inclusion cysts, since they are composed of thin layers of epidermal cells filled with epithelial debris. True cysts arising from sebaceous epithelial cells are uncommon.

Epidermal inclusion cysts are soft to firm, usually elevated, and are filled with an odorous cheesy material. Their most common sites of occurrence are the scalp, face, ears, neck, and back. They are usually covered by normal skin, which may show dimpling at the site of skin attachment. They frequently present as infected cysts.

Treatment consists of surgical excision.

B. Dermoid Cyst: Dermoid cysts are deeper than epidermal cysts. They are not attached to the skin but frequently are attached to or extend through underlying bony structures. They may appear in many sites but are most common around the nose or the orbit, where they may extend to meningeal structures, necessitating CT scans to determine their extent.

Treatment is by surgical excision, which may necessitate sectioning of adjacent bony structures.

Pigmented Nevi

Nevocellular nevi are groups of cells of probable neural crest origin which contain melanomas that form melanin more rapidly upon stimulation than surrounding tissue. These cells migrate to different parts of the skin to give different types of nevi. They may also be distinguished by their clinical presentation.

A. Junctional Nevi: Junctional nevi are well-defined pigmented lesions appearing in infancy. They are usually flat or slightly elevated and light brown to dark brown. They may appear on any part of the body, but most nevi seen on the palms, soles, and genitalia are of the junctional type. Histologically, a proliferation of melanocytes is present in the epidermis at the epidermal-dermal junction. It was formerly thought that these nevi give rise to malignant melanoma and that all junctional nevi should be excised for prophylactic reasons. However, most investigators now feel that the risk is very slight. If there is no change in their appearance, treatment is unnecessary. Any change such as itching, inflammation, darkening in color, halo formation, increase in size, bleeding, or ulceration calls for immediate treatment.

Surgical excision is the only safe method of treatment.

B. Intradermal Nevi: Intradermal nevi are the typical dome-shaped, sometimes pedunculated, fleshy to brownish pigmented moles that are characteristically seen in adults. They frequently contain hairs and may occur anywhere on the body.

Microscopically, melanocytes are present entirely within the dermis and, in contrast to junctional nevi, show little activity. They are rarely malignant and require no treatment except for aesthetic reasons.

Surgical excision is nearly always the treatment of choice. Pigmented nevi should never be treated without obtaining tissue for histologic examination.

C. Compound Nevi: Compound nevi exhibit the histologic features of both junctional and intradermal nevi in that melanocytes lie both at the epidermal-dermal junction and within the dermis. They are usually elevated, dome-shaped, and light- to dark-brown in color.

Because of the presence of nevus cells at the epidermal-dermal junction, the indications for treatment are the same as for junctional nevi. If treatment is indicated, surgical excision is the method of choice.

D. Spindle Cell-Epithelioma Cell Nevi: These nevi, formerly called benign juvenile melanomas, appear in children or adults. They vary markedly in vascularity, degree of pigmentation, and accompanying hyperkeratosis. Clinically, they simulate warts or hemangiomas rather than moles. They may increase in size rapidly, but the average lesion reaches only 6–8 mm in diameter, remaining entirely benign without invasion or metastases. Microscopically, the lesion can be confused with malignant melanoma by the inexperienced pathologist. The usual treatment is excisional biopsy.

E. Blue Nevi: Blue nevi are small, sharply defined, round, dark blue or gray-blue lesions that may occur anywhere on the body but are most commonly seen on the face, neck, hands, and arms. They usually appear in childhood as slowly growing, well-defined nodules covered by a smooth, intact epidermis. Microscopically, the melanocytes that make up this lesion are limited to (but may be found in all layers of) the dermis. An intimate association with the fibroblasts of the dermis is seen, giving the lesion a fibrotic appearance not seen in other nevi. This, together with extension of melanocytes deep into the dermis, may account for the blue rather than brown color.

Treatment is not mandatory unless the patient desires removal for aesthetic reasons or fear of cancer. Surgical excision is the treatment of choice.

F. Giant Hairy Nevi: Unlike most nevi arising from melanocytes, giant hairy nevi are congenital. They may occur anywhere on the body and may cover large areas. They may be large enough to cover the entire trunk (bathing trunk nevi). They are of special significance for several reasons: (1) Their large size is especially deforming from an aesthetic standpoint; (2) they show a definite predisposition for developing malignant melanoma; and (3) they may be associated with neurofibromas or melanocytic involvement of the leptomeninges and other neurologic abnormalities.

Microscopically, a varied picture is present. All of the characteristics of intradermal and compound nevi may be seen. Neurofibromas may also be present within the lesion. Malignant melanoma may arise anywhere within the large lesion; the reported rate of occurrence ranges from 1% to as high as 13.7% in one study. Malignant melanoma with metastases can arise in childhood and even in infancy.

The only full treatment is complete excision and skin grafting. Large lesions may require excision and grafting in stages. Some lesions are so large that excision is not possible and the most effective approach is using tissue expansion in combination with flaps. Split-thickness excision or dermabrasion has been successful when done in infancy.

Bauer BS, Vicari FA: An approach to excision of congenital giant pigmented nevi in infancy and early childhood. Plast Reconstr Surg 1988;82:1012.

Hemangioma

It is confusing to attempt to classify hemangiomas on the basis of their histology. For example, the histologic term capillary hemangioma is used for both the common involuting hemangioma of childhood that disappears by age 7 and the port wine stain that persists into adulthood. The term cavernous is used to designate several types of hemangiomas that behave quite differently. Some hemangiomas are true neoplasms arising from endothelial cells and other vascular elements (such as involuting hemangiomas of childhood, endotheliomas, and pericytomas). Others are not true neoplasms but rather malformations of normal vascular structures (eg, port wine stains, cavernous hemangiomas, and arteriovenous fistulas).

A simple classification based upon whether or not the hemangioma undergoes spontaneous involution is proposed in Table 44–3.

A. Involuting Hemangioma: Involuting hemangiomas are the most common tumors that occur in

Table 44–3. Proposed classification of hemangiomas based on appearance and clinical course of lesion.

Proposed Term	Terms in Common Use*
Involuting hemangioma	
Superficial	Strawberry nevus Nevus vasculosus Capillary hemangioma
Combined superficial and deep	Strawberry nevus Capillary hemangioma Capillary and cavernous hemangioma
Deep	Cavernous hemangioma
Noninvoluting hemangioma	
Port wine stain	Port wine stain Capillary hemangioma Nevus flammeus
Cavernous hemangioma	Cavernous hemangioma
Venous racemose aneurysm	Cavernous hemangioma
Arteriovenous fistula	Arteriovenous fistula

*Confusing because different terms are used to denote the same lesion and because the same term is sometimes used to denote different lesions.

childhood and constitute at least 95% of all the hemangiomas that are seen in infancy and childhood. They are true neoplasms of endothelial cells but are unique among neoplasms in that they undergo complete spontaneous involution.

Typically, they are present at birth or appear during the first 2–3 weeks of life. They grow at a rather rapid rate for 4–6 months; then growth ceases and spontaneous involution begins. Involution progresses slowly but is complete by 5–7 years of age.

Involuting hemangiomas appear on all body surfaces but are seen more often on the head and neck. They are seen twice as often in girls as in boys and show a predisposition for fair-skinned individuals.

Three forms of involuting hemangioma are seen: (1) superficial, (2) combined superficial and deep, and (3) deep. Superficial involuting hemangiomas appear as sharply demarcated, bright-red, slightly raised lesions with an irregular surface that has been described as resembling a strawberry. Combined superficial and deep involuting hemangiomas have the same surface characteristics, but beneath the surface, a firm bluish tumor is present that may extend deeply into the subcutaneous tissues. Deep involuting hemangiomas present as deep blue tumors covered by normal-appearing skin.

The histologic findings in involuting hemangiomas are quite different from those seen in other types of hemangiomas. There is a constant correlation between the histologic picture and the clinical course. During the growth phase, the lesion is composed of solid fields of closely packed round or oval endothelial cells. As would be expected during the growth phase, cellular division with mitotic figures is seen, so that the lesion is sometimes called a hemangioendothelioma by the pathologist. This term must not be used, however, since it is commonly used to denote the highly malignant angiosarcoma that is seen in adults.

As the phase of involution progresses, the histologic picture changes, with the solid fields of endothelial cells breaking up into closely packed, capillary-sized, vessel-like structures composed of several layers of soft endothelial cells supported by a sparse fibrous stroma. These vascular structures gradually become fewer and spaced more widely apart in a loose, edematous fibrous stroma. The endothelial cells continue to disappear, so that by the time involution is complete the histologic picture is entirely normal, with no trace of endothelial cells.

Treatment is not usually indicated, since the appearance following spontaneous regression is nearly always superior to the scars that follow surgical excision. Complete surgical excision of lesions that involve important structures such as the eyelids, nose, or lips results in unnecessary disfigurement that is difficult to repair.

Partial resection of a portion of a hemangioma of the brow or eyelid is indicated when the lesion is large enough to prevent light from entering the eye—a condition that will lead to blindness or amblyopia. The same type of treatment may be necessary for lesions of the mucosal surfaces of the lips when they project into the mouth and are traumatized by the teeth. In these cases, surgery should be very conservative—only enough of the lesion should be resected to alleviate the problem, and the remaining portions should be allowed to involute spontaneously.

In approximately 8% of cases, ulceration will occur. This may be accompanied by infection, which is treated by the use of compresses of warm saline or potassium permanganate and by the application of antibiotic powders and lotions. Bleeding from the ulcer is not common; when it does occur, it is easily controlled by the application of pressure. In rare cases, the platelet trapping of these lesions leads to the clinical picture of disseminated intravascular coagulopathy called **Kasabach-Merritt syndrome.**

After involution of large lesions, superficial scarring may be present or the involved skin may be thin, wrinkled, or redundant. These conditions may require conservative plastic surgery procedures.

The application of local agents such as dry ice to the surface of these lesions has been popular. This type of treatment has no effect on the deep portions of the hemangioma. It will destroy superficial lesions but results in severe scarring. Injections of sclerosing agents have minimal effect. There is no place for radiation therapy in the treatment of these benign lesions. Corticosteroids given systemically or intralesionally have been used with varying success. Anecdotal evidence exists in favor of compression to speed up the involution process and give a better final result.

B. Noninvoluting Hemangioma: Most noninvoluting hemangiomas are present at birth. In contrast to involuting hemangiomas, they do not undergo rapid growth during the first 4–6 months of life but grow in proportion to the growth of the child. They persist into adulthood and may cause severe aesthetic and functional problems. Some, such as arteriovenous fistulas, may cause death due to cardiac failure.

Unfortunately, treatment of noninvoluting hemangiomas is difficult and usually far from satisfactory.

Port wine stains are by far the most common of the noninvoluting hemangiomas. They may involve any portion of the body but most commonly appear on the face as flat patchy lesions that are reddish to purple in color. When present on the face, they are located in areas supplied by the sensory branches of the fifth cranial nerve. The light-red lesions may fade to a varying degree but persist into adulthood. Some of the deep red or purplish lesions that have a stippled appearance show a propensity for growth later in life, in which case they become raised and thickened, with nodules appearing on the surface.

Microscopically, port wine stains are made up of thin-walled capillaries that are arranged throughout the dermis. The capillaries are lined with mature flat endothelial cells. In the lesions that produce surface growth, groups of round proliferating endothelial cells and large venous sinuses are seen.

Results following treatment of the port wine stain have up to now been uniformly disappointing. Since most lesions occur on the face or neck, patients seek treatment for aesthetic reasons. The simplest and still most effective method of treatment is camouflaging. Unfortunately, this is difficult because the port wine stain is darker than the surrounding lighter skin.

Tattooing with skin-colored pigments may offer some measure of disguise in the lighter lesions but generally is unsatisfactory because the pigment deposited in the skin looks artificial and tends to be absorbed unevenly, producing a mottled appearance.

Superficial methods of treatment such as dry ice, liquid nitrogen, electrocoagulation, and dermabrasion are ineffective unless they destroy the upper layers of the skin, which produces severe scarring.

Radiation therapy, including the use of x-rays, radium, thorium X, and grenz x-rays, is to be condemned. If it is administered in doses high enough to destroy the vessels involved, it also destroys the surrounding tissues and the overlying skin and the cancer incidence after radiotherapy for skin hemangioma increases. Recent experience with the laser has been encouraging. In early or lighter red lesions, the pulsed dye and the argon laser are especially useful; its beam is selectively absorbed by red-pigmented material such as hemoglobin, and these lesions can be removed effectively. In darker and more advanced nodular lesions, the laser is less effective and probably contraindicated because of the severe scarring that develops and hyperpigmentation.

If the lesion is small, surgical excision with primary closure is possible. Unfortunately, most lesions are large. Sometimes the best choice is no treatment. Certain fast-growing capillary or primarily arterialized hemangiomas have been managed successfully with superselective embolization, either alone or in conjunction with surgery. This is performed under fluoroscopic control and with an expert team. There have been reports of slough of large portions of the face as a result of misdirected embolizations.

C. Cavernous Hemangioma: Cavernous hemangiomas are bluish or purplish lesions that are usually elevated. They may occur anywhere on the body but, like other hemangiomas, are more common on the head and neck. They are composed of mature, fully formed venous structures that are present in tortuous masses which have been described as feeling like a bag of worms.

Cavernous hemangiomas are usually present at birth but do not usually grow except to keep pace with normal body growth. In many cases, growth occurs later in life and may interfere with normal function.

Microscopically, cavernous hemangiomas are

made up of large dilated, closely packed vascular sinuses that are engorged with blood. They are lined by flat endothelial cells and may have muscular walls like normal veins.

Treatment is difficult. In only a few cases is the lesion small enough or superficial enough to permit complete surgical excision. Most lesions involve deeper structures—including muscle and bone—so that complete excision is impossible without radical surgery. Since most lesions are no more than aesthetic problems, radical surgery is rarely indicated. Occasionally, the injection of sclerosing agents directly into the venous channels may lead to some involution or may make surgical excision easier. Great care must be used so that areas of overlying skin do not slough.

PREMALIGNANT SKIN LESIONS

Actinic (Solar) Keratoses

Actinic keratoses are the most common of the precancerous skin lesions. They usually appear as small, single or multiple, slightly elevated, scaly or warty lesions ranging in color from red to yellow, brown, or black. Since they are related to sun exposure, they occur most frequently on the face and the backs of the hands in fair-skinned Caucasians whose skin shows evidence of actinic elastosis.

Microscopically, actinic keratoses consist of well-defined areas of abnormal epithelial cells limited to the epidermis. Approximately 15–20% of these lesions become malignant, in which case invasion of the dermis as squamous cell carcinoma occurs.

Since the lesions are limited to the epidermis, superficial treatment in the form of curettement and electrodesiccation or the application of chemical agents such as liquid nitrogen, phenol, bi- or trichloroacetic acid, or fluorouracil is curative. The application of fluorouracil (5-FU) cream is of particular benefit in preventive treatment in that it will destroy lesions of microscopic size—before they can be detected clinically—without causing damage to uninvolved skin.

Chronic Radiation Dermatitis & Ulceration

There are two distinct types of radiation dermatitis. The first and most common follows the acute administration of relatively high dosages of ionizing orthovoltage radiation over relatively short periods—almost always for the treatment of cancer. Dermatitis is characterized by an acute reaction that begins near the third week of therapy, when erythema, blistering, and sloughing of the epidermis start to occur. Burning and hyperesthesia are commonly present. This initial reaction is followed by scarring characterized by atrophy of the epidermis and dermis along with loss of skin appendages (sweat glands, sebaceous glands, and hair follicles). Marked fibrosis of the dermis occurs, with gradual endarteritis and occlusion of the dermal and subdermal vessels. Telangiectasia of the surface vessels is seen, and areas of both hypo- and hyperpigmentation occur.

The second type of radiation dermatitis follows chronic exposure to low doses of ionizing radiation over prolonged periods. It is usually seen in professional personnel who handle radioactive materials or administer x-rays or in patients who have been treated for dermatologic conditions such as acne or excessive facial hair. Therefore, the face and hands are most commonly involved. The acute reaction described above does not usually occur, but the same process of atrophy, scarring, and loss of dermal elements occurs. Drying of the skin becomes more pronounced, and deepening of the skin furrows is typically present.

In both types of radiation dermatitis, late changes such as the following may occur: (1) the appearance of hyperkeratotic growths on the skin surface, (2) chronic ulceration, and (3) the development of either basal cell or squamous cell carcinoma. Ulceration and cancer, however, are seen much less commonly in the first type of radiation dermatitis than in the second. When malignant growths appear, basal cell carcinomas are seen more frequently on the face and neck and squamous cell carcinomas more frequently on the hands and body.

Newer radiotherapeutic methods using megavoltage and cobalt techniques have a sparing effect on the skin. However, marked scarring and avascularity of deeper, more extensive areas may present more diffi cult problems.

Surgical excision is the treatment of choice. Excision should include all of the irradiated tissue including the area of telangiectasia, whenever possible, and the defect should be covered with an appropriate axial or musculocutaneous flap to provide a new blood supply.

Primary wound closure is feasible for only the smallest lesions, and even so at some risk. Free skin grafting is usually unsuccessful because of the damage to the vascular supply of the subcutaneous structures. Adjacent random flaps are unreliable because they depend upon blood supply from the surrounding irradiated area.

MALIGNANT LESIONS

1. INTRAEPIDERMAL CARCINOMA

Intraepidermal carcinoma includes Bowen's disease and erythroplasia of Queyrat.

Bowen's Disease

Bowen's disease is characterized by single or multiple, brownish or reddish plaques that may appear anywhere on the skin surface but often on covered surfaces. The typical plaque is sharply defined, slightly raised, scaly, and slightly thickened. The surface is often keratotic, and crusting and fissuring may be present. Ulceration is not common but when present suggests malignant degeneration with dermal invasion.

Histologically, hyperplasia of the epidermis is seen, with pleomorphic malpighian cells, giant cells, and atypical epithelial cells that are limited to the epidermis.

Treatment of small or superficial lesions consists of total destruction by curettement and electrodesiccation or by any of the other superficially destructive methods (cryotherapy, cytotoxic agents). Excision and skin grafting are preferred for larger lesions and for those that have undergone early malignant degeneration and invasion of the dermis.

Erythroplasia of Queyrat

Erythroplasia of Queyrat is almost identical to Bowen's disease both clinically and histologically but is confined to the glans penis and the vulva, where the lesions appear as red, velvety, irregular, slightly raised plaques. Treatment is as described for Bowen's disease.

2. BASAL CELL CARCINOMA

Basal cell carcinoma is the most common skin cancer. The lesions usually appear on the face and are more common in men than women. Since exposure to ultraviolet rays of the sun is a causative factor, basal cell carcinoma is most commonly seen in geographic areas where there is significant sun exposure and in people whose skins are most susceptible to actinic damage from exposure, ie, fair-skinned individuals with blue eyes and blond hair. It may occur at any age but is not common before age 40.

The growth rate of basal cell carcinoma is usually slow but nearly always steady and insidious. Several months or years may pass before the patient becomes concerned. Without treatment, widespread invasion and destruction of adjacent tissues may occur, producing massive ulceration. Penetration of the bones of the facial skeleton and the skull may occur late in the course. Basal cell carcinomas rarely metastasize, but death can occur because of direct intracranial extension or erosion of major blood vessels.

Typical individual lesions appear as small, translucent or shiny ("pearly") elevated nodules with central umbilication and rolled, pearly edges. Telangiectatic vessels are commonly present over the surface, and pigmentation is sometimes present. Superficial ulceration occurs early.

A less common type of basal cell carcinoma is the **sclerosing** or **morphea carcinoma,** consisting of elongated strands of basal cell cancer that infiltrate

the dermis, with the intervening corium being unusually compact. These lesions are usually flat and whitish or waxy in appearance and firm to palpation—similar in appearance to localized scleroderma.

The superficial **erythematous basal cell cancer** ("body basal") occurs most frequently on the trunk. It appears as reddish plaques with atrophic centers and smooth, slightly raised borders. These lesions are capable of peripheral growth and wide extension but do not become invasive until late.

Pigmented basal cell carcinomas may be mistaken for melanomas, because of the large number of melanocytes present within the tumor. They may also be confused with seborrheic keratoses.

Treatment

There are several methods of treating basal cell carcinoma. All may be curative in some lesions, but no one method is applicable to all. The special features of each basal cell cancer must be considered individually before proper treatment can be selected.

Since most lesions occur on the face, aesthetic and functional results of treatment are important. However, the most important consideration is whether or not therapy is curative. If the basal cell carcinoma is not eradicated by the initial treatment, continued growth and invasion of adjacent tissues will occur. This will result not only in additional tissue destruction but also in invasion of the tumor into deeper structures, making cure more difficult.

The principal methods of treatment are curettage and electrodesiccation, surgical excision, and radiation therapy. Chemosurgery, topical chemotherapy, and cryosurgery are not often used but may have value in selected cases.

A. Curettage and Electrodesiccation: Curettage plus electrodesiccation is the usual method of treatment for small lesions. After infiltration with suitable local anesthetic, the lesion and a 2- to 3-mm margin of normal-appearing skin around it are thoroughly curetted with a small skin curette. The resultant wound is then completely desiccated with an electrosurgical unit to destroy any tumor cells that may not have been removed by the curette. The process is then repeated once or twice if necessary. The wound is left open and allowed to heal secondarily.

When used as treatment for superficial basal cell carcinoma, curettage and electrodesiccation is a simple, quick, and inexpensive procedure that will cure nearly all superficial lesions. However, this method of treatment should not be used in the deeper infiltrative and morphea type lesions. These lesions should be treated by surgical excision, x-ray therapy, or chemosurgery.

B. Surgical Excision: Surgical excision, following the principles outlined earlier in this chapter, offers many advantages in the treatment of basal cell carcinoma: (1) Most lesions can be quickly excised in one procedure. (2) Following excision, the entire lesion can be examined by the pathologist, who can determine if the tumor has been completely removed. (3) Deep infiltrative lesions can be completely excised, and cartilage and bone can be removed if they have been invaded. (4) Lesions that occur in dense scar tissue or in other poorly vascularized tissues cannot be treated by curettage and desiccation, radiation therapy, or chemosurgery, since healing is poor. Excision and flap coverage may be the only method for treatment in these conditions. (5) Recurrent lesions in tissues that have been exposed to maximum safe amounts of radiation can be excised and covered.

Small to moderate-sized lesions can be excised in one stage under local anesthesia. The visible and palpable margins of the tumor are marked on the skin with marking ink. The width of excision is then marked 3–5 mm beyond these margins. If the margins of the basal cell carcinoma are vague, the width of excision will have to be wider to ensure complete removal of the lesion. The lines of incision are drawn around the lesion as a circle. This tissue is excised, taking care to leave a margin of normal-appearing subcutaneous tissue around the deep margins of the tumor. Frozen sections may be obtained at the time of excision to aid in determining whether tumor-free margins have been obtained. This is minimized with experience. It is better to err on the side of removing more normal tissue than necessary rather than to run the risk of including tumor at the margins. Closure of the wound is accomplished in the direction of minimal skin tension, usually along the skin lines. The dog-ears are removed appropriately.

Wounds resulting from the excision of some moderate-sized tumors and nearly all large tumors may necessitate for optimum reconstruction of function and appearance, the use of local, regional and free flaps. This can nearly always be performed in one stage.

The disadvantages of surgical excision are as follows: (1) Specialized training and experience are necessary to master the surgical techniques. (2) Whereas curettage and desiccation may be performed in the office, surgical excision requires specialized facilities. (3) In lesions with vague margins, an excessive amount of normal tissue may have to be excised to ensure complete removal. (4) Structures that are difficult to reconstruct, such as the eyelids, nasal tip, and lips, have to be sacrificed when they are extensively infiltrated and immediate reconstruction to cover vital structures is indicated. To overcome some of these objections, Mohs described in 1941 a new technique that allows for serial excisions and microscopic examination of chemically fixed tissue. Newer developments have obviated the cumbersome fixation techniques, but it may still take several hours to scan an area for suspected malignant cells. The procedure is nevertheless quite useful for recurrent lesions and in areas that deserve maximal preservation.

C. X-Ray Therapy: X-ray therapy is as effective as any other in the treatment of basal cell carcinoma. Its advantages are as follows: (1) Structures that are difficult to reconstruct, such as the eyelids, tear ducts, and nasal tip, can be preserved when they are invaded by but not destroyed by tumor. (2) A wide margin of tissue can be treated around lesions with poorly defined margins to ensure destruction of nondiscernible extensions of tumor. (3) It may be less traumatic than surgical excision to elderly patients with advanced lesions. (4) Hospitalization is not necessary.

The disadvantages are as follows: (1) Only well-trained, experienced physicians can obtain good results. (2) Expensive facilities are necessary. (3) Improperly administered radiation therapy may produce severe sequelae, including scarring, radiation dermatitis, ulceration, and malignant degeneration. (4) In hair-bearing areas, baldness will result. (5) It may be difficult to treat areas of irregular contour (ie, the ear and the auditory canal). (6) Repeated treatments over a period of 4–6 weeks may be necessary.

X-ray therapy should not be used in patients under age 40 except in unusual circumstances, and it should not be used in patients who have failed to respond to radiation therapy in the past.

3. SQUAMOUS CELL CARCINOMA

Squamous cell carcinoma is the second most common cancer of the skin in light-skinned racial groups and the most common skin cancer in darkly pigmented racial groups. As with basal cell carcinoma, sunlight is the most common causative factor in Caucasians, and most lesions in Caucasians occur in fair-skinned individuals. The most common sites of occurrence are the ears, the cheeks, the lower lip, and the backs of the hands. Other causative factors are chemical and thermal burns, scars, chronic ulcers, chronic granulomas (tuberculosis of the skin, syphilis), draining sinuses, contact with tars and hydrocarbons, and exposure to ionizing radiation. When a squamous cell carcinoma occurs in a burn scar, it is called a **Marjolin ulcer.** This lesion may appear many years after the original burn. It tends to be aggressive, and the prognosis is poor.

Since exposure to the sun is the greatest stimulus for the production of squamous cell carcinoma, most of these lesions are preceded by actinic keratosis on areas of the skin showing chronic solar damage. They may also arise from other premalignant skin lesions and from normal-appearing skin.

The natural history of squamous cell carcinoma may be quite variable. It may present as a slowly growing, locally invasive lesion without metastases or as a rapidly growing, widely invasive tumor with early metastatic spread. In general, squamous cell carcinomas that develop from actinic keratoses are more common and are of the slowly growing type, whereas those that develop from Bowen's disease, erythroplasia of Queyrat, chronic radiation dermatitis, scars, and chronic ulcers tend to be more aggressive. Lesions that arise from normal-appearing skin and from the lips, genitalia, and anal regions also tend to be aggressive.

Early squamous cell carcinoma usually appears as a small, firm erythematous plaque or nodule with indistinct margins. The surface may be flat and smooth or may be verrucous. As the tumor grows, it becomes raised, and, because of progressive invasion, becomes fixed to surrounding tissues. Ulceration may occur early or late but tends to appear earlier in the more rapidly growing lesions.

Histologically, malignant epithelial cells are seen extending down into the dermis as broad, rounded masses or slender strands. In squamous cell carcinomas of low-grade malignancy, the individual cells may be quite well differentiated, resembling uniform mature squamous cells having intercellular bridges. Keratinization may be present, and layers of keratinizing squamous cells may produce typical round "horn pearls." In highly malignant lesions, the epithelial cells may be extremely atypical; abnormal mitotic figures are common; intercellular bridges are not present; and keratinization does not occur.

As with basal cell carcinomas, the method of treatment that will eradicate squamous cell carcinomas and produce the best aesthetic and functional results varies with the characteristics of the individual lesion. Factors that determine the optimal method of treatment include the size, shape, and location of the tumor as well as the histologic pattern that determines its aggressiveness.

Treatment consists of surgery or irradiation. The advantages and disadvantages of each type of therapy are discussed above. Since basal cell carcinomas are relatively nonaggressive lesions that rarely metastasize, failure to eradicate the lesion may result only in local recurrence. Although this may result in extensive local tissue destruction, there is rarely a threat to life. Aggressive squamous cell carcinomas, on the other hand, may metastasize to any part of the body, and failure of treatment may have fatal consequences. For this reason, total eradication of each lesion is the imperative goal of treatment.

Because the overall incidence of lymph node metastasis is relatively low, most authorities agree that node resection is not indicated in the absence of palpable regional lymph nodes except in the case of very aggressive carcinomas of the genitalia and anal regions.

Boysen M et al: Experience with reconstructive surgery in 137 cases of head and neck cancer. Otolaryngology 1988;17:237.

Hanke CW: Lasers in dermatology. Indiana Med 1990; 83:394.

Lin AN, Carter DM, Balin AK: Nonmelanoma skin cancers in the elderly. Clin Geriatr Med 1989;5:161.

Lundell M, Holm LE, Silfversward C: Cancer incidence after radiotherapy for skin hemangioma: A retrospective cohort study in Sweden. J Natl Cancer Inst 1988; 80:1387.

Roenigk RK: Mohs' micrographic surgery. Mayo Clin Proc 1988;63:175.

Sloan GM et al: Intralesional corticosteroid therapy for infantile hemangiomas. Plast Reconstr Surg 1989;83:459.

Tan OT, Sherwood K, Gilchrest BA: Treatment of children with port-wine stains using the flashlamp-pulsed tunable dye laser. N Engl J Med 1989;320:416.

Yakes WF et al: Symptomatic vascular malformations: Ethanol embolotherapy. Radiology 1989;170:1059.

SOFT TISSUE INJURY

The plastic surgeon is often involved in emergency room assessment and treatment of soft tissue injuries. Many aspects of wound management must be considered in even a relatively simple facial laceration.

If possible, the following factors should be determined in patients with soft tissue injuries: (1) the type of wound or wounds (abrasion, contusion, etc); (2) the cause of injury; (3) the age of the injury; (4) the location of injured tissues; (5) the degree of contamination of the injured area before, during, and after trauma; (6) the nature and extent of associated injuries; and (7) the general health of the patient (eg, any chronic or acute illnesses or any allergies; any medications being taken).

The location of the wound must be noted because different healing characteristics are present in various types of skin. The face and scalp are highly vascular and therefore resist infection and heal faster than other areas, but there are many important structures in and around the face, and scars and defects are noticeable. Skin of the trunk, upper arms, and thighs is fairly thick and heals more slowly than facial or scalp skin and is more susceptible to infection. Scarring is less noticeable. The hands are a critical area because there are important structures near the surface, and the destruction caused by infection can be devastating. The lower legs are a particular problem area because the relatively poor blood supply can cause skin loss, and infection is more likely to occur.

Treatment
The type of wound must be determined so that proper treatment can be given. Contusions and swelling require ice packs for 24 hours, rest, and elevation. Abrasions should be cleaned and dressed in a sterile manner as for a skin graft donor site or must be washed daily until a dry scab forms or healing takes place. Ground-in dirt or gravel must be entirely scrubbed out or picked out with a small blade within

24 hours after injury, or foreign material will be sealed in and traumatic tattooing will result. Extensive local anesthesia may be required to accomplish this. Imbedded particulate matter from an explosion must be removed in a similar manner. Hematomas may be treated with ice bags and pressure until stable. Evacuation is then indicated if vital structures such as the ear or nasal septal cartilage are in danger of being injured or destroyed. Lacerations over bony prominences and various types of cuts require special care that will be detailed below. Treatment must be meticulous if optimal results are to be achieved. Puncture wounds and bites are notoriously innocuous in appearance but may result in severe destruction or tetanus or gas gangrene. Antibiotic coverage, irrigation, open treatment, and observation are indicated. Most bites on the face, however, can be cleaned and safely closed. Wounds that create flaps of skin or avulsions are difficult to manage. Careful debridement and judicious use of full- or split-thickness grafts from the avulsed tissue are recommended. Timing is the first factor to consider.

Wound contamination can be caused by bacteria on the surface of the wounding agent, such as rust on a nail or saliva on a tooth, or bacteria that enter the wound when the skin is broken. Bacteria driven into tissue become more established as time passes, and it is therefore important to know the age of the wound at the time of the presentation for treatment. Other injuries associated with cuts almost always take precedence in treatment. In general, wounds other than those on the face or scalp should not be closed primarily if they occurred 8–12 hours or longer before presentation unless they were caused by a very clean agent and have been covered by a sterile bandage in the interim. Delayed primary closure as described previously is an excellent and safe alternative. Nearly any facial wound up to 24 hours old can be safely closed with careful debridement, irrigation, and antibiotic coverage.

The surgeon must decide whether or not antibiotic treatment is indicated. In general, wounds treated appropriately and early do not call for antibiotic therapy. Antibiotics should be given for wounds with delayed presentation or those for which treatment is delayed by choice (eg, wounds with known contamination; wounds in compromised patients, such as very young or old persons, debilitated persons, or persons with general ill health; wounds in areas where infection may have serious consequences, such as the lower legs and the hands; and wounds in persons in whom bacteremia might have serious sequelae, such as those with prosthetic heart valves or orthopedic appliances). Antibiotics should be started before debridement and closure. Only a few days of coverage are necessary—usually until the wound is checked at 2–3 days and found to be free of infection. Penicillin or a substitute is appropriate for wounds involving the mouth, such as through-and-through lip lacerations and bites. Other wounds are usually contaminated by *Staphylococcus aureus,* and an antibiotic effective for penicillin-resistant *S aureus* is therefore appropriate. If gram-negative or anaerobic contamination is suspected, wound closure is risky, and hospitalization of the patient for treatment with parenteral antibiotics should be considered. Tetanus prophylaxis should be routinely given for patients who have not received current immunizations or who have wounds likely to lead to tetanus. Guidelines for this are detailed in Chapter 8.

Anesthesia is an important part of adequate soft tissue wound care and closure. Local anesthesia with either 0.5 or 1% lidocaine with epinephrine 1:200,000 or 1:100,000 is recommended for all wounds except those in areas of appendages, such as earlobes, toes, fingers, and the penis, where plain lidocaine should be used. This may be given through the wound edge before debridement and irrigation for maximum patient comfort. Complete epinephrine vasoconstrictor effect occurs within 7 minutes. Overdose of epinephrine and lidocaine injection into vessels or use of the drugs in patients sensitive to these agents should be avoided.

The importance of irrigation cannot be overstated. Over 90% of bacteria in a recently sustained and superficially contaminated wound can be eliminated by adequate irrigation. Ideally, a physiologic solution such as lactated Ringer's solution or normal saline should be forcefully ejected from a large syringe with a 19-gauge needle or from other equipment designed for this purpose such as a water-jet apparatus. The wound is irrigated once to remove surface clots, foreign material, and bacteria and is then debrided and irrigated again. Detergents and antiseptic solutions are toxic to exposed tissue and should not be used.

Debridement must include removal of all obviously devitalized tissues. In special areas such as the eyelids, ears, nose, lips, and eyebrows, debridement must be done cautiously, since the tissue lost by debridement may be difficult to replace. Where tissues are more abundant, such as in the cheek, chin, and forehead areas, debridement may be more extensive. Small irregular or ragged wounds in these areas can be excised completely to produce clean, sharply cut wound edges which, when approximated, will produce the finest possible scar. Because the blood supply in the face is plentiful, damaged tissues of questionable viability should be retained rather than debrided away. The chances for survival are good.

Following adequate anesthesia, debridement, and irrigation, the wound is ready for final assessment and closure. Lighting must be adequate, and appropriate instruments should be available. The patient and the surgeon must be positioned comfortably. The skin surrounding the wound is prepared with an antiseptic solution, and the area is draped. A final check of the depth and extent of the wound is made, and vital structures are inspected for injury. Hemostasis must be achieved by use of epinephrine, pressure, cautery, or suture ligature. Important structures in facial wounds include the parotid duct, lacrimal duct, and branches of the facial nerve. These should be repaired in the operating room by microsurgical techniques.

Layers of tissue—usually muscle—in the depth of the wound should be closed first with as few absorbable sutures as possible, since sutures are foreign material within the wound. If possible, dead space should be closed with judicious use of fine absorbable sutures. If dead space cannot be closed, external pressure or small drains are sometimes effective. Skin closure should begin at the most important points of the laceration (eg, the borders of the ears and nose; the vermilion border or margins of the lip; the margins of the eyebrow [which should never be shaved]; and the scalp hairline). Subcuticular sutures are very helpful. Skin edges can be approximated without tension or strangulation with 5-0 or 6-0 monofilament suture material as outlined earlier under wound closure.

Complicated lacerations, such as complex stellate wounds or avulsion flaps, often heal with excessive scarring. Because of the associated subcutaneous tissue injury, U-shaped or trap-door avulsion lacerations almost always become unsightly as a result of wound contracture. Small lacerations of this type are best excised and closed in a straight line initially; larger flaps that must be replaced usually require secondary revision. Extensive loss of skin is generally best treated by initial split-thickness skin grafting followed later by secondary reconstruction. Primary attempts to reconstruct with local flaps may fail because of unsuspected injury to these adjacent tissues. The decision to convert avulsed tissues to free grafts that may not survive and thus delay healing requires sound surgical judgment.

Small or moderate-sized closures on the face may be dressed with antibiotic ointment alone. The patient may cleanse the suture lines with hydrogen peroxide to clear away crusts and dirt and then reapply the ointment. Elsewhere, closures benefit from the protection of a sterile bandage. Pressure dressings are useful in preventing hematoma formation and severe edema that may result in poor wound healing. Dressings should be changed early and the wound inspected for hematoma or signs of infection. Hematoma evacuation, appropriate drainage, and antibiotic therapy based on culture and sensitivity studies may be required. Removal of sutures in 3–5 days, followed by splinting of the incision with sterile tape, will minimize scarring from the sutures themselves.

The final result of facial wound repair depends on the nature and location of the wounds, individual propensity to scar formation, and the passage of time. A year or more must often pass before resolution of scar contracture and erythema results in maximum improvement. Only after this time can a decision be made regarding the desirability of secondary scar revision.

In wounds involving the major joints the extracapsular soft tissue and the intracapsular structures should be considered individually to assess accurately the magnitude of the injury and to provide a prognosis. Open joint injuries that are single penetrating and without extensive soft tissue damage, permit uncomplicated joint and wound closure. Injuries that are single or multiple penetrations with extensive soft-tissue disruption (flaps, avulsions, degloving) often require secondary operations to attain closure. In injuries which show open periarticular fractures with extension through the adjacent intra-articular surface and with associated nerve or vascular injury requiring repair, the cornerstone for successful management is debridement, antibiotic therapy properly timed and performed, joint closure and aggressive treatment of the bony injury. Newer techniques such as free tissue transfer can expedite wound care, decrease morbidity and spare some limbs from amputation.

Collins DN, Temple SD: Open joint injuries: Classification and treatment. Clin Orthop 1989;No. 243:48.

FACIAL BONE FRACTURES

Because of the aesthetic and functional importance of the face, fractures of the facial bones—though rarely life-threatening—are best treated by surgeons who have extensive experience with facial injuries and reconstruction. Operation is most successful when performed in the acute setting, usually within the first week, because reconstruction becomes much more difficult if surgery is delayed.

Facial bone fractures are usually caused by trauma from a blunt instrument, such as a fist or club, or by violent contact with the steering wheel, dash-board, or windshield during an automobile accident. Particularly in the latter case, the patient should be assessed for associated injuries. For example, cervical spine injuries are present in up to 12% of automobile accident patients and should be treated before facial bone injuries. Injuries to the brain, eyes, chest, abdomen, and extremities must also be assessed and may require early treatment.

The diagnosis of facial fractures is made primarily on clinical examination. Ideally, the examination should be done immediately, so that swelling will not obscure the findings. The mechanism and the line of direction of injury are important. If conscious, the patient should be asked about previous facial injuries, areas of pain and numbness, whether the jaw opens properly and the teeth come together normally, and whether vision in all quadrants is normal.

Most facial fractures can be palpated, or at least the abnormal position of bones can be noted. Beginning along the mandibular rims, feel for irregularities of the facial bones. The dental occlusion is noted. With bimanual palpation, placing the thumbs inside the mouth, one can elicit bony crepitus if there is an associated fracture. The maxilla and mid face can be rocked forward and backward between the thumb and the index finger in the presence of a midfacial fracture. Nasal fractures may be detected by palpation. Irregularities and step-offs along the infraorbital border, lateral orbital rim, or zygomatic arch regions indicate a depressed zygomatic fracture.

Radiologic studies are only an adjunct to the diagnosis of facial fractures. Rarely is a significant fracture seen on x-ray that is not also clinically evident. Helpful views include the Waters and submento-vertex projections and oblique views of the mandible. If available, the panorex view of the mandible is very useful. CT scans of facial bones, with appropriate biplanar and three-dimensional reconstructions so that bones can be viewed through several planes, are helpful in assessing the extent of fractures in posterior areas such as the ethmoid area, posterior and inferior orbit, pterygoid plates, and base of the skull.

The bones of the nose are the most commonly fractured facial bones. Next in frequency are the mandible, the zygomatic malar bones, and the maxilla.

NASAL FRACTURES

Fractures may affect the nasal bones, cartilage, and septum. Fractures occur in two patterns, caused by lateral or head-on trauma.

With lateral trauma, the nasal bone on the side of the injury is fractured and displaced toward the septum; the septum is deviated and fractured; and the nasal bone on the side away from the injury is fractured and displaced away from the septum, so that the upper part of the nose, as a whole, is deviated. Depending upon the degree of violence, one or more of these displacements will be present, and the degree of comminution is variable.

Head-on trauma gives rise to telescoping and saddling of the nose and broadening of its upper half as a result of the depression and splaying of the fractured nasal bones. This of course produces severe damage to the septum, which usually buckles or actually suffers a fracture. The diagnosis of a fractured nose is made on clinical grounds alone, and x-rays are unnecessary.

Nasal fractures requiring reduction should be treated with a minimum of delay, for they tend to become fixed in the displaced position in a few days. The surgical approach depends on whether the fracture has resulted in deviation or collapse of the nasal

bones. Local anesthesia is preferred; either topical tetracaine or cocaine intranasally or lidocaine for infiltration of the skin can be used. The nasal bones may be disimpacted with intranasal forceps or a periosteal elevator and aligned by external molding or pressure. Collapsed nasal fractures can be repositioned with Walsham's nasal forceps, introduced into each nostril and placed on each side of the septum, which is then elevated to its proper position. A septal hematoma should be recognized and drained to prevent infection and subsequent necrosis of the cartilaginous septum with associated collapse of the entire nose. Compound fractures of the nose require prompt repair of the skin wound and, if possible, early reduction of the displaced nasal bones.

External splinting, which is essentially a protective dressing, and intranasal packing using nonadhering gauze are appropriate after reduction. The intranasal packing provides support for the septum in its reduced position and helps prevent development of a hematoma. It also provides counter pressure for the external splint immobilizing the nasal bones and prevents them from collapsing. The packing is usually removed within 48 hours.

In severe comminuted nasal fractures, the medial canthal ligaments, which are easily felt by applying lateral traction to the upper eyelid, may have dislodged. If they have been avulsed, they should be reattached in position to prevent late deformities. For these severe fractures involving the entire naso-orbital and ethmoid complex, the coronal approach, which offers wide exposure, allows for proper anatomic reduction of all small nasal fragments as well as repositioning of the canthal ligaments with transnasal wire and correction and elevation of the telescoped bone fragments at the root of the nose and glabella.

The lacrimal apparatus is commonly disrupted in these injuries and should be repaired and stented appropriately.

MANDIBULAR FRACTURES

Mandibular fractures are most commonly bilateral, generally occurring in the region of the mid body at the mental foramen, the angle of the ramus, or at the neck of the condyle. A frequent combination is a fracture at the mental region of the body with a condylar fracture on the opposite side. Displacement of the fragments results from the force of the external blow as well as the pull of the muscles of the floor of the mouth and the muscles of mastication. The diagnosis is suggested by derangement of dental occlusion associated with local pain, swelling, and often crepitation upon palpation. Appropriate x-rays confirm the diagnosis. Special views of the condyle, including tomograms, may be required. Sublingual hematoma and acute malocclusion are usually diagnostic of a mandibular fracture.

Restoration of functional dental occlusion is the most important consideration in treating mandibular fractures. In patients with an adequate complement of teeth, arch bars or interdental wires can be placed. Local nerve block anesthesia is preferable for this procedure, though certain patients may require general anesthesia. Intermaxillary elastic traction will usually correct minor degrees of displacement and bring the teeth into normal occlusion by overcoming the muscle pull. When the fracture involves the base of a tooth socket with suspected devitalization of the tooth, extraction of the tooth should be considered. Particularly in the incisor region, such devitalized teeth may be a source of infection, leading to the development of osteomyelitis and nonunion of the fracture.

Patients with more severe mandibular injuries require anatomic reduction and fixation of the fracture by the open, direct technique. These include compound, comminuted, and unfavorable fractures. An unfavorable fracture is one that is inherently unstable because muscle pull distracts the fracture segments. In this situation, intermaxillary fixation alone is insufficient. Edentulous patients also benefit from the open technique, although proper dentures or dental splints are useful to maintain normal occlusion.

Metal wire fixation of fractured segments and intermaxillary fixation for 6 weeks is a proved and popular method of fracture treatment. The recent resurgence in popularity of the screw-plate system is due to a number of advantages over wiring. The screw plate usually achieves rigid fixation in three dimensions, providing adequate stability; it eliminates the need for intermaxillary fixation in most cases; it is useful in complex, comminuted fractures; and it is quite easy to use after familiarity with the technique has been acquired.

With bilateral parasymphysial fractures, anterior stabilization of the tongue may be lost, so that it may fall back and obstruct the airway. Anterior stabilization and splinting must be accomplished early in these cases.

Open reduction is rarely advised in condylar fractures; simple intermaxillary fixation for 4–6 weeks is sufficient. Indications for open reduction are severely displaced fractures, which may prevent motion of the mandible because of impingement of the coronoid process on the zygomatic arch. In children, the fracture may destroy the growth center of the condyle, resulting in maldevelopment of the mandible and gross distortion.

ZYGOMATIC & ORBITAL FRACTURE

Fractures of the zygomatic bones may involve just the arch of the zygomatic bone or the entire body of the zygoma (the malar eminence) and the lateral wall and floor of the orbit. The so-called tripod fracture characteristically occurs at the frontozygomatic and zygomaticomaxillary sutures as well as at the arch. Displacement of the body of the zygoma results in flattening of the cheek and depression of the orbital rim and floor.

Important diagnostic signs are subconjunctival hemorrhage, disturbances of extraocular muscle function (which may be accompanied by diplopia), and loss of sensation in the upper lip and alveoli on the involved side as a result of injury to the infraorbital nerve. Reduction of a displaced zygomatic fracture is seldom an emergency procedure and may be delayed until the patient's general condition is satisfactory for anesthesia. Local anesthesia will suffice only for reduction of fractures of the zygomatic arch. More extensively displaced fractures usually require general anesthesia. At least two-point fixation with direct interosseous wiring is necessary for these fractures. Here again, delicate mini-plates have been used with success, providing anatomic reduction and rigid fixation.

Depressed fractures of the zygomatic arch can best be elevated using the Gillies technique. Through a temporal incision above the hairline, an instrument is passed beneath the superficial layer of the temporalis fascia and under the arch and the body of the zygoma. The fracture can also be elevated percutaneously with a hook in conjunction with overlying palpation to achieve accurate reduction.

Extensive disruption should be suspected in conjunction with the zygomatic fracture when significant diplopia and enophthalmos and posterior displacement of the globe are present. Orbital fat and extraocular muscles may herniate through the defect and become entrapped, giving rise to the signs and symptoms. A "blowout" fracture is similar disruption of the orbital floor due to blunt trauma to the globe but not associated with a fracture of the zygoma or orbital rim. Treatment in both cases demands exploration, reduction of herniated contents, and repair of the floor. The most direct approach is through a lower lid subciliary incision, which provides excellent visualization. A buccal transantral (Caldwell-Luc) approach can be used, and blind antral packing for support has been described. This is quite hazardous, because bony spicules may be pushed into the ocular globe and perhaps cause injury or blindness. In cases where there is extensive communication or loss of bony fragments of the floor, use of local autogenous bone or cartilage as a scaffold is ideal. A thin sheet of alloplastic material such as Silastic has also been satisfactory.

Even with careful anatomic reduction and repair of

the orbital floor, ocular problems—particularly enophthalmos—may persist. This may be due to an undiagnosed fracture, especially a medial ethmoidal blowout fracture. These can be properly evaluated with CT scanning. Treatment requires reduction and repair of the defect. The injury can at times cause ischemia of herniated soft tissue and subsequent atrophy and scarring. This may result in enophthalmos, which is almost impossible to resolve completely.

MAXILLARY FRACTURES

Maxillary fractures range in complexity from partial fractures through the alveolar process to extensive displacement of the midfacial structures in conjunction with fractures of the frontonasal bones and orbital maxillary region and total craniofacial separation. Hemorrhage and airway obstruction require emergency care, and in severe cases, trachcostomy is indicated. Mobility of the maxilla can be elicited by palpation in extensive fractures. "Dish-face" deformity of the retrodisplaced maxilla may be disguised by edema, and careful x-ray studies are necessary to determine the extent and complexity of the midfacial fracture. Treatment may have to be delayed because of other severe injuries. A delay of as long as 10–14 days may be safe before reduction and fixation, but the earliest possible restoration of maxillary position and dental occlusion is desirable to prevent late complications.

In the case of unilateral fractures or bilateral fractures with little or no displacement, splinting by intermaxillary fixation for 4 weeks may suffice. Fractures are usually displaced inferiorly or posteriorly and require direct surgical disimpaction and reduction. Early reduction may help control bleeding, as torn, stretched vessels are allowed to reestablish their normal tension. In certain severe cases, external traction may be necessary. Manipulation is directed toward restoring normal occlusion and maintaining the reduction with intermaxillary fixation to the mandible in association with direct fixation or supporting wires from other intact facial or cranial bones. Complicated fractures may require external fixation utilizing a head cap and intraoral splints in conjunction with multiple surgical incisions for direct wire fixation. Coexisting mandibular fractures usually necessitate open reduction and fixation at the same time.

Antonyshyn O, Gruss JS: Complex orbital trauma: The role of rigid fixation and primary bone grafting. Plast Reconstr Surg 1988;7:61.

Salyer KE.: *Teachings in Aesthetic Craniofacial Surgery.* Gower, 1989.

Thaller SR, Kawamoto HK: A histologic evaluation of fracture repair in the midface. Plast Reconstr Surg 1990; 85:196.

Thaller SR, Mabourakh S: Pediatric mandibular fractures. Ann Plast Surg 1991;26:511.

Yaremchuk MJ: Vascularized bone grafts for maxillofacial reconstruction. Clin Plast Surg 1989;16:29.

CONGENITAL HEAD & NECK ANOMALIES

CLEFT LIP & CLEFT PALATE

Cleft lip, cleft palate, and combinations of the two are the most common congenital anomalies of the head and neck. The incidence of facial clefts has been reported to be 1 in every 650–750 live births, making this deformity second only to clubfoot in frequency as a reported birth defect.

The cleft may involve the floor of the nostril and lip on one or both sides and may extend through the alveolus, the hard palate, and the entire soft palate. A useful classification based on embryologic and anatomic aspects divides the structures into the primary and the secondary palate. The dividing point between the primary palate anteriorly and the secondary palate posteriorly is the incisive foramen. Clefts can thus be classified as partial or complete clefts of the primary or secondary palate (or both) in various combinations. The most common clefts are left unilateral complete clefts of the primary and secondary palate and partial midline clefts of the secondary palate, involving the soft palate and part of the hard palate.

Most infants with cleft palate present some feeding difficulties, and breast feeding may be impossible. As a rule, enlarging the openings in an artificial nipple or using a syringe with a soft rubber feeding tube will solve difficulties in sucking. Feeding in the upright position helps prevent oronasal reflux or aspiration. Severe feeding and breathing problems and recurrent aspiration are seen in Pierre Robin syndrome, in which the palatal cleft is associated with a receding lower jaw and posterior displacement of the tongue, obstructing the oropharyngeal airway. This is a medical emergency and is a cause of sudden infant death syndrome (SIDS). Nonsurgical treatment includes pulling the tongue forward with an instrument and laying the baby prone with a towel under the chest to let the mandible and tongue drop forward. Insertion of a small (No. 8) nasogastric tube into the pharynx may temporarily prevent respiratory distress and may be used to supplement the baby's feedings. Several surgical procedures that bring the tongue and mandible forward have been described but should be employed only when conservative measures have been tried without success.

Treatment

Surgical repair of cleft lip is not considered an emergency. The optimal time for operation can be described as the widely accepted "rule of ten." This includes body weight of 10 lb (4.5 kg) or more and a hemoglobin of 10 g/dL or more. This is usually at some time after the 10th week of life. In most cases, closure of the lip will mold distortions of the cleft alveolus into a satisfactory contour. In occasional cases where there is marked distortion of the alveolus, such as in severe bilateral clefts with marked protrusion of the premaxilla, preliminary maxillary orthodontic treatment may be indicated. This may involve the use of carefully crafted appliances or simple constant pressure by use of an elastic band.

General endotracheal anesthesia via an orally placed endotracheal tube is the anesthetic technique of choice. A variety of techniques for repair of unilateral clefts have evolved over many years. Earlier procedures ignored anatomic landmarks and resulted in a characteristic "repaired harelip" look. The Millard rotation advancement operation that is now commonly used for repair employs an incision in the medial side of the cleft to allow the cupid's bow of the lip to be rotated down to a normal position. The resulting gap in the medial side of the cleft is filled by advancing a flap from the lateral side. This principle can be varied in placement of the incisions and results in most cases in a symmetric lip with normally placed landmarks. Bilateral clefts, because of greater deficiency of tissue, present more challenging technical problems. Maximum preservation of available tissue is the underlying principle, and most surgeons prefer approximation of the central and lateral lip elements in a straight line closure, rolling up the vermilion border of the lip (Manchester repair).

Secondary revisions are frequently necessary in the older child with a repaired cleft lip. A constant associated deformity in patients with cleft lip is distortion of the soft tissue and cartilage structures of the ala and dome of the nose. These patients often present with deficiency of growth of the structures of the mid face. This has been attributed to intrinsic growth disturbances and to external pressures from the lip and palate repairs. Some correction of these deformities, especially of the nose, can be done at the initial lip operation. More definitive correction is done after the cartilage and bone growth is more complete. These may include scar revisions and rearrangement of the cartilage structure of the nose. Recent approaches involve degloving of the nasal skin envelope with complete exposure of the abnormal cartilage framework. These are then rearranged in proper position with or without additional grafts. Maxillary osteotomies (Le Fort I with advancement) will substantially correct the midfacial depression. A tight upper lip due to severe tissue deficiency can be corrected by a two-stage transfer of a lower lip flap known as an Abbe flap.

Palatal clefts may involve the alveolus, the bony hard palate, or the soft palate, singly or in any combination. Clefts of the hard palate and alveolus may be either unilateral or bilateral, whereas the soft palate cleft is always midline, extending back through the uvula. The width of the cleft varies greatly, making the amount of tissue available for repair also variable. The bony palate, with its mucoperiosteal lining, forms the roof of the anterior mouth and the floor of the nose. The posteriorly attached soft palate is composed of five paired muscles of speech and swallowing.

Surgical closure of the cleft to allow for normal speech is the treatment of choice. The timetable for closure depends on the size of the cleft and any other associated problems. However, the defect should be closed before the child undertakes serious speech, usually before age 2. Closure at 6 months usually is performed without difficulty and also aids in the child's feeding. If the soft palate seems to be long enough, simple approximation of the freshened edges of the cleft after freeing of the tissues through lateral relaxing incisions may suffice. If the soft palate is too short, a pushback type of operation is required. In this procedure, the short soft palate is retrodisplaced closer to the posterior pharyngeal wall utilizing the mucoperiosteal flaps based on the posterior palatine artery.

Satisfactory speech following surgical repair of cleft palate is achieved in 70–90% of cases. Significant speech defects usually require secondary operations when the child is older. The most widely used technique is the pharyngeal flap operation, in which the palatopharyngeal space is reduced by attaching a flap of posterior pharyngeal muscle and mucosa to the soft palate. This permits voluntary closure of the velopharyngeal complex and thus avoids hypernasal speech. Various other kinds of pharyngoplasties have been useful in selected cases.

CRANIOFACIAL ANOMALIES

These are congenital deformities of the hard and soft tissues of the head. Particular problems of the brain, eye, and internal ear are treated by the appropriate specialist. The craniofacial surgeon often needs the collaboration of these specialists when operating on such patients.

Serious craniofacial anomalies are relatively rare, although mild forms often go undiagnosed or accepted as normal variants. A classification is therefore difficult, although many have been proposed. Tessier has offered a numerical classification based on clinical presentation. He considers a cleft to be the basis of the malformation, which involves both hard and soft tissues. Other classifications are based on embryologic and etiologic features. With greater understanding and continued investigation, classification efforts will no doubt be more satisfactory.

There are well-known chromosomal and genetic aberrations as well as environmental causes that can lead to craniofacial deformity. The cause in most cases, however, is unknown. Arrest in the migration and proliferation of neural crest cells and defects in differentiation characterize most of these deformities. We will describe some of the more common ones in brief terms.

Crouzon's syndrome (craniofacial dysostosis) and **Apert's syndrome** (acrocephalosyndactyly) are closely related, differing in the extremity deformities present in the latter. Both are autosomal dominant traits with variable expression. Both present with skull deformities due to premature closure of the cranial sutures. The cranial sutures most affected will determine the type of skull deformity. Exophthalmos, midfacial hypoplasia, and hypertelorism are also features of these two syndromes.

The facial organs and tissues proceed in great measure from the first and second branchial arches and the first branchial cleft. Disorders in their development lead to a spectrum of anomalies of variable severity. **Treacher-Collins syndrome** (mandibulofacial dysostosis) is a severe disorder characterized by hypoplasia of the malar bones and lower eyelids, colobomas, and antimongoloid slant of the palpebrae. The mandible and ears are often quite underdeveloped. The presentation is bilateral and is an autosomal dominant trait. A unilateral deformity known as **hemifacial microsomia** presents with progressive skeletal and soft tissue underdevelopment. The Goldenhar variant of hemifacial microsomia is a severe form associated with upper bulbar dermoids, notching of the upper eyelids, and vertebral anomalies.

Some of these patients show mental retardation, but in most cases intelligence is not affected. The psychosocial problems are serious and most often related to how the patients look. Within the past 2 decades, craniofacial surgery has progressed so that previously untreatable deformities can now be corrected. With the anatomic work of Le Fort as a basis—and guided by the incomplete attempts of Gillies and others—Paul Tessier, in the late 1960s, proposed a set of surgical techniques to correct major craniofacial deformities. Two basic concepts soon emerged from his work: (1) Large segments of the craniofacial skeleton can be completely denuded of their blood supply, repositioned, and yet survive and heal; and (2) the eyes can be translocated horizontally or vertically over a considerable distance with no adverse effect on vision. The tendency today is to operate at approximately 6–9 months of age (not later than 9 months) for cranial vault remodeling and fronto-orbital advancement.

A bicoronal scalp incision is utilized to expose the skull and facial bones with an intra- or extracranial approach. The cut bones are then reshaped, repositioned, and fixed with a combination of wires or miniplates and screws. The latter have the advantage of rigid fixation and less need to maintain large movements with bone grafts. Autogenous inlay and onlay bone grafts can be used to improve contour. The entire operation is usually completed in one stage, and complications are surprisingly few. Miniplates have been used extensively in the last few years. In infants, fixation with absorbable suture material such as Maxon can replace the usual steel wires and avoid any radiologic tracks.

Craniofacial surgery has improved the treatment not only of major congenital deformities but also of major complex facial fractures, chronic sequelae of trauma, isolated exophthalmos, fibrous dysplasia, and aesthetic facial sculpturing.

MICROTIA

Microtia is absence or hypoplasia of the pinna of the ear, with a blind or absent external auditory meatus.

The incidence of significant auricular deformity is about one in 8000 births and is usually spontaneous. Ten percent of these defects are bilateral, and boys are afflicted twice or three times as commonly as girls. Because the ear arises from the first and second branchial arches, the middle ear is always involved, and many patients have other disorders of the first and second arches. The inner ear structures are usually spared.

Generally, correction of conductive hearing by an otologist has not been long-lasting or helpful, and surgery for this problem is reserved for bilateral cases.

Reconstruction of the external ear usually involves a multistage procedure beginning at preschool age. Autogenous rib cartilage or cartilage from the opposite ear is used to construct a framework to replace the absent ear. The cartilage is imbedded under the skin in the appropriate area, and after adjustments are made in local tissue to reposition or recreate the earlobe and conchal cavity, the framework is elevated posteriorly and the resulting sulcus grafted to obtain projection. In cases where local tissue is poor or unavailable, the neighboring superficial temporalis fascia is dissected and placed over the cartilage framework. This is then skin-grafted with adequate tissue. The opposite (normal) ear is occasionally altered to provide better symmetry. Excellent results have been achieved. Silastic frameworks for ear cartilage have also been used, and although their use eliminates donor site problems, rates of infection and extrusion have been unacceptable.

Lesser deformities, such as overly large, prominent, or bent ears, are corrected by appropriate resection of skin and cartilage, "scoring" of the cartilage to alter its curve, and placement sutures to aid in contouring.

Bardach J, Salyer KE: *Surgical Techniques in Cleft Lip and Palate.* Year Book, 1987.

Marchac D, Renier D: New aspects of craniofacial surgery. World J Surg 1990;14:725.

McCarthy JG: The timing of surgical intervention in craniofacial anomalies. Clin Plast Surg 1990;17:161.

Salyer KE: *Teachings in Aesthetic Craniofacial Surgery.* Gowen Medical, 1989.

ANOMALIES OF THE HANDS & EXTREMITIES

The most common hand anomaly is syndactyly, or webbing of the digits. This may be simple, involving only soft tissue, or complex, involving fusion of bone and soft tissue. The fusion may be partial or complete. Surgical correction involves separation and repair with local flaps and skin grafts. Correction should be done before growth disturbance of the webbed digits takes place. Other anomalies such as extra digits (polydactyly), absence of digits (adactyly), or cleft hand (claw hand) may occur.

Flexion contractures of the hands or digits may require surgical release and appropriate skin grafting. Congenital ring constriction of the extremities may be associated also with congenital amputation. The ring constrictions are best treated by excision and Z-plasty.

Poland's syndrome consists of a variable degree of unilateral chest deformity—usually absence of the pectoralis major muscle—associated with hand brachysyndactyly. The hand deformity is treated according to the severity. The latissimus dorsi muscles can be transposed to replace the absent pectoralis major, simulating the sites of origin and insertion. In more severe cases and in women requiring breast and chest reconstruction, the transverse rectus abdominis island flap can be used to replace the deficit.

POSTABLATIVE RECONSTRUCTION

HEAD & NECK RECONSTRUCTION

Many of the tumors discussed in Chapter 15 require surgical excision as a primary form of therapy. This often involves removal of large areas of composite tissue, such as the floor of the mouth, the maxilla, part of the mandible, or the lymph-bearing tissue of the neck. Reconstruction after such resections can be very challenging and may require special skill.

As discussed previously, the use of musculocutaneous flaps and free flaps is very advantageous for coverage of extensive postablative defects, especially in the head and neck region. One- or two-stage procedures can be used.

Since no two surgical resections for tumor in the head and neck are identical, the key to effective treatment is preoperative planning. Probable extent of resection, areas that will require pre- or postoperative radiation therapy, incision and flaps created by neck dissections, and available donor areas must all be carefully assessed. Tissue attached to an adequate blood supply must be used to ensure early and watertight healing in the mouth and oropharynx, in areas of radiation injury, and over metal or other alloplastic implants.

Useful musculocutaneous flaps in the head and neck are the sternocleidomastoid, platysma, trapezius, pectoralis major, and latissimus dorsi muscles. Useful axial skin flaps can be obtained from the forehead, deltopectoral, and cervicohumeral areas. When these flaps are insufficient or unavailable for the reconstructive needs of the patient, free tissue transfer must be used. Many flaps with acceptable donor sites exist. The deep circumflex iliac vessels provide an osteocutaneous flap quite useful in mandible reconstruction. The forearm and scapular areas are also good sites for composite free flaps. Healing is quick, so that radiation, if necessary, may be started as early as one month after surgery.

Pearl RM et al: An approach to mandibular reconstruction. Ann Plast Surg 1988;21:401.

Stark RB: *Plastic Surgery of the Head and Neck.* Churchill Livingstone, 1987.

BREAST RECONSTRUCTION

Reconstruction of the female breast after mastectomy is becoming common in the USA as new techniques have become available and more women have become aware of this option. Most insurance carriers now pay for this procedure as part of the treatment for breast cancer. Even women with significant defects in the anterior chest wall as a result of radical mastectomy and radiation therapy can undergo reconstructive surgery if they are otherwise appropriate candidates.

Generally, women with stage I or II breast cancer and no evidence of active disease following mastectomy are considered for breast reconstruction. Although consultation with a plastic surgeon prior to mastectomy may be helpful and is advised, the decision regarding the type of mastectomy and postoperative adjunctive therapy is left up to the patient and her cancer surgeon. There is no evidence that reconstructive surgery in the breast area alters the course of disease or masks local recurrence.

A few centers perform immediate breast reconstruction at the time of mastectomy, but usually reconstruction is delayed. Immediate breast reconstruction does not interfere with adjunctive therapy.

When the pectoralis major muscle is intact and skin cover is adequate, a simple silicone gel bag implant beneath the pectoralis and serratus anterior muscles may be all that is required. When the pectoralis major and minor muscles have been removed and the overlying skin is very tight, scarred, or injured by radiation therapy, new skin and muscle must be brought in to cover an implant. The technique of using a latissimus dorsi musculocutaneous flap for this purpose has become highly refined and has produced reliable results. Based on its thoracodorsal pedicle, the origin of this muscle is detached and, along with a skin island, is swung on its insertion out onto the anterior chest wall, where it provides an anterior axillary fold and adequate coverage for an implant. The skin island is positioned within the reopened mastectomy incision or below it as indicated for contouring. Although the donor area scar can be significant, donor area morbidity is minimal. Other flaps used for this purpose are usually axial skin flaps, such as thoracoepigastric or musculocutaneous flaps based on the rectus abdominis muscle.

A transverse rectus abdominal flap based on the superior epigastric vessels coursing through the rectus abdominis muscle has been successfully used to provide adequate tissue so that an implant is not required. The incision at the donor site is similar to that of an abdominoplasty operation along the lower abdomen. This operation produces the most normal and natural breast in appearance and feel.

As mastectomy has become more limited by preservation of the innervated pectoralis major muscle, the only deficit appears to be skin. More recently, skin expanders have been introduced for breast reconstruction. A silicone bag with a separate valve is inserted under the chest skin and muscle. At intervals over about a 6-week period, the bag is progressively inflated through the valve and percutaneously until the chest skin and muscle are expanded to at least 25% more than the desired volume. The expander is then replaced by a permanent implant. The attractiveness of the procedure is readily apparent, and in some cases a skin expander is being inserted at the time of mastectomy. The disadvantages include the hemispheric expansion of the skin, which may result in a hard, rounded breast mound; the necessity for a second operation; and problems with infection, deflation, exposure of the prosthesis, and occasional skin necrosis when expansion is too rapid. Fortunately, these latter problems can be reduced to a minimum.

In some patients, the opposite (noncancerous) breast may be altered to better match the reconstructed breast. A breast that is hypertrophic may be reduced and a ptotic breast elevated.

The nipple-areola complex can also be reconstructed. This is generally done after breast reconstruction and any contralateral breast surgery is well healed, so that reliable and symmetric positioning of the nipple and areola can be achieved. The current technique is use of a full-thickness skin graft from the upper inner thigh near the groin crease for reconstruction of the areola and either borrowed skin from the opposite nipple or small local skin flaps for reconstruction of the nipple.

Prophylactic subcutaneous mastectomy or simple mastectomy is performed in some patients. Indications for the procedure are controversial and include high risk of cancer in the opposite breast, strong family history of breast cancer (particularly a mother or sister with premenopausal bilateral breast cancer). Other possible indications include intractable mastodynia, cancerophobia, and breasts that cannot be adequately evaluated because of severe fibrocystic disease. The risk of developing breast cancer after prophylactic mastectomy is reduced but not totally eliminated, since all breast tissue is not removed.

It should be stressed that prophylactic mastectomy and reconstruction is not a cosmetic procedure. Scarring, poor contour, and insensible areas may result, and implant problems are significant.

Adequate skin and muscle are readily available following this type of mastectomy. Incisions can be kept to a minimum and placed so they are well hidden around the areola or in the inframammary fold. The silicone implant is generally placed beneath the pectoralis and serratus anterior muscles to help avoid or minimize scar contracture.

Bostwick J III: Breast reconstruction after mastectomy. Semin Surg Oncol 1988;4:274

Hartrampf CR Jr: The transverse abdominal island flap for breast reconstruction: A 7-year experience. Clin Plast Surg 1988;15:703.

Lejour M, Jabri M, Deraemaecker R: Analysis of long-term results of 326 breast reconstructions. Clin Plast Surg 1988;15:689.

Vasconez LO, Lejour M, Gamboa-Bobadilla M: *Atlas of Breast Reconstruction.* Gower, 1991.

LOWER EXTREMITY RECONSTRUCTION

Probably the most difficult area for which to provide wound coverage and closure is the lower extremity, particularly the distal leg and foot areas. Tenuous and unstable skin grafts or poorly vascularized local or cross-leg skin flaps were once the only tissues available for resurfacing of these parts of the body. When large segments of bone were exposed or missing or when infection had become established, these grafts or flaps often were inadequate and amputation was the only recourse. Use of musculocutaneous flaps and particularly free flaps has greatly improved coverage in the lower extremities.

Generally, wound problems in the lower leg, ankle, and foot involve orthopedic injuries, such as compound ankle or distal tibial fractures. Incisions and metal screws and plates associated with open reduction and fixation of fractures may lead to increased scarring and make coverage more difficult. Other injuries requiring reconstruction are avulsion loss of the skin of the leg, heel, or sole of the foot and ischemic or venous stasis skin loss.

Treatment depends on the extent of tissue loss and the depth of the wound. Fairly extensive wounds around the knee and upper third of the leg can be covered with a (usually medial) gastrocnemius muscle flap and a split-thickness skin graft. The middle third of the leg can be covered in a similar manner by the soleus muscle in many cases. Large middle third and distal third defects are more difficult to reconstruct. Although there are small muscles that end in tendons in the foot, such as the peroneus brevis, flexor hallucis longus, and extensor digitorum muscles, they can provide only limited coverage. If there is a suitable recipient artery remaining in the leg, better coverage is generally provided by a free muscle flap such as the gracilis muscle for small and medium-sized defects or the latissimus dorsi muscle for larger defects.

Large areas of the heel or the sole of the foot are difficult to replace because skin in these regions is specially constructed to bear the weight of the body without shearing or breaking down. Free muscle flaps surfaced with skin graft can be used, but protective sensation is missing. The use of free neurovascular axial skin flaps, such as the inferior gluteal thigh flap and the deltoid flap, may help provide coverage with some sensation.

Small segments of missing tibia can be replaced by soft tissue coverage followed by bone grafting. Free microvascular fibula or iliac crest transplants have been used to replace larger segments of missing bone.

Osteomyelitis of the tibia or bones in the foot may be devastating and often uncontrollable. Probably because of poor vascularity in the area, even long-term antibiotic treatment has often failed to control bone infections in the leg. Recently, effective surgical treatment for bone infections has been developed. The bone is surgically debrided and replaced with a microvascular free muscle flap such as the gracilis muscle. Apparently, the muscle tissue with its excellent blood supply not only covers the exposed bone but assists natural defenses in controlling infection. Antibiotics are also used, but the well-vascularized muscle flap appears to be the deciding factor in control of infection. Bone grafts can be added later if needed.

Cronewett JL et al: Limb salvage despite extensive tissue loss: Free tissue transfer combined with distal revascularization. Arch Surg 1989;124:609.

Koshima I, Fukuda H, Soeda S: Free combined anterolateral thigh flap and vascularized iliac bone graft with double vascular pedicle. J Reconstr Microsurg 1989;5:55.

Meland NB et al: Experience with 80 rectus abdominis free-tissue transfers. Plast Reconstr Surg 1989;83:481.

Stevenson TR: Lower extremity reconstruction. West J Med 1991;154:205.

Yousif NJ, Ye Z: Analysis of cutaneous perfusion: An aid to lower extremity reconstruction. Clin Plast Surg 1991; 18(3):559.

PRESSURE SORES

Pressure sores—often less precisely called bedsores or decubitus ulcers—are another example of difficult wound problems that can be treated by plastic surgery. Pressure sores generally occur in patients who are bedridden and unable or unwilling to change position; patients who cannot change position because of a cast or appliance; and patients who have no sensation in an area that is not moved even though they may be ambulatory. The underlying cause of sores in these patients is ischemic necrosis resulting from prolonged pressure against tissue overlying bone, particularly bony prominences. There is also some evidence that local factors in denervated skin predispose to pressure breakdown.

Absence of normal protective reflexes must be compensated for. Prevention is clearly the best treatment for pressure sores. Casts and appliances must be well padded, and points of pressure or pain should be relieved. Bedridden patients must be turned to a new position at least every two hours. Water and air mattresses, sheepskin pads, and foam cushions may help relieve pressure but are not substitutes for frequent turning. The introduction of the flotation bed system (Clinitron) has greatly aided in the management of these patients. The pressure on the skin at any time is less than the capillary filling pressure, avoiding many ischemic problems. Paraplegics should not sit in one position for more than two hours. Careful daily examination should be made for erythema, the earliest sign of ischemic injury. Erythematous areas should be freed from all pressure. The use of electrical stimulations, biomaterials, and growth factors or additional modalities to expedite wound repair may soon become available.

Once pressure necrosis is established, it is important to determine whether underlying tissues such as fat and muscle are affected, since they are much more likely than skin to become necrotic. A small skin ulcer may be the manifestation of a much larger area of destruction below. If the area is not too extensive and if infection and abscess due to external or hematogenous bacteria are not present, necrotic tissue may be replaced by scar tissue. Continued pressure will not only prevent scar tissue from forming but will also extend the injury. A surface eschar or skin may cover a significant abscess.

If the pressure sore is small and noninfected, application of drying agents to the wound and removal of all pressure to the area may permit slow healing. Wounds extending down to bone rarely heal without surgery. Infected wounds must be debrided down to clean tissue. The objectives at operation are to debride devitalized tissue, including bone, and to provide healthy, well-vascularized padded tissue as a covering. All of the original tissue that formed the bed of the ulcer must be excised.

When the patient's nutritional status and general condition of health are optimal, definitive coverage can be performed. Coverage is usually accomplished with a muscle, musculocutaneous, or, sometimes, an axial or random pattern flap. Well-vascularized muscle appears to help control established low-grade bacterial contamination. The muscle flaps used for the more common bedsores are as follows: greater trochanter—tensor fasciae latae; ischium—gracilis, gluteus maximus, or hamstrings; sacrum—gluteus maximus. Occasionally, it is possible to provide sensibility to the area of a pressure sore with an innervated flap from above the level of paraplegia. The most common example is the tensor fasciae latae flap with the contained lateral femoral cutaneous nerve from L4 and L5, which is used to cover an ischial sore. Rarely, an innervated intercostal flap from the abdominal wall may be used to cover an insensible sacrum. The tissue expansion techniques should not be the primary surgery treatment of decubitus ulcers but can be used in difficult cases where available tissue is insufficient to close the wound.

Postoperatively, the donor and recipient areas must be kept free of pressure for 2–3 weeks to allow for complete healing. This puts significant demands on other areas of the body that may be equally at risk or may already have areas of breakdown. The use of the air-fluidized (Clinitron) bed has greatly aided such situations.

In spite of excellent padding provided by musculocutaneous flaps, recurrence of pressure sores is still a major problem, because the situation that caused the original breakdown usually still exists. Prevention of sores is even more important for these patients.

Braddom RL, Leadbetter MG: The use of a tissue expander to enlarge a graft for surgical treatment of a pressure ulcer in a quadriplegic: Case report. Am J Phys Med Rehabil 1989;68:70.

Bruck JC et al: More arguments in favor of myocutaneous flaps for the treatment of pelvic pressure sores. Ann Plast Surg 1991;25:85.

Moss RJ, La-Puma J: The ethics of pressure sore prevention and treatment in the elderly: A practical approach. J Am Geriatr Soc 1991;39:905.

AESTHETIC SURGERY

Surgery for aesthetic reconstruction has received publicity out of proportion to its importance amongst the various types of plastic surgery. This is probably because of its psychologic effects on the patient and its cost. In addition, some less well trained and even unscrupulous surgeons have given aesthetic surgery a dubious reputation. Nevertheless, aesthetic procedures are being requested today more commonly than ever. A skilled surgeon can perform such operations safely and with maximum benefit to the patient.

Patient selection is probably as important as any other factor. Not all patients are good candidates for aesthetic procedures, and such operations are contraindicated in others. Age or poor general health of the patient may be a reason for delay or avoidance of purely elective procedures. Two other major factors must be considered. The first factor is the anatomic feasibility of the procedure. Can the alterations be made successfully and safely? Which technique will best accomplish the goal? The second factor is the psychologic makeup of the patient. Does the patient fully understand the nature of the proposed procedure and its risks and consequences? Are the patient's expectations realistic? Cosmetic changes in appearance will generally not save a failing marriage, help to procure a new job, or substantially improve a person's station in life, and persons with such expectations should not undergo aesthetic surgery. Surgery should be postponed for persons experiencing severe stress, such as is associated with divorce, death of a loved one, or other periods of emotional instability.

The ideal candidate for cosmetic surgery is an adult or mature teenager who has a realistic idea of what is to be accomplished, is not under pressure from others to have the operation done, and does not expect major changes in interpersonal relations or career potential following surgery. Personal satisfaction is a valid reason for seeking aesthetic refinements.

The more common aesthetic procedures are discussed below. Some procedures involve correction of functional problems as well and are therefore not always considered purely cosmetic procedures.

RHINOPLASTY

Surgical alterations of nasal structures are done for relief of airway obstruction (usually secondary to trauma) and to reshape the nose because of undesirable characteristics, such as a prominent dorsal hump, bulbous or drooping tip, or overly large size. There is often a combination of problems.

Procedures are generally performed through intranasal incisions. The nasal skin is usually temporarily freed from its underlying bony and cartilaginous framework, so that the framework can be altered by removal, rearrangement, or augmentation of bone or cartilage. The skin is then redraped over the new foundation. The nasal septum and lower turbinate can also be altered to reestablish an open airway.

Surgery can be done under local or general anesthesia; in either case, topical and injectable vasoconstrictors and anesthetic agents are commonly used. Hospitalization may or may not be indicated. Nasal packing is often used for hemostasis and support of the nasal mucosa during initial healing, as incisions are usually only minimally sutured with absorbable sutures. External nasal splints are placed to control swelling and provide some protection, particularly if osteotomy of the nasal bones is performed.

Convalescence requires 10–14 days before most swelling and periorbital ecchymosis subside; however, several months are often required before completely normal sensation returns, and all swelling resolves.

Nasal procedures are very commonly performed, generally quite safe, and usually effective. Complications include bleeding, internal scarring, recurrence of airways obstruction, and irregularities of contour. Infections are rare except with the use of alloplastic nasal implants.

RHYTIDECTOMY
(Facelift)

The combined effects of gravity, exposure, and loss of elasticity due to aging result in varying degrees of wrinkles and sagging of skin along the cheeks, jawline, neck, and elsewhere in the facial area. These natural signs of aging can be removed to a great extent by a facelift procedure. Not all wrinkles can be removed, however; those in the forehead, around the eyes, in the nasolabial area, and around the lips are not significantly corrected without additional procedures.

Rhytidectomy generally includes a major procedure, with extensive incisions hidden just in front of and behind the ear, in the temporal scalp, and behind the ear in the occipital hairline. The skin of the lateral cheeks, jawline, and neck is dissected free in the subcutaneous plane. Excess skin is then trimmed away. Fat is often removed from the cheeks and submental area, and the platysma muscle that forms the foundation for the neck may be altered to give support and a youthful contour to the neck and submental angle. Drains are sometimes used as well as a padded circumferential dressing to protect the face and provide light pressure during healing. The introduction of fat aspiration procedures (liposuction) has been adapted to the neck and face region to give fine definition of the chin and jawline and to substantially correct the double-chin appearance.

Either local or general anesthesia may be used for this often lengthy (2–4 hours) and extensive procedure. Local vasoconstrictors are routinely given.

Complications include hematoma, skin slough, injury to branches of the facial nerve or great auricular nerve, scars, and asymmetry. Signs of aging often recur in one or more years.

BLEPHAROPLASTY

Blepharoplasty involves removal of a redundant skin of the upper and lower eyelids and removal of periorbital fat protruding through sagging orbital septa. It is done alone or as part of a facelift procedure.

Incisions are made in the upper lids surrounding previously marked redundant skin, which is removed. A subciliary incision is generally used in the lower lids. The orbicularis oculi muscle may be altered if necessary. The periorbital fat compartments are opened, and protruding fat is removed. The extent of redundant skin in the lower lid is gauged, and the skin is resected. External sutures are used. Minimal or no dressing is required.

Local anesthesia in the form of lidocaine with epinephrine is usually adequate. Swelling and ecchymosis subside in 7–10 days, and sutures are removed in 3–4 days.

Complications include bleeding, hematoma formation, epidermal inclusion cysts, ectropion, and asymmetry. Patients are usually satisfied with the results. Recurrence is much less of a problem than with facelift procedures.

MAMMOPLASTY

Aside from procedures related to breast cancer, surgery of the female breast is generally done for one of the following reasons: to increase the size of the breasts (augmentation mammoplasty), or to lift the breasts (mastopexy). Augmentation, lifting of the breasts, and correction of asymmetry are nearly always done for cosmetic reasons. Reduction of hypertrophied breasts may, however, be done for functional reasons, since such breasts can cause poor posture, back and shoulder pain, and discomfort due to grooves from brassiere straps.

Augmentation Mammoplasty

In procedures for augmentation of the breasts, a silicone bag implant filled with silicone gel, saline, air, or a combination of these substances is placed beneath the breast tissue in the submammary or subpectoral plane. Incisions are concealed in the periareolar margin, inframammary fold area, or axilla. Dissection is then carried out above or below the pectoralis major muscle, and the implant is placed in the pocket created. Drains are not generally used, and a padded dressing providing light pressure is applied.

The procedure can be done on an outpatient basis with local anesthesia, although this may not be satisfactory when subpectoral implants are used. General anesthesia is often used for augmentation procedures.

Although patient satisfaction is excellent in most cases, a significant rate of capsular contracture remains a problem in about 20%. Scar tissue around the implant may contract in variable degrees even in the same patient. Control of this process is difficult even though the best possible environment for healing is provided (ie, appropriate implants are used, infection is controlled, bleeding is not present, debris is removed, and movement is restricted). Implants placed in the subpectoral position appear to be associated with a lesser degree of capsular contracture and less severe deformity if contracture occurs.

Other complications include hematoma, infection, exposure of the implant, deflation or rupture of the implant, asymmetry of the breasts, and external scars. Breast function and sensation are usually not altered in any way.

Silicone gel has been used as an implant material for 30 years. Although the matter has recently become controversial, there is no definitive scientific evidence that silicone gel is carcinogenic or that it produces collagen type diseases.

Mastopexy

Mastopexy is another common procedure used for correction of sagging or ptotic breasts. Although some breasts develop in a ptotic manner, most cases are caused by normal relaxation of aging tissues, gravity and atrophy after pregnancy and lactation. It is not clear whether use of a brassiere alters this process in any significant manner. The degree of deformity is defined by the relationship of the areola to the inframammary fold and the direction of the nipple.

Correction may be done with simultaneous reduction or augmentation. An incision must be made around the areola, through the lower or lateral quadrant (to a variable extent), and usually within the inframammary fold in all but the most minimally deformed breasts. Significant scarring will occur.

General anesthesia, drains, and hospitalization are more commonly required for this procedure: Recovery requires 2–3 weeks.

Complications include bleeding; infection; tissue loss, altered sensation, or loss of function in the nipple-areola area; scars; and asymmetry of breasts.

Patient satisfaction with the results is often not as great as with other procedures. Satisfaction often depends on how well the patient is prepared to accept the resulting scars.

Reduction Mammoplasty

Reduction mammoplasty is similar to mastopexy, since nearly all hypertrophic breasts are ptotic and must be lifted during correction. Enlargement can occur during puberty or later in life. Massive breasts can become a significant disability to the patient.

Although various techniques have been developed for breast reduction, nearly all require a pedicle to carry the nipple areola to its new position and a circumareolar incision as well as an inverted @bl = incision beneath the areola. In gigantomastia, the nipple-areola is often removed as a free full-thickness graft and positioned appropriately. Most tissue is removed from the center and lower poles of the breast.

General anesthesia is nearly always required, as dissection and blood loss can be significant. Transfusions may be indicated as well as operative drains and hospitalization for several days.

Although problems with nipple-areola loss, bleeding, infection, asymmetry of breasts, and scarring may occur; these women are generally among the most satisfied and appreciative of patients.

ABDOMINOPLASTY & OTHER AESTHETIC PROCEDURES

Other procedures usually classified as aesthetic are abdominoplasty and other operations for removal of excess tissue from the lower trunk, thighs, and upper arms. Patients with sagging tissue due to aging, pregnancies, multiple abdominal operations, or significant weight loss are usually good candidates for body contour procedures. Surgery can benefit the occasional patient with an isolated excessive deposit of fat below the lower abdominal skin, in the thighs (trochanteric lipodystrophy), or elsewhere. The typical case of generalized obesity, however, is not amenable to surgical correction of contour deformity.

Abdominoplasty usually involves removal of a large ellipse of skin and fat down to the wall of the lower abdomen. Dissection is carried out in the same plane up to the costal margin. The naval is circumscribed and left in place. After the upper abdominal flap is stretched to the suprapubic incision, excess skin and fat are excised. The fascia of the abdominal wall midline can be plicated and thus tightened. The umbilicus is exteriorized through an incision in the flap at the proper level, and the wound is closed over drains with a long incision generally in an oblique line or W shape just above the os pubis and out to the area below the anterior iliac crests (so-called bikini line).

Spinal anesthesia is used in some cases. Hospitalization may be required for a few days. Blood transfusions are sometimes necessary.

Complications involve blood or serum collections beneath the flap, infection, tissue loss, and wide scars. Results are generally very good, with excellent patient satisfaction in properly selected cases.

Various surgical procedures have been devised to remove excess skin and fat from the upper arms, buttocks, and thighs. Unfortunately, nearly all of these procedures result in significant scarring, and there may be difficulty in achieving a smooth transition between the end point of the contour alteration and normal tissue. The use of a suction apparatus fitted with appropriate cannulas to remove localized excess fat deposits has become widespread. It is clear, however, that patient selection and judicious use of liposuction are necessary to avoid complications, including hypovolemia due to blood loss, hematoma formation, skin sloughs, and waviness and depressions in the operative site. Used with discretion, liposuction can offer definition to areas of the abdomen, flanks, thighs, and buttocks.

TELANGIECTASIAS
(Spider Veins)

When there is no trace of primary or secondary varicosities, most telangiectasias, or spider veins, are viewed as a cosmetic problem. However, one should be aware that in some cases spider veins may be an indication of deep venous valvular insufficiency. Factors that may play a role in the formation of spider veins include venostasis with decreased flow rate due to atony of the venous wall, chronic venous inflammation, hormonal influences, or venous compression at the saphenofemoral valve.

Treatment of spider veins is with sclerosing agents, which may include hypertonic saline, sodium tetradecol, and hydroxypolyethoxydodecan (Sclerovein). These agents are injected directly into the spider veins with the objective of creating intimal damage that will result in fibrosis and obliteration of the lumen. The technique is simple and effective, but when the sclerosing agent extravasates it might produce superficial skin necroses.

REFERENCES

Ives-Gerard I: *Body Sculpturing by Lipoplasty.* Churchill Livingstone, 1989.
Lewis JR Jr (editor). *The Art of Aesthetic Plastic Surgery.* Little, Brown, 1989.

Sheen JH: *Aesthetic Rhinoplasty.*Mosby, 1987.
Tardy EM, Brown RJ: *Surgical Anatomy of the Nose.* Raven Press, 1990.

Hand Surgery

45

Eugene S. Kilgore, MD, William P. Graham III, MD, & Robert E. Markison, MD

Both in industry and in the home, the hand is the most commonly injured part of the body. A disorder of the hand rarely jeopardizes life but often impairs vocational capacity.

INTRODUCTION

The prime functions of the hand are feeling (sensibility) and grasping. Sensibility is important on the radial sides of the index, long, and ring fingers and on the opposing ulnar side of the thumb, where one must feel and be able to pinch, pick up, and hold things. The ulnar side of the small finger and its metacarpal, upon which the hand usually rests, must register the sensations of contact and pain to avoid burns and other trauma.

Mobility is critical for grasping. The upper extremity is a cantilevered system extending from the shoulder to the fingertips. It must be adaptable to varying rates and kinds of movements. Stability of joints proximally is essential for good skeletal control distally.

The specialization of the thumb ray has endowed humans with superior aptitudes for defense, work, and dexterity. The thumb has exquisite sensibility and is a highly mobile structure of appropriate length, with a well-developed adductor and thenar (pronating) musculature. It is the most important digit of the hand, and every effort must be made to preserve its function.

The **position of function** of the upper extremity favors reaching the mouth and perineum as well as comfortable, forceful, and unfatiguing grip and pinch. The elbow is held at or near a right angle, the forearm neutral between pronation and supination, and the wrist extended 30 degrees with the fingers furled to almost meet the opposed (pronated) tip of the thumb (Figure 45–1A). This is the desired stance of the extremity if stiffness is likely to occur, and it should be adopted when joints are immobilized by splinting, arthrodesis, or tenodesis.

Opposite to the position of function is the **position of rest,** in which the flexed wrist extends the digits, making grip and pinch awkward, uncomfortable, weak, and fatiguing (Figure 45–1B). The forearm is usually pronated and the elbow may be extended.

This habitus is assumed, without intention, after injury, paralysis, and the onset of painful states; it is also called the position of the injury. Stiffening in this attitude jeopardizes function.

ANATOMY

All references to the forearm and hand should be made to the radial and ulnar sides (not lateral and medial), and to the volar (or palmar) and dorsal surfaces. The digits should be identified as the thumb, index finger, long finger, ring finger, and small finger, or referred to as rays I, II, III, IV, and V.

Skin is the elastic outer sleeve and glove of the arm and hand. Sacrifice of its surface area or elasticity by debridement and fibrosis can severely curtail range of motion and constrict circulation. In the adult hand, the dorsal skin stretches about 4 cm in the longitudinal and in the transverse planes when the fist closes, and the palmar skin stretches a similar amount when the palm is flattened and spread. The long finger can easily have 48 cm^2 of skin cover, and the whole hand (exclusive of digits) 210 cm^2.

Fascia anchors palmar skin to bone to make pinch and grip stable; the midlateral fibers of "Cleland's and Grayson's ligaments" keep the skin sleeve from twisting about the digit (Figure 45–2). In the form of sheaths and pulleys, fascia holds tendons in the concavity of arched joints to convey mechanical efficiency and power. The fascial sleeve of the forearm, hand, and digits must sometimes be slit along with skin to prevent or relieve congestion (eg, compartment syndrome). Any fascial compartment of the

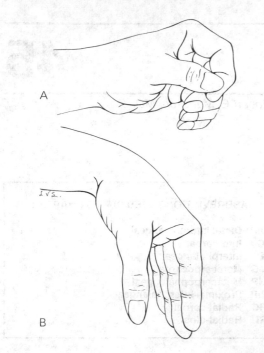

Figure 45–1. Positions of function **(A)** and rest (injury) **(B)**.

hand provides a space for infection or an avenue for its dissemination.

Each finger has four joints (MC, MP, PIP, and DIP—see accompanying box), any two of which may be fused and still leave adequate overall function. The thumb has only three joints (MC, MP, and IP), and every effort must be made to preserve at least two. The position of the wrist stretches and governs the efficiency of extrinsic muscle contraction. The wrist is the "key joint" of the hand, governing motion of the digits, and must be included in the immobiliza-

tion process required for any major digital problem. The stability of the digital joints and their planes of motion are governed by the length of the ligaments and the anatomy of their articulating surfaces. The longitudinal and transverse arches of the hand (Figure 45–3) are architectural prerequisites to gripping, pinching, and cupping and are maintained by the active contraction and passive tone of intact intrinsic muscles. The arches create the position of function. When the arches are collapsed, the hand assumes the position of injury or the clawed hand. Loss of these arches is most often initiated by edema. They may be preserved by splinting in the position of function, elevation without constriction, and early restoration of active and vigorous joint motion.

Each MP and IP joint has a distally anchored volar trapdoor called the volar plate (Figure 45–4) in addition to collateral ligaments stabilizing the joint in either side (Figure 45–5).

The extrinsic flexor tendons are contained in fibrous **sheaths** to prevent bowstringing and preserve mechanical efficiency as the digits furl into the palm. Pulleys (hypertrophied sections of the sheath) resist the points of greatest tendency to bowstring. Sheaths are inelastic and relatively avascular. Therefore, they crowd and congest any swollen, inflamed, or injured tendons and curtail glide by friction, constriction, and the generation of inelastic adhesions. **"No-man's-land"** is the zone from the middle of the palm to just beyond the PIP joint, wherein the superficialis and profundus lie ensheathed together and recovery of glide is so difficult after wounding (Figure 45–6).

Across the wrist, the dense volar carpal ligament closes the bony carpal canal (**carpal tunnel**) through which pass all eight finger flexors as well as the

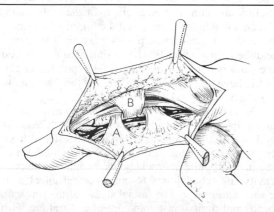

Figure 45–2. **A:** Cleland's ligament. **B:** Transverse retinacular ligament.

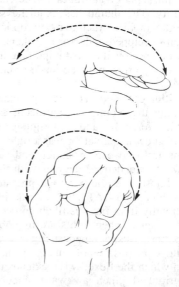

Figure 45–3. Longitudinal **(top)** and transverse **(bottom)** arches.

Extension

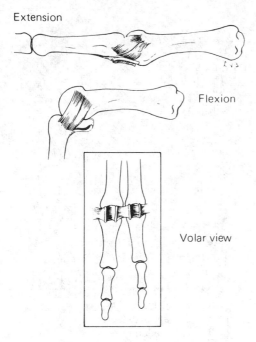

Flexion

Volar view

Figure 45–4. Volar plate.

flexor pollicis longus and median nerve (Figure 45–6). The **ulnar bursa** is the continuation of the synovium around the long flexors of the small finger through the carpal tunnel, encompassing the other finger flexors which interrupted their separate bursae at the midpalm level. The **radial bursa** is the synovium around the flexor pollicis longus continued through the carpal tunnel. These two bursae may intercommunicate. **Parona's space** is that tissue plane over the pronator quadratus in the distal forearm deep to the radial and ulnar bursae.

The extensor tendons are ensheathed in 6 compartments at the wrist beneath the extensor retinaculum (Figures 45–7 and 45–8), which predisposes to adhesions. Its role as a pulley is not vital and can be dispensed with.

The nerves of greatest importance to hand function are the musculocutaneous, radial, ulnar, and median. The importance of the musculocutaneous and radial nerves combined is forearm supination and of the radial nerve alone is innervation of the extensor muscles. The ulnar nerve innervates 15 of the 20 intrinsic muscles. The median nerve, by its sensory innervation, is "the eye of the hand"; through its motor innervation, it maintains most of the long flexors, the pronators of the forearm, and the thenar muscles. Figure

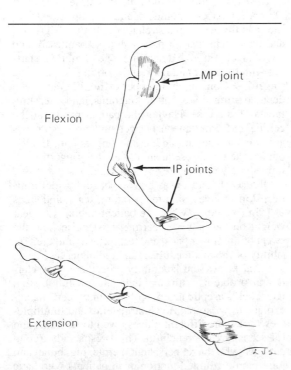

Figure 45–5. Collateral ligaments.

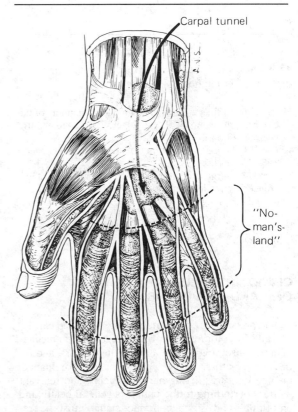

Figure 45–6. Carpal tunnel and no-man's-land.

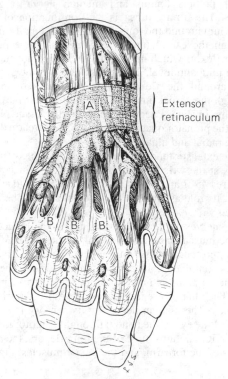

Figure 45–7. A: Extensor retinaculum over 6 tendon compartments. **B:** Juncturae tendinum (conexus intertendineus).

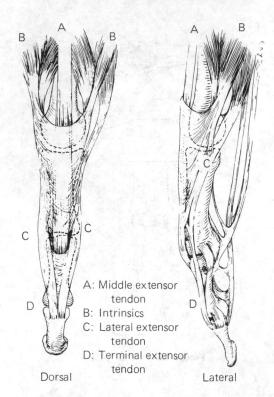

A: Middle extensor tendon
B: Intrinsics
C: Lateral extensor tendon
D: Terminal extensor tendon

Dorsal   Lateral

Figure 45–8. Extensor hood mechanism.

45–9 shows the sensory distribution of the ulnar, radial, and median nerves.

Harris C Jr, Rutledge GL Jr: The functional anatomy of the extensor mechanism of the finger. J Bone Joint Surg [Am] 1972;54:713.

Kauer JM: Functional anatomy of the wrist. Clin Orthop 1980;No. 149:9.

Lampe EW: Surgical anatomy of the hand: With special reference to infections and trauma. Clin Symp 1988;40:1.

Markison RE, Kilgore ES: The hand. In: *Clinical Surgery.* Davis J (editor). Mosby, 1987.

Spinner M: *Kaplan's Functional and Surgical Anatomy of the Hand.* Lippincott, 1984.

CLINICAL EVALUATION OF HAND DISORDERS

The presenting complaint must be recorded explicitly and in complete detail with regard to its mechanism of onset, evolution, aggravating factors, and relieving factors. Age, sex, hand dominance, occupation, preexisting hand problems, and relevant matters pertaining to the patient's general health and emotional and socioeconomic status must be recorded also.

The examination should follow an orderly routine. Observe the neck, shoulders, and both upper extremities and the action and strength of all muscle groups, and be certain that all parts can pass painlessly and coordinately through a normal range of motion, starting with the head and neck and working down to the fingertips. Compare both upper extremities and keep detailed immediate notes, diagrams, and measurements of the case. Having the patient reach for the ceiling and simultaneously open and close both fists and then spread and adduct the fingers and, finally, oppose the thumbs sequentially to each fingertip will immediately emphasize any abnormalities.

Observe habitus, wasting, hypertrophy, deformities, skin changes, skin temperature, scars, and signs of pain (including when the patient attempts to bear weight on the palms). Feel the wrist pulses and the sweat of the finger pads, and test reflexes and the sensibility of the median, ulnar, and radial nerves.

Serial x-rays and laboratory procedures may clarify a problem with an indolent evolution (eg, Kienböck's aseptic necrosis of the lunate, causing unexplained wrist pain). Contralateral and multiple-view x-rays in different planes (even tomograms and CT scans) are often helpful. This is especially true in patients who have persistent perplexing bone and joint pain or limited motion or in patients who have not attained adult growth. In the case of wrist prob-

flammatory conditions (eg, carpal tunnel syndrome, trigger finger).

Markison RE: Trauma to the extremities. In: *Current Therapy of Trauma.* Trunkey DD, Lewis FR (editors). BC Decker, 1986.

GENERAL OPERATIVE PRINCIPLES

A bloodless field (eg, by tourniquet ischemia) is essential for accurate evaluation, dissection, and management of tissues of the hand. This is achieved by elevating or exsanguinating the extremity and then inflating a padded blood pressure cuff around the arm to 100 mm Hg above systolic pressure. This is readily tolerated by the unanesthetized arm for 30 minutes and by the anesthetized arm for 2 hours.

Incisions (Figure 45–10) must be either zigzagged across lines of tension (eg, never cross perpendicularly to a flexion crease) or run longitudinally in "neutral" zones (eg, connecting the lateral limits of the flexion and extension creases of the digits); and, whenever possible, must be designed so that a healthy skin-fat flap is raised over the zone of repair of a tendon, nerve, or artery.

Proper evaluation and treatment of a fresh injury often requires extension of the wound. Normal structures can then be recognized and traced into the zone of injury, where blood and trauma so often make their identification difficult or impossible.

Constriction and tension by dressings must be avoided at all costs. The dressing should be applied evenly to the skin without wrinkles. The wound should be covered with a single layer of fine-mesh gauze followed by a wet spongy medium (fluffs, mechanic's waste, Rest-On, Kling, or Kerlix). Wet-

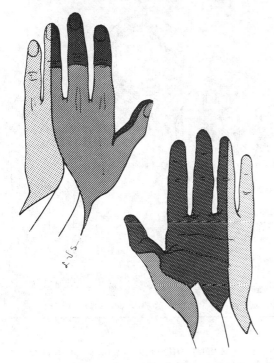

Figure 45–9. Sensory distribution in the hand. Dotted area, ulnar nerve; diagonal area, radial nerve; darker area, median nerve.

lems, arthrograms and arthroscopy may be of diagnostic value. MRI can also be quite helpful in the diagnosis of subtle carpal bone problems.

The diagnosis is often made by noting the response to therapy. This is particularly true in the case of local corticosteroids injected at the site of noninfectious in-

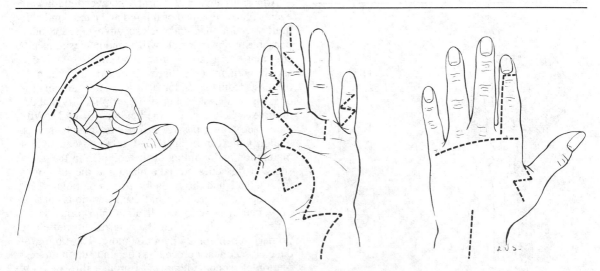

Figure 45–10. Proper placement of skin incisions.

ness facilitates the drainage of blood into the dressing, which should be applied with gentle pressure to curtail dead space.

Splinting and immediate elevation are paramount in controlling swelling and pain and favoring healing. In general, plaster (fast-setting) or fiberglass is preferred because of its adaptability to specific requirements. More often than not, the wrist requires immobilization along with any other part of the hand (Figure 45–11 and 45–12).

It must be appreciated that effective immobilization of a finger most often requires concomitant immobilization of one or more adjacent fingers, usually in the position of function. Straight splints such as tongue blades involve a hazard of digital stiffness and distortion and should not be used across the MP joint.

Persistence of pain signifies inadequate immobilization and, if throbbing is present, congestion. Congestion must be promptly relieved by elevation and sectioning of the cast and dressing and, if necessary, the skin and fascia.

Maneksha FR: Techniques and drugs for regional anesthesia in surgery of the hand. Orthop Rev 1987;16:417.

TENDON DISORDERS

Tendon disorders are most commonly due to trauma or to inflammatory or degenerative conditions. These may be restricted to one or more tendons or may be part of a generalized disorder involving

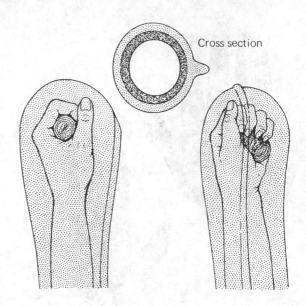

Figure 45–12. Casting.

other tissues and structures. Neoplastic and congenital disorders of the tendons are rare.

The prerequisites to successful tendon surgery are (1) that the tendons be covered with healthy padded and pliable skin; (2) that the joints to be moved by the tendons are supple and have an adequate passive range of motion; (3) that the muscles to the tendons be elastic, and that they be innervated or capable of being so; (4) that the patient be motivated and capable of responsibility for the rehabilitative effort; (5) that the surgeon have the appropriate training, skill, and technical facilities; and (6) usually, that the musculotendinous units involved not be spastic and the digits involved not irrevocably anesthetic.

Adhesions invariably form wherever tendons are even slightly inflamed or injured and can completely nullify tendon function; even so, adhesions are indispensable to repair. Rarely will a tendon reestablish its continuity or a tendon graft develop its own blood supply without some ingrowth of capillaries and fibroblasts from the tendon bed. Thus, it is not only the quantity of adhesions but also their pliability that determines whether or not the tendon will glide. With much active and passive effort over many months, tendon glide can be increased as a consequence of maturation and molding of the collagen in the adhesions. If this does not take place and the adhesions remain thick and short, tendon excursion fails.

Preoperative treatment of fresh lacerations consists of wound closure, immobilization, and prophylactic antibiotics. Such cases can be deferred for definitive primary repair for 24 hours or more. The timing of delayed secondary procedures depends upon the resolution of wound edema and fibrous callus (ie, how soft and pliable it is). After 6–8 weeks, tendons that

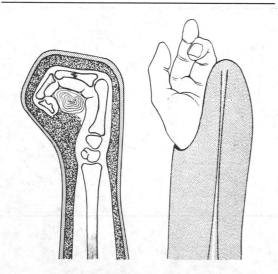

Figure 45–11. Casting.

retract over 2.5 cm may defy full excursion because the muscle elasticity has been lost or the tendon is recoiled and congealed in scar.

Tenorrhaphy must be done without surface trauma along the tendon or its bed. The juncture is made end-to-end or by weaving one tendon with the other, using nylon or wire sutures. A flexor tendon graft is anchored distally to bone (Figure 45–13). Tenodesis will occur if the surface of the tendon and the surface where adherence is desired are roughened. The position of immobilization needed to relieve tension on the tendon sutures is ideally determined when the wound is still open and the tendon juncture is in view. The duration of immobilization after tenorrhaphy is generally for no more than 3–4 weeks. Controlled early passive mobilization after tenorrhaphy may be initiated in the manner of Duran to forestall excessive tendon adherence. This requires very close supervision by the surgeon or therapist to avoid rupture of the repaired tendon.

The access to tenolysis should be through a wound offering effective exposure and placed where the immediate active and passive joint motion that must follow will not jeopardize healing of the wound by undue stretching or direct pressure. The most common causes of failure are immobilization of the tendon for longer than 24 hours after lysis; failure of the patient to move the tendon by repeated active contraction of the musculotendinous unit; carrying out a concomitant procedure requiring immobilization (eg, neurorrhaphy); and separation of the tendon.

Tendon lengthening is used to advance a tenorrhaphy beyond a point of constriction (eg, pulley) or to elongate a contracted musculotendinous unit.

The patient must understand that musculotendinous and joint mobilization after tendon surgery is a time-consuming process, often taking many weeks or months. Exercise—eg, squeezing a sponge after flexor tendon surgery—should be sufficient to make progress but not so much as to cause lingering pain and swelling. "Ball squeezing" has no place in getting tendons to glide early, since it blocks the movement of digital joints. Once glide has been achieved, however, ball squeezing may strengthen the muscles.

Diagnosis & Treatment of Tendon Injuries

Detailed circumstances of the injury must be studied to suspect the extent of damage. A puncture wound by glass, for example, can inflict deep injury out of proportion to the external evidence of the damage or the apparently intact function.

Tendon injury may be single or multiple and may be complicated by injury to nerve or bone. Diagnosis, treatment, and prognosis may be difficult. One must know the terminal joint that a given tendon moves, where overlap of function may mask the loss of action of a specific tendon, and how to block the action of tendons that conflict with functional testing of their fellow travelers.

Repeated testing will serve to confirm a tendon injury and differentiate unconscious or willful withholding of pertinent clinical information. The history, the habitus of the joints, and the results of specific tendon testing are the three crucial elements in the diagnosis of tendon deficits.

The state of the wound and the complexity of the injury are the principal issues the hand surgeon must weigh in choosing a primary or secondary tenorrhaphy and its type. Tidy wounds generally favor primary tenorrhaphy. Primary tenorrhaphy is defined as one that is done within 24–72 hours after injury.

When wounds are untidy, contaminated, or complicated by fracture or ischemia, formal tenorrhaphy may have to be delayed for weeks or months until the tendon bed is more favorable to healing and glide. However, interim tacking of the tendons—together, to tendon sheaths, or to bone—to maintain the fiber length of a muscle may be done as a preliminary procedure.

"Mallet" finger ("baseball" or "drop" finger) (Figure 45–14) is due to division or attenuation of the extensor to the distal phalanx. A distal joint that can be passively but not actively extended is diagnostic. The injury most commonly results from sudden forceful flexion of the digit when it is held in rigid extension. Either the extensor is partially or completely ruptured, or the dorsal lip of the bone is avulsed. Less frequently, the injury is due to direct trauma such as a laceration or a crush force. An x-ray should be taken to determine the presence and extent of any fracture.

Treatment may not be necessary if the loss of active extension is less than 15 degrees and any existing fracture is only a chip. More severe injury requires 6 weeks of continuous splinting in full distal joint extension (*not* hyperextension) with or without 40 degrees of PIP joint flexion. Joint fixation internally with fine Kirschner wire or externally with padded

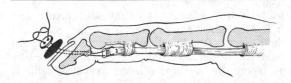

Figure 45–13. Flexor tenorrhaphy by advancement or graft. Pulleys are saved.

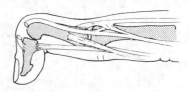

Figure 45–14. Mallet finger with swan-neck deformity.

aluminum, plastic, or even plaster splints is equally effective. A lacerated tendon should be delicately reapproximated. When a significantly displaced fracture fragment represents one-third or more of the surface of the joint, it should be reduced if necessary by wiring or pinning. In selected cases, smaller fracture fragments may be removed. If there is sufficient articular disruption, one may consider joint fusion. Tendon grafting is difficult and easily leads to a poor cosmetic and functional result. It should be done only rarely.

Swan-neck deformity (Figure 45–14) is a frequent complication of mallet finger, but it may also be the result of disparity of pull between the extrinsic flexors and extensor hood with or without attenuation of the DIP joint extensor. It is seen in congenitally hypermobile joints, spastic and rheumatoid states, and following resection of the superficialis tendon. The dorsal hood acts to extend the distal joint but is held back by its insertion at the base of the middle phalanx, which it therefore hyperextends ("PIP joint recurvatum"). This in turn increases the tension on the profundus, which hyperflexes the DIP joint. If the mallet deformity is 25 degrees or less and there is some active distal joint extension, it may be treated by undermining and elevating the extensor hood at the PIP joint and severing its insertion on the base of the middle phalanx. Otherwise, the deformity may be corrected by tethering PIP joint extension with one slip of the flexor digitorum superficialis threaded through the flexor pulley of the proximal phalanx with the PIP joint flexed 20 degrees, or by the Littler technique.

The **"buttonhole,"** or **"boutonnière," deformity** (Figure 45–15) appears as the opposite of the swan-neck deformity: hyperextension of the DIP joint and flexion of the PIP joint. There is attenuation or separation of the dorsal hood, so that the middle extensor tendon becomes ineffective and the lateral extensor tendons shift volar to the PIP joint axis and the joint buckles dorsally, and the entire extrinsic-intrinsic force on the hood passes onto the lateral extensor tendons, which flex the PIP joint and hyperextend the DIP joint. This deformity may develop suddenly or, more often, insidiously after closed blunt or open trauma over the dorsum of the PIP joint.

To avoid this complication, sutured extensor tendon lacerations and severe contusions over the PIP joint should always have the PIP joint alone splinted in extension for 3–4 weeks. A small, oblique Kirschner wire provides an alternative form of immobilization. Established deformities can be treated by such immobilization but more often require operative correction.

Tendon rupture, subluxation, and drift. The most frequent rupture of a healthy tendon is that of the distal joint extensor of one of the fingers as a result of sudden, forceful flexion (see mallet finger, above), or avulsion of the profundus from the distal phalanx in violent flexion. Other tendons rupture where they have been weakened by division and suture, partial transection, crushing, or attritional fraying over roughened bone. The synovial thickening, degenerative tendon nodularity, and roughening of articular bone seen in the rheumatoid hand easily dispose to rupture by mechanical abrasion and circulatory depletion of tendons. Much can be done prophylactically in rheumatoid disease by synovectomy, sectioning of constricting tendon sheaths, and resection of bony spurs and tendon nodules. If correction of any form of tendon rupture is indicated, the methods of doing so include suture, tendon graft, tendon transfer, or tenodesis.

The most common subluxations and drifts of tendons are twofold: (1) volar drift of the intrinsic tendons as they pass the PIP joint of the fingers, causing the "buttonhole" deformity (see above); and (2) ulnar drift of the extrinsic middle extensors (central slips) as they pass the MP joints. The latter may result from trauma that divides or attenuates the lateral expansion (sagittal band) of the extensor hood on the radial side of the central slip. It more commonly results from attenuation of the entire extensor hood over the MP joint as a consequence of marked distention of the joint space and thickening of the synovium in rheumatoid arthritis. Treatment of ulnar drift involves repositioning of the extensor tendon to a point central to the MP joint and holding it by appropriate reefing of the sagittal band fibers of the hood on the radial side.

Evaluation of Results

The excursion and force of centripetal pull of the operated tendon should be compared with the normal one in the opposite hand and objective measurements recorded at least once a month. It then becomes readily apparent whether or not progress is being made. If the conscientious patient makes no progress in 2–3 months, the impairment is probably static and the patient should be considered for further surgical treatment or released from care. Often, however, 6–12 months are required before maximal function is restored.

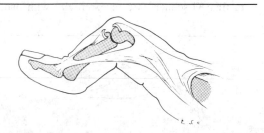

Figure 45–15. Buttonhole deformity.

Browne EZ Jr, Ribik CA: Early dynamic splinting for extensor tendon injuries. J Hand Surg 1989;14:72.

Louis DS, Hunter JM: Rehabilitation of the injured hand. Hand Clin 1989;5:507.

Dovelle S, Heeter PK: The Washington regimen: Rehabilitation of the hand following flexor tendon injuries. Phys Ther 1989;69:1034.

Imbriglia JE, Hunter J, Rennie W: Secondary flexor tendon reconstruction. Hand Clin 1989;5:395.

Manske PR: Flexor tendon healing. J Hand Surg 1988; 13:237.

Matthews JP: Early mobilization after flexor tendon repair. J Hand Surg [Br] 1989;14:363.

Schneider LH, Bush DC: Primary care of flexor tendon injuries. Hand Clin 1989;5:383.

Schneider LH, Bush DC: Primary care of flexor tendon injuries. Hand Clin 1989;5:383.

Singer M, Maloon S: Flexor tendon injuries: The results of primary repair. J Hand Surg 1988;13:269.

Strickland JW: Flexor tendon surgery: Part 1: Primary flexor tendon repair. J Hand Surg [Br] 1989;14(3):261.

Strickland JW: Flexor tendon surgery: Part 2: Free tendon grafts and tenolysis. J Hand Surg [Br] 1989;14(4):368.

FRACTURES, DISLOCATIONS, & LIGAMENTOUS INJURIES

The wrist and digits should be generally maintained in the position of function after reduction. Unstable alignment may require internal fixation to hold reduction. At all costs, avoid extremes of joint position and forceful pressure of external splints and plaster. Constant digital traction is hazardous because it leads to joint stiffness. To minimize stiffness, immobilization should be maintained for the shortest time consistent with adequate control of pain and tissue repair.

Elevation of the forearm and removal of all jewelry and snug clothing are essential to control edema. The patient's own responsibilities in this regard must be repeatedly explained. When swelling is excessive, it must be reduced and the soft tissues rendered pliable as soon as possible. Reduction of the displaced fracture or dislocated joint sometimes makes the soft tissues pliable again. A releasing incision of skin and fascia may be needed to overcome brawny induration. It can be closed later with a split-thickness skin graft.

Open injuries involving bones and joints require prophylactic antibiotics systemically and often in the wound or joint as well (see Chapter 8).

FRACTURED METACARPALS & PHALANGES

Fractures of **metacarpals** and **proximal** and **middle phalanges** tend to bow and to rotate. Rotation of a finger causes it to cross over an adjacent finger during flexion, thus blocking digital excursion, fist making, and grasp. Rotation is avoided by having the injured finger flexed alongside an adjacent finger.

Dorsal and volar bowing is caused by the pull of intrinsic and extrinsic flexor and extensor forces. These forces can be most effectively neutralized by immobilizing the wrist and the digits in the position of function. Reduction of bowing has the risk of added predisposition to joint stiffness and tenodesis incident to excessive manipulation or surgery. Therefore, if the bowing is less than 20–30 degrees, this risk must be weighed carefully, for such deformity may not be functionally significant. Greater angles of bowing of the phalanges must, however, be corrected by either closed or open methods. Angulation of up to 40 degrees can be tolerated in some metacarpal neck fractures.

The immobilized MP joints must be maintained in functional flexion. In the case of the ring and small fingers, this function means between 60 and 80 degrees of flexion. Malleable and rigid ready-made volar splints cannot be applied without a threat to this important angle of MP joint flexion or (equally harmful) a threat of too much compression of the soft tissue of the palm or a rotary deformity at the fracture site.

After closed or open reduction, a preferred method of immobilization is to furl the digits over a volar roll of soft gauze, which allows the position of function to be maintained (Figures 45–11 and 45–12). The forearm and pertinent digits are then wrapped in loosely applied cast padding followed by a light circumferential plaster cast, keeled for strength across the extended wrist. This immobilization is usually maintained for 3 weeks, although with rigid internal fixation it may be for only a few days. The patient should be seen every 2–3 days so that the cast can be removed for guarded active and passive joint motion under supervision of the surgeon.

Two basal metacarpal fractures deserve special mention:

(1) Bennett's intra-articular fracture is an impaction of the thumb metacarpal, causing an oblique fracture into the MC joint between the volar base and the dorsal base. The latter frequently subluxates dorsally. The ideal treatment when there is displacement is reduction by centrifugal pulling on the thumb and pressure volarward on the base of the metacarpal followed by fixation with a Kirschner wire. If satisfactory realignment is not achieved, open reduction is advocated.

(2) A spiral or displaced fracture of the **base of the fifth metacarpal** always deserves an immediate and repeated check on the function of the first dorsal interosseus muscle to establish the integrity of the deep motor branch of the ulnar nerve, which is easily injured by this fracture.

Distal phalangeal fractures are located at the tuft, shaft, or base. Pain is the prime reason for treatment, and it may be compounded if subungual hematoma is also present. Decompression relieves the pain. This can be done by drilling the nail with a 19-caliber hypodermic needle mounted on a syringe, or by burning a hole through the nail with the hot end of a safety pin or paper clip. This is quite painless if done gently, but in the anxious patient a digital nerve block may be required. Pain and swelling are best controlled by applying a well-padded forearm cast covering the injured finger with at least one adjacent finger or the injured thumb alone in boxing glove fashion. After 1–2 weeks, a digital guard can take the place of the cast.

Minute marginal **digital joint fractures** usually need no more than 1–2 days of immobilization. Stiffness and pain can be overcome by early mobilization. Fractures with involvement of one-fourth to one-third of the joint surface require careful reduction and immobilization for 3 weeks unless rigid internal fixation is resorted to, in which case guarded early motion may be initiated under supervision. In some cases, the fragment should be resected. Mangled joints should be set at a functional angle for fusion or, in select circumstances, the MP or PIP joints may be replaced by a Silastic implant if tendons are functioning.

In closed or open **crushing fractures** with a lot of swelling, the prime consideration should be preservation of the circulation, particularly venous return. Anatomic reduction of the bone is of secondary importance. Leaving a wound open or even slitting skin and fascia to loosen the tissues may be the best way to aid the circulation and may also make it possible to secure alignment and the position of function. Reduction is often well maintained by molding a roll of very wet, loose gauze to the injured digits or whole hand and then applying a well-cushioned boxing-glove type of forearm cast to the appropriate digits or the whole hand. Internal fixation is advisable in selected cases.

Open reduction is the technique of choice in injuries that present a gaping wound with exposed fractures. It is also the preferred technique in the following circumstances: (1) when perfect reduction is important for subsequent function, as in intra-articular fractures, or when indicated for the removal of a potentially troublesome displaced small fragment; (2) if it allows reduction with less soft tissue trauma than by closed reduction; (3) to facilitate internal fixation in difficult reductions; or (4) to allow early movement and prevent stiffness.

DISLOCATIONS

Dislocations of the wrist and fingers are less frequent than fractures. Swelling may completely mask the bone displacement, but motion is usually limited and painful. X-rays may be indispensable to the diagnosis. In the case of the wrist, multiple views and comparison of right and left may be necessary.

Dislocations are most easily reduced by accentuating the position that produced the deformity with simultaneous centrifugal traction on the distal segment followed by firm pressing of the displaced bone into its anatomic position. A reduction snap may be heard and is often promptly followed by excellent range of motion. A postreduction x-ray should usually be taken.

Limited progressive mobilization is usually advisable to avoid stiffness. It may start within 3–4 weeks for the wrist and a week for the digits. A concomitant fracture or an open dislocation would interdict mobilization so early. Compound dislocations require prophylactic treatment with antibiotics.

Open reduction is indicated whenever closed reduction requires much force. A chronic dislocation may defy even an open reduction without lysis and division of soft tissue or resection arthroplasty.

The most common dislocation about the digits is dorsal displacement of the distal segment on the proximal one. When ligaments are intact, reduction may be difficult. The most difficult is the dislocated MP joint of one of the fingers, which normally requires open reduction. It traps the head of the metacarpal in a noose formed by the lumbrical radially, the flexor tendons and pretendinous palmar fascia band ulnarly, the volar plate and collateral ligaments on the dorsum distally, and the transverse palmar fascia on the volar aspect proximally. Volar exposure with section of the fascia proximally or dorsal exposure with splitting of the volar plate makes reduction quite easy, although section of the ulnar collateral ligament must sometimes be added.

Dislocation of an IP joint is most often reduced immediately by the patient or a bystander and requires little or no immobilization. Resistance to flexion means inadequate reduction. Failure of reduction can mean that the displaced phalangeal head has escaped sideways from under the hood of the extensor mechanism, which then closes in between the head and the base of the more distal phalanx and locks the deformity. Recurrence of the dislocation usually means that the volar plate has been torn off at its origin distally. All of these difficulties require open procedures to restore normal anatomic relationships. Repair of the volar plate requires 3–4 weeks of immobility. One obliquely placed Kirschner wire provides sufficient fixation of the joint.

Chronic dislocations with erosion of the joint should be handled by replacing the joint with a Silastic prosthesis if the surrounding tendons are functionally intact; otherwise, the joints should be fused in the position of function. **Rheumatoid arthritis** causes a variety of insidious dislocations. The most common is at the MP joint, where **volar** and **ulnar drifting** of the proximal phalanx in relation to the metacarpal occurs due to the mean force of intrinsic-extrinsic tendon pull in association with pathologically attenuated joint capsules and ligaments. When intrinsic muscles atrophy and fibrose, these distortions may be irreducible without soft tissue surgery. At the PIP and DIP joint levels, the distortion may be of the **swan-neck** (PIP hyperextension and DIP flexion) or **buttonhole** type (PIP flexion and DIP hyperextension).

LIGAMENTOUS INJURIES

The ligaments of the **MP** and **PIP joints** are the most commonly injured. These vary from total ruptures to tears without any loss of stability. Either the ligament tears, or its bony attachment is avulsed, or both ligament and bone are torn. Those of the MP joint are usually due to violent abduction, whereas PIP ligaments rupture with equal proclivity on the radial or ulnar sides. Diagnosis may depend on stress x-ray view, often requiring a local lidocaine infiltration to block pain to show abnormal widening of a joint.

Except for the thumb, treatment of purely ligamentous injuries is seldom surgical. Splinting should often be brief to avoid excessive stiffness and pain, which may result. As long as there is intact intrinsic and extrinsic tendon function and the patient is careful to avoid further injury, early motion within 2–3 days of injury is often desirable. One finger can be splinted by loosely strapping it to an adjacent digit ("buddy-taping") for 2–4 weeks. The pain of these injuries is notoriously slow to resolve, irrespective of treatment.

Twisting injuries and falls may rupture the radial collateral ligament of the thumb by an adduction force; most commonly, however, the injury is an abduction force that tears the ulnar collateral ligament ("game-keeper's thumb"). Partial tears with limited instability may be treated by buddy-taping the thumb to the index finger for 4 weeks. Total tears should be sutured or reconstructed surgically.

If there is a sizable avulsed bone fragment in any of these injuries, it must be accurately reduced or, if it involves less than one-fourth of the surface area of the PIP or MP joint, removed. One may try local injections of small amounts of corticosteroid and lidocaine for chronic pain or try resection of scarred intrinsic muscle and the leading edge of the intermetacarpal ligament for intractable pain in the finger webs.

Burkhalter WE: Closed treatment of hand fractures. J Hand Surg 1989;14(2 Part 2):390.

Burkhalter WE: Hand fractures. Instr Course Lect 1990;39:249.

Campbell RM Jr: Operative treatment of fractures and dislocations of the hand and wrist region in children. Orthop Clin North Am 1990;21:217.

Culver JE: Sports-related fractures of the hand and wrist. Clin Sports Med 1990;9:85.

Hankin FM, Peel SM: Sport-related fractures and dislocations in the hand. Hand Clin 1990;6:429.

Kilgore ES: Dislocation of the digits, wrist and hand. In: *Current Practice of Emergency Medicine,* 2nd ed. Callahan ML (editor). BC Decker, 1991.

Putnam MD, Seitz WH Jr: Advances in fracture management in the hand and distal radius. Hand Clin 1989; 6:455.

Saunders SR: Physical therapy management of hand fractures. Phys Ther 1989;69:1065.

Wolfe SW, Dick HM: Articular fractures of the hand. Part I: Guidelines for assessment. Orthop Rev 1991;20:27.

Wolfe SW, Dick HM: Articular fractures of the hand. Part II: Guidelines for management. Orthop Rev 1991;20: 123.

HAND INFECTION

Pyogenic infections of the hand often develop and spread as a result of failure to preserve or restore good venous and lymphatic drainage following trauma. In order to prevent as well as to treat infection, it is necessary to control swelling and congestion of tissues and to avoid any dead space filled with stagnant blood or serum. Trauma and inflammation cause tissue tension by sequestration of edema fluid. This in turn impairs tissue oxygenation by compressing the blood vessels, and a vicious cycle may develop that can lead to necrosis within the constrictive sleeves of fascia and skin.

Acute swelling predisposes to infection, especially if there has been contamination through a puncture or an open wound. Tissues and structures with a limited blood supply—or a blood supply that is easily choked off—are most susceptible to infection. Tissues that have the least natural resistance to infection are those of tendon sheaths, joints, bone, and nail folds.

Prevention & Treatment of Pyogenic Infections

Constrictive clothing, jewelry, dressings, casts, and even a tightly closed wound can impair oxygenation. Comfortable immobilization and elevation of the hand above the level of the heart will help to control swelling. Throbbing pain is a symptom of excessive swelling that demands prompt mechanical relief and not analgesics. If pain, swelling, and induration progress despite other mechanical measures, immediate slitting of skin and fascia in one or more areas is mandatory. This is usually done either along the dorsoradial or the dorsoulnar side of the digits, the hand, and the midvolar or middorsal surface of the forearm and wrist, with care to avoid injury to nerves, major vessels, and tendons. A dorsal transverse skin incision over the heads of the metacarpals (sparing the veins) allows the MP joints of the swollen hand to flex and assume the functional position. Prophylactic local and systemic antibiotics are indicated for all contaminated wounds or whenever the circulation has been compromised in the presence of a wound. Antisludging treatment (eg, dextran 40) may also be considered. Clearly definable and easily recovered foreign bodies and nonviable tissue should be removed without endangering residual function. The evacuation of blood, serum, and foreign fluids can be facilitated by loosely fitting drains and wet dressings. Tetanus immunization should be given as indicated.

Adequate immobilization usually requires a splint of the wrist. In serious cases or uncooperative patients, the elbow should be splinted also and the patient kept flat in bed with the hand propped up on pillows. Without immobilization, the infection may be "milked" into uninvolved areas and progress farther.

The need for antibiotics is determined by the extent of the infection. If the process is already well localized, simple drainage may be all that is needed. Since 65% of pyogenic infections are due to *Staphylococcus aureus* (50%), or beta-hemolytic streptococci (15%), begin with antibiotics empirically while waiting for cultures. Cat bites cause infection with *Pasteurella multocida,* which is sensitive to penicillin.

When incision and drainage of an abscess is necessary, it should always be done at the point of maximum tenderness or the point of maximum fluctuation, where the overlying tissues are thinnest. The drainage wound should run parallel to and not across the paths of nerves, arteries, and veins. Wounds should be made long enough and should be zigzagged, when necessary, to avoid secondary contractures.

Cellulitis, Lymphangitis, & Adenitis

Cellulitis is manifested by local swelling, warmth, redness, and tenderness. It usually demands immobilization and elevation, and sometimes fasciotomy, in addition to antibiotics. Lymphangitis and adenitis are most often due to streptococci and require elevation and immobilization as well as antibiotics.

Pyogenic Granuloma

Pyogenic granuloma is a mound of granulation-like tissue 3–20 mm (or more) in diameter. It usually develops under a chronically moist dressing and may form around a suture knot. A small granuloma (6–7 mm in diameter) exposed to the air will soon dry up and epithelialize, whereas larger ones should be

scraped flush with the skin under local anesthesia and covered with a thin split-thickness skin graft. If the granuloma is adjacent to the nail and the nail is acting as a foreign body aggravating the reaction, the nail must be removed.

Pyoderma

Pyoderma (subepithelial abscess) is the forerunner of **collar-button abscess.** It develops within the skin in a hair follicle or infected blister or inflamed callus. Unattended, such problems commonly lead to this abscess, which becomes collar-button in configuration when it points into the subdermal fat. Treatment by means of incision, debridement of a blister or callus, drainage, water-soaked or zinc oxide dressings, rest, and elevation is usually sufficient.

Infections Around the Nail

The rigidity of the fingernail causes it to press upon and aggravate any inflammation of the soft tissues surrounding it. The nail fold is often traumatized and becomes secondarily inflamed, leading to a **paronychia** on the radial or ulnar side. The lesion is called an **eponychia** if it involves the base of the nail; a **"runaround"** if the entire fold is involved; and a subungual abscess if pus develops and extends under the nail plate. **Subonychia** is inflammation between the nail bed and the bony phalanx. Because of the early and unrelenting tissue tension that develops, these entities are quite painful. Abscess formation often results, occasionally at some distance proximal to the nail fold (paraeponychial abscess). Early treatment before abscess formation is by means of water-soaked or zinc oxide dressings, elevation immobilization, and antibiotics. Most abscesses can be drained painlessly with a needlepoint scalpel without drawing blood; the insensible necrotic skin cap should be cut through where it points, and drainage should be assured by applying zinc oxide ointment (Figure 45–16). Sagittal incisions that form a "trapdoor" of the eponychium should be reserved for the long-standing case in which a dense fibrous callus of the nail fold must be excised. Occasionally, the nail must be basally excised or totally avulsed, after which the

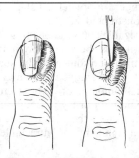

Figure 45–16. Incision and drainage of paronychia.

eponychial fold should be separated from the nail matrix by a thin, loose pack. Chronically wet nails of dishwashers may develop tissue changes and nail deformities best treated by removing the nail plate. Fungal infections should be diagnosed and treated, and the fingers should be protected from water or excessive sweating. Chronic or recurrent nail fold infections are often the telltale sign of deep-rooted anxiety and stress, which needs treatment along with the nail fold problem.

Space Infections

The skin and fascia compartmentalize certain areas of the hand and forearm, predisposing these spaces to increased tissue tension and the progression of infection to abscess formation. The treatment of early space infection involves elevation, immobilization, and antibiotics administered systemically. If this does not arrest the progression of symptoms and signs within a few hours—or if the space is already tense when first examined—incision and drainage are required. Recovery is expedited by an antibiotic drip into a deep space administered through a fine catheter, but there must always be a drain present to prevent development of a compartment syndrome.

A. Volar Digital Pulp (Fat Pad) Spaces of the Digits: (Figure 45–17.) Whether in the proximal, middle, or distal pad, any abscess that points to the center of the pad should be drained by an incision that is precisely central and runs longitudinally but does not cross the flexion crease. This preserves the important digital arteries and nerves. A **felon** pointing centrally should be drained centrally (Figure 45–18). Fishmouth, lateral, and transverse incisions have made far too many fingertips gangrenous or anesthetic. Division of the vertical fascial fibers on the pulp was recommended in the past but is rarely necessary and can irretrievably deprive the pad of the tethering it needs for stable pinching.

B. Web Spaces: The web spaces are the path of least resistance for pus from infected distal palm calluses, puncture wounds, and infections of the lumbrical canals. Infection and abscess formation in the dorsum of the thumb web may be the result of extension from the volar thenar space. A dorsal sagittal incision is usually most desirable between the fingers. A dor-

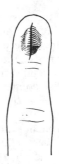

Figure 45–18. Incision of felon (distal fat pad infection).

sal incision in the web of the thumb may be zigzagged to prevent contracture (Figure 45–10).

C. Midpalmar Space: The midpalmar space becomes infected by direct puncture or by extension of infections from the flexor sheaths of rays II, III, or IV (Figure 45–6). Only the skin should be incised over the point of fluctuation. The rest of the dissection should be carried out by gentle spreading with a blunt clamp to avoid injury to arteries, nerves, and tendons. Infection spreads easily from this space along the lumbrical canals and to the thenar space.

D. Hypothenar and Thenar Spaces: A hypothenar space abscess is usually a product of a penetrating wound and should be drained where it points. The same is true for a thenar space abscess, which may point in the palm rather than the thumb web.

E. Space of Parona: This space lies over the pronator quadratus beneath the flexor muscles in the distal forearm. Infection here is usually due to extension of pus from the flexor sheaths of the thumb (radial bursa) or small finger (ulnar bursa). Drainage should be along the ulnar side of the forearm deep to the flexor tendons and the ulnar nerve and artery.

F. Dorsal Subaponeurotic and Subcutaneous Spaces: The subaponeurotic space lies deep to the extensor tendons on the back of the hand, and the subcutaneous space is superficial to it. Either or both may become infected by puncture, open injury, or extension of infection from the digits and web spaces. Drainage is best done through the dorsoradial side of ray II or the ulnar side of ray V. A superficial transverse incision, sparing the veins, may be made over the metacarpal heads for additional drainage and to allow flexion of the MP joints into the position of function.

Septic Tenosynovitis

Because circulation is limited and easily compromised, the flexor and extensor synovial tendon sheaths (bursae) are most susceptible to infection after contamination and are avenues for the spread of infection. The ulnar bursa extends from the level of the distal joint of the small finger to incorporate all

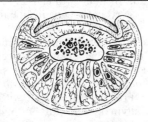

Figure 45–17. Cross section of distal phalanx.

flexors of the other fingers as they pass through the carpal tunnel. Here it often communicates with the radial bursa coming from the thumb. The bursae of the index, long, and ring fingers usually terminate at the mid palm. Intercommunication of bursae is variable. The 6 dorsal tendon compartments under the extensor retinaculum of the wrist have separate synovial bursae (Figure 45–7).

The cardinal sign of tenosynovitis is moderate to severe pain along a given synovial bursa when the tendon therein is made to glide a short distance actively and passively, thereby stretching the inflamed synovium. Passive motion of a flexor tendon must be performed by touching no more than the patient's fingernail, thus avoiding misdiagnosis by limiting the stimulus to motion of the synovial bursa. Ultrasonography of the distal palm can also be helpful when the diagnosis is unclear. The probe is held across the palm and reveals swelling of the involved tendon and fluid around the tendon at the proximal flexor sheath.

Only unresponsive, tensely swollen, and toxic cases need immediate incision and drainage. With rest, elevation, and antibiotics, it is safe to observe most cases for several hours. The preferred method of incision and drainage (Figure 45–19) is to make a short sagittal midline distal wound immediately over the tendon and introduce a small plastic catheter into the synovial bursa for irrigating with a solution of antibiotic mixed with lidocaine. Another catheter should be inserted for drainage through a counterincision in the more proximal portion of the involved sheath (eg, in the palm for digital flexor sheath infection and proximal to the extensor retinaculum for extensor compartment infections). These incisions do not cross flexion creases. The hand should then be elevated and immobilized in the position of function

and covered by continuously kept wet or zinc oxide dressings. Phlegmonous tenosynovitis usually requires opening of the entire synovial sheath (often through a lateral midaxial digital incision, or longitudinally across the wrist for extensor sheath infections) and, frequently, excision of necrotic tendon and sometimes amputation of a digit.

Bone & Joint Infections

The limited circulation of these structures makes them very susceptible to infection. Any open wound of bone or joint deserves immediate treatment as though infection were already established. Penetrating tooth wound infections (eg, **human or animal bite infections**) are among the most virulent. They often involve the dorsum of the MP and PIP joints as a result of striking a blow with a closed fist. In such cases, the hand should be immediately coated with zinc oxide over the wound, immobilized in a loosely padded boxing glove cast, elevated, and observed closely. Osteomyelitis responds well to a prolonged course of antibiotics and sequestrectomy where indicated.

Miscellaneous Infections

A. Streptococcal Gangrene: This is a very toxic process that causes rapid necrosis and requires emergency fasciotomy and excision of necrotic tissue, continuous compresses with silver sulfadiazine or zinc oxide ointment or 0.5% silver nitrate solution, and massive antibiotic therapy. Microaerophilic streptococcal infection (Meleney's phagedenic ulcer, sloughing ulcer) is a similar process that must be treated promptly in the same way.

B. Tuberculosis: Tuberculous infection of the hand is usually chronic and may be relatively painless. Some cultures take months to become positive. Tuberculosis commonly involves only one hand, which may be the only focus of infection in the body. Bones and joints may be infected, but the infection more commonly involves the tendon synovium, which becomes matted to the tendons. Treatment is by synovectomy and antituberculosis drug therapy for 6–12 months.

C. Leprosy: Leprous neuritis of the median and ulnar nerves causes sensory and motor loss to the hand. Crippling claw deformities develop as a result of intrinsic muscle palsy. Open sores appear on the hands as a result of trauma to anesthetic digits. Reconstructive surgery and occupational training are required.

D. Fungal Infections: Fungal infections involve primarily the nails. Tinea unguium (onychomycosis) may be caused by many organisms, including *Epidermophyton floccosum, Trichophyton,* and *Candida albicans.* Prolonged treatment with antifungal drugs—griseofulvin systemically or nystatin topically—may be necessary, along with daily applications of fungicidal agents such as tolnaftate. Removal

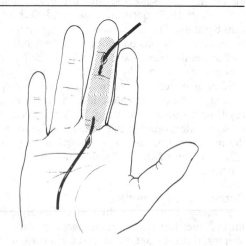

Figure 45–19. Drainage and irrigation for septic tenosynovitis. The antibiotic solution drips in through the distal catheter and drains out through the proximal one.

of the nail is advocated for chronic intractable cases associated with deformation of the nail.

E. Herpes Simplex: An inordinate amount of pain, with little or no swelling or induration, predating and accompanying the appearance of multiple tiny vesicles suggests herpes simplex. The vesicles may appear cyclically. They contain clear fluid and not pus, as do paronychias, with which they are frequently confused. Antibiotics are not indicated in this self-limited viral infection, nor is the application of photoactive dyes, which may be carcinogenic. Ether applied periodically to unroofed vesicles may shorten the clinical course. Acyclovir 5% ointment applied topically every 3 hours six times daily for 7 days decreases the severity and duration of symptoms but is of no value in prophylaxis.

F. Rare Infections: Gas gangrene, syphilis, deep fungal infections (eg, coccidioidomycosis, actinomycosis, blastomycosis, sporotrichosis), tularemia, anthrax, yaws, and glanders are diagnosed by means of a pertinent history of exposure, chronicity, and laboratory studies to identify the pathogen.

Burkhalter WE: Deep space infections. Hand Clin 1989; 5:553.

Canales FL, Newmeyer WL 3d, Kilgore ES Jr: The treatment of felons and paronychias. Hand Clin 1989;5:515.

Dellinger EP et al: Hand infections: Bacteriology and treatment. A prospective study. Arch Surg 1988;123:745.

Faciszewski T, Coleman DA: Human bite wounds. Hand Clin 1989;5:561.

Fowler JR: Viral infections. Hand Clin 1989;5:613.

Freeland AE, Senter BS: Septic arthritis and osteomyelitis. Hand Clin 1989;5:533.

Gunther SF, Levy CS: Mycobacterial infections. Hand Clin 1989;5:591.

Gunther SF: Chronic infections. Instr Course Lect 1990;39:547.

Gunther SF: Infections of the hand. Instr Course Lect 1990;39:527.

Hitchcock TF, Amadio PC: Fungal infections. Hand Clin 1989;5:599.

Mancini LH, Fort LK: Rehabilitation of the infected hand. Hand Clin 1989;5:635.

Neviaser RJ: Tenosynovitis. Hand Clin 1989;5:525.

Perry AW et al: Finger stick felons. Ann Plast Surg 1988;20:249.

Reyes FA: Infections secondary to intravenous drug abuse. Hand Clin 1989;5:629.

Snyder CC: Animal bite wounds. Hand Clin 1989;5:571.

Zubowicz VN, Gravier M: Management of early human bites of the hand. Plast Reconstr Surg 1991;88:111.

NONINFECTIOUS INFLAMMATORY DISORDER

The entities in this group have little in common except a greater or lesser degree of inflammatory or collagen reaction and change. They include wear-and-tear conditions, degenerative states, rheumatic and collagen disease, and gout. Pain is often the presenting complaint, and there may be a coexisting abnormality of appearance or mechanical function.

CONSTRICTIVE CONDITIONS

In stenosing tenosynovitis there is a disproportion between the clearance inside a tendon pulley or tunnel and the diameter of the tendon or tendons that must glide through it. Any pulley or tunnel may be implicated. The more common sites are as follows:

(1) The proximal digital pulleys in the distal palm, causing **trigger finger** or **thumb** (stenosing flexor tenosynovitis). There is local tenderness of the pulley; pain, which may be referred to the PIP joint; and (usually but not always) locking of the digit in flexion with a painful jog as it goes into extension (ie, as the bulge in the tendon or tendons passes through the tight pulley).

(2) The pulley over the radial styloid housing the abductor pollicis longus and extensor pollicis brevis, causing **De Quervain's tenosynovitis.** Local tenderness and pain occur if these tendons are actively or passively stretched (eg, Finkelstein's test).

(3) The volar carpal ligament, causing **carpal tunnel syndrome.** The "soft" median nerve is compressed against the ligament by the nine "hard" tendons in the tunnel deep to it. Mild compression causes disturbance of sleep by aching and numbness over the distribution of the nerve (most often the long and ring fingers, whose sensory fibers are closest to the ligament), but always sparing the small finger. Severe constriction causes constant hypesthesia as well as paralysis of the abductor pollicis brevis. Diagnosis is usually based on 6 factors: (1) the history; (2) a positive Phalen wrist flexion test; (3) altered sensibility on stroking the skin over the distribution of the median nerve; (4) a positive Tinel sign at the wrist; (5) weakness or atrophy of the abductor pollicis brevis; and (6) improvement following injection of the carpal canal with lidocaine and corticosteroids.

(4) Ulnar nerve compression (less common) occurs as the nerve passes behind the medial epicondyle (the cubital tunnel), between the heads of the flexor carpi ulnaris, or along Guyon's canal from the pisiform bone to the hook of the hamate. The diagnosis is based on a knowledge of the anatomy of innervation.

(5) Other nerve compression states include compression of the median nerve in the proximal forearm (pronator tunnel or anterior interosseous nerve syndromes) and compression of the radial nerve (Frohse's tunnel or posterior interosseous nerve syndromes).

Electromyography and nerve conduction studies may be helpful in evaluating nerve compressions.

These disorders may be congenital; may be due to chronic adaptive hypertrophy of tendon and pulley alike in response to work or repetitive activity; or may be due to tissue changes associated with aging. They can occur at any age. Other factors are distortion or scar caused by trauma; tumor; and rheumatoid synovitis or nodules.

Relief of these conditions can be achieved by local injections of triamcinolone or dexamethasone mixed with lidocaine *(never into a nerve)* or by means of surgical section of the constricting pulley or tunnel. Local injections may be tried three or four times at weekly intervals before resorting to surgery, which involves a hazard of sensitive scar or prolonged weakness. A disabling complication of surgery for De Quervain's tenosynovitis is a very painful neuroma of the radial nerve; of surgery for carpal tunnel syndrome, a painful neuroma of the palmar cutaneous nerve to the thenar eminence; and of release of a trigger phenomenon, a painful neuroma of the digital nerve. Immediate surgery is justified if the constriction is so tight that no tendon glide is possible and in cases of rapidly progressive or unrelenting motor or sensory nerve impairment, irreversible rheumatoid or nonspecific synovial thickening, or other space-consuming lesions.

Surgery must never be performed blindly or without a tourniquet. Adequate proximal and distal decompression is essential. When a nerve is decompressed, if the epineurial sheath is also found to be thickened or if there is an hourglass constriction, epineurotomy is in order.

Anderson B, Kaye S: Treatment of flexor tenosynovitis of the hand ("trigger finger") with corticosteroids. Arch Intern Med 1991;151:153.

Bonnici AV, Spencer JD: A survey of "trigger finger" in adults. J Hand Surg 1988;13:202.

Cho DS: The electrodiagnosis of the carpal tunnel syndrome. S D J Med 1989;42:5.

Luchetti R, Schoenhuber R, Landi A: Assessment of sensory nerve conduction in carpal tunnel syndrome before, during and after operation. J Hand Surg 1988;13:386.

Mesgarzadeh M et al: Carpal tunnel: MR imaging. Part II. Carpal tunnel syndrome. Radiology 1989;171:749.

Nau HE, Lange B, Lange S: Prediction of outcome of decompression for carpal tunnel syndrome. J Hand Surg 1988;13:391.

Okutsu I et al: Measurement of pressure in the carpal canal before and after endoscopic management of carpal tunnel syndrome. J Bone Joint Surg [Am] 1989;71:679.

Spinner RJ, Bachman JW, Amadio PC: The many faces of carpal tunnel syndrome. Mayo Clin Proc 1989;64:829.

Thorpe AP: Results of surgery for trigger finger. J Hand Surg 1988;13:199.

DUPUYTREN'S CONTRACTURE (Palmar Fasciitis)

The cause of Dupuytren's contracture, which is common particularly among white populations of Celtic origin, is not known. It occurs in one of three types (acute, subacute, and chronic), predominantly in males over 50 who have been in sedentary occupations, and is bilateral in about half of cases. There is a hereditary influence, and the incidence is higher among idiopathic epileptics, diabetics, alcoholics, and patients with chronic illnesses. The contracture may develop in women who do not work and (in laborers) in the hand that does the least work, so that it is not considered work-related. It is frequently found in the plantar fascia of the instep and occasionally in the penis (Peyronie's disease).

Dupuytren's contracture manifests itself most commonly in the palm by thickening, which may be nodular, and therefore mistaken for a callosity; or cord-like, and therefore mistaken for a tendon abnormality because it passes into the digits and restricts their extension. This process typically involves the longitudinal and vertical components of the fascia but at times seems to exist apart from anatomically distinct fascia. The skin may fuse with it and become raised and rock-hard, or it may be greatly shrunken and sometimes drawn into a deeply puckered crevasse. The disorder invades the palm at the expense of fat but is never adherent to vessels, nerves, or musculotendinous structures (although it may be adherent to flexor tendon sheaths). It has an unpredictable rate of progression, but the earlier it starts in life, the more destructive and recurrent it is apt to be.

Dupuytren's fasciitis may involve any digit or web space, but it affects predominantly the ring and small fingers. In long-standing cases the fingers may be drawn tightly into the palm, resulting in secondary contracture of joint capsule and ligaments, flexor sheaths, and atrophic muscles.

Surgery is indicated when the disorder has progressed sufficiently, especially when it causes any flexion contracture of the PIP joint. The patient must be warned about the increasing technical difficulty with progressive flexion and adduction contractures and the potential for recurrence after surgery. Fasciectomy is the surgical procedure that gives the best long-term results. In selected cases where only the longitudinal pretendinous fascial band is involved and the skin moves freely over it, subcutaneous fasciotomy done through a small longitudinal incision may release a contracture quite well with only a few days of postoperative disability. In the occasional case with acute and rapid onset of a tender nodule, local triamcinolone may be used for not only subjective but even objective relief.

Depending upon the amount of cutaneous shrinkage, skin grafts may be required for wound closure after fasciectomy. The overlying dermis has been implicated as an inductive mechanism in this process. Thus, skin grafting may diminish the recurrence rate in severe cases. The hopelessly contracted little finger must sometimes be amputated.

Motion should be started within 3–5 days after surgery. Dynamic splints and postoperative injection of corticosteroids into joints and the zone of surgery may help the well-motivated patient.

The complications of surgery are digital infarction and ischemic skin flaps, hematoma formation, fibrosis and stiffness, anesthesia or neuromatous pain, and recurrence of fasciitis and contracture. In general, the functional reward to the patient is great at any age.

Hill NA, Hurst LC: Dupuytren's contracture. Hand Clin 1989;5:349.

Murrell GA, Francis MJ, Howlett CR: Dupuytren's contracture: Fine structure in relation to aetiology. J Bone Joint Surg [Br] 1989;71:367.

Rombouts JJ et al: Prediction of recurrence in the treatment of Dupuytren's disease: Evaluation of a histologic classification. J Hand Surg 1989;14:644.

Sennwald GR: Fasciectomy for treatment of Dupuytren's disease and early complications. J Hand Surg 1990; 15:755.

Seyer AE, Hueston JT: Dupuytren's contracture. Hand Clin 1991;7:4.

DEGENERATIVE OSTEOARTHRITIS

Degenerative osteoarthritis is common in people over age 40. It affects women more often than men and involves primarily the digital IP joints and the basal (MC) joint of the thumb. Heberden's nodes of hypertrophic bone cause typical bossing with occasional associated dorsal ganglion (mucous cyst) formation of the distal joints. Such cysts may press on the nail matrix and cause longitudinal grooving of the fingernail. If they are excised, magnification should be used. The subjacent bony spur that is often present may be excised to prevent recurrence, but doing so may cause an acute arthritis flare. Joint deformity, pain, and stiffness may be treated by replacement of the joint with a prosthetic silicone rubber joint spacer or hinge (see below) or by joint fusion.

RHEUMATOID DISEASE

Rheumatoid disease is of unknown cause and is most commonly polycyclic. It affects all the tissues of mesenchymal origin in the hand, especially the synovial tissues. The x-ray changes vary from early marginal joint erosion with associated osteoporosis to advanced destructive changes and subluxation, particularly of the wrist and the MP and PIP joints. The disease often starts in the hands and involves the synovia of joints and tendons. Initially there is vague pain of insidious (sometimes acute) onset, swelling, stiffness, and local hyperthermia. In time, thickening of synovial tissues about the joints and tendons causes destruction and distortion. Tendons may rupture, especially where frayed by bone changes. Rheumatoid granulomatous nodules develop in the substance of tendons and tendon sheaths and subcutaneously over bony prominences. Stretched ligaments and retinacular tissues can no longer maintain the alignment of joints and tendons against the mean pulling forces, and a host of digital deformities may develop (swan-neck or boutonnière deformity, ulnar drift, and "intrinsic plus" deformity). With intrinsic muscle fibrosis and advanced joint destruction, many of these deformities become fixed.

The ideal management of these cases consists of combined medical and surgical supervision and guidance. It is always hoped that physical and emotional rest, heat, analgesia, therapeutic exercise, and anti-inflammatory agents (eg, aspirin, ibuprofen, corticosteroids, gold salts) will check the progression of disease. When these measures are not successful, surgical procedures (synovectomy, arthroplasty, tenoplasty, resection of nodules, arthrodesis, ulnar styloidectomy, etc) may forestall further destruction and preserve function and cosmetic appearance.

The problems amenable to surgical correction arc the following: (1) Boggy synovitis about flexor and extensor tendons. (2) Boggy synovitis of wrist or digital joints. (3) Rheumatoid nodules. (4) Tendon rupture (mainly of the extensors of the ring and small fingers, and the flexor of the thumb). (5) Constrictive conditions (stenosing tenosynovitis and median and ulnar nerve compression syndromes). (6) Joint erosions, subluxations, and fixed deformities.

Ertel AN: Flexor tendon ruptures in rheumatoid arthritis. Hand Clin 1989;5:177.

Ferlic DC: Boutonnière deformities in rheumatoid arthritis. Hand Clin 1989;5:215.

Odonovan TM, Ruby LK: The distal radioulnar joint in rheumatoid arthritis. Hand Clin 1989;5:249.

Philips CA: Management of the patient with rheumatoid arthritis. The role of the hand therapist. Hand Clin 1989;5:291.

Rheumatoid arthritis. Hand Clin 1989;5:111.

Stirrat CR: Treatment of tenosynovitis in rheumatoid arthritis. Hand Clin 1989;5:169.

Wood VE, Ichtertz DR, Yahiku H: Soft tissue metacarpophalangeal reconstruction for treatment of rheumatoid hand deformity. J Hand Surg 1989;14(2 Part 1):163.

Silicone Rubber Implants

Made of heat-vulcanized, medical-grade silicone elastomer stock, these implants ("joint spacers") were developed for arthritic joint and carpal bone replacement. They have been effectively time-tested for replacement of the MP and PIP joints (even the wrist joint), the trapezium, scaphoid, and lunate bones as well as the ulnar styloid and radial head. If there has been much soft tissue reconstruction, immobilization is continued for 4–6 weeks; if not, motion may be guardedly initiated in 3 or 4 days with 24-hour dynamic splinting for 3 weeks and nighttime dynamic splinting for an additional 3 weeks. The removal of carpal bones can be difficult and hazardous. Postoperative immobilization should be maintained for 4–6 weeks. Silicone rubber implants do not give the patient license to load (stress) the implant unduly, since disintegration may occur and even lead to extensive cystic degenerative bone changes. However, if proper respect is paid to their limited tolerance to excessive stress, these implants can give lifelong functional satisfaction.

SCLERODERMA, LUPUS ERYTHEMATOSUS, & SARCOIDOSIS

These systemic diseases of unknown cause have distinctive—though not necessarily pathognomonic—manifestations in the hands.

Scleroderma initially produces joint stiffness, hyperhidrosis, and Raynaud's phenomenon. Unchecked, it leads to marked tautness of skin and rigidity of joints with associated osteoporosis (even atrophy and ultimate resorption of the distal phalanges) and soft tissue calcifications.

Lupus erythematosus, which may be initiated or aggravated by certain drugs, foreign proteins, or psychic states, often causes polyarthritis indistinguishable from that of rheumatoid arthritis. It does not usually lead to similar joint destruction.

Sarcoidosis may produce digital nodules and articular swellings, and x-rays may show small punched-out lesions, particularly of the phalanges.

GOUT

Gout is a metabolic disorder of uric acid metabolism that affects about 1% of the population; approximately 50% of patients with gout have cheiragra (gouty hands).

The diagnosis is suggested by a rapid onset of severe pain and inflammatory signs about the joints and musculotendinous structures, simulating a phlegmonous infectious cellulitis with marked induration (eg, most dramatically seen about the elbow). The usual duration of an attack is 5–10 days. The serum uric acid is elevated in 75% of cases. Gout may coexist with rheumatoid disease or osteoarthritis. The diagnosis is confirmed by identification of uric acid crystals in joint fluid or tissue biopsy.

In time, typical tophi form, consisting of toothpaste-like infiltrates of urate crystals, arising in multilobulated form about soft tissue structures that have been invaded. X-rays show characteristic punched-out lesions at the margins of articular cartilage.

Prophylactic treatment of gouty arthritis consists of diet, colchicine, allopurinol (a urate-blocking agent) or probenecid (a uricosuric agent), and avoidance of stress. Colchicine, 0.6 mg/h with a glass of water for 6–8 doses or to the point of gastrointestinal distress, is the time-honored means of interrupting an attack, but phenylbutazone, corticotropin gel, and corticosteroids are also of value.

Surgical measures consist of drainage of abscessed tophi (seldom needed) and tophectomy. The latter procedure is more often of cosmetic than functional value. Tophectomy consists of removal of as much tophaceous material as can be fairly easily recovered. The surgeon should be careful not to destroy ligaments, tenoretinacular structures, nerves, and vessels in the process.

BURNS OF THE HAND

The hands are a common site of thermal (including frictional), electrical, chemical, and radiation burns. Function is imperiled in all instances by swelling and scar formation. Prompt measures to preserve existing function are often urgently required. Delay may lead to irreversible impairment and deformity. Burn therapy is covered in Chapter 14.

The urgent objective of treatment of burns of the hand is to restore mobility as soon as possible (within 1–3 weeks) by the following measures: (1) Control of swelling (by elevation, escharotomy, and fasciotomy). (2) Control of pain (by cold compresses, elevation, analgesics, and grafting). (3) Prevention of infection (by topical anti-infective agents), immediate or early grafting, and control of congestion. (4) Prompt (even primary) debridement followed by grafting as soon as oozing has stopped and the wound appears ready.

The burned hand should be covered with a clean (if possible, sterile), dry dressing and the patient transported as soon as possible to the hospital emergency department. First-degree burns are treated with cold compresses. Second-degree burns should be debrided if blisters are bulky or already broken. Burns involving loss of 2.5 cm^2 or more of skin may then be covered with a biologic dressing, if available, such as allograft (homograft) or xenograft (which are bacteriostatic) or amniotic membrane. All of these effectively control pain. Pigskin is an ideal xenograft (heterograft). If grafts are not available, an ideal emollient is silver sulfadiazine or a thick coating of zinc oxide ointment. Motion is encouraged from the beginning, whereas dependency and the "position of injury" are discouraged. Splinting at night may be useful. When the epithelium no longer weeps, lanolin may be applied after the hand has been soaked in water.

A deep second-degree burn or third-degree burn that involves one-third to one-half or more of the surface area of a digit, hand, or forearm usually causes enough swelling to threaten loss of function. Hand swelling is greatest on the dorsum, where the skin is loose and the space beneath will accommodate a lot of water. This forces MP joint extension and thumb adduction, creating "a claw hand in disguise." The burned part must be constantly and carefully watched. If elevation alone is not effective and the patient becomes less able than formerly to close the fist and touch the thumb to the little finger—or if throbbing pain progresses followed by numbness— then immediate bedside escharotomy with biologic dressing and prompt operating room debridement and grafting must be considered. Brawny induration must be prevented.

When motion is being lost or is already lost, it is far better to debride skin primarily or within the first week and have the hand grafted and mobilized within 10 days than to anxiously await for 3–4 weeks the possible survival of the burned skin at the expense of cicatrix formation and immobility.

After debridement with a dermatome or scalpel, the ooze usually precludes immediate grafting. This, therefore, should be deferred for 24 hours. Postage stamp, mesh, or sheet grafts that are thin (0.2–0.25 mm) are most apt to take and should be used over beds of equivocal graft-sustaining quality. Wet dressings protected by plastic and a padded boxing glove cast for 1 or 2 days are used for immobilization. If open treatment is used, a conscientious attendant must daily remove any serum collections from beneath the graft.

Prolonged splinting should be avoided as much as possible except when the patient is resting or sleeping. At these times the hand should be propped up comfortably on pillows to keep it higher than the level of the heart. Isoprene splinting material is ideal for this purpose because it can be sterilized and heat-molded to fit the patient. The position of function must be maintained in modeling any splint, and constrictive wrappings must never be used. Hanging the extremity by a noose is not to be done unless a long-arm cast is applied with the elbow at 90 degrees. Elastic bandages are also dangerously constrictive.

Burns severe enough to cause actual charring are usually associated with extensive second- and third-degree burns. The charred elements should be excised as soon as the general condition of the patient allows and the wounds should be closed as soon as possible.

Restoration of movement. The patient with a burned hand must be helped and encouraged to move every joint of the upper extremity as soon and as often after injury as possible.

Reconstructive Procedures

The proper initial care can prevent or limit many but not all of the functional disabilities caused by burns. The hand surgeon can do much by individualized procedures to reduce the extent of some of the disabilities. Resurfacing is accomplished with split-thickness grafts for appearance, with full-thickness grafts for release of flexion and web contractures, and with pedicle grafts when better padding is needed. Joints may be freed by capsulotomies and tenotomies, or they may be fixed permanently in a functional attitude by arthrodesis.

Cosmesis and function can be well served by amputation. A ray resection of a useless index finger may greatly compensate for a thumb web contracture.

Electrical Burns

High-voltage injuries to the extremity may be of great but hidden magnitude. Beneath the skin sleeve, extensive coagulation necrosis of vessels, nerves, and musculotendinous structures may be present, and its extent may not become manifest for several days. Electrical contact points usually have third-degree skin burns. The treatment parallels that described for injection injuries (see p 1160). It is not uncommon to have to amputate a hand or an arm that has been damaged by an electrical burn. Early decompression by incisions of the skin and underlying fascia may limit progressive injury secondary to congestion.

Frostbite

Rapid rewarming by immersion in water at 40–44 °C until there is flushing of digital skin (usually in 30 minutes) is the prime initial treatment. The pain associated with this must be controlled. There is no need for early surgical treatment unless a circumferential eschar curtailing blood flow calls for escharotomy. Children who suffer minor cases of frostbite may develop premature epiphyseal closures.

Bentivegna PE, Deane LM: Chemical burns of the upper extremity. Hand Clin 1990;6:253.

Brcic A: Primary tangential excision for hand burns. Hand Clin 1990;6:211.

Clarke HM et al: Acute management of pediatric hand burns. Hand Grossman JAI et al: Burns of the upper extremity. Hand Clin 1990;6(2):1.

Harrison DH, Parkhouse N: Experience with upper extremity burns. Hand Clin 1990;6:191.

Puddicombe BE, Nardone MA: Rehabilitation of the burned hand. Hand Clin 1990;6:281.

Sykes PJ: Severe burns of the hand: A practical guide to their management. J Hand Surg [Br] Vol 1991;16:6.

TUMORS & PSEUDOTUMORS OF THE HAND

Except for squamous cell carcinoma of the dorsal skin, cancer in the hand is rare. A variety of lesions are found in the hand, including hematomas, foreign bodies, scars, calluses, warts, nevi, cysts, bone bossings and exostoses, xanthomas, enchondromas, giant cell tumors, nerve tumors, fibromas, hemangiomas, carcinomas, and sarcomas. Squamous cell and basal cell carcinomas and melanomas are discussed in Chapters 44 and 47. The most commonly seen hand tumors are ganglions, warts, inclusion cysts, giant cell tumors of soft tissue, and enchondromas.

Ganglion & Mucous Cyst

Where there is a synovial lining, a protrusion may develop followed by later isolation of a closed pouch or cul-de-sac to form a cyst filled with the physiologic lubricant fluid of joints and tendons. The old concept of "mucoid degeneration" and development from embryologic cell rests has now been abandoned. If adsorption of water occurs, the cyst will have a jelly-like consistency. Sudden, forceful bending of a joint may cause extrusion of the synovium between ligamentous fibers and the sudden appearance of a cyst. More frequently, the cyst appears insidiously. Pain may be caused by tension within the cyst and pressure on adjacent tissues.

Most ganglions arise from the joints of the wrist, but any joint and tendon sheath can give rise to one. The path followed is along the tissue planes of least resistance. The length and pathway of a stalk are unpredictable. When there is protrusion through more than one fibrous tissue plane, the cyst may have an hourglass configuration.

A volar wrist ganglion always deserves a careful preoperative test of collateral arterial competency (Allen's test) to ensure good digital circulation if one artery must be divided in removing the ganglion. A flexor sheath ganglion at the base of a digit is usually like a "pebble in the shoe." It may be mistaken for a sesamoid.

Treatment of a ganglion is not indicated unless the patient insists. Puncture with a large-bore needle under lidocaine anesthesia followed by aspiration or simply squeezing out of the contents, and then injection of triamcinolone may sustain many in remission. Some claim "cure" by this procedure. Flexor sheath ganglions of the digit that are off center should not be

so treated, for in such cases the nerve and artery may be injured by the needle.

If surgery is required, the cyst should be removed without trauma to surrounding nerves or tendons down to the joint or tendon sheath, which is entered so that resection can be complete. Recurrence and complications usually occur when the surgeon fails to use a tourniquet and magnification, to explore adequately, and to visualize "satellite cysts" as the joint is entered.

Inclusion Cyst & Foreign Body Granuloma

Injury can carry viable epidermal cells deep to the dermis, into fat, or even into bone. With growth of these cells, keratinized cells accumulate into a ball or cyst which compresses the tissue in which it lies. Bone may become eroded. At surgery, an inclusion cyst looks like a pearl and has a soft thin wall that surrounds its cheesy contents. It will not recur if it is totally enucleated, which is usually easy to do. In contrast to this is a foreign body granuloma, which is adherent to surrounding tissues, has friable granulomatous tissue within it, and is often better curetted and drained rather than excised. The offending foreign body, if not absorbed, will be found and should be removed.

Posttraumatic Neuroma

This common lump only presents for treatment when it is painful. Such will be the case if it lies on a hard surface (eg, tendon or bone) at a point of pressure, or when it is trapped in scar tissue and subjected to stretching. (The treatment of neuromas is described in Chapter 38.)

Xanthoma (Giant Cell Tumor of Soft Tissue)

This is an insidiously growing, painless, nonfriable, hard, often multinodular tumor that arises from the fibrous flexor sheath or collateral ligaments or fascia. Even though benign, it extends under tendons and collateral ligaments and through joints. Unless all of the brownish-yellow tumor is removed, the tumor may recur.

Enchondroma, Giant Cell Tumor of Bone, & Aneurysmal Bone Cyst

Enchondromas constitute 90% of true bone tumors of the hand. The classic finding is calcific stippling of the lytic bone defect, most common in the proximal phalanges and distal half of the metacarpals. The carpal bones are spared. Aneurysmal bone cysts and giant cell tumors of bone are practically identical except for their vascularity. Pathologic fracture may be the presenting finding.

Treatment consists of curettement of the contents and wall of the lesion followed by packing of the hole with tiny cortical chips from the proximal third of the ulna.

Lipoma

This tumor usually occurs on the volar aspect of the digit or palm. If the proper plane is followed in the dissection, the lesion can be easily enucleated. Caution must be taken during dissection when the lesion is adjacent to major nerves.

Neurofibroma & Schwannoma

Neurofibromas are usually multiple (Recklinghausen's disease) and consist of thickened nerve sheath elements, that can be felt by running the fingers up and down the extremities and trunk. There is a rare tendency to malignant degeneration. The usual indication for resection of this tumor is cosmetic. It is usually not symptomatic. It should be enucleated under magnification so as to spare the nerve. If growth is rapid, cancer should be suspected and a long segment of the nerve resected or amputation contemplated. Schwannoma is usually solitary and is apt to be exquisitely painful.

Hemangioma

Hemangiomas in infants should never be treated by irradiation. The common strawberry angiomas will involute after their initial growth period. If the angioma is rapidly enlarging, it may be induced to involute by a course of corticosteroid therapy. In the older patient (and a few infants), surgical removal is the only means of treatment. Angiography may be helpful in determining the nature and extent of this group of tumors. They may be located primarily in skin, fat, or muscle; however, in the case of cavernous hemangiomas, may extend throughout all tissues and be impossible to totally remove without amputation or destroying digital or hand function.

Actinic Keratosis & Bowen's Disease

These lesions respond well to topical fluorouracil (5-FU), 2–5% solution in propylene glycol. Bowen's lesions are usually found on the dorsum of the hands in persons exposed chronically to sunlight, and they present as blotchy, hyperkeratotic, scaling, reddened areas.

Glomus Tumor

This rare tumor, comprised of blood vessels and unmyelinated nerves of a heat-regulating arteriovenous shunt, may cause extremely severe pain. It can develop anywhere but is most dramatic under the fingernail, where "pinpoint" pressure initiates the pain. Half of patients may have no symptoms, only a visible or palpable lesion. Treatment consists of meticulous dissection and total excision under magnification.

Binkovitz LA, Berquist TH, McLeod RA: Masses of the hand and wrist: detection and characterization with MR imaging. Am J Roentgenol 1990;154:323.

Johnson J, Kilgore E, Newmeyer W: Tumorous lesions of the hand. J Hand Surg 1985;10:284.

Rayner CR: Soft tissue tumors of the hand. J Hand Surg [Br] 1991;16(2):125.

COMPLEX INJURIES OF THE HAND

GENERAL PLAN OF MANAGEMENT

Sudden physical or functional loss of part or all of the hand or arm is a shocking experience that deserves special recognition and attention on the part of the surgeon. Psychologic and physical comfort should be given, and the patient must be spared alarming comments as well as any false hopes of replantation or salvage.

Amputation may be physical or functional. Injury and disease may functionally (though not physically) amputate by crushing, mangling, paralyzing, stiffening causing pain, or otherwise destroying all or part of the hand beyond hope of useful recovery. In such cases, salvage may be impossible and surgical amputation is justified to improve the overall physical and psychologic effectiveness of the patient.

Referral

When patients are referred, the injured part should be comfortably aligned and splinted without constriction. Bleeding should be controlled by compression or by ligation of the bleeder provided it is adequately exposed under tourniquet ischemia and loupe magnification to avoid injuring adjacent nerves. Wet dressings should be applied to open wounds to facilitate sequestration of blood and serum, and the extremity should be comfortably elevated. In the case of open injuries, prophylactic antibiotics should be given. An amputated part may be irrigated and, if possible, placed in a container or plastic bag on ice. Even if replantation is not feasible, tissue (eg, skin or bone) from the ablated part is sometimes of value in primary or secondary reconstructive procedure.

In Vivo Tissue Bank

A "nearly amputated," badly crushed, or mangled digit, hand, or arm may present a great challenge to good judgment and to the surgeon's technical skill in acting on a decision to attempt salvage. Viable structures and tissues can often be replanted or transferred to give maximal restoration of function, ie, the patient can serve as his or her own "in vivo tissue bank" if the surgeon keeps a functionally irretrievable digit or other forearm or hand structure alive, or as a free graft transfer, for use elsewhere in reconstruction.

Assessment of Problem

Complex injuries notoriously cause multilevel and multitissue involvement ("common wound"). All structures are congealed in the reactive process, culminating in a common scar (callus) with loss of structural independence.

The surgeon must individualize the treatment of complex hand injuries by considering such factors as age, occupation, hand dominance, economic status, cosmesis, emotional makeup, and general health. In other words, adequate salvage and maximal salvage are relative to the patient's needs, desires, and capacities. An extensive reconstructive effort is justified if, without it, there will be little or no function; but one must be careful not to destroy existing function and to spare the patient unwarranted disability and expense and disappointment by heroic efforts that might fail. It is sometimes best to remove part or all of the hand in the interest of the patient's overall psychologic and functional competence and productivity.

FOREIGN BODIES

Foreign bodies should be removed only if they interfere with function, threaten further tissue injury cause symptoms or anxiety, or result in dead space or infection. If removal is necessary, it is often facilitated by a period of observation and waiting (eg, 2–3 weeks) until congestion and bloody extravasation have cleared. In the meantime, the hand should be initially splinted, elevated, and, in some case, drained. Prophylactic antibiotics should be given. Roentgenograms are sometimes diagnostic.

Anderson MA, Newmeyer WL III, Kilgore ES Jr: Diagnosis and treatment of retained foreign bodies in the hand. Am J Surg 1982;144:63.

Russell RC et al: Detection of foreign bodies in the hand. J Hand Surg 1991;16:2.

AMPUTATION

Management of the Stump

The objective in treating an amputated part is to create a painless stump with soft tissue cover that will meet the functional needs of the patient and will have good sensibility and adequate stability and pliability. Digital amputation will either be transverse or will face obliquely to the dorsal, palmar, radial, or ulnar aspects of the digit (Figure 45–20). It may involve more than one phalanx.

When sufficient stump cover is not available locally, it must be obtained from grafts and flaps. The most predictable take is achieved by a thin (0.2–0.25 mm) split-thickness graft; this should always be the first choice if there is any doubt about blood supply, infection, or joint stiffness. Sutures are not needed

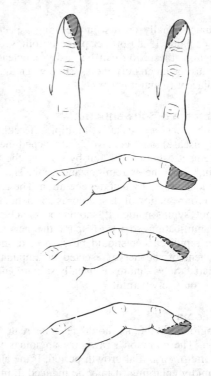

Figure 45–20. Distal digit amputation.

except in large grafts; however, initial immobilization and elevation of the wrist as well as the digit are vital in achieving a take of the graft.

Primary and secondary advancement or pedicle grafts should be considered when it is necessary to give better skin cover over palmar-oblique surfaces of all digits, the radial-oblique surface of the fingers, and the ulnar-oblique surface of the thumb (Figure 45–21); when one does not want to shorten digital bone or a transverse amputation surface; or when it is necessary to cover the body of the hand. Transverse digital stumps of infants will close by secondary intention with a result equal to or better than what can be achieved by surgery. In the case of the body of the hand, vascularized free flaps of muscle or skin are sometimes indicated.

Indications for Replantation

It is feasible to replant (revascularize) all or part of any amputated finger even to the level of the middistal phalanx, providing there is not excessive tissue destruction (eg, mangling). However, replantation may restore tissue perfusion but not always function, and the surgeon must consider each case carefully to decide whether replantation will benefit the patient and whether return of function can be achieved. Some patients may benefit from replantation for cosmetic reasons even if function cannot be restored. Factors to consider are age (especially physiologic

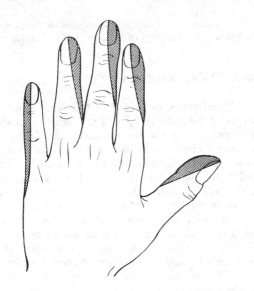

Figure 45–21. Areas requiring padded skin.

age), hand dominance, occupation, social and economic responsibilities, motivation, and ability to undergo the rehabilitative process.

Replantation should never be considered if the patient has severe coexisting injuries (eg, head trauma), significant chronic illness, or life threatening acute illness or if the amputated part is excessively crushed or mangled. Replantation should seldom be considered if the patient is over 50 years of age; if the extremity is severely contaminated, was avulsed rather than cut off, or had significant preexisting malfunction; if cooling of the amputated part has been delayed for 6 hours or more; or if only one finger is lost.

When the patient is referred to the replantation center, the amputated part should be immediately placed in a dressing inside a waterproof plastic bag that is surrounded with ice (not dry ice). The replantation surgeon should be notified immediately, and the patient should be told that the surgeon will determine the feasibility and advisability of replantation.

Ninety percent of replantations maintain viability. Failures occur in the first 2 weeks (50% in the first 4–5 days).

Indications for Amputation

Irreversible ischemia is the only absolute indication for amputation. The other major indication is where salvage of the digit or part of it will threaten the overall function of the hand, the extremity, or the patient. Such may be the case with an overwhelmingly injured or infected finger that is hopelessly stiff or painful and may jeopardize the function of the other good fingers, or with malignant tumor (eg, malignant melanoma).

Degloving Injuries

These injuries are usually caused by having a ring torn violently from a digit, eg, in falling from a fence and simultaneously hooking the ring on a prong. The skin, fat, and neurovascular bundles are ripped off, and flexor tendons may be avulsed along with the middle and distal phalanges. The other digits are usually not injured. The best treatment is usually to amputate. One has a choice of primary ray amputation through the metacarpal or amputation through the proximal phalanx. Salvage and reconstruction are possible only rarely and involve a great deal of time, with several major surgical procedures and some jeopardy to the function of adjacent normal digits.

Amputation of Rays III & IV

Amputation of the long or ring finger causes a gap through which material and liquids in the cupped hand will escape. This gap can be closed by removing the metacarpal at its proximal third (ray resection) and allowing the adjacent metacarpal heads to be approximated; or by the central transplantation of an adjacent osteotomized metacarpal onto the stump of the resected metacarpal (ray transfer). When the index, long, and ring fingers are gone, rotation osteotomy of the fifth metacarpal may be needed so that the small fingertip can comfortably oppose the thumb.

Thumb Amputation

Because most human skills are hampered by loss of part or all of the thumb, preservation, replantation, reconstruction, or replacement of a thumb has great functional merit. The prime objectives are the preservation of length, the proper placement for opposition, and provision of a stable strut against which the fingers can flex with force. Ideally, there should be sensibility where the thumb and fingers meet in pinch, and this can be provided with a neurovascular island pedicle transfer from the least important side of one of the fingers (eg, ulnar side of rays IV, III, or II or radial side or ray V). Not so urgent (but desirable) attainments are motion and power, particularly to control all the planes of movement of the MC joint. If this exists, bone-strutted tube pedicle thumb reconstruction—or a digital transfer (pollicization) on a neurovascular pedicle—can compensate remarkably for any loss. An alternative procedure is the free transfer of the first or second toe.

Prosthetic Devices

The loss of part or all of the hand can be compensated both functionally and cosmetically by a variety of prostheses. Their use involves careful adaptation to the requirements of the patient, who must receive appropriate training to ensure successs.

Doyle JR, Seitz WH Jr, McBride M: Replantation. Hand Clin 1989;5:415.

Feller AM, Graf P, Biemer E: Replantation surgery. World J Surg 1991;15:477.

Gaul JS, Nunley JA: Digital replantation. Surg Annu 1989;21:343.

Goldner RD, Urbaniak JR: Indications for replantation in the adult upper extremity. Occup Med 1989;4:525.

Iglesias M, Serrano A: Replantation of amputated segments after prolonged ischemia. Plast Reconstr Surg 1990; 85:425.

Terk KC et al: Replantation and revascularization of hands: Clinical analysis and functional results of 261 cases. J Hand Surg 1989;14:17.

Urbaniak JR: Replantation. In: *Operative Hand Surgery,* 2nd ed. Green DP (editor). Churchill Livingstone, 1988.

Whitney TM et al: Clinical results of bony fixation methods in digital replantation. J Hand Surg 1990;15:328.

WRINGER, CRUSH, & COMPRESSION INJURIES

In wringer injury, part or all of the extremity is dragged into and compressed by one or more machine-driven rollers. It is common in industries where rolls or sheets of material are drawn between rollers for threading, printing, or compressing purposes or where conveyor belts are used.

The arm is advanced until anatomic obstruction is met. Avulsion of skin and fat or a friction burn of the tissues (or both) may result. The thumb web is the first common obstruction, and the hand skin (more commonly, the loosely fixed dorsal skin) then becomes avulsed or burned. The next obstruction is the elbow, and the last the axilla.

Vessels, nerves, and muscles may be avulsed and bones may be dislocated or broken. The most common unrecognized complication is secondary congestion, which can lead to paralysis and severe muscle fibrosis (eg, Volkmann's contracture) and joint stiffness.

Most patients should be hospitalized, kept flat in bed with the extremity comfortably elevated, and observed hourly. Progressive throbbing pain leading to anesthesia and tightness of the skin and fascia sleeves of the finger, hand, or arm requires longitudinal slitting of skin and fascia. More than one muscle compartment may need decompression, and the pronator teres muscle and transverse carpal ligament must sometimes be sectioned to liberate the median nerve.

Skin avulsed by the wringer is usually in the form of a retrograde flap with imperiled circulation to it. One must judge the color by capillary filling of the flap; if this is poor or absent, debride all the fat from the flap and apply it as a full-thickness graft, or discard it completely in favor of a primary or delayed split-thickness skin graft. In most cases, fractures and dislocations should be reduced and aligned, but the overall circulation of the extremity is of more initial concern than definitive management of specific tissue and structural injuries. Abrasion burns are often third-degree and, if so, require debridement and grafting when the integrity of the circulation is restored.

INJECTION INJURIES

These injuries are caused by the sudden introduction of substances under high pressure (ie, hundreds or thousands of pounds per square inch). The substances include air or other gases; liquids such as water, paint, oil, and a host of chemicals in various solutions; and solids and semisolids such as grease and molten plastic. Accordingly, these accidents occur principally in industry. Air pressure hoses in gasoline service stations, aerosol bombs, and sandblast hoses are typical sources of gas-driven injuries. Paint guns, oil and grease guns, and nozzles that inject molten plastic at high temperatures (eg, 260 °C [500 °F]) are among the most common other sources of these injuries.

The history is the most important clue to the severity of the injury and the need for immediate treatment. While operating a high-pressure device, an individual suddenly feels a strange sensation which ranges from very painful to not painful at all. The patient may present a totally normal appearing hand with perhaps an almost undetectable pinpoint injection site; or the hand may be discolored or pale and cold, and tensely swollen due to the injected material.

Sometimes the injection is limited to a single digit, but often the great pressure forces the material to spread widely throughout the hand and even into the forearm. The greatest problems stem from the following: (1) The chemical irritant effect on all tissues, causing vascular thrombosis and toxic inflammation and necrosis. (2) The primary congestion effect of the material, leading within minutes or hours to secondary congestion due to the inflammatory response, all of which first interrupts microvascular venous flow and then leads to arterial arrest and gangrene. (3) Thermal burns (eg, from hot plastic). (4) Inability to remove enough of the offending material to forestall a short-term or long-term cicatricial foreign body response, which ultimately leads to fibrosis so extensive that it destroys the functions of sensation and mobility.

The examination should include an immediate x-ray to demonstrate, if possible, the distribution of material or gas in the hand; and a careful evaluation of sensibility, tenderness, induration, crepitation, color, temperature, and mobility. All such cases require immediate and continued unrelenting scrutiny, even if the part seems completely normal. With evidence of retained foreign material causing swelling, ischemia, or progressive throbbing pain, the hand must be immediately explored if for no other reason than to release the tourniquet effect of the skin and fascia induced by the congestion. It is impossible to remove all of the foreign material when it is widespread and invasive. As much should be removed as can be done by gentle scraping and teasing—and resecting that which lies in bloodless tissue—as long as one does not further damage the viable tissues to the point of greater congestion or ischemia and interfere with the normal process of demarcation and sequestration.

In addition to appropriate decompression and debridement, the hand must be drained and covered with compresses of zinc oxide, silver sulfadiazine, Ringer's solution, 0.5% silver nitrate solution, or povidone-iodine. The hand must be held in the posi-

tion of function and elevated, with the patient kept supine. Prophylactic antisludging agents (dextran 40), corticosteroids, antibiotics, and antitetanus medication must be administered. In most instances, hospitalization is urgent.

The objective is to minimize loss of function, and the most important initial effort must be to preserve circulation and avoid infection. If only one digit is involved and its functional fate is hopeless, amputation may be the most expeditious means of treatment.

REFERENCES

Amadio PC: Epidemiology of hand and wrist injuries in sports. Hand Clin 1990;6:379.

Bodell LS, Martin ML: Hand and wrist fractures in occupational medicine. Occup Med 1989;4:497.

Brand P: *Clinical Mechanics of the Hand.* Mosby, 1985.

Brandfonbrener AG: The epidemiology and prevention of hand and wrist injuries in performing artists. Hand Clin 1990;6:365.

Grabb WC, Smith JW: Hand and upper extremity plastic surgery. Part IV in: *Plastic Surgery: A Concise Guide to Clinical Practice,* 3rd ed, Little, Brown, 1980.

Green DP (editor): *Operative Hand Surgery,* 2nd ed. Churchill Livingstone, 1988.

Hunter JM et al: *Rehabilitation of the Hand,* 3rd ed. Mosby, 1990.

Lamb DW: *The Practice of Hand Surgery,* 2nd ed. Blackwell, 1989.

Lister G: *The Hand: Diagnosis and Indications,* 2nd ed. Churchill Livingstone, 1984.

Markison RE: Treatment of musical hands: Redesign of the interface. Hand Clin 1990;6:525.

Milford L: *The Hand,* 3rd ed. Mosby, 1988.

Omer GE Jr, Spinner M: *Management of Peripheral Nerve Problems.* Saunders, 1980.

Pitner MA: Pathophysiology of overuse injuries in the hand and wrist. Hand Clin 1990;6:355.

Prokop LL: Upper-extremity rehabilitation: conditioning and orthotics for the athlete and performing artist. Hand Clin 1990;6:517.

Teleisnik J: *The Wrist.* Churchill Livingstone, 1985.

Tubiana R: *The Hand.* Saunders, 1981–1988 (three volumes).

Watson N, Smith RJ: *Methods and Concepts in Hand Surgery.* Butterworths, 1986.

Wynn-Parry CB: *Rehabilitation of the Hand,* 4th ed. Butterworths, 1981.

Yoshimura M: Toe-to-hand transfer. Plast Reconstr Surg 1980;66:74.

46

Pediatric Surgery

Alfred A. deLorimier, MD, Michael R. Harrison, MD, & N. Scott Adzick, MD

CARE OF THE NEWBORN

Neonatal Intensive Care

The newborn infant with a surgically correctable lesion often has other disorders that threaten survival. The care of these babies—particularly the premature and small-for-gestational-age babies—has improved with the emergence of the intensive care nursery. Advances in the technology of infant monitoring and respiratory support have been dramatic. Tiny babies can receive ventilatory support from sophisticated infant respirators for prolonged periods in a precisely controlled microenvironment. Temperature is controlled by servoregulation, while pulse and blood pressure are continuously recorded. Ventilation is monitored by transcutaneous O_2 and CO_2 electrodes or by indwelling arterial catheters. The metabolic consequences of prematurity and intrauterine growth retardation are monitored by frequent measurement of glucose, calcium, electrolytes, and bilirubin in microliter quantities of blood. Nutritional requirements for growth and development can be provided by enteral or parenteral routes.

This kind of specialized care of critically ill newborns requires trained personnel and specialized equipment. The care of such babies is best accomplished in designated regional centers capable of providing pediatric surgical and neonatal intensive care.

Transportation of Newborn Surgical Patients

When transporting newborn infants for surgery, the following precautions must be observed: (1) Support normal body temperature by using an incubator maintained at 34 °C (93.2 °F) or by wrapping the baby in a plastic bag (or both). (2) Keep the airway clear by supplying a bulb syringe or suction device to aspirate mucus and vomitus. Intubate and ventilate the infant if there is impaired breathing. (3) Keep the stomach empty by giving nothing by mouth. Infants with intestinal obstruction should have a nasogastric tube placed in the stomach and should be aspirated at frequent intervals. (4) Provide intravenous glucose infusions to prevent hypoglycemia. An umbilical artery catheter inserted into the distal aorta may be used for monitoring blood gases. (5) Provide proper identification and pertinent medical information to be transported with the infant.

Determination of Gestational Age

Infants with surgically treatable lesions frequently weigh less than 2500 g. It is important to distinguish premature infants from intrauterine growth-retarded infants. Premature infants have a high incidence of hyaline membrane disease, whereas growth-retarded infants are subject to intrauterine asphyxia with meconium aspiration, pneumothorax, and hypoglycemia and frequently have major congenital anomalies. The gestational age of the infant is calculated from the date of the last normal menstrual period. The weight of the baby can be correlated with gestational age, and intrauterine growth retardation is defined as birth weight below the 25th percentile for gestational age. Clinical assessment of gestational age by morphologic and neurologic examination of the small infant is often more accurate than calculation from the menstrual history. Five signs may be useful in assessing gestational age. Infants of 36 weeks' gestational age or less have (1) fine fuzzy hair, (2) ears that lack cartilaginous support, (3) a breast nodule less than 3 mm in diameter, (4) testicles in the inguinal canal and a small scrotum with few rugae, and (5) skin on the feet with few transverse creases confined to the balls of the feet anteriorly.

Kliegman RM, Fanaroff AA: Developmental metabolism and nutrition. In: *Pediatric Anesthesiology* Gregory GA (editor). Churchill Livingstone, 1983.

Temperature Regulation

A. Simple Heat Loss: Infants and children have a relatively greater body surface area and a thinner subcutaneous fat layer than adults. Therefore, heat loss by conduction and radiation may be four times that of the adult. Infants respond to hypothermia by norepinephrine secretion, which increases the metabolic rate (particularly in the myocardium) and produces vasoconstriction with impaired tissue perfusion and increased lactic acid production. Hypothermia induces pulmonary vasoconstriction, resulting in right-to-left shunting in the ductus arteriosus and atrium, thus increasing hypoxia and acidosis. Shock and cardiac arrest may result. The neutral thermal environmental temperature is that temperature at which the oxygen consumption of the infant is minimal when the core temperature is normal, ie, when the gradient between the skin surface (particularly the face) and the environmental temperature is less than 1.5 °C (2.7 °F). The optimal environmental temperature is 34 °C (93.2 °F) (slightly higher for premature infants). Although environmental temperature can be servocontrolled from skin or rectal temperature, it is difficult to detect fever or hypothermia due to sepsis when this technique is used.

B. Effect of Drugs: Depressant and anesthetic drugs abolish the thermoregulatory response of the patient. Because environmental temperature is usually lower than body temperature (even in a heated operating room), body temperature falls. Hypothermia is associated with decreased oxygen consumption as long as the thermoregulatory mechanism is abolished by anesthesia. However, when anesthesia is discontinued and the body temperature is low, oxygen consumption must increase dramatically to correct the hypothermia, which is metabolically very expensive. High oxygen consumption during the interval when respiratory and cardiac responses are depressed can result in severe hypoxia, acidosis, and cardiorespiratory failure.

C. Prevention of Heat Loss: Infants should be transported to and from the x-ray department or operating room in a warm incubator, and the incubator temperature should be maintained when the baby is removed. In the operating room, the temperature of the infant must be continuously recorded by placing a thermistor in the rectum or esophagus. Body heat may be conserved by wrapping the extremities with sheet wadding and by using a circulating heating pad and infrared lamp, but these measures are often not enough in small infants. The operating room should be prewarmed and the temperature kept at about 20–27 °C (69–80.6 °F). Wet sponges and drapes exaggerate evaporative heat losses. Plastic drapes against the skin help contain body heat and keep the skin dry. When large volumes of blood are required, the blood should be warmed by circulating it through tubing immersed in warm water (37 °C [98.6 °F]) or prewarmed in the container before being transfused. One of the most effective means of regulating body temperature is to heat and humidify the gases during endotracheal anesthesia.

Coran AG: Perioperative care of the pediatric patient. Surg Annu 1991;1:315.
Donovan EF: Perioperative care of the surgical neonate. Surg Clin North Am 1985;65:1061.
Schwartz MZ et al: Complications of prematurity that may require surgical intervention. Arch Surg 1988;123:1135.
Warner BW et al: Multiple purpose central venous access in infants less than 1000 grams. J Perinat Med 1987;24:686.

Cardiorespiratory Management

A. Cardiorespiratory Resuscitation: Newborn infants with surgically treatable disease frequently are asphyxiated during birth. Causes of as-

phyxia include antepartum hemorrhage, prolonged labor, respiratory insufficiency due to aspiration pneumonitis, and congenital diaphragmatic hernia. The resulting hypoxia, hypercapnia, and acidosis produce generalized vasoconstriction. In particular, increased pulmonary vascular resistance occurs when the PO_2 falls below 50 mm Hg and the pH is less than 7.3. Normally, a right-to-left shunt of 20% of the cardiac output is present in newborn infants. During asphyxia, this shunt increases, and the existing hypoxia and acidosis may become greatly exaggerated. Cyanosis is an inadequate sign of hypoxia in the newborn, because fetal hemoglobin is 85% saturated at PO_2 levels of 42 mm Hg, whereas in the adult, hemoglobin is 85% saturated at PO_2 levels of 52 mm Hg. Therefore, in circumstances that produce asphyxia in the newborn, resuscitation must be accomplished before clinical signs are obvious.

At birth, the pharynx should be aspirated of mucus, amniotic fluid, or meconium. Respirations should be assisted or controlled with bag and mask, and prolonged respiratory support may require endotracheal intubation. A small air leak between the endotracheal tube and the airway is necessary to minimize laryngeal trauma. The required tube diameter may be 2.5–4 mm. The diameter of the tube should approximate that of the little finger or the nostril. The trachea from the glottis to the carina in the newborn is 5–7.5 cm long, and placement of the tube into the right or left bronchus must be avoided. An orotracheal tube is preferred to a nasotracheal one to minimize trauma and subsequent infection in the nasal passages. The ventilatory pressure must be carefully monitored to prevent rupture of the lung.

In the absence of abnormal diffusion or shunting, an inspired oxygen concentration of 40% will result in an arterial PO_2 of 110–116 mm Hg. The inspired oxygen concentration must be frequently monitored with an oxygen analyzer. Prolonged hyperoxia (arterial $PO_2 > 120$ mm Hg) may cause retrolental fibroplasia and pulmonary oxygen toxicity in premature infants. When an infant has pulmonary insufficiency and requires greater oxygen concentrations, with or without assisted ventilation, it is essential to repeatedly measure the arterial PO_2 and regulate the inspired oxygen concentration to keep the blood PO_2 between 60 and 80 mm Hg. Transcutaneous PO_2 electrodes and pulse oximetry make continuous monitoring of oxygen saturation possible.

The frequent monitoring of these infants is most easily accomplished by inserting a polyvinyl catheter through the umbilical artery into the distal aorta with the tip of the catheter positioned at L4 and confirmed radiographically. Indwelling arterial catheters can also be placed in the radial or temporal arteries either percutaneously or by cutdown. Blood pressure may be recorded by connecting the catheter to a strain gauge and recorder.

Respiratory acidosis is corrected by increasing alveolar ventilation; assisted ventilation will be needed if the P_{CO_2} exceeds 50 mm Hg. Metabolic acidosis is usually due to inadequate tissue perfusion because of hypovolemia or heart failure. If hypovolemia is present, volume replacement with lactated Ringer's solution or 5% albumin solution is indicated. A right atrial catheter can be used to monitor right heart pressure and detect adequate volume replacement or heart failure. If heart failure requires inotropic agents, their effectiveness will be enhanced by correcting acidosis. If the arterial pH is less than 7.2 and is primarily due to metabolic acidosis, sodium bicarbonate, 1–2 meq/kg, can be given slowly intravenously. After an equilibration period of 5–10 minutes, the pH and base deficit measurements should be repeated and the requisite amount of additional sodium bicarbonate given.

When asphyxia has been present for long periods, the resulting vasoconstriction may produce a decreased blood volume. Correction of hypoxia and acidosis can sometimes result in vasodilatation and hypovolemic shock. The blood volume must be replenished by transfusing lactated Ringer's solution, fresh frozen plasma, whole blood, or 5% albumin solution. The requirements for assisted ventilation, high oxygen concentrations, buffering, and volume replacement can be determined only by repeated evaluation of the patient's peripheral perfusion, blood pressure, right atrial pressure, urine output, and the P_{O_2}, P_{CO_2}, and pH status of the blood.

B. Assisted Ventilation: Following certain operations—particularly after thoracotomy or tight abdominal wall closure—lung volume is diminished and diaphragmatic motion greatly impaired. Assisted ventilation may be required for 24 hours or more.

This is best accomplished by firmly fixing an endotracheal tube in place and connecting it to either a modern infant ventilator or a system for continuous positive airway pressure (CPAP) breathing. CPAP breathing helps keep the terminal airways open and is particularly useful when alveolar collapse develops, such as in hyaline membrane disease or with persistent atelectasis. Chest percussion, instillation of saline into the endotracheal tube, and suctioning by careful sterile technique are necessary while the endotracheal tube is in place.

Most infant ventilators are time-cycled flow generators capable of delivering both CPAP and intermittent mandatory ventilation (IMV). IMV is a synthesis of simple mechanical ventilation and CPAP breathing that allows the baby to breathe independently between mandatory breaths provided by the ventilator while a continuous positive pressure is maintained on the airway.

The gas mixture flowing into the system should be carefully controlled by an air-oxygen mixing device, and the inspired oxygen concentration should be regulated to maintain the arterial P_{O_2} at 60–80 mm Hg. The gas should be humidified by using a heated neb-

ulizer. Absorption of fluid in the lung may be considerable, and parenteral fluid may have to be restricted. When the arterial P_{O_2} exceeds 80 mm Hg, the inspired oxygen concentration is gradually lowered toward room air, the end-expiratory pressure is lowered to 2 mm Hg, and the rate of IMV is then gradually decreased. In this way, the baby is gradually weaned from oxygen and mechanical ventilation, but CPAP of at least 2 mm Hg should be maintained until the endotracheal tube can finally be removed. Upon removal of the tube, the inspired oxygen concentration should be increased to 10% greater than that during the period of assistance until ventilation becomes normal.

C. Postoperative Position: Although the pain threshold of a young infant is quite high, the protective response to pain is to remain immobilized. The young infant breathes primarily with the diaphragm, and respiratory excursion becomes limited following the pain of an operative incision in the chest or abdomen. Therefore, it is important to rotate the young infant from side to side at least every hour to prevent atelectasis. It is usually necessary to restrain the arms to prevent dislodgment of the nasogastric and intravenous tubes. When the arms are restrained, it must be done in the lateral position with the two arms together—the arms must never be restrained on opposite sides of the crib, because the baby might aspirate vomitus.

Blood Loss & Replacement

A. Determination of Blood Loss: Defects in the coagulating mechanism may occur in newborn infants as a result of vitamin K deficiency, thrombocytopenia, and temporary hepatic insufficiency due to immaturity, asphyxia, or infection. Before operation, newborn infants should receive vitamin K_1, 1–2 mg intravenously or intramuscularly. If an extensive surgical procedure is anticipated, freshly drawn blood should be typed and cross-matched in case transfusion is required.

The blood volume of a newborn infant ranges from 50 to 100 mL/kg body weight (average, 85 mL/kg). This wide variation is due principally to the timing and technique of clamping the umbilical cord. By 1 month of age, premature and full-term infants have a blood volume of approximately 75 mL/kg.

The blood lost during operation varies greatly according to the extent of the operative procedure, the disease being treated, and the effectiveness of hemostasis. Mild blood loss, amounting to less than 10% of the blood volume, usually does not require transfusion. In a 3.5-kg infant, mild blood loss would be a volume up to 30 mL. Because blood loss greater than 10% should be corrected and because these volumes are quite small, it is imperative to develop methods for closely monitoring the amount of blood lost during operation. Dry sponges should be used and weighed shortly after use to minimize error from evaporation. The suction line, connected to a calibrated trap on the operating table, should be short to diminish the dead space of the tubing and to provide immediate data about accumulated blood loss. Visual observation may be used as a rough guide, but it tends to give a falsely low estimate of the loss.

B. Replacement of Blood Loss: Whenever an operation results in blood loss greater than 10% of blood volume, an indwelling plastic catheter must be placed in a vein and secured to prevent dislodgment under drapes. Procedures associated with loss of more than 20% of blood volume should be preceded by a venous catheter with the catheter tip directed into the right atrium. This catheter should be connected to a manometer for measuring central venous pressure and a three-way stopcock for taking samples for blood gas and pH measurements. Arterial pressure should be monitored by a Doppler blood pressure cuff on the arm. An umbilical artery catheter should be placed in the distal aorta of the newborn infant for continuous display of pressure. A transverse abdominal incision can be made above the umbilicus without interfering with the catheter.

In infants with hematocrits greater than 50%, blood loss may be replaced by infusing lactated Ringer's solution or fresh frozen plasma to compensate for losses of up to 25% of total blood volume. Greater blood losses should be replaced with freshly drawn whole blood or packed red cells. A transfusion of packed red blood cells at a volume of 10 mL/kg usually raises the hematocrit 3–4%. Transfusion of old blood may result in cardiac arrest and death as a result of hyperkalemia, hypocalcemia, acidosis, hypothermia, and air embolism. The transfused blood should be prewarmed to body temperature by running it through coiled tubing immersed in water at 37 °C (98.6 °F).

Citrate-phosphate-dextrose (CPD) is a better blood preservative because it maintains the carrying capacity and release of oxygen for a longer period than acid-citrate-dextrose (ACD) preservatives. After transfusion, metabolism of the citrate to bicarbonate may cause metabolic alkalosis. Heparinized blood diminishes the metabolic complications of ACD blood, but protamine sulfate may be required to correct a prolonged clotting time. Hypocalcemia—produced by complexing calcium with citrate—may be treated by giving 2 mL of 10% calcium gluconate for each 100 mL of CPD blood transfused.

With excessive blood loss, clotting factors and platelets can be depleted rapidly, and fresh frozen plasma and platelets of identical blood type should be available. A transfusion of 0.1 unit/kg of platelets raises the platelet count by approximately 25,000/μL.

Humidity

A high environmental humidity may be desired to liquefy viscid pulmonary secretions or to treat croup. An ultrasonically generated mist is the only effective means of getting water droplets as far as the larynx or upper trachea. The mist should be delivered through a face mask, hood, or incubator. Infants can absorb a significant volume of ultrasonic mist water, and they may develop pulmonary edema if not carefully monitored. Infants with an endotracheal tube or a tracheostomy must be given humidified gases to breathe.

Overgrowth of bacteria such as *Pseudomonas* will occur in the mist generator and incubator within a short time. Therefore, the incubator and generator should be changed and cleaned at least every 2 days. The fluid requirements of these babies are greatly decreased when high humidification is used. Body temperature may rise as a result of heat retention in an environment with high humidity.

Dziedzie K, Vidyasagar D: Pulse oximetry in neonatal intensive care. Clin Perinatol 1989;16:177.

FLUID & ELECTROLYTE MANAGEMENT

Fluid and electrolyte therapy requires a knowledge of normal basic requirements, preexisting deficits, and continuing losses (see Chapter 9). Special pediatric considerations are as follows.

Requirements for Newborn Infants

Normally, 5–10% of a newborn infant's birth weight is lost in the first 3–7 days. Part of the weight lost is meconium, vernix, and urine; however, the major component is excess total body water. During the first 4 days on oral feedings, a normal newborn infant will have a urine volume of 20–30 mL/kg/d and an insensible water loss of 20–25 mL/kg/d. The total urinary excretion of sodium, potassium, and chloride is less than 0.9 meq/kg. Oliguria and a shift in the potassium/nitrogen ratio due to increased aldosterone secretion do not occur following stress in the first few weeks of life. A sodium-excreting factor following stress has been postulated, since urinary retention of sodium and chloride does not occur when there are large extrarenal losses of these ions. The usual amount of water given during the first 4 days after birth is 80 mL/kg/d. However, when a newborn infant is cared for under infrared heat, the additional insensible water losses will increase requirements to 100–130 mL/kg/d. Normally, the maximum tolerance for sodium and chloride is 1.5 meq/kg/d; for potassium, 1 meq/kg/d. Therefore, maintenance fluid following operative procedures with small third-space losses performed in the first 4 days after birth should consist of 10% dextrose in 0.2% saline, given at a rate of 50–80 mL/kg/d. Potassium chloride or bicarbonate, 15 meq/L, and calcium gluconate, 200–400 mg/kg/d, are usually added to the solution. Additional potassium, calcium, bicarbonate, and glucose may be added according to the results of blood chemistry determinations and the clinical status of the patient. Following an operation such as laparotomy or thoracotomy, the fluid requirement may exceed 150 mL/kg/d for 2–3 days postoperatively. When these larger third-space losses occur, 5% dextrose in lactated Ringer's solution should be given.

Many stressed newborn infants develop low blood levels of potassium, calcium, magnesium, and glucose. A deficiency of any one of these will produce such signs as vomiting, abdominal distention, poor feeding, apneic spells, cyanosis, limpness, eye rolling, high-pitched cry, tremors, or convulsions. Convulsions and tetany due to hypocalcemia should be treated with intravenous 10% calcium solution (chloride, lactate, or gluconate) given at a rate of 1 mL/min while the ECG or heart sounds are being carefully monitored. Although hypocalcemia can be largely eliminated by adding calcium salts to intravenous solutions, caution is required, since subcutaneous infiltration may produce severe vasoconstriction and skin necrosis.

Hypoglycemia occurs frequently in infants with intrauterine growth retardation, respiratory distress, asphyxia, or central nervous system abnormalities. Hypoglycemia is defined as a blood glucose less than 20 mg/dL in the premature or low-birth-weight infant; less than 30 mg/dL in full-sized infants within the first 72 hours after birth; and less than 40 mg/dL thereafter in full-term infants. The treatment of hypoglycemia consists of giving 50% glucose, 1–2 mL/kg intravenously, followed by a continuous infusion of 10–15% glucose solutions at a rate equivalent to that needed for maintenance water requirements.

Requirements for Older Infants & Children

Three methods are available for determining the physiologic limits for water, based upon (1) total body weight, (2) body surface area, and (3) calculated basal caloric expenditure related to body weight.

The simplest method is to calculate fluid replacements on the basis of body weight. Daily maintenance fluid and electrolyte requirements are summarized in Table 46–1 and Figure 46–1. Maintenance requirements per kilogram decrease with increasing size. The physiologic limits of water replacement are 35 mL/kg above or below the mean daily requirements. Determining basal requirements on the basis of body surface area or caloric expenditure requires additional calculations. Surface area must be determined from nomograms by knowing the height and weight of the patient. With this method, 1500 mL/m^2/d is considered the usual minimum water requirement, with a physiologic range of 1200–3500 mL/m^2/d. In the caloric system, the minimum water requirement is considered to be 100 mL/100 kcal expended. The basic caloric requirements related to weight are as follows: up to 10 kg, 100 kcal/kg; 10–20 kg, 1000 kcal for the first 10 kg plus 50 kcal for each kilogram above 10; over 20 kg, 1500 kcal for the first 20 kg plus 20 kcal/kg over 20 kg. Additional

Table 46–1. Maintenance requirements.

Age: Size		Premature[1] <3 kg	Infants 3–10 kg	Children 11–20 kg	Children <20 kg
Water	(mL/kg/ 24 h)	125–150	100–125	75–100	40–75
Sodium	(meq/kg/ 24 h)	1–2	1–3	1–3	1–2
Potassium	(meq/kg/ 24 h)	1–2	1–3	1–3	1–2
Calories	(kcal/kg/ 24 h)	>125	>100	>75	>40
Protein	(g/kg/ 24 h)	3–4	3–3.5	2.5–3	1–2.5
Urinary output	(mL/kg/ 24 h)	1–3	1–3	1–3	1–3

[1]Newborns of any size require only half of the normal maintenance amounts for the first 1–2 days.

water should be given according to the state of hydration, body temperature, and estimated caloric expenditure above basal activity.

The normal daily sodium requirement is usually 1–3 meq/kg, but it may vary from 0.5 to 5 meq/kg in extreme cases. The usual range of potassium required is the same as that of sodium. The large reserve of calcium and magnesium in bone makes short-term intravenous replacement unnecessary except in cases requiring prolonged parenteral nutrition.

Continuing Losses

Continuing losses such as gastric juice, ileostomy output, pleural fluid, and third-space fluid must be replaced as rapidly as they occur, preferably within 4–8 hours. The electrolyte composition of some body fluids and solutions for replacement are shown in Table 46–2. During operative procedures, third-space losses in the injured serosal surfaces, bowel wall, and lumen should be replaced by giving lactated Ringer's solution, 5–15 mL/kg/h; the amount to be given depends upon the magnitude of the operative procedure. Eight to 24 hours postoperatively, 5% dextrose in Ringer's lactate is continued at a rate calculated to be 30–50% greater than average maintenance.

The status of hydration, the intake and output, and the weight of infants and small children should be assessed at frequent intervals. The orders for intravenous fluids should be rewritten at least every 8 hours.

When these ranges of tolerance for fluid and electrolytes are known, polyionic solutions can be made using concentrated electrolyte solutions. The volume of a repair solution is usually given at a rate close to maximal tolerance, and the glucose content should therefore be 5% to prevent osmotic diuresis. Maintenance solutions can be made with 10% glucose.

Preexisting Deficits

Existing deficits from external fluid losses such as vomiting, diarrhea, and third-space losses into the

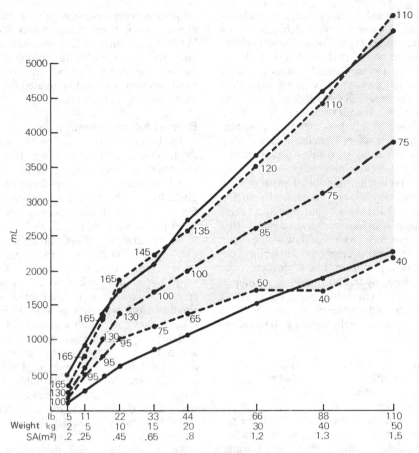

Figure 46–1. Comparison of two methods of calculating intravenous fluid requirements. Solid lines show the maximum (3000 mL/m^2) and minimum (1200 mL/m^2) fluid requirements by surface area. The broken lines show the mean (mL/kg) and the range (35 mL/kg) from the mean total fluid requirements. The surface area system underestimates the requirements in infants weighing less than 10 kg, probably because of errors in the nomograms.

Table 46–2. Replacement of abnormal losses of fluids and electrolytes.

Type of Fluid	Electrolyte Content				Replacement
	Na$^+$ (meq/L)	K$^+$ (meq/L)	Cl$^-$ (meq/L)	HCO$_3^-$ (meq/L)	
Gastric (vomiting)	50(20–90)	10(4–15)	90(50–150)	...	5% Dextrose in half-normal (0.45%) saline plus KCl 20–40 meq/L
Small bowel (ileostomy)	110(70–140)	5(3–10)	100(70–130)	20(10–40)	Lactated Ringer's
Diarrhea	80(10–140)	25(10–60)	90(20–120)	40(30–50)	Lactated Ringer's with or without HCO$_3^-$
Bile	145(130–160)	5(4–7)	100(80–120)	40(30–50)	Lactated Ringer's with or without HCO$_3^-$
Pancreatic	140(130–150)	5(4–7)	80(60–100)	80(60–110)	Lactated Ringer's with or without HCO$_3^-$
Sweat Normal	20(10–30)	4(3–10)	20(10–40)	...	...
Cystic fibrosis	90(50–130)	15(5–25)	90(60–120)	...	...

bowel lumen, peritoneal cavity, or large wounds require replacement. Patients with dehydration or shock will require rapid expansion of blood volume. A catheter should be placed in the right atrium via the jugular or subclavian vein. Central venous pressure, blood pH, and blood gases may be constantly monitored from this catheter. Lactated Ringer's solution, normal saline, or 5% albumin solution in amounts of 10–20 mL/kg should be given as rapidly as possible, while the right atrial pressure is maintained below 15 cm of water. If anemia exists, whole blood is substituted for these solutions as soon as the type and crossmatch are done. Following this initial expansion of the blood volume, rehydration is continued with 5% dextrose in lactated Ringer's solution at the maximum physiologically tolerated rate until a rise in central venous pressure occurs or urine flow has been established. Clinical improvement is determined by examination of skin perfusion, blood pressure, central venous pressure, hydration, pulse, urine output and specific gravity, hematocrit, blood electrolytes, arterial blood gases, and arterial pH.

Replacement of sodium deficits may also be calculated as follows:

$$\text{Sodium needed (meq)} = \left(\frac{140 - \text{Patient's}[Na^+]_s}{(\text{meq})} \right) \times \frac{60\% \text{ of body wt}}{(\text{kg})}$$

If dehydration is also present, sodium should be replaced by using normal saline solution. Hyponatremia associated with abnormal retention of water (edema) should be treated by restriction of water intake. Albumin replacement and diuretics may accelerate reversal of low serum sodium and edema fluid formation.

Significant acidosis (serum HCO_3^- > 3–15 meq/L or base deficit > 8) should be corrected with sodium bicarbonate. The replacement requirement is calculated by multiplying the base deficit (meq/L) by the estimated extracellular volume (30% total body weight in kilograms). The result is the required number of milliequivalents of $NaHCO_3$ that must be given intravenously over a period of 8–24 hours. A bolus injection of $NaHCO_3$ must be given slowly and must not exceed 1 meq/kg. If the magnitude of acidosis is known only by the serum bicarbonate level, a rule of thumb for $NaHCO_3$ replacement (in a concentration of 44.5 meq/50 mL) is 4 mL/kg, to raise the serum HCO_3^- by 5 meq/L.

Coran A, Drongowski R: Body fluid compartment changes following neonatal Surgery. J Pediatr Surg 1989;24:829.

NUTRITION

An infant requires calories at a rate of 100–150 kcal/kg/24 h and protein at a rate of 2–3 g/kg/24 h to achieve a normal weight gain of 10–15 g/kg/24 h (Table 46–1). These requirements decline with age but increase with sepsis, stress, and trauma. The catabolic state associated with prolonged starvation and the increased energy expenditures accompanying surgical conditions should be treated by providing adequate calories and protein.

Enteral Alimentation

The best means of providing calories and protein is through the gastrointestinal tract. If the gastrointestinal tract is functional, standard infant formulas, blenderized meals, or prepared elemental diets can be given by mouth, through nasogastric or nasojejunal feeding tubes, or through gastrostomy or jejunostomy tubes placed surgically.

The availability of nutritionally complete liquid diets of low viscosity allows continuous feeding through small-diameter catheters. Elemental diets made by mixing crystalline amino acids, oligosaccharides, and fats can be completely absorbed in the small intestine with little residue. Their use is limited because they cause diarrhea as a result of the high osmolality of full-strength formulas. This can be avoided by administering dilute solutions by continuous drip. Initially, the volume of dilute solution is gradually increased, and the concentration is then progressively increased in stepwise fashion—ie, half strength, two-thirds strength, three-fourths strength, and full strength. Formulas that remain below 500 mosm are best.

Small Silastic or polyethylene catheters such as those used for intravenous infusion can be passed through the nose or mouth into the stomach or jejunum and are well tolerated for long periods. These small catheters can also be placed in the stomach or jejunum surgically and brought through the abdominal wall for postoperative feeding. Silastic is superior to other plastics because it does not become more rigid when exposed to intestinal contents. Parenteral nutrition combined with enteral feeding is often necessary for infants with short bowel syndromes until intestinal adaptation occurs.

Parenteral Alimentation
(See also Chapter 10.)

The indications for parenteral alimentation include the following: (1) expected period of prolonged ileus, eg, following repair of gastroschisis or jejunal atresia; (2) intestinal fistulas; (3) supplementation of oral feedings, as in intractable diarrhea, short bowel syndrome, or various malabsorption syndromes; (4) intrauterine growth-retarded infants; (5) catabolic wasting states such as infections or tumors when gastric feedings are inadequate; and (6) treatment of necrotizing enterocolitis in infants who have feedings withheld for a prolonged time.

Concentrated solutions (> 15% glucose) thrombose peripheral vessels. Placement of a catheter into the superior vena cava or right atrium allows the large blood flow to dilute the solution immediately. The catheter may be placed percutaneously through the subclavian or internal jugular vein, or by cutdown over the external jugular, anterior facial, internal jugular, cephalic, or brachial vein. This should be performed with strict aseptic technique. The catheter should be of inert material such as Silastic tubing. The catheter should be sutured to the skin to prevent accidental dislodgment. Tunneling the catheter subcutaneously with a separate exit point on the chest wall may decrease the risk of infection. For long-term use, Broviac or Hickman catheters, with Dacron cuffs positioned at the exit site of the skin, are preferred to minimize infection and to prevent accidental dislodgment. The dressing should be changed daily and cleansed with iodine solution.

Intravenous alimentation solutions containing an amino acid source (2–5% crystalline amino acids or protein hydrolysate), glucose (10–40%), electrolytes, vitamins, and trace minerals are used. The electrolyte composition of the protein solution should be known, so that the desired composition of the final solution can be adjusted by appropriate additives according to the individual patient's requirements. A standard solution suitable for infants and young children must contain calcium, magnesium, and phosphate to allow for growth. Trace minerals are also added to the basic solution (Table 46–3).

These concentrated solutions must be infused at a constant rate with an infusion pump to avoid blood backing up the catheter and clotting and to prevent wide fluctuations of blood glucose and amino acid concentrations. To provide adequate calories, the volume of infusion is usually above that of maintenance water requirements. If it is necessary to restrict the volume of infusion, more concentrated glucose solutions can be made.

Complications of prolonged intravenous alimentation are numerous. The most frequent problem is sepsis, and immediate removal of the catheter usually results in prompt clinical improvement. Accidental dislodgment of the catheter is a problem that can be prevented by careful fixation with skin sutures and taping. Clotting in the catheter might be controlled by adding 1 unit of heparin per milliliter of solution. Emphasis on a constant rate of infusion will minimize hyper- or hypoglycemia. Analysis of serum electrolytes (including Ca^{2+} and PO_4^{3-}) may be necessary several times a week initially, but the interval is decreased to once a week when the patient is stable. Patients must be observed for ammonia intoxication and for vitamin or trace mineral deficiency.

These solutions are deficient in linoleic acid, an essential fatty acid. Linoleic acid deficiency is characterized by thrombocytopenia; thin, scaly, flushed skin; and a peculiarly firm subcutaneous fat. This can be prevented by giving Intralipid intravenously. Zinc deficiency presents as an exfoliative dermatitis involving the face, groin, fingers, and skin creases. It mimics acrodermatitis enteropathica. It can be corrected by adding more zinc to the solution. Progressive hepatomegaly and jaundice of uncertain origin occur after prolonged parenteral alimentation. This syndrome usually subsides when the parenteral solution is discontinued or when it is infused for a period of 12–14 hours and then the infusion is stopped for 8–12 hours.

The risks of central venous catheterization can be avoided by using less concentrated solutions of amino acids (2–3%) and glucose (< 12%) in combination with an emulsified fat solution (Intralipid) given through peripheral veins. Intralipid is a 10% or 20% soybean oil emulsified to 0.5 μm, stabilized with 1.2% egg yolk phospholipids, and 2.25% glycerin is added to make the solution isotonic. Intralipid contains 110 kcal/dL of solution. The solution contains 54% linoleic acid, an essential fatty acid. It may be given alone or concurrently with an amino acid–glucose solution through a side arm of the intravenous cannula placed close to the venous puncture site to minimize destabilization of the emulsion. Infusion pumps must be used to administer Intralipid as well as the standard solution to ensure the proper rate of infusion and to prevent one solution from backing up into the other. Intralipid 10% is started at a rate of 0.5 g/kg/d and is gradually increased to 4 g/kg/d. Infusions in excess of this may result in the fat overload syndrome: lipemic blood, seizures, congestive failure, hepatosplenomegaly with jaundice and abnormal liver function, thrombocytopenia, and renal failure. Large infusion volumes may be necessary to provide adequate calories through peripheral vessels. When peripheral vascular access is limited and infusion is frequently interrupted, caloric replacement by peripheral vein becomes less than optimal. For this reason, peripheral alimentation is most useful when the anticipated needs are short-term.

Chwals W et al: Measured energy expenditure in critically ill infants and young children. J Surg Res 1988;44:467.

Groner J, Brown M, Stallings V: Resting energy expenditure in children following major operative procedures. J Pediatr Surg 1989;24:825.

Holcomb GW 3d, Ziegler MM Jr: Nutrition and cancer in children. Surg Annu 1990;2:129.

Pierro A et al: Metabolism of intravenous fat emulsion in the surgical newborn. J Pediatr Surg 1989;24:95.

Ross P et al: Thrombus associated with central venous catheters in infants and children. J Pediatr Surg 1989;24:253.

Taylor L, O'Neill JA Jr: Total parenteral nutrition in the pediatric patient. Surg Clin North Am 1991;71:477.

Winthrop A et al: Analysis of energy and macronutrient balance in the postoperative infant. J Pediatr Surg 1989;24:686.

Table 46–3. Parenteral nutrition in infants and children.

Requirements		Solutions
Water	40–150 mL/kg/d	Amino acid solutions: final protein concentration of 2–4 g/dL.
Calories	40–150 kcal/kg/d	Dextrose in water: final dextrose concentration of 10–40 g/dL.
Protein	1–4 g/kg/d	Intravenous fat emulsion (Intralipid): commercially available; give 1–4
Nonprotein calories as glucose and fat to provide calorie:nitrogen ratio of 150–200:1		g/kg over 12–15 hours. Example of a standard solution: 2% amino acids in 35% dextrose in water plus Intralipid. This combination has a calorie:nitrogen ratio of 110:1.
Electrolytes		Electrolytes are ordered daily according to serum electrolyte levels and clinical picture. Amounts shown are examples of final concentrations in a standard solution; these can be adjusted with acetate by the pharmacist. Calcium and phosphate precipitation is determined by the protein content of the solution. For a 2.1–3% amino acid solution, the following calcium and phosphate concentrations are recommended:
Sodium	2–4 meq/kg/d	40 meq/L
Chloride	2–4 meq/kg/d	40 meq/L
Potassium	1–4 meq/kg/d	30 meq/L
Phosphate	0.4–3 meq/kg/d (0.5–1 mmol/kg/d)	20 meq/L
Calcium	0.5–3 meq/kg/d	8 meq/L
Magnesium	0.15–1 meq/kg/d	8 meq/L

	Ca(meq/L)	18	15	12	20	8	5
	PO$_4$(mmol/L)	5	6	8	10	15	40

Requirements		Solutions
Vitamins		Amounts shown are contained in a 5-mL vial of commercially available multivitamin infusion (M.V.I.). Add 2 mL to each liter of standard solution.
Vitamin A	1500–5000 IU/d	10,000 USP units
Vitamin C	35–60 IU/d	400 mg
Vitamin D	400 IU/d	1000 USP units
Vitamin E	5–30 IU/d	5 IU
Thiamine	0.3–2 mg/d	50 mg
Riboflavin	0.4–1.7 mg/d	10 mg
Pyridoxine	0.4–2 mg/d	15 mg
Niacin	5–20 mg/d	100 mg
Pantothenic acid	3–10 mg/d	25 mg
Vitamin K	...	2 mg/L	These vitamins may be added to standard solution in the concentrations shown or may be given separately.
Vitamin B$_{12}$	1–6 µg/d	10 µg/L
Folic acid	0.05–0.4 mg/d	0.5 mg/L
Biotin	35–200 µg/dL	50 µg/L
Trace Minerals		At left is an example of a stock additive solution prepared by the pharmacist to yield the indicated concentrations of elementary mineral per liter of standard solution. A commercially available product, Pediatric Trace Element Concentrate, can be used; 0.2 mL provides 100 µg of zinc, 20 mµ of copper, 6 µg of manganese, and 0.17 µg of chromium. The recommended dose of this product is 0.2 mL/kg/d.
Zinc	20–40 µg/kg/d	3 mg
Copper	15–20 µg/kg/d	1 mg
Manganese	5–20 µg/kg/d	1 mg
Chromium	0.2–0.5 µg/kg/d	0.03 mg
Iodine	5 µg/kg/d	0.5 mg
Fluoride	1 µg/kg/d	0.1 mg
Iron	0.1–0.2 mg/kg/d	5 mg/L in solution (or give intramuscularly weekly).
Linoleic acid	4% of total calories to prevent fatty acid deficiency.	Intralipid, 1–4 g/kg/d

LESIONS OF THE HEAD & NECK

DERMOID CYSTS

Dermoid cysts are congenital inclusions of skin and appendages commonly found on the scalp and eyebrows and in the midline of the nose, neck, and upper chest. They present as painless swellings that may be completely mobile or fixed to the skin and deeper structures. Dermoid cysts of the eyebrows and scalp may produce a depression in the underlying bone that appears as a smooth, punched-out defect on radiographs of the skull. These cysts contain a cheesy material that is produced by desquamation of the cells of the epithelial lining. Dermoid cysts of the neck may be confused with thyroglossal duct cysts, but they usually do not move with swallowing or protrusion of the tongue as thyroglossal cysts do. Dermoid cysts should be excised intact, since incomplete removal will result in recurrence. Those arising on the eyebrows should be excised through an incision within the hairline. The eyebrows should not be shaved.

BRANCHIOGENIC ANOMALIES

Branchiogenic anomalies include sinuses, cysts, cartilaginous rests, cervical fistulas (Figure 46–2), and cervical cysts. These lesions are remnants of the branchial apparatus present during the first month of fetal life. The primitive neck develops four external clefts and four pharyngeal pouches that are separated by a membrane. Between the clefts and pouches are branchial arches.

Preauricular sinuses, cysts, and cartilaginous rests probably arise from anomalous development of the auricle. Fistulas that arise above the hyoid bone and communicate with the external auditory canal represent persistence of the first branchial cleft. Fistulas that communicate between the anterior border of the sternocleidomastoid muscle and the tonsillar fossa are of second branchial origin, and those that extend into the piriform sinus are derived from the third branchial pouch. Fourth branchial fistulas have not been described.

A tract of branchial origin may form a complete fistula, or one end may be obliterated to form an external or internal sinus, or both ends may resorb, leaving an aggregate of cells forming a cyst. First branchial cleft tracts are always lined by squamous epithelium based on thick connective tissue. Cysts and sinuses of second or third branchial origin are lined by squamous, cuboidal, or ciliated columnar epithelium. Cervical fistulas and cysts have a prominent lymphoid stroma beneath the epithelial lining that may contain germinal centers and Hassall's corpuscles.

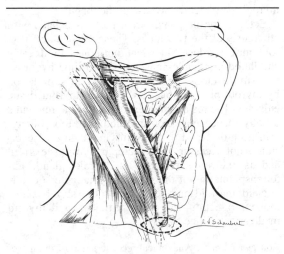

Figure 46–2. Branchiogenic fistula from second branchial cleft origin. The fistula extends along the anterior border of the sternocleidomastoid muscle and courses between the internal and external carotid arteries and cephalad to the hypoglossal nerve to enter the tonsillar fossa.

Clinical Findings

In the preauricular area, the anomalies may take the form of cysts, sinuses, skin tags, or cartilaginous nubbins. A sinus or fistulous opening along the anterior border of the sternocleidomastoid muscle is readily seen at birth and usually discharges a mucoid or purulent material. The patient may complain of a foul-tasting discharge in the mouth upon massaging the tract, but the internal orifice is rarely recognized. Lateral cervical cysts without an external sinus are usually not recognized in childhood but become evident in young adulthood. The cysts are characteristically found anterior and deep to the upper third of the sternocleidomastoid muscle, or they may be located within the parotid gland or pharyngeal wall, over the manubrium, or in the mediastinum. Branchiogenic anomalies occur with equal frequency on each side of the neck, and 10% are bilateral.

Differential Diagnosis

Granulomatous lymphadenitis due to mycobacterial infections may produce cystic lymph nodes and draining sinuses, but these are usually distinguishable by the chronic inflammatory reaction that preceded the purulent discharge. Hemangiomas, cystic hygromas, and lymphangiomas are soft, spongy tumor masses that might be confused with cervical cysts, but the latter have a firmer consistency. Cystic hygromas and lymphangiomas transilluminate, and cervical cysts do not. Carotid body tumors are quite firm, are located at the carotid bifurcation, and occur in older patients. Lymphomas produce firm masses in the area where branchial remnants occur, but multiple, matted nodes rather than a solitary cystic tumor distinguish these lesions. Mucoid material may be expressed from the openings of branchial sinuses or fistulas, and a firm cordlike tract may be palpable along its course.

Complications

The sinuses and cysts are prone to become repeatedly infected, producing cellulitis and abscesses. Very rarely, carcinoma may occur.

Treatment & Prognosis

Superficial skin tags and cartilaginous rests can be easily excised under sedation and local anesthesia. Preauricular sinus tracts may be very deceptive in their extent, and the surgeon should be prepared to proceed with extensive dissection under general anesthesia to completely excise these lesions. General anesthesia is required for proper excision of branchial fistulas and cysts. Cervical cysts are excised through transverse incisions directly over the mass.

Infected sinuses and cysts require initial incision and drainage. Perform excision of these tracts only when the acute inflammatory reaction has subsided.

Lin J-N, Wang KL: Persistent third branchial apparatus. J Pediatr Surg 1991;26:663.

Sonnino RE et al: Unusual pattern of congenital neck masses in children. J Pediatr Surg 1989;24:966.

Toi O et al: Branchial remnants: A review of 58 cases. J Pediatr Surg 1988;23:789.

THYROGLOSSAL DUCT REMNANTS

The thyroid gland develops from an evagination in the floor of the primitive pharynx, between the first pair of pharyngeal pouches, during the fourth week of gestation. If the anlage of the thyroid does not descend normally, the thyroid gland may form in the tongue or remain as a mass anywhere in the midline of the neck from the submandibular fossa to the pretracheal area. If the thyroglossal duct persists, the tract forms a cyst that usually communicates with the foramen cecum of the tongue. The thyroglossal duct descends through the second branchial arch anlage, the hyoid bone, prior to its fusion in the midline. Because of this, the tract of a persistent thyroglossal duct usually extends through the hyoid bone (Figure 46–3).

Thyroid follicles may be found in 30–40% of specimens. Three or more tracts are frequently present between the thyroglossal cysts and the base of the tongue.

Clinical Findings

The most common finding is a rounded, cystic mass of varying size in the midline of the neck just below the hyoid bone. The acute inflammatory reaction of an infection may herald the presence of a cyst. The fluid content of the cyst is usually under pressure and may give the impression of a solid tumor. Cysts and aberrant midline thyroid glands move with swallowing and with protrusion of the tongue. When a solid midline mass is detected, evidence of athyreosis should be sought, such as hypothyroidism and absence of the palpable lateral lobes of the normal thyroid.

Differential Diagnosis

Only lymph nodes, dermoid cysts, and enlarged delphian nodes containing metastases are confused with thyroglossal remnants in the midline of the neck. Dermoid cysts do not move with swallowing. Lingual thyroids may be confused with hypertrophied lingual tonsil or with a dermoid cyst, fibroma, angioma, sarcoma, or carcinoma of the tongue. These lesions and thyroglossal cysts may be distinguished from aberrantly located thyroid glands by needle aspiration or by radioiodine scintiscan.

Complications

Lingual thyroid glands may produce dysphagia, dysphonia, dyspnea, hemorrhage, or pain. Carcinoma develops more frequently in ectopic thyroid tissue than in normal thyroid glands. Thyroglossal cysts are prone to become infected, and spontaneous drainage or incision and drainage of an abscess will result in a chronically draining fistula. Excision of an ectopic thyroid usually removes all remaining thyroid tissue, producing subsequent hypothyroidism.

Treatment

Acute infection in thyroglossal tracts should be treated with local heat and antibiotics. Abscesses should be incised and drained. After complete subsidence of the inflammatory reaction, thyroglossal cysts and ducts should be excised. The mid portion of the hyoid bone should be removed en bloc with the thyroglossal tract to the base of the tongue.

Ectopic thyroid glands are usually associated with athyreosis of the two lobes. These remnants of thyroid may produce sufficient hormones until early childhood and adolescence, at which time hypothyroidism develops. Because of increased stimulation by thyrotropic hormone, the aberrant thyroid tissue enlarges. The residual hypertrophic thyroid remnants usually recede in response to administration of thyroid hormone, and in many instances surgical excision is not necessary. If an ectopic thyroid is excised and is the only remnant of thyroid gland, autotransplantation of the gland into the rectus or sternocleidomastoid muscle may be successful, but hormone production will be insufficient, and thyroid medication will be necessary.

Housawa M et al: Anatomical reconstruction of the thyroglossal duct. J Pediatr Surg 1991;26:766.

Pelausa ME, Forte V: Sistrunk revisited: A 10 year review of revision of thyroglossal duct surgery at Toronto's Hospital for Sick Children. J Otolaryngol 1989;18:325.

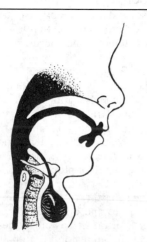

Figure 46–3. Thyroglossal cyst and duct course through the hyoid bone to the foramen cecum of the tongue.

MUSCULAR TORTICOLLIS

Infants with congenital muscular torticollis may initially develop a nontender, hard, fusiform swelling diffusely involving the sternocleidomastoid muscle. The muscle tumor may be present at birth but is usually not noticed until the second to sixth weeks of life. The tumor appears with equal frequency in both sexes and on each side of the neck. Rarely, there is more than one tumor in the muscle or both sternocleidomastoid muscles are involved. The tumor resolves in 6–7 weeks, and in about half of cases the sternocleidomastoid muscle becomes fibrotic. A history of breech delivery is present in 20–30% of these children. Older children (age 2–15) may develop sternocleidomastoid fibrosis and torticollis without an initial history of tumor formation.

The sternocleidomastoid tumor or fibrosis may be present with or without torticollis. When torticollis occurs, the sternocleidomastoid muscle is shortened, the mastoid process on the involved side is pulled down toward the clavicle and sternum, and the head is tilted and directed toward the opposite shoulder. The shoulder on the affected side is raised, and there may be cervical and thoracic scoliosis. The fusiform mass may be palpable in the affected sternocleidomastoid muscle, or the muscle may feel like a tight, hard band. Passive rotation of the head to the ipsilateral side of the involved muscle will be resisted and limited to varying degree, and the muscle will appear as a protuberant band. Because of persistent pressure when the patient is recumbent, the ipsilateral face and contralateral occiput will be flattened or hypoplastic.

If the torticollis is corrected late, the adjacent neck structures may also become shortened, and division of the sternocleidomastoid muscle will not be sufficient to correct the deformity. Delay in correction of the torticollis will produce permanent facial deformity.

The infant with a sternocleidomastoid tumor or fibrosis should be treated by forcefully rotating the neck and head in a full range of motion. This procedure should be performed at least four times a day even though it may be quite uncomfortable for the child. If the muscle continues to become progressively shortened, with facial and occipital skull deformity, both heads of the sternocleidomastoid muscle should be divided through a small transverse incision just above the clavicle. After the muscle is divided, the head should be turned to the ipsilateral side and any surrounding muscle or fascial contracture should also be divided. It is unnecessary to excise the tumor, which involves a risk of injuring the spinal accessory nerve. Only the platysma muscle and skin layers are closed. When postoperative pain has subsided, exercises to provide a full range of neck motion must be carried out. The use of a neck brace is rarely indicated.

Surgical division of the muscle must be performed early to prevent progressive facial and occipital flattening. This procedure does not reverse the bony changes that have already developed. Dividing the muscle produces permanent "hollowing" of the lower neck on the affected side.

Binder H et al: Congenital muscular torticollis: Results of conservative management with long-term follow-up in 85 cases. Arch Phys Med Rehabil 1987;68:222.

Bredenkamp JK et al: Congenital muscular torticollis. Arch Otolaryngol Head Neck Surg 1990;116:212.

Leung YK, Leung PC: The efficacy of manipulative treatment for sternomastoid tumors. J Bone Joint Surg [Br] 1987;69:473.

CERVICAL LYMPHADENOPATHY

1. PYOGENIC LYMPHADENITIS

Infections in the upper respiratory passages, scalp, ear, or neck produce varying degrees of secondary lymphadenitis. Most of the causative organisms are streptococci and staphylococci. In infants and young children, the clinical course of the suppurative lymphadenitis may greatly overshadow a seemingly insignificant or inapparent primary infection. Scalp or ear infections produce pre- or postauricular and suboccipital lymph node involvement; submental, oral, tonsillar, and pharyngeal infections affect the submandibular and deep jugular nodes.

With significant lymphadenitis, the regional lymph nodes become greatly enlarged and produce local pain and tenderness. Fever is high initially and then becomes intermittent and may persist for days or weeks. The regional nodes may remain enlarged and firm for prolonged periods, or they may suppurate and produce surrounding cellulitis and edema. Subsequently, the nodes may involute or a fluctuant abscess may form, resulting in redness and thinning of the overlying skin.

A smoldering lymphadenitis that neither resolves nor forms an abscess can be confused with granulomatous lymphadenitis, lymphoma, or metastatic tumor. After several weeks, there will usually be a reduction in the size and firmness of pyogenic adenitis. Excisional biopsy is occasionally required to differentiate these lesions.

In the acute phase, the patient should be treated with antistaphylococcal antibiotics. In the subacute or chronic phase, the presence of pus in the node may be confirmed by needle aspiration of the mass. When an abscess is present, a general anesthetic should be given and the abscess incised and drained.

2. GRANULOMATOUS LYMPHADENITIS

Although typical tuberculous cervical adenitis is very rare in the USA, atypical mycobacteria frequently cause chronic suppuration in the cervical, axillary, and inguinal lymph nodes.

Granulomatous lymphadenitis and caseation may occur in the regional nodes draining the inoculation site of BCG. **Cat-scratch disease** causes a caseating lymphadenitis in regional lymph nodes.

Children under age 6 are most frequently affected. The initial manifestation is a painless, progressive enlargement of the lymph nodes in the deep cervical chain and the parotid, suboccipital, submandibular, and supraclavicular nodes. The duration of lymphadenopathy is usually 1–3 months or longer. The nodes may be large and mobile or, with progressive disease, may become matted, fixed, and finally caseate to form a cold abscess. Incision or spontaneous breakthrough of the skin will result in a chronically draining sinus. In tuberculosis, both sides of the neck or multiple groups of nodes are infected, and the chest x-ray indicates pulmonary involvement. In atypical mycobacterial lymphadenitis, pulmonary disease is rare and the cervical adenitis is unilateral. The tuberculin skin test is weakly positive in over 80% of patients with atypical infection. Skin test antigens from the various strains of atypical mycobacteria are available.

Cat-scratch fever is usually acquired by a bite or scratch from a kitten. It is caused by a pleomorphic, gram-negative bacillus that requires a silver stain for detection in tissue. It is an acute illness characterized by fever, malaise, and occasionally a pustular lesion at the site of the scratch. Tender lymph node enlargement usually develops. Two to 4 weeks later, regional lymphadenitis persists, producing painful, fixed suppurative nodes that may develop into a chronically draining sinus.

The firm, rubbery, or fixed nodes resemble lymphoma or metastatic tumor (neuroblastoma or thyroid carcinoma) and may be distinguished only by excisional biopsy. A positive skin test helps differentiate granulomatous adenitis from malignant lymphadenopathy. A fluctuant node can be confused with branchial cleft or thyroglossal cysts.

Granulomatous lymphadenitis progresses to caseation and breakdown of the overlying skin in the great majority of affected children.

Atypical tuberculous lymphadenitis may be treated with rifampin, 10 mg/kg/d. If the infection seems to be progressing, the nodes should be excised. In adults ciprofloxacin and in children trimethoprim-sulfamethoxazole may shorten the course of cat-scratch disease and prevent suppuration.

The procedure of choice is surgical excision of involved nodes before caseation occurs. Once the nodes become fluctuant or a draining sinus forms, a wedge of involved skin should be excised and the underlying necrotic nodes should be curetted out (rather than excised), taking care not to injure neighboring nerves. The wound edges and skin should be closed primarily. The value of continuing chemotherapy is influenced by sensitivity tests on the cultured material. Excision and primary closure usually result in excellent healing with good cosmetic results.

Holley HP: Successful treatment of cat-scratch disease with ciprofloxacin. JAMA 1991;265:1563.

Moriarity RA, Margileth AM: Cat-scratch disease. Infect Dis Clin North Am 1987;1:575.

CONGENITAL DEFORMITIES OF THE CHEST WALL (Pectus Excavatum, Pectus Carinatum)

Anomalous development of the costal cartilages and sternum produces a variety of chest wall deformities. Failure of fusion of the two sternal bands during embryonic development produces congenital sternal cleft, which may involve the upper, lower, or entire sternum. This defect is usually associated with protrusion of the pericardium and heart (ectopia cordis) and congenital heart lesions.

Clinical Findings

Most affected children are noted to have the deformity at birth. In some cases, the defect does not occur until late childhood. Paradoxic motion in the area of the pectus excavatum is commonly seen in infants. The deformity may stabilize, but most cases progress in severity with age. The incidence in girls and boys is probably equal, but surgical consultation is requested three or four times more frequently in boys.

In pectus excavatum, the xiphoid is the deepest portion of the depression. The sternum curves posteriorly from the manubriosternal junction, though the manubrium may also be posteriorly directed. The costal cartilages, curving posteriorly to insert on the sternum, are deformed and fused. The third, fourth, and fifth ribs are usually affected, though the second through eighth costal cartilages and ribs may be involved. The severity of the defect varies greatly from a mild, insignificant depression to an extreme where the xiphoid bone is adjacent to the vertebrae. Chest x-ray shows the posterior depression and displacement of the heart to the left. Angiocardiograms may show impingement of the sternum on the right atrium or ventricle.

These patients are typically round-shouldered, with stooped posture, potbelly, and an asthenic appearance. They tend to be withdrawn and refuse to participate in sports activities, particularly if their deformity might be exposed. Many patients complain of easy fatigability or inability to compete in exertional activities. Cardiopulmonary function studies show impaired stroke volume and cardiac output during upright exercise. After the defect is repaired, parents and children comment upon the great improvement in the child's well-being and exercise tolerance.

Treatment & Prognosis

The operation is performed to improve both cosmetic appearance and cardiopulmonary function. Mild deformities should be left alone and the patient followed to observe for progression. Moderate to severe defects should be repaired, particularly when the patient or parent indicates a desire for improvement. The ideal age is 6–7 years. Operation in older children requires greater operative time, and a good result is easier to achieve in young children. Blood for transfusion should be available. Preoperatively, older children should be taught how to use a mechanical ventilator to assist in treating and preventing atelectasis postoperatively.

A stainless steel strut may be passed beneath the sternum and anchored by sutures to the fourth or fifth rib laterally on each side. This serves to ensure ideal position of the sternum and minimizes postoperative paradoxic motion and pain. The strut may be removed 6 or more months later.

The round-shouldered, slouched posture will persist postoperatively. An acquired habit of maintaining an erect posture is established by using a T-brace fitted for the patient. The brace must be worn during waking hours for at least 6 months. Exercises such as pull-ups and push-ups are initiated 6 weeks postoperatively.

Scherer LR et al: Surgical management of children and young adults with Marfan syndrome and pectus excavatum. J Pediatr Surg 1988;23:1169.
Shamberger R, Welch K: Surgical repair of pectus excavatum. J Pediatr Surg 1988;23:615.

SURGICAL RESPIRATORY EMERGENCIES IN THE NEWBORN

Respiratory distress may be produced by airway obstruction, displacement of lung volume, or pulmonary parenchymal insufficiency.

Certain aspects of respiration peculiar to the infant must be appreciated. Except during periods of crying, the newborn baby is an obligate nasal breather. The ability to breathe through the mouth may take weeks or months to acquire. Inspiration is accomplished

chiefly by diaphragmatic excursion, and the intercostal and accessory muscles contribute little to ventilation. Impaired inspiration results in retraction of the sternum, costal margin, and neck fossae; the resulting paradoxic motion may contribute to respiratory insufficiency. The airway is small and flaccid, so that it is readily occluded by mucus or edema, and it collapses readily under slight pressure. Dyspneic infants swallow large volumes of air, and the distended stomach and bowel may further impair diaphragmatic excursion.

Classification
A. Upper Airway:
1. Micrognathia–Pierre Robin syndrome.
2. Macroglossia–Muscular hypertrophy, hypothyroidism, lymphangioma.
3. Anomalous nasopharyngeal passage–Choanal atresia, Treacher-Collins syndrome, Apert's syndrome, and Crouzon's syndrome.
4. Tumors, cysts, or enlarged thyroid remnants in the pharynx or neck.
5. Laryngeal or tracheal stenosis, webs, cysts, tumors, or vocal cord paralysis.

B. Intrathoracic:
1. Atelectasis.
2. Pneumothorax and pneumomediastinum.
3. Pleural effusion or chylothorax.
4. Pulmonary cysts, sequestration, and tumors.
5. Tracheal stenosis with complete tracheal rings.
6. Tracheomalacia or bronchomalacia.
7. Congenital lobar emphysema.
8. Diaphragmatic hernia or eventration.
9. Esophageal atresia or tracheoesophageal fistula.
10. Vascular rings and sling (anomalous origin of left pulmonary artery).
11. Mediastinal tumors and cysts.

PIERRE ROBIN SYNDROME

Pierre Robin syndrome is a congenital defect characterized by micrognathia and glossoptosis, often associated with cleft palate. The small lower jaw and strong sucking action of the infant allow the tongue to be sucked back and occlude the laryngeal airway and may be life-threatening.

Most infants (mild cases) should be kept in the prone position during care and feeding. A nasogastric or gastrostomy tube may be necessary. Nasohypopharyngeal intubation is effective in preventing occlusion of the larynx. If conservative measures fail, prompt attention to maintaining an open airway by tracheostomy is indicated. Feeding by gastrostomy may be necessary. The tongue may be sutured forward to the lower jaw, but this frequently breaks down. In time, the lower jaw develops normally. These infants eventually learn how to keep the tongue from occluding the airway.

CHOANAL ATRESIA

Complete obstruction at the posterior nares owing to choanal atresia may be unilateral and relatively asymptomatic. It may be membranous (10%) or bony (90%). When it is bilateral, severe respiratory distress is manifested by marked chest wall retraction on inspiration and a normal cry.

There is arching of the head and neck in an effort to breathe, and the baby is unable to eat. The diagnosis is confirmed by inability to pass a tube through the nares to the pharynx. With the baby in a supine position, radiopaque material may be instilled into the nares and lateral x-rays of the head taken to outline the obstruction. A CT scan of the nasopharynx will define bone occlusion.

Emergency treatment consists of maintaining an oral airway by placing a nipple, with the tip cut off, in the mouth. The membranous or bony occlusion may then be perforated by direct transpalatal excision, or it may be punctured and enlarged with a Hegar dilator. The newly created opening must be stented with plastic tubing for 5 weeks to prevent stricture.

CONGENITAL PHARYNGEAL OR LARYNGEAL TUMORS, CYSTS, & STENOSES

Tumors affecting the airway of the pharynx include lingual thyroid and teratoma. The pharynx and larynx may be obstructed by hemangioma, lymphangioma, neurofibroma, and fibrosarcoma. Thyroglossal cysts, pharyngeal inclusion cysts, and laryngeal cysts may compromise breathing. Stenoses of the larynx result from fibrous webs, which are remnants of epithelial ingrowths during embryonic formation of the larynx. They may be located at the true cords or may be supraglottic.

Retractions of the chest occur on inspiration, and a prolonged expiratory wheeze may be noted. A hoarse, weak, or completely absent cry indicates involvement of the larynx. In the absence of other obvious causes of airway obstruction such as tumors of the neck, direct laryngoscopy and bronchoscopy should be performed.

The paramount concern of treatment is to provide an adequate airway; treatment of the obstructing lesion is of secondary importance. An endotracheal tube should be placed in the trachea and anchored with tape to the lips. Emergency tracheostomy may be required. A lingual thyroid can be made smaller by the administration of thyroid hormone. Heman-

gioendotheliomas may respond to adrenocorticosteroids, and they involute spontaneously within 1–2 years. Cavernous hemangiomas and lymphangiomas are extremely difficult to excise intact when adjacent normal structures are involved. Cysts of the pharynx may be aspirated or marsupialized until excision can be accomplished. Laryngeal webs may be excised by cup forceps or endoscopic laser.

Subglottic stenosis secondary to prolonged endotracheal intubation has been managed in a variety of ways, including tracheal dilation, local injection of corticosteroids, endotracheal stenting, and endotracheal electroresection or cryotherapy. The anterior cricoid split and insertion of a cartilage graft taken from the fifth rib produces excellent results.

Handley GH, Reilly JS: Nasal obstruction in children. Otolaryngol Clin North Am 1989;22:383.

Kaplan LC: The CHARGE association: Choanal atresia and multiple congenital anomalies. Otolaryngol Clin North Am 1989;22:661.

Kearns DB et al: Computed tomography in choanal atresia. J Laryngol Otol 1988;102:414.

White P, Forte V: Surgical management of nasal airway obstruction in children. J Otolaryngol 1989;18:155.

CONGENITAL TRACHEAL STENOSIS & MALACIA

There are three main types of congenital tracheal stenosis: generalized hypoplasia; funnel-like narrowing, usually tapering to a tight stenosis just above the carina; and segmental stenosis of various lengths that can occur at any level. Tracheomalacia is usually secondary to external compression by vascular rings or tumors. It is also associated with esophageal atresia.

The diagnostic approach to an infant with respiratory distress and possible distal tracheal obstruction must be carefully integrated with plans for management of the airway, because the compromised infant airway is easily occluded by edema or secretions. This is especially so in distal tracheal lesions, where an endotracheal or tracheostomy tube may not relieve the distal obstruction. The diagnostic value of every procedure must be weighed against the threat of precipitating airway obstruction. Tracheal lesions can be visualized using magnification radiographs, xerograms, or CT scans. Dynamic lesions, such as tracheomalacia and vascular compression syndromes, are best defined by videotape fluoroscopy or cineradiography with barium in the esophagus. Angiography may be necessary. Flow/volume curves can define the level of obstruction (intrathoracic versus extrathoracic) and the type of obstruction (stenosis versus malacia).

Although bronchoscopy and bronchography often provide the best delineation of tracheobronchial lesions, these more invasive procedures can precipitate acute obstruction from edema or inflammation. A ventilating infant bronchoscope with Hopkins optics should be kept above the critical area to avoid precipitating obstruction. If tracheobronchoscopy is performed, use only a small amount of contrast medium (micropulverized barium, 50% weight/volume, mixed in normal saline) or pass a Fogarty catheter, inflating a 1- or 2-mL balloon with 50% diatrizoate meglumine (Hypaque) to outline the extent of stenosis and to minimize tracheal irritation.

Stenotic and malacic lesions in infants and children should be managed as conservatively as possible, preferably without intubation. "Temporary" stenting of these lesions is seldom temporary, since the presence of the tube itself ensures continued trauma and irritation such that the tube cannot be removed without airway obstruction. If an infant or child cannot be managed without intubation, surgical correction must be considered. Resection with reconstruction has proved to be the treatment of choice for tracheal lesions. Tracheal reconstruction is feasible in infancy in selected cases, but the risks are high. Long tracheal stenosis—involving more than half the length of the trachea—is treated by incising the mid anterior trachea and suturing a rib cartilage graft from the fifth rib.

Brown WJ, Haddart SN: Tracheoaortopexy via midline sternotomy in tracheomalacia. J Pediatr Surg 1991; 26:660.
deLorimier AA et al: Tracheobronchial obstructions in infants and children: Experience with 45 cases. Ann Surg 1990;212:277.
Kiely E, Spitz L, Breeton R: Management of tracheomalacia by aortopexy. Pediatr Surg Int 1987;2:13.
Loeff DS et al: Congenital tracheal stenosis: A review of 22 patients from 1965 to 1987. J Pediatr Surg 1988;23:744.
Tsugawa C et al: Congenital stenosis involving a long segment of the trachea: Further experience in reconstructive surgery. J Pediatr Surg 1988;23:471.
Wells TR et al: Reconsideration of the anatomy of sling left pulmonary artery: The association of one form with bridging bronchus. J Pediatr Surg 1988;23:892.

ATELECTASIS

The airway of the unborn infant is normally filled with fluid that is formed in the lungs. This fluid flows out of the trachea to contribute to amniotic fluid. During asphyxia, the unborn baby may attempt to breathe, resulting in inhalation of amniotic fluid, meconium, or blood. When the airways are filled with this debris, they may become plugged at birth and prevent aeration of the lungs. Secretions of mucus may cause atelectasis in cases in which an endotracheal tube or tracheostomy tube has been used without humidified air or in infants with cystic fibrosis.

Prenatal asphyxia should be suspected when there is prolonged and difficult labor and when bradycardia occurs in the infant. Babies who are small for gestational age and depressed infants with low Apgar scores are particularly prone to aspiration. Meconium will be noted in the amniotic fluid and pharynx. With the onset of breathing, respirations will be labored, but chest wall retractions are not usually prominent. Chest x-rays will indicate lack of aeration in some areas or hyperaeration in areas where partial obstruction of the bronchus occurs. Bacterial pneumonia and sepsis frequently follow prolonged atelectasis.

An asphyxiated, meconium-stained, or depressed newborn infant should be treated by pharyngeal aspiration and immediate insertion of an endotracheal tube into the trachea. The trachea should also be aspirated of debris before ventilatory resuscitation is attempted. Bronchoscopy and direct aspiration of the plugged bronchus may be necessary. Increased concentrations of inspired oxygen with ultrasonic humidification should be given to maintain the peripheral arterial Po_2 at about 60–80 mm Hg. Intensive physical therapy with postural drainage and chest cupping will be needed. Because of the risk of pneumothorax, positive-pressure ventilation should be avoided unless it is required to maintain adequate oxygenation. Treatment with extracorporeal membrane oxygenation (ECMO) may be lifesaving for critically ill neonates with respiratory failure who have failed maximal medical therapy.

Krummel TM et al: Alveolar arterial oxygen gradients versus the neonatal pulmonary insufficiency index for prediction of mortality in ECMO candidates. J Pediatr Surg 1984;19:380.

CONGENITAL DIAPHRAGMATIC HERNIA & EVENTRATION OF THE DIAPHRAGM

Fusion of the transverse septum and pleuroperitoneal folds normally occurs during the eighth week of embryonic development. If diaphragmatic formation is incomplete, the pleuroperitoneal hiatus (foramen of Bochdalek) persists. The intestine normally returns from the umbilicus for rotation and fixation within the abdomen at the tenth week of gestation. If the bowel should herniate into the chest at this early stage, nonfixation of the mesentery and colon will occur. Since the transition from the glandular to the bronchial phase of pulmonary development occurs at about the 15th week of gestation, severe impairment of pulmonary development may occur when the bowel compresses the lung (Figure 46–4). Experimental studies have shown that pulmonary hypoplasia is due to the herniation of bowel and not just to an association of anomalies. The earlier in gestation the hernia occurs, the more severe the pulmonary hypoplasia.

Eventration of the diaphragm may be congenital or acquired. Congenital eventration may consist of only

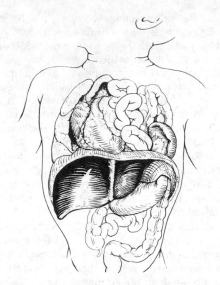

Figure 46–4. Congenital posterolateral (Bochdalek) diaphragmatic hernia. Bowel, spleen, and liver herniate into the chest and severely compromise lung development in utero and ventilation after birth. (Reproduced, with permission, from Schrock TR: *Handbook of Surgery,* 6th ed. Jones, 1978.)

pleural and peritoneal membranes, with attenuation of muscular and fibrous layers. The diaphragmatic serosal membranes may protrude slightly into the pleural space or may line it completely. When intact pleural membranes exist, the distinction between eventration and Bochdalek's hernia may be quite arbitrary. Varying degrees of pulmonary hypoplasia also occur with diaphragmatic eventration.

Acquired diaphragmatic eventration may occur as a result of direct injury to the phrenic nerve associated with brachial or cervical plexus trauma during birth or during thoracotomy.

Clinical Findings

Symptoms may appear immediately after birth or not until the infant is several months old. Severe respiratory distress may be characterized by gasping respirations with cyanosis. Pulmonary hypoplasia is the most frequent cause of death. The left side of the diaphragm is affected four or five times as frequently as the right. The abdomen is usually scaphoid. The chest on the side of the hernia may be dull to percussion, but bowel sounds are not usually appreciated. When the hernia is on the left, the heart sounds may be heard best on the right side of the chest. A chest x-ray will show bowel in the thorax, with a shift of the mediastinal structures to the opposite side.

Treatment

An endotracheal tube should be placed in the trachea and assisted ventilation controlled to prevent a positive pressure greater than 35 cm H_2O. A nasogastric tube should be placed in the stomach to aspirate swallowed air and to prevent distention of the herniated bowel, which would further compress the lungs. An umbilical artery catheter should be inserted to the level of the lower aorta, and metabolic acidosis must be corrected.

A transverse abdominal incision should be made and the herniated bowel reduced from the pleural space. The negative pressure between the bowel and the chest wall may make reduction difficult. This negative pressure may be broken by inserting a tube along the pleura and injecting air through it. A hernia sac should be sought and excised. Following reduction of the bowel, a chest tube should be placed in the pleural space and connected to a water seal and not to vacuum. No attempt should be made to expand the collapsed and hypoplastic lung by positive pressure. The diaphragmatic defect should be closed by nonabsorbable sutures. In many instances, a synthetic material is required to close large defects. The abdominal cavity may be too small and undeveloped to accommodate the intestine and permit closure of the abdominal wall muscle and fascial layers. In such cases, abdominal wall skin flaps should be mobilized and closed over the protruding bowel. The resulting ventral hernia can be repaired later when the infant is thriving. Continued respiratory support and treatment of hypoxia, hypercapnia, and acidosis are required postoperatively. Persistent pulmonary hypertension may result in right-to-left shunt and produce severe hypoxia in the lower aorta. Nitric oxide added to the ventilation gases can induce pulmonary vasodilation, improve pulmonary perfusion, and reverse the right-to-left shunt. The persistent fetal circulation physiology may be treated successfully in many cases by extracorporeal membrane oxygenation (ECMO). Hypoxic myocardiopathy may require infusion of dopamine to enhance cardiac output. Localized eventration may be approached better by means of a posterolateral thoracotomy.

Prognosis

The death rate depends upon the severity of pulmonary hypoplasia, the presence or absence of associated anomalies, and the quality of care provided for these critically ill infants. Surgical units that are immediately adjacent to obstetric services report death rates as high as 80%, because infants with severe pulmonary hypoplasia will be recognized and treated immediately. Infants who survive transfer to surgical centers remote from the delivery area usually have less severe disease, and the death rates reported from these facilities are usually under 50%. It seems unlikely that the death rate can be significantly reduced until pulmonary hypoplasia can be reversed by correcting the lesion before birth (ie, in utero). Diaphragmatic hernia can be accurately diagnosed before birth. Polyhydramnios is a common finding that prompts prenatal ultrasound evaluation. Even with optimal postnatal management, the death rate for fetuses with diaphragmatic hernia and polyhydramnios exceeds 80%. Prenatal repair has proved physiologically sound and technically feasible.

Adzick NS et al: Fetal diaphragmatic hernia: Ultrasound diagnosis and clinical outcome in 38 cases. J Pediatr Surg 1989;24:654.

Breaux CW et al: Improvement in survival of patients with congenital diaphragmatic hernia utilizing a strategy of delayed repair after medical and/or extracorporeal membrane oxygenation stabilization. J Pediatr Surg 1991;26:333.

deLorimier AA et al: Diaphragmatic hernia. In: *Pediatric Surgery*. Ashcraft KW, Holder TM (editors). Saunders, 1992.

Frostell C et al: Inhaled nitric oxide: A selective pulmonary vasodilator reversing hypoxic pulmonary vasoconstriction. Circulation 1991;83:2038.

Harrison MR et al: The fetus with diaphragmatic hernia. In: *The Unborn Patient. Prenatal Diagnosis and Treatment*. Harrison MR et al (editors). Saunders, 1991.

Newman KD: Extracorporeal membrane oxygenation and congenital diaphragmatic hernia: Should any infant be excluded? J Pediatr Surg 1990;25:1048.

Puri P (editor): Congenital diaphragmatic hernia. Mod Probl Paediatr 1989;24:142.

Wilson JM et al: Congenital diaphragmatic hernia: Predictors of severity in the ECMO era. J Pediatr Surg 1991;26:1028.

CONGENITAL LOBAR EMPHYSEMA

Lobar emphysema consists of massive hyperinflation of a single lobe; rarely, more than one lobe is affected. The upper and middle lobes are most frequently involved. There are three kinds of lobar emphysema: (1) hypoplastic emphysema, (2) polyalveolar lobe, and (3) bronchial obstruction.

Hypoplastic emphysema is distinguished by a segment, lobe, or whole lung that has a reduced number of bronchial branches with a diminished number and smaller size of blood vessels. The number of alveoli is abnormally decreased, but the air spaces are too large. The hyperlucent region seen on chest x-ray is normal or small in volume, and since it does not affect the surrounding normal lung, surgical treatment is unnecessary.

Polyalveolar lobe is characterized by a normal size and number of bronchial branches, but there is an abnormal number of alveoli from each respiratory unit. These alveoli are prone to expand excessively, producing emphysema, which encroaches on the surrounding normal lung and therefore requires removal.

Bronchial obstruction may occur either from deficient bronchial cartilage support, redundant mucosa, bronchial stenosis, mucous plug or bronchial compression by anomalous vessels, or other mediastinal lesions. With inspiration, the bronchus opens to allow air into the lung; but on expiration the bronchus collapses, trapping the air, and with each respiratory cycle there is progressive expansion of the lobe. Bronchial atresia results filling of the lobe with air by collateral ventilation from adjacent lung, but the lack of rapid air exodus results in air trapping.

In one-third of patients, respiratory distress is noted at birth; in only 5% of cases do symptoms develop after 6 months. Males are affected twice as frequently as females. The signs include progressive and severe dyspnea, wheezing, grunting, coughing, cyanosis, and difficulty with feedings. Increased dimensions of the chest and retractions may be seen. The chest is hyperresonant, and decreased breath sounds may be noted over the affected lobe. Chest x-rays show radiolucency of the emphysematous lobe, with bronchovascular markings extending to the lung periphery. Compression atelectasis of the adjacent lung, shift of the mediastinum, depression of the diaphragm, and anterior bowing of the sternum are usually seen. The emphysematous lobe may continue to expand, compressing adjacent lung and airways and asphyxiating the infant.

Occasionally, the emphysema may be due to a mucous plug in the bronchus that may be aspirated by bronchoscopy. Compression of the bronchus by mediastinal masses may be relieved by removal of the tumor or repair of anomalous vessels. Treatment of mildly symptomatic cases may not be necessary.

Many patients with lobar emphysema are severely symptomatic, and pulmonary lobectomy is necessary. Anesthesia should not be started until all personnel are ready for emergency thoracotomy. Excessive positive pressure ventilation should be avoided. The prognosis following surgical relief of the lobar emphysema is excellent. Some patients may show residual disease in the remaining lung. At long-term follow-up, lung volumes are normal, but the air flow rates are diminished.

Martinez-Frontanilla LA et al: Surgery of acquired lobar emphysema in the neonate. J Pediatr Surg 1984;19:375.

Tapper D et al: Polyalveolar lobe. J Pediatr Surg 1980;15:931.

LUNG CYSTS

Congenital lung cysts, which arise from anomalous development of the foregut, are classified as follows: (1) bronchogenic cyst, (2) cystic adenomatoid malformation, (3) pulmonary sequestration, and, (4) bronchopulmonary foregut malformations. Embryonic tissues that were destined to form bronchi and lung become anomalous isolated structures within or outside of the lung. Lung cysts produce symptoms from their size and position, resulting in compression of bronchi or lung parenchyma, or from infection and abscess formation within the cyst and surrounding normal lung.

Bronchogenic Cysts

Bronchogenic cysts are lined by cuboidal or ciliated columnar epithelium and are filled with mucoid material. Repeated infection in the cyst may produce squamous epithelial metaplasia. About one-half arise in the mediastinum and do not communicate with the bronchi. They appear as radiopaque masses on chest x-rays. When located within the lung parenchyma, the cysts usually communicate with the airways and consequently are prone to abscess formation. Bronchogenic cysts arise in the right lung three times more often than in the left. They are more common in the lower lobes but may be found in any lobe. Partial compression of bronchi produces hyperinflation of the involved lung, while complete obstruction produces atelectasis. Rupture of a cyst that communicates with bronchi may present as a tension pneumothorax. Treatment is by excision of the cyst, which may require lobectomy or, very rarely, pneumonectomy.

Cystic Adenomatoid Malformation

This lesion is considered a hamartoma in which multiple cysts are lined by a polypoid proliferation of bronchial epithelium surrounded by striated muscle and elastic tissue, but there is an absence of mucous glands and cartilage. Two types are described based upon the size of the cysts: (1) cysts greater than 5 mm in diameter, and (2) bulky lesions less than 5 mm in diameter that are more solid, with bronchial and alveolar-like spaces.

This cyst occurs with equal frequency in both lungs, with a slight predominance in the upper lobes. Many cases are identified in utero by ultrasound because of the development of polyhydramnios or fetal hydrops. A large mass compresses the fetal lung, resulting in pulmonary hypoplasia at birth. In addition, it may distort or obstruct the esophagus to produce polyhydramnios. Compression of venous return to the heart with exudation of protein into the lung fluid may cause fetal congestive heart failure, hydrops fetalis, and death in utero. Following birth, cystic adenomatoid malformation produces symptoms from displacement by the mass of normal lung and from infection in the cyst. Associated renal and nervous system anomalies may occur. Occasionally, multiple lobes are involved. The high fetal mortality rate associated with hydrops and very large masses compressing normal lung warrant resection in utero. Following birth, the discovery of cystic adenomatoid malformation is usually associated with pulmonary infection and abscess formation. Resection of the affected lobe is necessary.

Pulmonary Sequestration & Bronchopulmonary Foregut Malformation

These lesions may be extralobar or intralobar. A sequestration consists of normally developed bronchioles and alveoli without direct communication with the tracheobronchial tree. Sequestrations occur in the lower chest, most commonly on the left, adjacent to the mediastinum. They usually have a systemic arterial blood supply from the aorta, either above or below the diaphragm, and pulmonary venous drainage. Rarely, sequestrations may occur in the upper or middle lobes. Extralobar sequestration is usually asymptomatic and presents on chest x-ray as a radiopaque mass in the lower lung. Intralobar sequestrations communicate through the alveoli of normal surrounding lung, and therefore they are prone to infection and lung abscess formation.

On rare occasions, a sequestration will communicate with the esophagus or stomach, a condition termed bronchopulmonary foregut malformation. These anomalies usually present as unresolving lower lobe pneumonia with abscess. Treatment is by excision of the sequestration, but extensive inflammation involving the surrounding lower lobe may require lobectomy.

Neilson IR et al: Congenital adenomatoid malformation of the lung: Current management and prognosis. J Pediatr Surg 1991;26:975.

ESOPHAGEAL ANOMALIES

Classification (Figure 46–5)
A. With Esophageal Atresia:
1. With a blind proximal pouch and a fistula between the distal end of the esophagus and the trachea (85% of cases).
2. With a blind proximal esophageal pouch, no tracheoesophageal fistula, and a blind distal esophagus (10% of cases).
3. With fistulas between both proximal and distal esophageal segments and the trachea (0.5% of cases).
4. With a fistula between the proximal esophagus and the trachea and a blind distal esophagus without fistula (0.3% of cases).

B. Without Esophageal Atresia:
1. With an H type tracheoesophageal fistula (4–5% of cases).
2. With esophageal stenosis consisting of a membranous occlusion between the mid and distal thirds of the esophagus (rare).
3. With a laryngotracheoesophageal cleft

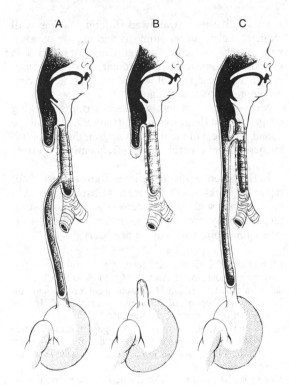

Figure 46–5. Congenital esophageal anomalies. The most common is esophageal atresia with a tracheoesophageal fistula to the distal segment *(A).* The second most common is esophageal atresia without a tracheoesophageal fistula *(B).* Tracheoesophageal fistula without esophageal atresia *(C)* is the third most common anomaly, and two-thirds of these fistulas are located above the first thoracic vertebra. (Reproduced, with permission, from Schrock TR: *Handbook of Surgery,* 6th ed. Jones, 1978.)

consisting of a linear communication between these structures (very rare).

Clinical Findings

Shortly after birth, the infant with esophageal atresia is noted to have excessive salivation and repeated episodes of coughing, choking, and cyanosis. Attempts at feeding result in choking, gagging, and regurgitation. Infants with tracheoesophageal fistula in addition to esophageal atresia will have reflux of gastric secretions into the tracheobronchial tree, with resulting severe chemical bronchitis and pneumonia. Pneumonic infiltrates are usually noted first in the right upper lobe.

A size 10F catheter should be passed into the esophagus by way of the nose or mouth; if esophageal atresia is present, the tube will not go down the expected distance to the stomach. Smaller tubes will coil in the upper esophageal pouch or may pass from the tracheoesophageal fistula to the stomach, giving a false impression of normal esophagus. Too much contrast material will result in aspiration. If a tracheo-

esophageal fistula connects to the lower esophageal segment, air will be present in the stomach and bowel. Absence of air below the diaphragm usually means that distal tracheoesophageal fistula is not present.

Tracheoesophageal fistula without esophageal atresia will produce repeated coughing, cyanosis, and pneumonia. These episodes are more apt to occur with swallowing of liquids than with solid foods. Abdominal distention is a prominent finding because the Valsalva effect of coughing and crying forces air through the fistula into the stomach and bowel. The diagnosis may be difficult. A cineesophagogram taken from a lateral position is required. The swallowed material should be a thin barium mixture or diatrizoate (Hypaque). The presence and position of the fistula can also be determined by bronchoscopy. A general anesthetic is used, and modern endoscopes with magnifying lenses readily locate the fistula. Two-thirds of the fistulas are located in the neck; the remainder are within the thorax.

Laryngotracheoesophageal cleft produces symptoms similar to those of tracheoesophageal fistula but of much greater severity. Laryngoscopy may show the cleft between the arytenoids extending down the larynx. Bronchoscopy is the best means of outlining the cleft.

Differential Diagnosis

Newborn infants may have transient dysphagia, with aspiration of feedings because of an uncoordinated swallowing mechanism. This usually subsides within the first 2 days after birth. Prolonged swallowing dysfunction may occur with brain anomaly or injury.

Treatment

Aspiration pneumonia must be treated before surgical treatment is begun. A sump suction catheter should be placed in the infant's upper esophageal pouch and connected to continuous suction. The head of the bed should be elevated. The infant should be placed in a humidified incubator, turned from side to side every hour, and stimulated to cry and cough. Ampicillin, 75 mg/kg, and gentamicin, 1.5 mg/kg, should be given every 8 hours intravenously. The position of the aortic arch should be determined, because a right aortic arch makes repair from the usual right thoracotomy hazardous. If the infant is fully mature and has no severe anomalies, extrapleural thoracotomy should be done for division of tracheoesophageal fistula and primary esophageal anastomosis. The operation should be staged for premature babies, those with associated severe anomalies, or those with short upper esophageal segments. The first stage consists of gastrostomy and transpleural division of the tracheoesophageal fistula. A sump suction catheter is maintained in the upper esophageal pouch, and feeding is done by gastrostomy until the infant has become strong enough to tolerate the second-stage procedure. A short upper pouch can be elongated with a 22–24F Hurst bougie two or three times per day over a period of 2–6 weeks. The second-stage procedure consists of an extrapleural thoracotomy followed by anastomosis of the two esophageal segments. A long distance between the two esophageal ends may be corrected by making one or more circumferential incisions in the muscularis of the proximal esophagus to allow the mucosa to stretch the desired length.

For infants with esophageal atresia and no tracheoesophageal fistula, cervical esophagostomy and gastrostomy is required. Feeding is through the gastrostomy tube until the infant weighs 9–11 kg, at which time a colon or gastric tube interposition is used to establish continuity between the cervical esophagus and the stomach. However, preoperative stretching by bougienage and intraoperative circumferential esophagomyotomy can produce sufficient esophageal lengthening to allow primary end-to-end esophageal reconstruction in most of these "long gap" atresias.

In infants with H type tracheoesophageal fistulas, the fistula is located above the thoracic inlet in two-thirds of cases. These fistulas may be divided through a left transverse cervical incision. Intrathoracic fistulas may be divided by an extrapleural right thoracotomy.

Esophageal webs respond readily to esophageal dilation. This is usually accomplished with Hurst or Maloney mercury-weighted bougies. Dilations are repeated until healing occurs without recurrence of the webs. Esophagoscopy and excision of portions of a tough or thick web, using biopsy forceps or the endoscopic laser, may be required in addition to dilation. A lower esophageal stricture containing cartilage will require excision and anastomosis.

Prognosis

The survival rate for a full-term infant without associated anomalies is excellent. However, deaths do occur as a result of pulmonary complications, severe associated anomalies, prematurity, and sepsis due to anastomotic disruption. Anastomotic leaks occur either because of technical problems or because of the extreme weakness of the distal esophageal wall. In performing the anastomosis, the extrapleural approach prevents the development of empyema and confines infection to a small localized area. Swallowing is a reflex response that must be reinforced early in infancy. If establishment of esophageal continuity is delayed for more than 4–6 weeks, it may take many months or years to teach the patient to swallow. Babies with cervical esophagostomy should be encouraged to suck, eat, and swallow during gastrostomy feedings.

Dysphagia may occur for months or years following successful repair of esophageal atresia. Stricture of the anastomosis may require one or more dilations with a filiform and follower or with antegrade or retrograde dilators. Swallowed foreign bodies will lodge at the site of anastomosis and require removal with esophagoscopy. Another cause of dysphagia may be neuromuscular incoordination, usually associated with esophageal anomalies. This frequent problem improves with age.

Most of these infants have an alarming, barking cough and rattling sound on respiration owing to chondromalacia of the tracheal rings at the site of tracheoesophageal fistula. This frequently improves with age.

Reflux esophagitis sometimes follows successful repair and may result in recurrent aspiration pneumonitis and esophagitis. Recurrent anastomotic stricture is usually due to gastroesophageal reflux. Antireflux fundoplication may be necessary.

Puntis JWL et al: Growth and feeding problems after repair of esophageal atresia. Arch Dis Child 1990;65:84.

deLorimier AA, Harrison MR: Esophageal replacement. In: *Pediatric Esophageal Surgery.* Ashcraft KW, Holder TM (editors). Grune & Stratton, 1986.

deLorimier AA, Harrison MR: Long gap esophageal atresia: Primary anastomosis after esophageal elongation by bougienage and esophagomyotomy. J Thorac Cardiovasc Surg 1980;79:138.

McKinnon LJ, Kosloske AM: Prediction and prevention of anastomotic complications of esophageal atresia and tracheoesophageal fistula. J Pediatr Surg 1990;25:778.

Pohlson EC et al: Improved survival with primary anastomosis in low birth weight neonates with esophageal atresia. J Pediatr Surg 1988;23:418.

VASCULAR RINGS

Tracheobronchial and esophageal compression by the great vessels may occur as a result of anomalies of the aortic arch or of abnormally located or enlarged pulmonary arteries. The genesis of aortic vascular rings may be understood if the embryo is considered to have two aortic arches, each with a carotid and subclavian artery and a ductus arteriosus (Figure 46–6). In the normal development of the aortic arch, the distal portion of the right arch is obliterated. There are five main types of vascular rings: (1) Persistence of both arches gives rise to double aortic arch (Figure 46–7); (2) obliteration of the left distal arch generates right aortic arch and persistent left ligamentum arteriosum; (3) obliteration of the right arch between the right carotid and subclavian arteries results in anomalous origin of the right subclavian artery; (4) incorporation of the right proximal arch into the left arch produces anomalous origin of the innominate artery; and (5) incorporation of the left proximal arch into right arch gives rise to an anomalous origin of the left common carotid artery.

When the left pulmonary artery arises from the right pulmonary artery, it encircles the right side of the trachea and courses between the trachea and

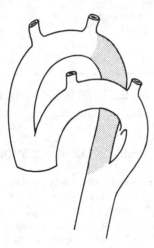

Figure 46–6. Normal embryonic aortic arch.

esophagus to the left lung. This sling effect produces significant compression of the lower trachea and proximal main bronchi. Complete tracheal rings with tracheal stenosis are frequently associated. Aneurysmal dilatation of the pulmonary artery usually occurs in association with ventricular septal defect and infundibular stenosis. Other forms of congenital heart defects are frequent. Each of these anomalies may compress and encircle the trachea and esophagus, producing respiratory distress and symptoms of obstruction on swallowing.

Clinical Findings

Affected infants have a characteristic inspiratory and expiratory wheeze, stridor, or croup. The head is held in an opisthotonic position to prevent compres-

sion of the trachea. If the head is forcibly flexed, the stridor is increased and apnea may occur. There may be hesitation on swallowing, with episodes of choking—so-called dysphagia lusoria. Chest x-rays may show compression of the trachea. Anteroposterior and lateral esophagograms show indentation of the esophagus at the level of T3 and T4. Echocardiograms can demonstrate the anomalous anatomy. When there is no esophageal indentation, a tracheogram or bronchoscopy may be necessary to demonstrate tracheal compression resulting from anomalous origin of the innominate or left common carotid artery. An angiocardiogram is not necessary for isolated aortic arch anomalies but is required for assessing congenital heart lesions associated with anomalies of the pulmonary artery. Esophagoscopy and bronchoscopy may be helpful in assessing the degree and level of compression.

Treatment

The aortic arch anomaly must be completely dissected and visualized through a left thoracotomy. The smallest component of a double aortic arch must be divided. An anomalous right subclavian artery is divided at its origin. The anomalous innominate or left carotid arteries are pulled forward by placing sutures between their adventitia and the sternum. The accompanying fibrous bands and sheaths constricting the trachea and esophagus must also be divided. Pulmonary artery slings are corrected by dividing the origin of the left pulmonary artery and anastomosing it to the main pulmonary artery anterior to the trachea. However, more than half of pulmonary slings are associated with complete tracheal ring stenosis, which will require preferential repair. Aneurysmal dilatation of the pulmonary artery is relieved by correcting the congenital heart defect; occasionally, the pulmonary artery requires reduction in size by direct surgical resection.

Occasionally, symptoms persist postoperatively because of deformed tracheocartilaginous rings. This may require tracheostomy and endotracheal intubation for a prolonged period of time. If tracheomalacia or stenotic tracheal rings are present, sleeve resection of the abnormal portion of the trachea and bronchi with anastomosis should be accomplished.

Filston H, Ferguson TB Jr, Oldham HN: Airway obstruction by vascular anomalies: Importance of telescopic bronchoscopy. Ann Surg 1987;205:541.

deLorimier AA: Vascular rings. In: *Current Therapy in Cardiovascular Surgery.* Grillo HC et al (editors). Decker, 1989.

GASTROESOPHAGEAL REFLUX

Studies of esophageal motility—including manometric measurements of the cardioesophageal junc-

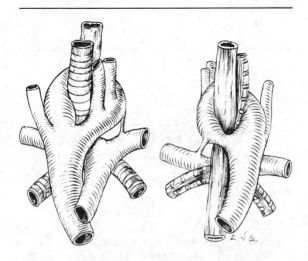

Figure 46–7. Anterior (left) and posterior views of double aortic arch constricting the trachea and esophagus.

tion—show absence of the high-pressure zone in the terminal esophagus in most newborn infants. Evolution to the normal adult pattern of peristalsis and cardioesophageal sphincter function occurs after several months. Until this happens, many infants experience varying degrees of regurgitation after feeding, referred to as **chalazia.** In rare severe cases, repeated gastric reflux may produce peptic esophagitis and interfere with development of a competent sphincter.

Symptoms consist of repeated effortless regurgitation of feedings, particularly when the baby is placed in a recumbent position. The baby will be hungry and will readily feed after regurgitating. Persistent regurgitation may result in poor weight gain; peptic esophagitis with appearance of blood in the vomitus; or occult bleeding, producing anemia. One cause for apnea and sudden infant death syndrome (SIDS) is regurgitation and aspiration. Lesser degrees of aspiration, particularly during sleep, may produce recurrent pneumonia. Stricture formation of the lower esophagus and metaplasia of the mucosa producing Barrett's esophagus are possible late effects.

Almost one-half of infants and children with gastroesophageal reflux have neurologic disorders related to perinatal asphyxia or congenital nervous system anomalies. Abnormal motility of the esophagus and gastric dysmotility and impaired gastric emptying are frequently present. Gastroesophageal reflux is associated with esophageal atresia, congenital diaphragmatic hernia, and omphalocele.

The symptoms are the same as those of esophageal hiatal hernia and incompetent cardioesophageal sphincter. The diagnosis is established by prolonged monitoring of lower esophageal pH.

Conservative treatment is successful in most cases. Feedings should be thickened with rice cereal, and reflux is lessened if the baby is maintained upright in an infant seat or in a prone position. Use of metaclopramide or bethanechol increases lower esophageal tone and diminishes reflux in most patients. If a prolonged trial of conservative therapy fails or if complications of reflux can be documented (ie, esophagitis, stricture, anorexia, recurrent aspiration pneumonia, failure to thrive), an antireflux procedure such as the Nissen or Thal fundoplication is indicated. Pyloroplasty may be required when there is associated impaired gastric emptying.

Andze GO et al: Diagnosis and treatment of gastroesophageal reflux in 500 children with respiratory symptoms. J Pediatr Surg 1991;26:295.

Cooper JE et al: Barrett's esophagus in children. J Pediatr Surg 1987;22:191.

Caniano DA et al: The failed antireflux procedure: Analysis of risk factors and morbidity. J Pediatr Surg 1990;25:1022.

Tuggle DW et al: The efficacy of Thal fundoplication in the treatment of gastroesophageal reflux: The influence of the central nervous system. J Pediatr Surg 1989;23:638.

Wheatley MJ et al: Redo fundoplication in infants and children with recurrent gastroesophageal reflux. J Pediatr Surg 1991;26:758.

GASTROINTESTINAL DISORDERS

HYPERTROPHIC PYLORIC STENOSIS

Pyloric stenosis results from hypertrophy of the circular and longitudinal muscularis of the pylorus and the distal antrum of the stomach (Figure 46–8). The cause is not known. The male/female incidence is 4:1. The disorder is more common in first-born infants and occurs four times more often in the offspring of mothers who had the disease as infants than in those whose fathers had the disease. If one monozygotic twin is affected, the other will have the disorder also in two-thirds of cases. A seasonal variation is noted in the occurrence of symptoms, with peaks in spring and fall.

Clinical Findings
A. Symptoms and Signs: The typical affected infant is full-term when born and feeds and grows well until 2 weeks after birth, at which time occasional regurgitation of some of the feedings occurs. Several days later, however, the vomiting becomes more frequent and projectile. The vomitus contains the previous feeding and no bile. Blood may be seen in the vomitus in 5% of cases, and coffee-ground or occult blood is frequently present. Shortly after vomiting, the infant acts starved and will feed again. The stools become infrequent and firm in consistency as dehydration occurs. The premature and weak, chronically starved infant does not have the strength for

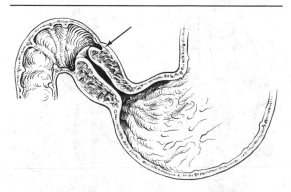

Figure 46–8. Hypertrophic pyloric stenosis. Note that the distal end of the hypertrophic muscle protrudes into the duodenum (arrow), accounting for the ease of perforation into the duodenum during pyloromyotomy.

projectile vomiting, and seemingly effortless regurgitation is the usual symptom.

Less frequently, symptoms occur earlier—even shortly after birth—or as much as 4 months later.

Weight loss follows progressive starvation. Jaundice with indirect hyperbilirubinemia occurs in fewer than 10% of cases. Gastric peristaltic waves can usually be seen moving from the left costal margin to the area of the pylorus. In over 95% of cases, the pyloric "tumor," or "olive," can be palpated when the infant is relaxed. Abdominal relaxation may be accomplished by sedating the infant or by feeding clear fluids and simultaneously aspirating the stomach contents with a nasogastric tube.

B. Imaging Studies: A gastrointestinal series is indicated only in the approximately 10% of cases in which a pyloric tumor cannot be palpated. Results of radiographic studies, preferably using small amounts of diatrizoate meglumine (Gastrografin), include the following diagnostic signs: (1) outlining of the narrow pyloric channel by a single "string sign" or "double track" owing to folds of mucosa; (2) a pyloric "beak" where the pyloric entrance from the antrum occurs; (3) the "shoulder" sign, in which the pyloric mass bulges into the antrum; (4) the pyloric "tit," where the contrast bulges on the lesser curvature between peristaltic waves; and (5) complete obstruction of the pylorus. Abdominal ultrasound will identify hypertrophic pyloric stenosis when the muscle thickness is greater than 4 mm and the length of the pylorus is greater than 16 mm. Ultrasound will miss 8% of infants with pyloric stenosis.

Differential Diagnosis

Repeated nonbilious vomiting in early infancy may be due to feeding problems, intracranial lesions, incompetence of the cardioesophageal sphincter (chalasia) with or without hiatal hernia, pylorospasm, duodenal stenosis, malrotation of the bowel, or adrenal insufficiency.

Complications

Repeated vomiting with inadequate intake of formula results in hypokalemic hypochloremic alkalosis, dehydration, and starvation. Gastritis and reflux esophagitis occur frequently and may contribute to an incompetent cardioesophageal sphincter. Aspiration of vomitus may produce pneumonia or suffocation.

Treatment & Prognosis

Conservative treatment with antispasmodics has been advocated by some but requires prolonged, constant vigilance and care to maintain nutrition and prevent aspiration of vomitus. After many months, pyloric hypertrophy may subside, with relief of obstructive symptoms.

The preferred operative treatment is Fredet-Ramstedt pyloromyotomy, which should be undertaken only after dehydration and hypokalemic hypochloremic alkalosis have been corrected. A nasogastric tube should be placed preoperatively to empty the stomach.

Postoperatively, nasogastric suction is continued for 8–12 hours. Following this, the infant is fed 10% dextrose solution, 30 mL initially; regular formula is then resumed, giving 45 mL every 3 hours for three feedings and then increasing the volume 15 mL at a time until the normal intake is being given. The hospital stay averages 2 days. Occasionally, an infant will vomit persistently, and prolonged nasogastric suction may be required for several days until normal motility returns. Careful management should result in no deaths and prompt recovery.

Forman HP et al: A rational approach to the diagnosis of hypertrophic pyloric stenosis. J Pediatr Surg 1990;25:262.

Keller H et al: Comparison of preoperative sonography with intraoperative findings in congenital hypertrophic pyloric stenosis. J Pediatr Surg 1987;22:950.

Wheeler RA et al: Feeding regimens after pyloromyotomy. Br J Surg 1990;77:1018.

INTESTINAL OBSTRUCTION IN THE NEWBORN

The cardinal signs and symptoms of intestinal obstruction are (1) polyhydramnios in the mother, (2) vomiting, (3) abdominal distention, and (4) failure to pass meconium. Polyhydramnios is related to the level of obstruction and occurs in approximately 45% of women who have infants with duodenal atresia and 15% of those who have infants with ileal atresia. When a tube is routinely passed into the stomach of a newborn, a volume of residual material greater than 40 mL is diagnostic of obstruction. Vomiting occurs early in upper intestinal obstruction, and it is bile-stained if the obstruction is distal to the ampulla of Vater. Abdominal distention is related to the level of obstruction, being most marked for distal obstructions. Meconium is passed in 30–50% of newborn infants with intestinal obstruction, but failure to pass meconium within the first 24 hours is distinctly abnormal.

Causes of neonatal intestinal obstruction include intestinal atresia or stenosis, annular pancreas, malrotation and peritoneal bands or volvulus, meconium ileus, Hirschsprung's disease, meconium plug syndrome, and neonatal small left colon syndrome. Atresia of the bowel occurs in the duodenum in 40%, in the jejunum in 20%, in the ileum in 20%, and in the colon in 10% of cases.

1. CONGENITAL DUODENAL OBSTRUCTION

Duodenal atresia and stenosis produce obstruction at the level of the ampulla of Vater. In 75% of cases, the bile is diverted to the proximal duodenum. Annular pancreas is almost always associated with hypoplasia of the duodenum at the level of the ampulla. The cause is failure of recanalization from the solid cord phase during intestinal development. In about half of cases, multiple congenital anomalies are present, including Down's syndrome in 30% and congenital heart disease in 20%. Birth weight is less than 2500 g in half of these infants.

Vomiting, usually including bile, occurs shortly after birth and during attempted feedings. The upper abdomen may be distended. Meconium is passed in over 50% of cases. Abdominal x-rays show a distended stomach and duodenum ("double bubble" sign). Gas in the small and large intestine indicates incomplete obstruction. Barium (in saline) enema identifies the presence or absence of malrotation, and it may be noted that the colon is unused (microcolon).

The abdomen is explored through a right upper transverse abdominal incision. The hepatic flexure may have to be mobilized to expose the duodenum. Although it is tempting to perform a Heineke-Mikulicz duodenoplasty for stenosis and webs, there is a risk of injuring the ampulla of Vater. A retrocolic, side-to-side duodenoduodenostomy is the procedure of choice. A gastrostomy should also be performed to decompress the stomach and duodenum and to check on the amount of residual material in the stomach during graded feedings.Commonly, the duodenum is hugely dilated above the obstruction, which results in impaired aboral progression of ingested feedings. This problem is resolved by excision of a portion of the antimesenteric wall of the bowel to make the lumen diameter normal (tapered duodenoplasty). Gastrojejunostomy should not be done, because the blind duodenal pouch may cause repeated vomiting. Mortality is related to prematurity and associated anomalies.

Spigland N, Yazbeck S: Complications associated with surgical treatment of congenital intrinsic duodenal obstruction. J Pediatr Surg 1990;25:1127.

2. ATRESIA & STENOSIS OF THE JEJUNUM, ILEUM, & COLON

Atresia and stenosis of the jejunum, ileum, and colon are caused by a mesenteric vascular accident in utero such as may result from hernia, volvulus, or intussusception, producing aseptic necrosis and resorption of the necrotic bowel. Although atresia may occur in any portion of the intestine, most cases occur in the proximal jejunum or distal ileum. A short area of necrosis may produce only stenosis or a membranous web occluding the lumen (type I). A more extensive infarct may leave a fibrous cord between the two bowel loops (type II), or the proximal and distal bowel may be completely separated with a V-shaped defect in the mesentery (Figure 46–9; type IIIa). Multiple atresias occur in 10% of cases (type IV). A type III variant (type IIIb) is commonly called apple-peel or Christmas tree atresia, in which there is a blind-ending proximal jejunum, absence of a long length of mid small bowel, and a terminal ileum coiled around its blood supply from the ileocolic vessels.

Vomiting of bile, abdominal distention, and failure to pass meconium indicate intestinal obstruction. Plain abdominal x-rays will give an estimate of how far along the intestine the obstruction exists; small bowel, however, cannot be distinguished from colon in the newborn. No contrast material should be given by mouth to newborn babies with complete intestinal obstruction. A barium (in saline) enema may be indicated to detect the level of obstruction and the coexistence of anomalous rotation or associated colon atresia. In obstructions that occur in the distal bowel

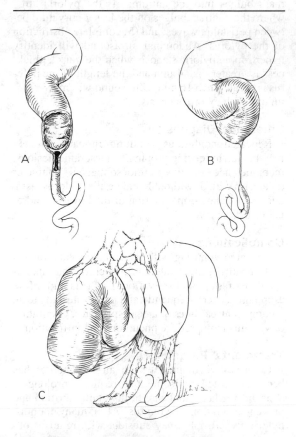

Figure 46–9. Types of intestinal atresia. ***A:*** A membranous web. ***B:*** Fibrous band connecting two blind ends. ***C:*** Complete separation of the two ends, with a V-shaped defect in the mesentery.

and appear relatively early in gestation, the colon is empty of meconium and appears abnormally narrow. When the obstruction is proximal or when it occurs late in pregnancy, meconium is passed into the colon. Barium enema will then outline a more generous-sized colon with its contents. Rarely, a microcolon is not just unused bowel but is due to Hirschsprung's disease. In older children with evidence of partial intestinal obstruction, a small bowel series may be indicated to identify intestinal stenosis.

A transverse upper abdominal incision is preferred. Infants with jejunal atresia usually have greatly dilated bowel from the stomach to the point of obstruction. This overly distended jejunum should be resected— to the ligament of Treitz, if necessary—since it is a source of persistent functional obstruction if it is retained. This same principle applies for membranous atresia, and the temptation to resect the web and perform a Heineke-Mikulicz resection should be resisted. If there is a long segment of abnormally dilated jejunum, the antimesenteric bowel wall should be resected to a normal diameter along with intestinal anastomosis. Infants born with extensive small bowel loss should have a Bianchi procedure, where the entire greatly dilated jejunum is divided longitudinally into two lengths of bowel. The end of the jejunum in continuity with the duodenum is anastomosed to the proximal end of the divided bowel.

In patients with ileal atresia, only the most distal blind end is bulbously dilated, and this should be excised. In order to prevent malabsorption, resection of the ileum should not be too extensive. A great discrepancy between the diameter of the segments of intestine proximal and distal to the atresia is the rule. Therefore, the preferred anastomosis will be end-to-oblique or end-to-side.

A gastrostomy is preferred to help in postoperative decompression and to provide graded feedings.

Atresia of the proximal colon should be treated by resection of the dilated bowel and ileocolostomy. Atresia of the distal colon may be treated by proximal end colostomy or by a Mikulicz side-to-side colostomy. Later, the continuity of the distal colon may be established by end-to-end anastomosis.

The high death rate is related to sepsis, malfunctioning proximal bowel and anastomosis, prematurity, and coexisting meconium peritonitis. In contrast to duodenal atresia, associated anomalies are unusual in small bowel and colon atresia.

Davenport M, Bianchi A: Congenital intestinal atresia. Br J Hosp Med 1990;44:174.

Puri P, Fujimoto T: New observations on the pathogenesis of multiple intestinal atresias. J Pediatr Surg 1988;23:221.

Shen-Schwarz S, Fitko R: Multiple gastrointestinal atresias with imperforate anus: Pathology and pathogenesis. Am J Med Genet 1990;36:451.

Thompson JS et al: Experience with intestinal lengthening

for the short-bowel syndrome. J Pediatr Surg 1991; 26:721.

Weber TM: Short bowel syndrome in children. Arch Surg 1991;126:841.

DISORDERS OF INTESTINAL ROTATION

The midgut of a 10-week-old fetus normally returns from the umbilicus to the abdominal cavity and undergoes counterclockwise rotation about the superior mesenteric artery axis. The duodenojejunal portion of gut rotates posterior to the superior mesenteric vessels for 270 degrees. The duodenojejunal junction becomes fixed at the ligament of Treitz and located to the left of and cephalad to the superior mesenteric artery. The cecocolic portion of the midgut also rotates 270 degrees counterclockwise, anterior to the superior mesenteric artery; and the cecum normally becomes fixed in the right lower abdomen.

Pathogenesis & Classification

Anomalies of rotation and fixation (twice as common in males as in females) include (1) nonrotation, (2) incomplete rotation, (3) reversed rotation, and (4) anomalous fixation of the mesentery.

A. Nonrotation: With nonrotation, the midgut is suspended from the superior mesenteric vessels; the small bowel is located on the right side of the abdomen and the large bowel in the left abdomen. No fixation occurs, and adhesive bands are not present. Because its base is so short, the mesentery is narrow, which predisposes to volvulus, with clockwise twisting of the bowel about the superior mesenteric vessels. This anomaly is usually found in patients with omphalocele, gastroschisis, and congenital diaphragmatic hernia.

B. Incomplete Rotation: Incomplete rotation may affect the duodenojejunal segment, the cecocolic segment, or both. Adhesive bands are usually present. In the most common form, the cecum is located near the origin of the superior mesenteric vessels, and dense peritoneal bands extend from the right flank to the cecum and obstruct the duodenum or other segments of the small bowel. Volvulus is very common (Figure 46–10).

C. Reversed Rotation: In reversed rotation, the bowel rotates varying degrees in a clockwise direction about the superior mesenteric axis. The duodenojejunal loop is anterior to the superior mesenteric artery. The cecocolic loop may be prearterial or may be rotated clockwise or counterclockwise in a retroarterial position. In either case, the cecum may be right-sided or left-sided. The most frequent anomaly is retroarterial clockwise rotation, which causes obstruction of the right colon.

D. Anomalous Fixation of Mesentery: Anomalies of mesenteric fixation account for internal mesenteric and paraduodenal hernias, mobile cecum, or

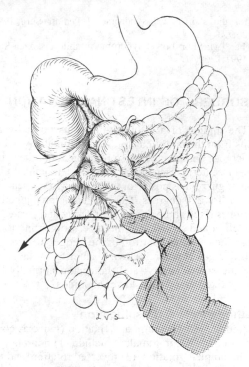

Figure 46–10. Malrotation of the midgut with volvulus. Note cecum at the origin of the superior mesenteric vessels. Fibrous bands cross and obstruct the duodenum as they adhere to the cecum. Volvulus is untwisted in a counterclockwise direction.

obstructing adhesive bands in the absence of anomalous bowel rotation. Excessive rotation of the duodenojejunaljunction results in superior mesenteric artery compression of the third portion of the duodenum (superior mesenteric artery syndrome).

Clinical Findings

Anomalies of intestinal rotation may cause symptoms related to intestinal obstruction, peptic ulceration, or malabsorption. Three-fourths of patients develop intestinal obstruction in infancy. Older patients may develop intermittent obstruction. The obstruction is in the duodenum or upper jejunum as a result of adhesive bands or midgut volvulus. Vomiting of bile occurs initially. Older patients may be thin and underweight because of chronic postprandial discomfort or malabsorption. With duodenal obstruction from bands, abdominal distention is not prominent. Volvulus, however, produces marked abdominal distention. Bloody stools and signs of peritonitis are manifestations of intestinal infarction. Plain abdominal x-rays may show a "double bubble" sign that mimics duodenal stenosis. Distribution of gas throughout the intestines may be normal. When volvulus with gangrene occurs, the bowel is distended with gas, and the intestinal walls are thickened. Bar-

ium enema demonstrates abnormal position of the cecum. With chronic intermittent symptoms of obstruction and a normal position of the cecum on barium enema, an upper gastrointestinal and small bowel series will show distention of the duodenum and narrowing at the point of obstruction.

Peptic ulcer occurs in 20% of patients, presumably as a result of antral and duodenal stasis. Malabsorption with steatorrhea may result from partial venous and lymphatic obstruction, which is associated with coarse rugal folds in the small bowel.

Treatment

Through a transverse upper abdominal incision, the entire bowel should be delivered from the abdominal cavity to assess the anomalous arrangement of the intestinal loops. Volvulus should be untwisted in a counterclockwise direction (Figure 46–10). The Ladd procedure is used for incomplete rotation with obstruction of the duodenum by congenital bands. It consists of division of the bands between the duodenum and proximal colon and the lateral abdominal wall. The appendix is removed. The cecum is then placed in the left lower quadrant and the duodenum moved to the right lateral abdomen.

For duodenal obstruction without anomalous rotation of the colon, the right colon should be mobilized to expose the duodenum, the ligament of Treitz is divided, and the duodenum is moved to the right lateral abdomen. A Kocher maneuver should be accomplished, with complete mobilization of the third and fourth portions of the duodenum. Upon completion of the above procedures, a gastrostomy should be performed and a Foley catheter threaded through it down the duodenum and jejunum. The balloon should then be inflated and withdrawn to the stomach. This maneuver will detect an intrinsic web partially obstructing the bowel, which may coexist with anomalies of rotation and fixation.

Prognosis

About 30% of infants treated for volvulus die from complications of midgut gangrene. Once the anomaly has been corrected, the long-term results are good. Some patients tend to form adhesions that cause recurrent intestinal obstruction. Recurrent volvulus is rare after the Ladd procedure. Constipation and intestinal dysmotility occur in many of these patients.

Millar A et al: The deadly vomit: Malrotation and midgut volvulus. J Pediatr Surg Int 1987;2:172.

Powell D, Othersen H, Smith C: Malrotation of the intestines in children: The effect of age on presentation and therapy. J Pediatr Surg 1989;24:777.

Rescorla F et al: Anomalies of intestinal rotation in childhood: Analysis of 447 cases. Surgery 1990;108:710.

Spigland N et al: Malrotation presenting beyond the neonatal period J Pediatr Surg 1990;25:1139.

MECONIUM ILEUS

In 20% of infants born with cystic fibrosis, the thick mucous secretions of the small bowel produce obstruction by inspissated meconium. This usually occurs in the mid ileum but may develop in the jejunum or colon. Although there is no clear correlation between pancreatic insufficiency and the development of inspissated meconium, meconium ileus also occurs in patients with pancreatic duct obstruction and pancreatic aplasia. Meconium obstruction with no apparent cause has also been described in newborn infants.

Meconium ileus may be complicated by volvulus of the heavy, distended loops of bowel. Depending upon how early in fetal life this occurs, the volvulus may progress to gangrene of the bowel, perforation with meconium peritonitis, or atresia of the ileum—singly or in combination (Figure 46–11).

Meconium ileus equivalent is intestinal obstruction from viscid mucous secretions occurring after the newborn period. All of these patients have cystic fibrosis. The age at onset varies from several days after birth to early adulthood, but most cases occur within the first year. Respiratory infection and fever with dehydration usually precede the obstruction.

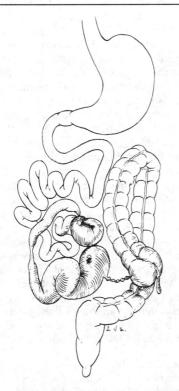

Figure 46–11. Complicated meconium ileus. Includes malrotation, volvulus of the heavy, meconium-filled bowel, and ischemic necrosis of the bowel, producing stenosis, atresia, or perforation with meconium peritonitis.

Paradoxically, these patients usually have symptoms of pancreatic insufficiency with steatorrhea before the onset of intestinal obstruction.

Clinical Findings

The infant typically has a normal birth weight. The abdomen is usually distended and may be large enough to cause dystocia. In most cases, no meconium is passed. Vomiting of bile occurs early. Loops of thick, distended bowel may be seen and felt. Plain abdominal x-rays show loops of bowel that vary greatly in diameter; the thick meconium gives a ground glass appearance. Air mixed with the meconium produces the soap bubble sign, which is usually located in the right lower quadrant. X-rays taken shortly after the infant has been placed in an upright position may fail to show air-fluid levels because the thick, viscid meconium fails to layer out rapidly. An x-ray contrast enema will show microcolon with some meconium flecks. Reflux of contrast medium through the ileocecal valve demonstrates a small terminal ileum containing inspissated mucus; more proximally, the bowel is progressively distended with packed meconium. In complicated meconium ileus, perforation may be detected by the presence of abdominal calcification or extraluminal air. The sweat chloride test is usually impractical in the newborn because very little sweat can be collected. The albumin content of meconium in babies with cystic fibrosis is high, whereas no protein is found normally. Histologic sections of resected bowel show an increase in number and size of the goblet cells, and the intestinal glands engorged with inspissated mucus.

Complications

The most common complication of cystic fibrosis is repeated pulmonary infection with chronic bronchopneumonia, bronchiectasis, atelectasis, and lung abscess. Malabsorption due to pancreatic insufficiency requires pancreatic enzyme replacement. Rectal prolapse and intussusception may be produced by passage of inspissated stools. Nasal polyps and chronic sinusitis are frequent. Biliary cirrhosis and bleeding varices from portal hypertension are late manifestations of bile duct obstruction by mucus.

Treatment

A nasogastric tube should be inserted into the stomach and connected to suction. Under fluoroscopic control, enemas containing full-strength diatrizoate meglumine (Gastrografin), which is hygroscopic, or acetylcysteine (Mucomyst), which is mucolytic, may disperse the meconium in uncomplicated cases. The infant must be well hydrated, and intravenous infusions must be continued during the procedure in order to prevent hypovolemia. Most patients, however, have bowel gangrene, atresia, or perforation due to volvulus and require a Mikulicz resection of the most dilated portion of the ileum.

Postoperatively, the proximal and distal loops of bowel are irrigated with acetylcysteine, and eventually the Mikulicz enterostomy can be closed.

The patient must be placed in an environment with high humidity to keep tracheobronchial secretions fluid. Ultrasonic mist is preferable. Postural drainage with cupping of the chest should be taught to the parents so that they will continue to maintain tracheobronchial toilet indefinitely. Long-term prophylactic antibiotics are not indicated, since infection with antibiotic-resistant *Pseudomonas* and *Klebsiella* organisms usually develops.

Pancreatic enzyme replacement in the form of pancreatin (Viokase) or pancrelipase (Cotazym) may be required. A low-fat formula in the newborn may give better absorption and growth than standard formulas.

Meconium ileus equivalent should be treated by nasogastric suction, diatrizoate meglumine or 4% acetylcysteine enemas, and 4% acetylcysteine instilled into the stomach. Respiratory infection and fever with dehydration usually are contributing factors to meconium ileus equivalent.

Prognosis

The most frequent cause of death is progressive respiratory insufficiency due to plugging of bronchi with mucus, which produces chronic bronchitis, atelectasis, pneumonia, and lung abscess. About 50% of affected children die by age 10 years. Chronic malabsorption develops as a result of pancreatic insufficiency and because the viscid mucus produces a barrier between the bowel lumen and the intestinal mucosa.

Caspi B et al: Prenatal diagnosis of cystic fibrosis: Ultrasonographic appearance of meconium ileus in the fetus. Prenat Diagn 1988;8:379.

Evans JS, George DE, Mollit D: Biliary infusion therapy in the inspissated bile syndrome of cystic fibrosis. J Pediatr Gastroenterol Nutr 1991;12:131.

Millar AJ, Rode H, Cywes S: Management of uncomplicated meconium ileus with T tube ileostomy. Arch Dis Child 1988;63:309.

Mornet E et al: Genetic differences between cystic fibrosis with and without meconium ileus. Lancet 1988;1:376.

Rescorla FJ et al: Changing patterns of treatment and survival in neonates with meconium ileus. Arch Surg 1989;124:837.

NECROTIZING ENTEROCOLITIS

Necrotizing enterocolitis is characterized by necrosis, ulceration, and sloughing of intestinal mucosa, which frequently progresses to full-thickness necrosis and perforation. Pneumatosis progresses from the submucosa through the muscular layer to the subserosa. The terminal ileum and right colon are usually affected first, followed in descending order of frequency by transverse and descending colon, appendix, jejunum, stomach, duodenum, and esophagus—in fact, the entire bowel may be necrotic. Eighty percent of cases occur in premature infants weighing less than 2500 g at birth, and 50% are under 1500 g. However, the disorder may also occur in full-term infants. Necrotizing enterocolitis more commonly appears within 1 week after birth in mature infants, while premature infants are more inclined to develop the condition later. Contrary to earlier impressions, there is no established relationship between necrotizing enterocolitis and stressful perinatal events, such as premature rupture of membranes with amnionitis, breech delivery, intrauterine bradycardia, umbilical vessel catheterization with or without exchange transfusion, respiratory distress syndrome, sepsis, omphalitis, and congenital heart disease. An associated patent ductus arteriosus is common. In older infants and children, necrotizing enterocolitis is usually preceded by malnutrition and gastroenteritis. The clustering of cases in nurseries suggests that an infectious agent is responsible. Usually the infant has been fed, and the presence of intraluminal nutrients seems to contribute to bacterial proliferation.

Clinical findings include increased gastric residual, bilious vomiting, abdominal distention, bloody stools, episodes of apnea and bradycardia, lethargy, and poor skin perfusion. When intestinal perforation occurs, guarding is evident on abdominal examination, but in weak premature infants this may not be obvious. Supine and cross-table lateral abdominal x-rays show small bowel distention early, followed by pneumatosis cystoides intestinalis and eventually gas within the portal vein. Perforation with free peritoneal air develops in 20% of cases. Infants who develop ascites without free air should have a paracentesis and examination of the fluid for bacteria, which would signify perforation. Abdominal wall erythema and a fixed abdominal mass are signs of bowel necrosis. The white blood count may be low or high, but thrombocytopenia is usually present.

Treatment includes cessation of feedings, nasogastric suction, systemic antibiotics, and correction of hypoxia, hypovolemia, acidosis, and electrolyte abnormalities. TPN should be started. Resection of necrotic bowel with ileostomy, colostomy, or primary anastomosis is necessary for bowel infarction. Critically ill very small infants can be treated by draining the peritoneal cavity, using local anesthesia. In one-third of cases, the disorder resolves without further treatment, and the overall survival rate is more than 50%. Stricturing of the bowel may occur as a late complication following healing.

Ein SH et al: A 13-year experience with peritoneal drainage under local anesthesia for necrotizing enterocolitis perforations. J Pediatr Surg 1990;25:1034.

Griffiths D et al: Primary anastomosis for necrotizing enterocolitis: A 12-year experience. J Pediatr Surg 1989;24:515.

Grosfeld J et al: Changing trends in necrotizing enterocolitis. Ann Surg 1991;214:300.

Radhakrishnan J et al: Colonic strictures following successful management of enterocolitis. J Pediatr Surg 1991;26:1043.

Spigland N et al: Surgical outcome of necrotizing enterocolitis. Pediatr Surg Int 1990;5:355.

HIRSCHSPRUNG'S DISEASE

Hirshsprung's disease (aganglionic megacolon) is due to failure in the cephalocaudal migration of the parasympathetic myenteric nerve cells into the distal bowel. Therefore, the absence of ganglion cells always begins at the anus and extends a varying distance proximally. The aganglionic bowel produces a functional obstruction, because the bowel does not have normal propulsive waves and contracts en masse in response to distention. Short-segment aganglionosis involving only the terminal rectum occurs in about 10% of cases; the disease extends to the sigmoid colon in 65%; more proximal colon in 10%; and the entire colon with small bowel involvement in 10–15%. Extensive involvement of the small bowel is rare.

Males are affected five times more frequently than females in cases in which the diseased segment is of the usual length. Females tend to have longer aganglionic segments. A familial association occurs in 5–10% of cases—more frequently when females are affected. The length of involvement tends to be consistent in familial cases. Other anomalies such as Down's syndrome are present also in 10–15% of patients.

Clinical Findings

A. Symptoms and Signs: The symptoms vary widely in severity but almost always occur shortly after birth. The infant passes little or no meconium within 24 hours. Thereafter, chronic or intermittent constipation usually occurs. Progressive abdominal distention, vomiting, reluctance to feed, diarrhea, listlessness, irritability, and poor growth and development follow. A rectal examination in the infant may be followed by expulsion of stool and flatus, with remarkable decompression of abdominal distention. However, foul-smelling diarrhea and abdominal distention should be considered to be Hirschsprung's disease until proved otherwise. In older children, chronic constipation and abdominal distention are characteristic. Passage of flatus and stool requires great effort, and the stools are small in caliber. These children are sluggish, with wasted extremities and flared costal margins. Rectal examination in older children usually reveals a normal or contracted anus and a rectum without feces. Impacted stools in the greatly dilated and distended sigmoid colon can be palpated across the lower abdomen.

B. Imaging Studies: Plain abdominal x-rays in infants show dilated loops of bowel, but it is difficult to distinguish small and large bowel in infancy. A barium (in saline) or a metrizamide enema x-ray should be performed. There should be no attempt to clean out the stool before barium enema, for this will obscure the change in caliber between aganglionic and ganglionic bowel. The barium enema may not show a transition zone in the first 6 weeks after birth, since the liquid stool can pass the aganglionic bowel and the proximal intestine may not be dilated. The aganglionic segment appears relatively narrow compared to the dilated proximal bowel. The proximal aganglionic intestine can be dilated by impacted stool or enema, giving a false impression of the level of the normal colon. Irregular, bizarre contractions that do not encircle the aganglionic portion of the bowel may also be recognized. The dilated proximal bowel may have circumferential, smooth, parallel contractions (similar in appearance to those of the jejunum) that are exaggerated contraction waves. Lateral x-rays should be taken of the pelvis to demonstrate the rectum, the transition zone, and the irregular contractions that may otherwise be obscured by the redundant sigmoid colon on anteroposterior views. Normally, the rectum is wider than the rest of the colon (except the cecum), and when the rectum is seen to be narrower than the proximal colon, the diagnosis is Hirshsprung's disease. X-ray examinations of the abdomen and lateral pelvis should be repeated after evacuation 24–48 hours later. The barium will be retained for prolonged periods, and saline enemas may be required to evacuate it. The delayed film may show the transition zone and the bizarre irregular contractions more clearly than the initial study.

C. Laboratory Findings: Definitive diagnosis is made by rectal biopsy. Mucosal biopsies may be taken from the posterior rectal wall with a suction biopsy capsule without anesthesia. Serial section may demonstrate the characteristic lack of ganglion cells and proliferation of nerve trunks in Meissner's plexus. If the findings are equivocal, it is necessary to remove a 1- × 2-cm full-thickness strip of mucosa and muscularis from the posterior rectum proximal to the dentate line under anesthesia. A sample of this size is sufficient for the pathologist to determine whether ganglion cells are or are not present in Meissner's plexus or in Auerbach's plexus. Manometric studies with show a failure of relaxation of the internal sphincter following rectal distention by a balloon.

Differential Diagnosis

Low intestinal obstruction in the newborn infant may be due to rectal or colonic atresia, meconium plug syndrome, or meconium ileus. Hirschsprung's disease in patients who develop enterocolitis and diarrhea may mimic other causes of diarrhea. Chronic constipation due to functional causes may suggest Hirschsprung's disease. Although functional constipation may occur early in infancy, the stools are normal in caliber, soiling is frequent, and enterocolitis is not usually a problem. In functional constipation, stool is palpable in the lower rectum, and a barium enema shows uniformly dilated bowel to the level of the anus. However, short segment Hirschsprung's disease may be difficult to differentiate, and rectal biopsy may be necessary. Segmental dilatation of the colon is a rare entity which causes constipation similar to that found in Hirschsprung's disease.

Complications

The death rate for untreated aganglionic megacolon in infancy may be as high as 80%. Nonbacterial, nonviral enterocolitis is the principal cause of death. This tends to occur more frequently in infants but may appear at any age. The cause is not known but seems to be related to the high-grade partial obstruction. There is no correlation between the length of aganglionosis and the occurrence of enterocolitis. Perforation of the colon and appendix may result from the distal bowel obstruction. Atresia of the distal small bowel or colon also develops secondary to bowel obstruction due to Hirschsprung's disease in utero.

Anastomotic leak with perirectal and pelvic abscess is the most serious problem following definitive surgical treatment (see below). This complication should be treated immediately by proximal colostomy until the anastomosis has healed. Necrosis of the pulled-through colon may occur if the bowel has not been mobilized sufficiently to prevent tension on the mesenteric blood supply. It is occasionally necessary to divide the inferior mesenteric artery. For this reason, a left transverse colostomy should be avoided (unless it is the position of the transition zone) because the collateral blood supply between the middle and left colic arteries may be divided.

Treatment

The large bowel obstruction and enterocolitis may be relieved initially by placing a large tube in the rectum and repeatedly washing out the colon contents with saline solution. Infants under 1 year of age should have a preliminary colostomy. Conservative measures with enemas may not prevent further obstruction and enterocolitis. The colostomy should be placed at the transition zone, and the presence of ganglion cells at the colostomy site must be confirmed by frozen section biopsy. In total aganglionic colon, an ileostomy is necessary. Because loop colostomies tend to prolapse in infants, it is preferable to divide the bowel, close the distal end, and bring the proximal colon through by suturing the seromuscular portion of the bowel wall to all abdominal wall layers.

Definitive operation should be performed when the patient weighs about 9 kg. Four operative procedures have proved effective.

A. Swenson Operation: In the Swenson procedure, the overly dilated and aganglionic colon and rectum are excised to within 1 cm of the mucocutaneous junction of the anus. The transected end of the normally ganglionated bowel is sutured end-to-end with the distal anorectal segment.

B. Duhamel Operation: In both the Duhamel and the Soave (see below) procedures, the overly dilated and aganglionic bowel is removed down to the rectum at the level of the pelvic peritoneal reflection. In the Duhamel operation, the rectum is oversewn, and the proximal bowel is brought between the sacrum and the rectum and sutured end-to-side to the rectum above the dentate line. The intervening spur of rectum and bowel is divided, and a side-to-side anastomosis is made with a stapler (Figure 46–12).

C. Soave Operation: The Soave operation consists of dissecting the mucosa out of the residual rectal stump, pulling the proximal bowel through, and suturing it to the rectum just above the dentate line.

D. Lynn Operation: Rectal myectomy is used for distal rectal (short-segment) aganglionosis. With lateral retractors in the dilated anal canal, a 1-cm transverse incision is made 1 cm above the dentate line through the rectal mucosa to the muscularis. The mucosa is dissected off the muscularis in a cephalad direction to the transition zone. A strip of muscularis 1 cm wide is removed to the transition zone. The rectal mucosa is reapproximated.

Prognosis

Although in the neonatal period the death rate is high in untreated infants, most patients who are properly treated for Hirschsprung's disease do very well. Problems with occasional incontinence and soiling may occur in a few cases. Episodic constipation and abdominal distention are more common, since the aganglionic internal anal sphincter is intact. Patients with these symptoms respond to anal dilation. Occasionally, an internal sphincterotomy may be necessary. Smaller children may still develop enterocolitis after definitive treatment, and they should be vigorously treated with a large rectal tube and enemas.

Doig CM: Hirschsprung's disease: A review. Int J Colorectal Dis 1991;6:52.

Foster P et al: Twenty-five years' experience with Hirschsprung's disease. J Pediatr Surg 1990;25;531.

Heitz PU, Komminoth P: Biopsy diagnosis of Hirschsprung's disease and related disorders. Curr Top Pathol 1990;81:257.

Mebis J et al: Neuropathology of Hirschsprung's Disease: En face study of microdissected intestine. Hepatogastroenterology 1990;37:596.

Morikawa Y et al: Motility of the anorectum after the Soave-Denda operation. Prog Pediatr Surg 1989;24:67.

Sherman J et al: A 40-year multinational retrospective study of 880 Swenson procedures. J Pediatr Surg 1989;24:883.

Stannard VA et al: Familial Hirschsprung's disease. J Pediatr Surg 1991;26:591.

Tam PK, Boyd GP: Origin, course, and endings of abnormal

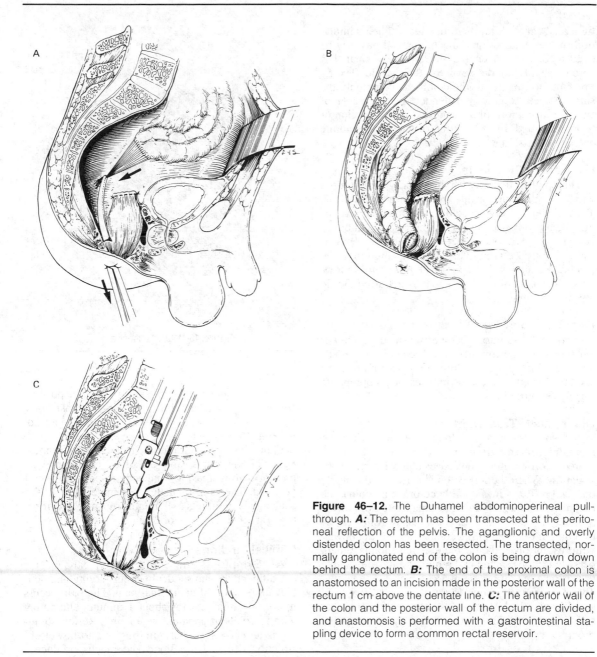

Figure 46–12. The Duhamel abdominoperineal pull-through. **A:** The rectum has been transected at the peritoneal reflection of the pelvis. The aganglionic and overly distended colon has been resected. The transected, normally ganglionated end of the colon is being drawn down behind the rectum. **B:** The end of the proximal colon is anastomosed to an incision made in the posterior wall of the rectum 1 cm above the dentate line. **C:** The anterior wall of the colon and the posterior wall of the rectum are divided, and anastomosis is performed with a gastrointestinal stapling device to form a common rectal reservoir.

enteric nerve fibres in Hirschsprung's disease defined by whole-mount immunohistochemistry. J Pediatr Surg 1990;25:457.

Vizi ES et al: Characteristics of cholinergic neuroeffector transmission of ganglionic and aganglionic colon in Hirschsprung's disease. Gut 1990;31:1046.

NEONATAL SMALL LEFT COLON SYNDROME (Meconium Plug Syndrome)

This problem of newborn infants consists of low intestinal obstruction associated with a left colon of narrow caliber and a dilated transverse and right colon. The infants are in most cases otherwise normal, though approximately 30–50% are born to diabetic mothers and are large for gestational age. Most are over 36 weeks gestational age and have normal birth weights. Two-thirds are male. Hypermagnesemia has been occasionally associated when the mother has been treated for eclampsia by magnesium sulfate injections. Little or no meconium is passed, and progressive abdominal distention is followed by vomiting.

Rectal examination may be normal or may reveal a

tight anal canal. After thermometer or finger stimulation of the rectum, some meconium and gas may be evacuated. Barium enema shows a very small left colon, usually to the level of the splenic flexure. Proximal to this point, the colon and commonly the small bowel are greatly distended. In about 30% of cases, a meconium plug is present at the junction of the narrow and dilated portion of the bowel, and the enema will dislodge it.

Differential Diagnosis

The small left colon syndrome may be confused with Hirschsprung's disease or meconium ileus. These lesions rarely cause obstruction at the level of the splenic flexure, and when the colon readily decompresses without further obstruction, Hirschsprung's disease is unlikely. Finding albumin in the meconium suggests meconium ileus. Careful follow-up with sweat chloride tests may be required to rule out meconium ileus.

Complications

If colonic distention becomes severe, the cecum or appendix may perforate. The difficulty in differentiating small left colon syndrome from meconium ileus and Hirschsprung's disease may lead to inappropriate surgical exploration.

Diagnosis & Treatment

A nasogastric tube should be inserted and intravenous fluids started. Barium or Hypaque enema is required to differentiate the causes of low intestinal obstruction. When the left colon is narrow and contrast material refluxes into the dilated proximal colon, the diagnosis is most likely the small left colon syndrome. The contrast enema is usually followed by evacuation of stool and decompression of the bowel, with resolution of the problem. A few infants remain persistently obstructed and require a colostomy at the transition zone. Subsequent rectal biopsy or anal manometry fails to show Hirschsprung's disease. In some infants, colostomy closure at 1 year of age results in recurrent obstruction due to hypotonia of the proximal bowel.

INTUSSUSCEPTION

Telescoping of a segment of bowel (intussusceptum) into the adjacent segment (intussuscipiens) is the most common cause of intestinal obstruction in children under 2 years (Figure 46–13). The process of intussusception may result in gangrene of the intussusceptum. The most common form is intussusception of terminal ileum into the right colon (ileocolic intussusception), but ileoileal, ileoileocolic, jejunojejunal, and colocolic intussusceptions also occur. In 95% of infants and children, a contributing cause is not found. The disease is most common in

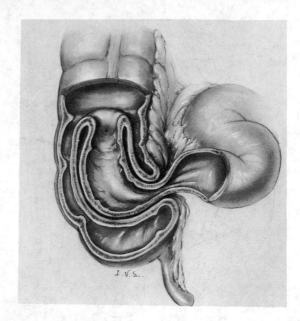

Figure 46–13. Intussusception.

midsummer and midwinter, and there is a positive correlation with adenovirus infections. In most cases, hypertrophied Peyer's patches are noted to be a leading edge. Mechanical factors such as Meckel's diverticulum, polyps, intramural hematoma (Henoch-Schönlein purpura), and intestinal lymphoma are present with increasing frequency in patients over 1 year old. The ratio of males to females is 3:1. The peak age is in infants 5–9 months of age; 80% of patients are under the age of 2 years.

Clinical Findings

A. Symptoms and Signs: The typical patient is a healthy child who suddenly begins crying and doubles up because of abdominal pain. The pain occurs in episodes that last for about 1 minute, alternating with intervals of apparent well-being. Reflex vomiting is an early sign, but vomiting due to bowel obstruction occurs late. Blood and mucus produce a "currant jelly" stool. In small infants—and in postoperative patients—the colicky pain may not be apparent; these babies become withdrawn, and the most prominent symptom is vomiting. Pallor and sweating are common signs during colic. A mass is usually palpable along the distribution of the colon. A hollow right lower quadrant may be noted. Occasionally, intussusception is palpable on rectal examination.

B. Laboratory Findings: The blood count usually shows polymorphonuclear leukocytosis and hemoconcentration.

C. Imaging Studies: The most important test is barium enema, which shows a characteristic obturation obstruction. Plain films of the abdomen may demonstrate evidence of mechanical intestinal obstruction or a soft tissue mass.

Complications

Repeated vomiting and bowel obstruction will produce progressive dehydration. Prolonged intussusception produces edema and hemorrhagic or ischemic infarction of the intussusceptum.

Treatment

Hypovolemia and dehydration must be corrected by fluids. A right atrial catheter for central venous pressure monitoring is indicated for very sick patients. Barium enema should not be attempted until the patient has been resuscitated enough to allow an operative procedure to be performed safely. The baby should be sedated with meperidine, 1–2 mg/kg, and secobarbital, 1–2 mg/kg. The barium is given under fluoroscopic control in an effort to distend the intussuscipiens and reduce the intussusceptum, which is successful in about 50% of cases. The enema bag must not be raised more than 75 cm above the patient. If the initial enema is unsuccessful, it should be repeated two or three times following evacuation of the barium before reduction by enema can be considered a failure. Barium enema will not reduce gangrenous bowel. There is increasing interest in reducing intussusception by insufflation of air into the rectum.

Operation is required for unsuccessful enema reduction or signs of bowel perforation and peritonitis. When no gangrene is present, reduction is accomplished by gentle retrograde compression of the intussuscipiens, not by traction on the proximal bowel. Resection of the intussusception is indicated if the bowel cannot be reduced or if the intestine is gangrenous. A Mikulicz resection may be necessary in critically ill patients.

The appendix is usually removed to prevent confusion in later years if abdominal pain occurs and a right lower quadrant scar is seen.

Prognosis

Intussusception recurs after 3% of barium enema reductions and 1% of operative reductions. In the hands of an experienced surgeon, the death rate should approach zero. Deaths do occur if treatment of gangrenous bowel is delayed.

Ang NT, Beasley SW: The leadpoint in intussusception. J Pediatr Surg 1990;25:640.

Barr LL et al: Significance of age, duration and the dissection sign in intussusception. Pediatr Radiol 1990;20:454.

Palder SB et al: Intussusception: Barium or air? J Pediatr Surg 1991;26:271.

West K et al: Intussusception: Current management in infants and children. Surgery 1987;102:704.

DUPLICATIONS OF THE GASTROINTESTINAL TRACT

Duplications may occur at any point along the gastrointestinal tract from the mouth to the anus. Duplications occur (in order of decreasing frequency) in the ileum (50% of cases), mediastinum, colon, rectum, stomach, duodenum, and neck. Intrathoracic and small bowel duplications are usually spherical; colonic duplications are commonly long and tubular (Figure 46–14). Characteristically, the intra-abdominal duplications are within the mesentery and have a common wall with the intestine. Combined thoracoabdominal duplications also occur in which the thoracic saccular component extends through the esophageal hiatus or a separate diaphragmatic opening to empty into the duodenum or jejunum. A thoracic duplication, associated with a cervical or thoracic vertebral anomaly, in which the duplication communicates with the subarachnoid space, is called a neurenteric cyst or enterogenous cyst. Associated cardiovascular, neurologic, skeletal, urologic, and gastrointestinal anomalies occur in more than a third of cases.

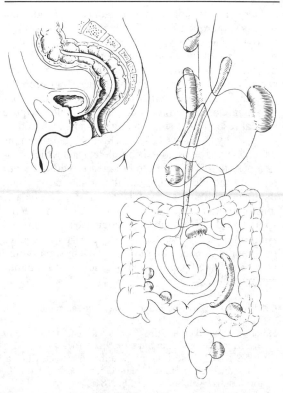

Figure 46–14. Duplications of the gastrointestinal tract. Duplications may be saccular or tubular. They usually arise within the mesentery, having a common wall with the intestine. Thoracoabdominal duplications arise from the duodenum or jejunum and extend through the diaphragm into the mediastinum.

Clinical Findings

A. Symptoms and Signs: Two-thirds of patients with duplications are symptomatic in the first year of life. Duplications of the neck and mediastinum produce respiratory distress by compression of the airway. Thoracic duplications may also ulcerate into the lung and lead to pneumonia or hemoptysis. Intestinal duplications usually produce abdominal pain owing to spastic contraction of the bowel, excessive distention of the duplication, or peptic ulceration resulting from ectopic gastric mucosa. Intestinal obstruction due to intussusceptions, volvulus, or encroachment on the lumen by an intramural cyst also occurs. An isolated asymptomatic mass may be the only finding. Peptic ulceration caused by ectopic gastric mucosa may produce massive gastrointestinal bleeding.

B. Imaging Studies: Studies include x-ray films of the chest and thoracolumbar spine, CT or MRI scans of the chest, barium enema, esophagography, and gastrointestinal series. If an intraspinal extension of a duplication is suspected, an MRI may be indicated. Ultrasonography may show a cystic or tubular mass within the mediastinum or abdomen.

Treatment

Duplications not intimately adherent to adjacent organs should be excised. Isolated spherical duplications can be excised with the adjacent segment of bowel and an end-to-end anastomosis of the bowel performed. Long tubular duplications can be decompressed by establishing an anastomosis between the proximal and distal ends of adjacent bowel. Noncommunicating duplications, which would require radical resection of surrounding structures, should be drained by a Roux-en-Y technique. Duplications which cannot be removed completely and which contain gastric mucosa should be opened (without jeopardizing the blood supply of the normal bowel) and the mucosal lining excised. During resection of a mediastinal duplication, extension of the lesion into the spine and abdomen must be recognized and removed. An intra-abdominal extension is closed at the level of the diaphragm, and complete excision by laparotomy is accomplished. Carcinoma may arise within duplications of the colon.

Gilchrist BF et al: Neurenteric cyst: Current management. J Pediatr Surg 1990;25:1231.

Holcomb GW 3d et al: Surgical management of alimentary tract duplications. Ann Surg 1989;209:167.

Ildstad S et al: Duplications of the alimentary tract: Clinical characteristics, preferred treatment, and associated malformations. Ann Surg 1988;208:184.

Mathur M et al: Histochemical pattern in alimentary tract duplications of children. Am J Gastroenterol 1991;86:1419.

OMPHALOMESENTERIC DUCT ANOMALIES

Anomalies of the omphalomesenteric duct (vitelline duct) are remnants of the embryonic yolk sac. When the entire duct remains intact, it is recognized as an **omphalomesenteric fistula.** When the duct is obliterated at the intestinal end but communicates with the umbilicus at the distal end, it is called an **umbilical sinus.** When the epithelial tract persists but both ends are occluded, an umbilical cyst or intra-abdominal **enterocystoma** may develop. The entire tract may be obliterated, but a fibrous band may persist between the ileum and the umbilicus (Figure 46–15).

The most common remnant of the omphalomesenteric duct is Meckel's diverticulum, which is

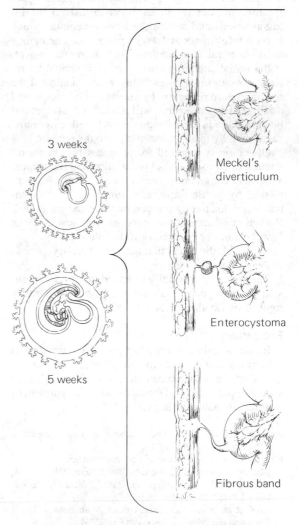

Figure 46–15. Omphalomesenteric duct anomalies arise from the primitive yolk sac. Remnants include Meckel's diverticulum, enterocystoma, and a fibrous band or fistulous tract between the ileum and the umbilicus.

present in 1–3% of the population. Meckel's diverticulum may be lined wholly (or in part) by small intestinal, colonic, or gastric mucosa, and it may contain aberrant pancreatic tissue. Heterotopic tissue is found in 5% of asymptomatic and 60% of symptomatic cases, where more than 60% contain gastric mucosa. In contrast to duplications and pseudodiverticula, Meckel's diverticulum is located on the antimesenteric border of the ileum, 10–90 cm from the ileocecal valve.

Clinical Findings

Meckel's diverticulum occurs with equal frequency in both sexes. It is usually asymptomatic and is seen as an incidental finding during operation for some other disease. Of those with Meckel's diverticulum, the lifelong risk of complications is 4%, and 40% of these cases occur in children under 10 years of age. Symptomatic omphalomesenteric remnants (male/female incidence 3:1) produce rectal bleeding in 40%, intussusception in 20%, diverticulitis or peptic perforation in 15%, umbilical fistula in 15%, intestinal obstruction in 7%, and abscess in 3% of cases. Tumors such as carcinoids, leiomyomas, leiomyosarcomas, and carcinomas are very rare.

Rectal bleeding associated with Meckel's diverticulum is due to peptic ulceration of ectopic gastric mucosa. Over 50% of these patients are under 2 years of age. The blood is mixed with stool and is most often dark red or bright red; tarry stools are unusual. A history of a previous episode of bleeding may be elicited in 40% of cases. Occult bleeding from Meckel's diverticulum is very rare. Younger patients tend to bleed very briskly and may exsanguinate rapidly.

Diverticulitis or free perforation will present with abdominal pain and peritonitis identical to acute appendicitis. The pain and tenderness occur in the lower abdomen, most commonly near the umbilicus. An almost pathognomonic sign is cellulitis of the umbilicus.

A mucoid, purulent, or enteric discharge and excoriation about the umbilicus characterize an umbilical sinus or omphalomesenteric fistula. Recurrent cellulitis or deep abdominal wall abscess about the umbilicus also occurs.

Intestinal obstruction may develop as a result of volvulus of the bowel about a persistent band between the umbilicus and the ileum or as a result of herniation of bowel between the mesentery and a persistent vitelline or mesodiverticular vessel. Obstruction is the most common presentation in adults. Infarction of the incarcerated hernia not uncommonly occurs and disturbs the blood supply to Meckel's diverticulum.

Contrast studies rarely outline the primary defect. Technetium Tc 99m pertechnetate may localize in gastric mucosa lining Meckel's diverticulum and may identify the source of hematochezia or melena. The retention of Tc 99m pertechnetate in the mucous and parietal cells is enhanced by giving cimetidine, 30 mg/kg intravenously 30 minutes before administration of the nuclide.

Treatment & Prognosis

After depleted blood volume has been restored and fluid and electrolyte disturbances have been corrected, the patient should be explored through a transverse abdominal incision. An omphalomesenteric remnant with a narrow base may be treated by amputation and closure of the bowel defect. In cases where the anomaly has a wide mouth with ectopic tissue or where an inflammatory or ischemic process involves the adjacent ileum, intestinal resection with the diverticulum and anastomosis may be necessary. Involvement of Meckel's diverticulum by tumor would require intestinal resection with the lymphatic pathways of the mesentery. Severe illness or death may occur if operation is delayed.

Fowler C et al: Hemoperitoneum from Meckel's diverticulum. J Pediatr Surg 1988;23:952.
St Vil D et al: Meckel's diverticulum in children: A 20-year review. J Pediatr Surg 1991;26:1289.
Turgeon DK, Barnett JL: Meckel's diverticulum. Am J Gastroenterol 1990;85:777.

ANORECTAL ANOMALIES
(Imperforate Anus)
(Figure 46–16)

The normal continence mechanism for bowel control consists of an internal sphincter composed of smooth muscle and the striated muscle complex from the levator ani and external sphincter. The striated muscles assume a funnel shape, originating from the pubis, pelvic rim, and sacrum. These muscles converge at the perineum while interdigitating with the internal and external sphincters. Most of the striated muscle complex consists of horizontal muscles that contract against the wall of the rectum and anus, while longitudinal muscle fibers run in a cephalocaudal direction and elevate the anus.

Anomalies of the anus result from abnormal growth and fusion of the embryonic anal hillocks. The rectum is normally developed, and the sphincter mechanism is usually intact. With proper surgical treatment, the sphincter will function normally.

Anomalies of the rectum develop as a result of faulty division of the cloaca into the urogenital sinus and rectum by the urorectal septum. In these anomalies, the internal sphincter and striated muscle complex are hypoplastic. Therefore, surgical repair results in varying degrees of continence. Commonly, there are associated sacral anomalies with impaired sensory and neuromuscular innervation and genitourinary anomalies.

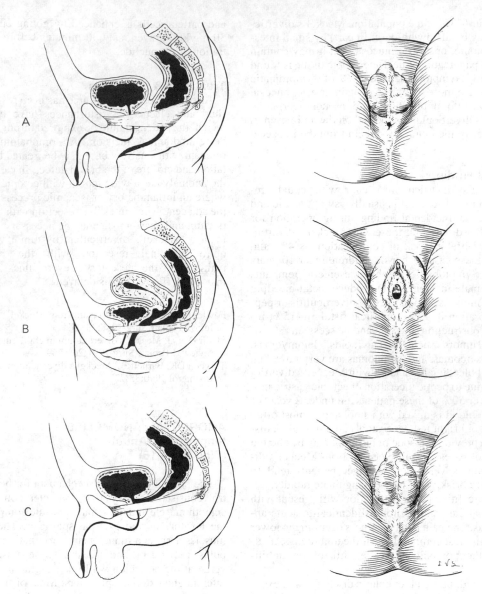

Figure 46–16. Three types of anorectal anomalies. **A:** Translevator anal atresia with anoperineal fistula. **B:** Supralevator anorectal atresia with rectovaginal fistula. **C:** Supralevator anorectal atresia with rectourethral fistula.

Classification

Physical examination of the perineum and imaging studies determine the extent of malformation of the anus or rectum. When an orifice is evident at the perineum or distal vagina, the anomaly is referred to as a low imperforate anus. The absence of an obvious orifice at the perineal level suggests a high imperforate anus (anorectal atresia). In most instances, with high imperforate anus, there is a communication (fistula) with the urethra or bladder in the male or with the upper vagina or bladder in the female.

A. Low Anomalies: In low anomalies, the anus may be ectopically placed anterior to the normal po-

sition, or it may be in the normal position with a narrow outlet due to stenosis or an anal membrane. There may be no opening in the perineum, but the skin at the anal area is heaped up and may extend as a band in the perineal raphe, completely covering the anal opening. A small fistula usually extends from the anus anteriorly to open in the raphe of the perineum, scrotum, or penis in the male or the vulva in the female.

B. High Anomalies: In high anomalies, the rectum may end blindly (10%), but more commonly there is a fistula to the urethra or bladder in the male or the upper vagina in the female. In the female, a very high fistula may extend between the two halves of a bicornuate uterus directly to the bladder.

Another form of high imperforate anus is a cloacal anomaly or urogenital sinus in which there is a common channel (vagina) with a short urethrovaginal fistula and a rectovaginal fistula.

Clinical Findings

A. Signs: The best means of establishing the type of anorectal anomaly is by physical examination. In low anomalies, an ectopic opening from the rectum can be detected in the perineal raphe in males or in the lower vagina, vestibule, or fourchette in females. A high anomaly exists when no orifice or fistula can be seen upon examination of the perineum or when meconium is found at the urethral meatus, in the urine, or in the upper vagina.

B. Imaging Studies: X-ray studies are sometimes useful when the clinical impression is unclear. The upside down lateral film of the pelvis with the baby inverted is an inaccurate method of establishing the lower extent of the rectum, because swallowed air may not have completely displaced the meconium from the rectum, or the striated muscle complex may be contracted, which obliterates the lumen and makes it look as if the gas in the rectum ends high in the pelvis. With crying or straining, the puborectalis muscle and rectum may actually descend below the ischium, giving a falsely low estimate of rectal height. Gas in the bladder clearly indicates a rectourinary fistula. Lower abdominal and perineal ultrasound, CT, and MRI have been advocated to define the pelvic anatomy, but they are rarely indicated. Anomalies of the vertebrae and the urinary tract occur in two-thirds of patients with high anomalies and in one-third of male patients with low anomalies. Vertebral abnormalities in females invariably indicate a high imperforate anus. Anomalies of the sacrum warrant an MRI scan of the lumbosacral area to identify spinal cord anomalies such as a tethered filum terminale.

Complications

Delay in diagnosis of imperforate anus may result in excessive large bowel distention and perforation of the cecum.

Associated anomalies are frequent and include esophageal atresia, anomalies of the gastrointestinal tract, agenesis of one or more sacral vertebrae—agenesis of S1, S2, or S3 is associated with corresponding neurologic deficits, resulting in neuropathic bladder and greatly impaired continence—genitourinary anomalies, and anomalies of the heart and lungs.

The presence of a rectourinary fistula allows reflux of urine into the rectum and colon, and absorption of ammonium chloride may cause acidosis. Colon contents will reflux into the urethra, bladder, and upper tracts, producing recurrent pyelonephritis. A divided sigmoid colostomy rather than a loop colostomy will prevent this until the fistula can be closed at a later date.

Treatment

A. Low Anomalies: Low anomalies are usually repaired from the perineal approach in the newborn period. The anteriorly placed anal opening is mobilized to the level of the levator ani and transferred to the normal position. After healing, the anal opening must be dilated daily for 6–8 months to prevent stricture formation and to allow for growth.

B. High Anomalies: These should be treated by preliminary sigmoid colostomy. If there is doubt about the diagnosis of a high or low anomaly, it is better to perform a colostomy than to attempt a perineal repair and have the anomaly prove to be a high one. The colostomy should be divided to prevent movement of stool into the distal loop, which would cause recurrent urinary tract infection. After the baby's weight reaches about 9 kg, a posterior sagittal anorectoplasty is performed; subsequently, the colostomy is closed. It is important to preserve the afferent and efferent nerves of the defecation reflex arc as well as the existing sphincter muscles.

In high anomalies, the anal sphincters are poorly developed—especially the internal sphincter. Therefore, continence is most dependent upon a functioning striated muscle complex, which requires conscious voluntary contraction.

Complications

Surgical complications include damage to the nervi erigentes, resulting in poor bladder and bowel control and failure of erection. Division of a rectourethral fistula some distance from the urethra produces a blind pouch, prone to recurrent infection and stone formation, while cutting the fistula too short may result in urethral stricture. Erroneously attempting to repair a high anomaly from the perineal approach may leave a persistent rectourinary fistula. An abdominoperineal pull-through procedure performed for a low anomaly invariably produces an incontinent patient who might otherwise have had an excellent prognosis.

Prognosis

Most patients with imperforate anus also have constipation as an inherent part of the disease. The colon and rectum are usually very dilated and have desultory motility. This is fortunate for individuals who have defective sphincter control, but it requires considerable attention to prevent obturation obstruction and constant soiling. Patients with low anomalies usually have good sphincter function. Children with high anomalies do not have an internal sphincter that provides continuous, unconscious, and unfatiguing control against soiling. However, in the absence of a lower spine anomaly, perception of rectal fullness, ability to distinguish between flatus and stool, and conscious voluntary control of rectal discharge by contraction of the striated muscle complex can be accomplished. When the stools become liquid, sphincter control is usually impaired in patients with high anomalies.

Langemeijer R, Molenaar JC: Continence after posterior sagittal anorectoplasty. J Pediatr Surg 1991;26:587.

Pena A: Atlas of surgical management of anorectal malformations. Springer-Verlag, 1990.

Pena A: Surgical management of anorectal malformations: A unified concept. Pediatr Surg Int 1988;3:82.

Templeton JM, Ditesheim JA: High imperforate anus: Quantitative results of long-term fetal continence. J Pediatr Surg 1985;20:645.

Whitehead WE, Shuster, MM: Anorectal physiology and pathophysiology. Am J Gastroenterol 1987;82:487.

LIVER & BILIARY TRACT DISORDERS

NEONATAL JAUNDICE, BILIARY ATRESIA, & HEPATITIS

Jaundice in the first week of infancy is usually due to indirect (unconjugated) hyperbilirubinemia. The causes include (1) "physiologic jaundice" due to immaturity of hepatic function; (2) Rh, ABO, and rare blood group incompatibilities, which produce hemolysis; and (3) infections.

Jaundice that persists beyond the first week in which the indirect and conjugated bilirubin levels are elevated presents difficult problems in diagnosis and treatment. The most frequent cause (60%) of prolonged jaundice in infancy is biliary atresia; various forms of hepatitis occur in 35%; and choledochal cyst is found in 5% of cases of obstructive jaundice.

Extrahepatic biliary atresia is the absence of patent bile ducts draining the liver. Familial cases and the frequent association with the polysplenia syndrome indicate a congenital onset. However, biliary atresia probably develops after birth because jaundice is not usually remarkable in the newborn period, but it becomes evident more than 2 weeks later. Furthermore, conjugated bilirubin is not cleared by the placenta, as unconjugated bilirubin is, and jaundice due to conjugated hyperbilirubinemia with biliary obstruction has not been recognized in newborn infants. The atretic ducts consist of solid fibrous cords that may contain occasional islands of biliary epithelium. The extent of duct involvement varies greatly.

In infants with extrahepatic biliary atresia, the liver develops progressive periportal fibrosis, and the liver cords eventually become disrupted by the cirrhotic process. Proliferation of the bile canaliculi, containing inspissated bile, and lakes of extravasated bile may also be noted.

Intrahepatic biliary atresia and biliary hypoplasia are rare. The extrahepatic bile ducts are patent, but liver biopsies show progressive disappearance of the intrahepatic portal ducts. Biliary hypoplasia associated with Alagille's syndrome (cardiovascular, skeletal, facial, and ocular anomalies) is associated with long survival, while other cases progress to cirrhosis with longevity of 3–5 years, with persistent or intermittent jaundice.

The infant who develops jaundice is usually fullterm with an uneventful neonatal course. Jaundice is first noted in 2 or 3 weeks. Stools may be normal or clay-colored, and the urine may be dark. The stools contain an increased quantity of fat but are of normal consistency and not frothy. The liver may be of normal size early, but it becomes enlarged with time. The infant with surgical obstructive jaundice develops a hard liver as a consequence of progressive cirrhosis; patients with hepatitis have an enlarged liver of softer consistency. Splenomegaly usually develops in all forms of prolonged jaundice in infancy.

Liver function tests are of no help in distinguishing obstructive jaundice from medical jaundice in infants. The bilirubin levels may vary considerably from day to day. Serum transaminase levels are often high in all forms of jaundice, and the serum albumin decreases and serum globulin increases after 4 months in medical or surgical jaundice.

Differential Diagnosis

Other causes of obstructive jaundice are choledochal cyst, inspissated bile syndrome, and hepatitis. A choledochal cyst is identified by the presence of a palpable mass in the right upper quadrant and ultrasonographic confirmation. Inspissated bile syndrome follows a hemolytic process in which a large bilirubin load is excreted into the bile ducts, where it becomes coalesced and impacted. This is recognized by abdominal ultrasound.

Hepatitis is most commonly of unknown cause. It may be due to a variety of infections, often of maternal origin, such as toxoplasmosis, cytomegalovirus, rubella syndrome, herpes simplex, coxsackievirus, and varicella. Serum should be tested for elevated antibody titers to these agents.

Serial scintiscans of the right upper abdomen should be obtained after injection of technetium 99m-labeled iminodiacetate compounds (IDA, HIDA, PIPIDA, DISIDA) to observe the intensity of uptake within the liver and evidence of secretion into the bowel. Needle biopsy of the liver may be safely performed at any age if bleeding and clotting tests are normal. A diagnosis based on needle biopsy is accurate in 60%, equivocal in 16%, and erroneous in 24% of cases. A diagnosis based on the combined results of HIDA scan, needle biopsy, abdominal exploration, cholangiography, and open liver biopsy is accurate in

98% of cases. Genetic metabolic diseases producing jaundice include alpha-antitrypsin deficiency, galactosemia, and cystic fibrosis.

Delayed treatment of patients with correctable forms of biliary atresia will result in progressive cirrhosis. Surgical exploration for neonatal jaundice is indicated as early in infancy as possible, when biliary atresia is the likely cause of jaundice.

Treatment

Preoperative care includes correction of anemia and administration of intravenous glucose and K vitamins. The operation should be scheduled in the morning so that the infant will be on a "nothing-by-mouth" regimen no longer than 6 hours. X-ray facilities should be made ready in the operating room, and the anesthetic period is made as short as possible. The gallbladder should be located and cannulated through a transverse abdominal incision. Diatrizoate (Hypaque) diluted to 25% should be gently instilled into the biliary tree; the surgeon should take care to prevent pressure that might disrupt the bile ducts. If x-rays show a patent common duct but no reflux into the liver, a rubber-shod bulldog clamp may be placed on the distal common duct and the cholangiogram repeated. During development of the x-ray films, a wedge of liver is obtained for biopsy. If atresia of the bile duct is found, the obliterated duct and surrounding fibrosis should be dissected off the portal vein into the hilum of the liver. A Roux-en-Y hepaticojejunostomy is performed to the perihilar liver capsule. A number of variations to this procedure, including use of an intussuscepted antireflux valve, are used to minimize postoperative cholangitis. The appendix may also be used as a conduit between the porta hepatis and the duodenum.

Prognosis

Following portoenterostomy, clearing of jaundice occurs in 80% of patients under 60 days of age but drops to 40% or less beyond 90 days. No persistently jaundiced patient lives 10 years. The survival for jaundice-free children at 10 years is 70%, and prognosis is dependent upon the extent of hepatic fibrosis, the presence of larger ductules at the porta hepatis, and a low incidence of cholangitis.

Patients with correctable forms of atresia may develop recurrent cholangitis. Most often, the cause of the cholangitis is unknown, but it could be related to anastomotic stricture or bile duct fibrosis with intrahepatic bile duct abscesses. Reexploration and revision of the anastomosis may be necessary. Preliminary jejunal diversion by an isolated skin jejunostomy loop may prevent cholangitis and sepsis in young infants. The average life span for infants with uncorrectable biliary atresia is 19 months. Death is due to progressive liver failure, bleeding from esophageal varices, or sepsis. Patients with uncorrectable atresia will develop progressive ascites, making

their care difficult; they eat poorly and become rapidly wasted. Palliation of ascites can be achieved by diuretics. Fat-soluble vitamin deficiency should be prevented by giving triple the usual dosages of these vitamins by mouth. The only hope for patients with end-stage liver disease is liver transplantation.

Crombleholme TM et al: Biliary appendico-duodenostomy: A non-refluxing conduit for biliary reconstruction. J Pediatr Surg 1989;24:665.

deLorimier AA, Harrison MR: Congenital biliary atresia. In: *Surgery of the Gall Bladder and Bile Ducts.* Way LW, Pellegrini CA (editors). Saunders, 1987.

Karrer FM: Biliary atresia registry: 1976 to 1989. J Pediatr Surg 1990;25:1076.

Laurent J et al: Long-term outcome after surgery for biliary atresia. Gastroenterology 1990;99:1793.

Ohya T, Mihano T, Kimura K: Indication for portoenterostomy based on 103 patients with Suruga II modification. J Pediatr Surg 1990;25:801.

Tagge DU et al: A long term experience with biliary atresia: Reassessment of prognostic factors. Ann Surg 1991;214:590.

CHOLEDOCHAL CYST

There are three kinds of congenital choledochal cysts: (1) segmental cystic dilatation of the common bile duct, which occasionally extends into the common, right, or left hepatic duct (type I); (2) cystic diverticulum arising from a common bile duct of normal caliber (type II); and (3) choledochocele (type III), a saccular dilatation of the terminal common bile duct within the duodenal wall at the ampulla of Vater. The last two types are rare. In almost all cases of the first two types, the pancreatic and common bile duct meet to form a common channel several centimeters above the ampulla of Vater but below the cyst. This anomalous union, a persistence of the embryonic hepaticopancreatic duct, allows regurgitation of pancreatic juice into the bile duct, which is thought to have an etiologic role in development of the cystic changes in the bile duct. The walls of choledochal cysts are fibrotic, with a varying amount of inflammatory reaction. The luminal surfaces have a metaplastic epithelial lining or none at all, which probably causes the commonly occurring strictures of cyst-to-intestine anastomoses.

Jaundice in early infancy associated with cystic structures at the liver hilum is probably a different disease from choledochal cyst in older children and adults. The clinical course and prognosis in these infants are the same as those of biliary atresia.

The clinical manifestations of type I and type II choledochal cyst are recurrent abdominal pain, episodic jaundice, and a right upper quadrant mass, though in most cases one of these features is missing. Spontaneous rupture of the cyst and recurrent pancreatitis may occur. The ratio of females to males is 3:1.

The diagnosis can be made from the clinical presentation plus liver function tests, abdominal ultrasonography, upper gastrointestinal tract barium studies, and operative cholangiograms.

Choledochoceles (type III) usually present after age 15 with abdominal pain as the principal complaint. There are two kinds: (1) saccular dilatation of the bile duct just proximal to the ampulla of Vater, and (2) a diverticulum beneath the duodenal mucosa that empties into the terminal bile duct. Many of these lesions are lined by duodenal mucosa, which suggests that they may more accurately be considered a form of duodenal duplication than a bile duct cyst. Some cases have been drained by endoscopic techniques, but a local operation to excise or drain the cyst is probably safer. In contrast with types I and II, adenocarcinoma is a rare complication of this lesion.

The treatment of choice is excision of the choledochal cyst. The duodenal end of the bile duct should be oversewn without injury to the anomalous entry of the pancreatic duct. The common hepatic duct should be anastomosed to a Roux-en-Y limb of jejunum. Side-to-side choledochoduodenostomy is not recommended, because it is followed by a high incidence of stricture of the anastomosis and recurrent cholangitis. Cholecystectomy should be performed regardless of the method used to treat the cyst. Biliary cirrhosis and portal hypertension may occur from prolonged ductal obstruction. Bile duct carcinoma is 20 times more frequent in patients with choledochal cyst than in the normal population, which is one reason why excision of the cyst is preferable to drainage.

Forbes A, Murray-Lyon IM: Cystic disease of the liver and biliary tract. Gut (September) 1991;(Suppl):S116.

Joseph VT: Surgical techniques and long-term results in the treatment of choledochal cyst. J Pediatr Surg 1990;25:782.

Karrer FM et al: Congenital biliary tract disease. Surg Clin North Am 1990;70:1403.

Lopez RR et al: Variation in management based on type of choledochal cyst. Am J Surg 1991;161:612.

Misra SP, Dwivedi M: Pancreaticobiliary ductal union. Gut 1990;31:1144.

Okada A et al: Congenital dilatation of the bile duct in 100 instances and its relationship with anomalous junction. Surg Gynecol Obstet 1990;171:291.

Savader SJ et al: Choledochal cysts: Classification and cholangiographic appearance. AJR Am J Roentgenol 1991;156:327.

Suda K, Matsumoto Y, Miyano T: Narrow duct segment distal to choledochal cyst. Am J Gastroenterol 1991;86:1259.

Yoshida H et al: Biliary malignancies occurring in choledochal cysts. Radiology 1989;173:389.

ABDOMINAL WALL DEFECTS

INGUINAL HERNIA & HYDROCELE

The processus vaginalis remains patent in over 80% of newborn infants. With increasing age, the incidence of patent processus vaginalis diminishes. At 2 years, 40–50% are open, and in adults 25% are persistently patent. Actual herniation of bowel into a widely patent processus vaginalis develops in 1–4% of children; 45% occur within the first year of life. Indirect inguinal hernia occurs four times more frequently in males. Direct and femoral hernias occur in children but are very rare.

Clinical Findings

The diagnosis of hernia in infants and children can be made only by the demonstration of an inguinal bulge originating from the internal ring. The bulge often cannot be elicited at will, and signs such as a large external ring, the "silk glove" sign, and thickening of the cord are not dependable. Under these circumstances, a reliable history alone may be sufficient. Hernias are found on the right side in 60% of cases, on the left side in 25%, and bilaterally in 15%. Indirect hernias are more common in premature infants, and they are more frequently bilateral than in older patients. The processus vaginalis may be obliterated at any location proximal to the testis or labium. When the bowel herniates into the scrotum, it is called complete indirect inguinal hernia; when it does not reach the level of the external ring, it is an incomplete inguinal hernia.

Incarcerated inguinal hernia accounts for approximately 10% of childhood hernias, and the incidence is highest in infants. In 45% of females with incarcerated hernia, the contents of the sac consist of various combinations of ovary, tube, and uterus. These structures are usually a sliding component of the sac.

Hydroceles almost always represent peritoneal fluid trapped in a patent processus vaginalis; hence, they are commonly called communicating hydroceles. A hydrocele is characteristically an oblong, nontender, soft mass that transilluminates.

Differential Diagnosis

A hydrocele under tension is often confused with incarcerated inguinal hernia. Transillumination of the scrotum or groin with a flashlight distinguishes fluid from bowel. The sudden appearance of fluid confined to the testicular area may represent a noncommunicating hydrocele secondary to torsion of the testis or testicular appendage or to epididymo-orchitis. Rectal examination and palpation of the peritoneal side of the inguinal ring may distinguish an incarcerated hernia from a hydrocele or other inguinoscrotal mass.

Complications

Failure to treat an inguinal hernia in infancy shortly after the diagnosis has been made may allow the hernia to become incarcerated and subsequently strangulated. About a third of incarcerated inguinal hernias in infancy show evidence of strangulation, and in 5% of cases the bowel is gangrenous. Compression of the spermatic vessels by an incarcerated hernia may produce hemorrhagic infarction of a testicle.

Treatment

Inguinal hernia in infancy and childhood should be repaired soon after diagnosis. In premature infants under constant surveillance in the hospital, hernia repair may be deferred until the baby is strong enough to be discharged. High ligation of the hernia sac by obliteration of the internal ring (leaving enough space for the spermatic cord), using sutures in the trasversalis fascia, is all that is required.

An incarcerated hernia in an infant can usually be reduced initially before operation. This is accomplished by sedation with meperidine, 2 mg/kg intramuscularly, and secobarbital, 2 mg/kg intramuscularly, and by elevation of the foot of the bed to keep intra-abdominal pressure from being exerted against the inguinal area. When the infant is well sedated, the hernia may be reduced by gentle pressure over the internal ring in a manner that milks the bowel into the abdominal cavity. During this time, nasogastric suction and intravenous fluid replacement should be started. If the bowel is not reduced within an hour, operation is required. If the hernia is reduced, operative repair may be delayed for 24 hours to allow edema in the tissues to subside. There should be little delay in reducing an incarcerated ovary and repair in females, as there is no risk of injuring the vas deferens or spermatic vessels. Bloody stools and edema and red discoloration of the skin around the groin suggest strangulated hernia, and reduction of the bowel should not be attempted. Emergency repair of incarcerated inguinal hernia is technically difficult because the edematous tissues are friable and tear readily. When gangrenous intestine is encountered, the hemorrhagic fluid in the sac should be prevented from entering the abdominal cavity. The gangrenous bowel should be resected and an end-to-end intestinal anastomosis performed. Black, hemorrhagic discoloration of the testis or ovary does not require excision of the gonad.

Boley SJ et al: The irreducible ovary: A true emergency. J Pediatr Surg 1991;26:1035.

Fonkalsrud EW, deLorimier AA, Clatworthy HW: Femoral and direct inguinal hernias in infants and children. JAMA 1976;192:597.

Grosfeld JL: Current concepts in inguinal hernia in infants and children. World J Surg 1989;13:506.

UNDESCENDED TESTIS (Cryptorchidism)

In the seventh month of gestation, the testicles normally descend into the scrotum. A fibromuscular band—the gubernaculum—extends from the lower pole of the testes to the scrotum, and this band probably acts by guiding the path for descent during differential growth of the fetus rather than by pulling the testes down. Undescended testis, or cryptorchidism, is a form of dystopia of the testis that occurs when there is arrested descent and fixation of the position of the testis retroperitoneally, in the inguinal canal, or just beyond the external ring. Continued descent of the testes may progress after birth, but descent comes to a halt before 1 year of age.

Another form of dystopia is ectopic testis, in which the gubernaculum may have guided the testis to the pubis, penis, perineum, or thigh or to a subcutaneous position superficial to the inguinal canal. In these instances, the testis has descended beyond the external ring of the inguinal canal, and the vascular supply is sufficiently developed to pose little difficulty in operative repair.

True cryptorchidism occurs in fewer than 0.5% of males. The right testis is affected in 45% of cases, the left testis in 30%, and both testes in 25%.

Dystopic testes must be distinguished from retractile testicles. The very active cremaster of children under 3 years of age—and the small size of the testis—allow it to retract to the external inguinal ring or within the inguinal canal. The retractile testis usually can be manipulated into the lower scrotum. At puberty, the retractile testis will remain permanently in the lower scrotum; it functions normally, and it requires no surgery.

The complications of dystopic testis include abnormal spermatogenesis, inguinal hernia, trauma, torsion, tumor, associated anomalies, and psychologic effects.

Normal spermatogenesis requires the critical cooler temperature range provided in the scrotum. When the testis remains undescended and subjected to normal body temperature, degenerative changes in the seminiferous tubules occur in which the lining cells become progressively atrophic and hyalinized, with peritubular fibrosis. Eventually, only the Sertoli cells of the tubules remain. Dystopia may affect the interstitial cells, and maximum testosterone production following administration of gonadotropin may be subnormal.

The degenerative changes begin to occur at 1 year of age. Unless the disorder is corrected, all bilaterally cryptorchid adult males are sterile.

A patent processus vaginalis is present in 95% of

patients with cryptorchidism, and approximately 25% develop a hernia.

The fixed position of the testis within the inguinal canal or in an ectopic position makes it particularly vulnerable to trauma. The lack of a broad attachment of the testis in an ectopic location makes it particularly prone to torsion and infarction.

Tumors of the testis develop in one per 50,000 adult males per year. Approximately 10% of these tumors occur in an undescended testis, and since fewer than 0.5% of males are born cryptorchid, the incidence of testicular carcinoma in undescended testes is 30–50 times higher than in the normal male population. The occurrence of tumors in undescended testes begins in teenagers, and operative repair does not lessen the risk of malignant change. The incidence of tumor occurring in the contralateral normally descended testis may also be higher than normal.

Anomalies associated with cryptorchidism occur in about 15% of cases and include a wide variety of syndromes, or they may be confined to the urinary and lower alimentary tracts. Fewer than 50% of the anomalies are associated with Klinefelter's syndrome, hypogonadotropic hypogonadism, or germinal cell aplasia. Other anomalies include the prune belly syndrome, horseshoe kidneys, renal agenesis or hypoplasia, exstrophy of the bladder, and ureteral reflux.

Treatment

Chorionic gonadotropin, 250 IU intramuscularly for infants less than 12 months of age or 500 IU for children 1–6 years old, given twice a week for 5 weeks, has been advocated to stimulate descent. Histologic damage can occur with excessive gonadotropin treatment. It is very doubtful that a true dystopic testis can respond, and descent with this treatment is used to identify patients with retractile testicles.

Orchidopexy is the surgical method for mobilizing the testis, based on the testicular vessels and the vas deferens, from the ectopic location to the scrotum. When the dystopic testis is not palpable preoperatively, 17% are absent, 33% are intra-abdominal, and 50% are in the inguinal canal or just beyond the inguinal ring. Very high testes with a short blood supply can be brought into the scrotum by multistage operations, allowing growth and lengthening of the blood supply between procedures. Testicles confined in the inguinal canal occur in 25% of cases, and most of these can be brought into the scrotum in one stage. Ectopic testicles located outside the inguinal canal, such as in the subcutaneous inguinal pouch, occur in over 50% of cases, and the testicular vessels are so well developed that scrotal placement is rarely a problem.

The ideal age for orchidopexy is less than 18 months old. The prognosis for fertility following orchidopexy in unilateral maldescent is 80%, whereas fertility after bilateral orchidopexy is about 50%.

Elder JS: The undescended testis: Hormonal and surgical management. Surg Clin North Am 1988;68:983.

Gough MH: Cryptorchidism. Br J Surg 1989;76:109.

Hawtrey CE: Undescended testis and orchiopexy: Recent observations. Pediatr Rev 1990;11:305.

Hazebroek FWJ et al: Luteinizing hormone-releasing-hormone nasal spray will not replace orchidopexy in the treatment of boys with undescended testis. J Pediatr Surg 1987;22:1177.

Hutson JM et al: Testicular descent: New insights into its hormonal control. Oxf Rev Reprod Biol 1990;12:1.

Palmer JM: The undescended testicle. Endocr Metabol Clin North Am 1991;20:231.

Testicular descent revisited. Lancet 1989;1:360.

UMBILICAL HERNIA

A fascial defect at the umbilicus is frequently present in the newborn, particularly in premature infants. The incidence is highest in blacks. In most children, the umbilical ring progressively diminishes in size and eventually closes. Fascial defects less than 1 cm in diameter close spontaneously by 5 years of age in 95% of cases. When the fascial defect is greater than 1.5 cm in diameter, it seldom closes spontaneously. Protrusion of bowel through the umbilical defect rarely results in incarceration in childhood. Surgical repair is indicated when the intestine becomes incarcerated, when the fascial defect is greater than 1 cm, in girls over 2 years of age, and in all children over 4 years of age.

OMPHALOCELE

Omphalocele is a congenital defect of the periumbilical abdominal wall in which the coelomic cavity is covered only by peritoneum and amnion. There are two kinds of omphalocele: fetal and embryonic. **Fetal omphalocele** is a small abdominal defect (< 4 cm wide) with herniation of bowel into a sac of amnion that has the umbilical vessels located at the apex of the sac. This is due to failure in development in the periumbilical abdominal wall after the first 8 weeks of gestation. Other anomalies are present in less than 10% of these patients. About 15% of congenital abdominal wall defects are fetal omphaloceles.

Embryonic omphalocele is due to failure of abdominal wall closure in the embryonic stage of development (before the eighth week). It is characterized by a wide abdominal wall defect, usually greater than 4 cm in width, in which the amnion does not protrude far beyond the abdomen, and the umbilical cord joins the abdominal wall at the perimeter of the defect rather than at the apex. Liver as well as bowel is herniated. Multiple anomalies are present in 50% of these cases, such as congenital heart defects (20%) (tetralogy of Fallot; atrial septal defect); trisomies 21, D, and E; diaphragmatic hernia; and renal anomalies.

Other associated anomalies include (1) **pentalogy of Cantrell,** in which the omphalocele is epigastric in position and there is a defect in the diaphragm and pericardium, allowing pericardial herniation of bowel, a split or shortened lower sternum, ventricular septal defect, and diverticulum from the heart—and a small thorax, which may result in pulmonary hypoplasia; (2) **Beckwith-Wiedemann syndrome,** in which a midabdominal omphalocele is associated with a baby who is large for gestational age and who has macroglossia, visceromegaly of the kidneys, adrenal glands, and pancreas, hypoglycemia in early infancy, and a high frequency of hepatoblastoma, Wilms' tumor, or adrenocortical carcinoma; and (3) **hypogastric omphalocele** associated with cloacal exstrophy and spinal dysraphism.

Treatment

Omphaloceles with small abdominal defects can be treated by excising the omphalocele sac and reapproximating the linea alba and skin.

Most large embryonic omphaloceles cannot be closed without staging the procedure. A nasogastric tube should be placed on suction to minimize intestinal distention. A central venous catheter is required to monitor central venous pressure and blood gases in anticipation of postoperative hypovolemia from third space losses and for TPN. An umbilical artery catheter can be maintained without interfering with the repair. A bladder catheter can be used to monitor intra-abdominal pressure. Without removing the amniotic sac, a silicone rubber sheet is formed into a tube (silo), which is sutured to the skin at the perimeter of the omphalocele membrane. The silo is progressively compressed to invert the amniotic sac and its contents into the abdomen and to bring the edges of the linea alba together by stretching the abdominal wall muscles. This requires a number of days. During the operation, the infant should be paralyzed and ventilated through an endotracheal tube. The intra-abdominal pressure produced by the silo should not exceed 20 cm water to avoid impairing venous return from the bowel and kidneys. When abdominal relaxation is sufficient to allow the rectus muscles to come together, the silo is removed, the amnion is left inverted into the abdominal cavity, and the defect in the linea alba is closed. Epigastric hernias may require a Teflon patch to avoid distortion of the costal arch.

Nonoperative management is advised for infants with severe associated anomalies. The amnion is covered with bactericidal silver sulfadiazine, and an eschar forms over the amnion. The membrane becomes vascularized beneath the eschar, and contraction of the wound with skin growth covers the defect.

The survival rate for infants with small omphaloceles is excellent. Deaths associated with embryonic omphaloceles are principally from wound dehiscence and ensuing infection and from associated anomalies.

See references at end of next section.

GASTROSCHISIS

Gastroschisis is a defect in the abdominal wall that usually is to the right of a normal insertion of the umbilical cord. It is probably produced by rupture of an embryonic omphalocele sac in utero. The remnants of the amnion are usually reabsorbed. The skin may continue to grow over the remnants of the amnion, and there may be a bridge of skin between the defect and the cord. The small and large bowel herniate through the abdominal wall defect. Having been bathed in the amnionic fluid, and with compression of the blood supply at the abdominal defect, the bowel wall has a very thick, shaggy membrane covering it. The loops of intestine are usually matted together, and the intestine appears to be abnormally short. The membrane thickens during delay in surgical closure and compromises the outcome. When the anomaly is discovered in utero by ultrasound, the mother should deliver at the hospital where the baby will be operated on.

Complications

Since the bowel has not been contained intra-abdominally, the abdominal cavity fails to enlarge, and it frequently cannot accommodate the protuberant bowel. Over 70% of the infants are premature, but associated anomalies occur in less than 10% of cases. Nonrotation of the midgut is present. Intestinal atresia occurs frequently, because segments of intestine that have herniated through the defect become infarcted in utero.

Treatment & Prognosis

Small defects may be closed primarily after manually stretching the abdominal cavity. Frequently, a staged approach is required. Initially, the bowel should be covered by forming a tube from silicone-coated fabric and incorporating the protuberant bowel into the tube (silo). The end of the tube is tied off. As edema and shaggy membrane of the protuberant intestine are absorbed, the bowel will readily reduce into the abdominal cavity. Reduction is aided by having the infant paralyzed and receiving endotracheal ventilation to relax the abdominal wall and allow it to stretch and accommodate the bowel. Total parenteral nutrition is supplied via a right atrial catheter. When the bowel has completely returned within the abdomen, the silicone-coated tube is removed and the abdominal wall is closed in layers. A gastrostomy is valuable in postoperative care of the baby, because gastrointestinal function is often slow to return.

The death rate for infants with gastroschisis has been greatly reduced by this technique. Poor gastrointestinal function and episodes of sepsis, presumably from compromised bowel, may occur. Total parenteral nutrition may be necessary for several weeks.

Adam AS, Corbally MT, Fitzgerald RJ: Evaluation of conservative therapy for exomphalos. Surg Gynecol Obstet 1991;172:394.

de Lorimier AA et al: Amnion inversion in the treatment of giant omphaloceles. J Pediatr Surg 1990;26:804.

Caniano DA et al: An individualized approach to the management of gastroschisis. J Pediatr Surg 1990;25:292.

Gilbert W, Nicolaides K: Fetal omphalocele: Associated malformations and chromosomal defects. Obstet Gynecol 1987;70:633.

Hughes MD et al: Fetal omphalocele: Prenatal US detection of concurrent anomalies and other predictors of outcome. Radiology 1989;173:371.

Meller JL, Reyes HM, Loeff DS: Gastroschisis and omphalocele. Clin Perinatol 1989;16:113.

Shak R, Wooley MM: Gastroschisis and intestinal atresia. J Pediatr Surg 1991;26:788.

Stringer MD et al: Controversies in the management of gastroschisis: A study of 40 patients. Arch Dis Child 1991;66:34.

Torfs C, Curry C, Roeper P: Gastroschisis. J Pediatr 1990;116:1.

Yaster M et al: Prediction of successful primary closure of congenital abdominal wall defects using intraoperative measurements. J Pediatr Surg 1989;24:1217.

TUMORS IN CHILDHOOD

NEUROBLASTOMA

Of all childhood neoplasms, neuroblastoma is exceeded only by leukemia and brain tumors in frequency. Two-thirds of cases occur within the first 5 years of life. This tumor is of neural crest origin and may originate anywhere along the distribution of the sympathetic chain. Neuroblastomas originate in the retroperitoneal area in 75% of cases; 55% arise from the adrenal gland. The biologic behavior varies with the age of the patient, the site of primary origin, and the extent of the disease (Table 46–4).

Clinical Findings

The most common finding is the presence of a mass, which may be primary or metastatic. Nonspecific symptoms include vomiting, diarrhea, constipation, weight loss, and fever. In infants, metastases confined to the liver or subcutaneous fat are frequent and bone metastases unusual. In older children, metastases to lymph nodes and bone are found in over 70% of cases at diagnosis. Pain in areas of bony involvement and in joints with associated myalgia and fever mimics rheumatic fever. Hypertension and diarrhea may occur as a result of catecholamine and vaso-

Table 46–4. Incidence of primary origin of neuroblastoma in relation to age.

Location of Primary	Infants (%)	All Ages (%)	Survival (%)
Neck	5	3	100
Mediastinum	33	16	85
Adrenal	37	55	20
Extra-adrenal	18	20	18
Pelvis	1.5	1.5	60
Unknown	5.5	4.5	<10

active intestinal peptide secretion. Abdominal neuroblastoma may be distinguished from other tumors by the hard, irregular surface of the tumor and the tendency to cross the midline. X-ray films show a soft tissue mass displacing surrounding structures, and calcification is present in 45% of tumors. For retroperitoneal tumors, an intravenous urogram shows displacement or compression of the adjacent kidney without distortion of the renal calices. CT scan of the area of tumor involvement helps to identify the relationship to surrounding structures. Chest x-ray, complete bone survey, bone scan, and bone marrow aspiration for histologic examination are indicated because of the frequency of bony metastases. About 70% of neuroblastomas produce norepinephrine and its metabolites. Dopamine and the breakdown products of excess norepinephrine production, vanillylmandelic acid (VMA) and homovanillic acid (HVA), should be measured in urine specimens at intervals so that the clinical course of the patient can be followed.

Prognostic Factors

Besides age, site of primary, and stage (Table 46–5), other prognostic factors include histologic grade (Shimada); elevated serum neuron-specific enolase in infants (poor prognosis); elevated serum ferritin (poor prognosis); and analysis of the tumor for

Table 46–5. Staging of neuroblastoma.

	Survival
I. Tumor confined to site of origin	100%
IIa. Unilateral tumor completely excised. Nodes negative.	80%
IIb. Unilateral tumor, complete or incomplete excision. Nodes positive.	70%
III. Tumor infiltrating across the midline, or a unilateral tumor with contralateral nodes positive.	40%
IV. Remote disease in bone, soft tissue, distant nodes.	15%
IVs. Infants with stage I or stage II primary and remote spread to liver, skin, or bone marrow.	85%

the presence of more than three copies of the N-*myc* oncogenes (poor prognosis).

Treatment

A localized neuroblastoma should be excised, and the local area of the tumor should be irradiated only when gross tumor remains. Unresectable neuroblastomas should be treated initially by chemotherapy and radiation therapy and then by surgical resection for residual tumor. Most neuroblastomas are radiosensitive and respond to 3000 cGy or less of radiation. Patients with disseminated disease should be treated with a combination of chemotherapeutic agents such as cyclophosphamide (Cytoxan), vincristine, dacarbazine, doxorubicin, cisplatin, and teniposide. Patients with stage III or stage IV tumors and more than three N-*myc* copies benefit from total body radiation followed by bone marrow transplantation.

Brodeur AE, Brodeur GM: Abdominal masses in children: Neuroblastoma, Wilms' tumor, and other considerations. Pediatr Rev 1991;12:196.

deLorimier AA et al: Neuroblastoma. In: *Current Genitourinary Cancer Surgery.* Crawford ED, Das B (editors). Lea & Febiger, 1990.

Haase G et al: Improvement in survival after excision of primary tumor in stage III neuroblastoma. J Pediatr Surg 1989;24:194.

Hiyama E: N-*myc* gene amplification and other prognosis-associated factors in neuroblastoma. J Pediatr Surg 1990;25:1095.

Nesbit ME Jr: Advances and management of solid tumors in children. Cancer 1990;65:696.

Shamberger RC et al: Surgical management of stage III and IV neuroblastoma. J Pediatr Surg 1991;26:1113.

Smith EI, Castleberry RP: Neuroblastoma. Curr Probl Surg 1990;27:573.

Smith EI et al: A surgical perspective on the current staging in neuroblastoma: The International Neuroblastoma Staging System Proposal. J Pediatr Surg 1989;24:386.

TUMORS OF THE KIDNEY

Renal neoplasms account for about 10% of malignant tumors in children. Eighty percent of patients are under 4 years of age. There are four histologically distinct malignant tumors. Nephroblastoma (Wilms's tumor), which accounts for 80%, consists of a variety of embryonic tissues such as abortive tubules and glomeruli, smooth and skeletal muscle fibers, spindle cells, cartilage, and bone. Wilms's tumor may be present at birth or, very rarely, may develop in adults up to the sixth decade. Nephroblastoma is considered a favorable histologic diagnosis because, with current multimodal treatment, the survival rate exceeds 85%. Unfavorable histologic diagnoses are anaplastic sarcoma (focal or diffuse), clear cell sarcoma, and rhabdoid tumors. Although this last group of neoplasms accounts for fewer than 10% of renal cancers,

it is responsible for more than 50% of deaths due to renal tumors in children.

The left kidney is affected in 50% of cases and the right kidney in 45%. In 5% of cases the tumors are bilateral; 60% are synchronous and 40% are metachronous. Associated anomalies and their incidence per 1000 cases are aniridia, 8.5; hemihypertrophy, 25; cryptorchidism, 28; and hypospadias, 18. Beckwith-Wiedemann syndrome and neurofibromatosis occur occasionally, and renal tumors may also occur in families.

Clinical Findings

Symptoms consist of abdominal enlargement in 60% of cases; pain in 20%; hematuria in 15%; malaise, weakness, anorexia, and weight loss in 10%; and fever in 3%. An abdominal mass, palpable in almost all cases, is usually very large, firm, and smooth, and it does not ordinarily extend across the midline. Hypertension, noted in over half of patients, may cause congestive heart failure. An intravenous urogram shows distortion of the calices and kidney. Nonopacification on the urogram indicates tumor extension into the ureter or renal vessels. Cystoscopy and retrograde urography are unnecessary.

Differential Diagnosis

Abdominal masses may also be caused by hydronephrotic, multicystic, or duplicated kidneys and by neuroblastoma, teratoma, hepatoma, and rhabdomyosarcoma. Ultrasonography, CT scanning, and intravenous urography can usually distinguish nephroblastoma from these other tumors. Caliceal distortion indicates renal origin. Calcification occurs in 10% of cases of nephroblastoma and tends to be more crescent-shaped, discrete, and peripherally situated than the calcification of neuroblastoma, which is finely stippled.

Complications

Extension of tumor into the renal vein and inferior vena cava can usually be detected by ultrasonography and MRI. These vessels should be carefully felt during abdominal exploration, and the tumor should be removed in such a way that tumor embolization will not occur. Metastases to the lungs should be sought by chest x-rays and CT scans and liver metastases by CT and isotope liver scans.

Treatment & Prognosis

The preferred treatment is immediate nephrectomy and excision of all surrounding tissues within Gerota's fascia, including retroperitoneal lymphadenectomy. Irradiation of the tumor bed is indicated if the tumor has extended beyond the capsule of the kidney to involve adjacent organs or lymph nodes. Large, necrotic, hemorrhagic tumors may require preoperative angiographic embolization to facilitate their extirpation. Very large tumors may be treated with radiation therapy and chemotherapy preoperatively to reduce their size. A significant reduction in size usually occurs in 7–10 days, after which nephrectomy can be readily performed. Nephrectomy is accomplished through a long transverse or thoracoabdominal incision.

Prognostic factors that influence survival include extension of tumor beyond the capsule, presence of lymph node metastases, and histologic pattern. Patients with differentiated tumors have a survival rate of 92%; those with focal anaplasia (found in fewer than 10% of microscopic fields), 60%; and those with diffuse anaplasia, 20%. Survival is rare with rhabdoid or clear cell sarcoma.

The stage of the disease is determined by the pathologic findings: Stage I is tumor confined to a kidney that has been completely excised; stage II is tumor extending beyond the kidney (perirenal tissues, renal vein or vena cava, biopsy or local spill in the flank) and completely excised; stage III is residual, nonhematogenous tumor confined to the abdomen (lymph node metastases, preoperative or intraoperative diffuse peritoneal deposits, residual tumor at the surgical margins, or unresectable tumor); stage IV is hematogenous metastases (lung, liver, bone, and brain); and stage V is bilateral renal involvement.

All patients should receive combination chemotherapy postoperatively, consisting of dactinomycin and vincristine. In addition, doxorubicin, 60 mg/m^2, should be given for stage III and IV nephroblastoma and for all cases with unfavorable histologic findings. The cardiotoxicity of doxorubicin is substantial, and the drug might be reserved for children with unfavorable prognostic factors. The role of radiotherapy to the tumor bed or the whole abdomen for extensive intra-abdominal spill remains to be determined.

Metastases in the lung or liver may be resected or treated with radiation therapy. Any residual tumor following radiation therapy, including multiple lesions, should be resected.

Nephroblastoma is bilateral in 5–10% of cases. These lesions may be treated by varying combinations of partial nephrectomy, irradiation, and chemotherapy. The cure rate is about 80%.

D'Angio GJ et al: Treatment of Wilms' tumor: Results of the Third National Wilms' Tumor Study. Cancer 1989;64:349.

Greenberg M et al: Preoperative chemotherapy for children with Wilms' tumor. J Pediatr Surg 1991;26:949.

Larsen E et al: Surgery only for the treatment of patients with stage I Wilms' tumor. Cancer 1990;66:264.

Longacker MT et al: Hyaluronic acid stimulating activity in the urine of Wilms' tumor patients. J Natl Cancer Inst 1990;82:135.

TERATOMA

Teratomas are congenital neoplasms derived from all three basic germ cells of the early embryo. Sites of origin (in order of frequency) are the ovaries, testes, anterior mediastinum, presacral and coccygeal regions, and retroperitoneum.

These tumors should be excised because of their malignant potential and the symptoms produced by their size. The most common malignant type is the yolk sac tumor (endodermal sinus tumor). Serum alpha-fetoprotein and chorionic gonadotropin levels can be monitored to detect the presence of recurrent germ cell tumors. Some malignant tumors respond to x-ray therapy. Regardless of the stage of disease, these tumors behave aggressively and should be treated adjunctively with a combination of cisplatin, vinblastine, and bleomycin or with dactinomycin, cyclophosphamide, and vincristine.

Ein SH: Malignant sacrococcygeal teratoma—endodermal sinus, yolk sac tumor—in infants and children: A 32-year review. J Pediatr Surg 1985;20:473.

Mann JR: Results of the United Kingdom Children's Cancer Study Group's Malignant Germ Cell Tumor Studies. Cancer 1989;63:1657.

Tapper D, Lack EE: Teratomas in infancy and childhood: A 54-year experience at the Children's Hospital Medical Center. Ann Surg 1983;198:398.

RHABDOMYOSARCOMA

Embryonal rhabdomyosarcoma has a favorable prognosis, while alveolar, monomorphous, and undifferentiated sarcomas have poor prognoses. Rhabdomyosarcoma may develop in any part of the body. Tumors arising in the orbit, the oral cavity, the face and neck, and the nontrigonal area of the bladder, vagina, and peri-testicular areas have a good prognosis. The prognosis is poor for tumors of the parameningeal areas (such as the nasopharynx, sinuses, middle ear, infratemporal fossa), prostate, trunk, extremities, and retroperitoneum. The prognosis also depends upon the histologic features, the site of the primary lesion, the group or stage of disease, and tumor size. Status of the disease after surgery also has a bearing. Group I tumors are confined to the site of origin and have been completely excised. Group II tumors have microscopic residual disease at the primary site following excision. Group III tumors have gross residual disease (IIIa), no residual disease but regional lymph node metastases (IIIb), or both gross residual tumor and regional lymph node spread (IIIc). Group IV (stage IV) tumors have metastases, either blood-borne or by lymphatics, to sites distant from the primary.

Stage I disease consists of group I, II, or III tumors arising from favorable sites of origin whether or not they are invasive, large, or incompletely excised. Stage II tumors originate in unfavorable sites, are less than 5 cm in diameter, have no nodal metastases, and are grouped as I, II, or IIIa. Stage III tumors arise from unfavorable sites, are greater than 5 cm in diameter, and may have regional lymph node metastases.

Treatment consists of resection of the primary tumor. Chemotherapy or radiation therapy, alone or in combination, may be indicated for large lesions that appear to be unresectable. Local recurrence and metastases to lung, liver, brain, and bone are common following apparent local control, and all patients therefore should receive postoperative chemotherapy. The regimen should consist of several drugs, including vincristine, dactinomycin (actinomycin D), and cyclophosphamide (VAC), ifosfamide, and etoposide. Local irradiation is used for residual primary disease and for metastases that have not responded to chemotherapy.

The 5-year survival for stage I tumors is 90%; for stage II, clinical group I or II, it is 77%; for stage II, clinical group III, it is 65%; and for stage III lesions (group I, II, or III), it is 55%. Stage IV tumors arising from favorable sites of origin are curable, while those from unfavorable sites have a very poor prognosis.

Bonilla JA, Healy GB: Management of malignant head and neck tumors in children. Pediatr Clin North Am 1989;36:1443.

Goren MP, Shapiro DN: Pediatric soft tissue sarcomas. Curr Opin Oncol 1990;2:481.

Hays D et al: Clinical staging and treatment results in rhabdomyosarcoma of the female genital tract among children and adolescents. Cancer 1988;61:1893.

Hays DM: Secondary surgical procedures to evaluate primary tumor status in patients with chemotherapy-responsive stage III and IV sarcomas. J Pediatr Surg 1990;25:1100.

Houghton PJ, Shapiro DN, Houghton JA: Rhabdomyosarcoma: From the laboratory to the clinic. Pediatr Clin North Am 1991;38:349.

Issa MM, Shortliffe LM: Pediatric genitourinary tumors. Curr Opin Oncol 1991,3.543.

McHenry CR et al: Vaginal neoplasms in infancy: The combined role of chemotherapy and conservative surgical resection. J Pediatr Surg 1988;23:842.

Prognostic factors in childhood rhabdomyosarcoma. Lancet 1989;2:959.

Rao BN, Etcubanas EE, Green AA: Present-day concepts in the management of sarcomas in children. Cancer Invest 1989;7:349.

BATTERED CHILD SYNDROME

Child abuse is any nonaccidental injury inflicted by a parent, guardian, or neighbor. It may be passive, in the form of emotional or nutritional deprivation, but it is most readily recognized in the active form characterized as "battered, bruised, beaten, broken, and burned." It is estimated that 1 million children per year in the USA suffer injuries that should be reported to the National Center on Child Abuse and Neglect. About 20–50% of children are rebattered after the first diagnosis, resulting in death in 5% and permanent physical damage in 35% when the syndrome is not recognized.

Etiology

The child abuser is usually a young, insecure, unstable person who had an unhappy childhood and who has unrealistic expectations of the child. Most (not all) of these individuals are of low socioeconomic status. The abuser may be a parent, guardian, baby-sitter, neighborhood child, or mother's boyfriend. Active traumatic abuse is usually perpetrated by the father, but passive neglect with failure to thrive from nutritional or emotional deprivation is usually attributable to the mother.

Clinical Findings

In most cases, the battered child is under 3 years of age and is the product of a difficult or premature pregnancy and labor, usually unwanted or illegitimate. Many battered children have congenital anomalies or are hyperkinetic and colicky. Usually, there is a discrepancy between the history supplied and the magnitude of the injury or else a reluctance to give a history. Contradictory histories or delay in bringing the child to medical attention—or many different emergency room visits in different hospitals for unusual reasons—should be regarded with suspicion. A past injury in the child or sibling and almost any injury in an infant under 1 year of age are likely to be the results of child abuse. The parents may be evasive or hostile. They may have open guilt feelings or may be capable of complete concealment. Usually, the innocent spouse is more protective of the abuser than of the child.

The child is usually withdrawn, apathetic, whimpering, and fearful and shows signs of neglect or failure to thrive. Multiple forms of injury will be noted at varying stages of healing. The child should be completely disrobed to enable the clinician to look for welts, bruises, lacerations, bite or belt wounds, stick or coat hanger marks on the head, trunk, buttocks, or extremities, and similar evidence of mistreatment. Cigarette, hot plate, match, or scalding burns may be evident. Subgaleal hematomas may be caused by pulled hair. Retinal hemorrhage or detachment may follow blows to the head. Abdominal injuries may produce ruptured liver, spleen, or pancreas or bowel perforation. Sexual abuse should be identified by determining whether the vaginal introitus or anus is bruised, lacerated, or enlarged and whether aspirated fluid contains sperm or prostatic acid phosphatase.

Even though no obvious fracture may be present, a skeletal roentgenographic survey should be performed. The bone most commonly fractured is the femur, followed by the humerus in the region of the diaphysis. Rib fractures and periosteal reactions in various stages of healing will be seen. Skull fractures are most commonly seen in infants less than 1 year old. Suture separation of the skull may indicate subdural hematoma. Neurologic injury may require a brain scan or MRI.

Management

The child should be admitted to the hospital to be protected until the home environment can be evaluated. Injuries should be documented radiologically and with photographs. The presence of sperm in the vagina or anal canal should be confirmed. Bleeding disorders should be evaluated by a platelet count, bleeding time, prothrombin time, and plasma thromboplastin test to make certain that multiple bruises are not due to coagulopathy. A serologic test for syphilis may be indicated as well as cultures (including pharyngeal) for gonorrhea.

Injuries should be treated. Consultation with ophthalmologists, neurologists, neurosurgeons, orthopedic surgeons, and plastic surgeons may be required.

It is required by law in every state for both the hospital and the physician to report child abuse, suspected as well as documented, to local authorities. The district attorney's office can inform the physi-

cian about details of the local law. The physician is the protector of the child and a consultant to the parents and must not assume the role of prosecutor or judge. The most difficult task is to notify the parents without confrontation, accusation, or anger that battering or neglect is suspected. The physician must tell the parents that the law requires reporting injuries that are unexplained or inadequately explained in view of the nature of the injury. A written referral should then be made to other professionals, such as child welfare personnel, social workers, or psychiatrists. The referral should describe the history of past injuries and the nature of current injuries, results of physical examination and laboratory and x-ray studies, and a statement about why nonaccidental trauma is suspected.

Prognosis

The abuser may require careful evaluation for possible psychosis by a psychiatrist. Child welfare personnel and social workers will have to assess the home environment and work with the parents to prevent future abuse. It may be necessary to place the child in a foster home, but approximately 90% of families can be reunited.

King J et al: Analysis of 429 fractures in 189 battered children. J Pediatr Anthrop 1989;8:585.

Kottmeier PK: The battered child. Pediatr Ann 1987; 16:343.

REFERENCES

Ashcraft KW, Holder TM (editors): *Pediatric Esophageal Surgery.* Grune & Stratton, 1986.

Ashcraft KW, Holder TM (editors): *Pediatric Surgery.* Saunders, 1992.

Gray SW, Skandalakis JE: *Embryology for Surgeons: The Embryological Basis for Treatment of Congenital Defects.* Saunders, 1972.

Harrison MR, Golbus MS, Filly RA: *The Unborn Patient: Prenatal Diagnosis and Treatment,* 2nd ed. Grune & Stratton, 1990.

Hays DM: *Pediatric Surgical Oncology.* Grune & Stratton, 1986.

Kelalis PP, King LR, Belman AB: *Clinical Pediatric Urology,* 2nd ed. 2 vols. Saunders, 1985.

Rudolph AM, Hoffman JIE (editors): *Pediatrics,* 19th ed. Appleton & Lange, 1990.

Welch KJ et al (editors): *Pediatric Surgery,* 4th ed. 2 vols. Year Book, 1985.

Oncology & Cancer Chemotherapy

47

Jeffrey Arbeit, MD, David C. Hohn, MD, Andrew Ridge, MD, Robert S. Warren, MD,
& Samuel D. Spivack, MD Karen K. Fu, MD, & Theodore L. Phillips, MD

INCIDENCE & CLASSIFICATION OF TUMORS

Samuel D. Spivack, MD

Approximately 1 million new cases of cancer are diagnosed each year in the USA, excluding non-melanoma skin cancer and carcinoma in situ of the cervix. Cancer is responsible for 22% of all deaths and (next to heart disease) is the second leading cause of death. The incidence of neoplasia by site and sex is shown in Table 47–1.

Although the term "tumor" originally denoted any mass or swelling, the present meaning is generally synonymous with neoplasm (a new pathologic growth of tissue). A neoplasm may be characterized as benign or malignant depending upon its histologic, gross, and clinical features. Malignant neoplasms usually show imperfect differentiation and structure atypical of the tissue of origin, an infiltrative growth pattern not contained by a true capsule, and relatively frequent and abnormal mitotic figures. Growth rarely ceases, although the rate of growth may be irregular, and many malignant tumors have a propensity for metastasis. Benign tumors generally lack these features, although they may be fatal as a result of impingement of other structures and impairment of function.

Neoplasms are classified according to their tissue of origin. Those from mesenchyme (muscle, bone, tendon, cartilage, fat, vessels, or lymphoid or connective tissue) are called sarcomas. Malignant tumors of epithelial origin are carcinomas and may be further classified, according to their histologic appearance, as adenocarcinomas (glandular), squamous (epidermoid), transitional, or undifferentiated. Tumors may be composed of one neoplastic cell type (although also containing nonneoplastic stromal elements such as blood vessels); may contain several neoplastic cell types of common derivation from the same germ cell layer (mixed tumors); or may derive from more than one embryonic germ cell layer (teratomas).

ETIOLOGIC FACTORS IN TUMOR FORMATION

Jeffrey Arbeit, MD

Quantity, structure, and function of specific molecules (eg, growth factors and their receptors, signal transducers, or tumor suppressor genes) are abnormal in cancer cells. Although the mutations occur sporadically and are most often of unknown cause, they may result from exposure to environmental carcinogens (eg, chemicals, foreign bodies, irradiation, viruses). Since changes are inherited by daughter cells, enough abnormal cells may accumulate to produce an invasive malignancy. The abnormalities of neoplasia will be reviewed by comparison with normal molecular physiology.

MOLECULAR PHYSIOLOGY OF THE NORMAL & NEOPLASTIC CELL

Specific molecules are responsible for cellular organization within tissues. Adhesion molecules determine cell shape and polarity. Others direct the attachment of cells to extracellular matrix and basement membranes. Growth factors (GFs) influence intra- and intercellular behavior. Growth factors may act on the cell of origin (autocrine function), nearby cells (paracrine function), or distant cells (endocrine function). Each growth factor binds to a surface molecule (growth factor receptor; GFR), which causes the receptor to send a signal into the cell, activating other molecules in the cytoplasm and the nucleus. Important cytoplasmic molecules in this chain include the juxtamembrane signal transducers, the intermediate filaments that control cell shape and locomotion, the molecules of the protein secretory and degradation pathways, and the protein synthetic machinery (eg, ribosomes, messenger RNA [mRNA], and associated proteins). mRNA, made in the nucleus from template DNA (transcribed), contains the genetic information that directly codes for specific proteins. In the nucleus, DNA is organized into regulatory segments

Table 47–1. Cancer incidence (in %) by site and sex.[1]

	Male	Female
Skin	3	2
Oral	4	2
Lung	22	10
Breast	...	26
Colon and rectum	14	16
Pancreas	3	3
Prostate	19	...
Uterus	...	11
Ovary	...	4
Urinary tract	9	4
Leukemia and lymphomas	8	7
All other	18	14

[1]Source: *CA–A Cancer Journal for Clinicians* 1986;36:9.

(promoters, enhancers) and protein coding sequences (open reading frames; ORFs). The open reading frames are further organized into exons and introns; the former code for structural units, protein, and RNA, whereas the latter are spliced out during RNA processing, allowing for diversity in genetic response. The nucleus contains proteins that replicate DNA, repair DNA to prevent mutations, or transcribe DNA. Communication between the nucleus and other parts of the cell is bidirectional. Signals from the nucleus (eg, mRNA) stimulate production of grwoth factors or growth factor receptors, which in turn send signals that alter nuclear proteins to change the rate of DNA synthesis or the rate of gene transcription (**gene expression**).

Mutations in DNA produce altered or lost genes. Single bases may be changed (point mutations), or segments of DNA may be lost (deletions) or rear-ranged (translocations). **Dominant mutations** result in increased production or lack of regulation of molecules and a gain in function. **Recessive mutations** result in loss of a molecule (due to premature termination of transcription) or structural problems. The consequent loss of function may be compensated by the normal product produced in diploid cells. Many molecules exist in structurally defined multi-unit complexes. **Dominant/negative** mutations produce an abnormal molecule that is able to complex with a normal counterpart, but the unit is inactive.

Many changes seen in cancer cells have counterparts in normal embryogenesis and organ development, lymphocyte blastogenesis, surgical wound healing, the metabolic response to trauma and sepsis, and organ regeneration or hypertrophy after injury or resection. The molecular alterations in cancer cells either exaggerate normal function, inappropriately express juvenile developmental patterns, or change important regulatory functions.

GROWTH FACTORS

Growth factors are small peptides that bind to specific cell membrane receptors. Binding produces an intracellular response that results either in growth and proliferation or in inhibition of function. The growth factors that influence solid tumor behavior are listed in Table 47–2. Autocrine growth factor production by cancer cells may stimulate tumor growth, while paracrine secretion may produce angiogenesis or fibroplasia (or both) by normal neighboring cells.

Table 47–2. Growth factors.

Acronym	Full Name	Normal Action	Relation to Neoplasia
PDGF	Platelet-derived growth factor	Stimulates growth of normal cells	Autocrine stimulation of breast cancer.
EGF	Epithelial growth factor		Increased serum levels in breast cancer correlate with more rapid growth and spread.
TGFα	Transforming growth factor alpha		Secreted by breast cancer cells. Secretion blocked by tamoxifen.
TGFβ	Transforming growth factor beta	Inhibits the growth of normal cells. Stimulates some tumor cells.	Secreted by colon cancers. Paracrine action inhibits growth of nearby crypt cells, allowing more growth of tumor cells.
FGF	Fibroblast growth factor	One of the principal angiogenesis factors	Present in intracellular matrix. Lysis of matrix by neoplasm releases FGF, which stimulates angiogenesis and fosters tumor growth.
IGF-1	Insulinlike growth factor	Responsible for growth hormone action. Inhibits peripheral insulin effects.	Several neoplasms (breast, hepatoma, colon) exhibit increased IGF-1 activity.
Bombesin			Produced by small cell lung cancers; increased numbers of bombesin receptors on the tumor cells results in growth stimulation.

GROWTH FACTOR RECEPTORS

Growth factor receptors have an extracellular domain, an alpha helical transmembrane segment, and an intracellular domain (Figure 47–1). The extracellular domain binds ligand (eg, growth factors); the transmembrane helix anchors the protein; and the intracellular domain (a tyrosine kinase) phosphorylates proteins on tyrosine residues using ATP. When the growth factor binds to its growth factor receptor, the receptor forms a dimer or oligomer with adjacent counterparts, and the activated receptors phosphorylate each other at multiple tyrosines. The latter are then used as attachment sites for associated signal transduction molecules. The fully assembled membrane complex sends signals to the nucleus. The molecules in the cytoplasm that receive and amplify the signals from this complex are unknown.

Growth factor receptors can be grouped into three classes depending on the structure of the extracellular and intracellular domains. In class I are the receptors EGF/TGFα, the oncoproteins of v-erb-B, and HER-2/neu. Class II is composed of the insulin and insulin-like growth factor receptors. Class III includes the platelet-derived growth factor (PDGF) and the fibroblast growth factor (FGF) receptor and the proto-oncogenes c-*fms*/CSF-1 and c-*kit*. Growth factor receptors encoded by oncogenes frequently have truncated extracellular domains or altered regulatory sites that leave the receptor continuously activated. Proliferation of cancers may be stimulated by this persistent signaling.

SIGNAL TRANSDUCTION

The signal transduction pathway, composed of the phosphatidylinositol/ITP$_3$/DAG/Ca^{2+} system, protein kinase C, and the GTP-binding proteins (ie, the *ras* proto-oncogenes) (Figure 47–1), is important in cancer physiology because it carries signals from growth factor receptors to the nucleus.

When ligand binds to growth factor receptor, phosphatidylinositol is split by phospholipase C into inositol triphosphate (ITP$_3$) and diacylglycerol (DAG) (Figure 47–1). ITP$_3$ releases Ca^{2+} from intracellular vesicles, which activates a number of enzymes and structure-motility proteins. It also directly stimulates a number of membrane proteins, including growth factor receptors and protein kinase C. Diacylglycerol and the tumor promoter 12-tetradecanoyl-13-phorbolacetate or phorbol myristate acetate both activate protein kinase C. Activated protein kinase C phosphorylates proteins on serine and threonine, which either stimulates or inhibits their activity (Figure 47–1). Stimulation of protein kinase C is responsible for the increase in c-*fos* and c-*myc* expression seen after many growth factors bind to their growth factor receptors. Growth factor receptors stimulate protein kinase C either by directly activating phospholipase C, which raises membrane diacylglycerol levels, or by activating G proteins, which subsequently stimulate phospholipase C and increase membrane diacylglycerol.

Proteins that bind guanosine triphosphate are referred to as G proteins; binding activates the protein. Activation stops when guanosine triphosphate is converted to guanosine diphosphate, a process stimulated by guanosine triphosphate-activating protein. The system can be regulated by modulating the time guanosine triphosphate is bound before it is degraded to guanosine diphosphate. The principal G proteins involved in signal transduction following growth factor receptor stimulation belong to the *ras* family, which are proto-oncogenes encoded by c-*Ha* (Harvey)-*ras*, c-*Ki* (Kirsten)-*ras*, or N-*ras*. When ligand binds to growth factor receptor, cytoplasmic ras protein binds guanosine triphosphate, translocates into the membrane, and then shuttles to phospholipase C or other as yet unidentified effectors and activates them. They in turn activate protein kinase C (Figure 47–1). The signal decays when ras guanosine triphosphate-activating protein activates guanosine triphosphate hydrolysis. Point mutations at codons 12, 13, or 61 alter critical amino acids at the guanosine triphosphate binding site, so guanosine triphosphate-activating protein is unable to stimulate hydrolysis of bound guanosine triphosphate, and the ras protein produces a continuous proliferative signal (Figure 47–1). The role of activated oncogenes such as *ras* in the genesis of solid malignancies is discussed below.

ONCOGENES

Oncogenes resulting from the action of RNA tumor viruses are acquired (transduced) from the host genome. During transduction, the structures of normal host genes, called proto-oncogenes, are mutated into oncogenes. Genes isolated from viruses have a prefix "v" (eg, v-*Ha-ras*); those from host DNA have a "c" ("cellular") prefix (eg, c-*Ha-ras*). Italic type is used in referring to the gene, whereas roman type is used to designate the **oncoprotein** encoded by the gene. Proto-oncogenes are expressed during cell proliferation and at defined periods in embryologic development. Proto-oncogenes may be reactivated during organ regeneration, wound healing, lymphocyte blastogenesis, etc (eg, during cellular proliferation). Oncogenes may be classified according to their intracellular location and the function of their encoded oncoproteins (Table 47–3). Oncogenes cause malignant transformation by overproduction of a normal or mutant oncoprotein.

Growth Factor Oncogenes

The only documented example of this kind of oncoprotein is the product of the *sis* (simian sarcoma

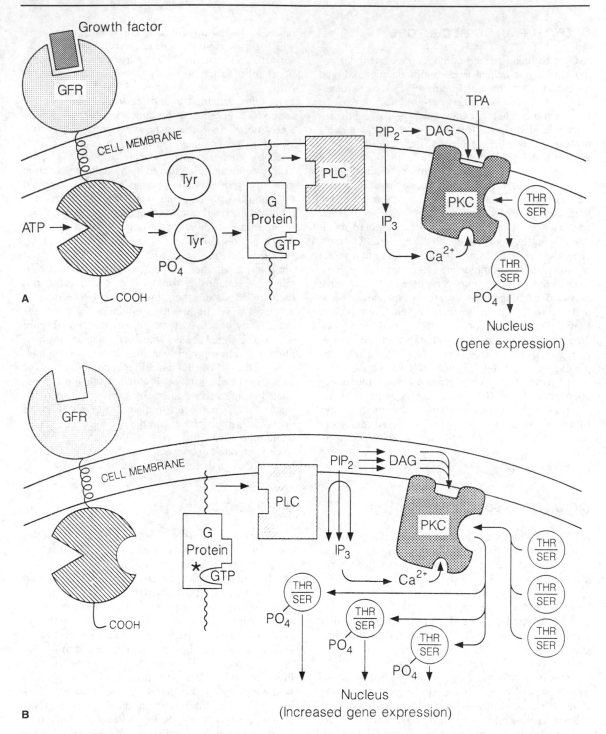

Figure 47–1. The signal transduction pathway in (A) normal cells and in (B) cancers with *ras* mutations. **A:** After a GF binds to its GFR, a cytoplasmic G protein binds GTP and attaches to the membrane via a fatty acid tail. The G protein then stimulates phospholipase C (PLC), which splits phosphoinositol bisphosphate (PIP$_2$) into ITP$_3$ and diacylglycerol (DAG). DAG diffuses in the membrane and activates protein kinase C (PKC) in conjunction with calcium released from cytoplasmic vesicles by ITP$_3$. The tumor promoter 12-o-tetradecanoylphorbol-13-acetate (TPA) directly activates PKC without calcium. Activated PKC phosphorylates proteins on threonine or serine and produces expression of proto-oncogenes, such as c-*fos* and c-*myc*. **B:** A G protein with a mutation at its GTP binding site, such as an activated ras oncoprotein, does not hydrolyze bound GTP and as a result is continuously "on." PLC and subsequently PKC are continuously stimulated without a GF binding to a GFR, producing a constant proliferative signal from the cell membrane to the nucleus.

virus) oncogene, a variant of platelet-derived growth factor. Constitutive production of this oncoprotein can cause malignant transformation. Receptor down-regulation is ineffective in decreasing the stimulus because the platelet-derived growth factor receptor is activated by the sis oncoprotein while still inside intracytoplasmic secretory vesicles.

Growth Factor Receptor Oncogenes

These oncogenes encode oncoproteins that belong to one of the three classes of growth factor receptors described above (Table 47–3). Important proteins in each of these subclasses include c-erb-B, HER-2/neu, c-kit, c-fms, and others. The former two are in the epidermal growth factor receptor family, whereas the latter two belong to the platelet-derived growth factor family. The prototypical example, the v-erb-B (avian erythroblastosis) protein, has a truncated extracellular domain but an intact transmembrane and cytoplasmic domain. This mutation is presumed to result in constitutive activation of growth factor receptor. The HER-2/neu gene encodes an oncoprotein similar to epidermal growth factor receptor. This gene has been found to be amplified in 30% of breast and ovarian carcinomas, and in each case tumors with this gene amplified have an increased frequency of lymph node metastasis and a decreased disease-free survival.

Signal Transduction Oncogenes

The ras family of oncogenes, the predominant members of this group, are the most common kind of oncogenes and are found in 20% of solid tumors. ras genes are frequently mutant in a variety of epithelial tumors. Mutant ras genes correlate with lymph node metastases in breast cancer. Mutant ras genes are also found in 50% of colon cancers, 35% of dysplastic colon polyps, and 15% of tubulovillous adenomas. The gene is usually normal in adjacent mucosa, implying that the ras mutation is not an early tumorigenic event.

c src, c raf, and c mos encode cytoplasmic signal transduction molecules that may function in the more distal part of the signaling pathway from the membrane receptor to the nucleus.

Nuclear Oncogenes

This group includes c-myc, c-myb, c-fos, c-erb-A, and c-jun (Table 47–3). The proteins encoded are predominantly transcription factors. They bind to enhancers and promoters upstream of target genes, attract other proteins sequentially, and form a complex that moves along the DNA molecule and transcribes the genetic code into messenger, transfer, and ribonuclear RNA.

c-myc expression is increased in a number of solid tumors, most notably breast and lung cancers. Its most interesting role, however, is in Burkitt's lymphomas and leukemias, where the c-myc gene is translocated from chromosome 8 and inserted next to the promoters for either the IgG or IgM light chains. This results in constitutive expression of the c-myc protein to high levels in the nucleus, which presumably stimulates proliferation of these cells. Another myc gene, N-myc, is associated with aggressive behavior in neuroblastomas regardless of stage. Determination of N-myc status may be useful in selecting patients for adjuvant therapy.

Tumor Suppressor Genes

The products of these genes are cell cycle regulators, adhesion proteins, developmental induction molecules, and others of unknown function. In general, both gene copies are lost in cancers, though some may be dominant-negatives, in which case the tumors are heterozygous. Furthermore, in most cases reintroduction of a normal gene copy will convert a malignant to a normal phenotype.

The existence of tumor suppressor genes was inferred from epidemiologic studies of epithelial cancers. Karyotype analysis and chromosome banding demonstrated that while many cancers had an abnormal number of chromosomes—usually more than the diploid 46—some had losses of specific chromosomes or translocations of parts of one chromosome to another (eg, the Philadelphia chromosome). Experimental fusion of normal and malignant cells demonstrated that the hybrid cells reverted toward normal, but tumorigenesis recurred when the normal chromosomes were spontaneously ejected from the hybrids.

Table 47–3. Location, classification, and functions of oncogenes and tumor suppressor genes.

Ligands	Membrane Receptors	Signal Transducers	Transcription Factors	Suppressor
sis	erb-B (neu)	N-ras	fos	Rb
	fms	Ha-ras	jun	p53
	kit	Ki-ras	erb-A	APC
	ros	src	c-myc	DCC
	trk	yes	N-myc	MCC
	ret	fgr		WAGR
	sea	abl		
	met	fes		
		A-raf		
		B-raf		
		mos		

Individual chromosomes were isolated in xenogeneic hybrids, and the genes they contained were identified and partially localized (ie, "mapped"). **Restriction-fragment-length polymorphisms (RFLPs)** are polymorphic genes (ie, there are multiple alleles in the population, so an individual stands a good chance of being heterozygous). The two alleles have a different pattern of restriction sites, places where DNA digesting enzymes can cut, so two fragments of different length appear when the DNA is analyzed on electrophoresis gels with a radioactive probe specific for the polymorphic allele. With computer-assisted programs, the inheritance of an RFLP can be charted within and across families. This establishes linkage of the RFLP with a particular cancer and the likelihood of a patient getting the disease given the presence of the RFLP.

Restriction-fragment-length polymorphisms are also informative about tumor suppressor function. In a typical analysis, peripheral blood monocytes and tumor tissue are studied. The monocytes retain two different bands while the tumor cells have just one, which means the tumor has lost heterozygosity and is **hemizygous** for the polymorphism compared with the monocytes. Since the restriction-fragment-length polymorphism is very near the suppressor oncogene, the latter has also been lost during tumorigenesis. The remaining single band often consists of a mutated gene that fails to encode a suppressor protein. The term "suppressor-recessive" derives from the ability of the cell to maintain a normal phenotype despite the loss of one parental gene. Cells become cancerous when both parental copies are lost, either as a result of missing chromosomal material or because of mutation.

Retinoblastoma

Patients with hereditary retinoblastoma (Rb) inherit an abnormal chromosome from one parent, a process called **germ-line mutation.** The condition is recessive, since a normal chromosome from the unaffected parent is also present. During the final weeks of gestation or in early infancy, another **somatic mutation** occurs in a retinal cell that inactivates the remaining normal *Rb* gene. Then, with loss of both parental suppressor oncogenes, the retinal cell undergoes malignant transformation. In the sporadic form of the disease, two somatic mutations inactivate both suppressor genes. Tumor tissue is homozygous for the *Rb* locus, while peripheral blood lymphocytes remain heterozygous. A portion of the long arm of chromosome 13 is absent in the tumors of these patients.

About 35% of these patients develop second primary tumors, most often osteogenic or soft tissue sarcomas. DNA from these tumors are also homozygous at the *Rb* locus. Furthermore, in many sporadic adult malignancies (eg, in breast, small-cell lung, and ovarian carcinomas and in sarcomas), the *Rb* gene is lost,

a situation associated with a poor prognosis and rapid metastasis.

pRb is a nuclear protein that while unphosphorylated suppresses the start of a new cell cycle in G_0 or G_1. Phosphorylation inactivates the protein and allows the cell cycle to begin. At the end of mitosis, pRb again becomes unphosphorylated and active. pRb has a "pocket" that binds several proteins, including p34 kinase, cyclin A, and E2F (Figure 47–2A). The first two molecules control entry into the cell cycle, while the last is a powerful transcription factor that turns on a number of genes crucial to growth and proliferation. Thus, pRb acts like a sponge to sequester and inactivate these proteins.

p53

Loss of the *p53* gene (by point mutation or chromosome deletion) occurs in many epithelial and mesenchymal tumors and is the single most common genetic change found in malignancy. *p53* is deleted or mutant in over 75% of colon cancers—a change absent in polyps, which implies that it occurs late in carcinogenesis. The *p53* gene undergoes point mutations in characteristic places. Where exposure to aflatoxin is common in China, over 95% of hepatomas have a mutant *p53* at codon 249.

p53 protein binds to the part of viral DNA (SV40, a DNA tumor virus) critical for DNA replication, preventing the protein complex that replicates DNA from binding to this segment. In the presence of mutant p53 that cannot bind, the viral DNA is rapidly reproduced. If p53 performs the same function at the numerous replication sites on human chromosomes, loss of the gene would predispose to cell proliferation (Figure 47–2B).

Wilms' Tumor

Wilms' tumors have lost a gene called *WAGR* (Wilms' tumor, aniridia, genitourinary abnormalities, retardation). The gene, located on the short arm of chromosome 11, has been cloned and found to be crucial in the development of the embryonic kidney, being especially active during ureteric induction by mesenchyme. Minicell fusion, which introduces a normal chromosome 11 into Wilms tumor cell lines, can reverse tumorigenicity.

Lung Cancer

In addition to losses of either *p53* or *Rb,* small-cell and squamous cell lung cancers consistently have deletions of part of the short arm of chromosome 3.

Colon Cancer

Hereditary familial adenomatous polyposis (FAP) is associated with deletions of chromosome 5, and 40% of sporadic colon cancers and 40% of dysplastic polyps contain deletions of the *FAP* locus. The loss of this locus in polyps suggests it is an early event in tumorigenic progression. Two genes have been

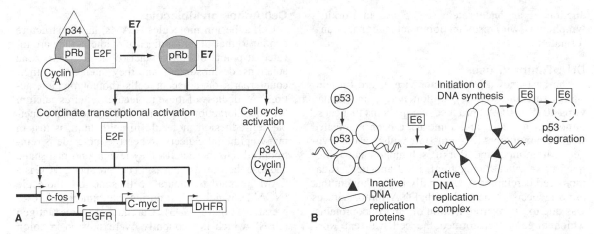

Figure 47–2. Models of the molecular mechanisms of two tumor suppressor gene products pRB and p53. In panel **A,** pRb is complexing with cyclin A, p34 kinase, and E2F. The first two molecules activate the cell cycle; E2F is a potent transcription factor that activates a number of genes required for cell proliferation. In the second panel the E7 oncoprotein of human papillomavirus (HPV) binds to pRb and disrupts the former complex, leading to cell cycle activation and proliferation. In panel **B,** p53 binds to an origin of replication in chromosomal DNA, preventing attachment of the multiprotein complex that replicates DNA. In the presence of the HPV E6 oncoprotein, p53 is degraded by the ubiquitin pathway, so the DNA is vacant, allowing the replication machinery to bind and new DNA synthesis to begin.

cloned that map to this locus. One, called "missing in colon carcinoma" *(MCC),* is probably a signal transducer with functions similar to those of a *ras*-guanosine triphosphate-activating protein. *MCC* is rarely mutant in familial adenomatous polyposis. Another gene, adenomatous polyposis coli *(APC),* is always mutant in familial adenomatous polyposis and is mutant in 25% of sporadic colon cancers. *APC* encodes for a huge protein of unknown function. Heterozygous individuals are affected, which suggests that this may be a dominant-negative mutant.

Additional deletions have been found on chromosomes 18 and 17 in cancers (but not polyps), which suggests that they are late events. The portion of chromosome 17 lost in these cancers contains *p53.* When present in cancers, *p53* is usually mutant. The gene on chromosome 18 has also been cloned. The "deletion colon carcinoma" *(DCC)* gene encodes a cell adhesion molecule that is lost during tumorigenesis.

OTHER MECHANISMS OF CARCINOGENESIS

Chemicals, foreign bodies, certain kinds of radiation, and viruses can also cause cancer. Tumorigenesis by these agents is important because it may shed light on spontaneous human carcinogenesis and because many are environmental carcinogens.

Chemical Carcinogenesis

The cause of many epithelial cancers (eg, lung,

esophageal, head and neck, gastric, pancreatic, and colon cancers) involves exposure to chemical carcinogens—high-fat diet, smoking, alcohol, etc. Animal studies indicate that chemical carcinogens produce cancers in two ways. The agent can be a **complete carcinogen,** in which case the tumor arises after a variable latent period following exposure; or it can be an "initiator," a factor that alters cells at suboptimal doses but requires repeated exposure to another agent termed a "promoter" (eg, 12-tetradecanoyl-13-phorbolacetate) for tumors to appear. Initiated cells remain dormant but with malignant potential; tumors can be promoted for up to a year after exposure to the initiator. Initiators are predominantly polycyclic hydrocarbons able to form electrophilic radicals after in vivo processing, whereupon they then bind tightly to DNA (adduct formation). The close proximity of these highly reactive chemical radicals and DNA induces point mutations at the binding site. The *ras* oncogene is frequently mutated by chemical carcinogens. The high incidence of *ras* gene mutations in colon cancer may result from the actions of carcinogens in feces.

Radiation Carcinogenesis

Ionizing radiation disrupts chromosomes. Genes are broken apart in the malignancy, which either destroys their protein coding functions or separates proximal regulatory elements from the protein coding regions. Destruction of encoded proteins could inactivate suppressor oncogenes, and cells could escape from proliferation control. Removal of the gene regulatory segments could lead to uncontrolled overproduction of an oncoprotein (eg, c-*myc* in Burkitt's lymphoma), with resultant dominant malignant transformation.

DNA Tumor Viruses

The best-known DNA tumor viruses are Epstein-Barr virus, adenovirus, papillomavirus, and simian virus 40 (SV40). All produce oncoproteins that cause tumors in animals, and some have been associated with human tumors (Epstein-Barr virus: nasopharyngeal carcinomas and Burkitt's lymphoma; papillomavirus: cervical, anogenital, head and neck squamous cell carcinomas). Originally it was thought that tumorigenesis associated with DNA tumor viruses was due to the overproduction of viral oncoproteins, which directly transformed the cell. Current work suggests that the DNA virus oncoproteins bind to tumor suppressor gene products, including pRb and p53. For example, the adenovirus E1A oncoprotein binds to pRb. The second transforming protein of adenovirus, E1B, binds to p53. The SV40 T antigen, a potent oncoprotein when expressed in animal cells, binds to pRb and p53. The E7 protein of the human papillomavirus (HPV) binds to pRb, while its E6 gene product binds to p53. When E1A binds to pRb, the sequestered host proteins that normally attach to the "pocket" are released (Figure 47–2A). These activate the cell cycle directly by release of p34 kinase and cyclin A and indirectly via E2F-enhanced transcription of proliferative genes (Figure 47–2A). HPV E6 binding to p53 facilitates the destruction of this tumor suppressor product by the ubiquitin pathway (Figure 47–2B). These viral oncoproteins produce rapid host cell proliferation and predispose to host cell malignancy by sequestering or inactivating secondary and tertiary growth control genes.

TUMOR METASTASIS

Many cancers remain localized and become large in the absence of distant spread; others metastasize when they are very small. Transformed cells in vitro are not necessarily tumorigenic when injected into nude mice, and tumorigenic cells frequently do not metastasize. However, when DNA from metastatic cells is introduced into nonmetastatic tumor cells, the recipients metastasize. The available evidence suggests that the metastatic phenotype is coordinated by genes that are turned on and others that are suppressed. The pattern of metastasis characteristic of specific tumors reflects the influence of other complex factors.

The proteins that are overproduced or down-regulated in metastatic tumor cells are grouped according to function as follows: cell adhesion molecules, angiogenic factors, proteins that interact with the extracellular matrix, and molecules that coordinate cell shape.

Cell Adhesion Molecules

Cell adhesion molecules (CAMs) have a structure similar to that of antibodies. In epithelia they are located at points of cell contact (tight junctions, zona adherens, desmosomes), and they interact with their counterparts on adjacent cells (homotypic interaction). A subclass of these molecules requires calcium for this interaction (cadherins). E-cadherin, a principal cell adhesion molecule in epithelium, is lost in many epithelial cancers. When the molecule is reintroduced into these cells, they regain a normal shape and lose their invasiveness. In colon cancer, DCC is a CAM related to neural cell adhesion molecule (NCAM), which is lost during late tumorigenic progression (Figure 47–3). Carcinoembryonic antigen (CEA), which is frequently overexpressed in colon cancers, is also a cell adhesion molecule. In embryogenesis, CEA is diffusely expressed on all surfaces of colonic epithelial cells, while later it is confined to the apical surface. In colon cancers, CEA is again diffusely expressed over the entire cell surface (Figure 47–3). Thus, colon tumorigenesis is accompanied by loss of a differentiated type of cell adhesion molecule and the reappearance of an embryonic molecule (Figure 47–3). This change might alter the adhesiveness of colon cancer, with cells facilitating invasiveness.

Another interesting cell adhesion molecule is CD44, which facilitates lymphocyte homing and matrix interaction. Highly metastatic rodent cells produce altered CD44.* When the genes for these meta-

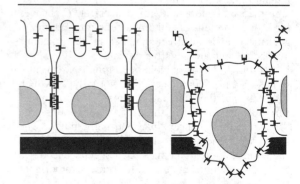

Figure 47–3. In the panel at left, an adult colonic epithelial cell is shown with its normal cell adhesion molecules, the "deleted in colon carcinoma" (DCC) gene product. During colonic tumorigenesis, this gene is lost from chromosome 18, and concomitantly CEA, an embryonic cell adhesionmolecule, is expressed diffusely over the entire cell membrane. CEA has less adhesiveness compared with DCC, and this property facilitates invasiveness of the tumor cell. Invasion through the basement membrane would be controlled by another set of molecules.

*CD is *c*luster of *d*ifferentiation. The term refers to antigenic epitopes found on lymphocytes.

static type CD44 molecules are put into localized tumorigenic cells, the latter begin to metastasize.

Other work suggests that the endothelium of various tissues expresses specific cell adhesion molecules that are coincidentally expressed by certain malignancies, entrapping systemic cells of particular cancers, and helping to explain preferential metastatic spread.

Angiogenic Factors

Among the angiogenic factors are bFGF, TGFβ, platelet-derived endothelial cell growth factor, and tumor necrosis factor. Experimental work in rodents suggests that tumor growth and metastasis may be inhibited by compounds that antagonize angiogenesis. In breast cancer, there is a correlation between metastases in node-negative patients and the amount of angiogenesis visible microscopically.

Extracellular Matrix Molecules

Local invasion by tumor cells involves proteolytic degradation of basement membrane and intracellular matrix and blood vessel invasion, which are coordinated by the products of many genes.

Type IV collagenase degrades the unique type IV collagen in basement membrane and is frequently increased in metastatic cancer cells. Since the endothelial basement membrane is the first barrier that cancer cells must penetrate, increased production of this enzyme may be a critical step. Metastatic cells also make more membrane-associated protease enzymes, including plasminogen activator, urokinase, and cathepsin B. Stimulation of the expression of c-*fos* leads to increased secretion of transin, another enzyme that degrades extracellular matrix. Another proteolytic enzyme, hyaluronidase stimulating factor, is secreted by Wilms tumor cells and is present in both the blood and the tumors of these patients.

Laminin, an important component of basement membrane, is a cruciate-shaped protein with multiple domains that interact with extracellular matrix components (eg, type IV collagen or heparan sulfate) or the laminin receptor. The central domain of laminin is homologous with EGF, and binding of laminin to its receptor produces a proliferative signal. Metastatic cancer cells have more laminin receptors, and they overproduce laminin, which can result in autocrine stimulation of proliferation. The principal extracellular adhesion protein is fibronectin. Attachment of cells to this molecule causes them to stop and adhere tightly to the underlying surface. Metastatic tumor cells have fibronectin receptors but produce less fibronectin, which makes them more mobile and less adherent.

Cytoskeletal Molecules

The product of the nm23 gene phosphorylates intracellular intermediate filaments that control cell shape. Highly metastatic mouse melanoma cells have

lost this gene product, and reintroduction of the molecule into these cells markedly decreases their metastatic potential. Thus, alterations of the cytoskeleton, by altering cell deformation or mobility, may affect metastatic potential.

MULTISTEP CARCINOGENESIS

The multiple discrete stages of carcinogenesis are beginning to be understood at the molecular level. Cells may first develop or inherit a mutation in one suppressor oncogene, which may produce a slight deregulation of proliferation. Alternatively, the initial event may be exposure to an environmental carcinogen or infection with a DNA tumor virus. The increased proliferation may increase the spontaneous rate of mutation. These mutations may then activate oncogenes such as growth factor receptors, signal transducers, or nuclear factors controlling transcription or the cell cycle. The further deregulated and enhanced cell proliferation may lead to unstable mitotic cell divisions, with loss of parts of chromosomes containing critical suppressor oncogenes that may be the last barrier before malignancy is achieved. Finally, additional mutations may result in overproduction of matrix-degrading enzymes and a decreased number of cell adhesion receptors, predisposing to metastases.

The molecular changes in colon cancer in human multistep carcinogenesis are the best-understood factors (Figure 47–4). Patients may inherit increased susceptibility to the disease governed by a mutant familial adenomatous polyposis product. Dominant/negative interference of the normal familial adenomatous polyposis function by this mutant may increase proliferation of the crypt stem cells, which transmit the mutation to daughter cells. Exposure to chemical carcinogens in the stool may produce *ras* mutations, which further increase cell growth by continuous activation of the signal transduction pathway (Figures 47–1 and 47–4). The combination of the two mutations, one inherited and the other epigenetic, may lead to mistakes in the replication of DNA or chromosome separation during mitosis, because faster cell cycling predisposes to fidelity errors. Allelic deletions during mitosis cause loss of chromosome segments, such as those that contain the *DCC* gene on chromosome 18. This may also be responsible for loss of the *p53* gene on chromosome 17, and additional effects of chemical carcinogens may produce additional mutations of this tumor suppressor at its hot spot codons 148–290. Induction of embryonic CAM CEA also occurs at some point in this progression (Figure 47–3). The important point is the diverse functions of the mutant or lost molecules. Two tumor suppressor genes *(FAP, p53),* one or two signal transduction molecules (ras, perhaps MCC), and two cell

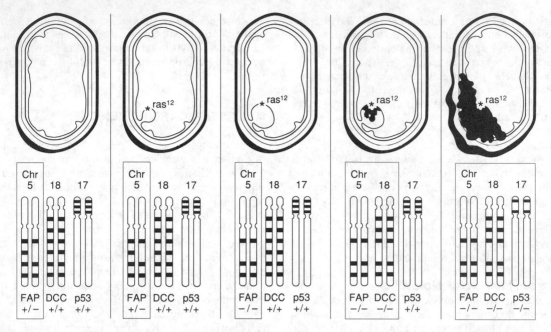

Figure 47–4. This series of panels depicts the hypothesized molecular progression of human colonic carcinogenesis. First, a mutation in the FAP gene is inherited. Then the *ras* gene is mutated by chemical carcinogens. The resulting accelerated proliferation leads to errors in mitosis, producing deletions in chromosomes 17 and 18. These deletions remove p53 and DCC function and result in an invasive malignancy. Not shown is the reexpression of CEA.

adhesion molecules (DCC, CEA) are mutated or reexpressed (Figure 47–4).

Thus malignancy is the result of an accumulation of critical mutations which produce a metastatic tumor. A corollary is that one specific oncogene or lost suppressor oncoprotein may be necessary but not sufficient to produce the complete malignant phenotype.

Aaronson SA: Growth factors and cancer. Science 1991; 254:1146.

Bos JL: *ras* Oncogenes in human cancer: A review. Cancer Res 1989;49:4682.

Cantley LC: Oncogenes and signal transduction. Cell 1991; 64:281.

Cross M: Growth factors in development, transformation and tumorigenesis. Cell 1991;64:271.

Groden J: Identification and characterization of the familial adenomatous polyposis coli gene. Cell 1991;66:589.

Fearon E: Identification of a chromosome 18q gene that is altered in colorectal cancers. Science 1990;247:49.

Hollstein M: p53 mutations in human cancers. Science 1991;253:49.

Kinzler K: Identification of FAP locus genes from chromosome 5q21. Science 1991;253:661.

Kinzler K: Identification of a gene that is located at chromosome 5q21 that is mutated in colorectal cancers. Science 1991;251:1366.

Lewin B: Oncogenic conversion by regulatory changes in transcription factors. Cell 1991;64:303.

Liotta LA: Cancer metastasis and angiogenesis: An imbalance of positive and negative regulation. Cell 1991;64: 327.

Malkin D: Germ line p53 mutations in a familial syndrome of breast cancer, sarcomas, and other neoplasms. Science 1990;250:1233.

Moore GE, Ed: Foreign body carcinogenesis. Cancer 1991; 67:2731.

Nowell PC: Cytogenetics of tumor progression. Cancer 1991;65:2172.

Pastan I, Fitzgerald D: Recombinant toxins for cancer treatment. Science 1991;254:1173. Rigas B, Ed: Oncogenes and suppressor genes: Their involvement in colon cancer. J Clin Gastroenterol 1990;12:494.

Shields PG, Harris CC: Molecular epidemiology and the genetics of environmental cancer. JAMA 1991;266:681.

Solomon E, Borrow J, Goddard AD: Chromosome aberrations and cancer. Science 1991;254:1153.

Takeichi M: Cadherin cell adhesion receptors as a morphogenetic regulator. Science 1991;251:1451.

Walsh JH et al: A: Autocrine growth factors and solid tumor malignancy. West J Med 1991;155:152.

Weinberg RA: Oncogenes, antioncogenes, and the molecular basis of multistep carcinogenesis. Cancer Res 1989; 49:3713.

Weinberg RA: The genetic bases of cancer. Arch Surg 1990;125:257.

Weinberg RA: Tumor suppressor genes. Science 1991;254: 1138.

zur Hausen H: Viruses in human cancers. Science 1991; 254:1167.

VALUE OF GRADING & STAGING IN MALIGNANT DISEASE

Samuel D. Spivack, MD

For most curable neoplasms, the first therapeutic attempt must be definitive if cure is to be achieved; this means that initial therapy must be radical enough to encompass and extirpate or sterilize all existing foci of disease. An accurate delineation of the stage and extent of disease is thus an important initial step in consideration of the most appropriate treatment for the patient.

Grading and staging of neoplasms are attempts to describe the degree of malignancy and the dissemination of the cancer. Histologic grading determines the degree of anaplasia of tumor cells, varying from grade I (very well differentiated) to grade IV (undifferentiated). Grading has prognostic value in some tumors (soft tissue sarcomas, transitional cell carcinoma of bladder, astrocytoma, and chondrosarcoma) but is of little predictive value in others (melanoma or osteosarcoma). Staging of cancer is based upon the extent of its spread rather than on histologic appearance and has been standardized for many cancers by use of the TNM system. T refers to the degree of local extension at the primary site, N to the clinical findings in regional nodes, and M to the presence of distant metastases. Some cancers are staged by clinical examination alone (eg, squamous cell carcinoma of the cervix), whereas for others (eg, transitional cell carcinoma of the bladder and adenocarcinoma of the colon) the stage is determined on the basis of findings in the resected surgical specimen. In both instances, there is an excellent correlation of stage with prognosis.

For many neoplasms, both the histologic grading and the clinical staging have relevance to the choice of treatment and prognosis. Nowhere is this more evident than for Hodgkin's disease and other lymphomas. Lymphocyte-predominant and nodular varieties clearly have a more favorable prognosis than lymphocyte-depleted and diffuse histologic types, and disease limited to lymph nodes is potentially cured by radiotherapy, whereas extranodal dissemination is generally best palliated by combination chemotherapy.

Staging laparotomy and splenectomy are useful in Hodgkin's disease and in clinical research trials for other lymphomas but do not help in determining therapy for clinical stage III (and IV) non-Hodgkin's lymphomas. These patients are not usually curable with total nodal radiotherapy and should therefore be treated with systemic combination chemotherapy, palliative radiotherapy to limited fields of involvement, or both. Useful studies to define clinical stage include chest x-rays, bipedal lymphangiography, CT scanning, and needle biopsy of bone marrow; laparoscopically directed percutaneous liver biopsy may be useful in selected patients.

Chabner BA: Staging of non-Hodgkin's lymphoma. Semin Oncol 1980;7:285.
Spiro SG: Diagnosis and staging. Recent Results Cancer Res 1984;92:16.

SURGERY FOR MALIGNANT DISEASES

David C. Hohn, MD

Surgical excision is the most effective means of removing the primary lesion of most solid neoplasms and achieves a higher rate of primary control than any other form of therapy. Resection of incurable but symptomatic tumors or bypass of unresectable tumors that obstruct the intestinal tract or bile ducts may provide worthwhile palliation. In a number of highly malignant tumors, where wide excision is impossible or would cause major deformity, excision with narrow margins combined with radiation and chemotherapy has been successfully employed.

Most common neoplasms involving single organs have been discussed in preceding chapters. Tumors that characteristically involve multiple organ systems or diverse body regions are presented here.

MALIGNANT MELANOMA

Over 600,000 new cases of skin cancer are detected annually in the USA, and 32000 of these are melanomas. While only 5% of skin cancers are melanomas, about two-thirds of all deaths from skin cancer are due to melanomas. The incidence of melanoma has been increasing for the past 2 decades, with a particularly sharp rise in the last 5 years. The 5-year survival rate has also increased from 50% to 80% during this 20-year period, presumably reflecting improved methods of diagnosis and treatment.

The incidence of cutaneous melanoma is much higher in whites than in blacks, equal in men and women, extremely low in children, and increased with age in adults.

Exposure to ultraviolet radiation appears to be associated with a higher incidence of melanoma, as is the case with other cutaneous cancers. There is increasing concern that depletion of ultraviolet-absorbing ozone in the stratosphere is behind a global increase in skin cancers. Familial clustering of melanoma has been recognized and has previously been attributed to environmental factors and phenotypes (fair skin). Recent research has demonstrated a clear familial association between dysplastic nevi and a high incidence of melanoma. Patients from melanoma-prone families who have dysplastic nevi appear to have a lifetime risk of melanoma approaching 100%, and periodic screening of these families is recommended. The risk of melanoma in patients with dysplastic nevi and no family history is uncertain.

Pigmented Lesions

The appearance of a new pigmented nevus should arouse suspicion of melanoma. About one-third of all melanomas arise from pigmented nevi. Since the average white adult has 15–20 nevi, it is imperative that clinicians be able to recognize the various benign pigmented skin lesions and have a clear idea of the indications for biopsy or excision. Recognition and early excision of atypical pigmented lesions are potentially lifesaving, since surgery is the only effective treatment.

Junctional nevi are usually small, circumscribed, light brown or black, flat or only slightly elevated, and rarely contain hair. They are found on all areas of the body, and moles of the mucous membranes, genitalia, soles, and palms are usually of this type. The nevus cells are located in the epidermis and at the dermal-epidermal junction.

Intradermal nevi range from small spots to extensive areas covering much of the body. The lesions show variable shape and surface configuration, are usually brown or black, and often are slightly elevated. Nevus cells are confined to the dermis, and the lesions are basically benign. Compound nevi have both junctional and intradermal elements. Blue nevi are circumscribed, flat or dome-shaped, bluish-black lesions, usually on the hands, face, or arms. Although benign, they may closely resemble nodular melanoma and require diagnostic excisional biopsy.

Dysplastic nevi are somewhat larger (5–12 mm) than common nevi. They have macular and papular components, are variegated in color (tan-brown) on a pink base, and have indistinct, irregular edges. Unlike common nevi, dysplastic nevi are most prevalent on covered body areas, though they can appear anywhere. Any suspicious lesions should be excised. An accurate family history should be obtained in such cases, and first-degree relatives should be examined.

Congenital nevi occur in about 1% of newborns, and most lesions are small. Along with dysplastic nevi, these lesions are now classified as precursors of melanoma. The estimated lifetime risk of melanoma developing in large congenital nevi (> 20 cm) is 5–20%, with some increased risk in smaller lesions as well. Prophylactic excision is cosmetically prohibitive in many cases, and these lesions must be carefully monitored for suspicious change.

Other pigmented lesions, including basal cell carcinomas, seborrheic keratoses, and actinic keratoses, occasionally resemble melanoma and require biopsy for diagnosis.

The features of pigmented lesions that should arouse a suspicion of melanoma and indicate the need for excisional biopsy are shown in Table 47–4. In general, benign lesions exhibit order and malignant lesions disorder in color, contour of border, and surface texture. If there is any doubt about the diagnosis, excisional biopsy with a margin of normal skin is indicated.

Clinical & Histologic Classification

The most widely used classification of melanoma is based on clinical and histologic features of the lesions. In order of frequency of occurrence, the major types of melanoma are superficial spreading melanoma, nodular melanoma, and lentigo maligna melanoma. Recognition of these different lesions is important, as management and prognosis may differ.

Melanomas have also been classified according to level of dermal invasion (Clark's levels; see Table 47–5) and total thickness of the lesion (Breslow; see Table 47–6). This latter method of classification has a particularly high correlation with type and extent of metastatic spread and with prognosis.

A. Superficial Spreading Melanoma: This is the most common type, and half arise from a preexisting mole. The typical lesion is slightly elevated and brown, with small discrete nodules of black, gray, blue, or pinkish hue. Although it may appear on any part of the body, this form of melanoma occurs most commonly on the back in both sexes and on the lower extremities in women. Once malignant change oc-

Table 47–4. Features suggestive of melanoma or melanomatous transformation of a nevus.

Color
    Irregular areas of tan, brown, or black, with focal
        shades of red, blue, or white.
    Darkening of a pigmented lesion.
    Development of pigmented satellite lesions.

Size
    Recent or rapid enlargement.
    Diameter greater than 10 mm.

Shape
    Irregular margin.
    Notching or indentation.

Surface
    Erosion or ulceration.
    Bleeding.
    Crusting.
    Irregular surface elevations.

Symptoms
    Pruritus.
    Inflammation with tenderness or pain.

Location
    Back.
    Lower extremities.
    Location subject to trauma or irritation.

Table 47–5. Staging of malignant melanoma. (After Clark.)

Level I =	In situ melanoma above the basement membrane.
Level II =	Invasion into the papillary dermis.
Level III =	Filling the papillary layer and extending to the junction of the papillary and reticular layers but not entering the reticular layer.
Level IV =	Into the reticular layer of the dermis.
Level V =	Subcutaneous tissue involvement.

curs, lesions exhibit lateral intraepithelial spread as well as deeper dermal invasion (Figure 47–5A).

Histologically, the malignant melanocytes are fairly uniform in appearance, with a prominent intraepidermal component and a variable degree of dermal invasion.

B. Nodular Melanoma: Nodular melanoma (Figure 47–5B) may develop at the site of a preexisting nevus and rapidly becomes a palpable, elevated, firm nodule. It may be dense black or reddish blue-black. Occasionally, amelanotic nodules develop. This type of melanoma may occur on any part of the body, and when it appears at a site not visible to the patient, the lesion may become quite large and ulcerate before it is noticed. A distinct convex nodular development indicates deep dermal invasion. This is the most dangerous kind of lesion in that it gives rise to the most obscure premonitory signs and is often in an advanced stage of malignancy when first detected. Histologically, the malignant cells arise from the epidermal-dermal junction and invade deeply into the dermis and subcutaneous tissue with relatively little lateral intradermal invasion.

C. Lentigo Maligna Melanoma: This form of melanoma usually occurs in older patients on an exposed surface of the body. It is seen most often as a large melanotic freckle ("Hutchinson's freckle") on the temple or malar region (Figure 47–5C). The lesion grows very slowly, often developing over a period of years. Clinically, it is the largest of the malignant moles, often reaching 5–6 cm in diameter. Initially, it is flat and cannot be felt, but as cancer develops it becomes slightly raised, with a palpable thickening. Discrete brown to black nodules may be scattered through it. Characteristically, the edge is quite irregular.

Table 47–6. Level of invasion, tumor thickness, and incidence of recurrence of metastasis. (After Breslow.)

Clark's Levels	Percentage With Recurrence or Metastasis at 5 Years	Thickness (mm)	Percentage With Recurrence or Metastasis at 5 Years
I	0%	<0.76	0%
II	4%	0.76–1.5	33%
III	33%	1.51–2.25	32%
IV	61%	2.26–3	69%
V	78%	>3	84%

The histologic changes of cancer tend to be scattered irregularly throughout the lesion. Malignant melanocytes seem to concentrate in the darker areas.

D. Classification by Depth of Invasion: Clark has classified melanomas by level of cutaneous invasion, and Breslow has correlated total tumor thickness with biologic behavior of melanoma. Survival varies inversely with either of these criteria, while the incidence of lymph node metastasis varies directly with the depth of invasion. Regardless of the type of melanoma, nodal and distant metastases are rare with level I and II lesions or lesions less than 0.75 mm thick. Lesions reaching levels III, IV, and V or lesions more than 1.5 mm thick have a high incidence of metastatic spread (Table 47–6). There is also a correlation between aggressiveness of the tumor type and level of invasion. Lentigo maligna melanoma rarely extends deeply, but large numbers of superficial spreading melanomas reach levels II and III, and nodular melanomas often involve level IV or level V. On the basis of the microstage classification, low-risk and high-risk primary lesions can be defined.

E. Anatomic Subsites and Risk of Recurrence: Recent studies have correlated poor survival rates and high risk of recurrence with specific locations of primary melanoma. High-risk areas include the upper back, the posterolateral arm, the posterior and lateral neck, and the posterior scalp (BANS region). Location and thickness are the most accurate predictors of prognosis.

Surgical Treatment

A. Primary Lesion: For most lesions, tissue diagnosis is best established by limited excisional biopsy. Full-thickness incisional or punch biopsy may be employed with large lesions, but partial-thickness "shave" biopsies should be avoided. Definitive treatment is primarily surgical but must be modified depending upon the type and location of the melanoma, the depth of invasion, and the presence of lymph node involvement. The risk of local recurrence correlates more with tumor thickness than with width of the surgical margin. Therefore, many authorities now advocate margins of 1–2 cm for thin melanomas and 2–3 cm for thicker lesions. Further reduction of margins may be warranted to spare uninvolved important structures such as eyes, ears, and facial nerves. Very wide and deep excisions may be necessary for definitive treatment of locally advanced melanomas.

Melanomas of fingers and toes should be managed by ray amputation without attempts at local excision.

B. Prophylactic Node Dissection: There is no definite proof that prophylactic node dissection improves survival rates. It is now generally accepted that superficial lesions showing less than 0.75 mm of invasion do not require node dissection. Management of intermediate-thickness lesions is less clear; however, a randomized trial of node dissection versus observation is nearing completion and should clarify the

A

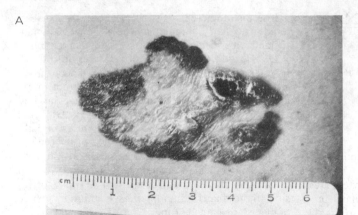

B

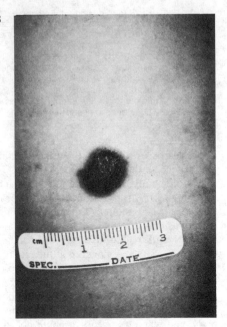

C

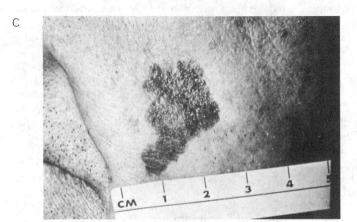

Figure 47–5. Types of melanoma. **A:** Superficial spreading melanoma (large advanced lesion). **B:** Nodular melanoma (note close resemblance to benign nevi). **C:** Lentigo maligna melanoma. (Courtesy of R Sagebiel.)

indications for node dissection. The incidence of both nodal and systemic metastases is high in patients with thick (> 4 mm) lesions, and most authorities recommend against prophylactic node dissection. Prophylactic node dissection should probably be avoided when (1) the lymphatic drainage of the primary site involves several different groups of regional lymph nodes, (2) there is serious concurrent disease, (3) the patient is over age 70, and (4) there are unresectable distant metastases. When truncal melanomas with multiple or uncertain routes of lymphatic drainage are present, lymphoscintigraphy is of value in planning node dissection.

C. Therapeutic Node Dissection: Clinically involved axillary and superficial inguinal lymph nodes should be treated with formal en bloc node group resection unless unresectable distant metastases are present. Deep inguinal node involvement carries a poor prognosis, but resection of these nodes adds morbidity. Therefore, deep node dissection should be confined to selected patients with no evi-

dence of distant disease, where it may prolong disease-free survival.

In occasional patients, resection of surgically accessible metastatic lesions or solitary pulmonary metastases may provide significant palliation and in rare cases may be curative.

Nonsurgical Treatment

Cutaneous melanoma and even visceral metastases may rarely undergo spontaneous regression, perhaps as a result of activation of immune mechanisms. Efforts to identify melanoma-associated antigens and to develop immunotherapeutic techniques are in progress. Responses have been reported with interferon, interleukin-2, and tumor-infiltrating lymphocyte (TIL) treatment.

Melanomas are unpredictably radioresistant, and radiotherapy is rarely used as definitive treatment. It has been used for palliation of metastatic lesions, for treatment of primary lesions in surgically inaccessible areas, and in lieu of surgery in elderly or high-risk patients. Encouraging response rates have been reported with fast neutrons and adjunctive hyperthermia.

Combining adjuvant chemotherapy with definitive surgery has not increased survival rates or the disease-free interval. Although treatment of disseminated melanoma with systemic chemotherapy has previously been of limited benefit, recently developed multiagent regimens incorporating dacarbazine (DTIC), *Vinca* alkaloids, and cisplatin have yielded response rates of 30–40%.

There is a growing experience with regional normothermic and hyperthermic perfusion of melanomas of the extremities with high concentrations of phenylalanine mustard and other drugs. The rate of response to therapy is high, and amputation can often be avoided in patients with local recurrence, satellitosis, or in-transit metastases—but survival is not prolonged. Long-term palliation may follow combinations of radiation, regional or systemic chemotherapy, immunotherapy, and surgery.

Prognosis

The most important factors in prognosis appear to be the size of the tumor and the depth of invasion. Small tumors with minimal invasion (< 0.7 mm) are usually curable by wide local excision. The prognosis is usually favorable in lentigo maligna melanoma and in superficial spreading melanomas without deep invasion. Most nodular melanomas, particularly if ulcerated and associated with deep invasion, have a poor prognosis.

Lesions of the extremities have a more favorable prognosis than those of the trunk, and women with malignant melanoma have better survival statistics at 5 and 10 years than men.

Aebersold P et al: Lysis of autologous melanoma cells by tumor-infiltrating lymphocytes: Association with clinical response. J Natl Cancer Inst 1991;83:932.

Amron DM, Moy RL: Stratospheric ozone depletion and its relationship to skin cancer. J Dermatol Surg Oncol 1991;17:370.

Balch CM: The role of elective lymph node dissection in melanoma: Rationale, results, and controversies. J Clin Oncol 1988;6:163.

Barth RJ, Venzon DJ, Baker AR: The prognosis of melanoma patients with metastases to two or more lymph node areas. Ann Surg 1991; 214:125.

Berd D et al: Treatment of metastatic melanoma with an autologous tumor-cell vaccine: Clinical and immunologic results in 64 patients. J Clin Oncol 1990;8:1858.

Calabro A, Singletary SE, Balch CM: Clinical behavior and patterns of relapse in 1001 consecutive patients with malignant melanoma regional nodal metastases. Arch Surg 1989;124:1051.

Coit D, Sauven P, Brennan M: Prognosis of thick cutaneous melanoma of the trunk and extremity. Arch Surg 1990;125:322.

Coit DG, Brennan MF: Extent of lymph node dissection in melanoma of the trunk or lower extremity. Ann Surg 1989;124:162.

Council on Scientific Affairs: Harmful effects of ultraviolet radiation. JAMA 1989;262:380.

Edwards MJ et al: Isolated limb perfusion for localized melanoma of the extremity. Arch Surg 1990;125:317.

Gorenstein LA et al: Improved survival after resection of pulmonary metastases from malignant melanoma. Ann Thorac Surg 1991;52:204.

Jacques DP, Coit DG, Brennan MF: Major amputation for advanced malignant melanoma. Surg Gynecol Obstet 1989;169:1.

Karakousis CP et al: Survival after groin dissection for malignant melanoma. Surgery 1991;109:119.

Koretz MJ et al: Randomized study of interleukin-2 (IL-2) alone vs. IL-2 plus lymphokine-activated killer cells for treatment of melanoma and renal cell cancer. Arch Surg 1991;126:898.

Legha SS: Current therapy for malignant melanoma. Semin Oncol 1989;16:34.

Lock-Andersen J, Rossing N, Drzseiecki KT: Preoperative cutaneous lymphoscintigraphy in malignant melanoma. Cancer 1989;63:77.

Mackie RM, Freudenberger T, Aitchison TC: Personal risk factor chart for cutaneous melanoma. Lancet 1989;2:487.

Markowitz JS et al: Prognosis after initial recurrence of cutaneous melanoma. Arch Surg 191;126:703.

Stern SJ, Guillamondegui OM: Mucosal melanoma of the head and neck. Head Neck Surg 1991;13:22.

Thompson LW: Skin cancer: Early detection. Semin Surg Oncol 1989;5:153.

Thorn M et al: Trends in survival from malignant melanoma: Remarkable improvement in 24 years. J Natl Cancer Inst 1989;81:611.

Veronesi U, Cascinelli N: Narrow excision (1-cm margin). Arch Surg 1991;126:438.

Vollmer RT: Malignant melanoma. A multivariate analysis of prognostic factors. Pathol Annu 1989;24(Part 1):383.

Wasselle J et al: Localization of malignant melanoma using monoclonal antibodies. Arch Surg 1991;126:481.

SOFT TISSUE SARCOMAS

Soft tissue sarcomas are derived from mesodermal connective and supporting tissues and are named according to the normal tissue in which they develop: fat, fibrous tissue, muscle, blood vessels, etc. These tumors are rare, constituting 1% of human cancers; they occur in all age groups; and they may arise in any area of the body. Although they have been traditionally classified according to tissue of origin, it is now evident that histologic grade and clinical stage are more important as prognostic indicators and in determining treatment approach. Soft tissue sarcomas rarely spread to lymph nodes, but hematogenous pulmonary metastases are common.

Most soft tissue sarcomas arise de novo and only rarely result from malignant degeneration of preexisting benign tumors; they occasionally arise in areas of radiation exposure. It has been suggested that trauma may predispose to the development of soft tissue sarcomas; however, most authorities regard such associations as coincidental rather than causal. Oncogenic viruses cause sarcomas in various animals, and although viral particles have been demonstrated in certain human sarcomas, there is no proof that viruses cause sarcoma in humans.

Certain diagnostic and therapeutic principles are common to most soft tissue sarcomas. Accurate diagnosis is essential and requires a representative sample of tissue. Incisional biopsy through a small incision is best for large lesions; wide excisional biopsy may be performed for small (ie, < 2 cm) superficial lesions. Needle biopsy and needle aspiration cytology have been increasingly used as an alternative to open biopsy. Many sarcomas are well circumscribed and encased in a pseudocapsule, offering the temptation of limited local excision to the unwary surgeon. Local recurrence invariably follows such efforts. These tumors not only invade locally but also spread extensively along musculofascial planes. En bloc excision with a margin of normal tissue is necessary. When tumors are close to major extremity vessels, en bloc excision including major vessels with vascular reconstruction may occasionally salvage the limb. Amputation is usually reserved for tumors that are otherwise unresectable or recur repeatedly.

Soft tissue sarcomas are relatively radiosensitive. Radiotherapy occasionally cures unresectable tumors or converts inoperable ones to a state of operability. It may also reduce local recurrence rates. A combination of wide local excision with postoperative irradiation for extremity sarcomas has yielded survival and recurrence rates comparable to those achieved with amputation. Chemotherapy has been dramatically successful in embryonal rhabdomyosarcomas and certain other tumors of childhood, and combinations including doxorubicin and ifosfamide have caused regression of metastatic sarcomas in adults. Although one major study demonstrated improved survival with adjuvant doxorubicin, cyclophosphamide, and methotrexate combined with definitive limb-sparing surgery or amputation in patients with soft tissue extremity sarcomas, several recent trials have failed to demonstrate such benefit. Several current trials in patients with high-grade sarcomas are evaluating preoperative (neoadjuvant) chemotherapy with continued treatment postoperatively only in the responders. Hyperthermic perfusion of extremity sarcomas with chemotherapeutic drugs combined with surgery or irradiation is also under investigation.

Pulmonary metastases occur frequently with all forms of sarcoma. These lesions are frequently confined to the lung, and pulmonary resection in such cases has yielded disease-free cure rates as high as 30%.

Sarcomas may arise in any type of soft tissue (adipose, fibrous, muscular, mesenchymal, histiocytic, neural, vascular, lymphatic, synovial). Many of these tumors are uncommon and beyond the scope of this text.

Liposarcomas

Liposarcomas are the most common sarcomas in humans. The average age at onset is about 50 years, and occurrence in children is rare. Although liposarcomas occur in all body areas, they are most frequent in the retroperitoneum and the lower extremities, with these two sites accounting for about two-thirds of cases. Four subtypes of liposarcoma are recognized: well-differentiated, myxoid, round cell, and pleomorphic. The latter types have the poorest prognosis. Liposarcomas cause few early symptoms and, in the retroperitoneum, may become massive before detection, displacing portions of the gastrointestinal tract or ureter. The widest possible surgical excision should be the initial treatment in most cases. In retroperitoneal tumors, however, the margins are often inadequate, and postoperative radiotherapy is frequently employed.

Many liposarcomas grow slowly and recur locally long after an apparently successful resection. Reoperation for even the most extensive recurrent liposarcomas may result in long periods of control and palliation. Respective 5- and 10-year survival rates are 50% and 35%.

Fibrosarcomas

Fibrosarcoma is the second most common sarcoma of soft tissue, and histologic differentiation from benign fibromatoses may be difficult. Many tumors formerly regarded as fibrosarcomas are now classified more accurately as leiomyosarcomas, liposarcomas, or malignant fibrous histiocytomas. Dermatofibrosarcoma, which recurs locally and metastasizes rarely, develops as a circumscribed protuberance arising from the skin of the trunk and is best treated by wide local excision. Fibrosarcomas also require wide total excision or, occasionally, amputation. Even deep fibrosarcomas of the buttock can occasionally be widely excised with adequate margins and amputation avoided.

Preoperative chemotherapy or irradiation (or both) may render a tumor more clearly circumscribed and permit a well-planned excision with the line of dissection in normal tissue. As in all other soft tissue sarcomas, shelling out of even the most obviously encapsulated lesion results in a high rate of local recurrence. Five- and 10-year survival rates as high as 62% and 50% have been reported.

Rhabdomyosarcomas

Embryonal rhabdomyosarcomas are the most frequently diagnosed forms of soft tissue sarcoma in children. These tumors respond to radiation therapy and chemotherapy, and use of multimodality treatment regimens has resulted in long-term survival in 70–90% of cases. These tumors are discussed in detail in Chapter 46.

Leiomyosarcomas

Leiomyosarcomas resemble fibrosarcomas and occur with greatest frequency in the uterus, stomach, and small intestine, where they appear as well-circumscribed defects. Leiomyosarcomas of the stomach may become enormous and fill the abdomen, though they have but a single origin from a small area of gastric or colonic wall. Despite apparent localization and encapsulation, recurrence even after wide excision is likely.

Musculoaponeurotic Fibromatoses (Desmoid Tumors)

The musculoaponeurotic fibromatoses are a group of nonmetastasizing, locally invasive dysplastic lesions of connective tissue. Included in this group are nodular fasciitis, plantar fibromatosis, and the lesions previously classified as desmoid tumors. Most of the "desmoid" lesions involve skeletal muscle and associated fascial layers. They most frequently occur in women in the abdominal wall during or following pregnancy, but they are almost as common in men and in extra-abdominal sites, including the head and neck, thigh, and shoulder. Lesions occasionally arise in surgical scars and in the mesenteries, and a familial form is associated with Gardner's syndrome. Wide excision with a margin of normal tissue is the recommended treatment. However, extremities and major vessels and nerves should be spared even if recurrence is likely. Local recurrences are common, and repeat excisional surgery is often required. These lesions may also respond to radiation therapy. Occasional cases have responded to treatment with antiestrogen therapy (tamoxifen) or to prostaglandin inhibitors.

Bevilacqua RG et al: Prognostic factors in primary retroperitoneal soft-tissue sarcomas. Arch Surg 1991;126:328.

Brennan MF: Management of extremity soft-tissue sarcoma. Am J Surg 1989;158:71.

Collin CF et al: Prognostic factors for local recurrence and survival in patients with localized extremity soft-tissue sarcoma. Semin Surg Oncol 1988;4:30.

Donaldson SS: Rhabdomyosarcoma: Contemporary status and future directions. Arch Surg 1989;124:1015.

Eilbert FR et al: Progress in the recognition and treatment of soft tissue sarcomas. Cancer 1990;65:660.

Elias AD, Antman KH: Adjuvant chemotherapy for soft tissue sarcoma: An approach in search of an effective regimen. Semin Oncol 1989;16:305.

Hoekstra HJ et al: A combination of intraarterial chemotherapy, preoperative and postoperative radiotherapy, and surgery as limb-saving treatment of primarily unresectable high-grade soft tissue sarcomas of the extremities. Cancer 1989;63:59.

Kettelhack C et al: Hyperthermic limb perfusion for malignant melanoma and soft tissue sarcoma. Eur J Surg Oncol 1990;16:370.

Kinsella TJ et al: Preliminary results of a randomized study of adjuvant radiation therapy in resectable adult retroperitoneal soft-tissue sarcomas. J Clin Oncol 1988;6:18.

Kinsella TJ et al: Treatment of high-risk sarcomas in children and young adults: Analysis of local control using intensive combined modality therapy. NCI Monogr 1988;6:291.

Lane RH, Stephens DH, Reiman HM: Primary retroperitoneal neoplasms: CT findings in 90 cases with clinical and pathologic correlation. AJR 1989;152:83.

Lanza LA et al: Response to chemotherapy does not predict survival after resection of sarcomatous pulmonary metastases. Ann Thorac Surg 1991;51:219.

Lawrence W Jr, Neifeld JP: Soft tissue sarcomas. Curr Probl Surg 1989;11:759.

London J et al: MR imaging of liposarcomas: Correlation of MR features and histology. J Comput Assist Tomogr 1989;13:832.

Mazanet R, Antman KH: Sarcomas of soft tissue and bone. Cancer 1991;68:464.

McKinnon JG et al: Management of desmoid tumors. Surg Gynecol Obstet 1989;169:104.

Neugut AI, Sordillo PP: Leiomyosarcomas of the extremities. J Surg Oncol 1989;40:65.

Robinson M et al: Treatment of extremity soft tissue sarcomas with surgery and radiotherapy. Radiother Oncol 1990;18:221.

Scott SM et al: Soft tissue fibrosarcoma. A clinicopathologic study of 132 cases. Cancer 1989;64:925.

Shiraki M et al: Pathologic analysis of advanced adult soft tissue sarcomas, bone sarcomas, and mesotheliomas. The Eastern Cooperative Oncology Group (ECOG) experience. Cancer 1989;64:484.

Stotter AT et al: The influence of local recurrence of extremity soft tissue sarcoma on metastasis and survival. Cancer 1990;65:1119.

Tepper JE: Role of radiation therapy in the management of patients with bone and soft tissue sarcomas. Semin Oncol 1989;16:281.

Tsujimoto M et al: Multivariate analysis for histologic prognostic factors in soft tissue sarcomas. Cancer 1988;62:994.

Zalupski M et al: Phase III comparison of doxorubicin and dacarbazine given by bolus versus infusion in patients with soft-tissue sarcomas: A Southwest Oncology Group Study. J Natl Cancer Inst 1991;83:926.

Kaposi's Sarcoma

Kaposi's sarcoma is a rare malignant disease characterized by flat purplish-red skin lesions that may also involve mucous membranes and occasionally the intestinal tract and other visceral organs. Although the precise cause is not known, two forms of the disease are now recognized. A nonaggressive form occurs sporadically and in elderly Ashkenazic Jews and Central Europeans. An aggressive form occurs primarily in immunosuppressed organ transplant patients or patients with AIDS and in the populations of Central Africa.

Patients with the aggressive form of the disease frequently have visceral involvement, with fever, chills, and lymphadenopathy, and survival is usually short. Zidovudine (AZT) has no antitumor activity but may extend survival in patients with AIDS. Interferon has shown antitumor activity and has been combined with AZT in current trials. Radiotherapy is effective for treatment of skin lesions (especially in the nonaggressive form). Surgery may be required for patients presenting with intestinal perforation, intussusception, or hemorrhage.

Kovacs JA et al: Combined zidovudine and interferon-alpha therapy in patients with Kaposi sarcoma and the acquired immunodeficiency syndrome (AIDS). Ann Intern Med 1989;111:280.

Krown SE, Metroka C, Wernz JC: Kaposi's sarcoma in the acquired immune deficiency syndrome: A proposal for uniform evaluation, response, and staging criteria. J Clin Oncol 1989;7:1201.

Spittle MF: Diagnosis and treatment of Kaposi's sarcoma. J Antimicrob Chemother 1989;23:127.

Volberding PA, Kaplan LD: Treatment of AIDS and its attendant malignancies. Prog Clin Biol Res 1989;288:459.

Ziegler JL et al: Kaposi's sarcoma: A comparison of classical, endemic, and epidemic forms. Semin Oncol 1984; 11:47.

SOLITARY METASTASES

Even though more than 80% of apparently solitary metastases are eventually found to be multiple, an occasional cure results from their excision. In patients with a solitary lung metastasis, lobectomy gives 5-year survival rates of 15–60% depending upon the tissue of origin, the histologic characteristics of the tumor, and the time of appearance of the metastasis. The best results have been achieved when the metastasis was discovered more than 2 years after treatment of the primary, and a few patients with limited multiple metastases may benefit from surgical excision. Reasonably good success (ie, 30% 5-year cure rate) has resulted from excision of liver metastases developing from adenocarcinoma of the colon (see Chapter 31). Surgery is much less successful for brain metastases. The prognosis for solitary bony metastases is poor, but occasional cures have followed removal or radiation of metastases from hypernephroma, testicular and gynecologic neoplasms, various sarcomas, and occasional intestinal tumors.

In patients with indolent, localized, bulky metastases, incomplete excision (debulking) may be of symptomatic benefit. Long-term palliation sometimes follows radiation therapy for metastases from certain radiosensitive tumors such as breast cancer, Wilms's tumor, seminoma, neuroblastoma, and some sarcomas.

Beattie EG: Surgical treatment of pulmonary metastases. Cancer 1984;54:2729.

Goya T et al: Surgical resection of pulmonary metastases from colorectal cancer: 10-year follow-up. Cancer 1989; 64:1418.

Patchell RA et al: A randomized trial of surgery in the treatment of single metastases to the brain. N Engl J Med 1990;322:494.

Steele G, Ravikumar TB: Resection of hepatic metastases from colorectal cancer: Biologic perspective. Ann Surg 1989;210:1127.

Volberding P: Therapy of Kaposi's sarcoma in AIDS. Semin Oncol 1984;11:60.

RADIATION THERAPY

Karen K. Fu, MD,
& Theodore L. Phillips, MD

Radiation therapy deals with the treatment of disease using ionizing radiation. Since most diseases treated by radiation therapy are malignant neoplasms, radiation therapy is actually a branch of oncology. Radiation therapy is the treatment of choice for the control of cancer in many sites. In other situations it is used—with curative intent—in conjunction with surgery or chemotherapy. It is also used for the relief of symptoms resulting from cancer.

In order to know when and how to apply radiation therapy, the radiation oncologist must be familiar with the biologic behavior of various forms of cancer and with the results obtainable by all treatment methods. The realization that cancer is the second most common cause of death and that over 60% of cancer patients will require radiation therapy during the course of their disease underscores the importance of this branch of medical science.

PHYSICAL PRINCIPLES & RADIATION SOURCES

The radiations commonly used in radiotherapy include x-rays, gamma (γ)-rays, electrons, and beta (β)-rays. X-rays and γ-rays are identical in properties but are produced by different sources. Electrons and β-rays also differ only in the source from which they are derived. X-rays, γ-rays, electrons, protons, and β-rays are referred to as low-LET (linear energy transfer) radiation. Other types of radiation—eg, neutrons, protons, alpha (α) particles, heavy ions, and pi mesons—are referred to as high-LET radiation. They have been used in the treatment of diseases in selective sites. All have the common property of producing ionization within tissue. Ionization and other effects, such as excitation and free radical formation, cause chemical changes in cellular components. The total amounts of energy absorbed are exceedingly small, and the biologic effects are caused by the sensitivity to ionization of certain portions of cells.

X-rays and γ-rays are electromagnetic radiations with neither mass nor charge; neutrons have mass but no charge; electrons, β-rays, protons, and heavy ions are charged particles. X-rays are derived from the interaction between moving electrons and matter, whereas γ-rays are emitted during the decay of radioactive isotopes (radium, ^{60}Co, etc). In biologic material, these rays give up energy by ejecting electrons from atomic orbits; in turn, the ejected electrons deposit energy in creating charged ions (ionization) within the target material. Most of the total ionization is caused by these secondary electrons. The distribution of the absorbed energy is related both to the absorption pattern of the primary radiation and the distance the secondary electrons travel within the tissue. When a beam of x-rays enters tissue, the energy absorption at first increases because the secondary electrons are building to a maximum. The depth of this maximum point beneath the surface increases with the energy of the x-rays. After a maximum, the energy absorption decreases in exponential fashion.

In the case of electron beams, the ionization within tissue is due in large part to the primary electrons. The energy is deposited fairly uniformly along the pathway of the electron. Such electrons travel a finite distance and then stop. With a monoenergetic electron beam, energy absorption in soft tissue is thus relatively constant from the surface to near the end of the electron's path, at which point the deposition of energy rises slightly and then falls abruptly to zero.

When fast neutrons interact with tissue, highly ionizing, heavily charged particles such as protons, α particles, and heavy recoils are released. The dose deposited by them decreases exponentially with depth of penetration. Most of the dose is contributed by the recoiling protons from hydrogen in tissue. The absorbed dose in fatty tissues, which are hydrogen-rich, is about 15% higher than that in muscle. The depth dose distribution of 14-MeV neutrons is similar to that of ^{60}Co γ-rays.

When charged particles heavier than electrons, such as protons, helium ions, heavy ions, and pions, pass through tissue, the dose deposited increases slowly with depth of penetration and gives rise to a sharp increase of dosage near the end of the range owing to the Bragg peak effect. The peak is very narrow. However, for radiotherapeutic applications, it can be broadened to any desired width with the use of a ridge filter. The dose at the peak compared with the dose at the entrance is reduced with increasing width of the Bragg peak, but it is never smaller than at the entrance, and the exit dose is negligible.

Figure 47–6 shows the depth-dose distributions of protons, electrons, x-rays and γ-rays. The different absorption characteristics of these radiation beams can be adapted to fit various clinical situations.

In modern radiotherapy, two or more radiation beams or rotating arcs are often combined to produce a more desirable distribution of absorbed energy than would result from a single beam. Furthermore, compensating or wedge-shaped filters are frequently used to compensate for body contour or to alter the shape of the absorption curve (Figure 47–7).

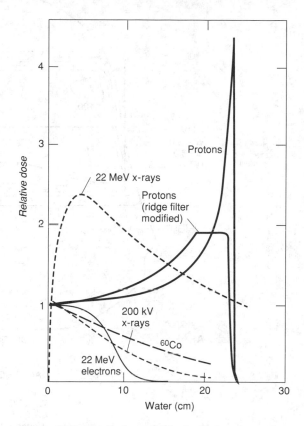

Figure 47–6. Depth-dose distributions of protons, electrons, x-rays, and γ-rays. (Redrawn from Raju MR, Richman C: Negative pion radiotherapy: Physical and radiobiological aspects. Curr Top Rad Res Q 1972;159–233.)

Currently, megavoltage (> 1 million volt) x-rays or γ-rays are used for radiotherapy of deeply situated lesions. The advantages of the higher energy radiations are (1) "skin sparing," (2) less absorption in bone, (3) decreased energy absorption by healthy tissue, and (4) greater penetration. "Skin sparing" derives from the fact that the absorbed energy or dose at any depth depends largely on the secondary electrons. With x-rays generated by a 250-kilovolt peak (kVp) x-ray machine, the secondary electrons travel such short distances that the maximum energy absorption is essentially at the surface. With higher energies, the secondaries travel many millimeters or even centimeters; therefore, energy absorption builds up and does not reach its maximum until a considerable depth has been reached. In the case of ^{60}Co γ-rays, the maximum energy deposition is at 5 mm; for x-rays from a 24-million-electron volt (MeV) betatron, the maximum is at 4 cm beneath the surface (Figure 47–8). Decreased absorption of megavoltage irradiation in bone compared with that in soft tissues is due to the difference in atomic number of the atoms within these two types of tissue. The fact that higher energy

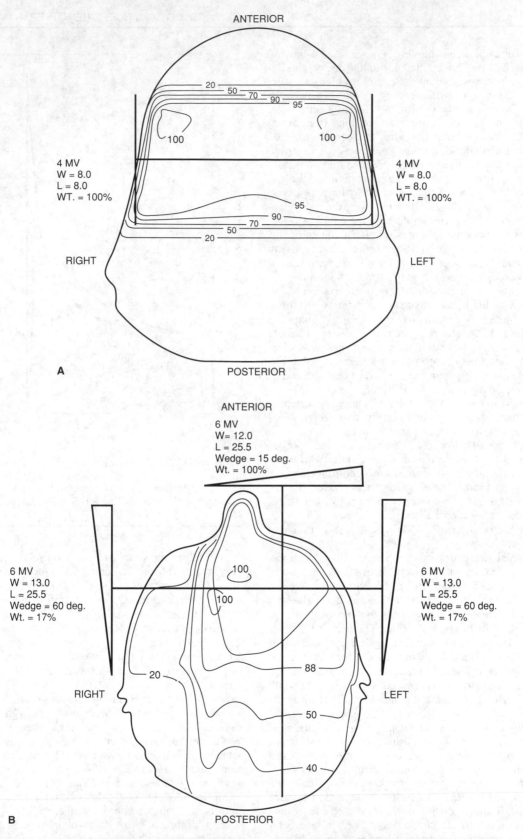

Figure 47–7. Isodose curves for several combinations of external radiation beams from linear accelerator x-rays. *A:* Two 4-MV x-ray beans 8 × 8 cm with opposed central axis. *B:* Three 6-MV x-ray beams 12 × 25.5 cm, 13 × 25.5 cm, and 13 × 25.5 cm, with central axis at right angles to each other utilizing 15-degree and 30-degree wedge filters. *C:* Two rotating 6-MV x-ray beams, 5 × 5 cm, with 30-degree wedge filters (one from 70–180 degrees, the other from 180–290 degrees). *D:* Six 18-MV x-ray beams 11 × 8 cm with central axis at 45- to 90-degree angles to each other.

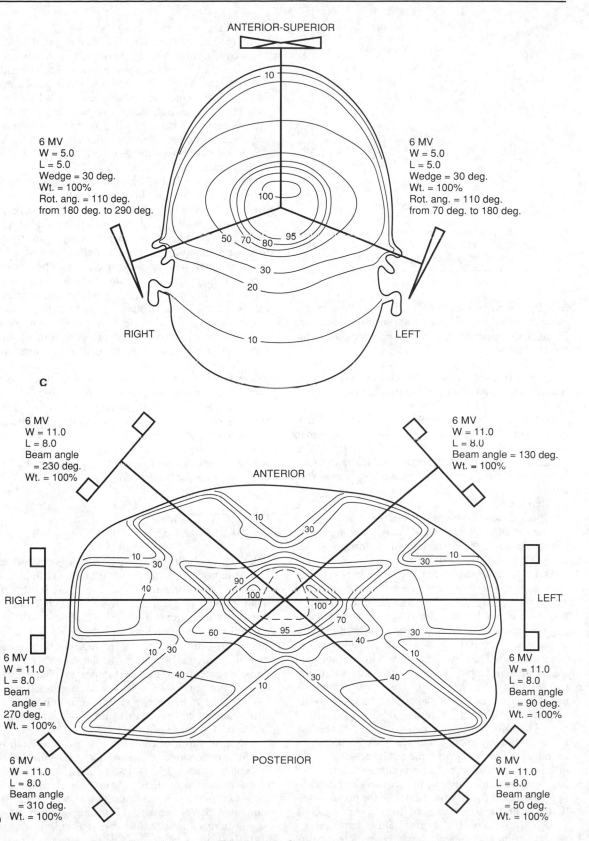

ANTERIOR-SUPERIOR

6 MV
W = 5.0
L = 5.0
Wedge = 30 deg.
Wt. = 100%
Rot. ang. = 110 deg.
from 180 deg. to 290 deg.

6 MV
W = 5.0
L = 5.0
Wedge = 30 deg.
Wt. = 100%
Rot. ang. = 110 deg.
from 70 deg. to 180 deg.

RIGHT

LEFT

C

6 MV
W = 11.0
L = 8.0
Beam angle
= 230 deg.
Wt. = 100%

6 MV
W = 11.0
L = 8.0
Beam angle = 130 deg.
Wt. = 100%

ANTERIOR

RIGHT

LEFT

6 MV
W = 11.0
L = 8.0
Beam
angle =
270 deg.
Wt. = 100%

6 MV
W = 11.0
L = 8.0
Beam angle
= 90 deg.
Wt. = 100%

6 MV
W = 11.0
L = 8.0
Beam angle
= 310 deg.
Wt. = 100%

POSTERIOR

6 MV
W = 11.0
L = 8.0
Beam angle
= 50 deg.
Wt. = 100%

D

Figure 47–7. Continued.

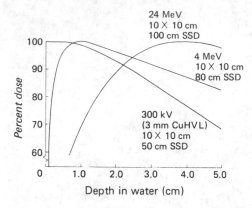

Figure 47–8. Comparison of the depth doses for x-ray beams of different energies. SSD = source-skin distance; CuHVL = copper half value layer.

radiations undergo less side-scatter and thus have a more sharply defined beam contributes to a decrease in radiation dose to healthy tissue surrounding the target volume.

Detailed discussion of the sources of external beam therapy is beyond the scope of this book, but a few broad statements about presently available equipment may be useful.

Orthovoltage machines produce x-rays with energies up to 300 kVp. At present, the most common sources for deep therapy are linear accelerators that produce x-rays with energies of 4–6 MeV. Linear accelerators producing x-rays or electron beams with energies up to 25 MeV are also now widely used. Less common but available in some centers are ^{60}Co machines, linear accelerators, and betatrons capable of energies of 35 or even 45 MeV. All photon or x-ray beams above 1 MeV are known as "megavoltage" beams.

Short-distance radiotherapy (brachytherapy) takes advantage of the rapid decrease in dose with distance from a radiation source. For this purpose, the radiation source may be placed within a cavity (intracavitary) or inserted directly into tissue (interstitial). One or more sources may be used, with the geometric arrangement dictated by the clinical circumstances of the particular lesion. In permanent interstitial implants, the sources are left in place permanently. In temporary interstitial implants and intracavitary insertions, the sources are removed after a prescribed period of time. They may be in the form of needles, narrow tubes, wires, or small seeds. To minimize the radiation exposure of medical personnel, an afterloading technique is commonly used. Interstitial afterloading nylon tubes or intracavitary afterloading applicators are usually inserted with the patient anesthetized in the operating room and subsequently loaded with radioactive sources after the patient recovers from anesthesia. Recently, remote control afterloading machines have become available in major medical centers. With this equipment, the radiation exposure to medical personnel is eliminated. The commonly used radioactive sources include iridium, cesium, and iodine. Radium, radon seeds, cobalt, yttrium, gold, americium, and palladium are used less often. Iodine-loaded eye plaques are used in the treatment of some small choroidal melanomas and retinoblastomas. Beta-ray applicators such as the ^{90}Sr-loaded eye applicator are used for the treatment of thin superficial lesions.

In the USA, brachytherapy has traditionally been delivered as continuous low-dose-rate (0.4–2.0 Gy/h) irradiation. Recently, there has been an increase in the use of remote control afterloading high-dose-rate (> 12 Gy/h) intracavitary brachytherapy in the treatment of a variety of cancers, including gynecologic, endobronchial, and esophageal cancers. The advantages of high-dose-rate remote afterloading techniques are elimination of radiation exposure of medical personnel, short patient immobilization time, elimination of complications resulting from prolonged bed rest, decreased patient discomfort, and the fact that treatment can be performed on an outpatient basis. However, the maximum doses tolerated with this technique are reduced, and for many sites the optional fractionation scheme is still under study.

Different tissues will actually absorb different amounts of energy when exposed to the same beam of radiation. The unit of absorbed dose is the gray (Gy), which represents the absorption of 1 joule (energy unit) per kilogram of matter. Ionizing radiation of all types can be measured in Gy (1 Gy = 100 rads).

BIOLOGIC BASIS OF RADIATION THERAPY

In radiobiology, cell death is usually defined as loss of reproductive integrity. Following radiation, a cell may appear physically intact and may be able to make protein or synthesize DNA or even undergo several mitoses, but if it has lost the ability to divide indefinitely it is considered dead. This definition of cell death—in terms of loss of reproductive integrity—is particularly relevant to the radiotherapy of tumors, since one of the most important characteristics of a tumor is its ability to divide indefinitely. The basic aim of radiotherapy of tumors is either to destroy them or to render them unable to divide and cause further spread of cancer.

The mechanism of radiation-induced cell death is not fully understood. However, the great bulk of radiobiologic data suggests that the most sensitive site of radiation injury in the cell is in the nucleus. Experiments on mammalian cells using a microbeam technique in which either the nucleus or cytoplasm could be selectively irradiated indicate that the nucleus is 100–1000 times more sensitive than the cytoplasm.

There is strong circumstantial evidence that the DNA of the chromosomes constitutes the primary target for radiation-induced cell lethality. Some studies have shown that radiation can cause breaks in one or both DNA strands and that the number of unrepaired double-strand breaks as well as the number of chromosomal aberrations corresponds to the fraction of cells killed.

In vitro studies of cell cultures have shown that cell death following irradiation appears to be a complex exponential function of dose—ie, a specified radiation dose kills a constant fraction of irradiated cells. Thus, the dose required to kill a given number of tumor cells depends on the number of tumor cells initially present and is related to the tumor size. Figure 47–9 shows typical survival curves for mammalian cells exposed to radiation plotted on a semilogarithmic scale. For densely ionizing radiation such as neutrons, the dose-response curve is a straight line (Figure 47–9 curve A). For sparsely ionizing radiation such as x-rays, the dose-response curve may have an initial shoulder followed by a portion that is straight or almost straight. The slope of the final straight portion of the survival curve is usually related to the D_o, or the dose required to reduce the surviving fractions to 37%. The D_o increases directly with cellular radioresistance. With the exception of lymphocytes and germinal cells, the D_o levels for most mammalian cells irradiated in vitro lie within the range of 110–240 cGy.

The survival curve for sparsely ionizing radiation shown in Figure 47–9 curve B is often referred to as a multitarget single-hit survival curve, which assumes that all cells in the population contain a number of targets (N) of uniform size; a target is inactivated by a single hit, and cell death occurs only when N targets have been hit. The multitarget survival curve can be described by the following equation:

$$\text{Surviving fraction} = 1 - [1 - e^{-D/D_o}]^N$$

The multitarget equation often gives a poor fit to survival data in the very low dose and very high dose regions for some cell lines and culture conditions. A two-component cell survival model describes radiation cell inactivation by a linear-quadratic equation:

$$\text{Surviving fraction} = e^{[-\alpha D - \beta D^2]}$$

According to this model, cell inactivation by radiation can result from single-hit (α) or double-hit (β) events. This two-component model appears to give a better fit for most mammalian cell survival data (curve C) than the multitarget equation (curve B). This model was developed from molecular and microdosimetric theories and equates the cellular surviving fraction with the product of two exponential terms depending upon the first and second order of the dose, respectively.

In vivo, other factors affect the end results of irra-

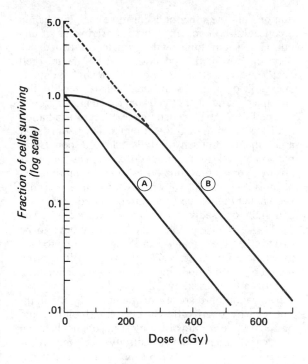

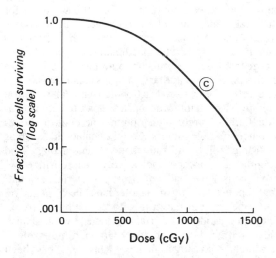

Figure 47–9. Cell survival curves following irradiation of cell cultures. **Curve A:** Survival curve for densely ionizing radiation. **Curve B:** Survival curve for sparsely ionizing radiation-multitarget single-hit model. **Curve C:** Survival curve for sparsely ionizing radiation-2-component linear-quadratic model.

diation, and the situation is far more complex than in a cell culture. Apparent growth or shrinkage of any normal tissue or tumor will depend upon the balance between new cell production and the natural cell death rate as well as upon cell killing by an outside agent. Two tumors with equal cellular sensitivities and an equal number of cells but different cell growth and cell loss rates may show the effect of irradiation at different times, and the clinician may be misled if a judgment about sensitivity is made too soon. Comparison of cell survival after doses given as single exposures versus the same doses given in multiple exposures separated by various time intervals has shown that in most cell systems, enhanced cellular repair and increased survival follow divided doses. The total dose with multiple exposures may have to be two to five times greater than a single dose to produce the same effect (Figure 47–10). Ways of improving the therapeutic ratio using various dose fractionation patterns are under study.

The radiation response of mammalian cells is influenced by many different chemical, biologic, and physical factors. One of the most important chemical factors influencing radiosensitivity is oxygen. Well-oxygenated cells are 2½–3 times as sensitive as anoxic cells. With few exceptions, normal tissues have an adequate oxygen supply. In animal tumors, up to 30% of cells are severely hypoxic, and the same presumably applies to human tumors. If it were not for the phenomenon called reoxygenation, hypoxia would tend to protect tumor cells. With fractionated radiation exposures, the death and subsequent loss of oxygenated cells permit hypoxic ones to come into position nearer a capillary and thus regain sensitivity. The effectiveness of fractionated clinical radiation therapy is probably due in large part to reoxygenation. Failure of reoxygenation may account for the resistance of some tumors. Certain compounds such as metronidazole, misonidazole, nimorazole, and etanidazole appear to selectively radiosensitize hypoxic cells. The results of most clinical trials evaluating the use of misonidazole have been negative, partly because of the drug's dose-limiting neurotoxicity. In a randomized trial conducted by the Danish Head and Neck Cancer Study Group, **nimorazole,** a less neurotoxic hypoxic cell sensitizer, has been shown to improve the local-regional control rate in patients irradiated for carcinoma of the supraglottic larynx and pharynx. Other trials using SR-2508, which is also less neurotoxic, have been completed recently in the United States and in Europe. The results are not yet available. Other compounds such as cysteine and the thiophosphate amifostine, which contain sulfhydryl groups, appear to offer preferential radioprotection to normal tissues. In addition,

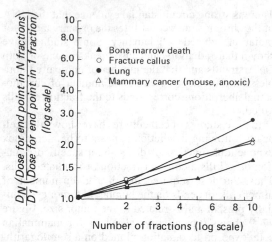

Figure 47–10. A demonstration of the effect of recovery between doses on radiation tolerance. The ratio of the dose for a given end point in N fractions to the dose for the same end point in one fraction is plotted against the number of fractions. Both are on logarithmic scales.

some chemotherapeutic agents such as dactinomycin, doxorubicin, cisplatin, and bleomycin are known to enhance radiation effects on normal tissues as well as tumors.

The radiosensitivity of mammalian cells also varies with the position in the cell cycle (cell age). This variation of radiosensitivity with cell cycle phase appears to be different for different cell lines.

Neutrons, helium ions, heavy ions, and pi mesons cause dense ionizations in tissues and are referred to as high-LET (linear energy transfer) radiation. The sensitivity of mammalian cells exposed to these types of radiation appears to be less dependent on the oxygen concentration and position in the cell cycle. These particles are currently under clinical investigation. Preliminary results suggest that high-LET radiation may be more effective than photons for the treatment of salivary gland tumors, bone tumors, and soft tissue sarcomas.

Many interrelated factors play a role in the clinical application of radiation therapy: (1) the inherent sensitivity of normal cells and tumor cells in the volume treated, (2) the total number of various types of cells present, (3) the ability of normal cells to migrate and tumor cells to metastasize, (4) the capability of repopulation of tumor versus normal tissue, (5) redistribution of cells in the cell cycle, (6) repair of sublethal damage in tumor and normal cells, (7) oxygen tension and reoxygenation, and (8) recruitment. The extent to which these factors affect the sparing of normal tissue cells and the killing of tumor cells forms the basis of radiation therapy.

---

* Therapeutic ratio = $\dfrac{\text{Damage to tumor}}{\text{Damage to normal tissue}}$

PRE- & POSTOPERATIVE RADIATION THERAPY

The rationale for combining radiation therapy and surgery in the treatment of cancer is that each method may compensate for deficiencies of the other. Irradiation may be used to sterilize the margins of a lesion; surgical resection may then be relied upon to remove the less radiosensitive central portion or extensions into bone and cartilage. Irradiation may, by killing the majority of cancer cells prior to resection, reduce the probability of seeding or dissemination of viable cancer cells during surgery. Postoperative radiation therapy is indicated when the surgical margins are close or positive, when there is microscopic or gross residual disease, or when the risk of local recurrence is great because of extensive tumor invasion. The use of such combined therapy is rational for highly invasive, poorly differentiated cancers with a high risk of spread and in situations where adequate surgical resection is impossible for anatomic reasons.

Pre- or postoperative radiation therapy may also be given to regional lymph nodes. This is not combination therapy in the sense that both methods are applied to the same area; rather, the radiation is used to extend the definitive therapy beyond the limits of the surgical excision. An example of such combination therapy is the irradiation of cervical lymph nodes following total laryngectomy for advanced carcinoma of the larynx.

SELECTION & MANAGEMENT OF RADIATION THERAPY PATIENTS

Specific indications for the selection of patients for curative radiation therapy are listed in Table 47–7. In general, the smaller, superficial, exophytic lesions are most amenable to radiation therapy; large, avascular, necrotic tumors and those with bone involvement are less likely to be controlled permanently by radiation therapy alone. Radiation should be used when it offers either a higher cure rate or the same cure rate as surgery, with fewer side effects or a better functional result. Radiation therapy may occasionally be used instead of surgery if the patient's general condition contraindicates a radical operation.

Palliation involves the relief of symptoms by the use of a specific treatment method. Patients selected for palliative treatment with radiation should have a local problem, present or impending, that can be relieved or significantly delayed in onset by treatment. Palliative radiotherapy may be employed for pain due to local invasion or bone involvement, obstruction of hollow organs, involvement of functioning areas in the brain or spinal cord, irritation or ulceration of mucosal surfaces such as those of the bronchi or bladder, or local ulcerating, infected tumor masses. In certain cancers, such as those arising in the oral or pharyngeal mucosa, the dosage required for palliation is essentially the same as that used for cure. Palliation of obstructive or brain lesions also requires large doses. Lasting palliation of bone pain can often be achieved with substantially lower doses.

The proper selection of patients for radiation therapy requires close cooperation between the surgeon, radiation oncologist, and medical oncologist. A combined plan, involving two or three methods of treatment, may offer the best chance of cure or palliation. It is usually best if the patient is seen jointly by all members of the oncology team and the treatment planned as a joint effort from the beginning.

A patient being considered for radiation therapy should have a thorough medical evaluation, including history, physical examination, and laboratory tests. Significant medical problems should be attended to and housing and transportation problems solved before treatment is undertaken. The most frequent problem arising during radiation therapy is the maintenance of adequate food and fluid intake. Patients irradiated around the head and neck often lose appetite because of changes in saliva and impaired taste sensation. Specially prepared foods and suitable encouragement may be of value. Special diets may be needed for patients with bowel problems. Changes in diet or use of medications for the control of symptoms resulting from irradiation should never be taken without first consulting the radiotherapist, since the severity of the reaction is used as a guide to treatment.

Cancer patients are often ill and subject to numerous concomitant medical problems. Acute myocardial infarction, serum hepatitis, acute appendicitis, perforation of a peptic ulcer, and many other unrelated major medical or surgical problems may occur in patients undergoing radiation therapy. The tendency to ascribe such problems to the irradiation should be resisted so that definitive therapy will not be delayed.

NEW RADIOTHERAPY MODALITIES

To further improve the therapeutic ratio, several new radiotherapy modalities are currently under active clinical investigation: (1) altered fractionation, (2) high-LET particle radiotherapy, (3) hyperthermia, (4) intraoperative radiotherapy, (5) radiosurgery, (6) radioimmunotherapy, and (7) three-dimensional conformal radiotherapy. The current status of each of these modalities is discussed in the following paragraphs.

Altered Fractionation

Time-dose fractionation has been the subject of intense research interest since the early days of radiotherapy. Over the years, there have been many attempts to optimize radiotherapy fractionation

Table 47–7. Role of radiotherapy in the treatment of specific neoplastic diseases.

	Role of Radiotherapy	Dosage[1]	Results
Skin cancer Basal cell carcinoma Squamous cell carcinoma	Curative treatment alternative to surgery for lesions not invading the bone. Treatment of choice for lesions of the eyelids and over cartilage.	Size-dependent: 40 Gy in ten fractions over 2 weeks to 45 Gy in 15 fractions over 3 weeks for lesions up to 2–3 cm in size; 50–70 Gy in 20–35 fractions over 4–7 weeks for larger lesions.	Five-year local control rate: 96–99% for basal cell carcinoma; 92–94% for squamous cell carcinoma.
Malignant melanoma	Curative treatment alternative to surgery for lentigo maligna and lentigo maligna melanoma. Treatment of patients refusing surgery. Postoperatively for microscopic or gross residual disease. Palliation of unresectable and metastatic disease.	45–50 Gy in 10–15 fractions over 2–3 weeks, depending on lesion size, for lentigo maligna. 6 Gy per fraction in two fractions per week to a total dose of 30 Gy in five fractions over 2.5 weeks postoperatively for microscopic residual disease in head and neck melanoma. 50 Gy in 20 fractions over 4 weeks or 32 Gy in four fractions over 4 weeks are equally effective for palliative treatment of skin or lymph node metastases.	Local control with primary radiotherapy for lentigo maligna: 90%. Two-year actuarial local-regional control with postoperative adjuvant radiotherapy in head and neck melanoma: 90–95%. Response rate to palliative radiotherapy for skin or soft tissue or lymph node metastases: ≈ 24% complete and 58% overall.
Breast cancer	Control of local disease after gross excision or lumpectomy for ductal carcinoma in situ as an alternative to mastectomy.	45–50 Gy to the breast ± 10–15 Gy boost to a total dose of 60 Gy to the lumpectomy site.	Ten-year actuarial local control rate: 86%. Ten-year actuarial survival: 94%.
	Control of local-regional disease after gross excision or lumpectomy as an alternative to mastectomy and axillary lymphadenectomy for stage T1 and T2 disease.	45–50 Gy to the breast and regional nodes ± 10–20 Gy boost to a total dose of 60–65 Gy to the lumpectomy site.	Local control rate: 80–98%. Five-year disease-free survival: 69–95%. Ten-year disease-free survival: 52–93%.
	Postoperative radiotherapy reduces local-regional recurrence after mastectomy and chemotherapy for locally advanced disease: lesions >5 cm, four or more positive nodes, skin involvement, positive margins, and poorly differentiated carcinomas.	45–50 Gy to the chest wall ± regional lymph nodes.	Local-regional control after chemotherapy, surgery, and radiotherapy: 88–98%.
	Combined with chemotherapy in the treatment of advanced inoperable lesions.	50 Gy to the breast ± 20–30 Gy boost with external beam radiotherapy or interstitial implants (or both) to gross disease.	Five-year local control: 50–75%.
	Combined with chemotherapy ± hyperthermia in the treatment of local-regional recurrence after mastectomy.	With no prior radiotherapy, 45–50 Gy to chest wall ± regional lymph nodes plus 10–15 Gy boost to gross disease. With prior radiotherapy, dose is individualized.	Five-year local control probability of 71% and survival rate of 35% have been reported with comprehensive irradiation of the chest wall and regional lymph nodes. For chest wall recurrence, complete responses of 64–94% have been achieved with radiotherapy ± hyperthermia compared to 24–47% with radiotherapy alone.
Bone tumors Ewing's sarcoma	Control of primary tumor.	40–45 Gy to involved bone and a generous margin ± 15–20 Gy boost with a reduced field to a total dose of 55–60 Gy to the tumor in conjunction with chemotherapy.	Local control rate: 90–95%. Five-year disease-free survival: 55–73% with localized disease at presentation. Disease-free survival: 75–85% for limited disease involving distal extremities; 25–35% for large central lesions.

(continued)

Table 47–7. Role of radiotherapy in the treatment of specific neoplastic diseases. (continued)

	Role of Radiotherapy	Dosage[1]	Results
	Palliation of lung metastases.	13.5 Gy in 10 fractions over 2 weeks to whole lung plus chemotherapy.	
Osteosarcoma	Treatment of disease in unresectable sites, eg, the spine and the base of the skull.	Doses in excess of 65–70 Gy are necessary for palliation.	
Chondrosarcoma	Treatment of disease in unresectable sites, eg, the spine and the base of the skull.	65–75 Gy with photon or particle photon (helium or neon) irradiation.	Local control: 45%; actuarial survival: 41% at 5 years, 36% at 10 years with photon irradiation. Actuarial local control rate: 68%; survival rate 70% at 3 years with charged particle (helium or neon) irradiation alone or mixed with photons, 91% at 5 years with proton irradiation.
Multiple myeloma	Local control of solitary plasmacytoma. Palliation of symptomatic lesions.	40–50 Gy for apparently solitary plasmacytoma. 20–30 Gy for palliation of bone pain.	Local control: 77%; 5-year survival 50–60%; 10-year survival 15–20% for solitary plasmacytoma, 20% complete and 70% partial pain relief.
Giant cell tumor	Treatment of lesions in sites not suitable for resection, eg, vertebra, sacrum.	45–55 Gy	Local control rate: 75–90%.
Eosinophilic granuloma	Local control of solitary lesions.	6–10 Gy	Local control rate: 75–100%.
Soft tissue sarcomas	Combined with limb-sparing surgery in the treatment of resectable lesions of the extremity. No demonstrated value in retroperitoneal sarcoma.	Preoperative: 50 Gy ± 15 Gy boost to the tumor bed with intraoperative brachytherapy or postoperative external beam irradiation.	Five-year actuarial local control rate: 97%; disease-free survival: 71%.
		Postoperative: 64–66 Gy with reduced fields after 50 Gy.	Five-year actuarial local control rate: 91%; disease-free survival: 81%.
	Treatment of unresectable disease.	70–80 Gy with reduced fields after 50 Gy and 60–65 Gy.	No evidence of disease rate: 50% for lesions <5 cm and 29% for lesions 5–17 cm in size. 59% 5-year local control rate for locally advanced disease treated with high-LET charged particle radiotherapy.
Rhabdomyosarcoma	Combined with surgery and chemotherapy for childhood rhabdomyosarcomas.	45–50 Gy for microscopic disease and 50–60 Gy for gross residual disease.	Local control with doses >40 Gy: 90% for group I, 90% for group II, 70% for group III, and 59% for group IV. Five-year survival: 82–88% for group I, 77–90% for group II, 64% for group III, and 20% for group IV.
Desmoid tumors (aggressive fibromatosis)	Given postoperatively for macroscopic or microscopic residual disease after resection. Used alone for unresectable disease.	50–60 Gy	Local control rate: 70–90%.
Central nervous system tumors Malignant gliomas	Postoperative radiotherapy ± chemotherapy prolongs useful survival.	60 Gy	Astrocytoma with anaplastic foci: median survival, 36.2 months; 3-year actuarial survival, 45%; 5-year survival, 18%. Glioblastoma multiforme: median survival, 8.6 months; 3-year survival, 4%.

(continued)

Table 47–7. Role of radiotherapy in the treatment of specific neoplastic diseases. (continued)

	Role of Radiotherapy	Dosage[1]	Results
Astrocytomas (low-grade)	Role of radiotherapy is controversial. Postoperative radiotherapy is probably indicated after incomplete resection or after biopsy only for lesions in unresectable sites.	50–54 Gy	Five-year survival: 41–68%. Survival for thalamic and hypothalamic tumors: 60–70%.
Optic nerve glioma	Radiotherapy is indicated for symptomatic progressive disease with intracranial extension and for tumors of the optic chiasm.	50 Gy	Five-year survival: 75–100%.
Brain stem glioma	Radiotherapy is the primary treatment modality.	54 Gy with conventional fractionation at 1.8 Gy per fraction per day. 72 Gy with hyperfractionation at 1 Gy per fraction twice daily.	Five-year overall survival: 20–30% with conventional fractionated radiotherapy. Three-year actuarial survival: 60% for adults and 36% for children with hyperfractionated radiotherapy.
Medulloblastoma	Postoperative craniospinal radiotherapy after subtotal or total resection.	54 Gy to posterior fossa, 36 Gy to the spinal axis.	Survival 53–71% at 5 years; 41–63% at 10 years.
Ependymoma	Postoperative radiotherapy improves survival.	55–60 Gy for adults, 45–50 Gy for children. Prophylactic spinal irradiation for high-grade infratentorial tumors.	Five-year survival: 60–70% for differentiated tumors and 15–30% for anaplastic tumors.
Oligodendroglioma	Postoperative radiotherapy improves survival.	55–60 Gy with reduced fields after 45–50 Gy.	Five-year survival: >65–90%.
Craniopharyngioma	Postoperative radiotherapy after incomplete resection. Radiotherapy alone for inoperable lesions.	54–55 Gy	Five- to 10-year survival: 72–90% after incomplete resection and postoperative radiotherapy.
Meningioma	Postoperative radiotherapy after incomplete resection prolongs the interval before recurrence and may improve survival.	50–54 Gy	Progression-free survival: 70–90% at 5 years; 60–77% at 10 years.
Pineal tumors	Cranial ± spinal radiotherapy is indicated after biopsy or subtotal resection and shunt.	45–54 Gy to the brain for adults with dose reduction for children; 25–36 Gy to the spinal axis.	Five-year survival: 45–75%.
Neurilemmoma, schwannoma, neurinoma	Postoperative radiotherapy after subtotal resection reduces recurrence rate.	50–54 Gy	Actuarial recurrence rate at 15 years: 6% with postoperative radiotherapy versus 59% with subtotal resection only.
Pituitary adenoma	Radiotherapy is often effective in controlling the hypersecretion and mass effects of large tumors. Particle radiotherapy and radioactive implants have been used in the treatment of small intrasellar tumors.	45–50 Gy	Control rate: 77–90% for acromegaly; 52–100% for Cushing's disease. Recurrence-free survival for adenomas with mass effect: 93% at 5 years with radiotherapy alone; 96% at 5 years and 86% at 10 years with surgery ± radiotherapy.
Malignant lymphoma	Radiotherapy ± chemotherapy may prolong survival of patients with primary CNS lymphoma. Palliative treatment of AIDS-related CNS lymphoma.	40–50 Gy whole brain ± 10–15 Gy boost to the primary site. 40 Gy over 3 weeks for AIDS-related lymphoma.	With radiotherapy alone, survival is 28% at 2 years and 0–20% at 5 years. With combined radiotherapy and chemotherapy, a 3-year actuarial survival of 71% has been reported. Prognosis with AIDS-related CNS lymphoma is extremely poor.
Metastatic carcinomas	Palliation.	30 Gy over 2 weeks to whole brain ± additional boost in selective patients.	One-year survival: <20%.

(continued)

Table 47–7. Role of radiotherapy in the treatment of specific neoplastic diseases. (continued)

	Role of Radiotherapy	Dosage[1]	Results
Neuroblastoma	Postoperative radiotherapy combined with chemotherapy is beneficial for patients over 1 year of age with stage III disease with lymph node metastases. Palliative treatment of symptomatic metastases unresponsive to chemotherapy. Total body irradiation is sometimes used as part of a preparatory regimen for bone marrow transplant in patients with stage IV disease treated with aggressive chemoradiotherapy with curative intent.	15–30 Gy at 1.5–2.0 Gy per fraction depending on the age of the patient and the site of disease. Palliation can be achieved with a single dose of 5 Gy or 15–20 Gy with fractionated doses. Total dose for total body irradiation ranged from 7.5 to 12 Gy in one to six fractions over 1–5 days.	Survival is 90% or more for stage I, 80–90% or more for stage II, and 73% for stage III disease treated with multimodality therapy. A 2-year actuarial relapse-free survival of 25% after aggressive chemoradiotherapy followed by autologous bone marrow transplant has been reported by the Children's Cancer Study Group. Survival for stage IV-S patients is 93% in low-risk patients and 32% in high-risk patients.
Thyroid carcinomas	Postoperative radiotherapy ± radioactive iodine (^{131}I) in the treatment of microscopic or gross residual disease for locally invasive or recurrent papillary, follicular, and medullary carcinomas. Palliative treatment of anaplastic, giant cell, or spindle cell carcinomas and symptomatic metastases. [?THYROID LYMPHOMA]	60–70 Gy postoperatively depending on the amount of disease present. Hyperfractionated radiotherapy has been combined with chemotherapy in the treatment of anaplastic carcinoma following biopsy or thyroidectomy.	10-year survival: 90–95% for papillary carcinoma; 60–75% for follicular carcinoma, and ≈50% for medullary carcinoma. Median survival of anaplastic carcinoma is approximately 4–5 months.
Ocular and intraorbital tumors Retinoblastoma	External beam radiotherapy is used for multifocal lesions or lesions close to the macula or the optic nerve with the goal of preserving vision. Radioactive eye plaques have been used for solitary lesions and for localized recurrences following external beam radiotherapy.	45–50 Gy with external beam irradiation. With radioactive eye plaques, a dose of 40–50 Gy is delivered to the tumor apex.	Cure rates of 85–90% with either radiotherapy or surgery have been reported. Rate of preservation of vision with external beam radiotherapy ± photocoagulation or cryotherapy are approximately 95%, 86%, 85%, 69%, and 25% for Reese-Ellsworth group I, II, III, IV, and V tumors, respectively.
Rhabdomyosarcoma	Radiotherapy combined with chemotherapy following biopsy is the treatment of choice.	50–60 Gy	Five-year disease-free survival: 94%
Ocular melanoma	Radioactive eye plaques or external beam particle radiotherapy with protons or helium ions as an alternative to enucleation.	70 Gy equivalent with particle radiotherapy. 70 Gy at 1 mm beyond the apex of tumor with radioactive eye plaques.	Over 90% of the eyes treated are retained, with vision preserved in >50%.
Orbital lymphoma	Treatment of choice for localized primary orbital lymphoma.	36–40 Gy	Local control rate is ≈ 97%.

(continued)

Table 47–7. Role of radiotherapy in the treatment of specific neoplastic diseases. (continued)

	Role of Radiotherapy	Dosage[1]	Results
Head and neck cancer	Primary treatment for carcinoma of the nasopharynx. Preferred treatment for stage I-II carcinoma of the larynx, tongue, floor of mouth, oropharynx, and hypopharynx with preservation of organ function. Combined with surgery ± chemotherapy for moderately advanced operable disease. Used alone or combined with chemotherapy or other treatment modifiers for advanced inoperable or recurrent disease. Postoperative radiotherapy for salivary gland tumors with high risk of local recurrence. Neutron or heavy ion radiotherapy for inoperable salivary gland tumors. Used alone or combined with surgery ± chemotherapy for paranasal sinus carcinoma.	65–75 Gy for gross disease, 60 Gy for high-risk subclinical disease, 45–54 Gy for low-risk microscopic disease. Higher tumor doses can be achieved with hyperfractionated radiotherapy or interstitial implant boost with acceptable late normal tissue.	Five-year local control rates vary according to the primary site, the size and extent of the primary lesion, and the size and number of the involved lymph nodes. The control rate for stage I carcinoma of the vocal cord is 90–95%. Early carcinomas of the tongue, the floor of the mouth, the tonsil, the soft palate, the nasopharynx, the supraglottic larynx, and the hypopharynx can be controlled by radiotherapy in about 80–90% of cases. Local-regional control rates exceeding 70% can be achieved with combined surgery and radiotherapy ± chemotherapy in moderately advanced operable disease. Control rates with radiotherapy alone or combined with chemotherapy for advanced inoperable disease are lower.
Lung cancer Non-small cell carcinoma	Used postoperatively when there are hilar or mediastinal lymph node metastases or positive surgical margins. Used preoperatively in superior sulcus carcinomas. Definitive treatment of inoperable disease. Palliation of symptomatic metastases.	50–66 Gy with postoperative radiotherapy depending on the amount of residual disease present. 60–70 Gy with definitive radiotherapy.	Five-year survival: 20–56% with surgery ± postoperative radiotherapy; 15–34% with preoperative radiotherapy ± surgery; and 23–28% with radiotherapy alone in superior sulcus carcinomas; 16–32% with radiotherapy alone in patients with early-stage technically operable disease. Two-year survival: 10–29%; local control with doses over 60 Gy: 60% or more with radiotherapy alone for inoperable disease.
Small cell carcinoma	Combined with chemotherapy as the primary treatment. The role of prophylactic cranial irradiation is controversial.	45–50 Gy with conventional fractionated or, more recently, accelerated hyperfractionated radiotherapy. For prophylactic cranial irradiation, a dose of 24–30 Gy is delivered to patients achieving complete response after chemotherapy and thoracic irradiation.	Median survival with chemotherapy ± conventional fractionated radiotherapy: 48–97 weeks. Two-year actuarial survival of 53% has been reported with concurrent chemotherapy and accelerated hyperfractionated radiotherapy.
Thymomas	Postoperative radiotherapy reduces local recurrence after surgery for invasive thymomas. Definitive radiotherapy ± chemotherapy is used for unresectable disease.	45–50 Gy with postoperative radiotherapy. Doses of 50–60 Gy or higher may be necessary for long-term local control of unresectable disease.	Local control: 55–84% with postoperative radiotherapy for invasive thymomas after complete resection; 60–80% with doses over 49 Gy for unresectable invasive thymomas treated with radiotherapy alone. Overall 5-year survival: 46–75%.
Gastrointestinal tract neoplasms Squamous cell carcinoma of the esophagus	Primary treatment modality for squamous cell carcinoma of the proximal third of the esophagus. Combined with surgery ± chemotherapy for resectable carcinoma of the middle third. Combined with chemotherapy for inoperable disease with curative or palliative intent.	40–60 Gy with pre- or postoperative radiotherapy. 50–66 Gy ± chemotherapy with definitive radiotherapy.	Overall 5-year survival is less than 10% in the majority of the series regardless of treatment method. Two-year survival with chemoradiotherapy: 22–48%. Palliation of dysphagia or pain can be achieved in 60–80% of patients treated with full-course radiotherapy.

(continued)

Table 47–7. Role of radiotherapy in the treatment of specific neoplastic diseases. (continued)

	Role of Radiotherapy	Dosage[1]	Results
Stomach	Preoperative radiotherapy ± chemotherapy may render borderline resectable lesions resectable. Intraoperative radiotherapy can improve the survival of patients with stage II-IV disease. Postoperative radiotherapy ± chemotherapy may reduce local-regional recurrence in high-risk patients and in patients with residual disease after surgery. Radiotherapy ± chemotherapy is used in the palliation of advanced incurable disease.	28–35 Gy with intraoperative radiotherapy. 45–55 Gy ± chemotherapy with pre- or postoperative radiotherapy.	Five-year survival of resectable gastric carcinoma with surgery ± intraoperative radiotherapy and surgery alone: 87%, 93%, for stage I; 84%, 62% for stage II; 62%, 37% for stage III; and 15% and 0% for stage IV disease. Five-year survival with radiotherapy ± chemotherapy for locally advanced gastric carcinoma: 0–20%.
Colon	Role of radiotherapy remains unestablished. Retrospective studies suggest improved local control with postoperative radiotherapy in high-risk patients.	45–50 Gy delivered postoperatively.	Local failure rates with surgery alone and with surgery ± postoperative radiotherapy of 11% and 6% for B2 disease; 30% and 5% for B3 disease; 32% and 25% for C2 disease; 49% and 43% for C3 disease; and corresponding survival rates of 70% and 60% for B2 disease; 64% and 78% for B3 disease; 45% and 57% for C2 disease; 38% and 49% for C3 disease have been reported.
Rectum	Postoperative radiotherapy ± chemotherapy improves the local-regional control and survival of patients with modified Astler-Coller stage B2, B3, and C1–3 disease. Radiotherapy ± chemotherapy may render borderline resectable disease resectable and provide palliation and sometimes long-term local control for advanced inoperable disease. Endocavitary radiotherapy may be used as a surgical alternative for small well-differentiated to moderately well-differentiated carcinomas less than 10 cm from the anal verge and for elderly or poor-risk patients and those who refuse colostomy.	Postoperative radiotherapy: 45–50 Gy ± additional boost is small intestine can be excluded, combined with chemotherapy. Dose of preoperative radiotherapy in patients presenting with resectable disease has been variable. In patients presenting with initially unresectable disease, preoperative radiotherapy with 45–55 Gy ± 10–20 Gy intraoperative radiotherapy ± chemotherapy has been used. A dose of 60–65 Gy or higher is often necessary for local control of unresected [UNRESECTABLE??] disease. With endocavitary radiotherapy, four treatments of 30 Gy each separated by a 2-week interval are delivered with superficial x-rays using the Papillon technique.	Most studies suggest that postoperative radiotherapy ± chemotherapy can decrease local failure rates by as much as 20% after resection of modified Astler-Coller stage B2, B3 and C1–3 disease. Two randomized trials also showed a survival benefit in patients treated with combined modality compared to surgery alone or surgery combined with postoperative radiotherapy or surgery combined with postoperative chemotherapy. A large randomized trial by the European Organization for Research on Treatment of Cancer showed improved local control but not survival with preoperative radiotherapy. Five-year survival rates for patients irradiated after subtotal resection are about 24%. In patients with initially unresectable disease, 50–70% may become resectable after preoperative radiotherapy exceeding 45 Gy. Long-term local control can be achieved in 25–35% of these patients. A 5-year survival rate of 78% has been reported for selected patients with early favorable lesions in the lower rectum treated with endocavitary radiotherapy alone.

(continued)

Table 47–7. Role of radiotherapy in the treatment of specific neoplastic diseases. (continued)

	Role of Radiotherapy	Dosage[1]	Results
Anus	Radiotherapy alone can be curative in early lesions. Radiotherapy combined with chemotherapy is curative with organ function preservation in more advanced disease.	60–65 Gy with radiotherapy alone. Doses in the range of 30–50 Gy have been used in combination with chemotherapy.	Local control of 80% and 5-year survival of 79% for selected early lesions treated with radiotherapy alone have been reported. The local control rate with combined modality therapy is about 85%. Five-year survivals of 55% and cause-specific survivals of 69% have been reported recently.
Pancreas	Postoperative radiotherapy combined with chemotherapy improves survival for resectable disease. Palliative radiotherapy is combined with fluorouracil for inoperable disease.	40–50 Gy postoperative radiotherapy ± fluorouracil for resectable lesions. 45–50 Gy ± intraoperative radiotherapy of 20 Gy and fluorouracil for unresectable disease.	Two- and 5-year survival rates were 42% and 14% with and 15% and 5% without postoperative radiotherapy ± fluorouracil in a randomized trial by the Gastrointestinal Tumor Study Group. Two-year survival with combined radiotherapy and fluorouracil for unresectable disease is about 6–12%.
Biliary tract	Postoperative radiotherapy may improve local control and survival rates after curative resection in high-risk patients. Significant palliation and occasionally long-term survival can be achieved with radiotherapy ± chemotherapy for unresectable or incompletely resected disease.	45–50 Gy with postoperative radiotherapy ± chemotherapy. Higher doses may be delivered to the primary tumor using intraoperative radiotherapy or brachytherapy boost or external beam particle therapy.	Median survival of 29 months with surgery alone and 63 months with surgery ± postoperative radiotherapy have been reported in patients receiving curative surgery. Median survival of patients irradiated for locally advanced disease is in the range of 6–18 months.
Female genital tract Ovary	Intraperitoneal ^{32}P may be used as adjunctive therapy for microscopic residuum in unfavorable stage I disease. External beam abdominopelvic irradiation is effective in controlling microscopic and small (<2 cm) residual disease after surgery in stage IB, II, and III disease, though most of these patients are now treated with combination chemotherapy.	With intraperitoneal radiotherapy, 15 mCi Of ^{32}P is usually instilled. With external beam radiotherapy, a dose of 30 Gy at 1.0–1.5 Gy per day is delivered to the whole abdomen and pelvis, and the pelvis is boosted with reduced fields to a total dose of 45–50 Gy. The dose to the liver is limited to 22.5–25 Gy and to the kidneys to 18–20 Gy. Lower doses are used when abdominopelvic irradiation is delivered after chemotherapy.	Five-year survival following external beam abdominopelvic irradiation: 63.5–94% for stage I, 45–85% for stage II disease. Overall 5-year survival for stage III disease is approximately 30%.
Dysgerminoma	Radiotherapy in moderate doses can be curative for this exquisitely radiosensitive tumor. However, stage IB, II, and III are now treated by combination chemotherapy after conservative surgery with preservation of fertility. Radiotherapy is the preferred treatment for intra-abdominal disease after complete surgery when preservation of fertility is not an issue.	20–25 Gy for microscopic and 30–35 Gy for macroscopic disease. Smaller fraction sizes of 1.0–1.5 Gy per fraction per day are used with abdominopelvic irradiation.	Survival of children with disease confined to the pelvis or with minimal abdominal involvement is 95–100%. Tumor rupture or extensive metastases reduce survival. The overall survival rate is 75–85%.

(continued)

Table 47–7. Role of radiotherapy in the treatment of specific neoplastic diseases. (continued)

	Role of Radiotherapy	Dosage[1]	Results
Uterus	Postoperative radiotherapy and, less often, preoperative radiotherapy can reduce the incidence of pelvic and vaginal recurrence in stage I endometrial carcinoma when the tumor is poorly differentiated or when there is deep myometrial invasion or enlargement of the uterus to over 8 cm. Pre- and postoperative radiotherapy for stage II endometrial carcinoma. Radiotherapy alone or combined with surgery for stage III and radiotherapy alone or combined with systemic therapy for stage IV endometrial carcinoma. Pre- or postoperative radiotherapy may reduce pelvic recurrence in uterine sarcoma.	45–50 Gy external beam irradiation to the pelvis ± intracavitary brachytherapy for stage I disease. A combination of external beam radiotherapy to the pelvis and intracavitary brachytherapy to the uterus and vagina is usually used for stage II–IV disease. Dose depends on the amount of tumor present.	Five-year actuarial survival: 82–95% for stage I, 60–83% for stage II, 25–40% for stage III, and 5% for stage IV endometrial carcinoma.
Cervix	Except for young patients, radiotherapy is the primary treatment of choice for most patients with invasive carcinoma. Extrafascial hysterectomy is performed after radiotherapy in the treatment of some bulky endocervical cancer.	Intracavitary brachytherapy alone for stage IA disease. A dose of 75–80 Gy is delivered to point A in two insertions. A combination of external beam irradiation and intracavitary brachytherapy is used to deliver a total dose of 50–60 Gy to the parametrial tissues and 85–90 Gy to point A for stage IB–III disease.	Control of disease in the pelvis: 94–98% for stage I, 84–94% for stage IIA, 75–82% for stage IIB, 63–64% for stage III, and 32–34% for stage IV disease. Five-year survival: 88–91% for stage I, 61–83% for stage II, 33–45% for stage III, and 14–19% for stage IV disease.
Vagina	Radiotherapy is the treatment of choice for most carcinomas of the vagina.	Stage I disease may be treated with intracavitary ± interstitial brachytherapy alone. A dose of 60–70 Gy is delivered to the entire vaginal mucosa, and an additional 20–30 Gy is delivered to the tumor area. For stage II–IV disease, a dose of 40–50 Gy is delivered to the pelvis with external beam radiotherapy followed by additional 30–40 Gy to the tumor with intracavitary or interstitial brachytherapy.	Five-year actuarial survival: 80–90% for stage I, 50–60% for stage II, 30–40% for stage III, and 5% for stage IV disease.
Vulva	Most vulvar cancers are treated by surgery ± radiotherapy. Radiotherapy may be used in the primary treatment of patients who are medically inoperable or have refused surgery and in the palliation of advanced disease. Postoperative radiotherapy is indicated when there are close or positive surgical margins, multiple lymph node involvement, or extracapsular spread.	For localized inoperable disease, a dose of 40–45 Gy is delivered to the vulva and the pelvic and inguinal nodes, followed by an additional 25–30 Gy through an interstitial implant to the primary and 20–25 Gy through an electron beam to the inguinal nodes. Small superficial lesions may be treated with external electron beam or interstitial implant alone to a dose of ≈65 Gy. Postoperative radiotherapy usually delivers 45–50 Gy to the pelvis and vulva, with additional boost to the positive margins through an interstitial implant or external electron beam irradiation and additional boost to the inguinal areas through external electron beam irradiation to a total dose of 60–65 Gy for microscopic and 65–70 Gy for gross residual disease.	The 5-year survival is ≈80–90% for patients without lymph node metastases and 30–50% for those with positive nodes. Five-year survival of 70% for stage I and II and 39% for stages III and IV was reported in one series using high-energy electron beam irradiation following biopsy, though 24% of the patients developed ulcers and 5% developed extensive tissue necrosis. In a randomized trial of postoperative elective irradiation to the pelvis and inguinal areas versus observation following radical vulvectomy and bilateral inguinal lymphadenectomy in patients with invasive vulvar cancer with positive inguinal nodes, the 2-year survival and regional lymph node recurrent rates were 68% and 11.9% for the irradiated group and 54% and 25.4% for the nonirradiated group.

(continued)

Table 47–7. Role of radiotherapy in the treatment of specific neoplastic diseases. (continued)

	Role of Radiotherapy	Dosage[1]	Results
Male genital tract Testis	Postoperative radiotherapy to the para-aortic, ipsilateral renal hilar and pelvic lymph nodes is indicated for stage I and IIA seminoma. The use of "consolidation" radiotherapy after chemotherapy for stages IIB, III, and IV seminoma is controversial and should probably be reserved for overt disease progression.	25–30 Gy for stage I and IIA and 35 Gy for more bulky disease at 1.25–1.5 Gy per fraction per day.	Three-year disease-free survival after radical orchiectomy and postoperative radiotherapy: 97% for stage I, 86% for stage II seminoma.
Seminoma	Postoperative radiotherapy to the para-aortic, ipsilateral renal hilar and pelvic lymph nodes is indicated for stage I and IIA seminoma. The use of "consolidation" radiotherapy after chemotherapy for stages IIB, III, and IV seminoma is controversial and should probably be reserved for overt disease progression.	25–30 Gy for stage I and IIA and 35 Gy for more bulky disease at 1.25–1.5 Gy per fraction per day.	Three-year disease-free survival after radical orchiectomy and postoperative radiotherapy: 97% for stage I, 86% for stage II seminoma.
Nonseminomatous tumors	Surgery and chemotherapy are the primary therapy. Radiotherapy is used for palliation of brain or bone metastases.	30 Gy in 10 fractions over 2 weeks for palliation.	
Prostate	Radiotherapy is an alternative to surgery for stages A and B disease. Radiotherapy ± hormonal therapy is used and in the definitive treatment of stage C disease and palliation of stage D disease.	Minimum tumor dose to the prostate: 65 Gy for stage A and B disease and 70 Gy for stage C disease. 45–50 Gy to the pelvis for intermediate to high-grade, bulky stage B and stage C disease.	Five-year survival: 74–100% for stage A and B, 52–78% for stage C disease. Ten-year survival: 42–70% for stage A and B and 32–47% for stage C disease. Fifteen-year survival: 35–38% for stage A and B, 18–27% for stage C disease.
Penis	Radiotherapy is an alternative to surgery in patients who desire preservation of organ function and may be the treatment of choice for early disease.	A variety of techniques including radioactive mold, interstitial implant, and external beam irradiation have been used to deliver 60–70 Gy to the tumor.	Local control rate: 32–100% overall, 44–100% for stage I–II and 33–39% for stage III–IV disease with radiotherapy alone.
Urinary tract Kidney: Wilms' tumor	Combined with chemotherapy in the treatment of stage III–V disease and stage II disease with unfavorable histology.	12–38 Gy depending on age, site, histology and amount of tumor present.	Results of the Third National Wilms Tumor Study showed 4-year relapse-free survivals of 89–92% for stage I, 87–89% for stage II, 74–84% for stage III, and 72–78% for stage IV disease.
Bladder	The role of radiotherapy combined with chemotherapy in the definitive treatment of T2 and T3 disease following transurethral resection as an alternative to radical cystectomy is under investigation. Radiotherapy is combined with chemotherapy in the palliation of unresectable or metastatic disease.	45 Gy to the pelvis with additional boost to 65 Gy to the tumor ± chemotherapy.	Local control: 51–88% after concurrent chemotherapy and radiotherapy; 65% after neoadjuvant ± concurrent chemotherapy and radiotherapy. Survival: 64% for T2 and 24% for T3–4 disease at 4 years after concurrent chemotherapy and radiotherapy; 89% for T2 and 50% for T3–4 disease at 3 years after neoadjuvant ± concurrent chemotherapy and radiotherapy.

(continued)

Table 47–7. Role of radiotherapy in the treatment of specific neoplastic diseases. (continued)

	Role of Radiotherapy	Dosage[1]	Results
Female urethra	Treatment of choice for early disease. Combined with surgery for advanced resectable disease. Palliation of advanced unresectable and recurrent disease after surgery.	Small lesions may be treated with interstitial implant alone with a dose of 60–70 Gy. Larger lesions are usually treated with a combination of external beam irradiation and interstitial implant to deliver 45–50 Gy to the pelvis and inguinal nodes and 70–80 Gy to the tumor.	Five-year disease-free survival after radiotherapy alone: 32–69% overall; 64–100% for distal lesions; 0–60% for proximal lesions.
Malignant lymphoma and leukemias Hodgkin's disease	Radiotherapy is the most effective single agent for Hodgkin's disease. Stages I and IIA can be treated with subtotal nodal irradiation alone. Stages IB, IIB, and IIIA can be treated with subtotal or total nodal irradiation alone or combined with chemotherapy. Stages IIIB and IV are treated with chemotherapy ± low dose radiotherapy to areas of initial bulky disease. Bulky mediastinal disease is usually treated with combined chemotherapy and radiotherapy.	40–44 Gy to gross disease, 25–36 Gy to microscopic or minimal disease.	Five-year survival: 94–96% for stage I–IIA; 80–90% for stage IB, IIB, and IIIA; 66–84% for stage IIIB and IV disease.
Non-Hodgkin's lymphoma	Stage I disease can be cured with radiotherapy alone. Stage II disease is usually treated with combination chemotherapy ± radiotherapy to involved areas. Stage III and stage IV disease are primarily managed with chemotherapy; radiotherapy is sometimes given to areas of initial bulky disease following chemotherapy. CNS and bone lesions are usually treated with radiotherapy ± chemotherapy. Total body irradiation is used in the preparative regimen in bone marrow transplantation for aggressive or recurrent disease.	40–50 Gy to gross disease; 25–36 Gy to microscopic disease or minimal residual disease after chemotherapy.	Five-year survival rates of 80–100% with radiotherapy alone for stage I–II nodular lymphomas and 5-year disease-free survival of 72–82% with combination chemotherapy and radiotherapy for stage I–II large cell lymphomas have been reported.
Acute lymphoblastic leukemia (ANLL)	Cranial irradiation is used to prevent CNS relapse following chemotherapy in high-risk patients (WBC>25,000/μL, T cell immunophenotype, or presence of Philadelphia chromosome on presentation) and in patients with overt CNS involvement. Testicular irradiation is used for testicular infiltration during or after chemotherapy. Low-dose radiotherapy provides rapid palliation of pain or other symptoms from leukemic infiltration of bones, joints, and soft tissues. Total body irradiation is used in the preparative regimen for bone marrow transplant following chemotherapy-induced second or subsequent remission after relapse.	18 Gy in 10–12 fractions ± intrathecal methotrexate for CNS prophylaxis; 24 Gy in 12–16 fractions to the cranium and 14–15 Gy in ten fractions to the spine for overt CNS disease after remission induction with systemic and intrathecal chemotherapy. A dose of 24–25 Gy at 1.5–2.0 Gy per fraction is usually used for testicular relapse. A dose of 6–10 Gy at 1.5–2.0 Gy per fraction per day may be sufficient for the relief of symptoms from bone or joint or soft tissue involvement.	Five-year leukemia-free survival rates of 70–75% can now be achieved.

(continued)

Table 47–7. Role of radiotherapy in the treatment of specific neoplastic diseases. (continued)

	Role of Radiotherapy	Dosage[1]	Results
Acute nonlymphoblastic leukemias (ANLL) and chronic myologenous leukemias (CML)	Total body irradiation is used in the preparative regimen for bone marrow transplantation. Splenic irradiation is used in the palliation of pain from massive splenomegaly due to leukemic infiltration.	Dose fractionation for total body irradiation varies at different centers. Current regimens include 2 Gy per fraction twice daily to a total of 12 Gy or 1.2 Gy per fraction three times daily to a total of 13.2 Gy. Doses of 0.50–.75 Gy per fraction per day for 4–5 days may be sufficient for splenic irradiation as white cell or platelet counts can drop precipitously after doses of less than 1 Gy.	Survival rates of 65% at 3–8 years after bone marrow transplantation in first remission of ANLL in children have been reported.
Benign diseases Keloids	Postoperative radiotherapy beginning 24–48 hours after excision can prevent recurrence.	15 Gy in three to five fractions using electrons or superficial x-rays.	73–90% control rate.
Graves' ophthalmopathy	Radiotherapy to the orbit can reduce soft tissue swelling, decrease proptosis, and improve ocular mobility and visual acuity.	20 Gy	About 65–68% of patients will have good to excellent response.
Pterygium	Postoperative radiotherapy can decrease vascularization at the operative site and reduce recurrence.	10 Gy per fraction per week for 3 weeks with superficial beta ray irradiation using strontium 90 applicator beginning within 24 hours after excision.	Over 95% with no recurrence.
Heterotopic bone formation	Postoperative radiotherapy prevents heterotopic bone formation following total hip arthroplasty.	10 Gy in five fractions per week or a single dose of 7 Gy within 72 hours after surgery.	Over 95% with no recurrence.

[1]Delivered at a rate of 1.8–2.0 Gy per fraction per day, five fractions per week.

schedules. Conventional fractionated radiotherapy consists of 1.8–2.5 Gy per fraction, five or six daily fractions per week, to a total dose of 60–75 Gy over 6–8 weeks. With hyperfractionation, the dose per fraction is decreased, the number of fractions per week and the total dose are increased, and the overall time of therapy is less than or the same as that of conventional fractionation. With accelerated fractionation, the dose per fraction is less than or the same as that of conventional fractionation, the number of fractions per week is increased, the total dose is greater than or the same as that of conventional fractionation, and the overall therapeutic time is decreased. With hypofractionation, the dose per fraction is increased, the number of fractions per week is decreased, and the total dose and overall therapeutic time are less than or the same as those of conventional fractionation. In split-course radiotherapy, a planned break—usually 1 or 2 weeks—is introduced during the treatment course to allow healing of acute reactions before further treatment is delivered.

The principal objective of altered fractionation is to improve the therapeutic ratio. During a course of fractionated radiotherapy, tissues can repair sublethal damage, redistribute over the different phases of the cell cycle, and repopulate between fractions. Tumor cells that are initially hypoxic may be reoxygenated and become more radiosensitive. Various normal tissues and tumors differ in their capacities to repair radiation damage, redistribute among the different cell cycle phases, and regenerate and reoxygenate, and for these reasons they respond differently to fractionated radiotherapy. The differential response of tumors and normal tissues with fractionated radiotherapy offers an opportunity for improving the therapeutic ratio through manipulations of time, dose, and fractionation. Currently, the most commonly used altered fractionation schemes consist of hyperfractionation or accelerated fractionation or a combination of the two.

The primary rationale for hyperfractionation is that there is greater sparing of late-responding normal tissues such as the lung, brain, and spinal cord than of early- or acute-responding normal tissues such as skin, mucous membranes, intestinal epithelium, and bone marrow and tumors—and with decrease of dose per fraction. Thus, with hyperfractionation, one can improve the therapeutic ratio by reducing late normal tissue toxicities through a decrease of the dose per fraction and to increase tumor control through an increase of the total dose. The primary rationale for accelerated fractionation is that shortening the overall treatment time minimizes tumor repopulation during fractionated radiotherapy and thus increases tumor control. Since little if any regeneration occurs in late-responding normal tissues, a reduced overall treatment time will not affect late normal tissue injury. Since the dose per fraction in an accelerated fractionation scheme is usually decreased or unchanged from conventional fractionation, late normal tissue injury is decreased or unchanged. However, an acute normal tissue reaction may increase during hyperfractionated as well as accelerated fractionated radiotherapy.

During the past 2 decades, altered fractionation radiotherapy has been tried in a variety of tumor sites, including the head and neck, brain, lung, bladder, prostate, breast, lymphoma, melanoma, soft tissue sarcomas, and metastatic tumors. Most of these trials were nonrandomized. Randomized clinical trials thus far suggest improved local-regional control in T3N1 or N0 carcinoma of the oropharynx with hyperfractionated radiotherapy and improved local-regional control as well as increased survival rates in bladder cancer and in malignant gliomas with accelerated hyperfractionated radiotherapy. Clinical trials evaluating the relative efficacy of various fractionation schemes alone or combined with chemical or biologic treatment modifiers are in progress.

Particle Radiotherapy

At present, particle radiotherapy machines are very costly and are available in only a few centers worldwide. Particle radiotherapy is done with neutrons, protons, pions, and heavy ions such as helium, neon, carbon, and silicon. Radiotherapy using neutrons, pions, and heavy ions is referred to as high-LET radiotherapy. Compared with low-LET photon radiation, high-LET radiations are biologically more effective and less oxygen- and cell cycle-dependent, and there is less repair of sublethal damage. Furthermore, protons, pions, and heavy ions have a more favorable depth-dose distribution than neutrons or photons. Randomized trials of neutron radiotherapy in England and in the United States have shown significant improvement in local-regional control as well as survival compared with conventional photon radiotherapy for inoperable salivary gland tumors. Overall pooled data from the literature indicate a local-regional control rate of 67% with fast neutrons versus 24% with photons or electrons for inoperable and recurrent salivary gland tumors. Other randomized trials suggest an advantage for mixed neutron and photon beam irradiation compared with photon irradiation alone for metastatic squamous cell carcinoma in cervical lymph nodes and locally advanced carcinoma of the prostate. However, other randomized trials comparing neutron irradiation alone or mixed neutron and photon irradiation with photon irradiation for advanced squamous cell carcinoma of the head and neck, malignant gliomas, and lung cancer have been negative. Nonrandomized studies also suggest an improved local control rate with neutron radiotherapy compared with photons or electrons in the treatment of inoperable soft tissue sarcomas, osteogenic sarcomas, and chondrosarcomas. In the past, neutron radiotherapy has been limited by the use of physics laboratory-based cyclotrons, low-energy neutron beams with poor dose distribution, primitive beam delivery systems, immobile horizontal beam positions, fixed cone collimators, and lack of adequate radiation field verification methods and external blocks. Clinical trials have recently been completed using high-energy, isocentric, hospital-based neutron beams with multileaf collimation systems and CT treatment planning for improved dose distribution for advanced squamous cell carcinoma of the head and neck, lung cancer, and advanced carcinoma of the prostate. The results are not yet available.

Protons and helium ion radiotherapy have been used in the treatment of uveal melanoma and selected benign intracranial lesions (pituitary adenomas and arteriovenous malformations) and of selected malignant tumors at the base of the skull or adjacent to the spinal cord, including chordomas, chondrosarcomas, meningiomas, and craniopharyngiomas. For uveal melanoma, the local control rate is 96% and the 5-year survival rate is approximately 80%. The local control rates for skull-base chondrosarcomas and chordomas are 91% and 65%, respectively.

Phase I/II studies of high-LET charged particle radiotherapy have been performed with negative π mesons and with neon, carbon, and silicon ions. Promising results have been reported for locally advanced paranasal sinus tumors, salivary gland tumors, soft tissue and bone sarcomas, prostate cancer, and locally advanced or recurrent nasopharyngeal cancer. Phase III trials now in progress at the University of California, Lawrence Berkeley Laboratory, will compare neon ion versus photon radiotherapy for prostate cancer and neon ions versus helium ions for selected tumor sites, including bone and soft tissue sarcomas, carcinoma of the nasopharynx and paranasal sinuses, locally advanced melanoma, and salivary gland tumors and juxtaspinal chordoma and chondrosarcomas.

Hyperthermia

Hyperthermia at temperatures above 41–42 °C has a direct cytotoxic effect on both normal and tumor cells. Hyperthermia is particularly effective against hypoxic cells and cells in the S phase of the cell cycle, which are both radioresistant. Hyperthermia has a radiosensitizing effect and inhibits the repair of sublethal radiation damage. In addition, hyperthermia has been shown to potentiate the cytotoxicity of a number of chemotherapeutic agents, including bleomycin, cisplatin, and mitomycin. Thus, hyperthermia may be potentially advantageous when combined with radiotherapy or chemotherapy.

Hyperthermia has been combined with radiotherapy in the treatment of advanced or recurrent breast cancer, head and neck cancer, malignant melanoma, cervical cancer, and soft tissue sarcomas. Nonrandomized clinical trials have consistently shown a higher complete response rate with hyperthermia combined with radiotherapy than with radiotherapy alone. One randomized trial compared radiotherapy alone with radiotherapy plus hyperthermia in N3 (fixed and inoperable) metastatic squamous cell carcinoma in cervical lymph nodes. The complete response rate was 82% with hyperthermia combined with radiotherapy versus only 37% with radiotherapy alone. Two-year actuarial local control and survival were also better for the group receiving radiotherapy and hyperthermia. A randomized phase III trial by the Radiation Therapy Oncology Group (RTOG) for superficial tumors showed an actuarial local control rate of 80% for radiotherapy combined with hyperthermia versus 15% with radiotherapy alone for lesions less than 3 cm but no significant difference in larger lesions. Phase III clinical trials now in progress at the European Society of Hyperthermic Oncology (ESHO) will compare hyperthermia combined with radiotherapy with radiotherapy alone in previously untreated locally advanced breast cancer, neck nodes, and recurrent or metastatic melanoma. Another RTOG phase II/III trial is evaluating interstitial radiotherapy alone versus interstitial thermoradiotherapy for recurrent, persistent, or metastatic tumors suitable for implantation.

Intraoperative Radiotherapy

Intraoperative radiotherapy involves the administration of radiotherapy to microscopic or gross residual disease after surgical resection during an operative procedure. Intraoperative radiotherapy can be delivered either as a large single dose using external beam radiotherapy with electrons or superficial x-rays or as intraoperative brachytherapy. This technique allows the delivery of radiation to target sites exposed by the operative procedure while minimizing radiation to adjacent normal tissues. Normal tissues such as the stomach and small intestine can be excluded from the radiation field. It is also possible to spare critical normal tissues (such as the spinal cord) underneath the tumor volume by selecting appropriate energy of the electron beam or using protective shields.

With external beam intraoperative radiotherapy, a dose of 10–15 Gy is used for microscopic residual disease and a dose of 20 Gy or more for gross residual disease, usually in combination with pre- or postoperative conventional external beam radiotherapy. Ideally, intraoperative radiotherapy is best performed with a dedicated radiotherapy machine in the operating suite. Currently, however, in most institutions, intraoperative radiotherapy is performed in the radiation oncology department. The patient is transported from the operating room to the radiation oncology department, maintained under portable anesthesia, and monitored by closed-circuit television during the procedure. Following intraoperative radiotherapy, the patient is returned to the operating room for completion of the operative procedure.

External beam intraoperative radiotherapy alone or in combination with conventional external beam radiotherapy has been used in the treatment of advanced or recurrent carcinoma of the stomach, pancreas, rectum, bladder, lung, retroperitoneal soft tissue sarcomas, gynecologic tumors, periaortic lymph nodes, head and neck cancers, biliary or gallbladder carcinomas, brain tumors, and pediatric tumors. A prospective comparative study from Japan suggested improved survival statistics with intraoperative radiotherapy compared with resection alone for patients with stage II–IV gastric carcinoma. The 5-year survival rates were 87% for stage I, 84% for stage II, 62% for stage III, and 15% for stage IV disease treated with resection plus intraoperative radiotherapy and 93%, 62%, 37%, and 0%, respectively, with resection alone. The National Cancer Institute also conducted two randomized trials of intraoperative radiotherapy in carcinoma of the pancreas. The first trial compared conventional external beam radiotherapy with intraoperative radiotherapy alone after surgical resection. The local control and disease-free survival rates in patients surviving the surgery were improved with intraoperative radiotherapy, though median survival was 12 months for both groups. The second trial evaluated conventional external beam radiotherapy plus fluorouracil alone or combined with intraoperative radiotherapy in patients with unresectable disease. The median survival was 8 months for both arms. Another randomized trial from the National Cancer Institute compared intraoperative radiotherapy plus postoperative conventional external beam radiotherapy with postoperative conventional external beam radiotherapy alone after resection of retroperitoneal soft tissue sarcomas. There was a suggestion of improved local control with intraoperative radiotherapy, though median survival was not significantly different. Nonrandomized studies from the Massachusetts General Hospital and the Mayo Clinic suggest an advantage in local control as well as survival in locally advanced or recurrent rectal carcinoma.

Intraoperative brachytherapy is delivered either as a temporary or a permanent interstitial implant. With temporary interstitial implants, the afterloading nylon catheters are placed under direct vision over the tumor bed and secured in place with absorbable sutures. They are fastened to the skin surface with plastic buttons. They are loaded with ribbons carrying ^{192}Ir seeds 7–10 days postoperatively. With permanent interstitial implants, ^{125}I seeds are inserted directly into the residual tumor with a trocar, or Vicryl sutures carrying ^{125}I seeds are placed over the tumor bed and secured in place with surgical clips or sutures. The dose delivered depends on the amount of disease present and the dose of prior or subsequent external beam radiotherapy. Intraoperative brachytherapy alone or combined with external beam irradiation has been used in the treatment of advanced or recurrent head and neck cancer; soft tissue sarcomas; pediatric tumors; carcinoma of the pancreas, bladder, biliary tract, or gallbladder; and lung cancer—as well as advanced or recurrent pelvic malignancies.

Radiosurgery

Radiosurgery is a procedure whereby a high dose of radiation, usually in a single fraction (10–25 Gy), can be delivered to a small target volume (about 3 cm) without clinically significant radiation exposure to adjacent normal tissues. Stereotactic techniques are used for accurate localization of the target and measurement of its dimensions. Three-dimensional treatment planning is then used to deliver the dose to the target volume using multiple radiation beams directed at the target. Various techniques and radiation sources, including ^{60}Co γ-ray units, protons, helium ion, and neutron beams and modified ^{60}Co or linear accelerator x-rays have been used to deliver high doses of radiation .

Radiosurgery has been used to treat a variety of benign lesions, including arteriovenous malformations and acoustic neurinomas; and malignant tumors, including low-grade or anaplastic astrocytomas, glioblastoma multiforme, and other primary or metastatic intracranial tumors. Radiosurgery has hitherto been used chiefly in the treatment of inoperable or surgically inaccessible arteriovenous malformations. The technique has been successful in reducing the risk of intracranial hemorrhage. Objective responses with angiographic demonstration of normalization of circulation time, disappearance of pathologic vessels in the previous nidi, and normalization or disappearance of draining veins have been described. The angiographic complete response rate is in the range of 65–95% at 2 years for arteriovenous malformations with a maximum diameter of 3 cm. With careful treatment planning and delivery, the procedure is safe and well tolerated. However, occasional acute reactions have been reported, including headaches, elevated temperature, and an increased risk of seizures. Permanent complications occur in less than 5% of patients. The efficacy of radiosurgery in the treatment of malignant intracranial tumors is currently under investigation.

Radioimmunotherapy

Radioimmunotherapy involves the systemic administration of radiolabeled antibodies directed against tumor-associated or tumor-specific antigen. By targeting and binding antigen on the tumor cell surface, radioimmunoglobins provide a more selective means of delivering therapeutic doses of radiation to the tumor. The radiation is delivered as continuous low-dose-rate irradiation, which may have additional radiobiologic advantages compared with fractionated high-dose-rate external beam radiotherapy. Clinical radioimmunotherapy thus far has employed ^{131}I and ^{90}Yt monoclonal or polyclonal antibodies derived from different species (rabbit, pig, baboon, and horse) or human-murine chimeric antibodies produced by genetic engineering. Clinical trials have investigated the use of radioimmunotherapy in the treatment of hepatocellular carcinoma, Hodgkin's disease, and non-Hodgkin's lymphomas, chronic lymphocytic leukemia, breast cancer, ovarian carcinoma, and malignant gliomas. An early phase I/II study by the RTOG using external beam radiotherapy and chemotherapy followed by ^{131}I antiferritin-specific radioimmunoglobin produced a 41% partial remission and a 7% complete remission rate in patients with hepatoma. Survival and response depended on the alpha-fetoprotein (AFP) status. The median survival was 5 months in AFP-positive patients and 10.5 months in AFP-negative ones. In a subsequent randomized trial, following induction treatment with combined external beam radiotherapy and chemotherapy, patients were stratified by AFP status and randomized to receive chemotherapy consisting of doxorubicin and fluorouracil or ^{131}I antiferritin radioimmunotherapy and allowing crossover treatment if tumor progression occurred. There were no significant differences between the two treatment groups in partial remission or survival rates. However, remission was achieved with ^{131}I antiferritin in seven of 11 patients following chemotherapy failure. Tumors that were initially nonresectable became resectable in 7% of the patients (AFP-positive or AFP-negative) who received ^{131}I antiferritin. In another phase I/II study by the RTOG, ^{131}I antiferritin radioimmunotherapy led to a 40% partial remission rate and one complete remission in 37 patients with Hodgkin's disease who failed MOPP-ABVD or other chemotherapy. Partial or complete remissions have also been reported with radioimmunotherapy in intrahepatic cholangiocarcinoma, chronic lymphocytic leukemia, non-Hodgkin's lymphoma, and ovarian carcinoma. Thus far, major normal tissue toxicity has been limited to the bone marrow.

Three-Dimensional Conformal Radiotherapy

Three-dimensional conformal radiotherapy involves the use of computerized imaging techniques and three-dimensional computerized treatment planning systems and computer-driven treatment delivery systems, such as multileaf collimators and on-line verification systems in external beam radiotherapy. The objective of three-dimensional conformal radiotherapy is to conform the spatial distribution of high radiation doses to the contour of the tumor volume while decreasing the volume of the surrounding normal tissues receiving high radiation doses. With three-dimensional conformal radiotherapy, it is possible to increase the dose to the tumor and improve local tumor control without increasing the rate of complications in normal tissues. Currently, three-dimensional conformal radiotherapy is used by some in the treatment of carcinoma of the prostate, head and neck, and lung and in malignant brain tumors. Clinical trials of the RTOG to establish the proper dose level and treatment technique as well as to evaluate the efficacy of this new modality are now in progress for a number of tumor sites.

TOXICITY & COMPLICATIONS OF RADIOTHERAPY

Any cancer can be locally destroyed by radiation if the dose is sufficient. In clinical practice, the dose-limiting factor is the damage unavoidably sustained by nearby normal tissues. With properly trained radiation oncologists and modern equipment, the incidence of clinically significant complications is low.

The acute reactions and late complications of radiotherapy depend on many factors: (1) the type of normal tissues irradiated, (2) the total dose delivered, (3) the dose per fraction, (4) the overall treatment time, (5) the volume of tissue irradiated, (6) the use of adjuvant chemotherapy or other treatment modifiers, (7) the use of operative treatment, (8) the patient's age, and (9) the presence of underlying diseases such as diabetes mellitus, collagen vascular disease, ataxia-telangiectasia, and superimposed infection. Acute reactions are manifestations of stem cell depletion in tissues with rapid cell turnover rates such as the skin, mucous membranes, intestinal epithelium, and bone marrow. Late complications usually result from damage to the parenchymal cells or the connective vascular tissue. Late normal tissue injury may be manifested as early as 6 weeks to 3 months or as late as several years after radiotherapy. The clinical symptoms and signs of acute and late radiation injury depend on the tissue and organ irradiated. For example, acute reactions consisting of erythema, increased pigmentation, dry or moist desquamation, and epilation and late complications consisting of ulceration, edema, and fibrosis can occur after irradiation of the skin and subcutaneous tissues. Acute reactions consisting of nausea, vomiting, and diarrhea and late complications consisting of chronic ulceration, bleeding, malabsorption, fibrosis, and stenosis can occur after gastrointestinal irradiation. The incidence of radiation toxicity increases with the magnitude of the dose per fraction, the total dose, and the volume irradiated and with a decrease of overall treatment time. Chemotherapeutic agents such as doxorubicin, dactinomycin, fluorouracil, bleomycin, and cisplatin

are known to increase the effects of radiation on normal tissues. Radioprotectors such as WR-2721 and certain biologic response modifiers such as recombinant human granulocyte colony-stimulating factor (G-CSF) and interleukin-1 may reduce acute or late normal tissue radiation toxicity. Surgery may also reduce the normal tissue tolerance to radiation. Children and elderly patients tolerate radiation less well than other segments of the population. Patients with underlying vascular or collagen diseases are more prone to develop radiation complications. Patients with ataxia-telangiectasia are deficient in the repair of DNA damage from ionizing radiation and have increased radiation sensitivity. The severity of acute or late radiation reactions may also be aggravated by superimposed infections.

Table 47–8 shows the tolerance doses to whole organ irradiation after a single dose or fractionated doses of radiotherapy. The tolerance doses ($TD_{5/5}$ and $TD_{50/5}$) refer to 5% and 50% incidences of severe to life-threatening complications occurring within 5 years after radiotherapy.

Management of the acute reactions and late complications of radiotherapy depends on the tissue or organ involved and the severity of the reaction. Acute skin reactions may be managed with topical moisturizing or steroid creams, cornstarch, aluminum acetate solution compresses, loose clothing, and avoidance of trauma. Acute mucositis and dysphagia associated with head and neck irradiation may be alleviated with analgesics, topical anesthetics, salt and baking soda mouth rinses, and antibiotics or antifungal agents for superimposed infection. Antinauseant and antidiarrheal drugs and corticosteroid suppositories or enemas may alleviate symptoms from irradiation of the gastrointestinal tract. Pyridium may reduce dysuria from acute radiation cystitis.

Late reactions affecting normal tissues are usually managed conservatively. Analgesics are used for pain relief and antibiotics for infection. Corticosteroids may be beneficial during the acute phase of late reactions. Exercises and elastic stockings may reduce arm and leg edema from subcutaneous fibrosis and impaired lymphatic drainage. Hyperbaric oxygenation is sometimes effective in facilitating the healing of soft tissue or bone necrosis. It may sometimes be impossible to distinguish radiation ulcer or radionecrosis from tumor recurrence. Unfortunately, soft tissue or bone necrosis may be aggravated by repeated biopsies or trauma. Occasionally, severe late normal tissue toxicity, including chronic ulcer, radionecrosis of soft tissues or bone, hemorrhage, intestinal obstruction or stenosis, chronic gastroenteritis, and cystitis may require surgical resection of the involved tissue or organ. Construction of a pericardial window or pericardiectomy may be necessary for radiation pericarditis. Symptoms due to impaired endocrine function are treated with hormonal replacement.

Table 47–8. Tolerance doses (TD$_{5/5}$–TD$_{50/5}$) to whole organ irradiation.[1]

Single Dose (cGy)		Fractionated Dose (cGy)	
Lymphoid tissues	200–500	Testes	100–200
Bone marrow	200–1000	Ovary	600–1000
Ovary	200–600	Eye (lens)	600–1200
Testes	200–1000	Lung	2000–3000
Eye (lens)	200–1000	Kidney	2000–3000
Lung	700–1000	Liver	3500–4000
Gastrointestinal tract	500–1000	Skin	3000–4000
Colon and rectum	1000–2000	Thyroid	3000–4000
Kidney	1000–2000	Heart	4000–5000
Heart	1800–2000	Lymphoid tissue	4000–5000
Liver	1500–2000	Bone marrow	4000–5000
Mucosa	500–2000	Gastrointestinal tract	5000–6000
Vasculoconnective tissue systems	1000–2000	Vasculoconnective tissue systems	5000–6000
Skin	1500–2000	Spinal cord	5000–6000
Peripheral nerve	1500–2000	Peripheral nerve	6500–7700
Spinal cord	1500–2000	Mucosa	6500–7700
Brain	1500–2000	Brain	6000–7000
Bone and cartilage	>3000	Bone and cartilage	>7000
Muscle	>3000	Muscle	>7000

[1]Modified from Rubin P: The law and order of radiation sensitivity. In: *Radiation Tolerance of Normal Tissues,* vol 23. Vaeth JM, Myer JL (editors). Karger, 1989.

RADIATION THERAPY OF SPECIFIC DISEASES

Table 47–7 is an outline of radiotherapy of specific diseases. It is intended only as a general guide to the place of radiation therapy and the dosage levels used, the areas or volumes treated, and the results obtainable. It is not intended for use as a manual of radiation therapy. In clinical practice, treatment planning is varied for each patient and each disease. Treatment plans, including the daily and total dose to be delivered, are often altered during the course of treatment depending upon the response of the lesion and the effects on the patient. A discussion sufficiently detailed to permit conduct of treatment for a specific patient is beyond the scope of this discussion.

Modern cancer therapy often employs a multimodality approach. For optimal management, all physicians who are to be responsible for the care of a cancer patient should be consulted before any procedure—even biopsy—is performed. Seeing the intact, untouched lesion can be of immense help in planning definitive treatment, whether it be surgery, radiation therapy, chemotherapy, or a combination of various treatment modalities. To excise the evidence and then refer the patient elsewhere for treatment imposes a severe handicap upon the therapist and the patient.

Ang KK, Byers RM: Adjuvant therapy for patients with colon and rectal cancer. JAMA 1990;264:1444.

Ang KK et al: Regional radiotherapy as adjuvant treatment for head and neck malignant melanoma. Arch Otolaryngol Head Neck Surg 1990;116:169.

Cummings BJ et al: Epidermoid anal cancer: Treatment by radiation alone or by radiation and 5-fluorouracil with and without mitomycin C. Int J Radiat Oncol Biol Phys 1991;21:1115.

Fisher B et al: Eight-year results of a randomized clinical trial comparing total mastectomy and lumpectomy with or without irradiation in the treatment of breast cancer. N Engl J Med 1989;320:822.

Hall EJ: *Radiobiology for the Radiologist,* 3rd ed. Harper & Row, 1988.

Halperin EC et al: *Pediatric Radiation Oncology.* Raven Press, 1989.

Hanks GE et al: Outcome for lymph node dissection negative T-1b, T-2 (A2, B) prostate cancer treated with external beam radiation therapy in RTOG 77-06. Int J Radiat Oncol Biol Phys 1991;21:1099.

Khan FM: *The Physics of Radiation Therapy.* William & Wilkins, 1984.

Koh WJ et al: Fast neutron radiation for inoperable and recurrent salivary gland cancers. Am J Clin Oncol 1989;12:316.

Krook JE et al: Effective surgical adjuvant therapy for high-risk rectal carcinoma. N Engl J Med 1991;324:709.

Larson DA, Gutin PH: Introduction to radiosurgery. Neurosurg Clin North Am 1990;1:897.

Leibel SA et al: The biological basis for conformal three-dimensional radiation therapy. Int J Radiat Oncol Biol Phys 1991;21:805.

Linstadt DE et al: Neon ion radiotherapy: Results of the phase I/II clinical trial. Int J Radiat Oncol Biol Phys 1991;20:761.

Moss WT, Cox JD: *Radiation Oncology: Rationale, Technique, Results,* 6th ed. Mosby, 1989.

Order S et al: A randomized prospective trial comparing full dose chemotherapy to ^{131}I antiferritin: An RTOG study. Int J Radiat Oncol Biol Phys 1991;20:953.

Overgaard J et al: Nimorazole as a hypoxic radiosensitizer in the treatment of supraglottic larynx and pharynx carcinoma: First report from the Danish Head and Neck Cancer Study (DAHANCA) protocol 5-85. Radiother Oncol 1991;20:143.

Perez CA, Brady LW: *Principles and Practice of Radiation Oncology,* 2nd ed. Lippincott, 1992.

Rubin P: Law and order of radiation sensitivity: Absolute versus relative. Front Radiat Ther Oncol 1989;23:7.

Sneed PK, Phillips TL: Combining hyperthermia and radiation: How beneficial? Oncology 1991;5:99.

Suit H, Urie M: Proton beams in radiation therapy. J Natl Cancer Inst 1992;84:144.

Suit HD et al: The treatment of patients with stage M0 soft tissue sarcoma. Clin Oncol 1988;6:854.

Tepper JE, *Fractionation in Radiation Therapy,* vol 2, No. 1. Saunders, 1992.

Willett CG et al: Intraoperative electron beam radiation therapy for primary locally advanced rectal and rectosigmoid carcinoma. Clin Oncol 1991;9:843.

Wang CC: *Clinical Oncology: Indications, Techniques, and Results.* PSG Publishing, 1988.

CANCER IMMUNOLOGY & IMMUNOTHERAPY

Robert S. Warren, MD

The immune system is seen as occupying a controlling role in host resistance to malignant tumor growth. Evidence for this view is the high incidence of cancers in diseases associated with impaired cellular or humoral immunity (Table 47–9). For example, patients with primary immunodeficiency syndromes have a 50% chance of acquiring non-Hodgkin's lymphoma. Leukemia is also more common in these patients (15%), though the incidence of the common epithelial malignancies is only slightly higher. Immunologic reconstitution by bone marrow transplantation at an early age can prevent the development of non-Hodgkin's lymphoma in congenitally immunodeficient children.

AIDS is associated with a 100-fold greater risk of Kaposi's sarcoma, an uncommon malignancy in the general population. Patients with Kaposi's sarcoma associated with AIDS also demonstrate an unusual distribution of these tumors, with more frequent involvement of the face, gastrointestinal tract, and lymph nodes. Non-Hodgkin's lymphoma is more

Table 47–9. Diseases predisposing to the development of cancer.

A. Primary immunodeficiency syndromes
   1. Ataxia-telangiectasia
   2. Wiskott-Aldrich syndrome
   3. Common variable immunodeficiency
   4. Severe combined immunodeficiency (SCID)
B. Acquired immunodeficiency syndrome (AIDS)
C. Organ transplant recipients
D. Patients receiving immunosuppressive therapy for autoimmune or collagen-vascular diseases
E. Patients receiving chemotherapy

common in patients with AIDS than in the general population and tends to be more aggressive, with a higher frequency of extranodal involvement (bone marrow, central nervous system). There is an increased incidence of squamous cell cancers of the genitalia in females and the anorectum in males with AIDS, frequently in association with human papillomavirus (HPV) infection. As the survival of AIDS patients increases in response to AZT and other therapies, an increased incidence of other malignancies not commonly affecting this young age group is anticipated.

Recipients of solid organ transplants receive life-long immunosuppressive therapy, and their risk of acquiring cancer is three times that of age-matched controls. The incidence of squamous carcinomas involving sun-exposed areas of the skin and lip is 18 times greater, and the rate of squamous carcinoma of modified skin (anus, vulva) and the uterine cervix, non-Hodgkin's lymphoma, and hepatobiliary cancers is also much higher. In one study of 4241 cadaveric renal transplant recipients, the overall incidence of cancer after 17 years was 55%. Recent data suggest that replacement of azathioprine with cyclosporine for immunosuppression does not decrease the overall incidence of cancer in transplant patients, though the types of malignancies change, ie, there are fewer squamous cancers and more cases of lymphoma and Kaposi's sarcoma. Patients with rheumatoid arthritis or other autoimmune disorders receiving immunosuppressive therapy are also more susceptible to malignancies similar to those seen in renal transplant recipients (a preponderance of skin cancers and non-Hodgkin's lymphoma), though the magnitude of the increase is not as great.

Second malignancies are more common in patients undergoing cancer chemotherapy with alkylating agents, particularly in children. Acute leukemia is the most frequent second malignancy, with non-Hodgkin's lymphoma and bladder cancer being less common. The second malignancies develop an average of 4–6 years after treatment of the primary cancer.

The mechanisms responsible are unknown. Some studies have suggested that increased proliferation of latent oncogenic viruses may be involved (eg, HPV inducing anal cancer; HTLV-1 and AIDS lymphoma; hepatitis B virus and hepatocellular carcinoma). The immune surveillance hypothesis suggests that failure of immune mechanisms to recognize and eliminate transformed or mutated malignant cells represents the principal defect.

IMMUNOTHERAPY

Better understanding of cellular and humoral immune mechanisms in the past decade has led to a different approach to cancer treatment. Terms for these new therapies include biologic therapy, immunotherapy, adoptive immunotherapy, active specific immunotherapy, and serotherapy. The strategy common to all is to enhance the endogenous host antineoplastic capacity through manipulation of the immune system.

Antibodies in Cancer Treatment (Serotherapy)

The use of monoclonal antibodies in cancer therapy is predicated on the presence of tumor-associated antigens on the surface of malignant cells, which distinguishes them from normal tissues. These antigens are classified as follows: oncofetal antigens, such as carcinoembryonic antigen (CEA), alpha-fetoprotein (AFP), or human chorionic gonadotropin (hCG), which are present on cells of a given tumor type (eg, breast or gastrointestinal cancers); differentiation antigens, which characterize a particular state of differentiation in many tissues; or tissue-specific antigens. Growth factor receptors and protein products of oncogenes may also serve as targets of monoclonal antibody therapy.

Monoclonal antibodies that selectively react with human tumor-associated antigens have been used for diagnosis, for monitoring of disease progression, and for antitumor therapy. Monoclonal antibody coupled to gamma-emitting radioisotopes has been used to detect occult foci of metastatic disease. Imaging is accomplished preoperatively using a gamma camera or intra-operatively with a hand-held gamma probe. The use of iodinated antibodies has been limited by in vivo deiodination, so technetium 99m- or indium 111-labeled antibodies are more commonly used. Radioimmunolocalization using monoclonal antibody directed against CEA or the tumor antigen TAG-72 in colon cancers may help in the management of about 10% of patients undergoing curative surgery.

The therapeutic use of monoclonal antibodies was first studied using unconjugated antibodies, whose antitumor effect was thought to occur through activation of cell-mediated antibody-dependent mechanisms. Other monoclonal antibodies may block binding of tumor growth factors to their cellular receptors or may target protein products of oncogenes that are overexpressed in certain tumors (eg, HER2/neu in breast cancer). Unfortunately, tumor responses to unconjugated antibody therapy are uncommon and transient. To improve their efficacy, monoclonal antibodies have been conjugated to high-energy beta-emitting radioisotopes (eg, iodine-125, iodine-131, yttrium-90, rhenium-186 and -188). Radiolabeled antibody conjugates need not be internalized by the cell to effect killing. Furthermore, they affect antigen-negative cells within a radius of 1 mm from the site of binding, which overcomes the problem of heterogeneity of antigen expression within tumors.

Alternatively, monoclonal antibodies may be conjugated to plant, bacterial, or fungal toxins (eg, ricin A, diphtheria toxin) to produce a hybrid molecule that exhibits the selectivity of the monoclonal antibody and the tremendous potency of the toxin (frequently one molecule of toxin per cell is enough for killing). Clinical trials are under way using a number of radioimmunoconjugates or immunotoxins, and efforts are being made to improve the efficacy of antibody conjugates by enhancing specificity, by improving antigen expression by target cells, and by the use of immunoglobulin fragments of unconjugated antibodies with better tissue uptake.

Another problem that has been encountered with the repeated use of mouse monoclonal antibody in humans is development of a human anti-mouse antibody response (HAMA). To limit the HAMA response, "humanized" antibodies have been generated by recombinant DNA technology. A monoclonal antibody is constructed consisting of the constant region derived from a human gene and the variable region derived from a mouse gene. These chimeric monoclonal antibodies express the antigen-combining site of the mouse antibody but are much less likely to induce the HAMA response in humans since the majority of the chimeric antibody is of human origin. Furthermore, designer antibody-toxin conjugates can be genetically engineered and expressed in bacteria, permitting the production of large amounts of immunotoxins economically.

Nonspecific Immunotherapy

Although human cancers elicit a host immune response, spontaneous regression of human tumors is rare. In an effort to augment the endogenous host defenses, a number of agents have been tested as nonspecific immunomodulators. The earliest efforts were by the orthopedic surgeon William Coley (c 1910), who noted the occasional regression of tumors in patients who developed febrile illnesses. Coley administered preparations of attenuated or heat-killed bacteria (Coley's toxins) and produced a few spectacular clinical results. The appeal of this approach waned with the development of radiation therapy and chemotherapy, but interest in nonspecific immunotherapy revived in the 1970s after Mathe (1969) reported that acute lymphocytic leukemia responded to the administration of bacille Calmette-Guérin (BCG). In addition to BCG, *Corynebacterium parvum,* levamisole, and thymosin have been used clinically to nonspecifically activate antitumor immunity. The results have been disappointing with a few exceptions: intralesional BCG has an effect in melanoma, but clinical utility is limited; intravesical BCG is very effective in the treatment of superficial bladder cancers, replacing cystectomy as the first line of therapy in this disease; and levamisole in combination with fluorouracil is effective adjuvant chemotherapy following resection of Dukes B_2 or C colon carcinoma.

Cytokines

BCG and other nonspecific immunomodulators exert antineoplastic effects by inducing production of one or more cytokines, the protein hormones of the immune system (Table 47–10). The predominant cellular sources of these cytokines are T-lymphocytes and cells of the reticuloendothelial system (circulating monocytes, tissue macrophages). Several cytokines are either directly cytotoxic toward tumor cells or enhance cellular or humoral antitumor activity. Others have proinflammatory effects (TNF, IL-1, IL-6, IL-8) or function as endogenous anti-inflammatory hormones (IL-4, IL-10, TGFβ). The availability of

Table 47–10. Human cytokines.

Cytokine	Important Biologic Actions
Interferon α (IFNα)	Direct cytotoxic activity against some tumor cells. Also antiviral; up-regulates class I major histocompatibility antigens (MHC) on target cells; enhances natural killer (NK) lymphocyte activity.
Interferon β (IFNβ)	Activates monocytes and macrophages to release other cytokines. Includes both class I and class II MHC antigens; enhances NK cell activity; antiviral.
Interferon γ (IFNγ)	Activates monocytes and macrophages to release other cytokines. Includes both class I and class II MHC antigens; enhances NK cell activity; antiviral.
Tumor necrosis factor α (TNFα)	Cytotoxic for many tumor cells in vitro; promotes proliferation of certain nontransformed cells in culture. Procoagulant activity leads to hemorrhagic necrosis of murine tumors in vivo. Proximal mediator of many of the metabolic and hemodynamic effects of gram-negative and gram-positive sepsis. Also called "cachectin," but role in cancer cachexia not well established. Angiogenic; stimulates class II MHC expression.
Colony-stimulating factors	G-CSF, M-CSF, and GM-CSF support the growth of granulocytes, monocytes, or both types of progenitor cells, respectively. These agents augment antibody-dependent cell-mediated tumor cytotoxicity, which is useful in the management of chemotherapy-induced leukopenia.
Interleukins	Many of the interleukins were designated by terms which characterize one or more of their frequently multiple biologic activites. By convention, these proteins have been designated interleukins to reflect their functions as intercellular signals between leukocytes. However, as with TNF and the interferon, these proteins exert their varied actions on many types of cells outside of the immune system as well.
IL-1	Lymphocyte-activating factor. Enhances proliferative response to mitogens; induces similar pattern of hormone release and metastatic effects to TNFα. Antagonist to the IL-1 receptor proteins protects rabbits and mice from bacterial septic shock.

(continued)

Table 47–10. Human cytokines. (continued)

Cytokine	Important Biologic Actions
IL-2	T and B lymphocyte growth factor. Induces TNF, IL-1, and IFNγ in vivo. Induces lymphokine-activated killer (LAK) activity by resting or activated T cells.
IL-3	Enhances hematopoietic stem cell proliferation. May be useful in diminishing the pancytopenia associated with chemotherapy.
IL-4	Down-regulates TNF, IL-1, and IL-6 production by activated macrophages but also augments cytolytic T cell activity and LAK activity; B cell growth factor.
IL-5	Eosinophil growth factor.
IL-6	Most potent inducer of hepatic acute-phase protein synthesis. Stimulates T cell proliferation in presence of IL-1 and induces B cell differentiation. Autocrine growth factor in multiple myeloma and renal cell carcinoma.
IL-7	Enhances mitogen-stimulated T cell proliferation and growth of B cell precursors; enhances CTL and LAK generation.
IL-8	Chemotactic factor for neutrophils.
IL-9	Stimulates T cell proliferation.
IL-10	Down-regulates macrophage production of proinflammatory cytokines (IL-1, IL-6, TNFα, IL-8).
IL-11	Enhances proliferation of pluripotent stem cells; augments antigen-specific antibody response.
IL-12	Co-stimulates for lymphocyte activities in the presence of IL-2 or other cytokines (IFNα, IFN8, IL-1).

large quantities of these hormones as a result of recombinant DNA technology has permitted extensive testing in humans. The most successful cytokine has been IFNα, which produces response rates of 80% in hairy cell leukemia and 75% in chronic myelogenous leukemia, but it exerts less activity (10–20%) against solid tumors such as melanoma and renal cell carcinoma. Tumor necrosis factor (TNF) is cytotoxic toward many kinds of human tumors in culture, but phase I and phase II human trials (Table 47–11) revealed severe side effects: fever, metabolic acidosis, hypoglycemia, and hypotension. In addition to its antineoplastic activity, TNF is a key mediator of the acute hemodynamic and metabolic changes in sepsis. Other cytokines probably exert similar pleiotropic effects in vivo, acting upon multiple targets outside the immune system (eg, hepatocytes, endothelial cells, skeletal muscle, central nervous system), which may limit their clinical safety. Clinical trials are under way to test the antineoplastic efficacy of IL-1, IL-3, and IL-4. Cytokines may also find a therapeutic role in combination with chemotherapy. Alternatively, certain cytokines (G-CSF, M-CSF, GM-CSF) are being used to reverse the pancytopenia associated with high-dose chemotherapy.

Table 47–11. Establishment of the utility of a new antineoplastic agent requires a sequence of clinical studies to determine first the tolerance and toxicity of the agent and then its antitumor activity.

Phase I	The investigational drug is given at a low initial dose (based on animal studies) to a small group of patients who have either failed standard therapy or for whom no effective therapy exists. The dose is then escalated until the dose-limiting toxicity is reached. This establishes the maximally tolerated dose (MTD).
Phase II	A larger number of patients who qualify for the study on the same basis as phase I subjects are given the previously established MTD. This will determine the response rate for a given tumor type.
Phase III	A prospective randomized trial is conducted with previously untreated patients given either the investigational drug or standard therapy for a given tumor type. This study assumes that phase II results compare favorably with historical controls.

Adoptive Immunotherapy

The cytokine IL-2 stimulates the proliferation of lymphocytes activated by specific tumor antigens. Given in high doses, IL-2 was found to induce the regression of advanced tumors in mice. In an attempt to enhance IL-2 activity, a novel approach to immunotherapy was developed: Circulating lymphocytes harvested from the patient were stimulated by IL-2 to proliferate in culture, and these autologous lymphokine-activated killer cells (LAK) were returned to the patient with additional IL-2. This regimen produced objective regression rates in renal cell carcinoma and melanoma of about 35%, with many durable responses. To enhance therapeutic specificity, tumor-infiltrating lymphocytes (TIL) rather than circulating lymphocytes were used, based upon the premise that TIL cells should represent a population of lymphocytes with increased recognition of tumor antigens. Studies by Rosenberg et al demonstrated that TILs harvested from a tumor expanded in culture in the presence of IL-2 and then returned to the patient to maintain their immunologic memory and home in to sites of tumor. One interesting modification of this approach is to insert the gene for TNF into TILs by molecular genetic methods, thus targeting cells capable of secreting high local concentrations of TNF to the tumor. The results of the first efforts with gene therapy in humans are eagerly awaited.

Tumor Vaccines: Active Specific Immunotherapy

Augmentation of antitumor immunity through the use of autologous tumor cell vaccines or by immunization of the cancer patient with purified cellular components shared by many tumors (eg, GM2, a ganglioside common to the plasma membrane of many melanomas) has yet to produce worthwhile results.

Current efforts are directed at finding tumor antigens that are more immunogenic. A novel approach so far confined to animal studies is to transfect tumor cells with various cytokines (IFN-8, G-CSF, TNFα) before vaccination. The cytokine-secreting cells are more likely to trigger an immune response toward otherwise weakly immunogenic tumor cells.

Antisense Oligonucleotides

Antisense oligonucleotides are short segments of chemically synthesized DNA which, by virtue of their nucleotide sequence, have the property of binding specifically to complementary messenger RNA molecules and thereby preventing the translation of specific gene products. Antisense oligonucleotides have been found to inhibit virus replication and oncogene expression in cultured cells. One potential application may be to target tumor cell genes involved in multidrug resistance, abnormal growth factor receptors, or genes important in metastasis.

DeJager L et al: Long-term complete remission in bladder carcinoma in situ with intravesical BCG overview analysis of six phase II trials. Urology 1991;38:507.

Dolnick, BJ: Antisense agents in cancer research and therapeutics. Cancer Invest 1991;9:185.

Kawakami Y et al: Shared human melanoma antigens. J Immunol 1992;148:638.

Penn I: Cancer in the immunosuppressed organ recipient. Transplantation 1991;23:1771.

Rock CS, Lowry SF: Tumor necrosis factor alpha. J Surg Res 1991;51:434.

Rosenberg SA: Immunotherapy and gene therapy of cancer. Cancer Res 1991;51:5074. Rosenberg SA et al: Experience with the use of high-dose interleukin-2 in the treatment of 652 cancer patients. Ann Surg 1989;210:474.

Rosenberg SA et al: Gene transfer into humans: Immunotherapy of patients with advanced melanoma, using tumor-infiltrating lymphocytes modified by retroviral gene transduction. N Engl J Med 1990;323:570.

Slamon DJ et al: Studies of the Hers/neu protooncogene in human breast and ovarian cancer. Science 1989;244:707.

Shalaby MR et al: Development of humanized bispecific antibodies reactive with cytotoxic lymphocytes and tumor cells overexpressing the HER2 protooncogene. J Exp Med 1992;175:217.

Stickney DR et al: Bifunctional antibody: A binary radiopharmaceutical delivery system for imaging colorectal carcinoma. Cancer Res 1991;51:6650.

Vaickus L, Foon KA: Overview of monoclonal antibodies in the diagnosis and therapy of cancer. Cancer Invest 1991;9:195.

CANCER CHEMOTHERAPY

Samuel D. Spivack, MD

SCIENTIFIC BASIS OF CHEMOTHERAPY

Selective Toxicity: The Qualitative Approach

A basic goal of cancer chemotherapy is the development of agents that have selective toxicity against replicating tumor cells but which at the same time spare replicating host tissues. Such an ideal drug has not yet been found, and only the hormones and asparaginase (and, to a lesser extent, mitotane and streptozocin) approach this goal. Although these drugs have important side effects, their toxicity is not primarily directed against normal replicating cells.

The Quantitative Kinetic Approach

Since in most instances qualitative metabolic differences between normal and neoplastic cells have not been discovered, the chemotherapist must plan according to quantitative differences in the proliferative kinetics of normal and neoplastic cell growth if tumor regression without major host toxicity is to be achieved. Early bacteriologists, in their study of germicidal agents, formulated the concept of the logarithmic order of cell kill. According to this theory, any particular treatment will kill a certain fraction of cells independently of the total number of cells present (provided the growth rate is constant). Thus, "cure," in the sense of killing the last remaining tumor cells, is more readily achieved by drugs when the total tumor cell burden is small. For example, a drug that is 99% efficient kills 2 logs of cells regardless of the total number of cells present and will reduce a tumor cell population of 100 to a single remaining cell, whereas it will leave 10,000 remaining cells of an initial tumor cell number of 1 million.

The quantitative evaluation of drug effects on normal and neoplastic tissues was furthered by the development of an in vivo assay system to allow measurement of the dose-response relationship of a variety of agents against both neoplastic and normal hematopoietic stem cells. At least two cell survival curves have been observed. The first curve shows decimation of both normal and neoplastic cells to almost the same degree, whereas the other shows a much greater decimation of tumor cells than of normal stem cells. The selectivity of the agents in the second class was attributed to a differential effect of the agents, which attacked proliferating cells in the mitotic cycle while sparing resting cells not in mitotic division. Thus arose the classification of forms of therapy into (1) cell cycle-specific (CCS) agents, which attack only actively proliferating cells engaged in DNA synthesis and the mitotic cycle; and (2) cell cycle-nonspecific (CCNS) agents, which kill both normal and tumor cells regardless of their proliferative state.

The important implications of these data are borne out by evidence in experimental tumor systems and to some extent in humans: (1) Differences in sensitivity of normal hematopoietic precursors and neoplastic cells are a function of the difference in their proliferative states and not a result of any inherent qualitative biochemical differences between the two cell types. (2) Injured or stimulated marrow or normal tissue that is proliferating as rapidly as neoplastic tissue will be affected to the same extent as neoplastic tissue.

As a general rule, any tissue, normal or neoplastic, manifests an early logarithmic phase of exponential growth during which most cells are in active mitosis. When a certain bulk is achieved, there is a transition to a later steady state plateau phase of growth during which a lesser fraction of cells is in the proliferative cycle. To maximize the therapeutic effects of CCS antineoplastic agents, resting cells must be induced to enter the proliferative cycle without at the same time increasing normal tissue vulnerability. This implies a reduction of tumor bulk with a reentry from the plateau phase into the log phase of exponential growth. Methods for reducing tumor bulk presently include treatment by CCNS agents such as x-ray or mechlorethamine and removal of gross tumor masses at surgery, but these stratagems all too often have attendant toxicities.

These concepts have suggested an approach to "curative" sequential chemotherapy of advanced tumors using a CCNS agent followed by a CCS agent in repeated courses.

While this is an idealized approach to curative therapy, similar principles have resulted in cure of laboratory-induced neoplasms, and such concepts form the basis for several successful new antileukemic regimens—particularly for childhood leukemia. Clearly, this approach will be improved by a better understanding of human tumor cell kinetics in individual patients; by new knowledge about the dose, duration, and site of action of antitumor agents; by the development of new marrow-sparing agents; and by appropriately synergistic combinations of drugs as well as better means of measuring their effects on microscopic tumor deposits.

A new technique for growing tumor stem cells with clonogenic or colony-forming capability has recently been developed. The clonogenic cells are obtained from a fresh tumor biopsy specimen and can be grown in soft agar and tested against standard and new anticancer drugs for inhibition of clonogenicity. This technique may simplify the identification of clinically effective drugs. It is 99% accurate in predicting lack of clinical response, which suggests that the assay may be most useful in avoiding fruitless clinical trials. Further studies using the tumor stem cell assay will focus on the use of drug combinations.

If the results of prospective studies follow the pattern predicted by this assay, the design of future trials and individual patient treatment will be radically altered from the present empiric approach.

Elion GB: Selectivity: Key to chemotherapy. Cancer Res 1985:45:2943.

Helson L: How much progress has been achieved in cancer therapy? Biomed Pharmacother 1988;42:629.

Macdonald EA: Cost-effectiveness of cancer chemotherapy: Risks/benefit ratio: Socio-economic and ethical considerations. Cancer Treat Rev 1987;14:345.

GUIDELINES FOR THE INSTITUTION OF CANCER CHEMOTHERAPY

Establish the Diagnosis

A firm diagnosis of neoplastic disease must be made before treatment is started. This will usually (and preferably) include a histologic diagnosis, but in some instances the diagnosis may be based solely on analysis of exfoliative cytology. In rare instances, a biochemical parameter (eg, chorionic gonadotropin) in a consistent clinical setting may constitute a rationale for institution of therapy, though tissue diagnosis is always preferable. In emergency situations (eg, superior vena cava syndrome), it may be necessary to institute therapy without histologic or biochemical documentation; in such cases, diagnostic procedures are required after clinical stabilization has been achieved.

Delineate the Stage & Extent of Disease

This objective can frequently be achieved by correlating symptoms and the known natural history of the neoplasm with appropriate radiologic, chemical, and surgical staging data. The lymphomas are staged according to the modified Ann Arbor classification; many solid tumors are best staged by the TNM system.

Establish the Goal of Therapy

The histologic diagnosis and extent of the disease frequently define the goal of therapy as either curative or palliative with or without the likelihood of prolonged survival and frequently determine the most appropriate treatment—surgery, radiotherapy, chemotherapy, or a combination of these methods.

Thus, the therapeutic objective should be based upon what can be accomplished by each mode of therapy. For example, the following disseminated cancers are curable by chemotherapy: most postgestational choriocarcinomas, many Wilms tumors and seminomas, some childhood acute lymphoblastic leukemias, adult and childhood lymphomas, and some testicular carcinomas in young men. For other neoplasms, chemotherapy may afford significant palliation and prolongation of life, even in advanced stages of breast, ovarian, endometrial, prostate, thyroid, and oat cell cancers and for acute leukemia, lymphomas, myeloma, and macroglobulinemia. Some patients with colon or gastric carcinoma, sarcomas, and head and neck tumors may be relieved of symptoms by chemotherapy, but survival cannot yet be prolonged. Most patients with disseminated melanoma and lung, renal, and pancreatic carcinoma are not objectively benefited by systemic chemotherapy.

Measure Antitumor Response

After treatment is started, serial observations of objectively measured parameters are essential to judge the antitumor response (measurable mass, tumor product, or remote effect) and to monitor the toxicity of treatment. For example, in the treatment of gestational trophoblastic disease, assay of chorionic gonadotropin measures a tumor product that correlates directly with the number of neoplastic cells and will reveal subclinical amounts (10^6 cells or less) of tumor which must continue to receive chemotherapy. The sensitivity of this assay is largely responsible for the 90% cure rate of trophoblastic disease. In contrast, a "complete clinical remission" of acute leukemia (a normal bone marrow) occurs with a tumor cell mass of 10^9; most solid tumors contain 10^{10}–10^{11} (10–100 g) of tumor cells before the mass can be detected clinically.

Currently useful markers for testicular tumors include the beta subunit of human chorionic gonadotropin, carcinoembryonic antigen (CEA), and alpha-fetoprotein (AFP). A rising CEA titer measured serially may also predict in a nonquantitative manner the recurrence or progression of colonic carcinoma, and AFP may indicate the presence of hepatocellular carcinoma. Other tumor products—such as monoclonal paraproteins (myeloma, macroglobulinemia, occasional lymphomas), 5-hydroxyindoleacetic acid (carcinoid), and acid phosphatase or prostate-specific antigen (prostatic cancer)—and ectopic hormone production (oat cell carcinomas) may correlate positively with the presence and proliferation of specific neoplasms. Estrogen and progesterone receptors should be measured in tissue from breast carcinoma, since the findings predict responsiveness to hormone manipulations for metastatic disease. Radionuclide, CT, and ultrasound scanning provide serial noninvasive measurements of tumor response to therapy. Only rarely should a second-look laparotomy be required to determine the status of a previously treated abdominal neoplasm.

Acceptable Drug Toxicity

The degree of toxicity that is acceptable depends on the probability and risks of achieving the therapeutic goal, other clinical characteristics of the individual patient, and the availability of supportive facilities to manage the anticipated toxicity.

Status of Patient

The patient's subjective and functional status must always be considered in formulating and instituting a therapeutic program. Subjective symptoms of disease usually parallel objective parameters of progression or regression of the neoplasm. When this is not so, other factors such as unrecognized drug toxicity, unreliable parameters of tumor response, and the masking of disease progression by certain forms of therapy (eg, corticosteroids) must be considered. The Karnofsky performance index (Table 47–12) is useful for following the functional status of the patient and is as important as objectively measurable parameters, especially when the goal of treatment is palliation.

The above considerations apply generally to cancer chemotherapy. Experimental drugs or treatment protocols may be considered if all of the following criteria are met: (1) Proved methods of effective therapy have been exhausted. (2) Data collection and dissemination of the information obtained will contribute toward answering the questions asked in the protocol. (3) The patient's human rights are fully protected, and informed consent has been obtained. (4) There is a reasonable expectation that the treatment will do more good than harm.

Balducci L et al: Systemic treatment of cancer in the elderly. Arch Gerontol Geriat 1988;7:119.

Kemeny MM, Brennan MF: The surgical complications of chemotherapy in the cancer patient. Curr Probl Surg 1987;24:609.

Phister JE, Jue SG, Cusack BJ: Problems in the use of anticancer drugs in the elderly. Drugs 1989;37:551.

Thiel HJ, Fietkau R, Sauer R: Malnutrition and the role of nutritional support for radiation therapy patients. Recent Results Cancer Res 1988;108:205.

CHEMOTHERAPEUTIC AGENTS
(See Tables 47–13 and 47–14)

Chemotherapeutic Agents With Selective Toxicity

Only the adrenocortical hormones, sex hormones, and asparaginase have demonstrated a predictable selective killing power of tumor cells based on metabolically exploitable differences between neoplastic and normal tissue.

A. Glucocorticoids: The glucocorticoids exert a "lympholytic" effect that can repeatedly induce remission of acute lymphoblastic leukemia, especially in combination with vincristine. This lympholytic effect, which does not depend on the mitotic activity of the tumor, is also useful in chronic lymphocytic leukemia, lymphomas, and myeloma.

The adrenal corticosteroids are also beneficial for certain hormonally sensitive tumors such as breast and prostatic cancer. They improve cerebral edema accompanying brain tumors, palliate hemolytic anemias associated with chronic lymphocytic leukemia and the lymphomas, and correct hypercalcemia associated with various neoplasms. Their antineoplastic effects are less if they are given on an intermittent schedule; large daily doses for the shortest time necessary to produce the desired effect are preferred. Toxicity may be metabolic (hyperglycemia, sodium retention, potassium wasting), gastrointestinal (peptic ulceration), or immunosuppressive (increased susceptibility to infection). Myopathies, psychosis, hypertension, and osteoporosis are important side effects of long-term administration.

B. Estrogens: The estrogenic steroids were used in the early 1940s for prostatic carcinoma and represented one of the first successful attempts at rational cancer chemotherapy. Shortly thereafter, estrogens were found useful in postmenopausal patients with breast cancer. Diethylstilbestrol, the most widely used estrogen, is potent, inexpensive, and effective when given orally but may cause gastrointestinal disturbances, fluid retention, feminization in males, and uterine bleeding. It may also cause hypercalcemia and "tumor flare" of disseminated breast carcinoma.

C. Synthetic Progestational Agents: These drugs are useful in pharmacologic doses for disseminated or uncontrolled carcinoma of the endometrium and occasionally for hypernephroma and breast cancer.

D. Androgens: The androgens are used princi-

Table 47–12. Karnofsky performance index.

	%	
Able to carry on normal activity. No special care is needed.	100	Normal. No complaints. No evidence of disease.
	90	Able to carry on normal activity. Minor signs or symptoms of disease.
	80	Normal activity with effort. Some signs or symptoms of disease.
Unable to work. Able to live at home and care for most personal needs. A varying amount of assistance is needed.	70	Cares for self. Unable to carry on normal activity or to do active work.
	60	Requires occasional assistance but is able to care for most of his needs.
	50	Requires considerable assistance and frequent medical care.
Unable to care for self. Requires equivalent of institutional or hospital care. Disease may be progressing rapidly.	40	Disabled. Requires special care and assistance.
	30	Severely disabled. Hospitalization is indicated, although death is not imminent.
	20	Very sick. Hospitalization necessary.
	10	Very sick. Hospitalization necessary.
	0	Moribund. Fatal processes progressing rapidly.
		Dead.

Table 47–13. Solid tumors responsive to chemotherapy.

Neoplasm	Current Drugs of Choice	Other Useful Agents
Hodgkin's disease	MOPP: mechlorethamine, Oncovin (vincristine), prednisone, procarbazine, alternating with doxorubicin, bleomycin, vincristine, and dexamethasone	Carmustine or lomustine, dacarbazine.
Non-Hodgkin's lymphoma	Cyclophosphamide, vincristine, prednisone, doxorubicin in combinations	Bleomycin, procarbazine, carmustine, or lomustine
Multiple myeloma	Melphalan plus prednisone	Cyclophosphamide, procarbazine, vincristine, carmustine, doxorubicin
Squamous cell carcinoma of head and neck	Methotrexate, bleomycin, cisplatin	Alkylators
Squamous cell carcinoma of lung	Cisplatin plus vinblastine or etoposide	Doxorubicin, cyclophosphamide, methotrexate, procarbazine in combinations
Squamous cell carcinoma of cervix	Bleomycin plus mitomycin plus vincristine; cisplatin plus fluorouracil	Alkylators, doxorubicin, methotrexate
Transitional cell carcinoma of bladder	Cisplatin plus mitomycin plus vinblastine	Doxorubicin, intravesical thiotepa
Malignant melanoma	Dacarbazine	Carmustine, hydoxyurea, vincristine
Adenocarcinoma of gastrointestinal origin	Fluorouracil	Doxorubicin, mitomycin
Adenocarcinoma of breast	CMF: cyclophosphamide, methotrexate, fluorouracil; or doxorubicin plus cyclophosphamide. Hormonal manipulations.	Mitomycin, vincristine; bleomycin plus vinblastine
Adenocarcinoma of ovary	Cyclophosphamide plus cisplatin	Other alkylators, altretamine, fluorouracil, methotrexate
Renal cell carcinoma	Progestagens, interferon	Lomustine, glucocorticoids, androgens, vinblastine
Testicular carcinoma	Vinblastine plus bleomycin plus cisplatin	Doxorubicin, alkylators, methotrexate, vincristine, dactinomycin, plicamycin, etoposide
Endometrial carcinoma	Doxorubicin plus cyclophosphamide	Progestagens
Prostatic carcinoma	Estrogen, leuprolide plus flutamide	Prednisone, fluorouracil, doxorubicin, estramustine
Various soft tissue sarcomas	Doxorubicin plus dacarbazine or methotrexate in high doses plus leucovorin calcium	Cyclophosphamide plus vincristine plus dactinomycin
Insulinoma	Streptozocin	
Adrenocortical carcinoma	Mitotane	Aminoglutethimide (for hypersecretion)
Carcinoid	Fluorouracil plus streptozocin	(?)Mitomycin; octreotide acetate for functional syndromes
Wilms' tumor	Dactinomycin with surgery plus radiotherapy	Vincristine, doxorubicin
Neuroblastoma	Cyclophosphamide, vincristine, doxorubicin	Dactinomycin, procarbazine
Choriocarcinoma, postgestational	Methotrexate or vincristine plus dactinomycin	Vinblastine, mercaptopurine, alkylators
Thyroid carcinoma	Radioiodine plus thyroid suppression	Doxorubicin (?)cisplatin
Esophageal squamous carcinoma	Cisplatin plus fluorouracil with concomitant radiotherapy	Mitomycin

pally in the treatment of disseminated breast cancer, especially in pre- and perimenopausal (1–4 years) women. They also have a role in the stimulation of erythropoiesis in anemic patients with several neoplastic and myelophthisic diseases. The toxic effects of androgens include excessive virilization of women, prostatism in men, and fluid retention; tumor flare and hypercalcemia occur occasionally. The halogenated androgens, which are effective when given orally, can produce cholestatic jaundice, though the parenteral nonhalogenated compounds do not do so.

E. Antihormones: Tamoxifen is an antiestrogen nonsteroidal agent that blocks estrogen receptor sites on tumor cells and antagonizes estrogen stimulation of hormone-dependent tumors such as breast and perhaps renal carcinoma. Nausea, hot flashes, and mild thrombocytopenia are toxicities associated with oral administration.

Table 47–14. Response, dosage, and toxicity of cancer chemotherapeutic drugs when used as single agents.

Agent	Response >50%	Response in 30–50%	Response <30%	Route	Toxicity	Usual Adult Dose[1]	Specificity[2]
Hormones							
Glucocorticoids	Hypercalcemia, Hodgkin's disease and other lymphomas (in combination), tumor edema of brain.	Breast carcinoma, multiple myeloma.	Hypernephroma.	Orally. (IV and IM preparations also available.)	Moon facies, sodium retention, potassium wasting, hyperglycemia, peptic ulcer, immunosuppression, hypertension, osteoporosis, myopathy. Moon facies, sodium retention, potassium wasting.	Prednisone: 1–2 mg/kg/d for brief intervals (<6 weeks if possible); then maintain at minimal required daily dosage.	Not known
Estrogens	Prostatic carcinoma.	Breast carcinoma.		Orally, IV, IM.	Sodium retention, feminization, uterine bleeding, nausea and vomiting.	Diethylstilbestrol: 5–25 mg/d for breast; 2.5–5 mg/d for prostate. Ethinyl estradiol: 3 mg/d for breast.	Not known
Progestagens		Endometrial carcinoma.	Hypernephroma.	Orally, IM.	Sodium retention.	Hydroxyprogesterone: 1 g 2–3 times weekly IM. Medroxyprogesterone: 200–600 mg orally twice weekly.	Not known
Androgens		Myelophthisic and refractory anemias; breast carcinoma.	Hypernephroma.	Orally, IM.	Sodium retention, masculinization; cholestatic jaundice with oral preparations.	Testosterone propionate: 100 mg 2–3 times weekly. Fluoxymesterone: 10–40 mg/d orally.	Not known
Tamoxifen	Postmenopausal breast carcinoma (receptor assay-positive).			Orally.	Nausea, vomiting, hot flashes; rarely, hypercalcemia.	20–60 mg/d in divided doses.	CCNS
Estramustine phosphate	Prostatic carcinoma.			Orally.	Nausea, vomiting; rarely, marrow suppression.	14 mg/kg/d in divided doses.	CCNS
Alkylators							
Mechlorethamine	Hodgkin's disease, neoplastic effusions.	Non-Hodgkin's lymphoma.	Melanoma; cervical, head and neck, bronchogenic carcinoma.	IV, intracavitary.	Nausea and vomiting, marrow depression, ulcer if extravasated, hypogonadism, fetal anomalies, alopecia.	1 g/m² every 3–5 weeks; 2–4 mg/kg/d orally for 10 days.	CCNS
Cyclophosphamide	Burkitt's lymphoma, Hodgkin's disease, other lymphomas.	Multiple myeloma, neuroblastoma, breast carcinoma, ovarian carcinoma.	Oat cell carcinoma of lung, cervical carcinoma, Ewing's sarcoma.	IV, orally.	Nausea and vomiting, marrow depression, alopecia, hemorrhagic cystitis.	1 g/m² every 3–5 weeks; 2–4 mg/kg/d orally for 10 days.	(?)CCNS

(continued)

Table 47–14. Response, dosage, and toxicity of cancer chemotherapeutic drugs when used as single agents. (continued)

Agent	Response >50%	Response in 30–50%	Response <30%	Route	Toxicity	Usual Adult Dose[1]	Specificity[2]
Chlorambucil	Hodgkin's disease	Non-Hodgkin's lymphomas, breast carcinoma ovarian carcinoma.	(?)Cervical carcinoma.	Orally.	Marrow depression, gastroenteritis.	0.1–0.2 mg/kg/d.	CCNS
Melphalan		Myeloma, ovarian carcinoma.		Orally.	Marrow depression (occasionally pro onged), gastroenteritis.	0.25 mg/kg/d orally for 4 days every 6 weeks; 2–4 mg/d as maintenance.	CCNS
Thiotepa		Ovarian carcinoma, neoplastic effusions.		IV, intracavitary.	Marrow depression.	0.8 mg/kg IV as single dose every 4–6 weeks; 0.8 mg/kg by intracavitary injection.	CCNS
Ifosfamide		Testicular carcinoma and oat cell carcinoma of lung.	Non-oat cell carcinoma of lung, cervical cancer.	IV.	Marrow depression, cystitis, neurotoxicity.	Ifosfamide, 2–5 g/m², with mesna, 3 g/m², for 24–36 hours every 3–4 weeks.	CCNS
Altretamine (hexamethylmelamine)		Ovarian carcinoma		Orally.	Nausea, vomiting, marrow suppression.	150 mg/m² for 21 days.	CCS
Nitrosoureas Carmustine, lomustine		Primary and metastatic brain tumors, meningeal carcinomatosis, Hodgkin's disease, other ymphomas.	Melanoma.	Carmustine IV, lomustine orally	Nausea and vomiting, prolonged marrow depression, local phlebitis.	Carmustine: 75–100 mg/m² IV daily for 2 days every 4–6 weeks. Lomustine: 130 mg/m² orally every 6 weeks.	CCNS
Streptozocin	Insulinoma.			IV.	Nephrotoxicity, gastroenteritis.	1 g/m² every 3–4 weeks.	CCNS
Inorganic metallic salt Cisplatin	Ovarian and testicular carcinomas.		Squamous carcinoma, transitional carcinoma.	IV.	Nausea and vomiting, bone marrow depression, nephrotoxicity, ototoxicity.	80–100 mg/m² every 3 weeks with mannitol diuresis. (Use lower dose when renal function is impaired.)	CCNS
Carboplatin	Ovarian carcinoma.		Various squamous and transitional cell carcinomas.	IV.	Nausea and vomiting, bone marrow depression, nephropathy.	300 mg/m² every 3–4 weeks.	CCNS

(continued)

Table 47–14. Response, dosage, and toxicity of cancer chemotherapeutic drugs when used as single agents. (continued)

Agent	Response >50%	Response in 30–50%	Response <30%	Route	Toxicity	Usual Adult Dose[1]	Specificity[2]
Structural analogues							
Methotrexate	Choriocarcinoma, Burkitt's lymphoma.	Squamous carcinoma of head and neck, testicular, breast carcinoma.	Various brain tumors, squamous cell carcinoma of lung.	Orally, IV, intrathecally.	Ulcerative mucositis, gastroenteritis, dermatitis, marrow depression, hepatitis, abortion.	40–60 mg/m² IV weekly; 20–40 mg IV twice weekly; 5–15 mg intrathecally weekly; 2.5–5 mg/d orally. Higher doses with leucovorin calcium.	CCS
Fluorouracil		Breast carcinoma, colon and rectal carcinoma.	Other carcinomas of gastrointestinal origin; ovarian, prostatic carcinoma.	Orally, IV, intra-arterial infusion.	Atrophic dermatitis, gastroenteritis, mucositis, marrow depression, neuritis.	15–20 mg/kg IV weekly for at least 6 weeks; 15 mg/kg orally weekly.	CCS
Mercaptopurine		Choriocarcinoma (postgestational).		Orally.	Bone marrow depression.	2.5 mg/kg/d.	CCS
Cytotoxic antibiotics							
Dactinomycin	Wilms' tumor, choriocarcinoma.	Testicular carcinoma.	Soft tissue sarcomas.	IV.	Nausea and vomiting, stomatitis, gastroenteritis, proctitis, marrow depression, ulcer if extravasated, alopecia; radiation potentiator.	0.01 mg/kg/d for 5 days every 4–6 weeks, or 0.04 mg/kg as single dose IV weekly.	CCNS
Fludarabine phosphate	Chronic lymphocytic leukemia, well-differentiated lymphomas.			IV.	Severe marrow depression.	25 mg/m²/d for 5 days every month.	CCS
Doxorubicin	Histiocytic and Hodgkin's lymphoma.	Transitional cell carcinoma of bladder, breast carcinoma.	Various sarcomas.	IV.	Alopecia, marrow depression, myocardiopathies, ulcer if extravasated; stomatitis. Radiation potentiator.	60 mg/m² every 3 weeks to maximum total dose of 550 mg/m².	CCNS
Plicamycin			Gastric and pancreatic carcinomas.	IV.	Nausea and vomiting, bone marrow depression, ulcer if extravasated.	20 mg/m² every 6 weeks.	CCNS
Bleomycin		Lymphomas, testicular carcinomas.	Squamous cell carcinoma of head, neck.	IV, IM, SC.	Allergic dermatitis, pulmonary fibrosis, fever, mucositis.	15 mg twice weekly; total cumulative dosage should not exceed 150 mg/m².	CCS
Vinca alkaloids							
Vinblastine	Hodgkin's disease.	Choriocarcinoma.	Breast, testicular carcinoma, non-Hodgkin's lymphomas.	IV.	Marrow depression, alopecia, ulcer if extravasated, nausea and vomiting, neuropathy.	0.1–0.2 mg/kg IV weekly.	CCS

(continued)

Table 47–14. Response, dosage, and toxicity of cancer chemotherapeutic drugs when used as single agents. (continued)

Agent	Response >50%	Response in 30–50%	Response <30%	Route	Toxicity	Usual Adult Dose[1]	Specificity[2]
Vincristine	Hodgkin's disease, other lymphomas, Wilms' tumor, neuroblastoma, medulloblastoma, choriocarcinoma.		Ewing's sarcoma; testicular, breast carcinoma; brain tumors; (?) multiple myeloma.	IV.	Alopecia, neuropathy (peripheral and autonomic), ulcer if extravasated.	1.5 mg/m² weekly or less often. No individual dosage should exceed 2 mg.	CCS
Miscellaneous agents							
Mitotane	Hypersecretion in adrenocortical carcinoma.	Reduction of tumor mass in adrenocortical carcinoma.		Orally.	Gastroenteritis, dermatitis, CNS abnormalities.	5–12 g daily	CCNS
Aminoglutethimide	Hypersecretion in adrenal carcinoma.			Orally.	Nausea, vomiting, somnolence.	250 mg 3–4 times daily with steroid replacement.	CCNS
Procarbazine	Hodgkin's disease.		Lymphomas; oat cell, large-cell lung carcinoma.	Orally.	Marrow depression, gastroenteritis, dermatitis, CNS abnormalities.	50–150 mg/m²/d to toxicity or response; maintain with 50–100 mg/d orally.	CCNS
Dacarbazine			Melanoma, soft tissue sarcomas.	IV.	Gastroenteritis, marrow depression, hepatitis, phlebitis, alopecia; ulcer if extravasated.	150–250 mg/m²/d IV for 5 days every 4–6 weeks.	CCNS
Hydroxyurea			Melanoma, brain tumors.	Orally.	Nausea, vomiting, bone marrow depression.	300 mg/m²/d for 5 days.	CCS
Etoposide	Testicular carcinoma (in combination with cisplatin).	Small-cell carcinoma of lung, lymphoma.		IV, orally (irregular absorption).	Hypotension with rapid IV administration, hematopoietic suppression, alopecia, nausea, neuropathy.	100 mg/m² IV daily for 5 days.	CCS
Paclitaxel (Taxol)		Ovarian carcinoma.	Breast carcinoma, lung carcinoma.	IV.	Marrow suppression, neuropathy, hypersensitivity, myalgias, bradycardia, hypotension, nausea, alopecia, liver enzyme elevation.	135 mg/m²/24 h every 3 weeks.	CCS

[1]Modifications of drug dosages: If white count is over 4500/µL and platelet count is >150,000/µL, give full dose; if white count is >150,000/µL, give full dose; if white count is <3000/µL and platelet count is <75,000/µL, give 0–25% of full dose; if white count is 3500–4500/µL and platelet count is 100,000–150,000/µL, give 75% of full dose. See text.

[2]CCS = cell cycle-specific; CCNS = cell cycle-nonspecific.

ANTICANCER DRUGS: GENERIC AND TRADE NAMES

Allopurinol (Zyloprim)
Altretamine (Hexalen; formerly
   hexamethylmelamine)
Aminoglutethimide (Cytadren)
Asparaginase (Elspar)
Bleomycin (Blenoxane)
Busulfan (Myleran)
Carboplatin (Paraplatin)
Carmustine (BiCNU)
Chlorambucil (Leukeran)
Cisplatin (Platinol)
Cyclophosphamide (Cytoxan)
Cyproterone acetate (Androcur)
Cytarabine (Cytosar-U)
Dacarbazine (DTIC-Dome)
Dactinomycin (Cosmegen)
Daunorubicin (Cerubidine)
Doxorubicin (Adriamycin)
Estramustine phosphate (Emcyt)
Etoposide (VePesid)
Fludarabine phosphate (Fludara)
Fluorouracil (Efudex)
Flutamide (Eulexin)

Hydroxyurea (Hydrea)
Ifosfamide (Ifex)
Interferon alfa-2a (Roferon-A)
Interferon alfa-2b (Intron A)
Leuprolide (Lupron)
Lomustine (CeeNU)
Mechlorethamine (Mustargen)
Melphalan (Alkeran)
Mercaptopurine (Purinethol)
Methotrexate (Folex)
Mitomycin (Mutamycin)
Mitotane (Lysodren)
Mitoxantrone (Novantrone)
Paclitaxel (Taxol)
Plicamycin (Mithracin; formerly
   mithramycin)
Procarbazine (Matulane)
Streptozocin (Zanosar)
Tamoxifen (Nolvadex)
Thioguanine (as such)
Thiotepa (as such)
Vinblastine sulfate (Velban)
Vincristine sulfate (Oncovin)

Antiandrogens include cyproterone acetate, a steroidal congener that possesses potent progestational actions; and flutamide, a nonsteroidal anilide that acts by inhibiting androgen-binding tumor tissue. These drugs may be of benefit in advanced prostatic carcinoma no longer responsive to hormonal manipulations that were effective in the past. Cyproterone has orphan drug status in the United States.

Reactivation of tumors responsive to prior castration or estrogen therapy or, in 30–40% of patients, failure to respond, may be due to persistent androgens of adrenal origin. Therefore, a new antihormonal strategy has been developed to achieve complete androgen blockade by using a luteinizing hormone-releasing hormone (LHRH) agonist or surgical castration to block testicular androgens in association with a pure antiandrogen (flutamide) in order to neutralize adrenal androgens.

Some investigators believe that complete androgen blockade is the treatment of choice in an effort to achieve more complete remissions of longer duration for metastatic prostatic cancer and to minimize the appearance of androgen-resistant cell clones. Several randomized clinical trials currently in progress are comparing LHRH agonists alone with such treatment in combination with flutamide. In early results, the combination appears superior.

The discovery of gonadotropin-releasing hormone and its analogues has made it possible to suppress Leydig cell function in humans. Efficacy in the treatment of prostatic cancer has been shown with LHRH agonists with the elimination of estrogenic side effects. Leuprolide is such an agonist; it is a synthetic nonapeptide that can achieve medical castration and appears to be as effective as diethylstilbestrol with fewer side effects. Leuprolide is available at present only in an injectable form; an intranasal preparation is being developed.

The Alkylators

The alkylators, whose prototype is mechlorethamine, react with nucleophilic substances within the cell to form cross-links at the guanine residues of parallel double DNA strands. With the possible exception of cyclophosphamide, the alkylators are CCNS drugs and affect both resting and dividing cells; both normal and malignant cells are injured.

Mechlorethamine is the alkylator of choice in the treatment of Hodgkin's disease, either singly or in combination with other drugs.

For Burkitt's lymphoma, **cyclophosphamide** may be curative, and it is also the agent of choice for undifferentiated small cell carcinoma of the lung. Cyclophosphamide has a unique role in childhood acute leukemia, in which other alkylators are ineffective. For most purposes, however, equivalent doses of the various alkylators produce equivalent responses, and there is cross-resistance among the alkylators except for the nitrosoureas (see below). The choice of alkylators thus rests upon the desired route and mode of administration and variations in toxicity.

Chlorambucil has had its major use in chronic lymphocytic leukemia, Hodgkin's disease, and Waldenström's macroglobulinemia. Its major advantage is its narrow spectrum of toxicity (hematopoietic only) and ease of administration (oral). **Melphalan** is usually given for multiple myeloma, but this may be merely traditional; **busulfan** is customarily used in chronic myelocytic leukemia and in polycythemia vera; all alkylators are equally effective against ovarian carcinoma.

Mechlorethamine is a vesicant if extravasated. Cyclophosphamide and thiotepa are much less irritating if applied directly to tissues, because they must first be metabolized to the active form. The immediate effects of intravenous alkylator administration are nausea and vomiting beginning within 30 minutes and persisting for 8–10 hours; premedication with a phenothiazine is preventive. The important delayed effects of alkylators are principally on rapidly proliferating tissues (hematopoietic, gonadal, skin, and gastrointestinal), with bone marrow suppression being the most prominent. In the marrow, cell necrosis begins at 12 hours; the nadir of blood count depression is at 7–10 days; and marrow regeneration time limits the administration of mechlorethamine to intervals of 4–6 weeks.

Some alkylators cause relatively characteristic adverse reactions. Examples are alopecia and hemorrhagic cystitis associated with cyclophosphamide and melanosis and pulmonary fibrosis with busulfan. All alkylators can cause hypospermia, menstrual irregularities, and fetal anomalies.

Thiotepa is discussed in Table 47–14.

Ifosfamide, a structural isomer of cyclophosphamide, has a broader range of activity and may have an improved therapeutic index owing to its lower myelosuppressive potential. This advantage is offset by severe urothelial toxicity. Ifosfamide is, therefore, generally given in conjunction with mesna (a urothelium protector) and has been used in salvage therapy for testicular carcinomas, soft tissue sarcomas, and lung carcinoma. The drug may also have a role in gynecologic tumors and lymphomas.

Altretamine
(Hexamethylmelamine)

Altretamine is a substituted melamine structurally similar to the ethyleneimonium intermediates in the hydrolysis of mechlorethamine, but it does not appear to share cross-resistance with alkylators. Instead, it probably functions as an antimetabolite to impair synthesis of nucleotide. The drug may have limited use in lung and breast cancer, but its major role is as a second-line drug used singly or in combination chemotherapy of ovarian cancer, where response rates of up to 40% are reported in alkylator-resistant patients.

The Nitrosoureas

Carmustine (BCNU) and **lomustine** (CCNU) are cell cycle-nonspecific synthetic chemicals that act much like the classic alkylators but have several unique and exploitable properties, including lipid solubility, and delayed onset of marrow suppression compared to the alkylators (see above). Moreover, there appears to be no cross-resistance with other alkylators. These drugs are effective in Hodgkin's disease but less so in non-Hodgkin's lymphomas; they appear promising for metastatic and primary central nervous system neoplasms because of their lipid solubility. Carmustine is administered intravenously; lomustine is given orally.

Streptozocin, a nitrosourea antibiotic derived from *Streptomyces,* has been useful in treating metastatic insulinoma; 16 of 23 treated patients in one series experienced a reduction of hyperinsulinism, and several had objective decreases in tumor mass. Toxicities are primarily renal and gastrointestinal. Marrow function is not usually impaired.

Structural Analogues
(Antimetabolites)

The antimetabolites are specific cytotoxic agents closely related to substrates normally utilized by cells for metabolism and growth. The structural analogues interfere with nucleic acid synthesis to impair proliferation of normal and neoplastic cells. They are generally CCS drugs, with proliferating cells being more vulnerable to their effects than are resting cells.

A. Methotrexate: Methotrexate competitively inhibits dihydrofolate reductase; acquired resistance to methotrexate results from increased dihydrofolate reductase activity, since the rate of enzyme synthesis exceeds the rate of methotrexate uptake by resistant cells.

Methotrexate toxicity may be hematologic, gastrointestinal, hepatic, or dermatologic. These effects may be alleviated or prevented by the prompt administration (preferably within 1 hour, but no longer than several hours) of leucovorin calcium (folinic acid, citrovorum factor). One treatment regimen has used leucovorin calcium to "rescue" the marrow after administration of toxic doses, though it is not yet certain that the antitumor effect is more pronounced. Methotrexate may be administered orally, intramuscularly, intravenously, or intrathecally; it is bound to plasma protein and excreted in the urine. Hepatic or renal failure is a contraindication; leukopenia, thrombocytopenia, stomatitis, and gastroenteritis with diarrhea are the toxic side effects that may require reduction in dosage.

Although methotrexate has been used for over 30 years, critical questions regarding dosage and scheduling have not been fully answered. Intermittent (twice-weekly) administration is superior to daily administration for maintenance of remission in childhood acute leukemia. In acute leukemia, "resistance" to methotrexate is relative and may be overcome by revising the schedule of administration and dosage. Intrathecal methotrexate is effective for central nervous system leukemia deposits even when marrow disease has become "resistant." Methotrexate can cure most cases of gestational choriocarcinoma. It has been used extensively in the treatment of epithelial neoplasia of the head and neck and is useful in breast cancer, testicular tumors, lung cancer, medulloblastomas, and other brain tumors.

B. Fluorouracil: Fluorouracil (5-FU) is a thymine analogue that in vivo interferes with thymidylate synthetase, an enzyme involved in the formation of thymidylic acid, a DNA precursor. The agent is first metabolized to 2'-deoxy-5-fluorouridine. This compound itself is now available (as floxuridine; FUDR) for use by perfusion, but it has not been shown to have a clear advantage over fluorouracil. Fluorouracil is metabolized principally in the liver. Its major toxicities include stomatitis, enteritis, and marrow suppression; significant atrophic dermatitis is occasionally reported; neurotoxicity is rare.

Fluorouracil has been most useful in breast and colonic adenocarcinoma, but it is also beneficial against pancreatic, gastric, ovarian, and prostatic cancer. The preferred schedule of administration is once weekly rather than the 4-day loading dose schedule initially advocated, since the latter is more toxic without being more effective. The dosage should be in the range of 15–20 mg/kg intravenously once a week as tolerated.

Since antimetabolites such as methotrexate and fluorouracil act only on rapidly proliferating cells, they damage the cells of mucosal surfaces such as the gastrointestinal tract. Methotrexate has similar effects on the skin. These toxicities are at times more significant than those that have occurred in the bone marrow, and they should be looked for routinely when these agents are used.

Erythema of the buccal mucosa is an early sign of mucosal toxicity. If therapy is continued beyond this point, oral ulceration will develop. In general, it is wise to discontinue therapy at the time of appearance of early oral ulceration. This finding usually heralds the appearance of similar but potentially more serious ulceration at other sites lower in the gastrointestinal tract. Therapy can usually be reinstituted when the oral ulcer heals (within 1 week to 10 days). The dose of drug used may need to be modified downward at this point, with titration to an acceptable level of effect on the mucosa.

C. Mercaptopurine and Thioguanine: Mercaptopurine (6-MP) and thioguanine (6-TG) are purine antagonists; mercaptopurine is the analogue of hypoxanthine and thioguanine the analogue of guanine. Although the actions of these two drugs are quite similar and they share cross-resistance, they are probably not identical. Thioguanine (but not mercaptopurine) is synergistic with cytarabine for induction of remission in acute myelocytic leukemia. Mercaptopurine is metabolized via the xanthine oxidase pathway, which is blocked by allopurinol. Therefore, the dosage of mercaptopurine must be reduced to 25% of the usual dosage if allopurinol is administered concomitantly. Full doses of thioguanine may be given in conjunction with allopurinol.

The purine analogues suppress purine synthesis through pseudofeedback inhibitory mechanisms that inhibit formation and interconversion of the intermediary compounds. The major toxicity is marrow suppression, which may be delayed in onset for several weeks. The major clinical role is in induction and maintenance of remission in the acute leukemias and in blastic transformation of chronic myelocytic leukemia. These may be of some benefit in lymphomas and ovarian carcinoma.

D. Fludarabine Phosphate: Fludarabine phosphate is an adenine nucleoside analogue that shows promising therapeutic activity in the clinical treatment of lymphocytic hematologic malignancies, especially those with a low proliferative index. The mechanism of action is felt to be through inhibition of DNA synthesis by inhibiting both DNA polymerase and ribonucleotide reductase. The drug has significant antitumor activity in patients with chronic lymphocytic leukemia and may achieve bone marrow remissions in that disease—a significant advantage over usually employed alkylators such as chlorambucil or combinations such as cyclophosphamide, vincristine, and prednisone. It is anticipated that fludarabine will soon be available as a standard agent in the treatment of chronic lymphocytic leukemia and other indolent lymphoproliferative diseases.

Cytotoxic Antibiotics

These agents, the first of which was dactinomycin, were isolated in the 1940s by Waksman from soil strains of bacteria of the *Streptomyces* class.

A. Dactinomycin: Dactinomycin is an inhibitor of DNA-dependent synthesis of RNA by ribosomes. Its toxicities include hematopoietic suppression, ulcerative stomatitis, and gastroenteritis. It causes intense local tissue necrosis if extravasated. The drug is retained for a considerable time intracellularly, and acquired resistance is thought to correlate with poor cellular uptake or poor retention of the drug. The major application of dactinomycin is in sequential combination with radiation therapy for Wilms' tumor; maintenance long-term administration of the drug adds significantly to the salvage obtained with combinations of surgery, radiation therapy, and adjuvant short-term courses of the drug. Dactinomycin is of proved value in trophoblastic cancer, soft tissue sarcomas, and testicular carcinoma, especially in combination with alkylators and antimetabolites. The optimal scheduling and combination of drugs with dactinomycin is not known, but the most customary regimen has been in courses of several days at dosages of 15 μg/kg/d intravenously repeated after 2–4 weeks as toxicity allows.

B. Doxorubicin: Doxorubicin and daunorubicin are tumoricidal anthracycline antibiotics that intercalate between adjacent base pairs of double-stranded DNA. Toxicity includes marrow suppression, alopecia, and mucositis. Severe local tissue necrosis occurs if the drug is extravasated. Doxorubicin is excreted mainly through the bile and must be used in reduced dosage in patients whose hepatic function is impaired. Both drugs have delayed cardiac toxicity. The problem is greater with doxorubicin, because this drug has a major role in the treatment of sarcomas, breast cancer, lymphomas, and certain other solid tumors; the use of daunorubicin is limited to the treatment of acute leukemias. Recent studies of left ventricular function indicate that some reversible changes in cardiac dynamics occur in most patients by the time they have received 300 mg/m². Serial echocardiographic measurements can detect these abnormalities. Echocardiographic measurement of left ventricular ejection fraction appears most useful in this regard. Alternatively, the left ventricular voltage can be measured serially by electrocardiography. Doxorubicin should not be used in elderly patients with significant intrinsic cardiac disease, and no patient should receive a total dose in excess of 550 mg/m². Patients who have had prior chest or mediastinal radiotherapy may be more prone to develop doxorubicin heart disease. ECGs should be obtained serially. The appearance of a high resting pulse rate may herald the appearance of overt cardiac toxicity. Unfortunately, toxicity may be irreversible or fatal at high dosage levels. At lower dosages (eg, 350 mg/m²), the symptoms and signs of cardiac failure generally respond well to digitalis, diuretics, and cessation of doxorubicin therapy.

The anthracycline derivative mitoxantrone has displayed a spectrum of antitumor efficacy similar to that of doxorubicin but with less cardiac toxicity and milder alopecia. The dose-limiting side effect is granulocytopenia when the drug is administered every 3 weeks; when lower daily doses are given for 5 consecutive days, mucositis is the major toxic effect.

C. Plicamycin: Plicamycin (mithramycin) is useful in the treatment of hypercalcemia resistant to hydration and corticosteroids, and the dosage may be less than that required for tumoricidal activity though still within the toxic range. Its major usefulness is in embryonal cell carcinoma and other testicular tumors, and its toxicity includes marrow suppression, hepatic and gastrointestinal injury, and complex coagulopathies.

D. Bleomycin: Bleomycin is an antitumor antibiotic that in clinical use as an anticancer drug is a mixture of various fractions differing in the amine moiety. The principal mode of action appears to be scission of DNA strands or inhibition of ligase, which impairs cell division. The most serious toxic effects are pulmonary interstitial pneumonitis and fibrosis, which may be fatal and are usually dose-related, occurring with a cumulative dosage greater than 150 mg/m² or less if given in conjunction with prior pulmonary radiation. Generally, older patients or those with preexisting lung disease are most susceptible.

Bleomycin hypersensitivity pneumonitis with eosinophilia may occur at any dosage and may respond to corticosteroid administration—in contrast to fibrosing pneumonitis, for which corticosteroids are not as effective.

Other bleomycin toxicities include anaphylactic and acute febrile reactions, stomatitis, and dermatitis with hyperpigmentation and desquamation of palms, soles, and pressure areas. The drug is marrow-sparing and may be administered by the intravenous, intramuscular, or subcutaneous routes, though the intravenous route is usual. Its major usefulness is in testicular neoplasia, squamous carcinomas, lymphomas, and cervical carcinoma, and it may be used intrapleurally to sclerose malignant effusions.

E. Mitomycin: Mitomycin is a useful agent against gastric and pancreatic adenocarcinoma and shows promise against breast cancer.

The Plant Alkaloids

The plant alkaloids include the periwinkle *(Vinca rosea)* derivatives vincristine and vinblastine—closely related compounds with widely different toxicities and somewhat different spectra of activity. Both *Vinca* alkaloids are bound to cytoplasmic precursors of the mitotic spindle in S phase, with polymerization of the microtubular proteins that comprise the mitotic spindle.

A. Vinblastine: Vinblastine sulfate is a major agent against Hodgkin's disease and testicular carcinoma and has lesser efficacy in the non-Hodgkin lymphomas. The toxicity of vinblastine is primarily marrow suppression, but gastroenteritis, neurotoxicity, and alopecia also occur—the latter much less commonly than with vincristine. The drug is usually given once a week. Severe local ulceration may occur if the drug extravasates into the subcutaneous tissues.

B. Vincristine: Vincristine sulfate is primarily neurotoxic and may induce peripheral, autonomic, and, less commonly, cranial neuropathies. The peripheral neuropathy can be manifested by sensory, motor, or autonomic symptoms or a combination of such symptoms. In its mildest form it consists of paresthesias ("pins and needles") of the fingers and toes. Occasional patients develop acute jaw or throat pain after vincristine therapy. This may be a form of trigeminal neuralgia. With continued vincristine therapy, the paresthesias extend to the proximal interphalangeal joints; hyporeflexia appears in the lower extremities; and significant weakness develops in the quadriceps muscle group. At this point, it is wise to discontinue vincristine therapy until the neuropathy has subsided somewhat. Peroneal weakness should be avoided lest symptomatic footdrop and impairment of gait occur.

Constipation is the most common symptom of the autonomic neuropathy that occurs with vincristine therapy. This symptom should always be dealt with prophylactically—ie, patients receiving vincristine should be started on stool softeners and mild cathartics at the same time therapy is instituted. If this potential complication is neglected, severe impaction may result in association with an atonic bowel.

More serious autonomic involvement can lead to acute intestinal obstruction, with signs indistinguishable from those of an acute abdomen. Bladder neuropathies are uncommon but may be severe.

Alopecia occurs in 20% of patients, but hematologic suppression is unusual. Vincristine is extremely effective in inducing remissions in acute lymphoblastic leukemia, especially in combination with prednisone, and is quite active in all forms of lymphoma. It is one of the most effective agents against childhood tumors, choriocarcinoma, and various sarcomas. Because of its lack of significant overlapping toxicity with most other chemotherapeutic agents, vincristine is receiving wide use in combination with other agents. The optimal dosage and scheduling for this agent remain to be elucidated; weekly administration is customary but may not be the best regimen.

C. Paclitaxel (Taxol): This is one of the most promising new agents against cancer. There is growing evidence of its activity against ovarian and breast cancer and possible activity against lung cancer. The drug binds to the microtubules and causes disarray in the formation of the mitotic spindle. It is an extract of the bark of the western yew tree, which is difficult to isolate and formulate from the bark. Therefore, intense efforts are under way to synthesize the drug, both to provide for better formulation and because current stands of Pacific yew would not be adequate to provide sufficient drug to treat a major patient population.

The 24-hour infusion schedule has been the most commonly used schedule of administration in investigative trials, with bronchospasm and hypotension being associated with the diluent necessary because of the limited aqueous solubility of taxol. Peripheral neuropathy has been another major effect, and neutropenia has also been a prominent toxic reaction. If the problems of synthesis can be overcome and if the toxicity can be ameliorated, paclitaxel may be one of the most interesting and challenging new drugs to enter clinical trials for cancer.

Miscellaneous Compounds

Mitotane is a DDT congener that may cause adrenocortical necrosis and therefore plays a useful role in reducing excessive steroid output in 70% of patients with adrenocortical carcinoma; in about 35%, an objective decrease in tumor mass is also recorded. Toxicities include dermatitis, gastroenteritis, and central nervous system abnormalities.

Aminoglutethimide is a derivative of glutethimide, a sedative-hypnotic drug that causes adrenal insufficiency with chronic use. Aminoglutethimide blocks adrenal steroidogenesis by inhibiting the enzymatic conversion of cholesterol to pregnenolone, thus reducing mineralocorticoid, glucocorticoid, and sex steroid production. The "medical adrenalectomy" thus induced can be beneficial for breast and prostatic cancers, though the degree of benefit is not precisely defined as yet. Toxicities include somnolence, nausea and vomiting, and, occasionally, skin rash. Supplemental mineralocorticoids and glucocorticoids must be administered with aminoglutethimide.

Estramustine phosphate combines an estradiol and an alkylator. It is used in prostatic carcinoma. It is not yet clear whether this complex will prove to be superior to either agent used alone, but the approach may lead to similar combinations in the future. Toxicities of oral administration include nausea and vomiting, thrombophlebitis, and mild hematopoietic suppression.

Procarbazine is a monoamine oxidase inhibitor whose exact mechanism of action is uncertain. It may cause both oxidation and alkylation of cellular constituents. Procarbazine is effective in Hodgkin's disease and may have some effect in various solid tumors, including oat cell carcinoma of the lung and melanoma. It finds wide use in combination chemotherapy as part of the MOPP regimen for Hodgkin's disease, and higher-dosage regimens are also being evaluated in the treatment of other solid tumors. Doses are limited because of hematologic, central nervous system, or gastrointestinal side effects, though tolerance to gastrointestinal side effects may develop. Occasional drug dermatitis is also reported.

Dacarbazine is a synthetic derivative of the triazene class that has both antimetabolite and alkylator-like activity. Dacarbazine has significant activity against melanoma and, in combination with doxorubicin, against various sarcomas. Toxicities, in addition to those listed in Table 47–14, may include a flu-like syndrome with myalgias.

Asparaginase is an enzyme that has been partially purified and derived from several sources, including guinea pig serum and cultures of *Escherichia coli*. It catalyzes the hydrolysis of *l*-asparagine to *l*-aspartic acid and ammonia. Certain tumor cells, especially lymphoblasts, require exogenous asparagine for protein synthesis and optimal growth, while most normal mammalian cells are able to synthesize sufficient endogenous asparagine. Asparaginase has proved efficacy only in acute lymphoblastic leukemia, but it has stimulated great interest because it exploits rarely found biochemical differences between normal and neoplastic tissue. Toxicity has proved to be severe and includes the expected allergic effects of intravenous administration of a foreign protein as well as pancreatitis and hepatic dysfunction.

Cisplatin is a heavy metal antitumor agents whose mechanism of action is unknown. Major acute toxicities may include severe vomiting and renal tubular necrosis and may be minimized by careful hydration and mannitol administration to promote brisk diuresis during the infusion of cisplatin. Other toxicities include high-frequency ototoxicity and bone marrow suppression, with leukopenia, thrombocytopenia, and anemia. The drug is usually given as a 2-hour infusion in a covered bottle (because it is light-sensitive). Major uses include testicular, bladder, and ovarian carcinomas and, in combination with fluorouracil, esophageal squamous carcinoma.

Carboplatin is a new platinum analogue with a spectrum of antineoplastic activity similar to that of cisplatin. It has reduced neurotoxicity, ototoxicity, and nephrotoxicity but causes more bone marrow suppression. Because there is less nausea and a because shorter period of intravenous hydration is required, this analogue may allow easier administration of outpatient platinum therapy.

Etoposide, a podophyllotoxin derivative (an extract of mandrake root), was found to have cytolytic properties when used in treating venereal warts. Antimitotic effects are related to breakage in single-stranded DNA. The drug shows significant activity as a single agent against small-cell lung cancer and lymphomas and is an important component of potentially curative "salvage therapy" combinations against testicular carcinoma in combination with ifosfamide. The principal toxicity of etoposide is hematopoietic suppression, chiefly leukopenia with a nadir in white blood count at 7–14 days and recovery by 21 days. Nausea, vomiting, alopecia, and (occasionally) peripheral neuropathy may also occur. Hypotension and anaphylactic reactions have been reported, especially with rapid intravenous administration. The drug should be given by slow intravenous infusion over 30–60 minutes. Oral administration is also effective, with the dosage approximately double the intravenous dose.

Alpha interferons. Clinical experience with alpha interferons has shown marked therapeutic activity in patients with hairy cell leukemia. There is also a potential role for interferon in combination with cytotoxic drugs for the treatment of multiple mycloma, and interferon appears to be effective in cutaneous T cell lymphomas and chronic lymphocytic leukemia. It may also be effective in chronic myelocytic leukemia; and among the solid tumors, melanoma, renal carcinoma, and ovarian carcinoma have all shown modest benefit in early trials. Toxicity consists primarily of flu-like symptoms (chills, fever, and malaise), central nervous symptoms (somnolence and confusion), hypotension, and granulocytopenia—all dose-related and rapidly reversible with cessation of therapy.

Differentiation-Promoting Agents

Differentiation-promoting therapy represents a unique new approach in the treatment of neoplasia. The capacity of a vitamin A-related retinoid compound to promote morphologic and functional differentiation of acute promyelocytic leukemia in vitro and in vivo without causing cytotoxicity may repre-

sent a major advance and a new avenue of approach through the utilization of agents that modify the genetic encoding of proteins to promote normal proliferation and differentiation. Vitamin A derivatives such as beta-carotene and 13-cis-retinoic acid may also be useful in preventing formation of epithelial head and neck tumors and in reversing the premalignant dysplastic lesion of oral leukoplakia. In addition to the significance of these specific benefits, this work represents another new approach to cancer through the field of chemoprevention of neoplasia.

Castaigne S et al: All-*trans* retinoic acid as a differentiation therapy for acute promyelocytic leukemia: I. Clinical results. Blood 1990;76:1704.

Current developments and future direction with ifosfamide: An update. Semin Oncol 1992;19(1 Suppl 1):1.

Garewal HS et al: Response of oral leukoplakia to beta carotene. J Clin Oncol 1990;8:1715.

Greenberg ER et al: A clinical trial of beta carotene to prevent basal cell and squamous cell carcinomas of the skin. N Engl J Med 1990;323:789.

Holmes FA et al: Phase two study of taxol in patients with metastatic breast cancer. Proc Am Soc Clin Oncol 1991;10:60.

Hong WK et al: Prevention of second primary tumors with isotretinoin in squamous cell carcinoma of the head and neck. N Engl J Med 1990;323:795.

Keating MJ: Fludarabine phosphate in the treatment of chronic lymphocytic leukemia. Semin Oncol 1990;17(5 Suppl 8):49.

McGuire WP et al: Taxol: A unique antineoplastic agent with significant activity in advanced ovarian epithelial neoplasms. Ann Intern Med 1989;111:273.

Ostrowsky MJ: Intracavitary therapy with bleomycin for the treatment of malignant pleural effusions. J Surg Oncol 1989;Suppl 1:7.

Van Echo DA, Egorin MJ, Aisner J: The pharmacology of carboplatin. Semin Oncol 1989;16(Suppl 5):1.

SURGICAL ADJUVANT CHEMOTHERAPY

It has been suggested that surgical or radiotherapeutic (CCNS) measures that reduce tumor bulk and increase the growth fraction of a tumor might increase tumor sensitivity to chemotherapeutic agents (CCS) without increasing marrow sensitivity. Thus, chemotherapeutic agents given after operation might improve results when there is no clinical evidence of residual disease but recurrence is statistically likely. In 1957, in order to test the validity of this reasoning, the National Surgical Adjuvant Breast Project began trials in which patients with clinically curable breast cancer were randomly given thiotepa for 2 days after radical mastectomy; controls received no chemotherapy. There was no significant difference in recurrence rates between treated and control patients in any category after 5 years, but premenopausal women with four or more positive axillary nodes who were treated demonstrated a recurrence rate 40% lower than that of the control group 18–36 months postoperatively. A controlled study of patients treated with melphalan intermittently for periods up to 2 years again showed significant benefit—in lengthening of the disease-free interval—for the treated group of premenopausal women with four or more histologically involved axillary nodes. A later study using a combination of cyclophosphamide, methotrexate, and fluorouracil as adjuvant treatment after mastectomy has confirmed a reduction in recurrence rate for the premenopausal treated group at 5 years. The doxorubicin-cyclophosphamide combination has prolonged the disease-free interval of pre- and postmenopausal patients. Whether this benefit will be sustained and accompanied by lengthened survival awaits further observations. Nevertheless, adjuvant chemotherapy with cyclophosphamide, methotrexate, and fluorouracil in premenopausal women is now widely accepted. While such therapy clearly benefits the average patient, toxic complications may be serious, and a small but statistically significant number of treated patients develop a second cancer.

In 1985, the National Institutes of Health Consensus Conference on the Adjuvant Therapy of Breast Cancer suggested that certain "high-risk" patients might be considered for adjuvant chemotherapy outside the context of a clinical trial. The risk factors include involvement of axillary nodes, large primary tumor size equal to or greater than 2.5 cm, negative estrogen receptor assay, poor histologic differentiation, high proliferative mitotic index, and younger patients. In May 1988, the National Cancer Institute further extended the scope of adjuvant therapy for breast cancer by issuing a Clinical Alert which concluded that adjuvant hormonal or cytotoxic chemotherapy can have a beneficial impact on the natural history of node-negative breast cancer patients. Current recommendations for adjuvant therapy outside of research trials include the following:

(1) Tamoxifen is indicated for at least 2 years for the postmenopausal low-risk patient with a receptor-positive tumor.

(2) For the premenopausal, receptor-positive, low-risk patient, tamoxifen also appears to prolong disease-free survival.

(3) For both pre- and postmenopausal high-risk patients, adjuvant chemotherapy with a regimen such as cyclophosphamide, methotrexate, fluorouracil, and prednisone results in improved disease-free survival.

This is not an edict for the treatment of all node-negative breast cancer patients; those with small carcinomas (< 1 cm) were not evaluated in these studies and should be treated primarily within the confines of a clinical trial designed to elucidate the benefit, if any, of adjuvant therapy in that favorable subset of patients.

Adjuvant chemotherapy with fluorouracil is also undergoing evaluation for colorectal neoplasms. Based upon a clinical update issued by the National Cancer Institute in October 1989, there is a recommendation for consideration of patients for adjuvant therapy on a protocol study of resected Dukes B and C colorectal carcinoma. The protocol includes the combination of levamisole (an anthelmintic drug) and fluorouracil for a 1-year course of treatment. This regimen reduced cancer recurrence in both Dukes B and Dukes C patients and improved survival in Dukes C patients in comparison with no adjuvant therapy and did so at acceptable toxicity.

Adjuvant chemotherapy has been of documented worth in Wilms' tumor and neuroblastoma and may be of benefit in stage II–IIIB Hodgkin's disease in conjunction with radiation therapy. Adjuvant therapy of osteosarcoma with high-dose methotrexate-leucovorin rescue or doxorubicin after amputation has improved disease-free survival rates. However, for incompletely understood reasons, current statistics for amputation alone have also shown improved disease-free survival rates, presumably because of improved roentgenographic and radionuclide techniques that can detect early metastatic disease. Randomized studies are under way to elucidate the role of adjuvant chemotherapy in osteosarcoma. Among other tumors that seem promising candidates for controlled studies of adjuvant chemotherapy are ovarian carcinoma, testicular tumors, and certain other soft tissue sarcomas.

Rhabdomyosarcoma in children can now be treated effectively by wide local excision (avoiding amputation) followed by irradiation and repeated cyclic therapy with dactinomycin and vincristine.

PALLIATION OF EMESIS CAUSED BY CHEMOTHERAPY

Nausea and vomiting are among the most frequent and disabling toxicities of cancer chemotherapy. Protracted bouts of retching have caused some patients to withdraw from potentially curative therapy, especially regimens containing cisplatin. Phenothiazines are among the safest effective antiemetics for adults receiving moderately emetogenic drugs such as fluorouracil, methotrexate, and moderate doses of cyclophosphamide. Prochlorperazine may be given in 10-mg doses orally or intramuscularly every six hours; absorption from suppositories is somewhat unpredictable. The major adverse reaction is agitation, which can usually be controlled by concomitant administration of diphenhydramine. For more potent emetogenic regimens such as cisplatin and high-dose cyclophosphamide, metoclopramide (Reglan), 2 mg/kg given slowly intravenously over a 10- to 30-minute period every 2 hours, is effective and well tolerated.

Marihuana derivatives such as tetrahydrocannabinol (THC) are about as effective as oral prochlorperazine but less effective than metoclopramide against strongly emetic drugs such as cisplatin. Tetrahydrocannabinol is available in the USA to oncologists working in institutions that have completed an investigative new drug application for protocol trials. This agent seems to be better tolerated and more effective in younger patients and is relatively contraindicated in elderly patients or those with cardiovascular or psychiatric disabilities.

Haloperidol is useful against strongly emetogenic drugs such as cisplatin, mechlorethamine, and doxorubicin. Cardiovascular side effects are fewer than with phenothiazines; sedation is the most common side effect. The usual dosage is 2 mg parenterally before chemotherapy is administered. Another agent useful against strongly emetogenic drugs is lorazepam, 1–2 mg parenterally before administration of chemotherapeutic agents.

Ondansetron is a serotonin antagonist that has just become available in the United States for intravenous use to prevent nausea and vomiting due to cancer chemotherapy. An oral formulation is available in many other countries. Ondansetron antagonizes the depolarizing action of serotonin, both at receptors on afferent vagal nerve terminals in the upper gastrointestinal tract and in the chemoreceptor trigger zone of the central nervous system. The drug has no significant antidopamine activity and is, therefore, seldom associated with adverse extrapyramidal effects. Placebo-controlled trials have shown that ondansetron has antiemetic activity in patients receiving potent emetogenic drugs such as cisplatin and is a more effective antiemetic than metaclopramide. Adverse effects include diarrhea and headache, and the recommended dosage has been 0.15 mg/kg intravenously over 15 minutes, given three times 4 hours apart, beginning 30 minutes before the chemotherapy.

Cubeddu LX et al: Efficacy of ondansetron (GR38032F) and the role of serotonin in cisplatin-induced nausea and vomiting. N Engl J Med 1990;322:810

Einhorn LH et al: Ondansetron: A new antiemetic for patients receiving cisplatin chemotherapy. J Clin Oncol 1990;8:731.

LATE COMPLICATIONS OF CHEMOTHERAPY

The increasing effectiveness of chemotherapy in prolonging survival has meant that treated patients are often at increased risk of developing a second malignant growth. The most frequent second cancer is acute myelogenous leukemia; other second drug- or radiation-associated cancers are sporadic. Acute myelogenous leukemia has been observed in up to 2% of long-term survivors of Hodgkin's disease treated with radiotherapy and MOPP and in patients with ovarian carcinoma or myeloma treated with melphalan. Despite this problem, the risk/benefit ratio is strongly in favor of the initial therapeutic regimen. However, the risks of adjuvant alkylator therapy of stage I breast carcinoma may exceed benefits if the incidence of leukemia exceeds 2%. There is evidence that certain drugs (melphalan, procarbazine) are more carcinogenic or leukemogenic than other alkylators, such as cyclophosphamide, and other classes of drugs, such as antimetabolites.

INFUSION & PERFUSION THERAPY

Selective arterial infusion has been used to deliver higher concentrations of drugs to the tumor than could be tolerated by systemic administration. One worker gave fluorouracil by hepatic arterial infusion to 200 patients with hepatic metastases, most of whom had failed to respond to intravenous fluorouracil. About 60% of the patients objectively improved and survived an average of 8.7 months; nonresponders lived an average of 2½ months.

Regional perfusion is an experimental technique that has given promising results in the following situations: (1) melanoma of an extremity perfused with mechlorethamine, phenylalanine mustard, or dacarbazine; (2) head and neck tumors perfused through the carotid artery with alkylators, fluorouracil, or methotrexate; and (3) hepatomas and metastatic adenocarcinoma in liver infused via the hepatic artery with fluorouracil and other drugs.

Recently, the development of a totally implanted drug delivery system for hepatic arterial chemotherapy has been shown to be safe and effective. A Silastic cannula is placed by laparotomy, and a pump is implanted subcutaneously; the pump can be refilled percutaneously. In a small preliminary series, 11 of 13 patients responded to floxuridine via continuous infusion for a median period of 6 months. This implanted system should facilitate further investigation of regional hepatic chemotherapy.

Another intravascular approach to palliation of abdominal neoplasms is transcatheter occlusion by Gelfoam or coil embolization. This technique is used most often for renal cell carcinoma but is also useful for dearterializing hepatic tumors by embolic occlusion of the hepatic artery.

MANAGEMENT OF VESICANT DRUG EXTRAVASATIONS

Infiltration of chemotherapeutic agents may cause severe local tissue necrosis. The greatest problems occur with mechlorethamine, vincristine, vinblastine, dactinomycin, doxorubicin, daunorubicin, plicamycin, mitomycin, and dacarbazine. As soon as infiltration is suspected, intravenous administration should be discontinued and a record made of the approximate amount, volume, and extent of extravasation. No drug is injected locally. The patient is instructed to apply ice for 20 minutes four times a day for 72 hours. This causes local vasoconstriction and decreases fluid absorption in the initial hours after injury. Although initially the lesion may show only local induration and then superficial blistering, this may be misleading, as the ultimate extent may include chronic ulceration, painful fibrosis, and injury to muscles and tendons, which may impair hand function. Within 72 hours, the patient should be evaluated by a plastic surgeon, who should follow the patient closely. With this approach, only 12 of 50 patients have required surgery. If extreme pain or tissue necrosis is present, surgical excision of the area of infiltration—particularly of the subcutaneous tissues—should be performed promptly. For established ulcers with tissue fibrosis, however, adequate treatment usually requires wide excision down to the level of healthy tissue. In the forearm or the dorsum of the hand, removal of extensor tendons and immediate coverage with a meshed split-thickness skin graft may be required. The use of flaps is avoided whenever possible.

To avoid extravasation, a properly flowing intravenous infusion should be established before injection of the drug. A convenient route of vascular access in cancer patients is the Silastic catheter surgically placed in the cephalic or jugular vein and positioned in the superior vena cava with the distal end tunneled beneath the skin to an accessible exit point on the lower chest wall. The Dacron wool cuff becomes infiltrated by connective tissue, which secures the catheter in position and forms a barrier to infection of the tunnel. Drugs, blood products, fluids, and parenteral nutrition solutions may be administered through the catheter. Blood may be withdrawn; this avoids the pain and complications of difficult venipunctures. These catheters may remain in place for prolonged periods with a low rate of infection, so that the problems of drug extravasation, phlebitis, and difficult venous access may be avoided. A totally implantable system of intravenous access is also available (Portocath, Infusa-port).

COMBINATION CHEMOTHERAPY

Combinations of drugs that block multiple biosynthetic pathways are given in an attempt to exert a synergistic effect on the tumor. The drugs of a combination are selected to avoid overlapping toxicity. This approach has been of greatest value where no single agent is highly effective. Thus, vincristine plus prednisone or cytarabine plus thioguanine produces more complete remissions of acute leukemia than either agent alone, and toxicity is not increased. Survival is prolonged in proportion to the duration of re-

mission, which documents the importance of achieving complete remission.

The cyclic administration of mechlorethamine, vincristine (Oncovin), prednisone, and procarbazine ("MOPP") produces 81% complete remissions of Hodgkin's disease in untreated stage III and stage IV; 76% complete remissions after radiotherapy alone; and 50% complete remissions after prior radiotherapy and chemotherapy. Seventy percent of complete responders were alive after 5 years, and 50% were continuously free of disease during that period. Single-agent therapy with these drugs is much less successful. Improved—but less striking—results have also followed chemotherapy of non-Hodgkin's lymphoma. The combination of cyclophosphamide, vincristine, and prednisone ("CVP") produces about 60% complete remissions with a median duration of 5 months.

In breast cancer, the combination of an alkylator (usually thiotepa or, more recently, cyclophosphamide) with methotrexate and fluorouracil and with varying combinations of testosterone and prednisone has given a 50–60% response rate. Approximately 80% of patients with visceral and skin metastases have responded to a five-drug program: daily oral cyclophosphamide and prednisone; weekly intravenous fluorouracil after a 4-day loading dose regimen; and methotrexate and vincristine for 8 weeks (if possible), with maintenance at more widely spaced intervals with varying dosages. Another highly effective combination is doxorubicin and cyclophosphamide. In general, for appropriate candidates, combinations of effective cytotoxic agents are preferable to single-agent chemotherapy for breast cancer.

The treatment of testicular cancers is representative of an era of chemotherapeutic and radiotherapeutic progress since the development in 1960 by Li and others of combination chemotherapy (chlorambucil, methotrexate, and dactinomycin) for patients with disseminated disease. Nonseminomatous testicular carcinomas have recently been treated successfully with varying combinations of bleomycin, vinblastine, and cisplatin. Samuels reported an overall 75% response rate, with a 45% complete remission rate, to a regimen of vinblastine and bleomycin. Einhorn and Donohue treated 50 patients with a triple combination of bleomycin, vinblastine, and cisplatin with 75% complete and 26% partial remissions. Toxicity was significant, but remissions lasted for six months to more than 30 months. The majority of patients in remission longer than 2 years appeared to be cured.

BONE MARROW AUTOTRANSPLANTATION FOR SOLID TUMORS

Autologous bone marrow transplantation is currently undergoing clinical trials for patients with metastatic solid tumors—in particular, breast cancer. Autologous bone marrow transplantation may be curative for leukemias and high-grade lymphomas and is now under intense scrutiny as a modality of definitive therapy for common solid tumors. Such disciplinary effort with treatment represents a major multidisciplinary effort with a significant financial outlay—currently $100,000 per transplant—and significant risks of morbidity and mortality (5%). The goal of such therapy must therefore be the achievement of long-term disease-free survival in a significant proportion of patients. In both the laboratory and clinical settings, there is evidence that intensive doses of chemotherapy induce a higher response rate in many solid tumors; myelosuppression is the dose-limiting toxicity for almost all chemotherapy agents used against solid tumors. Removal of the patient's own bone marrow prior to the administration of very high-dose chemotherapy and subsequent reinfusion of that bone marrow when cytotoxic drugs have been cleared from the circulation makes possible the administration of dosages that would otherwise be associated with a high incidence of life-threatening infections.

Although the long-term results for breast cancer are not yet definitive, it would appear that the response rate is higher than might be expected from standard drugs used in conventional dosages and combinations. The 2-year disease-free survival, however, appears to be between 25% and 50%. Thus, the full potential of high-dose chemotherapy to affect the duration of survival of patients with breast cancer remains to be demonstrated in properly controlled clinical trials. It is anticipated that this will be done in the adjuvant setting, where the effect of high-dose chemotherapy should be much greater among patients with a smaller tumor burden.

Alternatively, through the use of colony-stimulating factors, it may also be possible to achieve greater dose intensification and benefits comparable to autologous bone marrow transplantation at a lesser cost.

Frei E et al: Bone marrow autotransplantation for solid tumors: Prospects. J Clin Oncol 1989;7:515.

EVALUATION & MANAGEMENT OF PATIENTS WITH AN UNKNOWN PRIMARY CARCINOMA

Samuel D. Spivack, MD

About 15% of cancer patients present with metastatic tumor from an unknown primary site of origin. The most common sources are the pancreas and the lung. If the presenting metastasis is a squamous carcinoma, the primary is most often in the lung, but occa-

sionally an occult nasal, oropharyngeal, or laryngeal primary is found that may be treated with curative intent if evaluation reveals no dissemination beyond regional nodes.

For adenocarcinomas or undifferentiated carcinomas, an extensive search for the primary may be unrevealing until late in the course of the illness. The objectives of care are to palliate symptoms from the metastases and to identify the primary source, especially in the case of more treatable (often hormonally responsive) tumors such as those of the breast, prostate, uterus, and thyroid. Extensive radiologic and endoscopic evaluation is justified in the search for a primary source of a solitary metastasis, but it usually produces little benefit for patients with multiple sites of dissemination; palliative therapy of symptoms caused by the metastases is usually more important. Unusual sites of metastatic presentation include the skin (usually from a lung, colon, or kidney primary), intraocular structures (usually from a female breast primary), and the lower female genital tract (usually from an ovarian or uterine primary).

Electron microscopy may be helpful in detecting melanosomes in melanoma or specific inclusion bodies of APUD (*Amine Precursor Uptake and Decarboxylation*) in endocrine tumors. Hormone receptor proteins may be of value in defining breast or endometrial carcinoma, and lymphocyte markers for T and B cells help to support a diagnosis of malignant lymphoma. Each of these techniques requires special fixation or handling of fresh tissue. Serum markers (carcinoembryonic antigen [CEA], alpha-fetoprotein [AFP], human chorionic gonadotropin [hCG], and acid phosphatase) may also be useful in suggesting the origin of cancers.

Several recent reports have described young men with poorly differentiated and rapidly growing neoplasms, usually in a midline distribution (retroperitoneal or mediastinal) and in most cases accompanied by findings of marker substances (β-hCG or AFP) in serum or intracellularly by immunocytochemical methods. Whether these tumors arise from germ cell rests or by conversion of somatic cells to neoplasms expressing features of a germ cell tumor is currently unknown. It is, however, important to recognize that the extragonadal germ cell cancer syndrome is highly treatable by chemotherapeutic agents as used for testicular carcinoma and shows a good response rate even when widely disseminated tumor is present.

Unless the above data reveal a chemosensitive tumor, treatment of widely disseminated neoplasm of uncertain primary origin should be directed to symptomatic palliation. Chemotherapeutic combinations such as FAM (fluorouracil, Adriamycin [doxorubicin], and mitomycin) have not been particularly useful in these cases, but local surgical extirpation or radiotherapy of solitary nodal metastases can provide significant benefit, especially if the lesion is a well-differentiated squamous carcinoma located in the upper cervical or midcervical nodes. Improved survival rates can also be achieved by resection of solitary pulmonary or hepatic metastases, depending upon the site of origin of the primary tumor and the disease-free interval before the occurrence of the solitary lesion.

de Braud F et al: Metastatic squamous cell carcinoma of an unknown primary localized to the neck: Advantages of an aggressive treatment. Cancer 1989;64:510.

Greco FA, Hainsworth JD: The management of patients with adenocarcinoma and poorly differentiated carcinoma of unknown primary site. Semin Oncol 1989;16(4 Suppl six):116.

Greenberg BR, Lawrence HJ: Metastatic cancer with unknown primary. Med Clin North Am 1988;72:1055.

Guthrie TH Jr: Treatable carcinoma of unknown origin. Am J Med Sci 1989;298:74.

Haskell CM et al: Metastasis of unknown origin. Curr Probl Cancer 1988;12:5.

Le Chevalier T et al: Early metastatic cancer of unknown primary origin at presentation: A clinical study of 302 consecutive autopsied patients. Arch Int Med 1988;148:2035.

Merchut MP: Brain metastases from undiagnosed systemic neoplasms. Arch Int Med 1989;149:1076.

Ringenberg QS et al: Malignant ascites of unknown origin. Cancer 1989;64:753.

Strnad CM et al: Peritoneal carcinomatosis of unknown primary site in women: A distinctive subset of adenocarcinoma. Ann Intern Med 1989;111:213.

PARANEOPLASTIC SYNDROMES
(Table 47–15)

Samuel D. Spivack, MD

A cancer produces symptoms largely because the primary tumor mass or its metastases interfere with normal organ functions. It may also produce remote effects on other organs not directly involved with the neoplasm. These remote effects are termed paraneoplastic syndromes. Functioning endocrine tumors (see Chapters 16 and 34) are expected to produce systemic effects, but many other kinds of tumor can also produce paraneoplastic syndromes. Even if fever, malignant cachexia, and anemia of chronic disease are excluded, paraneoplastic syndromes occur in about 10% of patients with cancer, and occasionally they represent the first sign of the disease.

Endocrine, gastrointestinal, neurologic, hematologic, dermatologic, renal, and rheumatologic dysfunctions have been described. The endocrine effects are understood best, since many cancers produce true hormones or substances that mimic the physiologic effects of hormones. Similar mechanisms are thought to operate through growth factor production and reg-

Table 47–15. Common paraneoplastic syndromes.

	Common Causes
Endocrine	
ACTH/Cushing's	Lung, adrenal cancers
Inappropriate ADH secretion	Lung cancer
Hypercalcemia	Breast, lung, kidney, prostate cancers, myeloma
Adult onset rickets	Soft tissue and bone tumors
Hypoglycemia	Insulinomas, sarcomas, hepatomas
Neurologic	
Encephalomyelitis	Lung cancer
Opsoclonus	Lung, breast, uterine cancers, pediatric neuroblastoma
Neuropathies and neuromuscular syndromes	Myeloma, breast, lung, ovarian cancers, thymomas
Cerebellar atrophy	Breast, ovarian cancers
Hematologic	
Erythrocytosis	Hypernephroma, Wilms's tumor, hepatoma
Granulocytosis	GI, lung, brain tumors, melanoma
Eosinophilia	Lymphomas, melanoma, brain tumors
Thrombocytosis	Leukemias, lymphomas
DIC	Pancreas, lung, stomach, prostate cancers
Migratory thrombophlebitis	GI, lung, breast, ovarian, prostate cancers
Dermatologic	
Acanthosis nigricans	Gastric, abdominal cancers
Leser-Trelat keratoses	Lymphomas, GI cancers
Bazex's acrokeratosis	Head and neck, GI, lung cancers
Flushing	Carcinoid tumor
Dermatomyositis	All types of cancer
Pruritus	Lymphomas
Miscellaneous	
Fever	Lymphoma, hypernephroma, hepatoma
Nonmetastatic hepatic dysfunction	Hypernephroma
Hypertrophic osteoarthropathy	Lung cancer, tumors metastatic to chest
Amyloidosis	Myeloma, lymphoma, hypernephroma

ulation of growth factor receptor levels. Antibodies against tumor antigens that cross-react with normal tissues mediate neurologic syndromes, and immune complex deposition is believed to cause some paraneoplastic disorders. However, in many cases the cause of paraneoplastic syndromes is unknown.

The remote symptoms that characterize a paraneoplastic syndrome may create the impression that a localized cancer has metastasized, and constitutional symptoms due to treatable problems such as infection may be erroneously attributed to a paraneoplastic syndrome, resulting in a delay in starting therapy. Rarely, a paraneoplastic symptom represents the initial manifestation of a curable malignant tumor. Recrudescence of symptoms may herald tumor recurrence after initial treatment, serving as a tumor marker. Thus, prompt recognition and evaluation of paraneoplastic syndromes is important.

Disabling symptoms may respond to treatment of the primary cancer, debulking surgery to remove most of a tumor, or medications that interfere with a tumor's humoral effects.

The diagnosis of a paraneoplastic syndrome is not secure until direct tumor invasion, obstruction, vascular compromise, treatment-related toxicity, or fluid and electrolyte disorders have been excluded as causes of the signs or symptoms.

Abeloff MD: Paraneoplastic syndromes: A window on the biology of cancer. N Engl J Med 1987;317:1598.

Antel JP, Moumdjian R: Paraneoplastic syndromes: A role for the immune system. J Neurol 1989;236:1.

Axelrod L, Ron D: Insulin-like growth factor II and the riddle of tumor-induced hypoglycemia. N Engl J Med 1988;319:1477.

Dropcho EJ: The remote effects of cancer on the nervous system. Neurol Clin 1989;7:579.

Ellis DL et al: Melanoma, growth factors, acanthosis nigricans, the sign of Leser-Trelat, and multiple acrochordons. N Engl J Med 1987;317:1582.

Hildebrand J: Signs, symptoms, and significance of paraneoplastic neurological syndromes. Oncology 1989; 3:57.

Kornguth SE: Neuronal proteins and paraneoplastic syndromes. N Engl J Med 1989;321:1607.

Naschitz JE, Abrahamson J, Yeshurun D: Clinical significance of paraneoplastic syndrome. Oncology 1989;46: 40.

Odell WD: Paraendocrine syndromes of cancer. Adv Intern Med 1989;34:325.

Sons HU: Pulmonary embolism and cancer: Predisposition to venous thrombosis and embolism as a paraneoplastic syndrome. J Surg Oncol 1989;40:100.

PAIN PALLIATION IN CANCER

Samuel D. Spivack, MD

Malignant disease may cause pain by obstruction of a hollow viscus, by destruction of the supporting architecture of weight-bearing bones, by infiltration of nerve roots or plexuses by tumor, and by infiltrative growth within a closed compartment such as periosteum, fascia, or a visceral capsule. Pain may sometimes be controlled by decreasing tumor bulk by radiation therapy, surgery, and chemotherapy. Radiation therapy is most effective for bony metastases; surgery may bypass an obstruction of bowel or biliary tract; and regional intra-arterial chemotherapy can reduce liver pain of hepatic metastases in 50–70% of selected patients.

All too often, however, these measures are only temporarily or partially effective, and nonspecific symptomatic treatment of pain is required. Aspirin and acetaminophen are the most effective nonnarcotics and, combined with codeine, are useful for ambulatory patients. Narcotic analgesics such as morphine or hydromorphone are often required in terminal cancer, and the fear of producing drug addiction should never prevent their administration to such patients. In patients with persistent or recurrent pain, a regular schedule of administration at 3- to 4-hour intervals may afford better palliation than larger doses at less frequent intervals. Methadone has a relatively long duration of action (6–8 hours) and a good oral/parenteral potency ratio. Liquid preparations are sometimes preferable, though there seems to be no advantage to hospice mixture or Brompton's cocktail (a mixture of heroin, cocaine, phenothiazine, and ethyl alcohol) as compared with aqueous morphine solutions.

Neurosurgical and anesthetic measures are appropriate in patients who have not responded to other palliative measures or who have neuroanatomically localized pain that can be eradicated without producing major neurologic dysfunction. Dorsal rhizotomy is appropriate for segmental somatic pain of thoracoabdominal dermatomes but would be a poor choice for pain in an extremity because of the concomitant loss of sensory function resulting from the procedure. Percutaneous cordotomy is an effective procedure for unilateral pain located in segments lower than the upper thoracic area. Thalamotomy may be useful in control of head and facial pain, as may tractotomy as well (trigeminal or spinal thalamic). Somatic nerve and autonomic plexus blocks may be useful when a more effective surgical procedure is refused or otherwise unavailable.

Breitbart W: Psychiatric management of cancer pain. Cancer 1989;63:2336.

Elliott K, Foley KM: Neurologic pain syndromes in patients with cancer. Neurol Clin 1989;7:333.

Foley KM: Controversies in cancer pain. Medical perspectives. Cancer 1989;63(11 Suppl):2257.

Hanks GW: Controlled-release morphine (MST Contin) in advanced cancer: The European experience. Cancer 1989;63(11 Suppl):2378.

Inturrisi CE: Management of cancer pain: Pharmacology and principles of management. Cancer 1989;63(11 Suppl):2308.

Miser AW, Miser JS: The treatment of cancer pain in children. Pediatr Clin North Am 1989;36:979.

Portenoy RK: Cancer pain. Epidemiology and syndromes. CA 1989;63(11 Suppl):2298.

Portenoy RK: Practical aspects of pain control in the patient with cancer. Can J Clin 1988;38:327.

BACTERIAL SEPSIS IN CANCER PATIENTS

Samuel D. Spivack, MD

Infection is the cause of death in 60–75% of patients with leukemia or lymphoma and 40–50% of patients with solid tumors. In some instances, this is due to impaired host defense mechanisms (leukemia, lymphoma, myeloma); in others, it is due to myelosuppressive and immunosuppressive effects of cancer therapy or progressive cancer with cachexia.

In patients with acute leukemia or granulocytopenia (granulocyte count < 600/μL), infection is a medical emergency. Fever is virtually pathognomonic of infection—usually with gram-negative organisms—in these patients.

Appropriate cultures (eg, blood, sputum, urine, cerebrospinal fluid) should always be obtained before therapy is started, but bactericidal antibiotics must usually be started before results are available. Gram stains may demonstrate a predominant organism.

In the absence of granulocytopenia and in nonleukemic patients, the empiric combination of a cephalosporin antibiotic and tobramycin has proved exceedingly useful for patients with acute bacteremia. Therapy with combinations of this nature must be given judiciously, as they are of very broad spectrum; they should always be replaced by the most appropriate antibiotics as soon as culture data become available. The combination of cephalosporin and kanamycin is ineffective against *Pseudomonas* infection. In the current era of intensive chemotherapy of cancer, *Pseudomonas* bacteremia is now the most frequent infection in granulocytopenic patients and is all too often fulminant and fatal within 72 hours. Prompt institution of combination therapy with tobramycin and ticarcillin may offer the best chance of cure. Because of drug interactions, these two compounds cannot be mixed but must be administered separately. This combination is of lesser efficacy against *Escherichia coli* sepsis and should not be used for that purpose. Initial treatment of febrile patients with acute leukemia or granulocytopenia should consist of three drugs: cephalothin, tobramycin, and ticarcillin. If a causative organisms is isolated, the combination is replaced with the best agent or agents; otherwise, the combination is continued until the infection has resolved.

Granulocyte transfusions have recently proved to have significant value for granulocytopenic cancer patients with sepsis; however, until recently, the complex procurement procedures limited their availability. Untreated patients with chronic myelogenous leukemia can serve as excellent granulocyte donors for cancer patients with granulocytopenia. Although collection is ideally carried out with a blood cell separator, simple leukapheresis techniques may also be of value with chronic myelogenous leukemia donors. Use of normal donors requires a blood cell separator or filtration-leukapheresis device. Optimal use of normal granulocyte transfusion appears to require at least four daily transfusions (in addition to antibiotics) to localize infection.

Hematopoietic growth factors represent a major new development in the amelioration of neutropenia after chemotherapy. Recombinant granulocyte colony-stimulating factor (G-CSF; filgastrim) is a human glycoprotein hormone that has been produced clinically in a nonglycosylated form through recombinant DNA technology. It acts on precursor cells to promote formation of the differentiated granulocytic neutrophil. Another colony-stimulating factor derived from the granulocyte macrophage is GM-CSF (sargramostim), which stimulates granulocyte, macrophage, and eosinophil colony formation and acts in combination with erythropoietin to stimulate a burst of erythroid activity as well. G-CSF has rapidly gained a role in the amelioration of neutropenia after chemotherapy. Results of a randomized controlled G-CSF trial have shown that the severity and duration of neutropenia were reduced, leading to a reduction of 50% in the incidence of infections or suspected infections. GM-CSF is approved only for use in hastening the recovery of autologous bone marrow transplantation following very intensive chemotherapy or a combination of chemotherapy with radiation. Adverse effects of G-CSF include mild or moderate bone pain in about 20% of patients who receive it, the bone pain resolving promptly with cessation of treatment and frequently even with continuation of therapy. The usual administration is by subcutaneous injection at a starting dose of 5 μg/kg/d, beginning 3 or 4 days after chemotherapy for up to 2 weeks or until the neutrophil count is 10,000/μL. As a practical matter, the daily dosage of C-CSF is either 300 μg or 480 μg, which are the two available vial sizes.

Applebaum FR: The clinical use of hematopoietic growth factors. Semin Hematol 1989;26:7.

Banerjee C et al: Bacillus infections in patients with cancer. Arch Int Med 1988;148:1769.

Del Favero A et al: Septicaemia due to gram-positive cocci in cancer patients. J Antimicrob Chemother 1988;21 (Suppl):157.

Fainstein V, Elting LS, Bodey GP: Bacteremia caused by non-sporulating anaerobes in cancer patients: A 12-year experience. Medicine 1989;68:151.

Gabrilove JL et al: Effect of granulocyte colony stimulating factor on neutropenia and associated morbidity due to chemotherapy for transitional cell carcinoma of the urothelium. N Engl J Med 1988;318:1414.

Groopman JE: Clinical applications of colony stimulating factors. Semin Oncol 1988;15(Suppl 6):27.

Groopman JE, Molina JM, Scadden DT: Hematopoietic

growth factors, biology and clinical applications. N Engl J Med 1989;321:1449.

Karabinis A et al: Risk factors for candidemia in cancer patients: A case-control study. J Clin Microbiol 1988; 26:429.

Komshian SV et al: Fungemia caused by *Candida* species and *Torulopsis glabrata* in the hospitalized patient: Frequency, characteristics, and evaluation of factors influencing outcome. Rev Infect Dis 1989;11:379.

Viscoli C: Aspects of infections in children with cancer. Recent Results Cancer Res 1988;108:71.

PALLIATION OF LOCAL COMPLICATIONS OF NEOPLASIA*

Samuel D. Spivack, MD

Effusions

At least half of all patients with lung or breast cancer will develop a pleural effusion at some time during the illness. Ascites is a common complication of ovarian carcinoma. Lymphomas may be associated with chylous or nonchylous effusion of either or both sites. One-fourth of all effusions are neoplastic in origin, and where pulmonary infarction is unlikely, most bloody effusions are from neoplasm. The diagnosis in malignant pleural effusions can be established by cytologic study of the fluid and pleural biopsy with the Cope needle.

Diuretics may be sufficient to control neoplastic ascitic effusions. However, when recurrent accumulations of fluid cause dyspnea, abdominal distention, or pericardial tamponade, palliative control should be attempted.

A. Pleural Effusions: Control of pleural effusions is best achieved by obliteration of the pleural space with sclerosing agents such as mechlorethamine, bleomycin, or tetracycline. The lung must be fully expanded, and negative intrathoracic pressure must be applied to appose the pleural surfaces for several days, with a large thoracostomy tube connected to water-sealed drainage. If the lung is not expandable—because of endobronchial obstruction with massive atelectasis, fibrothorax with "trapped lung," or massive intraparenchymal replacement by tumor—obliteration of the pleural space is contraindicated.

Intrapleural bleomycin is useful for controlling malignant pleural effusion when administered in a 60–mg dose. Side effects and toxicity of bleomycin tend to be mild, and the drug can safely be administered to myelosuppressed patients. When the pleural surfaces are apposed, freshly prepared bleomycin, 60- mg in 50 mL saline, is instilled intrapleurally through the clamped chest tube and the patient is positioned for 1 minute each in the prone, left decubitus, supine, right decubitus, and knee-chest positions to distribute the drug. After 4 hours, the tube is unclamped and drainage reestablished for 24–48 hours or until no further fluid is forthcoming. The procedure may be repeated in 3–4 weeks if the first attempt is unsuccessful.

Up to 90% of pleural effusions can be palliated with this technique. If the attempt fails, tetracycline, 0.5–1 g, can be used in similar fashion.

B. Ascitic Effusions: Ascites is generally best treated by attempting to control the underlying disease, usually ovarian carcinoma or malignant lymphoma. Mechlorethamine frequently induces chemical peritonitis. Thiotepa and bleomycin do not have a vesicant action on tissues and are thus more gentle. Spironolactone, 100–150 mg daily in divided doses, is occasionally useful as a diuretic in controlling ascites. For selected patients, the peritoneovenous shunt (LeVeen) may control ascites.

C. Pericardial Effusions: Pericardial effusions are best treated by irradiation except when previous radiotherapy has included the proposed field or when the effusion is due to a radioresistant tumor. Impending tamponade must always be anticipated and treated by pericardiocentesis, creation of a pericardial window, or pericardiectomy. If needle pericardiocentesis is performed for a malignant effusion, thiotepa may be instilled into the pericardial cavity (in systemic doses) at the termination of the procedure. Mechlorethamine should not be used, since it induces too severe an inflammatory response.

Caval Obstruction

The superior vena cava syndrome has long been considered to be a potentially life-threatening oncologic emergency. It is characterized by venous congestion and distention of tributaries of the superior vena cava, and thus the clinical presentation is with edema of the face and arms—frequently associated with dyspnea and the hazard of central venous thrombosis or cerebral edema. The syndrome may occur with various diseases, most commonly bronchogenic carcinoma and the malignant lymphomas. In the past, all superior vena caval obstructions were treated by radiation therapy with the addition of an alkylator, but the current tendency is for a precise tissue diagnosis to be obtained whenever possible and without delay, followed by institution of an appropriate chemotherapeutic combination or radiotherapy, depending upon the cause of the superior vena caval obstruction. CT scan with CT digital phlebography is the most valuable technique to define the site and extent of obstructing thrombus in the superior vena cava. Needle aspiration cytology of a lymph node or of the mass may divulge a histologic diagnosis. Mediasti-

---

*Spinal cord compression and cerebral edema are discussed in Chapter 3.

noscopy is still a controversial procedure, since complications such as bleeding may occur.

Bony Lytic Lesions

Palliation of metastases to weight-bearing bones is best achieved by irradiation. If pathologic fracture is impending, prophylactic fixation can minimize illness, especially in areas such as the femoral neck that are susceptible to considerable stress. Prolonged bed rest should be avoided whenever possible, for in addition to the usual complications, patients with bony disease are prone to develop hypercalcemia, and this tendency is accentuated by immobilization. Supportive bracing is often a useful adjunct for vertebral involvement.

Metabolic Complications of Neoplasia

A. Hypercalcemia Associated With Neoplastic Disease: Hypercalcemia occurs most commonly with myeloma, breast carcinoma, and lung carcinoma and is occasionally seen in patients with prostatic carcinoma, lymphomas, and leukemia. It has also been reported with a wide variety of metastatic or disseminated neoplasms. Symptoms include confusion, somnolence, nausea and vomiting, constipation, dehydration with polyuria, and general clinical deterioration that can easily be mistaken for progressive disease or direct neurologic involvement by tumor. The true nature of this metabolic complication may easily be overlooked, resulting in hypercalcemic death secondary to cardiac, neurologic, and renal toxicity. Hypercalcemia may be due to elaboration of a parathyroid hormone-like substance by tumor (lung carcinoma), to osteolytic sterols (as secreted by breast tumors), or to increased bone resorption by invasion and neoplastic destruction of bone (as in myeloma).

The mainstay of therapy to reduce calcium is hydration with isotonic saline (to promote a diuresis of 2–3 L/24 h) in addition to appropriate tumoricidal therapy, mobilization of the bedridden, institution of a low-calcium diet devoid of dairy products, and appropriate treatment of bacterial infections. If the patient was receiving androgens or estrogens for breast carcinoma, they should be withdrawn. Chelating agents such as sodium citrate promote renal excretion of calcium, and potent diuretics such as furosemide or ethacrynic acid also inhibit calcium resorption by the renal tubule. These measures, however, may not be appropriate in patients with impaired renal function or congestive heart failure or may not be sufficient of themselves, and other measures such as glucocorticoids (prednisone, 60–100 mg/d) may be required. The corticosteroids appear to act by reducing calcium resorption from bone. Oral phosphate is often rapidly effective, but intravenous phosphates are too hazardous to be recommended. Mithramycin, 25 μg/kg intravenously, is a prompt and effective agent for marked hypercalcemia. It may be the drug of choice where vigorous hydration is not possible because of renal failure or fluid overload; preexisting pancytopenia is a relative contraindication. Salmon calcitonin, 4 MRC units/kg intramuscularly every 12 hours, will also produce a rapid fall in serum calcium concentration in conjunction with other measures discussed above.

Among the newer agents with promising efficacy in controlling the hypercalcemia of malignancy is pamidronate, a highly effective second-generation bisphosphonate derivative that has just been released for clinical use. Adverse reactions include transient mild fever and local pain at the infusion site. Dosage is according to the severity of the hypercalcemia and ranges from 60 mg for moderate hypercalcemia to 90 mg for severe hypercalcemia, the dose being given as a single intravenous 24-hour infusion. If hypercalcemia recurs, re-treatment may be considered after a minimum of 7 days have elapsed. Another new and effective drug for hypercalcemia is gallium nitrate, which inhibits bone resorption and has a median duration of activity of 11 days. One drawback to its use is the schedule of administration, which is a continuous 5-day infusion. Nephrotoxicity is a potential adverse effect of the drug.

B. Hyperuricemia in Neoplastic Disease: Hyperuricemia is a potentially lethal result of high nucleic acid turnover associated with some cancers—especially after effective cytotoxic therapy. Uric acid nephropathy is related to intraluminal precipitation of uric acid in the distal renal tubule and collecting duct, with progressive intrarenal obstruction and failure. This sequence of events can often be avoided by maintaining satisfactory hydration and alkalinization of the urine to pH 7.0 by oral sodium bicarbonate (6–12 g/d) or by giving acetazolamide (0.5–1 g/d). Although allopurinol does not replace these measures, the preventive use of this drug (300–800 mg/d) should be considered in patients with leukemia, lymphomas, and myeloproliferative disorders. If mercaptopurine is being given, the dose must be reduced to one-fourth to one-third of usual when allopurinol is started. Peritoneal dialysis or hemodialysis may be required to treat established urate uropathy in conjunction with the above measures.

C. Fever in Neoplastic Disease: Fever is common when bulky liver metastases are present and is a constitutional symptom of disseminated lymphomas. Fever in these instances may be mediated by prostaglandins and can often be suppressed by indomethacin, 25 mg orally three times daily. Indomethacin is more effective than aspirin or acetaminophen. A thorough search for infection must be carried out before fever is assumed to be a result of neoplasm.

PSYCHOLOGIC SUPPORT OF THE PATIENT WITH NEOPLASTIC DISEASE

Samuel D. Spivack, MD

In this chapter, specific neoplastic problems and their palliation have been discussed. Successful management of the patient with these problems requires a coordinated effort in organizing specific methods of therapy by the physician in charge. Because continuity of care is an important factor in delivering frequently diverse therapies, any physician who undertakes primary management of patients with neoplastic diseases assumes an obligation that may extend from initial diagnosis to terminal care. Given the wide variations in the clinical course of malignant neoplasia, the need for effective management may thus extend from a brief time to many years. During this period, rapport with the patient and family based upon skillful treatment, effective and honest communication, and humane care and consideration will be among the major palliative benefits offered by the physician. Such a relationship can support hope despite the statistical unlikelihood of long survival, because the patient's anxieties and fears are usually of abandonment, dependency, pain, and loss of individuality or of dignity rather than of impending death.

HOME CARE OF THE PATIENT WITH ADVANCED CANCER

Samuel D. Spivack, MD

Some patients with advanced cancer and their families may prefer that the terminal phase of illness be spent in the home, with its comforts and access to relatives and friends. Careful assessment of the patient's physical and emotional needs must be considered by

Table 47–16. Checklist of supplies and potential equipment needs for home care.

Bedroom
1. Adjustable electric bed with egg-crate mattress or sheepskin pad.
2. Bedside commode, bedpan, urinal, and catheter equipment.
3. Oxygen tank, valve, humidifier, and mask.
4. Oral suction equipment.
5. Rubber doughnut or foam pillow.

Bathroom
1. Shower stool or bath bench and grab bars.
2. Elevated toilet seat.
3. Ostomy care supplies and disposable enemas.

Mobility aids
1. Wheelchair (collapsible).
2. Four-point walker or cane.

Medications
1. Analgesics
   a. Oral tablets or liquids (eg, morphine sulfate solution. Brompton's mixture. Schlesinger's solution).
   b. Parenteral premeasured narcotics in disposable syringes with needles and alcohol sponges (eg, Tubex).
   c. Suppositories (eg, hydromorphone (Dilaudid), 3 mg).
2. Antiemetics (eg, oral, parenteral, or suppository forms of phenothiazines).
3. Mouth care supplies (eg, hydrogen peroxide, viscous lidocaine, glycerin swabs, nystatin suspension or lozenges for candidiasis).
4. Nutritional liquid dietary supplements.

the physician before discharge from the hospital. It is important to ensure a smooth transition to home care by obtaining in advance all required equipment and supportive assistance (Table 47–16). Home care is not appropriate for all patients but must be individually determined. The physician in charge should ideally be the coordinator of all supportive personnel—including visiting nurses, the dietitian, home health aides, priests and ministers, and medical social workers—rather than delegating this responsibility to others who do not have an established therapeutic relationship with the patient and family. In many instances, the guidance thus provided is more significant and more beneficial than the specialized technical therapies discussed throughout this chapter. Quality of care is best secured by acting upon the principle that much can yet be done for the patient even when little can be done against the neoplasm.

48   Organ Transplantation

Nancy L. Ascher, MD, Fraser M. Keith, MD, Juliet Melzer, MD,
Oscar Salvatierra, Jr., MD, Nicholas J. Feduska, MD, & John P. Roberts, MD

The development of human organ transplantation is one of the truly outstanding medical achievements of this century. Working as a team, surgeons, nephrologists, and immunologists can totally rehabilitate most transplanted patients. Before the availability of renal transplantation and hemodialysis, all patients with end-stage renal failure succumbed to the illness. Although hemodialysis can prolong survival and provide partial rehabilitation for many patients with end-stage renal disease, only renal transplantation can truly restore them to a normal life-style. The success of renal transplantation was followed by heart and liver transplantation, and pancreatic transplantation is currently making the transition from experimental to therapeutic status.

KIDNEY TRANSPLANTATION

The principal biologic impediment to successful transplantation of an organ from one human to another human (**allograft**) is the immunologic rejection reaction that results from the genetic dissimilarity between the two individuals. It is rarely possible to perform a transplant between a genetically identical pair (monozygotic twins) (**isograft**). Transplantation of an organ between species (**xenograft**) has never been successful.

It was not until the early 1960s that practical immunosuppression became available with the advent of azathioprine and its combined use with prednisone. The success of this regimen ushered in a period of great enthusiasm and utilization of kidney allograft transplants.

There have been many other developments during the ensuing years, including refinement of surgical procedures, optimal utilization of living related and cadaver kidneys, and improvements in immunosuppression. This led to the performance of over 9000 kidney transplants in 1988 in the USA, of which approximately 30% were from living related donors and 70% from cadavers. These transplants were per-

formed with graft and patient survival rates far better than those achieved 2 decades earlier.

Renal diseases responsible for renal failure currently treated by transplantation are chronic glomerulonephritis, 50%; diabetic nephropathy, 30%; chronic pyelonephritis, 8%; malignant nephrosclerosis, 6%; polycystic kidney disease, 5%; and other renal disease, 6%. In patients age 10 and younger with end-stage renal disease, the incidence of glomerulonephritis is only 30%, and congenital nonobstructive and obstructive uropathies are more common than in adults (30%).

IMMUNOLOGIC RESPONSE

HLA Histocompatibility Antigens

The host response to the donor's histocompatibility antigens is the major biologic obstacle to successful transplantation. A single chromosomal complex of closely linked genes makes up the code for the major histocompatibility antigens. The **major histocompatibility complex (MHC)** in humans is called the **HLA system** (originally for human leukocyte antigen) and occupies a segment of the short arm of the sixth chromosome. The HLA system is now known to include at least seven histocompatibility loci: **HLA-A, HLA-B, HLA-C, HLA-D, HLA-DR, HLA-DQ,** and **HLA-DP.** Each HLA gene locus is highly polymorphic, so that about 8–50 separate antigens are controlled by each locus. The HLA chromosomal complex, including the HLA antigens, is termed a **haplotype,** which is the portion of the phenotype determined by closely linked genes of a single chromosome inherited from one parent.

Histocompatibility antigens are classified in groups according to function and biochemistry as class I antigens (at the A, B, and C loci) and class II antigens (at the D and DR loci). Class I antigens are composed of a 44,000-MW heavy chain carrying the alloantigenic specificity and a 12,000-MW light chain associated with β_2-microglobulin. Class II antigens are composed of a 33,000-MW alpha chain and a 28,000-MW beta chain that carries the HLA specificities. Although both class I and class II antigens can elicit an immunologic response, class I antigens act as targets of cytotoxic T cells, and class II antigens have an important function in antigen presentation in vivo and in stimulation in vitro of the proliferative response of the mixed lymphocyte culture (MLC). Class I and class II antigens are also distributed differently on cells. Class I antigens are present on virtually all nucleated cells in the body, including T and B lymphocytes and platelets; class II antigens are expressed only on B lymphocytes, monocytes, macrophages, some types of endothelial cells, and activated T lymphocytes, but are not expressed on platelets or unstimulated T cells. In the kidney, class I antigens are present on glomeruli, the vasculature, and tubules. In contrast, class II antigens appear to be located primarily on interstitial dendritic cells.

Lymphocytes are categorized as T or B cells. The cellular response directed against mismatched HLA antigens is T cell-dependent. Functional T cell subsets are generally divided into (1) helper T lymphocytes, which preferentially recognize class II antigens; (2) cytotoxic T lymphocytes, which preferentially recognize class I antigens; and (3) suppressor cells, which act to enhance graft survival. Allograft rejection is a complex event that results from the cytodestructive effects of activated helper T cells, cytotoxic T cells, B lymphocytes, antibodies, and activated macrophages. Activation of helper T cells by class II antigens stimulates the release of various factors, including interleukin-2 and macrophage-stimulating lymphokine. Cytotoxic T lymphocytes stimulated by class I antigens develop interleukin-2 receptors. Subsequently, stimulated macrophages and other accessory cells release interleukin-1, which in turn also influences the release of interleukin-2. Interleukin-2 then interacts with specific interleukin-2 receptors on activated helper and cytotoxic T cells, initiating DNA synthesis and eventual clonal proliferation of receptor-bearing cells. In addition, the continued viability of activated T cell clones is interleukin-2-dependent. In essence, the activation of helper T cells by alloantigens and interleukin-1 stimulates the release of a variety of lymphokines from helper T cells, and this process in turn activates macrophages, cytotoxic T cells, and antibody-releasing B cells. Although cytotoxic T cells are the dominant cell type infiltrating the allograft during rejection, helper T cells are most important in initiating the process.

The humoral response is also important, especially for class I antigens. Recipients who mount a primary immune response against class I antigens, manifested by the presence of cytotoxic antibodies in the serum, can produce an overwhelming secondary antibody response upon reexposure to the same antigens. The existence of cytotoxic anti-HLA antibody in a recipient at the time of transplantation (with a graft bearing antigen against which the antibodies are directed) results in an immediate destructive hyperacute rejection reaction, involving fixation of antibody to the donor vascular endothelium, formation of platelet and fibrin plugs, and ischemic necrosis of the organ. In practice, this is avoided by performing before surgery a complement-mediated cytotoxic cross-match with pretransplant recipient sera against T lymphocytes from the potential donor.

Histocompatibility Testing, Cross-Matching, & Blood Group Compatibility

When donor and recipient are identical twins, there is no antigenic difference, and grafts are accepted without immunosuppressive therapy, but such transplants are rare. Grafts from HLA-identical siblings give the next best results and constitute the most common privileged immunologic situation in transplantation. Nevertheless, even though there may be perfect matching for the major histocompatibility antigens in an HLA-identical sibling match, immunosuppression is required because of incompatibilities at minor histocompatibility loci. Parents, offspring, and half of siblings will share one HLA haplotype plus many minor antigens, since they have one identical chromosome.

HLA histocompatibility testing is primarily of value in searching for HLA-identical siblings; it has not proved valuable in choosing between parents, offspring, or HLA-non-identical siblings as donors—except to identify the zero-haplotype match sibling. Since cadaver organs are donated by an unrelated person, it is not surprising that many experts question the value of HLA matching for cadaver kidney transplantation. The HLA system is the most polymorphic genetic system known, and it is very unlikely that one will find perfectly matched cadaver kidney donors for prospective recipients. Nevertheless, six-antigen-match (at the A, B, and DR loci) cadaver kidneys do appear to provide better graft survival compared with lesser matched grades.

Regardless of the results of tissue typing and antigen matching, it is essential to determine whether a recipient has preformed antibodies against antigens on the tissues of a potential donor, since their presence would result in an immediate (hyperacute) rejection reaction. These antibodies can be identified by cross-matching the patient's serum against the donor's lymphocytes. Preexisting antibodies have usually developed because of prior exposure to foreign histocompatibility antigens, such as by blood transfusion, pregnancy, or previous transplantation.

Although histocompatibility and cross-match testing are important, an absolute prerequisite before kidney transplantation is the presence of ABO blood group compatibility.

Brent L et al: The role of immunology in the development of clinical transplantation. Immunol Lett 1989;21:81.

Gale RP, Reisner Y: Graft rejection and graft-versus-host disease: Mirror images. Lancet 1986;1:1468.

Gilkes WR, Gore SM, Bradley BA: Matchability in kidney transplantation. Tissue Antigens 1988;32:121.

Koene RA et al: Variable expression of major histocompatibility antigens: Role in transplantation immunology. Kidney Int 1986;30:1.

Kupiec-Weglinski JW, Tilney NL: Lymphocyte migration patterns in organ allograft recipients. Immunol Rev 1989; 108:63.

Mitchison NA: T cells in transplantation immunity. Immunol Lett 1989;21:15.

Opelz G: Influence of HLA matching on survival of second kidney transplants in cyclosporine-treated recipients. Transplantation 1989;47:823.

Opelz G: The role of HLA matching and blood transfusions in the cyclosporine era. Collaborative transplant study. Transplant Proc 1989;21:609.

The Influence of Blood Transfusions on Graft Survival

A. Pretransplant Blood Transfusions: Random third-party blood transfusions given before a first cadaver kidney transplant have a beneficial effect on graft survival in patients treated with immunosuppression using azathioprine and prednisone. The improved graft survival occurs whether or not the patients form cytotoxic antibodies in response to the transfusions. The mechanism of the beneficial effect is still speculative.

Pretransplant transfusions do not benefit recipients of cadaver organs who are treated with cyclosporine preceded by antilymphocyte globulin (sequential therapy) as the primary mode of immunosuppression. A number of multicenter trials report no difference in graft survival rates among patients treated with cyclosporine who did or did not receive pretransplant transfusions, but other reports, including those from our center, showed improved graft survival rates following pretransplant transfusions when sequential therapy was not utilized.

B. Donor-Specific Blood Transfusions (DST): Living related one-haplotype donor-recipient pairs with a high stimulating MLC have in our experience resulted in a 56% 1-year graft survival rate. In order to select MLC-incompatible related donor-recipient pairs that would experience better graft survival rates, and in an effort to alter the recipient's immune response, patients have received transplants after receiving transfusions from their prospective kidney donors (donor-specific transfusions) before transplantation. Graft survival rates for these patients were 94%, 90%, and 83% at 1, 2, and 5 years, respectively, using azathioprine immunosuppression.

The DST approach has also been applied with promising results with transplants involving poorly matched living nonrelated donors.

Most promising has been recent experience combining DST with the most effective cyclosporine protocol (sequential therapy). Graft enhancement with DST appears to be maximized with an immunosuppressive regimen that allows lower doses of both cyclosporine and prednisone than in non-DST-treated patients. Graft survival in a series of more than 50 patients at this center is essentially 100% at 2 years. Further experience and follow-up will be needed to confirm these early results.

Thus, it appears that MLC-incompatible living related donors, and perhaps living nonrelated donors as well, can now be selected with prospects of excellent graft survival. The posttransplant course of most recipients who receive donor-specific transfusions has been similar to that of two-haplotype matched transplants, and consequently they have required less aggressive corticosteroid therapy. Avoidance of potentially unsuccessful living related transplants is very important. For the potential kidney donor, the process of blood donation has been harmless, compared to the risk of donating a kidney that would probably be rejected.

The Influence of Presensitization on Cadaver Graft Survival Rate

The effect of previous blood transfusions and other methods of recipient sensitization on cadaver renal allograft survival has been controversial. Patients with end-stage renal failure often require transfusions and as a result develop antibodies. The more antibodies that form, the more likely that a donor kidney will be incompatible on cross-match. In our series, graft survival rate seems to be the same as in a nonimmunized recipient as long as extended testing of all reactive sera is carried out. The favorable graft survival rate of the hyperimmunized group is consistent with the theory that if potential recipients have been permitted to form cytotoxic antibodies to histocompatibility antigens, then cross-match tests will select only those kidneys with antigens to which recipients respond less readily.

The obvious disadvantage of presensitization is that it is more difficult to find a compatible cadaver donor, and hence the period of waiting for a transplant is prolonged. In general, the duration of the waiting period correlates directly with the level of antibodies. High levels of antibodies do not negate the possibility of a transplant, and in fact a number of successful transplants have been reported in patients with antibody levels as high as 100%.

Lagaaij EL et al: Effect of one-HLA-DR-antigen-matched and completely HLA-DR-mismatched blood transfusions on survival of heart and kidney allografts. N Engl J Med 1989;321:701.

Melzer VS et al: The beneficial effect of pretransplant blood transfusions in cyclosporine-treated cadaver renal allograft recipients. Transplantation 1987;43:61.

Salvatierra O: Current strategy for donor-specific blood transfusions, including a pre- and posttransplant role for azathioprine. Transplant Proc 1988;20:37.

Immunosuppressive Drug Therapy

The best current immunosuppressive protocol appears to be sequential (quadruple) therapy. This entails initial use of prednisone, azathioprine, and antilymphocyte (or antithymoblast) globulin. The latter drug is used only for induction until approximately 7 days post operation, with introduction of cyclosporine at 5 days post operation (2 days of overlap). If renal function is not good at 5 days (serum creatinine < 2.5 mg/dL), cyclosporine introduction and the 2-day overlap of these two medications is delayed. Subsequent tapering of prednisone and cyclosporine dosage levels is then achieved with time. Rejection episodes are initially treated with increased steroid dosages or, in the absence of an immediate response, with monoclonal or polyclonal antibodies as later described.

The primary drugs used for immunosuppression today are azathioprine, corticosteroids (prednisone), cyclosporine, and antilymphocyte or antithymocyte globulins. As a working hypothesis, it is assumed that the closer the histocompatibility match, the less immunosuppression by drugs will be required to achieve graft acceptance. Use of immunosuppressive agents even in lower doses imposes an increased risk of death and complications due to viral, fungal, and bacterial infections.

A. Azathioprine: Azathioprine is one of the mercaptopurine class of drugs and inhibits nucleic acid synthesis. Patients are maintained indefinitely on daily doses of 1 mg/kg or less, with the dosage adjusted in accordance with the white cell count. The drug may cause depression of the bone marrow elements (leukocytes and platelets) and may cause jaundice. In the face of untoward effects or in the presence of infections, the drug is temporarily discontinued or reduced. Azathioprine is never given in increased doses during an acute rejection episode, and the dosage may have to be reduced during rejection when renal function is poor.

B. Corticosteroids (Prednisone): Prednisone, which is used in almost all transplant recipients, is usually given in association with azathioprine and cyclosporine. The dosage must be regulated carefully so as to prevent complications such as infection, the development of cushingoid features, hypertension, increased bruisability, and acne. At our center, the initial maintenance prednisone dosage is 0.5 mg/kg/d. This dosage is then further decreased in the outpatient clinic until maintenance levels of about 10 mg/d for adults are obtained. In recent years, most transplant centers have used corticosteroids less aggressively than before; this has resulted in fewer problems with infection and in improved patient survival rates.

The exact site of action of corticosteroids on the immune response is not known, but it is believed that they inhibit the inflammatory aspect of rejection.

High daily doses of prednisone in children inhibit growth. This may be circumvented by alternate-day treatment, administering the drug once in the morning every other day. This dosage regimen is usually started after the initial 6-month period of daily corticosteroid administration, before which time there is the greatest risk of graft loss secondary to rejection. The exact dosage has not been precisely defined, but an initial 2 mg/kg in children on alternate days has permitted growth.

Therapy for a rejection episode may consist of increasing the prednisone dosage to 2–3 mg/kg and then tapering the dosage to a maintenance level, or of intravenous administration of larger doses of corticosteroids for a brief period, followed by tapering of dosages to maintenance levels. In general, immunosuppressive therapy should not be increased after the second rejection episode, nor should it be increased after the first rejection episode if renal function does not return to normal or near normal.

C. Cyclosporine: Cyclosporine is a cyclic undecapeptide isolated from a fungus. It is a potent immunosuppressant and the first compound identified that can inhibit immunocompetent lymphocytes specifically and reversibly. Cyclosporine is probably just the first of a new generation of important immunosuppressants. Its primary mechanism of action appears to be inhibition of the production and release of interleukin-2 by T helper cells. In addition, it also interferes with the release of interleukin-1 by macrophages, as well as with proliferation of B lymphocytes. Blood levels must be carefully monitored, for the drug is nephrotoxic and hepatotoxic and may also increase the incidence of neoplasms, particularly lymphomas.

The graft survival rate at 1 year for recipients of cadaver kidney transplants treated with cyclosporine is greater than 80%—better than the 55–60% rates with conventional immunosuppression (without cyclosporine). Cyclosporine has a major role in kidney transplantation involving related individuals. One-year graft survival rates of more than 90% have been reported for recipients of one-haplotype-matched related transplants in which recipients were treated with cyclosporine and did not receive donor-specific transfusions. The combination of DST with sequential quadruple therapy appears to allow the use of lower cyclosporine and prednisone dosages.

D. Antithymoblast or Antilymphocyte Globulin (ALG) and Antithymocyte Globulin (ATG): Antilymphoblast globulin and antithymocyte globulin are important adjunctive immunosuppressants. They are effective, particularly in induction of immunosuppressive therapy and in the treatment of corticosteroid-resistant rejection. Both ALG and ATG can be made by immunizing horses, rabbits, or sheep, but the main source at present is horses. Lymphocytes from human peripheral blood, spleen, lymph nodes, or thymus serve as the immunogen. In the Minnesota antilymphoblast preparation, a human T cell lymphoblastoid cell line is used. After immunization, the serum is recovered and the active globulin fraction is isolated. Some workers have used cultured lymphoblasts for immunization. The IgG fraction is purified and then given intramuscularly or intravenously.

E. Monoclonal Antibody Therapy: The focus of antirejection therapy has been to develop more specific therapy to control the rejection process. An example of such an agent is the monoclonal antibody OKT3, which is secreted by a hybridoma produced by the technique developed by Kohler and Milstein. OKT3 may have some advantages over ALG or ATG preparations in management of rejection in that it specifically blocks T cell generation and function. Because it is a monoclonal antibody and reacts with a defined antigen, it can be consistently produced with a defined activity and without unwanted reactivities. OKT3 efficacy may be greatest in the treatment of steroid-resistant rejection, where excellent results have been obtained and where further high-dose steroids are obviated.

Carpenter CB: Immunosuppression in organ transplantation. N Engl J Med 1990;322:1224.

Hiesse C et al: Multiple drug combinations with "low-dose" cyclosporine for renal transplantation: Multivariate analysis of risk factors determining short-term graft survival within one renal transplant center. Transpl Int 1988; 1:149.

Kahan BD et al: Pharmacodynamics of cyclosporine. Transplant Proc 1986;18(Suppl 5):238.

Kahan BD: The impact of cyclosporine on the practice of renal transplantation. Transplant Proc 1989;21(3 Suppl 1):63.

Lafferty KJ et al: Prevention of rejection by treatment of the graft: An overview. Prog Clin Biol Res 1986;224:87.

Lorber MI et al: Hepatobiliary and pancreatic complications of cyclosporine therapy in 466 renal transplant recipients. Transplantation 1987;43:35.

Martinelli GP et al: Pretransplant conditioning with donor-specific transfusion effect in the absence of sensitization. Transplantation 1987;42:140.

Sommer BG, Henry M, Ferguson RM: Sequential anti-lymphoblast globulin and cyclosporine for renal transplantation. Transplantation 1987;43:85.

SOURCES OF DONOR KIDNEYS

The three sources of kidneys for renal transplantation are living related donors, cadaver donors, and living nonrelated donors. Of all the patients who are acceptable candidates for transplantation, only about 30% have a willing and medically suitable living related donor. The donor must be ABO-compatible with the recipient. Living donors should be in good health both physically and psychologically. Above all, the living donor should be a volunteer and must clearly understand the nature of the procedure so that informed consent to the operation can be given. Donors must be of legal age.

Living Donors

Over the last decade, more than 10,000 people have donated kidneys for transplantation. In young donors, the remaining kidney hypertrophies and in a few months provides 75–80% of the original renal function. Follow-up studies on donors show that they have good renal function and suffer no ill effects from the procedure, either physically or psychologically. Women with one kidney do not have an increased incidence of urinary infections during pregnancy. Some transplant surgeons have advocated removal of the right kidney in women of childbearing age because of the increased chance of the gravid uterus partially obstructing the right ureter during pregnancy.

The main risk to a donor is the anesthesia and the operation itself. The death rate is estimated to be 0.1%—about the same risk as in driving 8–10 thousand miles a year in an automobile.

The most common complication following nephrectomy, except for minor atelectasis, is wound infection, which occurs in less than 1% of cases and is usually superficial.

After the donor has been judged to be a true volunteer and the risks and complications have been explained, special studies are undertaken in the hospital. A detailed history is taken, and a physical examination is performed. The routine workup includes chest x-ray, ECG, urinalysis, complete blood count, fasting blood glucose, serum bilirubin, creatinine clearance, and blood urea nitrogen. If these are normal, an excretory urogram is performed; if that is normal, a renal arteriogram is performed. Kidneys with multiple renal arteries may be transplanted, but care must be taken in the anastomosis of small accessory vessels. When there are multiple renal veins, the smaller veins may be ligated, since there is free communication of the veins within the kidney. If the arteriogram is normal, the patient is an acceptable donor.

Cadaver Donors

Since only 30% of recipients have a suitable living donor, the only way to provide transplantation to most patients is to use cadaver kidneys, which are in short supply, or kidneys from living nonrelated donors. It is essential to the success of the procedure that the transplanted organ be of good quality. This means that the organ must be removed before or immediately after cardiac arrest. Brain death must be established in cadaver donors before organs can be removed. Most states have legislation to the effect that a patient can be declared dead if irreversible cessation of brain function has occurred. The kidneys may be removed for transplantation up to 1 hour after cardiac arrest, provided intra-aortic flush with iced solution is used for in situ cooling of the kidneys. It is also important that the donor have relatively normal renal function at the time of death. Phenoxybenzamine or another vasodilator drug is often given to prevent renal vasospasm during the agonal phase.

There are two techniques for short-term preservation of kidneys: simple hypothermia and continuous pulsatile perfusion. With simple hypothermia, the organs are flushed with an appropriate solution, the most common at present being UW and Collins' solution. These solutions contain appropriate amounts of osmotically active but nonpermeable solutes such as glucose, mannitol, or sucrose, and their main beneficial effect is to prevent cellular swelling during hypothermic storage. Kidneys can be successfully preserved by cold storage alone, especially if warm ischemia was minimal during organ removal. However, after 30 hours, there appears to be a progressively increasing incidence of acute tubular necrosis—over 80% in organs preserved for 48 hours. The technique of simple hypothermia is the method of choice for small transplant units that perform fewer than 25 transplants per year.

With continuous hypothermic pulsatile perfusion preservation, kidneys can be stored for up to 3 days and perhaps longer, with a low incidence of acute tubular necrosis. This method of preservation eases the logistical problems involved in transplantation, since patients awaiting kidneys often live a long distance from the transplant center. Another advantage of pulsatile perfusion is that the sudden influx of a large number of cadaver organs can be easily managed.

Patients who are hyperimmunized with high levels of antibodies have a better chance of extended cross-match testing with perfusion preservation and therefore better graft survival. In addition, the presence of a low ATN rate with perfusion preservation allows maximum efficacy of cyclosporine with little risk of nephrotoxicity or permanent nonfunction of cadaver kidneys.

Enough kidneys and other organs for transplantation will not be available until there is greater public acceptance and support for organ donation. Many US citizens now carry Uniform Donor Cards that comply with the Uniform Anatomical Gift Act, which has been adopted by all 50 states. In addition in many states, persons may record the desire to donate an organ when they renew the driver's license; this is considered a legal document. The generally accepted age range for cadaver donors is 1–55 years, although donors up to age 70 years have been accepted after close scrutiny of the donor's general medical status. The cadaver donor must have evidence of good kidney function and must be free of systemic infection, cancer (except for primary brain tumors), and other diseases that could be transferred from the donor to the recipient by the transplant. HIV and hepatitis screening are mandatory.

SELECTION OF RECIPIENTS

During the early years of renal transplantation, most of the patients accepted for transplantation were in the younger age group from 15 to 45 years. In recent years, the age range has been extended in both directions—children below age 1 and adults up to age 70. Children between ages 5 and 15 do as well as adults below age 50. Children below age 5—and especially below age 1—seem to have a higher death rate but do well in centers specializing in infant transplantation. Infants and small children do poorly on dialysis. Although transplantation is not contraindicated in the elderly, the success rate is lower in these patients because associated diseases are more common; resistance to infection is less; and the surgical risks are greater. It appears that success rates for older patients may be improved by the use of sequential immunosuppression, so the number of older patients currently being accepted for transplantation is increasing.

The ideal recipient is one who has no serious infections or lower urinary tract disease, with minimal and reversible systemic disease secondary to renal failure. Recipients with the following primary renal diseases have been successfully transplanted: glomerulonephritis, pyelonephritis, polycystic kidney disease, malignant hypertension, reflux pyelonephritis, Goodpasture's syndrome, congenital renal hypoplasia, renal cortical necrosis, Fabry's syndrome, and Alport's syndrome. Successful transplants have been achieved in patients with certain systemic diseases in which the kidney is one of the end organs (cystinosis, systemic lupus erythematosus, and insulin-dependent juvenile diabetes). Renal transplantation is generally contraindicated in oxalosis because the disease recurs in the transplant quickly.

When the bladder is found to be unsuitable for ureteral implantation, a Bricker conduit has been used to obtain satisfactory urinary drainage. However, most long-term defunctionalized bladders can still be utilized for ureteral reimplantation. Patients with a history of peptic ulcer disease may be accepted for transplantation, but those with active or recurring ulcers refractory to medical therapy should first be treated surgically for this problem.

Emotional instability or psychosis has been thought to be a contraindication to transplantation, but successful transplantation may cure these patients if their emotional difficulties were due to uremia or poor response to dialysis. Unfortunately, there is no way to tell if the psychiatric symptoms are a manifestation of the renal disease.

Advanced retinopathy due to uncontrolled hypertension and peripheral neuropathy secondary to uremia often improve after transplantation. Diabetic retinopathy often stabilizes or improves after transplantation, so transplantation is frequently recommended for diabetics with renal disease before they reach end-stage disease.

The decision to accept patients in the poorer risk groups is usually based on the available dialysis facilities and the number of cadaver kidneys offered for transplantation.

Once a patient has been selected as a transplant candidate, either hemodialysis or chronic ambulatory peritoneal dialysis is usually started. If the patient is to receive a transplant from a living related donor, dialysis may not be necessary before the transplant is performed. Recipients awaiting a cadaver kidney will usually require dialysis.

Bilateral nephrectomy prior to transplantation was common in the 1960s but has been performed less frequently in recent years. The indications for preliminary nephrectomy are (1) severe hypertension uncontrolled by dialysis or medication, (2) anatomic abnormalities of the urinary tract with or without infection (eg, hydronephrosis, ureteral reflux), and (3) polycystic kidney disease with documented recurring infections or recurring episodes of gross hematuria requiring transfusions. Only 6% of recipients require preliminary bilateral nephrectomy.

There is no good evidence that splenectomy is of value before transplantation with current cyclosporine immunosuppressive protocols.

Broyer M: Kidney transplantation in children: Data from the EDTA registry. Transplant Proc 1989;21:1985.

Dyer PA et al: Evidence that matching for HLA antigens significantly increases transplant survival in 1001 renal transplants performed in the northwest region of England. Transplantation 1989;48:131.

Howard RJ et al: Kidney transplantation in older patients. Transplant Proc 1989;21:2020.

Land W: Kidney transplantation: State of the art. Transplant Proc 1989;21:1425.

Mattern WD et al: Selection of ESRD treatment: An international study. Am J Kidney Dis 1989;13:457.

Najarian JS, Sutherland DE: Transplantation in diabetic patients. Contrib Nephrol 1989;70:56.

Najarian JS et al: Long-term survival following kidney transplantation in 100 type I diabetic patients. Transplantation 1989;47:106.

Surman OS: Psychiatric aspects of organ transplantation. Am J Psychiatry 1989;146:972.

Sun CH et al: Serum erythropoietin levels after renal transplantation. N Engl J Med 1989;321:151.

Thorogood J et al: The impact of center variation on the HLA-DR matching effect in kidney graft survival. Transplantation 1989;48:231.

OPERATIVE TECHNIQUES

Great care should be taken in removal of the living donor kidney. The major difference between nephrectomy for transplantation and nephrectomy for disease is that the quality of the donor kidney must be preserved. This means that every attempt should be made to minimize renal ischemia and damage to the ureter. Renal ischemia may be minimized by hydrating the donor and administering an osmotic diuretic to promote a urine flow rate of 3–4 mL/min at the time of nephrectomy. Since the blood supply for the ureter arises from the renal artery, the ureter should not be skeletonized and dissected high in the renal pedicle.

Recipient Operation

The surgical technique of renal transplantation involves anastomoses of the renal artery and vein and ureter (Figure 48–1). In adults, the transplant kidney is placed in the iliac fossa through an oblique lower abdominal incision. The iliac and hypogastric arteries and the iliac vein are mobilized as indicated for the proposed specific anastomosis. An end-to-side anastomosis is performed between renal vein and iliac vein; an end-to-end anastomosis can be performed between the renal artery and hypogastric artery, unless the latter is too arteriosclerotic. In that case, the renal artery is anastomosed end-to-side to the common (or external) iliac artery. When multiple arteries are present in cadaver donors, the kidneys are transplanted with anastomoses of a Carrell patch of donor aorta containing the multiple renal arteries to the common (or external) iliac artery.

In small children and infants, a midline abdominal incision is used, and the cecum and ascending colon are mobilized medially, exposing the aorta and vena cava. End-to-side anastomoses of the renal vessels to the vena cava and aorta are then accomplished; the

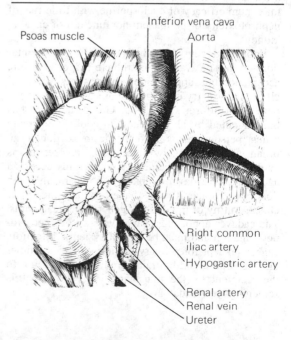

Figure 48–1. Technique of renal transplantation.

kidney is secured in its retroperitoneal location by approximating the previously divided posterior parietal peritoneum over the transplanted kidney.

Many centers have been reluctant to use small pediatric cadaver kidneys, and when used, pediatric kidneys have often been transplanted en bloc with the donor aorta and vena cava anastomosed to the recipient's iliac vessels, along with double ureteral anastomoses. We prefer to transplant pediatric cadaver kidneys as single units with the arterial anastomosis consisting of a Carrell patch of donor aorta and a Carrell patch of the vena cava for the venous anastomoses. Direct anastomoses of the small renal vessels to the larger recipient vessels too often result in thromboses. The en bloc transplantation of both kidneys into one recipient provides a larger functioning renal mass that more closely approximates the immediate needs of the recipient, but a single small kidney hypertrophies so fast that its function soon matches the recipient's needs.

Urinary tract continuity can be established by pyeloureterostomy, ureteroureterostomy, or ureteroneocystostomy. We have used ureteroneocystostomy by a modified Politano-Leadbetter submucosal tunnel technique in 3500 renal transplants with very few complications.

POSTOPERATIVE MANAGEMENT & COMPLICATIONS

Recipients who have received transplants from living donors usually undergo immediate diuresis and natriuresis. The magnitude is related to how hydrated the patient was before transplantation. The diuresis and natriuresis occur because the transplanted kidney is vasodilated, but the glomerular filtration rate as measured by inulin clearance is rarely above that expected for a single kidney. The kidney has been found to have a low PAH (para-aminohippurate) extraction ratio and a low filtration fraction but a normal TmPAH. How long vasodilatation persists after transplantation is not known.

Once this phase has passed, the patient maintains a relatively stable weight, although the weight may increase because of increased appetite and food intake. At our center, the urethral catheter is usually left in place from 5 to 7 days to ensure healing of the bladder incision. Most recipients may be started on a solid food diet with no added salt on the first to third postoperative days.

Kidney transplantation can be followed by a variety of postoperative complications that must be recognized and treated early for optimal results. A number of these problems are unique to the operation or to transplantation in general. In 3500 consecutive transplants performed at our center, the incidence of vascular complications was less than 1%. The most common vascular complication is renal artery stenosis, which is usually associated with rejection involving the renal artery. This may result in severe hypertension. It may be treated surgically or in some cases by percutaneous transluminal balloon angioplasty. Urologic complications occur in fewer than 2% of patients, most often urinary extravasation from the cystotomy closure, ureteral necrosis, or ureteral obstruction. These complications can be kept to a minimum by attention to technical details during donor nephrectomy and graft implantation. Early surgical treatment is necessary to avoid infection and loss of the graft. Lymphocele of the transplant bed, formerly a common problem, has now become rare with careful ligation of the adjacent lymphatics during preparation of the recipient blood vessels. Large lymphoceles may obstruct the ureter or vasculature of the transplanted kidney, and they occasionally become infected. Sterile lymphoceles may be drained into the peritoneal cavity, while infected lymphoceles should be drained externally.

Many complications of transplantation are consequences of immunosuppressive therapy, and they have become less frequent now that immunosuppression is less aggressive. Pulmonary and gastrointestinal complications are most common. Others include cushingoid changes, cataracts, aseptic necrosis of bone, steroid diabetes, and increased frequency of tumors (mainly malignant lymphomas). Pyelonephritis may affect either the transplant or the native kidneys. Preliminary nephrectomy is indicated in patients with an increased risk of pyelonephritis, such as those with vesicoureteral reflux or a history of recurrent infections or calculi.

Cyclosporine may produce nephrotoxicity, hypertension, and hepatotoxicity and, less commonly, hirsutism, tremor, gastrointestinal symptoms, gingival hyperplasia, and neoplasia. Acute nephrotoxicity and hypertension can be obviated by careful monitoring of cyclosporine blood levels, but the long-term effects of cyclosporine therapy are not yet known.

Bacterial pneumonia is now the most common pulmonary complication. Infections with viruses, *Pneumocystis carinii,* and *Aspergillus* are seen much less often than previously. Bacterial pneumonia can usually be treated effectively with antibiotics selected on the basis of drug sensitivity studies.

Gastrointestinal complications may affect all levels of the intestine, and the diagnosis is often difficult because of the masking effect of immunosuppressive drugs. *Candida* esophagitis occurs with a higher frequency in diabetic patients and usually responds to oral nystatin.

Peptic ulcer may develop after transplantation despite vigorous prophylactic use of antacids and drugs such as cimetidine or ranitidine. The problem is greatest in the early months following transplantation. Three out of four patients with peptic ulcer disease present with gastrointestinal hemorrhage. Factors related to the occurrence of peptic ulcer are treatment of an acute rejection episode (ie, when corticosteroid dosage is increased) and the presence of sepsis or hepatitis. The incidence of peptic ulcer has decreased by nearly half in the past decade (from 11% to 6%) as the intensity of corticosteroid therapy has been decreased, and the use of H_2 blocking agents has been liberalized. Further reductions in corticosteroid dosages are now possible as nonulcerogenic drugs such as cyclosporine have become a mainstay of current immunosuppressive protocols with a marked reduction in the incidence of peptic ulcer disease. The mortality rate of peptic ulcer was once very high (about 50%), whether patients were treated surgically or medically. However, the patients who died often had multisystem disease, with sepsis being the primary cause of death. Medical therapy to prevent peptic ulcers in transplant recipients must therefore be aggressive, and surgical therapy should be performed promptly if medical therapy fails. Prophylactic ulcer operations should be limited to patients with an antecedent history of peptic ulcer refractory to medical therapy.

Hepatitis and **pancreatitis** are other gastrointestinal complications that may occur in transplant patients. Hepatitis may be caused by viral infections (hepatitis B virus, cytomegalovirus) or may be a complication of immunosuppressive drugs (eg, azathioprine). Pancreatitis can also be a direct complication of immunosuppressive drugs (eg, prednisone, azathioprine), but some cases result from gallstone disease. The current incidence of posttransplant pancreatitis is about 1%. The incidence of pancreatitis is no greater in the early months following transplantation than later. More than half of cases of pancreatitis occur in patients with a normally functioning transplant, and only one-fourth occur in association with treatment for rejection. In general, patients with pancreatitis have higher serum cholesterol and triglyceride levels and a higher incidence of nephrosclerosis as the cause of renal disease. Patients with posttransplant pancreatitis have survival rates of 74% and 50% at 1 and 5 years, respectively, compared with 96% and 87% for patients who did not have pancreatitis.

Gottesdiener KM: Transplanted infections: Donor-to-host transmission with the allograft. Ann Intern Med 1989; 110:1001.

Metselaar HJ, Weimar W: Cytomegalovirus infection and renal transplantation. J Antimicrob Chemother 1989;23 (Suppl E):37.

Stoffel M et al: Treatment of cytomegalovirus pneumonitis with ganciclovir in renal transplantation. Transpl Int 1988;1:181.

GRAFT REJECTION

The major hazard for the postoperative allograft recipient is rejection. Most rejections occur within the first 3 months. There are four kinds of rejection:

(1) Hyperacute rejection is due to preformed cytotoxic antibodies against donor lymphocytes or renal cells. This reaction begins soon after completion of the anastomosis, and complete graft destruction occurs in 24–48 hours. Initially, the graft is pink and firm, but it then becomes blue and soft, with evidence of diminished blood flow. There is no effective method of treating this reaction, and patients who have preformed antibodies against donor cells should not be transplanted with a kidney from that donor. Pretransplant crossmatch testing can eliminate this type of rejection.

(2) Accelerated rejection usually appears within 5 days after a period of good function. It is believed to be related to subliminal preformed cytotoxic antibodies against donor cells not detected by the usual cytotoxicity techniques. It has also been suggested that sensitized cells could bring about this reaction.

(3) Acute rejection is the most common type of rejection episode during the first 3 months after transplantation. It is primarily an immune cellular reaction against foreign antigens and is characterized by oliguria, weight gain, hypertension, and blood chemical evidence of impaired renal function. Fever and tenderness and enlargement of the graft are less common with cyclosporine immunosuppressive protocols than was the case with prednisone and azathioprine therapy. This type of rejection process may be reversed by increasing the dosage of corticosteroids. If this is unsuccessful, an ALG or ATG preparation or a monoclonal OKT3 preparation can be used.

(4) Chronic rejection is a late cause of renal deterioration mediated by humoral factors. It is most often diagnosed on the basis of slowly decreasing renal function in association with proteinuria and hypertension. Chronic rejection is resistant to corticosteroid therapy, and graft loss will eventually occur, although perhaps not for several years after renal function begins to deteriorate.

Diagnosis

There is no single study that will pinpoint a rejection crisis. However, an elevation of blood urea nitrogen and serum creatinine appears to be the most consistent and reliable means of detecting renal deterioration secondary to rejection. The glomerular filtration rate as measured by creatinine clearance also declines. The urine shows an increase in protein and lymphocytes, and urinary sodium is low. Renal studies with iodipamide I 131 (^{131}I Hippuran) or pertechnetate Tc 99m may be used to confirm rejection and exclude urologic causes of renal function impairment.

Renal ultrasonography is often the first test to help

diagnose rejection and to exclude ureteral obstruction as a cause of deterioration of renal function. Prominence of renal pyramids and loss of renal sinus fat are findings consistent with rejection.

Magnetic resonance imaging (MRI) may also be helpful in diagnosing rejection and in distinguishing between rejection and cyclosporine nephrotoxicity. MRI reveals changes in tissue water content and blood flow, variables affected by rejection and cyclosporine nephrotoxicity. With rejection, corticomedullary differentiation is lost, while it is preserved with cyclosporine nephrotoxicity.

The diagnosis is made by analysis of the total clinical and laboratory findings. Although a rejection crisis will be experienced by most patients (HLA-identical siblings tend to have very few), they can usually be successfully treated so the patient will survive with normal renal function. After the first rejection episode, others are less frequent. There is evidence that a blocking antibody is formed that prevents host cells from attacking the graft's vascular endothelium. Whatever the mechanism, most grafts that are lost are rejected within the first 3 months; very few grafts are lost after 2 years.

Since most rejection reactions occur within the first 3 months, the death rate from immunosuppressive drugs is highest during this period.

Differential Diagnosis

There are a number of considerations in the differential diagnosis of rejection, including ureteral obstruction. With the current use of cyclosporine as a major component of immunosuppressive therapy, cyclosporine nephrotoxicity must be excluded as a cause of renal dysfunction. If a high cyclosporine blood level is present, cyclosporine nephrotoxicity is the most likely explanation; this can be confirmed if serum creatinine levels decrease after reducing the cyclosporine dosage. If the diagnosis remains unclear, a renal biopsy is helpful in confirming the presence of rejection.

Antibodies as a barrier to kidney transplantation. Lancet 1989;1:357

Hayry P et al: Local events in graft rejection. Transplant Proc 1989;21:3716.

HEART TRANSPLANTATION

Fraser Keith, MD

The first successful human heart allograft was performed in 1967. At that time, however, immunosuppression with azathioprine and steroids was inadequate to prevent significant numbers of deaths and morbidity from rejection and infection, and the procedure remained confined to an experimental state in selected institutions worldwide. The advent of cyclosporine in 1981 resulted in improved survival, and in 1985 heart transplantation was federally designated as no longer experimental. In 1988, there were 2500 heart transplants performed worldwide—1600 of them in 118 centers in the United States. The 1-year survival rate is 80% and the 5-year survival rate is 74%.

Selection of Donors

Cardiac donors should be men aged 40 or below or women 45 or below with established brain death. They should be ABO-compatible with the recipient and within 20% of the recipient's body weight. There should be no history of preexistent or intercurrent cardiac disease, which can most often be ruled out by echocardiography. Preferably, there should be no history of cardiac arrest and the donor should be receiving less than 10 µg/kg/min of dopamine. There should be no evidence of transmissible disease, and donors must have no evidence of bacterial infection and be hepatitis antigen-negative and HIV-negative. Donors should be free of a history of cancer except for primary brain tumor.

At donor cardiectomy, which is performed in conjunction with the harvesting of kidney and usually liver or pancreas, the heart is arrested with cold potassium cardioplegia and stored in a balanced electrolyte solution at 4 °C. Optimal function is obtained when the heart is implanted with less than 4 hours of ischemia. Because of the shortage of donor organs, donor age has been raised and ischemic time extended in some institutions.

Selection of Recipients

Patients for cardiac transplantation should have end-stage cardiac disease for which there is no other surgical option, should have received maximal medical treatment, and should have a life expectancy of less than 1 year. Most of heart transplant candidates have idiopathic dilated cardiomyopathy or ischemic cardiomyopathy. Patients should be less than 55 years of age, have a short duration of illness, have no systemic disease that will be worsened by the immunosuppressive regimen (infection, insulin-dependent diabetes, severe peripheral vascular disease, poorly controlled hypertension), as well as no underlying renal insufficiency that cannot be attributed to low cardiac output. Patients should have pulmonary vascular resistance of less than 5 Wood units, since levels above this or a pulmonary artery systolic pressure of greater than 50 mm Hg or a transpulmonary gradient (mean pulmonary artery pressure – pulmonary capillary wedge pressure) of greater than 15 mm Hg are associated with inadequate donor heart function. A history of compliance with a complex medical regimen and a strong social support system are necessary for long-term success.

The recipient's serum is cross-matched against a random panel of lymphocytes from a number of donors. If the percentage of reactive antibodies is greater than 15%, then a prospective cross-match between the donor and the potential recipient is necessary. Although human leukocyte antigen (HLA) typing is performed, there is only time for a retrospective cross-match. A higher survival rate is reported with one or no HLA-DR antigen mismatches compared with two DR antigen mismatches.

Operative Technique

The operative technique originally developed by Lower and Shumway continues to be used and is shown in Figure 48–2. The recipient heart is removed, and the dilated right and left atria are trimmed. The left atrial anastomosis is performed first and then the right, each with one continuous suture. The aortic and then pulmonary artery anastomoses are then performed. Topical cooling is continued, and the addition of blood cardioplegia after the atrial anastomoses may improve graft function. The implant time is generally 45–60 minutes, and "payback" time of support on total cardiopulmonary bypass after cross-clamp removal is determined by the total ischemic time and visual assessment of cardiac function. The heart rate is supported by atrial pacing or isoproterenol.

Immunosuppression

Triple immunosuppression with corticosteroids, azathioprine, and cyclosporine is the cornerstone of most immunosuppressive protocols and has allowed lower doses of each drug with fewer drug-related complications. Perioperative induction immunosuppressive therapy may include the three drugs mentioned or may employ T lymphocyte cytolytic therapy with antithymocyte globulin (ATG), antilymphoblast globulin (ALG), or murine antihuman lymphocyte monoclonal antibody (OKT3) in order to avoid the renal toxicity sometimes associated with early high-dose cyclosporine. Rejection is diagnosed on endomyocardial biopsy, which is performed regularly, since rejection may occur in the absence of clinical symptoms. Rejection is treated with pulsed steroids (1 g of methylprednisolone daily for 3 days) and resistant rejection with ATG, ALG, or OKT3.

Follow-Up Care

Transplant recipients must be carefully monitored for infection and rejection. Endomyocardial biopsies are performed every other month for the first year, then every 3 months. The incidence of rejection episodes is 0.5–1.5 per patient for the first year. The major infection rate is 1.5 episodes per patient for the first year and then declines. Accelerated coronary atherosclerosis occurs in 30–40% of patients within 5 years after transplantation. The only treatment of severe accelerated coronary atherosclerosis is retransplantation. Progressive renal dysfunction may occur over time and is probably related to the total cyclosporine dose. Patients with decreasing creatinine clearance can be converted to azathioprine and steroids alone with stabilization of renal function but with a higher incidence of rejection.

Alcerman EL, Wexler L: Angiographic implications of cardiac transplantation. Am J Cardiol 1989;64:16E.

Dein JR et al: Cardiac retransplantation in the cyclosporine era. Ann Thorac Surg 1989;48:350.

Heck CF, Shumway SJ, Kaye MP: The registry of the international society for heart transplantation: Sixth official report—1989. J Heart Transplant 1989;8:271.

Hosenpud JD et al: Abnormal exercise hemodynamics in cardiac allograft recipients 1 year after cardiac transplantation. Relation to preload reserve. Circulation 1989; 80:525.

Kirklin JK et al: Pulmonary vascular resistance and the risk of heart transplantation. J Heart Transplant 1988;7:331.

Labovitz AJ et al: Exercise capacity during the first year after cardiac transplantation. Am J Cardiol 1989;64:642.

Lagaaij EL et al: Effect of one-HLA-DR-antigen-matched and completely HLA-DR-mismatched blood transfusions on survival of heart and kidney allografts. N Engl J Med 1989;321:701.

Murali S et al: Hemodynamic abnormalities following cardiac transplantation: Relationship to hypertension and survival. Am Heart J 1989;118:334.

Renlund DG et al: Survival following cardiac transplantation: What are acceptable standards? West J Med 1987; 146:627.

Rose EA et al: Humoral immune responses after cardiac transplantation: Correlation with fatal rejection and graft atherosclerosis. Surgery 1989;106:203.

COMBINED HEART-LUNG TRANSPLANTATION

Fraser Keith, MD

Combined heart-lung transplantation was first performed in 1981. Initially it was felt that rejection of both organs would be evident in the myocardial biopsy. However experience has shown that rejection is dissimilar in the two organs, with heart rejection occurring infrequently and lung rejection, evidenced by obliterative bronchiolitis and arteritis, being a more severe problem. The current indication for heart-lung transplantation is end-stage disease in both organs or end-stage disease in one with poor function in the other prohibiting single organ transplantation. Examples are primary pulmonary hypertension, congenital heart disease with Eisenmenger's physiology, fi-

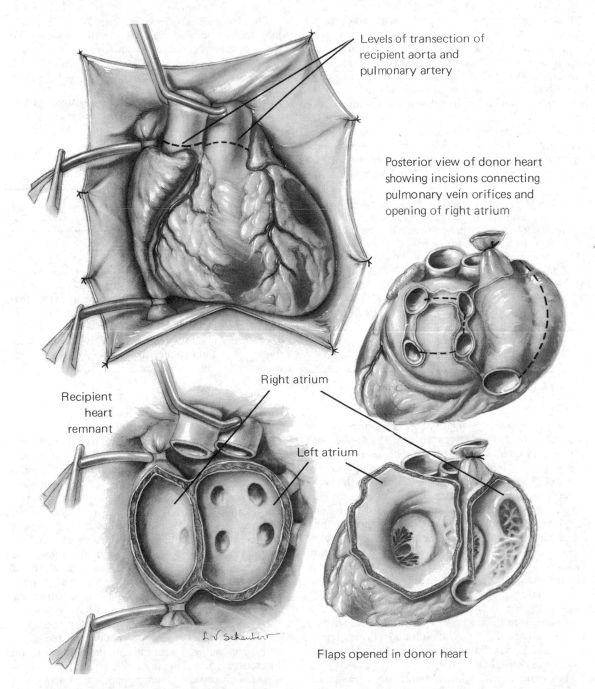

Levels of transection of recipient aorta and pulmonary artery

Posterior view of donor heart showing incisions connecting pulmonary vein orifices and opening of right atrium

Recipient heart remnant

Right atrium

Left atrium

Flaps opened in donor heart

Figure 48–2. ***Top left:*** Recipient heart showing levels of transection across aorta and pulmonary artery. ***Lower left:*** Implantation site with recipient heart removed. ***Top right:*** Posterior view of donor heart showing lines of incision connecting pulmonary vein orifices and opening the right atrium in preparation for implantation. ***Lower right:*** Flaps opened in donor heart in preparation for implantation.

brotic lung disease and cor pulmonale, and cystic fibrosis.

The operation consists of en bloc heart-lung transplantation with anastomosis of the trachea, right atrium, and aorta of the donor. Lung perfusion or total body perfusion has allowed long distance procurement, making heart-lung transplantation more practical.

Immunosuppression consists of cyclosporine and azathioprine with no steroids initially in order to promote tracheal wound healing. Heart-lung transplantation currently results in a 70% 1-year survival rate.

Griffith BD et al: Heart-lung transplantation: Lessons learned and future hopes. Ann Thorac Surg 1987;43:6.
Jamieson SW et al: Operative technique for heart-lung transplantation. J Thorac Cardiovasc Surg 1984;87:930.
McGregor CGA et al: Isolated pulmonary rejection after combined heart-lung transplantation. J Thorac Cardiovasc Surg 1985;90:623.

LUNG TRANSPLANTATION

Fraser Keith, MD

Single lung transplantation became clinically successful through a systematic approach by the Toronto Lung Transplant Group to the problem of bronchial disruption, which had made previous attempts unsuccessful. The addition of an omental wrap to the bronchial anastomosis and the avoidance of steroids during the first 3 weeks allowed bronchial healing and clinical success. Candidates for lung transplantation have end-stage fibrotic lung disease, are oxygen-dependent, and are likely to die of their disease within 12–18 months. Lung donors are scarce, but the use of one lung for transplantation does not preclude using the heart for another recipient. Long-distance procurement of lungs has been possible since institution of a regimen consisting of pulmonary artery flush with cold Euro-Collins solution following prostaglandin E_1 via the central venous line to promote pulmonary vasodilatation.

For patients with bilateral pulmonary sepsis, such as cystic fibrosis or bronchiectasis, or patients with emphysema and normal heart function, double lung transplantation has been carried out in a few patients. The advantage is that the patient does not have the potential complications of heart transplant and rejection. Another innovative approach to the lung transplant patient with a normal heart is the operation where a heart-lung block is placed in a patient with end-stage lung disease and a normal heart, and the recipient's heart is extracted and donated to a patient in need of an isolated heart transplantation.

The Toronto experience reports 12 of 16 single lung transplants and eight of the first nine double lung transplants surviving hospitalization.

Cooper JD: Lung transplantation. Ann Thorac Surg 1989; 47:28.
Pearson FG: Lung transplantation. Ann Surg 1989;124:535.
Stevens JH, Raffin TA, Baldwin JC: Status of transplantation of the human lung. Surg Gynecol Obstet 1989;169: 179.

LIVER TRANSPLANTATION

Nancy Ascher, John Roberts, MD

After many years of experimental effort, Dr Thomas Starzl performed the first human liver transplantation in 1963. The subsequent twenty-five years have seen markedly improved results (70–90% 1-year patient survival) and markedly increased activity in the field (more than 1500 liver transplants performed in the United States in 1988).

INDICATIONS

Since the introduction of clinical liver transplantation, the list of indications has rapidly expanded and the list of contraindications has diminished. The diseases for which liver transplant is most often indicated in adults include chronic active hepatitis, primary biliary cirrhosis, sclerosing cholangitis, autoimmune hepatitis, and alcoholic liver disease. Less common indications are Wilson's disease, α_1-antitrypsin deficiency, Budd-Chiari syndrome, and hemochromatosis. Alcoholic cirrhosis, a subject of considerable controversy, is now recognized as an accepted indication for liver transplant if the patient has demonstrated the ability to abstain from alcohol and is clearly committed to continued abstinence. Early reports indicating poor results in alcoholic recipients have been challenged recently by data indicating no difference in their outcomes.

Although chronic active hepatitis B is a frequent indication for liver transplantation (particularly in Europe), there are conflicting reports about the rate and severity of recurrent disease. It appears that nearly every patient with chronic hepatitis B infection and up to 20% of patients with acute hepatitis B infection become reinfected with hepatitis B after transplantation. The severity of the recurrent disease ranges from a new chronic carrier state to fulminant liver failure. A number of approaches have been tried in an attempt to decrease the rate of recurrent hepatitis, including the use of alpha interferon, hyperimmune globulin, and modification of immunosuppression, but none have been successful.

There is controversy also concerning the role of liver transplantation in the treatment of cancer in adults. In primary hepatocellular carcinoma or cholangiocarcinoma confined to the liver and biliary tree without nodal involvement, 5-year survival rates of 30–40% have been achieved; with nodal involvement, the results are poorer. An exception to these relatively poor results is seen with liver transplantation for fibrolamellar carcinoma, where survival exceeds 50%. The high rate of recurrence in cholangiocarcinoma has led the Pittsburgh group to perform cluster transplants in which the liver, pancreas, duodenum, and distal stomach are resected with transplantation of liver, pancreas, and small bowel as one unit. Follow-up of these patients has been short, but the results are promising. The rationale for cluster transplantation is to resect the nodal drainage shared by these organs.

The most common indication for transplantation in children is extrahepatic biliary atresia. Other common diagnoses are chronic active hepatitis, α_1-antitrypsin deficiency, tyrosinemia, and other inborn errors of metabolism.

Portal vein thrombosis, which at one time was a contraindication to transplant, is now managed by using vein grafts to bypass thrombosed vessels. Most transplant surgeons will perform liver transplantation if either the superior mesenteric vein, the portal vein, or the splenic vein is patent. Current absolute contraindications to transplantation are active substance abuse, positive HIV status in the recipient, and evidence of severe irreversible central nervous system disease.

DONOR SELECTION

The donors for liver transplantation are usually young trauma victims who have sustained an irreversible brain injury and have an intact circulation but are being kept alive on a respirator. Contraindications to donation are (1) HIV-positive status, (2) evidence of systemic infection or malignancy, and (3) massive and irreversible hepatic injury. It is not required that the liver size and blood type of the donor and recipient match; blood group incompatibility does not contraindicate donation, and livers can be pared down to accommodate a smaller recipient. Restrictions on donor age have been relaxed because the function of transplanted organs from older donors has been good.

The technique of preserving the liver grafts after removal from the donor is based on decreasing metabolic requirements by keeping the graft cold. Blood is flushed from the organ to prevent vascular occlusion; preservation solution is infused; and the organ is kept on ice at 40 °C. The University of Wisconsin (UW) preservation solution contains high-molecular-weight sugar molecules that do not diffuse into the cell, which keeps the cells from swelling. These sugars and glutamine act as free oxygen radical scavengers, which are thought to prevent injury upon reperfusion of the graft. The UW solution has extended the period of safe in vitro liver preservation from 10 hours to more than 36 hours. The distance a donor liver can be transported is thus expanded, and the extended preservation time has allowed surgeons to pare down livers safely in the cold.

OPERATIVE TECHNIQUE

In general, liver transplantation is an orthotopic procedure: The host liver is removed and the donor organ placed in an orthotopic position. The operation is performed in three phases: the dissection phase, during which the attachments of the diseased liver are dissected and the vascular structures are prepared for resection; the anhepatic phase, which extends from the time the host liver is removed until the time the donor liver is revascularized; and the reperfusion phase, during which blood is circulating through the new organ and the biliary tree is reconstructed.

Vascular instability during the anhepatic phase is avoided using venovenous bypass or preloading to overcome decreased venous return when vena caval flow is interrupted. Recipient portal vein and hepatic artery thrombosis are not contraindications to transplantation; donor iliac vein and artery can be used to bypass thrombosed or stenotic vessels.

The development of the pared-down liver technique to provide tissue for one or two recipients from a single donor organ has expanded the donor pool for small recipients. Although the results are not as good as with unaltered grafts, it seems likely that they will improve with time. The use of a segment (ie, left lateral segment) from a living related liver donor has recently become a reality and undoubtedly will often be resorted to in the future.

The current methods of biliary drainage—choledochocholedochostomy (if the recipient duct is intact) or choledochojejunostomy (if it is not intact)—have decreased the incidence of postoperative biliary leaks and sepsis. The indications for choledochojejunostomy include biliary atresia, sclerosing cholangitis, cholangiocarcinoma, size discrepancy between donor and recipient duct, and excessive bleeding from the recipient duct.

The method of rearterialization of the donor organ depends on the specific arterial supply to the graft. The incidence of aberrant vessels to the right lobe (from the superior mesenteric artery) and to the left lobe (from the left gastric artery) is over 20%. The celiac axis conduit may be used alone if the only variant is a replaced left hepatic artery. If a replaced right hepatic artery exists, the superior mesenteric orifice can be anastomosed to the splenic artery orifice or it can be used as the conduit itself with anastomosis of its most proximal end to the orifice of the celiac axis.

There is renewed interest in heterotopic liver transplantation with the new graft placed beneath the recipient liver. The heterotopic approach is best accomplished with a naturally small or pared-down donor organ because of space limitations when the host liver is not removed. The heterotopic graft requires portal inflow. Whether these grafts will flourish in the absence of vascular compromise to the host liver is unknown. Studies in animals indicate that a heterotopic graft requires both a source of portal inflow and decreased vascular inflow to the native organ in order to avoid atrophy of the allograft.

IMMUNOSUPPRESSIVE THERAPY

The use of cyclosporine as an immunosuppressive agent has greatly improved the results of liver transplantation. Most centers use triple-drug therapy (cyclosporine, prednisone, azathioprine) to take advantage of the synergy between several agents while minimizing toxicity. The dose of each drug is individualized according to the patient's sensitivity and toxicity. There is controversy about whether antilymphocyte preparations (OKT3 or ALG-antilymphocyte globulin) should be reserved for treatment of rejection or should be used for prophylaxis (to prevent rejection). In one controlled trial using OKT3 as prophylaxis, a benefit in prevention of rejection was shown without increased mortality or morbidity.

Efforts are under way to develop more powerful immunosuppressive agents with more specific effects. Starzl recently reported promising results with a new agent, FK-506, which is similar to cyclosporine in that it inhibits interleukin-2 production and release but is more potent. The agent has been used successfully in first-time transplant recipients and in individuals who are losing their grafts to rejection while receiving conventional immunosuppressive therapy. Given its potency and moderate lack of specificity, opportunistic infections would be anticipated to be a problem with FK-506. Randomized controlled trials will be necessary to determine the role of this immunosuppressive agent.

COMPLICATIONS

Complications following liver transplantation fall into two groups: technical complications occurring as a result of the transplant procedure and complications resulting from the host immune response or the results of immunosuppressive drugs. Technical complications include bleeding, primary nonfunction of the liver, hepatic artery thrombosis, portal vein thrombosis, biliary stenosis and leaks, and intra-abdominal in-

fection. Immune-related complications include rejection and opportunistic infections of viral, fungal, or bacterial origin, nephrotoxicity, bone marrow suppression, and steroid toxicity.

Primary nonfunction refers to a condition where the new liver does not function and death results unless a second transplant is performed. The incidence varies from 1% up to 20%. This entity occurs as a spectrum ranging from severe dysfunction to conditions where some aspects of liver function remain intact while others do not. The incidence may also reflect the availability of second livers; transplant surgeons with an ample supply of donor organs may be more likely to decide that a poorly functioning graft will not recover. The cause of primary nonfunction is poorly understood: donor injury before retrieval, preservation technique, and recipient immunologic response have all been suggested as contributing factors. Hepatic artery and portal vein thrombosis are fortunately rare early after transplant, as the consequences are often serious without retransplantation. Biliary stenosis or leak are frequent complications (5–20%) but are rarely lethal. The incidence of complications following choledochocholedochostomy is the same as for choledochojejunostomy. These complications can often be successfully treated with transhepatic tube drainage or nasobiliary drainage rather than reoperation.

Rejection—the most frequent complication of liver transplantation—occurs in about 60% of patients. It is characterized by specific histologic findings and usually is associated with abnormalities in liver function tests, though the latter may be nonspecific. The histologic features include a mixed portal infiltrate with injury to bile duct epithelia and inflammation of the central vein endothelia (endothelitis). The hepatic parenchyma is a late target for the rejection response. The pattern of injury mirrors the distribution of major histocompatibility complex (MHC) antigens on the surfaces of the affected cells. Bile duct epithelium and central vein endothelium are rich in class I and class II antigens, whereas there is a relative paucity of class I antigens and no class II antigens on hepatocytes. Rejection can be differentiated histologically from other causes of hepatic dysfunction—such as hepatitis—and graded according to its severity. When diagnosed early and treated aggressively, rejection rarely culminates in a need for retransplantation. Because the principal rejection target is the bile duct epithelium, severe unrelenting rejection is often manifested by destruction and disappearance of bile ducts (vanishing bile duct syndrome). The treatment for rejection depends on its severity. Mild rejection is treated with additional corticosteroids; moderate to severe rejection is treated with an antilymphocyte preparation.

Cytomegalovirus (CMV) infection is an the opportunistic infection seen in about 50% of liver transplant recipients. It is usually mild, consisting of fever, leukopenia, malaise, and viremia, but 15% of patients develop a more serious picture with pneumonitis or hepatitis. Patients most at risk for severe CMV disease are those without previous CMV exposure who receive a liver or blood products from a CMV-positive donor. Treatment for CMV is with ganciclovir. Although relapse is common (20%), repeat treatment is usually successful.

Epstein-Barr virus (EBV) is another common viral pathogen in these patients. Although the systemic illness with EBV infection is usually mild, it may be associated with development of a lymphoproliferative disorder known as "posttransplant lymphoma." Treatment consists of prolonged acyclovir administration and a decrease in immunosuppression.

Since fungal infections may occur, nystatin is used prophylactically to decrease gastrointestinal colonization by *Candida albicans*.

FUTURE DIRECTION OF LIVER TRANSPLANTATION

Developments over the past 25 years have made liver transplantation a common treatment for end-stage liver disease. Although liver donation has steadily increased, there is a marked discrepancy between the number of potential donors and the number of recipients, which will stimulate further developments. For example, living related hepatic transplantation using the left lateral segment may become common. Furthermore, hepatocyte transplantation has a potential role in patients with enzyme deficiencies such as α_1-antitrypsin (α_1-antiprotease) deficiency. The optimal technique for cellular transplant and the optimal immunosuppression regimen for this procedure are unknown. Xenotransplantation (the use of organs from other species) would provide additional donor material. The specific mechanisms of xenograft rejection and the appropriate treatment to prevent rejection are still obscure. Previous attempts at xenotransplantation have been uniformly unsuccessful because of uncontrolled rejection.

Disease prevention is another major area that could change liver transplantation. For example, increasing understanding of hepatitis C may lead to the development of a vaccine that could eliminate the need for transplantation in many patients.

Adler M et al: Relationship between the diagnosis, preoperative evaluation, and prognosis after orthotopic liver transplantation. Ann Surg 1988;208:196.

Ascher NL et al: Infection and rejection of primary hepatic transplant in 93 consecutive patients treated with triple immunosuppressive therapy. Surg Gynecol Obstet 1988; 167:474.

Auxiliary liver transplantation. Lancet 1989;1:533.

Broelsch CE et al: Liver transplantation, including the concept of reduced-size liver transplants in children. Ann Surg 1988;208:410.

Busuttil RW et al: The first 100 liver transplants at UCLA. Ann Surg 1987;206:387.

Colonna JO II et al: Infectious complications in liver transplantation. Arch Surg 1988;123:360.

Council on Scientific Affairs: Introduction to the management of immunosuppression. JAMA 1987;257:1781.

Emond JC et al: Liver transplantation in the management of fulminant hepatic failure. Gastroenterology 1989;96:1583.

Esquivel CO et al: Transplantation for primary biliary cirrhosis. Gastroenterology 1988;94:1207.

Iwatsuki S et al: Liver transplantation in the treatment of bleeding esophageal varices. Surgery 1988;104:697.

Jamieson NV: A new solution for liver preservation. Br J Surg 1989;76:107.

Kalyoglu M et al: extended preservation of the liver for clinical transplantation. Lancet 1988;1:617.

Krom RAF et al: The first 100 liver transplantations at the Mayo Clinic. Mayo Clin Proc 1989;64:84.

Kusne S et al: Infections after liver transplantation. Medicine 1988;67:132.

Letourneau JG et al: Biliary complications after liver transplantation in patients with preexisting sclerosing cholangitis. Radiology 1988;167:349.

Lewis JH et al: Liver transplantation: Intraoperative changes in coagulation factors in 100 first transplants. Hepatology 1989;9:710.

Makowka L, Van Thiel DH: Liver transplantation. Gastroenterol Clin North Am (March) 1988;17. [Entire issue.]

Marsh JW Jr et al: Orthotopic liver transplantation for primary sclerosing cholangitis. Ann Surg 1988;207:21.

Millikan WJ Jr et al: Change in hepatic function, hemodynamics, and morphology after liver transplant: Physiological effect of therapy. Ann Surg 1989;209:513.

Millis JM et al: Orthotopic liver transplantation for biliary atresia: Evolution of management. Arch Surg 1988;123:1237.

Motschman TL et al: Blood bank support of a liver transplantation program. Mayo Clin Proc 1989;64:103.

O'Grady JG, Williams R: Present position of liver transplantation and its impact on hepatological practice. Gut 1988;29:566.

Rakela J et al: Acute hepatic failure: The emerging role of orthotopic liver transplantation. Mayo Clin Proc 1989; 64:424.

Rettke SR et al: Anesthesia approach to hepatic transplantation. Mayo Clin Proc 1989;64:224.

Roberts JP et al: Liver transplantation today. Ann Rev Med 1989;40:287.

Shaw BW et al: Venous bypass in clinical liver transplantation. Ann Surg 1984;200:524.

Starzl TE et al: FK 506 for liver, kidney, and pancreas transplantation. Lancet 1989;2:1000.

Starzl TE et al: Liver transplantation in older patients N Engl J Med 1987;316:484.

Sterioff S et al: Retrieval of donor livers. Mayo Clin Proc 1989;64:112.

Stock PG et al: Biopsy-guided immunosuppressive therapy in the treatment of liver transplant rejection: An individualized approach. Clin Trans 1987;1:179.

Stock PG et al: Factors influencing early survival after liver transplantation. Am J Surg 1989;157:215.

Wood RP et al: Complications requiring operative interven

tion after orthotopic liver transplantation. Am J Surg 1988;156:513.

PANCREATIC TRANSPLANTATION

Juliette Melzer, MD

Although pancreatic transplantation involves transplantation of a nonessential organ as compared with the liver, heart, or kidney, it has enormous potential in the management of patients with insulin-dependent diabetes. In this disease, even though insulin and diet are carefully controlled, vascular changes in small arteries continue relentlessly. Many patients develop severe retinopathy at an early age, leading to blindness, renal disease and uremia, and peripheral vascular disease with severe neuropathy or limb loss.

There are approximately 1 million patients with type I (insulin-dependent) diabetes mellitus in the USA, and an additional 10,000 new cases occur each year. Hence, the potential usefulness of pancreatic transplants for treating these patients is obvious. Currently, whole organ pancreas transplantation with implantation of a duodenal cuff containing the pancreatic duct into the bladder appears to be the most promising. With this technique under coverage of cyclosporine therapy, about 65% of transplant patients survive for 1 year.

Much research has dealt with the transplantation of isolated pancreatic islet cells, which could eventually become the procedure of choice. Numerous studies have documented reversal of experimental diabetes by pancreatic islet cell transplantation in a variety of animal models and by several routes of administration. The feasibility of this procedure in humans would be enhanced if the islet cells could be successfully preserved before transplantation and if graft sites more accessible and less hazardous than the portal vein or the peritoneal cavity could be shown to be useful.

Bilous RW et al: The effects of pancreas transplantation on the glomerular structure of renal allografts in patients with insulin-dependent diabetes. N Engl J Med 1989; 321:80.

Cook DW, Sasaki T: Current status of pancreas transplantation. West J Med 1989;150:309.

Lloyd RV et al: Pancreas transplantation: An immunohistochemical analysis of pancreatic hormones and HLA-DR expression. Mod Pathol 1989;2:323.

Patel B, Wolverson MK, Mahanta B: Pancreatic transplant rejection: Assessment with duplex US. Radiology 1989; 173:131.

Sutherland DE: Coming of age for pancreas transplantation. West J Med 1989;150:314.

Sutherland DE et al: Long-term outcome of pancreas transplants functioning at one year. Transplant Proc 1989; 21:2845.

Squifflet JP, Moudry K, Sutherland DE: Is HLA matching relevant in pancreas transplantation: A registry analysis. Transplant Int 1988;1:26.

Stratta RJ et al: Early diagnosis and treatment of pancreas allograft rejection. Transplant Int 1988;1:6.

Tattersall R: Is pancreas transplantation for insulin-dependent diabetics worthwhile? N Engl J Med 1989;321:112.

Wright FH et al: Function of pancreas allografts more than 1 year following transplantation. Arch Surg 1989; 124:796.

REFERENCES

Calne RY: *Color Atlas of Liver Transplantation.* Medical Economics Books, 1985.

Castaneda-Zuniga WR (editor): *Radiologic Diagnosis of Renal Transplant Complications.* Univ Minnesota Press, 1985.

Egan TM, Kaiser LR, Cooper JD: Lung transplantation. Curr Probl Surg (Oct) 1989;26:675.

Stites DP, Stobo JD, Wells JV (editors) *Basic & Clinical Immunology,* 6th ed. Appleton & Lange, 1987.

Tilney, NL: Renal transplantation. Curr Probl Surg (Sept) 1989;26:603.

Appendix

Marcus A. Krupp, MD

TABLE OF CONTENTS

CHEMICAL CONSTITUENTS OF BLOOD & BODY FLUIDS

Validity of Numerical Values in Reporting Laboratory Results

The value reported from a clinical laboratory after determination of the concentration or amount of a substance in a specimen represents the best value obtainable with the method, reagents, instruments, and technical personnel involved in obtaining and processing the material.

Accuracy is the degree of agreement of the determination with the "true" value (eg, the known concentration in a control sample). **Precision** denotes the reproducibility of the analysis and is expressed in terms of variation among several determinations on the same sample. Reliability is a measure of the congruence of accuracy and precision.

Precision is not absolute but is subject to variation inherent in the complexity of the method, the stability of reagents, the accuracy of the primary standard, the sophistication of the equipment, and the skill of the technical personnel. Each laboratory should maintain data on precision (reproducibility) that can be expressed statistically in terms of the standard deviation from the mean value obtained by repeated analyses of the same sample. For example, the precision in determination of cholesterol in serum in a good laboratory may be the mean value ± 5 mg/dL. The 95% confidence limits are ± 2 SD, or ± 10 mg/dL. Thus, any value reported is "accurate" within a range of 20 mg/dL. Thus, the reported value 200 mg/dL means that the true value lies between 190 and 210 mg/dL. For the determination of serum potassium with a variance of 1 SD of ± 0.1 mmol/L, values ± 0.2 mmol could be obtained on the same specimen. A report of 5.5 could represent at best the range 5.3–5.7 mmol/L. That is, the two results—5.3 mmol/L and 5.7 mmol/L—might be obtained on analysis of the same sample and still be within the limits of precision of the test.

Physicians should obtain from the laboratory the values for the variation of a given determination as a basis for deciding whether one reported value represents a change from another on the same patient.

Interpretation of Laboratory Tests

Normal values are those that fall within 2 SD of the mean value for the normal population. This normal range encompasses 95% of the population. Many factors may affect values and influence the normal range; by the same token, various factors may produce values that are normal under the prevailing conditions but outside the 95% limits determined under other circumstances. These factors include age; race; sex; environment; posture; diurnal and other cyclic variations; fasting or postprandial state, foods eaten; drugs; and level of exercise.

Normal or reference values vary with the method employed, the laboratory, and conditions of collection and preservation of specimens. The normal values established by individual laboratories should be clearly expressed to ensure proper interpretation.

Interpretation of laboratory results must always be related to the condition of the patient. A low value may be the result of deficit or of dilution of the substance measured, eg, low serum sodium. Deviation from normal may be associated with a specific disease or with some drug consumed by the subject—eg, elevated serum uric acid levels may occur in patients with gout or may be due to treatment with chlorothiazides or with antineoplastic agents. (See Tables 1 and 2.)

Values may be influenced by the method of collection of the specimen. Inaccurate collection of a 24-hour urine specimen, variations in concentration of the randomly collected urine specimen, hemolysis in a blood sample, addition of an inappropriate anticoagulant, and contaminated glassware or other apparatus are examples of causes of erroneous results.

Table 1. Drugs interfering directly with chemical tests.*

Many drugs and metabolites react with ferric chloride and affect tests for ketone bodies, phenylpyruvic acid, homogentistic acid, and melanogen. Dyes (eg, methylene blue, phenazopyridine, BSP, phenolsulfonphtalein, indigo-carmine, indocyanine green, azure A) color plasma and urine; they affect most colorimetric procedures. Some drugs act as indicators (eg, phenolphthalein, vegetable laxatives) and affect tests carried out at a particular pH.

Test	Drug	Effect†	Cause
Serum			
Bilirubin	Caffeine, theophylline.	−	Color reaction depressed.
Calcium	Edetate calcium disodium.	−	Interferes with dye-binding methods; no effect on flame methods.
Chloride	Bromide.	+	Reacts like chloride.
Cholesterol	Bromide.	+	Enhances color when iron reagent used.
	Metandienone.	+	Interferes with Zimmerman reaction.
Creatinine	Ascorbic acid, salicylates, barbiturates, methyldopa.	+	Interfere wtih alkaline picrate method.
Glucose	Dextran.	+	Copper complex in copper reduction methods.
Iron	Intravenous iron dextran.	+	Total iron increased.
Iron-binding capacity (unsaturated)	Intravenous iron dextran.	−	Available transferrin saturated.
Protein	Dextran.	−	Hemodilution.
Quinidine	Triamterene.	+	Interfering fluorescence.
Uric acid	Ascorbic acid, theophylline.	+	Phosphotungstic acid reduced.
Urine			
Catecholamines	Erythromycin, methyldopa, tetracyclines, quinine, quinidine, salicylates, hydralazine, B vitamins (high doses).	+	Interfering fluorescence.
Chloride	Bromide.	+	Reacts like chloride.
Creatinine	Nitrofuran derivatives.	+	React with color reagent.
Glucose (Benedict's test)	Some vaginal powders.	+	Contain glucose: urine contaminated.
	Drugs excreted as glucuronates.	+	Reduce Benedict's reagent.
	Salicylates.	+	Excreted as salicyluric acid.
	Ascorbic acid (high doses).	+	Reduces Benedict's reagent.
	Chloral hydrate.	+	Metabolites reduce.
	Nitrofuran derivatives.	+	Metabolites reduce.
	Cephalothin.	+	Black-brown color.
5-HIAA	Phenothiazines.	−	Inhibit color reaction.
	Mephenesin, methocarbamol.	+	Similar color reaction.
Adrenocortical steroids 17-hydroxysteroids, 17-ketogenic steroids,	Meprobamate, phenothiazines, spironolactone, penicillin G.	+	Similar color reactions.
17-ketosteroids	Cortisone.	+	Mainly 17-hydroxy- and 17-ketogenic steroids.
Phenolsulfonphthalein	Dyes and BSP.	+	Interfering colors.
Pregnanediol	Methenamine mandelate.	+	Unknown.
Protein	Tolbutamide.	+	Metabolite precipitated by salicylsulfonic acid; by heat and acetic acid.
Uric acid	Theophylline, ascorbic acid.	+	Phosphotungstic acid reduced.
Vanillylmandelic acid	Methenamine mandelate.	+	Similar color.

*Slightly modified and reproduced, with permission, from Lubran M: The effects of drugs on laboratory values. Med Clin North Am 1969;53:211.

†Plus (+) indicates a false-positive or enhanced effect; minus (−), a false-negative or diminished effect.

Table 2. Some drugs affecting prothrombin time (Quick one-stage test) of patients receiving anticoagulant therapy with coumarin or phenindione derivatives.

Prothrombin Time Increased By	Prothrombin Time Decreased By
Acetaminophen	Aminoglutethimide
Allopurinol	Antihistamines
ρ-Aminosalicylic acid	Azathioprine
Amiodarone	Barbiturates
Androgens	Carbamazepine
Antibiotics (tetracyclines, some cephalosporins [especially cefamandole, cefaperazone, moxalactam], erythromycin, chloramphenicol, metronidazole, sulfonamides)	Contraceptives, oral
	Cyclophosphamide
	Digitalis (in cardiac failure)
	Diuretics
	Ethchlorvynol
	Glutethimide
Chloral hydrate	Griseofulvin
Cholestyramine	Mercaptopurine
Cimetidine	Phenytoin
Clofibrate	Rifampin
Disulfiram	Vitamin K (in polyvitamin preparations and some diets)
Glucagon	Xanthines (eg, caffeine)
Heparin (Quick test increased; no effect on prothrombin-proconvertin [P and P] test)	
Hydroxyzine	
Indomethacin	
Mefenamic acid	
Methimazole	
Metronidazole	
Nalidixic acid	
Naproxen	
Oxyphenbutazone	
Phenylbutazone	
Phenyramidol	
Phenytoin	
Propylthiouracil	
Quinidine	
Quinine	
Salicylates (>1 g/d)	
Sulfinpyrazone	
Thyroid hormones	
Tricyclic antidepressants	

Note: Whenever an unusual or abnormal result is obtained, all possible sources of error must be considered before responding with therapy based on the laboratory report. Laboratory medicine is a specialty, and experts in the field should be consulted whenever results are unusual or in doubt.

Effect of Meals & Posture on Concentration of Substances in Blood

A. Meals: The usual normal values for blood tests have been determined by assay of "fasting" specimens collected after 8–12 hours of abstinence from food. With few exceptions, water is usually permitted as desired.

Few routine tests are altered from usual fasting values if blood is drawn 3–4 hours after breakfast. When blood is drawn 3–4 hours after lunch, values are more likely to vary from those of the true fasting state (ie,

as much as +31% for AST [SGOT], –5% for lactate dehydrogenase, and lesser variations for other substances). Valid measurement of triglyceride in serum or plasma requires abstinence from food for 10–14 hours.

B. Posture: Plasma volume measured in a person who has been supine for several hours is 12–15% greater than in a person who has been up and about or standing for an hour or so. It follows that measurements performed on blood obtained after the subject has been lying down for an hour or more will yield lower values than when blood has been obtained after the same subject has been upright. An intermediate change apparently occurs with sitting.

Values in the same subject change when position changes from supine to standing as follows: increase in total protein, albumin, calcium, potassium, phosphate, cholesterol, triglyceride, AST (SGOT), the phosphatases, total thyroxine, hematocrit, erythrocyte count, and hemoglobin. The greatest change occurs in concentration of total protein and enzymes (+11%) and calcium (+3% to +4%). In a series of studies, change from the upright to the supine position resulted in the following decreases: total protein, –0.5 g; albumin, –0.4 to –0.6 g; calcium, –0.4 mg; cholesterol, –10 to –25 mg; total thyroxine, –0.8 to –1.8 μg; and hematocrit, –4% to –9%, reflecting hemodilution as interstitial fluid reenters the circulation.

A tourniquet applied for 1 minute instead of 3 minutes produced the following changes in reported values: total protein, +5%; iron, +6.7%; cholesterol, +5%; AST (SGOT), +9.3%; and bilirubin, +8.4%. Decreases were observed for potassium, –6%; and creatinine, –2.3%.

Validity of Laboratory Tests

The clinical value of a test is related to its specificity and sensitivity and the incidence of the disease in the population tested.

Sensitivity means percentage of positive results in patients with the disease. The test for phenylketonuria is highly sensitive: a positive result is obtained in all who have the disease (100% sensitivity). The carcinoembryonic antigen (CEA) test has low specificity: only 72% of those with carcinoma of the colon test positive when the disease is extensive, and only 20% are positive with early disease. Lower sensitivity occurs in the early stages of many diseases—in contrast to the higher sensitivity in well-established disease.

Specificity means percentage of negative results among people who do not have the disease. The test for phenylketonuria is highly specific: 99.9% of normal individuals give a negative result. In contrast, the CEA test for carcinoma of the colon has a variable specificity: about 3% of nonsmoking individuals give a false-positive result (97% specificity), whereas 20% of smokers give a false-positive result (80% specific ity). The overlap of serum thyroxine levels between hyperthyroid patients and those taking oral contraceptives or those who are pregnant is an example of a change in specificity from that prevailing in a different set of individuals.

The **predictive value** of a positive test defines the percentage of positive results that are true positives. This is related fundamentally to the incidence of the disease. In a group of patients on a urology service, the incidence of renal disease is higher than in the general population, and the serum creatinine level will have a higher predictive value in that group than for the general population.

Formulas for definitions:

$$\text{Sensitivity} = \frac{\text{True positive}}{\text{True positive} + \text{false negative}} \times 100$$

$$\text{Specificity} = \frac{\text{True negative}}{\text{True negative} + \text{false positive}} \times 100$$

$$\text{Predictive value} = \frac{\text{True positive}}{\text{True positive} + \text{false positive}} \times 100$$

Before ordering a test, attempt to determine whether test sensitivity, specificity, and predictive value are adequate to provide useful information. To be useful, the result should influence diagnosis, prognosis, or therapy; lead to a better understanding of the disease process; and benefit the patient.

SI Units (Système International d'Unités)

A "coherent" system of measurement has been developed by an international organization designated the General Conference of Weights and Measures. An adaptation has been tentatively recommended by the Commission on Quantities and Units of the Section on Clinical Chemistry, International Union of Pure and Applied Chemistry. SI units are in use in some European countries, and the conversion to SI will continue if the system proves to be helpful in understanding physiologic mechanisms.

Eight fundamental measurable properties of matter (with authorized abbreviations shown in parentheses) were selected for clinical use.

length: metre (m)
mass: kilogram (kg)
amount of substance: mole (mol)
time: second (s)
thermodynamic temperature: kelvin (K)
electric current: ampere (A)
luminous intensity: candela (cd)
catalytic activity: katal (kat)

Derived from these are the following measurable properties:

mass concentration: kilogram/litre (kg/L)
mass fraction: kilogram/kilogram (kg/kg)
volume fraction: litre/litre (L/L)
volume: cubic metre (m^3); for clinical use, the unit will be the litre (L)
substance concentration: mole/litre (mol/L)
molality: mole/kilogram (mol/kg)
mole fraction: mole/mole (mol/mol)
pressure: pascal (Pa) = newton/m^2

Number	Name	Symbol
10^{12}	tera	T
10^9	giga	G
10^6	mega	M
10^3	kilo	k
10^2	hecto	h
10^1	deca	da
10^{-1}	deci	d
10^{-2}	centi	c
10^{-3}	milli	m
10^{-6}	micro	μ
10^{-9}	nano	n
10^{-12}	pico	p
10^{-15}	femto	f
10^{-18}	atto	a

Decimal factors are as follows:

"Per"—eg, "per second"—is often written as the negative exponent. Per second thus becomes $\bullet s^{-1}$; per meter squared, $\bullet m^{-2}$; per kilogram, $\bullet kg^{-1}$. *Example:* $cm/s = cm \bullet s^{-1}$; $g/m^2 = g \bullet m^{-2}$; etc.

In anticipation that the SI system may be adopted in the USA in the next several years, values are reported here in the traditional units with equivalent SI units following in parentheses.

COMMON CLINICAL VALUES IN TRADITIONAL & SI MEASUREMENTS*

Albumin, Serum or Plasma

See Proteins, Serum or Plasma.

Aminotransferases, Serum

Normal (varies with method): AST (SGOT), 6–25 IU/L at 30 °C; SMA, 10–40 IU/L at 37 °C; SMAC, 0–41 IU/L at 37 °C. ALT (SGPT), 3–26 IU/L at 30 °C; SMAC, 0–45 IU/L at 37 °C.

A. Precautions: Avoid hemolysis. Remove serum from clot promptly.

B. Physiologic Basis: Aspartate aminotransferase (AST; SGOT), alanine aminotransferase (ALT; SGPT), and lactic dehydrogenase are intracellular enzymes involved in amino acid or carbohydrate me-

---

*The values listed below and in the following section have been gleaned from many sources. Values will vary with method and individual laboratory.

tabolism: These enzymes are present in high concentrations in muscle, liver, and brain. Elevations of concentrations of these enzymes in the blood indicate necrosis or disease, especially of these tissues.

C. Interpretation:

1. Elevated after myocardial infarction (especially AST); acute infectious hepatitis (ALT usually elevated more than AST); cirrhosis of the liver (AST usually elevated more than ALT); and metastatic or primary liver neoplasm. Elevated in transudates associated with neoplastic involvement of serous cavities. AST is elevated in muscular dystrophy, dermatomyositis, and paroxysmal myoglobinuria.

2. Decreased with pyridoxine (vitamin B_6) deficiency (often as a result of repeated hemodialysis), renal insufficiency, and pregnancy.

D. Drug Effects on Laboratory Results: Elevated by a host of drugs, including anabolic steroids, androgens, clofibrate, erythromycin (especially estolate) and other antibiotics, isoniazid, methotrexate, methyldopa, phenothiazines, oral contraceptives, salicylates, acetaminophen, phenacetin, indomethacin, acetohexamide, allopurinol, dicumarol, carbamazepine, chlordiazepoxide, desipramine, imipramine, codeine, morphine, meperidine, tolazamide, propranolol, guanethidine, pyridoxine, and drugs that produce spasm of the sphincter of Oddi.

Ammonia, Blood

Normal (Conway): 10–110 µg/dL whole blood. (SI: 12–65 µmol/L.)

A. Precautions: Do not use anticoagulants containing ammonia. Suitable anticoagulants include potassium oxalate, edetate calcium disodium, and heparin that is ammonia-free. The determination should be done immediately after drawing blood. If the blood is kept in an ice-water bath, it may be held for up to 1 hour.

B. Physiologic Basis: Ammonia present in the blood is derived from two principal sources: (1) In the large intestine, putrefactive action of bacteria on nitrogenous materials releases significant quantities of ammonia. (2) In the process of protein metabolism, ammonia is liberated. Ammonia entering the portal vein or the systemic circulation is rapidly converted to urea in the liver. Liver insufficiency may result in an increase in blood ammonia concentration, especially if protein consumption is high or if there is bleeding into the bowel.

C. Interpretation: Blood ammonia is elevated in hepatic insufficiency or with liver bypass in the form of a portacaval shunt, particularly if protein intake is high or if there is bleeding into the bowel.

D. Drug Effects on Laboratory Results: Elevated by methicillin, ammonia cycle resins, chlorthalidone, and spironolactone. Decreased by

monoamine oxidase inhibitors and oral antimicrobial agents.

Amylase, Serum

Normal (varies with method): 80–180 Somogyi units/dL serum. (One Somogyi unit equals amount of enzyme that will produce 1 mg of reducing sugar from starch at pH 7.2.) 0.8–3.2 IU/L.

A. Precautions: If storage for more than 1 hour is necessary, blood or serum must be refrigerated.

B. Physiologic Basis: Normally, small amounts of amylase (diastase)—molecular weight about 50,000, originating in the pancreas and salivary glands—are present in the blood. Inflammatory disease of these glands or obstruction of their ducts results in regurgitation of large amounts of enzyme into the blood and increased excretion via the kidney.

C. Interpretation:

1. Elevated in acute pancreatitis, pseudocyst of the pancreas, obstruction of pancreatic ducts (carcinoma, stone, stricture, duct sphincter spasm after morphine), and mumps. Occasionally elevated in renal insufficiency, in diabetic acidosis, and in inflammation of the pancreas from a perforating peptic ulcer. Rarely, combination of amylase with an immunoglobulin produces elevated serum amylase activity (macroamylasemia) because the large molecular complex (molecular weight at least 160,000) is not filtered by the glomerulus.

2. Decreased in acute and chronic hepatitis, in pancreatic insufficiency, and, occasionally, in toxemia of pregnancy.

D. Drug Effects on Laboratory Results: Elevated by morphine, codeine, meperidine, methacholine, sodium diatrizoate, and cyproheptadine. Perhaps elevated by pentazocine and thiazide diuretics. Pancreatitis may be induced by indomethacin, furosemide, chlorthalidone, ethacrynic acid, corticosteroids, histamine, salicylates, and tetracyclines. Decreased by barbiturate poisoning.

Amylase, Urine

Normal (varies with method): 40–250 Somogyi units/h.

A. Precautions: If the determination is delayed more than 1 hour after collecting the specimen, urine must be refrigerated.

B. Physiologic Basis: See Amylase, Serum. If renal function is adequate, amylase is rapidly excreted in the urine. A timed urine specimen (2, 6, or 24 hours) should be collected and the rate of excretion determined.

C. Interpretation: Elevation of the concentration of amylase in the urine occurs in the same situations in which serum amylase concentration is elevated. Urinary amylase concentration remains elevated for up to 7 days after serum amylase levels have returned to normal following an attack of pancreatitis. Thus, the determination of urinary amylas may be useful if the patient is seen late in the course of an attack of pancreatitis. An elevated serum amylase with a normal or low urine amylase excretory rate may be seen in the presence of renal insufficiency or with macroamylasemia.

Bilirubin, Serum

Normal: Total, 1.1–1.2 mg/dL (SI: 3.5–19 µmol/L). Direct (glucuronide), 0.1–0.4 mg/dL. Indirect (unconjugated), 0.2–0.7 mg/dL. (SI: direct, up to 7 µmol/L; indirect, up to 12 µmol/L.)

A. Precautions: The fasting state is preferred to avoid turbidity of serum. For optimal stability of stored serum, samples should be frozen and stored in the dark.

B. Physiologic Basis: Destruction of hemoglobin yields bilirubin, which is conjugated in the liver to the diglucuronide and excreted in the bile. Bilirubin accumulates in the plasma when liver insufficiency exists, biliary obstruction is present, or the rate of hemolysis increases. Rarely, abnormalities of enzyme systems involved in bilirubin metabolism in the liver (eg, absence of glucuronyl transferase) result in abnormal bilirubin concentrations.

C. Interpretation:

1. Direct and indirect forms of serum bilirubin are elevated in acute or chronic hepatitis; biliary tract obstruction (cholangiolar, hepatic, or common ducts); toxic reactions to many drugs, chemicals, and toxins; and Dubin-Johnson and Rotor's syndromes.

2. Indirect serum bilirubin is elevated in hemolytic diseases or reactions and absence or deficiency of glucuronyl transferase, as in Gilbert's disease and Crigler-Najjar syndrome.

3. Direct and total bilirubin can be significantly elevated in normal and jaundiced subjects by fasting 24–48 hours (in some instances even 12 hours) or by prolonged caloric restriction.

D. Drug Effects on Laboratory Results: Elevated by acetaminophen, chlordiazepoxide, novobiocin, and acetohexamide. Many drugs produce either hepatocellular damage or cholestasis.

Calcium, Serum

Normal: Total, 8.5–10.3 mg/dL or 4.2–5.2 meq/L. Ionized, 4.2–5.2 mg/dL or 2.1–2.6 meq/L. (SI: total, 2.1–2.6 mmol/L; ionized, 1.05–1.3 mmol/L.)

A. Precautions: Glassware must be free of calcium. The patient should be fasting. Serum should be promptly separated from the clot.

B. Physiologic Basis: Endocrine, renal, gastrointestinal, and nutritional factors normally provide for precise regulation of calcium concentration in plasma and other body fluids. Since some calcium is bound to plasma protein, especially albumin, determination of the plasma albumin concentration is necessary before the clinical significance of abnormal serum calcium levels can be interpreted accurately.

C. Interpretation:

1. Elevated in hyperparathyroidism, secretion of parathyroid-like hormone by malignant tumors, vitamin D excess, milk-alkali syndrome, osteolytic disease such as multiple myeloma, invasion of bone by metastatic cancer, Paget's disease of bone, Boeck's sarcoid, immobilization, and familial hypocalciuria. Occasionally elevated with hyperthyroidism and with ingestion of thiazide drugs.

2. Decreased in hypoparathyroidism, vitamin D deficiency (rickets, osteomalacia), renal insufficiency, hypoproteinemia, malabsorption syndrome (sprue, ileitis, celiac disease, pancreatic insufficiency), severe pancreatitis with pancreatic necrosis, and pseudohypoparathyroidism.

Calcium, Urine (Daily Excretion)

Ordinarily there is a moderate continuous urinary calcium excretion of 50–150 mg/24 h, depending upon the intake. (SI: 1.2–3.7 mmol/24 h.)

A. Procedure: The patient should remain on a diet free of milk and cheese for 3 days prior to testing; for quantitative testing, a neutral ash diet containing about 150 mg calcium per day is given for 3 days. Quantitative calcium excretion studies may be made on a carefully timed 24-hour urine specimen.

B. Interpretation: On the quantitative diet, a normal person excretes 125 ± 50 mg (1.8–4.4 mmol) of calcium per 24 hours. In hyperparathyroidism, the urinary calcium excretion usually exceeds 200 mg/24 h (5 mmol/d). Urinary calcium excretion is almost always elevated when serum calcium is high.

Cholesterol, Serum or Plasma

Normal: 150–280 mg/dL. (SI: 3.9–7.2 mmol/L.) See Table 3.

A. Precautions: The fasting state is preferred.

B. Physiologic Basis: Cholesterol concentrations are determined by metabolic functions, which are influenced by heredity, nutrition, endocrine function, and integrity of vital organs such as the liver and kidney. Cholesterol metabolism is intimately associated with lipid metabolism.

C. Interpretation:

Table 3. Lipidemia: Ranges of population (USA) for serum concentrations of cholesterol (C), triglyceride (TG), low-density lipoprotein cholesterol (LDL-C), and high-density lipoprotein cholesterol (HDL-C).*

Age	C (mg/dL)	TG (mg/dL)	LDL-C (mg/dL) Upper Limit	HDL-C (mg/dL)	
				Male	Female
<29	120–240	10–140	170	45 ± 12	55 ± 12
30–39	140–270	10–150	190		
40–49	150–310	10–160	190		
>49	160–330	10–190	210		

*Reproduced, with permission, from Krupp MA et al: *Physician's Handbook*, 21st ed. Lange, 1985.

1. **Elevated** in familial hypercholesterolemia (xanthomatosis), hypothyroidism, poorly controlled diabetes mellitus, nephrotic syndrome, chronic hepatitis, biliary cirrhosis, obstructive jaundice, hypoproteinemia (idiopathic, with nephrosis or chronic hepatitis), and lipidemia (idiopathic, familial).

2. **Decreased** in acute hepatitis and Gaucher's disease. Occasionally decreased in hyperthyroidism, acute infections, anemia, malnutrition, and apolipoprotein deficiency.

D. Drug Effects on Laboratory Results: Elevated by bromides, anabolic agents, trimethadione, and oral contraceptives. Decreased by cholestyramine resin, haloperidol, nicotinic acid, salicylates, thyroid hormone, estrogens, clofibrate, chlorpropamide, phenformin, kanamycin, neomycin, and phenyramidol.

Creatine Kinase (CK) or Creatine Phosphokinase (CPK), Serum

Normal (varies with method): 10–50 IU/L at 30 °C.

A. Precautions: The enzyme is unstable, and the red cell content inhibits enzyme activity. Serum must be removed from the clot promptly. If assay cannot be done soon after drawing blood, serum must be frozen.

B. Physiologic Basis: CPK splits creatine phosphate in the presence of ADP to yield creatine and ATP. Skeletal and heart muscle and brain are rich in the enzyme.

C. Interpretation:

1. **Elevated** in the presence of muscle damage such as with myocardial infarction, trauma to muscle, muscular dystrophies, polymyositis, severe muscular exertion (jogging), hypothyroidism, and cerebral infarction (necrosis). Following myocardial infarction, serum CK concentration increases rapidly (within 3–5 hours), and it remains elevated for a shorter time after the episode (2 or 3 days) than does AST or LDH.

2. **Not elevated** in pulmonary infarction or parenchymal liver disease.

Creatine Kinase Isoenzymes, Serum

See Table 4.

A. Precautions: As for CK (see above).

B. Physiologic Basis: CK consists of three proteins separable by electrophoresis. Skeletal muscle is characterized by isoenzyme MM, myocardium by isoenzyme MB, and brain by isoenzyme BB.

C. Interpretation: CK isoenzymes are increased in serum. CK-MM is elevated in injury to skeletal muscle, myocardial muscle, and brain; in muscle disease (eg, dystrophies, hypothyroidism, dermatomyositis, polymyositis); in rhabdomyolysis; and after severe exercise. CK-MB is elevated soon (within 2–4 hours) after myocardial infarction and for up to 72 hours afterward (high levels are prolonged with extension of infarct or new infarction); also elevated in extensive rhabdomyolysis or muscle injury, severe muscle disease, Reye's syndrome, or Rocky Mountain spotted fever. CK-BB is occasionally elevated in severe shock, in some carcinomas (especially oat cell carcinoma or carcinoma of the ovary, breast, or prostate), or in biliary atresia.

Creatine, Urine (24 Hours)

Normal: See Table 5.

A. Precautions: Collection of the 24-hour specimen must be accurate. The specimen may be refrigerated or preserved with 10 mL of toluene or 10 mL of 5% thymol in chloroform.

B. Physiologic Basis: Creatine is an important constituent of muscle, brain, and blood; in the form of creatine phosphate, it serves as a source of high-energy phosphate. Normally, small amounts of creatine are excreted in the urine, but in states of elevated catabolism and in the presence of muscular dystrophies, the rate of excretion is increased.

C. Interpretation:

1. **Elevated** in muscular dystrophies such as progressive muscular dystrophy, myotonia atrophica, and myasthenia gravis; muscle wasting, as in acute poliomyelitis, amyotrophic lateral sclerosis, and myositis; starvation and cachectic states; hyperthyroidism; and febrile diseases.

2. **Decreased** in hypothyroidism, amyotonia congenita, and renal insufficiency.

Creatinine, Serum or Plasma

Normal: 0.7—1.5 mg/dL. (SI: 60—132 µmol/L.)

A. Precautions: None.

B. Physiologic Basis: Endogenous creatinine is excreted by filtration through the glomerulus and by tubular secretion at a rate about 20% greater than

Table 4. Creatine kinase isoenzymes.

Isoenzyme		Normal Levels % of Total
(Fastest)	Fraction 1, BB	0
	Fraction 2, MB	0–3
(Slowest)	Fraction 3, MM	97–100

Table 5. Urine creatine and creatinine, normal values (24 hours).[1]

	Creatine	Creatinine
Newborn	4.5 mg/kg	10 mg/kg
1–7 months	8.1 mg/kg	12.8 mg/kg
2–3 years	7.9 mg/kg	12.1 mg/kg
4–4½ years	4.5 mg/kg	14.6 mg/kg
9–9½ years	2.5 mg/kg	18.1 mg/kg
11–14 years	2.7 mg/kg	20.1 mg/kg
Adult male	0–50 mg	25 mg/kg
Adult female	0–100 mg	21 mg/kg

[1]SI factors: creatine, mg/24 h × 7.63 – µmol/24 h; creatinine, mg/24 h × 8.84 = µmol/24 h.

clearance of inulin. The Jaffe reaction measures chromogens other than creatinine in the plasma. Because the chromogens are not passed into the urine, the measurement of creatinine in the urine is about 20% less than chromogen plus creatinine in plasma, providing, fortuitously, a compensation for the amount secreted. Thus, inulin and creatinine clearances for clinical purposes are comparable and creatinine clearance is an acceptable measure of glomerular filtration rate—except that with advancing renal failure, creatinine clearance exceeds inulin clearance owing to the secretion of creatinine by remaining renal tubules.

C. Interpretation: Creatinine is elevated in acute or chronic renal insufficiency, urinary tract obstruction, and impairment of renal function induced by some drugs. Materials other than creatinine may react to give falsely high results with the alkaline picrate method (Jaffe reaction): acetoacetate, acetone, β-hydroxybutyrate, α-ketoglutarate, pyruvate, glucose, bilirubin, hemoglobin, urea, and uric acid. Values below 0.7 mg/dL are of no known significance.

D. Drug Effects on Laboratory Results: Elevated by ascorbic acid, salicylates, barbiturates, sulfobromophthalein, methyldopa, and phenolsulfonphthalein, all of which interfere with the determination by the alkaline picrate method.

Creatinine, Urine

Normal: See Table 5.

Glucose, Serum or Plasma

Normal: Fasting "true" glucose, 65–110 mg/dL. (SI: 3.6–6.1 mmol/L.)

A. Precautions: If determination is delayed beyond 1 hour, sodium fluoride, about 3 mg/mL blood, should be added to the specimen. The filtrates may be refrigerated for up to 24 hours. Errors in interpretation may occur if the patient has eaten sugar or received glucose solution parenterally just prior to the collection of what is thought to be a "fasting" specimen.

B. Physiologic Basis: The glucose concentration in extracellular fluid is normally closely regulated, with the result that a source of energy is available to tissues, and no glucose is excreted in the urine. Hyperglycemia and hypoglycemia are nonspecific signs of abnormal glucose metabolism.

C. Interpretation:

1. Elevated in diabetes, hyperthyroidism, adrenocortical hyperactivity (cortical excess), hyperpituitarism, and hepatic disease (occasionally).

2. Decreased in hyperinsulinism, adrenal insufficiency, hypopituitarism, hepatic insufficiency (occasionally), functional hypoglycemia, and hypoglycemic agents.

D. Drug Effects on Laboratory Results: Elevated by corticosteroids, chlorthalidone, thiazide diuretics, furosemide, ethacrynic acid, triamterene, in-

domethacin, oral contraceptives (estrogen-progestin combinations), isoniazid, nicotinic acid (large doses), phenothiazines, and paraldehyde. Decreased by acetaminophen, phenacetin, cyproheptadine, pargyline, and propranolol.

γ-Glutamyl Transpeptidase or Transferase, Serum

Normal: Males, < 30 mU/mL at 30 °C. Females, < 25 mU/mL at 30 °C. Adolescents, < 50 mU/mL at 30 °C.

A. Precautions: Avoid hemolysis.

B. Physiologic Basis: γ-Glutamyl transferase (GGT) is an extremely sensitive indicator of liver disease. Levels are often elevated when transaminases and alkaline phosphatase are normal, and it is considered more specific than both for identifying liver impairment due to alcoholism.

The enzyme is present in liver, kidney, and pancreas and transfers C-terminal glutamic acid from a peptide to other peptides or λ-amino acids. It is induced by alcohol.

C. Interpretation: Elevated in acute infectious or toxic hepatitis, chronic and subacute hepatitis, cirrhosis of the liver, intrahepatic or extrahepatic obstruction, primary or metastatic liver neoplasms, and liver damage due to alcoholism. It is elevated occasionally by congestive heart failure and rarely in postmyocardial infarction, pancreatitis, and pancreatic carcinoma.

Iron, Serum

Normal: 50–175 μg/dL. (SI: 9–31.3 μmol/L.)

A. Precautions: Syringes and needles must be iron-free. Hemolysis of blood must be avoided. The serum must be free of hemoglobin.

B. Physiologic Basis: Because of diurnal variation with highest values in the morning, fasting morning blood specimens are desirable. Iron concentration in the plasma is determined by several factors, including absorption from the intestine, storage in intestine, liver, spleen, and marrow; breakdown or loss of hemoglobin; and synthesis of new hemoglobin.

C. Interpretation:

1. Elevated in hemochromatosis, hemosiderosis (multiple transfusions, excess iron administration), hemolytic disease, pernicious anemia, and hypoplastic anemias. Often elevated in viral hepatitis. Spuriously elevated if patient has received parenteral iron during the 2–3 months prior to determination.

2. Decreased in iron deficiency; with infections, nephrosis, and chronic renal insufficiency; and during periods of active hematopoiesis.

Iron-Binding Capacity, Serum

Normal: Total, 250–410 μg/dL. (SI: 45–73 μmol/L.) Percent saturation, 20–55%.

A. Precautions: None.

B. Physiologic Basis: Iron is transported as a

complex of the metal-binding globulin transferrin (siderophilin). Normally, this transport protein carries an amount of iron that represents about 30–40% of its capacity to combine with iron.

C. Interpretation of Total Iron-Binding Capacity:

1. Elevated in iron deficiency anemia, with use of oral contraceptives, in late pregnancy, and in infants. Occasionally elevated in hepatitis.

2. Decreased in association with decreased plasma proteins (nephrosis, starvation, cancer), chronic inflammation, and hemosiderosis (transfusions, thalassemia).

D. Interpretation of Saturation of Transferrin:

1. Elevated in iron excess (iron poisoning, hemolytic disease, thalassemia, hemochromatosis, pyridoxine deficiency, nephrosis, and, occasionally, hepatitis).

2. Decreased in iron deficiency, chronic infection, cancer, and late pregnancy.

Lactate Dehydrogenase (LDH), Serum, Serous Fluids, Spinal Fluid, or Urine

Normal (varies with method): Serum, 55–140 IU/L at 30 °C; SMA, 100–225 IU/L at 37 °C; SMAC, 60–200 IU/L at 37 °C. Serous fluids, lower than serum. Spinal fluid, 15–75 units (Wroblewski); 6.3–30 IU/L. Urine, less than 8300 units/8 h (Wroblewski).

A. Precautions: Any degree of hemolysis must be avoided because the concentration of LDH within red blood cells is 100 times that in normal serum. Heparin and oxalate may inhibit enzyme activity. Remove serum from clot promptly.

B. Physiologic Basis: LDH catalyzes the interconversion of lactate and pyruvate in the presence of NADH or $NADH_2$. It is distributed generally in body cells and fluids.

C. Interpretation: Elevated in all conditions accompanied by tissue necrosis, particularly those involving acute injury of the heart, red cells, kidney, skeletal muscle, liver, lung, and skin. Marked elevations accompany hemolytic anemias, the anemias of vitamin B_{12} and folate deficiency, and polycythemia rubra vera. The course of rise in concentration over 3–4 days followed by a slow decline during the following 5–7 days may be helpful in confirming the presence of myocardial infarction; however, pulmonary infarction, neoplastic disease, and megaloblastic anemia must be excluded. Although elevated during the acute phase of infectious hepatitis, enzyme activity is seldom increased in chronic liver disease.

D. Drug Effects on Laboratory Results: Decreased by clofibrate.

Lactate Dehydrogenase (LDH) Isoenzymes, Serum

Normal: See Table 6.

Table 6. Lactate dehydrogenase isoenzymes.

Isoenzyme		Percentage of Total (and Range)
(Fastest)	1 (α_1)	28 (15–30)
	2 (α_2)	36 (22–50)
	3 (β)	23 (15–30)
	4 (γ_1)	6 (0–15)
(Slowest)	5 (γ_2)	6 (0–15)

A. Precautions: As for LDH (see above).

B. Physiologic Basis: LDH consists of five separable proteins, each made of tetramers of two types, or subunits, H and M. The five isoenzymes can be distinguished by kinetics, electrophoresis, chromatography, and immunologic characteristics. By electrophoretic separation, the mobility of the isoenzymes corresponds to serum proteins α_1, α_2, β, γ_1, and γ_2. These are usually numbered 1 (fastest-moving), 2, 3, 4, and 5 (slowest moving). Isoenzyme 1 is present in high concentrations in heart muscle (tetramer H H H H) and in erythrocytes and kidney cortex; isoenzyme 5, in skeletal muscle (tetramer M M M M) and liver.

C. Interpretation: In myocardial infarction, the α isoenzymes are elevated—particularly LDH 1—to yield a ratio of LDH 1:LDH 2 of greater than 1. Similar α isoenzyme elevations occur in renal cortex infarction and with hemolytic anemias.

LDH 5 and 4 are relatively increased in the presence of acute hepatitis, acute muscle injury, dermatomyositis, and muscular dystrophies.

D. Drug Effects on Laboratory Results: Decreased by clofibrate.

Lipase, Serum

Normal: 0.2—1.5 units.

A. Precautions: None. The specimen may be stored under refrigeration up to 24 hours prior to the determination.

B. Physiologic Basis: A low concentration of fat-splitting enzyme is present in circulating blood. In the presence of pancreatitis, pancreatic lipase is released into the circulation in higher concentrations, which persist, as a rule, for a longer period than does the elevated concentration of amylase.

C. Interpretation: Serum lipase is elevated in acute or exacerbated pancreatitis and in obstruction of pancreatic ducts by stone or neoplasm.

Magnesium, Serum

Normal: 1.8–3 mg/dL or 1.5–2.5 meq/L. (SI: 0.75–1.25 mmol/L.)

A. Precautions: None.

B. Physiologic Basis: Magnesium is primarily an intracellular electrolyte. In extracellular fluid, it affects neuromuscular irritability and response. Magnesium deficit may exist with little or no change in extracellular fluid concentrations. Low magnesium levels in plasma have been associated with tetany, weakness, disorientation, and somnolence.

C. Interpretation:

1. Elevated in renal insufficiency and in overtreatment with magnesium salts.

2. Decreased in chronic diarrhea, acute loss of enteric fluids, starvation, chronic alcoholism, chronic hepatitis, hepatic insufficiency, excessive renal loss (diuretics), and inadequate replacement with parenteral nutrition. May be decreased in and contribute to persistent hypocalcemia in patients with hypoparathyroidism (especially after surgery for hyperparathyroidism) and when large doses of vitamin D and calcium are being administered.

Phosphatase, Acid, Serum

Normal values vary with method: 0.1–0.63 Sigma units.

A. Precautions: Do not draw blood for assay for 24 hours after prostatic massage or instrumentation. For methods that measure enzyme activity, complete the determination promptly, since activity declines quickly; avoid hemolysis. For immunoassay methods, the enzyme is stable for 3–4 days when the serum is refrigerated or frozen.

B. Physiologic Basis: Phosphatases active at pH 4.9 are present in high concentration in the prostate gland, erythrocytes, platelets, reticuloendothelial cells, liver, spleen, and kidney. A variety of isoenzymes have been found in these tissues and serum and account for different activities operating against different substrates.

C. Interpretation: In the presence of carcinoma of the prostate, the prostatic fraction of acid phosphatase may be increased in the serum, particularly if the cancer has spread beyond the capsule of the gland or has metastasized. Palpation of the prostate will produce a transient increase. Total acid phosphatase may be increased in Gaucher's disease, malignant tumors involving bone, renal disease, hepatobiliary disease, diseases of the reticuloendothelial system, and thromboembolism. Fever may cause spurious elevations.

Phosphatase, Alkaline, Serum

Normal values vary with method.

A. Precautions: Serum may be kept in the refrigerator for 24–48 hours, but values may increase slightly (10%). The specimen will deteriorate if it is not refrigerated. Do not use fluoride or oxalate.

B. Physiologic Basis: Alkaline phosphatase is present in high concentration in growing bone, in bile, and in the placenta. In serum, it consists of a mixture of isoenzymes not yet clearly defined. The isoenzymes may be separated by electrophoresis; liver alkaline phosphatase migrates faster than bone and placental alkaline phosphatase, which migrate together.

C. Interpretation:

1. Elevated in—

a. Children (normal growth of bone).

b. Osteoblastic bone disease-Hyperparathyroidism, rickets and osteomalacia, neoplastic bone disease (osteosarcoma, metastatic neoplasms), ossification as in myositis ossificans, Paget's disease (osteitis deformans), and Boeck's sarcoid.

c. Bile duct or cholangiolar obstruction due to stone, stricture, or neoplasm.

d. Hepatic disease resulting from drugs such as chlorpromazine and methyltestosterone.

e. Pregnancy.

2. Decreased in hypothyroidism and in growth retardation in children.

D. Drug Effects on Laboratory Results: Elevated by acetohexamide, tolazamide, tolbutamide, chlorpropamide, allopurinol, sulfobromophthalein, carbamazepine, cephaloridine, furosemide, methyldopa, phenothiazine, and oral contraceptives (estrogen-progestin combinations).

Phosphorus, Inorganic, Serum

Normal: Children, 4–7 mg/dL. (SI: 1.3–2.3 mmol/L.) Adults, 3–4.5 mg/dL. (SI: 1–15. mmol/L.)

A. Precautions: Glassware cleaned with phosphate cleansers must be thoroughly rinsed. The fasting state is necessary to avoid postprandial depression of phosphate associated with glucose transport and metabolism.

B. Physiologic Basis: The concentration of inorganic phosphate in circulating plasma is influenced by parathyroid gland function, action of vitamin D, intestinal absorption, renal function, bone metabolism, and nutrition.

C. Interpretation:

1. Elevated in renal insufficiency, hypoparathyroidism, and hypervitaminosis D.

2. Decreased in hyperparathyroidism, hypovitaminosis D (rickets, osteomalacia), malabsorption syndrome (steatorrhea), ingestion of antacids that bind phosphate in the gut, starvation or cachexia, chronic alcoholism (especially with liver disease), hyperalimentation with phosphate-poor solutions, carbohydrate administration (especially intravenously), renal tubular defects, acid-base disturbances, diabetic ketoacidosis (especially during recovery), and genetic hypophosphatemia. Occasionally decreased during pregnancy and with hypothyroidism.

Proteins, Serum or Plasma (Includes Fibrinogen)

Normal: See Interpretation, below.

A. Precautions: Serum or plasma must be free of hemolysis. Since fibrinogen is removed in the process of coagulation of the blood, fibrinogen determinations cannot be done on serum.

B. Physiologic Basis: Concentration of protein determines colloidal osmotic pressure of plasma. The concentration of protein in plasma is influenced by the nutritional state, hepatic function, renal function, occurrence of disease such as multiple myeloma, and metabolic errors. Variations in the fractions of plasma proteins may signify specific disease.

C. Interpretation:

1. Total protein, serum-Normal: 6–8 g/dL. (SI: 60–80 g/L.) See albumin and globulin fractions, below, and Table 7.

2. Albumin, serum or plasma-Normal: 3.5–5.5 g/dL. (SI: 33–55 g/L.)

a. Elevated in dehydration, shock, hemoconcentration, and administration of large quantities of concentrated albumin "solution" intravenously.

b. Decreased in malnutrition, malabsorption syndrome, acute or chronic glomerulonephritis, nephrosis, acute or chronic hepatic insufficiency, neoplastic diseases, and leukemia.

3. Globulin, serum or plasma-Normal: 2–3.6 g/dL. (SI: 20–36 g/L.) (See Tables 8 and 9.)

a. Elevated in hepatic disease, infectious hepatitis, cirrhosis of the liver, biliary cirrhosis, and hemochromatosis; disseminated lupus erythematosus; plasma cell myeloma; lymphoproliferative disease; sarcoidosis; and acute or chronic infectious diseases, particularly lymphogranuloma venereum, typhus, leishmaniasis, schistosomiasis, and malaria.

b. Decreased in malnutrition, congenital agammaglobulinemia, acquired hypogammaglobulinemia, and lymphatic leukemia.

4. Fibrinogen, plasma-Normal: 0.2–0.6 g/dL. (SI: 2–6 g/L.)

a. Elevated in glomerulonephritis, nephrosis (occasionally), and infectious diseases.

b. Decreased in disseminated intravascular coagulation (accidents of pregnancy such as placental ablation, amniotic fluid embolism, and violent labor; meningococcal meningitis; metastatic carcinoma of the prostate and occasionally of other organs; and leukemia), acute and chronic hepatic insufficiency, and congenital fibrinogenopenia.

Thyroxine (T_4), Total (TT_4), Serum

Normal: Radioimmunoassay (RIA), 5–12 μg/dL (SI: 65–156 and nmol/L); competitive binding protein (CPB) (Murphy-Pattee), 4–11 μg/dL (SI: 51–142 nmol/L).

A. Precautions: None.

B. Physiologic Basis: The total thyroxine level

Table 7. Protein fractions as determined by electrophoresis.

	Percentage of Total Protein
Albumin	52–68
α_1 globulin	2.4–4.4
α_2 globulin	6.1–10.1
β globulin	8.5–14.5
γ globulin	10–21

Table 8. Gamma globulins by immunoelectrophoresis.

IgA	90–450 mg/dL
IgG	700–1500 mg/dL
IgM	40–250 mg/dL
IgD	0.3–40 mg/dL
IgE	0.006–0.16 mg/dL

does not necessarily reflect the physiologic hormonal effect of thyroxine. Levels of thyroxine vary with the concentration of the carrier proteins (thyroxine-binding globulin and prealbumin), which are readily altered by physiologic conditions such as pregnancy and by a variety of diseases and drugs. Any interpretation of the significance of total T_4 depends upon knowing the concentration of carrier protein either from direct measurement or from the result of the erythrocyte or resin uptake of triiodothyronine (T_3) (see below). It is the concentration of free T_4 and of T_3 that determines hormonal activity.

C. Interpretation:

1. Elevated in hyperthyroidism, with elevation of thyroxine-binding proteins, and at times with active thyroiditis or acromegaly.

2. Decreased in hypothyroidism (primary or secondary) and with decreased concentrations of thyroxine-binding proteins.

D. Drug Effects on Laboratory Results: Increased by ingestion of excess T_4. A variety of drugs alter concentration of thyroxine-binding proteins (see below), with parallel changes in total T_4 concentration. Decreased by ingestion of T_3, which inhibits thyrotropin secretion, with resultant decrease in T_4 secretion and concentration. T_4 synthesis may be decreased by aminosalicylic acid, corticosteroids, lithium, the thiouracils, methimazole, and sulfonamides. Total T_4 concentration may be reduced as a result of displacement from carrier protein-binding sites by aspirin, chlorpropamide, phenytoin, halofenate, and tolbutamide. Cholestyramine may reduce T_4 concen-

Table 9. Some constituents of globulins.

Globulin	Representative Constituents
α_1	Thyroxine-binding globulin Transcortin Glycoprotein Lipoprotein Antitrypsin
α_2	Haptoglobin Glycoprotein Macroglobulin Ceruloplasmin
β	Transferrin Lipoprotein Glycoprotein
γ	γG γD γM γE γA

tration by interfering with its enterohepatic circulation.

Thyroxine, Free, Serum

Normal (equilibrium dialysis): 0.8–2.4 ng/dL. (SI: 0.01–0.03 nmol/L.) May be estimated from measurement of total thyroxine and resin T_3 uptake.

A. Precautions: None.

B. Physiologic Basis: The metabolic activity of T_4 is related to the concentration of free T_4. T_4 is apparently largely converted to T_3 in peripheral tissue. (T_3 is also secreted by the thyroid gland.) Both T_4 and T_3 seem to be active hormones.

C. Interpretation:

1. Elevated in hyperthyroidism and at times with active thyroiditis.

2. Decreased in hypothyroidism.

D. Drug Effects on Laboratory Results: Elevated by ingestion of excess T_4. Decreased by T_3, thiouracils, and methimazole.

Thyroxine-Binding Globulin (TBG), Serum

Normal (radioimmunoassay): 2–4.8 mg/dL.

A. Precautions: None.

B. Physiologic Basis: TBG is the principal carrier protein for T_4 and T_3 in the plasma. Variations in concentration of TBG are accompanied by corresponding variations in concentration of T_4 with intrinsic adjustments that maintain the physiologically active free hormones at proper concentration for euthyroid function. The inherited abnormalities of TBG concentration appear to be X-linked.

C. Interpretation:

1. Elevated in pregnancy, in infectious hepatitis, and in hereditary increase in TBG concentration.

2. Decreased in major depleting illness with hypoproteinemia (globulin), nephrotic syndrome, cirrhosis of the liver, active acromegaly, estrogen deficiency, and hereditary TBG deficiency.

D. Drug Effects on Laboratory Results: TBG or binding capacity increased by pregnancy, estrogens and progestins (including oral contraceptives), chlormadinone, perphenazine, and clofibrate. Decreased by androgens, anabolic steroids, cortisol, prednisone, corticotropin, and oxymetholone.

Triiodothyronine (T_3) Uptake, Serum; Resin (RT_3U) or Thyroxine-Binding Globulin Assessment (TBG Assessment)

Normal: RT_3U, as percentage of uptake of ^{125}I-T_3 by resin, 25–36%; RT_3U ratio (TBG assessment) expressed as ratio of binding of ^{125}I-T_3 by resin in test serum/pooled normal serum, 0.85–1.15.

A. Precautions: None.

B. Physiologic Basis: When serum thyroxine-binding proteins are normal, more TBG binding sites will be occupied by T_4 in T_4 hyperthyroidism, and fewer binding sites will be occupied in hypothyroidism. ^{125}I-labeled T_3 added to serum along with a sec-

ondary binder (resin, charcoal, talc, etc) is partitioned between TBG and the binder. The binder is separated from the serum, and the radioactivity of the binder is measured for the RT_3U test. Since the resin takes up the non-TBG-bound radioactive T_3, its activity varies inversely with the numbers of available TBG sites, ie, RT_3U is increased if TBG is more nearly saturated by T_4 and decreased if TBG is less well saturated by T_4.

C. Interpretation:

1. RT_3U and RT_3U ratio are **increased** when available sites are decreased, as in hyperthyroidism, acromegaly, nephrotic syndrome, severe hepatic cirrhosis, and hereditary TBG deficiency.

2. RT_3U and RT_3U ratio are **decreased** when available TBG sites are increased, as in hypothyroidism, pregnancy, the newborn, infectious hepatitis, and hereditary increase in TBG.

D. Drug Effects on Laboratory Results: RT_3U and RT_3U ratio are elevated by excess T_4, androgens, anabolic steroids, corticosteroids, corticotropin, anticoagulant therapy (heparin and warfarin), oxymetholone, phenytoin, phenylbutazone, and large doses of salicylate. RT_3U and RT_3U ratio are decreased by T_3 therapy; by estrogens and progestins, including oral contraceptives; and by thiouracils, chlormadinone, perphenazine, and clofibrate.

Transaminases

See Aminotransferases, above.

Triglycerides, Serum

Normal: < 165 mg/dL. (SI: < 165 g/L.) See also Table 3.

A. Precautions: Subject must be in a fasting state (preferably for at least 16 hours). The determination may be delayed if the serum is promptly separated from the clot and refrigerated.

B. Physiologic Basis: Dietary fat is hydrolyzed in the small intestine, absorbed and resynthesized by the mucosal cells, and secreted into lacteals in the form of chylomicrons. Triglycerides in the chylomicrons are cleared from the blood by tissue lipoprotein lipase (mainly adipose tissue), and the split products are absorbed and stored. Free fatty acids derived mainly from adipose tissue are precursors of the endogenous triglycerides produced by the liver. Transport of endogenous triglycerides is in association with β-lipoproteins, the very low density lipoproteins. In order to ensure measurement of endogenous triglycerides, blood must be drawn in the postabsorptive state.

C. Interpretation: Concentration of triglycerides, cholesterol, and lipoprotein fractions (very low density, low-density, and high-density) is interpreted collectively. Disturbances in normal relationships of these lipid moieties may be primary or secondary in origin.

1. Elevated (hyperlipoproteinemia)-

a. Primary-Type I hyperlipoproteinemia (exogenous hyperlipidemia), type III hyperbetalipoproteinemia, type II broad beta hyperlipoproteinemia, type IV hyperlipoproteinemia (endogenous hyperlipidemia), and type V hyperlipoproteinemia (mixed hyperlipidemia).

b. **Secondary-**Hypothyroidism, diabetes mellitus, nephrotic syndrome, chronic alcoholism with fatty liver, ingestion of contraceptive steroids, biliary obstruction, and stress.

2. **Decreased (hypolipoproteinemia)-**

a. **Primary-**Tangier disease (α-lipoprotein deficiency), abetalipoproteinemia, and a few rare, poorly defined syndromes.

b. **Secondary-**Malnutrition, malabsorption, and, occasionally, with parenchymal liver disease.

Urea Nitrogen & Urea, Blood, Plasma, or Serum

Normal: Blood urea nitrogen, 8–25 mg/dL (SI: 2.9–8.9 mmol/L). Urea, 21–53 mg/dL (SI: 3.5–9 mmol/L).

A. **Precautions:** *Do not use* ammonium oxalate or "double oxalate" as anticoagulant, for the ammonia will be measured as urea.

B. **Physiologic Basis:** Urea, an end product of protein metabolism, is excreted by the kidney. The urea concentration in the glomerular filtrate is the same as in the plasma. Tubular reabsorption of urea varies inversely with rate of urine flow. Thus, urea is a less useful measure of glomerular filtration than is creatinine, which is not reabsorbed. Blood urea nitrogen varies directly with protein intake and inversely with the rate of excretion of urea.

C. **Interpretation:**

1. **Elevated in-**

a. Renal insufficiency-Nephritis, acute and chronic; acute renal failure (tubular necrosis); and urinary tract obstruction.

b. Increased nitrogen metabolism associated with diminished renal blood flow or impaired renal function-Dehydration (from any cause) and upper gastrointestinal bleeding (combination of increased protein absorption from digestion of blood plus decreased renal blood flow).

c. Decreased renal blood flow-Shock, adrenal insufficiency, and occasionally congestive heart failure.

2. **Decreased** in hepatic failure, nephrosis not complicated by renal insufficiency, and cachexia.

D. **Drug Effects on Laboratory Results:** Elevated by many antibiotics that impair renal function, guanethidine, methyldopa, indomethacin, isoniazid, propranolol, and potent diuretics (decreased blood volume and renal blood flow).

Uric Acid, Serum or Plasma

Normal: Males, 3–9 mg/dL (SI: 0.18–0.53 mmol/L); females, 2.5–7.5 mg/dL (SI: 0.15–0.45 mmol/L).

A. **Precautions:** If plasma is used, lithium oxa-

late should be used as the anticoagulant; potassium oxalate may interfere with the determination.

B. **Physiologic Basis:** Uric acid, an end product of nucleoprotein metabolism, is excreted by the kidney. Gout, a genetically transmitted metabolic error, is characterized by an increased plasma or serum uric acid concentration, an increase in total body uric acid, and deposition of uric acid in tissues. An increase in uric acid concentration in plasma and serum may accompany increased nucleoprotein catabolism (blood dyscrasias, therapy with antileukemic drugs), use of thiazide diuretics, or decreased renal excretion.

C. **Interpretation:**

1. **Elevated** in gout, preeclampsia-eclampsia, leukemia, polycythemia, therapy with antileukemic drugs and a variety of other agents, renal insufficiency, glycogen storage disease (type I), Lesch-Nyhan syndrome (X-linked hypoxanthine-guanine phosphoribosyltransferase deficit), and Down's syndrome. The incidence of hyperuricemia is greater in Filipinos than in whites.

2. **Decreased** in acute hepatitis (occasionally), treatment with allopurinol, and treatment with probenecid.

D. **Drug Effects on Laboratory Results:** Elevated by salicylates (low doses), thiazide diuretics, ethacrynic acid, spironolactone, furosemide, triamterene, and ascorbic acid. Decreased by salicylates (large doses), methyldopa, clofibrate, phenylbutazone, cinchophen, sulfinpyrazone, and phenothiazines.

Uric Acid, Urine

Normal: 350–600 mg/24 h on a standard purine-free diet. (SI: 2.1–3.6 mmol/24 h.) Normal urinary uric acid/creatinine ratio for adults is 0.21–0.59; maximum of 0.75 for 24-hour urine while on purine-free diet.

A. **Precautions:** Diet should be free of high-purine foods prior to and during 24-hour urine collection. Strenuous activity may be associated with elevated purine excretion.

B. **Physiologic Basis:** Elevated serum uric acid may result from overproduction or diminished excretion.

C. **Interpretation:**

1. **Elevated** renal excretion occurs in about 25–30% of cases of gout due to increased purine synthesis. Excess uric acid synthesis and excretion are associated with myeloproliferative disorders. Lesch-Nyhan syndrome (hypoxanthine-guanine phosphoribosyltransferase deficit) and some cases of glycogen storage disease are associated with uricosuria.

2. **Decreased** in renal insufficiency, in some cases of glycogen storage disease (type I), and in any metabolic defect producing either lactic acidemia or β-hydroxybutyric acidemia. Salicylates in doses of less than 2–3 g/d may produce renal retention of uric acid.

Friedman RB et al: Effects of diseases on clinical laboratory tests. Clin Chem 1980;26(Suppl 4):1D.

Hansten PD: Important drug interactions. In: *Basic & Clinical Pharmacology*, 4th ed. Katzung BG (editor). Appleton & Lange, 1989.

Lippert H, Lehmann HP: *SI Units in Medicine: An Introduction to the International System of Units With Conversion Tables and Normal Ranges.* Urban & Schwarzenberg, 1978.

Lundberg GD, Iverson C, Radulescu G (editors): Now read this: The SI units are here. (Editorial.) JAMA 1986;255:2329.

Powsner EK: SI quantities and units for American medicine. JAMA 1984;252:1737.

Scully RE et al: Normal reference laboratory values: Case records of the Massachusetts General Hospital. N Engl J Med 1986;314:39.

Sonnenwirth AC, Jarett L: *Gradwohl's Laboratory Methods and Diagnosis,* 8th ed. Vols 1 and 2. Mosby, 1980.

NORMAL LABORATORY VALUES

(Blood [B], Plasma [P], Serum [S], Urine [U]) HEMATOLOGY

Bleeding time: Ivy method, 1–7 minutes (60–420 seconds). Template method, 3–9 minutes (180–540 seconds).

Cellular measurements of red cells: Average diameter = 7.3 μm (5.5–8.8 μm).

Mean corpuscular volume (MCV): Men, 80–94 fL; women, 81–99 fL (by Coulter counter).

Mean corpuscular hemogloblin (MCH): 27–32 pg.

Mean corpuscular hemoglobin concentration (MCHC):32–36 g/dL red blood cells (32–36%).

Color, saturation, and volume indices: 1 (0.9–1.1).

Clot retraction: Begins in 1–3 hours; complete in 6–24 hours. No clot lysis in 24 hours.

Coagulation time (Lee-White): At 37 °C, 6–12 minutes; at room temperature, 10–18 minutes.

Fibrinogen split products: Negative > 1:4 dilution.

Fragility of red cells: Begins at 0.45–0.38% NaCl; complete at 0.36–0.3% NaCl.

Hematocrit (PCV): Men, 40–52%; women, 37–47%.

Hemoglobin: [B] Men, 14–18 g/dL (2.09–2.79 mmol/L as Hb tetramer); women, 12–16 g/dL (1.86–2.48 mmol/L). [S] 2–3 mg/dL.

Partial thromboplastin time: Activated, 25–37 seconds.

Platelets: 150,000–400,000/μL (0.15–0.4 × 10^{12}/L).

Prothrombin: [P] 75–125%. Less than 2 seconds deviation from control. (See Table 2.)

Red blood count (RBC): Men, 4.5–6.2 million/μL (4.5–6.2 × 10^{12}/L); women, 4–5.5 million/μL (4–5.5 × 10^{12}/L).

Reticulocytes: 0.2–2% of red cells.

Sedimentation rate: Less than 20 mm/h (Westergren); 0–10 mm/h (Wintrobe).

White blood count (WBC) and differential: 5000–10,000/μL (5–10 × 10^9/L).

Myelocytes	0 %
Juvenile neutrophils	0 %
Band neutrophils	0–5 %
Segmented neutrophils	40–60%
Lymphocytes	20–40%
Eosinophils	1–3 %
Basophils	0–1 %
Monocytes	4–8 %
Lymphocytes: Total, 1500–4000/μL	
B cell	5–25%
T cell	60–88%
Suppressor	10–43%
Helper	32–66%
H:S	

BLOOD, PLASMA, OR SERUM CHEMICAL CONSTITUENTS
(Values vary with method used.)

Acetone and acetoacetate: [S] 0.3–2 mg/dL (3–20 mg/L).

Aldolase: [S] Values vary with method used.

α-Amino acid nitrogen: [S, fasting] 3–5.5 mg/dL (2.2–3.9 mmol/L).

Aminotransferases:

Aspartate aminotransferase (AST; SGOT) (varies with method used): [S] 6–25 IU/L at 30°C; SMA, 10–40 IU/L at 37 °C; SMAC, 0–41 IU/L at 37 °C.

Alanine aminotransferase (ALT; SGPT) (varies with method used): [S] 3–26 IU/L at 30°C; SMAC, 0–45 IU/L at 37 °C.

Ammonia: [B] < 110 μg/dL (mol/L) (diffusion method). Do not use anticoagulant containing ammonium oxalate.

Amylase: [S] 80–180 units/dL (Somogyi). Values vary with method used.

α₁-Antitrypsin: [S] > 180 mg/dL.

Ascorbic acid: [P] 0.4–1.5 mg/dL (23–85 μmol/L).

Base, total serum: [S] 145–160 meq/L (145–160 mmol/L).

Bicarbonate: [S] 24–28 meq/L (24–28 mmol/L).

Bilirubin: [S] Total, 0.2–1.2 mg/dL (3.5–20.5 μmol/L). Direct (conjugated), 0.1–0.4 mg/dL (< 7 μmol/L). Indirect, 0.2–0.7 mg/dL (mol/L).

Calcium: [S] 8.5–10.3 mg/dL (2.1–2.6 mmol/L). Values vary with albumin concentration.

Calcium, ionized: [S] 4.25–5.25 mg/dL; 2.1–2.6 meq/L (1.05–1.3 mmol/L).

β-Carotene: [S, fasting] 50–300 μg/dL (0.9–5.58 μmol/L).

Ceruloplasmin: [S] 25–43 mg/dL (1.7–2.9 μmol/L).

Chloride: [S or P] 96–106 meq/L (96–106 mmol/L).

Cholesterol: [S or P] 150–265 mg/dL (3.9–6.85 mmol/L). (See Lipid fractions.) Values vary with age.

Cholesteryl esters: [S] 65–75% of total cholesterol.

CO$_2$ content: [S or P] 24–29 meq/L (24–29 mmol/L).

Complement: [S] C3 (β$_{1C}$), 90–250 mg/dL. C4 (β$_{1E}$), 10–60 mg/dL. Total (CH$_{50}$), 75–160 mg/dL.

Copper: [S or P] 100–200 μg/dL (16–31 μmol/L).

Cortisol: [P] 8:00 AM, 5–25 μg/dL (138–690 nmol/L); 8:00 PM < 10 μg/dL (275 nmol/L).

Creatine kinase (CK): [S] 10–50 IU/L at 30°C. Values vary with method used.

Creatine kinase isoenzymes: See Table 4.

Creatinine: [S or P] 0.7–1.5 mg/dL (62–132 μmol/L).

Cyanocobalamin: [S] 200 pg/mL (148 pmol/L).

Epinephrine: [P] Supine, < 100 pmol/L).

Ferritin: [S] Adult women, 20–120 ng/mL; men, 30–300 ng/mL. Child to 15 years, 7–140 ng/mL.

Folic acid: [S] 2–20 ng/mL (4.5–45 nmol/L). [RBC] > 140 ng/mL (> 318 nmol/L).

Glucose: [S or P] 65–110 mg/dL (3.6–6.1 mmol/L).

Haptoglobin: [S] 40–170 mg of hemoglobin-binding capacity.

Iron: [S] 50–175 μg/dL (9–31.3 μmol/L).

Iron-binding capacity: [S] Total, 250–410 μg/dL (44.7–73.4 μmol/L). Percent saturation, 20–55%.

Lactate: [B, special handling] Venous, 4–16 mg/dL (0.44–1.8 mmol/L).

Lactate dehydrogenase (LDH): (Varies with method.) [S] 55–140 IU/L at 30 °C; SMA, 100–225 IU/L at 37 °C; SMAC, 60–200 IU/L at 37 °C.

Lipase: [S] < 150 U/L.

Lipid fractions: [S or P] Desirable levels: HDL cholesterol, > 40 mg/dL; LDL cholesterol, < 180 mg/dL; VLDL cholesterol, < 40 mg/dL. (To convert to mmol/L, multiply by 0.026.)

Lipids, total: [S] 450–1000 mg/dL (4.5–10 g/L).

Magnesium: [S or P] 1.8–3 mg/dL (0.75–1.25 mmol/L).

Norepinephrine: [P] Supine, < 500 pg/mL (< 3 nmol/L).

Osmolality: [S] 280–296 mosm/kg water (280–296 mmol/kg water).

Oxygen:

Capacity: [B] 16–24 vol%. Values vary with hemoglobin concentration.

Arterial content: [B] 15–23 vol%. Values vary with hemoglobin concentration.

Arterial % saturation: 94–100% of capacity.

Arterial Po_2 (Pao_2): 80–100 mm Hg (10.67–13.33 kPa) (sea level). Values vary with age.

Paco_2: [B, arterial] 35–45 mm Hg (4.7–6 kPa).

pH (reaction): [B, arterial] 7.35–7.45 (H$^+$ 44.7–45.5 nmol/L).

Phosphatase, acid: [S] 1–5 units (King-Armstrong) 0.1–0.63 units (Bessey-Lowry).

Phosphatase, alkaline: [S] Adults, 5–13 units (King-Armstrong). 0.8–2.3 (Bessey-Lowry); SMA, 30–85 IU/L at 37 °C; SMAC, 30–115 IU/L at 37 °C.

Phospholipid phosphorus: [S] 5–12 mg/dL (1.45–2 g/L).

Phosphorus, inorganic: [S, fasting] 3–4.5 mg/dL (1–1.5 mmol/L).

Potassium: [S or P] 3.5–5 meq/L (3.5–5 mmol/L).

Protein:

Total: [S] 6–8 g/dL (60–80 g/L).

Albumin. [S] 3.5–5.5 g/dL (35–55 g/L).

Globulin: [S] 2–3.6 g/dL (20–36 g/L).

Fibrinogen: [P] 0.2–0.6 g/dL (2–6 g/L).

Separation by electrophoresis: See Table 7.

Prothrombin clotting time: [P] By control.

Pyruvate: [B] 0.6–1 mg/dL (70–114 μmol/L).

Serotonin: [B] 5–20 μg/dL (0.2–1.14 μmol/L).

Sodium: [S or P] 136–145 meq/L (136–145 mmol/L).

Specific gravity: [B] 1.056 (varies with hemoglobin and protein concentration). [S] 1.0254–1.0288 (varies with protein concentration).

Sulfate: [S or P] As sulfur, 0.5–1.5 mg/dL (156–468 μmol/L).

Transferrin: [S] 200–400 mg/dL (23–45 μmol/L).

Triglycerides: [S] < 165 mg/dL (1.9 mmol/L). (See Lipid fractions.)

Urea nitrogen: [S or P] 8–25 mg/dL (2.9–8.9 mmol/L). Do not use anticoagulant containing ammonium oxalate.

Uric acid: [S or P] Men, 3–9 mg/dL (0.18–0.54 mmol/L); women, 2.5–7.5 mg/dL (0.15–0.45 mmol/L).

Vitamin A: [S] 15–60 μg/dL (0.53–2.1 μmol/L).

Vitamin B$_{12}$: [S] 200 pg/mL (148 pmol/L).

Vitamin D: [S] Cholecalciferol (D$_3$): 25-Hydroxycholecalciferol, 8–55 ng/mL (19.4–137 nmol/L); 1,25-dihydroxycholecalciferol, 26–65 pg/mL (62–155 pmol/L); 24,25-dihydroxycholecalciferol, 1–5 ng/mL (2.4–12 nmol/L).

Volume, blood (Evans blue dye method): Adults, 2990–6980 mL. Women, 46.3–85.5 mL/kg; men, 66.2–97.7 mL/kg.

Zinc: [S] 50–150 μg/dL (7.65–22.95 μmol/L).

HORMONES, SERUM OR PLASMA

Pituitary:

Growth hormone (GH): [S] Adults, 1–10 ng/mL (46–465 pmol/L) (by RIA).

Thyroid-stimulating hormone (TSH): [S] < 10 µU/mL.

Follicle-stimulating hormone (FSH): [S] Prepubertal, 2–12 mIU/mL; adult men, 1–15 mIU/mL; adult women, 1–30 mIU/mL; castrate or postmenopausal, 30–200 mIU/mL (by RIA).

Luteinizing hormone (LH): [S] Prepubertal, 2–12 mIU/mL; adult men, 1–15 mIU/mL; adult women, < 30 mIU/mL; castrate or postmenopausal, > 30 mIU/mL.

Corticotropin (ACTH): [P] 8:00–10:00 AM, up to 100 pg/mL (22 pmol/L).

Prolactin: [S] 1–25 ng/mL (0.4–10 nmol/L).

Somatomedin C: [P] 0.4–2 U/mL.

Antidiuretic hormone (ADH; vasopressin); [P] Serum osmolality 285 mosm/kg, 0–2 pg/mL; > 290 mosm/kg, 2–12+ pg/mL.

Adrenal:

Aldosterone: [P] Supine, normal salt intake, 2–9 ng/dL (56–250 pmol/L); increased when upright.

Cortisol: [S] 8:00 AM, 5–20 µg/dL (0.14–0.55 µmol/L); 8:00 PM, < 10 µg/dL (0.28 µmol/L).

Deoxycortisol: [S] After metyrapone, > 7 µg/dL (> 0.2 µmol/L).

Dopamine: [P] < 135 pg/mL.

Epinephrine: [P] < 0.1 ng/mL (< 0.55 nmol/L).

Norepinephrine: [P] < 0.5 µg/L (< 3 nmol/L).

See also Miscellaneous Normal Values.

Thyroid:

Thyroxine, free (FT_4): [S] 0.8–2.4 ng/dL (10–30 pmol/L).

Thyroxine, total (TT_4): [S] 5–12 µg/dL (65–156 nmol/L) (by RIA).

Thyroxine-binding globulin capacity: [S] 12–28 µg T_4/dL (150–360 nmol T_4/dL).

Triiodothyronine (T_3): [S] 80–220 ng/dL (1.2–3.3 nmol/L).

Reverse triiodothyronine (rT_3): [S] 30–80 ng/dL (0.45–1.2 nmol/L).

Triiodothyronine uptake (RT_3U): [S] 25–36%; as TBG assessment (RT_3U ratio), 0.85–1.15.

Calcitonin: [S] < 100 pg/mL (< 29.2 pmol/L).

Parathyroid: Parathyroid hormone levels vary with method and antibody. Correlate with serum calcium.

Islets:

Insulin: [S] 4–25 µU/mL (29–181 pmol/L).

C-peptide: [S] 0.9–4.2 ng/mL.

Glucagon: [S, fasting] 20–100 pg/mL.

Stomach:

Gastrin: [S, special handling] Up to 100 pg/mL (47 pmol/L). Elevated, > 200 pg/mL.

Pepsinogen I: [S] 25–100 ng/mL.

Kidney:

Renin activity: [P, special handling] Normal sodium intake: Supine, 1–3 ng/mL/h; standing, 3–6 ng/mL/h. Sodium depleted: Supine, 2–6 ng/mL/h; standing, 3–20 ng/mL/h.

Gonad:

Testosterone, free: [S] Men, 10–30 ng/dL; women, 0.3–2 ng/dL. (1 ng/dL = 0.035 nmol/L.)

Testosterone, total: [S] Prepubertal, < 100 ng/dL; adult men, 300–1000 ng/dL; adult women, 20–80 ng/dL; luteal phase, up to 120 ng/dL.

Estradiol (E_2): [S, special handling] Men, 12–34 pg/mL; women, menstrual cycle 1–10 days, 24–68 pg/mL; 11–20 days, 50–300 pg/mL; 21–30 days, 73–149 pg/mL (by RIA). (1 pg/mL = 3.6 pmol/L.)

Progesterone: [S] Follicular phase, 0.2–1.5 mg/mL; luteal phase, 6–32 ng/mL; pregnancy, > 24 ng/mL; men, < 1 ng/mL = 3.2 nmol/L.)

Placenta:

Estriol (E_3): [S] Men and nonpregnant women, < 0.2 µg/dL (< 7 nmol/L) (by RIA).

Chorionic gonadotropin: [S] Beta subunit: Men, < 9 mIU/mL; pregnant women after implantation, > 10 mIU/mL.

NORMAL CEREBROSPINAL FLUID VALUES

Appearance: Clear and colorless.

Cells: Adults, 0–5 mononuclears/µL; infants, 0–20 mononuclears/µL.

Glucose: 50–85 mg/dL (2.8–4.7 mmol/L). (Draw serum glucose at same time.)

Pressure (reclining): Newborns, 30–90 mm H_2O; children, 50–100 mm H_2O; adults, 70–200 mm H_2O (avg = 125 mm H_2O).

Proteins: Total, 20–45 mg/dL (200–450 mg/L) in lumbar cerebrospinal fluid. IgG, 2–6 mg/dL (0.02–0.06 g/L).

Specific gravity: 1.003–1.008.

RENAL FUNCTION TESTS

p-Aminohippurate (PAH) clearance (RPF): Men, 560–830 mL/min; women, 490–700 mL/min.

Creatinine clearance, endogenous (GFR): Approximates inulin clearance (see below).

Filtration fraction (FF): Men, 17–21%; women, 17–23%. (FF = GFR/RPF.)

Inulin clearance (GFR): Men, 110–50 mL/min; women, 105–132 mL/min (corrected to 1.73 m^2 surface area).

Maximal glucose reabsorptive capacity (Tm_{GEE}): Men, 300–450 mg/min; women, 250–350 mg/min.

Table 10. Therapeutic serum levels of some commonly used drugs.[1,2]

Drug		Therapeutic Range		
		Peak	**Trough**	
Antibiotics	Amikacin	20–30 µg/mL	1–8 µg/mL	>30 µg/mL
	Kanamycin	20–30 µg/mL	1–8 µg/mL	>30 µg/mL
	Gentamicin	5–10 µg/mL	<2 µg/mL	>12 µg/mL
	Tobramycin	5–10 µg/mL	<2 µg/mL	>12 µg/mL
	Netilmicin	6–10 µg/mL	<2 µg/mL	>12 µg/mL
	Chloramphenicol	15–20 µg/mL	…	>25 µg/mL

Drug		Therapeutic Range	Toxic Level
Antiarrhythmics	Digoxin	0.8–2 ng/mL	2.5 ng/mL
	Digitoxin	10–22 ng/mL	35 ng/mL
	Lidocaine	1.5–5 µg/mL	>7 µg/mL
	Procainamide	4–10 µg/mL	>16 µg/mL
	Procainamide (N-acetylprocainamide)	10–30 µg/mL	>30 µg/mL
	Quinidine	2–5 µg/mL	>10 µg/mL
	Disopyramide	3–5 µg/mL	>7 µg/mL
Antiepileptics	Phenytoin	10–20 µg/mL	>20 µg/mL
	Phenobarbital	15–40 µg/mL	>40 µg/mL
	Primidone	5–12 µg/mL	>15 µg/mL
	Ethosuximide	40–100 µg/mL	>150 µg/mL
	Valproic acid	50–100 µg/mL	>100 µg/mL
	Carbamazepine	8–12 µg/mL	>15 µg/mL
Antidepressants	Amitriptyline	120–150 ng/mL	>500 ng/mL
	Desipramine	150–250 ng/mL	>500 ng/mL
	Imipramine	150–250 ng/ml	>500 ng/mL
	Nortriptyline	50–150 ng/mL	>500 ng/mL
	Lithium	0.6–1.4 meq/L	>2 meq/L
Others	Theophylline	10–20 µg/mL	>20 µg/mL
	Aspirin	100–250 µg/mL	>300 µg/mL
	Acetaminophen	…	>250 µg/mL

[1]See also Holford NHG: Clinical interpretation of drug concentrations. In: *Basic & Clinical Pharmacology*, 5th ed. Katzung BG (editor). Appleton & Lange, 1993.

[2]Plasma drug concentrations should be monitored when the drug has a narrow therapeutic range and the toxic level is near the upper range of the therapeutic range; when the therapeutic range is difficult to assess clinically; when the drug is given to achieve a therapeutic effect quickly and subsequent dosage must be modified; and when compliance with the prescribed dosage is in question.

Maximal $_{PAH}$ excretory capacity (Tm$_{PAH}$): 80–90 mg/min.

Osmolality: On normal diet and fluid intake: Range 500–850 mosm/kg water. Achievable range, normal kidney: Dilution 40–80 mosm; concentration (dehydration) up to 1400 mosm/kg water (at least three to four times plasma osmolality).

Specific gravity of urine: 1.003–1.030.

MISCELLANEOUS NORMAL VALUES (Urine [U], Feces (F)

Adrenal hormones and metabolites:

Aldosterone: [U] 2–26 µg/24 h (5.5–72 nmol). Values vary with sodium and potassium intake.

Catecholamines: [U] Total, < 100 µg/24 h. Epinephrine, < 10 µg/24 h (< 55 nmol); norepinephrine, < 100 µg/24 h (< 591 nmol). Values vary with method used.

Cortisol, free: [U] 20–100 µg/24 h (0.55–2.76 µmol).

11,17-Hydroxycorticoids: [U] Men, 4–12 mg/24 h; women, 4–8 mg/24 h. Values vary with method used.

17-Ketosteroids: [U] Under 8 years, 0–2 mg/24 h; adolescents, 2–20 mg/24 h. Men, 10–20 mg/24 h; women, 5–15 mg/24 h. Values vary with method used. (1 mg = 3.5 µmol.)

Metanephrine: [U] < 1.3 mg/24 h (< 6.6 µmol) or < 2.2 µg/mg creatinine. Values vary with method used.

Vanillylmandelic acid (VMA): [U] Up to 7 mg/24 h (< 35 µmol).

Fat: [F] Less than 30% dry weight.

Lead: [U] < 80 µg/24 h (< 0.4 µmol/d).

Porphyrins:

Delta-aminolevulinic acid: [U] 1.5–7.5 mg/24 h (11.4–57.2 µmol).

Coproporphyrin: [U] < 230 µg/24 h (< 345 nmol).

Uroporphyrin: [U] < 40 µg/24 h (< 60 nmol).

Porphobilinogen: [U] < 2 mg/24 h (< 8.8 µmol).

Urobilinogen: [U] 0–2.5 mg/24 h (< 4.23 µmol).

Urobilinogen: [F] 40–280 mg/24 h (68–474 µmol).

Index

NOTE: Page numbers in bold face type indicate a major discussion. A *t* following a page number indicates tabular material and an *i* following a page number indicates an illustration. Drugs are listed under their generic names. When a drug trade name is listed, the reader is referred to the generic name.